Appropriate nursing diagnoses presented for every drug

High Alert header highlights drugs that pose the greatest risk if administered improperly

Nursing diagnoses
- Infection, risk for (uses)
- Knowledge, deficient (teaching)
- Mobility, impaired physical (uses)

Implementation
PO route
- Give all medications PO if possible, avoiding IM inj, since bleeding may occur
- Give with meals to reduce GI upset; nausea is common
- For several days before transplant surgery, patients should be placed in protective isolation

IV route
- Prepare in biologic cabinet using gown, gloves, mask; give after diluting 100 mg/10 ml sterile water for inj; rotate to dissolve; may dilute with 50 ml or more saline or give in saline given over >30 min (intermittent inf)

Y-site compatibilities: D₅W, NaCl 0.45%

Subheadings indicate various administration routes

Patient/family education
- Teach patient to take as prescribed, do not miss doses; if dose is missed on daily regimen, skip dose; if on multiple dosing/day, take as soon as remembered
- Teach patient that therapeutic response may take 3-4 mo in rheumatoid arthritis, to continue with prescribed exercise, rest, other medications; that product is needed for life in renal transplant
- Instruct patient to report fever, rash, severe diarrhea, chills, sore throat, fatigue, since serious infections may occur; or clay-colored stools and cramping (hepatotoxicity)
- Advise patient to use contraceptive measures during treatment for 12 wk after ending therapy; product is teratogenic
- Advise patient to avoid vaccinations
- Tell patient to avoid crowds and persons with known infections to reduce risk of infection
- Instruct patient not to use OTC medications without approval of prescriber
- Advise patient to use soft-bristled toothbrush to prevent bleeding

Evaluation
Positive therapeutic outcome
- Absence of graft rejection
- Immunosuppression in autoimmune disorders
- Increased joint mobility without pain in rheumatoid arthritis

---

! HIGH ALERT

warfarin (Rx)
(war'far-in)
Coumadin, Jantoven, warfarin sodium, Warfilone ✦
Func. class.: Anticoagulant

Pregnancy category X

Do not confuse:
Coumadin/Cardura/Compazine

Action: Interferes with blood clotting by indirect means; depresses hepatic synthesis of vit K–dependent coagulation factors (II, VII, IX, X)

Canadian drugs identified with a maple-leaf icon

Therapeutic outcome: Prevention of clotting

Uses: Antiphospholipid antibody syndrome, deep vein thrombosis, prevention or treatment of venous thrombosis, pulmonary emboli, thromboembolic complications associated with atrial fibrillation or cardiac valve replacement, after MI to reduce risk of death

Dosage and routes
Adult: PO/IV 2.5-10 mg/day titrated to INR
Geriatric: PO/IV 2-10 mg/day
Child: PO/IV 0.2 mg/kg/day titrated to INR

Geriatric, pediatric, and other special doses included throughout

Available forms: Tabs 1, 2, 2.5, 3, 4, 5, 6, 7.5, 10 mg; 5.4 mg powder for inj

Adverse effects
CNS: Fever, dizziness, fatigue, headache, lethargy
CV: Angina, chest pain, edema, hypotension, syncope
GI: Diarrhea, nausea, vomiting, anorexia, stomatitis, cramps, **hepatitis,** cholestatic jaundice
GU: **Hematuria**
HEMA: **Hemorrhage, agranulocytosis, leukopenia, eosinophilia,** ecchymosis, anemia, petechiae
INTEG: Rash, dermatitis, urticaria, alopecia, pruritus
MISC: Epistaxis, hemoptysis, mouth ulcers, taste disturbances, priapism, dyspnea
MS: Bone fractures
SYST: **Anaphylaxis,** coma, cholesterol, microembolisms, **exfoliative dermatitis, purple toe syndrome**

Common and life-threatening adverse effects grouped by body system

Contraindications: Pregnancy X, breast-feeding, hypersensitivity, hemophilia, leukemia with bleeding, peptic ulcer disease, thrombocytopenic purpura, hepatic disease (severe), malignant hypertension, subacute bacterial endocarditis, acute nephritis, blood dyscrasias,

---

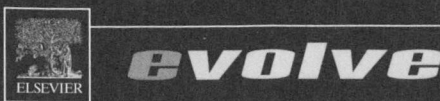

ELSEVIER

evolve

⫶• To access your Online Resources, visit:
http://evolve.elsevier.com/nursingdrugupdates/Skidmore/NDG

Evolve® Online Resources for *Mosby's Drug Guide for Nurses,*
ninth edition, offers the following features:

- **Drug Monographs**
  Includes full monographs for drugs new to this edition.

- **FDA Alerts**
  Provides updates on drug recalls, labeling changes, new
  interactions, and safety warnings.

- **Recently Approved Drugs**
  Offers a table of drugs approved by the FDA after publication
  of the book, including links to approved product inserts.

- **Color Pill Atlas**
  Provides full-color photographs identifying the most
  commonly prescribed medications and dosages.

- **Drug Name Safety Information**
  Links to organizations and resources involved in reducing
  medication errors caused by drug name confusion.

- **English-to-Spanish Translation**
  Provides Spanish translations and pronunciations for common
  drug phrases and terms.

- **Drug Dosage Calculators**
  Features 30 handy clinical calculators, including several IV
  and PO dosage calculators, and an IV dose rate calculator.

http://evolve.elsevier.com/nursingdrugupdates/Skidmore/NDG

Mosby's Drug Guide for Nurses, Ninth Edition, Companion CD-ROM

Use *Mosby's Drug Guide for Nurses, Ninth Edition, Companion CD-ROM* to find drug information fast! This five-in-one CD-ROM provides you with NCLEX® examination review questions for 60 key drugs, patient teaching guides, a calculation tutorial, a drug card creator, and calculators.

This Companion CD-ROM includes:

- **NCLEX® Examination Review Questions for 60 Key Drugs**
  Includes complete, printable information for the 60 key drugs in the book, matched with 356 NCLEX® examination review questions.

- **Patient Teaching Guides**
  Contains English and Spanish patient teaching guides for select key drugs.

- **Calculation Tutorial**
  Provides calculations and conversions paired with practice problems and answers.

- **Drug Card Creator**
  Features a blank drug card template that is fully customizable and printable.

- **Calculators**
  Contains 30 handy clinical calculators, including several IV and PO dosage calculators, and an IV dose rate calculator.

Contact Us
For further information, visit us at http://us.elsevierhealth.com or call us at (800) 545-2522.

Mini CD-ROM
This mini CD-ROM will work in your CD-ROM drive. Place it on the inner ring of the tray, as shown, and follow the on-screen installation instructions.

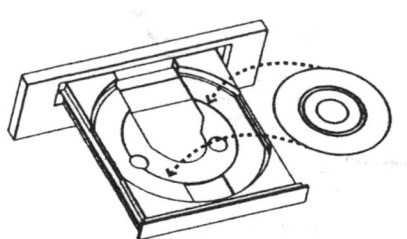

This mini-CD does
not work in:
    Floppy Drives
    Slot Drives
    Zip Drives
    Stereos
Insert this mini-CD
into your CD-ROM
drive as shown at left.

Important
No credit or refund will be issued on this book if the CD envelope has been opened, torn, or otherwise tampered with.

Companion CD-ROM for *Skidmore, Mosby's Drug Guide for Nurses*, Ninth Edition
This CD is designed to run on both PC and Macintosh.

Microsoft Windows Users

Your computer should meet the following minimum requirements:
Windows XP SP2, or 32-bit Vista operating system (64-bit versions are not currently supported)
Intel Pentium 4 processor (or equivalent ×86 chipset) / 1 GHz or greater
512 MB RAM (256 MB or lower may be sluggish)
Minimum 800 × 600 pixels screen resolution (1024 × 768 recommended)
16-Bit color
16× or faster CD-ROM drive / 8× or faster DVD-ROM

Instructions

If your system does not support Auto-run, double-click "**Skidmore.exe**" from My Computer >
CD/DVD-ROM to begin.

Macintosh Users

Your computer should meet the following minimum requirements:

MAC OS 10.4.x and 10.5.x operating system
Intel-based processor or PowerPC G4/G5 (867 MHz or higher)
512 MB RAM (256 MB or lower may be sluggish)
Minimum 800 × 600 pixels screen resolution (1024 × 768 recommended)
16-Bit color
16× or faster CD-ROM drive / 8× or faster DVD-ROM

Instructions

A CD icon labeled "**Skidmore**" will appear on the screen once inserted. Double-click
"**Skidmore**," then "**Skidmore.exe**" to launch software.
   OR
Insert CD and copy contents to your hard drive. Open the newly copied folder and "**Skidmore**"
run to launch software.

ONLINE TECHNICAL SUPPORT

Technical support for this product is available 24 hours a day, seven days a week, excluding
holidays. Before calling, make sure that your computer meets the minimum system requirements
to run this software. Inside the United States, call (800) 692-9010. Outside the United States, call
(314) 447-8094. You may also fax your questions to (314) 447-8078 or via e-mail at:
technical.support@elsevier.com

Copyright © 2011, 2009, 2007, 2005, 2003, 2001, 1999, 1997, 1996 by Mosby, Inc., an affiliate
of Elsevier Inc.
Part Number: 9996073858

ISBN: 978-0-323-08104-7

Mosby's

Drug
Guide
for Nurses

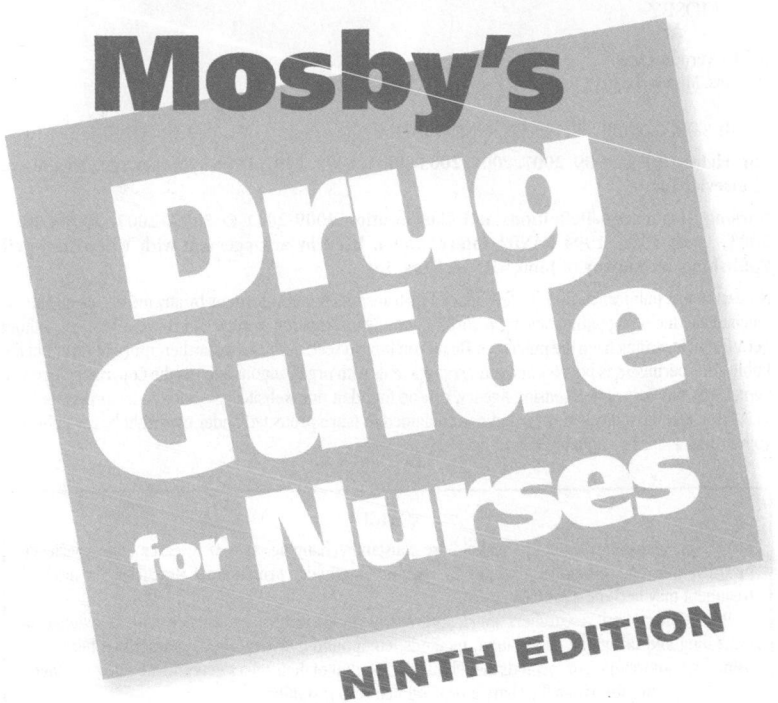

Mosby's Drug Guide for Nurses

NINTH EDITION

Linda Skidmore-Roth, RN, MSN, NP
Consultant
Littleton, Colorado

Formerly, Nursing Faculty
New Mexico State University
Las Cruces, New Mexico
El Paso Community College
El Paso, Texas

ELSEVIER
MOSBY

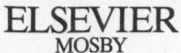

3251 Riverport Lane
St. Louis, Missouri 63043

MOSBY'S DRUG GUIDE FOR NURSES, NINTH EDITION ISBN: 978-0-323-08104-7

NOTICES

Knowledge and best practice in this field are constantly changing. As new research and experience broaden our understanding, changes in research methods, professional practices, or medical treatment may become necessary.

Practitioners and researchers must always rely on their own experience and knowledge in evaluating and using any information, methods, compounds, or experiments described herein. In using such information or methods they should be mindful of their own safety and the safety of others, including parties for whom they have a professional responsibility.

With respect to any drug or pharmaceutical products identified, readers are advised to check the most current information provided (i) on procedures featured or (ii) by the manufacturer of each product to be administered, to verify the recommended dose or formula, the method and duration of administration, and contraindications. It is the responsibility of practitioners, relying on their own experience and knowledge of their patients, to make diagnoses, to determine dosages and the best treatment for each individual patient, and to take all appropriate safety precautions.

To the fullest extent of the law, neither the Publisher nor the authors, contributors, or editors, assume any liability for any injury and/or damage to persons or property as a matter of products liability, negligence or otherwise, or from any use or operation of any methods, products, instructions, or ideas contained in the material herein.

International Standard Book Number 978-0-323-08104-7

Acquisitions Editor: Nancy O'Brien
Associate Developmental Editor: Angela Perdue
Publishing Services Manager: Pat Joiner-Myers
Senior Project Manager: Mary Pohlman
Senior Book Designer: Teresa McBryan

Printed in the United States of America

Last digit is the print number: 9   8   7   6   5   4   3   2   1

Consultants

Timothy L. Brenner, PharmD, BCOP
Clinical Pharmacy Specialist
UPMC Cancer Centers
Pittsburgh, Pennsylvania

Claudia Chiesa, PhD
Marana, Arizona

David S. Chun, PharmD, BCPS
Richmond Heights, Missouri

Jeffrey J. Fong, PharmD, BCPS
Assistant Professor of Pharmacy Practice
Massachusetts College of Pharmacy and Health
  Sciences
Worcester, Massachusetts

Amanda Gross, RPh
Clinical Pharmacist
University of Colorado Hospital
Aurora, Colorado

Dana H. Hamamura, PharmD
Clinical Pharmacist, Emergency Department
University of Colorado Hospital
Aurora, Colorado

Rose Knapp, NDP, RN, APRN-C
Assistant Professor of Nursing/Pharmacology
New York University
New York, New York

Michael J. Koronkowski, PharmD, CGP
Clinical Assistant Professor, Geriatrics
University of Illinois, College of Pharmacy
Chicago, Illinois

Shalini S. Lynch, PharmD
Assistant Clinical Professor of Pharmacy
University of California, San Francisco, School
  of Pharmacy
San Francisco, California

Michele Matthews, PharmD
Assistant Professor
Massachusetts College of Pharmacy
Clinical Pharmacist
Brigham and Women's Hospital
Boston, Massachusetts

Sandra Meeker, MSN, RN
Assistant Professor
University of Mary Hardin Baylor
Belton, Texas

Joshua J. Neumiller, PharmD, CDE, CGP, FASCP
Assistant Professor
Washington State University
Spokane, Washington

Christopher T. Owens, PharmD, BCPS
Associate Professor and Chair
Idaho State University College of Pharmacy
Pocatello, Idaho

Brenda Pavill, PhD, RN, FNP, IBCLC
Associate Professor
University of North Carolina at Wilmington
Wilmington, North Carolina

Adam B. Pesaturo, PharmD, BCPS
Critical Care Pharmacist
Baystate Medical Center
Springfield, Massachusetts

Kimberly A. Pesaturo, PharmD, BCPS
Assistant Professor of Pharmacy Practice
Massachusetts College of Pharmacy and Health
  Sciences
Worcester, Massachusetts

Sarah Reidunn Pool, MS, RN
Nurse Manager
Mayo Clinic
Rochester, Minnesota

Randolph Eldon Regal, BS, PharmD, RPh
Clinical Associate Professor, Adult Internal
  Medicine
University of Michigan
Ann Arbor, Michigan

Sheila M. Seed, PharmD, RPh, MPH
Assistant Professor of Pharmacy Practice
Massachusetts College of Pharmacy and Health
  Sciences
Worcester, Massachusetts

Stephen M. Setter, PharmD, DVM, CDE, CGP, FASCP
Associate Professor of Pharmacotherapy
Elder Services/Visiting Nurses Association
Washington State University
Spokane, Washington

Travis E. Sonnett, PharmD
Clinical Assistant Professor
Washington State University
Pullman, Washington

Patricia R. Teasley, MSN, RN
Nursing Programs Coordinator/Professor
Central Texas College
Killeen, Texas

Juanita C. Widener, MAEd, BSN, RN
Instructor of Nursing
Bainbridge College
Bainbridge, Georgia

NCLEX Writer

Susan McGregor-Huyer, RN, MSN, CHPN, CLNC
MH Consultants
University of Phoenix
Mahtomedi, Minnesota

Preface

Mosby's Drug Guide for Nurses, ninth edition, is the most in-depth handbook available for nursing students! Since its first publication in 1996, more than 100 U.S. and Canadian pharmacists and consultants have reviewed the book's content closely. Today, *Mosby's Drug Guide for Nurses* is more up-to-date than ever—with features that make it easy to find critical information fast!

NEW FEATURES
- There are 25 recent FDA-approved drugs for 2011 located throughout the book and in Appendix A, and there are 15 recent FDA-approved drugs for 2012 located behind the index.
- The latest NANDA nursing diagnoses are included.
- A mini CD-ROM is included that features over 350 NCLEX® examination review questions, patient teaching guides, and drug information for the 60 key drugs that students will encounter most in clinicals. A comprehensive calculation tutorial, a drug card creator, and dosage calculators are also on the CD.

NEW FACTS
This edition features thousands of new drug facts, including:
- New drugs and new dosage information
- Newly researched adverse effects
- New Black Box Warnings
- The latest precautions, interactions, and contraindications
- IV therapy updates
- Revised nursing considerations
- Updated patient/family education guidelines
- Updates on key new drug research

ORGANIZATION
This handbook is organized into four main sections:
- A four-color insert of drug mechanisms and drug administration
- Individual drug monographs (in alphabetical order by generic name)
- Drug Categories
- Appendixes

The guiding principle behind this book is to provide fast, easy access to drug information and nursing considerations. Every detail—from the cover, binding, and paper to the typeface, two-color design, and appendixes—has been carefully chosen with the user in mind.

Here's what you'll find in each section of the handbook:

Color Insert

Mechanisms-of-Action and Sites-of-Action Illustrations

These 16 detailed, full-color illustrations are added to help enhance the understanding of the mechanism or site of action for the following drugs and drug classes:

- ACE inhibitors
- Adrenocortical steroids
- Anticholinergic bronchodilators
- Antidepressants
- Antidiabetic agents
- Antifungal agents
- Antiinfective agents
- Antiretroviral agents
- Benzodiazepines
- Diuretics
- Drugs used to treat GERD
- Laxatives
- Narcotic agonist-antagonist analgesics
- Narcotic analgesics
- Phenytoin
- Sympatholytics

Photo Atlas of Drug Administration

This practical resource for students and practitioners lists standard precautions and provides 30 full-color illustrations depicting the physical landmarks and administration techniques used for **IV**, IM, SUBCUT, and ID drug delivery.

Also included in the color insert are standard precautions and the 2011 Recommended Childhood and Adolescent Immunization Schedule for the United States.

Individual Drug Monographs

This book includes monographs for more than 4000 generic and trade medications—those most commonly administered by students. Common trade names are given for all drugs regularly used in the United States and Canada, with drugs available only in Canada identified by a maple leaf icon (✻).

Each monograph provides the following information, whenever possible, for safe, effective administration of each drug:

High-alert status: Identifies drugs with the most potential to cause harm to patients if administered incorrectly.

"Tall Man" lettering: Uses the capitalization of distinguishing letters to avoid medication errors and is required by the FDA for drug manufacturers.

Key drug status: Identifies drugs of special prominence within their functional class that are often encountered by students during clinicals. These drugs are denoted with a special CD icon (💿) to direct the user to additional materials on the CD.

Pronunciation: Helps the nurse master complex generic names.

Rx, OTC: Identifies prescription or over-the-counter drugs.

Functional and chemical classifications: Helps the nurse recognize similarities and differences among drugs in the same functional but different chemical classes.

Pregnancy category: FDA pregnancy categories **A, B, C, D,** or **X** are noted at the beginning of each monograph, as well as under Precautions or Contraindications depending on FDA category. Appendix E provides a detailed explanation of each category.

Controlled substance schedule: Includes schedules for the United States and Canada.

Do not confuse: Presents drug names that might easily be confused within each appropriate monograph.

Action: Describes pharmacologic properties concisely.

Therapeutic outcome: Details all possible results of medication use.

Uses: Lists the conditions the drug is used to treat.

Unlabeled uses: Describes drug uses that may be encountered in practice but are not yet FDA approved.

Dosages and routes: Lists all available and approved dosages and routes for adult, pediatric, and geriatric patients.

Available forms: Includes tablets, capsules, extended release, injectables (**IV**, IM, SUBCUT), solutions, creams, ointments, lotions, gels, shampoos, elixirs, suspensions, suppositories, sprays, aerosols, and lozenges.

Adverse effects: Groups these reactions by alphabetical body system, with common side effects *italicized* and life-threatening reactions in **bold type** for emphasis.

Contraindications: Lists conditions under which the drug absolutely should not be given, including FDA pregnancy safety categories **D** or **X.**

Precautions: Lists conditions that require special consideration when the drug is prescribed, including FDA pregnancy safety categories **A, B,** and **C.**

Black Box Warnings: Identifies FDA warnings that highlight serious and life-threatening adverse effects.

Pharmacokinetics/pharmacodynamics: Features a quick-reference chart of concise facts of pharmacokinetics (absorption, distribution, metabolism, excretion, half-life) and pharmacodynamics (onset, peak, duration).

Interactions: Lists confirmed drug, food, herb, and lab test interactions.

Nursing considerations: Identifies key nursing considerations for each step of the nursing process: Assessment, Nursing Diagnoses, Implementation, Patient/Family Education, and Evaluation, including positive therapeutic outcomes. Instructions for giving drugs by various routes (e.g., **IV**, PO, IM, SUBCUT, topically, rectally) appear under Implementation, with route subheadings in bold.

Compatibilities: Lists syringe, Y-site, and additive compatibilities and incompatibilities. If no compatibilities are listed for a drug, the necessary compatibility testing has not been done and that compatibility information is unknown. To ensure safety, assume that the drug may not be mixed with other drugs unless specifically stated.

Nursing Alert icon ◆: Highlights situations in which the patient could potentially be at risk.

Treatment of overdose: Lists drugs and treatments for overdoses where appropriate.

Drug Categories

The Drug Categories section, following the individual drug monographs, provides general information about the various functional classes to promote learning about the similarities and differences among drugs in the same functional class. It summarizes action, uses, adverse effects, contraindications, precautions, pharmacokinetics, interactions, and nursing considerations for each functional class.

Appendixes

Selected new drugs: Includes comprehensive information on 25 key drugs approved by the FDA during the last 12 months.

Ophthalmic, nasal, topical, and otic products: Provides essential information for 140 ophthalmic, nasal, topical, and otic products commonly used today, grouped by chemical drug class.

Vaccines and toxoids: Features an easy-to-use table with generic and trade names, uses, dosages and routes, and contraindications for 39 key vaccines and toxoids.

Combination products: Provides details on the forms and uses of more than 600 combination products.

Abbreviations and pregnancy categories: Lists abbreviations alphabetically with their meanings and explains the five FDA pregnancy categories.

The following sources were consulted in the preparation of this edition:

Blumenthal M: *The Complete German Commission E Monographs: Therapeutic Guide to Herbal Medicines,* Austin, 1998, American Botanical Council.

Brunton L, Lazo J, Parker K: *Goodman and Gilman's The Pharmacological Basis of Therapeutics,* ed 11, New York, 2006, McGraw-Hill.

Clinical Pharmacology [database online], Tampa, 2010, Gold Standard, Inc. http://www.clinicalpharmacology.com. Updated March 2010.

Gahart BL: *Intravenous Medications,* ed 26, St. Louis, 2010, Mosby.

McKenry LM, Tessier E, Hogan MA: *Mosby's Pharmacology in Nursing,* ed 22, St. Louis, 2006, Mosby.

Acknowledgments

I am indebted to the nursing and pharmacology consultants who reviewed the manuscript and pages and thank them for their criticism and encouragement. I would also like to thank Nancy O'Brien and Angela Perdue, my editors, whose active encouragement and enthusiasm have made this book better than it might otherwise have been. I am likewise grateful to Mary Pohlman and Graphic World Inc. for the coordination of the production process and assistance with the development of the new edition.

Linda Skidmore-Roth

Contents

Insert: Selected New Drugs for 2012

cabazitaxel	liraglutide
carglumic acid	lurasidone
ceftaroline	pegloticase
dabigatran	sipuleucel-T
dalfampridine	tocilizumab
denosumab	ulipristal
eribulin	vilazodone
fingolimod	

Evolve Website Contents

- Content Updates
- Calculators
- Canadian Controlled Substance Chart
- Canadian Recommended Immunization Schedules for Infants and Children
- Color Pill Atlas
- Controlled Substance Chart
- Drug Name Safety
- English-to-Spanish Translations
- FDA Alerts
- Herbal Products
- High-Alert Canadian Medications
- High-Alert Drugs
- Rarely Used Drugs
- Recently Approved Drugs
- Weblinks

COLOR INSERT

Immunization Schedules for Children and Adolescents

Standard Precautions

Mechanisms and Sites of Action

Photo Atlas of Drug Administration

Recommended Childhood and Adolescent Immunization Schedule—United States, 2011

Immunization Schedule for Persons Aged 0-6 Years

Vaccine ▼ Age ▶	Birth	1 month	2 months	4 months	6 months	12 months	15 months	18 months	19-23 months	2-3 years	4-6 years
Hepatitis B[1]	HepB	HepB				HepB					
Rotavirus[2]			RV	RV	RV[2]						
Diphtheria, Tetanus, Pertussis[3]			DTaP	DTaP	DTaP		DTaP				DTaP
Haemophilus influenzae type b[4]			Hib	Hib	Hib[4]	see footnote[3]	Hib				
Pneumococcal[5]			PCV	PCV	PCV	PCV				PPSV	PPSV
Inactivated Poliovirus[6]			IPV	IPV	IPV		IPV				IPV
Influenza[7]						Influenza (Yearly)					
Measles, Mumps, Rubella[8]						MMR					MMR
Varicella[9]						Varicella					Varicella
Hepatitis A[10]						HepA (2 doses)			see footnote[8] see footnote[9]	HepA Series	
Meningococcal[11]										MCV4	MCV4

Range of recommended ages for all children

Range of recommended ages for certain high-risk groups

This schedule includes recommendations in effect as of December 21, 2010. Any dose not administered at the recommended age should be administered at a subsequent visit, when indicated and feasible. The use of a combination vaccine generally is preferred over separate injections of its equivalent component vaccines. Considerations should include provider assessment, patient preference, and the potential for adverse events. Providers should consult the relevant Advisory Committee on Immunization Practices statement for detailed recommendations: **http://www.cdc.gov/vaccines/pubs/acip-list.htm.** Clinically significant adverse events that follow immunization should be reported to the Vaccine Adverse Event Reporting System (VAERS) at **http://www.vaers.hhs.gov** or by telephone, 800-822-7967.

Immunization Schedule for Persons Aged 7-18 Years

Vaccine ▼ Age ▶	7–10 years	11–12 years	13–18 years
Tetanus, Diphtheria, Pertussis[1]		Tdap	Tdap
Human Papillomavirus[2]	see footnote [2]	HPV (3 doses)(females)	HPV series
Meningococcal[3]	MCV4	MCV4	MCV4
Influenza[4]		Influenza (Yearly)	
Pneumococcal[5]		Pneumococcal	
Hepatitis A[6]		HepA Series	
Hepatitis B[7]		Hep B Series	
Inactivated Poliovirus[8]		IPV Series	
Measles, Mumps, Rubella[9]		MMR Series	
Varicella[10]		Varicella Series	

Range of recommended ages for all children

Range of recommended ages for catch-up immunization

Range of recommended ages for certain high-risk groups

This schedule includes recommendations in effect as of December 21, 2010. Any dose not administered at the recommended age should be administered at a subsequent visit, when indicated and feasible. The use of a combination vaccine generally is preferred over separate injections of its equivalent component vaccines. Considerations should include provider assessment, patient preference, and the potential for adverse events. Providers should consult the relevant Advisory Committee on Immunization Practices statement for detailed recommendations: **http://www.cdc.gov/vaccines/pubs/acip-list.htm**. Clinically significant adverse events that follow immunization should be reported to the Vaccine Adverse Event Reporting System (VAERS) at **http://www.vaers.hhs.gov** or by telephone, 800-822-7967.

STANDARD PRECAUTIONS

The following precautions are used in the care of all patients regardless of their diagnosis or disease. They are also applied when handling or cleaning equipment or supplies that are potentially contaminated.

1. Wear gloves any time that you may contact blood, any moist body fluid (except sweat), secretions, excretions, nonintact skin, or mucous membranes.

2. Remove your gloves, wash your hands, and reapply clean gloves if your gloves become soiled with infective material.

3. Even if you are wearing gloves, remove them, wash your hands, and apply clean gloves *immediately before* contact with mucous membranes or nonintact skin.

4. Wear a protective cover gown of waterproof material if your clothing is likely to have substantial contact with infective material or if splashing of body fluids is likely.

5. Wear a face shield or goggles to protect your eyes if splashing of secretions is likely.

6. Any time a face shield or goggles are worn, wear a surgical mask to protect the mucous membranes of your nose and mouth. A surgical mask may be worn during certain sterile procedures without protective eyewear. However, protective eyewear is *never* worn without a surgical mask.

7. Handle needles, razors, broken glass, and other sharp objects with care. Needles should never be recapped. All sharps should be disposed of in a puncture-resistant sharps container.

8. Wash your hands before and after each patient contact.

9. Wash your hands before you apply and after you remove gloves. Do not assume that hand washing is unnecessary because gloves were worn. Do not wash your hands with gloves on them.

10. Gloves are used for the care of one patient only, then discarded.

11. Follow your facility policy for disposal of gloves and other contaminated items. These items are generally not disposed of in open trash containers. Facilities have designated disposal sites for these biohazardous waste materials.

12. Use resuscitation barrier devices as an alternative to mouth-to-mouth resuscitation.

13. Linen should be handled in a manner that prevents contamination of the outside of the container. Linen from isolation rooms was previously double bagged. Double bagging is no longer recommended since all linen is handled as potentially infectious. Double bag linen only if the outside of the bag becomes contaminated during the bagging process.

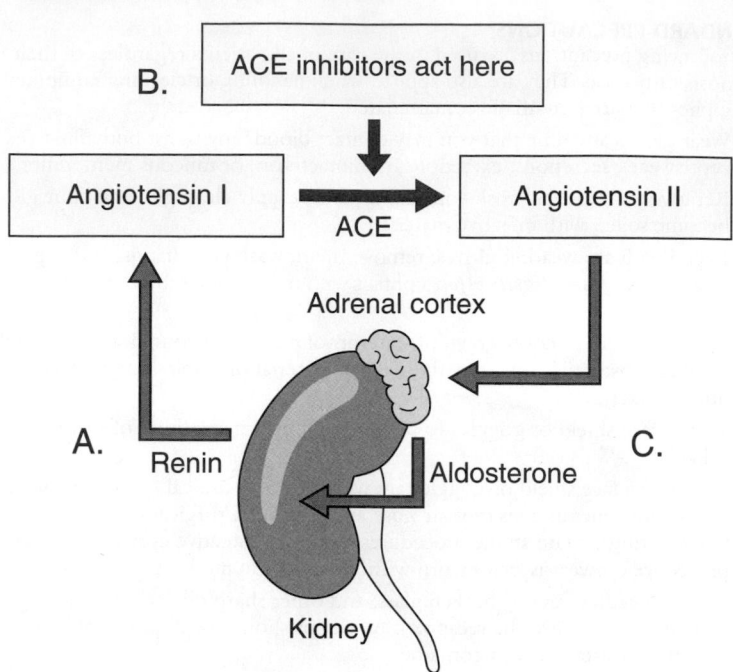

Plate 1 The renin-angiotensin-aldosterone system plays a major role in regulating B/P. Any condition that decreases renal blood flow, reduces B/P, or stimulates β_1-adrenergic receptors prompts the kidneys to release renin **(A)**. Renin acts on angiotensinogen, which is converted to angiotensin I, a weak vasoconstrictor. Angiotensin-converting enzyme (ACE) converts angiotensin I to angiotensin II, which causes systemic and renal blood vessels to constrict **(B)**. Systemic vasoconstriction increases peripheral vascular resistance, raising the B/P. Renal vasoconstriction decreases glomerular filtration, resulting in sodium and water retention and increasing blood volume and B/P. In addition, angiotensin II acts on the adrenal cortex, causing it to release aldosterone **(C)**. This makes the kidneys retain additional sodium and water, which further increases the B/P. ACE inhibitors, such as captopril, enalapril, and lisinopril, block the action of ACE. As a result, angiotensin II cannot form, which prevents systemic and renal vasoconstriction and the release of aldosterone. (From Prosser S, Worster B, Dewar K: *Applied Pharmacology for Nurses and Other Health Care Professionals*, St. Louis, 2000, Mosby.)

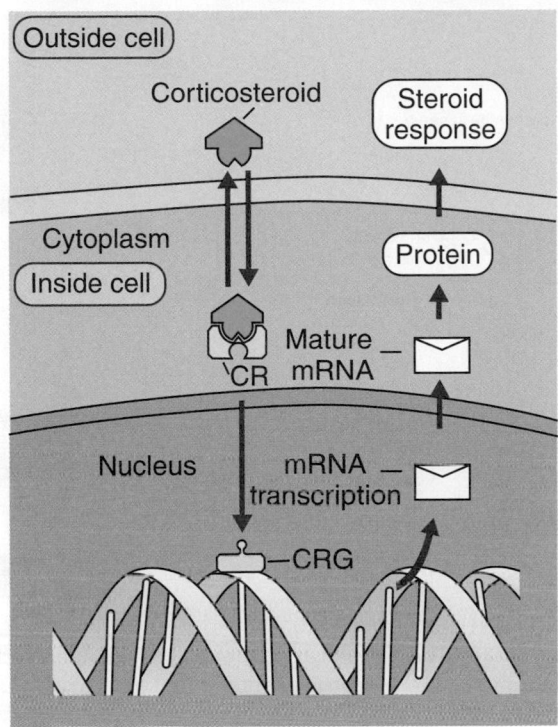

Plate 2 Adrenocortical steroids (also called corticosteroids) are available in many forms, such as predniSONE, and produce a wide range of effects, such as immunosuppression and antiinflammation. Here is how these drugs work at the cellular level.

Corticosteroids are hormones that are naturally produced by the body (endogenous hormones). Synthetic corticosteroids work much the same as the endogenous hormones. When a corticosteroid enters a cell, it binds to corticosteroid receptors (CRs) in the cell's cytoplasm, forming a complex. The complex moves to the nucleus, where it causes the transcription of corticosteroid responsive genes (CRGs) to messenger ribonucleic acid (mRNA), eventually translating to a protein that produces a steroid response in target tissues. (From Taylor: *Mosby's Crash Course Pharmacology*, St. Louis, 1998, Mosby.)

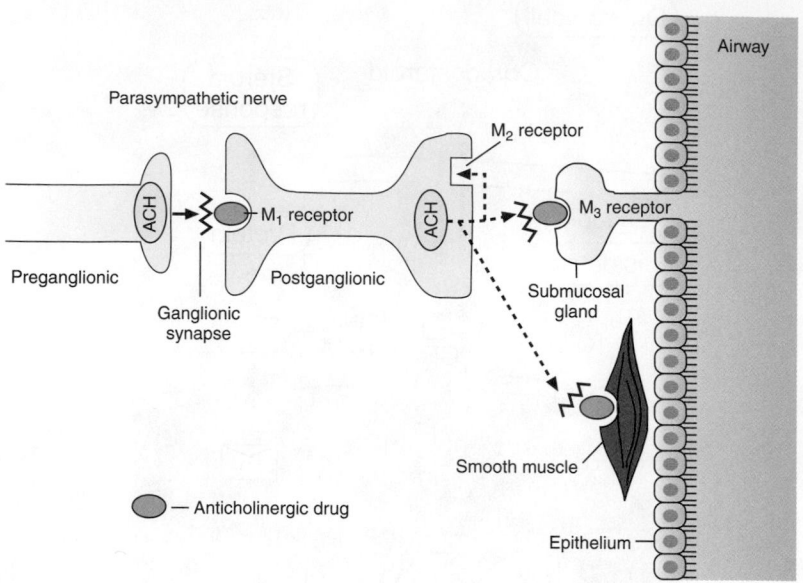

Plate 3 Anticholinergic bronchodilators, such as ipratropium, work by blocking muscarinic-1 (M_1) receptors on postganglionic parasympathetic nerve endings and muscarinic-3 (M_3) receptors on the cell membranes of bronchial smooth muscles and submucosal glands. Normally, stimulation of the M_1 and M_3 receptors by acetylcholine (ACH) causes bronchoconstriction and mucus secretion from submucosal glands. Anticholinergic bronchodilators block these specific muscarinic receptors from the effects of acetylcholine, causing bronchial smooth muscle relaxation, bronchodilatation, and decreased mucus production. (From Gardenhire OS: *Rau's Respiratory Care Pharmacology,* ed 7, St. Louis, 2008, Mosby.)

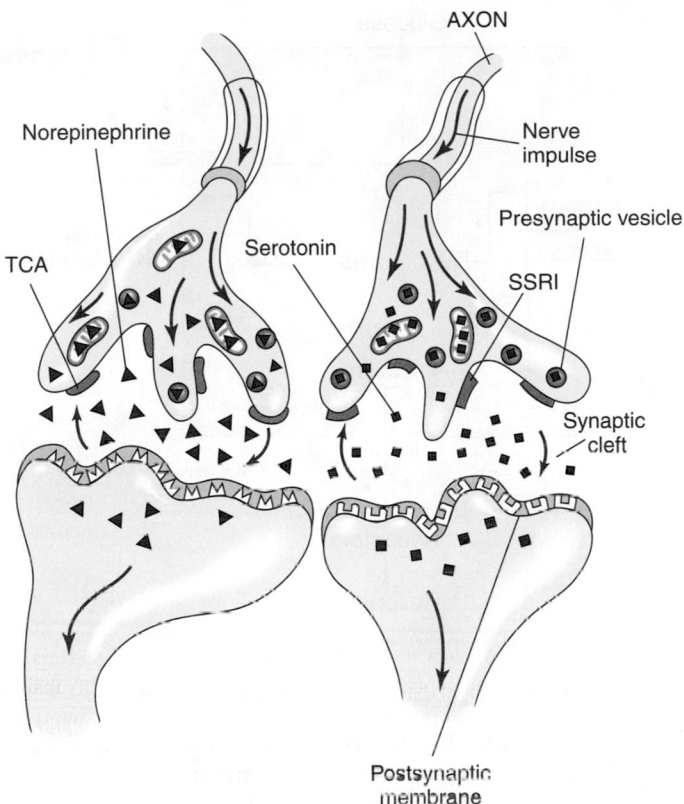

Plate 4 Depression is thought to occur when levels of neurotransmitters, such as norepinephrine and serotonin, are reduced at postsynaptic receptor sites. These neurotransmitters affect a wide array of functions, including mood, obsessions, appetite, and anxiety. Antidepressants work by increasing the availability of these neurotransmitters at postsynaptic membranes and by enhancing and prolonging their effects. As a result, these agents improve mood, reduce anxiety, and minimize obsessions.

Antidepressants typically are classified as tricyclic antidepressants (TCAs), monoamine oxidase inhibitors (not shown), selective serotonin reuptake inhibitors (SSRIs), and atypical antidepressants (not shown). TCAs, such as amitriptyline and desipramine, primarily block norepinephrine reuptake at presynaptic membranes, thereby increasing the norepinephrine concentration at synapses and making more available at postsynaptic receptors.

SSRIs, such as fluoxetine and paroxetine, selectively inhibit serotonin uptake at presynaptic membranes. This action leads to increased serotonin availability at postsynaptic receptors. (From Gutierrez K: *Pharmacotherapeutics: Clinical Decision Making in Nursing,* ed 2, Philadelphia, 2008, Saunders.)

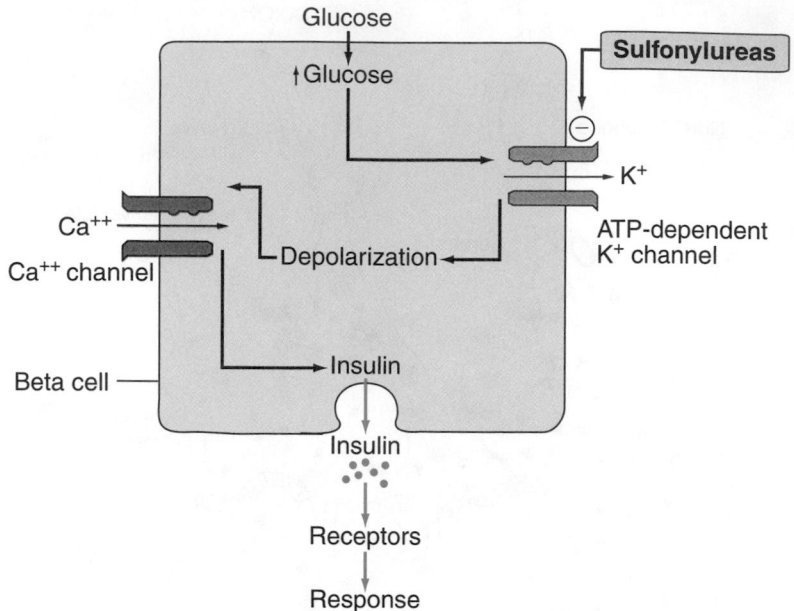

Plate 5 Diabetes mellitus takes two forms: type 1 diabetes characterized by a complete lack of insulin and type 2 diabetes marked by insufficient insulin secretion, insulin resistance in peripheral tissues, or both. Normally, the beta cells in the pancreatic islets of Langerhans are responsible for secreting insulin. The rise of glucose levels in the beta cell triggers adenosine triphosphate (ATP)-dependent potassium (K^+) channels in the membranes of beta cells to close. Then the beta cells depolarize and calcium (Ca^{++}) enters the cell through Ca^{++} channel, and insulin is released from the cell. When circulating insulin engages with insulin receptors on cell membranes, it facilitates the movement of glucose into the cell, among other actions.

Type 1 diabetes is treated with the use of exogenous insulin, which mimics natural insulin in the body. Insulin takes many forms with varying degrees of onset, peak, and duration, including rapid, regular, intermediate, and long acting.

Type 2 diabetes is usually treated with oral agents. Sulfonylureas, such as glyburide, block ATP-dependent K^+ channels in the cell membranes of beta cells, ultimately resulting in the release of insulin. (From Taylor: *Mosby's Crash Course Pharmacology,* St. Louis, 1998, Mosby.)

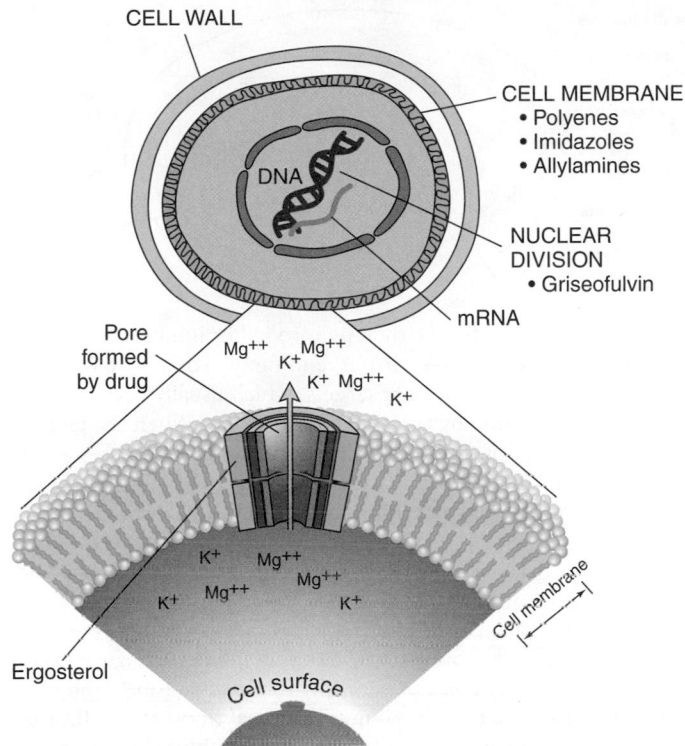

Plate 6 Antifungal agents primarily affect fungi at one of two sites: the cell membrane or the cell nucleus. Most of these agents, such as polyene, imidazole, and allylamine antifungals, act on the fungal cell membrane. Polyene antifungals, such amphotericin B, bind to ergosterol and increase cell membrane permeability. Imidazole antifungals, such as fluconazole and ketoconazole, interfere with ergosterol synthesis by inhibiting the cytochrome P_{450} enzyme system, altering the cell membrane, and inhibiting fungal growth. Allylamine antifungals, such as terbinafine, inhibit the enzyme squaline epoxidase, which disrupts ergosterol production—and cell membrane integrity. When cell membrane permeability increases, cellular components, including potassium (K^+) and magnesium (Mg^{++}), leak out. Loss of these cellular components leads to cell death.

Another antifungal agent, griseofulvin, directly affects the fungal nucleus, interfering with mitosis. By binding to structures in the mitotic spindle, it prevents cells from dividing, which eventually leads to their death. (From Gutierrez K: *Pharmacotherapeutics: Clinical Decision Making in Nursing,* ed 2, Philadelphia, 2008, Saunders.)

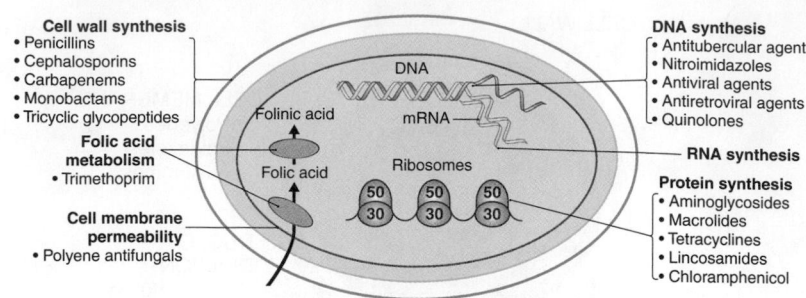

Cell wall synthesis
- Penicillins
- Cephalosporins
- Carbapenems
- Monobactams
- Tricyclic glycopeptides

Folic acid metabolism
- Trimethoprim

Cell membrane permeability
- Polyene antifungals

DNA

Folinic acid

mRNA

Folic acid

Ribosomes

50 30 50 30 50 30

DNA synthesis
- Antitubercular agent
- Nitroimidazoles
- Antiviral agents
- Antiretroviral agents
- Quinolones

RNA synthesis

Protein synthesis
- Aminoglycosides
- Macrolides
- Tetracyclines
- Lincosamides
- Chloramphenicol

Plate 7 The goal of antiinfective therapy is to kill or inhibit the growth of microorganisms such as bacteria, viruses, and fungi. To achieve this goal, antiinfective agents must reach their targets, which usually occurs through absorption and distribution by the circulatory system. When the target is reached, a drug can kill or suppress microorganisms by:
- Inhibiting cell wall synthesis or activating enzymes that disrupt the cell wall, which leads to cellular weakening, lysis, and death. Penicillins (ampicillin), cephalosporins (cefazolin), carbapenems (imipenem), monobactams (aztreonam), and tricyclic glycopeptides (vancomycin) act in this way.
- Altering cell membrane permeability through direct action on the cell wall, which allows intracellular substances to leak out and destabilizes the cell. Polyene antifungals (amphotericin) work by this mechanism.
- Altering protein synthesis by binding to bacterial ribosomes (50/30) or affecting ribosomal function, which leads to cell death or slowed growth respectively. Aminoglycosides (gentamicin), macrolides (erythromycin), tetracyclines (doxycycline), lincosamides (clindamycin), and the miscellaneous antiinfective chloramphenicol use this action.
- Inhibiting DNA or RNA, including messenger RNA (mRNA), synthesis by binding to nucleic acids or interacting with enzymes required for their synthesis. Antitubercular agents (rifampin), nitroimidazoles (metronidazole), antiviral agents (acyclovir), antiretroviral agents (stavudine), and quinolones (ciprofloxacin) act like this.
- Inhibiting the metabolism of folic acid and folinic acid or other cellular components that are essential for bacterial cell growth. The miscellaneous antiinfective trimethoprim employs this mechanism of action. (From Page C et al: *Integrated Pharmacology*, ed 3, St. Louis, 2006, Mosby.)

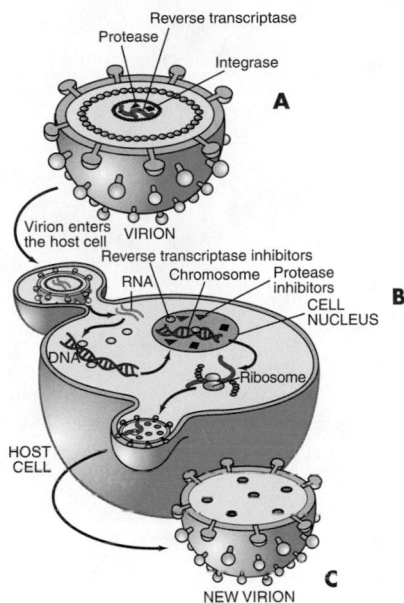

Plate 8 When viruses reproduce, the infectious viral particle, or virion (**A**), enters the host cell. The virion attaches to the cell's surface and then inserts itself into the host cell (**B**). Once inside, the virion uncoats, and the enzyme reverse transcriptase makes two copies of the viral RNA: one copy is identical; the other is a mirror image. These two copies form double-stranded viral DNA that enters the host cell's nucleus, where it inserts itself into the host cell's DNA with the help of the enzyme integrase. Then viral DNA reprograms the host cell to produce additional viral RNA, which begins the process of forming new viruses. Specifically, messenger RNA (mRNA) instructs ribosomal RNA (rRNA) to produce a new chain of proteins and enzymes that are used to form new viruses. Protease cuts the chains, creating individual proteins. These combine with new RNA to create new virions, which bud and are released from the host cell (**C**).

Antiretroviral agents target specific enzymes during viral reproduction. Nucleoside reverse transcriptase inhibitors, such as stavudine, interfere with the action of reverse transcriptase by mimicking naturally occurring nucleosides. Nucleotide reverse transcriptase inhibitors, such as tenofovir, block reverse transcriptase by competing with the natural substrate deoxyadenosine triphosphate and by causing DNA chain termination. Nonnucleoside reverse transcriptase inhibitors, such as delavirdine, work by directly binding to reverse transcriptase. As a result, no viral DNA is available to insert itself into the host cell's DNA. Protease inhibitors, such as indinavir, bind to and interfere with the action of protease; thus, the new chain of proteins formed by rRNA cannot be cut into individual proteins to make new viruses. (From Gutierrez K: *Pharmacotherapeutics: Clinical Decision Making in Nursing,* ed 2, Philadelphia, 2008, Saunders.)

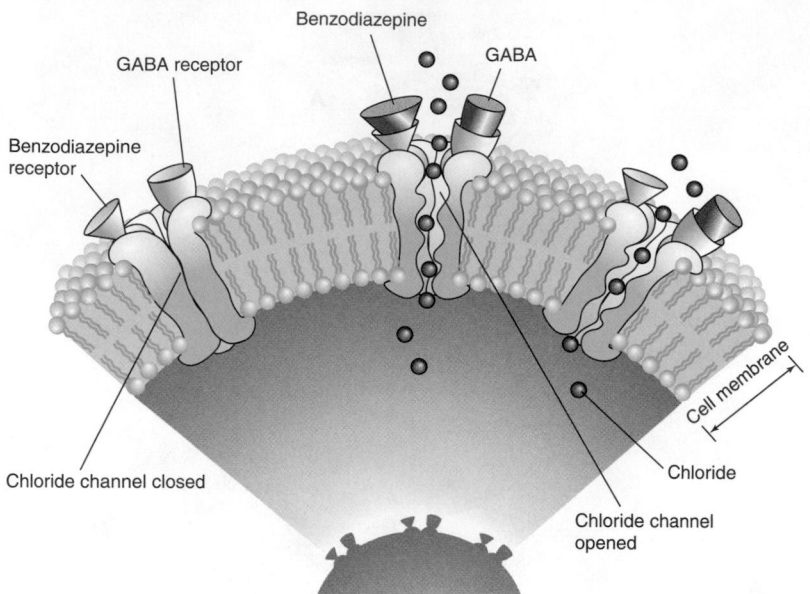

Plate 9 Benzodiazepines reduce anxiety by stimulating the action of the inhibitory neurotransmitter, gamma-aminobutyric acid (GABA), in the limbic system. The limbic system plays an important role in the regulation of human behavior. Dysfunction of GABA neurotransmission in the limbic system may be linked to the development of certain anxiety disorders.

The limbic system contains a highly dense area of benzodiazepine receptors that may be linked to the antianxiety effects of benzodiazepines. These benzodiazepine receptors are located on the surface of neuronal cell membranes and are adjacent to GABA receptors. The binding of a benzodiazepine to its receptor enhances the affinity of a GABA receptor for GABA. In the absence of a benzodiazepine, the binding of GABA to its receptor causes the chloride channel in the cell membrane to open, which increases the influx of chloride into the cell. This influx of chloride results in hyperpolarization of the neuronal cell membrane and reduces the neuron's ability to fire, which is why GABA is considered an inhibitory neurotransmitter.

A benzodiazepine acts only in the presence of GABA. When it binds to a benzodiazepine receptor, it prolongs the time that the chloride channel remains open. This results in greater depression of neuronal function and a reduction in anxiety. (From Gutierrez K: *Pharmacotherapeutics: Clinical Decision Making in Nursing,* ed 2, Philadelphia, 2008, Saunders.)

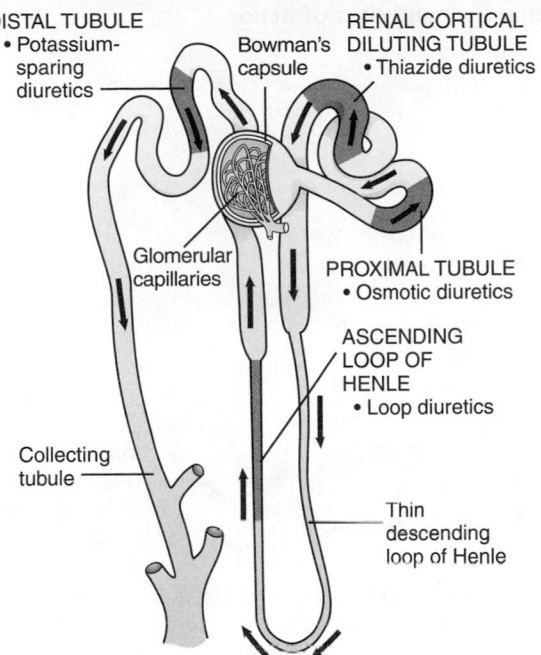

DISTAL TUBULE
• Potassium-sparing diuretics

Bowman's capsule

RENAL CORTICAL DILUTING TUBULE
• Thiazide diuretics

Glomerular capillaries

PROXIMAL TUBULE
• Osmotic diuretics

ASCENDING LOOP OF HENLE
• Loop diuretics

Collecting tubule

Thin descending loop of Henle

Plate 10 Diuretics act primarily to increase water and sodium excretion by the kidneys, thereby increasing urine output. In the process, chloride, potassium, and other electrolytes may also be excreted. Most diuretics act by blocking sodium, water, and chloride reabsorption by peritubular capillaries in the nephrons. As a result, water and electrolytes remain in the convoluted tubules to be excreted as urine. The increased water and electrolyte excretion reduces blood volume—and ultimately blood pressure.

Diuretics belong to four major subclasses:

1. Thiazide diuretics, such as hydrochlorothiazide, act in the early portion of the distal convoluted tubule, called the cortical diluting segment. These drugs block sodium, chloride, and water reabsorption and promote their excretion along with potassium.

2. Loop diuretics, such as furosemide, act primarily in the thick ascending limb of the loop of Henle, blocking sodium, water, and chloride reabsorption. Then these substances are excreted along with potassium.

3. Potassium-sparing diuretics, such as spironolactone, act in the late portion of the distal convoluted tubule and collecting tubule. Here, they inhibit the action of aldosterone, leading to sodium excretion and potassium retention. Although triamterene and amiloride, two other potassium-sparing diuretics, act at the same site, they do not affect aldosterone. Instead, these drugs directly block the exchange of sodium and potassium, leading to decreased sodium reabsorption and decreased potassium excretion.

4. Osmotic diuretics, such as mannitol, work in the proximal convoluted tubule. As their name implies, these diuretics increase the osmotic pressure of the glomerular filtrate, inhibiting the passive reabsorption of water, sodium, and chloride. (From Gutierrez K: *Pharmacotherapeutics: Clinical Decision Making in Nursing,* ed 2, Philadelphia, 2008, Saunders.)

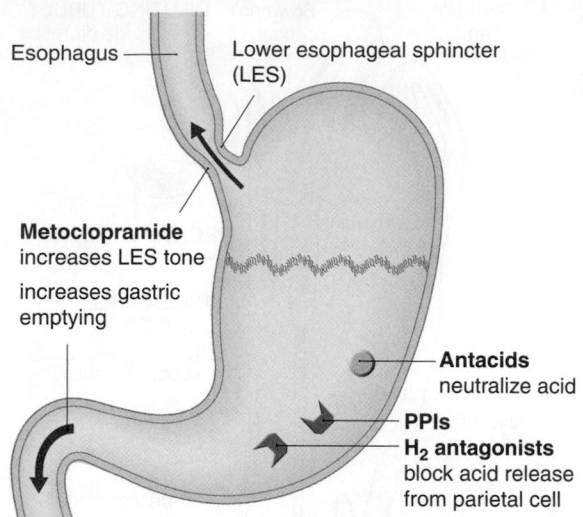

Esophagus — Lower esophageal sphincter (LES)

Metoclopramide increases LES tone

increases gastric emptying

Antacids neutralize acid

PPIs
H₂ antagonists block acid release from parietal cell

Plate 11 Gastroesophageal reflux disease (GERD) occurs when acidic stomach contents regurgitate into the esophagus, causing heartburn. The disorder may result from a weakness or incompetence of the lower esophageal sphincter (LES). Because the malfunctioning LES makes the reflux leave the stomach and reenter the esophagus slowly, the esophageal mucosa is exposed to the acid for a long time. Because the enzymatic action of parietal cells in the stomach makes the reflux highly acidic, GERD causes irritation and possible erosion of the esophageal mucosa.

Treatment of GERD can employ drugs from several classes: histamine (H_2) antagonists, proton pump inhibitors (PPIs), the miscellaneous GI agent metoclopramide, and antacids. H_2 antagonists, such as cimetidine, act in parietal cells of the stomach. Normally, H_2-receptor stimulation results in gastric acid secretion. By blocking these receptors, H_2 antagonists decrease the amount and acidity of gastric secretion, including secretion that occurs with fasting, food consumption at night, and stomach distension.

PPIs, such as esomeprazole, also suppress gastric acid secretion. However, they do it by inhibiting the hydrogen-potassium-adenosine triphsophatase enzyme system, which is located on the surface of parietal cells and controls their gastric acid secretion. PPIs block acid secretion that results from fasting or abdominal distension caused by food ingestion.

Metoclopramide increases the tone and motility of the upper GI tract. It works by stimulating the release of acetylcholine from GI nerve endings, which improves LES tone and leads to decreased reflux. The drug also stimulates gastric emptying, which reduces gastric contents.

Antacids, such as aluminum hydroxide, act primarily in the stomach by chemically combining with the hydrogen ions (H^+) in gastric acid and raising the pH of gastric contents. They do not prevent reflux. However, they make the reflux less acidic, so it causes less damage to the esophageal mucosa. (From Page C et al: *Integrated Pharmacology*, ed 3, St. Louis, 2006, Mosby.)

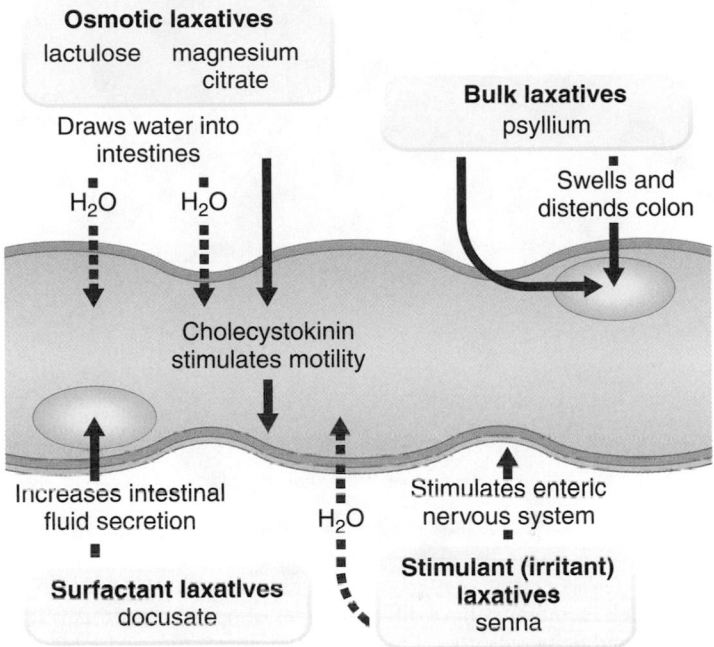

Plate 12 Laxatives ease or stimulate defecation. Typically, they are classified by their mechanism of action as bulk-forming, osmotic, stimulant, or surfactant laxatives.

Bulk-forming laxatives, such as psyllium, act in the small and large bowel. Because ingredients in these laxatives are undigestible, they remain within the stool and increase the fecal mass by drawing in water. These agents also enhance bacterial growth in the colon, further adding to the fecal mass.

Osmotic laxatives, such as lactulose, draw water into the intestinal lumen, causing the fecal mass to soften and swell. This osmotic action may be enhanced by the metabolism of colonic bacteria to lactate and other organic acids. These acids decrease colonic pH and increase colonic motility.

Stimulant (or irritant) laxatives, such as senna, act on the intestinal wall to increase water and electrolytes in the intestinal lumen. In addition, they directly irritate the colon, increasing motility.

Surfactant laxatives (or fecal softeners), such as docusate, reduce the surface tension of the stool, allowing water to enter it. These laxatives may also help to increase water and electrolyte excretion into the intestinal lumen, softening and increasing the fecal mass. (From Page C et al: *Integrated Pharmacology*, ed 3, St. Louis, 2006, Mosby.)

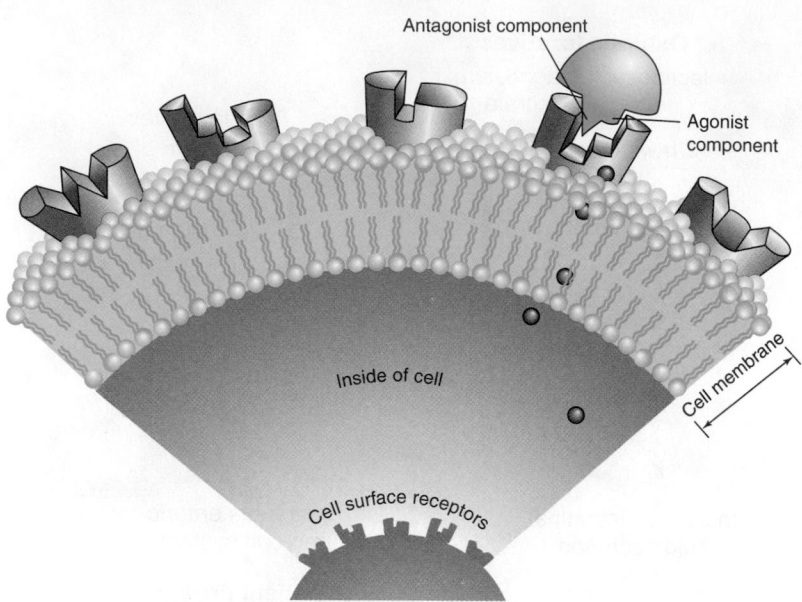

Plate 13 Cell membranes have different types of opioid receptors, such as mu, kappa, and delta receptors. Opioid agonist-antagonists work by stimulating one type of receptor, while simultaneously blocking another type. As agonists, they work primarily by activating kappa receptors to produce analgesia and such other effects as CNS and respiratory depression, decreased GI motility, and euphoria. As antagonists, they compete with opioids at mu receptors, helping to reverse or block some of the other effects of agonists. (From Gutierrez K: *Pharmacotherapeutics: Clinical Decision Making in Nursing,* ed 2, Philadelphia, 2008, Saunders.)

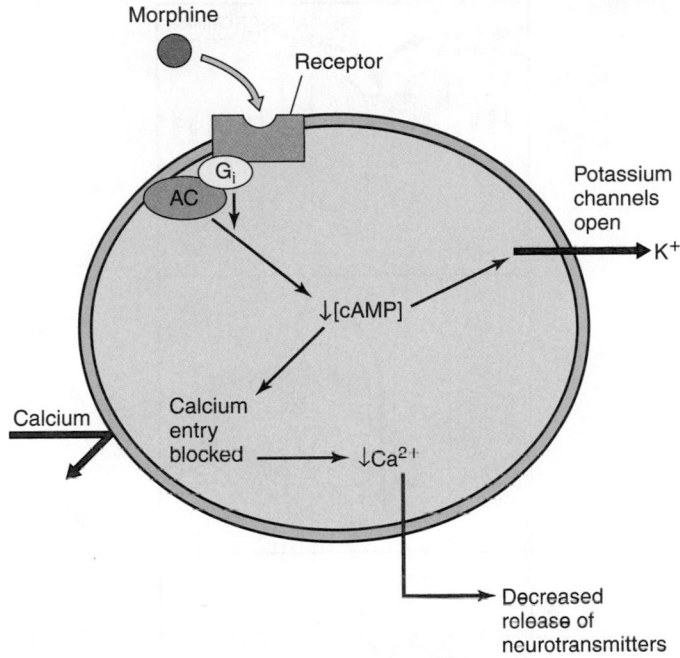

Plate 14 Narcotic analgesics bind to three types of opioid receptors: mu, kappa, and delta receptors. They produce analgesia primarily by activating mu receptors. However, they also engage with and activate kappa and delta receptors, producing other effects, such as sedation and vasomotor stimulation.

When morphine or another narcotic analgesic binds to opioid receptors, activation occurs. The receptors send signals to the enzyme adenyl cyclase (AC) to slow activity by way of G proteins (G_i). Decreased adenyl cyclase activity causes reduced production of cyclic adenosine monophosphate (cAMP). A secondary messenger substance, cAMP is important for regulating cell membrane channels. A reduced cAMP level allows fewer potassium ions to leave the cell and blocks calcium ions from entering the cell. This ion imbalance—especially the reduced intracellular calcium level—ultimately decreases the release of neurotransmitters from the cell, thereby blocking or reducing pain impulse transmission. (From Minneman KP, Wecker L: *Brody's Human Pharmacology: Molecular to Clinical,* ed 4, St. Louis, 2005, Mosby.)

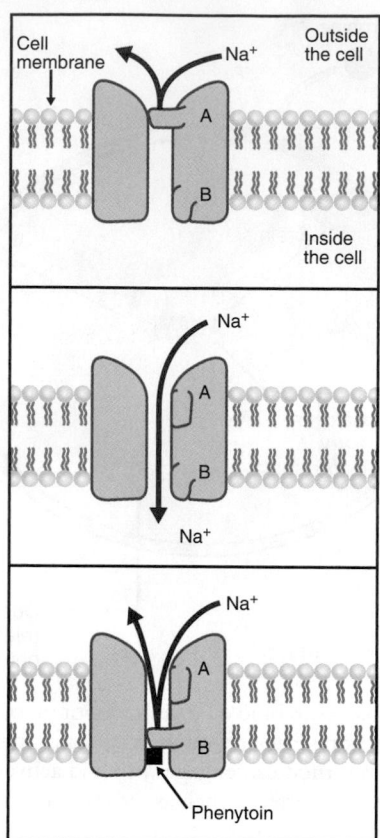

Plate 15 Phenytoin, which is used to treat tonic-clonic seizures, acts in the motor cortex and brain stem, where the tonic phase of tonic-clonic seizures originates. By altering sodium transport across neuronal cell membranes, phenytoin stabilizes the cell membrane, reduces repetitive firing of the neurons, and halts or limits the spread of seizures. The first illustration shows a neuronal cell membrane in its resting state. The activation gate (**A**) of the sodium channel in the cell membrane is closed and blocks sodium (Na^+) from entering the cell. In the second illustration, a nerve impulse has caused depolarization and opening of the activation gate, allowing Na^+ to move into the cell. In the third illustration, depolarization continues and an inactivation gate (**B**) moves into the channel. This prevents Na^+ from moving into the cell. Phenytoin prolongs the inactivated state of the sodium channel by preventing reopening of the inactivation gate. By further preventing Na^+ from entering the cell, phenytoin slows impulse transmission, and thus slows the rate at which neurons fire. (From Minneman KP, Wecker L: *Brody's Human Pharmacology: Molecular to Clinical,* ed 4, St. Louis, 2005, Mosby.)

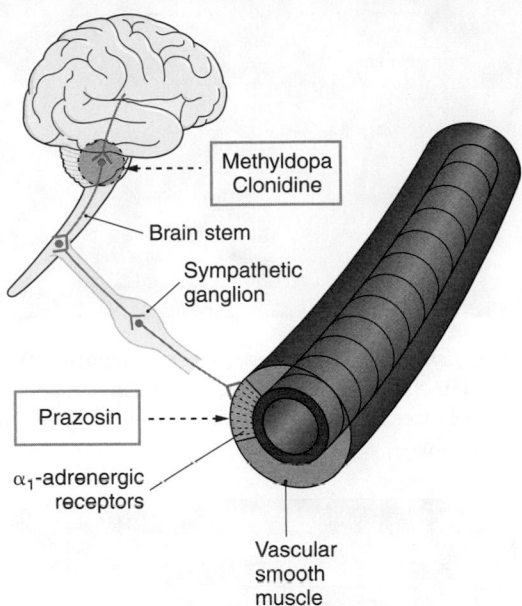

Plate 16 Sympatholytics inhibit sympathetic nervous system (SNS) activity, which plays a major role in regulating B/P. Normally when the SNS is stimulated, nerve impulses travel from the cardiovascular center of the CNS to the sympathetic ganglia. From there, the impulses travel along postganglionic fibers to specific effector organs, such as the heart and blood vessels. SNS stimulation also triggers the release of norepinephrine, which acts primarily at alpha-adrenergic receptors.

Sympatholytics fall into two subclasses: central-acting α_2 agonists and peripheral-acting α_1-adrenergic antagonists. Central-acting α_2 agonists, such as methyldopa and clonidine, stimulate α_2-adrenergic receptors in the cardiovascular center of the CNS and reduce activity in the vasomotor center of the brain, interfering with sympathetic stimulation of the heart and blood vessels. This causes blood vessel dilatation and decreased cardiac output, which leads to reduced B/P.

Peripheral-acting α_1-adrenergic antagonists, such as prazosin, inhibit the stimulation of α_1-adrenergic receptors by norepinephrine in vascular smooth muscle, interfering with SNS-induced vasoconstriction. As a result, the blood vessels dilate, reducing peripheral vascular resistance and venous return to the heart. These effects, in turn, lead to decreased B/P. (From Prosser S, Worster B, Dewar K: *Applied Pharmacology for Nurses and Other Health Care Professionals,* St. Louis, 2000, Mosby.)

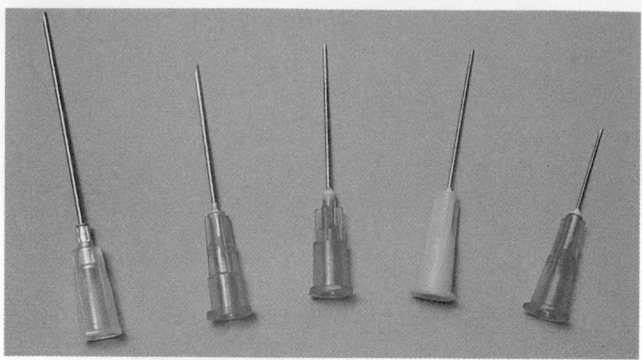

Plate 17 Needles. *Left to right:* 19 gauge, 1½-inch length; 20 gauge, 1-inch length; 21 gauge, 1-inch length; 23 gauge, 1-inch length; and 25 gauge, ⅝-inch length. (From Potter PA, Perry AG: *Fundamentals of Nursing,* ed 7, St. Louis, 2009, Mosby.)

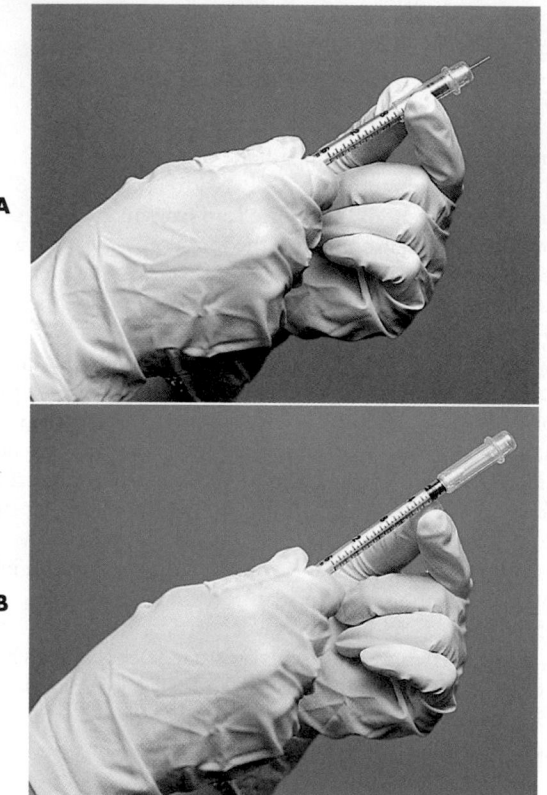

Plate 18 Needle with plastic guard to prevent needle sticks. **A,** Position of guard before injection. **B,** After injection, the guard locks in place, covering the needle. (From Potter PA, Perry AG: *Fundamentals of Nursing,* ed 7, St. Louis, 2009, Mosby.)

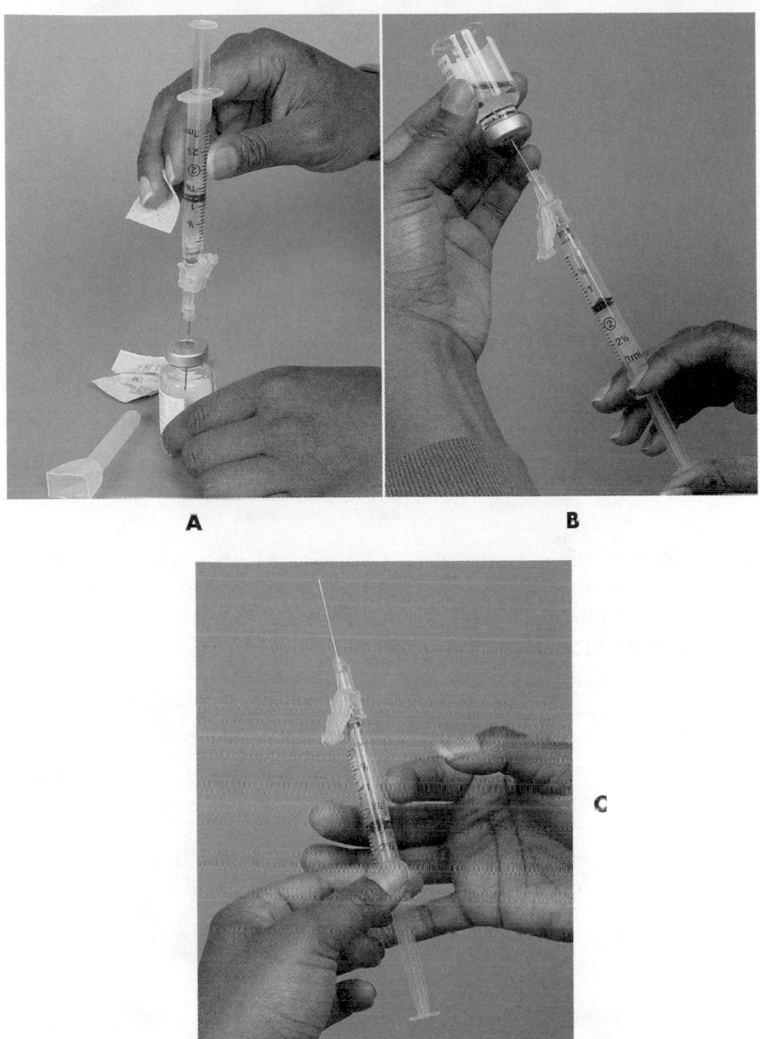

A

B

C

Plate 19 Preparing an injection from a vial. Remove needle cap from syringe. Pull back on the plunger to draw amount of air into syringe equivalent to volume of medication to be aspirated from vial. **A,** Insert tip of needle, with bevel pointing up, through center of rubber seal. Apply pressure to tip of needle during insertion. **B,** Allow air pressure to fill syringe gradually with medication. Pull back slightly on plunger if necessary. **C,** Remove remaining air from syringe by holding it and needle upright. Tap barrel to dislodge air bubbles. Draw back slightly on plunger and then push plunger upward to eject air. Do not eject fluid. (From Potter PA, Perry AG: *Fundamentals of Nursing,* ed 6, St. Louis, 2005, Mosby.)

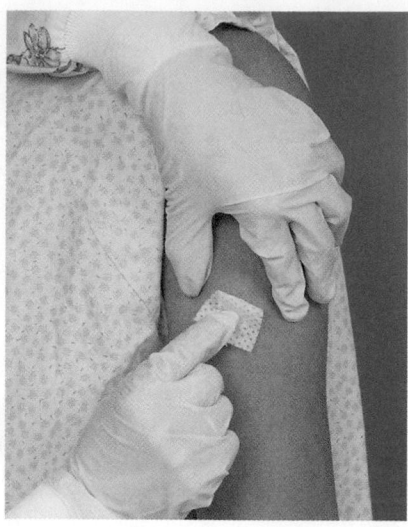

Plate 20 Administering an injection. Cleanse site with antiseptic swab. Apply swab at center of site and rotate outward in circular direction for about 5 cm (2 in). (From Potter PA, Perry AG: *Fundamentals of Nursing,* ed 7, St. Louis, 2009, Mosby.)

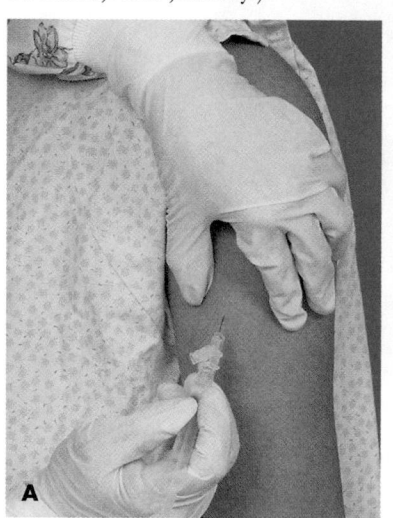

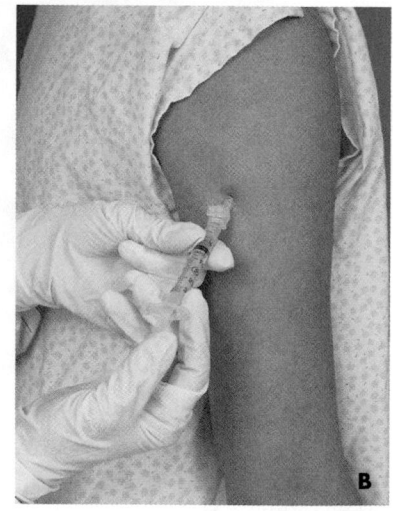

Plate 21 A, For a subcutaneous injection, hold the syringe between the thumb and forefinger of the dominant hand as a dart, with the palm down. **B,** After injecting the needle at a 45- to 90-degree angle, grasp lower end of syringe barrel with nondominant hand to end of plunger. Avoid moving syringe while slowly pulling back on plunger to aspirate drug. If blood appears in syringe, remove needle, discard medication and syringe, and repeat procedure. *Exception:* Do not aspirate when giving heparin. (From Potter PA, Perry AG: *Fundamentals of Nursing,* ed 7, St. Louis, 2009, Mosby.)

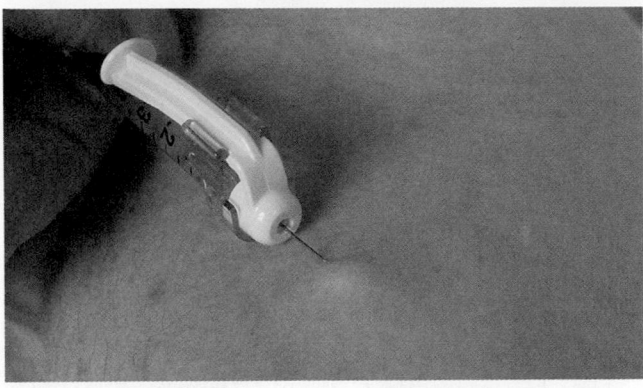

Plate 22 For an intradermal injection, note formation of small bleb approximately 6 mm (¼ in) in diameter at injection site. (From Potter PA, Perry AG: *Fundamentals of Nursing,* ed 7, St. Louis, 2009, Mosby.)

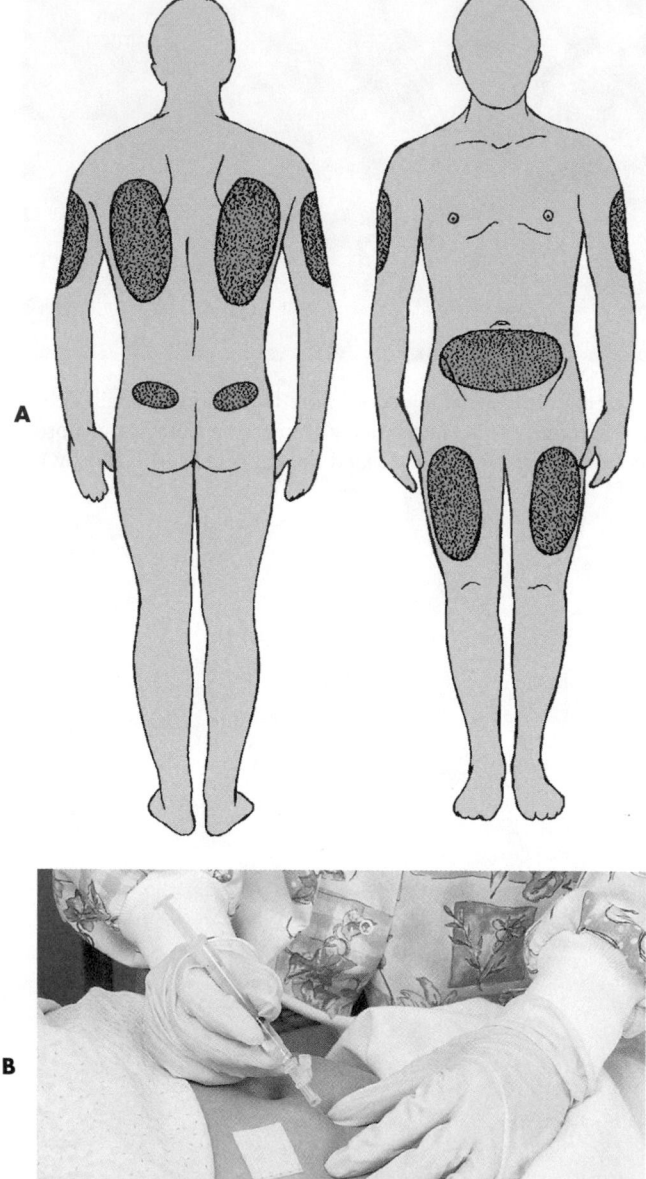

Plate 23 A, Sites recommended for subcutaneous injections.
B, Giving subcutaneous injection in the abdomen. (From
Potter PA, Perry AG: *Fundamentals of Nursing,* ed 6,
St. Louis, 2005, Mosby.)

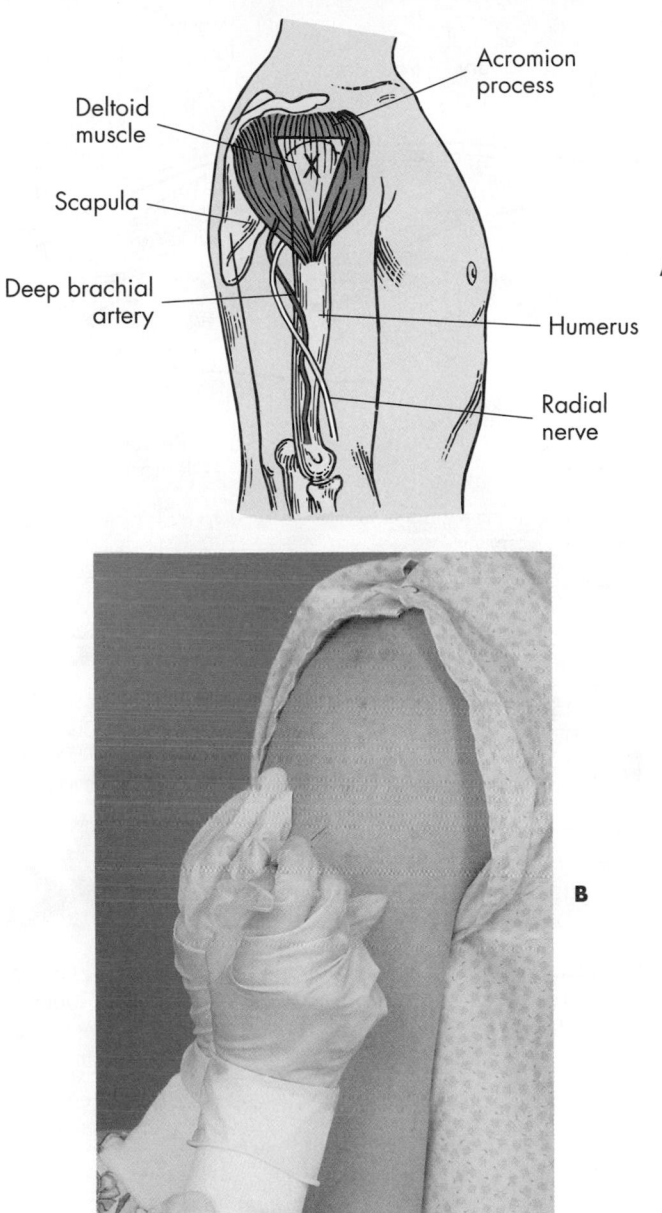

Plate 24 A, Landmarks for IM injection into the deltoid muscle. **B,** Giving IM injection in deltoid muscle. (From Potter PA, Perry AG: *Fundamentals of Nursing,* ed 7, St. Louis, 2009, Mosby.)

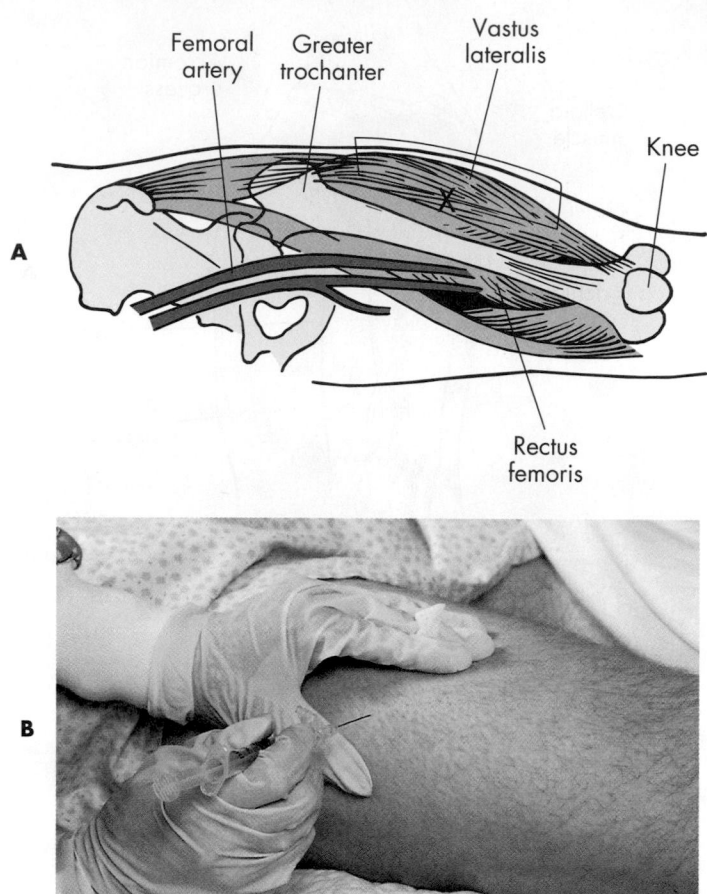

Plate 25 A, Landmarks for IM injection in vastus lateralis. **B,** Giving IM injection in vastus lateralis site. (From Potter PA, Perry AG: *Fundamentals of Nursing,* ed 7, St. Louis, 2009, Mosby.)

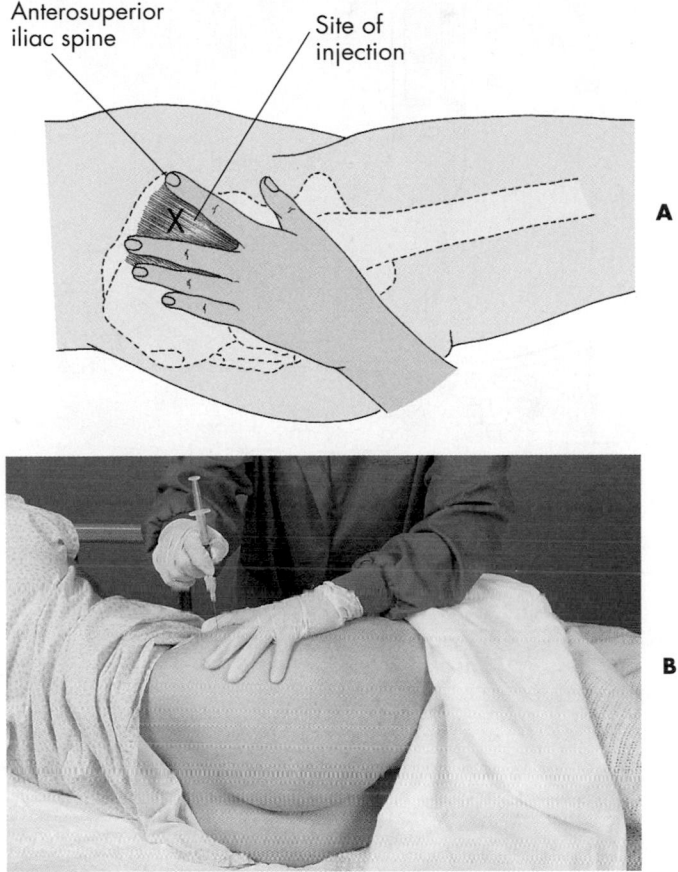

Anterosuperior
iliac spine

Site of
injection

A

B

Plate 26 A, Anatomical view of ventrogluteal site. **B,** Giving IM injection
into ventrogluteal muscle to avoid major nerves and blood vessels. (From
Potter PA, Perry AG: *Fundamentals of Nursing,* ed 7, St. Louis, 2009,
Mosby.)

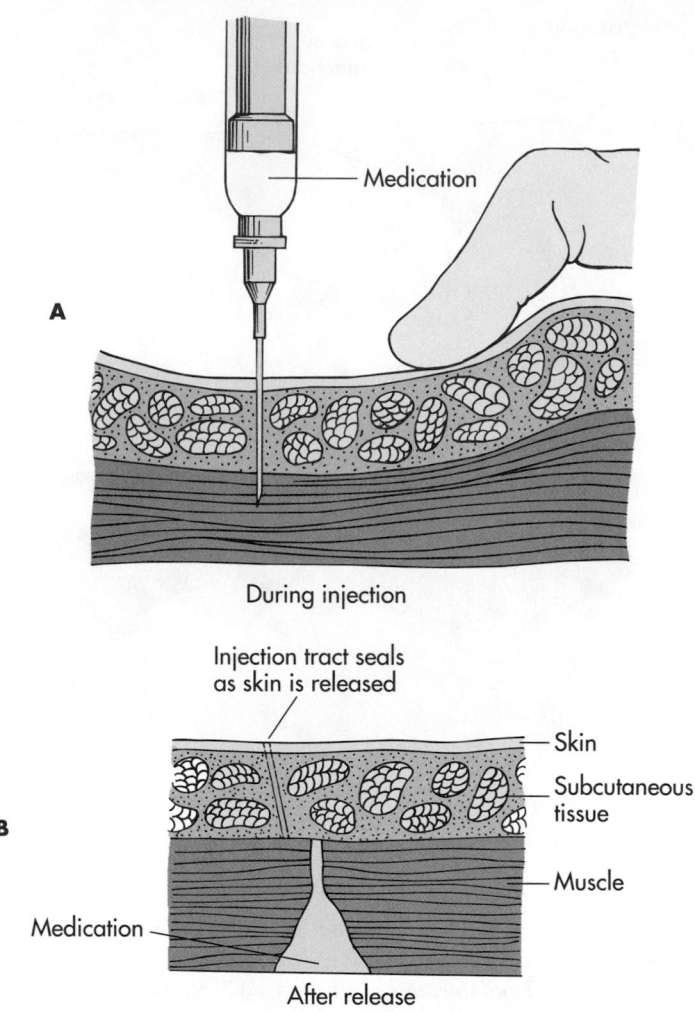

A

Medication

During injection

Injection tract seals
as skin is released

B

Skin

Subcutaneous
tissue

Muscle

Medication

After release

Plate 27 Z-track method of injection. **A,** Pulling on overlying skin during
IM injection moves tissues to prevent later tracking. **B,** The Z-track left after
injection prevents the deposit of medication through sensitive tissue. (From
Potter PA, Perry AG: *Fundamentals of Nursing,* ed 7, St. Louis, 2009,
Mosby.)

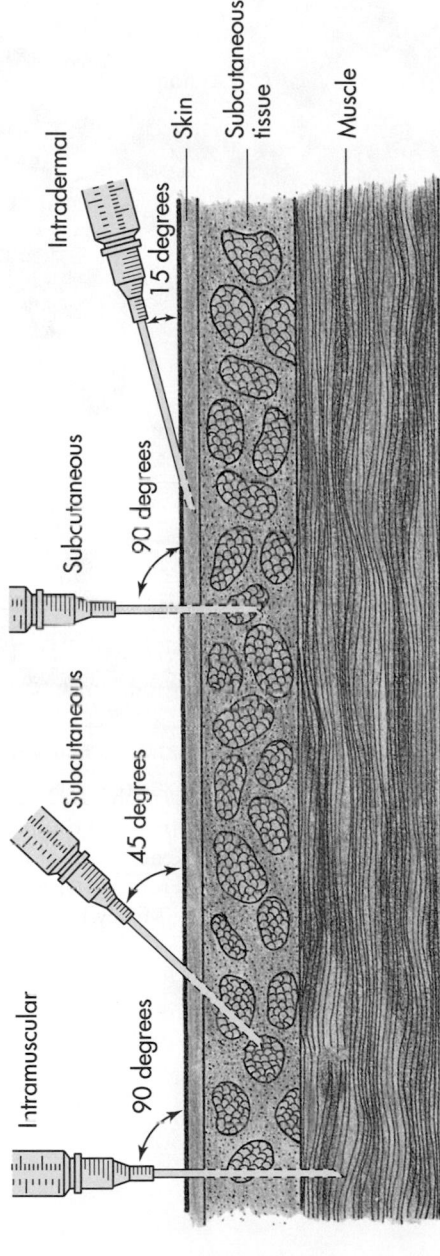

Plate 28 Comparison of angles of insertion for IM (90 degrees), SUBCUT (45 degrees and 90 degrees), and ID (15 degrees) injections. (From Potter PA, Perry AG: *Fundamentals of Nursing*, ed 7, St. Louis, 2009, Mosby.)

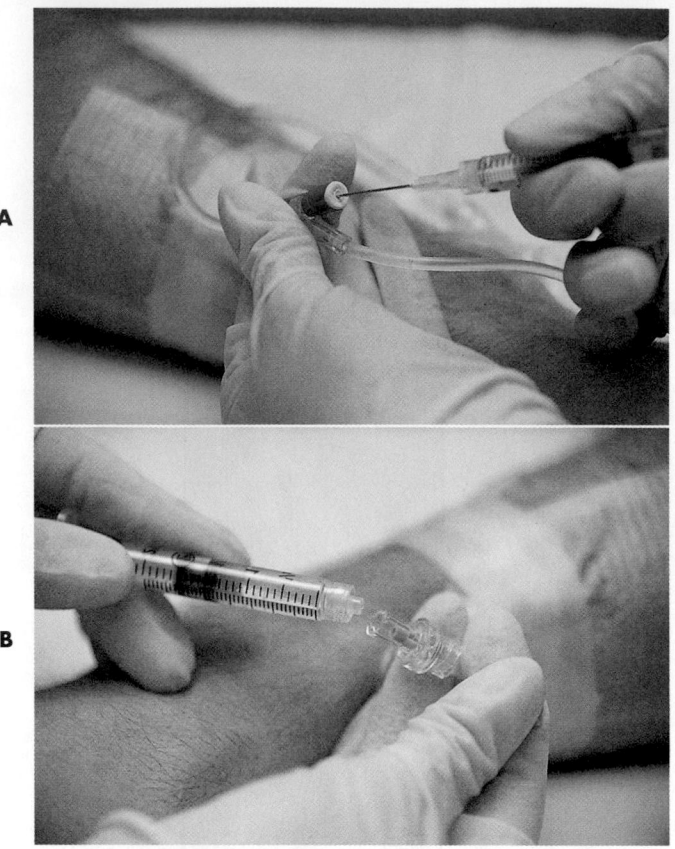

Plate 29 Administering medication by **IV** bolus (push). **A,** Needle system: Insert small-gauge needle of syringe containing prepared drug through center of injection port. **B,** Needleless system: Remove cap of needleless injection port. Connect tip of syringe directly. (From Potter PA, Perry AG: *Fundamentals of Nursing,* ed 5, St. Louis, 2001, Mosby.)

Continued

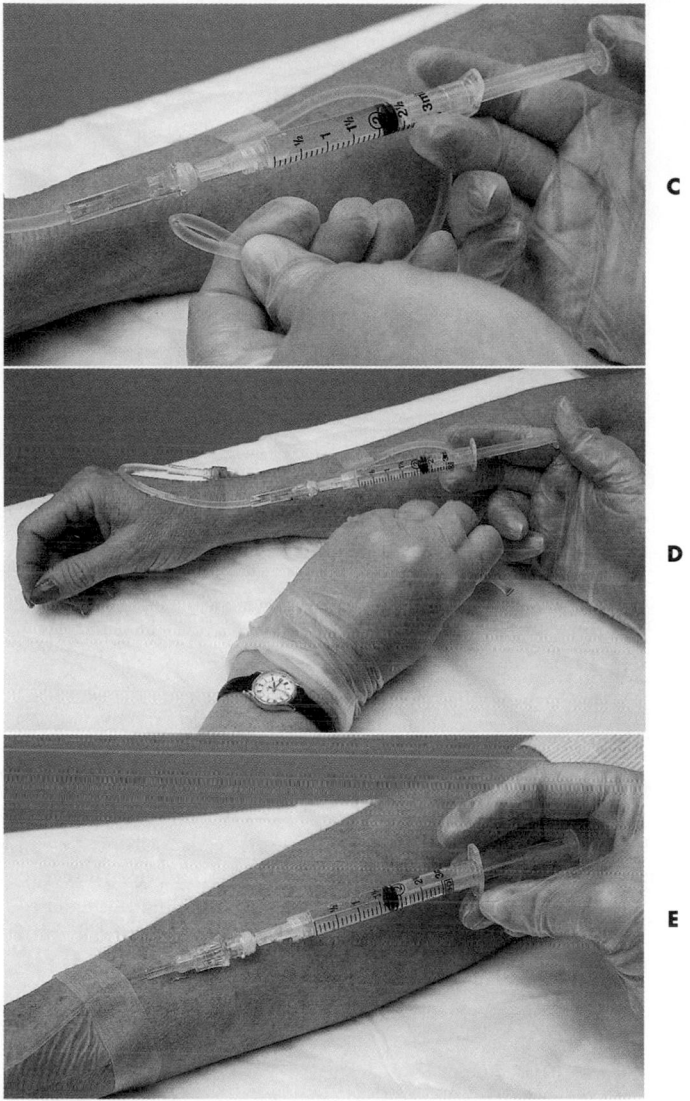

C

D

E

Plate 29 C, Occlude **IV** line by pinching tubing just above injection port.
Pull back gently on syringe's plunger to aspirate blood return. **D,** After
noting blood return, continue to occlude tubing and inject medication
slowly over several minutes (read directions on drug package). Use watch to
time administration. **E, IV** lock: Insert needle of syringe containing prepared
drug through center of diaphragm. (From Potter PA, Perry AG:
Fundamentals of Nursing, ed 6, St. Louis, 2005, Mosby.)

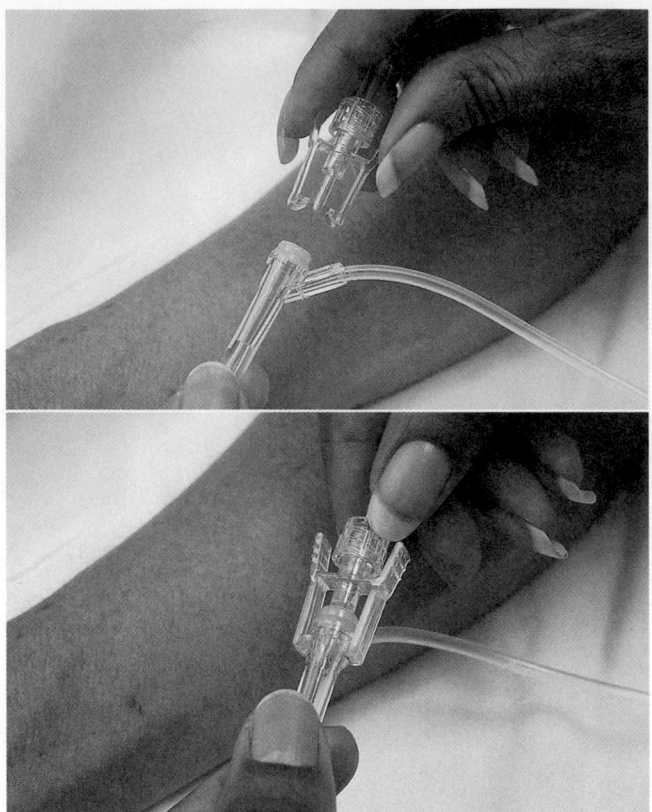

Plate 30 Administering **IV** medication by piggyback, volume administration sets of miniinfusors (syringe pump). Use needle-lock device to secure needle of secondary piggyback line through injection port of main line. (From Potter PA, Perry AG: *Fundamentals of Nursing,* ed 6, St. Louis, 2005, Mosby.)

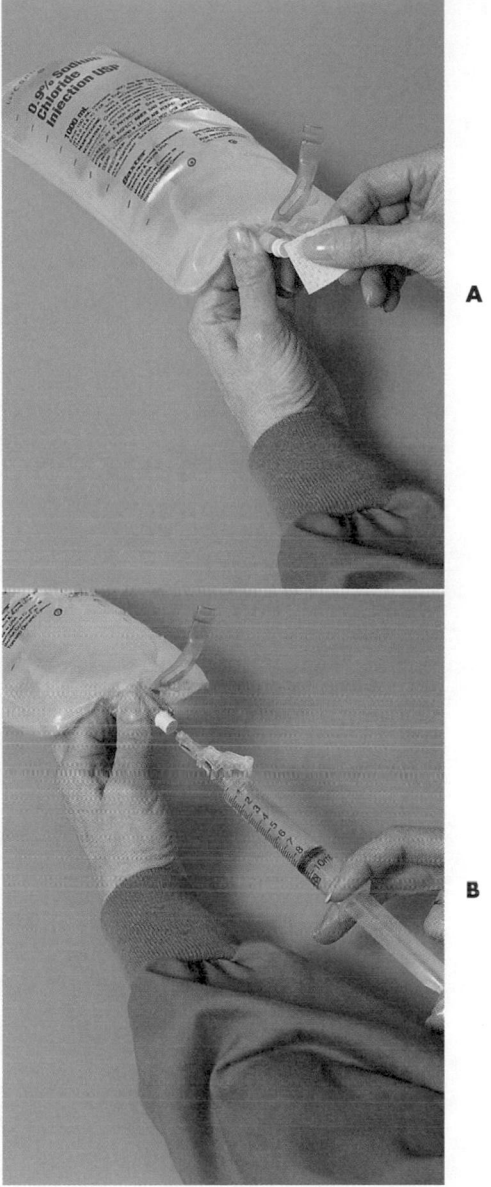

Plate 31 Adding medications to **IV** fluid containers. **A,** Wipe off port or injection site with alcohol or antiseptic swab. **B,** Remove needle cap from syringe, insert needle of syringe through center of injection port or site, and inject medication. (From Potter PA, Perry AG: *Fundamentals of Nursing*, ed 7, St. Louis, 2009, Mosby.)

abacavir (Rx)
(aba-ka'veer)
Ziagen
Func. class.: Antiretroviral
Chem. class.: Nucleoside reverse transcriptase inhibitor (NRTI)

Pregnancy category C

Action: A synthetic, nucleoside analog with inhibitory action against HIV; inhibits replication of HIV by incorporating into cellular DNA by viral reverse transcriptase, thereby terminating the cellular DNA chain

Therapeutic outcome: Decreased symptoms of HIV

Uses: In combination with other antiretroviral agents for HIV-1 infection (not to be used with lamivudine or tenofovir)

Dosage and routes
Adult: PO 300 mg bid or 600 mg daily with other antiretrovirals
Adolescents and children ≥3 mo: PO 8 mg/kg bid, max 300 mg bid with other antiretrovirals

Hepatic dose
Adult: (Child-Pugh 5-6) PO oral/sol 200 mg bid

Available forms: Tabs 300 mg; oral sol 20 mg/ml

Adverse effects
CNS: Fever, headache, malaise, insomnia, paresthesia
*GI: Nausea, vomiting, diarrhea, anorexia, cramps, abdominal pain, increased AST, ALT, **hepatotoxicity***
HEMA: **Granulocytopenia, anemia,** lymphopenia
INTEG: Rash, urticaria, hypersensitivity reactions
META: **Lactic acidosis**
MISC: Increased CPK, **fatal hypersensitivity reactions**
RESP: Dyspnea

Precautions: Pregnancy C, breastfeeding, child <3 mo, granulocyte count <1000/mm³ or Hgb <9.5 g/dl, severe renal disease, impaired hepatic function

Black Box Warning: Hypersensitivity, lactic acidosis, moderate to severe hepatic disease

Pharmacokinetics
Absorption	Rapid/extensive (PO)
Distribution	50% plasma protein binding, extravascular space, then erythrocytes
Metabolism	To inactive metabolite
Excretion	Kidneys, feces
Half-life	1½-2 hr

Pharmacodynamics
Unknown

Interactions
Individual drugs
Alcohol: increased abacavir levels; do not use with alcohol
Ribavirin: possible lactic acidosis
Methadone: decreased levels of methadone
Tipranavir: decreased abacavir levels
Drug/lab test
Increased: glucose, triglycerides

NURSING CONSIDERATIONS
Assessment
• Assess for symptoms of HIV and possible infection, increased temp
• Assess for lactic acidosis (elevated lactate levels, increased liver function tests) and severe hepatomegaly with steatosis; discontinue treatment and do not restart
⬥ Assess for fatal hypersensitivity reactions: fever, rash, nausea, vomiting, fatigue, cough, dyspnea, diarrhea, abdominal discomfort; treatment should be discontinued and not restarted
⬥ Assess for pancreatitis: abdominal pain, nausea, vomiting, elevated liver enzymes; product should be discontinued because condition can be fatal
• Monitor CBC, differential, platelet count qmo; withhold product if WBC is <4000/mm³ or platelet count is <75,000/mm³; notify prescriber of results; monitor viral load and CD4 counts during treatment
• Monitor renal function studies; BUN, serum uric acid, urine CCr before, during therapy; these may be elevated throughout treatment
• Monitor temp q4hr; may indicate beginning of infection
• Monitor liver function tests before, during therapy (bilirubin, AST, ALT, amylase, alkaline phosphatase, creatine phosphokinase, creatinine prn or qmo)

Nursing diagnoses
• Infection, risk for (uses)
• Injury, risk for (adverse reactions)
• Knowledge, deficient (teaching)

Adverse effects: *italic* = common, **bold** = life-threatening

Implementation
PO route
- Give on empty stomach, q12hr around the clock
- Give in combination with other antiretrovirals with or without food
- Store in cool environment; protect from light; do not freeze

Patient/family education
- Advise patient to report signs of infection: increased temp, sore throat, flulike symptoms; to avoid crowds and those with known infections
- Instruct patient to report signs of anemia: fatigue, headache, faintness, shortness of breath, irritability
- Advise patient to report bleeding; avoid use of razors or commercial mouthwash
- Inform patient that product is not a cure but will control symptoms
- Inform patient that major toxicities may necessitate discontinuing product
- Instruct patient to use contraception during treatment
- Caution patient to avoid OTC products or other medications without approval of prescriber
- Caution patient not to have any sexual contact without use of a condom; needles should not be shared; blood from infected individual should not come in contact with another's mucous membranes
- Give Medication Guide and Warning Card; discuss points on guide
- Advise patient to stop product if skin rash, fever, cough, shortness of breath, GI symptoms occur and notify prescriber immediately; advise all health care providers that allergic reactions have occurred with this product

Evaluation
Positive therapeutic outcome
- Increased CD4 count, decreased viral load

---

abatacept (Rx)
(ab-a-ta'sept)
Orencia
Func. class.: Antirheumatic agent (disease modifying); biologic response modifier

Pregnancy category C

Action: A selective costimulation modulator, inhibits T-lymphocytes, inhibits tumor necrosis factor (TNF-α), interferon-γ, interleukin-2, which are involved in immune and inflammatory reactions

Therapeutic outcome: Decreased pain, inflammation in joints

Uses: Polyarticular juvenile rheumatoid arthritis; acute, chronic rheumatoid arthritis that has not responded to other disease-modifying agents, may use in combination with DMARDs; do not use with TNF antagonists (adalimumab, etanercept, infliximab) or anakinra

Dosage and routes
- Give at 2, 4 wk after first infusion
Adult >100 kg: **IV** INF 1 g
Adult 60-100 kg: **IV** INF 750 mg
Adult <60 kg: **IV** INF 500 mg

Juvenile rheumatoid arthritis (JRA)/juvenile idiopathic arthritis (JIA)
Child ≥6 yr/adolescent >100 kg: **IV** INF 1000 mg over 30 min q4wk starting at wk 8
Child >6 yr/adolescent >75 kg: **IV** INF 750 mg over 30 min q2wk × 2 doses, then 750 mg over 30 min q4wk starting at wk 8

Available forms: Lyophilized powder, single-use vials 250 mg

Adverse effects
CNS: Headache, asthenia, dizziness
CV: Hypertension, hypotension
GI: Abdominal pain, dyspepsia, nausea
INTEG: Rash, *inj site reaction,* flushing, urticaria, pruritus
RESP: Pharyngitis, cough, URI, non-URI, *rhinitis,* wheezing
SYST: **Anaphylaxis, malignancies, angioedema**

Contraindications: Hypersensitivity, TB, viral hepatitis

Precautions: Pregnancy **C**, breastfeeding, children, geriatric, recurrent infections, COPD

Pharmacokinetics
Absorption	Unknown
Distribution	Unknown
Metabolism	Unknown
Excretion	Unknown
Half-life	Terminal 13-16 days, steady state 60 days

Pharmacodynamics
Unknown

Interactions
Individual drugs
Anakinra: do not use

 Alert   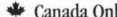 Canada Only   Drug on CD   * "Tall Man" lettering (See Preface)

Drug classifications

Corticosteroids, immunosuppressives: do not use concurrently

TNF antagonists (adalimumab, etanercept, infliximab): do not use

Vaccines: do not give concurrently; immunizations should be brought up to date before treatment

NURSING CONSIDERATIONS
Assessment
- Assess for latent/active TB before beginning treatment
- Assess for pain, stiffness, ROM, swelling of joints during treatment
- Assess for inj site pain, swelling
- Monitor patient's overall health on each visit; product should not be given with active infections

Nursing diagnoses
- Knowledge, deficient (teaching)
- Pain, chronic (uses)

Implementation
- To reconstitute, remove plastic flip top from vial and wipe the top with alcohol wipe; insert syringe needle into vial and direct stream of sterile water for inj on the wall of vial; rotate vial until mixed; vent with needle to rid foam after reconstitution 25 mg/ml; further dilute in 100 ml from a 100 ml infusion bag/bottle; withdraw the needed volume (2 vials remove 20 mg; 3 vials remove 30 ml, 4 vials remove 40 ml); slowly add the reconstituted Orencia sol from each vial into the infusion bag/bottle using the same disposable syringe supplied; mix gently, discard unused portions of vials; do not use if particulate is present or if discolored; give over 30 min; use non–protein binding filter (0.2-1.2 mcg)
- Do not admix with other sol or medications
- Store in refrigerator; do not use expired vials

Patient/family education
- Teach patient that product must be continued for prescribed time to be effective
- Advise patient to use caution when driving; dizziness may occur
- Advise patient not to have vaccinations while taking this product
- Discuss with patient information included in packaging

Evaluation
Positive therapeutic outcome
- Decreased inflammation, pain in joints; decreased erythrocyte sedimentation rate (ESR)

abobotulinumtoxinA
(ay-boh-bot'yoo-li-num-tox'in-A)
Dysport
Func. class.: Dermatological agent

Dosage and routes
Cervical dystonia
Adult: IM 500 units divided among affected muscles and repeated q12wk or longer

Facial wrinkles
Adult <65 yr: IM 50 units administered in 5 equal aliquots of 10 units each, may last up to 4 months

Uses: Cervical dystonia, facial wrinkles

Contraindications: Hypersensitivity to this product or bovine products, infection

acarbose (Rx)
(a-kar'bose)
Precose
Func. class.: Oral antidiabetic
Chem. class.: α Glucosidase inhibitor
Pregnancy category B

Do not confuse:
Precose/PreCare

Action: Delays the digestion/absorption of ingested carbohydrates by inhibiting α-glucosidase, results in a smaller rise in blood glucose after meals; does not increase insulin production

Therapeutic outcome: Decreased blood glucose levels in diabetes mellitus

Uses: Type 2 diabetes mellitus, alone or in combination with a sulfonylurea, metformin

Dosage and routes
Initial dose
Adult >60 kg: PO 25 mg tid with first bite of meal

Maintenance dose
Adult: PO May be increased to 50-100 mg tid; dosage adjustment at 4-8 wk intervals
Adult <60 kg: PO Max 50 mg tid

Available forms: Tabs 25, 50, 100 mg

Adverse effects
GI: Abdominal pain, diarrhea, flatulence, increased serum transaminase level

Contraindications: Hypersensitivity, breastfeeding, diabetic ketoacidosis, cirrhosis, inflammatory bowel disease, ileus, colonic ulceration, partial intestinal obstruction,

Adverse effects: *italic* = common, **bold** = life-threatening

chronic intestinal disease, serum creatinine >2 mg/dl

Precautions: Pregnancy **B**, children, renal/hepatic disease

Pharmacokinetics

Absorption	Poor systemic
Distribution	Unknown
Metabolism	GI tract
Excretion	Kidneys as intact drug
Half-life	Elimination 2 hr

Pharmacodynamics

Onset	Unknown
Peak	1 hr
Duration	Unknown

Interactions
Individual drugs
Digoxin: decreased acarbose effect
Insulin, phenytoin: increased hypoglycemia
Isoniazid: increased hyperglycemia
Drug classifications
Calcium channel blockers, corticosteroids, diuretics, estrogens, oral contraceptives, phenothiazines, progestins, sympathomimetics: increased hyperglycemia; digestive enzymes, intestinal absorbents, thiazide diuretics, loop diuretics, corticosteroids: decreased effect of acarbose
Sulfonylureas, insulin: increased hypoglycemia
Drug/herb
Alfalfa, aloe, basil, bay, bilberry, bitter melon, black cohosh, buchu, burdock, chromium, coenzyme Q10, coriander, eyebright (po), fenugreek, garlic, ginseng, glucomannan, glucosamine, goat's rue, gymnema, horehound, horse chestnut, jambul, myrrh, myrtle, raspberry, Siberian ginseng: increased hypoglycemia
Bee pollen, blue cohosh, broom, chromium, elecampane, eucalyptus, gotu kola, senega: decreased hypoglycemia
Drug/lab test
Increased: AST, bilirubin
Decreased: calcium, vit B_6

NURSING CONSIDERATIONS
Assessment
• Assess for hypoglycemia (weakness, hunger, dizziness, tremors, anxiety, tachycardia, sweating), hyperglycemia; even though this product does not cause hypoglycemia, if on a sulfonylurea or insulin, hypoglycemia may be additive; if hypoglycemia occurs, treat with glucose or if severe, **IV** dextrose or IM glucagon
• Monitor 1 hr postprandial glucose for establishing effectiveness, then glycosylated Hgb q3mo
• Monitor AST, ALT q3mo × 1 yr, and periodically thereafter, if elevated dose, may need to be reduced or discontinued; obtain glycosylated Hgb periodically
• Assess for stress, surgery, or other trauma that may require change in dose

Nursing diagnoses
• Knowledge, deficient (teaching)
• Noncompliance (teaching)
• Nutrition: less than body requirements, imbalanced (adverse reactions)
• Nutrition: more than body requirements, imbalanced (uses)

Implementation
• Give tid with first bite of each meal 3 times/day
• Provide storage in tight container in cool environment

Patient/family education
• Teach patient the symptoms of hypoglycemia, hyperglycemia and what to do about each
• Instruct that medication must be taken as prescribed; explain consequences of discontinuing the medication abruptly; that insulin may need to be used during stress such as trauma, surgery, fever
• Tell patient to avoid OTC medications, herbal products unless approved by prescriber
• Teach patient that diabetes is a lifelong illness; product will not cure condition; that diet and exercise regimen must be followed
• Instruct patient to carry/wear emergency ID as diabetic
• Teach not to breastfeed
• Inform that GI side effects may occur

Evaluation
Positive therapeutic outcome
• Improved signs, symptoms of diabetes mellitus (decreased polyuria, polydipsia, polyphagia; clear sensorium, absence of dizziness, stable gait)

acebutolol (Rx)
(a-se-byoo' toe-lole)
Monitan ✦, Sectral
Func. class.: Antihypertensive
Chem. class.: Selective β_1-blocker; group II
antidysrhythmic (II)

Pregnancy category B

Action: Competitively blocks stimulation of
β-adrenergic receptors within vascular smooth
muscle (decreases rate of SA node discharge,
increases recovery time), slows conduction of
AV node resulting in decreased heart rate
(negative chronotropic effect), which decreases O_2 consumption in myocardium
because of β_1-receptor antagonism; also
decreases renin-aldosterone-angiotensin
system at high doses, inhibits β_2-receptors in
bronchial system (high doses)

Therapeutic outcome: Decreased B/P,
heart rate, AV conduction; control of dysrhythmias

Uses: Mild to moderate hypertension, management of PVCs

Dosage and routes
Hypertension
Adult: PO 400 mg daily or in 2 divided
doses; may be increased to desired response;
maintenance 200-1200 mg daily in 2 divided
doses
Geriatric: PO Max 800 mg daily

Ventricular dysrhythmia
Adult: PO 200 mg bid, may increase
gradually; usual range 600-1200 mg daily;
should be tapered over 2 wk before discontinuing
Geriatric: PO Max 800 mg daily

PVC management
Adult: PO 200 mg bid, may increase
gradually; usual range 600-1200 mg daily in
divided doses
Geriatric: PO max 800 mg daily

Renal dose
Adult: PO CCr 25-50 ml/min, reduce dose by
50%; if <25 ml/min reduce dose by 75%

Available forms: Caps 200, 400 mg; tabs
100, 200, 400 mg ✦

Adverse effects
*CNS: Insomnia, fatigue, dizziness, mental
changes,* memory loss, hallucinations, depression, lethargy, drowsiness, strange dreams,
catatonia, headache

CV: **Profound hypotension, bradycardia,
CHF,** cold extremities, postural hypotension,
2nd- or 3rd-degree heart block, edema
EENT: Sore throat; dry, burning eyes
ENDO: Increased hypoglycemic response to
insulin
GI: Nausea, diarrhea, vomiting, **mesenteric
arterial thrombosis, ischemic colitis,**
flatulence
GU: Impotence, decreased libido, dysuria,
nocturia, polyuria
HEMA: **Agranulocytosis, thrombocytope-
nia, purpura**
INTEG: Rash, flushing, pruritus, sweating,
alopecia, dry skin
MISC: Facial swelling, weight gain, decreased
exercise tolerance
MS: Joint pain, cramping
RESP: **Bronchospasm,** dyspnea, wheezing,
cough

Contraindications: Hypersensitivity to
this agent or β-blockers; cardiogenic shock,
heart block (2nd or 3rd degree), sinus bradycardia, CHF, cardiac failure

Precautions: Pregnancy **B,** breastfeeding,
children, major surgery, diabetes mellitus,
renal/hepatic/thyroid disease, COPD, asthma,
well-compensated heart failure, peripheral
vascular disease, abrupt discontinuation

Black Box Warning: Abrupt discontinuation

Pharmacokinetics

Absorption	Well absorbed, rapid
Distribution	Crosses placenta, enters breast milk (small amounts), minimal CNS; protein binding 26%
Metabolism	Liver to diacetolol
Excretion	Urine
Half-life	8-13 hr diacetolol, 3-4 hr acebutolol

Pharmacodynamics

	PO (ANTIHYPER-TENSIVE)	PO (ANTIDYS-RHYTHMIAS)
Onset	1-1½ hr	1 hr
Peak	2-4 hr	4-6 hr
Duration	12-24 hr	10-12 hr

Interactions
Individual drugs
Calcium, cholestyramine, colestipol: decreased
antihypertensive effect
Cimetidine, diltiazem, hydrALAZINE, methyldopa, prazosin, respirine, verapamil:
bradycardia, increased hypotension

Adverse effects: *italic* = common, **bold** = life-threatening

Ergots: increased peripheral ischemia

Insulin: increased hypoglycemia

Drug classifications

Anticholinergics, cardiac glycosides, diuretics, other antihypertensives, calcium channel blockers: increased hypotension, bradycardia

Calcium channel blockers, diuretics: increased hypotension

Calcium channel blockers, cardiac glycosides, diuretics: bradycardia

NSAIDs: decreased antihypertensive effect

Oral sulfonylureas: attenuated effects

Theophyllines, β_2-agonists: decreased bronchodilatation

Drug/herb

Aconite: increased toxicity, death

Aloe, betel palm, buckthorn bark/berry, butterbur, cascara sagrada bark, cola tree, figwort, guarana, hawthorn, lily of the valley, motherwort, plantain, rhubarb root, senna leaf/fruits: increased acebutolol effect

Coenzyme Q10, yohimbe: decreased antihypertensive effect

St. John's wort: decreased acebutolol effect

Drug/lab test

Positive: antinuclear antibodies titer

Increased: serum lipoprotein levels, BUN, potassium, triglyceride, uric acid, LDH, AST, ALT, blood glucose, alkaline phosphatase

NURSING CONSIDERATIONS

Assessment

• Monitor B/P during beginning treatment, periodically thereafter; pulse q4hr; note rate, rhythm, quality; apical/radial pulse before administration; notify prescriber of any significant changes (pulse <50 bpm)

• Check for baselines in renal, liver function tests before therapy begins

• Assess for edema in feet, legs daily, monitor I&O, daily weight; check for jugular vein distention, crackles bilaterally, dyspnea (CHF)

• Monitor skin turgor, dryness of mucous membranes for hydration status, especially geriatric

Nursing diagnoses

• Cardiac output, decreased (side effects)

• Injury, risk for (side effects)

• Knowledge, deficient (teaching)

• Noncompliance (teaching)

Implementation

PO route

• Given before meals, at bedtime; tablet may be crushed or swallowed whole; give with food to prevent GI upset; reduced dosage in renal dysfunction; check pulse before giving, hold dose and notify prescriber if pulse is <60 bpm

• Store protected from light, moisture; place in cool environment

Patient/family education

◆ Teach patient not to discontinue product abruptly, severe cardiac reactions may occur, taper over 2 wk; may cause precipitate angina if stopped abruptly

• Advise patient that product may mask signs of hypoglycemia or alter blood glucose levels

• Teach patient not to use OTC products containing α-adrenergic stimulants (such as nasal decongestants, cold preparations); to avoid alcohol, smoking; to limit sodium intake as prescribed

• Teach patient how to take pulse and B/P at home, advise when to notify prescriber

• Instruct patient to comply with weight control, dietary adjustments, modified exercise program

• Tell patient to carry/wear emergency ID to identify product(s) that patient is taking, allergies; tell patient that product controls symptoms but does not cure

• Caution patient to avoid hazardous activities if dizziness or drowsiness is present; that product may cause sensitivity to cold

• Teach patient to report symptoms of CHF: difficult breathing, especially on exertion or when lying down, night cough, swelling of extremities or bradycardia, dizziness, confusion, depression, fever

• Teach patient to take product as prescribed, not to double or skip doses; take any missed doses as soon as remembered if several hours until next dose

• Advise patient to continue with required lifestyle changes (exercise, diet, weight loss, stress reduction)

Evaluation

Positive therapeutic outcome

• Decreased B/P in hypertension (after 1-2 wk)

• Absence of dysrhythmias

Treatment of overdose: Lavage, **IV** atropine for bradycardia, **IV** theophylline for bronchospasm, digoxin, O_2, diuretic for cardiac failure, hemodialysis, **IV** glucose for hypoglycemia, **IV** diazepam (or phenytoin) for seizures

acetaminophen (OTC)
(a-seat-a-mee'noe-fen)
Abenol ✦, Acephen, Aceta, Apo-Acetaminophen ✦, Apra, Atasol ✦, Children's Feverall, Equaline Children's Pain Relief, Equaline Infant's Pain Relief, Exdol ✦, Genapap, Genebs, Good Sense Acetaminophen, Good Sense Children's Pain Relief, Header Children's Pain Reliever, Infantaire, Mapap, Panadol, Q-Pap, Q-Pap Children's, Redutemp, Robigesic ✦, Rounax ✦, Silapap, Tapanol, T-Painol, Tylenol, Walgreen's Acetaminophen, Walgreen's Non-Aspirin, XS Pain Reliever
Func. class.: Nonopioid analgesic
Chem. class.: Nonsalicylate, paraaminophenol derivative

Pregnancy category B

Action: May block pain impulses peripherally that occur in response to inhibition of prostaglandin synthesis; does not possess antiinflammatory properties; antipyretic action results from inhibition of prostaglandins in the CNS (hypothalamic heat-regulating center)

Therapeutic outcome: Decreased pain, fever

Uses: Mild to moderate pain or fever; arthralgia, dental pain, dysmenorrhea, headache, myalgia, osteoarthritis

Dosage and routes
Adult and child >12 yr: PO/RECT 325-650 mg q4-6hr prn, max 4 g/day
Child 1-12 yr: PO 10-15 mg/kg q4-6hr, max 5 doses/24 hr; RECT 10-20 mg/kg/dose q4-6hr
Neonates: RECT 10-15 mg/kg/dose q6-8hr

Available forms: Rectal supp 80, 120, 125, 325, 600, 650 mg; chewable tabs 80, 160 mg; caps 500 mg; elix 120, 160, 325 mg/5 ml; liquid 160 mg/5 ml, 500 mg/15 ml; sol 100 mg/1 ml, 120 mg/2.5 ml granules 80 mg/packet, 80 mg/cap; tabs 160, 325, 500, 650 mg

Adverse effects
CNS: Stimulation, drowsiness
GI: Nausea, vomiting, abdominal pain; **hepatotoxicity, hepatic seizure (overdose), GI bleeding**
GU: **Renal failure** (high, prolonged doses)
HEMA: **Leukopenia, neutropenia, hemolytic anemia (long-term use), thrombocytopenia, pancytopenia**
INTEG: Rash, urticaria
SYST: Hypersensitivity
TOXICITY: **Cyanosis, anemia, neutropenia, jaundice, pancytopenia, CNS stimulation, delirium followed by vascular collapse, seizures, coma, death**

Contraindications: Hypersensitivity; intolerance to tartrazine (yellow dye #5), alcohol, table sugar, saccharin, depending on product

Precautions: Pregnancy **B**, breastfeeding, geriatric, anemia, renal/hepatic disease, chronic alcoholism

Pharmacokinetics
Absorption	Well absorbed (PO), variable (RECT)
Distribution	Widely distributed; crosses placenta in low concentrations
Metabolism	Liver 85%-95%; metabolites are toxic at high levels
Excretion	Kidneys—metabolites, breast milk
Half-life	3-4 hr

Pharmacodynamics
	PO	RECT
Onset	½-1 hr	½-1 hr
Peak	1-3 hr	1-3 hr
Duration	3-4 hr	3-4 hr

Interactions
Individual drugs
Alcohol, carbamazepine, diflunisal, isoniazid, rifabutin, rifampin, sulfinpyrazone: increased hepatotoxicity; decreased effect
Colestipol, cholestyramine: decreased absorption of acetaminophen
Warfarin: hypoprothrombinemia; long-term use, high doses of acetaminophen
Zidovudine: increased bone marrow suppression
Drug classifications
Barbiturates, hydantoins: decreased effect; increased hepatotoxicity
NSAIDs, salicylates: increased renal adverse reactions
Drug/herb
St. John's wort: decreased acetaminophen effect
Drug/lab test
Interference: chemstrip G, Dextrostix, Visidex II, 5-HIAA

NURSING CONSIDERATIONS
Assessment
• Monitor liver function studies: AST, ALT, bilirubin, creatinine before therapy if long-

term therapy is anticipated; may cause hepatic toxicity at doses >4 g/day with chronic use
- Monitor renal function studies: BUN, urine creatinine, occult blood; albumin indicates nephritis
- Monitor blood studies: CBC, pro-time if patient is on long-term therapy
- Check I&O ratio; decreasing output may indicate renal failure (long-term therapy)
- Assess for fever and pain: type of pain, location, intensity, duration, temp, diaphoresis
- Assess for chronic poisoning: rapid, weak pulse; dyspnea; cold, clammy extremities; report immediately to prescriber
- Assess hepatotoxicity: dark urine, clay-colored stools, yellowing of skin and sclera; itching, abdominal pain, fever, diarrhea if patient is on long-term therapy
- Assess allergic reactions: rash, urticaria; if these occur, product may have to be discontinued

Nursing diagnoses
- Injury, risk for (side effects)
- Knowledge, deficient (teaching)
- Mobility, impaired physical (uses)
- Pain, acute (uses)
- Pain, chronic (uses)

Implementation
PO route
- Administer to patient crushed or whole; chewable tabs may be chewed
- Give with food or milk to decrease gastric symptoms; give 30 min before or 2 hr after meals; absorption may be slowed
- Shake suspension well

Patient/family education
◆ Teach patient not to exceed recommended dosage; acute poisoning with liver damage may result; acute toxicity includes symptoms of nausea, vomiting, and abdominal pain; prescriber should be notified immediately
- Inform patient that toxicity may occur when used with other combination products
- Advise patient not to use with alcohol or herbals without prescriber approval
- Teach patient to recognize signs of chronic overdose: bleeding, bruising, malaise, fever, sore throat
- Inform patient that urine may become dark brown as a result of phenacetin (metabolite of acetaminophen)
- Tell patient to notify prescriber for pain or fever lasting more than 3 days

Evaluation
Positive therapeutic outcome
- Decreased pain, use pain scoring
- Decreased fever

Treatment of overdose: Product level q4hr, gastric lavage, activated charcoal; administer oral acetylcysteine to prevent hepatic damage (*see acetylcysteine monograph*, p. 43)

*acetaZOLAMIDE (Rx)
(a-set-a-zole'-a-mide)
Apo-Acetazolamide ✿, acetaZOLAMIDE, Damazide, Diamox, Diamox Sequels
Func. class.: Diuretic carbonic anhydrase inhibitor; antiglaucoma agent, antiepileptic
Chem. class.: Sulfonamide derivative

Pregnancy category C

Do not confuse:
acetaZOLAMIDE/acetoHEXAMIDE, Diamox/Dobutrex/Trimox

Action: Decreases the aqueous humor in the eye, which lowers intraocular pressure by the inhibition of carbonic anhydrase; also inhibits carbonic anhydrase activity in proximal renal tubules to decrease reabsorption of water, sodium, potassium, bicarbonate; decreases carbonic anhydrase activity in CNS, increasing seizure threshold; prevents uric acid or cysteine buildup in the renal system by the decrease in pH, causing alkaline urine

Therapeutic outcome: Decreased intraocular pressure; control of seizures; prevention and treatment of acute mountain sickness; prevention of uric acid/cysteine renal stones; decreased edema in lung tissue and peripherally; decreased B/P

Uses: Open-angle glaucoma, closed-angle glaucoma (preoperatively if surgery delayed), epilepsy (petit mal, grand mal, mixed), edema in CHF, product-induced edema, acute altitude sickness

Unlabeled uses: Urine alkalinization, metabolic alkalosis in mechanical ventilation, decrease CSF production in infants with hydrocephalus, familial periodic paralysis, nystagmus

Dosage and routes
Closed-angle glaucoma
Adult: PO/**IV** 250 mg q4hr or 250 mg bid, to be used for short-term therapy

Open-angle glaucoma
Adult: PO/**IV** 250 mg-1 g/day in divided doses for amounts over 250 mg or 500 mg SR bid

Edema in CHF
Adult: **IV** 250-375 mg/day in AM
Child: **IV** 5 mg/kg/day in AM

Seizures
Adult: PO/**IV** 8-30 mg/kg/day in 1-4 divided doses, usual range 375-1000 mg/day; ER not recommended in seizures
Child: PO/**IV** 8-30 mg/kg/day in divided doses tid or qid, or 300-900 mg/m²/day, not to exceed 1 g/day

Altitude sickness
Adult: PO 250 mg q8-12hr; EXT REL 500 mg q12-24hr, start therapy 24-48 hr prior to ascent and ≥48 hr after arrival at high altitude

Renal dose
Adult: PO/**IV** CCr 10-50 ml/min, give dose q12hr; CCr <10 ml/min, avoid use
Geriatric: PO 250 mg bid; use lowest effective dose

Urine alkalinization (unlabeled)
Adult: PO 5 mg/kg/dose, repeat 2-3× over 24 hr

Available forms: Tabs 125, 250 mg; ext rel caps 500 mg; inj 500 mg

Adverse effects
CNS: Drowsiness, paresthesia, anxiety, depression, headache, dizziness, confusion, stimulation, fatigue, **seizures**
EENT: Myopia, tinnitus
ENDO: Hyperglycemia
GI: Nausea, vomiting, anorexia, diarrhea, melena, weight loss, **hepatic insufficiency, cholestatic jaundice, fulminant hepatic necrosis,** taste alterations, **bleeding**
GU: Frequency, polyuria, **uremia,** glucosuria, hematuria, dysuria, crystalluria, renal calculi
HEMA: **Aplastic anemia, hemolytic anemia, leukopenia, thrombocytopenia, purpura, pancytopenia**
INTEG: Rash, pruritus, urticaria, fever, **Stevens-Johnson syndrome,** photosensitivity, flushing
META: Hypokalemia, hyperchloremic acidosis, hyponatremia, sulfonamide-like reactions

Contraindications: Hypersensitivity to sulfonamides, severe renal/hepatic disease, electrolyte imbalances (hyponatremia, hypokalemia), hyperchloremic acidosis, Addison's disease, long-term use in closed-angle glaucoma, adrenalcortical insufficiency

Precautions: Pregnancy **C**, breastfeeding, hypercalciuria, COPD

Pharmacokinetics

Absorption	GI tract—65% if fasting, 75% with food; **IV**—complete
Distribution	Crosses placenta; widely distributed
Metabolism	None
Excretion	Kidneys, unchanged (80% within 24 hr); breast milk
Half-life	2½-5½ hr

Pharmacodynamics

	PO	PO–EXT REL	IV
Onset	1½ hr	2 hr	2 min
Peak	2-4 hr	3-6 hr	15 min
Duration	8-12 hr	18-24 hr	4-5 hr

Interactions
Individual drugs
CycloSPORINE: increased toxicity
Diflunisal: increased side effects
Flecainide: increased action of flecainide
Lithium: increased excretion of lithium
Memantine: increased action of memantine
Methenamine: decreased acetaZOLAMIDE effect
Phenytoin: increased action of phenytoin
Primidone: decreased primidone level
Procainamide: increased action of procainamide
Quinidine: increased action of quinidine
Drug classifications
Amphetamines: increased action
Anticholinergics: increased anticholinergic action
Salicylates: increased toxicity
Procainamide: increased action of procainamide
Quinidine: increased action of quinidine
Drug/lab test
Decreased: thyroid iodine uptake
False positive: urinary protein, 17-hydroxysteroids

NURSING CONSIDERATIONS
Assessment
• Assess patient for tinnitus, hearing loss, ear pain; periodic testing of hearing is needed when high doses of this product are given by **IV** route
• Monitor manifestations of hypokalemia: *RENAL:* acidic urine, reduced urine osmolality, nocturia, polyuria, polydipsia; *CARDIAC:* hypotension, broad T wave, U wave, ectopy, tachycardia, weak pulse; *NEURO:* muscle weakness, altered LOC, drowsiness, apathy,

Adverse effects: *italic* = common, **bold** = life-threatening

lethargy, confusion, depression; *GI:* anorexia, nausea, cramps, constipation, distention, paralytic ileus; *RESP:* hypoventilation, respiratory muscle weakness
• Monitor for CNS, GI, cardiovascular, integumentary, neurologic manifestations of hypocalcemia: *CNS:* personality changes, anxiety, disturbances, depression, psychosis, nausea, vomiting; *GI:* constipation, abdominal pain from muscle spasm; *CV:* decreased contractility, decreased cardiac output, hypotension, lengthened ST segment, prolonged QT interval; *INTEG:* scaling eczema, alopecia, hyperpigmentation; *NEURO:* tetany, muscle twitching, cramping, grimacing, seizure, altered deep tendon reflexes, spasm
• Monitor for manifestations of hypomagnesemia: *CNS:* agitation; *NEURO:* muscle twitching, paresthesias, hyperactive reflexes, positive Babinski's reflex, dysphagia, nystagmus, seizures, tetany; *GI:* nausea, vomiting, diarrhea, anorexia, abdominal distention; *CARDIAC:* ectopy, tachycardia, broad, flat, or inverted T waves, depressed ST segment, prolonged QT, decreased cardiac output, hypotension
• Monitor for manifestations of hyponatremia: *CV:* increased B/P, cold, clammy skin, hypovolemia or hypervolemia, vomiting, diarrhea, abdominal cramps; *NEURO:* lethargy, increased intracranial pressure, confusion, headache, seizures, coma, fatigue, tremors, hyperreflexia
• Monitor for manifestations of hyperchloremia: *NEURO:* weakness, lethargy, coma; *RESP:* deep, rapid breathing
• Assess fluid volume status: I&O ratio and record, count or weigh diapers as appropriate, distended neck veins, crackles in lung, color, quality, and specific gravity of urine, skin turgor, adequacy of pulses, moist mucous membranes, bilateral lung sounds, peripheral pitting edema; dehydration symptoms of decreasing output, thirst, hypotension, dry mouth, and mucous membranes should be reported
• Monitor electrolytes: potassium, sodium, calcium, magnesium; also include BUN, blood pH, ABGs, uric acid, CBC, blood glucose
• Assess B/P before and during therapy with patient lying, standing, and sitting as appropriate; orthostatic hypotension can occur rapidly
• Monitor blood, urine glucose in diabetic patients; glucose levels may be increased
• Assess for eye pain, change in vision when using product for intraocular pressure

• Assess neurologic status when using product for seizures
• Assess for decreased symptoms of acute mountain sickness: headache, nausea, vomiting, dizziness, fatigue, drowsiness, shortness of breath, insomnia
• Assess for cross-sensitivity between other sulfonamides and this product

Nursing diagnoses
• Fluid volume, deficient (side effects)
• Fluid volume, excess (uses)
• Knowledge, deficient (teaching)
• Sensory perception, disturbed (uses)

Implementation
• Give in AM to avoid interference with sleep
• Administer fluids 2-3 L/day to prevent renal calculi, unless contraindicated
• Potassium replacement if potassium level is <3.0 ml/dl

PO route
• Do not crush or chew ext rel caps; caps may be opened and sprinkled on food
• Give with food, if nausea occurs, crush tabs and mix with sweet substance to counteract bitter taste

IV route
• Do not use solution that is yellow or has a precipitate or crystals
• Dilute 500 mg of product/5 ml or more sterile water for inj; use within 24 hr

IV, direct route
• Give over 1 min or more

Intermittent IV infusion route
• May be added to NS, D_5W, $D_{10}W$, 0.45% NaCl; give over 4-8 hr

Additive compatibilities: Cimetidine, ranitidine

Additive incompatibilities: Multivitamins

Patient/family education
• Teach patient to take the medication early in the day to prevent nocturia
• Instruct patient to take with food or milk if GI symptoms of nausea and anorexia occur
• Teach patient to maintain a record of weight on a weekly basis and notify prescriber of weight loss of >5 lb
• Caution patient that this product causes a loss of potassium, so food rich in potassium should be added to the diet; refer to a dietitian for assistance in planning
• Advise patient to wear protective clothing and sunscreen in the sun to prevent photosensitivity
• Teach patient not to use alcohol or any OTC medications without prescriber's approval; serious product reactions may occur

- Emphasize the need to contact prescriber immediately if muscle cramps, weakness, nausea, dizziness, or numbness occurs
- Teach patient to take own B/P and pulse and record
- Teach patient to continue taking medication even if feeling better; this product controls symptoms but does not cure the condition
- Teach patient to see ophthalmologist periodically; glaucoma is a slow process
- Advise patient to increase fluids to 2-3 L/day if not contraindicated
- Instruct patient to report nausea, vertigo, rapid weight gain, change in stools

Evaluation
Positive therapeutic outcome
- Decreased intraocular pressure
- Decreased edema
- Decreased seizures
- Prevention of mountain sickness
- Prevention of uric acid/cysteine stones

Treatment of overdose: Lavage if taken orally, monitor electrolytes, administer dextrose in saline, monitor hydration, CV, renal status

---

acetylcholine ophthalmic
See Appendix B

---

acetylcysteine (Rx)
(a-se-teel-sis'tay-een)
Acetadote, Mucomyst ✦, Parvolex ✦
Func. class.: Mucolytic; antidote—acetaminophen
Chem. class.: Amino acid ʟ-cysteine
Pregnancy category B

Action: Decreases viscosity of secretions in respiratory tract by breaking disulfide links of mucoproteins; serves as a substrate of glutathione, which is necessary to inactivate toxic metabolites in acetaminophen overdose

Therapeutic outcome: Decreased hepatotoxicity from acetaminophen overdose (PO); decreased viscosity of mucus in respiratory disorders (inh)

Uses: Acetaminophen toxicity, bronchitis, cystic fibrosis, COPD, atelectasis

Unlabeled uses: Prevention of contrast media nephrotoxicity

Dosage and routes
Mucolytic
Adult and child: INSTILL 1-20 ml (10%-20% sol) q2-6hr prn, or 3-5 ml (20% sol) or 6-10 ml (10% sol) tid or qid; nebulization (face, mask, mouthpiece, tracheostomy) 1-10 ml of a 20% sol or 2-20 ml of a 10% sol q2-6hr; nebulization (tent, croupette) may require large dose, up to 300 ml/treatment

Acetaminophen toxicity
Adult and child: PO 140 mg/kg, then 70 mg/kg q4hr × 17 doses to total 1330 mg/kg; **IV** loading dose 150 mg/kg over 60 min (dilution 150 mg/kg in 200 ml of D₅); maintenance dose 1:50 mg/kg over 4 hr (dilution 50 mg/kg in 500 ml D₅); maintenance dose 2:100 mg/kg over 16 hr (dilution 100 mg/kg in 1000 ml D₅)

Available forms: Oral sol 10%, 20%; inj 20% (200 mg/ml)

Adverse effects
CNS: *Dizziness, drowsiness,* headache, fever, chills
CV: Hypotension, flushing, tachycardia
EENT: *Rhinorrhea,* tooth damage
GI: *Nausea,* stomatitis, constipation, vomiting, anorexia, **hepatotoxicity,** diarrhea
INTEG: Urticaria, rash, fever, clamminess, pruritus
RESP: **Bronchospasm,** burning, **hemoptysis,** chest tightness, cough

Contraindications: Hypersensitivity, increased intracranial pressure, status asthmaticus

Precautions: Pregnancy **B,** breastfeeding, hypothyroidism, Addison's disease, CNS depression, brain tumor, asthma, renal/hepatic disease, COPD, psychosis, alcoholism, seizure disorders, bronchospasms, asthma, anaphylactoid reactions, fluid restriction, weight <40 kg

Pharmacokinetics	
Absorption	Extensive (PO), locally (inh)
Distribution	Unknown
Metabolism	Liver
Excretion	Kidneys
Half-life	5.6 hr (adult), 11 hr (newborn)

Pharmacodynamics		
	PO	INH
Onset	Unknown	5-10 min
Peak	Unknown	Unknown
Duration	Up to 4 hr	1 hr

Adverse effects: *italic* = common, **bold** = life-threatening

Interactions
Individual drugs

Iron, copper, rubber: do not use with acetylcysteine

Amphotericin B, chlortetracycline, chymotrypsin, erythromycin lactobionate, hydrogen peroxide, iodized oil, oxytetracycline, sodium ampicillin, tetracycline, trypsin: do not mix with antibiotics

Drug classifications

Nitrates: increased effect

NURSING CONSIDERATIONS
Assessment
Mucolytic use

• Assess cough: type, frequency, character, including sputum

• Assess characteristics, rate, rhythm of respirations, increased dyspnea, sputum; discontinue if bronchospasm occurs; ABGs for increased CO_2 retention in asthma patients

• Monitor VS, cardiac status including checking for dysrhythmias, increased rate, palpitations

Antidotal use

• Assess liver function tests, acetaminophen levels, pro-time, glucose, electrolytes; inform prescriber if dose is vomited or vomiting is persistent; provide adequate hydration; decrease dosage in hepatic encephalopathy

• Assess for nausea, vomiting, rash; notify prescriber if these occur

Nursing diagnoses

• Airway clearance, ineffective (uses) (mucolytic)

• Gas exchange, impaired (uses) (mucolytic)

• Injury, risk for (uses) (antidote)

• Knowledge, deficient (teaching)

• Poisoning, risk for (uses) (antidote)

Implementation

• Give decreased dosage to geriatric patients; their metabolism may be slowed; give gum, hard candy, frequent rinsing of mouth for dryness of oral cavity

• Use only if suction machine is available

PO route (Antidotal use)

• Lavage, then give within 24 hr; give with cola or soft drink to disguise taste; can be given with H_2O through tubes; use within 1 hr

Direct Intratracheal INSTILL

• Use ½-1 hr before meals for better absorption, to decrease nausea; only after patient clears airway by deep breathing, coughing

• Give by syringe 2-3 doses of 1-2 ml of 10%-20% sol up to q1hr; 20% sol diluted with NS or water for injection; may give 10% sol undiluted

• Store in refrigerator: use within 96 hr of opening

• Provide assistance with inhaled dose: bronchodilator if bronchospasm occurs; wash face and rinse mouth after use to remove sticky feeling

• Use mechanical suction if cough insufficient to remove excess bronchial secretions

IV route

• Dilute with D_5, 0.45% NaCl

Incompatibilities: Rubber, metals, stability with other products unknown

Patient/family education
Mucolytic use

• Tell patient to avoid driving or other hazardous activities until patient is stabilized on this medication; avoid alcohol, other CNS depressants; will enhance sedating properties of this product

• Teach patient that unpleasant odor will decrease after repeated use; that discoloration of solution after bottle is opened does not impair its effectiveness; avoid smoking, smoke-filled rooms, perfume, dust, environmental pollutants, cleaners

• Teach patient to report vomiting, as dose may need to be repeated

Evaluation
Positive therapeutic outcome

• Absence of purulent secretions when coughing (mucolytic use)

• Clear lung sounds bilaterally (mucolytic use)

• Absence of hepatic damage (acetaminophen toxicity)

• Decreasing blood toxicology (acetaminophen toxicity)

---

acyclovir ◉ (Rx)
(ay-sye′kloe-veer)
Avirax ✦, Zovirax
Func. class.: Antiviral
Chem. class.: Acyclic purine nucleoside analog

Pregnancy category B

Action: Interferes with DNA synthesis by conversion to acyclovir triphosphate, causing decreased viral replication, time of lesional healing

Therapeutic outcome: Decreased amount and time of healing of lesions

Uses: Mucocutaneous herpes simplex virus, herpes genitalis (HSV-1, HSV-2), varicella infections, herpes zoster, herpes simplex encephalitis

Dosage and routes
Renal dose
Adult and child: PO/**IV** CCr >50 ml/min 100% dose q8hr; CCr 25-50 ml/min 100% dose q12hr; CCr 10-25 ml/min 100% dose q24hr; CCr 0-10 ml/min 50% of dose q24hr

Herpes simplex
Adult: PO 200 mg q4hr
Adult and child >12 yr: **IV** INF 5 mg/kg over 1 hr q8hr × 5 days
Child <12 yr: **IV** INF 250 mg/m² or 30 mg/kg/day divided q8hr over 1 hr × 5 days

Genital herpes
Adult: PO 200 mg q4hr 5 times a day while awake × 5 days to 6 mo depending on whether initial, recurrent, or chronic; **IV** 5 mg/kg q8hr × 5 days

Herpes simplex encephalitis
Adult: **IV** 10 mg/kg over 1 hr q8hr × 10 days
Child 3 mo-12 yr: **IV** 20 mg/kg q8hr × 10 days
Child birth-3 mo: **IV** 10 mg/kg q8hr × 10 days

Herpes zoster
Adult: PO 800 mg q4hr while awake × 7-10 days; **IV** 10 mg/kg q8hr × 7 days

Varicella-zoster
Adult and child >40 kg: PO 800 mg qid × 5 days; **IV** (unlabeled) 20 mg/kg/day q8hr × 5 days (immunocompetent); 10 mg/kg/day q8hr × 7-10 days (immunocompromised)
Child ≥2 yrs: PO 20 mg/kg qid × 5 days

Mucosal/cutaneous herpes simplex infections in immunosuppressed patients
Adult and child >12 yr: **IV** 5 mg/kg q8hr × 7 days
Child <12 yr: **IV** 10 mg/kg q8hr × 7 days

Available forms: Caps 200 mg; tabs 400, 800 mg; inj **IV** 500 mg; oral susp

Adverse effects
CNS: Tremors, confusion, lethargy, hallucinations, **seizures,** *dizziness, headache,* encephalopathic changes
EENT: Gingival hyperplasia
GI: Nausea, vomiting, diarrhea, increased ALT, AST, abdominal pain, glossitis, colitis
GU: **Oliguria, proteinuria, hematuria,** vaginitis, moniliasis, **glomerulonephritis, acute renal failure,** changes in menses, polydipsia
HEMA: **Thrombotic thrombocytopenia purpura, hemolytic uremic syndrome** (immunocompromised patient)
INTEG: Rash, urticaria, pruritus, pain or phlebitis at **IV** site, unusual sweating, alopecia
MS: Joint pain, leg pain, muscle cramps

Contraindications: Hypersensitivity to this product or ganciclovir, famciclovir, penciclovir, valacyclovir, or valganciclovir

Precautions: Pregnancy **B,** breastfeeding, renal/hepatic disease, electrolyte imbalance, dehydration, neurologic disease

Pharmacokinetics	
Absorption	Minimal (PO)
Distribution	Widely distributed, crosses placenta; CSF concentration 50% plasma; protein binding 9%-33%
Metabolism	Liver, minimal
Excretion	Kidneys, 95% unchanged
Half-life	2.0-3.5 hr, increased in renal disease

Pharmacodynamics		
	PO	IV
Onset	Unknown	Rapid
Peak	1½-2½ hr	Infusion's end
Duration	Unknown	Unknown

Interactions
Individual drugs
Interferon: increased synergistic effect
Mycophenolate, probenecid: increased neurotoxicity, nephrotoxicity
Zidovudine: increased CNS side effects
Zoster vaccine: avoid concurrent use

NURSING CONSIDERATIONS
Assessment
• Monitor for signs of infection, type of lesions, area of body covered, purulent drainage
• Check I&O ratio; report hematuria, oliguria, fatigue, weakness; may indicate nephrotoxicity; check for protein in urine during treatment
• Monitor any patient with compromised renal system, since product is excreted slowly in poor renal system function; toxicity may occur rapidly
• Monitor liver studies: AST, ALT

Adverse effects: *italic* = common, **bold** = life-threatening

- Monitor blood studies: WBC, RBC, Hct, Hgb, bleeding time; blood dyscrasias may occur; product should be discontinued
- Monitor renal studies: urinalysis, protein, BUN, creatinine, CCr; increased BUN, creatinine indicates renal failure and nephrotoxicity
- Obtain C&S before product therapy; product may be taken as soon as culture is taken; repeat C&S after treatment; determine the presence of other sexually transmitted diseases
- Monitor bowel pattern before, during treatment; if severe abdominal pain with bleeding occurs, product should be discontinued
- Assess allergies before treatment, reaction of each medication; place allergies on chart in bright red letters; allergic reaction: burning, stinging, swelling, redness, rash, vulvitis, pruritus
- Assess neurologic status in herpes encephalitis

Nursing diagnoses
- Infection, risk for (uses)
- Knowledge, deficient (teaching)

Implementation
PO route
- Do not break, crush, or chew caps
- Give with food to lessen GI symptoms; may give without regard to meals with 8 oz of water
- Store at room temperature in dry place
- May be taken orally before infection occurs or when itching or pain occurs, usually before eruptions
- Must be taken at equal intervals around the clock
- Shake suspension before use

IV route
- Provide increased fluids to 3 L/day to decrease crystalluria
- Give by int inf after reconstituting with 10 ml sterile water for injection/500 mg of product (50 mg/ml); shake; dilute in 0.9% NaCl, LR, D_5W, D_5/0.25% NaCl, D_5/0.45% NaCl, D_5/0.9% NaCl (7 mg/ml); give over at least 1 hr (constant rate) by infusion pump to prevent nephrotoxicity; do not reconstitute with sol containing benzyl alcohol or parabens; check infusion site for redness, pain, induration; rotate sites
- Lower dosage in acute or chronic renal failure
- Store at room temperature for up to 12 hr after reconstitution; if refrigerated, sol may show a precipitate that clears at room temperature; yellow discoloration does not affect potency

Y-site compatibilities: Allopurinol, amikacin, ampicillin, amphotericin B cholesteryl sulfate complex, cefamandole, cefazolin, cefonicid, cefoperazone, ceforanide, cefotaxime, cefoxitin, ceftazidime, ceftizoxime, ceftriaxone, cefuroxime, cephapirin, chloramphenicol, cimetidine, clindamycin, cotrimoxazole, dexamethasone sodium phosphate, dimenhyDRINATE, diphenhydrAMINE, doxycycline, DOXOrubicin, erythromycin, famotidine, filgrastim, fluconazole, gallium, gentamicin, granisetron, heparin, hydrocortisone sodium succinate, hydromorphone, imipenem/cilastatin, lorazepam, magnesium sulfate, melphalan, methylPREDNISolone sodium succinate, metoclopramide, metronidazole, multivitamin infusion, nafcillin, oxacillin, paclitaxel, penicillin G potassium, pentobarbital, perphenazine, piperacillin, potassium chloride, propofol, ranitidine, remifentanil, sodium bicarbonate, tacrolimus, teniposide, tetracycline, theophylline, thiotepa, ticarcillin, tobramycin, trimethoprim-sulfamethoxazole, vancomycin, zidovudine
Y-site incompatibilities: DOBUTamine, DOPamine, ondansetron, verapamil
Additive compatibilities: Fluconazole
Additive incompatibilities: Blood products, protein-containing solutions, DOBUTamine, DOPamine

Patient/family education
PO route
- Teach patient that product may be taken orally before infection occurs or when itching or pain occur, usually before eruptions; that partners need to be told that patient has herpes; they can become infected, so condoms must be worn to prevent reinfections; that product does not cure infection, just controls symptoms and does not prevent infection to others
- ⬥ Tell patient to report sore throat, fever, fatigue; may indicate superinfection; that product must be taken at equal intervals around the clock to maintain blood levels for duration of therapy
- Tell patient to notify prescriber of side effects: bruising, bleeding, fatigue, malaise; may indicate blood dyscrasias
- Tell patient to seek dental care during treatment to prevent gingival hyperplasia
- Teach female patients with genital herpes to have regular Pap smears to prevent undetected cervical cancer

Evaluation
Positive therapeutic outcome
- Absence of itching, painful lesions
- Crusting and healed lesions

Treatment of overdose: Discontinue product, hemodialysis, resuscitate if needed

acyclovir topical
See Appendix B

adalimumab (Rx)
(add-a-lim'yu-mab)
Humira
Func. class.: Antirheumatic agent (disease modifying), immunomodulator

Pregnancy category B

Do not confuse:
Humira/Humalin

Action: A form of human IgG1 monoclonal antibody specific for human tumor necrosis factor (TNF); elevated levels of TNF are found in patients with rheumatoid arthritis

Therapeutic outcome: Decreased pain, inflammation in joints, better ROM

Uses: Reduction in signs and symptoms and inhibiting progression of structural damage in patients with moderate to severe active rheumatoid arthritis in patients ≥18 years of age who have not responded to other disease-modifying agents, JRA, psoriatic arthritis, Crohn's disease, moderate-severe plaque psoriasis

Dosage and routes
Rheumatoid arthritis/ankylosing spondylitis/psoriatic arthritis
Adult: SUBCUT 40 mg every other wk

Juvenile rheumatoid arthritis (JRA)
Child ≥4 yr/adolescent ≥30 kg: SUBCUT 40 mg every other wk
Child ≥4 yr/adolescent ≥15 kg to <30 kg: SUBCUT 20 mg every other wk

Crohn's disease
Adult: SUBCUT 160 mg given as 4 inj on day 1, or 2 inj on days 1 and 2, then 80 mg at wk 2 and 40 mg every other wk, starting at wk 4

Plaque psoriasis
Adult: SUBCUT 80 mg baseline as 2 inj, then 40 mg every other week starting 1 wk after dose × 16 wk

Available forms: Inj 40 mg/0.8 ml

Adverse effects
CNS: Headache
CV: Hypertension
EENT: Sinusitis
GI: Abdominal pain, nausea, hepatic damage
INTEG: Rash, *inj site reaction*
MISC: Flulike symptoms, UTI, hypertension, back pain, lupuslike syndrome, risk of cancer, antibody development to this drug, **risk of infection (TB, invasive fungal infections, other opportunistic infections); may be fatal**
RESP: URI, **pulmonary fibrosis**

Contraindications: Hypersensitivity

Black Box Warning: Active infections

Precautions: Pregnancy **B**, breastfeeding, children, geriatric, CNS demyelinating disease, lymphoma, latent TB, CHF, hepatitis B carriers

Pharmacokinetics
Absorption	Unknown
Distribution	Unknown
Metabolism	Unknown
Excretion	Unknown
Half-life	Terminal 2 wk

Pharmacodynamics
Unknown

Interactions
Drug classification
Vaccines: do not give concurrently; immunization should be brought up to date before treatment

NURSING CONSIDERATIONS
Assessment
- Assess for pain, stiffness, ROM, swelling of joints during treatment
- Check for inj site pain, swelling; usually occur after 2 inj (4-5 days)
- ◆ Check for infections, stop treatment if present, some serious infections, including sepsis, may occur; patients with active infections should not be started on this product

Nursing diagnoses
- Activity intolerance (uses)
- Knowledge, deficient (teaching)
- Mobility, impaired physical (uses)
- Pain, chronic (uses)

Implementation
- Do not admix with other sol or medications, do not use filter, protect from light

Adverse effects: *italic* = common, **bold** = life-threatening

Patient/family education
• Teach patient about self-administration if appropriate: inj should be made in thigh, abdomen, upper arm; rotate sites at least 1 inch from old site; do not inject in areas that are bruised, red, hard
• Advise patient that if medication is not taken when due, inject next dose as soon as remembered and inject next dose as scheduled

Evaluation
Positive therapeutic outcome
• Decreased inflammation, pain in joints

---

adefovir (Rx)
(add-ee-foh′veer)
Hepsera
Func. class.: Antiviral
Pregnancy category C

Action: Inhibits hepatitis B virus DNA polymerase by competing with natural substrates and by causing DNA termination after its incorporation into viral DNA; causes viral DNA death

Therapeutic outcome: Improving liver function tests, lessening symptoms of chronic hepatitis B

Uses: Chronic hepatitis B

Dosage and routes
Adult: PO 10 mg daily, optimal duration unknown

Renal dose
Adult: PO CCr ≥50 ml/min 10 mg q24hr; CCr 30-49 ml/min 10 mg q48hr; CCr 10-29 ml/min 10 mg q72hr; hemodialysis 10 mg q7 days following dialysis

Available forms: Tabs 10 mg

Adverse effects
CNS: Headache
GI: Dyspepsia, abdominal pain, nausea, vomiting, diarrhea, hepatomegaly
GU: Hematuria, glycosuria, **nephrotoxicity**
MISC: Fever, rash, weight loss

Contraindications: Hypersensitivity

Precautions: Pregnancy **C**, breastfeeding, children, geriatric

Black Box Warning: Severe renal disease, impaired hepatic disease, lactic acidosis, HIV

Pharmacokinetics
Absorption	Rapidly from GI tract
Distribution	Unknown
Metabolism	Unknown
Excretion	Kidneys 45%
Half-life	7.48 hr

Pharmacodynamics
Onset	Unknown
Peak	1¾ hr
Duration	Unknown

Interactions
Individual drugs
Acetaminophen, aspirin, indomethacin: increased granulocytopenia
Acetaminophen, acyclovir, adriamycin, amphotericin B, cimetidine, dapsone, DOXOrubicin, fluconazole, flucytosine, ganciclovir, indomethacin, interferon, morphine, pentamidine, phenytoin, probenecid, trimethoprim, vinBLAStine, vinCRIStine: increased serum concentrations, toxicity
Drug classifications
Benzodiazepines, nucleoside analogs (experimental), sulfonamides: increased serum concentrations, toxicity

Black Box Warning: NNRTIs, NRTIs

Drug/lab test
Increased: ALT, AST, amylase, creatine kinase

NURSING CONSIDERATIONS
Assessment
◆ Assess for nephrotoxicity: increasing CCr, BUN
• Assess for HIV before beginning treatment because HIV resistance may occur in chronic hepatitis B patients
◆ Assess for lactic acidosis, severe hepatomegaly with stenosis
• Assess geriatric patients more carefully; may develop renal, cardiac symptoms more rapidly
• Assess for exacerbations of hepatitis after discontinuing treatment, monitor liver function tests

Nursing diagnoses
• Infection, risk for (uses)
• Knowledge, deficient (teaching)

Implementation
• Give by mouth without regard to food
• Store in cool environment; protect from light

Patient/family education
• Advise patient that optimal duration of treatment is unknown, that drug is not a cure; transmission may still occur

---

◆ Alert   ✤ Canada Only   🌐 Drug on CD   * "Tall Man" lettering (See Preface)

- Advise patient to avoid use with other medications unless approved by prescriber
- Advise patient to notify prescriber of decreased urinary output
- Avoid breastfeeding

Evaluation
Positive therapeutic outcome
- Decreased symptoms of chronic hepatitis B, improving liver function tests

---

! HIGH ALERT

adenosine (Rx)
(ah-den'oh-seen)
Adenocard, Adeno-jec, Adenoscan
Func. class.: Antidysrhythmic—miscellaneous
Chem. class.: Endogenous nucleoside
Pregnancy category C

Do not confuse:
Adenocard/adenosine phosphate

Action: Slows conduction through AV node, can interrupt reentry pathways through AV node, and can restore normal sinus rhythm in patients with paroxysmal supraventricular tachycardia (PSVT)

Therapeutic outcome: Normal sinus rhythm in patients diagnosed with SVT

Uses: SVT, as a diagnostic aid to assess myocardial perfusion defects in CAD; Wolff-Parkinson-White (WPW) syndrome

Dosage and routes
Antidysrhythmic
Adult and child >50 kg: IV BOL 6 mg; if conversion to normal sinus rhythm does not occur within 1-2 min, give 12 mg by rapid **IV** BOL; may repeat 12 mg dose again in 1-2 min
Infant and child <50 kg: IV BOL 0.05 mg/kg; if not effective, increase dose by 0.05 mg/kg q2min to a max of 0.3 mg/kg/dose or 12 mg

Diagnostic use
Adult: IV 140 mcg/kg/min × 6 min

Wolff-Parkinson-White (WPW)
Adult/adolescent/child ≥50 kg: IV BOL 6 mg by rapid INF, follow with saline flush; then **IV** BOL 12 mg if needed

Available forms: Inj 3 mg/ml (vial); 6 mg/2 ml (vial)

Adverse effects
CNS: Light-headedness, dizziness, arm tingling, numbness, apprehension, blurred vision, headache

CV: Chest pain/pressure, **atrial tachydysrhythmias,** sweating, palpitations, hypotension, *facial flushing*
GI: Nausea, metallic taste, throat tightness, groin pressure
RESP: Dyspnea, chest pressure, hyperventilation, **bronchospasm (asthmatics)**

Contraindications: Hypersensitivity, 2nd- or 3rd-degree heart block, AV block, sick sinus syndrome, atrial flutter, atrial fibrillation, ventricular tachycardia

Precautions: Pregnancy C, breastfeeding, children, geriatric, asthma

Pharmacokinetics
Absorption	Complete bioavailability
Distribution	Erythrocytes, cardiovascular endothelium
Metabolism	Liver, converted to inosine and adenosine monophosphate
Excretion	Kidneys
Half-life	10 sec

Pharmacodynamics
Onset	Rapid
Peak	Unknown
Duration	1-2 min

Interactions
Individual drugs
Caffeine, theophylline: decreased effects of adenosine
Carbamazepine: increased heart block
Digoxin: increased ventricular fibrillation
Dipyridamole: increased effects of adenosine
Smoking: increased tachycardia
Drug/herb
Aconite: increased toxicity, death
Aloe, broom, chronic buckthorn use, cascara sagrada (chronic use), figwort, fumitory, goldenseal, kudzu, licorice, rhubarb, senna: increased effect
Coltsfoot, guarana: decreased effect
Horehound: increased serotonin effect

NURSING CONSIDERATIONS
Assessment
- Monitor I&O ratio, electrolytes (potassium, sodium, chloride)
- Assess cardiopulmonary status: pulse, respiration, ECG intervals (PR, QRS, QT); check for transient dysrhythmias (PVCs, PACs, sinus tachycardia, AV block)
- Assess respiratory status: rate, rhythm, lung fields for crackles, watch for respiratory depression; bilateral crackles may occur in

Adverse effects: italic = common, bold = life-threatening

CHF patient; if increased respiration, increased pulse occurs, product should be discontinued
• Assess CNS effects: dizziness, confusion, paresthesias; product should be discontinued

Nursing diagnoses
• Cardiac output, decreased (uses)
• Gas exchange, impaired (adverse reactions)
• Knowledge, deficient (teaching)

Implementation
IV, direct (bolus) route
• Give **IV** BOL undiluted; give 6 mg or less by rapid inj; if using an **IV** line, use port near insertion site, flush with 0.9% NaCl (50 ml); warm to room temperature before giving
Intermittent INF (diagnostic testing)
• Use 30 ml vial, undiluted, by peripheral vein at a rate of 140 mcg/kg/min over 6 min for a total dose of 0.84 mg/kg, inject Thalium 201 as close to venous access as possible after 3 min of infusion
Solution compatibilities: D_5LR, D_5W, LR, 0.9% NaCl
• Store at room temperature; sol should be clear; discard unused product

Patient/family education
• Tell patient to report facial flushing, dizziness, sweating, palpitations, chest pain
• Instruct patient to rise from sitting or standing slowly to prevent orthostatic hypotension

Evaluation
Positive therapeutic outcome
• Normal sinus rhythm
• Diagnosis of perfusion defect

---

albumin, normal serum 5%/ 25% (Rx)
(al-byoo'min)
Albuminar 5%, Albutein 5%, Buminate 5%, Plasbumin 5%, Albuminar 25%, Albutein 25%, Buminate 25%, Flexbumin 25%, Plasbumin 25%
Func. class.: Blood derivative—plasma volume expander
Chem. class.: Placental human plasma

Pregnancy category C

Action: Exerts colloidal oncotic pressure, which expands volume of circulating blood by pulling fluid from extravascular to intravascular spaces, and maintains cardiac output

Therapeutic outcome: Restoration of plasma volume by extravascular to intravascular fluid shift

Uses: Restores plasma volume in burns, hyperbilirubinemia, shock, hypoproteinemia, prevention of cerebral edema, cardiopulmonary bypass procedures, ARDS, hemorrhage; also replacement in nephrotic syndrome

Dosage and routes
Burns
Adult: **IV** dose to maintain plasma albumin at 30-50 g/L, use 5% sol initially, then 25% sol after 24 hr

Shock
Adult: **IV** 500 ml of 5% sol q30min, as needed
Child: 0.5-1 g/kg/dose, 5% sol, may repeat as needed; max 6 g/kg/day

Hypoproteinemia
Adult: **IV** 1000-2000 ml of 5% sol/day, max 5-10 ml/min or 25-100 g of 25% sol/day; max 3 ml/min, titrated to patient response
Child/infant: **IV** 0.5-1 g/kg/dose over 2-4 hr, may repeat q1-2days

Hyperbilirubinemia/ erythroblastosis fetalis
Infant: **IV** 1 g of 25% sol/kg 1-2 hr before transfusion

Available forms: Inj 50, 250 mg/ml (5%, 25%)

Adverse effects
CNS: Fever, chills, flushing, headache
CV: **Fluid overload,** hypotension, erratic pulse, tachycardia
GI: Nausea, vomiting, increased salivation
INTEG: Rash, urticaria
RESP: Altered respirations, **pulmonary edema**

Contraindications: Hypersensitivity, CHF, severe anemia, renal insufficiency, pulmonary edema

Precautions: Pregnancy **C,** decreased salt intake, decreased cardiac reserve, lack of albumin deficiency, renal/hepatic disease, chronic anemia

Pharmacokinetics	
Absorption	Complete bioavailability
Distribution	Intravascular spaces
Metabolism	Liver
Excretion	Unknown
Half-life	Terminal, 21 days

Pharmacodynamics	
Onset	15-30 min
Peak	Unknown
Duration	Unknown

 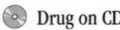

Interactions
Drug/lab test
Increased: alkaline phosphatase

NURSING CONSIDERATIONS
Assessment
- Monitor blood studies: Hct, Hgb; if serum protein declines, dyspnea, hypoxemia can result; check for decreasing B/P, erratic pulse, respiration
- ◆ Monitor CVP: pulmonary wedge pressure will increase if overload occurs; I&O ratio: urinary output may decrease; CVP reading: distended neck veins indicate circulatory overload; shortness of breath, anxiety, insomnia, expiratory crackles, frothy blood-tinged sputum, cough, cyanosis indicate pulmonary overload
- Assess for allergy: fever, rash, itching, chills, flushing, urticaria, nausea, vomiting, hypotension; requires discontinuation of infusion, use of new lot if therapy reinstituted; premedicate with diphenhydrAMINE

Nursing diagnoses
- Fluid volume, deficit (uses)
- Fluid volume, excess (adverse reactions)
- Injury, risk for (uses)
- Knowledge, deficient (teaching)

Implementation
IV route
- Check type of albumin; some are stored at room temperature, some need to be refrigerated; use only amber-colored sol without precipitate; solution should be clear, use within 4 hr of opening
- Give **IV** slowly to prevent fluid overload; 5% sol may be given undiluted; 25% sol may be given diluted (D_5W, 0.9% NaCl) or undiluted; give over 4 hr, use infusion pump
- Provide adequate hydration before, during administration; whole blood may need to be given to prevent anemia; monitor hydration during treatment
- 5% sol may be used in hypovolemic/intravascular depletion
- 25% sol may be used in sodium/fluid restriction

Y-site compatibilities: Diltiazem
Solution compatibilities: LR, NaCl, Ringer's, D_5W, $D_{10}W$, $D_{2\frac{1}{2}}W$, dextrose/saline, dextran$_6$ D_5, dextran$_6$ NaCl 0.9%, dextrose/Ringer's, dextrose/LR

Patient/family education
- Explain use, reason for albumin; provide information on what to report to prescriber (hypersensitivity, fluid overload)

Evaluation
Positive therapeutic outcome
- Increased B/P, decreased edema (shock, burns)
- Increased serum albumin levels
- Increased plasma protein (hypoproteinemia)

---

albuterol 🍁 (Rx)
(al-byoo′ter-ole)
AccuNeb, Airet, albuterol, Gen-Salbutamol 🍁, Novo-Salmol 🍁, Proair HFA, Proventil, Proventil HFA, Ventodisk 🍁, Ventolin HFA, Vospire ER
Func. class.: Bronchodilator
Chem. class.: Adrenergic β_2-agonist, sympathomimetic, bronchodilator
Pregnancy category C

Do not confuse:
albuterol/atenolol, Proventil/ Prinivil, Salbutamol/salmeterol, Ventolin/Vantin

Action: Causes bronchodilatation by action on β_2 (pulmonary) receptors by increasing levels of cyclic adenosine monophosphate (cAMP), which relaxes smooth muscle; produces bronchodilatation; CNS, cardiac stimulation, increased diuresis, and increased gastric acid secretion; longer acting than isoproterenol

Therapeutic outcome: Increased ability to breathe because of bronchodilatation

Uses: Prevention of exercise-induced asthma, acute bronchospasm, bronchitis, emphysema, bronchiectasis, reversible airway obstruction

Unlabeled uses: Hyperkalemia in dialysis patients

Dosage and routes
To prevent exercise-induced bronchospasm
Adult: INH (metered dose inhaler) 2 puffs 15 min before exercising

Other respiratory conditions
Adult and child ≥12 yr: INH (metered dose inhaler) 2 puffs q4hr; PO 2-4 mg tid-qid, max 32 mg/day, depending on formulation; NEB/IPPB PO 2.5 mg q6-8hr
Geriatric: PO 2 mg tid-qid, may increase gradually to 8 mg tid-qid
Child 2-12 yr: INH (metered dose inhaler) 0.1 mg/kg tid (max 2.5 mg tid-qid); NEB/IPPB 0.1-0.15 mg/kg/dose tid-qid or 1.25 mg tid-qid for child 10-15 kg or 2.5 mg tid-qid >15 kg

---

*Adverse effects: *italic* = common, **bold** = life-threatening*

Available forms: Aerosol 90 mcg/actuation; tabs 2, 4 mg; oral sol 2 mg/5 ml; ext rel 4, 8 mg; inh sol 0.5, 0.83, 1, 2, 5 mg/ml; powder for inh (Ventodisk) 200, 400 mcg; inh caps 200 mcg; 100 mcg/spray, 80 inh/canister, 200 inh/canister

Adverse effects
CNS: Tremors, anxiety, insomnia, headache, dizziness, stimulation, *restlessness,* hallucinations, flushing, irritability
CV: Palpitations, tachycardia, hypertension, angina, hypotension, dysrhythmias
EENT: Dry nose, irritation of nose and throat
GI: Heartburn, nausea, vomiting
MISC: Flushing, sweating, anorexia, bad taste/smell changes, hypokalemia
MS: Muscle cramps
RESP: Cough, wheezing, dyspnea, **bronchospasm,** dry throat

Contraindications: Hypersensitivity to sympathomimetics, tachydsrhythmias, severe cardiac disease, heart block

Precautions: Pregnancy **C**, breastfeeding, exercise-induced bronchospasm (aerosol) in children <12 yr, cardiac/renal disease, hyperthyroidism, diabetes mellitus, hypertension, prostatic hypertrophy, closed-angle glaucoma, seizures, hypoglycemia, seizure disorder

Pharmacokinetics
Absorption	Well absorbed (PO)
Distribution	Unknown
Metabolism	Liver extensively, tissues
Excretion	Unknown, breast milk
Half-life	3-4 hr

Pharmacodynamics
	PO	PO–EXT REL	INH
Onset	½ hr	½ hr	5-15 min
Peak	2½ hr	2-3 hr	1-1½ hr
Duration	4-6 hr	12 hr	4-6 hr

Interactions
Individual drugs
Atomoxetine, selegiline: increased CV effects
Drug classifications
Adrenergics: increased action of albuterol; do not use together
β-Adrenergic blockers: block therapeutic effect
Antidepressants (tricyclic): increased chance of hypertension; do not use together
Bronchodilators (aerosol): increased action of bronchodilator
Diuretics (potassium-losing): increased ECG changes/hypokalemia

MAOIs: increased chance of hypertensive crisis; do not use together
Oxytocics: severe hypotension; do not use together
Theophylline: toxicity
Drug/herb
Black tea, green tea, cola nut, guarana, yerba maté: increased stimulation
Drug/food
Caffeine products, chocolate: increased stimulation

NURSING CONSIDERATIONS
Assessment
• Assess respiratory function: vital capacity, forced expiratory volume, ABGs, lung sounds; heart rate, rhythm; B/P, sputum (baseline and during therapy)
• Determine that patient has not received theophylline therapy before giving dose, to prevent additive effect; client's ability to self-medicate
• Monitor for evidence of allergic reactions; paradoxic bronchospasm; withhold dose; notify prescriber if bronchospasm occurs

Nursing diagnoses
• Airway clearance, ineffective (uses)
• Gas exchange, impaired (uses)
• Knowledge, deficient (teaching)

Implementation
PO route
• Do not break, crush, or chew ext rel tabs
• Give PO with meals to decrease gastric irritation; oral sol for children (no alcohol, sugar)
• In geriatric patients, a spacing device is advised
Aerosol route
• Give after shaking metered dose inhaler; have patient exhale and place mouthpiece in mouth, inhale slowly while depressing inhaler, hold breath, remove inhaler, exhale slowly; allow at least 1 min between inhalations; avoid using near flames or source of heat
• Track number of inhalations used and discard when labeled inhalations have been used
• Store in light-resistant container; do not expose to temperatures >86° F (30° C)
Nebulizer/IPPB route
• Dilute 5 mg/ml sol/2.5 ml 0.9% NaCl for inhalation; other solutions do not require dilution for nebulizer O_2 flow or compressed air 6-10 L/min

Patient/family education
• Tell patient not to use OTC medications before consulting prescriber; excess stimula-

tion may occur; instruct patient to use this medication before other medications and allow at least 5 min between each to prevent overstimulation; to limit caffeine products such as chocolate, coffee, tea, and cola

• Teach patient to use inhaler; review package insert with patient; to avoid getting aerosol in eyes or blurring may result; to wash inhaler in warm water and dry daily; to rinse mouth after using; to avoid smoking, smoke-filled rooms, persons with respiratory infections

⬥ Teach patient that if paradoxic broncho-spasm occurs to stop product immediately and notify prescriber

• Instruct patient on administration of dose, not to use more than prescribed; serious side effects may occur; if taking PO regularly and dose is missed, take when remembered; space other doses on new time schedule; do not double doses

• In geriatric patients, a spacing device is advised

Evaluation
Positive therapeutic outcome
• Absence of dyspnea and wheezing after 1 hr
• Improved airway exchange
• Improved ABGs

Treatment of overdose: Administer a β₁-adrenergic blocker, **IV** fluids

---

❗ HIGH ALERT

aldesleukin, IL-2 (Rx)
(al-dess-loo'kin)
Proleukin
Func. class.: Antineoplastics—miscellaneous
Chem. class.: Interleukin-2, human recombinant, cytokine

Pregnancy category C

Do not confuse:
aldesleukin/oprelvekin, Proleukin/Oprelvekin/Prokine

Action: Enhancement of lymphocyte mitogenesis and stimulation of IL-2–dependent cell lines; enhancement of lymphocyte cytotoxicity; induction of killer cell activity; induction of interferon-γ production; results in activation of cellular immunity and cytokines and inhibition of tumor growth

Therapeutic outcome: Prevention of rapid growth of malignant cells

Uses: Metastatic renal cell carcinoma in adults, phase II for HIV in combination with zidovudine, melanoma (metastatic)

Unlabeled uses: Acute myelogenous leukemia (AML), cutaneous T-cell lymphoma (CTCL), HIV, Hansen's disease (leprosy), mycosis fungoides, non-Hodgkin's lymphoma

Dosage and routes
Renal cell cancer/malignant melanoma
Adult: **IV** INF 600,000 international units/kg (0.037 mg/kg) over 15 min q8hr × 14 doses; off 9 days; repeat schedule for another 14 doses, for a maximum of 28 doses/course

Available forms: Powder for inj 22 million international units/vial

Adverse effects
CNS: Mental status changes, *dizziness,* sensory dysfunction, syncope, motor dysfunction, fever, chills, headache, impaired memory, depression, sleep disturbances, hallucinations, rigors, neuropathy
CV: Hypotension, sinus tachycardia, dysrhythmias, bradycardia, PVCs, PACs, myocardial ischemia, **myocardial infarction, cardiac arrest,** capillary leak syndrome, **CVA**
EENT: Reversible visual changes
GI: Nausea, vomiting, *diarrhea,* stomatitis, anorexia, GI bleeding, dyspepsia, constipation, **intestinal perforation/ileus,** jaundice, ascites
GU: **Oliguria/anuria, proteinuria, hematuria,** dysuria, **renal failure**
HEMA: Anemia, **thrombocytopenia, leukopenia, coagulation disorders, leukocytosis, eosinophilia**
INTEG: Pruritus, *erythema, rash,* dry skin, **exfoliative dermatitis,** purpura, petechiae, urticaria
MS: Arthralgia, myalgia
RESP: Pulmonary congestion, dyspnea, **pulmonary edema, respiratory failure,** tachypnea, pleural effusion, wheezing, **apnea**
SYST: Infection

Contraindications: Hypersensitivity, abnormal thallium stress test or pulmonary function tests, organ allografts

Black Box Warning: Cardiac/pulmonary disease, coma

Precautions: Pregnancy C, breastfeeding, children, CNS metastases, bacterial infections, renal/hepatic disease, anemia, thrombocytopenia

Black Box Warning: Capillary leak syndrome, infection

Adverse effects: *italic* = common, **bold** = life-threatening

Pharmacokinetics

Absorption	Complete bioavailability
Distribution	Rapid extracellular, intravascular
Metabolism	Kidneys (convoluted tubules)
Excretion	Kidneys
Half-life	85 min

Pharmacodynamics

Onset	4 wk
Peak	Unknown
Duration	≤12 mo

Interactions
Individual drugs
Indomethacin, methotrexate, asparaginase, DOXOrubicin: increased toxicity
Drug classifications
Aminoglycosides: increased toxicity
Antihypertensives: increased hypotension
Cytotoxic chemotherapy: increased toxicity
Glucocorticosteroids: decreased tumor effectiveness
Psychotropics: unpredictable reactions
Drug/lab test
Increased: bilirubin, BUN, serum creatinine, transaminase, alkaline phosphatase, hypomagnesemia, acidosis hypocalcemia, hypophosphatemia, hypokalemia, hyperuricemia, hypoalbuminemia, hypoproteinemia, hyponatremia, hyperkalemia, alkalosis (toxic effect of product)

NURSING CONSIDERATIONS
Assessment
• Monitor CBC, differential, platelet count weekly; withhold product if WBC is <2000/mm^3 or platelet count is <75,000/mm^3; notify prescriber of these results; transfusion of RBCs, platelets may be required
◆ Identify capillary leak syndrome (CLS), including a drop in mean arterial pressure (2-12 hr after initiating therapy); hypotension and hypoperfusion will occur; if B/P <90 mm Hg, monitor ECG, CVP in cardiac patients
• Monitor renal function studies: BUN, serum uric acid, urine CCr, electrolytes before, during therapy; I&O ratio; report fall in urine output to <30 ml/hr
• Monitor temp q4hr; fever may indicate beginning infection
• Check liver function tests before, during therapy: bilirubin, AST, ALT, alkaline phosphatase, LDH as needed or monthly
• Monitor ECG; watch for ST-T wave changes, low QRS and T, possible dysrhythmias (sinus tachycardia, PVCs)

• Monitor baselines in pulmonary function; document FEV >2 L or ≥75% before therapy; check daily VS, pulse oximetry, dyspnea, crackles, ABGs, watch for respiratory failure, intubate if necessary
• Obtain stress thallium study before therapy; document normal ejection fraction, unimpaired wall motion
• Assess for bleeding: hematuria, guaiac, bruising or petechiae, mucosa, or orifices q8hr
• Assess for GI symptoms: frequency of stools, cramping
• Assess for acidosis, signs of dehydration: rapid respirations, poor skin turgor, decreased urine output, dry skin, restlessness, weakness
• Assess for cardiac status: B/P, pulse, character, rhythm, rate, ABGs, ECG
• Assess for infection: sore throat; antibiotics may be prescribed prophylactically

Nursing diagnoses
• Body image, disturbed (adverse reactions)
• Infection, risk for (adverse reactions)
• Injury, risk for (adverse reactions)
• Knowledge, deficient (teaching)

Implementation
Intermittent IV infusion route
• Give by intermittent **IV** INF after diluting 22 million international units (1.3 mg)/1.2 ml sterile (1.1 mg/ml) H$_2$O for inj at side of vial and swirl, do not shake; dilute dose with 50 ml D$_5$W and give over 15 min; use plastic bag; do not use an in-line filter; give through Y-tube or 3-way stopcock
• Give DOPamine 1-5 kg/min before onset of hypotension; decreased dose preserves kidney output
• Give hydrocortisone, dexamethasone, or sodium bicarbonate (1 mEq/1 ml) for extravasation, apply ice compresses
• Store any diluted product in refrigerator; do not freeze; administer within 48 hr; bring to room temperature before infusing; discard unused portion
Y-site compatibilities: Amikacin, **IV** fat emulsion, gentamicin, morphine, piperacillin, potassium chloride, ticarcillin, tobramycin, TPN #145, amphotericin B, calcium gluconate, diphenhydrAMINE, DOPamine, fluconazole, foscarnet, heparin, magnesium sulfate, metoclopramide, ondansetron, ranitidine, trimethoprim/sulfamethoxazole

Patient/family education
• Teach patient to avoid use of products containing aspirin or ibuprofen, razors, commercial mouthwash because bleeding may

occur; to report symptoms of bleeding, hematuria, tarry stools
• Tell patient to report signs of anemia: fatigue, headache, irritability, faintness, shortness of breath
• Tell patient to report any changes in breathing or coughing even several months after treatment
• Advise patient that contraception will be necessary during treatment; teratogenesis may occur
• Teach patient to report signs/symptoms of infection: fever, chills, sore throat; patient should avoid crowds or persons with known infections
• Advise patient to avoid alcohol, NSAIDs, salicylates; GI bleeding may occur
• Advise patient that visual problems may occur but are reversible

Evaluation
Positive therapeutic outcome
• Decreased spread of malignancy

---

alemtuzumab (Rx)
(al-em-tuz'uh-mab)
Campath
Func. class.: Antineoplastic—miscellaneous
Chem. class.: Monoclonal antibody
Pregnancy category C

Action: Composed of recombinant DNA-derived humanized monoclonal antibody (campath-1H), binds to CD52 antigen that is present on surface of B and T lymphocytes, causes lysis of leukemic cells

Therapeutic outcome: Decreased in number of white blood cells

Uses: B-cell chronic lymphocytic leukemia that has been treated with alkylating agents and that has failed fludarabine therapy, graft-versus-host disease (GVHD)

Dosage and routes
Adult: **IV** 3 mg over 2 hr daily; when tolerated, increase to 10 mg; when 10 mg tolerated, increase to 30 mg daily; maintenance is 30 mg/day 3 ×/wk on alternate days for 12 wk; titration usually takes 3-7 days; max single dose 30 mg; max weekly dose 90 mg

Available forms: Sol for inj 30 mg/ml

Adverse effects
CNS: Dizziness, insomnia, depression, headache, tremor, somnolence, fatigue, drowsiness, weakness

CV: Hypo/hypertension, tachycardia, edema, chest pain, supraventricular tachycardia
GI: Anorexia, diarrhea, constipation, *nausea, stomatitis, vomiting, abdominal pain, dyspepsia*
HEMA: **Anemia, neutropenia, thrombocytopenia, pancytopenia,** purpura, epistaxis
INTEG: Rash, local reaction, pruritus
MISC: Rigors, fever, *infusion reactions,* **sepsis, risk for fatal infection**
MS: Back pain
RESP: Cough, pneumonia, rhinitis, **bronchospasm,** dyspnea, pharyngitis

Contraindications: Hypersensitivity

Black Box Warning: Active systemic infection, immunodeficiency

Precautions: Pregnancy **C,** breastfeeding, children

Black Box Warning: Infusion-related reaction

Pharmacokinetics
Absorption	Unknown
Distribution	Unknown; steady state 6 wk
Metabolism	Unknown
Excretion	Unknown
Half-life	12 days

Pharmacodynamics
Unknown

Interactions
Individual drugs
Radiation: increased bone marrow depression
Drug classifications
Live virus vaccines: decreased antibody reaction
Other neoplastics: increased bone marrow depression
Drug/lab test
Diagnostic tests using antibodies

NURSING CONSIDERATIONS
Assessment
• Assess CBC, platelets qwk or more often if myelosuppression occurs; assess CD4+ after therapy until recovery of >200 cells/mcL
• Assess for symptoms of infection; chills, fever, headache, may be masked by product fever; do not administer product if infection is present
• Assess CNS reaction: LOC, mental status, dizziness, confusion

---

Adverse effects: *italic* = common, **bold** = life-threatening

- Assess cardiac status: lung sounds; ECG before and during treatment, especially in those with cardiac disease
- Assess for bone marrow depression: bruising, bleeding, blood in stools, urine, sputum, emesis

Nursing diagnoses
- Body image, disturbed (adverse reactions)
- Infection, risk for (adverse reactions)
- Injury, risk for (adverse reactions)
- Knowledge, deficient (teaching)
- Nutrition: less than body requirements, imbalanced (side effects)

Implementation
IV route
- Do not give **IV** push or bolus
- Withdraw amount needed; do not shake ampule; use 5 μm filter prior to dilution, check for particulate matter and discoloration; dilute with 100 ml sterile 0.9% NaCl or D$_5$W, invert to mix, do not add other products or infuse in same **IV** tubing
- Store reconstituted sol for ≤8 hr at room temperature, do not freeze; protect from light

Patient/family education
- Instruct patient to take acetaminophen for fever
- Advise patient to avoid hazardous tasks, since confusion, dizziness may occur
- Instruct patient to report signs of infection: sore throat, fever, diarrhea, vomiting

Evaluation
Positive therapeutic outcome
- Decreased in production of malignant lymphocytes

---

alendronate (Rx)
(al-en'droe-nate)
Fosamax
Func. class.: Bone-resorption inhibitor
Chem. class.: Bisphosphonate

Pregnancy category C

Do not confuse:
Fosamax/Flomax

Action: Decreases rate of bone resorption and may directly block dissolution of hydroxyapatite crystals of bone; inhibits normal and abnormal bone resorption, mineralization, inhibits osteoclast activity

Therapeutic outcome: Decreased symptoms of osteoporosis, Paget's disease

Uses: Treatment and prevention of osteoporosis in postmenopausal women, treatment of osteoporosis in men, Paget's disease, treatment of corticosteroid-induced osteoporosis in postmenopausal women not receiving estrogen, or in men who are continuing corticosteroid treatment with low bone mass

Dosage and routes
Osteoporosis in postmenopausal women
Adult and geriatric: PO 10 mg daily or 70 mg qwk

Osteoporosis in men
Adult: PO 10 mg/day or 70 mg qwk

Paget's disease
Adult and geriatric: PO 40 mg daily × 6 mo, consider retreatment for relapse

Prevention of osteoporosis
Adult: PO 5 mg daily or 35 mg qwk

Corticosteroid-induced osteoporosis in postmenopausal women (not receiving estrogen)
Adult: PO 10 mg daily

Corticosteroid-induced osteoporosis in men or premenopausal women (not receiving estrogen)
Adult: PO 5 mg daily

Renal dose
Adult: PO CCr ≤35 ml/min, not recommended

Available forms: Tabs 5, 10, 35, 40, 70 mg; oral sol 70 mg/75 ml

Adverse effects
CNS: Headache
CV: **Atrial fibrillation**
GI: Abdominal pain, constipation, nausea, vomiting, esophageal ulceration, acid reflux, dyspepsia, **esophageal perforation,** diarrhea
META: Hypophosphatemia, hypocalcemia
MS: Bone pain, osteonecrosis of the jaw
SYST: **Angioedema, Stevens-Johnson syndrome, toxic epidermal necrolysis**

Contraindications: Hypersensitivity to bisphosphonates, delayed esophageal emptying, inability to sit or stand for 30 min, hypocalcemia

Precautions: Pregnancy **C,** breastfeeding, children, CCr <35 ml/min, esophageal disease, ulcers, gastritis, poor dental health

---

A

Pharmacokinetics	
Absorption	Bioavailability 60%
Distribution	Mainly to bones; protein binding 78%
Metabolism	Unknown
Excretion	Via kidneys after bound to bone
Half-life	>10 yrs

Pharmacodynamics	
Unknown	

Interactions
Individual drugs
Ranitidine (**IV**): increased alendronate effect
Drug classifications
Aminoglycosides, antacids, calcium supplements: decreased absorption
H$_2$ blockers, proton pump inhibitors (PPIs), gastric mucosal agents, NSAIDs, salicylates: adverse GI reactions
Drug/food
Caffeine, food, orange juice: decreased product absorption

NURSING CONSIDERATIONS
Assessment
◆ Assess for serious reactions: angioedema, Stevens-Johnson syndrome, toxic epidermal necrolysis, atrial fibrillation
• Assess dental status, regular dental exams should be done; dental extractions (cover with anti-infectives) prior to procedure
• Hormonal status if a woman, prior to treatment
• For osteoporosis: bone density testing
• For Paget's disease: increased skull size, bone pain, headache
• Monitor renal studies and Ca, P, Mg, K
• Assess for hypercalcemia: paresthesia, twitching, laryngospasm, Chvostek's, Trousseau's signs
• Monitor alkaline phosphatase; level of 2 × upper limit of normal is indicated for Paget's disease

Nursing diagnoses
• Injury, risk for (uses)
• Knowledge, deficient (teaching)

Implementation
• Give PO for 6 mo to be effective in Paget's disease; take with 8 oz of water 30 min before 1st food, beverage, or medication of the day
• Patient to remain upright for 30 min after dose to prevent esophageal irritation
• Store in cool environment out of direct sunlight

Patient/family education
• Teach patient to remain upright for 30 min after dose to prevent esophageal irritation; if dose is missed, skip dose, do not double doses or take later in day
• Teach patient to take in AM, only before food, other meds, to take with 6-8 oz of water (not mineral water)
• Teach patient to take calcium, vit D if instructed by provider
• Teach patient to use weight-bearing exercise to increase bone density
• Teach patient to let provider know if pregnancy is planned or suspected or if nursing
• Advise to maintain good oral hygiene

Evaluation
Positive therapeutic outcome
• Increased bone mass, absence of fractures

alfuzosin (Rx)
(al-fyoo'zoe-sin)
Uroxatral
Func. class.: Antiadrenergic
Chem. class.: Quinazoline
Pregnancy category B

Action: Binds preferentially to α_{1A}-adrenoceptor subtype located mainly in the prostate, relaxing smooth muscles

Therapeutic outcome: Resolution of symptoms of benign prostatic hyperplasia

Uses: Symptoms of benign prostatic hyperplasia

Dosage and routes
Adult: PO EXT REL 10 mg daily, taken after same meal each day

Available forms: Ext rel tabs 10 mg

Adverse effects
CNS: Dizziness, headache, fatigue, flushing
CV: Postural hypotension (dizziness, lightheadedness, fainting) within a few hours of administration, chest pain, tachycardia, angina
GI: Nausea, abdominal pain, dyspepsia, constipation, diarrhea, liver injury, jaundice
GU: Impotence, priapism
INTEG: Rash, urticaria, **angioedema,** pruritus
MISC: Body pain in general, xerostomia, rhinitis
RESP: Upper respiratory tract infection, pharyngitis, bronchitis, sinusitis

Contraindications: Hypersensitivity, moderate to severe hepatic impairment, not indicated for use in women or children, breastfeeding (but not used in women)

Precautions: Pregnancy **B**, geriatric, coronary artery disease, coronary insufficiency, mild hepatic disease, mild/moderate/severe renal disease, history of QT prolongation or coadministration with medications known to prolong QT interval, torsades de pointes, syncope, surgery, prostate cancer, orthostatic hypotension, ocular surgery, CAD, dysrhythmias, angina

Pharmacokinetics

Absorption	Unknown
Distribution	Moderately protein bound (82%-90%)
Metabolism	Liver (by CYP3A4 enzyme)
Excretion	Urine
Half-life	10 hr

Pharmacodynamics
Unknown

Interactions
Individual drugs
Alcohol: possible increased effects of alfuzosin
Doxazosin, itraconazole, ketoconazole, prazosin, ritonavir, terazosin: do not take concurrently
Drug classifications
Beta-blockers, nitrates, phosphodiesterase 5 inhibitors: increased hypotension
CYP3A4 inhibitors (ketoconazole, itraconazole, ritonavir): do not take concurrently

NURSING CONSIDERATIONS
Assessment
• Assess for prostatic hyperplasia: change in urinary patterns, baseline and throughout treatment
• Monitor CBC with differential and liver function tests; B/P and heart rate; QT prolongation
• Monitor BUN, uric acid, urodynamic studies (urinary flow rates, residual volume)
• Monitor I&O ratios, weight daily, edema; report weight gain or edema

Nursing diagnoses
• Urinary elimination, impaired (uses)
• Knowledge, deficient (teaching)

Implementation
• Swallow tabs whole; do not break, crush, or chew tabs
• Store in tight container in cool environment

Patient/family education
• Advise not to drive or operate machinery for 4 hr after first dose or after dosage increase

Evaluation
Positive therapeutic outcome
• Decreased symptoms of benign prostatic hyperplasia

---

aliskiren (Rx)
(a-lis'kir-en)
Tekturna
Func. class.: Antihypertensive
Chem. class.: Direct renin inhibitor

Pregnancy category
C (1st trimester)
D (2nd/3rd trimesters)

Action: Renin inhibitor that acts on the renin-angiotensin system (RAS)

Therapeutic outcome: Decrease in B/P

Uses: Hypertension, alone or in combination with other antihypertensives

Dosage and routes
Adult: PO 150 mg/day, may increase to 300 mg/day if needed, max 300 mg/day

Available forms: Tabs 150, 300 mg

Adverse effects
CNS: Headache, dizziness
CV: Orthostatic hypotension, hypotension
GI: Diarrhea
GU: Renal stones, increased uric acid
INTEG: Rash
META: Hyperkalemia
MISC: Angioedema

Contraindications: Hypersensitivity

Black Box Warning: Pregnancy **D** (2nd/3rd trimester)

Precautions: Pregnancy **C** (1st trimester), breastfeeding, children, geriatric, angioedema, aortic/renal artery stenosis, cirrhosis, CAD, dialysis, hyper/hypokalemia, hyponatremia, hypotension, hypovolemia, renal/hepatic disease, surgery, diabetes, seizures

Pharmacokinetics

Absorption	Poorly, bioavailability 2.3%
Distribution	Steady state 7-8 days
Metabolism	Unknown
Excretion	91% unchanged in the feces
Half-life	Unknown

Pharmacodynamics

Onset	Unknown
Peak	1-3 hr
Duration	Unknown

 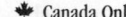

A

Interactions
Individual drugs
Atorvastatin, ketoconazole: increased aliskiren levels
Warfarin: decreased levels of warfarin
Drug classifications
ACE inhibitors, angiotensin receptor antagonists: increased potassium levels
Diuretics, other antihypertensives: increased hypotension
Drug/food
High-fat meal: decreased absorption
Drug/lab test
Increased: uric acid, CPK, BUN, serum creatinine
Decreased: Hct, Hgb

NURSING CONSIDERATIONS
Assessment
- Monitor blood tests: CBC with differential; Hct, Hgb may be decreased; uric acid, serum creatinine, BUN may be increased; potassium, hyperkalemia may occur
- Assess for allergic reactions: angioedema may occur
- Monitor daily dependent edema in feet, legs; weight, B/P, orthostatic hypotension

Nursing diagnoses
- Cardiac output, decreased (uses)
- Knowledge, deficient (teaching)
- Noncompliance (teaching)

Implementation
- PO; do not use with a high-fat meal
- Give daily with a full glass of water, titrate up to achieve correct dose
- Do not discontinue abruptly
- Store in tight container at room temperature

Patient/family education
- Teach patient the importance of complying with dosage schedule even if feeling better
- Instruct patient to notify if pregnancy is planned or suspected; if pregnant, product will need to be discontinued
- Teach patient how to take B/P and normal reading for age group
- Advise patient that if dose is missed, take as soon as possible; if it is almost time for the next dose, take only that dose; do not double dose
- Instruct patient not to use OTC products, including herbs, supplements unless approved by prescriber
- Advise patient to report to prescriber immediately: dizziness, faintness, chest pain, palpitations, uneven or rapid heart beat, headache, severe diarrhea, swelling of tongue or lips, trouble breathing, difficulty swallowing, tightening of the throat
- Caution patient not to operate machinery or perform hazardous tasks if dizziness occurs
- Advise patient to avoid faintness; do not get up or stand up rapidly

Evaluation
Positive therapeutic outcome
- Decrease in B/P

alitretinoin (Rx)
(al-ee-tret′i-noyn)
Panretin
Func. class.: Retinoid, 2nd generation, topical antineoplastic
Pregnancy category D

Action: Controls cellular differentiation and proliferation of neoplastic and healthy cells by binding to retinoid receptors

Therapeutic outcome: Decreased size and number of lesions

Uses: Kaposi's sarcoma cutaneous lesions

Dosage and routes
Adult: TOP Apply enough gel to cover lesions with a generous coating, allow to dry for 3-5 min before covering with clothing, do not apply near mucosal areas, apply as long as benefit occurs, do not rub gel into lesion

Available forms: Topical gel 0.1%

Adverse effects
INTEG: Rash, stinging, pain, warmth, redness, erythema, blistering, crusting, peeling, dermatitis, pain

Contraindications: Pregnancy **D**, hypersensitivity to retinoids

Precautions: Breastfeeding, eczema, sunburn, geriatric, cutaneous T-cell lymphoma

Pharmacokinetics	
Absorption	Small amounts
Distribution	Unknown
Metabolism	Unknown
Excretion	Kidneys
Half-life	Unknown

Pharmacodynamics
Unknown

Interactions
Individual drugs
DEET: do not use around DEET (an insect repellant)

Adverse effects: *italic* = common, **bold** = life-threatening

NURSING CONSIDERATIONS
Assessment
- Assess part of body involved, including time involved, what helps or aggravates condition, cysts, dryness, itching
- Assess for dermal toxicity that may start as erythema, then edema; product may need to be discontinued and restarted

Nursing diagnoses
- Body image, disturbed (uses)
- Knowledge, deficient (teaching)
- Skin integrity, impaired (uses)

Implementation
- Apply bid initially to lesions, can be increased to tid-qid according to tolerance, discontinue for a few days if severe reactions occur
- Store at room temperature
- Wash hands after application

Patient/family education
- Instruct patient to avoid application on normal skin, and to avoid getting cream in eyes, nose, other mucous membranes
- Advise patient to avoid sunlight, sunlamps or to use protective clothing or sunscreen to prevent burns
- Advise patient that treatment may cause warmth, stinging, dryness; peeling will occur
- Caution patient that product does not cure condition; only relieves symptoms; that therapeutic results may be seen in 2-3 wk but may not be optimal until after 6 wk

Evaluation
Positive therapeutic outcome
- Decrease in size and number of lesions

---

allopurinol (Rx)
(al-oh-pure'i-nole)
Aloprim, allopurinol, Apo-Allopurinol ✤, Lopurin, Purinol ✤, Zyloprim
Func. class.: Antigout drug, antihyperuricemic
Chem. class.: Xanthine enzyme inhibitor

Pregnancy category C

Do not confuse:
allopurinol/apresoline, Lopurin/Lupron, Zyloprim/Zovirax

Action: Inhibits the enzyme xanthine oxidase, reducing uric acid synthesis

Therapeutic outcome: Decreasing serum uric acid levels, decreasing joint pain

Uses: Chronic gout, hyperuricemia associated with malignancies, recurrent calcium oxalate calculi, uric acid calculi

Dosage and routes
Increased uric acid levels in malignancies
Adult: PO 600-800 mg/day in divided doses, for 2-3 days; start up to 1-2 days prior to chemotherapy; **IV** INF 200-400 mg/m²/day, max 600 mg/day 24-48 hr prior to chemotherapy, may be divided at 6-, 8-, 12-hr intervals
Child 6-10 yr: PO 300 mg/day, adjust dose after 48 hr
Child <6 yr: PO 150 mg/day, adjust dose after 48 hr
Child: **IV** INF 200 mg/m²/day, initially as a single dose or divided q6-12hr

Gout (mild)
Adult: PO 100-300 mg/day, increase qwk based on uric acid levels, max 800 mg/day, maintenance dose 100-200 mg bid-tid

Gout (moderate-severe)
Adult: PO 400-600 mg/day in a single dose or divided bid-tid, max 800 mg/day, doses >300 mg should be given in divided doses

Recurrent calculi
Adult: PO 200-300 mg/day in a single dose or divided bid-tid, max 300 mg/dose, 800 mg/day

Uric acid nephropathy prevention
Adult and child >10 yr: PO 600-800 mg daily × 2-3 days

Renal dose
Adult: PO/**IV** CCr 10-20 ml/min 100-200 mg/day; CCr 3-9 ml/min 100 mg/day or 100 mg every other day; CCr, 3 ml/min 100 mg q24hr or longer or 100 mg every third day

Available forms: Tabs, scored, 100, 300 mg; inj 500 mg/vial

Adverse effects
CNS: Headache, drowsiness, neuritis, paresthesia
EENT: Retinopathy, cataracts, epistaxis
GI: Nausea, vomiting, anorexia, malaise, metallic taste, cramps, peptic ulcer, diarrhea, stomatitis
HEMA: **Agranulocytosis, thrombocytopenia, aplastic anemia, pancytopenia, leukopenia, bone marrow suppression, eosinophilia**
INTEG: Fever, chills, dermatitis, pruritus, purpura, erythema, ecchymosis, alopecia, rash, **Stevens-Johnson syndrome**

 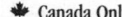

MISC: Myopathy, arthralgia, hepatomegaly, **cholestatic jaundice, renal failure, exfoliative dermatitis**

Contraindications: Hypersensitivity

Precautions: Pregnancy C, breastfeeding, children, renal/hepatic disease

Pharmacokinetics

Absorption	80%
Distribution	Widely distributed
Metabolism	Liver to oxypurinol
Excretion	Kidneys
Half-life	1-2 hr

Pharmacodynamics

	PO	IV
Onset	Unknown	Unknown
Peak	1½ hr	Up to 30 min
Duration	Unknown	Unknown

Interactions
Individual drugs
Ammonium chloride potassium/sodium phosphate, vit C: increased kidney stone formation
Ampicillin, amoxicillin: increased risk of rash
Azathioprine: increased bone marrow depression
Mercaptopurine: increased bone marrow depression
Rasburicase: increased xanthine nephropathy, calculi
Theophylline: increased action of theophylline
Drug classifications
ACE inhibitors: increased hypersensitivity
Anticoagulants (oral): increased action of oral anticoagulants
Antidiabetics (oral): increased action of antidiabetics
Antineoplastics: increased bone marrow suppression
Diuretics (thiazide): increased hypersensitivity

NURSING CONSIDERATIONS
Assessment
• Assess for pain including location, characteristics, onset/duration, frequency, quality, intensity or severity of pain, precipitating factors
• Monitor uric acid levels q2wk; normal uric acid levels are 6 mg/dl or less; check I&O ratio; increase fluids to 2 L/day to prevent stone formation, toxicity
• Monitor CBC, AST, BUN, creatinine before starting treatment, monthly; check blood glucose in diabetic patients receiving oral antidiabetic agents
• Monitor nutritional status: discourage organ meat, sardines, salmon, legumes, gravies (high-purine foods), alcohol

Nursing diagnoses
• Knowledge, deficient (teaching)
• Nutrition: more than body requirements, imbalanced (uses)

Implementation
PO route
• Give with meals to prevent GI symptoms; crush and mix with food or fluids for patients with swallowing difficulties
• Increased fluid intake to 2 L/day
• Give a few days before antineoplastic therapy if using for hyperuricemia associated with malignancy
IV infusion route
• Reconstitute 30-ml vial with 25 ml of sterile water for inj; dilute to desired conc with 0.9% NaCl for inj or D$_5$ for inj, begin inf within 10 hr
Solution incompatibilities: Amikacin, amphotericin B, carmustine, cefotaxime, chlorproMAZINE, cilastatin, cimetidine, clindamycin, cytarabine, dacarbazine, DAUNOrubicin, diphenhydrAMINE, DOXOrubicin, doxycycline, droperidol, floxuridine, gentamicin, haloperidol, hydrOXYzine, idarubicin, imipenem, mechlorethamine, meperidine, metoclopramide, methylPREDNISolone, minocycline, nalbuphine, netilmicin, ondansetron, prochlorperazine, promethazine, sodium bicarbonate, streptozocin, tobramycin, vinorelbine

Patient/family education
• Tell patient to increase fluid intake to 2 L/day; to avoid taking large doses of vit C; kidney stone formation may occur; to maintain a diet enhancing urine alkalinity (e.g., milk, other dairy products); if taking for calcium oxalate stones, reduce dairy products, refined sugar, sodium, meat
• Tell patient to report skin rash, stomatitis, malaise, fever, aching; product should be discontinued
• Advise patient to avoid hazardous activities if drowsiness or dizziness occurs; response may take several days to determine
• Tell patient to avoid alcohol, caffeine; these substances increase uric acid levels and decrease allopurinol levels
• Teach patient to report side effects and adverse reactions to prescriber, including rash, itching, nausea, vomiting

Evaluation
Positive therapeutic outcome
- Decreased pain in joints
- Decreased stone formation in kidney
- Decreased uric acid level to 6 mg/dl

almotriptan (Rx)
(al-moh-trip'tan)
Axert
Func. class.: Antimigraine agent
Chem. class.: 5-HT$_1$ receptor agonist, triptan

Pregnancy category C

Action: Binds selectively to the vascular 5-HT$_{1B/1D/1F}$ receptor subtype, exerts antimigraine effect; causes vasoconstriction in cranial arteries

Therapeutic outcome: Absence of migraines

Uses: Acute treatment of migraine with or without aura (Adults/adolescents/child ≥12 yr)

Dosage and routes
Adult/adolescents/child ≥12 yrs: PO 6.25-12.5 mg, may repeat dose after 2 hr; do not give more than 2 doses/24 hr, 25 mg/day, or 4 treatment cycles within any 30-day period

Renal/hepatic dose
Adult: PO 6.25 mg initially, max 12.5 mg

Available forms: Tabs 6.25, 12.5 mg

Adverse effects
CNS: Tingling, hot sensation, burning, feeling of pressure, tightness, numbness, dizziness, sedation, headache, anxiety, fatigue, cold sensation, **seizures**
CV: Flushing, palpitations, tachycardia, **coronary artery vasospasm, MI, ventricular fibrillation, ventricular tachycardia**
EENT: Throat, mouth, nasal discomfort; vision changes
GI: Nausea, xerostomia
INTEG: Sweating
MS: Weakness, neck stiffness, myalgia
RESP: Chest tightness, pressure

Contraindications: Hypersensitivity, cluster headache, hemiplegia, vascular migraine, ischemic heart disease or risk for, peripheral vascular syndrome; concurrent use of ergotamine-containing preparations, uncontrolled hypertension, basilar or hemiplegic migraine; concurrent MAOI therapy or within 2 wk

Precautions: Pregnancy **C**, breastfeeding, children <18 yr, geriatric, postmenopausal women, men >40 yr, risk factors for coronary artery disease, MI, hypercholesterolemia, obesity, diabetes, impaired renal/hepatic function, sulfonamide hypersensitivity

Pharmacokinetics
Absorption	Well absorbed (~70%)
Distribution	35% protein bound
Metabolism	Liver (metabolite); metabolized by MAO-A, CYP2D6, CYP3A4
Excretion	Urine, feces
Half-life	3-4 hr

Pharmacodynamics
Onset	Unknown
Peak	1-3 hr
Duration	3-4 hr

Interactions
Individual drugs
Ergot: increased vasospastic effects
Ketoconazole: increased plasma concentration of almotriptan
Drug classifications
5-HT$_1$ agonists, ergot derivatives: increased vasospastic effects
CYP2D6 inhibitors: increased almotriptan effect; do not use together
MAOIs: increased almotriptan effect; do not use together
Drug/herb
Butterbur, feverfew: increased almotriptan effect

NURSING CONSIDERATIONS
Assessment
- Assess B/P, signs/symptoms of coronary vasospasms
- Assess for tingling, hot sensation, burning, feeling of pressure, numbness, flushing
- Assess for stress level, activity, recreation, coping mechanisms
- Assess neurologic status: LOC, blurring vision, nausea, vomiting, tingling in extremities preceding headache
- Assess for ingestion of tyramine-containing foods (pickled products, beer, wine, aged cheese), food additives, preservatives, colorings, artificial sweeteners, chocolate, caffeine, which may precipitate these types of headaches

Nursing diagnoses
- Knowledge, deficient (teaching)
- Pain, acute (uses)

Implementation

- Swallow tabs whole; do not break, crush, or chew tabs
- Provide quiet, calm environment with decreased stimulation from noise, bright light, excessive talking

Patient/family education

- Instruct patient to use contraception while taking product, notify prescriber if pregnancy is planned or suspected, avoid breastfeeding
- Advise patient to have dark, quiet environment available
- Inform patient that product does not prevent or reduce number of migraine attacks
- Advise patient to report chest pain, drowsiness, dizziness, tingling, flushing, pressure

Evaluation

Positive therapeutic outcome

- Decrease in severity of migraine

Treatment of overdose: Gastric lavage followed by activated charcoal; clinical and ECG monitoring for ≥20 hr after overdose

---

alprazolam (Rx)

(al-pray′zoe-lam)
Apo-Alpraz ✦, Niravam, Novo-Alprazol ✦, Nu-Alpraz ✦, Xanax, Xanax XR
Func. class.: Antianxiety/sedative/hypnotic
Chem. class.: Benzodiazepine, short/intermediate acting

Pregnancy category D

Controlled substance schedule IV

Do not confuse:
alprazolam/lorazepam, Xanax/Lanoxin/Tylox/Zantac

Action: Depresses subcortical levels of CNS, including limbic system, reticular formation

Therapeutic outcome: Decreased anxiety

Uses: Anxiety, panic disorders with or without agoraphobia, anxiety with depressive symptoms

Unlabeled uses: Premenstrual dysphoric disorders, insomnia, PMS, alcohol withdrawal syndrome

Dosage and routes
Anxiety disorder
Adult: PO 0.25-0.5 mg tid, may increase q3-4days if needed, max 4 mg/day in divided doses

Geriatric: PO 0.125-0.25 mg bid; increase by 0.125 mg as needed
Panic disorder
Adult: PO 0.5 mg tid, may increase up to 1 mg/day q3-4days, max 10 mg/day; EXT REL TABS (Xanax XR) give daily in AM 0.5-1 mg initially, maintenance 1-10 mg daily

Premenstrual dysphoric disorders (unlabeled)
Adult: PO 0.25 mg bid-qid, starting on day 16-18 of menses, taper over 2-3 days when menses occurs

Hepatic dose
Reduce dose by 50%

Insomnia (unlabeled)
Adult: PO 0.25-0.5 mg at bedtime

Available forms: Tabs 0.25, 0.5, 1, 2 mg; ext rel tabs (Xanax XR) 0.5, 1, 2, 3 mg; orally disintegrating tabs 0.25, 0.5, 1, 2 mg; oral solution, 1 mg/ml

Adverse effects
CNS: Dizziness, drowsiness, confusion, headache, anxiety, tremors, stimulation, fatigue, depression, insomnia, hallucinations, memory impairment, poor coordination
CV: Orthostatic hypotension, **ECG changes, tachycardia,** hypotension
EENT: Blurred vision, tinnitus, mydriasis
GI: Constipation, dry mouth, nausea, vomiting, anorexia, diarrhea, weight gain/loss, increased appetite
GU: Decreased libido
INTEG: Rash, dermatitis, itching

Contraindications: Pregnancy **D**, breastfeeding, hypersensitivity to benzodiazepines, closed-angle glaucoma, psychosis, addiction

Precautions: Geriatric, debilitated, hepatic disease, obesity, severe pulmonary disease

Pharmacokinetics

Absorption	Slow, complete
Distribution	Widely distributed; crosses placenta; crosses blood-brain barrier, protein binding 80%
Metabolism	Liver, to active metabolites
Excretion	Kidneys, breast milk
Half-life	12-15 hr

Pharmacodynamics

	PO	ORAL DISINTEGRATING
Onset	1 hr	
Peak	1-2 hr	1.5-2 hr
Duration	4-6 hr, therapeutic response 2-3 days	

Adverse effects: *italic* = common, **bold** = life-threatening

Interactions
Individual drugs
Alcohol: increased CNS depression
Cigarette smoking: decreased drug level
CYP3A4 inhibitors (cimetidine, disulfiram, erythromycin, fluoxetine, isoniazid, itraconazole, ketoconazole, metoprolol, propoxyphene, propranolol, valproic acid): increased action of alprazolam
Levodopa: decreased action of levodopa
Rifampin: decreased action of alprazolam
Drug classifications
Anticonvulsants, antihistamines: increased CNS depression
CYP3A4 inducers (barbiturates): decreased action of alprazolam
Sedative/hypnotics, opioids: increased CNS depression
Xanthines: decreased sedation
Drug/herb
Cat's claw, chamomile, cowslip, echinacea, goldenseal, hops, kava, licorice, Queen Anne's lace, skullcap, St. John's wort, valerian, wild cherry: increased CNS depression
Drug/food
Grapefruit juice: increased product level
Drug/lab test
Increased: ALT, AST, alkaline phosphatase

NURSING CONSIDERATIONS
Assessment
🔹 Assess mental status: mood, sensorium, anxiety, affect, sleeping pattern, drowsiness, dizziness, especially geriatric; physical dependency, withdrawal symptoms: anxiety, panic attacks, agitation, seizures, headache, nausea, vomiting, muscle pain, weakness; suicidal tendencies; indications of increasing tolerance and abuse; withdrawal seizures may occur after rapid decrease in dose or abrupt discontinuation; short duration of action makes it the product of choice in the geriatric
• Monitor B/P (with patient lying, standing), pulse; if systolic B/P drops 20 mm Hg, hold product, notify prescriber
• Monitor blood studies: CBC during long-term therapy; blood dyscrasias have occurred rarely; decreased hematocrit, neutropenia may occur
• Monitor hepatic studies: AST, ALT, bilirubin, creatinine LDH, alkaline phosphatase, if on long-term treatment
• Monitor I&O; indicate renal dysfunction if on long-term treatment

Nursing diagnoses
• Anxiety (uses)
• Injury, risk for (adverse reactions)
• Knowledge, deficient (teaching)

Implementation
• Give with food or milk for GI symptoms; high fat meal will decrease absorption; tab may be crushed, if patient is unable to swallow medication whole, and mixed with foods or fluids; may divide total daily dose into more times/day, if anxiety occurs between doses
• Give sugarless gum, hard candy, frequent sips of water for dry mouth
• Discontinue, decrease by 0.5 mg q3days
• Place orally disintegrating tabs on tongue to dissolve and swallow
• Give ext rel tab in AM

Patient/family education
• Tell patient that product may be taken with food or fluids, and tabs may be crushed or swallowed whole
• Tell patient not to use for everyday stress or longer than 4 mo unless directed by prescriber; not to take more than prescribed amount; may be habit forming; not to double doses or skip doses; memory impairment is a sign of long-term use
• Tell patient to avoid OTC preparations unless approved by prescriber; alcohol and CNS depressants will increase CNS depression
• Tell patient to avoid driving, activities that require alertness, since drowsiness may occur; to avoid alcohol ingestion or other psychotropic medications; to rise slowly or fainting may occur, especially geriatric; that drowsiness may worsen at beginning of treatment
• Tell patient not to discontinue medication abruptly after long-term use; withdrawal symptoms include vomiting, cramping, tremors, seizures

Evaluation
Positive therapeutic outcome
• Decreased anxiety, restlessness, sleeplessness (short-term treatment only)

Treatment of overdose: Lavage, VS, supportive care, flumazenil

A

! HIGH ALERT

alteplase (Rx)
(al-ti-plaze')

Activase, Activase rt-PA ❦, Lysatec rt-PA ❦, Cathflo, tissue plasminogen activator, t-PA

Func. class.: Thrombolytic enzyme
Chem. class.: Tissue plasminogen activator (TPA)

Pregnancy category C

Do not confuse:
alteplace/Altace

Action: Produces fibrin conversion of plasminogen to plasmin; able to bind to fibrin, convert plasminogen in thrombus to plasmin, which leads to local fibrinolysis, limited systemic proteolysis

Therapeutic outcome: Lysis of thrombi in MI, pulmonary emboli (life threatening)

Uses: Lysis of obstructing thrombi associated with acute MI; conditions requiring thrombolysis (e.g., PE, unclotting arteriovenous shunts, acute ischemic CVA), central venous catheter occlusion

Unlabeled uses: Arterial thromboembolism, deep vein thrombosis (DVT), occlusion prophylaxis, percutaneous coronary intervention (PCI)

Dosage and routes
Pulmonary embolism
Adult: **IV** 100 mg over 2 hr, then heparin

Acute ischemic stroke
Adult: **IV** 0.9 mg/kg, max 90 mg; give as INF over 1 hr, give 10% of dose **IV** BOL over 1st min

Myocardial infarction (standard infusion)
Adult >65 kg: **IV** a total of 100 mg, given over 3 hr; 6-10 mg given **IV** BOL over 1-2 min, then the remaining 50-54 mg over the remainder of the hr, during 2nd, 3rd hr 20 mg is given by cont **IV** INF (20 mg/hr)
Adult <65 kg: **IV** 1.25 mg/kg over 3 hr; 60% in first 1 hr (10% as a bolus), remaining 40% over next 2 hr

Myocardial infarction (accelerated infusion)
Adult >67 kg: 100 mg total dose: give 15 mg **IV** BOL, then 50 mg over 30 min, then 35 mg over 60 min
Adult <67 kg: 15 mg **IV** BOL: then 0.75 mg/kg over 30 min (max 50 mg); 0.5 mg/kg over the next 60 min (max 35 mg)

Occlusion prophylaxis (unlabeled)
Adult >30 kg: Max 2 mg in 2 ml; may use up to 2 doses (120 min apart)

Available forms: Powder for inj 50 mg (29 million international units/vial), 100 mg (58 million international units/vial), lyophilized powder for injection 2 mg

Adverse effects
CV: **Sinus bradycardia, ventricular tachycardia, accelerated idioventricular rhythm, bradycardia, recurrent ischemic stroke,** hypotension
INTEG: Urticaria, rash
SYST: **GI, GU, intracranial, retroperitoneal bleeding, surface bleeding, anaphylaxis,** fever

Contraindications: Hypersensitivity, active internal bleeding, recent CVA, severe uncontrolled hypertension, intracranial/intraspinal surgery/trauma (within 3 mo), aneurysm, brain tumor, platelets <100,000 mm³

Precautions: Pregnancy **C**, breastfeeding, children, geriatric, neurologic deficits, mitral stenosis, recent GI/GU bleeding, diabetic retinopathy, subacute bacterial endocarditis, arrhythmias, diabetic hemorrhage retinopathy

Pharmacokinetics	
Absorption	Complete
Distribution	Unknown
Metabolism	>80% liver
Excretion	Kidneys
Half-life	35 min

Pharmacodynamics	
Onset	Immediate
Peak	30-45 min
Duration	4 hr

Interactions
Individual drugs
Abciximab, aspirin, clopidogrel, dipyridamole, eptifibatide, heparin, plicamycin, ticlopidine, tirofiban, valproic acid: increased bleeding
Nitroglycerin: decreased effect
Drug classifications
Anticoagulants (oral), cephalosporins (some), NSAIDs, salicylates: increased bleeding
Drug/herb
Agrimony, alfalfa, angelica, anise, basil, bay, bilberry, black haw, bogbean, bromelain, buchu, cat's claw, chondroitin, cinchona bark, dong quai, evening primrose, fenu-

Adverse effects: *italic* = common, **bold** = life-threatening

greek, feverfew, garlic, ginger, ginkgo, ginseng, green tea, horse chestnut, Irish moss, kelp, kelpware, khella, lovage, lungwort, meadowsweet, motherwort, mugwort, nettle, papaya, parsley (large amounts), pau d'arco, pineapple, poplar, prickly ash, safflower, saw palmetto, tonka bean, turmeric, wintergreen, yarrow: increased risk of bleeding

Chamomile, coenzyme Q10, flax, glucomannan, goldenseal, guar gum: decreased anticoagulant effect

Drug/lab test
Increased: pro-time, APTT, TT

NURSING CONSIDERATIONS
Assessment
• Monitor VS q15min, B/P, pulse, respirations (including peripheral), neurologic signs, temp at least q4hr; temp >104° F (40° C) indicates internal bleeding; monitor rhythm closely; ventricular dysrhythmias may occur with hyperfusion; monitor heart, breath sounds, neurologic status, and peripheral pulses
⬥ Assess for bleeding during first hr of treatment and 24 hr after procedure: hematuria, hematemesis, bleeding from mucous membranes, epistaxis, ecchymosis, puncture sites; guaiac all body fluids and stools; obtain blood studies (Hct, platelets, PTT, pro-time, TT, APTT) before starting therapy; pro-time or APTT must be less than 2 times control before starting therapy; TT or pro-time q3-4hr during treatment; obtain CPK-MB to identify product effectiveness
• Assess hypersensitivity: fever, rash, facial swelling, dyspnea, itching, chills; mild reaction may be treated with antihistamines; report to prescriber
• Monitor ECG; on monitor, watch for segment changes, changes in rhythm: sinus bradycardia, ventricular tachycardia, accelerated idioventricular rhythm may occur due to reperfusion; cardiac enzymes, radionuclide myocardial scanning/coronary angiography

Nursing diagnoses
• Injury, risk for (adverse reactions)
• Pain, chronic (uses)
• Tissue perfusion, ineffective (uses)

Implementation
Intermittent IV infusion route
• Give after reconstituting with provided diluent; add appropriate amount of sterile water for inj (no preservatives); 20-mg vial/20 ml or 50-mg vial/50 ml (1 mg/ml); mix by slow inversion or dilute with 0.9% NaCl, D₅W

to a concentration of 0.5 mg/ml further dilution; 1.5 to <0.5 mg/ml may result in precipitation of product; use 18-G needle; flush line with NaCl after administration; use reconstituted **IV** sol within 8 hr or discard, within 6 hr of coronary occlusion for best results
⬥ Do not use 150 mg or more total dose; intracranial bleeding may occur
• Give heparin therapy after thrombolytic therapy is discontinued and when thrombi time, ACT, and APTT less than 2 times control (about 3-4 hr)
• Avoid invasive procedures, inj, rec temp; apply pressure for 30 sec to minor bleeding sites; 30 min to sites of atrial puncture, followed by pressure dressing; inform prescriber if this does not attain hemostasis; apply pressure dressing
• Store powder at room temperature or refrigerate; protect from excessive light

Y-site compatibilities: Lidocaine, metoprolol, propranolol
Y-site incompatibilities: DOBUTamine, DOPamine, heparin, nitroglycerin
Additive compatibilities: Lidocaine, morphine, nitroglycerin

Patient/family education
• Teach patient reason for alteplase, signs and symptoms of bleeding, allergic reactions, when to notify prescriber

Evaluation
Positive therapeutic outcome
• Lysis of pulmonary thrombi
• Adequate hemodynamic state
• Absence of congestive heart failure

aluminum hydroxide (OTC)
AlternaGEL, Alugel ✤, aluminum hydroxide, Alu-Tab, Amphojel, Basal gel ✤, Dialume
Func. class.: Antacid, hypophosphatemic, antiulcer
Chem. class.: Aluminum product, phosphate binder

Pregnancy category C

Action: Neutralizes gastric acidity, binds phosphates in GI tract; these phosphates are excreted

Therapeutic outcome: Decreased acidity, healing of ulcers; decreased phosphate levels in chronic renal failure

Uses: Adjunct in peptic, gastric, duodenal ulcers; antacid; hyperphosphatemia in chronic renal failure; reflux esophagitis, hyperacidity, heartburn, stress ulcer prevention in critically ill, GERD

Unlabeled uses: GI bleeding

Dosage and routes
Antacid
Adult: SUSP PO 600 mg 1 hr after meals, at bedtime; chewed, max 6 times per day

Hyperphosphatemia
Adult: PO 300-600 mg tid
Child: PO 50-150 mg/kg/day in 4-6 divided doses

GI bleeding (unlabeled)
Infant: PO 2-5 ml/dose q1-2hr
Child: PO 5-15 ml/dose q1-2hr

Available forms: Caps 500 mg; tabs 600 mg; susp 320 mg/5 ml, 450 mg/5 ml, 600 mg/5 ml; 675 mg/5 ml

Adverse effects
GI: *Constipation,* anorexia, **obstruction,** fecal impaction
META: *Hypophosphatemia,* hypercalciuria

Contraindications: Hypersensitivity to this product or aluminum products

Precautions: Pregnancy **C,** breastfeeding, geriatric, fluid restriction, decreased GI motility, GI obstruction, dehydration, renal disease, sodium-restricted diets

Pharmacokinetics
Absorption	Not usually absorbed
Distribution	Widely distributed if absorbed; crosses placenta
Metabolism	Unknown
Excretion	Feces, kidneys (small amounts), breast milk
Half-life	Unknown

Pharmacodynamics
Onset	20-40 min
Peak	½ hr
Duration	1-3 hr

Interactions
Individual drugs
Allopurinol, amprenavir, delavirdine, diflunisal, digoxin, gabapentin, gatifloxacin, isoniazid, ketoconazole, penicillamine, phenytoin, quinidine, ticlopidine, warfarin: decreased effect of each of these drugs

Drug classifications
Cephalosporins, corticosteroids, H_2 antagonists, iron salts, phenothiazines, quinolones, tetracyclines, thyroid hormones: decreased effect of each of these drug classifications
Drug/herb
Buckthorn, cascara sagrada, castor, Chinese rhubarb: decreased action of these herbs
Drug/food
High-protein meal: decreased product effect

NURSING CONSIDERATIONS
Assessment
• Assess pain symptoms: location, duration, intensity, alleviating precipitating factors
• Monitor phosphate levels, since product is bound in GI system; urinary pH, calcium, electrolytes; hypophosphatemia: anorexia, weakness, fatigue, bone pain, hyperreflexia
• Monitor constipation; increase bulk in diet if needed

Nursing diagnoses
• Constipation (adverse reactions)
• Knowledge, deficient (teaching)
• Pain, chronic (uses)

Implementation
• 2 tsp (10 ml) will neutralize 20 mEq of acid; 2 tabs will neutralize 16 mEq of acid
PO route
• Give laxatives or stool softeners if constipation occurs, especially geriatric
• Give after shaking suspension; follow with water to facilitate passage
• Tab may be chewed if patient is unable to swallow—drink 8 oz of water after chewing; or by nasogastric tube if patient unable to swallow
• Give with 8 oz of water for hyperphosphatemia unless contraindicated
• Give 1 hr before or after other medications to prevent poor absorption
• Give 15 ml 30 min after meals and at bedtime (esophagitis)
NG tube route
• May be given as prescribed q1-2hr and given by gastric tube after diluting with water (peptic ulcer)

Patient/family education
• Instruct patient to increase fluids to 2000 ml/day unless contraindicated
• Instruct patient to avoid phosphate-containing foods (most dairy products, eggs, fruits, carbonated beverages) during product therapy; to add cheese, corn, pasta, plums, prunes, lentils after product (hypophosphatemia)

- Instruct patient not to use for prolonged periods if serum phosphate is low or if on a low-sodium diet; CHF patients should check for sodium content and use sodium-reduced products
- Instruct patient that stools may appear white or speckled; constipation may result; to report black tarry stools, which indicate gastric bleeding
- Instruct patient to check with prescriber after 2 wk of self-prescribed antacid use; may be used for 4-6 wk after symptoms subside or as prescribed
- Instruct patient to separate other medications by 2 hr

Evaluation
Positive therapeutic outcome
- Absence of pain, decreased acidity
- Increased pH of gastric secretions
- Decreased phosphate levels

---

alvimopan (Rx)
(al-vi′moe-pan)
Entereg
Func. class.: Functional GI disorder agent
Chem. class.: Peripheral μ-opioid receptor antagonist

Pregnancy category B

Action: Acts within the GI tract, antagonizes opioid-induced GI dysfunction

Therapeutic outcome: Resolution of ileus

Uses: Ileus, post-operative

Dosage and routes
Ileus, post-operative
Adult: PO 12 mg given ½-5 hrs before surgery, then 12 mg bid the day after surgery, max 7 days (15 doses)

Available forms: Caps 12 mg

Adverse effects
CV: **MI**
GI: Dyspepsia, flatulence, constipation
GU: Urinary retention
MISC: **Anemia,** hypokalemia
MS: Back pain

Contraindications: Hypersensitivity

Black Box Warning: No more than 15 doses

Precautions: Pregnancy **B,** breastfeeding, renal/hepatic disease, children, GI obstruction, MI, complete GI obstruction surgery

Pharmacokinetics

Absorption	High fat meal decreases absorption
Distribution	Protein binding 80%-94%
Metabolism	Unknown
Excretion	Kidneys (35%)
Half-life	Terminal 10-18 hr

Pharmacodynamics
Unknown

INTERACTIONS
Individual drugs
Amiodarone, bepridil, cycloSPORINE, diltiazem, itraconazole, quinidine, quinine, spironolactone, verapamil: increased alvimopan effect
Methylnaltrexone: duplicate therapy
Drug classifications
Opiate agonists: increased GI adverse reactions; do not give if opiate agonists were taken for ≥7 days
Opiate antagonists: duplicate therapy

NURSING CONSIDERATIONS
Assessment
- Monitor Hgb/Hct, serum potassium

Nursing diagnoses
- Knowledge, deficient (teaching)

Implementation
- Use in hospital only; therapeutic doses of opiates should not be used for >7 consecutive days
- Must register in EASE program
- Do not give >15 doses (short-term hospital only)
- Give without regard to food
- Store at room temperature

Patient/family education
- Instruct the patient in the reason for the product

Evaluation
Positive therapeutic outcome
- Resolution of ileus

---

amantadine (Rx)
(a-man'ta-deen)
amantadine HCl, Symmetrel
Func. class.: Antiviral, antiparkinsonian agent
Chem. class.: Tricyclic amine

Pregnancy category C

Do not confuse:
amantadine/ranitidine/rimantadine, Symmetrel/Synthroid

Action: Prevents uncoating of nucleic acid in viral cell, preventing penetration of virus to host; causes release of dopamine from neurons

Therapeutic outcome: Resolution of infection, lessening of parkinsonism symptoms

Uses: Prophylaxis or treatment of influenza type A, extrapyramidal reactions, parkinsonism, Parkinson's disease

Unlabeled uses: Neuroleptic malignant syndrome, MS-associated fatigue

Dosage and routes
Influenza type A
Adult and child >12 yr: PO 200 mg/day in single dose or divided bid; max 400 mg/day

Geriatric: PO no more than 100 mg/day
Child 9-12 yr: PO 100 mg bid
Child 1-9 yr: PO 5 mg/kg/day divided bid-tid, not to exceed 150 mg/day

Extrapyramidal reaction/parkinsonism
Adult: PO 100 mg bid, up to 400 mg/day in EPS; give for 1 wk, then 100 mg as needed up to 400 mg in parkinsonism

Renal dose
Adult: PO CCr 40-50 ml/min 100 mg/day; CCr 30 ml/min 200 mg 2 ×/wk; CCr 20 ml/min 100 mg 3 ×/wk; CCr 10 ml/min 100 mg alternating with 200 mg q7days

MS-associated fatigue (unlabeled)
Adult: PO 200 mg daily or 100 mg bid

Neuroleptic malignant syndrome (unlabeled)
Adult: PO 100 mg bid × 3 wk

Available forms: Caps 100 mg; syr 50 mg/5 ml

Adverse effects
CNS: Headache, dizziness, drowsiness, fatigue, *anxiety,* psychosis, *depression, hallucinations,* tremors, *seizures,* confusion, *insomnia*
CV: Orthostatic hypotension, CHF
EENT: Blurred vision
GI: Nausea, vomiting, constipation, dry mouth, anorexia
GU: Frequency, retention
HEMA: Leukopenia, agranulocytosis
INTEG: Photosensitivity, dermatitis, livedo reticularis

Contraindications: Breastfeeding, child <1 yr, hypersensitivity, eczematic rash

Precautions: Pregnancy **C,** geriatric, epilepsy, CHF, orthostatic hypotension, psychiatric disorders, renal/hepatic disease, peripheral edema

Pharmacokinetics	
Absorption	Unknown
Distribution	Crosses placenta
Metabolism	Not metabolized
Excretion	Urine unchanged (90%), breast milk
Half-life	11-15 hr

Pharmacodynamics	
Onset	48 hr
Peak	2-4 hr
Duration	Unknown

Interactions
Individual drugs
Atropine: increased anticholinergic response
Intranasal influenzae vaccine: decreased effect of vaccine; avoid use 2 wk before or 48 hr after amantadine
Metoclopramide: decreased amantadine effect
Triamterene, hydrochlorothiazide: decreased excretion of amantadine
Drug classifications
Anticholinergics (other): increased anticholinergic response
CNS stimulants: increased CNS stimulation
Phenothiazines: decreased amantadine effect
Drug/herb
Belladonna, henbane: increased anticholinergic response
Pheasant's eye, quinine, scopolia root: increased action/side effects
Kava: decreased action

NURSING CONSIDERATIONS
Assessment
- Monitor I&O ratio; report frequency, hesitancy; serum BUN, creatinine baseline
- Assess CHF, confusion, mottling of skin
- Assess bowel pattern before, during treatment
- Assess skin eruptions, photosensitivity after administration of product

Adverse effects: *italic* = common, **bold** = life-threatening

- Assess respiratory status: rate, character, wheezing, tightness in chest
- Assess allergies before initiation of treatment, reaction of each medication
- Assess signs of infection
- Assess hematologic status for leukopenia, agranulocytosis
- Assess for livedo reticularis: mottling of the skin, usually red, edema, itching in lower extremities
- Assess for Parkinson's disease: gait, tremors, akinesia, rigidity
- Assess for toxicity: confusion, behavioral changes, hypotension, seizures

Nursing diagnoses
- Infection, risk for (uses)
- Knowledge, deficient (teaching)

Implementation
- Give before exposure to influenza; continue for 10 days after contact
- Give at least 4 hr before bedtime to prevent insomnia
- Give after meals for better absorption, to decrease GI symptoms
- Give in divided doses to prevent CNS disturbances: headache, dizziness, fatigue, drowsiness
- Store in tight, dry container
- Caps may be opened and mixed with food

Patient/family education
- Advise patient to change body position slowly to prevent orthostatic hypotension
- Teach about aspects of product therapy: need to report dyspnea, weight gain, dizziness, poor concentration, dysuria, behavioral changes
- Advise patient to avoid hazardous activities if dizziness, blurred vision occurs
- Advise patient to take product exactly as prescribed; parkinsonian crisis may occur if product is discontinued abruptly; do not double dose; if a dose is missed, do not take within 4 hr of next dose
- Teach to avoid alcohol; do not breastfeed

Evaluation
Positive therapeutic outcome
- Absence of fever, malaise, cough, dyspnea in infection; tremors, shuffling gait in Parkinson's disease

Treatment of overdose: Withdraw
product, maintain airway, administer epinephrine, aminophylline, O_2, **IV** corticosteroids, physostigmine

---

ambrisentan (Rx)
(am-bri-sen'tan)
Letairis ✤
Func. class.: Antihypertensive
Chem class.: Vasodilator/endothelin receptor antagonist

Pregnancy category X

Action: Endothelin-1 receptor antagonist; endothelin-1 is vasoconstrictor

Therapeutic outcome: Decreased shortness of breath, dizziness

Uses: Pulmonary arterial hypertension, alone or in combination with other antihypertensives

Dosage and routes
Adult: PO 5 mg/day; may increase to 10 mg if needed

Available forms: Tabs 5, 10 mg

Adverse effects
CNS: Headache, fever, flushing
CV: Orthostatic hypotension, hypotension, peripheral edema
EENT: Sinusitis, rhinitis
GI: Abdominal pain, constipation
GU: Decreased sperm counts
HEMA: Anemia
INTEG: Rash
RESP: Pharyngitis, dyspnea

Contraindications: Breastfeeding, hypersensitivity

Black Box Warning: Pregnancy X

Precautions: Children, women, geriatric, hepatitis, anemia, heart failure, jaundice, peripheral edema

Black Box Warning: Hepatic disease

Pharmacokinetics	
Absorption	Rapidly
Distribution	Protein binding 99%
Metabolism	By CYP3A4, CYP2C19
Excretion	Unknown
Half-life	Terminal 15 hr

Pharmacodynamics	
Onset	Unknown
Peak	2 hr
Duration	Unknown

Interactions
Individual drugs
Cimetidine, clopidogrel, efavirenz, felbamate, fluoxetine, modafinil, oxcarbazepine, ticlopidine: possibly increased ambrisentan

---

Fosphenytoin, griseofulvin, nevirapine, phenytoin, rifabutin, rifampin, rifapentine: need for ambrisentan dosage change

Mefloquine, nicardipine, propafenone, quinidine, ranolazine, tacrolimus, testosterone: decreased ambrisentan absorption

Drug classifications

Antihypertensives (other), diuretics, MAOIs: increased hypotension

Barbiturates: need for ambrisentan dosage change

CYP3A4 inhibitors (amprenavir, aprepitant, atazanavir, clarithromycin, conivaptan, cycloSPORINE, dalfopristin, danazol, darunavir, erythromycin, estradiol, imatinib, itraconazole, ketoconazole, nefazodone, nelfinavir, propoxyphene, quinupristin, ritonavir, RU-486, saquinavir, tamoxifen, telithromycin, troleandomycin, zafirlukast), CYP2C19/CYP3A4 (chloramphenicol, delavirdine, fluconazole, fluvoxamine, isoniazid, voriconazole): increased ambrisentan

Drug/herb

St. John's wort: need for ambrisentan dosage change

Drug/food

Grapefruit products: avoid use

Drug/lab test

Decreased: Hct, Hgb
Increased: LFTs

NURSING CONSIDERATIONS
Assessment

• Monitor blood tests: CBC with differential; Hct, Hgb may be decreased
• Monitor daily edema in feet, legs; weight, B/P, orthostatic hypotension
• Monitor hepatic function tests: AST, ALT, bilirubin
• Assess pregnancy status before giving this product; pregnancy category **X**

Nursing diagnoses

• Activity intolerance (uses)
• Breathing pattern, ineffective (uses)
• Knowledge, deficient (teaching)

Implementation

• Do not break, crush, or chew tabs
• Give daily with a full glass of water without regard to food
• Do not discontinue abruptly
• Only those facilities enrolled in the LEAP program may administer this product
• Store in tight container at room temperature

Patient/family education

• Teach patient the importance of complying with dosage schedule even if feeling better
• Instruct patient to notify if pregnancy is planned or suspected; if pregnant, product will need to be discontinued
• Advise patient that if a dose is missed, take as soon as possible; if it is almost time for the next dose, take only that dose; do not double dose
• Instruct patient not to use OTC products, including herbs, supplements unless approved by prescriber
• Advise patient to report to prescriber immediately: dizziness, faintness, chest pain, palpitations, uneven or rapid heart rate, headache
• Caution patient not to operate machinery or perform hazardous tasks if dizziness occurs
• Advise patient to avoid faintness; do not get up or stand up rapidly

Evaluation
Positive therapeutic outcome

• Decrease in B/P
• Decreased shortness of breath

amifostine (Rx)
(a-mi-foss'teen)
Ethyol
Func. class.: Cytoprotective agent for cisplatin

Pregnancy category C

Action: Binds and detoxifies damaging metabolites of cisplatin, alkylating agents, DNA-reactive agents, and ionizing radiation by converting this product by alkaline phosphatase in tissue to an active free thiol compound

Therapeutic outcome: Decreased toxic reaction from cisplatin

Uses: Used to reduce renal toxicity when cisplatin is given in ovarian cancer non-small cell lung cancer; reduces xerostomia (dry mouth) in radiation therapy for head, neck cancer

Unlabeled uses: To prevent or reduce cisplatin-induced neurotoxicity, cyclophosphamide-induced granulocytopenia; prevent or reduce toxicity of radiation therapy; reduce toxicity of paclitaxel, myelodysplastic syndrome (MDS)

Dosage and routes
Bone marrow suppression prophylaxis/nephrotoxicity prophylaxis/neurotoxicity prophylaxis (unlabeled)
Adult: **IV** 100-340 mg/m^2/day over 15 min prior to each dose of chemotherapy/radiation

Adverse effects: *italic* = common, **bold** = life-threatening

Reduction of renal damage with cisplatin

Adult: IV 910 mg/m² daily, within ½ hr before chemotherapy; give over 15 min; may reduce dose to 740 mg/m² if higher dose is poorly tolerated

Myelodysplastic syndrome (MDS) (unlabeled)

Adult: IV 100 mg/m² 3 ×/wk, max 300 mg/m² 3 ×/wk

Xerostomia

Adult: IV 200 mg/m² daily over 3 min as INF 15-30 min before radiation therapy

Available forms: Powder for inj lyophilized 500 mg/vial

Adverse effects

CNS: Dizziness, somnolence, loss of consciousness
CV: Hypotension
EENT: Sneezing
GI: Nausea, vomiting, hiccups, diarrhea
INTEG: Flushing, feeling of warmth
MISC: Hypocalcemia, rash, chills, **anaphylaxis, toxic epidermal necrolysis, Stevens-Johnson syndrome, exfoliative dermatitis,** *erythema multiforme*

Contraindications: Breastfeeding, hypersensitivity to mannitol, aminothiol; hypotension, dehydration

Precautions: Pregnancy **C**, children, geriatric, CV disease

Pharmacokinetics

Absorption	Complete
Distribution	Unknown
Metabolism	To free thiol compound
Excretion	Unknown
Half-life	5-8 min

Pharmacodynamics

Unknown

Interactions
Drug classifications
Antihypertensives: increased hypotension

NURSING CONSIDERATIONS
Assessment

• Assess for xerostomia: mouth lesion, dry mouth during therapy
• Assess fluid status before administration; administer antiemetic before administration to prevent severe nausea and vomiting; also, dexamethasone 20 mg **IV** and a serotonin antagonist such as ondansetron, dolasetron, or granisetron
• Monitor calcium levels before, during treatment; may cause hypocalcemia; calcium supplements may be given for hypocalcemia
• Monitor blood pressure before and q5min during infusion; antihypertensive should be discontinued 24 hr prior to infusion if severe hypotension occurs, give **IV** 0.9% NaCl to expand fluid volume, place in modified Trendelenburg position

Nursing diagnoses
• Injury, risk for (uses)
• Knowledge, deficient (teaching)

Implementation
Intermittent IV infusion route
• Give by **IV** intermittent inf after reconstituting with 9.7 ml of sterile 0.9% NaCl, further dilute with 0.9% NaCl to a concentration of 5-40 mg/ml, give at a rate over 15 min within ½ hr of chemotherapy
• Patient to be in supine position during infusion

Y-site compatibilities: Amikacin, aminophylline, ampicillin, ampicillin/ sulbactam, aztreonam, bleomycin, bumetanide, buprenorphine, butorphanol, calcium gluconate, carboplatin, carmustine, cefazolin, cefonicid, cefotaxime, cefotetan, cefoxitin, ceftazidime, ceftizoxime, ceftriaxone, cefuroxime, cimetidine, ciprofloxacin, clindamycin, cyclophosphamide, cytarabine, dacarbazine, dactinomycin, DAUNOrubicin, dexamethasone, diphenhydrAMINE, DOBUtamine, DOPamine, DOXOrubicin, doxycycline, droperidol, enalaprilat, etoposide, famotidine, floxuridine, fluconazole, fludarabine, fluorouracil, furosemide, gallium, gentamicin, granisetron, haloperidol, heparin, hydrocortisone, hydromorphone, idarubicin, ifosfamide, imipenem-cilastatin, leucovorin, lorazepam, magnesium sulfate, mannitol, mechlorethamine, meperidine, mesna, methotrexate, methylPREDNISolone, metoclopramide, metronidazole, mezlocillin, mitomycin, mitoxantrone, morphine, nalbuphine, netilmicin, ondansetron, piperacillin, plicamycin, potassium chloride, promethazine, ranitidine, sodium bicarbonate, streptozocin, teniposide, thiotepa, ticarcillin, ticarcillin/clavulanate, tobramycin, trimethoprim/sulfamethoxazole, trimetrexate, vancomycin, vinBLAStine, vinCRIStine, zidovudine
Additive incompatibilities: Do not mix with other products or solutions

---

Patient/family education

- Teach reason for medication and expected results
- Teach that side effects may cause severe nausea, vomiting, decreased B/P, chills, dizziness, somnolence, hiccups, sneezing

Evaluation

Positive therapeutic outcome

- Absence of renal damage

amikacin (Rx)

(am-i-kay'sin)
amikacin sulfate, Amikin
Func. class.: Antibiotic
Chem. class.: Aminoglycoside

Pregnancy category D

Do not confuse:

Amikin/**Amicar**

Action: Interferes with protein synthesis in bacterial cell by binding to ribosomal subunit, which causes misreading of genetic code; inaccurate peptide sequence forms in protein chain, causing bacterial death

Therapeutic outcome: Bactericidal effects for the following organisms: *Pseudomonas aeruginosa, Escherichia coli, Enterobacter, Acinetobacter, Providencia, Citrobacter, Staphylococcus, Serratia, Proteus*

Uses: Severe systemic infections of CNS, respiratory, GI, urinary tract, bone, skin, soft tissues caused by *Staphylococcus, Pseudomonas aeruginosa, Escherichia coli, Enterobacter, Acinetobacter, Providencia Citrobacter, Serratia, Proteus, Klebsiella pneumoniae*

Unlabeled uses: *Mycobacterium avium* complex (intrathecal or intraventricular) in combination; aerosolization, actinomycotic mycetoma

Dosage and routes

Severe systemic infections
Adult and child: IV INF 15 mg/kg/day in 2-3 divided doses q8-12hr in 100-200 ml D₅W over 30-60 min, not to exceed 1.5 g; use for 7-10 days; decreased dosages are needed in poor renal function as determined by blood levels, renal function studies; pulse dosing (once-daily dosing) may be used with some infections; IM 15 mg/kg/day in divided doses q8-12hr; daily or extended internal dosing as an alternative dosing regimen
Infant: **IV**/IM 10 mg/kg initially, then 7.5 mg/kg q12hr

Neonate: IM/**IV** 10 mg/kg initially, then 7.5 mg/kg q12hr
Premature neonate: **IV** 10 mg/kg initially, then 7.5 mg/kg q8-12hr

Severe urinary tract infections
Adult: IM 15 mg/kg/day divided q8-12hr

Hemodialysis
Adult: IM/**IV** 7.5 mg/kg followed by 5 mg/kg 3 ×/wk after each dialysis session (for TIW dialysis)

TB or other mycobacterial infection
Adult and adolescent: **IV** 7.5-15 mg/kg divided q12-24hr as part of a multiple-drug regimen
Child: **IV** 15-30 mg/kg/day divided q12-24hr as part of a multiple-drug regimen, max 1.5 g/day

Renal dose
Adult: **IV**/IM 7.5 mg/kg initially, then increased as determined by blood levels, renal function studies

Available forms: Inj IM, **IV** 50, 250 mg/ml

Adverse effects

CNS: Confusion, depression, numbness, tremors, **seizures,** muscle twitching, **neurotoxicity,** dizziness, vertigo, tinnitus, **neuromuscular blockade with respiratory paralysis**
CV: Hypotension or hypertension, palpitations
EENT: Ototoxicity, deafness, visual disturbances
GI: Nausea, vomiting, anorexia, increased ALT, AST, bilirubin, hepatomegaly, **hepatic necrosis,** splenomegaly
GU: **Oliguria, hematuria, renal damage, azotemia, renal failure, nephrotoxicity**
HEMA: **Agranulocytosis, thrombocytopenia, leukopenia, eosinophilia, anemia**
INTEG: Rash, burning, urticaria, dermatitis, alopecia

Contraindications: Pregnancy **D,** mild to moderate infections, hypersensitivity to aminoglycosides, sulfites

Precautions: Neonates, breastfeeding, geriatric, myasthenia gravis, Parkinson's disease

Black Box Warning: Hearing impairment, renal/neuromuscular disease

Pharmacokinetics

Absorption	Well absorbed (IM), completely absorbed (**IV**)
Distribution	Widely distributed in extracellular fluids, poor in CSF; crosses placenta
Metabolism	Minimal; liver
Excretion	Mostly unchanged (79%) in kidneys, removed by hemodialysis
Half-life	2-3 hr, prolonged up to 7 hr in infants; increased in renal disease

Pharmacodynamics

	IM	IV
Onset	Rapid	Rapid
Peak	15-30 min	1-2 hr
Duration	Unknown	Unknown

Interactions
Individual drugs
Acyclovir, amphotericin B, cycloSPORINE, vancomycin: nephrotoxicity

Cidofovir: do not use together

DimenhyDRINATE, ethacrynic acid: increased masking of ototoxicity

Indomethacin: increased serum trough and peak

Drug classifications
Anesthetics, nondepolarizing neuromuscular blockers: increased neuromuscular blockade, respiratory depression

Cephalosporins: inactivation of amikacin, nephrotoxicity

Drug/herb
Lysine (large amounts): increased toxicity

Acidophilus: do not use with antiinfectives

Drug/lab test
Increased: BUN, ALT, AST, bilirubin, LDH, alkaline phosphatase, creatinine

Decreased: calcium, sodium, potassium, magnesium

NURSING CONSIDERATIONS
Assessment
• Assess patient for previous sensitivity reaction

• Assess patient for signs and symptoms of infection, including characteristics of wounds, sputum, urine, stool, WBC >10,000/mm³, earache, temp; obtain baseline information before and during treatment

• Obtain C&S tests before beginning product therapy to identify if correct treatment has been initiated

• Assess for allergic reactions: rash, urticaria, pruritus

• Identify urine output; if decreasing, notify prescriber (may indicate nephrotoxicity); also notify prescriber of increased BUN and creatinine, urine CCr <80 ml/min; lower dosage should be given in renal impairment; urinalysis daily for protein, cells, casts; nephrotoxicity may be reversible if product stopped at first sign

• Monitor blood studies: AST, ALT, CBC, Hct, bilirubin, LDH, alkaline phosphatase; Coombs' test monthly if patient is on long-term therapy

• Monitor electrolytes: potassium, sodium, chloride, magnesium monthly if patient is on long-term therapy

• Assess bowel pattern daily; if severe diarrhea occurs, product should be discontinued

• Monitor for bleeding: ecchymosis, bleeding gums, hematuria, stool guaiac daily if on long-term therapy

• Assess for overgrowth of infection: perineal itching, fever, malaise, redness, pain, swelling, drainage, rash, diarrhea, change in cough, sputum

• Obtain weight before treatment; calculation of dosage is usually based on ideal body weight, but may be calculated on actual body weight

• Monitor VS during infusion, watch for hypotension, change in pulse

• Assess **IV** site for thrombophlebitis including pain, redness, swelling q30min; change site if needed; apply warm compresses to discontinued site

• Obtain serum peak, drawn 30-60 min after **IV** infusion or 60 min after IM injection; trough level drawn just before next dose; 20-30 mcg/ml, trough 4-8 mcg/ml, blood level should be 2-4 times bacteriostatic level

• Urine pH if product is used for UTI; urine should be kept alkaline

◆ Deafness by audiometric testing, ringing, roaring in ears, vertigo; assess hearing before, during, after treatment

• Dehydration: high specific gravity, decrease in skin turgor, dry mucous membranes, dark urine

• Vestibular dysfunction: nausea, vomiting, dizziness, headache; product should be discontinued if severe

Nursing diagnoses
• Diarrhea (side effects)
• Infection, risk for (uses)
• Injury, risk for (side effects)
• Knowledge, deficient (teaching)

Implementation
IM route
• Give deeply in large muscle mass, rotate inj sites

Intermittent **IV** infusion route
• Dilute 500 mg of product in 100-200 ml of **IV** D$_5$W, D$_5$NaCl, or 0.9% NaCl and give over ½-1 hr; flush after administration with D$_5$W or 0.9% NaCl

Syringe compatibilities: Clindamycin, doxapram

Y-site compatibilities: Acyclovir, amifostine, amiodarone, amsacrine, aztreonam, cisatracurium, cyclophosphamide, dexamethasone, diltiazem, enalamprilat, esmolol, filgrastim, fluconazole, fludarabine, foscarnet, furosemide, granisetron, idarubicin, IL-2, labetalol, lorazepam, magnesium sulfate, melphalan, midazolam, morphine, ondansetron, paclitaxel, perphenazine, remifentanil, sargramostim, teniposide, thiotepa, TPN #54, #61, #91, #203, #204, #212, vinorelbine, warfarin, zidovudine

Patient/family education
• Teach patient to report sore throat, bruising, bleeding, joint pain; may indicate blood dyscrasias (rare)
• Advise patient to contact prescriber if vaginal itching, loose foul-smelling stools, furry tongue occur; may indicate superinfection
• Advise patient to report hypersensitivity: rash, itching, trouble breathing, facial edema and notify prescriber

Evaluation
Positive therapeutic outcome
• Absence of signs/symptoms of infection: WBC <10,000/mm^3, temp WNL; absence of red draining wounds; absence of earache
• Reported improvement in symptoms of infection

Treatment of overdose: Withdraw product; administer epinephrine, O$_2$, hemodialysis, exchange transfusion in the newborn; monitor serum levels of product; may give ticarcillin or carbenicillin

---

amiloride (Rx)
(a-mill'oh-ride)
Amiloride HCl, Midamor
Func. class.: Potassium-sparing diuretic
Chem. class.: Pyrazine
Pregnancy category B

Do not confuse:
amiloride/amlodipine

Action: Inhibits sodium, potassium ATPase in the distal tubule, cortical collecting duct resulting in inhibition of sodium reabsorption and decreasing potassium secretion

Therapeutic outcome: Diuretic and antihypertensive effect while retaining potassium

Uses: Edema in CHF in combination with other diuretics; for hypertension, adjunct with other diuretics to maintain potassium; polyuria due to lithium administration

Unlabeled uses: Ascites

Dosage and routes
Adult: PO 5-10 mg daily in 1-2 divided doses; may be increased to 10-20 mg daily if needed

Ascites (unlabeled)
Adult: PO 10 mg/day, max 40 mg

Available forms: Tabs 5 mg

Adverse effects
CNS: Headache, dizziness, fatigue, weakness, paresthesias, tremor, depression, anxiety
CV: Orthostatic hypotension, dysrhythmias, angina
EENT: Blurred vision, increased intraocular pressure
ELECT: **Hyperkalemia,** dehydration
GI: Nausea, diarrhea, dry mouth, *vomiting, anorexia,* cramps, constipation, abdominal pain, jaundice
GU: Polyuria, dysuria, frequency, impotence
HEMA: **Aplastic anemia, neutropenia**
INTEG: Rash, pruritus, alopecia, urticaria
MS: Cramps
RESP: Cough, dyspnea, shortness of breath

Contraindications: Anuria, hypersensitivity, impaired renal function

Black Box Warning: Hyperkalemia

Precautions: Pregnancy **B,** breastfeeding, geriatric, dehydration, diabetes, acidosis

Pharmacokinetics	
Absorption	Variable (10%-15%)
Distribution	Widely distributed
Metabolism	Unchanged in urine (50%), in feces (40%)
Excretion	Renal; breast milk
Half-life	6-9 hr

Pharmacodynamics	
Onset	2 hr
Peak	6-10 hr
Duration	24 hr

Adverse effects: *italic* = common, **bold** = life-threatening

Interactions
Individual drugs
CycloSPORINE, tacrolimus: increased hyperkalemia

Lithium: increased lithium toxicity
Drug classifications
ACE inhibitors, diuretics (potassium-sparing), potassium products, salt substitutes: increased hyperkalemia

Antihypertensives: increased action

NSAIDs: decreased effectiveness of amiloride
Drug/herb
Arginine: fatal hypokalemia

Bearberry, gossypol, licorice: increased hypokalemia

Cucumber, dandelion, horsetail, licorice, nettle, pumpkin, Queen Anne's lace: increased amiloride effect

Khella: increased hypotension

St. John's wort: increased severe photosensitivity
Drug/food
Potassium foods: increased hyperkalemia
Drug/lab test
Interference: GTT

NURSING CONSIDERATIONS
Assessment
• Monitor manifestations of hyperkalemia: *MS:* fatigue, muscle weakness; *CARDIAC:* dysrhythmias, hypotension; *NEURO:* paresthesias, confusion; *RESP:* dyspnea

• Monitor for manifestations of hyponatremia: *CV:* increased B/P, cold, clammy skin, hypovolemia or hypervolemia; *GI:* anorexia, nausea, vomiting, diarrhea, abdominal cramps; *NEURO:* lethargy, increased ICP, confusion, headache, seizures, coma, fatigue, tremors, hyperreflexia

• Monitor for manifestations of hyperchloremia: *NEURO:* weakness, lethargy, coma; *RESP:* deep rapid breathing

• Assess fluid volume status: I&O ratios and record weight, distended red veins, crackles in lung, color, quality, and specific gravity of urine, skin turgor, adequacy of pulses, moist mucous membranes, bilateral lung sounds, peripheral pitting edema; dehydration symptoms of decreasing output, thirst, hypotension, dry mouth and mucous membranes should be reported

• Monitor electrolytes: potassium, sodium, calcium, magnesium; also include BUN, ABGs, uric acid, CBC, blood glucose

• Assess B/P before, during therapy with patient lying, standing, and sitting as appropriate; orthostatic hypotension can occur rapidly

Nursing diagnoses
• Fluid volume, deficient (side effects)
• Fluid volume, excess (uses)
• Knowledge, deficient (teaching)

Implementation
• Give in AM to avoid interference with sleep
• With food; if nausea occurs, absorption may be increased

Patient/family education
• Teach patient to take medication early in the day to prevent nocturia

• Instruct patient to take with food or milk if GI symptoms of nausea and anorexia occur

• Teach patient to maintain a weekly record of weight and notify prescriber of weight loss >5 lb

• Caution patient that this product causes an increase in potassium levels, so foods high in potassium should be avoided; refer to dietitian for assistance, planning

• Caution patient not to exercise in hot weather or stand for prolonged periods since orthostatic hypotension will be enhanced

• Teach patient not to use alcohol or any OTC medications without prescriber's approval; serious product reactions may occur

• Emphasize the need to contact prescriber immediately if muscle cramps, weakness, nausea, dizziness, or numbness occurs

• Teach patient to take own B/P and pulse and record

• Advise patient that dizziness and confusion may occur; avoid driving or other hazardous activities if alertness is decreased

• Teach patient to continue taking medication even if feeling better; this product controls symptoms but does not cure the condition

• Advise patient with hypertension to continue other medical treatment (exercise, weight loss, relaxation techniques, cessation of smoking)

Evaluation
Positive therapeutic outcome
• Prevention of hypokalemia (diuretic use)
• Decreased edema
• Decreased B/P
• Increased diuresis

Treatment of overdose: Lavage if taken orally; monitor electrolytes; administer **IV** fluids; monitor hydration, CV, renal status

amino acid (Rx)
(a-mee'noe)
Injection: FreAmine, HepatAmine
Solution: Aminess, Aminosyn, Branch
Amin, FreAmine III, NephrAmine,
Novamine, ProcalAmine, Ren Amin,
Travasol, Troph Amine
Func. class.: Caloric agent
Chem. class.: Nitrogen product

Pregnancy category C

Action: Needed for anabolism to maintain structure; decreases catabolism, promotes healing

Therapeutic outcome: Positive nitrogen balance, decreased catabolism

Uses: Hepatic encephalopathy, cirrhosis, hepatitis, nutritional support in cancer trauma; to prevent nitrogen loss when adequate nutrition by mouth, gastric, or duodenal tube cannot be used; intestinal obstruction, short bowel syndrome, severe malabsorption

Dosage and routes
Amino acid injection
Adult: **IV** 80-120 g/day; 500 ml of amino acids/500 ml D_{50} given over 24 hr

Amino acid solution
Adult: **IV** 1-1.5 g/kg/day titrated to patient's needs
Child: **IV** 2-3 g/kg/day titrated to patient's needs

Available forms: Inj; many strengths, types

Adverse effects
CNS: Dizziness, headache, confusion, **loss of consciousness**
CV: Hypertension, **CHF, pulmonary edema**
ENDO: Hyperglycemia, rebound hypoglycemia, electrolyte imbalances, hyperosmolar syndrome, hyperosmolar hyperglycemic nonketotic syndrome, alkalosis, acidosis, hypophosphatemia, hyperammonemia, dehydration, hypocalcemia
GI: Nausea, vomiting, liver fat deposits, abdominal pain, jaundice
GU: Glycosuria, osmotic diuresis
INTEG: Chills, flushing, warm feeling, rash, urticaria, extravasation necrosis, phlebitis at inj site

Contraindications: Hypersensitivity, severe electrolyte imbalances, anuria, severe liver damage, maple syrup urine disease, PKU

Precautions: Pregnancy C, children, renal disease, diabetes mellitus, CHF

Absorption	Complete bioavailability
Distribution	Widely distributed
Metabolism	Anabolism
Excretion	Kidney to urea nitrogen
Half-life	Unknown

Pharmacodynamics
Unknown

Interactions
Drug classifications
Tetracycline: decreased protein-sparing effects (inj only)

NURSING CONSIDERATIONS
Assessment
• Monitor electrolytes (potassium, sodium, calcium, chloride, magnesium), blood glucose, ammonia, phosphate, ketones; renal, liver function studies: BUN, creatinine, ALT, AST, bilirubin; urine glucose q6hr using Chemstrips, which are not affected by infusion substances; if BUN increases over 15%, therapy may need to be discontinued
• Check inj site for extravasation: redness along vein, edema at site, necrosis, pain; for a hard, tender area
• Monitor respiratory function q1hr: auscultate lung fields bilaterally for crackles; monitor respirations for quality, rate, rhythm that indicates fluid overload
• Monitor temp q4hr for increased fever, indicating infection; if infection is suspected, infusion is discontinued and tubing, bottle, catheter tip cultured; blood catheter may be obtained
◆ Monitor for impending hepatic coma: asterixis, confusion, fetor, lethargy
• Hyperammonemia: nausea, vomiting, malaise, tremors, anorexia, seizures; increased ammonia, ketone levels may occur

Nursing diagnoses
• Infection, risk for (adverse reactions)
• Injury, risk for (uses, adverse reactions)
• Knowledge, deficient (teaching)
• Nutrition: less than body requirements, imbalanced (uses)

Implementation
Continuous IV route
• Give up to 40% protein and dextrose (up to 12.5%) via peripheral vein; stronger solutions require central **IV** administration; TPN only mixed with dextrose to promote protein synthesis
• Use immediately after mixing in pharmacy under strict aseptic technique using laminar

Adverse effects: *italic* = common, **bold** = life-threatening

flowhood; use infusion pump, in-line filter (0.22 µm) unless mixed with fat emulsion and dextrose (3 in 1)

⬥ Use careful monitoring technique; do not speed up infusion; pulmonary edema, glucose overload will result

• Storage depends on type of solution; consult manufacturer

• Change dressing and **IV** tubing to prevent infection q24-48hr or q5-7days if transparent dressing is used

Y-site compatibilities: Amikacin, aminophylline, amoxicillin, ampicillin, ascorbic acid inj, atracurium, azlocillin, aztreonam, bumetanide, buprenorphine, calcium gluconate, carboplatin, cefamandole, cefazolin, cefonicid, cefoperazone, cefotaxime, cefotetan, cefoxtin, ceftazidime, ceftizoxime, ceftriaxone, cefuroxime, cephalothin, cephapirin, chloramphenicol, chlorproMAZINE, cimetidine, clindamycin, clonazepam, dexamethasone, diazepam, digoxin, diphenhydrAMINE, DOBUTamine, DOPamine, doxycycline, droperidol, enalaprilat, epinephrine, erythromycin lactobionate, famotidine, fentanyl, flucloxacillin, fluconazole, folic acid, foscarnet, gentamicin, granisetron, haloperidol, heparin, hydrocortisone, hydromorphone, hydrOXYzine, idarubicin, ifosfamide, IL-2, imipenem/cilastatin, insulin (regular), isoproterenol, kanamycin, leucovorin, levorphanol, lidocaine, lorazepam, magnesium sulfate, mannitol, meperidine, mesna, methicillin, metronidazole, mezlocillin, miconazole, morphine, moxalactam, multivitamins, nafcillin, netilmicin, nitroglycerin, norepinephrine, octreotide, ofloxacin, ondansetron, oxacillin, paclitaxel, penicillin G, penicillin G potassium, pentobarbital, phenobarbital, piperacillin, potassium chloride, prochlorperazine, ranitidine, salbutamol, sargramostim, tacrolimus, thiotepa, ticarcillin, ticarcillin/clavulanate, tobramycin, trimethoprim/sulfamethoxazole, urokinase, vancomycin, vecuronium, zidovudine

Y-site incompatibilities: Cephradine
Additive compatibilities: Amikacin, aminophylline, aztreonam, calcium gluconate, cefamandole, cefazolin, cefepime, cefotaxime, cefoxitin, cefsulodin, ceftazidime, ceftriaxone, cefuroxime, cimetidine, clindamycin, cyanocobalamin, cyclophosphamide, cycloSPORINE, cytarabine, DOPamine, epoetin, erythromycin, famotidine, folic acid, fosphenytoin, furosemide, heparin, insulin (regular), isoproterenol, lidocaine, meperidine, metaraminol, methicillin, methotrexate, methyldopate, methylPREDNISolone, metoclopramide, morphine, nafcillin, netilmicin, nizatidine,

norepinephrine, ondansetron, oxacillin, penicillin G potassium, penicillin G sodium, phytonadione, polymyxin B, sodium bicarbonate, tacrolimus, tobramycin, vancomycin

Patient/family education
• Teach reason for use of amino acids as part of nutrition (TPN)
• Instruct patient to report at once to prescriber if chills, sweating are experienced

Evaluation
Positive therapeutic outcome
• Weight gain
• Decreased jaundice in liver disorders
• Increased LOC

aminophylline (theophylline ethylenediamine) (Rx)
(am-in-off'i-lin)
Phyllocontin, Truphylline
Func. class.: Bronchodilator, spasmolytic
Chem. class.: Xanthine, ethylenediamine

Pregnancy category C

Action: Exact mechanism unknown; relaxes smooth muscle of respiratory system by blocking phosphodiesterase, which increases cyclic AMP; increased cyclic AMP alters intracellular calcium ion movements; produces bronchodilatation, increased pulmonary blood flow, relaxation of respiratory tract

Therapeutic outcome: Increased ability to breathe

Uses: Apnea in infancy for respiratory/myocardial stimulation, bronchial asthma, bronchospasm associated with chronic bronchitis, emphysema, bradycardia

Unlabeled uses: Methotrexate toxicity, sleep apnea, status asthmaticus

Dosage and routes
Adult: PO 6 mg/kg, then 3 mg/kg q6hr × 2 doses, then 3 mg/kg q8hr maintenance, max 900 mg/day or 13 mg/kg; PO in CHF 6 mg/kg, then 2 mg/kg q8hr × 2 doses, then 1-2 mg/kg q12hr maintenance; **IV** 4.7 mg/kg, then 0.55 mg/kg/hr × 12 hr, then 0.36 mg/kg/hr maintenance; **IV** in CHF 4.7 mg/kg, then 0.39 mg/kg/hr × 12 hr; then 0.08-0.16 mg/kg/hr maintenance
Geriatric and in cor pulmonale: PO 6 mg/kg, then 2 mg/kg q6hr × 2 doses, then 2 mg/kg q8hr maintenance; **IV** 4.7 mg/kg, 0.47 mg/kg/hr × 12 hr, then 0.24 mg/kg/hr maintenance

Child 9-16 yr: PO 6 mg/kg, then 3 mg/kg q4hr × 3 doses, then 3 mg/kg q6hr maintenance, max 18 mg/kg/day 12-16 yr, or 20 mg/kg/day 9-12 yr; **IV** 4.7 mg/kg, then 0.79 mg/kg/hr × 12 hr, then 0.63 mg/kg/hr maintenance

Child 6 mo-9 yr: PO 4 mg/kg q4hr × 3 doses, then 4 mg/kg q6hr maintenance, max 24 mg/kg/day; **IV** 4.7 mg/kg, then 0.95 mg/kg/hr × 12 hr, then 0.79 mg/kg/hr maintenance

Infants 6-52 wk: Dose (0.2 × age in wk) ÷ 5 × kg = 24 hr dose in mg

Neonates up to 40 wk premature postconception age: PO/**IV** 1 mg/kg q12hr

Neonates at birth or 40 wk postconception age: PO/**IV** >8 wk postnatal 1-3 mg/kg q6hr; 4-8 wk postnatal 1-2 mg/kg q8hr; up to 4 wk postnatal 1-2 mg/kg q12hr

Hepatic disease
Adult: PO 6 mg/kg, then 2 mg/kg q8hr × 2 doses, then 1-2 mg/kg q12hr maintenance; **IV** 4.7 mg/kg, then 0.39 mg/kg/hr × 12 hr, then 0.08-0.16 mg/kg/hr maintenance

Available forms: Inj 250 mg/10 ml, 500 mg/20 ml, 100 mg/100 ml in 0.45% NaCl; 200 mg/100 ml in 0.45% NaCl; rectal supp 250 mg, 500 mg; oral liq 105 mg/5 ml; tabs 100, 200 mg; cont rel tabs 225, 350 mg

Adverse effects
CNS: Anxiety, restlessness, insomnia, *dizziness,* **seizures,** headache, light-headedness, muscle twitching, tremors
CV: Palpitations, sinus tachycardia, hypotension, flushing, dysrhythmias, edema
GI: Nausea, vomiting, diarrhea, dyspepsia, anal irritation (suppositories), epigastric pain, reflux, anorexia
GU: Urinary frequency, SIADH
INTEG: Flushing, urticaria
MISC: Hyperglycemia
RESP: Tachypnea, increased respiratory rate

Contraindications: Hypersensitivity to xanthines, tachydysrhythmias

Precautions: Pregnancy **C,** breastfeeding, children, geriatric, CHF, cor pulmonale, hepatic disease, diabetes mellitus, hyperthyroidism, hypertension, seizure disorder, irritation of the rectum or lower colon, alcoholism, active peptic ulcer disease

Pharmacokinetics

Absorption	Well absorbed (PO), slow (PO–EXT REL), erratic (RECT)
Distribution	Widely distributed; crosses placenta
Metabolism	Liver to caffeine
Excretion	Kidneys
Half-life	3-12 hr, increased in renal disease, CHF, geriatric patients, smokers

Pharmacodynamics

	PO	PO–EXT REL	IV
Onset	15-60 min	Unknown	Immediate
Peak	1-2 hr	4-7 hr	Infusion's end
Duration	6-8 hr	8-12 hr	6-8 hr

Interactions
Individual drugs
Allopurinol (high doses), cimetidine, clarithromycin, disulfiram, erythromycin, fluvoxamine, interferon, mexiletine: decreased metabolism, increased toxicity of aminophylline
Carbamazepine, isoniazid: increased or decreased aminophylline levels
Halothane: increased risk of dysrhythmias
Ketoconazole, phenytoin, rifampin: decreased aminophylline effect
Lithium: decreased effect of lithium
Smoking: increased metabolism, decreased effect
Drug classifications
Barbiturates, β-adrenergic blockers: decreased effect of aminophylline
Benzodiazepines, corticosteroids, diuretics (loop), fluoroquinolones, influenza vaccines, oral contraceptives: increased aminophylline levels
Corticosteroids, influenza vaccines: increased aminophylline toxicity
Diuretics (loop): may increase or decrease aminophylline levels
Dose-dependent reversal of neuromuscular blockade
Fluoroquinolones: decreased metabolism, increased toxicity
Sympathomimetics: increased CNS, CV adverse reactions
Tetracyclines: increased adverse reactions
Drug/herb
Cola tree, ginseng, guarana, horsetail, Siberian ginseng, tea (black, green), yerba maté: increased effects
St. John's wort: decreased effects
Drug/food
High-carbohydrate, low protein diet: decreased elimination

Adverse effects: *italic* = common, **bold** = life-threatening

Low-carbohydrate, high-protein diet, charcoal-broiled beef: increased elimination
Xanthines: increased effect

Drug/lab test
Increased: plasma free fatty acids

NURSING CONSIDERATIONS
Assessment
• Monitor theophylline blood levels (therapeutic level is 10-20 mcg/ml); toxicity may occur with small increase above 20 mcg/ml, especially geriatric; determine whether theophylline was given recently (24 hr); check for toxicity: nausea, vomiting, anxiety, restlessness, insomnia, tachycardia, dysrhythmias, seizures; notify prescriber immediately
• Monitor I&O; diuresis will occur; dehydration may result in geriatric or children in whom diuresis is great
• Monitor respiratory rate, rhythm, depth; auscultate lung fields bilaterally; notify prescriber of abnormalities; check ECG for tachycardia, PVCs, PACs in patients with cardiac problems
• Monitor allergic reactions: rash, urticaria; if these occur, product should be discontinued, prescriber notified

Nursing diagnoses
• Activity intolerance (uses)
• Airway clearance, ineffective (uses)
• Injury, risk for (uses, adverse reactions)
• Knowledge, deficient (teaching)

Implementation
• Give around the clock to maintain blood (theophylline) levels
• If switching from **IV** to PO, give controlled-release dose at time of **IV** infusion discontinuation; if giving tab (immediate release), discontinue **IV** and wait >4 hr
• If GI upset occurs, take with 8 oz of water or food
• Increase fluids to 2 L/day
PO route
• Do not break, crush, or chew enteric-coated or cont rel tabs
• Avoid giving with food
Rectal route
• Rectal dose if patient is unable to take PO; retain rectal dose for ½ hour
IV route
• May be diluted for **IV** inf in 100-200 ml in D_5W, $D_{10}W$, $D_{20}W$, 0.9% NaCl, 0.45% NaCl, LR
• Give loading dose over ½ hr, max rate of inf 25 mg/min, use infusion pump; after loading dose, give by cont inf
• Avoid IM inj; pain and tissue damage may occur

• Only clear sol; flush **IV** line before dose; store diluted sol for 24 hr if refrigerated
Syringe compatibilities: Heparin, metoclopramide, pentobarbital, thiopental
Y-site compatibilities: Allopurinol, amifostine, amphotericin B sulfate complex, inamrinone, aztreonam, ceftazidime, cimetidine, cladribine, DOXOrubicin liposome, enalaprilat, esmolol, famotidine, filgrastim, fluconazole, fludarabine, foscarnet, gallium, granisetron, heparin sodium with hydrocortisone sodium succinate, labetalol, melphalan, meropenem, netilmicin, paclitaxel, pancuronium, piperacillin/tazobactam, potassium chloride, propofol, ranitidine, remifentanil, sargramostim, tacrolimus, teniposide, thiotepa, tolazoline, vecuronium
Y-site incompatibilities: DOBUTamine, hydrALAZINE, ondansetron
Additive compatibilities: Amobarbital, bretylium, calcium gluconate, chloramphenicol, cibenzoline, cimetidine, dexamethasone, diphenhydrAMINE, DOPamine, erythromycin lactobionate, esmolol, floxacillin, flumazenil, furosemide, heparin, hydrocortisone, lidocaine, mephentermine, meropenem, methyldopate, metronidazole/sodium bicarbonate, nitroglycerin, pentobarbital, phenobarbital, potassium chloride, ranitidine, secobarbital, sodium bicarbonate, terbutaline
Additive incompatibilities: Ascorbic acid, bleomycin, cephalothin, cefotaxime, chlorproMAZINE, cimetidine, clindamycin, codeine, dimenhyDRINATE, DOBUTamine, DOXOrubicin, doxycycline, epinephrine, erythromycin gluceptate, hydrALAZINE, hydrOXYzine, insulin, isoproterenol, meperidine, methicillin, morphine, nafcillin, nitroprusside, norepinephrine, oxytetracycline, papaverine, penicillin G, pentazocine, phenobarbital, phenytoin, prochlorperazine, promazine, promethazine, sulfiSOXAZOLE, tetracycline, vancomycin

Patient/family education
• Teach patient to take doses as prescribed, not to skip dose; to check OTC medications, current prescription medications for ephedrine, which will increase CNS stimulation; advise patient not to drink alcohol or caffeine products (tea, coffee, chocolate, colas), which will increase action
• Teach patient to avoid hazardous activities; dizziness may occur
• Teach patient if GI upset occurs, to take product with 8 oz of water or food; absorption may be decreased

---

- Teach patient to remain in bed 15-20 min after rect supp is inserted to prevent removal
- Instruct patient to avoid smoking because it increases metabolism; decreases blood levels and terminal half-life; dosage may need to be increased
- Teach patient to obtain blood levels of product every few months to prevent toxicity; not to change brands, since effect may not be the same
- Teach patient to increase fluids to 2 L/day to decrease viscosity of secretions
- Advise patient to report toxicity: nausea, vomiting, anxiety, insomnia, rapid pulse, seizures, flushing, headache, diarrhea

Evaluation
Positive therapeutic outcome
- Decreased dyspnea
- Respiratory stimulation in infants
- Clear lung fields bilaterally

⚠ HIGH ALERT

amiodarone (Rx)
(a-mee-oh'da-rone)
Cordarone, Pacerone
Func. class.: Antidysrhythmic (Class III)
Chem. class.: Iodinated benzofuran derivative

Pregnancy category D

Do not confuse:
amiodarone/inamrinone, Cordarone/Inocor

Action: Prolongs action potential duration and effective refractory period, noncompetitive α- and β-adrenergic inhibition; increases PR and QT intervals, decreases sinus rate, decreases peripheral vascular resistance

Therapeutic outcome: Decreased amount and severity of ventricular dysrhythmias

Uses: Severe ventricular tachycardia, supraventricular tachycardia, ventricular fibrillation not controlled by 1st-line agents

Dosage and routes
Ventricular dysrhythmias
Adult: PO loading dose 800-1600 mg/day for 1-3 wk; then 600-800 mg/day × 1 mo; maintenance 400 mg/day; **IV** loading dose (first rapid) 150 mg over the first 10 min then slow 360 mg over the next 6 hr; maintenance 540 mg given over the remaining 18 hr, decrease rate of the slow infusion to 0.5 mg/min

Child: PO loading dose 10-15 mg/kg/day in 1-2 divided doses for 4-14 days then 5 mg/kg/day (not recommended in children)
Child and infant: **IV**/INTRAOSSEOUS 5 mg/kg as a bolus (PALS guidelines)
Perfusion tachycardia: **IV** 5 mg/kg loading dose given over 20-60 min

Supraventricular tachycardia
Adult: PO 600-800 mg/day × 7 days or until desired response, then 400 mg/day × 21 days, then 200-400 mg/day maintenance
Child: PO 10 mg/kg/day (800 mg/1.72 m²/day) × 10 days or until desired response, then 5 mg/kg/day (400 mg/1.72 m²/day) × 21-28 days, then 2.5 mg/kg/day (200 mg/1.72 m²/day) (not recommended in children)

Available forms: Tabs 100, 200, 400 mg; inj 50 mg/ml

Adverse effects
CNS: Headache, dizziness, involuntary movement, tremors, peripheral neuropathy, malaise, fatigue, ataxia, paresthesias, insomnia
CV: Hypotension, **bradycardia, sinus arrest, CHF, dysrhythmias, SA node dysfunction**
EENT: Blurred vision, halos, photophobia, **corneal microdeposits,** dry eyes
ENDO: Hyper/hypothyroidism
GI: Nausea, vomiting, diarrhea, abdominal pain, anorexia, constipation, **hepatotoxicity**
INTEG: Rash, photosensitivity, blue-gray skin discoloration, alopecia, spontaneous ecchymosis, **toxic epidermal necrolysis,** urticaria
MISC: Flushing, abnormal taste or smell, edema, abnormal salivation, coagulation abnormalities
MS: Weakness, pain in extremities
RESP: **Pulmonary fibrosis,** pulmonary inflammation, **ARDS, gasping syndrome in neonates**

Contraindications: Pregnancy **D,** breastfeeding, neonates, infants, severe sinus node dysfunction, hypersensitivity, 2nd- or 3rd-degree cardiogenic shock

Black Box Warning: AV block, bradycardia

Precautions: Goiter, Hashimoto's thyroiditis, electrolyte imbalances, CHF, severe respiratory disease, children

Black Box Warning: Cardiac arrhythmias, pneumonitis, pulmonary fibrosis, severe hepatic disease

---

Adverse effects: *italic* = common, **bold** = life-threatening

Pharmacokinetics

Absorption	Slow, variable (PO) up to 65%
Distribution	Body tissues; crosses placenta
Metabolism	Liver
Excretion	Bile, kidney (minimal)
Half-life	15-100 days

Pharmacodynamics

	PO
Onset	1-3 wk
Peak	Unknown
Duration	Up to months

Interactions
Individual drugs
CycloSPORINE, dextromethorphan, digoxin, disopyramide, flecainide, methotrexate, phenytoin, procainamide, quinidine, theophylline: increased blood levels, increased toxicity
Warfarin: increased bleeding
Drug classifications
β-Adrenergic blockers, calcium channel blockers: increased bradycardia
Drug/herb
Aconite: increased toxicity, death
Aloe, broom, buckthorn (chronic use), cascara sagrada (chronic use), Chinese rhubarb, figwort, fumitory, goldenseal, kudzu, licorice, senna: increased effect
Coltsfoot: decreased effect
Horehound: increased serotonin effect
Drug/food
Grapefruit juice: toxicity
Drug/lab test
Increased: T_4

NURSING CONSIDERATIONS
Assessment
- Monitor I&O ratio; monitor electrolytes: potassium, sodium, chloride
- Monitor chest x-ray, thyroid function tests
- Monitor liver function studies: AST, ALT, bilirubin, alkaline phosphatase
- Monitor ECG continuously to determine product effectiveness; measure PR, QRS, QT intervals; check for PVCs, other dysrhythmias; monitor B/P continuously for hypo/hypertension; check for rebound hypertension after 1-2 hr
- Monitor for dehydration or hypovolemia
- Assess for CNS symptoms: confusion, psychosis, numbness, depression, involuntary movements; if these occur, product should be discontinued

- Assess for hypothyroidism: lethargy, dizziness, constipation, enlarged thyroid gland, edema of extremities, cool, pale skin
- Monitor hyperthyroidism: restlessness, tachycardia, eyelid puffiness, weight loss, frequent urination, menstrual irregularities, dyspnea, warm, moist skin
- ◆ Assess for pulmonary toxicity including ARDS, pulmonary fibrosis: dyspnea, fatigue, cough, fever, chest pain; product should be discontinued if these occur
- Monitor cardiac rate, respiration: rate, rhythm, character, chest pain, ventricular tachycardia, supraventricular tachycardia or fibrillation
- Assess sight and vision before treatment and throughout therapy; microdeposits on the cornea may cause blurred vision, halos, and photophobia

Nursing diagnoses
- Cardiac output, decreased (uses)
- Gas exchange, impaired (adverse reactions)
- Knowledge, deficient (teaching)

Implementation
Start with patient hospitalized and monitored
PO route
- Give reduced dosage slowly with ECG monitoring only
- Loading dose with food to decrease nausea
Intermittent IV infusion route
- 1000 mg/24 hr during loading/maintenance
- Initial loading: add 3 ml (150 mg) 100 ml D_5W (1.5 mg/ml) give over 10 min
- Loading inf: add 18 ml (900 mg) 500 ml D_5W (1.8 mg/ml) give over next 6 hr
- Maintenance inf: Give remainder of loading inf 540 mg over 18 hr (0.5 mg/min)
Continuous infusion route
- After 24 hr, give 1-6 mg/ml at 0.5 mg/ml, max 30 mg/min
Y-site compatibilities: Amikacin, bretylium, clindamycin, DOBUTamine, DOPamine, doxycycline, erythromycin, esmolol, gentamicin, insulin (regular), isoproterenol, labetalol, lidocaine, metaraminol, metronidazole, midazolam, morphine, nitroglycerin, norepinephrine, penicillin G potassium, phentolamine, phenylephrine, potassium chloride, procainamide, tobramycin, vancomycin
Additive compatibilities: DOBUTamine, lidocaine, potassium chloride, procainamide, verapamil
Solution compatibilities: D_5W, 0.9% NaCl

Patient/family education

- Instruct patient to report side effects immediately to prescriber
- Instruct patient that skin discoloration is usually reversible, but skin may turn bluish on neck, face, arms when used for long periods
- Advise patient that dark glasses may be needed for photophobia
- Instruct patient to use sunscreen and protective clothing to prevent burning associated with photosensitivity
- Instruct patient to take medication as prescribed, not to double doses
- Instruct patient to complete follow-up appointment with health care provider including pulmonary function studies, chest x-ray, ophthalmic examinations

Evaluation

Positive therapeutic outcome

- Decreased ventricular tachycardia
- Decreased supraventricular tachycardia or fibrillation

Treatment of overdose: Administer O_2, artificial ventilation, ECG, DOPamine for circulatory depression, diazepam or thiopental for seizures, isoproterenol

amitriptyline (Rx)

(a-mee-trip'ti-leen)

amitriptyline HCl, Apo-Amitriptyline ✦
Func. class.: Antidepressant—tricyclic
Chem. class.: Tertiary amine

Pregnancy category C

Do not confuse:
amitriptyline/nortriptyline

Action: Blocks reuptake of norepinephrine, serotonin into nerve endings that increase action of norepinephrine, serotonin in nerve cells

Uses: Major depression

Unlabeled uses: Neuropathic pain, prevention of cluster/migraine headaches, fibromyalgia

Therapeutic outcome: Decreased symptoms of depression after 2-3 wk

Dosage and routes
Depression
Adult: PO 75 mg/day in divided doses; may increase to 150 mg daily, not to exceed 300 mg/day
Geriatric and adolescent: PO 10-25 mg at bedtime; may be increased to 100 mg/day

Cluster/migraine headaches (unlabeled)
Adult: PO 50-300 mg/day

Pain (unlabeled)
Adult: PO 75-300 mg/day

Fibromyalgia/insomnia (unlabeled)
Adult: PO 10-50 mg nightly

Available forms: Tabs 10, 25, 50, 75, 100, 150 mg

Adverse effects

CNS: Dizziness, drowsiness, confusion, headache, anxiety, tremors, stimulation, weakness, insomnia, nightmares, EPS (geriatric), increased psychiatric symptoms, **seizures**
CV: Orthostatic hypotension, **ECG changes, tachycardia, hypertension,** palpitations, dysrhythmias
EENT: Blurred vision, tinnitus, mydriasis, ophthalmoplegia
GI: Constipation, dry mouth, weight gain, nausea, vomiting, **paralytic ileus,** increased appetite, cramps, epigastric distress, jaundice, **hepatitis,** stomatitis
GU: Urinary retention
HEMA: **Agranulocytosis, thrombocytopenia, eosinophilia, leukopenia, aplastic anemia**
INTEG: Rash, urticaria, sweating, pruritus, photosensitivity

Contraindications: Hypersensitivity to tricyclics, recovery phase of MI

Precautions: Pregnancy C, breastfeeding, geriatric, seizure disorders, prostatic hypertrophy, schizophrenia, psychosis, severe depression, increased intraocular pressure, closed-angle glaucoma, urinary retention, cardiac disease, renal/hepatic disease, hyperthyroidism, electroshock therapy, elective surgery

Black Box Warning: Child <12 yr, suicidal patients

Pharmacokinetics

Absorption	Well absorbed
Distribution	Widely distributed; crosses placenta
Metabolism	Liver, extensively
Excretion	Kidneys, breast milk
Half-life	10-46 hr

Pharmacodynamics

	PO
Onset	45 min
Peak	2-12 hr
Duration	Unknown

Adverse effects: *italic* = common, **bold** = life-threatening

Interactions
Individual drugs
Alcohol: increased CNS depression

Amiodarone, procainamide, quinidine: increased QT prolongation

Carbamazepine: increased amitriptyline levels, increased toxicity

Cimetidine, fluoxetine: increased levels, increased toxicity

Clonidine: decreased effects

Guanethidine: decreased effects

Drug classifications
Antidepressants, antidysrhythmics (class IC), phenothiazines: increased amitriptyline levels, toxicity

Antidysrhythmics (class IA, III), tricyclic antidepressants: increased QT prolongation

Antithyroid agents: increased risk of agranulocytosis

Barbiturates, benzodiazepines, CNS depressants, opioids, sedative/hypnotics, sympathomimetics (direct acting): increased CNS effects

MAOIs: hypertensive crisis, seizures, hyperpyretic crisis

Oral contraceptives: increased effects, toxicity

Sympathomimetics (indirect acting): decreased effects

Drug/herb
Belladonna, henbane, jimsonweed, scopolia: increased anticholinergic effect

Chamomile, hops, kava, lavender, skullcap, valerian: increased CNS depression

SAM-e, St. John's wort: serotonin syndrome

Scopolia, jimsonweed: increased amitriptyline action

Yohimbe: increased hypertension

Drug/lab test
Increased: serum bilirubin, blood glucose, alkaline phosphatase

NURSING CONSIDERATIONS
Assessment
- Monitor B/P (with patient lying, standing), pulse q4hr; if systolic B/P drops 20 mm Hg, hold product, notify prescriber; take VS q4hr in patients with cardiovascular disease
- Monitor blood studies: CBC, leukocytes, differential, cardiac enzymes if patient is receiving long-term therapy
- Monitor hepatic studies: AST, ALT, bilirubin
- Check weight weekly; appetite may increase with product
- Assess ECG for flattening of T wave, bundle branch block, AV block, prolongation of QTc interval, dysrhythmias in cardiac patients
- Assess for EPS primarily in geriatric: rigidity, dystonia, akathisia
- Assess mental status: mood, sensorium, affect, suicidal tendencies; increase in psychiatric symptoms: depression, panic
- Monitor urinary retention, constipation; constipation is more likely to occur in children or geriatric
- Assess for withdrawal symptoms: headache, nausea, vomiting, muscle pain, weakness; do not usually occur unless product was discontinued abruptly
- Identify alcohol consumption; if alcohol is consumed, hold dose until morning

Nursing diagnoses
- Coping, ineffective (uses)
- Injury, risk for (side effects)
- Knowledge, deficient (teaching)
- Noncompliance (teaching)

Implementation
- Give with food or milk for GI symptoms
- Crush if patient is unable to swallow medication whole
- Give dosage at bedtime if oversedation occurs during day; may take entire dose at bedtime; geriatric may not tolerate once/day dosing
- Store at room temperature; do not freeze

Patient/family education
- Teach patient that therapeutic effects may take 2-3 wk
- Instruct patient to use caution in driving or other activities requiring alertness because of drowsiness, dizziness, blurred vision; to avoid rising quickly from sitting to standing, especially geriatric; management of anticholinergic effects
- Advise patient to avoid alcohol ingestion, other CNS depressants; overheating
- Teach patient not to discontinue medication quickly after long-term use; may cause nausea, headache, malaise
- Advise patient to wear sunscreen or large hat, since photosensitivity occurs; hyperthermia can occur
- Teach patient to increase fluids, bulk in diet if constipation, urinary retention occur, especially geriatric
- Teach patient to use gum, hard sugarless candy, or frequent sips of water for dry mouth
- Instruct patient to use contraception during treatment

Evaluation
Positive therapeutic outcome
- Decreased depression
- Absence of suicidal thoughts

Treatment of overdose: ECG monitoring, lavage, administer anticonvulsant, sodium bicarbonate

amlodipine (Rx)
(am-loe'di-peen)
Norvasc
Func. class.: Antianginal, calcium channel blocker, antihypertensive
Chem. class.: Dihydropyridine

Pregnancy category C

Do not confuse:
amlodipine/amiloride, Norvasc/Navane

Action: Inhibits calcium ion influx across cell membrane during cardiac depolarization; produces relaxation of coronary vascular smooth muscle and peripheral vascular smooth muscle; dilates coronary vascular arteries; increases myocardial oxygen delivery in patients with vasospastic angina

Therapeutic outcome: Decreased angina pectoris, dysrhythmias, B/P

Uses: Chronic stable angina pectoris, hypertension, variant angina (Prinzmetal's angina); may coadminister with other antihypertensives, antianginals

Dosage and routes
Coronary artery disease
Adult: PO 5-10 mg daily
Geriatric: PO 5 mg daily, may increase; max 10 mg/day

Hypertension
Adult: PO 5 mg daily initially, max 10 mg/day
Geriatric: PO 2.5 mg/day; may increase to 5 mg/day, max 10 mg/day

Hepatic dose/geriatric
Adult: PO 2.5 mg/day, may increase to 10 mg/day (antihypertensive); 5 mg/day, may increase to 10 mg/day (antianginal)

Available forms: Tabs 2.5, 5, 10 mg

Adverse effects
CNS: Headache, fatigue, dizziness, asthenia, anxiety, depression, insomnia, paresthesia, somnolence
CV: Peripheral edema, bradycardia, hypotension, palpitations, syncope, chest pain
GI: Nausea, vomiting, diarrhea, gastric upset, constipation, flatulence, anorexia, gingival hyperplasia, dyspepsia, dysphagia
GU: Nocturia, polyuria, sexual difficulties
INTEG: Rash, pruritus, urticaria, hair loss

MISC: Flushing, muscle cramps, cough, weight gain, tinnitus, epistaxis

Contraindications: Hypersensitivity to this product, severe aortic stenosis, severe obstructive coronary artery disease

Black Box Warning: Hypersensitivity to dihydropyridine

Precautions: Pregnancy C, breastfeeding, children, geriatric, CHF, hypotension, hepatic injury

Pharmacokinetics

Absorption	Well absorbed up to 90%
Distribution	Crosses placenta, protein binding 95%
Metabolism	Liver, extensively
Excretion	Kidneys to metabolites (90%)
Half-life	30-50 hr; increased in geriatric, hepatic disease

Pharmacodynamics

Onset	Unknown
Peak	6-10 hr
Duration	24 hr

Interactions
Individual drugs
Alcohol, fentanyl, quinidine: increased hypotension
Diltiazem: increased amlodipine level
Lithium: increased neurotoxicity
Drug classifications
Antihypertensives, nitrates: increased hypotension
NSAIDs: decreased antihypertensive effect
Drug/herb
Barberry, betel palm, burdock, goldenseal, khat, khella, lily of the valley, plantain: increased effect
Yohimbe: decreased effect
Drug/food
Grapefruit juice: increased hypotension

NURSING CONSIDERATIONS
Assessment
• Assess fluid volume status: I&O ratio and record, weight; CHF: distended red veins, crackles in lung; color, quality and specific gravity of urine, skin turgor, adequacy of pulses, moist mucous membranes, bilateral lung sounds, peripheral pitting edema; dehydration symptoms of decreasing output, thirst, hypotension, dry mouth and mucous membranes should be reported

Adverse effects: *italic* = common, **bold** = life-threatening

- Assess for angina: intensity, location, duration of pain
- Monitor B/P and pulse; if B/P drops, call prescriber
- Monitor ALT, AST, bilirubin daily; if these are elevated, hepatotoxicity is suspected
- Monitor if platelet count is <150,000/mm^3; product is usually discontinued and another product started
- Monitor cardiac status: B/P, pulse, respiration, ECG

Nursing diagnoses
- Cardiac output, decreased (uses)
- Knowledge, deficient (teaching)

Implementation
- Give once a day, without regard to meals

Patient/family education
- Advise patient to avoid hazardous activities until stabilized on product, dizziness is no longer a problem
- Instruct patient to avoid alcohol and OTC products unless directed by prescriber
- Advise patient to comply in all areas of medical regimen: diet, exercise, stress reduction, smoking cessation, product therapy; to notify prescriber of irregular heartbeat, shortness of breath, swelling of feet, face, and hands, severe dizziness, constipation, nausea, hypotension
- Teach patient to use as directed even if feeling better; may be taken with other cardiovascular products (nitrates, β-blockers)
- Advise to avoid large amounts of grapefruit juice or alcohol

Evaluation
Positive therapeutic outcome
- Decreased anginal pain
- Decreased B/P
- Increased exercise tolerance

Treatment of overdose: Defibrillation, β-agonists, **IV** calcium inotropic agents, diuretics, atropine for AV block, vasopressor for hypotension

---

amoxapine (Rx)
(a-mox′a-peen)
amoxapine, Asendin
Func. class.: Antidepressant
Chem. class.: Dibenzoxazepine derivative, secondary amine

Pregnancy category C

Do not confuse:
amoxapine/amoxicillin/Amoxil

Action: Blocks reuptake of norepinephrine, serotonin into nerve endings, thereby increasing action of norepinephrine, serotonin in nerve cells

Therapeutic outcome: Decreased symptoms of depression after 2-3 wk

Uses: Depression with anxiety or agitation

Dosage and routes
Adult: PO 50 mg bid-tid; may increase to 100 mg tid on third day of therapy; not to exceed 300 mg/day unless lower doses have been given for at least 2 wk; may be given daily dose at bedtime; not to exceed 600 mg/day in hospitalized patients
Geriatric: PO 25 mg bid-tid, may increase by 25 mg/wk, up to 300 mg/day in divided doses

Available forms: Tabs 25, 50, 100, 150 mg

Adverse effects
CNS: Dizziness, drowsiness, confusion, headache, anxiety, tremors, stimulation, weakness, insomnia, nightmares, EPS (geriatric), increased psychiatric symptoms, paresthesia, impairment of sexual functioning, **neuroleptic malignant syndrome, seizures**
CV: Orthostatic hypotension, ECG changes, tachycardia, hypertension, palpitations, **dysrhythmias**
EENT: Blurred vision, tinnitus, mydriasis, ophthalmoplegia
GI: Dry mouth, constipation, nausea, vomiting, **paralytic ileus,** increased appetite, cramps, epigastric distress, jaundice, **hepatitis,** stomatitis, weight gain
GU: Urinary retention, **acute renal failure**
HEMA: **Agranulocytosis, thrombocytopenia, eosinophilia, leukopenia**
INTEG: Rash, urticaria, sweating, pruritus, photosensitivity
META: Increased prolactin levels

Contraindications: Hypersensitivity to tricyclics, recovery phase of MI, seizure

---

disorders, prostatic hypertrophy, closed-angle glaucoma

Precautions: Pregnancy **C**, geriatric, severe depression, increased intraocular pressure, urinary retention, cardiac/hepatic disease, hyperthyroidism, electroshock therapy, elective surgery, schizophrenia, urinary retention

Black Box Warning: Suicidal patients, children

Pharmacokinetics

Absorption	Well absorbed
Distribution	Widely distributed, crosses placenta, steady state 2-7 days
Metabolism	Liver, extensively
Excretion	Kidneys, breast milk
Half-life	8 hr; metabolite 30 hr

Pharmacodynamics

Onset	1-2 wk
Peak	90 min
Duration	6-12 wk

Interactions
Individual drugs
Cimetidine, fluoxamine, paroxetine, sertraline: increased amoxapine levels, increased toxicity of amoxapine
Clonidine, epinephrine, norepinephrine: increased hypertensive effect
Mibefradil, bepridil, flecainide, probucol, propafenone, ranolazine: increased QT prolongation
Drug classifications
Barbiturates: decreased amoxapine effect
CNS depressants: increased CNS depression
◆MAOIs: hypertensive crisis, seizures, hyperpyretic crisis
Tricyclics, phenothiazines, class IA/III antidysrhythmics: increased QT prolongation
Drug/herb
Chamomile, hops, kava, lavender, skullcap, St. John's wort, valerian: increased CNS depression
Belladonna, corkwood, henbane, jimsonweed: increased anticholinergic effect
SAM-e, scopolia: increased amoxapine action
Drug/lab test
Increased: blood glucose, liver function tests
Decreased: blood glucose, WBC

NURSING CONSIDERATIONS
Assessment
- Monitor B/P (with patient lying, standing), pulse q4hr; if systolic B/P drops 20 mm Hg,

hold product, notify prescriber; take vital signs q4hr in patients with cardiovascular disease
- Assess ECG for flattening of T wave, bundle branch block, AV block, dysrhythmias in cardiac patients
- Monitor blood studies: CBC, leukocytes, differential, cardiac enzymes, LFTs, thyroid function tests if patient is receiving long-term therapy
- Monitor blood level: therapeutic 20-100 ng/ml
- Monitor hepatic studies: AST, ALT, bilirubin
- Check weight weekly; appetite may increase with product
- Assess for EPS primarily in geriatric: rigidity, dystonia, akathisia
- Assess mental status: mood, sensorium, affect, suicidal tendencies; increase in psychiatric symptoms: depression, panic; confusion (geriatric)
- Monitor urinary retention, constipation; constipation is more likely to occur in children and geriatric
- Assess for withdrawal symptoms: headache, nausea, vomiting, muscle pain, weakness; do not usually occur unless product was discontinued abruptly
- Identify alcohol consumption; if alcohol is consumed, hold dose until morning

Nursing diagnoses
- Coping, ineffective (uses)
- Injury, risk for (side effects)
- Knowledge, deficient (teaching)
- Noncompliance (teaching)

Implementation
- Give with food or milk for GI symptoms
- Crush if patient is unable to swallow medication whole
- Store at room temperature; do not freeze

Patient/family education
- Teach patient that therapeutic effects may take 2-3 wk
- Instruct patient to use caution in driving or other activities requiring alertness because of drowsiness, dizziness, blurred vision; to avoid rising quickly from sitting to standing, especially geriatric
- Teach patient to avoid alcohol ingestion, other CNS depressants, may potentiate effects
- Teach patient not to discontinue medication quickly after long-term use: may cause nausea, headache, malaise
- Teach patient to wear sunscreen or large hat, since photosensitivity occurs
- Teach patient to increase fluids, bulk in diet if constipation, urinary retention occur, especially geriatric

Adverse effects: *italic* = common, **bold** = life-threatening

- Advise patient to take gum, hard sugarless candy, or frequent sips of water for dry mouth

Evaluation
Positive therapeutic outcome
- Decreased depression
- Absence of suicidal thoughts

Treatment of overdose: ECG monitoring, induce emesis, lavage, activated charcoal, administer anticonvulsant

amoxicillin (Rx)
(a-mox-i-sill'in)
amoxicillin, Apo-Amoxi ✤, Moxtag, Novamoxin ✤, Nu-Amoxi ✤
Func. class.: Antiinfective, antiulcer
Chem. class.: Aminopenicillin

Pregnancy category B

Do not confuse:
amoxicillin/amoxapine

Action: Interferes with cell wall replication of susceptible organisms by binding to the bacterial cell wall; the cell wall, rendered osmotically unstable, swells and bursts from osmotic pressure; bactericidal, lysis mediated by bacterial cell wall autolysis

Therapeutic outcome: Bactericidal effects for the following organisms: effective for gram-positive cocci (*Staphylococcus aureus, Streptococcus pyogenes, Streptococcus faecalis, Streptococcus pneumoniae*), gram-negative cocci (*Neisseria gonorrhoeae, Neisseria meningitidis*), gram-negative bacilli (*Haemophilus influenzae, Proteus mirabilis, Salmonella*), in combination for *Helicobacter pylori*, gram-positive bacilli (*Corynebacterium diphtheriae, Listeria monocytogenes, Escherichia coli*)

Uses: Infections of respiratory tract, skin, gastrointestinal tract, genitourinary tract, otitis media, meningitis, septicemia, sinusitis, and bacterial endocarditis prophylaxis in combination with other products used for treatment of *Helicobacter pylori*

Unlabeled uses: Lyme disease, anthrax treatment and prophylaxis

Dosage and routes
Renal disease
Adult: PO CCr 10-30 ml/min 250-500 mg q12hr; CCr <10 ml/min 250-500 mg q24hr; do not use 875 mg strength if CCr <50 ml/min

Systemic infections
Adult: PO 750 mg-1.75 g daily in divided doses q8hr or q12hr
Child: PO 20-50 mg/kg/day in divided doses q8hr

Gonorrhea/urinary tract infections
Adult: PO 3 g given with 1 g probenecid as a single dose; followed by tetracycline or erythromycin

Chlamydia trachomatis
Adult: PO 500 mg/day × 1 wk

Bacterial endocarditis prophylaxis
Adult: PO 2 g 1 hr prior to procedure
Child: PO 50 mg/kg/hr 1 hr prior to procedure, max 2 g

Helicobacter pylori
Adult: PO 1000 mg bid given with lansoprazole 30 mg bid, clarithromycin 500 mg bid × 2 wk; or 1000 mg bid given with omeprazole 20 mg bid, clarithromycin 500 mg bid × 2 wk; or 1000 mg tid given with lansoprazole 30 mg tid × 2 wk

Available forms: Caps 250, 500 mg; chewable tabs 125, 200, 250, 400 mg; tabs 500, 875 mg; susp pedidrops 50 mg/ml; susp 125, 200, 250, 400 mg/5 ml

Adverse effects
CNS: Headache, **seizures,** agitation, confusion, dizziness
GI: Nausea, vomiting, diarrhea, increased AST, ALT, abdominal pain, glossitis, colitis, **pseudomembranous colitis**
HEMA: Anemia, increased bleeding time, **bone marrow depression, granulocytopenia, hemolytic anemia**
INTEG: Urticaria, rash
SYST: **Anaphylaxis, respiratory distress, serum sickness, Stevens-Johnson syndrome**

Contraindications: Hypersensitivity to penicillins

Precautions: Pregnancy **B,** breastfeeding, neonates, hypersensitivity to cephalosporins, severe renal disease, acute lymphocytic leukemia

Pharmacokinetics	
Absorption	Well absorbed (90%)
Distribution	Readily in body tissues, fluids, CSF; crosses placenta
Metabolism	Liver (30%)
Excretion	Breast milk, kidney, unchanged (70%)
Half-life	1-1.3 hr

 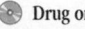

Pharmacodynamics	
Onset	½ hr
Peak	2 hr
Duration	Unknown

Interactions
Individual drugs
Methotrexate: increased methotrexate levels
Probenecid: increased amoxicillin levels, decreased renal excretion
Warfarin: increased anticoagulant effects
Drug classifications
Contraceptives (oral): decreased contraceptive effectiveness
Drug/herb
Acidophilus: do not use with antiinfectives, separate by several hours
Khat: decreased absorption, separate by 2 hr
Drug/lab test
False positive: urine glucose, urine protein, direct Coombs' test

NURSING CONSIDERATIONS
Assessment
• Assess patient for previous sensitivity reaction to penicillins or other cephalosporins; cross-sensitivity between penicillins and cephalosporins is common
• Assess patient for signs and symptoms of infection, including characteristics of wounds, sputum, urine, stool, WBC >10,000/mm^3, earache, fever; obtain baseline information and monitor symptoms during treatment
• Obtain C&S before beginning product therapy to identify if correct treatment has been initiated
• Assess for allergic reactions during treatment: rash, urticaria, pruritus, chills, fever, joint pain; angioedema may occur a few days after therapy begins; epinephrine and resuscitation equipment should be available for anaphylactic reactions
• Identify urine output; if decreasing, notify prescriber (may indicate nephrotoxicity); also, increased BUN, creatinine, urinalysis, protein, blood
• Monitor blood studies: AST, ALT, CBC, Hct, bilirubin, LDH, alkaline phosphatase, Coombs' test monthly if patient is on long-term therapy
• Monitor electrolytes: potassium, sodium, chloride monthly if patient is on long-term therapy
• Assess bowel pattern daily; diarrhea, cramping, blood in stools; if severe diarrhea occurs, notify prescriber; product should be discontinued; pseudomembranous colitis may occur

• Monitor for bleeding: ecchymosis, bleeding gums, hematuria, stool guaiac daily if on long-term therapy
• Assess for overgrowth of infection: perineal itching, fever, malaise, redness, pain, swelling, drainage, rash, diarrhea, change in cough, sputum

Nursing diagnoses
• Diarrhea (side effects)
• Infection, risk for (uses)
• Injury, risk for (side effects)
• Knowledge, deficient (teaching)
• Noncompliance (teaching)

Implementation
PO route
• Give in even doses around the clock; if GI upset occurs, give with food; product must be given for 10-14 days to ensure organism death and prevent superinfection; store in tight container
• The caps may be opened and contents taken with fluids
• Shake susp well before each dose, may be used alone or mixed in drinks, use immediately; susp may be stored in refrigerator for 14 days

Patient/family education
⚕ Teach patient to report sore throat, bruising, bleeding, joint pain; may indicate blood dyscrasias (rare)
• Advise patient to contact prescriber if vaginal itching, loose foul-smelling stools, diarrhea, sore throat, fever, fatigue, furry tongue occur; may indicate superinfection or agranulocytopenia
• Instruct patient to take all medication prescribed for the length of time ordered; not to double dose; chew form is available
• Advise patient to notify prescriber of diarrhea with blood or pus, which may indicate pseudomembranous colitis

Evaluation
Positive therapeutic outcome
• Absence of signs/symptoms of infection (WBC <10,000/mm^3, temp WNL, absence of red draining wounds or earache)
• Prevention of endocarditis
• Resolution of ulcer symptoms

Treatment of anaphylaxis: Withdraw product, maintain airway, administer epinephrine, aminophylline, O$_2$, **IV** corticosteroids

Adverse effects: *italic* = common, **bold** = life-threatening

amoxicillin/clavulanate (Rx)
(a-mox-i-sill'in)
Augmentin, Augmentin ES-600,
Augmentin XR, Clavulin ✤
Func. class.: Broad-spectrum antiinfective
(extended spectrum)
Chem. class.: Aminopenicillin-β-lactamase
inhibitor

Pregnancy category B

Action: Interferes with cell wall replication
of susceptible organisms; the cell wall, rendered osmotically unstable, swells and bursts
from osmotic pressure; lysis mediated by
bacterial cell wall autolytic enzymes, combination increases spectrum of activity against
β-lactamase resistance organisms

Therapeutic outcome: Bactericidal
effects for the following organisms: *Escherichia coli, Proteus mirabilis, Haemophilus
influenzae, Streptococcus faecalis, Streptococcus pneumoniae;* and β-lactamase–
producing organisms: *Neisseria gonorrhoeae,
Neisseria meningitidis, Shigella, Salmonella,
Enterococcus, Streptococcus*

Uses: Infections of respiratory tract, skin,
genitourinary tract; otitis media, sinusitis, and
endocarditis prophylaxis

Dosage and routes
Adult: PO 250-500 mg q8hr or 500-875 mg
q12hr depending on severity of infection
Child ≤40 kg: PO 20-90 mg/kg/day in
divided doses q8-12hr

Renal dose
Adult: PO CCr 10-30 ml/min dose q12hr;
CCr <10 ml/min dose q24hr; do not use 875
mg strength if CCr <30 ml/min; Augmentin XR
is contraindicated in renal disease

Available forms: Tabs 250, 500, 875
mg/125 mg clavulanate; chewable tabs 125,
200, 250, 400 mg; powder for oral susp 125,
200, 250, 400 mg/5 ml; (XR) ext rel tabs 1000
mg amoxicillin/62.5 mg clavulanate; (ES)
powder for oral susp 600 mg amoxicillin; 42.9
mg clavulanate 5 ml

Adverse effects
CNS: Headache, fever, **seizures**
GI: Nausea, diarrhea, vomiting, increased
AST, ALT, abdominal pain, glossitis, colitis,
black tongue, **pseudomembranous colitis**
GU: Oliguria, proteinuria, hematuria, *vagini-
tis, moniliasis,* **glomerulonephritis**
HEMA: Anemia, **bone marrow depression,
granulocytopenia, leukopenia, eosino-
philia,** thrombocytopenic purpura

INTEG: Rash, urticaria, dermatitis, **toxic
epidermal necrolysis**
META: Hyperkalemia, hypokalemia, alkalosis,
hypernatremia
SYST: **Anaphylaxis, respiratory distress,
serum sickness, superinfection, Stevens-
Johnson syndrome**

Contraindications: Hypersensitivity to
penicillins

Precautions: Pregnancy **B,** breastfeeding,
neonates, hypersensitivity to cephalosporins,
GI/renal disease

Pharmacokinetics
Absorption	Well absorbed (90%)
Distribution	Readily in body tissues, fluids, CSF; crosses placenta
Metabolism	Liver (30%)
Excretion	Breast milk; kidney, unchanged (70%), removed by hemodialysis
Half-life	1-1.3 hr

Pharmacodynamics
Onset	½ hr
Peak	2 hr
Duration	Unknown

Interactions
Individual drugs
Allopurinol: increased skin rash
Probenecid: increased amoxicillin levels
Warfarin: increased anticoagulant effect
Drug classifications
Contraceptives (oral): decreased contraceptive
effectiveness
Drug/herb
Acidophilus: do not use with antiinfectives;
separate by several hours
Khat: decreased absorption, separate by 2 hr
Drug/lab test
False positive: urine glucose, urine protein,
direct Coombs' test

NURSING CONSIDERATIONS
Assessment
• Assess patient for previous sensitivity reaction to penicillins or other cephalosporins;
cross-sensitivity between penicillins and
cephalosporins is common
• Assess patient for signs and symptoms of
infection, including characteristics of wounds,
sputum, urine, stool, WBC >10,000/mm^3,
earache, fever; obtain baseline information
and during treatment

- Complete C&S before beginning product therapy to identify if correct treatment has been initiated
- Assess for anaphylaxis: rash, urticaria, pruritus, chills, dyspnea, laryngeal edema, fever, joint pain; angioedema may occur a few days after therapy begins; epinephrine and resuscitation equipment should be available for anaphylactic reaction
- Identify urine output; if decreasing, notify prescriber (may indicate nephrotoxicity)
- Monitor renal studies: urinalysis, protein, blood, BUN, creatinine
- Monitor blood studies: AST, ALT, CBC, Hct, bilirubin, LDH, alkaline phosphatase, Coombs' test monthly if patient is on long-term therapy
- Monitor electrolytes: potassium, sodium, chloride monthly if patient is on long-term therapy
- Assess bowel pattern daily; diarrhea, cramping, blood in stools, report to prescriber; if severe diarrhea occurs, product should be discontinued; may indicate pseudomembranous colitis
- Monitor for bleeding: ecchymosis, bleeding gums, hematuria, stool guaiac daily if on long-term therapy
- Assess for overgrowth of infection: perineal itching, fever, malaise, redness, pain, swelling, drainage, rash, diarrhea, change in cough, sputum

Nursing diagnoses
- Diarrhea (side effects)
- Infection, risk for (uses)
- Injury, risk for (side effects)
- Knowledge, deficient (teaching)
- Noncompliance (teaching)

Implementation
PO route
- Give in even doses around the clock; if GI upset occurs, give with food; product must be taken for 10-14 days to ensure organism death and prevent superinfection; store in tight container; cap can be opened and mixed with food or liquid; chewable tabs should be chewed
- Administer only as directed; two 250-mg tabs not equivalent to one 500-mg tab due to strength of clavulanate
- Shake susp well before each dose; may be used alone or mixed in drinks, use immediately; susp may be stored in refrigerator for 10 days

Patient/family education
⊕ Teach patient to report sore throat, bruising, bleeding, joint pain; may indicate blood dyscrasias (rare)

- Advise patient to contact prescriber if vaginal itching, loose foul-smelling stools occur; may indicate superinfection
- Instruct patient to take all medication prescribed for the length of time prescribed
- Advise patient to notify prescriber of diarrhea with blood or pus, which may indicate pseudomembranous colitis
- Advise patient to use alternative contraceptive measures if using oral contraceptives

Evaluation
Positive therapeutic outcome
- Absence of signs/symptoms of infection (WBC <10,000/mm^3, temp WNL)
- Reported improvement in symptoms of infection

Treatment of anaphylaxis: Withdraw product, maintain airway, administer epinephrine, aminophylline, O_2, **IV** corticosteroids

---

AMPHOTERICIN B

amphotericin B deoxycholate (Rx)
(am-foh-tehr'ih-sin de-ox-ee-kohl'ate)
Fungizone
amphotericin B cholesteryl (Rx)
Amphotec
amphotericin B lipid based (Rx)
Abelcet
amphotericin B liposome (Rx)
AmBisome
Func. class.: Antifungal
Chem. class.: Amphoteric polyene
Pregnancy category B

Action: Increased cell membrane permeability in susceptible organisms by binding sterols in fungal cell membrane, causing leakage of cell components and cell death

Therapeutic outcome: Fungistatic against histoplasmosis, blastomycosis, coccidioidomycosis, cryptococcosis, aspergillosis, zygomycosis, candidiasis, sporotrichosis, cryptococcal meningitis, mucormycosis caused by mucormycosis, *Rhizopus, Absidia, Entomorphthera, Basidobolus*

Uses: Treatment of severe, possibly fatal fungal infections (**IV**); treatment of topical fungal infections

Unlabeled uses: Candiduria (bladder irrigation), funguria

Dosage and routes
Fungizone
Adult: **IV** give test dose of 1 mg (not required); then 0.25 mg/kg, increase daily slowly to 0.5 mg/kg, may give 1 mg/kg/day or 1.5 mg/kg/day, alternate day dosing may be used

Child: **IV** 0.25 mg/kg infused initially, increase by 0.25 mg/kg every other day to max of 1 mg/kg/day

Adult and child: TOP apply 2-4 × daily

Adult and child: PO 1 ml qid

Amphotec
Adult and child: **IV** 3-4 mg/kg/day, max 7.5 mg/kg/day

Abelcet
Adult and child: **IV** 5 mg/kg/day as a 1 mg/ml INF given 2.5 mg/kg/hr

AmBisome
Fungal infections
Adult and child: **IV** 3-5 mg/kg q24hr

Visceral leishmaniasis: 3 mg/kg q24hr days 1-5

Available forms: Amphotericin deoxycholate: inj 50-mg vial, oral susp 100 mg/ml; cream, ointment, lotion 3%; amphotericin B cholesteryl: powder for inj 50 mg/20 ml, 100 mg/50 ml; amphotericin B lipid complex: susp for inj 100 mg/20 ml vial; amphotericin B liposome: powder for inj 50 mg vial

Adverse effects
CNS: Headache, fever, chills, peripheral nerve pain, paresthesias, peripheral neuropathy, **seizures,** dizziness
EENT: Tinnitus, deafness, diplopia, blurred vision
GI: Nausea, vomiting, anorexia, diarrhea, cramps, **hemorrhagic gastroenteritis, acute liver failure**
GU: Hypokalemia, axotemia, hyposthenuria, **renal tubular acidosis,** nephrocalcinosis, **permanent renal impairment, anuria, oliguria**
HEMA: Normochromic and normocytic anemia, **thrombocytopenia, agranulocytosis, leukopenia, eosinophilia,** hypokalemia, hyponatremia, hypomagnesemia

INTEG: Burning, irritation, pain, necrosis at inj site with extravasation, flushing, dermatitis, skin rash (topical route)
MS: Arthralgia, myalgia, generalized pain, weakness, weight loss
SYST: **Stevens-Johnson syndrome, toxic epidermal necrolysis, exfoliative dermatitis**

Contraindications: Hypersensitivity, severe bone marrow depression

Precautions: Pregnancy **B,** breastfeeding, children, renal disease, anemia, hypokalemia, hypomagnesium, infections

Black Box Warning: Fungal infection

Pharmacokinetics

Absorption	Complete bioavailability (**IV**), rapidly absorbed (TOP)
Distribution	Body tissues
Metabolism	Liver
Excretion	Kidneys, detectable for several weeks
Half-life	Initial 24-48 hr, terminal 15 days

Pharmacodynamics

	IV	TOP
Onset	Immediate	Unknown
Peak	1-2 hr	Unknown
Duration	Unknown	Unknown

Interactions
Individual drugs
Cisplatin, cycloSPORINE, polymyxin B, vancomycin: increased nephrotoxicity
Digoxin: increased hypokalemia
Drug classifications
Nephrotoxic antibiotics: increased nephrotoxicity
Glucocorticoids, thiazides, skeletal muscle relaxants: increased hypokalemia
Drug/herb
Acidophilus: do not use with antiinfectives; separate by several hours
Gossypol: increased risk of nephrotoxicity

NURSING CONSIDERATIONS
Assessment
- Monitor VS q15-30min during first inf; note changes in pulse, B/P
- Monitor blood studies: Hgb, Hct, potassium, sodium, calcium, magnesium q2wk; BUN, creatinine weekly; decreased Hgb, Hct, and magnesium are common with increased potassium
- Monitor weight weekly; if weight increases over 2 lb/wk, edema is present; renal damage should be considered

- Monitor for renal toxicity: increasing BUN, serum creatinine; if BUN is >40 mg/dl or if serum creatinine >3 mg/dl, product may be discontinued or dosage reduced; I&O ratio: watch for decreasing urinary output, change in specific gravity; discontinue product to prevent permanent damage to renal tubules; provide hydration of 2-3 L/day
- Monitor for hepatotoxicity: increasing AST, ALT, alkaline phosphatase, bilirubin
- Monitor for allergic reaction: dermatitis, rash; product should be discontinued, antihistamines (mild reaction) or epinephrine (severe reaction) administered; check inj site for thrombophlebitis
- Monitor for hypokalemia: anorexia, drowsiness, weakness, decreased reflexes, dizziness, increased urinary output, increased thirst, paresthesias; if these occur, product should be decreased or discontinued and potassium administered

Topical route
- Monitor for allergic reaction: burning, stinging, swelling, redness

Nursing diagnoses
- Infection, risk for (uses)
- Injury, risk for (adverse reaction)
- Knowledge, deficient (teaching)

Implementation
Topical route
- Provide enough medication to cover lesions completely; do not cover with occlusive dressing; apply liberally and rub thoroughly into affected area; administer after cleansing with soap, water before each application; dry well (as ordered); wear gloves during application
- Store at room temperature in dry place

Deoxycholate
Intermittent IV infusion route
- Give after diluting 50 mg in 10 ml sterile water (no preservatives) (5 mg-1 ml); shake well, further dilute with 500 ml of D₅W to concentration of 0.1 mg/ml; do not use other diluents or sol; use large needle (20G); change needle for each step; wear gloves
- Use test dosage of 1 mg/20 ml D₅W; give over 10-30 min; if no reaction, product is administered as ordered
- Administer **IV** using in-line filter (mean pore diameter >1 μm) using distal veins; check for extravasation, necrosis q8hr; use an infusion pump; administer over 6 hr; rapid inf may result in circulation collapse; may also be given through central line
- Give acetaminophen and diphenhydrAMINE

30 min before inf to reduce fever, chills, headache
- Give product only after C&S confirm organism, product needed to treat condition; make sure product is used in life-threatening infections
- Store protected from moisture and light; diluted sol is stable for 24 hr at room temperature, 1 wk refrigerated

Syringe compatibilities: Heparin
Y-site compatibilities: Aldesleukin, diltiazem, DOXOrubicin liposome, famotidine, remifentanil, tacrolimus, teniposide, thiotepa, zidovudine
Y-site incompatibilities: Enalaprilat, fludarabine, foscarnet, ondansetron
Additive compatibilities: Fluconazole, heparin, hydrocortisone, methylPREDNISolone, sodium bicarbonate
Solution compatibilities: D₅W

Cholesteryl
Liposomal complex
IV route
- Reconstitute with 12 ml sterile water/50 ml vial (4 mg/ml), shake, use 5-micron filter, dilute in D₅W (1-2 mg/ml), give over 2 hr

Lipid complex
IV route
- Shake vial until dissolved, withdraw dose using 18-G needle, replace needle from syringe with product using 5-micron filter needle (use needle for 4 vials or less), empty contents in **IV** of D₅W (1 mg/ml), give at 2.5 mg/kg/hr, use infusion pump

Patient/family education
Topical route
- Teach patient that skin and clothing may become discolored; to use asepsis (hand washing) before, after each application to prevent further infection
- Instruct patient to apply with glove to prevent further infection; not to cover with occlusive dressing; to continue even if condition improves
- Teach patient to avoid use of OTC creams, ointments, lotions, unless directed by prescriber
- Instruct patient to report increased itching, burning, rash, redness; ointment may irritate most hairy areas; to report if condition worsens

IV route
- Advise patient that long-term therapy may be needed to clear infection (2 wk-3 mo depending on type of infection)
- Teach patient side effects and when to notify prescriber

Adverse effects: *italic* = common, **bold** = life-threatening

Evaluation
Positive therapeutic outcome
- Decreased in size, number of lesions (TOP)
- Decreased fever, malaise, rash
- Negative C&S for infecting organism

---

ampicillin (Rx)
(am-pi-sill'in)
Ampicin ✤, Apo-Ampi ✤,
NovoAmpicillin ✤, Nu-Ampi ✤,
Omnipen, Penbriten ✤, Principen
Func. class.: Broad-spectrum antiinfective
Chem. class.: Aminopenicillin

Pregnancy category B

Do not confuse:
Omnipen/imipenem

Action: Interferes with cell wall replication of susceptible organisms; the cell wall, rendered osmotically unstable, swells and bursts from osmotic pressure, lysis mediated by cell wall autolysis

Therapeutic outcome: Bactericidal effects for the following organisms: effective for gram-positive cocci *(Streptococcus aureus, Streptococcus pyogenes, Streptococcus faecalis, Streptococcus pneumoniae),* gram-negative cocci *(Neisseria gonorrhoeae),* gram-negative bacilli *(Haemophilus influenzae, Proteus mirabilis, Salmonella, Shigella, Listeria monocytogenes),* gram-positive bacilli

Uses: Infections of respiratory tract, skin, skin structures, genitourinary tract; otitis media, meningitis, septicemia, sinusitis, and endocarditis prophylaxis

Dosage and routes
Renal dose
Adult and child: CCr 30-50 ml/min q6-8hr; CCr 10-30 ml/min dose q8-12hr; CCr <10 ml/min dose q12hr

Systemic infections
Adult and child ≥40 kg (88 lb): PO 250-500 mg q6hr; **IV**/IM 2-8 g daily in divided doses q4-6hr
Child <40 kg: PO 50-100 mg/kg/day in divided doses q6-8hr; **IV**/IM 100-200 mg/kg/day in divided doses q6-8hr

Bacterial meningitis
Adult: IM/**IV** 500 mg-3 g q6hr, max 14 g/day
Child: IM/**IV** 200-400 mg/kg/day in divided doses q6hr, max 12 g/day

Gonorrhea
Adult and child ≥ 45 kg (99 lb): PO 3.5 g given with 1 g probenecid as a single dose

Prevention of bacterial endocarditis
Adult: IM/**IV** 2 g 30 min before procedure
Child: IM/**IV** 50 mg/kg 30 min before procedure, max 2 g

GI/GU infections other than caused by N. gonorrhoeae
Adult and child >20 kg: PO 250-500 mg q6hr, may use larger dose for more serious infections
Child ≤20 kg: PO 50-100 mg/kg/day in divided doses q6hr

Available forms: Powder for inj 125, 250, 500 mg, 1, 2, 10 g; **IV** inf 500 mg, 1, 2 g; caps 250, 500 mg; powder for oral susp, 125, 250, 500 mg/5 ml

Adverse effects
CNS: Lethargy, hallucinations, anxiety, depression, twitching, **coma, seizures**
GI: Nausea, vomiting, diarrhea, **pseudomembranous colitis,** stomatitis
GU: Oliguria, proteinuria, hematuria, *vaginitis, moniliasis,* **glomerulonephritis**
HEMA: Anemia, increased bleeding time, **bone marrow depression, granulocytopenia, leukopenia, eosinophilia**
INTEG: Rash, urticaria, **toxic epidermal necrolysis**
SYST: **Anaphylaxis, serum sickness, Stevens-Johnson syndrome**

Contraindications: Hypersensitivity to penicillins

Precautions: Pregnancy **B,** breastfeeding, neonates, hypersensitivity to cephalosporins, renal disease

Pharmacokinetics	
Absorption	Moderate, in duodenum (35%-50%)
Distribution	Readily in body tissues, fluids, CSF; crosses placenta
Metabolism	Liver (30%)
Excretion	Breast milk; kidney unchanged (70%), removed by dialysis
Half-life	50-110 min

Pharmacodynamics			
	PO	IM	IV
Onset	Rapid	Rapid	Rapid
Peak	2 hr	1 hr	Infusion's end
Duration	Unknown	Unknown	Unknown

⬥ Alert   ✤ Canada Only   ⊙ Drug on CD   ✳ "Tall Man" lettering (See Preface)

Interactions
Individual drugs
Allopurinol: increased ampicillin-induced skin rash
Probenecid: increased ampicillin levels, decreased renal excretion
Drug classifications
Contraceptives (oral): decreased contraceptive effectiveness
Drug/herb
Acidophilus: do not use with antiinfectives; separate by several hours
Khat: decreased absorption, separate by 2 hr
Drug/lab test
Increased: AST, ALT
Decreased: conjugated estrone in pregnancy, conjugated estriol
False positive: urine glucose, urine protein, direct Coombs' test

NURSING CONSIDERATIONS
Assessment
• Assess patient for previous sensitivity reaction to penicillins or other cephalosporins; cross-sensitivity between penicillins and cephalosporins is common
• Assess patient for signs and symptoms of infection, including characteristics of wounds, sputum, urine, stool, WBC >10,000/mm³, earache, fever; obtain baseline information and during treatment
• Obtain C&S before beginning product therapy to identify if correct treatment has been initiated
• Assess for allergic reactions: rash, urticaria, pruritus, chills, fever, joint pain; angioedema may occur a few days after therapy begins; epinephrine and resuscitation equipment should be on unit for anaphylactic reaction; also, check for ampicillin rash: pruritic, red, raised
◆ Identify urine output; if decreasing, notify prescriber (may indicate nephrotoxicity)
• Monitor renal studies: urinalysis, protein, blood, BUN, creatinine
• Monitor blood studies: AST, ALT, CBC, Hct, bilirubin, LDH, alkaline phosphatase, Coombs' test monthly if patient is on long-term therapy
• Monitor electrolytes: potassium, sodium, chloride monthly if patient is on long-term therapy
• Assess bowel pattern daily; if severe diarrhea occurs, product should be discontinued; may indicate pseudomembranous colitis
• Monitor for bleeding: ecchymosis, bleeding gums, hematuria, stool guaiac daily if on long-term therapy

• Assess for overgrowth of infection: perineal itching, fever, malaise, redness, pain, swelling, drainage, rash, diarrhea, change in cough, sputum

Nursing diagnoses
• Diarrhea (side effects)
• Infection, risk for (uses)
• Injury, risk for (side effects)
• Knowledge, deficient (teaching)
• Noncompliance (teaching)

Implementation
PO route
• Give in even doses around the clock; product must be taken for 10-14 days to ensure organism death and prevent superinfection; store caps in tight container
• Tabs may be crushed or caps opened and mixed with water
• Shake susp well before each dose; store in refrigerator for 2 wk or 1 wk at room temperature
IM route
• Reconstitute with 125 mg/0.9-1.2 ml; 250 mg/0.9-1.9 ml; 500 mg/1.2-1.8 ml; 1 g/2.4-7.4 ml; 2 g/6.8 ml
• Give deep in large muscle mass
IV route
• Reconstitute with 125 mg/0.9-1.2 ml; 250 mg/0.9-1.9 ml; 500 mg/1.2-1.8 ml; 1 g/2.4-7.4 ml; 2 g/6.8 ml
• Give by direct **IV** over 3-5 min in lower dosages (125-500 mg) or over 15 min in higher dosages (1-2 g)
• Give by intermittent inf after diluting with 0.9% NaCl, LR, D₅W, D₅/0.45% NaCl; use 50 ml of sol and dilute to concentration of <30 mg/ml
Syringe compatibilities: Chloramphenicol
Syringe incompatibilities: Erythromycin, gentamicin, kanamycin, lincomycin, metoclopramide, oxytetracycline, streptomycin, tetracycline
Y-site compatibilities: Acyclovir, amifostine, allopurinol, aztreonam, cyclophosphamide, DOXOrubicin liposome, enalaprilat, esmolol, famotidine, filgrastim, fludarabine, foscarnet, granisetron, heparin, regular insulin, labetalol, magnesium sulfate, melphalan, meperidine, morphine, multivitamins, oflaxacin, perphenazine, phytonadione, potassium chloride, propofol, remifentanil, thiotepa, tolazoline, vit B with C
Y-site incompatibilities: Calcium gluconate, epinephrine, fluconazole, hetastarch, hydromorphone, hydrALAZINE,

Adverse effects: *italic* = common, **bold** = life-threatening

ondansetron, sargramostim, verapamil, vinorelbine

Additive compatibilities: Clindamycin, erythromycin, floxacillin, furosemide, tacrolimus, teniposide, theophylline, verapamil

Additive incompatibilities: Amikacin, aztreonam, chlorproMAZINE, DOPamine, gentamicin, hydrALAZINE, hydrocortisone, prochlorperazine

Patient/family education

⬥ Teach patient to report sore throat, bruising, bleeding, joint pain; may indicate blood dyscrasias (rare)

• Advise patient to contact prescriber if vaginal itching, loose foul-smelling stools, furry tongue occur; may indicate superinfection

• Instruct patient to take all medication prescribed for the length of time ordered

• Advise patient to notify prescriber of diarrhea with blood or pus, which may indicate pseudomembranous colitis

• Tab may be crushed; cap may be opened and mixed with water

Evaluation

Positive therapeutic outcome

• Absence of signs/symptoms of infection (WBC <10,000, temp WNL)

• Reported improvement in symptoms of infection

Treatment of anaphylaxis: Withdraw product, maintain airway, administer epinephrine, aminophylline, O₂, **IV** corticosteroids

---

ampicillin/sulbactam (Rx)

(am-pi-sill'in/sul-bak'tam)

Unasyn

Func. class.: Broad-spectrum antiinfective
Chem. class.: Aminopenicillin

Pregnancy category B (ampicillin)

Action: Interferes with cell wall replication of susceptible organisms; the cell wall, rendered osmotically unstable, swells and bursts from osmotic pressure; lysis due to cell wall autolytic enzymes; this combination extends the spectrum of activity and inhibits β-lactamase that may inactivate ampicillin

Therapeutic outcome: Bactericidal against *Staphylococcus aureus, Klebsiella, Bacteroides fragilis, Enterobacter, Acinetobacter calcoaceticus, Pneumococcus, Enterococcus, Streptococcus, Escherichia coli, Proteus mirabilis, Neisseria meningitidis,*

Neisseria gonorrhoeae, Shigella, Salmonella, and *Haemophilus influenzae* organisms; use only with β-lactamase–producing strain of infection

Uses: Skin infections, intraabdominal infections, pneumonia, gynecologic infections, soft tissue infections, otitis media, sinusitis, meningitis, septicemia

Dosage and routes

Adult and child >40 kg: IM/**IV** 1 g ampicillin and 0.5 g sulbactam to 2 g ampicillin, and 1 g sulbactam q6hr, not to exceed 4 g/day sulbactam

Child <40 kg: **IV** 100-200 mg/kg/day (ampicillin component) divided q6hr, max 8 g/day

Renal dose

Adult ≥40 kg: IM/**IV** CCr 15-29 ml/min dose q12hr; CCr 5-14 ml/min dose q24hr

Available forms: Powder for inj 1.5 g (1 g ampicillin, 0.5 g sulbactam), 3 g (2 g ampicillin, 1 g sulbactam), 10 g (10 g ampicillin, 5 g sulbactam)

Adverse effects

CNS: Lethargy, hallucinations, anxiety, depression, twitching, **coma, seizures**

GI: Nausea, vomiting, diarrhea, increased AST, ALT, abdominal pain, glossitis, colitis, **pseudomembranous colitis,** hepatic necrosis/failure

GU: Oliguria, proteinuria, hematuria, *vaginitis, moniliasis,* **glomerulonephritis,** dysuria

HEMA: Anemia, increased bleeding time, **bone marrow depression, granulocytopenia, leukopenia, eosinophilia**

SYST: **Anaphylaxis, serum sickness, toxic epidermal necrolysis, Stevens-Johnson syndrome**

Contraindications: Hypersensitivity to penicillins, ampicillin, or sulbactam

Precautions: Pregnancy B, breastfeeding, neonates, hypersensitivity to cephalosporins, renal disease

Pharmacokinetics	
Absorption	Well absorbed (IM)
Distribution	Readily in body tissues, fluids, CSF; crosses placenta
Metabolism	Liver (10%-50%)
Excretion	Breast milk; kidney unchanged (75%)
Half-life	50-110 min (ampicillin)

 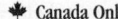

Pharmacodynamics

	IM	IV
Onset	Rapid	Immediate
Peak	1 hr	Infusion's end
Duration	Unknown	Unknown

Interactions
Individual drugs
Allopurinol: ampicillin-induced skin rash
Disulfiram: increased ampicillin level
Methotrexate: increased methotrexate level
Probenecid: increased ampicillin levels,
    decreased renal excretion
Drug classifications
Contraceptives (oral): decreased contraceptive
    effectiveness
Drug/herb
Acidophilus: do not use with antiinfectives;
    separate by several hours
Khat: decreased absorption; separate by 2 hr
Drug/lab test
False positive: urine glucose, urine protein

NURSING CONSIDERATIONS
Assessment
• Assess patient for previous sensitivity reaction to penicillins or cephalosporins; cross-sensitivity between penicillins and cephalosporins is common
• Assess patient for signs and symptoms of infection; including characteristics of wounds, sputum, urine, stool, WBC >10,000/mm³, earache, fever; obtain baseline information and during treatment
• Complete C&S before beginning product therapy to identify if correct treatment has been initiated
• Assess for allergic reactions: rash, urticaria, pruritus, chills, fever, joint pain; angioedema may occur a few days after therapy begins; epinephrine and resuscitation equipment should be on unit for anaphylactic reaction
◆ Identify urine output; if decreasing, notify prescriber (may indicate nephrotoxicity)
• Assess renal studies: urinalysis, protein, BUN, creatinine
• Monitor blood studies: AST, ALT, CBC, Hct, bilirubin, LDH, alkaline phosphatase, Coombs' test monthly if patient is on long-term therapy
• Monitor electrolytes: potassium, sodium, chloride monthly if patient is on long-term therapy
• Assess bowel pattern daily; if severe diarrhea occurs, product should be discontinued; may indicate pseudomembranous colitis
• Monitor for bleeding: ecchymosis, bleeding gums, hematuria, stool guaiac daily if on long-term therapy
• Assess for superinfection: perineal itching, fever, malaise, redness, pain, swelling, drainage, rash, diarrhea, change in cough, sputum

Nursing diagnoses
• Diarrhea (adverse reactions)
• Infection, risk for (uses)
• Injury, risk for (adverse reactions)
• Knowledge, deficient (teaching)
• Noncompliance (teaching)

Implementation
IM route
• Reconstitute by adding 3.2 ml/1.5 g or 6.4 ml/3 g; use sterile water, 0.5% or 2% lidocaine; give within 1 hr of preparation; give deep in large muscle mass
• Give after C&S completed; on empty stomach
IV route
• Give **IV** after diluting 1.5 g/3.2 ml sterile H₂O for inj; or 3 g/6.4 ml (250 mg ampicillin/125 mg sulbactam); allow to stand until foaming stops; give directly over 15-30 min; dilute further in 50 ml or more of D₅W, D₅/10.45% NaCl, 10% invert sugar in water, LR, 6% sodium lactate, isotonic NaCl; administer within 1 hr after reconstitution; give as an intermittent inf over 15-30 min
Y-site compatibilities: Amifostine, aztreonam, cefepime, enalaprilat, famotidine, filgrastim, fluconazole, fludarabine, granisetron, heparin, regular insulin, meperidine, morphine, paclitaxel, remifentanil, tacrolimus, teniposide, theophylline, thiotepa
Y-site incompatibilities: Idarubicin, ondansetron, sargramostim
Additive compatibilities: Aztreonam
Additive incompatibilities: Aminoglycosides

Patient/family education
• Teach patient to report sore throat, bruising, bleeding, joint pain, persistent diarrhea; may indicate blood dyscrasias (rare) or superinfection
• Advise patient to contact prescriber if vaginal itching, loose foul-smelling stools, furry tongue occur; may indicate superinfection
• Instruct patient to use another form of contraception other than oral contraceptives
◆ To report immediately pseudomembranous colitis: fever, diarrhea with pus, blood, or mucus; may occur up to 4 wk after treatment
• To wear or carry emergency ID if allergic to penicillin products

Adverse effects: *italic* = common, **bold** = life-threatening

Evaluation
Positive therapeutic outcome
- Absence of signs/symptoms of infection (WBC <10,000/mm³, temp WNL, absence of red draining wounds, earache)
- Reported improvement in symptoms of infection

Treatment of overdose: Withdraw product, maintain airway, administer epinephrine, aminophylline, O_2, **IV** corticosteroids for anaphylaxis

anagrelide (Rx)
(a-na'gre-lide)
Agrylin
Func. class.: Antiplatelet
Chem. class.: Imidazoquinazolinone
Pregnancy category C

Action: Reduces platelet count (mechanism not clear) and prevents early platelet shape changes in response to aggregating agents, thus inhibiting platelet aggregation

Therapeutic outcome: Inhibition of platelet aggregation

Uses: Chronic myelogenous leukemia (CML), thrombocytosis, polycythemia vera

Dosage and routes
Adult: PO 0.5 mg qid or 1 mg bid, may be adjusted after 1 wk, max 10 mg/day or 2.5 mg single dose; maintenance: titrate to lowest dose to maintain platelets <600,000/mcL; dosage range 1.5-3 mg/day

Available forms: Caps 0.5, 1.0 mg

Adverse effects
CNS: Headache, dizziness, **seizures,** paresthesia, **CVA,** fever
CV: Postural hypotension, tachycardia, palpitations, **CHF, MI, cardiomyopathy, cardiomegaly, complete heart block, atrial fibrillation, arrhythmia,** chest pain
EENT: Amblyopia, diplopia, tinnitus
GI: Diarrhea, abdominal pain, nausea, flatulence, vomiting, anorexia, constipation, pancreatitis
GU: Dysuria
HEMA: Anemia, **thrombocytopenia, ecchymosis, lymphadenoma**
INTEG: Rash, photosensitivity
MISC: Edema, pain
MS: Asthenia, back pain
RESP: Dyspnea

Contraindications: Hypersensitivity

Precautions: Pregnancy **C,** breastfeeding, child <16 yr, cardiac/renal/hepatic disease, hypotension, abrupt discontinuation, females

Pharmacokinetics
Absorption	Unknown
Distribution	Unknown
Metabolism	Liver, extensively
Excretion	Feces/urine
Half-life	Terminal half-life 3-4 days

Pharmacodynamics
Onset	Unknown
Peak	1 hr
Duration	>24 hr

Interactions
Individual drugs
Abciximab, aspirin, cimetidine, ciprofloxacin, eptifibatide, tirofiban, ticlopidine: increased bleeding risk
Sucralfate: decreased absorption, decreased plasma concentrations
Drug classifications
Anticoagulants, NSAIDs, SSRIs, thrombolytics: increased bleeding risk
Drug/herb
Arginine: gastric irritation
Bogbean, dong quai: increased effect
Bilberry, saw palmetto: decreased effect
Feverfew, ginger, ginkgo, green tea: increased bleeding risk
Drug/food
Grapefruit or grapefruit juice: avoid use
Decreased: absorption

NURSING CONSIDERATIONS
Assessment
- Monitor B/P, pulse baseline, during treatment until stable; take B/P with patient lying, standing; orthostatic hypotension is common
- Assess cardiac status: chest pain, what aggravates or ameliorates condition
- Monitor platelet counts q2days × 1 wk, and qwk thereafter; response should begin after 1-2 wk; Hgb, WBC

Nursing diagnoses
- Cardiac output, decreased (uses)
- Knowledge, deficient (teaching)

Implementation
- May give with food, monitor closely for dosage adjustment, there is better absorption on empty stomach
- Store at room temperature

 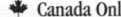

Patient/family education
• Teach patient that this medication is not a cure
• Advise patient that product may have to be taken continuously in evenly spaced doses only as directed; if a dose is missed, take one when remembered up to 4 hr; do not double doses
• Inform patient that it is necessary to quit smoking to prevent excessive vasoconstriction
• Advise patient to rise slowly from sitting or lying down to prevent orthostatic hypotension
• Caution patient not to use alcohol or OTC medication unless approved by prescriber; avoid grapefruit or juice
• Caution patient to avoid hazardous activities until stabilized on medication; dizziness may occur
• Teach patient to report cardiac reactions, increased bruising/bleeding
• Advise patient to use contraception (female, child-bearing age)
• Teach patient to inform health care provider before surgery of medication use
• Advise patient not to double dose; if dose is missed, take as soon as remembered; if close to next dose, omit dose

Evaluation
Positive therapeutic outcome
• Absence of thrombocythemia

anakinra (Rx)
(an-ah-kɪn'rah)
Kineret
Func. class.: Antirheumatic agent (disease modifying), immunomodulator
Chem. class.: Recombinant form of human interleukin-1 receptor antagonist (IL-1Ra)

Pregnancy category B

Action: A form of human interleukin-1 receptor antagonist (IL-1Ra) produced by DNA technology; blocks activity of IL-1, resulting in decreased cartilage degradation and decreased bone resorption

Therapeutic outcome: Decreased pain, inflammation

Uses: Reduction in signs and symptoms of moderate to severe active rheumatoid arthritis in patients 18 years of age or older who have not responded to other disease-modifying agents

Dosage and routes
Adult: SUBCUT 100 mg daily

Renal dose
Adult: SUBCUT 100 mg every other day

Available forms: Inj, 100 mg/0.67 ml prefilled glass syringe

Adverse effects
CNS: Headache
EENT: Sinusitis
GI: Abdominal pain, nausea, diarrhea
HEMA: **Neutropenia**
INTEG: Rash, *inj site reaction,* allergic reaction
MISC: Flulike symptoms
MS: *Worsening of RA, arthralgia*
RESP: URI

Contraindications: Hypersensitivity to *Escherichia coli*–derived proteins or this product, sepsis

Precautions: Pregnancy **B,** breastfeeding, children, geriatric, renal impairment, active infections

Pharmacokinetics	
Absorption	Well absorbed (SUBCUT)
Distribution	Unknown
Metabolism	Unknown
Excretion	Unknown
Half-life	4-6 hr

Pharmacodynamics	
Onset	Unknown
Peak	3-7 hr
Duration	Unknown

Interactions
Drug classifications
Antibody reactions: decreased
Etanercept, TNF blocking agents: increased risk of severe infection
Vaccines: do not coadminister; immunizations should be brought up to date before treatment

NURSING CONSIDERATIONS
Assessment
• Assess pain, stiffness, ROM, swelling of joints during treatment
• Assess for inj site pain, swelling; usually occur after 2 inj (4-5 days)
• Assess for infections, stop treatment if present

Nursing diagnoses
• Injury, risk for (side effects)
• Knowledge, deficient (teaching)
• Mobility, impaired physical (uses)
• Pain, chronic (uses)

Adverse effects: *italic* = common, **bold** = life-threatening

Implementation
- Do not use if cloudy or discolored or if particulate is present; protect from light
- Do not admix with other sol or medications, do not use filter

Patient/family education
- Teach patient about self-administration if appropriate: inj should be made in thigh, abdomen, upper arm; rotate sites at least 1 in from old site
- Advise patient to notify prescriber if pregnancy is planned or suspected, avoid breastfeeding

Evaluation
Positive therapeutic outcome
- Decreased inflammation, pain in joints

---

anastrozole (Rx)
(an-ass-stroh′zole)
Arimidex
Func. class.: Antineoplastic
Chem. class.: Aromatase inhibitor

Pregnancy category X

Action: Highly selective nonsteroidal aromatase inhibitor that lowers serum estradiol concentrations; many breast cancers have strong estrogen receptors

Therapeutic outcome: Prevention of rapidly growing malignant cells

Uses: Advanced breast carcinoma that has not responded to other therapy in estrogen-receptor-positive patients (usually postmenopausal); patients with advanced disease on tamoxifen, adjunct therapy in early breast cancer

Dosage and routes
Adult: PO 1 mg daily

Available forms: Tabs 1 mg

Adverse effects
CNS: Hot flashes, headache, light-headedness, depression, dizziness, confusion, insomnia, anxiety
CV: Chest pain, hypertension, thrombophlebitis, edema, **MI, CVA, cerebral infarction**
GI: Nausea, vomiting, altered taste leading to anorexia, diarrhea, constipation, abdominal pain, dry mouth
GU: Vaginal bleeding, pruritus vulvae, vaginal dryness, pelvic pain, UTI
HEMA: Leukopenia
INTEG: Rash, **Stevens-Johnson syndrome**
MS: Bone pain, myalgia, asthenia, bone loss, osteoporosis, arthralgia, fractures

RESP: Cough, sinusitis, dyspnea, **pulmonary embolism**

Contraindications: Pregnancy **X**, hypersensitivity, breastfeeding

Precautions: Children, geriatric, cardiac/hepatic disease, females, osteoporosis

Pharmacokinetics
Absorption	Adequately absorbed
Distribution	Unknown
Metabolism	Liver
Excretion	Feces, urine
Half-life	50 hr

Pharmacodynamics
Onset	Unknown
Peak	4-7 hr
Duration	Unknown

Interactions
Drug/lab test
Increased: GGT, AST, ALT, alkaline phosphatase, cholesterol, LDL

NURSING CONSIDERATIONS
Assessment
- Monitor CBC, differential, platelet count weekly; withhold product if WBC is <4000/mm^3 or platelet count is <75,000/mm^3; notify prescriber of results; monitor calcium levels (hypercalcemia is common)
- Assess for tumor flare: increase in bone, tumor pain during beginning treatment; give analgesics as ordered to decrease pain
- Assess for bleeding: hematuria, guaiac, bruising or petechiae, mucosa or orifices, q8hr; no rectal temp

Nursing diagnoses
- Injury, risk for (adverse reactions)
- Knowledge, deficient (teaching)

Implementation
- Do not break, crush, or chew enteric products
- Give with food or fluids for GI upset; repeat dose may be needed if vomiting occurs
- Store in light-resistant container at room temperature

Patient/family education
- Instruct patient to report any complaints, side effects to health care prescriber; if dose is missed, do not double next dose
- Advise patient that vaginal bleeding, pruritus, hot flashes, can occur, and are reversible after discontinuing treatment
- Inform patient about who should be told about tamoxifen therapy

---

- Advise patient to report vaginal bleeding immediately; that tumor flare—increase in size of tumor, increased bone pain—may occur and will subside rapidly; may take analgesics for pain
- Caution patient to use sunscreen and protective clothing to prevent burns because photosensitivity is common
- Teach patient that hair loss may occur during treatment; a wig or hairpiece may make patient feel better; new hair may be different in color, texture
- Inform patient that rash or lesions are temporary and may become large during beginning therapy

Evaluation
Positive therapeutic outcome
- Decreased spread of malignant cells in breast cancer

---

anidulafungin (Rx)
(a-nid-yoo-luh-fun'jin)
Eraxis
Func. class.: Antifungal, systemic
Chem. class.: Echinocandin

Pregnancy category C

Action: Inhibits fungal enzyme synthesis; causes direct damage to fungal cell wall

Therapeutic outcome: Decreased symptoms of candida infection, negative culture

Uses: *Esophageal candidiasis, Candida albicans, C. glabrata, C. parapsilosis, C. tropicalis*

Dosage and routes
Candidemia and other candida infections
Adult: **IV** loading dose 200 mg on day 1, then 100 mg/day until 14 days or more since last positive culture

Esophageal candidiasis
Adult: **IV** loading dose 100 mg on day 1, then 50 mg/day for at least 14 days and for at least 7 days after symptoms are resolved

Available forms: Powder for injection, lyophilized 50, 100 mg

Adverse effects
Candidemia/other candida infections
CNS: **Seizures,** dizziness, *headache*
CV: Deep vein thrombosis, **atrial fibrillation, right bundle branch block,** hypoten-

sion, **sinus arrhythmia, thrombophlebitis superficial, ventricular extrasystoles (rare)**
GI: Nausea; anorexia; vomiting; diarrhea; increased AST, ALT
META: Hypokalemia
Esophageal candidiasis
CNS: Headache
GI: Nausea, anorexia, vomiting, diarrhea, **hepatic necrosis**
HEMA: **Neutropenia, thrombocytopenia, leukopenia, coagulopathy**
INTEG: Rash
META: Hypocalcemia, hyperglycemia, hyperkalemia, hypernatremia, hypomagnesium (rare)
MS: Back pain, rigors

Contraindications: Hypersensitivity to this product or other echinocandins

Precautions: Pregnancy C, breastfeeding, children, severe hepatic disease

Pharmacokinetics
Absorption	Unknown
Distribution	Steady state after loading dose, protein binding 84%
Metabolism	Unknown
Excretion	Unknown
Half-life	Distribution 0.5-1 hr, terminal 40-50 hr

Pharmacodynamics
Unknown

Interactions
Individual drugs
CycloSPORINE: increased plasma concentrations
Drug/lab test
Increased: amylase, bilirubin, CPK, creatinine, ECG, QT prolongation, lipase
Decreased: platelets, magnesium, potassium, transferase, urea

NURSING CONSIDERATIONS
Assessment
- Assess for infection, clearing of cultures during treatment; obtain culture baseline and throughout; product may be started as soon as culture is taken
- Monitor CBC (RBC, Hct, Hgb), differential, platelet count periodically; notify prescriber of results
- Monitor renal studies: BUN, serum uric acid, urine CCr, electrolytes before and during therapy

---

Adverse effects: *italic* = common, **bold** = life-threatening

- Monitor hepatic studies before and during treatment: bilirubin, AST, ALT, alk phosphatase, as needed
- Assess for bleeding: hematuria, heme-positive stools, bruising or petechiae, mucosa or orifices; blood dyscrasias can occur
- Assess for GI symptoms: frequency of stools, cramping, if severe diarrhea occurs, electrolytes may need to be given

Nursing diagnoses
- Infection, risk for (uses)
- Injury, risk for (adverse reactions)
- Knowledge, deficient (teaching)

Implementation
IV route
- Reconstitute with provided dilutent 50 mg vial/5 ml (3.33 mg/ml), dilute with D_5 of 0.9% NaCl, only to a concentration of 0.5 mg/ml, run at no more than 1.1 mg/ml
- Do not use if cloudy or precipitated; do not admix
- Store at room temperature, away from light, do not freeze; diluted sol must be used within 24 hr

Patient/family education
- Advise patient to notify prescriber if pregnancy is suspected or planned; use nonhormonal form of contraception while taking this product
- Instruct patient to avoid breastfeeding while taking this product
- Advise patient to inform prescriber of kidney or liver disease
- Advise patient to report bleeding
- Teach patient to report signs of infection: increased temp, sore throat, flulike symptoms
- Teach patient to notify prescriber of nausea, vomiting, diarrhea, jaundice, anorexia, clay-colored stools, dark urine; heptatotoxicity may occur

Evaluation
Positive therapeutic outcome
- Decreased symptoms of candida infection, negative culture

❗ HIGH ALERT

anistreplase (Rx)
(an-is-tre-plaze')
anisoylated plasminogen, APSAC, Eminase
Func. class.: Thrombolytic enzyme
Chem. class.: Plasminogen activator
Pregnancy category C

Action: Promotes thrombolysis by promoting conversion of plasminogen to plasmin; complex is a combination of plasminogen and streptokinase

Therapeutic outcome: Thrombolysis in coronary arteries

Uses: Management of acute MI; for lysis of coronary artery thrombi; ST-elevation MI (STEMI) for lysis of coronary artery thrombi as soon as possible or within 12 hr of symptoms or within 24 hr if ischemia symptoms persist

Dosage and routes
Adult: **IV** INJ 30 units over 2-5 min as soon as possible after onset of symptoms

Available forms: Powder, lyophilized 30 units/vial

Adverse effects
CNS: Headache, fever, sweating, agitation, dizziness, paresthesia, tremor, vertigo, **intracranial hemorrhage, stroke**
CV: Hypotension, **dysrhythmias,** conduction disorders
GI: Nausea, vomiting
HEMA: Decreased Hct, **GI, GU, intracranial, retroperitoneal,** surface bleeding; **thrombocytopenia**
INTEG: Rash, urticaria, phlebitis at site, itching, flushing
MS: Low back pain, arthralgia, myalgia
RESP: Altered respirations, dyspnea, **bronchospasm, lung edema,** pulmonary bleeding
SYST: **Anaphylaxis (rare),** bleeding

Contraindications: Hypersensitivity, active internal bleeding, intraspinal or intracranial surgery, neoplasms of CNS, severe, uncontrolled hypertension, cerebral embolism, thrombosis, hemorrhage, hypersensitivity to this product or streptokinase, previous hemorrhagic stroke, recent trauma/history of CVA

Precautions: Pregnancy **C,** breastfeeding, geriatric, arterial emboli from left side of heart, ulcerative colitis/enteritis, renal/hepatic disease, hypocoagulation, COPD, subacute

---

bacterial endocarditis, rheumatic valvular disease, intraarterial diagnostic procedure or surgery (10 days), recent major surgery, previous streptokinase/anistreplase in last 12 mo

Pharmacokinetics

Absorption	Complete bioavailability
Distribution	Unknown
Metabolism	Binds to plasmin
Excretion	Kidneys
Half-life	105 min

Pharmacodynamics

Onset	Unknown
Peak	45 min
Duration	Unknown

Interactions
Individual drugs
Abciximab, aspirin, clopidogrel, dipyridamole, eptifibatide, heparin, plicamycin, ticlopidine, tirofiban, valproic acid: increased bleeding risk

Aminocaproic acid, aprotinen, tranexamic acid: decreased action of anistreplase
Drug classifications
Anticoagulants, antiplatelets, cephalosporins (some), NSAIDs: increased bleeding risk
Drug/herb
Agrimony, alfalfa, angelica, anise, basil, bay, bilberry, black currant, black haw, bladderwrack, bogbean, boldo, borage, bromelain, buchu, capsaicin, cat's claw, chaparral, chondroitin, cinchona bark, clove oil, curcumin, dandelion, dong quai, evening primrose, fenugreek, feverfew, garlic, ginger, ginkgo, ginseng, guggul, horse chestnut, Irish moss, kava, kelp, kelpware, khella, licorice, lovage, lungwort, meadowsweet, motherwort, mugwort, nettle, papaya, parsley (large amounts), pau d'arco, pineapple, poplar, prickly ash, red clover, safflower, saw palmetto, tanshen, tonka bean, turmeric, wintergreen, yarrow: increased risk of bleeding

Chamomile, coenzyme Q10, flax, glucomannan, goldenseal, guar gum: decreased anticoagulant effect
Drug/lab test
Increased: pro-time, APTT, TT
Decreased: fibrinogen, plasminogen

NURSING CONSIDERATIONS
Assessment
- Monitor VS, B/P, pulse, respirations, neurologic signs, temp at least q4hr, temp >104° F (40° C) or indicators of internal bleeding
- Assess for hypersensitivity: fever, rash, itching, chills; mild reaction may be treated with antihistamines; hypersensitivity reactions/ dyspnea, wheezing, facial swelling should be treated with epinephrine
- ◆ Monitor bleeding during first hr of treatment (hematuria, hematemesis, bleeding from mucous membranes, epistaxis, ecchymosis), continue to monitor for 24 hr after treatment; blood studies (Hct, platelets, PTT, pro-time, TT, APTT) before starting therapy; pro-time or APTT must be <2 × control before starting therapy; TT or pro-time q3-4hr during treatment
- Monitor ECG, treat bradycardia, ventricular changes; assess neurologic status, neurologic change may indicate intracranial bleeding; cardiac enzymes, radionuclide, myocardial scanning/coronary angiography

Nursing diagnoses
- Injury, risk for (uses, adverse reactions)
- Knowledge, deficient (teaching)
- Tissue perfusion, ineffective (uses)

Implementation
- Give heparin therapy after thrombolytic therapy is discontinued, TT or APTT <2 × control (about 3-4 hr)
- Avoid invasive procedures: inj, rect temp; about 10% of patients have high streptococcal antibody titers, requiring increased loading doses
- Treat fever with acetaminophen
- Provide pressure for 30 sec to minor bleeding sites, 30 min to sites of arterial puncture followed by dressing; inform prescriber if hemostasis not attained; apply pressure dressing
IV, direct route
- Give after reconstituting single-dose vial/ 5 ml sterile water for inj (not bacteriostatic water), and roll (not shake) to enhance reconstitution, try to minimize foaming; give over 2-5 min by direct IV, give within ½ hr of reconstitution or discard, do not add other meds to vial or syringe; give within 6 hr of thrombi identification for best results; cryoprecipitate or fresh frozen plasma if bleeding occurs; store powder in refrigerator; use within 30 min after reconstitution
Incompatibilities: Do not mix with other products in sol or syringe

Patient/family education
- Teach patient action of product and expected outcome; alert patient to possible hypersensitivity reactions and symptoms to report
- Advise patient bed rest is needed during entire course of treatment; handle patient as little as possible during therapy

Evaluation
Positive therapeutic outcome
- Absence of thrombolysis in MI
- Improved ventricular function

⚠ HIGH ALERT

antihemophilic factor VIII (AHF) (Rx)
(an-tee-hee-moe-fill'ik)
Alphanate, antihemophilic factor, Bioclate, Helixate FS, Hemofil M, Humate-P, Hyate:C, Koate-DVI, Kogenate, Kogenate FS, Monoclate-P, Recombinate, ReFacto
Func. class.: Hemostatic, blood factor
Chem. class.: Factor VIII

Pregnancy category C

Do not confuse:
Kogenate/Kogenate-2

Action: Necessary for clotting. Activates factor X in conjunction with activated factor IX; transforms prothrombin to thrombin

Therapeutic outcome: Control of hemorrhage or excessive bleeding in factor VIII deficiency

Uses: Hemophilia A, patients with acquired circulating factor VIII inhibitors, factor VIII deficiency; prevention of surgical bleeding, risk of thrombosis (von Willebrand disease)

Dosage and routes
Depends on severity of deficiency and level of antihemophilic factor

Massive hemorrhage
Adult and child: **IV** 40-50 units/kg, then 20-25 units/kg q8-12hr

Bleeding (overt)
Adult and child: **IV** 15-25 units/kg, then 8-15 units/kg q8-12hr × 4 days

Hemorrhage near vital organs
Adult and child: **IV** 25 units/kg, then 15 units/kg q8hr × 2 days, then 4 units/kg q8hr × 2 days

Minor hemorrhage
Adult and child: **IV** 8-10 units/kg q24hr × 2-3 days or 8 units/kg q12hr × 2 days, then q24hr × 2 days

Joint bleeding
Adult and child: **IV** 15 units/kg q8-12hr × 1-2 days

Available forms: Inj 250, 500, 1000, 1500 units/vial (number of units noted on label)

Adverse effects
CNS: Headache, *lethargy, chills, fever, flushing,* loss of consciousness
CV: *Hypotension,* tachycardia
GI: Nausea, vomiting, abdominal cramps, jaundice, constipation, diarrhea, anorexia, **viral hepatitis**
HEMA: **Thrombosis, hemolysis, risk of hepatitis B, risk of HIV**
INTEG: Rash, flushing, *urticaria,* stinging at inj site
MISC: **Anaphylaxis,** blurred vision, back pain
RESP: **Bronchospasm,** rhinitis, dyspnea, nosebleeds, wheezing

Contraindications: Hypersensitivity to mouse, hamster, bovine, porcine protein, breastfeeding, HIV

Precautions: Pregnancy C, neonates/infants, hepatic disease, blood types A, B, AB, factor VIII inhibitor, viral infection

Pharmacokinetics	
Absorption	Complete availability
Distribution	Plasma
Metabolism	Not metabolized
Excretion	No excretion
Half-life	Biphasic 4 hr, 15 hr

Pharmacodynamics	
Onset	Immediate
Peak	Unknown
Duration	12 hr

Interactions
Drug classifications
Anticoagulants, NSAIDs, salicylates: increased bleeding

NURSING CONSIDERATIONS
Assessment
- Monitor blood studies (coagulation factors assay by % normal): 5% prevents spontaneous hemorrhage, 30%-50% for surgery, 80%-100% for severe hemorrhage; blood group of

---

patient, donors (if applicable; most factor VIII not from specific blood group donors)
• Monitor I&O, urine color; notify prescriber if urine becomes orange, red; change in urine color signifying hemolytic reaction; patients other than blood type O are more at risk
• Monitor pulse: discontinue infusion if significant increase
• Obtain test for factor VIII inhibitors before starting treatment, may require concomitant antiinhibitor coagulant complex therapy; Hct, Coombs' test with blood types A, B, AB
• Assess for allergy: fever, rash, itching, jaundice, wheezing, tachycardia, nausea, vomiting; give diphenhydrAMINE (Benadryl); continue therapy if reaction is mild, discontinue if severe; notify prescriber
❖ Monitor bleeding at ankles, knees, elbows, other joints; check for rebleeding after 15-30 min

Nursing diagnoses
• Injury, risk for (uses, adverse reactions)
• Knowledge, deficient (teaching)
• Tissue perfusion, ineffective (uses)

Implementation
• Give hepatitis A/B vaccination at birth if diagnosed with hemophilia

IV route
• Administer after dilution with warm NS, D_5W, LR; give within 3 hr
• To prepare, administer factor VIII concentrates at first sign of danger; rotate gently to mix
• Warm to room temperature using plastic syringe to reconstitute

IV infusion route
• Administer by **IV** inf: give at ≤2 ml/min if concentration >34 units/ml; or over 3 min if concentration is <34 units/ml; filter before using
• Store in refrigerator; do not freeze; after reconstitution, do not refrigerate; give within 3 hr

Additive compatibilities: Do not mix with other products in sol or syringe

Patient/family education
• Advise patient to report any signs of bleeding: gums, under skin, urine, stools, emesis; review methods to prevent bleeding; to be checked q2-3mo for HIV screen
• Instruct patient to avoid salicylates/NSAIDs; increases bleeding tendencies, decreases clotting
• Instruct patient to prepare, administer factor VIII concentrates at first sign of danger
• Instruct patient to advise health professionals of treatment for hemophilia

• Advise patient that immunization for hepatitis B may be given first
• Instruct patient to report hives, urticaria, chest tightness, hypotension; may be monoclonal antibody–derived factor VII; signs of viral hepatitis, AIDS
• Advise patient to carry/wear emergency ID describing disease process, products used

Evaluation
Positive therapeutic outcome
• Absence of bleeding
• Prevention of rebleeding

apraclonidine ophthalmic
See Appendix B

aprepitant (Rx)
(ap-re′pi-tant)
Emend
Func. class.: Antiemetic   miscellaneous
Pregnancy category B

Action: Selective antagonist of human substance P/neurokinin 1 (NK_1) receptors decreasing emetic reflex

Therapeutic outcome: Decreased nausea, vomiting during chemotherapy

Uses: Prevention of nausea, vomiting associated with cancer chemotherapy (highly emetogenic/moderately emetogenic) including high-dose cisplatin; used in combination with other antiemetics; postop nausea, vomiting

Dosage and routes
Highly emetogenic
Adult: PO day 1 (1 hr prior to chemotherapy) aprepitant 125 mg with 12 mg dexamethasone PO with 32 mg ondansetron **IV**; day 2 aprepitant 80 mg with 8 mg dexamethasone PO; day 3 aprepitant 80 mg with 8 mg dexamethasone PO; day 4 only dexamethasone 8 mg PO

Moderately emetogenic
Adult: PO day 1 125 mg aprepitant with dexamethasone 12 mg PO, with ondansetron 8 mg PO × 2; days 2 and 3 80 mg aprepitant only

Prevention of postop nausea/ vomiting
Adult: PO 40 mg within 3 hr of induction of anesthesia

Available forms: Caps 40, 80, 125 mg

Adverse effects: *italic* = common, **bold** = life-threatening

Adverse effects

CNS: Headache, dizziness, insomnia, anxiety, depression, confusion, peripheral neuropathy
CV: Bradycardia, tachycardia, DVT, hypertension
GI: Diarrhea; constipation; abdominal pain; anorexia; gastritis; increased AST, ALT; *nausea;* vomiting; heartburn
GU: Increased BUN, serum creatine, proteinuria, dysuria
HEMA: Anemia, **thrombocytopenia, neutropenia**
INTEG: Pruritus, rash, urticaria
MISC: Asthenia, fatigue, dehydration, fever, hiccups, tinnitus, alopecia
SYST: **Anaphylaxis**

Contraindications: Hypersensitivity

Precautions: Pregnancy **B**, breastfeeding, children, geriatric, hepatic disease

Pharmacokinetics

Absorption	Unknown
Distribution	95% protein bound
Metabolism	Liver (CYP3A4 enzymes to an active metabolite)
Excretion	Not in kidneys
Half-life	10-12 hr

Pharmacodynamics
Unknown

Interactions
Individual drugs
Paroxetine: decreased action of both products
Drug classifications
CYP2C9 substrates (phenytoin, TOLBUTamide, warfarin), oral contraceptives: decreased action
CYP3A4 inhibitors (clarithromycin, diltiazem, itraconazole, ketoconazole, nefazodone, nelfinavir, ritonavir, troleandomycin): increased aprepitant action
CYP3A4 inducers (carbamazepine, phenytoin, rifampin): decreased aprepitant action
CYP3A4 substrates (alprazolam, cisapride, dexamethasone, docetaxel, etoposide, ifosfamide, irinotecan, methylPREDNISolone, midazolam, paclitaxel, pimozide, triazolam, vinBLAStine, vinCRIStine, vinorelbine): increased action
Drug/food
Grapefruit juice: decreased effect

NURSING CONSIDERATIONS
Assessment
• Assess for hypersensitive reactions: pruritus, rash, urticaria, anaphylaxis

• Assess for absence of nausea, vomiting during chemotherapy
• Advise those on warfarin to have clotting monitored closely during 2-wk period following administration of aprepitant

Nursing diagnoses
• Knowledge, deficient (teaching)

Implementation
• Give PO on 3-day schedule
• Take first dose 1 hr prior to chemotherapy
• Store at room temperature

Patient/family education
• Teach to report diarrhea, constipation
• Advise to take only as prescribed
• Advise to report all medication to prescriber prior to taking this medication
• Instruct to use nonhormonal form of contraception while taking this agent

Evaluation
Positive therapeutic outcome
• Absence of nausea, vomiting during cancer chemotherapy

arformoterol (Rx)
(ar-for-moe′ter-ole)
Brovana
Func. class.: Long-acting adrenergic β₂-agonist, sympathomimetic, bronchodilator

Pregnancy category C

Action: Causes bronchodilation by action on β₂ (pulmonary) receptors by increasing levels of cyclic cAMP, which relaxes smooth muscle; produces bronchodilation, CNS, cardiac stimulation, as well as increased diuresis and gastric acid secretion; longer acting than isoproterenol

Therapeutic outcome: Absence of dyspnea, wheezing after 1 hr, improved airway exchange, improved ABGs

Uses: COPD, including chronic bronchitis, emphysema

Dosage and routes
COPD
Adult: NEB 15 mcg, bid, AM, PM

Available forms: Inh sol 15 mcg/2 ml

Adverse effects
CNS: Tremors, anxiety, insomnia, headache, dizziness, stimulation, *restlessness,* hallucinations, flushing, irritability
CV: Palpitations, **tachycardia**, hypo/hypertension, angina, **dysrhythmias**
EENT: Dry nose, irritation of nose and throat

GI: Heartburn, nausea, vomiting
MISC: Flushing, sweating, anorexia, bad taste/smell changes, hypokalemia, **anaphylaxis**
MS: Muscle cramps
RESP: Cough, wheezing, dyspnea, **bronchospasm,** dry throat

Contraindications: Hypersensitivity to sympathomimetics, this product, or racemic formoterol; tachydysrhythmias, severe cardiac disease, heart block, children

Black Box Warning: Actively deteriorating COPD

Precautions: Pregnancy **C,** breastfeeding, cardiac disorders, hyperthyroidism, diabetes mellitus, hypertension, prostatic hypertrophy, closed-angle glaucoma, seizures, hypoglycemia

Pharmacokinetics

Absorption	Unknown
Distribution	Crosses placenta, protein binding 52%-65%
Metabolism	Direct conjugation by CYP2D6, CYP2C19, extensively
Excretion	Urine 63%, feces 11%
Half-life	Terminal (COPD) 26 hr

Pharmacodynamics

Onset	5 min
Peak	1-1½ hr
Duration	4-6 hr

Interactions
Individual drugs
Oxytoxics: increased severe hypotension
Theophylline: increased toxicity
Drug classifications
Adrenergics, MAOIs, tricyclics: increased action of arformoterol; do not use together
Nebulized bronchodilators: increased action of nebulized bronchodilators
Other β-blockers: decreased arformoterol action
Potassium-losing diuretics: increased ECG changes/hypokalemia
Drug/herb
Caffeine (cola nut, green/black tea, guarana, yerba maté, coffee, chocolate): increased stimulation

NURSING CONSIDERATIONS
Assessment
• Assess respiratory function: vital capacity, forced expiratory volume, ABGs; lung sounds, heart rate and rhythm, B/P, sputum (baseline and peak)

• Determine that patient has not received theophylline therapy or other bronchodilators before giving dose
• Assess patient's ability to self-medicate
• Assess for allergic reactions; anaphylaxis may occur
• Assess paradoxical bronchospasm; hold medication, notify prescriber if bronchospasm occurs

Nursing diagnoses
• Airway clearance, ineffective (uses)
• Knowledge, deficient (teaching)

Implementation
• Must be used by nebulization
• Store in refrigerator

Patient/family education
• Teach patient to use exactly as prescribed, that death has resulted from asthma with products similar to this one
• Advise patient not to use OTC medications; excess stimulation may occur

Evaluation
Positive therapeutic outcome
• Absence of dyspnea, wheezing after 1 hr, improved airway exchange, improved ABGs

---

⚠ HIGH ALERT

argatroban (Rx)
(are-ga-troe'ban)
Argatroban
Func. class.: Anticoagulant
Chem. class.: Thrombin inhibitor
Pregnancy category B

Do not confuse:
argatroban/Aggrastat

Action: Direct inhibitor of thrombin that is derived from L-arginine; it reversibly binds to the thrombin active site

Therapeutic outcome: Absence or decrease of thrombosis

Uses: Thrombosis, prophylaxis or treatment; anticoagulation prevention/treatment of thrombosis in heparin-induced thrombocytopenia (HIT); percutaneous coronary intervention (PCI) in those with a history of HIT

Dosage and routes
Heparin-induced thrombocytopenia or heparin-induced thrombocytopenia and thrombosis syndrome
Adult: CONT **IV** INF 2 mcg/kg/min (1 mg/ml); adjust dose until steady-state aPPT is

1.5-3 × initial baseline, not to exceed 100 sec, max dose 10 mcg/kg/min

Percutaneous coronary intervention (PCI) in HIT
Adult: IV INF 25 mcg/kg/min and a BOL of 350 mcg/kg given over 3-5 min, check ACT 5-10 min after BOL is completed, proceed if ACT >300 sec; if ACT <300 sec, give another 150 mcg/kg BOL and increase infusion rate to 30 mcg/kg/min; recheck ACT in 5-10 min; if ACT >450 sec, decrease infusion rate to 15 mcg/kg/min; recheck ACT in 5-10 min; once ACT is therapeutic, continue for duration of procedure

Hepatic dose
Adult: CONT INF 0.5 mcg/kg/min, adjust rate based on APTT

Available forms: Inj 100 mg/ml (2.5 ml) (must dilute 100-fold)

Adverse effects
CNS: Fever, **intracranial bleeding,** headache
CV: **Atrial fibrillation, ventricular tachycardia, coronary thrombosis, MI, myocardial ischemia, coronary occlusion, bradycardia,** chest pain, hypotension
GI: Nausea, vomiting, abdominal pain, diarrhea, **GI bleeding**
GU: **Hematuria,** abnormal kidney function, UTI
HEMA: **Hemorrhage**
RESP: Pneumonia, dyspnea, coughing, hemoptysis
SYST: **Sepsis**

Contraindications: Hypersensitivity, overt major bleeding

Precautions: Pregnancy **B,** breastfeeding, children, intracranial bleeding, renal function impairment, hepatic disease, severe hypertension, after lumbar puncture, spinal anesthesia, major surgery, congenital or acquired bleeding, GI ulcers

Pharmacokinetics	
Absorption	Unknown
Distribution	To extracellular fluid, 54% plasma protein binding
Metabolism	Liver
Excretion	Feces
Half-life	39-51 min

Pharmacodynamics
Unknown

Interactions
Individual drugs
Clopidogrel, dipyridamole, heparin, ticlodipine, warfarin: increased bleeding risk
Drug classifications
Antiplatelets, glycoprotein IIb/IIIa antagonists (abciximab, eptifibatide, tirofiban), NSAIDs, other anticoagulants, salicylates, thrombolytics (alteplase, reteplase, streptokinase, tenecteplase, urokinase): increased risk of bleeding
Drug/herb
Agrimony, alfalfa, angelica, anise, basil, bay, bilberry, black currant, black haw, bogbean, buchu, cat's claw, chondroitin, dong quai, fenugreek, feverfew, fish oils, garlic, ginger, ginkgo, ginseng, horse chestnut, Irish moss, kava, kelp, kelpware, khella, licorice, lovage, lungwort, meadowsweet, motherwort, mugwort, nettle, papaya, parsley, pau d'arco, pineapple, poplar, prickly ash, safflower, saw palmetto, senega, skullcap, turmeric, wintergreen: increased risk of bleeding
Chamomile, coenzyme Q10, flax, glucomannan, goldenseal, guar gum: decreased anticoagulant effect

NURSING CONSIDERATIONS
Assessment
• Obtain baseline APTT before treatment; do not start treatment if APTT ratio ≥2.5, then APTT 4 hr after initiation of treatment and at least daily thereafter; if APTT above target, stop inf for 2 hr, then restart at 50%, take APTT in 4 hr; if below target, increase inf rate by 20%, take APTT in 4 hr, do not exceed inf rate of 0.21 mg/kg/hr without checking for coagulation abnormalities
• Monitor APTT, which should be 1.5-3 × control
 Assess for bleeding gums, petechiae, ecchymosis, black tarry stools, hematuria/epistaxis, B/P, vaginal bleeding, and possible hemorrhage
• Fever, skin rash, urticaria

Nursing diagnoses
• Cardiac output, decreased (uses)
• Diarrhea (adverse reactions)
• Knowledge, deficient (teaching)

Implementation
• Avoid all IM inj that may cause bleeding
IV infusion route
• Dilute in 0.9% NaCl, D₅, LR to a final conc 1 mg/ml; dilute each 2.5-ml vial 100-fold by mixing with 250 ml of diluents, mix by re-

peated inversion of the diluent bag for 1 min; may be slightly hazy
- Dosage adjustment may be made after review of APTT, not to exceed 10 mcg/kg/min

Patient/family education
- Advise patient to use soft-bristle toothbrush to avoid bleeding gums, avoid contact sports, use electric razor, avoid IM inj
- Instruct patient to report any signs of bleeding: gums, under skin, urine, stools

Evaluation
Positive therapeutic outcome
- Absence or decrease of thrombosis

---

aripiprazole (Rx)
(a-rip-ip-pra′zol)
Abilify, Abilify Discmelt
Func. class.: Antipsychotic/neuroleptic

Pregnancy category C

Action: Exact mechanism unknown; may be mediated through both dopamine type 2 (D_2) and serotonin type 2 (5-HT_2) antagonism

Therapeutic outcome: Decreased excitement, hallucinations, delusions, paranoia, reorganization of patterns of thought, speech

Uses: Schizophrenia and bipolar disorder (adults and adolescents), agitation, mania, major depressive disorder, short-term mania or mixed episodes of bipolar disorder

Dosage and routes
Schizophrenia
Adult: PO 10-15 mg/day; if needed, dosage may be increased to 30 mg daily after 2 wk; maintenance 15 mg/day, periodically reassess

Major depressive disorder
Adult: PO 2-5 mg/day as an adjunct to other antidepressant treatment; adjust by 5 mg at ≥1 wk (range 2-15 mg/day)

Agitation in bipolar disorder/schizophrenia
Adult: IM 9.75 mg as a single dose; may start with a lower dose

Bipolar disorder
Adult: 15 mg/day, may increase to 30 mg/day if needed

Available forms: Tabs 2, 5, 10, 15, 20, 30 mg; inj 9.75 mg/1.3 ml; orally disintegrating tab 10,15 mg; oral sol 1 mg/ml

Adverse effects
CNS: Drowsiness, insomnia, agitation, anxiety, headache, **seizures, neuroleptic**
malignant syndrome, *light-headedness, akathisia, asthenia, tremor,* **stroke, suicidal ideation,** dystonia
CV: Orthostatic hypotension, **tachycardia**
EENT: Blurred vision, rhinitis
GI: Constipation, *nausea,* vomiting, jaundice, weight gain
INTEG: Rash
META: Hypoglycemia
RESP: Cough
SYST: **Death in geriatric patients with dementia**

Contraindications: Hypersensitivity, breastfeeding, seizure disorders

Precautions: Pregnancy C, geriatric, renal/cardiac/hepatic disease

Black Box Warning: Children, dementia, suicidal ideation

Pharmacokinetics
Absorption	Unknown
Distribution	Protein binding, 90%
Metabolism	Liver, extensively to major active metabolism
Excretion	Unknown
Half-life	Unknown

Pharmacodynamics
Unknown

Interactions
Individual drugs
Alcohol: increased sedation
Carbamazepine: decreased effects of aripiprazole
Erythromycin, fluoxetine, ketoconazole, quinidine, paroxetine: increased effects of aripiprazole, reduce dose
Famotidine, valproate: decreased aripiprazole level
Lithium: increased EPS
Drug classifications
Antipsychotics: increased EPS
CNS depressants: increased sedation
CYP3A4/CYP2D6 inhibitors: increased effects of aripiprazole, reduce dose
CYPA34 inducers: decreased effects of aripiprazole; increase dose
Drug/herb
Betel palm, kava: increased EPS
Cola tree, hops, nettle, nutmeg: increased neuroleptic effect

NURSING CONSIDERATIONS
Assessment
- Assess mental status before initial administration

Adverse effects: *italic* = common, **bold** = life-threatening

- Check for swallowing of PO medication; check for hoarding or giving of medication to other patients
- Monitor I&O ratio; palpate bladder if urinary output is low
- Monitor bilirubin, CBC, liver function tests qmo
- Assess affect, orientation, LOC, reflexes, gait, coordination, sleep pattern disturbances
- Monitor B/P standing and lying; also pulse, respirations; take q4hr during initial treatment; establish baseline before starting treatment; report drops of 30 mm Hg; watch for ECG changes
- Assess for dizziness, faintness, palpitations, tachycardia on rising
- Assess for EPS, including akathisia (inability to sit still, no pattern to movements), tardive dyskinesia (bizarre movements of the jaw, mouth, tongue, extremities), pseudoparkinsonism (rigidity, tremors, pill rolling, shuffling gait)

🔷 Assess for neuroleptic malignant syndrome: hyperthermia, increased CPK, altered mental status, muscle rigidity
- Assess skin turgor daily
- Assess for constipation, urinary retention daily; if these occur, increase bulk and water in diet

Nursing diagnoses
- Knowledge, deficient (teaching)
- Noncompliance (teaching)
- Sensory perception, disturbed (uses)
- Thought processes, disturbed (uses)

Implementation
- Administer reduced dose in geriatric
- Decreased stimulus by dimming lights, avoiding loud noises
- Supervise ambulation until patient is stabilized on medication; do not involve in strenuous exercise program because fainting is possible; patient should not stand still for a long time
- Store in tight, light-resistant container

Patient/family education
- Advise patient that orthostatic hypotension may occur and to rise from sitting or lying position gradually
- Advise patient to avoid hot tubs, hot showers, tub baths; hypotension may occur
- Instruct patient to avoid abrupt withdrawal of this product; EPS may result; product should be withdrawn slowly
- Teach patient to avoid OTC preparations (cough, hayfever, cold) unless approved by prescriber, because serious product interactions may occur; avoid use with alcohol, CNS depressants; increased drowsiness may occur
- Advise patient to avoid hazardous activities if drowsy or dizzy
- Explain importance of compliance with product regimen
- Advise patient, family to report impaired vision, tremors, muscle twitching, urinary retention
- Instruct patient to take extra precautions to stay cool in hot weather, that heat stroke may occur

Evaluation
Positive therapeutic outcome
- Decreased in emotional excitement, hallucinations, delusions, paranoia; reorganization of patterns of thought, speech

Treatment of overdose: Lavage if orally ingested; provide airway; *do not induce vomiting*

---

ascorbic acid
(vitamin C) (OTC, Rx)
(as-kor′bic)
Apo-C 🍁, ascorbic acid, Ascorbicap, C-Span, Cebid, Cecon, Cecore 500, Cemill, Cenolate, Cetane, Cevalin, Cevi-Bid, Ce-Vi-Sol, Flavorcee, Mega-C/A Plus, Ortho/CS, Sunkist
Func. class.: Vitamin C, water-soluble vitamin

Pregnancy category C

Action: Needed for wound healing, collagen synthesis, antioxidant, carbohydrate metabolism

Therapeutic outcome: Replacement and supplementation of vit C

Uses: Vit C deficiency, scurvy, delayed wound and bone healing, chronic disease, before gastrectomy, dietary supplement

Unlabeled uses: Common cold prevention

Dosage and routes
RDA
Neonates and up to 6 mo: PO 30 mg/day
Infants 6 mo-1 yr: PO 35 mg/day
Child 1-3 yr: PO 40 mg/day
Child 4-10 yr: PO 45 mg/day
Child 11-14 yr: PO 50 mg/day
Child 14-18 yr: PO 65 mg/day (females), 75 mg/day (males)
Adult: PO 50-500 mg/day

Scurvy
Adult: PO/SUBCUT/IM/**IV** 100 mg-250 mg daily × 2 wk, then 50 mg or more daily
Child: PO/SUBCUT/IM/**IV** 100-300 mg daily × 2 wk, then 35 mg or more daily

Wound healing/chronic disease/fracture
May be given with zinc
Adult: SUBCUT/IM/**IV**/PO 200-500 mg daily for 1-2 mo
Child: SUBCUT/IM/**IV**/PO 100-200 mg added doses for 1-2 mo

Urine acidification
Adult: 4-12 g daily in divided doses
Child: 500 mg q6-8hr

Available forms: Tabs 25, 50, 100, 250, 500, 1000, 1500 mg; effervescent tabs 1000 mg; chewable tabs 100, 250, 500 mg; time-release tabs 500, 750, 1000, 1500 mg; time-release caps 500 mg; crystals 4 g/tsp; powder 4 g/tsp; liquid 35 mg/0.6 ml; sol 100 mg/ml; syr 20 mg/ml, 500 mg/5 ml; inj SUBCUT, IM, **IV** 100, 250, 500 mg/ml

Adverse effects
CNS: Headache, insomnia, dizziness, fatigue, flushing
GI: Nausea, vomiting, diarrhea, anorexia, heartburn, cramps
GU: Polyuria, urine acidification, oxalate or urate renal stones, dysuria
HEMA: **Hemolytic anemia in patients with G6PD**
INTEG: Inflammation at inj site

Contraindications: Tartrazine, sulfite sensitivity; G6PD deficiency

Precautions: Pregnancy **C**, gout, diabetes, renal calculi (large doses)

Pharmacokinetics	
Absorption	Readily absorbed (PO)
Distribution	Widely distributed; crosses placenta
Metabolism	Oxidation
Excretion	Kidneys, inactive; breast milk
Half-life	Unknown

Pharmacodynamics
Unknown

Interactions
Drug/lab test
False positive: negatives in glucose tests (Clinitest, Tes-Tape)
False negative: occult blood (large dose), urine bilirubin, leukocyte determination

NURSING CONSIDERATIONS
Assessment
• Assess nutritional status for inclusion of foods high in vit C: citrus fruits, cantaloupe, tomatoes
• Assess for vit C deficiency before, during, and after treatment; scurvy (gingivitis, bleeding gums, loose teeth); poor bone development
• Monitor I&O ratio, polyuria; in patients receiving large doses, renal stones may occur; urine pH (acidification)
• Monitor ascorbic acid levels throughout treatment if continued deficiency is suspected
• Assess inj sites for inflammation, pain, redness, thrombophlebitis if in large doses

Nursing diagnoses
• Knowledge, deficient (teaching)
• Nutrition: less than body requirements, imbalanced (uses)

Implementation
PO route
• Swallow time rel tabs or caps whole; do not break, crush, or chew
• Mix oral sol with foods or fluids
IM route
• Not to be diluted; give deep in large muscle mass
IV, direct route
• Give undiluted by *direct* **IV** 100 mg over at least 1 min, rapid inf may cause fainting
Intermittent IV infusion route
• Give by intermittent inf after diluting with D_5W, $D_{10}W$, 0.9% NaCl, 0.45% NaCl, LR, Ringer's sol, dextrose/saline, dextrose/Ringer's combinations; temp will increase pressure in ampules; wrap with gauze before breaking
Syringe compatibilities: Metoclopramide, aminophylline, theophylline
Syringe incompatibilities: Cefazolin, doxapram
Additive compatibilities: Amikacin, calcium chloride, calcium gluceptate, calcium gluconate, cephalothin, chloramphenicol, chlorproMAZINE, colistimethate, cyanocobalamin, diphenhydrAMINE, heparin, kanamycin, methicillin, methyldopa, penicillin G potassium, polymyxin B, prednisoLONE, procaine, prochlorperazine, promethazine, verapamil
Additive incompatibilities: Bleomycin, cephapirin, nafcillin, sodium bicarbonate, warfarin
Y-site compatibilities: Warfarin

Patient/family education
• Teach patient necessary foods to be included in diet that are rich in vit C: citrus

Adverse effects: *italic* = common, **bold** = life-threatening

fruits, cantaloupe, tomatoes, chili peppers (red)

• Teach patient that smoking decreases vit C levels; not to exceed prescribed dose; increases will be excreted in urine, except time release

• Teach patient not to exceed RDA recommended dose, urinary stones may occur

• Teach patient using ascorbic acid for acidification of urine to test urine pH periodically

Evaluation
Positive therapeutic outcome

• Absence of anorexia, irritability, pallor, joint pain, hyperkeratosis, petechiae, poor wound healing

• Reversal of scurvy: bleeding gums, gingivitis, loose teeth

---

asenapine (Rx)
(a-sen′a-peen)
Saphris
Func. class.: Antipsychotic
Chem. class.: Benzisoxazole derivative

Pregnancy category C

Action: Unknown; may be mediated through both dopamine type 2 (D2) and serotonin type 2 (5-HT2A) antagonism

Therapeutic outcome: Decrease in delusions, hallucinations

Uses: Bipolar 1 disorder, schizophrenia

Dosage and routes
Schizophrenia
Adult: SL 5 mg bid, max 20 mg/day

Bipolar 1 disorder

Adult: SL 10 mg bid, may decrease to 5 mg bid as needed, max 20 mg/day

Available forms: SL tab 5, 10 mg

Adverse effects
CNS: EPS, pseudoparkinsonism, akathisia, dystonia, tardive dyskinesia, drowsiness, insomnia, agitation, anxiety, headache, **seizures, neuroleptic malignant syndrome,** dizziness
CV: Orthostatic hypotension, **sinus tachycardia, heart failure, QT prolongation, stroke, bundle branch block**
GI: Nausea, vomiting, *constipation,* weight gain, increased appetite
GU: Hyperprolactinemia, hyperglycemia, hyponatremia
HEMA: **Thrombocytopenia**

Contraindications: Breastfeeding, hypersensitivity

Precautions: Pregnancy **C**, children, geriatric patients, cardiac/renal/hepatic disease, breast cancer, Parkinson's disease, dementia, seizure disorder, CNS depression, agranulocytosis, QT prolongation, torsades de pointes, suicidal ideation, substance abuse

Pharmacokinetics
Absorption	Unknown
Distribution	Protein binding 95%
Metabolism	Liver
Excretion	Unknown
Half-life	Terminal 24 hr

Pharmacodynamics
Onset	Unknown
Peak	½-1½ hr
Duration	Unknown

Interactions
Individual drugs
Alcohol: increased sedation
Bepridil, haloperidol, methadone, chloroquine, clarithromycin, droperidol, erythromycin, grepafloxacin, halofantrine, pentamidine, probucol, sparfloxacin: increased QT prolongation
Carbamazepine: increased asenpine excretion
Drug classifications
Other CNS depressants: increased sedation
CYP2D6 inhibitors/substrates (SSRIs), other antipsychotics: increased EPS
Class IA/ III antidysrhythmics, some phenothiazines, β-agonists, local anesthetics, tricyclics: increased QT prolongation
CYP2D6 inducers (carbamazepine, barbiturates, phenytoins, rifampin): decreased asenpine action
Drug/herb
Kava: increased CNS depression
Betel palm, kava: increased EPS
Drug/lab test
Increase: prolactin levels

NURSING CONSIDERATIONS
Assessment
⊕ Assess mental status before initial administration; watch for suicidal thoughts and behaviors

• Assess for affect, orientation, LOC, reflexes, gait, coordination, sleep pattern disturbances

• Monitor for B/P standing and lying; also pulse, respirations; take these q4hr during initial treatment; establish baseline before starting treatment; report drops of 30 mm Hg;

---

watch for ECG changes; QT prolongation may occur
• Monitor for dizziness, faintness, palpitations, tachycardia on rising
• Assess for EPS, including akathisia, tardive dyskinesia (bizarre movements of the jaw, mouth, tongue, extremities), pseudoparkinsonism (rigidity, tremors, pill rolling, shuffling gait)
• Assess for neuroleptic malignant syndrome: hyperthermia, increased CPK, altered mental status, muscle rigidity
• Assess for serious reactions in geriatric patients: heart failure, sudden death
• Assess for constipation daily; increase bulk and water in diet if needed
• Assess for weight gain, hyperglycemia, metabolic changes in diabetes

Nursing diagnoses
• Knowledge, deficit (teaching)
• Noncompliance (teaching)

Implementation
PO route
• Reduce dose in geriatric patients
• Give anticholinergic agent on order from prescriber, to be used for EPS
• Avoid use with CNS depressants
• SL tab: remove tab, place tab under tongue, after it dissolves, swallow, advise not to chew, crush or swallow tabs, not to eat or drink for 10 min
• Supervise ambulation until patient is stabilized on medication; do not involve in strenuous exercise program because fainting is possible; patient should not stand still for a long time
• Increase fluids to prevent constipation
• Store in tight, light-resistant container

Patient/family education
• Caution patient that orthostatic hypotension may occur and to rise from sitting or lying position gradually
• Teach patient to avoid hot tubs, hot showers, tub baths; hypotension may occur
• Advise patient to avoid abrupt withdrawal of this product; EPS may result; product should be withdrawn slowly
• Advise patient to avoid OTC preparations (cough, hay fever, cold) unless approved by prescriber; serious product interactions may occur; avoid use of alcohol; increased drowsiness may occur
• Advise patient to avoid hazardous activities if drowsy or dizzy
• Advise patient about compliance with product regimen

• Advise patient that heat stroke may occur in hot weather; take extra precautions to stay cool
• Advise patient to use contraception, inform prescriber if pregnancy is planned or suspected

Evaluation
Positive therapeutic outcome
• Therapeutic response: decrease in emotional excitement, hallucinations, delusions, paranoia; reorganization of patterns of thought, speech

Treatment of overdose: Lavage if orally ingested; provide airway; *do not induce vomiting*

---

aspirin ⊗ (OTC)
(as′pir-in)
acetylsalicylic acid, Acuprin, Apo-ASA ✦, Apo-Asen ✦, Arthrinol ✦, Arthrisin ✦, Artria S.R., A.S.A., Aspergum, Aspirin ✦, Aspir-Low, Aspirtab, Astrin ✦, Bayer Aspirin, Coryphen ✦, Easprin, Ecotrin, 8 Hour Bayer Timed Release, Empirin, Entrophen ✦, Halfprin, Norwich Extra-Strength, Novasen ✦, PMS-ASA ✦, Sloprin, St. Joseph Children's Supasa ✦, Therapy Bayer, ZORprin
Func. class.: Nonopioid analgesic
Chem. class.: Salicylate

Pregnancy category D (3rd trimester)

Action: Blocks pain impulses in CNS, reduces inflammation by inhibition of prostaglandin synthesis; antipyretic action results from vasodilatation of peripheral vessels; decreases platelet aggregation

Therapeutic outcome: Decreased pain, inflammation, fever; absence of MI, transient ischemic attacks, thrombosis

Uses: Mild to moderate pain or fever including rheumatoid arthritis, osteoarthritis, thromboembolic disorders, transient ischemic attacks, rheumatic fever, post-MI, prophylaxis of MI, ischemic stroke, angina; acute MI

Unlabeled uses: Prevention of cataracts (long-term use), prevention of pregnancy loss in women with clotting disorders

Dosage and routes
Arthritis
Adult: PO 3 g/day in divided doses q4-6hr
Child >25 kg (55 lb): PO or rectal 90-130 mg/kg/day in divided doses

Adverse effects: *italic* = common, **bold** = life-threatening

Kawasaki disease (unlabeled)
Child: PO 80-100 mg/kg/day in 4 divided doses, maintenance 3-8 mg/kg/day as a single dose × 8 wk, given with gamma globulin

MI, stroke prophylaxis
Adult: PO 160-325 mg/day

Pain/fever
Adult: PO/RECT 325-650 mg q4hr prn, max 4 g/day
Child 2-11 yr: PO 10-15 mg/kg/dose q4hr, max 4 g/day

Thromboembolic disorders
Adult: PO 325-650 mg/day or bid

Transient ischemic attacks (risk)
Adult: PO 50-325 mg/day (grade 1A)

Prevention of recurrent MI
Adult: PO 75-162 mg/day

CABG
Adult: PO 325 mg/day starting 6 hr post-procedure, continue for 1 yr

PTCA
Adult: PO 325 mg 2 hr presurgery

Evolving MI with ST segment elevation (STEMI)
Adult: PO 160-325 mg non-enteric, chewed and swallowed immediately, maintenance 75-162 mg qd

Available forms: Tabs 81, 325, 500, 650, 800 mg; chewable tabs 81 mg; supp 300, 600, mg; gum 227 mg; enteric coated tabs 81, 325, 500, 975 mg; ext rel 800 mg; del rel tabs 325 mg

Adverse effects
CNS: Stimulation, drowsiness, dizziness, confusion, **seizures,** headache, flushing, hallucinations, **coma**
CV: Rapid pulse, pulmonary edema
EENT: Tinnitus, hearing loss
ENDO: Hypoglycemia, hyponatremia, hypokalemia
GI: Nausea, vomiting, **GI bleeding,** diarrhea, heartburn, anorexia, **hepatitis**
HEMA: **Thrombocytopenia, agranulocytosis, leukopenia, neutropenia, hemolytic anemia,** increased pro-time, PTT, bleeding time
INTEG: Rash, urticaria, bruising
RESP: Wheezing, hyperpnea
SYST: **Reye's syndrome (children), anaphylaxis, laryngeal edema**

Contraindications: Pregnancy **D** (3rd trimester), breastfeeding, children <12 yr, children with flulike symptoms, hypersensitivity to salicylates, tartrazine (FDC yellow dye #5), GI bleeding, bleeding disorders, vit K deficiency, peptic ulcer, acute bronchospasm, agranulocytosis, increased intracranial pressure, intracranial bleeding, nasal polyps, urticaria

Precautions: Abrupt discontinuation, acetaminophen/NSAIDs hypersensitivity, acid/base imbalance, alcoholism, ascites, asthma bone marrow suppression, geriatric patients, dehydration, G6PD deficiency, gout, heart-failure, anemia, renal/hepatic disease, pre/postoperatively, gastritis

Pharmacokinetics

Absorption	Well absorbed, small intestine (PO); erratic (enteric); slow (RECT)
Distribution	Rapidly, widely distributed; crosses placenta, protein binding 90%
Metabolism	Liver, extensively
Excretion	Inactive metabolites, kidney; breast milk
Half-life	15-20 min (low doses); 9 hr (high doses)

Pharmacodynamics

	PO	RECT
Onset	15-30 min	Slow
Peak	1-2 hr	4-5 hr
Duration	4-6 hr	6-7 hr

Interactions
Individual drugs
Alcohol, cefamandole, clopidogrel, eptifibatide, heparin, plicamycin, ticlopidine, tirofiban: increased risk of bleeding
Ammonium chloride, nizatidine: increased salicylate level
Insulin, methotrexate, phenytoin, valproic acid, warfarin: increased effects of each specific product
Nitroglycerin: increased hypotension
Probenecid: decreased effects of probenecid
Spironolactone, sulfinpyrazone: decreased effects
Drug classifications
ACE inhibitors: decreased antihypertensive effect
Antacids, corticosteroids, steroids, urinary alkalizers: decreased effects of aspirin
Anticoagulants, thrombolytics: increased risk of bleeding
Diuretics (loop), sulfonylamides, NSAIDs, β-blockers: decreased effect of each specific product

---

NSAIDs, antiinflammatories, steroids: increased gastric ulcers

Penicillins, oral hypoglycemics, sulfonamides, thrombolytic agents: increased effects of each specific product

Salicylates: decreased blood glucose levels

Urinary acidifiers: increased salicylate levels

Drug/herb
Anise, arnica, bilberry, bogbean, chamomile, chondroitin, clove, dong quai, fenugreek, feverfew, garlic, ginger, ginkgo, ginseng *(Panax)*, horse chestnut, Irish moss, licorice, pansy, red clover: increased risk of bleeding

Arginine, gossypol: gastric irritation

Drug/food
Foods acidifying urine may increase aspirin levels

Drug/lab test
Increased: coagulation studies, liver function studies, serum uric acid, amylase, CO_2, urinary protein

Decreased: serum potassium, cholesterol

Interference: VMA, 5-IIIAA, xylose tolerance test, TSH

NURSING CONSIDERATIONS
Assessment
- Assess for pain: character, location, intensity, ROM before and 1 hr after administration
- Monitor liver function studies: AST, ALT, bilirubin, creatinine if patient is on long-term therapy
- Monitor renal function studies: BUN, urine creatinine if patient is on long-term therapy
- Monitor blood studies: CBC, Hct, Hgb, pro-time if patient is on long-term therapy
- Check I&O ratio; decreasing output may indicate renal failure (long-term therapy)
- ◆ Assess hepatotoxicity: dark urine, clay-colored stools, yellowing of the skin and sclera, itching, abdominal pain, fever, diarrhea if patient is on long-term therapy
- Assess for allergic reactions: rash, urticaria; if these occur, product may have to be discontinued; patients with asthma, nasal polyps, allergies; severe allergic reactions may occur
- Assess for ototoxicity: tinnitus, ringing, roaring in ears; audiometric testing needed before, after long-term therapy
- Monitor salicylate level: therapeutic level 150-300 mcg/ml for chronic inflammation
- Check edema in feet, ankles, legs
- Identify prior product history; there are many product interactions

Nursing diagnoses
- Injury, risk for (side effects)
- Knowledge, deficient (teaching)
- Mobility, impaired physical (uses)
- Pain, acute (uses)
- Pain, chronic (uses)

Implementation
PO route
- Do not break, crush, or chew enteric product
- Administer to patient crushed or whole; chewable tab should be chewed
- Give with food or milk to decrease gastric symptoms; separate by 2 hr of enteric product; absorption may be slowed
- Give antacids 1-2 hr after enteric products
- Give with 8 oz of water and have patient sit upright for 30 min after dose; discard tabs if vinegar-like smell is present; avoid if allergic to tartrazine
- Give ½ hr before planned exercise

Patient/family education
- Teach patient to report any symptoms of renal/hepatic toxicity, visual changes, ototoxicity, allergic reactions, bleeding (long-term therapy)
- Instruct patient to take with 8 oz of water and sit upright for 30 min after dose to facilitate product passing into the stomach; to discard tabs if vinegar-like smell is present; to avoid if allergic to tartrazine
- Instruct patient not to exceed recommended dosage; acute poisoning may result
- Advise patient to read label on other OTC products; many contain aspirin
- Inform patient that the therapeutic response takes 2 wk (arthritis)
- Teach patient to report tinnitus, confusion, diarrhea, sweating, hyperventilation
- Advise patient to avoid alcohol ingestion; GI bleeding may occur
- Advise patient with allergies, nasal polyps, asthma, that allergic reactions may develop
- Instruct patient to read labels on other OTC products; may contain salicylates
- Teach patient not to give to children or teens with flulike symptoms or chicken pox; Reye's syndrome may develop

Evaluation
Positive therapeutic outcome
- Decreased pain
- Decreased inflammation
- Decreased fever
- Absence of MI
- Absence of transient ischemic attacks, thrombosis

Treatment of overdose: Lavage, activated charcoal, monitor electrolytes, VS

atazanavir (Rx)
(at-a-za-na′veer)
Reyataz
Func. class.: Antiretroviral
Chem. class.: Protease inhibitor
Pregnancy category B

Action: Inhibits human immunodeficiency virus (HIV-1) protease, which prevents maturation of the infectious virus

Therapeutic outcome: Decreasing symptoms of HIV

Uses: HIV-1 infection in combination with other antiretroviral agents

Dosage and routes
Antiretroviral-naive patients
Adult: PO 400 mg daily
Child ≥6 yr/adolescent ≥39 kg: PO 300 mg with ritonavir 100 mg qd
Child ≥6 yr/adolescent 32-39 kg: PO 250 mg with ritonavir 100 mg qd
Child ≥6 yr/adolescent 25-32 kg: PO 200 mg with ritonavir 100 mg qd

Antiretroviral-experienced patients
Adult: PO 300 mg daily and ritonavir 100 mg daily
Child ≥6 yr/adolescent ≥39 kg: PO 300 mg with ritonavir 100 mg qd
Child ≥6 yr/adolescent 32-39 kg: PO 250 mg with ritonavir 100 mg qd
Child ≥6 yr/adolescent 25-32 kg: PO 200 mg with ritonavir 100 mg qd

Hepatic dose
Adult: PO (Child-Pugh B) 300 mg daily; (Child-Pugh C) do not use

Available forms: Caps 100, 150, 200, 300 mg

Adverse effects
CNS: Headache, depression, dizziness, insomnia, peripheral neuropathy
GI: Diarrhea, abdominal pain, nausea, vomiting, **hepatotoxicity**
INTEG: Rash, **Stevens-Johnson syndrome***, photosensitivity*
MISC: Fatigue, fever, arthralgia, back pain, cough, lipodystrophy, pain, gynecomastia, nephrolithiasis

Contraindications: Hypersensitivity

Precautions: Pregnancy **B**, breastfeeding, children, geriatric, liver disease, alcoholism, antimicrobial resistance, AV block, diabetes, dialysis, elderly, females, hemophilia, hypercholesterolemia, immune reconstitution syndrome, lactic acidosis, pancreatitis

Pharmacokinetics
Absorption	Rapid, increased with food
Distribution	86% protein bound
Metabolism	Liver extensively by CYP3A4
Excretion	27% excreted unchanged in urine/feces (minimal)
Half-life	7 hr

Pharmacodynamics
Onset	Unknown
Peak	2 hr
Duration	Unknown

Interactions
Individual drugs
Chlorazepate, clarithromycin, cycloSPORINE, diazepam, irinotecan, midazolam, pimozide, sildenafil, sirolimus, tacrolimus, triazolam, warfarin: increased levels resulting in increased toxicity
Didanosine, efavirenz, rifampin: decreased atazanavir levels
Indinavir: increased hyperbilirubinemia
Drug classifications
Antacids, H₂-receptor antagonists, proton pump inhibitors: decreased atazanavir levels
Antidepressants (tricyclics), antidysrhythmics, ergots, calcium channel blockers, HMG-CoA reductase inhibitors, immunosuppressants: increased levels resulting in increased toxicity
Contraceptives (oral), estrogens: increased effects
CYP3A4 substrates, CYP3A4 inhibitors: increased atazanavir levels
CYP3A4 inducers: decreased atazanavir levels
Drug/herb
St. John's wort: decreased atazanavir levels
Drug/lab test
Increased: AST, ALT, total bilirubin, amylase, lipase, CK
Decreased: Hgb, neutrophils, platelets

NURSING CONSIDERATIONS
Assessment
◆ Assess for hepatic failure
• Assess for signs of infection, anemia
• Monitor liver function studies: ALT, AST, bilirubin
• Monitor bowel pattern before, during treatment; if severe abdominal pain with

 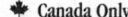

bleeding occurs, product should be discontinued; monitor hydration
• Monitor viral load, CD4 count throughout treatment
• Assess skin eruptions, rash, urticaria, itching
• Identify allergies before treatment, reaction of each medication; place allergies on chart

Nursing diagnoses
• Injury, risk for (uses, adverse reactions)
• Knowledge, deficient (teaching)

Implementation
• Administer with food; take 2 hr before or 1 hr after antacid or didanosine

Patient/family education
• Advise to take as prescribed with other antiretrovirals as prescribed; if dose is missed, take as soon as remembered up to 1 hr before next dose; do not double dose; do not share with others
• Teach that product must be taken daily to maintain blood levels for duration of therapy
• Teach that photosensitivity may occur; use protective clothing or stay out of the sun
• Instruct to notify prescriber if diarrhea, nausea, vomiting, rash occur; dizziness, light-headedness, ECG may be altered
• Inform that product interacts with many products and St. John's wort; advise prescriber of all products, herbal products used
• Advise that redistribution of body fat may occur; the effect is not known
• Teach that product does not cure HIV-1 infection or prevent transmission to others, only controls symptoms
• Advise that if taking sildenafil with atazanavir, there may be an increased risk of phosphodiesterase type 5 inhibitor-associated adverse events, including hypotension and prolonged penile erection; notify physician promptly of these symptoms

Evaluation
Positive therapeutic outcome
• Increasing CD4 counts; decreased viral load, resolution of symptoms of HIV-1 infection

atenolol (Rx)
(a-ten'oh-lole)
Apo-Atenolol ✦, atenolol ✦, Novo-Atenol ✦, Tenormin
Func. class.: Antihypertensive
Chem. class.: β-Blocker; β₁-, β₂-blocker (high doses)

Pregnancy category D

Do not confuse:
atenolol/**albuterol**/Altenol, Tenormin/thiamine/Imuran

Action: Competitively blocks stimulation of β-adrenergic receptor within vascular smooth muscle; produces negative chronotropic activity (decreases rate of SA node discharge, increases recovery time), slows conduction of AV node, decreases heart rate, negative inotropic activity, decreases O₂ consumption in myocardium; also decreases renin-aldosterone-angiotensin system at high doses, inhibits β₂-receptors in bronchial system at higher doses

Therapeutic outcome: Decreased B/P, heart rate, prevention of angina pectoris, MI

Uses: Mild to moderate hypertension; prophylaxis of angina pectoris; suspected or known MI (**IV** use)

Dosage and routes
Adult: PO 25-50 mg daily, increasing q1-2wk to 100 mg daily; may increase to 200 mg daily for angina or up to 100 mg for hypertension
Child: PO 0.8-1 mg/kg/dose initially, range 0.8-1.5 mg/kg/day, max 2 mg/kg/day
Geriatric: PO 25 mg/day initially

Renal dose
Adult: PO CCr 15-35 ml/min, max 50 mg/day; CCr <15 ml/min max 25 mg/day; hemodialysis 25-50 mg after dialysis

Available forms: Tabs 25, 50, 100 mg

Adverse effects
CNS: Insomnia, fatigue, dizziness, mental changes, memory loss, hallucinations, depression, lethargy, drowsiness, strange dreams, catatonia
CV: **Profound hypotension, bradycardia, CHF,** *cold extremities, postural hypotension, 2nd- or 3rd-degree heart block*
EENT: Sore throat, dry burning eyes, blurred vision, stuffy nose
ENDO: Increased hypoglycemic response to insulin
GI: Nausea, diarrhea, vomiting, **mesenteric arterial thrombosis, ischemic colitis**

Adverse effects: *italic* = common, **bold** = life-threatening

GU: Impotence, decreased libido
HEMA: Agranulocytosis, thrombocytopenia, purpura
INTEG: Rash, fever, alopecia
RESP: Bronchospasm, dyspnea, wheezing, pulmonary edema

Contraindications: Pregnancy **D,** hypersensitivity to β-blockers, cardiogenic shock, 2nd- or 3rd-degree heart block, sinus bradycardia, cardiac failure, Raynaud's disease, pulmonary edema

Precautions: Major surgery, breastfeeding, diabetes mellitus, renal disease, thyroid disease, CHF, COPD, asthma, well-compensated heart failure, dialysis, myasthenia gravis

Black Box Warning: Abrupt discontinuation

Pharmacokinetics

Absorption	50%-60% (PO)
Distribution	Crosses placenta; protein binding (5%-15%)
Metabolism	Not metabolized
Excretion	Breast milk, kidneys (50%), feces (50%—unabsorbed product)
Half-life	6-9 hr

Pharmacodynamics

	PO	IV
Onset	1 hr	Rapid
Peak	2-4 hr	5 min
Duration	24 hr	Unknown

Interactions
Individual drugs
Digoxin, diltiazem, hydralazine, methyldopa, prazosin, reserpine, verapamil: increased hypotension, bradycardia
Ephedrine, pseudoephedrine: increased hypertension
Insulin, theophylline, dopamine: decreased effect of each of these drugs
Drug classifications
Amphetamines: increased hypertension
Anticholinergics, cardiac glycosides, antihypertensives: increased hypotension, bradycardia
Antidiabetic agents (oral) MAOIs: decreased effect of each of these drugs
Sympathomimetics (cough, cold preparations): mutual inhibition
Drug/herb
Betel palm, butterbur, cola tree, figwort, fumitory, guarana, hawthorn, jaborandi tree,

lily of the valley, motherwort, plantain: increased atenolol effect
Coenzyme Q10, yohimbe: decreased atenolol effect
Drug/lab test
Increased: uric acid, potassium, triglyceride, blood glucose, BUN, ANA titer

NURSING CONSIDERATIONS
Assessment
• Monitor B/P during beginning treatment, periodically thereafter; pulse q4hr; note rate, rhythm, quality: apical/radial pulse before administration; notify prescriber of any significant changes (pulse <50 bpm); ECG
• Check for baselines in renal, liver function tests before therapy begins
• Assess for edema in feet, legs daily; monitor I&O, daily weight; check for jugular vein distention, crackles bilaterally, dyspnea (CHF)

Nursing diagnoses
• Cardiac output, decreased (uses)
• Injury, risk for (side effects)
• Knowledge, deficient (teaching)
• Noncompliance (teaching)

Implementation
PO route
• Given before meals, at bedtime; tablet may be crushed or swallowed whole; give with food to prevent GI upset; reduced dosage in renal dysfunction; take at same time each day
• Store protected from light, moisture; place in cool environment
IV route
• Give **IV** direct over 5 min or diluted in 10-50 ml D₅W, 0.9% NaCl, and give at prescribed rate
Y-site compatibilities: Acyclovir, amphotericin, bliposome, daptomycin, diltiazem, ertapenem, granisetron, hydromorphone, linezolid, lorazepam, meperidine, meropenem, morphine, ondansetron, palonosetron, piperacillin/tazobactam, tacrolimus, tirofiban, voriconazole

Patient/family education
⬥ Teach patient not to discontinue product abruptly; taper over 2 wk (angina) as directed; may cause precipitate angina if stopped abruptly; take at same time each day
• Teach patient not to use OTC products containing α-adrenergic stimulants (such as nasal decongestants, OTC cold preparations); to limit alcohol, smoking; to limit sodium intake as prescribed
• Teach patient how to take pulse and B/P at home; advise when to notify prescriber

 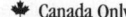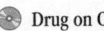

- Instruct patient to comply with weight control, dietary adjustments, modified exercise program
- Advise patient to carry/wear emergency ID for products, allergies, conditions being treated; tell patient product controls symptoms but does not cure
- Caution patient to avoid hazardous activities if dizziness, drowsiness is present
- Teach patient to report symptoms of CHF: difficult breathing, especially on exertion or when lying down, night cough, swelling of extremities or bradycardia, dizziness, confusion, depression, fever
- Teach patient to take product as prescribed, not to double doses, skip doses; take any missed doses as remembered if at least 6 hr until next dose
- Advise to change position slowly
- Advise patient that product may mask symptoms of hypoglycemia in diabetic patients
- Advise patient to use contraception while taking this product

Evaluation
Positive therapeutic outcome
- Decreased B/P in hypertension (after 1-2 wk)
- Absence of dysrhythmias
- Absence of MI
- Decreased angina/pain
- Increased activity tolerance

Treatment of overdose: Lavage, **IV** atropine for bradycardia, **IV** theophylline for bronchospasm, digoxin, O₂, diuretic for cardiac failure, hemodialysis, **IV** glucose for hyperglycemia, **IV** diazepam (or phenytoin) for seizures

---

atomoxetine (Rx)
(at-o-mox′eh-teen)
Strattera
Func. class.: Psychotherapeutic—miscellaneous

Pregnancy category C

Action: A selective norepinephrine reuptake inhibitor; may inhibit the presynaptic norepinephrine transporter; exact mechanism of action is unknown

Therapeutic outcome: Decreased hyperactivity, impulsivity, increased attention, organization, ability to complete tasks

Uses: Attention deficit hyperactivity disorder

Dosage and routes
Child ≤70 kg: PO 0.5 mg/kg, increase after 3 days to a target daily dose of 1.2 mg/kg in AM or evenly divided doses AM, late afternoon; max 1.4 mg/kg/day or 100 mg daily, whichever is less
Adult and child >70 kg: PO 40 mg daily, increase after 3 days to a target daily dose of 80 mg in AM or evenly divided doses AM, late afternoon; max 100 mg daily

Maintenance
Adolescent ≤15 yr and child ≥6 yr: PO 1.2-1.8 mg/kg/day

Initial dose titration with strong CYP2D6 inhibitors
Adult and child >6 yr weighing >70 kg: PO 40 mg/day each AM or 2 evenly divided doses, titrate to target of 80 mg/day if symptoms do not improve after 4 wk and dose is well tolerated

Hepatic dose
(Child-Pugh B) reduce dose by 50%
(Child-Pugh C) reduce dose by 75%

Available forms: Caps 10, 18, 25, 40, 60, 80, 100 mg

Adverse effects
CNS: Insomnia, dizziness, headache, irritability, crying, mood swings, fatigue, hypoesthesia, lethargy, paresthesia
CV: Palpitations, hot flushes, tachycardia, increased B/P
ENDO: Growth retardation
GI: Dyspepsia, nausea, anorexia, dry mouth, weight loss, vomiting, diarrhea, constipation, **hepatic injury**
GU: Urinary hesitancy, retention, dysmenorrhea, erectile disturbance, ejaculation failure, impotence, prostatitis, abnormal orgasm, male pelvic pain
INTEG: **Exfoliative dermatitis,** sweating, rash
MISC: Cough, rhinorrhea, dermatitis, ear infection

Contraindications: Hypersensitivity, closed-angle glaucoma, arteriosclerosis, cardiac disease, cardiomyopathy, heart failure, jaundice, MAOI therapy

Precautions: Pregnancy C, breastfeeding, hypertension, hepatic disease, angioedema, bipolar disorder, dysrhythmias, CAD, hypo/hypertension

Black Box Warning: Children <6 yr, suicidal ideation

Pharmacokinetics	
Absorption	Unknown
Distribution	Protein binding, 98%
Metabolism	Liver
Excretion	Kidneys
Half-life	Unknown

Pharmacodynamics

Unknown

Interactions
Individual drug
Albuterol: increased cardiovascular effects
Drug classifications
CYP2D6 inhibitors (amiodarone, cimetidine [weak], citalopram, clomiPRAMINE, delavirdine, escitalopram, fluoxetine, gefitinib, imatinib, paroxetine, propafenone, quinidine [potent], ritonavir, sertraline, thioridazine, venlafaxine): increased effects of atomoxetine
⬥MAOIs or within 14 days of MAOIs, vasopressors: hypertensive crisis
Pressor agents: increased cardiovascular effects

NURSING CONSIDERATIONS
Assessment
- Monitor VS, B/P; check patients with cardiac disease more often for increased B/P
- Monitor height, growth rate q3mo in children; growth rate may be decreased
⬥ Assess mental status: mood, sensorium, affect, stimulation, insomnia, aggressiveness, suicidal ideation
- Assess appetite, sleep, speech patterns
- Assess for attention span, decreased hyperactivity in ADHD persons

Nursing diagnoses
- Coping, ineffective (uses)
- Coping, compromised family (uses)
- Knowledge, deficient (teaching)
- Thought processes, disturbed (uses)

Implementation
- Swallow whole; do not break, crush, or chew
- Give without regard to food
- Provide gum, hard candy, frequent sips of water for dry mouth

Patient/family education
- Advise patient to avoid OTC preparations unless approved by prescriber
- Advise patient to avoid alcohol ingestion
- Advise patient to avoid hazardous activities until stabilized on medication
- Advise patient to get needed rest; patients will feel more tired at end of day; do not take dose late in day, insomnia may occur
- Advise to report suicidal ideation

Evaluation
Positive therapeutic outcome
- Decreased hyperactivity (ADHD)

atorvastatin (Rx)
(a-tore′va-stat-in)
Lipitor
Func. class.: Antilipidemic
Chem. class.: HMG-CoA reductase inhibitor
Pregnancy category X

Action: Inhibits HMG-CoA reductase enzyme, which reduces cholesterol synthesis, high doses lead to plaque regression

Therapeutic outcome: Decreased cholesterol levels and LDLs, increased HDLs

Uses: As an adjunct in primary hypercholesterolemia (types Ia, Ib), dysbetalipoproteinemia, elevated triglyceride levels; prevention of cardiovascular disease by reduction of heart risk in those with mildly elevated cholesterol

Dosage and routes
Adult: PO 10-20 mg daily, usual range 10-80, dosage adjustments may be made in 2-4 wk intervals, max 80 mg/day; patients requiring >45% reduction in LDL may be started at 40 mg daily
Child 10-17 yr: 10 mg qd, max 20 mg qd (heterozygous familial hypercholesterolemia in adolescent boys/postmenarchal girls)

Available forms: Tabs 10, 20, 40, 80 mg

Adverse effects
CNS: Headache, asthenia, **Lou Gehrig's disease (ALS)**
EENT: Lens opacities
GI: Abdominal cramps, constipation, diarrhea, heartburn, nausea, dyspepsia, *flatus,* **liver dysfunction,** pancreatitis, increased serum transaminase
GU: Impotence
INTEG: Rash, pruritus, alopecia
MISC: Hypersensitivity
MS: Myalgia, **rhabdomyolysis,** arthralgia
RESP: Pharyngitis, sinusitis

Contraindications: Pregnancy **X**, breastfeeding, hypersensitivity, active liver disease

Precautions: Past liver disease, alcoholism, severe acute infections, trauma, severe metabolic disorders, electrolyte imbalance

Pharmacokinetics

Absorption	Unknown
Distribution	Unknown
Metabolism	Liver
Excretion	Bile, feces, kidneys
Half-life	14 hr

Pharmacodynamics
Unknown

Interactions
Individual drugs
Clofibrate, cycloSPORINE, erythromycin, gemfibrozil, niacin: increased risk of rhabdomyolysis
Colestipol: decreased action of atorvastatin
Digoxin: increased action of digoxin
Erythromycin: increased levels of atorvastatin
Warfarin: increased action of warfarin
Drug classifications
Antifungals (azole): possible rhabdomyolysis
Contraceptives (oral): increased levels
Drug/herb
Glucomannan: increased effect
Gotu kola, St. John's wort: decreased effect
Drug/food
Grapefruit juice: possible toxicity
Oatbran may reduce effectiveness
Drug/lab test
Increased: bilirubin, alkaline phosphatase
Interference: thyroid function tests

NURSING CONSIDERATIONS
Assessment
• Assess nutrition: fat, protein, carbohydrates; nutritional analysis should be completed by dietitian before treatment
• Assess for muscle pain, tenderness; obtain CPK if these occur, product may need to be discontinued
• Monitor bowel pattern daily; diarrhea may be a problem
• Monitor triglycerides, cholesterol at baseline and throughout treatment; LDL and VLDL should be watched closely; if increased, product should be discontinued
• Monitor liver function studies q1-2mo during the first 1½ yr of treatment; AST, ALT, liver function tests may be increased
• Monitor renal studies in patients with compromised renal system: BUN, I&O ratio, creatinine
• Assess eyes via ophthalmic exam 1 mo after treatment begins, annually

Nursing diagnoses
• Diarrhea (adverse reactions)
• Knowledge, deficient (teaching)
• Noncompliance (teaching)

Implementation
• Administer total daily dose at any time of day
• Store in cool environment in airtight, light-resistant container

Patient/family education
• Inform patient that compliance is needed for positive results to occur, not to double doses
• Teach patient that risk factors should be decreased: high-fat diet, smoking, alcohol consumption, absence of exercise
• Advise patient to notify prescriber if the GI symptoms of diarrhea, abdominal or epigastric pain, nausea, vomiting; chills, fever, sore throat; muscle pain, weakness occur
• Advise patient that treatment will take several years
• Advise patient that blood work and eye exam will be necessary during treatment
• Advise not to take if pregnant
• Advise patient to stay out of the sun, use protective clothing, or use sunscreen to prevent photosensitivity (rare)

Evaluation
Positive therapeutic outcome
• Decreased cholesterol levels, serum triglyceride
• Improved ratio of HDLs

---

atovaquone (Rx)
(a-toe'va-kwon)
Mepron
Func. class.: Antiprotozoal
Chem. class.: Aromatic diamide derivative; analog of ubiquinone
Pregnancy category C

Action: Interferes with DNA/RNA synthesis in protozoa, specifically ATP and nucleic acid synthesis

Therapeutic outcome: Antiprotozoal for *Pneumocystis jiroveci* only

Uses: *P. jiroveci* infections in patients intolerant of trimethoprim/sulfamethoxazole (co-trimoxazole), prophylaxis, *Toxoplasma gondii,* toxoplasmosis

Dosage and routes
Acute, mild, moderate
Pneumocystis jiroveci *pneumonia (PCP)*
Adult and adolescent 13-16 yr: PO 750 mg bid with food tid for 21 days

Pneumocystis jiroveci *pneumonia prophylaxis*
Adult and adolescent: PO 1500 mg daily with meal

Available forms: Susp 750 mg/5 ml

Adverse effects
CNS: Dizziness, headache, anxiety, insomnia, asthenia, fever
CV: Hypotension
GI: Nausea, vomiting, diarrhea, anorexia, increased AST and ALT, **acute pancreatitis,** constipation, abdominal pain
HEMA: Anemia, **leukopenia, neutropenia, thrombocytopenia, methemoglobinemia**
INTEG: Pruritus, urticaria, *rash,* oral monilia, sweating
META: Hyperkalemia, hypoglycemia, hyponatremia
OTHER: Cough, dyspnea

Contraindications: Hypersensitivity or history of developing life-threatening allergic reactions to any component of the formulation, benzyl alcohol sensitivity

Precautions: Pregnancy **C,** breastfeeding, GI/hepatic disease, neonates, respiratory insufficiency

Pharmacokinetics
Absorption	Poor; increased when taken with fatty foods
Distribution	Unknown
Metabolism	Hepatic recycling
Excretion	Feces, unchanged (94%)
Half-life	2-3 days

Pharmacodynamics
Onset	Unknown
Peak	1-8 hr
Duration	Unknown

Interactions
Individual drugs
Rifampin, rifabutin, tetracycline: decreased effectiveness of atovaquone
Drug classifications
Use cautiously with highly protein-bound products with narrow therapeutic indices

NURSING CONSIDERATIONS
Assessment
• Assess for *Pneumocystis jiroveci:* monitor WBC, bilateral lung sounds, sputum for C&S; these should be checked before, periodically during, after treatment; after collection of 1st sputum, therapy may begin
• Monitor for symptoms of hyponatremia: *CV:* increased B/P, cold, clammy skin, hypovolemia or hypervolemia; *GI:* anorexia, nausea, vomiting, diarrhea, abdominal cramps; *NEURO:* lethargy, increased ICP, confusion, headache, seizures, coma, fatigue, tremors, hyperreflexia
• Monitor for symptoms of hypoglycemia/hyperglycemia in diabetic patients
• Monitor blood studies: blood glucose, CBC, platelets; I&O ratio; ECG for cardiac dysrhythmias, check B/P; liver function tests: AST, ALT
• Monitor for signs of infection; anemia; monitor bowel pattern before, during treatment
• Monitor respiratory status: rate, character, wheezing, dyspnea; ABGs, chest films
• Assess for dizziness, confusion, hallucination
• Assess for allergies before treatment, reaction of each medication; place allergies on chart; notify all people giving products

Nursing diagnoses
• Diarrhea (adverse reactions)
• Infection, risk for (uses)
• Knowledge, deficient (teaching)

Implementation
• Give with food (preferably fatty); increased absorption of the product and higher plasma concentrations will occur; give tid × 3 wk
• Give oral suspension after shaken
• Take all contents of foil pouch

Patient/family education
• Instruct patient to take with food, preferably fatty foods, to increase plasma concentrations
• Advise patient to take product exactly as prescribed

Evaluation
Positive therapeutic outcome
• Decreased temperature
• Ability to breathe
• Three negative sputum cultures

 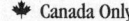

⚠ HIGH ALERT

atropine 🔷 (Rx)
(a′troe-peen)

Atreza, atropine sulfate, Atro-Pen, Sal-Tropine

Func. class.: Antidysrhythmic, anticholinergic parasympatholytic, mydriatic
Chem. class.: Belladonna alkaloid

Pregnancy category C

Do not confuse:
atropine/Akarpine

Action: Blocks acetylcholine at parasympathetic neuroeffector sites; increases cardiac output, heart rate by blocking vagal stimulation in heart; dries secretions by blocking vagus

Therapeutic outcome: Drying of secretions, increased heart rate, cycloplegia, mydriasis

Uses: Bradycardia <40-50 bpm, bradydysrhythmia, reversal of anticholinesterase agents, insecticide poisoning, blocking cardiac vagal reflexes, decreasing secretions before surgery, antispasmodic with GU and biliary surgery, bronchodilator

Dosage and routes
Bradycardia/bradydysrhythmias
Adult: **IV** BOL 0.5-1 mg given q3-5min, not to exceed 2 mg
Child: **IV** BOL 0.01-0.03 mg/kg up to 0.4 mg or 0.3 mg/m², may repeat q4-6hr, min dose 0.1 mg to avoid paradoxical reaction

Organophosphate poisoning
Adult and child: IM (Atro-Pen)/**IV** 2 mg qhr until muscarinic symptoms disappear; may need 6 mg qhr
Adult and child ≥90 lb, usually >10 yr: 2 mg IM (Atro-Pen)
Child 40-90 lb, usually 4-10 yr: 1 mg IM (Atro-Pen)
Child 15-40 lb, 6 mo-4 yr: 0.05 mg IM (Atro-Pen)

Presurgery
Adult and child >20 kg: SUBCUT/IM/**IV** 0.4-0.6 mg before anesthesia
Child <20 kg: IM/SUBCUT 0.01 mg/kg up to 0.4 mg ½-1 hr preop, max 0.6 mg/dose

Available forms: Inj 0.05, 0.1, 0.3, 0.4, 0.5, 0.8, 1 mg/ml; tabs 0.4 mg; inj prefilled autoinjectors (Atro-Pen) 0.5, 1, 2 mg

Adverse effects
CNS: Headache, dizziness, involuntary movement, confusion, psychosis, anxiety, **coma,** flushing, drowsiness, insomnia, weakness, delirium (geriatric)

CV: Hypo/hypertension, paradoxic bradycardia, angina, PVCs, **tachycardia,** ectopic ventricular beats
EENT: Blurred vision, photophobia, glaucoma, eye pain, pupil dilatation, nasal congestion
GI: Dry mouth, nausea, vomiting, abdominal pain, anorexia, constipation, **paralytic ileus,** abdominal distention, altered taste
GU: Retention, hesitancy, impotence, dysuria
INTEG: Rash, urticaria, contact dermatitis, dry skin, flushing
MISC: Suppression of breastfeeding, decreased sweating

Contraindications: Hypersensitivity to belladonna alkaloids, closed-angle glaucoma, GI obstructions, myasthenia gravis, thyrotoxicosis, ulcerative colitis, prostatic hypertrophy, tachycardia/tachydysrhythmias, asthma, acute hemorrhage, severe hepatic disease, myocardial ischemia

Precautions: Pregnancy C, breastfeeding, child <6 yr, geriatric, renal disease, CHF, hyperthyroidism, COPD, hypertension, intraabdominal infections, Down syndrome, spastic paralysis, gastric ulcer

Pharmacokinetics	
Absorption	Well absorbed (PO, SUBCUT, IM)
Distribution	Crosses blood-brain barrier, placenta
Metabolism	Liver
Excretion	Kidneys, unchanged (70%-90%); breast milk
Half-life	13-40 hr

Pharmacodynamics				
	PO	IM/ SUBCUT	IV	OPHTH
Onset	½ hr	15 min	2-4 min	½ hr
Peak	½-1 hr	30 min	2-4 min	30-60 min
Duration	4-6 hr	4-6 hr	4-6 hr	1-2 wk

Interactions
Individual drugs
Amantadine: increased anticholinergic effects
Ketoconazole, levodopa: decreased absorption
Potassium chloride (oral): mucosal lesions
Drug classifications
Antacids: decreased absorption of atropine
Antidepressants (tricyclic), antiparkinson agents: increased anticholinergic effect
Drug/herb
Aconite: increased toxicity, death
Aloe, buckthorn (chronic use), cascara sagrada (chronic use), figwort, fumitory,

Adverse effects: *italic* = common, **bold** = life-threatening

goldenseal, jimsonweed, kudzu, licorice, rhubarb, scopolia, senna: increased effect
Black root: forms insoluble complex
Coltsfoot: decreased effect
Horehound: increased serotonin effect

NURSING CONSIDERATIONS
Assessment
• Monitor I&O ratio; check for urinary retention and daily output in geriatric or postoperative patients
• Monitor ECG for ectopic ventricular beats, PVC, tachycardia in cardiac patients
• Monitor for bowel sounds; check for constipation; abdominal distention and constipation may occur
• Monitor respiratory status: rate, rhythm, cyanosis, wheezing, dyspnea, engorged neck veins
• Monitor cardiac rate: rhythm, character, B/P continuously
• Monitor allergic reaction: rash, urticaria

Nursing diagnoses
• Cardiac output, decreased (uses)
• Constipation (adverse reactions)
• Knowledge, deficient (teaching)

Implementation
PO route
• PO 30 min before meals
• Give increased bulk, water in diet if constipation occurs (anticholinergic effect)
IM route
• Expect atropine flush 15-20 min after inj; it may occur in children and is not harmful
IV route
• Give **IV** undiluted or diluted with 10 ml sterile H_2O; give at a rate of 0.6 mg/min; give through Y-tube or 3-way stopcock; do not add to **IV** sol; may cause paradoxic bradycardia lasting 2 min
Syringe compatibilities: Benzquinamide, butorphanol, chlorproMAZINE, cimetidine, dimenhyDRINATE, diphenhydrAMINE, droperidol, fentanyl, glycopyrrolate, heparin, hydromorphone, hydrOXYzine, meperidine, metoclopramide, midazolam, milrinone, morphine, nalbuphine, pentazocine, perphenazine, prochlorperazine, promazine, promethazine, propiomazine, ranitidine, scopolamine, sufentanil, vit B with C
Y-site compatibilities: Amrinone, etomidate, famotidine, heparin, hydrocortisone sodium succinate, meropenem, nafcillin, potassium chloride, sufentanil, vit B/C
Additive compatibilities: DOBUTamine, furosemide, meropenem, netilmicin, sodium bicarbonate, verapamil

Patient/family education
• Advise patient not to perform strenuous activity in high temperatures; heat stroke may result
• Instruct patient to take as prescribed; not to skip doses
• Instruct patient to report change in vision; blurring or loss of sight; trouble breathing; sweating; flushing, chest pain, allergic reactions, constipation, urinary retention
• Caution patient not to operate machinery if drowsiness occurs
• Advise patient not to take OTC products without approval of physician

Evaluation
Positive therapeutic outcome
• Decreased dysrhythmias
• Increased heart rate
• Decreased secretions, GI, GU spasms
• Bronchodilatation

Treatment of overdose: O_2, artificial ventilation, ECG; administer DOPamine for circulatory depression; administer diazepam or thiopental for seizure; assess need for antidysrhythmics

---

atropine ophthalmic
See Appendix B

❗ HIGH ALERT

azacitidine (Rx)
(a-za-sie-ti'deen)
Vidaza
Func. class.: Antineoplastic hormone
Chem. class.: DNA demethylation agent
Pregnancy category D

Do not confuse:
azacitidine/azathioprine

Action: Cytotoxic by producing damage to double-strand DNA during DNA synthesis

Therapeutic outcome: Improved blood counts in refractor anemia

Uses: Myelodysplastic syndrome (MDS)

Dosage and routes
Adult: SUBCUT 75 mg/m^2 daily × 7 days, q4wk, premedicate with antiemetic, dose may be increased to 100 mg/m^2 if no response is seen after 2 treatment cycles, minimum treatment 4 cycles

Available forms: Powdered for inj, lyophilized 100 mg

♦ Alert   � Canada Only   🔘 Drug on CD   * "Tall Man" lettering (See Preface)

Adverse effects
CNS: Anxiety, depression, dizziness, fatigue, headache
CV: Cardiac murmur, hypotension, tachycardia, peripheral edema
GI: Diarrhea, nausea, vomiting, anorexia, constipation, abdominal pain, distention, tenderness, hemorrhoids, mouth hemorrhage, tongue ulceration, stomatitis, dyspepsia, **hepatotoxicity, hepatic coma**
GU: **Real failure, renal tubular acidosis**, dysuria, UTI
HEMA: **Leukopenia, anemia, thrombocytopenia, neutropenia**, ecchymosis
INTEG: Irritation at site, rash, sweating, pyrexia
META: Hypokalemia

Contraindications: Pregnancy **D,** hypersensitivity to this product or mannitol, advanced malignant hepatic tumors

Precautions: Breastfeeding, children, geriatric, renal/hepatic disease; baseline albumin <30 g/L; a man should not father a child while taking this product

Pharmacokinetics

Absorption	Rapid
Distribution	Unknown
Metabolism	Liver
Excretion	Urine
Half-life	35-49 min

Pharmacodynamics

Onset	Unknown
Peak	½ hr
Duration	Unknown

Interactions
Drug classifications
Antineoplastics, other: increased bone marrow depression

NURSING CONSIDERATIONS
Assessment
• Assess for CNS symptoms: fever, headache, chills, dizziness
• Monitor hematologic response with patients with baseline WBC = to 3×10^9/L, absolute neutrophil count (ANC) = 1.5×10^9/L, and platelets = 75×10^9/L, adjust dose; ANC < 0.5 $\times 10^9$/L, platelets < 25×10^9/L, give 50% dose next course; ANC 0.5-1.5 $\times 10^9$/L, platelets 25-50 $\times 10^9$/L, give 67% next course
• Assess buccal cavity q8hr for dryness, sores, or ulceration, white patches, oral pain, bleeding, dysphagia

• Assess for signs of bone marrow depression: bruising, bleeding, blood in stools, urine, sputum, emesis

Nursing diagnoses
• Body image, disturbed (adverse reactions)
• Infection, risk for (adverse reactions)
• Injury, risk for (adverse reactions)
• Knowledge, deficient (teaching)

Implementation
• Administer antiemetics and dexamethasone 10 mg at least ½ hr before antineoplastics
SUBCUT route
• Reconstitute with 10 ml sterile water for inj (25 mg/ml), inject diluent slowly into vial, invert vial, 2-3 times and gently rotate; sol will be cloudy, use immediately; divide doses greater than 4 ml into 2 syringes, resuspend the contents 2-3 times and gently roll syringe between the palms for 30 sec immediately prior to administration
• Rotate injection site
• Increase patient's fluid intake to 2-3 L/day to prevent dehydration, unless contraindicated
• Assist patient with rinsing of mouth tid-qid with water, club soda; brushing of teeth bid-tid with soft brush or cotton-tipped applicator for stomatitis; use unwaxed dental floss
• Provide a nutritious diet with iron, vitamin supplement, low fiber, few dairy products

Patient/family education
• Instruct patient to avoid foods with citric acid or hot or rough texture if stomatitis is present; to drink adequate fluids
• Instruct patient to report stomatitis; any bleeding, white spots, ulcerations in mouth; tell patient to examine mouth daily, report symptoms
• Advise patient to use contraception during therapy
• Advise patient not to father a child while receiving this product

Evaluation
Positive therapeutic outcome
• Improvement in blood counts in refractory anemia, or refractory anemia with excess blasts

azathioprine (Rx)
(ay-za-thye'oh-preen)
Azasan, Imuran
Func. class.: Immunosuppressant
Chem. class.: Purine antagonist

Pregnancy category D

Do not confuse:
Imuran/Imferon/Elmiron/IMDUR/
Enduron/Tenormin

Action: Produces immunosuppression by inhibiting purine synthesis, DNA, RNA in cells

Therapeutic outcome: Absence of graft rejection, slowing of rheumatoid arthritis

Uses: Renal transplants to prevent graft rejection, often used with corticosteroids, cytotoxics; refractory rheumatoid arthritis, glomerulonephritis, nephrotic syndrome, bone marrow transplant

Unlabeled uses: Myasthenia gravis, chronic ulcerative colitis, Crohn's disease, Behçet's syndrome

Dosage and routes
Renal dose
CCr 10-50 ml/min 75% of dose; CCr <10 ml/min 50% of dose

Prevention of rejection
Adult and child: **IV** 3-5 mg/kg/day, then maintenance (PO) of at least 1-3 mg/kg/day

Refractory rheumatoid arthritis
Adult: PO 1 mg/kg/day; may increase dosage after 2 mo by 0.5 mg/kg/day; not to exceed 2.5 mg/kg/day

Available forms: Tabs 50, 75, 100 mg; inj **IV** 100 mg

Adverse effects
GI: Nausea, vomiting, stomatitis, esophagitis, **pancreatitis, hepatotoxicity, jaundice**
HEMA: **Leukopenia, thrombocytopenia, anemia, pancytopenia,** bleeding
INTEG: Rash, alopeia
MISC: Raynaud's symptoms, **serum sickness**
MS: Arthralgia, muscle wasting

Contraindications: Pregnancy **D**, breast-feeding, hypersensitivity

Precautions: Severe renal/hepatic disease, geriatric, thiopurine methyltransferase deficiency

Black Box Warning: Bone marrow suppression, neoplastic disease

Pharmacokinetics
Absorption	Readily (PO)
Distribution	Crosses placenta
Metabolism	Liver to mercaptopurine
Excretion	Kidney, minimal
Half-life	3 hr

Pharmacodynamics
	PO	IV
Onset	Unknown	Unknown
Peak	4 hr	Unknown
Duration	Unknown	Unknown

Interactions
Individual drugs
Do not admix with other products
Allopurinol: increased action of azathioprine
Cotrimoxazole: increased leukopenia
CycloSPORINE: increased myelosuppression
Warfarin: decreased action of warfarin
Drug classifications
ACE inhibitors: increased leukopenia
Antineoplastics: increased myelosuppression
Vaccines: decreased immune response
Drug/herb
Astragalus, echinacea, melatonin, safflower: increased immunosuppression
Ginseng, maitake, mistletoe, schisandra, St. John's wort, turmeric: decreased effect
Drug/lab test
Increased: liver function tests
Decreased: uric acid
Interference: CBC, diff count

NURSING CONSIDERATIONS
Assessment
- Assess symptoms of rheumatoid arthritis: pain in joints, stiffness, poor range of motion, inflammation before and during treatment
- Monitor blood studies: Hgb, WBC, platelets during treatment monthly; if leukocytes are <3000/mm^3 or platelets <100,000/mm^3, product should be discontinued or reduced; decreased Hgb level may indicate bone marrow suppression
- Monitor liver function studies: alkaline phosphatase, AST, ALT, amylase, bilirubin; and for hepatotoxicity: dark urine, jaundice, itching, light-colored stools; product should be discontinued
- Monitor I&O, weight daily, report decreasing urine output, toxicity may occur
- Assess for infection: increased temp, WBC; sputum, urine

 Alert　　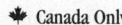 Canada Only　　 Drug on CD　　* "Tall Man" lettering (See Preface)

Nursing diagnoses
- Infection, risk for (uses)
- Knowledge, deficient (teaching)
- Mobility, impaired physical (uses)

Implementation
PO route
- Give all medications PO if possible, avoiding IM inj, since bleeding may occur
- Give with meals to reduce GI upset; nausea is common
- For several days before transplant surgery, patients should be placed in protective isolation
IV route
- Prepare in biologic cabinet using gown, gloves, mask; give after diluting 100 mg/10 ml of sterile water for inj; rotate to dissolve; may further dilute with 50 ml or more saline or glucose in saline given over >30 min (intermittent inf)

Solution compatibilities: D₅W, NaCl 0.9%, NaCl 0.45%

Patient/family education
- Teach patient to take as prescribed, do not miss doses; if dose is missed on daily regimen, skip dose; if on multiple dosing/day, take as soon as remembered
- Teach patient that therapeutic response may take 3-4 mo in rheumatoid arthritis, to continue with prescribed exercise, rest, other medications; that product is needed for life in renal transplant
- Instruct patient to report fever, rash, severe diarrhea, chills, sore throat, fatigue, since serious infections may occur; or clay-colored stools and cramping (hepatotoxicity)
- Advise patient to use contraceptive measures during treatment for 12 wk after ending therapy; product is teratogenic
- Advise patient to avoid vaccinations
- Tell patient to avoid crowds and persons with known infections to reduce risk of infection
- Instruct patient not to use OTC medications without approval of prescriber
- Advise patient to use soft-bristled toothbrush to prevent bleeding

Evaluation
Positive therapeutic outcome
- Absence of graft rejection
- Immunosuppression in autoimmune disorders
- Increased joint mobility without pain in rheumatoid arthritis

azelaic acid topical
See Appendix B

azelastine (Rx)
(ay′ze-lass-teen)
Optivar
Func. class.: Leukotriene synthesis inhibitor
Chem. class.: Phthalazinone derivative

Pregnancy category C

Action: Inhibits the synthesis and release of leukotrienes; antagonizes action of acetylcholine, histamine, serotonin

Therapeutic outcome: Decreased nasal stuffiness, itching, swollen eyes

Uses: Seasonal allergic rhinitis

Dosage and routes
Adult and child ≥12 yr: NASAL 2 sprays/nostril bid

Available forms: Spray 137 mcg/actuation

Adverse effects
CNS: Sedation (more common with increased dosages), drowsiness
MISC: Weight increase, myalgia

Contraindications: Hypersensitivity

Precautions: Pregnancy C

Pharmacokinetics
Absorption	Unknown
Distribution	Unknown
Metabolism	Liver, extensively
Excretion	Feces
Half-life	25-42 hr

Pharmacodynamics
Onset	Unknown
Peak	4-5 hr
Duration	Unknown

Interactions
Individual drugs
Alcohol: increased CNS depression
Drug classifications
CNS depressants, opioids, sedative/hypnotics: increased CNS depression

NURSING CONSIDERATIONS
Assessment
- Assess respiratory status: rate, rhythm, increase in bronchial secretions, wheezing, chest tightness; provide fluids to 2 L/day to decrease secretion thickness

Adverse effects: *italic* = common, **bold** = life-threatening

Nursing diagnoses

- Airway clearance, ineffective (uses)
- Knowledge, deficient (teaching)
- Noncompliance (teaching, overuse)

Implementation

- Remove cap/safety clip from spray pump
- Prime pump if using for first time, push 4 times quickly, away from face, blow your nose, then place tip of pump into one nostril, while holding other nostril closed, tilt head forward, and spray into nostril
- Put cover/safety clip back on

Patient/family education

- Teach patient all aspects of product uses; to notify prescriber if confusion, sedation occur; to avoid driving and other hazardous activity if drowsiness occurs; to avoid alcohol and other CNS depressants that may potentiate effect
- Caution patient not to exceed recommended dosage; dysrhythmias may occur

Evaluation

Positive therapeutic outcome

- Absence of runny or congested nose

---

azelastine nasal agent
See Appendix B

---

azelastine ophthalmic
See Appendix B

---

azithromycin (Rx)
(ay-zi-thro-my'sin)
Zithromax, Zmax
Func. class.: Antiinfective
Chem. class.: Macrolide (azalide)

Pregnancy category B

Do not confuse:
azithromycin/erythromycin, Zithromax/Zinacef

Action: Binds to 50S ribosomal subunits of susceptible bacteria and suppresses protein synthesis; much greater spectrum of activity than erythromycin; more effective against gram-negative organisms

Therapeutic outcome: Bacteriostatic against the following susceptible organisms: *Moraxella catarrhalis, Streptococcus pneumoniae, Streptococcus pyogenes, Staphylococcus aureus, Haemophilus influenzae, Clostridium, Legionella pneumophila, Chlamydia trachomatis, Mycoplasma;* no effect on methicillin-resistant *S. aureus;* in children: acute otitis media *(H. influenzae, M. catarrhalis, S. pneumoniae)* PO, acute pharyngitis/tonsillitis (group A streptococcal) PO; acute skin/soft tissue infections (PO); community-acquired pneumonia *(C. pneumoniae, H. influenzae, M. pneumoniae, S. pneumoniae)* PO; pharyngitis/tonsillitis *(S. pyogenes)*

Uses: Mild to moderate infections of the upper respiratory tract, in children: acute otitis media, lower respiratory tract; uncomplicated skin and skin structure infections, nongonococcal urethritis, or cervicitis; prophylaxis of disseminated *Mycobacterium avium* complex (MAC)

Dosage and routes
Most infections
Adult: PO 500 mg on day 1, then 250 mg daily on days 2-5 for a total dose of 1.5 g
Child 2-15 yr: PO 10 mg/kg on day 1, then 5 mg/kg × 4 days

Pelvic inflammatory disease
Adult: PO/**IV** 500 mg **IV** q24hr × 2 doses, then 500 mg PO q24hr × 7-10 days

Cervicitis/chlamydia/chancroid/ nongonococcal urethritis/syphilis
Adult: PO 1 g single dose

Gonorrhea
Adult: PO 2 g single dose

Endocarditis, prophylaxis
Adult: PO 500 mg 1 hr prior to procedure
Child: PO 15 mg/kg 1 hr prior to procedure

Community-acquired pneumonia
Adult: PO/**IV** 500 mg **IV** q24hr × 2 doses, then 500 mg PO q24hr × 7-10 days

Disseminated MAC infections
Adult: PO 600 mg/day in combination with ethambutol

Lower respiratory tract infections, acute skin/soft tissue infections, acute pharyngitis/tonsillitis
Child: PO 3-day regimen, 10 mg/kg daily × 3 days

Acute otitis media
Child: PO 30 mg/kg as a single dose or 10 mg/kg daily × 3 days or 10 mg/kg as a single dose on day 1, max 500 mg/day, then 5 mg/kg on days 2-5, max 250 mg/day

Prevention of acute otitis media
Child: PO 10 mg/kg qwk × 6 mo

Available forms: Tabs 250, 500, 600 mg; powder for inj 500 mg; powder for oral susp 1 g/packet; susp 100, 200 mg/5 ml

---

◆ Alert   ♣ Canada Only   ⊙ Drug on CD   * "Tall Man" lettering (See Preface)

Adverse effects
CNS: Dizziness, headache, vertigo, somnolence, myasthenia gravis
CV: Palpitations, chest pain
EENT: Hearing loss, tinnitus, loss of smell (anosmia)
GI: Nausea, vomiting, diarrhea, **hepatotoxicity,** abdominal pain, stomatitis, heartburn, dyspepsia, flatulence, melena, **cholestatic jaundice, pseudomembranous colitis,** tongue discoloration
GU: Vaginitis, moniliasis, nephritis
HEMA: Anemia
INTEG: Rash, urticaria, pruritus, photosensitivity
SYST: **Angioedema, Stevens-Johnson syndrome, toxic epidermal necrolysis**

Contraindications: Hypersensitivity to azithromycin, erythromycin, or any macrolide

Precautions: Pregnancy **B**, breastfeeding, child <6 mo for otitis media, child <2 yr for pharyngitis, geriatric, renal/hepatic/cardiac disease, tonsillitis

Pharmacokinetics

Absorption	Rapid, (PO) up to 50%
Distribution	Widely distributed
Metabolism	Unknown, minimal metabolism
Excretion	Unchanged (bile); kidneys, minimal
Half-life	11-70 hr

Pharmacodynamics

	PO	IV
Onset	Unknown	Unknown
Peak	2-4 hr	End of infusion
Duration	24 hr	24 hr

Interactions
Individual drugs
Bromocriptine, carbamazepine, cycloSPORINE, digoxin, disopyramide, methylPREDNISolone, phenytoin, theophylline, triazolam: increased effects of specific products
Ergotamine: toxicity
♦ Pimozide: dysrhythmias; fatal reaction
Triazolam: decreased clearance of triazolam
Drug classifications
Aluminum, magnesium antacids: decreased levels of azithromycin
Anticoagulants (orals): increased effect of oral anticoagulants
Drug/herb
Acidophilus: do not use with antiinfectives; separate by several hours

Drug/lab test
Increased: bilirubin, alkaline phosphatase, CPK, BUN, creatinine, AST, ALT

NURSING CONSIDERATIONS
Assessment
- Assess for signs and symptoms of infection: drainage, fever, increased WBC >10,000/mm^3, urine culture positive, sore throat, sputum culture positive
- Monitor respiratory status: rate, character, wheezing, tightness in chest; discontinue product if these occur
- Monitor allergies before treatment, reaction of each medication; place allergies on chart, notify all people giving products; skin eruptions, itching
- Monitor I&O ratio, renal studies; report hematuria, oliguria in renal disease; check urinalysis, protein, blood
- Monitor liver studies: AST, ALT, bilirubin, LDH, alkaline phosphatase; CBC with differential
- Monitor C&S before product therapy; product may be taken as soon as culture is taken; C&S may be repeated after treatment
- Monitor bowel pattern before, during treatment
- Assess for superinfection: sore throat, mouth, tongue; fever, fatigue, diarrhea, anogenital pruritus

Nursing diagnoses
- Diarrhea (adverse reactions)
- Infection, risk for (uses)
- Knowledge, deficient (teaching)

Implementation
PO route
- Provide adequate intake of fluids (2 L) during diarrhea episodes
- Give with a full glass of water; give susp 1 hr before or 2 hr after meals; tabs may be taken without regard to food; do not give with fruit juices
- Store at room temperature
- Reconstitute 1 g packet for susp with 60 ml water, mix, rinse glass with more water and have patient drink to consume all medication; packets not for pediatric use
- Do not take aluminum/magnesium-containing antacids or food simultaneously with this product
IV route
- Reconstitute 500 mg product/4.8 ml sterile water for inj (100 mg/ml), shake, dilute with ≥250 ml 0.9% NaCl, 0.45% NaCl, or LR to 1-2 mg/ml; diluted solution is stable for 24 hr or 7 days if refrigerated

Adverse effects: *italic* = common, **bold** = life-threatening

- Give 500 mg or more/1 hr, never give IM or as a bol

Patient/family education

- Instruct patient to report sore throat, black furry tongue, fever, loose foul-smelling stool, vaginal itching, discharge, fatigue; may indicate superinfection
- Caution patient not to take aluminum/magnesium-containing antacids or food simultaneously with this product; blood levels of azithromycin will be decreased
- Instruct patient to notify prescriber of diarrhea stools, dark urine, pale stools, yellow discoloration of eyes or skin, severe abdominal pain; cholestatic jaundice is a severe adverse reaction
- Teach patient to complete dosage regimen; to notify prescriber if symptoms continue
- Teach patient to notify prescriber if pregnancy is suspected
- Inform patient that sunburns may occur; wear protective clothing and sunscreen

Evaluation
Positive therapeutic outcome
- C&S negative for infection
- WBC within 5000-10,000/mm^3

azithromycin ophthalmic
See Appendix B

bacitracin topical
See Appendix B

baclofen 😎 (Rx)
(bak'loe-fen)
Lioresal, Lioresal Intrathecal
Func. class.: Skeletal muscle relaxant, central acting
Chem. class.: GABA, chlorophenyl derivative
Pregnancy category C

Do not confuse:
Lioresal/Lotensin

Action: Inhibits synaptic responses in CNS by stimulating GABAb receptor subtype, which decreases neurotransmitter function, decreasing frequency, severity of muscle spasms

Therapeutic outcome: Decreased spasticity of muscles

Uses: Spasticity in spinal cord injury, multiple sclerosis

Dosage and routes
Adult: PO 5 mg tid × 3 days, then 10 mg tid × 3 days, then 15 mg tid × 3 days, then 20 mg tid × 3 days, then titrated to response, max 80 mg/day; IT use implantable intrathecal INF pump; use screening trial of 3 separate BOL doses if needed 24 hr apart (50 mcg/ml, 75 mcg/1.5 ml, 100 mcg/2 ml); patients who do not respond to 100 mcg should not be considered for chronic IT therapy; initial double screening dose that produced result and give over 24 hr, increase by 10%-30% q24hr only; maintenance 1200-1500 mcg/day
Child 2-7 yr: PO 10-15 mg/day divided q8hr; titrate every 3 days by 5-15 mg/day to max 40 mg/day
Child ≥8 yr: As above, max 60 mg/day
Child: IT initial test dose same as adult; for small children, initial dose of 25 mcg/dose may be used; 25-1200 mcg/day infusion, titrated to response in screening phase
Geriatric: PO 5 mg bid-tid

Available forms: Tabs 10, 20 mg; intrathecal inj 10 mg/20 ml (500 mcg/ml), 10 mg/5 ml (2000 mcg/ml); pharmacy can prepare extemporaneous liquid preparations

Adverse effects
CNS: Dizziness, weakness, fatigue, drowsiness, headache, disorientation, insomnia, paresthesias, tremors, **seizures, coma; life-threatening CNS depression, CNS infection (IT)**
CV: Hypotension, chest pain, palpitations, edema; **cardiovascular collapse (IT)**
EENT: Nasal congestion, blurred vision, mydriasis, tinnitus
GI: Nausea, constipation, vomiting, increased AST, alkaline phosphatase, abdominal pain, dry mouth, anorexia
GU: Urinary frequency, hematuria
INTEG: Rash, pruritus
RESP: Dyspnea, respiratory failure (IT)

Contraindications: Hypersensitivity

Precautions: Pregnancy **C**, breastfeeding, geriatric, peptic ulcer, renal/hepatic disease, stroke, seizure disorder, diabetes mellitus

Black Box Warning: Abrupt discontinuation

Pharmacokinetics
Absorption	Well (PO)
Distribution	Widely, crosses placenta
Metabolism	Liver, partially
Excretion	Kidney, unchanged 70%-80%
Half-life	2½-4 hr

Pharmacodynamics	
	PO/IT
Onset	0.5-1 hr
Peak	4 hr
Duration	4-8 hr

Interactions
Individual drugs
Alcohol: CNS depression
Drug classifications
Antidepressants (tricyclics), barbiturates, MAOIs, opioids, sedative/hypnotics: increased CNS depression
Antihypertensives: increased hypotension
Drug/herb
Chamomile, hops, kava, skullcap, valerian: increased CNS depression
Drug/lab test
Increased: AST, ALT, alkaline phosphatase, blood glucose

NURSING CONSIDERATIONS
Assessment
• Monitor B/P, weight, blood glucose, and hepatic function periodically
• Check for increased seizure activity in patients with epilepsy; this product decreases seizure threshold, monitor ECG
• Check I&O ratio; check for urinary retention, frequency, hesitancy
• Allergic reactions: rash, fever, respiratory distress; severe weakness, numbness in extremities
• Assess CNS depression: dizziness, drowsiness, psychiatric symptoms
• Check dosage, as individual titration is required

Nursing diagnoses
• Injury, risk for (adverse reactions)
• Knowledge, deficient (teaching)
• Mobility, impaired physical (uses)

Implementation
PO route
• Give with meals for GI symptoms; gum, frequent sips of water for dry mouth
• Store in airtight container at room temperature
IT route
• Titration is based on response
• Test dose: Dilute to a concentration of 50 mcg/ml, give over 1 min or more
• Observe for decrease in muscle spasticity
• If response is not adequate, give 2 additional test doses (75 mcg/1.5 ml and 100 mcg/2 ml), maintenance infusion via implantable pump 500-2000 mcg/ml

Patient/family education
• Give test doses 24 hr apart
• Advise patient not to discontinue medication quickly; hallucinations, spasticity, tachycardia will occur; product should be tapered off over 1-2 wk
IT route
• Advise patient not to take with alcohol, other CNS depressants
• Caution patient to avoid hazardous activities if drowsiness or dizziness occur while taking this product
• Advise patient to avoid using OTC medication (cough preparations, antihistamines) unless directed by prescriber

Evaluation
Positive therapeutic outcome
• Decreased pain, spasticity

Treatment of overdose: Induce emesis of conscious patient, activated charcoal, dialysis, physostigmine to reduce life-threatening CNS side effects

balsalazide (Rx)
(ball-sal'a-zide)
Colazal
Func. class.: GI antiinflammatory
Chem. class.: Salicylate derivative
Pregnancy category B

Do not confuse:
Colazal/Clozaril

Action: Delivered intact to the colon, bioconverted to 5-ASA

Therapeutic outcome: Decreased inflammation in colon

Uses: Active, mild to moderate ulcerative colitis (adult and child)

Dosage and routes
Adult: PO 2250 mg (three 750 mg cap) tid × 8-12 wk, max 6.75 g/day
Adolescent and child 5-12 yr: PO 2250 mg (three 750 mg cap) tid × 8 wk

Available forms: Caps 750 mg

Adverse effects
CNS: Headache, insomnia, fatigue, fever, dizziness
EENT: Dry mouth, dry eyes, rhinitis, sinusitis, watery eyes, blurred vision
GI: Nausea, vomiting, abdominal pain, diarrhea
MS: Arthralgia, back pain, myalgia
SYST: **Anaphylaxis**

Adverse effects: *italic* = common, **bold** = life-threatening

Contraindications: Hypersensitivity to salicylates/5-aminosalicylates

Precautions: Pregnancy **B**, breastfeeding, child <14 yr, pyloric stenosis, renal disease, colitis, hepatitis

Pharmacokinetics

Absorption	Low, variable
Distribution	Protein binding 99%
Metabolism	Unknown
Excretion	Feces, as metabolites
Half-life	Unknown

Pharmacodynamics
Unknown

Interactions
Individual drugs
Azathioprine, warfarin: increased effect
Mercaptopurine, thioguanine: increased myelosuppression
Thioguanine: decreased effect
Varicella virus, live: avoid use
Drug classifications
SSRIs: increased bleeding
Drug/lab test
Increased: AST, ALT, GGT, LDH, bilirubin, alkaline phosphatase
False positive: urinary glucose test

NURSING CONSIDERATIONS
Assessment
• Monitor kidney function studies: BUN, creatinine, urinalysis (long-term therapy)
• Assess for allergic reaction: rash, dermatitis, urticaria, pruritus, dyspnea, bronchospasm
• Assess for myelosuppression: CBC

Nursing diagnoses
• Injury, risk for (uses)
• Knowledge, deficient (teaching)

Implementation
• Give with food in evenly divided doses; swallow tab whole or open cap, sprinkle on applesauce
• Use with resuscitative equipment available; severe allergic reactions may occur
• Give total daily dose evenly spaced to minimize GI intolerance
• Store in tight, light-resistant container at room temperature

Patient/family education
• Advise patient to notify prescriber if symptoms do not improve, if colitis symptoms worsen, if rash, hives, or respiratory problems occur

Evaluation
Positive therapeutic outcome
• Absence of fever, mucus in stools; resolution of symptoms of ulcerative colitis

---

⚠ **HIGH ALERT**

basiliximab (Rx)
(bas-ih-liks'ih-mab)
Simulect
Func. class.: Immunosuppressant
Chem. class.: Murine/human monoclonal antibody (interleukin-2) receptor antagonist

Pregnancy category B

Action: Binds to and blocks the IL-2 receptor, which is selectively expressed on the surface of activated T-lymphocytes; impairs the immune system to antigenic challenges

Therapeutic outcome: Prevention of graft rejection

Uses: Acute allograft rejection in renal transplant patients when used with cycloSPORINE and corticosteroids

Dosage and routes
Adult/child >35 kg: **IV** 20 mg × 2 doses; first dose within 2 hr before transplant surgery; second dose given 4 days after transplantation
Child 2-15 yr: **IV** 12 mg/m² × 2 doses; first dose within 2 hr before transplant surgery; second dose given 4 days after transplantation

Available forms: Powder for inj 10, 20 mg

Adverse effects
CNS: Pyrexia, chills, tremors, headache, insomnia, weakness, dizziness
CV: Chest pain, angina, **cardiac failure,** hypo/hypertension, edema
GI: Vomiting, nausea, diarrhea, constipation, abdominal pain, GI bleeding, gingival hyperplasia, stomatitis
INTEG: Acne, pruritus
META: Acidosis, hypercholesterolemia, hyperuricemia, hypo/hyperkalemia, hypocalcemia, hypophosphatemia
MISC: Infection, moniliasis, **anaphylaxis,** anemia, allergic reaction, dysuria, CMV infection, candidiasis
MS: Arthralgia, myalgia
RESP: Dyspnea, wheezing, cough, **pulmonary edema**

Contraindications: Hypersensitivity, exposure to viral infections, breastfeeding

---

Precautions: Pregnancy **B**, children, geriatric

Black Box Warning: Infections

Pharmacokinetics

Absorption	Unknown
Distribution	Unknown
Metabolism	Unknown
Excretion	Unknown
Half-life	7 days (adult)
	9½ days (child)

Pharmacodynamics

Onset	Unknown
Peak	½ hr (adults)
Duration	Unknown

Interactions
Drug classifications
Immunosuppressants: Increased immunosuppression
Drug/herb
Astragalus, echinacea, melatonin, safflower: increased immunosuppression
Ginseng, maitake, mistletoe, schisandra, St. John's wort, turmeric: decreased effect
Drug/lab test
Increased: BUN, cholesterol, uric acid, creatinine, potassium, calcium, blood glucose, Hgb, Hct
Decreased: Hgb, Hct, platelets, magnesium, phosphate

NURSING CONSIDERATIONS
Assessment
• Assess for infection, increased temp, WBC, sputum, urine
• Monitor blood studies: Hgb, WBC, platelets during treatment qmo; if leukocytes are <3000/mm³, product should be discontinued
• Monitor liver function studies: alkaline phosphatase, AST, ALT, bilirubin
• Assess hepatotoxicity: dark urine, jaundice, itching, light-colored stools; product should be discontinued
⬥ Assess for anaphylaxis, hypersensitivity: dyspnea, wheezing, rash, pruritus, hypotension, tachycardia; if severe hypersensitivity reactions occur, product should not be used again

Nursing diagnoses
• Infection, risk for (adverse reactions)
• Knowledge, deficient (teaching)

Implementation
• Administer all medications PO if possible; avoid IM inj, since infection may occur

IV route
• After adding 5 ml sterile water for inj, shake gently to dissolve, reconstitute to a vol of 50 ml with 0.9% NaCl or D_5, gently invert bag, do not shake, do not admix

Patient/family education
• Instruct patient to report fever, chills, sore throat, fatigue, since serious infection may occur; avoid crowds, persons with known upper respiratory infections; use contraception during treatment

Evaluation
Positive therapeutic outcome
• Absence of graft rejection

---

beclomethasone (Rx)
(be-kloe-meth'a-sone)
Beclodisk ✦, Beclovent, QVAR
Func. class.: Synthetic glucocorticoid (long acting)
Chem. class.: Beclomethasone diester

Pregnancy category C

Do not confuse:
beclomethasone/betamethasone

Action: Prevents inflammation by suppression of migration of polymorphonuclear leukocytes, fibroblasts, reversal of increased capillary permeability and lysosomal stabilization; does not suppress hypothalamus and pituitary function

Therapeutic outcome: Decreased inflammation and normal immunity

Uses: Seasonal, perennial allergic/vasomotor rhinitis, nasal polyps, chronic steroid-dependent asthma

Dosage and routes
Adult and child >12 yr: INH 48-80 mcg bid (alone) or 40-160 mcg bid (with inhaled corticosteroids), max 320 bid
Child 5-12 yr: INH 40 mcg bid, max 80 mcg bid

Available forms: Oral inh 40, 80, 250✦ mcg /metered spray

Adverse effects
CNS: Headache
EENT: Candidal infection of oral cavity, hoarseness, sore throat
GI: Dry mouth, dyspepsia
MISC: **Angioedema adrenal insufficiency,** facial edema, Churg-Strauss syndrome (rare)
RESP: **Bronchospasm,** wheezing, cough

Adverse effects: *italic* = common, **bold** = life-threatening

Contraindications: Hypersensitivity, status asthmaticus (primary treatment), nonasthmatic bronchial disease, bacterial, fungal, viral infections of mouth, throat, lungs

Precautions: Pregnancy **C**, breastfeeding, child <12, nasal disease/surgery

Pharmacokinetics

Absorption	Locally only
Distribution	Not distributed
Metabolism	Lungs, liver (by CYP3A)
Excretion	Feces, urine
Half-life	2.8 hr

Pharmacodynamics

	INH	NASAL
Onset	1-4 wk	10 min
Peak	Unknown	Unknown
Duration	Unknown	Unknown

NURSING CONSIDERATIONS
Assessment

• Assess adrenal suppression: 17-KS, plasma cortisol for decreased levels, adrenal function periodically for HPA axis suppression during prolonged therapy; monitor growth and development
• Assess blood studies, neutrophils, decreased platelets; WBC with diff baseline and q3mo; if neutrophils <1000/mm³, discontinue treatment
• Check nasal passages during long-term treatment for changes in mucus; check for burning, stinging; assess for glucocorticoid withdrawal: dizziness, hypotension, fatigue, muscle/joint pain; notify prescriber immediately
• Assess respiratory status: rest, rhythm, characteristics; auscultate lung bilaterally before and throughout treatment
• Assess for fungal infections in mucous membranes

Nursing diagnoses

• Airway clearance, ineffective (uses)
• Knowledge, deficient (teaching)
• Noncompliance (teaching)
• Oral mucous membrane, impaired (adverse reactions)

Implementation

• Give PO, using a spacer device for proper dose
• Use after cleaning aerosol top daily with warm water; dry thoroughly
• Store in cool environment; do not puncture or incinerate container

Inhalation route

• Shake inhaler, invert, tilt head backward, insert nozzle into nostril, away from septum; hold other nostril closed and depress activator, inhale through nose, exhale through mouth
• Shake oral aerosol well, use spacer

Patient/family education

• Teach patient to gargle/rinse mouth after each use to prevent oral fungal infections
• Teach patient that in times of stress, systemic corticosteroids may be needed to prevent adrenal insufficiency; do not discontinue oral product abruptly, taper slowly
• Teach patient to continue using product even if mild nasal bleeding occurs; is usually transient
• Teach patient method of administration after providing written instructions from manufacturer
• Clean inhaler by wiping with dry cloth

Evaluate
Positive therapeutic outcome
• Decrease in runny nose, improved symptoms of bronchial asthma

---

beclomethasone nasal agent
See Appendix B

---

benazepril (Rx)
(ben-a'za-pril)
Lotensin
Func. class.: Antihypertensive
Chem. class.: ACE inhibitor

Pregnancy category D

Action: Selectively suppresses renin-angiotensin-aldosterone system; inhibits ACE, preventing conversion of angiotensin I to angiotensin II

Therapeutic outcome: Decreased B/P in hypertension

Uses: Hypertension, alone or in combination with thiazide diuretics

Unlabeled uses: CHF

Dosage and routes
Adult: PO 10 mg daily initially, then 20-40 mg/day divided bid or daily (without a diuretic); 5 mg PO daily (with a diuretic); max 80 mg daily
Geriatric: PO 5-10 mg/day initially

B

Renal dose
Adult: PO 5 mg daily with CCr <30 ml/min; increase as needed to max of 40 mg/day

Available forms: Tabs 5, 10, 20, 40 mg

Adverse effects
CNS: Anxiety, hypertonia, insomnia, paresthesia, headache, dizziness, fatigue
CV: Hypotension, postural hypotension, syncope, palpitations, angina
GI: Nausea, constipation, vomiting, gastritis, diarrhea, melena
GU: Increased BUN, creatinine, decreased libido, impotence, urinary tract infection
INTEG: Rash, flushing, sweating
META: Hyperkalemia, hyponatremia
***MISC:* Angioedema**
MS: Arthralgia, arthritis, myalgia
RESP: Cough, asthma, bronchitis, dyspnea, sinusitis

Contraindications: Breastfeeding, children, hypersensitivity to ACE inhibitors

Black Box Warning: Pregnancy **D**

Precautions: Impaired renal/liver function, dialysis patients, hypovolemia, blood dyscrasias, CHF, COPD, asthma, geriatric, bilateral renal artery stenosis

Pharmacokinetics

Absorption	<40%
Distribution	Unknown; crosses placenta
Metabolism	Liver metabolites; protein binding 97%
Excretion	Kidney, breast milk (minimal)
Half-life	10-11 hr (metabolite); increased in renal disease

Pharmacodynamics

Onset	Unknown
Peak	½-1 hr
Duration	Unknown

Interactions
Individual drugs
Alcohol: increased hypotension (large amounts)
Azathioprine: increased myelosuppression
Digoxin, lithium: increased serum levels
Drug classifications
Antihypertensives, diuretics, nitrates, phenothiazines: increased hypotension
Diuretics (potassium-sparing), potassium supplements: increased hyperkalemia
NSAIDs: decreased hypotensive effects

Drug/herb
Aconite: increased toxicity, death
Astragalus, cola tree: increased or decreased antihypertensive effect
Barberry, betony, black catechu, black cohosh, bloodroot, broom, burdock, cat's claw, dandelion, goldenseal, hawthorn, Irish moss, Jamaican dogwood, kelp, khella, mistletoe, parsley: increased antihypertensive effect
Coltsfoot, guarana, khat, licorice, pineapple, yohimbe: decreased antihypertensive effect
Drug/lab test
Increased: AST, ALT, alkaline phosphatase, bilirubin, uric acid, blood glucose
False positive: ANA titer
Positive: ANA titer

NURSING CONSIDERATIONS
Assessment
- Monitor blood studies: neutrophils, decreased platelets
- Monitor B/P at peak/trough level of product, check for orthostatic hypotension, syncope; if changes occur, dosage change may be required
- Monitor renal studies: protein, BUN, creatinine; watch for increased levels that may indicate nephrotic syndrome and renal failure; monitor urine for protein; monitor renal symptoms: polyuria, oliguria, frequency, dysuria
- Establish baselines in renal, liver function tests before therapy begins
- Check potassium levels throughout treatment, although hyperkalemia rarely occurs
- Assess for allergic reactions: rash, fever, pruritus, urticaria; product should be discontinued if antihistamines fail to help

Nursing diagnoses
- Cardiac output, decreased (uses)
- Injury, risk for (side effects)
- Knowledge, deficient (teaching)
- Noncompliance (teaching)

Implementation
- Store in air-tight container at 86° F (30° C) or less
- Severe hypotension may occur after 1st dose of this medication; decreased hypotension may be prevented by reducing or discontinuing diuretic therapy 3 days before beginning benazepril therapy

Patient/family education
- Instruct patient not to discontinue product abruptly; advise patient to tell all persons associated with care

---

Adverse effects: *italic* = common, **bold** = life-threatening

- Teach patient not to use OTC products (cough, cold, allergy) unless directed by prescriber; serious side effects can occur; xanthines such as coffee, tea, chocolate, cola can prevent action of product
- Emphasize the importance of complying with dosage schedule, even if feeling better; to continue with medical regimen to decrease B/P: exercise, cessation of smoking, decreasing stress, diet modifications
- Emphasize the need to rise slowly to sitting or standing position to minimize orthostatic hypotension, not to exercise in hot weather because increased hypotension can occur
- Teach patient to notify prescriber of mouth sores, sore throat, fever, swelling of hands or feet, irregular heartbeat, chest pain, coughing, shortness of breath
- Caution patient to report excessive perspiration, dehydration, vomiting, diarrhea; may lead to fall in B/P
- Caution patient that product may cause dizziness, fainting, light-headedness; may occur during first few days of therapy; to avoid activities that may be hazardous
- Teach patient how to take B/P; teach normal readings for age group; ensure patient takes own B/P
- Advise patient to notify prescriber of pregnancy, product will need to be discontinued

Evaluation
Positive therapeutic outcome
- Decreased B/P in hypertension

Treatment of overdose: 0.9% NaCl **IV** inf, hemodialysis

⚠ HIGH ALERT

bendamustine (Rx)
(ben-da-muss'teen)
Treanda
Func. class.: Antineoplastic alkylating agent
Chem. class.: Nitrogen mustard

Pregnancy category Unknown

Action: Cross-linking DNA which causes single strand and double strand breaks, inhibits several mitotic checkpoints, combines alkylating and antimetabolite properties

Therapeutic outcome: Improvement in blood counts and morphology

Uses: Chronic lymphocytic leukemia, non-Hodgkin's lymphoma

Dosage and routes
Chronic lymphocytic leukemia
Adult: **IV** INF 100 mg/m^2 over 30 min on days 1, 2, q28days up to 6 cycles

Non-Hodgkin's lymphoma
Adult: **IV** INF 120 mg/m^2 over 60 min on days 1, 2, q21days up to 8 cycles

Available forms: Powder for inj 100 mg

Adverse effects
CNS: Asthenia, fatigue, fever, headache
CV: Hypertension, **hypertensive crisis**
GI: Nausea, vomiting, diarrhea, hyperbilirubinemia, constipation, stomatitis, anorexia
GU: **Renal failure**
HEMA: **Thrombocytopenia, leukopenia, anemia, lymphocytopenia, neutropenia, secondary malignancy, toxic epidermal necrolysis, tumor lysis syndrome**
INTEG: Bulbous rash, pruritus
META: Hyperuricemia
SYST: **Anaphylaxis,** infection, dehydration, **severe skin toxicities**

Contraindications: Pregnancy category unknown, hypersensitivity to this product or mannitol, children, hepatic disease, renal impairment, breastfeeding

Precautions: Hyperuricemia, infusion-related reactions, myelosuppression, infection, skin reactions

Pharmacokinetics	
Absorption	Unknown
Distribution	Protein binding 95%
Metabolism	Hydrolysis via cytochrome P450 1A2; two metabolites are produced
Excretion	90% unchanged (feces)
Half-life	40 min

Pharmacodynamics
Unknown

INTERACTIONS
Individual drugs
Cimetidine: increased toxicity
Clozapine: do not use due to risk of agranulocytosis
Drug classifications
Anticoagulants, aspirin, NSAIDs, platelet inhibitors, thrombolytics: increased risk of bleeding
Antineoplastics (other), radiation: increased toxicity
CYP1A2 inducers (barbiturates, carbamazepine, rifampin): decreased bendamustine

---

CYP1A2 inhibitors (atazanavir, cimetidine, ciprofloxacin, enoxacin, ethyl estradiol, fluvoxamine, mexiletine, norfloxacin, tacrine, thiabendazole, zileuton): increased bendamustine

Myelosuppressive agents: increased myelosuppression

Vaccines (live): increased adverse reactions, decreased antibody reaction

Drug/lab test
Increased: LFTs

NURSING CONSIDERATIONS
Assessment
• Assess CBC, differential, platelet count weekly; withhold product if WBC is <1000 or platelet count is <75,000; notify prescriber of results
• Monitor hepatic studies: AST, ALT, bilirubin
• Monitor renal studies: BUN, serum uric acid, urine CCr before, during therapy; I&O ratio; report fall in urine output of 30 ml/hr; electrolytes
• Assess for cold, cough, fever (may indicate beginning infection)
• Assess bleeding: hematuria, guaiac, bruising, petechiae, mucosa, orifices q8hr
• Assess for tumor-lysis syndrome

Nursing diagnoses
• Infection, risk for (adverse reactions)
• Injury, risk for (adverse reactions)
• Knowledge, deficient (teaching)
• Nutrition, less than body requirements, imbalanced (adverse reactions)

Implementation
• Give blood transfusions or RBC colony-stimulating factors to counter anemia
• Give antiemetic 30-60 min before giving product to prevent vomiting
• Give all medications PO, if possible avoid IM inj if platelets are <100,000/mm³
• Store reconstituted sol in refrigerator for 24 hr, or room temperature for 3 hr; protect from light; store vials at room temperature
Intermittent IV INF route
• Prepare in biologic cabinet wearing gown, gloves, mask; avoid contact with skin; can cause burning and staining the skin brown; use cytotoxic handling procedures
• After diluting 100 mg product/20 ml sterile water for inj (5 mg/ml), sol should be clear, colorless to pale yellow, completely dissolve in 5 min; if particulate is present, do not use
• Give within 30 min of reconstitution, withdraw the volume needed and further dilute in 500 ml NS or D$_{2.5\%/0.45\%}$ NS to a final conc

0.2-0.6 mg/ml; doses ≤100 mg/m², give over 30 min; doses >100 mg/m², give over 60 min

Patient/family education
• Advise patient to avoid use of aspirin, ibuprofen, razors, commercial mouthwash
• Instruct patient to report signs of anemia (fatigue, irritability, shortness of breath, faintness)
• Instruct patient to report signs of infection

Evaluation
Positive therapeutic outcome
• Improvement in blood counts and morphology

benzocaine topical
See Appendix B

benztropine 🚫 (Rx)
(benz'troe-peen)
Apo-Benztropin ✣, benztropine mesylate, Cogentin
Func. class.: Cholinergic blocker, antiparkinson agent
Chem. class.: Tertiary amine
Pregnancy category C

Action: Blockade of central acetylcholine receptors in the CNS; neurotransmitters are balanced

Therapeutic outcome: Decreased involuntary movements

Uses: Parkinsonian symptoms, EPS associated with neuroleptic products, acute dystonia, hypersalivation

Dosage and routes
Drug-induced extrapyramidal symptoms
Adult: IM/**IV** 1-4 mg daily/bid; give PO dose as soon as possible; PO 1-2 mg bid/tid; increase by 0.5 mg q5-6days
Child: IM/**IV** 0.02-0.05 mg/kg/dose 1-2 × 1 day
Geriatric: PO 0.5 mg daily/bid, increase by 0.5 mg q5-6days; max 4 mg/day

Parkinsonian symptoms
Adult: PO 1-2 mg daily, in 1-2 divided doses; increased 0.5 mg q5-6days titrated to patient response; max 6 mg daily

Acute dystonic reactions
Adult: IM/**IV** 1-2 mg, may increase to 1-2 mg bid (PO)

Adverse effects: *italic* = common, **bold** = life-threatening

Available forms: Tabs 0.5, 1, 2 mg; inj 1 mg/ml

Adverse effects

CNS: Confusion, anxiety, restlessness, irritability, delusions, hallucinations, headache, sedation, depression, incoherence, dizziness, memory loss; delirium (geriatric)

CV: Palpitations, tachycardia, hypotension, bradycardia

EENT: Blurred vision, photophobia, dilated pupils, difficulty swallowing, dry eyes, mydriasis, increased intraocular tension, closed-angle glaucoma

GI: Dryness of mouth, constipation, nausea, vomiting, abdominal distress, **paralytic ileus,** epigastric distress

GU: Hesitancy, retention, dysuria

INTEG: Rash, urticaria, dermatoses

MISC: Increased temperature, flushing, decreased sweating, **hyperthermia, heat stroke,** numbness of fingers

MS: Muscular weakness, cramping

Contraindications: Hypersensitivity, closed-angle glaucoma, myasthenia gravis, GI/GU obstruction, child <3 yr, peptic ulcer, megacolon, prostate hypertrophy

Precautions: Pregnancy **C**, breastfeeding, children, geriatric, tachycardia, renal/hepatic disease, product abuse history, dysrhythmias, hypo/hypertension, psychiatric patients

Pharmacokinetics

Absorption	Well (PO, IM), completely (**IV**) absorbed
Distribution	Unknown
Metabolism	Unknown
Excretion	Unknown
Half-life	Unknown

Pharmacodynamics

	IM/IV	PO
Onset	15 min	1 hr
Peak	Unknown	Unknown
Duration	6-10 hr	6-10 hr

Interactions

Individual drugs

Disopyramide, quinidine: increased anticholinergic effects

Drug classifications

Antidepressants (tricyclic), antihistamines, phenothiazines: increased anticholinergic effects

Antidiarrheals: decreased absorption

Drug/herb

Black catechu: increased constipation

Butterbur, jimsonweed: increased benztropine effect

Jaborandi, kava, pill-bearing spurge: decreased benztropine effect

NURSING CONSIDERATIONS

Assessment

• Monitor I&O ratio; retention commonly causes decreased urinary output, distention, frequency, incontinence

• Assess for parkinsonism, EPS: shuffling gait, muscle rigidity, involuntary movements, loss of balance, pill rolling, muscle spasms, drooling before and during treatment

• Monitor for urinary hesitancy, retention; palpate bladder if retention occurs

• Monitor for constipation, cramping, pain in abdomen, abdominal distention; increase fluids, bulk, exercise if this occurs

• Assess for tolerance over long-term therapy; dosage may have to be increased or changed

• Assess for mental status: affect, mood, CNS depression, worsening of mental symptoms during early therapy

• Assess for benztropine "buzz" or "high," patients may imitate EPS

Nursing diagnoses

• Knowledge, deficient (teaching)

• Mobility, impaired physical (uses)

• Noncompliance (teaching)

Implementation

PO route

• Give with or after meals to prevent GI upset; may give with fluids other than water; hard candy, frequent drinks, gum to relieve dry mouth

• Give at bedtime to avoid daytime drowsiness in patient with parkinsonism

• May be crushed and mixed with food

• Store at room temperature

IM route

• Give in large muscle mass for dystonic symptoms

IV route

• Give parenteral dose with patient recumbent to prevent postural hypotension; give undiluted 1 mg/1 min

Syringe compatibilities: Chlorpro-MAZINE, fluphenazine, metoclopramide, perphenazine, thiothixene

Y-site compatibilities: Fluconazole, tacrolimus

Patient/family education

• Teach patient to use caution in hot weather; product may increase susceptibility to stroke

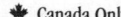

since perspiration is decreased; patient should remain indoors
- Advise patient not to discontinue this product abruptly; to taper off over 1 wk to prevent withdrawal symptoms (insomnia, involuntary movements, anxiety, tachycardias)
- Caution patient to avoid driving or other hazardous activities; drowsiness, dizziness may occur
- Teach patient to avoid OTC medication: cough, cold preparations with alcohol, antihistamines unless directed by prescriber; increased CNS depression may occur
- Advise patient to rise from sitting or recumbent position slowly to minimize orthostatic hypotension
- Teach patient to use good oral hygiene; to use sugarless gum, hard candy, frequent sips of water to decrease dry mouth; if dry mouth continues, saliva substitutes may be prescribed
- Instruct patient that doses should not be doubled, but missed dose may be taken up to 2 hr before next dose

Evaluation
Positive therapeutic outcome
- Absence of involuntary movements (pill rolling, tremors, muscle spasms)

betamethasone (Rx)
(bay-tah-meth′ah-sone)
Betnelan ✤, Betnesol ✤, Celestone, Cel-U Jec, Selestoject ✤
Func. class.: Corticosteroid, synthetic; glucocorticoid, long acting

Pregnancy category C

Do not confuse:
betamethasone/beclomethasone

Action: Decreases inflammation by suppression of migration of polymorphonuclear leukocytes, fibroblasts, reversal of increased capillary permeability and lysosomal stabilization

Therapeutic outcome: Decreased inflammation and normal immunity

Uses: Immunosuppression, severe inflammation, prevention of neonatal respiratory distress syndrome (by administration to mother)

Dosage and routes
Adult: PO 0.6-7.2 mg daily; IM/IV 0.6-7.2 mg daily in joint or soft tissue (sodium phosphate)
Child: PO 17.5 mcg/kg/day in 3 divided doses; IM 17.5 mcg/kg/day in 3 divided doses

every 3rd day or 5.8-8.75 mcg/kg/day as a single dose (adrenal insufficiency)

Other uses
Child: PO 62.5-250 mcg/kg/day in 3 divided doses; IM 20.8-125 mcg/kg/day of the base q12-24hr

Available forms: Tabs 500, 600 mcg; effervescent tabs 500 mcg ✤; syr 600 mcg/5 ml; ext rel tab 1 mg; sol for inj (phosphate) 3 mg/ml; susp for inj (phosphate/acetate) 6 mg/ml

Adverse effects
CNS: Depression, flushing, sweating, headache, bruising, mood changes
CV: Hypertension, **circulatory collapse, thrombophlebitis, embolism,** tachycardia, **necrotizing angiitis, CHF**
EENT: Fungal infections, increased intraocular pressure, blurred vision
GI: Diarrhea, nausea, abdominal distention, **GI hemorrhage,** increased appetite, **pancreatitis**
HEMA: **Thrombocytopenia**
INTEG: Acne, poor wound healing, bruising, petechiae
MS: Fractures, osteoporosis, weakness

Contraindications: Psychosis, hypersensitivity, idiopathic thrombocytopenia, acute glomerulonephritis, amebiasis, fungal infections, nonasthmatic bronchial disease, child <2 yr, AIDS, TB, threadworm, high doses in traumatic brain injury

Precautions: Pregnancy C, breastfeeding, diabetes mellitus, glaucoma, osteoporosis, seizure disorders, ulcerative colitis, CHF, myasthenia gravis, renal disease, esophagitis, peptic ulcer

Pharmacokinetics

Absorption	Well absorbed (PO); systemic (TOP)
Distribution	Crosses placenta
Metabolism	Liver, extensively
Excretion	Kidney, breast milk
Half-life	3-5 hr, adrenal suppression 3-4 days

Pharmacodynamics

	PO	IM	IV	TOP
Onset	1-2 hr	Unknown	Rapid	Unknown
Peak	2 hr	4-8 hr	4-8 hr	Unknown
Duration	3 days	1-1½ days	1-1½ days	Unknown

Interactions
Individual drugs
Alcohol, indomethacin: increased GI bleeding

Amphotericin B, piperacillin, ticarcillin: increased hypokalemia

CYP3A4 inhibitors (erythromycin, ketoconazole, indinavir, itraconazole, ritonavir, saquinavir): increased effects of betamethasone

Insulin: increased need for insulin

Isoniazid: decreased effect

Phenytoin, rifampin: decreased action; increased metabolism

Somatrem, somatropin: decreased effects

Drug classifications
Anticoagulants: decreased effect

Barbiturates: decreased action; increased metabolism

Fluoroquinolones: increased tendon rupture

Hypoglycemic agents: increased need for hypoglycemic agents

NSAIDs, salicylates: increased GI bleeding

Salicylates, oral contraceptives: decreased effects

Thiazides, loop diuretics: increased hypokalemia

Toxoids/vaccines: decreased immune response

Drug/herb
Aloe, buckthorn, cascara sagrada, Chinese rhubarb, senna: increased hypokalemia

Goldenseal, hawthorn, hops, lemon balm, licorice, lily of the valley, mistletoe, perilla, pheasant's eye, squill: increased corticosteroid effect

Drug/food
Grapefruit juice should be avoided

Drug/lab test
Increased: cholesterol, sodium, blood glucose, uric acid, calcium, urine glucose

Decreased: calcium, potassium, T_4, T_3, thyroid ^{131}I uptake test, urine 17-OHCS, 17-KS, PBI

False negative: skin allergy tests

NURSING CONSIDERATIONS
Assessment
Systemic route

• Monitor potassium, blood glucose, urine glucose while on long-term therapy; hypokalemia and hyperglycemia; check weight daily; notify prescriber of weekly gain >5 lb

• Monitor B/P q4hr, pulse; notify prescriber if chest pain occurs

• Monitor I&O ratio; be alert for decreasing urinary output and increasing edema

• Check plasma cortisol levels during long-term therapy (normal level: 138-635 nmol/L [SI units] when drawn at 8 AM); adrenal function periodically for HPA axis suppression

• Assess for symptoms of infection: increased temp, WBC even after withdrawal of medication; product masks infection symptoms

• Assess for symptoms of potassium depletion: paresthesias, fatigue, nausea, vomiting, depression, polyuria, dysrhythmias, weakness

• Monitor for edema, hypo/hypertension, cardiac symptoms

• Assess for mental status: affect, mood, behavioral changes, aggression

Topical route

• Check temp; if fever develops, product should be discontinued

• Assess for systemic absorption: increased temp, inflammation, irritation

Nursing diagnoses
• Infection, risk for (adverse reactions)
• Knowledge, deficient (teaching)
• Noncompliance (teaching)

Implementation
PO route

• Give with food or milk to decrease GI symptoms

IM route

• Give IM inj deep in large mass, rotate sites, avoid deltoid, use 21-G needle; in one dose in AM to prevent adrenal suppression; avoid SUBCUT administration; may damage tissue

Inhalation route

• Give inh with water to decrease possibility of fungal infections; titrated dose; use lowest effective dose

• Use after cleaning aerosol *top* daily with warm water; dry thoroughly

• Store in cool environment; do not puncture or incinerate container

Topical route

• Apply only to affected areas; do not get in eyes; apply medication, then cover with occlusive dressing (only if prescribed), seal to normal skin, change q12hr; systemic absorption may occur

• Apply only to dermatoses; do not use on weeping, denuded, or infected area

• Cleanse before applying product; use treatment for a few days after area has cleared

• Store at room temperature

IV route

• Give **IV** (only sodium phosphate product); give over >1 min; may be given by **IV** inf in compatible sol after shaking susp (parenteral)

• Give titrated dose; use lowest effective dose

Y-site compatibilities: Heparin, hydrocortisone, potassium chloride, vit B/C

◆ Alert　　♣ Canada Only　　💿 Drug on CD　　* "Tall Man" lettering (See Preface)

Patient/family education
Systemic route
- Advise patient that long-term therapy may be needed to clear infection (1-2 mo depending on type of infection); that emergency ID as corticosteroid user should be carried or worn; dosage adjustment may be needed
⬥ Instruct patient to notify prescriber if therapeutic response decreases; caution patient not to discontinue abruptly; adrenal crisis can result
- Instruct patient to avoid OTC products unless directed by prescriber
- Teach patient all aspects of product usage, including cushingoid symptoms
- Teach patient symptoms of adrenal insufficiency: nausea, anorexia, fatigue, dizziness, dyspnea, weakness, joint pain

Topical route
- Caution patient to avoid sunlight on affected area; burns may occur

Evaluation
Positive therapeutic outcome
- Ease of respirations, decreased inflammation (systemic)
- Absence of severe itching, patches on skin, flaking (topical)

---

betamethasone topical
See Appendix B

---

betamethasone (augmented) topical
See Appendix B

---

betaxolol ophthalmic
See Appendix B

---

bethanechol 🚫 (Rx)
(be-than′e-kol)
bethanechol chloride, Urebeth, Urecholine
Func. class.: Urinary tract stimulant, cholinergic
Chem. class.: Synthetic choline ester

Pregnancy category C

Action: Stimulates muscarinic acetylcholine receptors directly; mimics effects of parasympathetic nervous system stimulation; stimulates gastric motility, micturition; increases lower esophageal sphincter pressure

Therapeutic outcome: Absence of continued urinary retention

Uses: Urinary retention (postoperative, postpartum), neurogenic atony of bladder with retention

Unlabeled uses: Ileus

Dosage and routes
Adult: PO 10-50 mg bid-qid; SUBCUT 5 mg tid-qid prn
Child: PO 0.3-0.6 mg/kg/day divided in 3-4 doses/day

Test dose
Adult: SUBCUT 2.5 mg repeated 15-30 min intervals × 4 doses to determine effective dose

Ileus (unlabeled)
Adult: PO/SUBCUT 10-20 mg tid-qid; before meals (PO)

Available forms: Tabs 5, 10, 25, 50 mg; inj SUBCUT 5 mg/ml

Adverse effects
CNS: Dizziness, headache, malaise
CV: Hypotension, bradycardia, reflex tachycardia, **cardiac arrest, circulatory collapse**
EENT: Miosis, increased salivation, lacrimation, blurred vision
GI: Nausea, bloody diarrhea, belching, vomiting, cramps, fecal incontinence
GU: Urgency
INTEG: Rash, urticaria, flushing, increased sweating
RESP: **Acute asthma, dyspnea, bronchoconstriction**

Contraindications: Hypersensitivity, severe bradycardia, asthma, severe hypotension, hyperthyroidism, peptic ulcer, parkinsonism, seizure disorders, CAD, COPD, coronary occlusion, mechanical obstruction, peritonitis, recent urinary or GI surgery, GI/GU obstruction

Precautions: Pregnancy C, breastfeeding, child <8 yr, hypertension

Pharmacokinetics	
Absorption	Poorly absorbed (PO); well absorbed (SUBCUT)
Distribution	Does not cross blood-brain barrier
Metabolism	Unknown
Excretion	Kidneys
Half-life	Unknown

Adverse effects: *italic* = common, **bold** = life-threatening

Pharmacodynamics		
	PO	SUBCUT
Onset	30-90 min	5-15 min
Peak	1 hr	15-30 min
Duration	1-6 hr	2 hr

Interactions
Individual drugs
Procainamide, quinidine: decreased action of procainamide and quinidine
Drug classifications
Anticholinergics: decreased action
Anticholinesterase agents, cholinergic agonists: increased action, increased toxicity
Ganglionic blockers: increased severe hypotension
Drug/herb
Jaborandi: increased cholinergic effect
Jimsonweed, scopolia: decreased effects
Drug/lab test
Increased: AST, lipase/amylase, bilirubin

NURSING CONSIDERATIONS
Assessment
• Monitor B/P, pulse, respirations; observe after parenteral dose for 1 hr
• Check I&O ratio; check for urinary retention or incontinence; if bladder emptying does not occur, notify prescriber; catheterization may be needed
• Assess for bradycardia, hypotension, bronchospasm, headache, dizziness, seizures, sweating, cramping, respiratory depression; product should be discontinued if toxicity occurs; administer atropine

Nursing diagnoses
• Injury, risk for (adverse reactions)
• Knowledge, deficient (teaching)
• Urinary elimination, impaired (uses)

Implementation
PO route
• Give increased doses if tolerance occurs as prescribed
• To avoid nausea and vomiting, take on an empty stomach; 1 hr before or 2 hr after meals
• Store at room temperature
SUBCUT route
◆ Give parenteral dose by SUBCUT route; use of IM, **IV** may result in cardiac arrest or cholinergic crisis (diarrhea with blood, cramping, hypotension, circulatory collapse)
◆ Administer only with atropine sulfate available for cholinergic crisis; give only after all other cholinergics have been discontinued
• Do not use sol with a precipitate or if discolored

Patient/family education
• Instruct patient to take product exactly as prescribed; 1 hr before meals or 2 hr after meals; do not double doses; if dose is missed, take within 1 hr of scheduled dose
• Caution patient to make position changes slowly; orthostatic hypotension may occur
• Instruct patient to report cramping, diarrhea with blood, flushing to prescriber

Evaluation
Positive therapeutic outcome
• Absence of urinary retention
• Absence of abdominal distention

Treatment of overdose: Administer atropine 0.6-1.2 mg **IV** or IM (adult)

⚠ HIGH ALERT

bevacizumab (Rx)
(beh-va-kiz′you-mab)
Avastin
Func. class.: Antineoplastic—miscellaneous
Chem. class.: Monoclonal antibody

Pregnancy category C

Action: DNA-derived monoclonal antibody selectively binds to and inhibits activity of human vascular endothelial growth factor to reduce microvascular growth and inhibition of metastatic disease progression

Therapeutic outcome: Decreased tumor size

Uses: Metastatic carcinoma of the colon or rectum in combination with 5-FU **IV**, metastatic breast cancer, renal cell carcinoma, glioblastoma

Unlabeled uses: Adjunctive in breast, renal/pancreatic/neovascular/ovarian cancer, (wet) macular degeneration

Dosage and routes
Colorectal cancer
Adult: **IV** INF 5 mg/kg q14days given over 90 min; if well tolerated, the next infusion may be given over 60 min; if 60 min infusions are well tolerated, subsequent infusions may be given over 30 min

Metastatic breast cancer (previously received chemotherapy)
Adult: **IV** 10 mg/kg on days 1, 15 with paclitaxel 90 mg/m² on days 1, 8, 15, given q28days

---

Metastatic breast cancer (have not received chemotherapy)
Adult: **IV** 7.5 mg/kg or 15 mg/kg with docetaxel (100 mg/m² **IV**), repeat q3wk

Metastatic renal cell carcinoma
Adult: **IV** 10 mg/kg q2wk with interferon alfa 9 million units SC 3 × per wk, up to 52 wk

Available forms: Inj 25 mg/ml

Adverse effects

CNS: Asthenia, dizziness, **intracranial hemorrhage (malignant glioma)**
CV: **Deep vein thrombosis,** hypo/hypertension, **hypertensive crisis**
GI: Nausea, vomiting, anorexia, diarrhea, constipation, abdominal pain, colitis, stomatitis, **GI hemorrhage/perforation**
GU: Proteinuria, urinary frequency/urgency, **nephrotic syndrome**
HEMA: **Leukopenia, neutropenia, thrombocytopenia, microangiopathic hemolytic anemia**
META: Bilirubinemia, hypokalemia
MISC: **Exfoliative dermatitis, hemorrhage,** non-GI fistula formation, alopecia
RESP: Dyspnea, upper respiratory infection

Contraindications: Hypersensitivity

Precautions: Pregnancy **C**, breastfeeding, children, geriatric, CHF, blood dyscrasias, CV disease, hypertension

Black Box Warning: GI perforation wound dehiscence

Pharmacokinetics	
Absorption	Unknown
Distribution	Steady state 100 days
Metabolism	Unknown
Excretion	Unknown
Half-life	20 days

Pharmacodynamics	
Onset	Unknown
Peak	Unknown
Duration	Steady state 100 days

Interactions
Individual drugs
Sunitab: avoid concurrent use; microangiopathic hemolytic anemia may occur

NURSING CONSIDERATIONS
Assessment
• Monitor B/P q3-4wk
• Assess for symptoms of infection; may be masked by product
• Monitor CNS reaction: dizziness, confusion

• Assess GU status (proteinuria); nephrotic syndrome may occur; monitor urinalysis for increasing protein level; products should be held if protein ≥2 g/24 hr
◆ Assess for GI perforation, serious bleeding, nephrotic syndrome, hypertensive crisis; product should be discontinued permanently; or surgery, product should be discontinued temporarily

Nursing diagnoses
• Body image, disturbed (adverse reactions)
• Infection, risk for (adverse reactions)
• Injury, risk for (adverse reactions)
• Knowledge, deficient (teaching)

Implementation
IV route
• Do not give by **IV** bolus or **IV** push
• Give as **IV** inf over 90 min for first dose and 60 min thereafter, if well tolerated

Patient/family education
• Instruct patient to avoid hazardous tasks, since confusion, dizziness may occur
• Instruct patient to report signs of infection: sore throat, fever, diarrhea, vomiting
• Advise patient not to become pregnant while taking this product, or for several months after discontinuing treatment
• Advise patient to notify prescriber if pregnant or planning a pregnancy

Evaluation
Positive therapeutic outcome
• Decrease in size of tumors

bicalutamide (Rx)
(bi-kal-yut′ah-mide)
Casodex
Func. class.: Antineoplastic hormone
Chem. class.: Nonsteroidal antiandrogen
Pregnancy category X

Action: Competitively inhibits the action to androgens by binding to cytosol androgen receptors in target tissue

Therapeutic outcome: Prevention of growth of malignant cells

Uses: Stage D-2 metastatic prostate cancer in combination with luteinizing hormone-releasing hormone (LHRH) analog

Dosage and routes
Adult: PO 50 mg daily with LHRH

Available forms: Tabs 50 mg

Adverse effects

CNS: Dizziness, paresthesia, insomnia, anxiety, neuropathy, headache

CV: Hot flashes, hypertension, chest pain, **CHF,** edema

GI: Diarrhea, constipation, nausea, vomiting, increased liver enzyme test, anorexia, dry mouth, melena, abdominal pain

GU: Nocturia, hematuria, UTI, impotence, gynecomastia, urinary incontinence, frequency, dysuria, retention, urgency, breast tenderness, decreased libido

INTEG: Rash, sweating, dry skin, pruritus, alopecia

MISC: Infection, anemia, dyspnea, bone pain, headache, asthenia, *back pain,* flulike symptoms

Contraindications: Pregnancy **X,** women, hypersensitivity

Precautions: Breastfeeding, geriatric, renal/hepatic disease

Pharmacokinetics

Absorption	Well absorbed
Distribution	Unknown
Metabolism	Liver
Excretion	Urine, feces
Half-life	5.2 days

Pharmacodynamics

Onset	Unknown
Peak	31½ hr
Duration	Unknown

Interactions

Drug classifications

Anticoagulants: increased anticoagulation

Drug/lab test

Increased: AST, ALT, bilirubin, BUN, creatinine

Decreased: Hgb, WBC

NURSING CONSIDERATIONS

Assessment

• Assess for diarrhea, constipation, nausea, vomiting

• Assess for hot flashes, gynecomastia; assure patient that these are common side effects

• Monitor prostate specific antigen (PSA) liver function tests

Nursing diagnoses

• Injury, risk for (uses, adverse reactions)

• Knowledge, deficient (teaching)

Implementation

• Give at same time each day (for both products) either AM or PM with or without food

• Give only with LHRH treatment

Patient/family education

• Teach patient to recognize and report signs of anemia, renal/hepatic toxicity

• Advise patient that hair may be lost, but is reversible after therapy is discontinued

• Advise patient not to use other products unless approved by prescriber

• Advise patient to use contraception

Evaluation

Positive therapeutic outcome

• Decreased tumor size, spread of malignancy

---

bimatoprost ophthalmic
See Appendix B

---

bisacodyl (Rx, OTC)
(bis-a-koe′dill)

Bisac-Evac, Bisaco-Lax, Bisacolax ♣, Carter's Little Pills, Dacodyl, Deficol, Dulcagen, Dulcolax, Feen-a-Mint, Fleet Laxative, Laxit ♣, Modane, Reliable Gentle Laxative, Therelax

Func. class.: Laxative, stimulant

Chem. class.: Diphenylmethane

Pregnancy category C

Action: Acts directly on intestine by increasing motor activity; thought to irritate colonic intramural plexus; increases water in the colon

Therapeutic outcome: Decreased constipation

Uses: Short-term treatment of constipation, bowel or rectal preparation for surgery, examination

Dosage and routes

Adult ≥12 yr: PO 5-15 mg in PM or AM; may use up to 30 mg for bowel or rectal preparation; RECT 10 mg (single dose), 30 ml enema

Child 6-11 yr: PO 5 mg as a single dose; RECT 5 mg as a single dose

Available forms: Tabs 5 mg; enteric coated tabs 5 mg; supp 5, 10 mg; enema 10 mg/30 ml

Adverse effects

CNS: Muscle weakness

GI: Nausea, vomiting, anorexia, cramps, diarrhea, rectal burning (supp)

META: Protein-losing enteropathy, alkalosis, hypokalemia, **tetany,** electrolyte and fluid imbalances

---

Contraindications: Hypersensitivity, rectal fissures, abdominal pain, nausea, vomiting, appendicitis, acute surgical abdomen, ulcerated hemorrhoids, acute hepatitis, fecal impaction, intestinal/biliary tract obstruction

Precautions: Pregnancy C, breastfeeding

Pharmacokinetics

Absorption	Poor
Distribution	Unknown
Metabolism	Liver, minimally
Excretion	Kidneys
Half-life	Unknown

Pharmacodynamics

	PO	RECT
Onset	6-10 hr	15-60 min
Peak	Unknown	Unknown
Duration	Unknown	Unknown

Interactions
Drug classifications
Antacids, gastric acid pump inhibitors, H₂-blockers: increased gastric irritation
Drug/herb
Flax, lily of the valley, pheasant's eye, senna, squill: increased laxative action
Drug/food
Milk: increased gastric irritation

NURSING CONSIDERATIONS
Assessment
• Monitor blood, urine electrolytes if used often by patient; check I&O ratio to identify fluid loss
• Assess cramping, rectal bleeding, nausea, vomiting; if these symptoms occur, product should be discontinued; identify cause of constipation; identify whether fluids, bulk, or exercise missing from lifestyle

Nursing diagnoses
• Constipation (uses)
• Diarrhea (side effects)
• Knowledge, deficient (teaching)
• Noncompliance (teaching)

Implementation
PO route
• Swallow tabs whole; do not break, crush, or chew
• Give alone with water only for better absorption; do not take within 1 hr of antacids, milk
• Administer in AM or PM (oral dose)

Rectal route
• Lubricate before insertion, patient should retain for ½ hr

Patient/family education
• Discuss with the patient that adequate fluid and bulk consumption is necessary
• Advise patient that normal bowel movements do not always occur daily
• Teach patient not to use in presence of abdominal pain, nausea, vomiting; tell patient to notify prescriber if constipation unrelieved or if symptoms of electrolyte imbalance occur: muscle cramps, pain, weakness, dizziness, excessive thirst

Evaluation
Positive therapeutic outcome
• Decreased constipation within 3 days

---

bismuth subsalicylate (OTC)
(bis'meth sub-sa-li'si-late)
Bismatrol, Kaopectate, Kao-Tin, Kapectolin, K-pec Peptic Relief, Pepto-Bismol, Pepto-Bismol Maximum Strength, Pink Bismuth
Func. class.: Antidiarrheal/weak antacid
Chem. class.: Salicylate
Pregnancy category C

Do not confuse:
Kaopectate/Kayoxalate

Action: Inhibits prostaglandin synthesis responsible for GI hypermotility, intestinal inflammation; stimulates absorption of fluid and electrolytes; binds toxins produced by *Escherichia coli*

Therapeutic outcome: Absence of loose, watery stools

Uses: Diarrhea (cause undetermined); prevention of diarrhea when traveling; may be included to treat *Helicobacter pylori*, heartburn, indigestion, nausea

Dosage and routes
Antidiarrheal
Adult: PO 2 tab or 30 ml/15 ml extra/max strength q30min or 2 tabs q6min, max 4.2 g/24 hr
Antiulcer (unlabeled)
Adult: PO 524 mg q30-60min or 1048 mg q1hr, max 4.2 g/24 hr; given with metronidazole or tetracycline

Available forms: Tabs 262 mg; chewable tabs 262, mg; susp 87 mg/5 ml, 130 mg/15 ml, 262 mg/15 ml, 525 mg/15 ml

Adverse effects: *italic* = common, **bold** = life-threatening

Adverse effects

CNS: Confusion, twitching, neurotoxicity (high dose)

EENT: Hearing loss, tinnitus, metallic taste, blue gums, black tongue (chew tabs)

GI: Increased fecal impaction (high doses), dark stools, constipation, diarrhea, nausea

HEMA: Increased bleeding time

Contraindications: Child <3 yr; children, flulike symptoms; history of GI bleeding; renal disease, varicella, hypersensitivity to this product or salicylates

Precautions: Pregnancy C, breastfeeding, geriatric, anticoagulant therapy, gout, diabetes mellitus, immobility, bleeding disorders, previous hypersensitivity to NSAIDs, *Clostridium difficile*–associated diarrhea when used with antiinfectives for *H. pylori*

Pharmacokinetics

Absorption	Salicylate >90%
Distribution	None
Metabolism	None
Excretion	Feces (unchanged)
Half-life	Unknown

Pharmacodynamics

Onset	1 hr
Peak	2 hr
Duration	4 hr

Interactions
Individual drugs
Methotrexate: increased toxicity
Tetracycline: decreased absorption
Drug classifications
Anticoagulants (oral): increased effect of anticoagulants
Antidiabetics (oral): increased effect of antidiabetics
Quinolones: decreased absorption of quinolones
Salicylates: increased risk of salicylate toxicity
Drug/herb
Nutmeg: increased antidiarrheal effect
Sarsaparilla: increased bismuth absorption
Drug/lab test
Interference: radiographic studies of GI system

NURSING CONSIDERATIONS
Assessment
• Monitor skin turgor; dehydration may occur in severe diarrhea; monitor electrolytes (potassium, sodium, chloride) if diarrhea is severe or continues long term
• Assess bowel pattern (frequency, consistency, shape, volume, color) before product therapy, after treatment; check weight, bowel sounds; identify factors contributing to diarrhea (bacteria, diet, medications, tube feedings)

Nursing diagnoses
• Constipation (adverse reactions)
• Diarrhea (uses)
• Knowledge, deficient (teaching)

Implementation
• Shake susp before use; chewable tabs should not be swallowed whole

Patient/family education
• Teach patient to stop use if symptoms do not improve within 2 days or become worse, or if diarrhea is accompanied by high fever
• Teach patient to increase fluids for rehydration
• Tell patient to chew or dissolve chewable tabs in mouth; do not swallow whole; shake susp before using
• Tell patient to avoid other salicylates unless directed by prescriber; not to give to children because of possibility of Reye's syndrome
• Tell patient that stools may turn gray; tongue may darken; impaction may occur in debilitated patients

Evaluation
Positive therapeutic outcome
• Decreased diarrhea

bisoprolol (Rx)
(bis-oh'pro-lole)
Zebeta
Func. class.: Antihypertensive
Chem. class.: β_1-Blocker (selective)
Pregnancy category C

Do not confuse:
Zebeta/Diabeta/Zetia

Action: Preferentially and competitively blocks stimulation of β_1-adrenergic receptor within cardiac muscle (decreases rate of SA node discharge, increases recovery time), slows conduction of AV node, decreases heart rate, which decreases O_2 consumption in myocardium; decreases renin-aldosterone-angiotensin system; inhibits β_2-receptors in bronchial and vascular smooth muscle at high doses

Therapeutic outcome: Decreased B/P, heart rate

Uses: Mild to moderate hypertension

Unlabeled uses: Stable angina, stable CHF

Dosage and routes
Renal/hepatic dose
Adult: PO 2.5 mg, titrate upward

Hypertension
Adult: PO 5 mg/day, may increase if necessary to 20 mg once daily, max 40 mg/day; may need to reduce dose in presence of renal or hepatic impairment

Angina (unlabeled)
Adult: PO 5-20 mg/day

Heart failure (unlabeled)
Adult: PO 1.25 mg/day × 48 hr, then 2.5 mg/day for 1st mo, then 5 mg/day

Available forms: Tabs 5, 10 mg

Adverse effects
CNS: Vertigo, headache, insomnia, fatigue, dizziness, mental changes, memory loss, hallucinations, depression, lethargy, drowsiness, strange dreams, catatonia, peripheral neuropathy
CV: **Ventricular dysrhythmias, profound hypotension, bradycardia, CHF,** cold extremities, postural hypotension, **2nd- or 3rd-degree heart block**
EENT: Sore throat, dry burning eyes
ENDO: Increased hypoglycemic response to insulin
GI: Nausea, diarrhea, vomiting, **mesenteric arterial thrombosis,** ischemic colitis, flatulence, gastritis, gastric pain
GU: Impotence, decreased libido
HEMA: **Agranulocytosis, thrombocytopenia,** purpura, **eosinophilia**
INTEG: Rash, flushing, alopecia, pruritus, sweating
MISC: Facial swelling, weight gain, decreased exercise tolerance
MS: Joint pain, arthralgia
RESP: **Bronchospasm,** dyspnea, wheezing, cough, nasal stuffiness

Contraindications: Hypersensitivity to β-blockers, cardiogenic shock, heart block (2nd or 3rd degree), sinus bradycardia, CHF, cardiac failure

Precautions: Pregnancy **C,** breastfeeding, children, major surgery, diabetes mellitus, renal/hepatic/thyroid/peripheral vascular/aortic or mitral valve disease, COPD, asthma, well-compensated heart failure, myasthenia gravis

Black Box Warning: Abrupt discontinuation

Pharmacokinetics
Absorption	Well absorbed
Distribution	Unknown; protein binding (30%)
Metabolism	Liver, inactive metabolites
Excretion	Urine, unchanged (50%)
Half-life	9-12 hr

Pharmacodynamics
Onset	Unknown
Peak	2-4 hr
Duration	24 hr

Interactions
Individual drugs
Amiodarone, digoxin: increased bradycardia
Guanethidine, reserpine: increased hypotension
Drug classifications
ACE inhibitors, α-blockers, calcium channel blockers, diuretics: increased antihypertensive effect
Antidiabetics: increased antidiabetic effect
Calcium channel blockers: increased myocardial depression
Ergots: increased peripheral ischemia
NSAIDs, salicylates: decreased antihypertensive effects
Drug/herb
Aconite: increased toxicity, death
Betel palm, butterbur, cola tree, figwort, fumitory, guarana, hawthorn, lily of the valley, motherwort, plantain: increased β-blocking effect
Coenzyme Q10, St. John's wort, yohimbe: decreased β-blocking effect
Drug/lab test
Increased: AST, ALT, blood glucose, BUN, uric acid, potassium, lipoprotein, ANA titer
Interference: glucose/insulin tolerance tests

NURSING CONSIDERATIONS
Assessment
• Monitor B/P during beginning treatment, periodically thereafter; pulse q4hr: note rate, rhythm, quality; apical/radial pulse before administration; notify prescriber of any significant changes (pulse <50 bpm)
• Check for baselines in renal, liver function tests before therapy begins
• Assess for edema in feet, legs daily, monitor I&O, daily weight; check for jugular vein distention, crackles, bilaterally, dyspnea (CHF)
• Monitor skin turgor, dryness of mucous membranes for hydration status, especially geriatric

Nursing diagnoses
• Cardiac output, decreased (uses)
• Injury, risk for (side effects)
• Knowledge, deficient (teaching)
• Noncompliance (teaching)

Implementation
• Give daily; give with food to prevent GI upset; may be crushed
• Store protected from light, moisture; place in cool environment

Patient/family education
• Teach patient not to discontinue product abruptly; may cause precipitate angina if stopped abruptly; evaluate noncompliance
• Teach patient not to use OTC products containing α-adrenergic stimulants (such as nasal decongestants, cold preparations); to avoid alcohol, smoking and to limit sodium intake as prescribed
• Teach patient how to take pulse and B/P at home; advise when to notify prescriber
• Instruct patient to comply with weight control, dietary adjustments, modified exercise program
• Tell patient to carry/wear emergency ID to identify product being taken, allergies; tell patient product controls symptoms but does not cure
• Caution patient to avoid hazardous activities if dizziness, drowsiness present
• Teach patient to take product as prescribed, not to double doses, skip doses; take any missed doses as soon as remembered if at least 8 hr until next dose
• Advise patient to report bradycardia, dizziness, confusion, depression, fever, cold extremities
• Teach patient if diabetic, may mask signs of hypoglycemia, or alter blood glucose levels

Evaluation
Positive therapeutic outcome
• Decreased B/P in hypertension (after 1-2 wk)

Treatment of overdose:
Lavage, **IV** atropine for bradycardia, **IV** theophylline for bronchospasm, digoxin, O_2, diuretic for cardiac failure, hemodialysis, **IV** glucose for hypoglycemia, **IV** diazepam (or phenytoin) for seizures

---

! HIGH ALERT

bivalirudin (Rx)
(bye-val-i-rue′din)
Angiomax
Func. class.: Anticoagulant
Chem. class.: Thrombin inhibitor

Pregnancy category B

Action: Direct inhibitor of thrombin that is highly specific; able to inhibit free and clot-bound thrombin

Therapeutic outcome: Anticoagulation in percutaneous transluminal coronary angioplasty (PTCA), used with aspirin; heparin-induced thrombocytopenia with thrombosis syndrome

Uses: Unstable angina in patients undergoing PTCA, used with aspirin; heparin-induced thrombocytopenia; heparin-induced thrombocytopenia with thrombosis syndrome

Dosage and routes
PCI/PTCA
Adult: **IV** BOL 0.75 mg/kg, then **IV** INF 1.75 mg/kg/hr for 4 hr; another **IV** INF may be used at 0.2 mg/kg/hr for ≤20 hr; this product is intended to be used with aspirin (325 mg daily) adjusted to body weight

HIT/HITTS
Adult: **IV** BOL 0.75 mg/kg, then cont INF 1.75 mg/kg/hr for duration of procedure

Renal dose
Adult: **IV** GFR 30-59 ml/min, give 1.75 mg/kg/hr; GFR 10-29 ml/min, give 1 mg/kg/hr; dialysis-dependent patients, give 0.25 mg/kg/hr

Available forms: Inj, lyophilized 250 mg vial

Adverse effects
CNS: Headache, insomnia, anxiety, nervousness
CV: Hypo/hypertension, bradycardia
GI: Nausea, vomiting, abdominal pain, dyspepsia
HEMA: **Hemorrhage,** thrombocytopenia
MISC: Pain at inj site, pelvic pain, urinary retention, fever
MS: Back pain

Contraindications: Hypersensitivity, active bleeding, cerebral aneurysm, intracranial hemorrhage, recent surgery, CVA

Precautions: Pregnancy **B**, breastfeeding, children, geriatric, renal function impairment, hepatic disease, asthma, blood dyscrasias, thrombocytopenia, GI ulcers, hypertension

---

Pharmacokinetics	
Absorption	Unknown
Distribution	No protein binding
Metabolism	Unknown
Excretion	Kidneys
Half-life	25 min

Pharmacodynamics	
Onset	Unknown
Peak	Unknown
Duration	1 hr

Interactions
Drug classifications
Anticoagulants, thrombolytics: increased risk
of bleeding
Drug/herb
Agrimony, alfalfa, angelica, anise, bilberry,
black haw, bogbean, buchu, cat's claw,
chamomile, chondroitin, devil's claw, dong
quai, evening primrose, fenugreek, feverfew,
fish oils, garlic, ginger, ginkgo, ginseng,
horse chestnut, Irish moss, kava, kelp,
kelpware, khella, licorice, lovage, lungwort,
meadowsweet, motherwort, mugwort, nettle,
papaya, parsley (large amounts), pau
d'arco, pineapple, poplar, prickly ash, red
clover, safflower, saw palmetto, senega,
skullcap, tonka bean, turmeric, wintergreen,
yarrow: increased risk of bleeding
Coenzyme Q10, flax, glucomannan, goldenseal,
guar gum: decreased anticoagulant effect

NURSING CONSIDERATIONS
Assessment
⬥ Assess for fall in B/P or Hct that may indi-
cate hemorrhage
• Assess for fever, skin rash, urticaria
• Assess bleeding: check arterial and venous
sites, IM inj sites, catheters; all punctures
should be minimized

Nursing diagnoses
• Cardiac output, decreased (uses)
• Knowledge, deficient (teaching)

Implementation
• Prior to PTCA, give with aspirin, 325 mg
IV direct 1 mg/kg as a bolus; then intermittent
infusion
Intermittent IV infusion route
• To each 250-mg vial add 5 ml of sterile
water for inj, swirl until dissolved, further
dilute reconstituted vial with 50 ml of D₅W or
0.9% NaCl (5 mg/ml); the dose is adjusted to
body weight, run at 2.5 mg/kg/hr, do not
admix before or during administration
• Give reduced dose in renal impairment

Patient/family education
• Explain reason for product and expected
results

Evaluation
Positive therapeutic outcome
• Anticoagulation in PTCA

! HIGH ALERT

bleomycin (Rx)
(blee-oh-mye'sin)
Blenoxane
Func. class.: Antineoplastic, antibiotic
Chem. class.: Glycopeptide
Pregnancy category D

Action: Inhibits synthesis of DNA, RNA,
protein; derived from *Streptomyces
verticillus;* phase specific in the G₂ and M
phases; a nonvesicant, sclerosing agent

Therapeutic outcome: Prevention of
rapidly growing malignant cells

Uses: Cancer of head, neck, penis, cervix,
vulva of squamous cell origin, Hodgkin's/non-
Hodgkin's disease, lymphosarcoma, reticulum
cell sarcoma, testicular carcinoma, as a
sclerosing agent for malignant pleural effusion

Dosage and routes
Adult and child: IM/SUBCUT/**IV** 0.25-0.5
units/kg q1-2wk or 10-20 units/m²; then 1
unit/day or 5 units/wk; may also be given by
cont INF; max total dose, 400 units in lifetime

Hodgkin's disease (test dose)
Adult and child (unlabeled):
IM/**IV**/SUBCUT 52 units for first 2 doses
followed by 24 hr observation

Malignant pleural effusion
Adult: 60 units diluted in 100 ml of 0.9%
NaCl intrapleural inj given through a thoracotomy tube following drainage of excess pleural
fluid and complete lung expansion, remove
after 4 hr

Available forms: Powder for inj 15, 30
units/vial

Adverse effects
CNS: Pain at tumor site, headache, confusion
*GI: Nausea, vomiting, anorexia, stomatitis,
weight loss,* ulceration of mouth, lips
***IDIOSYNCRATIC REACTION:** Hypotension,
confusion, fever, chills, wheezing*
*INTEG: Rash, hyperkeratosis, nail changes,
alopecia,* pruritus, acne, striae, peeling,
hyperpigmentation

Adverse effects: *italic* = common, **bold** = life-threatening

RESP: **Fibrosis, pneumonitis,** wheezing, **pulmonary toxicity**
SYST: **Anaphylaxis,** radiation recall, Raynaud's phenomenon

Contraindications: Pregnancy **D**, breast-feeding, hypersensitivity, prior idiosyncratic reaction

Precautions: Renal/hepatic/respiratory disease, patients >70 yr old

Black Box Warning: Fever, pulmonary fibrosis

Pharmacokinetics

Absorption	Well absorbed (IM, SUBCUT, intrapleural, intraperitoneal)
Distribution	Widely distributed
Metabolism	Liver, 30%
Excretion	Kidneys, unchanged (50%)
Half-life	2 hr; increased in renal disease

Pharmacodynamics

Unknown

Interactions
Individual drugs
Fosphenytoin, phenytoin: decreased phenytoin levels
Radiation: increased toxicity, bone marrow suppression
Drug classifications
Anesthetics (general), antineoplastics: increased toxicity
Live virus vaccines: avoid concurrent use
Drug/lab test
Increased: uric acid

NURSING CONSIDERATIONS
Assessment
• Assess buccal cavity q8hr for dryness, sores or ulceration, white patches, oral pain, bleeding, dysphagia; obtain prescription for viscous lidocaine (Xylocaine)
🔴 Assess symptoms indicating anaphylaxis: rash, pruritus, urticaria, purpuric skin lesions, itching, flushing, wheezing, hypotension; have emergency equipment available
• Assess pulmonary function tests; chest x-ray before, during therapy; monitor q2wk during treatment; pulmonary diffusion capacity for carbon monoxide (DLCO) monthly; if <40% of pretreatment value, stop treatment
• Monitor CBC, differential, platelet count weekly; withhold product if WBC <4000/mm^3 or platelet count <100,000/mm^3; notify prescriber of results if WBC <20,000/mm^3, platelets <150,000/mm^3

• Monitor temp q4hr (may indicate beginning of infection)
• Monitor liver function tests before, during therapy (bilirubin, AST, ALT, LDH) as needed or monthly
• Assess for bleeding: hematuria, stool guaiac, bruising or petechiae, mucosa or orifices q8hr; inflammation of mucosa, breaks in skin
• Treat pulmonary infection prior to treatment; identify dyspnea, crackles, unproductive cough, chest pain, tachypnea
• Identify effects of alopecia on body image; discuss feelings about body changes; if edema in feet, joint pain, stomach pain, shaking present, prescriber should be notified; identify inflammation of mucosa, breaks in skin

Nursing diagnoses
• Body image, disturbed (adverse reactions)
• Infection, risk for (adverse reactions)
• Injury, risk for (adverse reactions)
• Knowledge, deficient (teaching)

Implementation
• Avoid contact with skin; very irritating; wash completely to remove
• Give fluids **IV** or PO before chemotherapy to hydrate patient
• Give antacid before oral agent; give antiemetic 30-60 min before giving product and prn to prevent vomiting; give antibiotics for prophylaxis of infection
• Provide liquid diet: carbonated beverages, gelatin may be added if patient is not nauseated or vomiting
• Rinse mouth tid-qid with water, club soda; brush teeth bid-qid with soft brush or cotton-tipped applicators for stomatitis; use unwaxed dental floss
IM/SUBCUT route
• IM test dose in lymphoma
• Reconstitute with 1-5 ml sterile water for inj; D$_5$W, 0.9% NaCl, rotate inj sites
IV route
• Product should be prepared by experienced personnel using proper precautions
• Two test doses 2-5 units before initial dose in lymphoma; monitor for anaphylaxis
• Give by direct **IV** after reconstituting 15 units or less/5 ml or more of D$_5$W or 0.9% NaCl; give 15 units or less/10 min through Y-tube or 3-way stopcock initial dose; monitor for anaphylaxis
Intermittent IV infusion route
• Administer after diluting 50-100 ml 0.9% NaCl, D$_5$W and giving at prescribed rate
Intrapleural route
• Give 60 units/50-100 ml of 0.9% NaCl,

administered by physician through thoracotomy tube

Syringe compatibilities: Cisplatin, cyclophosphamide, DOXOrubicin, droperidol, fluorouracil, furosemide, heparin, leucovorin, methotrexate, metoclopramide, mitomycin, vinBLAStine, vinCRIStine

Y-site compatibilities: Allopurinol, amisostine, aztreonam, cisplatin, cyclophosphamide, DOXOrubicin, DOXOrubicin liposome, droperidol, filgrastim, fludarabine, fluorouracil, granisetron, heparin, leucovorin, melphalan, methotrexate, metoclopramide, mitomycin, ondansetron, paclitaxel, piperacillin/tazobactam, sargramostim, teniposide, thiotepa, vinBLAStine, vinCRIStine, vinorelbine

Additive compatibilities: Amikacin, cephapirin, dexamethasone, diphenhydrAMINE, fluorouracil, gentamicin, heparin, hydrocortisone, phenytoin, streptomycin, tobramycin, vinBLAStine, vinCRIStine

Additive incompatibilities: Aminophylline, ascorbic acid inj, carbenicillin, cefazolin, cephalothin, diazepam, hydrocortisone, methotrexate, mitomycin, nafcillin, penicillin G sodium, terbutaline

Solution compatibilities: 0.9% NaCl

Patient/family education

• Teach patient to avoid use of products containing aspirin or ibuprofen, razors, commercial mouthwash; bleeding may occur; to report symptoms of bleeding (hematuria, tarry stools)

• Instruct patient to report signs of anemia (fatigue, headache, irritability, faintness, shortness of breath)

• Instruct patient to report any changes in breathing or coughing even several months after treatment; to avoid crowds and persons with respiratory tract or other infections

• Inform patient that hair may be lost during treatment; a wig or hairpiece may make patient feel better; new hair may be different in color, texture

• Caution patient not to have any vaccinations without the advice of the prescriber; serious reactions can occur

• Advise patient contraception is needed during treatment and for several months after completion of therapy

Evaluation
Positive therapeutic outcome

• Prevention of rapid division of malignant cells

boric acid otic
See Appendix B

bortezomib (Rx)
(bor-tez′oh-mib)
Velcade
Func. class.: Antineoplastic—miscellaneous
Chem. class.: Proteasome inhibitor

Pregnancy category D

Action: Reversible inhibitor of chymotrypsin-like activity in mammalian cells; causes a delay in tumor growth by disrupting normal homeostatic mechanisms

Therapeutic outcome: Decreased growth and spread of malignant cells

Uses: Multiple myeloma previously untreated or when at least two other treatments have failed; mantle cell lymphoma

Dosage and routes
Multiple myeloma (previously untreated)
Adult: **IV** BOL Give for 9 6-wk cycles; cycle 1-4, 1.3 mg/m^2/dose given on days 1, 4, 8, 11, then a 10-day rest period (days 12-21) and again on days 22, 25, 29, 32, then a 10-day rest period (days 33-42) given with melphalan (9 mg/m^2/day on days 1-4) and predniSONE (60 mg/m^2/day on days 1-4); this 6-wk cycle is considered one course; in cycles 5-9, give bortezomib 1.3 mg/m^2/dose on days 1, 8, 22, 29 with melphalan (9 mg/m^2/day on days 1-4) and predniSONE (60 mg/m^2/day on days 1-4); this 6-wk cycle is considered one course; at least 72 hr should elapse between consecutive doses

Mantle cell lymphoma
Adult: **IV** BOL 1.3 mg/m^2/dose (days 1, 4, 8, 11) followed by 10-day rest period (days 12 to 21); max 8 cycles

Neuropathic pain
Grade 1 with pain or grade 2, reduce to 1 mg/m^2; grade 2 with pain or grade 3, hold product until toxicity resolves, then start at 0.7 mg/m^2 qwk; grade 4 hematologic toxicities, withhold use

Available forms: Lyophilized powder for inj 3.5 mg

Adverse effects
CNS: Anxiety, insomnia, dizziness, headache, peripheral neuropathy, rigors, paresthesia
CV: Hypotension, edema

Adverse effects: *italic* = common, **bold** = life-threatening

GI: Abdominal pain, constipation, diarrhea, dyspepsia, nausea, vomiting, anorexia
HEMA: Anemia, **neutropenia, thrombocytopenia**
MISC: Dehydration, weight loss, herpes zoster, rash, pruritus, blurred vision
MS: Fatigue, malaise, weakness, arthralgia, bone pain, muscle cramps, myalgia, back pain, tumor lysis syndrome
RESP: Cough, pneumonia, dyspnea, URI

Contraindications: Pregnancy **D**, hypersensitivity to this product, boron, or mannitol

Precautions: Peripheral neuropathy, breastfeeding, children, geriatric, renal/hepatic disease, hypotension

Pharmacokinetics

Absorption	Unknown
Distribution	Protein binding 83%
Metabolism	P450 enzymes (3A4, 2D6, 2C19, 2C9, 1A2)
Excretion	Unknown
Half-life	9-15 hr

Pharmacodynamics
Unknown

Interactions
Individual drugs
3TC, amiodarone, atanavir, chloramphenicol, cisplatin, colchicine, cycloSPORINE, d4T, dapsone, ddI, didanosine, disulfiram, docetaxel, gold salts, INH, iodoquinal, isoniazid, lamivudine, metronidazole, nitrofurantoin, oxaliplatin, paclitaxel, penicillamine, phenytoin, ritonavir, stavudine, sulfasalazine, thalidomide, vinBLAStine, vinCRIStine, zacatabine ddc, ZDV, zidovudine, and others: increased peripheral neuropathy

Drug classifications
Antihypertensives: increased hypotension
Antivirals, statins, HMG-CoA reductase inhibitors: increased peripheral neuropathy
Oral hypoglycemics: increased hypo/hyperglycemia
Products that induce or inhibit CYP3A4: increased toxicity or decreased efficacy

NURSING CONSIDERATIONS
Assessment
• Assess hematologic status: platelets, CBC throughout treatment
• Monitor for extravasation at inj site

Nursing diagnoses
• Injury, risk for (uses, adverse reactions)
• Knowledge, deficient (teaching)

Implementation
• Reconstitute each vial with 3.5 ml 0.9% NaCl
• Use protective clothing during handling, preparation; avoid contact with skin

Patient/family education
• Teach to use contraception while on this product, avoid breastfeeding
• Advise to monitor blood glucose levels if diabetic
• Instruct to contact prescriber if new or worsening peripheral neuropathy, severe vomiting, diarrhea
• Advise to avoid driving, operating machinery until effect is known
• Advise to avoid using other medications unless approved by prescriber

Evaluation
Positive therapeutic outcome
• Improvement of multiple myeloma symptoms

---

bosentan (Rx)
(boh-sen-tan)
Tracleer
Func. class.: Vasodilator
Chem. class.: Endothelin receptor antagonist
Pregnancy category X

Action: Peripheral vasodilation occurs via antagonism of the effect of endothelin on endothelium and vascular smooth muscle

Therapeutic outcome: Decreased pulmonary arterial hypertension

Uses: Pulmonary arterial hypertension with WHO class III, IV symptoms

Unlabeled uses: Septic shock to improve microcirculatory blood flow

Dosage and routes
Adult >40 kg and child >12 yr: PO 62.5 mg bid × 4 wk, then 125 mg bid
Adult <40 kg and child >12 yr: PO 62.5 mg bid

Available forms: Tabs 62.5, 125 mg

Adverse effects
CNS: Headache, flushing, fatigue, fever
CV: Hypo/hypertension, **hypertensive crisis**, palpitations, edema of lower limbs
GI: Abnormal liver function, dyspepsia, **hepatotoxicity**, diarrhea

HEMA: **Anemia, leukopenia, neutropenia, lymphopenia, thrombocytopenia**
INTEG: Pruritus, **Stevens-Johnson syndrome, toxic epidermal necrolysis,** rash
MISC: Anaphylaxis, oligospermia, tumor lysis syndrome
SYST: **Secondary malignancy**

Contraindications: Pregnancy **X**, hypersensitivity, CVA, CAD

Precautions: Breastfeeding, children, geriatric, mitral stenosis, impaired hepatic function

Pharmacokinetics

Absorption	50% absorbed
Distribution	Protein binding >98%
Metabolism	Liver (metabolites); metabolized CYP2C9, CYP3A4, and possibly CYP2C19; steady state 3-5 days
Excretion	Biliary
Half-life	5 hr

Pharmacodynamics
Unknown

Interactions
Individual drugs
CycloSPORINE A, glyBURIDE: do not coadminister
CycloSPORINE A, ketoconazole: increased bosentan level
CycloSPORINE: decreased cycloSPORINE level
GlyBURIDE: glyBURIDE level decreased significantly, bosentan also decreased, increased liver function tests
Ketoconazole: increased bosentan level
Simvastatin: decreased effects
Warfarin: decreased anticoagulation
Drug classifications
Contraceptives (hormonal), statins: decreased effects
CYP2C9, CYP3A4 inhibitors: increased bosentan effects
Drug/lab test
Increased: ALT, AST
Decreased: Hgb, Hct

NURSING CONSIDERATIONS
Assessment
• Assess B/P, pulse during treatment until stable
• Assess hepatic tests: AST, ALT, bilirubin; liver enzymes may increase; if ALT/AST >3 and ≤5 × ULN, decrease dose or interrupt treatment and monitor AST/ALT q2wk; if >2 × ULN, and bilirubin >2 × ULN or signs of hepatitis, hepatic disease, stop treatment

• Assess blood studies: Hct, Hgb may be decreased
• Assess hepatic involvement: vomiting, jaundice; product should be discontinued

Nursing diagnoses
• Knowledge, deficient (teaching)
• Tissue perfusion, ineffective (uses)

Implementation
• Store at room temperature

Patient/family education
• Instruct patient to report jaundice, dark urine, joint pain, fatigue, malaise, bruising, easy bleeding; may indicate blood dyscrasias
• Caution patient to avoid pregnancy; to use nonhormonal form of contraception

Evaluation
Positive therapeutic outcome
• Decrease in pulmonary hypertension

brimonidine ophthalmic
See Appendix B

brinzolamide ophthalmic
See Appendix B

bromfenac ophthalmic
See Appendix B

bromocriptine (Rx)
(broe-moe-krip'teen)
Apo-Bromocriptine ❋, Cycloset, Parlodel, Parlodel Snap Tabs, PMS-Bromocriptine
Func. class.: Antiparkinsonian agent; DOPamine receptor agonist
Chem. class.: Ergot alkaloid derivative
Pregnancy category B

Do not confuse:
Parlodel/pindolol/Provera

Action: Inhibits prolactin release by activating postsynaptic dopamine receptors; activation of striatal dopamine receptors may be reason for improvement in Parkinson's disease

Therapeutic outcome: Decreased involuntary movements in Parkinson's disease; decreased breastfeeding; decreased hormone levels in acromegaly; absence of amenorrhea in hyperprolactinemia

Adverse effects: *italic* = common, **bold** = life-threatening

Uses: Parkinson's disease, amenorrhea/galactorrhea caused by hyperprolactinemia, infertility, acromegaly, pituitary adenomas, adjunct in type 2 diabetes

Unlabeled uses: Neuroleptic malignant syndrome, alcoholism, premenstrual syndrome, mastalgia, cocaine withdrawal, premenstrual breast syndromes

Dosage and routes
Hyperprolactinemia
Adult: PO 1.25-2.5 mg with meals; may increase by 2.5 mg q3-7days; usual dosage 2.5-15 mg/day

Acromegaly
Adult: PO 1.25-2.5 mg/day × 3 days at bedtime; may increase by 1.25-2.5 mg q3-7days; usual range 20-30 mg/day; max 100 mg/day

Type 2 diabetes (Cycloset only)
Adult: PO (initially) 0.8 mg qd in AM within 2 hr of waking, titrate by 0.8 mg/day no more than qwk to max 1.6-4.8 mg/day

Parkinson's disease
Adult: PO 1.25 mg bid with meals; may increase q2-4wk by 2.5 mg/day; not to exceed 100 mg/day, levodopa should be continued while bromocriptine is being instituted

Pituitary adenoma
Adult: PO 1.25 mg bid-tid, may increase over several weeks to 10-20 mg/day

Neuroleptic malignant syndrome (unlabeled)
Adult: PO 2.5-5 mg 2-6 ×/day

Cocaine withdrawal (unlabeled)
Adult: PO 0.625 mg qid × 42 days

Alcoholism (unlabeled)
Adult: PO 7.5 mg/day

Mastalgia (unlabeled)
Adult: PO 2.5-7.5 bid, starting 10-14 days prior to menses, discontinue when menses begins

Available forms: Caps 5 mg; tabs 2.5 mg; Cycloset tabs 0.8 mg

Adverse effects
CNS: Headache, depression, restlessness, anxiety, nervousness, confusion, **seizures,** hallucinations, *dizziness,* fatigue, drowsiness, abnormal involuntary movements, psychosis
CV: Orthostatic hypotension, decreased B/P, palpitations, extrasystole, **shock,** dysrhythmias, bradycardia, **MI**
EENT: Blurred vision, diplopia, burning eyes, nasal congestion

GI: Nausea, vomiting, anorexia, cramps, constipation, diarrhea, dry mouth, GI hemorrhage
GU: Frequency, retention, incontinence, diuresis
INTEG: Rash on face, arms, alopecia, coolness, pallor of fingers, toes, peripheral edema

Contraindications: Hypersensitivity to ergot, bromocriptine; severe ischemic disease, severe peripheral vascular disease, uncontrolled hypertension, preeclampsia, migraine

Precautions: Pregnancy **B,** breastfeeding, children, hepatic/renal disease, pituitary tumors, peptic ulcer disease, sulfite hypersensitivity, pulmonary fibrosis, dementia, GI bleeding, bipolar disorder

Pharmacokinetics
Absorption	Poorly absorbed
Distribution	Unknown
Metabolism	Liver, completely
Excretion	85%-98% feces
Half-life	4 hr (initial); 50 hr (terminal)

Pharmacodynamics
Onset	½-1½ hr
Peak	1-3 hr
Duration	8-12 hr

Interactions
Individual drugs
Alcohol: increased disulfiram-like reaction
Haloperidol, loxapine, methyldopa, metoclopramide, reserpine: decreased levels of bromocriptine
Levodopa: increased neurologic effects
Drug classifications
Antihypertensives: increased hypotension
Contraceptives (oral), estrogens, MAOIs, phenothiazines, progestins: decreased levels of bromocriptine
Drug/herb
Chaste tree fruit, kava: decreased bromocriptine effect
Horehound: increased serotonin effect
Drug/lab test
Increased: growth hormone, AST, ALT, BUN, CK, uric acid, alkaline phosphatase

NURSING CONSIDERATIONS
Assessment
• Assess symptoms of Parkinson's disease (EPS): shuffling gait, muscle rigidity, involuntary movements, pill rolling, muscle spasms, drooling before, during treatment

- Assess for resolution of symptoms of neuroleptic malignant syndrome: decreased temp, seizures, sweating, pulse
- Monitor for change in size of soft tissue volume in acromegaly
- Monitor B/P; establish baseline, compare with other readings; this product decreases B/P; patient should remain recumbent for 2-4 hr after first dose; supervise ambulation

Nursing diagnoses
- Knowledge, deficient (teaching)
- Mobility, impaired physical (uses)

Implementation
- Give with meals or milk to prevent GI symptoms; crush tab if patient has swallowing difficulty
- Give at bedtime so dizziness, orthostatic hypotension do not occur
- Store at room temperature in air-tight container

Patient/family education
- Advise patient to change position slowly to prevent orthostatic hypotension
- Tabs may be crushed and mixed with food
- Caution patient to use contraceptives during treatment with this product; pregnancy may occur; to use methods other than oral contraceptives
- Teach patient that therapeutic effect for Parkinson's disease may take 2 mo: galactorrhea, amenorrhea
- Caution patient to avoid hazardous activity if dizziness, drowsiness occurs during treatment start-up
- Advise patient to avoid alcohol and OTC medication unless approved by prescriber
- Teach patients with acromegaly to notify prescriber immediately if severe headache, nausea, vomiting, blurred vision occur; indicates change in or enlargement of tumor
- Advise patient to report symptoms of MI immediately

Evaluation
Positive therapeutic outcome
- Parkinson's disease: decreased slow movements, decreased drooling
- Decreased breast engorgement with accompanied pain, tenderness
- Acromegly: decreased growth hormone levels

bromitpheniramine (OTC, Rx)
(brome-fen-eer'a-meen)
Bidhist, BPM, brompheniramine, Brove X, Brove X CT, J-Tan, J-Tan PD, Lo Hist 12, Lodrane 24, Tana Cof-XR, VaZol
Func. class.: Antihistamine
Chem. class.: Alkylamine, H_1-receptor antagonist

Pregnancy category C

Action: Acts on blood vessels, GI, respiratory system by competing with histamine for H_1-receptor site; decreases allergic response by blocking histamine

Therapeutic outcome: Absence of allergy symptoms and rhinitis

Uses: Allergy symptoms, rhinitis, urticaria

Dosage and routes
Adult and child >12 yr: PO 4-8 mg q6-8hr, max 48 mg/day; TIME REL 6-12 mg bid-tid, max 48 mg/day
Child 6-12 yr: PO 2 mg q6-8hr, max 24 mg/day; EXT REL 6-12 mg/day
Child 2-6 yr: 1 mg q6-8hr (max 12 mg/day)

Available forms: Tabs 4 mg; elix 2 mg/5 ml; caps 4 mg; chew tab 12 mg; ext rel tab 6 mg; ext rel cap 12 mg; liquid 8 mg, 12 mg/5 ml

Adverse effects
CNS: Dizziness, drowsiness, poor coordination, fatigue, anxiety, euphoria, confusion, paresthesia, neuritis; paradoxical excitation (child, geriatric)
CV: Hypotension, palpitations, tachycardia
EENT: Blurred vision, dilated pupils, tinnitus, nasal stuffiness, dry nose, throat, mouth
GI: Nausea, vomiting, anorexia, constipation, diarrhea
GU: Retention, dysuria, frequency, impotence
HEMA: **Thrombocytopenia, agranulocytosis, hemolytic anemia** (rare)
INTEG: Photosensitivity
RESP: Increased thick secretions, wheezing, chest tightness

Contraindications: Hypersensitivity to H_1-receptor antagonists, acute asthma attack, lower respiratory tract disease, child <2 yr

Precautions: Pregnancy **C**, breastfeeding, increased intraocular pressure, renal/cardiac disease, hypertension, bronchial asthma, seizure disorder, stenosed peptic ulcers, hyperthyroidism, prostatic hypertrophy, bladder neck obstruction, closed-angle glaucoma

Adverse effects: *italic* = common, **bold** = life-threatening

Pharmacokinetics

Absorption	Well absorbed (PO, IM)
Distribution	Widely distributed; crosses blood-brain barrier
Metabolism	Liver, extensively
Excretion	Kidneys, metabolite; breast milk (minimal)
Half-life	12-34 hr

Pharmacodynamics

	PO	SUBCUT/IM	IV
Onset	15-30 min	30 min	Immediate
Peak	2-5 hr	Unknown	Unknown
Duration	6-12 hr	8-12 hr	8-12 hr

Interactions
Individual drugs
Alcohol: increased CNS depression
Aminophylline, insulin, pentobarbital: products are incompatible
Drug classifications
Barbiturates, opiates, sedative/hypnotics, tricyclics: increased CNS depression
MAOIs: increased anticholinergic effect
Drug/herb
Corkwood, henbane leaf: increased anticholinergic effect
Hops, Jamaican dogwood, kava, khat, senega: increased antihistamine effect
Drug/lab test
Interference: skin allergy tests (discontinue antihistamines before testing)

NURSING CONSIDERATIONS
Assessment
• Assess respiratory status: rate, rhythm, increase in bronchial secretions, wheezing, chest tightness; provide fluids to 2 L/day to decrease secretion thickness
• Monitor I&O ratio: be alert for urinary retention, frequency, dysuria, especially geriatric; product should be discontinued if these occur
• Monitor CBC during long-term therapy; blood dyscrasias may occur but are rare
Nursing diagnoses
• Airway clearance, ineffective (uses)
• Injury, risk for (side effects)
• Knowledge, deficient (teaching)
• Noncompliance (teaching, overuse)
Implementation
• May give with food to prevent GI upset; absorption is not altered by food
• Store in tight, light-resistant container

Patient/family education
• Teach patient all aspects of product use; to notify prescriber if confusion, sedation, hypotension occur; to avoid driving or other hazardous activity if drowsiness occurs; to avoid alcohol or other CNS depressants that may potentiate effect
• Instruct patient not to exceed recommended dosage; dysrhythmias may occur
• Teach patient hard candy, gum, frequent rinsing of mouth may be used for dryness
Evaluation
Positive therapeutic outcome
• Absence of runny or congested nose, rashes

budesonide (Rx)
(byoo-des'oh-nide)
Entocort EC, Pulmicort, Pulmicort Flexhaler, Pulmicort Respules, Rhinocort, Rhinocort Aqua
Func. class.: Glucocorticoid

Pregnancy category C

Action: Prevents inflammation by depression of migration of polymorphonuclear leukocytes, fibroblasts, reversal of increased capillary permeability and lysosomal stabilization; does not suppress hypothalamus and pituitary function

Uses: Rhinitis; prophylaxis for asthma; Crohn's disease

Dosage and routes
Rhinitis (Rhinocort, Rhinocort Aqua)
Adult and child >6 yr: 1 spray (32 mcg/spray) in each nostril daily in AM; may increase to 2 sprays (32 mcg/spray) per nostril qd
Asthma
Adult and child ≥6 yr: INH 400-600 mcg/day; 720 mcg/day
Crohn's disease
Adult: PO 9 mg daily AM × 8 wk

Available forms: Dry powder for INH 90, 180 mg/actuation (Pulmicort Flexhaler); inh susp 0.25 mg/2 ml, 0.5 mg/2 ml (Pulmicort Respules); 32 mcg/actuation (Rhinocort Aqua); tab 3 mg

Adverse effects
CNS: Headache, insomnia, hypertonia, syncope, dizziness, drowsiness
CV: Chest pain, hypertension, sinus tachycardia, palpitation

 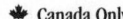

EENT: *Sinusitis, pharyngitis,* rhinitis, oral candidiasis
ENDO: Adrenal insufficiency, growth suppression in children
GI: Dry mouth, dyspepsia, nausea, vomiting, abdominal pain
MISC: Ecchymosis, fever, *hypersensitivity,* flulike symptoms, epistaxis, dysuria
MS: Back pain, myalgias, fractures
RESP: Nasal irritation, cough, nasal bleeding, *respiratory infections,* **bronchospasm**

Contraindications: Hypersensitivity, status asthmaticus

Precautions: Pregnancy **C**, inhaled form (**B**); breastfeeding, children, TB, fungal, bacterial, systemic viral infections, ocular herpes simplex, nasal septal ulcers; hepatic disease (caps)

Pharmacokinetics

Absorption	39%
Distribution	In airways, protein binding 85%-90%
Metabolism	Liver
Excretion	In urine (60%), small amounts in feces, enters breast milk
Half-life	2-3.6 hr

Pharmacodynamics

Onset	Respules 2-8 days, Rhinocort Aqua 10 hr
Peak	Respules 4-6 wk, Rhinocort Aqua 2 wk
Duration	Unknown

Interactions
Avoid using with products metabolized by CYP3A4 inhibition
Individual drugs
Cimetidine, ketoconazole: decreased budesonide metabolism
Varicella live vaccine: avoid concurrent use in pediatric patients
Drug/herb
Aloe, buckthorn, Chinese rhubarb, licorice, senna, St. John's wort: increased hypokalemia

NURSING CONSIDERATIONS
Assessment
• Assess respiratory status: rate, rhythm, increase in bronchial secretions, wheezing, chest tightness; provide fluids to 2 L/day to decrease thickness of secretions; check for oral candidiasis

• For bronchospasm, stop treatment and give bronchodilator
• With viral infections, corticosteroid use can mask infections
• For increased intraocular pressure, discontinue use if increase occurs

Nursing diagnoses
• Airway clearance, ineffective (uses)
• Injury, risk for (uses)
• Knowledge, deficient (teaching)

Implementation
PO route (Crohn's disease)
• Swallow caps whole; do not break, crush, or chew
• May repeat 8-wk course if needed; may taper to 6 mg/day for 2 wk before cessation
INH route (asthma)
• Use scissors to open pouch
• Store at 59°-86° F (15°-30° C); keep away from heat, open flame

Patient/family education
• Teach patient to notify prescriber of pharyngitis, nasal bleeding, oral candidiasis
• Instruct patient not to exceed recommended dose; adrenal suppression may occur
• Teach patient to carry/wear emergency ID identifying steroid use
• Instruct patient to read and follow package directions
• Instruct patient to prevent exposure to infections, especially viral
• Advise to use good oral hygiene if using by nebulizer or inhaler
• Teach patient to avoid breastfeeding

Evaluation
Positive therapeutic outcome
• Absence of asthma, rhinitis

---

budesonide nasal agent
See Appendix B

---

bumetanide (Rx)
(byoo-met'a-nide)
Bumex
Func. class.: Loop diuretic, antihypertensive
Chem. class.: Sulfonamide derivative
Pregnancy category C

Do not confuse:
Bumex/Buprenex/Permax

Action: Acts on the ascending loop of Henle in the kidney to inhibit the reabsorption of the electrolytes sodium and chloride, causing

Adverse effects: *italic* = common, **bold** = life-threatening

excretion of sodium, calcium, magnesium, chloride, water, and some potassium; also decreases reabsorption of sodium and chloride and increases the excretion of potassium in the distal tubule of the kidney; responsible for antihypertensive effect and peripheral vasodilatation

Therapeutic outcome: Decreased edema in lung tissue and peripherally; decreased B/P

Uses: Edema in congestive heart failure, renal/hepatic disease, ascites, heart failure

Dosage and routes
Adult: PO 0.5-2 mg daily may give 2nd or 3rd dose at 4-5 hr intervals; max 10 mg/day; may be given on alternate days or intermittently; IM/**IV** 0.5-1 mg; may give 2nd or 3rd dose at 2-3 hr intervals; max 10 mg/day
Child: PO/IM/**IV** 0.02-0.1 mg/kg q12hr, max 10 mg/day

Available forms: Tabs 0.5, 1, 2 mg; inj 0.25 mg/ml

Adverse effects
CNS: Headache, fatigue, weakness, vertigo
CV: Hypotension, chest pain, ECG changes, **circulatory collapse,** dehydration
EENT: Loss of hearing
ELECT: Hypokalemia, hypochloremic alkalosis, hypomagnesia, hyperuricemia, hypocalcemia, hyponatremia
ENDO: Hyperglycemia
GI: Nausea, diarrhea, dry mouth, vomiting, anorexia, cramps, **acute pancreatitis,** upset stomach, abdominal pain, **jaundice**
GU: Polyuria, **renal failure,** *glycosuria,* premature ejaculation
HEMA: **Thrombocytopenia, leukopenia, granulocytopenia,** hemoconcentration
INTEG: Rash, pruritus, purpura, **Stevens-Johnson syndrome,** sweating, photosensitivity
MS: Muscular cramps, stiffness, arthritis

Contraindications: Hypersensitivity to sulfonamides, anuria, hepatic coma

Black Box Warning: Electrolyte imbalance

Precautions: Pregnancy **C,** breastfeeding, neonates, severe renal disease, ascites, hepatic cirrhosis, blood dyscrasias, ototoxicity, hyperuricemia, hypokalemia

Black Box Warning: Dehydration

Pharmacokinetics

	PO/IM	
Absorption	Rapidly, completely absorbed	
	PO/IM/IV	
Distribution	Crosses placenta, protein binding >91%	
Metabolism	Liver (30%-40%)	
Excretion	Breast milk, urine (50% unchanged), feces (20%)	
Half-life	1-1½ hr; 6-15 hr neonates	

Pharmacodynamics

	PO	IM	IV
Onset	½-1 hr	40 min	5 min
Peak	1-2 hr	1-2 hr	½ hr
Duration	3-6 hr	4-6 hr	3-6 hr

Interactions
Individual drugs
Digoxin: increased toxicity
Indomethacin: decreased diuretic and antihypertensive effects of bumetanide
Lithium: decreased renal clearance causing increased toxicity
Metolazone: increased diuresis, electrolyte loss
Probenecid: decreased diuretic effect
Drug classifications
Aminoglycosides: increased ototoxicity
Antidiabetics: decreased antidiabetic effects
NSAIDs: decreased diuretic effect
Potassium-wasting products: increased hypokalemia
Drug/herb
Aloe, cucumber, dandelion, horsetail, pumpkin, Queen Anne's lace: increased diuretic effect
Khella: increased hypotension
St. John's wort: severe photosensitivity

NURSING CONSIDERATIONS
Assessment
• Assess patient for tinnitus, hearing loss, ear pain; periodic testing of hearing is needed when high doses of this product are given by **IV** route
• Monitor for manifestations of hypokalemia: *RENAL:* acidic urine, reduced urine osmolality, nocturia, polyuria, polydipsia; *CV:* hypotension, broad T wave, U wave, ectopy, tachycardia, weak pulse; *NEURO:* muscle weakness, altered LOC, drowsiness, apathy, lethargy, confusion, depression; *GI:* anorexia, nausea, cramps, constipation, distention, paralytic ileus; *RESP:* hypoventilation, respiratory muscle weakness
• Monitor for manifestations of hypocalcemia: *CNS:* personality changes, anxiety, distur-

bances, depression, psychosis; *GI:* nausea, vomiting, constipation, abdominal pain from muscle spasm; *CV:* decreased contractility, decreased cardiac output, hypotension, lengthened ST segment, prolonged QT interval; *INTEG:* scaling eczema, alopecia, hyperpigmentation; *NEURO:* tetany, muscle twitching, cramping, grimacing, seizure, altered deep tendon reflexes, spasm
- Monitor for manifestations of hypomagnesemia: *CNS:* agitation; *NEURO:* muscle twitching, paresthesias, hyperactive reflexes, positive Babinski's reflex, dysphagia, nystagmus, seizures, tetany; *GI:* nausea, vomiting, diarrhea, anorexia, abdominal distention; *CV:* ectopy, tachycardia, broad, flat, or inverted T waves, depressed ST segment, prolonged QT, decreased cardiac output, hypotension
- Monitor for manifestations of hyponatremia: *CV:* increased B/P, cold, clammy skin, hypo/hypervolemia; *GI:* anorexia, nausea, vomiting, diarrhea, abdominal cramps; *NEURO:* lethargy, increased ICP, confusion, headache, seizures, coma, fatigue, tremors, hyperreflexia
- Monitor for manifestations of hyperchloremia: *NEURO:* weakness, lethargy, coma; *RESP:* deep rapid breathing
- Assess fluid volume status: I&O ratio and record, distended red veins, crackles in lung, color, quality and specific gravity of urine, skin turgor, adequacy of pulses, moist mucous membranes, bilateral lung sounds, peripheral pitting edema; dehydration symptoms of decreasing output, thirst, hypotension, dry mouth and mucous membranes should be reported; if urinary output decreases or azotemia occurs, product should be discontinued
- Monitor electrolytes: potassium, sodium, calcium, magnesium; also include BUN, blood pH, ABGs, uric acid, CBC, blood glucose; severe electrolyte imbalances should be corrected before starting treatment
- Assess B/P before and during therapy with patient lying, standing, and sitting as appropriate; orthostatic hypotension can occur rapidly
- Monitor for digoxin toxicity (anorexia, nausea, vomiting, confusion, paresthesia, muscle cramps) in patients taking digoxin; lithium toxicity in those taking lithium

Nursing diagnoses
- Fluid volume, deficient (side effects)
- Fluid volume, excess (uses)
- Knowledge, deficient (teaching)
- Urinary elimination, impaired (side effects)

Implementation
- Give in AM to avoid interference with sleep
- Potassium replacement if potassium level is <3.0 mg/dl whole, or use oral solutions; product may be crushed if patient is unable to swallow

PO route
- With food, if nausea occurs; absorption may be reduced; the safest dosage schedule is on alternate days

IV route
- Do not use solution that is yellow or has a precipitate or crystals

IV, direct route
- Give undiluted through Y-tube or 3-way stopcock; give 20 mg or less/min

Intermittent IV infusion route
- May be added to 0.9% NaCl, D_5W, $D_{10}W$, $D_{20}W$, invert sugar 10% in electrolyte #1, LR, sodium lactate ⅙ mol/L; use within 24 hr to ensure compatibility; give through Y-tube or 3-way stopcock; give at 4 mg/min or less; use infusion pump

Syringe compatibility: Doxapram
Y-site compatibilities: Allopurinol, amifostine, aztreonam, cefepime, cisatracurium, cladribine, diltiazem, filgrastim, granisetron, lorazepam, morphine, piperacillin/tazobactam, propofol, remifentanil, teniposide, thiotepa, vinorelbine
Additive compatibilities: Floxacillin, furosemide

Patient/family education
- Teach patient to take the medication early in the day to prevent nocturia
- Instruct the patient to take with food or milk if GI symptoms of nausea and anorexia occur
- Teach patient to maintain weekly record of weight and notify prescriber of weight loss of >5 lb
- Caution the patient that this product causes a loss of potassium, so food rich in potassium should be added to the diet; refer to a dietitian for assistance in planning
- Caution the patient not to exercise in hot weather or stand for prolonged periods since orthostatic hypotension will be enhanced
- Teach patient not to use alcohol or any OTC medications without prescriber's approval; serious product reactions may occur
- Emphasize the need to contact prescriber immediately if muscle cramps, weakness, nausea, dizziness, or numbness occur
- Teach patient to take own B/P and pulse and record
- Caution the patient that orthostatic hypotension may occur; patient should rise slowly

Adverse effects: *italic* = common, **bold** = life-threatening

from sitting or reclining positions and lie down if dizziness occurs
• Teach patient to continue taking medication even if feeling better; this product controls symptoms but does not cure the condition
• Advise the patient with hypertension to continue other medical treatment (exercise, weight loss, relaxation techniques, cessation of smoking)

Evaluation
Positive therapeutic outcome
• Decreased edema
• Decreased B/P
• Increased diuresis

---

buprenorphine (Rx)
(byoo-pre-nor'feen)
Buprenex, Subutex
Func. class.: Opioid analgesic, partial agonist
Chem. class.: Thebaine derivative

Pregnancy category C

Controlled substance schedule V (parenteral); schedule III (tablet)

Do not confuse:
Buprenex/Bumex

Action: Inhibits ascending pain pathways in limbic system, thalamus, midbrain, hypothalamus by binding to opiate receptor sites; this alters pain perception and response; generalized CNS depression

Therapeutic outcome: Relief of pain

Uses: Moderate to severe pain

Unlabeled uses: Cocaine, opiate agonist withdrawal

Dosage and routes
Adult: IM/**IV** 0.3 mg q6hr prn; may repeat dose after ½ hr; reduce dosage in geriatric, may repeat after 30-60 min; EPIDURAL (unlabeled) 4 mcg/kg or 2 mcg/kg (epidural injection), remove over 48 hr
Child 2-12 yr: IM/**IV** 2-6 mcg/kg q4-6hr

Available forms: Inj 0.3 mg/ml (1-ml vials); SL tab 2, 8 mg as base

Adverse effects
CNS: Drowsiness, dizziness, confusion, headache, sedation, euphoria, **increased intracranial pressure,** amnesia
CV: Palpitations, bradycardia, change in B/P, tachycardia
EENT: Tinnitus, blurred vision, *miosis, diplopia*

GI: Nausea, vomiting, anorexia, constipation, cramps, dry mouth
GU: Increased urinary output, dysuria, urinary retention
INTEG: Rash, urticaria, bruising, flushing, diaphoresis, pruritus
RESP: **Respiratory depression,** dyspnea, hypo/hyperventilation

Contraindications: Hypersensitivity

Precautions: Pregnancy **C,** breastfeeding, substance abuse/alcoholism, increased intracranial pressure, MI (acute), severe heart disease, respiratory depression, renal/hepatic/pulmonary disease, hypothyroidism, Addison's disease, addiction (opioid)

Pharmacokinetics

Absorption	Well absorbed (IM)
Distribution	Crosses placenta
Metabolism	Liver, extensively by CYP3A4
Excretion	Kidneys, feces, breast milk
Half-life	2.2 hr (**IV**); 37 hr (SL)

Pharmacodynamics

	IM	IV
Onset	10-15 min	Immediate
Peak	1 hr	5 min
Duration	6 hr	6 hr

Interactions
Individual drugs
Alcohol: increased respiratory depression, hypotension, sedation
Drug classifications
Antihistamines, antipsychotics, CNS depressants, MAOIs, sedatives/hypnotics, skeletal muscle relaxants: increased respiratory depression, hypotension
CYP3A4 inducers (carbamazepine, phenobarbital, phenytoin, rifampin): decreased buprenorphine effect
CYP3A4 inhibitors (erythromycin, indinavir, ketoconazole, ritonavir, saquinavir): increased buprenorphine effect
Opioids: increased CNS depression
Drug/herb
Corkwood: increased anticholinergic effect
Gotu kola, Jamaican dogwood, kava, lavender, mistletoe, nettle, pokeweed, poppy, senega, St. John's wort, valerian: increased CNS depression

NURSING CONSIDERATIONS
Assessment
• Assess pain characteristics: location, intensity, type, severity before medication administration and after treatment

---

 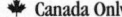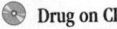

- Monitor VS after parenteral route; note muscle rigidity, product history, liver, kidney function tests, respiratory dysfunction: respiratory depression, character, rate, rhythm; notify prescriber if respirations are <10/min
- Monitor CNS changes: dizziness, drowsiness, hallucinations, euphoria, LOC, pupil reaction; withdrawal in opioid-dependent persons; if dependence occurs within 2 wk of discontinuing product, withdrawal symptoms will occur
- Monitor allergic reactions: rash, urticaria
- Monitor bowel pattern; severe constipation can occur

Nursing diagnoses
- Breathing pattern, ineffective (adverse reactions)
- Knowledge, deficient (teaching)
- Pain, acute (uses)
- Pain, chronic
- Sensory perception, disturbed (adverse reactions)

Implementation
- Give by inj (IM, **IV**), only with resuscitative equipment available; give slowly to prevent rigidity
- Long-term use is not recommended
IM route
- Give deep in large muscle mass; rotate sites of inj
IV route
- Give **IV** direct undiluted over 3-5 min (0.3 mg/2 min); give slowly
Syringe compatibility: Glycopyrrolate, haloperidol, heparin, midazolam
Y-site compatibilities: Allopurinol, amifostine, aztreonam, cefepime, cisatracurium, cladribine, filgrastim, granisetron, melphalan, piperacillin/tazobactam, propofol, remifentanil, teniposide, thiotepa, vinorelbine
Additive compatibilities: Atropine, bupivacaine, diphenhydrAMINE, droperidol, glycopyrrolate, haloperidol, hydrOXYzine, promethazine, scopolamine
Additive incompatibilities: Diazepam, floxacillin, furosemide, lorazepam

Patient/family education
- Instruct patient to report any symptoms of CNS changes, allergic reactions
- Caution patients to avoid CNS depressants: alcohol, sedative/hypnotics for at least 24 hr after taking this product
- Advise that tolerance may result when used for extended periods, but long-term use is not recommended
- Advise to avoid driving, other hazardous activities until reaction is known

- Discuss with patient that dizziness, drowsiness, and confusion are common; to avoid getting up without assistance; to avoid hazardous activities
- Discuss in detail all aspects of the product

Evaluation
Positive therapeutic outcome
- Relief of pain

Treatment of overdose: Naloxone 0.4 mg ampule diluted in 10 ml 0.9% NaCl, give by direct **IV** push 0.02 mg q2min (adult)

---

*buPROPion (Rx)
(byoo-proe'pee-on)
Aplenzin, Budeprion SR, Budeprion XL buPROPion, Wellbutrin, Wellbutrin SR, Wellbutrin XL, Zyban
Func. class.: Antidepressant—miscellaneous, smoking deterrent
Chem. class.: Aminoketone

Pregnancy category B

Do not confuse:
buPROPion/busPIRone, Zyban/Diovan/Zagam

Action: Inhibits reuptake of dopamine

Therapeutic outcome: Decreased symptoms of depression after 2-3 wk

Uses: Depression (Wellbutrin), smoking cessation (Zyban); seasonal affective disorder

Unlabeled uses: Neuropathic pain, enhancement of weight loss, attention deficit hyperactivity disorder (ADHD)

Dosage and routes
Depression
Adult: PO 100 mg bid initially, then increase after 3 days to 100 mg tid if needed; may increase after 1 mo to 150 mg tid; XL/ER/SR, initially 150 mg AM, increase to 300 mg/day if initial dose is tolerated; Aplenzin 174 mg qAM; may increase to 348 mg qAM on day 4; may increase to 522 mg after several weeks if needed
Geriatric: PO 50-100 mg/day, may increase by 50-100 mg q3-4days

Smoking cessation
Adult: PO 150 mg bid, begin with 150 mg daily × 3 days then 300 mg/day; continue for 7-12 wk, max 300 mg/day

Available forms: Tabs 75, 100 mg; sus rel tabs (SR) 100, 150 mg; ext rel tab (XL) 100, 150, 200, 300 mg (SR-12 hr, XL-24 hr); ext rel tab (Aplenzin) 174, 348, 522 mg

---

Adverse effects: *italic* = common, **bold** = life-threatening

Adverse effects

CNS: Headache, agitation, confusion, **seizures,** delusions, *insomnia, sedation, tremors,* dizziness, akinesia, bradykinesia, **suicidal ideation**
CV: **Dysrhythmias,** *hypertension,* palpitations, *tachycardia,* hypotension, **complete AV block, QRS prolongation (overdose)**
EENT: Blurred vision, auditory disturbance
GI: Nausea, vomiting, dry mouth, anorexia, diarrhea, increased appetite, *constipation*
GU: Impotence, frequency, retention, *menstrual irregularities,* altered taste
INTEG: Rash, pruritus, *sweating,* **Stevens-Johnson syndrome**
MISC: Weight loss or gain

Contraindications: Hypersensitivity, eating disorders, seizure disorder

Precautions: Pregnancy **B,** breastfeeding, geriatric, renal/hepatic disease, recent MI, cranial trauma, seizure disorders

Black Box Warning: Children <18 yr, suicidal thinking/behavior (young adults)

Pharmacokinetics

Absorption	Well absorbed; bioavailability poor
Distribution	Unknown
Metabolism	Liver extensively
Excretion	Kidneys
Half-life	14 hr, steady state 1½-5 wk

Pharmacodynamics

Onset	Up to 4 wk
Peak	Unknown
Duration	Unknown

Interactions
Individual drugs

Alcohol, levodopa, theophylline: increased risk of seizures
Carbamazepine, cimetidine, phenobarbitol, phenytoin: decreased buPROPion effect
Cimetidine: increased buPROPion levels
Ritonavir: increased buPROPion toxicity

Drug classifications

Antidepressants, benzodiazepines, MAOIs, phenothiazines, steroids (systemic): increased risk of seizures
CYP2D6/CYP2B6 inhibitors: increased buPRO-Pion effect
CYP450, CYP2D6 products: decreased buPRO-Pion effects
MAOIs: acute toxicity

Drug/herb

Belladonna, corkwood, jimsonweed: increased anticholinergic effect
Hops, kava, lavender: increased CNS depression

NURSING CONSIDERATIONS
Assessment

- Monitor B/P (with patient lying, standing), pulse q4hr; if systolic B/P drops 20 mm Hg hold product, notify prescriber; take vital signs q4hr in patients with CV disease
- Assess smoking cessation progress after 7-12 wk, if progress has not been made, product should be discontinued
- Assess for increased risk of seizures; if patient has used CNS depressant or CNS stimulants, dosage of buPROPion should not be exceeded
- Monitor blood studies: CBC, leukocytes, differential, cardiac enzymes if patient is receiving long-term therapy
- Monitor hepatic studies: AST, ALT, bilirubin if on long-term treatment
- Check weight weekly; appetite may increase with product
- Assess ECG for flattening of T wave, bundle branch block, AV block, dysrhythmias in cardiac patients
- Assess for EPS primarily in geriatric: rigidity, dystonia, akathisia
- Assess mental status: mood, sensorium, affect, suicidal tendencies; increase in psychiatric symptoms: depression, panic
- Monitor urinary retention, constipation; constipation is more likely to occur in children or geriatric
- Identify alcohol consumption; if alcohol was consumed, hold dose

Nursing diagnoses

- Coping, ineffective (uses)
- Injury, risk for (side effects)
- Knowledge, deficient (teaching)
- Noncompliance (teaching)

Implementation

- Give with food or milk for GI symptoms
- Give sugarless gum, hard candy, or frequent sips of water for dry mouth
- When switching to Aplenzin from Wellbutrin, Wellbutrin SR, or XL use these equivalents: 174 buPROPion HBr = 150 mg buPROPion HL4; 348 mg buPROPion HBr = 300 mg buPROPion HCl; 522 mg buPROPion HBr = 450 mg buPROPion HCl
- Store at room temperature; do not freeze

Patient/family education
- Teach patient that therapeutic effects may take 2-3 wk; not to increase dose without prescriber's approval; that treatment for smoking cessation lasts 7-12 wk
- Teach patient to use caution in driving or other activities requiring alertness because of drowsiness, dizziness, blurred vision; to avoid rising quickly from sitting to standing, especially geriatric
- Teach patient to avoid alcohol ingestion; alcohol may increase risk of seizures, obtain approval for other products
- Teach patient to increase fluids, bulk in diet if constipation, urinary retention occur, especially geriatric; notify prescriber immediately if urinary retention occurs
- Teach patient to take gum, hard sugarless candy, or frequent sips of water for dry mouth
- Advise patient not to use with nicotine patches unless directed by prescriber, may increase B/P
- ⭑ Teach patient that risk of seizures increases when dose is exceeded, or if patient has seizure disorder; suicidal ideas, behavior, hostility, depression may occur in children or young adults
- Teach patient to notify prescriber if pregnancy is suspected or planned

Evaluation
Positive therapeutic outcome
- Decrease in depression
- Absence of suicidal thoughts
- Smoking cessation

Treatment of overdose: ECG monitoring, induce emesis, lavage, activated charcoal, administer anticonvulsant

---

*busPIRone (Rx)
(byoo-spye′rone)
BuSpar, BuSpar Dividose, VanSpar
Func. class.: Antianxiety, sedative
Chem. class.: Azaspirodecanedione

Pregnancy category B

Do not confuse:
busPIRone/buPROPion

Action: Acts by inhibiting the action of serotonin (5-HT) by binding to serotonin and dopamine receptors; also increases norepinephrine metabolism; has shown little potential for abuse, a good choice in substance abuse

Therapeutic outcome: Decreased anxiety

Uses: Management and short-term relief of generalized anxiety disorders

Dosage and routes
Adult: PO 5 mg tid; may increase by 5 mg/day q2-3days; max 60 mg/day

Available forms: Tabs 5, 7.5, 10, 15, 30 mg

Adverse effects
CNS: Dizziness, headache, depression, stimulation, insomnia, nervousness, lightheadedness, numbness, paresthesia, incoordination, tremors, excitement, involuntary movements, confusion, akathisia, nightmares, hostility
CV: Tachycardia, palpitations, hypo/hypertension, **CVA, CHF, MI**
EENT: Sore throat, tinnitus, blurred vision, nasal congestion, red, itching eyes, change in taste, smell
GI: Nausea, dry mouth, diarrhea, constipation, flatulence, increased appetite, rectal bleeding
GU: Frequency, hesitancy, menstrual irregularity, change in libido
INTEG: Rash, edema, pruritus, alopecia, dry skin
MISC: Sweating, fatigue, weight gain, fever
MS: Pain, weakness, muscle cramps, spasms
RESP: Hyperventilation, chest congestion, shortness of breath

Contraindications: Hypersensitivity, child <18 yr

Precautions: Pregnancy **B,** breastfeeding, geriatric, impaired renal/hepatic function

Pharmacokinetics
Absorption	Rapidly absorbed
Distribution	Protein binding 86%
Metabolism	Liver, extensively
Excretion	Feces
Half-life	2-3 hr

Pharmacodynamics
Onset	Unknown
Peak	40-90 min
Duration	Unknown

Interactions
Individual drugs
Alcohol: increased CNS depression; avoid use
Carbamazepine, dexamethasone, phenobarbitol, phenytoin, rifampin: decreased busPIRone effect
Erythromycin, itraconazole, ketoconazole, nefazodone, ritonavir: increased busPIRone levels

---

Adverse effects: *italic* = common, **bold** = life-threatening

Drug classifications
Products metabolized by CYP450, 3A4: increased busPIRone levels
MAOIs, procarbazine: increased B/P, do not use together
Products induced by CYP3A4: decreased busPIRone action
Psychotropics: increased CNS depression, avoid use
Selective serotonin reuptake inhibitors: increase serotonin syndrome

Drug/herb
Cowslip, kava, Queen Anne's lace, valerian: increased CNS depression

Drug/food
Grapefruit juice: increased peak concentration of busPIRone

NURSING CONSIDERATIONS
Assessment
• Assess anxiety reaction: inability to sleep, apprehension, dread, foreboding, or uneasiness related to unidentified source of danger
• Assess for previous product dependence or tolerance; if patient is product dependent or tolerant, amount of medication should be restricted
• Monitor B/P (lying, standing), pulse; if systolic B/P drops 20 mm Hg, hold product, notify prescriber; check I&O; may indicate renal dysfunction
• Monitor mental status: mood, sensorium, affect, sleeping patterns, drowsiness, dizziness, suicidal tendencies; withdrawal symptoms when dose is reduced or product discontinued
• Assess for CNS reaction, some reactions may be unpredictable

Nursing diagnoses
• Anxiety (uses)
• Knowledge, deficient (teaching)
• Noncompliance (teaching)

Implementation
• Give with food or milk for GI symptoms (avoid grapefruit juice); sugarless gum, hard candy, frequent sips of water for dry mouth
• May be crushed

Patient/family education
• Teach patient that product may be taken consistently with or without food; if dose is missed take as soon as remembered; do not double doses
• Caution patient to avoid OTC preparations unless approved by the prescriber; to avoid alcohol ingestion and other psychotropic medications unless prescribed; that 1-2 wk of therapy may be required before therapeutic

effects occur; to avoid large amounts of grapefruit juice
• Caution patient to avoid driving and activities requiring alertness since drowsiness may occur; until medication response is known, tell patient that drowsiness may worsen at beginning of treatment
• Instruct patient not to discontinue medication abruptly after long-term use; if dose is missed, do not double
• Advise patient to rise slowly or fainting may occur, especially in geriatric

Evaluation
Positive therapeutic outcome
• Increased well-being
• Decreased anxiety, restlessness, sleeplessness, dread

! HIGH ALERT

busulfan (Rx)
(byoo-sul'fan)
Busulfex, Myleran
Func. class.: Antineoplastic alkylating agent
Chem. class.: Nitrosourea

Pregnancy category D

Do not confuse:
Myleran/Leukeran

Action: Changes essential cellular ions to covalent bonding with resultant alkylation; this interferes with normal biologic function of DNA; activity is not phase specific; action is due to myelosuppression

Therapeutic outcome: Prevention of rapid growth of malignant cells in chronic myelocytic leukemia

Uses: Chronic myelocytic leukemia, bone marrow ablation, stem cell transplant preparation in CML

Dosage and routes
Chronic myelocytic (granulocytic) leukemia
Adult: PO 4-8 mg/day initially; reduce dose if WBC levels reach 30,000-40,000/mm³; stop if WBC ≤20,000/mm³; maintenance 1-3 mg/day
Child: PO 0.06-0.12 mg/kg or 1.8-4.6 mg/m²; discontinue if WBC ≤20,000/mm³

Allogenic hemopoietic stem cell transplantation in chronic myelogenous leukemia
Adult: **IV** 0.8 mg/kg over 2 hr, q6hr × 4 days (total 16 doses); give cyclophosphamide

IV 60 mg/kg over 1 hr/day for 2 days, starting after 16th dose of busulfan

Available forms: Tabs 2 mg; sol for inj 6 mg/ml

Adverse effects
PO route
CV: Hypotension, **thrombosis,** *chest pain,* **tachycardia, atrial fibrillation, heart block,** pericardial effusion, **cardiac tampon-ade** (high dose with cyclophosphamide)
GI: Anorexia, constipation, dry mouth, nausea, vomiting, *diarrhea*
RESP: **Alveolar hemorrhage,** atelectasis, cough, hemoptysis, hypoxia, pleural effusion, pneumonia, sinusitis, **pulmonary fibrosis**
IV route
CNS: **Cerebral hemorrhage, coma, sei-zures,** *anxiety, depression, dizziness, headache,* encephalopathy, weakness, mental changes
EENT: Pharyngitis, epistaxis, cataracts
GI: Diarrhea, nausea, vomiting, weight loss
GU: Impotence, sterility, amenorrhea, gyneco-mastia, **renal toxicity,** hyperuremia, adrenal insufficiency–like syndrome
HEMA: **Thrombocytopenia, leukopenia, pancytopenia, severe bone marrow depression**
INTEG: Dermatitis, hyperpigmentation, alopecia
MISC: **Chromosomal aberrations**
RESP: **Irreversible pulmonary fibrosis,** pneumonitis

Contraindications: Pregnancy **D** (3rd trimester), breastfeeding, radiation, chemo-therapy, blastic phase of chronic myelocytic leukemia, hypersensitivity

Precautions: Child-bearing-age men and women, leukopenia, thrombocytopenia, anemia, hepatotoxicity, renal toxicity, seizures, tumor lysis syndrome, hyperkalemia, hyper-phosphatemia, hypocalcemia, hyperuricemia

Black Box Warning: Neutropenia, second-ary malignancy, thrombocytopenia

Pharmacokinetics	
Absorption	Rapidly absorbed
Distribution	Unknown; crosses placenta
Metabolism	Liver, extensively
Excretion	Kidneys, breast milk
Half-life	2.5 hr

Pharmacodynamics
Unknown

Interactions
Individual drugs
Acetaminophen, itraconazole: decreased busulfan clearance
Cyclophosphamide: cardiac tamponade
Phenytoin: decreased busulfan level
Radiation: increased toxicity, bone marrow suppression
Thioguanine: hepatotoxicity
Drug classifications
Anticoagulants, salicylates: increased risk of bleeding
Antineoplastics: increased toxicity, bone marrow suppression
Live virus vaccines: decreased antibody reac-tion
Drug/lab test
False positive: breast, bladder, cervix, lung cytology tests

NURSING CONSIDERATIONS
Assessment
• Monitor CBC, differential, platelet count weekly; withhold product if WBC <4000/mm^3 or platelets <75,000/mm^3; notify prescriber of results if WBC <15,000/mm^3, platelets <150,000/mm^3; institute thrombocytopenia precautions
• Monitor pulmonary function tests, chest x-ray films before, during therapy; chest film should be obtained q2wk during treatment; check for dyspnea, crackles, nonproductive cough, chest pain, tachypnea; pulmonary fibrosis may occur up to 10 yr after treatment with busulfan
• Assess for increased uric acid levels, swell-ing, joint pain primarily in extremities; patient should be well hydrated to prevent urate deposits
• Monitor renal function studies: BUN, serum uric acid, urine CCr before, during therapy; I&O ratio; report fall in urine output of 30 ml/hr; check for decreased hyperuricemia
• Monitor for cold, fever, sore throat (may indicate beginning infection); identify edema in feet, joint or stomach pain, shaking; pre-scriber should be notified
• Assess for bleeding: hematuria, guaiac, bruising or petechiae, mucosa or orifices q8hr; no rectal temps

Nursing diagnoses
• Body image, disturbed (adverse reactions)
• Infection, risk for (adverse reactions)
• Injury, risk for (adverse reactions)
• Knowledge, deficient (teaching)

Implementation

- Give 1 hr before or 2 hr after meals to lessen nausea and vomiting; give at same time daily
- Increased fluid intake to 2-3 L/day to prevent urate deposits, calculus formation
- Administer antibiotics for prophylaxis of infection; may be prescribed since infection potential is high
- Store in tight container

IV route
- Prepare in biologic cabinet using gloves, gown, mask; dilute with 10 times volume of product using D_5W or 0.9% NaCl (0.5 ml/ml); when withdrawing product, use needle with 5-micron filter provided, remove amount needed, remove filter, and inject product into diluent; always add product to diluent, not vice versa; stable for 8 hr at room temperature using D_5W or 0.9% NaCl; give by central venous catheter over 2 hr q6hr × 4 days, use infusion pump, do not admix
- Give antiemetic before **IV** route
- Give phenytoin before **IV** to prevent seizures in those with seizure disorders

Patient/family education

- Teach patient to avoid use of products containing aspirin or ibuprofen, razors, commercial mouthwash since bleeding may occur; to report symptoms of bleeding (hematuria, tarry stools)
- Instruct patient to report signs of anemia (fatigue, headache, irritability, faintness, shortness of breath)
- Instruct patient to report any changes in breathing or coughing even several months after treatment; to avoid crowds and persons with respiratory tract or other infections
- Teach patient that hair loss may occur; discuss the use of wigs or hair pieces
- Caution patient not to have any vaccinations without the advice of the prescriber; serious reactions can occur
- Advise patient that contraception is needed during treatment and for several months after the completion of therapy

Evaluation

Positive therapeutic outcome
- Decreased leukocytes to normal limits
- Absence of sweating at night
- Increased appetite, increased weight

butoconazole vaginal antifungal

See Appendix B

butorphanol (Rx)

(byoo-tor'fa-nole)

Stadol

Func. class.: Mixed opiate analgesic

Chem class.: Opioid antagonist, partial agonist

Pregnancy category C

Controlled substance schedule IV

Do not confuse:
Stadol/Haldol/Sotalol

Action: Depresses pain impulse transmission at the spinal cord level by interacting with opioid receptors

Therapeutic outcome: Relief of pain

Uses: Moderate to severe pain, general anesthesia induction/maintenance, headache, migraine, preanesthesia

Dosage and routes

Adult: IM 1-4 mg q3-4hr prn; **IV** 0.5-2 mg q3-4hr prn; nasal spray in 1 nostril q3-4hr; may give another dose 1-1½ hr later; may repeat q3-4hr

Geriatric: **IV** ½ adult dose at 2× the interval; intranasal may repeat q1-2hr

Severe pain

Adult: Intranasal 1 spray in each nostril q3-4hr

Renal dose

Adult: Intranasal max 1 mg, followed by 1 mg in 90-120 min; IM/**IV** give 50% of dose (0.5 mg **IV**, 1 mg IM); do not repeat within 6 hr

Available forms: Inj 1, 2 mg/ml; intranasal 10 mg/ml

Adverse effects

CNS: Drowsiness, dizziness, confusion, headache, sedation, euphoria, weakness, hallucinations

CV: Palpitations, bradycardia, hypotension

EENT: Tinnitus, blurred vision, miosis, diplopia, nasal congestion, unpleasant taste

GI: Nausea, vomiting, anorexia, constipation, cramps

GU: Increased urinary output, dysuria, urinary retention

INTEG: Rash, urticaria, bruising, flushing, diaphoresis, pruritus

***RESP:* Respiratory depression,** pulmonary hypertension, upper respiratory infection, sinusitis

Contraindications: Hypersensitivity to this product or preservative, addiction (opioid), CHF, MI

Precautions: Pregnancy **C**, breastfeeding, child <18 yr, addictive personality, increased ICP, respiratory depression, renal/hepatic disease, bowel impaction

Pharmacokinetics

Absorption	Well absorbed (IM, nasal); complete (**IV**)
Distribution	Crosses placenta, protein binding 80%
Metabolism	Liver, extensively
Excretion	Feces (10%-15%); kidneys, unchanged (small amounts)
Half-life	2-9 hr

Pharmacodynamics

	IM	IV	NASAL
Onset	5-10 min	1 min	15 min
Peak	½ hr	5 min	1-2 hr
Duration	3-4 hr	2-4 hr	4-5 hr

Interactions
Individual drugs
Alcohol: increased respiratory depression, hypotension, sedation
Drug classifications
Antipsychotics, CNS depressants, opioids, sedative/hypnotics, skeletal muscle relaxants: increased respiratory depression, hypotension
MAOIs: do not use 2 wk before butorphanol, fatal reaction
Drug/herb
Chamomile, Jamaican dogwood, kava, lavender, mistletoe, nettle, pokeweed, poppy, senega, skullcap, St. John's wort, valerian: increased CNS depression
Corkwood: increased anticholinergic effect

NURSING CONSIDERATIONS
Assessment
• Monitor VS after parenteral route; note muscle rigidity, product history, liver, kidney function tests, respiratory dysfunction: respiratory depression, character, rate, rhythm; notify prescriber if respirations are <10/min
• Monitor CNS changes: dizziness, drowsiness, hallucinations, euphoria, LOC, pupil reaction
• Monitor allergic reactions: rash, urticaria

Nursing diagnoses
• Injury, risk for (adverse reactions)
• Knowledge, deficient (teaching)
• Pain, acute (uses)
• Pain, chronic (uses)
• Sensory perception, disturbed (adverse reactions)

Implementation
• Store in light-resistant container at room temperature
IM route
• Give deeply in large muscle mass; rotate inj sites
Intranasal route
• Give 1 spray in nostril
• Remove clip and cover, prime before using until spray appears; pump must be reprimed q48hr; close nostril with finger and spray once quickly; have patient sniff
IV route
• Give **IV** undiluted at a rate of <2 mg/>3-5 min; titrate to patient response
Syringe compatibilities: Atropine, chlorproMAZINE, cimetidine, diphenhydrAMINE, droperidol, fentanyl, hydrOXYzine, meperidine, methotrimeprazine, metoclopramide, midazolam, morphine, pentazocine, perphenazine, prochlorperazine, promethazine, scopolamine, thiethylperazine
Syringe incompatibilities: DimenhyDRINATE, pentobarbital
Y-site compatibilities: Allopurinol, amifostine, aztreonam, cefepime, cisatracurium, cladribine, DOXOrubicin liposome, enalaprilat, esmolol, filgrastim, fludarabine, granisetron, labetalol, melphalan, paclitaxel, piperacillin/tazobactam, propofol, remifentanil, sargramostim, teniposide, thiotepa, vinorelbine

Patient/family education
• Instruct patient to report any symptoms of CNS changes, allergic reactions; to avoid CNS depressants: alcohol, sedative/hypnotics for at least 24 hr after taking this product
• Discuss with patient that dizziness, drowsiness, and confusion are common; to avoid getting up without assistance, hazardous activities
• Discuss in detail all aspects of the product
Nasal route
• Teach patient to blow nose to clear both nostrils before using
• Patient should replace clip and cover after use; caution patient not to shake medication

Evaluation
Positive therapeutic outcome
• Pain relief

Adverse effects: *italic* = common, **bold** = life-threatening

Treatment of overdose: Narcan 0.2-0.8 **IV**, O_2, **IV** fluids, vasopressors

---

calcitonin (rDNA) (Rx)
(kal-sih-toh'nin)
Fortical
calcitonin (salmon) (Rx)
Calcimir, Miacalcin, Miacalcin Nasal Spray, Osteocalcin, Salmonine
Func. class.: Parathyroid agents (calcium regulator)
Chem. class.: Polypeptide hormone

Pregnancy category C

Action: Decreases bone resorption, blood calcium levels by direct action on bone, GI system, and kidney; increases deposits of calcium in bones; renal excretion of calcium occurs; opposes parathyroid hormone

Therapeutic outcome: Lowered calcium level, decreasing symptoms of Paget's disease

Uses: Paget's disease, postmenopausal osteoporosis, hypercalcemia

Dosage and routes
rDNA
Paget's disease
Adult: SUBCUT 0.5 mg/day initially; may require 0.5 mg bid × 6 mo, then decrease until symptoms reappear

Salmon
Postmenopausal osteoporosis
Adult: SUBCUT/IM 100 international units/day; nasal 200 international units (1 spray) alternating nostrils daily, activate pump before 1st dose

Paget's disease
Adult: SUBCUT/IM 100 international units daily, maintenance 50-100 international units daily or every other day

Hypercalcemia
Adult: SUBCUT/IM 4 international units/kg q12hr, increase to 8 international units/kg q12hr if response is unsatisfactory

Available forms: Inj 200 international units/ml; nasal spray 200 international units/actuation

Adverse effects
CNS: Headache, **tetany,** chills, weakness, dizziness, fever
CV: Chest pressure
EENT: Nasal congestion, eye pain
GI: Nausea, diarrhea, vomiting, anorexia, abdominal pain, salty taste, epigastric pain
GU: Diuresis, nocturia, urine sediment, frequency
INTEG: Rash, flushing, pruritus of earlobes, edema of feet, inj site reaction
MS: Swelling, tingling of hands, backache
RESP: Dyspnea
SYST: **Anaphylaxis**

Contraindications: Hypersensitivity to this product or fish

Precautions: Pregnancy **C,** breastfeeding, children, renal disease, osteogenic sarcoma, pernicious anemia

Pharmacokinetics
Absorption	Completely absorbed
Distribution	Unknown
Metabolism	Rapid; kidneys, tissue, blood
Excretion	Kidneys, inactive metabolite
Half-life	1 hr

Pharmacodynamics
	SUBCUT
Onset	15 min
Peak	4 hr
Duration	8-24 hr

Interactions
Individual drugs
Lithium: decreased lithium effect

NURSING CONSIDERATIONS
Assessment
• Assess for GI symptoms, polyuria, flushing, head swelling, tingling, headache; may indicate hypercalcemia; nervousness, irritability, twitching, seizures, spasm, paresthesia indicate hypocalcemia during beginning of treatment
• Identify nutritional status; check diet for sources of vit D (milk, some seafood), calcium (dairy products, dark green vegetables), phosphates
• Monitor BUN, creatinine, uric acid, chloride, electrolytes, urine pH, urinary calcium, magnesium, phosphate, urinalysis (calcium should be kept at 9-10 mg/dl; vit D 50-135 international units/dl), alkaline phosphatase baseline and q3-6mo; check urine sediment for casts throughout treatment; monitor urine hydroxyproline in Paget's disease, biochemical markers of bone formation/absorption, radiologic evidence of fracture; bone density (osteoporosis)
• Assess for increased product level, since toxic reactions occur rapidly; have parenteral calcium or gluconate on hand if calcium level drops too low; check for tetany (irritability,

paresthesia, nervousness, muscle twitching, seizure, tetanic spasm)

Nursing diagnoses
- Injury, risk for (adverse reactions)
- Knowledge, deficient (teaching)
- Pain, chronic (uses)

Implementation
- Store at <77° F (25° C); protect from light

SUBCUT route (human)
- Give by SUBCUT route only; rotate inj sites; use within 6 hr of reconstitution; give at bedtime to minimize nausea, vomiting

IM route (salmon)
- After test dose of 10 international units/ml, 0.1 ml intradermally; watch 15 min; give only with epinephrine and emergency meds available
- IM inj in deep muscle mass slowly; rotate sites; preferred route if volume is >2 ml

Nasal route
- Use alternating nostrils for nasal spray; allow to warm to room temperature, prime to get full spray

Patient/family education
- Teach method of inj if patient will be responsible for self-medication
- Instruct patient to notify prescriber for hypercalcemic relapse: renal calculi, nausea, vomiting, thirst, lethargy, deep bone or flank pain
- Teach patient that warmth and flushing occur and last 1 hr
- Provide a low-calcium diet as prescribed (Paget's disease, hypercalcemia)
- Advise patients with osteoporosis to increase calcium and vit D in diet and to continue with moderate exercise to prevent continued bone loss
- Advise patients to report difficulty swallowing or change in side effects to prescriber immediately

Evaluation
Positive therapeutic outcome
- Calcium levels 9-10 mg/dl
- Decreasing symptoms of Paget's disease, including pain
- Decreased bone loss in osteoporosis

calcitriol (Rx)
(kal-si-tree'ole)
Calcijex, Rocaltrol, Vitamin D₃
Func. class.: Parathyroid agent (calcium regulator)
Chem. class.: Vitamin D hormone
Pregnancy category C

Do not confuse:
calcitriol/Calciferol

Action: Increases intestinal absorption of calcium, provides calcium for bones, increases renal tubular resorption of phosphate

Therapeutic outcome: Calcium at normal level

Uses: Hypocalcemia in chronic renal disease, hyperparathyroidism, pseudohypoparathyroidism

Dosage and routes
Hypocalcemia
Adult: **IV** 0.5 mcg tid, initially; may increase by 0.25-0.5 mcg/dose q2-4wk; 0.5-3 mcg tid maintenance

Predialysis
Adult: PO 0.25 mcg/day, max 0.5 mcg/day

Hypocalcemia during chronic dialysis
Adult: PO 0.5-3 mcg/day

Renal osteodystrophy
Adult: PO 0.25 mcg every other day to 3 mcg/day
Child: PO 0.014-0.041 mcg/kg/day

Hypoparathyroidism
Adult: PO 0.25-2.7 mcg/day
Child: PO 0.04-0.08 mcg/kg/day

Available forms: Caps 0.25, 0.5 mcg; inj 1 mcg/ml; oral sol 1 mcg/ml

Adverse effects
CNS: Drowsiness, headache, vertigo, fever, lethargy, hallucinations
CV: Palpitations, hypertension
EENT: Blurred vision, photophobia
GI: Nausea, diarrhea, vomiting, jaundice, anorexia, dry mouth, constipation, cramps, metallic taste
GU: Polyuria, hypercalciuria, hyperphosphatemia, hematuria, thirst
MS: Myalgia, arthralgia, decreased bone development, weakness
SYST: Anaphylaxis

Contraindications: Hypersensitivity, hyperphosphatemia, hypercalcemia, vit D toxicity

Precautions: Pregnancy **C**, breastfeeding, renal calculi, CV disease

Pharmacokinetics

Absorption	Well absorbed
Distribution	To liver, crosses placenta
Metabolism	Liver
Excretion	Bile
Half-life	3-6 hr, undergoes hepatic recycling, excreted in bile

Pharmacodynamics

Onset	2-6 hr
Peak	10-12 hr
Duration	Up to 5 days

Interactions
Individual drugs
Cholestyramine, mineral oil: decreased absorption of calcitriol
Phenytoin: increased vit D metabolism
Verapamil: increased dysrhythmias
Drug classifications
Antacids (magnesium): increased hypermagnesemia
Calcium supplements, diuretics (thiazide): increased hypercalcemia
Cardiac glycosides: increased dysrhythmias
Vitamin D products: increased toxicity
Vitamins (fat-soluble): decreased calcitriol absorption
Drug/food
Large amounts of high-calcium foods may cause hypercalcemia
Drug/lab test
False: increased cholesterol
Interference: alkaline phosphatase, electrolytes

NURSING CONSIDERATIONS
Assessment
• Assess GI symptoms, polyuria, flushing, head swelling, tingling, headache; may indicate hypercalcemia
• Identify nutritional status; check diet for sources of vit D (milk, some seafood), calcium (dairy products, dark green vegetables), phosphates
• Monitor BUN, creatinine, uric acid, chloride, electrolytes, urine pH, urinary calcium, magnesium, phosphate, urinalysis (calcium should be kept at 9-10 mg/dl; vit D 50-135 international units/dl), alkaline phosphatase baseline and q3-6mo

◆ Assess for increased product level, since toxic reactions occur rapidly; have calcium chloride on hand if calcium level drops too low; check for tetany

Nursing diagnoses
• Injury, risk for (adverse reactions)
• Knowledge, deficient (teaching)
• Pain, chronic (uses)

Implementation
PO route
• Do not break, crush, or chew caps
• Give with meals for GI symptoms
IV route
• Give by direct **IV** over 1 min

Patient/family education
• Teach patient the symptoms of hypercalcemia (renal stones, nausea, vomiting, anorexia, lethargy, thirst, bone or flank pain) and about foods rich in calcium
• Advise patient to avoid products with sodium: cured meats, dairy products, cold cuts, olives, beets, pickles, soups, meat tenderizers in chronic renal failure
• Advise patient to avoid products with potassium: oranges, bananas, dried fruit, peas, dark green leafy vegetables, milk, melons, beans in chronic renal failure
• Advise patient to avoid OTC products containing calcium, potassium, or sodium in chronic renal failure
• Instruct patient to avoid all preparations containing vit D
• Instruct patient to monitor weight weekly; maintain fluid intake

Evaluation
Positive therapeutic outcome
• Calcium levels 9-10 mg/dl

calcium carbonate (Rx)
(PO-OTC, **IV**-Rx)

Alka-Mints, Amitone, Apo-Cal ✤, Calcarb, Calci-Chew, Calcilac, Calci-Mix, Calcite ✤, Calglycine ✤, Cal-Plus, Calsan ✤, Caltrate, Caltrate Jr., Chooz, Dicarbosil, Equilet, Liquid-Cal, Maalox Antacid Caplets, Mallamint, Mylanta Lozenges ✤, Nephro-Calci, Nu-Cal ✤, Os-Cal, Oysco, Oystercal, Oyst-Cal, Rolaids Calcium Rich, Surpass, Surpass Extra Strength, Titralac, Tums, Tums E-X

Func. class.: Antacid, calcium supplement
Chem. class.: Calcium product

calcium acetate (OTC)
(kal′see-um ass′e-tate)

Calphron, PhosLo

Pregnancy category C

Do not confuse:
Os-Cal/Asacol

Action: Neutralizes gastric acidity

Therapeutic outcome: Neutralized gastric acidity; calcium at normal levels

Uses: Antacid, calcium supplement; not suitable for chronic therapy, hyperphosphatemia, hypertension in pregnancy, osteoporosis, prevention/treatment of hypocalcemia, hyperparathyroidism

Dosage and routes
Antacid
Adult: PO 0.5-1.5 g or 2 pieces of gum 1 hr before meals and at bedtime

Hyperphosphatemia
Adult: PO 1 g or more in divided doses

Hypertension in pregnancy
Adult: PO 500 mg tid during 3rd trimester

Prevention of hypocalcemia, depletion, osteoporosis
Adult: PO 1200 mg daily

Available forms: Calcium carbonate: chewable tabs 350, 420, 450, 500, 750, 1000, 1250 mg; tabs 500, 600, 650, 667, 1000, 1250, 1500 mg; gum 300, 450, 500 mg; susp 1250 mg/5 ml; caps 1250 mg; powder 6.5 g/packet; calcium acetate: tabs 250 mg (65 mg Ca), 667 mg (169 mg Ca), 668 mg (169 mg Ca), 1 g (250 mg Ca); caps 500 mg (125 mg Ca)

Adverse effects
GI: Constipation, anorexia, nausea, vomiting, flatulence, diarrhea, rebound hyperacidity, eructation
GU: Calculi, hypercalciuria

Contraindications: Hypersensitivity, hypercalcemia, hyperparathyroidism, bone tumors

Precautions: Pregnancy **C**, breastfeeding, geriatric, fluid restriction, decreased GI motility, GI obstruction, dehydration, renal disease

Pharmacokinetics
Absorption	⅓ absorbed by small intestines, must have adequate vit D for absorption
Distribution	Unknown
Metabolism	Unknown
Excretion	Feces, urine, crosses placenta
Half-life	Unknown

Pharmacodynamics
Onset	20 min
Peak	Unknown
Duration	20-180 min

Interactions
Individual drugs
Atenolol, etidronate, phenytoin, risedronate, ketoconazole: decreased levels of each drug
Digoxin: increased toxicity from hypercalcemia
Quinidine: increased quinidine levels
Drug classifications
Amphetamines: increased levels of amphetamines
Calcium channel blockers, fluoroquinolones, iron products, salicylates, tetracyclines: decreased levels of each specific product
Thiazide diuretics: increased hypercalcemia
Drug/herb
Lily of the valley, pheasant's eye, shark cartilage, squill: increased side effect, action
Drug/lab test
False increase: chloride
False decrease: magnesium, oxalate, lipase
False positive: benzodiazepines

NURSING CONSIDERATIONS
Assessment
• Monitor Ca$^+$ (serum, urine); Ca$^+$ should be 8.5-10.5 mg/dl, urine Ca$^+$ should be 150 mg/day, monitor weekly
◆ Assess for milk-alkali syndrome: nausea, vomiting, disorientation, headache
• Assess for constipation; increase bulk in the diet if needed
• Assess for hypercalcemia: headache, nausea, vomiting, confusion; hypocalcemia: paresthesia, twitching, colic, dysrhythmias, Chvostek's/Trousseau's sign
• Assess those taking digoxin for toxicity

Adverse effects: *italic* = common, **bold** = life-threatening

- Assess those taking for abdominal pain, heartburn, indigestion before, after administration

Nursing diagnoses
- Knowledge, deficient (teaching)
- Nutrition, less than body requirements, imbalanced (uses)

Implementation
PO route
- Administer as antacid 1 hr after meals and at bedtime
- Administer as supplement 1½ hr after meals and at bedtime
- Administer only with regular tablets or capsules; do not give with enteric-coated tablets
- Administer laxatives or stool softeners if constipation occurs

Patient/family education
- Advise patient to increase fluids to 2 L unless contraindicated, to add bulk to diet for constipation; notify prescriber of constipation
- Advise patient not to switch antacids unless directed by prescriber, not to use as antacid for >2 wk without approval by prescriber
- Teach patient that therapeutic dose recommendations are figured as elemental calcium
- Advise to avoid excessive use of alcohol, caffeine, tobacco
- Teach to avoid spinach, cereals, dairy products in large amounts

Evaluation
Positive therapeutic outcome
- Absence of pain, decreased acidity
- Decreased hyperphosphatemia in renal failure (Acetate)

CALCIUM SALTS

calcium chloride (Rx)
calcium gluceptate (Rx)
calcium gluconate (Rx)
Kalcinate
calcium lactate
(PO-OTC, **IV**-Rx)
Cal-Lac
Func. class.: Electrolyte replacement—calcium product

Pregnancy category C

Action: Cation needed for maintenance of nervous, muscular, skeletal systems, enzyme reactions, normal cardiac contractility, coagulation of blood; affects secretory activity of endocrine, exocrine glands

Therapeutic outcome: Calcium at normal level, absence of increased magnesium, potassium

Uses: Prevention and treatment of hypocalcemia, hypermagnesemia, hypoparathyroidism, neonatal tetany, cardiac toxicity caused by hyperkalemia, lead colic, hyperphosphatemia, vit D deficiency, osteoporosis prophylaxis, calcium antagonist toxicity (calcium channel blocker toxicity)

Dosage and routes
Calcium chloride
Adult: **IV** 500 mg-1 g q1-3days as indicated by serum calcium levels; give at <1 ml/min; **IV** 200-800 mg injected in ventricle of heart

Calcium gluceptate
Adult: **IV** 5-20 ml; IM 2-5 ml

Calcium gluconate
Adult: PO 0.5-2 g bid-qid; **IV** 0.5-2 g at 0.5 ml/min (10% sol); max **IV** dose 3 g
Child: PO/**IV** 500 mg/kg/day in divided doses

Calcium lactate
Adult: PO 325 mg-1.3 g tid with meals
Child: PO 500 mg/kg/day in divided doses

Available forms: Many; check product listings

Adverse effects
CV: Shortened QT interval, heart block, hypotension, bradycardia, dysrhythmias; **cardiac arrest (IV)**
GI: Vomiting, nausea, constipation, diarrhea, dehydration
HYPERCALCEMIA: Drowsiness, lethargy, muscle weakness, headache, constipation, **coma,** anorexia, nausea, vomiting, polyuria, thirst
INTEG: Pain, burning at **IV** site, severe venous thrombosis, necrosis, extravasation

Contraindications: Hypercalcemia, digoxin toxicity, ventricular fibrillation, renal calculi

Precautions: Pregnancy C, breastfeeding, children, renal disease, respiratory disease, cor pulmonale, digitalized patient, respiratory failure

---

Pharmacokinetics

Absorption	Complete bioavailability (**IV**)
Distribution	Readily extracellular; crosses placenta, protein binding 40-50%
Metabolism	Liver
Excretion	Feces (80%), kidney (20%), breast milk
Half-life	Unknown

Pharmacodynamics

	PO	IV
Onset	Unknown	Immediate
Peak	Unknown	Rapid
Duration	Unknown	½-1½ hr

Interactions
Individual drugs
Atenolol, digoxin, phenytoin, tetracyclines, thyroid, verapamil: decreased effect of each of these drugs
Drug classifications
Antacids: milk-alkali syndrome (renal disease)
Diuretics (thiazide): increased hypercalcemia
Fluoroquinolones: decreased absorption of fluoroquinolones when calcium is taken PO
Iron salts: decreased absorption of iron when calcium is taken PO
Drug/herb
Lily of the valley, pheasant's eye, shark cartilage, squill: increased side effects, action
Drug/lab test
False: decreased magnesium
Decreased: 17-OHCS
Increased: 11-OHCS

NURSING CONSIDERATIONS
Assessment
• Monitor ECG for decreased QT interval and T-wave inversion: in hypercalcemia, product should be reduced or discontinued
• Monitor calcium levels during treatment (9-10 mg/dl is normal level), urine calcium if hypercaluria occurs
• Assess cardiac status: rate, rhythm, CVP (PWP, PAWP if being monitored directly)
• Assess digitalized patients closely, an increase in calcium increases digoxin toxicity risk

Nursing diagnoses
• Injury, risk for (uses, adverse reactions)
• Knowledge, deficient (teaching)

Implementation
PO route
• Give PO with or following meals to enhance absorption
• Store at room temperature

IV route
• Administer **IV** undiluted or diluted with equal amounts of 0.9% NaCl for inj to a 5% sol; give 0.5-1 ml/min
• Give through small-bore needle into large vein; if extravasation occurs, necrosis will result (**IV**); IM inj may cause severe burning, necrosis, and tissue sloughing; warm sol to body temp before administering (only gluconate/gluceptate)
• Provide seizure precautions: padded side rails, decreased stimuli (noise, light); place airway suction equipment, padded mouth gag if calcium levels are low
• Patient should remain recumbent 30 min after IV dose
Calcium chloride
Syringe compatibilities: Milrinone
Y-site compatibilities: DOBUTamine, epinephrine, esmolol, inamrinone, morphine, paclitaxel
Additive compatibilities: Amikacin, amphotericin B, ampicillin, ascorbic acid, bretylium, ceftriaxone, cephapirin, chloramphenicol, DOPamine, hydrocortisone, isoproterenol, lidocaine, methicillin, norepinephrine, penicillin G potassium, penicillin G sodium, pentobarbital, phenobarbital, verapamil, vit B/C
Calcium gluceptate
Additive compatibilities: Ascorbic acid inj, isoproterenol, lidocaine, norepinephrine, phytonadione, sodium bicarbonate
Calcium gluconate
Syringe compatibilities: Aldesleukin, allopurinol, amifostine, aztreonam, cefazolin, cefepime, ciprofloxacin, cladribine, DOBUTamine, enalaprilat, epinephrine, famotidine, filgrastim, granisetron, heparin/hydrocortisone, labetalol, melphalan, midazolam, netilmicin, piperacillin/tazobactam, potassium chloride, prochlorperazine, propofol, sargramostim, tacrolimus, teniposide, thiotepa, tolazoline, vinorelbine, vit B/C
Additive compatibilities: Amikacin, aminophylline, ascorbic acid inj, bretylium, cephapirin, chloramphenicol, corticotropin, dimenhyDRINATE, erythromycin, furosemide, heparin, hydrocortisone, lidocaine, magnesium sulfate, methicillin, norepinephrine, penicillin G potassium, penicillin G sodium, phenobarbital, potassium chloride, tobramycin, vancomycin, verapamil, vit B/C

Patient/family education
• Caution patient to add food high in vit D content; to add calcium-rich foods to diet: dairy products, shellfish, dark green leafy

Adverse effects: *italic* = common, **bold** = life-threatening

vegetables; decrease oxalate-rich and zinc-rich foods: nuts, legumes, chocolate, spinach, soy
• Advise patient to prevent injuries, avoid immobilization

Evaluation
Positive therapeutic outcome
• Decreased twitching, paresthesias, muscle spasms
• Absence of tremors, seizures, dysrhythmias, dyspnea, laryngospasm, negative Chvostek's sign, negative Trousseau's sign

RARELY USED

canakinumab
(kan-a-kin-ue-mab)
Ilaris
Func. class.: Monoclonal antibody

Dosage and routes
Adult: SUBCUT: 150 mg q8wk, slowly inject a vial with 1 ml preservative-free sterile water for injection

Uses: Cryopyrin-associated periodic syndromes (CAPS)

Contraindications: Hypersensitivity

candesartan (Rx)
(can-deh-sar'tan)
Atacand
Func. class.: Antihypertensive
Chem. class.: Angiotensin II receptor (Type AT$_1$)

Pregnancy category
C (1st trimester),
D (2nd/3rd trimesters)

Action: Blocks the vasoconstrictor and aldosterone-secreting effects of angiotensin II; selectively blocks the binding of angiotensin II to the AT$_1$ receptor found in tissues

Therapeutic outcome: Decreased B/P

Uses: Hypertension, alone or in combination; CHF NYHA Class II-IV and ejection fraction ≤40%

Dosage and routes
Adult: PO (single agent) 16 mg daily initially in patients who are not volume depleted, range 8-32 mg/day; with diuretic or volume depletion, 2-32 mg/day as a single dose or divided bid

Renal dose
Adult: PO give lowest possible dose

Available forms: Tabs 4, 8, 16, 32 mg

Adverse effects
CNS: Dizziness, fatigue, headache
CV: Chest pain, peripheral edema, hypotension
EENT: Sinusitis, rhinitis, pharyngitis
GI: Diarrhea, nausea, abdominal pain, vomiting
GU: **Renal failure**
MS: Arthralgia, pain
RESP: Cough, upper respiratory infection
SYST: Angioedema

Contraindications: Hypersensitivity

Black Box Warning: Pregnancy D (2nd/3rd trimesters)

Precautions: Pregnancy C (1st trimester), breastfeeding, children, geriatric, hypersensitivity to ACE inhibitors, volume-depletion, renal/hepatic impairment

Pharmacokinetics
Absorption	Well absorbed
Distribution	Bound to plasma proteins
Metabolism	Extensive
Excretion	Feces, urine, breast milk
Half-life	9 hr

Pharmacodynamics
Onset	Unknown
Peak	2 hr
Duration	24 hr

Interactions
Individual drugs
Lithium: increased lithium level
Potassium: increased hypokalemia
Drug classifications
α-blockers, ACE inhibitors, β-blockers, calcium channel blockers: increased hypotension
Diuretics (potassium sparing): increased hypokalemia
NSAIDs, salicylates: decreased effect
Drug/herb
Aconite: increased toxicity, death
Astragalus, cola tree: increased or decreased antihypertensive effect
Barberry, betony, black catechu, black cohosh, bloodroot, broom, burdock, cat's claw, dandelion, goldenseal, Irish moss, Jamaican dogwood, kelp, khella, mistletoe, parsley, Queen Anne's lace, rue: increased antihypertensive effect
Coltsfoot, guarana, khat, licorice, yohimbe: decreased antihypertensive effect

NURSING CONSIDERATIONS
Assessment
- Assess B/P, pulse q4hr; note rate, rhythm, quality
- Monitor electrolytes: potassium, sodium, chloride; total CO_2
- Obtain baselines in renal, liver function tests before therapy begins
- Assess blood studies: BUN, creatinine, liver function tests before treatment
- Monitor for edema in feet, legs daily
- Assess for skin turgor, dryness of mucous membranes for hydration status; for angioedema: facial swelling, dyspnea
- Assess for pregnancy; this product can cause fetal death when given in pregnancy
- Assess for adverse reactions, especially in renal disease

Nursing diagnoses
- Fluid volume, deficient (side effects)
- Knowledge, deficient (teaching)
- Noncompliance (teaching)

Implementation
- Administer without regard to meals

Patient/family education
- Teach patient not to take the product if breastfeeding or pregnant, or have had an allergic reaction to this product
- If a dose is missed, instruct patient to take as soon as possible, unless it is within an hour before next dose
- Advise patient to comply with dosage schedule, even if feeling better
- Teach patient to notify prescriber of fever, swelling of hands or feet, irregular heartbeat, chest pain
- Advise patient excessive perspiration, dehydration, diarrhea may lead to fall in blood pressure—consult prescriber if these occur
- Inform patient that product may cause dizziness, fainting; light-headedness may occur
- Caution patient to rise slowly to sitting or standing position to minimize orthostatic hypotension
- Advise patient to avoid all OTC medications unless approved by prescriber; to inform all health care providers of medication use
- Teach proper technique for obtaining B/P and acceptable parameters

Evaluation
Positive therapeutic outcome
- Decreased B/P

capecitabine (Rx)
(cap-eh-sit'ah-bean)
Xeloda
Func. class.: Antineoplastic, antimetabolite
Chem. class.: Fluoropyrimidine carbamate

Pregnancy category D

Do not confuse:
Xeloda/Xenical

Action: Competes with physiologic substrate of DNA synthesis, thus interfering with cell replication in the S phase of cell cycle (before mitosis); also interferes with RNA and protein synthesis; product is converted to 5-fluorouracil (5-FU)

Therapeutic outcome: Decreasing symptoms of breast cancer

Uses: Monotherapy for paclitaxel-anthracycline-resistant metastatic breast, colorectal cancer when 5-FU monotherapy is preferred; treatment of patients with colorectal cancer who have undergone complete resection of their primary tumor

Unlabeled uses: Pancreatic cancer

Dosage and routes:
Adult: PO 2500 mg/m²/day in 2 divided doses q12hr at end of meal × 2 wk, then 1 wk rest period; given in 3-wk cycles; may be combined with docetaxel, when capecitabine dose is lowered; follow the NCIC (National Cancer Institute of Canada) common toxicity criteria

Renal dose
Adult: PO CCr 30-50 ml/min; decrease initial dose to 75% of usual dose

Available forms: Tabs 150, 500 mg

Adverse effects
CNS: Dizziness, headache, *paresthesia, fatigue,* insomnia
GI: Nausea, vomiting, anorexia, diarrhea, stomatitis, abdominal pain, constipation, dyspepsia, **intestinal obstruction, necrotizing enterocolitis**
HEMA: **Neutropenia, lymphopenia, thrombocytopenia,** anemia
INTEG: Hand and foot syndrome, dermatitis, nail disorder
MISC: Hyperbilirubinemia, eye irritation, edema, myalgia, limb pain, *pyrexia,* dehydration
RESP: Cough, dyspnea

Contraindications: Pregnancy **D,** infants, hypersensitivity to 5-FU, severe renal impairment (CCr <30 ml/min)

Adverse effects: *italic* = common, **bold** = life-threatening

Precautions: Renal/hepatic disease, breastfeeding, children, geriatric

Pharmacokinetics

Absorption	Readily, food decreased
Distribution	Unknown
Metabolism	Liver, extensively
Excretion	Kidneys
Half-life	45 min

Pharmacodynamics

Onset	Unknown
Peak	1½ hr
Duration	Unknown

Interactions
Individual drugs
Leucovorin: increased toxicity
Phenytoin: increased phenytoin level
Drug classifications
Antacids (aluminum, magnesium): increased capecitabine

Black Box Warning: Anticoagulants: increased risk of bleeding

Food/drug
Increased absorption; give within 30 min of a meal

NURSING CONSIDERATIONS
Assessment
• Assess buccal cavity q8hr for dryness, sores or ulceration, white patches, pain, bleeding, dysphagia; obtain prescription for viscous lidocaine (Xylocaine)
• Assess symptoms indicating severe allergic reaction: rash, pruritus, urticaria, purpuric skin lesions, itching, flushing; product should be discontinued
• Monitor CBC, differential, platelet count weekly; withhold product if WBC <4000/mm^3 or platelet count is <100,000/mm^3; notify prescriber of results if WBC <20,000/mm^3, platelet count <150,000/mm^3
• Monitor temp q4hr (may indicate beginning of infection)
• Assess for hand/foot syndrome: paresthesia, tingling, painful/painless swelling, blistering, erythema with severe pain of hands/feet
• Assess for toxicity: severe diarrhea, nausea, vomiting, stomatitis
• Assess GI symptoms: frequency of stools, cramping; if severe diarrhea occurs, fluids/electrolytes may need to be given
• Monitor liver function tests before and during therapy (bilirubin, AST, ALT, LDH) as needed or monthly; note jaundice of skin or sclera, dark urine, clay-colored stools, itchy skin, abdominal pain, fever, diarrhea
• Assess for bleeding: hematuria, stool guaiac, bruising or petechiae, mucosa or orifices q8hr; inflammation of mucosa, breaks in skin

Nursing diagnoses
• Body image, disturbed (adverse reactions)
• Infection, risk for (adverse reactions)
• Injury, risk for (adverse reactions)
• Knowledge, deficient (teaching)

Implementation
• Give antiemetic 30-60 min before giving product to prevent vomiting and prn; give antibiotics for prophylaxis of infection
• Provide liquid diet: carbonated beverages; gelatin may be added if patient is not nauseated or vomiting
• Help patient to rinse mouth tid-qid with water or club soda, brush teeth bid-qid with soft brush or cotton-tipped applicators for stomatitis, use unwaxed dental floss

Patient/family education
• Contraceptive measures are recommended during therapy; product is teratogenic to fetus
• Advise patient to avoid use of products containing aspirin or ibuprofen, razors, commercial mouthwash, since bleeding may occur; to report symptoms of bleeding (hematuria, tarry stools)
• Instruct patient to report signs of anemia (fatigue, headache, irritability, faintness, shortness of breath)
• Advise patient not to become pregnant while taking this product; to avoid using while breastfeeding
• Advise patient not to double dose, if dose is missed
• Advise patient to report immediately severe diarrhea, vomiting, stomatitis, fever ≥100° F, hand/foot syndrome, anorexia

Evaluation
Positive therapeutic outcome
• Prevention of rapid division of malignant cells

---

captopril **(Rx)**
(kap'toe-pril)
Capoten, Novo-Captopril ✷
Func. class.: Antihypertensive
Chem. class.: Angiotensin-converting enzyme (ACE) inhibitor
Pregnancy category D

Do not confuse:
captopril/Capitrol/carvedilol

 Alert   ✷ Canada Only   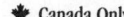 Drug on CD   * "Tall Man" lettering (See Preface)

Action: Selectively suppresses renin-angiotensin-aldosterone system; inhibits ACE; prevents conversion of angiotensin I to angiotensin II

Therapeutic outcome: Decreased B/P in hypertension; decreased preload, afterload in CHF

Uses: Hypertension, CHF, left ventricular dysfunction (LVD) after MI, diabetic nephropathy

Dosage and routes
Malignant hypertension
Adult: PO 25 mg increasing q2hr until desired response; max 450 mg/day

Hypertension
Adult: Initial dose: PO 12.5-25 mg bid-tid; may increase to 50 mg bid-tid at 1-2 wk intervals; usual range 25-150 mg bid-tid; max 450 mg
Child: PO 0.3-0.5 mg/kg/dose, titrate up to 6 mg/kg/day in 2-4 divided doses
Neonate: PO 0.05-0.1 mg/kg bid-tid, may increase as needed

CHF
Adult: PO 25 mg bid-tid; may increase to 50 mg bid-tid; after 14 days may increase to 150 mg tid if needed

LVD after MI
Adult: PO 50 mg tid, may begin treatment 3 days after MI; give 6.25 mg as a single dose, then 12.5 mg tid, increase to 25 mg tid for several days, then 50 mg tid

Diabetic nephropathy
Adult: PO 25 mg tid

Renal dose
Adult: PO CCr >50 ml/min, no change; CCr 10-50 ml/min, decrease dose by 25%; CCr <10 ml/min, decrease dose by 50%

Available forms: Tabs 12.5, 25, 50, 100 mg

Adverse effects
CNS: Fever, chills
CV: Hypotension, postural hypotension, *tachycardia,* angina
GI: Loss of taste, increased liver function tests
GU: Impotence, dysuria, nocturia, proteinuria, **nephrotic syndrome, acute reversible renal failure,** polyuria, oliguria, frequency
HEMA: **Neutropenia, agranulocytosis, pancytopenia, thrombocytopenia,** anemia
INTEG: Rash, pruritus
MISC: **Angioedema,** hyperkalemia
RESP: **Bronchospasm,** *dyspnea, cough*

Contraindications: Breastfeeding, children, hypersensitivity, heart block, potassium-sparing diuretics, bilateral renal artery stenosis, angioedema

Black Box Warning: Pregnancy **D**

C

Precautions: Dialysis patients, hypovolemia, leukemia, scleroderma, LE, blood dyscrasias, CHF, diabetes mellitus, renal/hepatic disease, thyroid disease, COPD, asthma

Pharmacokinetics	
Absorption	Well absorbed
Distribution	Widely distributed; crosses placenta, excreted in breast milk (small amounts)
Metabolism	Liver (50%)
Excretion	Kidneys, unchanged (50%)
Half-life	2 hr increase in renal disease

Pharmacodynamics	
Onset	¼-1 hr
Peak	1 hr
Duration	6-12 hr

Interactions
Individual drugs
Alcohol (acute ingestion): increased hypotension (large amounts)
Digoxin, lithium: increased serum levels, toxicity
Insulin: increased hypoglycemia
Drug classifications
Antacids, NSAIDs, salicylates: decreased captopril effect
Antidiabetics (oral): increased hypoglycemia
Antihypertensives, diuretics, nitrates, phenothiazines: increased hypotension
Diuretics (potassium-sparing), potassium supplements: increased toxicity, do not use
Sympathomimetics: do not use
Drug/herb
Aconite: increased toxicity, death
Astragalus, cola tree: increased or decreased antihypertensive effect
Barberry, betony, black catechu, black cohosh, bloodroot, broom, burdock, cat's claw, dandelion, goldenseal, Irish moss, Jamaican dogwood, kelp, khella, mistletoe, parsley: increased antihypertensive effect
Coltsfoot, guarana, khat, licorice, yohimbe: decreased antihypertensive effect
Drug/lab test
Increased: AST, ALT, alkaline phosphatase, bilirubin, uric acid, glucose
False positive: urine acetone, ANA titer

Adverse effects: *italic* = common, **bold** = life-threatening

NURSING CONSIDERATIONS
Assessment
- May be crushed and mixed with food
- Monitor blood studies: decreased platelets; WBC with diff baseline, periodically q3mo, if neutrophils <1000/mm³, discontinue treatment
- Monitor B/P, check for orthostatic hypotension, syncope; if changes occur, dosage change may be required
- Monitor renal studies: protein, BUN, creatinine; watch for increased levels that may indicate nephrotic syndrome and renal failure; monitor renal symptoms: polyuria, oliguria, frequency, dysuria
- Establish baselines in renal, liver function tests before therapy begins and check periodically; monitor for increased liver function studies; watch for increased uric acid, glucose
- Check potassium levels throughout treatment, although hyperkalemia rarely occurs
- Check for edema in feet, legs daily; monitor weight daily in CHF
- Assess for allergic reactions: rash, fever, pruritus, urticaria; product should be discontinued if antihistamines fail to help

Nursing diagnoses
- Cardiac output, decreased (uses)
- Injury, risk for (side effects)
- Knowledge, deficient (teaching)
- Noncompliance (teaching)

Implementation
- Store in air-tight container at 86° F (30° C) or less
- Severe hypotension may occur after first dose of this medication; decreasing hypotension may be prevented by reducing or discontinuing diuretic therapy 3 days before beginning captopril therapy
- Administer 1 hr before or 2 hr after meals
- May crush tab and dissolve in water, give within ½ hr, make sure tab is completely dissolved

Patient/family education
- Caution patient not to discontinue product abruptly; advise patient to tell all persons associated with care
- Teach patient not to use OTC products (cough, cold, allergy) unless directed by prescriber; serious side effects can occur; xanthines such as coffee, tea, chocolate, cola can prevent action of product
- Teach patient importance of complying with dosage schedule, even if feeling better; to continue with medical regimen to decrease

B/P: exercise, cessation of smoking, decreasing stress, diet modifications
- Emphasize the need to rise slowly to sitting or standing position to minimize orthostatic hypotension; not to exercise in hot weather or increased hypotension can occur
- Teach patient to notify prescriber of mouth sores, sore throat, fever, swelling of hands or feet, irregular heartbeat, chest pain, coughing, shortness of breath
- Caution patient to report excessive perspiration, dehydration, vomiting, diarrhea; may lead to fall in B/P
- Caution patient that product may cause dizziness, fainting, light-headedness; may occur during first few days of therapy; to avoid activities that may be hazardous
- Teach patient how to take B/P, and teach normal readings for age-group; ensure patient takes regularly
- Advise patient to tell prescriber if pregnancy is suspected or planned

Evaluation
Positive therapeutic outcome
- Decreased B/P in hypertension

Treatment of overdose: 0.9% NaCl **IV** infusion, hemodialysis

carbachol ophthalmic
See Appendix B

carbamazepine (Rx)
(kar-ba-maz′e-peen)
Apo-Carbamazepine ✦, Carbatrol, Epitol, Equetro, Novo-Carbamaz ✦, Tegretol, Tegretol CR ✦, Tegretol-XR, Teril
Func. class.: Anticonvulsant
Chem. class.: Iminostilbene derivative

Pregnancy category D

Do not confuse:
Tegretol/Toradol

Action: Exact mechanism unknown; appears to decrease polysynaptic responses and block posttetanic potentiation

Therapeutic outcome: Absence of seizures; decreased trigeminal neuralgia pain

Uses: Tonic-clonic, complex-partial, mixed seizures; trigeminal neuralgia; bipolar disorder

Unlabeled uses: Neurogenic pain, psychotic behavior with dementia, diabetic neuropathy, agitation, hiccups

Dosage and routes
Seizures
Adult and child >12 yr: PO 200 mg bid; may be increased by 200 mg/day in divided doses q6-8hr; maintenance 800-1200 mg/day; max 1600 mg/day (adult); max child 12-15 yr 1000 mg/day; max child >15 yr 1200 mg/day; adjustment is needed to minimum dose to control seizures; EXT REL give bid; RECT administration of oral SUSP 200 mg/10 ml or 6 mg/kg as a single dose

Child 6-12 yr: PO tabs 100 mg bid or SUSP 50 mg qid; may increase by <100 mg qwk, max 1000 mg/day; EXT REL tabs daily-bid

Child <6 yr: PO 10-20 mg/kg/day in 2-3 divided doses, may increase qwk

Trigeminal neuralgia
Adult: PO 100 mg/bid; may increase 100 mg q12hr until pain subsides; max 1200 mg/day; maintenance is 200-400 mg bid

Bipolar disorder
Adult: PO (Equetro only) 200 mg bid, may adjust dose by 200 mg daily to desired response; max 1600 mg/day

Agitation due to dementia (unlabeled)
Adult: PO 100 mg bid, may increase to 250-300 mg/day

Hiccups (unlabeled)
Adult: PO 200 mg tid

Available forms: Chewable tabs 100, 200 mg; tabs 200 mg; oral susp 100 mg/5 ml; ext rel tabs 100, 200, 400 mg; ext rel caps (Carbatrol) 200, 300 mg

Adverse effects
CNS: Drowsiness, dizziness, confusion, fatigue, **paralysis,** headache, hallucinations, **worsening of seizures,** unsteadiness, speech disturbances

Black Box Warning: Suicidal ideation

CV: **Hypertension, CHF,** hypotension, aggravation of CAD, dysrhythmias, **AV block**
EENT: Tinnitus, dry mouth, blurred vision, diplopia, nystagmus, conjunctivitis
ENDO: Syndrome of inappropriate antidiuretic hormone (SIADH) (geriatric)
GI: Nausea, constipation, diarrhea, anorexia, vomiting, abdominal pain, stomatitis, glossitis, increased liver enzymes, **hepatitis, hepatic porphyria**
GU: Frequency, retention, albuminuria, glycosuria, impotence, increased BUN, **renal failure**
HEMA: **Thrombocytopenia,** leukopenia, **agranulocytosis, leukocytosis, aplastic anemia, eosinophilia,** increased pro-time
INTEG: Rash, **Stevens-Johnson syndrome,** urticaria, photosensitivity, **toxic epidermal necrolysis**
RESP: Pulmonary hypersensitivity (fever, dyspnea, pneumonitis)

Contraindications: Pregnancy **D,** hypersensitivity to carbamazepine or tricyclics, AV or bundle branch block

Black Box Warning: Bone marrow depression

Precautions: Glaucoma, renal/hepatic/cardiac disease, psychosis, breastfeeding, child <6 yr, alcoholism, hepatic porphyria

Black Box Warning: Hematologic disease, agranulocytosis, leukopenia, neutropenia, thrombocytopenia, Asian patients

Pharmacokinetics
Absorption	Slow; completely absorbed
Distribution	Widely distributed; protein binding 76%
Metabolism	Extensively, liver, metabolized by CYP3A4
Excretion	Urine, feces, breast milk
Half-life	18-65 hr, then 8-29 hr after first month

Pharmacodynamics
Onset	Slow
Peak	4-5 hr
Duration	Unknown

Interactions
Individual drugs
Benzodiazepines, darunavir, delavirdine, doxycycline, felbamate, haloperidol, nefazodone, oxcarbazepine, phenobarbitol, phenytoin, primidone: decreased effect of these products

Cimetidine, clarithromycin, danzol, diltiazem, erythromycin, fluoxetine, fluvoxamine, isoniazid, propoxyphene, valproic acid, verapamil, voriconazole: increased carbamazepine levels

Cisplatin, DOXOrubicin, felbamate, phenobarbitol, phenytoin, primidone, rifampin, theophylline: increased carbamazepine levels

Contraceptives (oral): decreased effect of oral contraceptives

Desmopressin, lithium, hypressin, vasopressin: increased effects of each specific product

Doxycycline: decreased effect of doxycycline
Lithium: increased CNS toxicity
Phenobarbital: increased effect

Adverse effects: *italic* = common, **bold** = life-threatening

Phenytoin: increased and decreased plasma levels; decreased carbamazepine plasma levels

Thyroid hormones: decreased effect of thyroid hormones

Valproic acid: decreased plasma levels; increased half-life of carbamazepine

Warfarin: decreased effect of warfarin

Drug classifications

CYP3A4 inducers: decreased carbamazepine levels

CYP3A4 inhibitors: increased carbamazepine levels

⚠️MAOIs: fatal reaction; do not use together

Drug/herb

Ginkgo, quinine: increased anticonvulsant action

Ginseng, santonica: decreased anticonvulsant action

Drug/food

Grapefruit juice: increased peak concentration of carbamazepine

NURSING CONSIDERATIONS
Assessment

• Assess for seizures: character, location, duration, intensity, frequency, presence of aura

• Assess for trigeminal neuralgia: facial pain including location, duration, intensity, character, activity that stimulates pain

• Monitor liver function tests (AST, ALT) and urine function tests, BUN, urine protein periodically during treatments

• Assess blood studies: RBC, Hct, Hgb, reticulocyte counts qwk for 4 wk then q3-6mo if on long-term therapy; if myelosuppression occurs, product should be discontinued

• Check blood levels during treatment or when changing dose; therapeutic level 4-12 mcg/ml

• Assess for blood dyscrasias: fever, sore throat, bruising, rash, jaundice, epistaxis (long-term treatment only)

⚠️ Assess mental status: mood, sensorium, affect, behavioral changes, suicidal thoughts/behaviors

Nursing diagnoses

• Injury, risk for (side effects)
• Knowledge, deficient (teaching)

Implementation

• Do not break, crush, or chew ext rel tabs and caps

• Ext rel caps may be opened and beads mixed with food

• Chewable tabs should be chewed, not swallowed whole

• Give with food for GI symptoms

• Shake oral susp before use

• Mix an equal amount of water, D_5W, 0.9% NaCl when giving by NG tube, flush tube with 100 ml of above sol

Patient/family education

• Teach patient to carry/wear emergency ID stating patient's name, products taken, condition, prescriber's name, phone number

• Caution patient to avoid driving, other activities that require alertness until stabilized on medication

• Teach patient not to discontinue medication quickly after long-term use

• Teach patient to use a nonhormonal type of contraception to prevent harm to the fetus

• Advise patient to use sunscreen to prevent burns

• Teach patient to take exactly as prescribed; do not double or omit doses

• Teach patient to report immediately chills, rash, light-colored stools, dark urine, yellowing of skin/eyes, abdominal pain, sore throat, mouth, ulcers, bruising, blurred vision, dizziness

Evaluation

Positive therapeutic outcome

• Decreased seizure activity

Treatment of overdose: Lavage, VS

---

carbidopa-levodopa (Rx)
(kar-bi-doe′pa lee-voe-doe′pa)
Atamet, carbidopa/levodopa, Sinemet, Sinemet CR
Func. class.: Antiparkinsonism agent
Chem. class.: Catecholamine

Pregnancy category C

Action: Decarboxylation of levodopa to periphery is inhibited by carbidopa; more levodopa is made available for transport to brain and conversion to dopamine in the brain

Therapeutic outcome: Absence of involuntary movements

Uses: Parkinson's disease, parkinsonism resulting from carbon monoxide, chronic manganese intoxication, cerebral arteriosclerosis

Unlabeled uses: Restless legs syndrome

Dosage and routes
Beginning therapy for those not taking levodopa
Adult: PO 25 mg carbidopa/100 mg levodopa tid, may increase daily or every other day by 1 tab to desired response (8 tabs/day); EXT

REL tabs carbidopa 50 mg/levodopa 200 mg bid

For those not taking levodopa ER
Adult: PO 50 mg carbidopa/200 mg levodopa bid

For those taking levodopa ER
Adult: Begin treatment with 10% more levodopa/day given PO q4-8hr, may increase or decrease dose q3days

For those taking levodopa <1.5 g/day
Adult: PO 25 mg carbidopa/100 mg levodopa tid-qid, may increase daily to desired response

For those taking levodopa >1.5 g/day
Adult: PO 25 mg carbidopa/250 mg levodopa tid-qid, may increase daily to desired response

Restless legs syndrome (RLS) (unlabeled)
Adult: PO carbidopa 25 mg/levodopa 100 mg, 1 tab at bedtime, may repeat if awakening within 2 hr or 50 mg carbidopa/200 mg levodopa SUS REL tab 1-2 tabs 1 hr before bedtime

Available forms: Tabs 10 mg carbidopa/100 mg levodopa, 25 mg carbidopa/100 mg levodopa, 25 mg carbidopa/250 mg levodopa; ext rel tab 25 mg/100 mg, 50 mg/200 mg carbidopa/levodopa (Sinemet CR); oral disintegrating tab (Parcopa) 10 mg carbidopa/100 mg levodopa, 25 mg carbidopa/100 mg levodopa, 25 mg carbidopa/250 mg levodopa

Adverse effects
CNS: Involuntary choreiform movements, hand tremors, fatigue, headache, anxiety, twitching, numbness, weakness, confusion, agitation, insomnia, nightmares, psychosis, hallucination, hypomania, severe depression, dizziness
CV: Orthostatic hypotension, tachycardia, hypertension, palpitation
EENT: Blurred vision, diplopia, dilated pupils
GI: Nausea, vomiting, anorexia, abdominal distress, dry mouth, flatulence, dysphagia, bitter taste, diarrhea, constipation
HEMA: **Hemolytic anemia, leukopenia, agranulocytosis**
INTEG: Rash, sweating, alopecia
MISC: Urinary retention, incontinence, weight change, dark urine

Contraindications: Hypersensitivity, closed-angle glaucoma, malignant melanoma, history of malignant melanoma, or undiagnosed skin lesions resembling melanoma

Precautions: Pregnancy **C**, breastfeeding, diabetes, renal/cardiac/hepatic/respiratory disease, MI with dysrhythmias, open-angle glaucoma, seizures, peptic ulcer, depression

C

Pharmacokinetics

Absorption	Well absorbed (PO); ER dose slow
Distribution	Widely distributed
Metabolism	Liver, extensively
Excretion	Kidneys, metabolites
Half-life	Levodopa (1 hr); carbidopa (1-2 hr)

Pharmacodynamics

	PO	PO-ER
Onset	Unknown	Unknown
Peak	1 hr	2½ hr
Duration	6-24 hr	Unknown

Interactions
Individual drugs
Metoclopramide: increased effects of levodopa
Papaverine, pyridoxine: decreased effects of levodopa
Drug classifications
Antacids: increased effects of levodopa
Anticholinergics, benzodiazepines, hydantoins: decreased effects of levodopa
MAOIs: hypertensive crisis
Drug/herb
Kava, octacosanol: increased Parkinson's symptoms
Indian snakeroot: decreased action; increased EPS
Drug/food
Protein: decreased absorption of levodopa
Drug/lab test
Increased: AST, ALT, bilirubin, LDH, alkaline phosphatase, BUN
Decreased: VMA, BUN, creatinine
False increase: uric acid, urine protein
False positive: urine ketones (dipstick), Coombs' test
False negative: urine glucose

NURSING CONSIDERATIONS
Assessment
- Assess B/P, respiration, orthostatic B/P
- Monitor I&O ratio; retention commonly causes decreased urinary output, distention, frequency, incontinence; palpate bladder if retention occurs
- Assess for muscle twitching, blepharospasm that may indicate toxicity

---

Adverse effects: *italic* = common, **bold** = life-threatening

• Monitor renal, liver, hematopoietic studies; also for diabetes, acromegaly during long-term therapy

• Assess for parkinsonism: shuffling gait, muscle rigidity, involuntary movements, pill rolling, muscle spasms, drooling before and during treatment

• Monitor for constipation, cramping, pain in abdomen, abdominal distention; increase fluids, bulk, exercise if this occurs

• Assess for tolerance over long-term therapy; dose may have to be increased or changed

• Assess for mental status: affect, mood, CNS depression, worsening of mental symptoms during early therapy

Nursing diagnoses

• Knowledge, deficient (teaching)

• Mobility, impaired physical (uses)

Implementation

PO route

• Swallow ext rel tabs whole; do not break, crush, or chew

• Give product until NPO before surgery; check with prescriber for continuing product

• Adjust dosage depending on patient response

• Give with meals or after meals to prevent GI symptoms; limit protein taken with product

• Give only after MAOIs have been discontinued for 2 wk; if previously on levodopa, discontinue for at least 8 hr before change to levodopa-carbidopa

Patient/family education

• Teach patient to change positions slowly to prevent orthostatic hypotension

• Teach patient to report side effects: twitching, eye spasms, grimacing, protrusion of tongue, personality changes that indicate overdose

• Instruct patient to use product exactly as prescribed; if product is discontinued abruptly, parkinsonian crisis may occur; do not double doses; take missed dose as soon as remembered up to 2 hr before next dose

• Teach patient that urine, sweat may darken and is harmless

• Advise patient to use physical activities to maintain mobility and lessen spasms

• Instruct patient that OTC medications should not be used unless approved by prescriber

• Advise patient that drowsiness, dizziness are common; to avoid hazardous activities until response is known

• Explain that sips of water, hard candy, or gum may lessen dry mouth

• Teach patient to take with meals to prevent GI symptoms; to limit protein intake, which impairs product's absorption

Evaluation

Positive therapeutic outcome

• Decrease in akathisia

• Improved mood

• Decreased involuntary movements

❗ HIGH ALERT

carboplatin (Rx)

(kar'boe'pla-tin)

Paraplatin, Paraplatin-AQ ✦

Func. class.: Antineoplastic alkylating agent

Chem. class.: Platinum coordination compound

Pregnancy category D

Do not confuse:

carboplatin/cisplatin, Paraplatin/platinol

Action: Produces interstrand DNA crosslinks and to a lesser extent DNA-protein cross-links; activity is not cell cycle phase specific

Therapeutic outcome: Prevention of rapidly growing malignant cells

Uses: Initial treatment of ovarian cancer in combination with other agents; palliative treatment of recurrent ovarian carcinoma after treatment with other antineoplastic agents

Dosage and routes

(single agent)

Adult: IV INF initially 300 mg/m^2 given with cyclophosphamide, q4-6wk; refractory tumors 360 mg/m^2 single dose, may repeat q4wk, as needed; do not repeat until neutrophils >2000 mm^3 and platelets >100,000/mm^3

Renal dose

Adult: IV INF CCr 41-59 ml/min 250 mg/m^2, CCr 16-40 ml/min 200 mg/m^2; do not use in CCr <15 ml/min

Available forms: Lyophilized powder for inj 50, 150, 450 mg vials; aqueous sol for inj 50 mg/5 ml vial, 150 mg/15 ml vial, 450 mg/45 mg vial, 600 mg/60 ml vial

Adverse effects

CNS: **Seizures, central neurotoxicity,** peripheral neuropathy, dizziness, confusion

CV: Cardiac abnormalities

EENT: Tinnitus, hearing loss, *vestibular toxicity,* visual changes

GI: Severe nausea, vomiting, diarrhea, weight loss, mucositis, anorexia, constipation, taste change

---

HEMA: **Thrombocytopenia, leukopenia, pancytopenia, neutropenia, anemia,** bleeding
INTEG: Alopecia, dermatitis, rash, erythema, pruritus, urticaria
META: Hypomagnesemia, hypocalcemia, hypokalemia, hyponatremia, hyperuremia
SYST: **Anaphylaxis**

Contraindications: Pregnancy **D**, hypersensitivity to this product, platinum products, mannitol; significant bleeding, aluminum products used to prepare or administer carboplatin

Black Box Warning: Severe bone marrow depression

Precautions: Geriatric patients, radiation therapy within 1 mo, other cancer, chemotherapy within 1 mo, breastfeeding, liver disease

Black Box Warning: Anemia, infection

Pharmacokinetics

Absorption	Complete
Distribution	Unknown
Metabolism	Liver
Excretion	Kidneys
Half-life	Initial 1-2 hr; postdistribution 2½-6 hr; increased in renal disease

Pharmacodynamics

Onset	½ hr
Peak	Unknown
Duration	4-6 hr

Interactions
Individual drugs
Amphotericin B: increased nephrotoxicity or ototoxicity
Aspirin: increased risk of bleeding
Phenytoin: decreased levels
Radiation: increased toxicity, bone marrow suppression
Drug classifications
Aminoglycosides: ototoxicity, increased nephrotoxicity
Antineoplastics, bone marrow–suppressing products: increased bone marrow suppression
Myelosuppressives: increased myelosuppression
NSAIDs: increased risk of bleeding
Thrombolytic agents: increased risk of bleeding
Drug/lab test
Increased: AST, BUN, alkaline phosphatase, bilirubin, creatinine

NURSING CONSIDERATIONS
Assessment
• Monitor CBC, differential, platelet count weekly; withhold product if neutrophil count is <2000/mm^3 or platelet count is <100,000/mm^3; notify prescriber of results if WBC <20,000/mm^3, platelets <150,000/mm^3
• Assess for anaphylaxis: pruritus, wheezing, tachycardia; notify physician after discontinuing products; resuscitation equipment should be available
• Monitor renal function studies: BUN, creatinine, serum uric acid, urine CCr before, during therapy; I&O ratio; report fall in urine output to <30 ml/hr
• Monitor temp q4hr (may indicate beginning of infection)
• Monitor liver function tests before, during therapy (bilirubin, AST, ALT, LDH) as needed or monthly; note jaundice of skin or sclera, dark urine, clay-colored stools, itchy skin, abdominal pain, fever, diarrhea
• Assess for bleeding: hematuria, stool guaiac, bruising or petechiae, mucosa or orifices q8hr; inflammation of mucosa, breaks in skin
• Identify dyspnea, crackles, unproductive cough, chest pain, tachypnea
• Identify effects of alopecia on body image; discuss feelings about body changes

Nursing diagnoses
• Body image, disturbed (adverse reactions)
• Infection, risk for (adverse reactions)
• Injury, risk for (adverse reactions)
• Knowledge, deficient (teaching)

Implementation
• Antiemetic 30-60 min before giving product to prevent vomiting, and prn
IV route
• Give **IV** after diluting 10 mg/ml of sterile water for inj, D$_5$W, 0.9% NaCl (10 mg/ml); then further dilute with the same sol 1-4 mg/ml; give over 15 min or more (intermittent inf)
• Give **IV** inf over 5-6 hr; do not use needles or **IV** administration sets containing aluminum; may cause precipitate or loss of potency; diuretic (furosemide 40 mg **IV**) after inf
• Store protected from light at room temperature; reconstituted sol is stable for 8 hr at room temperature
Y-site compatibilities: Allopurinol, amifostine, aztreonam, cefepime, cladribine, DOXOrubicin liposome, filgrastim, fludarabine, granisetron, melphalan, ondansetron, paclitaxel, piperacillin/tazobactam, propofol,

---

Adverse effects: *italic* = common, **bold** = life-threatening

sargramostim, teniposide, thiotepa, vinorelbine
Additive compatibilities: Cisplatin, etoposide, floxuridine, ifosfamide, ifosfamide/etoposide, paclitaxel
Additive incompatibilities: Fluorouracil, mesna
Solution compatibilities: D_5/0.2% NaCl, D_5/0.45% NaCl, D_5/0.9% NaCl, 0.9% NaCl, D_5W, sterile water for inj
Solution incompatibilities: Sodium bicarbonate

Patient/family education

• Advise patient to report ringing/roaring in the ears, numbness, tingling in face, extremities, weight gain
• Teach patient to avoid use of products containing aspirin or ibuprofen, NSAIDs, alcohol, razors, commercial mouthwash, since bleeding may occur; to report symptoms of bleeding (hematuria, tarry stools)
• Instruct patient to report signs of anemia (fatigue, headache, irritability, faintness, shortness of breath); sore throat, bleeding, bruising, chills, back pain, blood in stools, dyspnea
• Instruct patient to report any changes in breathing or coughing even several months after treatment; to avoid crowds and persons with respiratory tract or other infections
• Advise patient that hair may be lost during treatment; a wig or hairpiece may make patient feel better; new hair may be different in color, texture
• Caution patient not to have any vaccinations without the advice of the prescriber; serious reactions can occur
• Teach patient that contraception is needed during treatment and for several months after the completion of therapy; not to breastfeed during treatment; to notify prescriber if pregnancy is planned or suspected

Evaluation
Positive therapeutic outcome
• Prevention of rapid division of malignant cells

---

carboprost (Rx)
(kar′boe-prost)
Hemabate, Prostin/15M ❦
Func. class.: Oxytocic, abortifacient
Chem. class.: Prostaglandin

Pregnancy category C

Action: Stimulates uterine contractions, causing complete abortion in approximately 16 hr

Therapeutic outcome: Loss of fetus; decreased postpartum bleeding

Uses: Abortion between 13 and 20 wk gestation; postpartum hemorrhage caused by uterine atony not controlled by other methods

Dosage and routes
To induce abortion
Adult: IM 250 mcg, then 250 mcg q1½-3½hr, may increase to 500 mcg if no response, max 12 mg total dose

Postpartum hemorrhage
Adult: IM 250 mcg, repeat at 15-90 min intervals, max total dosage 2 mg

Available forms: Inj 250 mcg/ml

Adverse effects
CNS: Fever, chills, headache
GI: Nausea, vomiting, diarrhea

Contraindications: Hypersensitivity, severe renal/hepatic/cardiac/respiratory disease, PID

Precautions: Pregnancy C, asthma, anemia, jaundice, diabetes mellitus, seizure disorders, past uterine surgery

Pharmacokinetics	
Absorption	Well absorbed (nasal)
Distribution	Widely distributed (extracellular fluid)
Metabolism	Liver—rapidly
Excretion	Kidneys
Half-life	3-9 min

Pharmacodynamics	
Onset	Unknown
Peak	16 hr
Duration	Unknown

Interactions
Drug classifications
Oxytocics: increased effects

NURSING CONSIDERATIONS
Assessment
• Monitor B/P, pulse; watch for change that may indicate hemorrhage
• Monitor respiratory rate, rhythm, depth; notify physician of abnormalities
• For length, duration of contraction; notify physician of contractions lasting over 1 min or absence of contractions
• Assess for incomplete abortion; pregnancy must be terminated by another method; product is teratogenic

Nursing diagnoses
• Knowledge, deficient (teaching)

Implementation
• Give IM inj in deep muscle mass; rotate inj sites if additional doses are given
• Have crash cart available on unit

Patient/family education
• Advise patient to report increased blood loss, abdominal cramps, increased temp, or foul-smelling lochia

Evaluation
Positive therapeutic outcome
• Loss of fetus
• Control of bleeding

---

carisoprodol (Rx)
(kar-i-soe-proe′dole)
carisoprodol, Soma, Soprodol 350, Vanadom
Func. class.: Skeletal muscle relaxant, central acting
Chem. class.: Meprobamate congener

Pregnancy category C

Do not confuse:
Soma/Soma compound

Action: Depresses CNS by blocking interneuronal activity in descending reticular formation of spinal cord, producing sedation

Therapeutic outcome: Relaxation of skeletal muscles

Uses: Relieving pain, stiffness in musculoskeletal disorders

Dosage and routes
Adult and child >12 yr: PO 350 mg tid and at bedtime, max 3 wk

Available forms: Tabs 350 mg

Adverse effects
CNS: Dizziness, weakness, drowsiness, headache, tremor, depression, insomnia, ataxia, irritability, **seizures**

CV: Postural hypotension, tachycardia
EENT: Diplopia, temporary loss of vision
GI: Nausea, vomiting, hiccups, epigastric discomfort
HEMA: Eosinophilia
INTEG: Rash, pruritus, fever, facial flushing, **erythema multiforme**
RESP: Asthmatic attack
SYST: **Angioedema, anaphylaxis**

Contraindications: Hypersensitivity

Precautions: Pregnancy C, breastfeeding, geriatric, renal/hepatic disease, addictive personality

Pharmacokinetics
Absorption	Well absorbed
Distribution	Crosses placenta
Metabolism	Liver, extensively, substrate of CYP2C19
Excretion	Kidney, unchanged; breast milk
Half-life	8 hr

Pharmacodynamics
Onset	½ hr
Peak	4 hr
Duration	4-6 hr

Interactions
Individual drugs
Alcohol: increased CNS depression
Meprobamate: do not use together
Drug classifications
Antidepressants (tricyclic), barbiturates, opioids, sedative/hypnotics: increased CNS depression
Drug/herb
Chamomile, kava, skullcap, valerian: increased CNS depression
Drug/lab test
Increased: AST, alkaline phosphatase, blood glucose

NURSING CONSIDERATIONS
Assessment
• Monitor ROM, atrophy, stiffness, and pain in muscles; assess throughout treatment
• Monitor ECG in seizure patients; poor seizure control has occurred with patients taking this product
• Assess for idiosyncratic reaction within a few min or hr of administration (disorientation, restlessness, weakness, euphoria, blurred vision); patient should be reassured that reaction is temporary
• Check for allergic reactions: rash, fever

Adverse effects: *italic* = common, **bold** = life-threatening

Nursing diagnoses
- Injury, risk for (adverse reactions)
- Knowledge, deficient (teaching)
- Mobility, impaired physical (uses)

Implementation
- Give with meals for GI symptoms
- Have patient use gum, frequent sips of water for dry mouth
- Store in tight container at room temperature
- Use for short term (2-3 wk), potential for habituation

Patient/family education
- Caution patient not to take with alcohol, other CNS depressants
- Advise patient to avoid altering activities while taking this product
- Caution patient to avoid hazardous activities if drowsiness or dizziness occurs
- Caution patient to avoid using OTC medication such as cough preparations, antihistamines, unless directed by prescriber

Evaluation
Positive therapeutic outcome
- Decreased pain, spasticity

Treatment of overdose: Activated charcoal, lavage, dialysis

⚠ HIGH ALERT

carmustine (Rx)
(kar-mus'teen)
BiCNU, Gliadel
Func. class.: Antineoplastic alkylating agent
Chem. class.: Nitrosourea

Pregnancy category D

Action: Alkylates DNA, RNA; inhibits enzymes that allow synthesis of amino acids in proteins; also responsible for cross-linking DNA strands; activity is not cell cycle phase specific

Therapeutic outcome: Prevention of rapidly growing malignant cells

Uses: Brain tumors such as glioblastoma, medulloblastoma, astrocytoma, ependymoma, metastic brain tumors; multiple myeloma (with prednisone), non-Hodgkin's, Hodgkin's disease, other lymphomas; GI, breast, bronchogenic, and renal carcinomas; wafer, as adjunct to surgery/radiation in newly diagnosed high-grade malignant glioma patients; in recurrent glioblastoma multiforme patients as adjunct to surgery

Unlabeled uses: Malignant melanoma

Dosage and routes
Adult: **IV** 75-100 mg/m^2 over 1-2 hr × 2 days or 150-200 mg/m^2 × 1 dose q6-8wk or 40 mg/m^2/day × 5 days q6wk; if WBC 3000-3999/mm^3 give 50% of dose; if WBC is 2000-2999/mm^3 and platelet count is 25,000-75,000/mm^3 give 25% of dose; withhold dose if WBC <2000/mm^3 and platelets <25,000/mm^3
Adult: Intracavitary 8 wafers inserted into resection cavity

Available forms: Powder for inj 100 mg; wafer 7.7 mg intracavitary

Adverse effects
GI: Nausea, vomiting, anorexia, stomatitis, **hepatotoxicity**
GU: Azotemia, **renal failure**
HEMA: **Thrombocytopenia, leukopenia, myelosuppression, anemia**
INTEG: Pain, burning, hyperpigmentation at inj site
RESP: **Fibrosis, pulmonary infiltrate**
SYST: **Secondary malignant neoplastic disease**

Contraindications: Pregnancy **D**, breast-feeding, hypersensitivity, leukopenia, thrombocytopenia

Precautions: Dental disease, extravasation, females, infection, leukopenia, neutropenia, secondary malignancy, thrombocytopenia

Black Box Warning: Bone marrow suppression, pulmonary fibrosis

Pharmacokinetics

Absorption	Completely absorbed
Distribution	Readily penetrates CSF
Metabolism	Liver, rapid
Excretion	Kidneys, breast milk
Half-life	Unknown

Pharmacodynamics
Unknown

Interactions
Individual drugs
Aspirin: increased risk of bleeding
Cimetidine, radiation: increased toxicity
Digoxin: decreased effects of digoxin
Phenytoin: decreased effects of phenytoin
Drug classifications
Anticoagulants: increased risk of bleeding
Antineoplastics: increased toxicity
Live vaccines: increased adverse reactions; decreased antibody reaction

---

 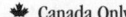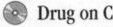

Myelosuppressive agents: increased myelosuppression

NURSING CONSIDERATIONS
Assessment
- Assess buccal cavity q8hr for dryness, sores or ulceration, white patches, pain, bleeding, dysphagia; obtain prescription for viscous lidocaine (Xylocaine)
- Assess symptoms indicating severe allergic reaction: rash, pruritus, urticaria, purpuric skin lesions, itching, flushing; product should be discontinued
- Monitor CBC, differential, platelet count weekly; withhold product if WBC <4000/mm³ or platelet count is <100,000/mm³; notify prescriber of results if WBC <20,000/mm³, platelets <150,000/mm³
- Monitor renal function studies: BUN, creatinine, urine CCr before and during therapy; I&O ratio; report fall in urine output to <30 ml/hr
- Monitor temp q4hr (may indicate beginning of infection)
- Monitor liver function tests before, during therapy (bilirubin, AST, ALT, LDH) as needed or monthly; note yellowing of skin or sclera, dark urine, clay-colored stools, itchy skin, abdominal pain, fever, diarrhea; hepatotoxicity can be serious and fatal
- Assess for bleeding: hematuria, stool guaiac, bruising or petechiae, mucosa or orifices q8hr; inflammation of mucosa, breaks in skin
- Monitor pulmonary function tests, chest x-ray films before, during therapy; chest film should be obtained q2wk during treatment; monitor for dyspnea, cough, pulmonary fibrosis; infiltrate occurs after high doses or several low-dose courses
- Identify effects of alopecia on body image; discuss feelings about body changes

Nursing diagnoses
- Body image, disturbed (adverse reactions)
- Infection, risk for (adverse reactions)
- Injury, risk for (adverse reactions)
- Knowledge, deficient (teaching)

Implementation
- Blood transfusion or RBC colony-stimulating factors to counter anemia may be required
- Give fluids **IV** or PO before chemotherapy to hydrate patient
- Provide antiemetic 30-60 min before giving product to prevent vomiting, and prn; antibiotics for prophylaxis of infection
- Provide liquid diet (carbonated beverages); gelatin may be added if patient is not nauseated or vomiting

- Give all medications PO, if possible; avoid IM inj if platelets <100,000/mm³
Wafer route
- Foil pouches may be kept at room temperature for 6 hr, if unopened
- If wafers are broken in several pieces, do not use
IV route
- Prepare in biologic cabinet wearing gown, gloves, mask; avoid contact with skin
- Administer after diluting 100 mg/3 ml ethyl alcohol (provided); then further dilute 27 ml sterile water for inj; then dilute with 100-500 ml 0.9% NaCl or D₅W; give over 1 hr or more; use only glass containers; reduce rate if discomfort is felt
- Flush **IV** line after carmustine with 10 ml 0.9% NaCl to prevent irritation at site
- Store reconstituted sol in refrigerator for 24 hr or room temperature for 8 hr
Y-site compatibilities: Amifostine, aztreonam, cefepime, filgrastim, fludarabine, granisetron, melphalan, ondansetron, piperacillin/tazobactam, sargramostim, teniposide, thiotepa, vinorelbine
Additive incompatibilities: Sodium bicarbonate

Patient/family education
- Teach patient to avoid use of products containing aspirin or ibuprofen, razors, commercial mouthwash, since bleeding may occur; to report symptoms of bleeding (hematuria, tarry stools)
- Advise patient to avoid foods with citric acid, hot flavor, or rough texture if stomatitis is present
- Instruct patient to report signs of anemia (fatigue, headache, irritability, faintness, shortness of breath); avoid smoking
- Advise patient that hair may be lost during treatment; a wig or hairpiece may make patient feel better; new hair may be different in color, texture
- Caution patient not to have any vaccinations without the advice of the prescriber; serious reactions can occur
- Advise patient that contraception is needed during treatment and for several months after completion of therapy; product has teratogenic properties

Evaluation
Positive therapeutic outcome
- Prevention of rapid division of malignant cells

carteolol ophthalmic
See Appendix B

carvedilol (Rx)
(kar-veh'dee-lol)
Coreg, Coreg CR
Func. class.: Antihypertensive α/β-blocker
Pregnancy category C

Do not confuse:
carvedilol/Captopril/Carteolol

Action: A mixture of nonselective β-blocking and α-blocking activity; decreases cardiac output, exercise-induced tachycardia, reflex orthostatic tachycardia; causes reduction in peripheral vascular resistance and vasodilatation

Therapeutic outcome: Decreased B/P in hypertension

Uses: Essential hypertension alone or in combination with other antihypertensives, CHF, LV dysfunction following MI, cardiomyopathy

Dosage and routes
Essential hypertension
Adult: PO 6.25 mg bid × 7-14 days if tolerated well, then increase to 12.5 mg bid × 7-14 days if tolerated well, may be increased if needed to 25 mg bid, max 50 mg daily; EXT REL cap 20 mg/day, may increase after 7-14 days to 40 mg/day

Congestive heart failure
Adult: PO 3.125 mg bid × 2 wk; if well tolerated, give 6.25 mg bid × 2 wk, then double q2wk to max dose 25 mg bid <85 kg or 80 mg bid >85 kg; EXT REL cap (Coreg CR) 10 mg/day × 2 wk

Cardiomyopathy
Adult: PO 6.25-25 mg bid

Available forms: Tabs 3.125, 6.25, 12.5, 25 mg; ext rel cap 10, 20, 40, 80 mg

Adverse effects
CNS: Dizziness, somnolence, insomnia, ataxia, hyperesthesia, paresthesia, vertigo, depression, fatigue, weakness, headache
CV: Bradycardia, postural hypotension, dependent edema, peripheral edema, **AV block, extrasystoles,** hypo/hypertension, palpitations, peripheral ischemia, **CHF, pulmonary edema**
GI: Diarrhea, abdominal pain, increased alkaline phosphatase, increased ALT/AST
GU: Decreased libido, *impotence,* UTI

MISC: Injury, back pain, viral infection, hypertriglyceridemia, **thrombocytopenia, hyperglycemia**
RESP: Rhinitis, pharyngitis, dyspnea, **bronchospasm**

Contraindications: Hypersensitivity, asthma, class IV decompensated cardiac failure, 2nd- or 3rd-degree heart block, cardiogenic shock, severe bradycardia, pulmonary edema

Precautions: Pregnancy C, breastfeeding, children, geriatric, cardiac failure, hepatic injury, peripheral vascular disease, anesthesia, major surgery, diabetes mellitus, thyrotoxicosis, emphysema, chronic bronchitis, renal disease

Black Box Warning: Abrupt discontinuation

Pharmacokinetics

Absorption	Readily and extensively absorbed
Distribution	>98% protein binding
Metabolism	Extensively liver
Excretion	Via bile into feces
Half-life	Terminal half-life 7-10 hr, increased in the geriatric, hepatic disease

Pharmacodynamics
Unknown

Interactions
Individual drugs
Alcohol (acute ingestion), cimetidine: increased toxicity
Clonidine: decreased heart rate, B/P
Digoxin: increased concentrations of digoxin
Reserpine, levodopa: increased hypotension, bradycardia
Rifampin: decreased levels of carvedilol
Drug classifications
Antihypertensives, nitrates: increased toxicity
Antidiabetic agents: increased hypoglycemia
Calcium channel blockers: increased conduction disturbance
MAOIs: increased bradycardia, hypotension
NSAIDs, thyroid hormones: decreased levels of carvedilol
Drug/herb
Aconite: increased toxicity, death
Astragalus, cola tree: increased or decreased antihypertensive effect
Barberry, betony, black catechu, black cohosh, bloodroot, broom, burdock, cat's claw, dandelion, goldenseal, hawthorn, Irish

moss, Jamaican dogwood, kelp, khella, mistletoe, parsley: increased antihypertensive effect

Coltsfoot, guarana, khat, licorice: decreased antihypertensive effect

Drug/lab test
Increased: ANA titer, blood glucose, potassium, triglycerides, uric acid

NURSING CONSIDERATIONS
Assessment
• Monitor renal studies including protein, BUN, creatinine; watch for increased levels that may indicate nephrotic syndrome; obtain baselines in renal and liver function tests before beginning treatment; if liver function tests are elevated, product should be discontinued
• Monitor I&O, weight daily
• Monitor B/P during beginning treatment and periodically thereafter; pulse q4hr, note rate, rhythm, quality
• Monitor apical/radial pulse before administration; notify prescriber of significant changes, pulse <50 bpm hold product, notify prescriber
• Assess for edema in feet and legs daily, fluid overload: dyspnea, weight gain, jugular vein distention, fatigue, crackles

Nursing diagnoses
• Cardiac output, decreased (uses)
• Injury, risk for (adverse reactions)
• Knowledge, deficient (teaching)
• Noncompliance (teaching)

Implementation
• Give PO before meals, at bedtime; tablets may be crushed or swallowed whole, give with food to decrease orthostatic hypotension; do not break, crush, or chew ext rel cap
• Administer reduced dosage in renal dysfunction

Patient/family education
• Teach patient not to break, crush, or chew ext rel cap
• Instruct patient to comply with dosage schedule even if feeling better, that improvement may take several weeks
• Teach patient to rise slowly to sitting or standing position to minimize orthostatic hypotension
• Encourage patient to report bradycardia, dizziness, confusion, depression, fever, weight gain, shortness of breath, cold extremities, rash, sore throat, bleeding, bruising
• Teach patient to take pulse at home; advise when to notify prescriber
◆ Encourage patient not to discontinue product abruptly, taper over 1-2 wk

• Advise patient to avoid hazardous activities until stabilized on medication; dizziness may occur
• Advise patient to avoid all OTC medications unless approved by prescriber
• Advise patient to carry/wear emergency ID with product name, prescriber at all times
• Advise patient to inform all health care providers of products, supplements taken

Evaluation
Positive therapeutic outcome
• Decreased B/P
• Decreased symptoms of CHF or angina

cefaclor
See cephalosporins—2nd generation

cefadroxil
cefazolin
See cephalosporins—1st generation

cefdinir
cefditoren pivoxil
cefepime
cefotaxime
See cephalosporins—3rd generation

cefotetan
cefoxitin
See cephalosporins—2nd generation

cefpodoxime
See cephalosporins—3rd generation

cefprozil
See cephalosporins—2nd generation

ceftazidime
ceftibuten
ceftizoxime
ceftriaxone
See cephalosporins—3rd generation

Adverse effects: *italic* = common, **bold** = life-threatening

cefuroxime
See cephalosporins—2nd generation

! HIGH ALERT

celecoxib (Rx)
(cel-eh-cox'ib)
Celebrex
Func. class.: Nonsteroidal antiinflammatory, antirheumatic
Chem. class.: COX-2 inhibitor

Pregnancy category
C (1st/2nd trimesters),
D (3rd trimester)

Do not confuse:
Celebrex/Celexa/Cerebra/Cerebyx

Action: Inhibits prostaglandin synthesis by selectively inhibiting cyclooxygenase 2 (COX-2), an enzyme needed for biosynthesis

Therapeutic outcome: Decreased pain, inflammation

Uses: Acute, chronic rheumatoid arthritis, osteoarthritis, familial adenomatous polyposis (FAP), acute pain, primary dysmenorrhea, ankylosing spondylitis, juvenile rheumatoid arthritis (JRA)

Unlabeled uses: Colorectal adenoma prophylaxis

Dosage and routes
Do not exceed recommended dose, deaths have occurred

Acute pain/primary dysmenorrhea
Adult: PO 400 mg initially, then 200 mg if needed on first day, then 200 mg bid prn on subsequent days, if needed; start with ½ dose in poor CYP2C9 metabolizers

Osteoarthritis
Adult: PO 200 mg/day as a single dose or 100 mg bid; start with ½ dose in poor CYP2C9 metabolizers

Rheumatoid arthritis
Adult: PO 100-200 mg bid; start with ½ dose in poor CYP2C9 metabolizers

Ankylosing spondylitis
Adult: PO 200 mg daily or in divided dose (bid); start with ½ dose in poor CYP2C9 metabolizers

FAP
Adult: PO 400 mg bid; start with ½ dose in poor CYP2C9 metabolizers

Juvenile rheumatoid arthritis (JRA)
Adolescent and child ≥2 yr
(>25 kg): PO 100 mg bid; start with ½ dose in poor CYP2C9 metabolizers
Child ≥2 yr (10-25 kg): PO 50 mg bid; start with ½ dose in poor CYP2C9 metabolizers

Colorectal adenoma prophylaxis (unlabeled)
Adult: PO 400 mg bid × 6 mo

Hepatic dose
(Child-Pugh class II)
Adult: PO reduce dose by 50%

Available forms: Caps 50, 100, 200, 400 mg

Adverse effects
CNS: Fatigue, anxiety, depression, nervousness, paresthesia, dizziness, insomnia
CV: **Stroke, MI, tachycardia, CHF,** angina, palpitations, dysrhythmias, hypertension, fluid retention
EENT: Tinnitus, hearing loss, blurred vision, glaucoma, cataract, conjunctivitis, eye pain
GI: Nausea, anorexia, vomiting, constipation, dry mouth, diverticulitis, gastritis, gastroenteritis, hemorrhoids, hiatal hernia, stomatitis, **GI bleeding/ulceration**
GU: **Nephrotoxicity: dysuria, hematuria, oliguria, azotemia, cystitis,** UTI
HEMA: **Blood dyscrasias,** epistaxis, bruising, anemia, **platelet aggregation**
INTEG: Purpura, rash, pruritus, sweating, erythema, petechiae, photosensitivity, alopecia, **serious sometimes fatal Stevens-Johnson syndrome, toxic epidermal necrolysis**
RESP: Pharyngitis, shortness of breath, pneumonia, coughing

Contraindications: Pregnancy **D** (3rd trimester), hypersensitivity to salicylates, iodides, other NSAIDs, sulfonamides

Black Box Warning: CABG

Precautions: Pregnancy **C** (1st/2nd trimester), breastfeeding, children <18 yr, geriatric, renal/hepatic disease, hypertension, severe dehydration, bleeding, GI, cardiac disorders, PVD, asthma

Black Box Warning: Peptic ulcer disease, MI, stroke

C

Pharmacokinetics

Absorption	Well absorbed (PO)
Distribution	Crosses placenta, protein binding 87%
Metabolism	Liver by CYP2C9
Excretion	Feces/kidneys, small amount
Half-life	11 hr

Pharmacodynamics

Onset	Unknown
Peak	3 hr
Duration	Unknown

Interactions
Individual drugs
Aspirin: decreased effectiveness; increased adverse reactions
Fluconazole: increased celecoxib level
Furosemide: decreased effect of furosemide
Lithium: increased toxicity
Warfarin: increased anticoagulant effects
Drug classifications
ACE inhibitors: may decrease effects of ACE inhibitors
Anticoagulants, antiplatelets, SSRIs, salicylates, thrombolytics: increased risk of bleeding
Antineoplastics: increased risk of hematologic toxicity
Bisphosphonates: increased toxicity
Glucocorticoids, NSAIDs: increased adverse reactions
Thiazide diuretics: decreased effectiveness of diuretics
Drug/herb
Arginine, gossypol: increased gastric irritation
Bearberry, bilberry: increased celecoxib effect
Bogbean, garlic, ginger, gingko, saw palmetto, turmeric: increased bleeding risk
St. John's wort: severe photosensitivity
Drug/lab test
Increased: ALT, AST, BUN

NURSING CONSIDERATIONS
Assessment
• Assess for pain of rheumatoid arthritis, osteoarthritis; check ROM, inflammation of joints, characteristics of pain
◆ Monitor blood counts during therapy; watch for decreasing platelets; if low, therapy may need to be discontinued, restarted after hematologic recovery; for blood dyscrasias (thrombocytopenia): bruising, fatigue, bleeding, poor healing
• Assess FAP patient for decreasing number of polyps

Nursing diagnoses
• Injury, risk for (side effects)
• Knowledge, deficient (teaching)
• Mobility, impaired physical (uses)
• Pain, acute (uses)
• Pain, chronic (uses)

Implementation
• Do not break, crush, chew, or dissolve caps; caps may be opened and mixed with applesauce, ingest immediately with water
• Administer with food or milk to decrease gastric symptoms
• Do not increase dose

Patient/family education
◆ Do not exceed recommended dose; notify prescriber, immediately of chest pain, skin eruptions, stop product
• Teach patient that product must be continued for prescribed time to be effective; to avoid other NSAIDs, sulfonamides
• Caution patient to report bleeding, bruising, fatigue, malaise, since blood abnormalities do occur; to report GI symptoms: black tarry stools, cramping
• Teach patient to take with a full glass of water to enhance absorption
• Teach patient to check with prescriber to determine when product should be discontinued before surgery; advise patient to notify prescriber if pregnancy is planned or suspected
• Advise patient to report possible respiratory infection: fever, shortness of breath, coughing, painful swallowing

Evaluation
Positive therapeutic outcome
• Decreased pain in arthritic conditions
• Decreased inflammation in arthritic conditions
• Decreased number of polyps (FAP)

cephalexin
See cephalosporins—1st generation

CEPHALOSPORINS— 1ST GENERATION

cefadroxil (Rx)
(sef-a-drox'ill)
cefadroxil, Duricef
cefazolin (Rx)
(sef-a'zoe-lin)
Ancef, cefazolin
cephalexin (Rx)
(sef-a-lex'in)
Apo-Cephalex ✤, cephalexin, Keflex,
Novo-Lexin ✤, Nu-Cephalex ✤, Panixine
cephradine (Rx)
(sef'ra-deen)
cephradine, Velosef
Func. class.: Antiinfective
Chem. class.: Cephalosporin (1st generation)

Pregnancy category B

Do not confuse:
cephalexin/cefaclor

Action: Inhibits bacterial cell wall synthesis, rendering cell wall osmotically unstable, leading to cell death by binding to cell wall membrane, lysis mediated by cell wall autolytic enzymes

cefadroxil
Therapeutic outcome: Bactericidal effects for the following: gram-negative bacilli *Escherichia coli, Proteus mirabilis, Klebsiella* (UTI only); gram-positive organisms *Streptococcus pneumoniae, Streptococcus pyogenes, Staphylococcus aureus*

Uses: Upper, lower respiratory tract, urinary tract, skin infections; otitis media; tonsillitis, UTI

cefazolin
Therapeutic outcome: Bactericidal effects for the following: gram-negative organisms *Haemophilus influenzae, Escherichia coli, Proteus mirabilis, Klebsiella;* gram-positive organisms *Staphylococcus aureus*

Uses: Upper, lower respiratory tract, urinary tract, skin infections; bone, joint, biliary, genital infections; endocarditis, surgical prophylaxis, septicemia

cephalexin
Therapeutic outcome: Bactericidal effects for the following: gram-negative organisms *Haemophilus influenzae, Escherichia coli, Proteus mirabilis, Klebsiella;* gram-positive organisms *Streptococcus pneumoniae, Streptococcus pyogenes, Staphylococcus aureus*

Uses: Upper, lower respiratory tract, urinary tract, skin, bone infections; otitis media

cephradine
Therapeutic outcome: Bactericidal effects for the following: gram-negative bacilli *Haemophilus influenzae, Escherichia coli, Proteus mirabilis, Klebsiella;* gram-positive organisms *Streptococcus pneumoniae, Streptococcus pyogenes, Staphylococcus aureus*

Uses: Serious respiratory tract, urinary tract, skin infections; otitis media

Dosage and routes
cefadroxil
Adult: PO 1-2 g daily or q12hr in divided doses, give a loading dose of 1 g initially
Child: PO 30 mg/kg/day in divided doses bid

Renal dose
Adult: PO CCr 25-50 ml/min, 500 mg q12hr; CCr 10-24 ml/min 500 mg q24hr, CCr <10 ml/min 500 mg q36hr

Available forms: Caps 500 mg; tabs 1 g; oral susp 125, 250, 500 mg/5 ml
cefazolin
Life-threatening infections
Adult: IM/**IV** 1-2 g q6hr, max 12 g/day
Child >1 mo: IM/**IV** 100 mg/kg in 3-4 divided doses, max 6 g/day

Mild/moderate infections
Adult: IM/**IV** 250 mg-1 g q8hr
Child >1 mo: IM/**IV** 25-50 mg/kg in 3-4 equal doses

Renal dose
Adult: IM/**IV** following loading dose CCr 35-54 ml/min dose q8hr; CCr 10-34 ml/min 50% of dose q12hr; CCr <10 ml/min 50% of dose q18-24hr
Child: IM/**IV** CCr >70 ml/min, no dosage adjustment; CCr 40-70 ml/min following loading dose, reduce dose to 7.5-30 mg/kg q12hr; CCr 20-39 ml/min, give 3.125-12.5 mg/kg after loading dose q12hr; CCr 5-19 ml/min, 2.5-10 mg/kg after loading dose q24hr

Available forms: Inj 250, 500 mg, 1, 5, 10, 20 g; infusion 500 mg, 1 g/50 ml vial
cephalexin
Moderate infections
Adult: PO 250-500 mg q6hr, max 4 g/day
Child: PO 25-50 mg/kg/day in 4 equal doses, max 4 g/day

Moderate skin infections
Adult: PO 500 mg q12hr

Endocarditis prophylaxis
2 g 1 hr before procedure

Severe infections
Adult: PO 500 mg-1 g q6hr
Child: PO 50-100 mg/kg/day in 4 equal doses, max 4 g/day

Renal dose
Adult: PO CCr 10-40 ml/min 250-500 mg, then 250-500 mg q8-12hr; CCr <10 mg/min 250-500 mg, then 250-500 mg q12-24hr

Available forms: Caps 250, 500 mg; tabs 250, 500 mg, 1 g; oral susp 125, 250 mg/5 ml

cephradine
Adult: PO 250 mg-1 g q6-12hr
Child >1 yr: PO 6-12 mg/kg q6hr

Renal dose
Adult: PO CCr >20 ml/min 500 mg q6hr; CCr 5-20 ml/min 250 mg q6hr

Available forms: Caps 250, 500 mg; oral susp 125, 250 mg/5 ml

Side effects/adverse reactions
CNS: Headache, dizziness, weakness, paresthesia, fever, chills, **seizures** (high doses)
GI: Nausea, vomiting, *diarrhea, anorexia,* pain, glossitis, bleeding; increased AST, ALT, bilirubin, LDH, alkaline phosphatase; abdominal pain, **pseudomembranous colitis**
GU: Proteinuria, vaginitis, pruritus, candidiasis, increased BUN, **nephrotoxicity, renal failure**
HEMA: **Leukopenia, thrombocytopenia, agranulocytosis,** anemia, **neutropenia, lymphocytosis, eosinophilia, pancytopenia, hemolytic anemia**
INTEG: Rash, urticaria, dermatitis
RESP: Dyspnea
SYST: **Anaphylaxis, serum sickness,** superinfection, **Stevens-Johnson syndrome**

Contraindications: Hypersensitivity to cephalosporins, infants <1 mo

Precautions: Pregnancy **B**, breastfeeding, hypersensitivity to penicillins, renal disease

cefadroxil

Pharmacokinetics

Absorption	Well absorbed
Distribution	Widely distributed; crosses placenta
Metabolism	Not metabolized
Excretion	Unchanged by kidneys; enters breast milk
Half-life	1½-2 hr

Pharmacodynamics

	PO
Onset	Rapid
Peak	1½-2 hr
Duration	12-24 hr

cefazolin

Pharmacokinetics

Absorption	Well absorbed
Distribution	Widely distributed; crosses placenta
Metabolism	Not metabolized
Excretion	Unchanged by kidneys; enters breast milk
Half-life	1½-2½ hr

Pharmacodynamics

	IM	IV
Onset	Rapid	10 min
Peak	1-2 hr	Infusion's end
Duration	6-12 hr	Unknown

cephalexin

Pharmacokinetics

Absorption	Well absorbed
Distribution	Widely distributed; crosses placenta
Metabolism	Not metabolized
Excretion	Kidneys, unchanged; enters breast milk
Half-life	½-1 hr; increased in renal disease

Pharmacodynamics

Onset	15-30 min
Peak	1 hr
Duration	6-12 hr

cephradine

Pharmacokinetics

Absorption	Well absorbed
Distribution	Widely distributed; crosses placenta
Metabolism	Not metabolized
Excretion	Kidneys, unchanged; enters breast milk
Half-life	1-2 hr

Pharmacodynamics

	PO/IM	IV
Onset	Rapid	Immediate
Peak	1-2 hr	Infusion's end
Duration	6-12 hr	

Adverse effects: *italic* = common, **bold** = life-threatening

Interactions
Individual drugs
Probenecid: increased toxicity
Drug classifications
Aminoglycosides, diuretics (loop): increased toxicity
Anticoagulants: increased protime; use cautiously
Drug/herb
Acidophilus: do not use with antiinfectives; separate by several hours
Drug/lab test
Increased: AST, ALT, alkaline phosphatase, LDH, BUN, creatinine, bilirubin
False positive: urinary protein, direct Coombs' test, urine glucose
Interference: cross-matching

NURSING CONSIDERATIONS
Assessment
- Assess patient for previous sensitivity reaction to penicillins or other cephalosporins; cross-sensitivity between penicillins and cephalosporins is common
- Assess patient for signs and symptoms of infection including characteristics of wounds, sputum, urine, stool, WBC >10,000/mm^3, earache, fever; obtain baseline information and during treatment
- Obtain C&S before beginning product therapy to identify if correct treatment has been initiated
- Assess for anaphylaxis: rash, urticaria, pruritus, chills, fever, joint pain; angioedema may occur a few days after therapy begins; epinephrine and resuscitation equipment should be available for anaphylactic reaction
- Identify urine output; if decreasing, notify prescriber (may indicate nephrotoxicity); also check for increased BUN, creatinine
- Monitor blood studies: AST, ALT, CBC, Hct, bilirubin, LDH, alkaline phosphatase, Coombs' test monthly if patient is on long-term therapy
- Monitor electrolytes: potassium, sodium, chloride monthly if patient is on long-term therapy
- Assess bowel pattern daily; if severe diarrhea occurs, product should be discontinued; may indicate pseudomembranous colitis
- Monitor for bleeding: ecchymosis, bleeding gums, hematuria, stool guaiac daily if on long-term therapy
- Assess for superinfection: perineal itching, fever, malaise, redness, pain, swelling, drainage, rash, diarrhea, change in cough, sputum

Nursing diagnoses
- Diarrhea (side effects)
- Fluid volume, risk for, deficient (side effects)
- Infection, risk for (uses)
- Injury, risk for (side effects)
- Knowledge, deficient (teaching)
- Noncompliance (teaching)

cefadroxil
Implementation
- Give in even doses around the clock; if GI upset occurs, give with food; product must be given for 10-14 days to ensure organism death and prevent superinfection
- Shake susp, refrigerate, discard after 2 wk

cefazolin
Implementation
IM route
- Reconstitute 250-500 mg of product with 2 ml sterile or bacteriostatic water for inj, or 0.9% NaCl; reconstitute 1 g of product with 2.5 ml; give deep in large muscle mass, massage
IV route
- Check for irritation, extravasation, phlebitis daily, change site q72hr
- For direct **IV** dilute in 10 ml of sterile water for inj; give over 5 min
- For intermittent inf dilute reconstituted sol (500 mg or 1 mg) in 50-100 ml D$_5$W, D$_{10}$W, D$_5$/0.25% NaCl, D$_5$/0.45% NaCl, D$_5$/0.9% NaCl, D$_5$/LR, or LR, 0.9% NaCl; give over 30-60 min; may be refrigerated up to 96 hr or stored 24 hr at room temperature
Syringe compatibilities: Heparin, vit B complex
Syringe incompatibilities: Ascorbic acid inj, cimetidine, lidocaine, vit B/C
Y-site compatibilities: Acyclovir, allopurinol, amifostine, atracurium, aztreonam, calcium gluconate, cyclophosphamide, diltiazem, enalaprilat, esmolol, famotidine, filgrastim, fluconazole, fludarabine, foscarnet, heparin, labetalol, lidocaine, magnesium sulfate, melphalan, meperidine, midazolam, morphine, multivitamins, ondansetron, pancuronium, perphenazine, regular insulin, sargramostim, tacrolimus, teniposide, theophylline, thiotepa, vecuronium, vit B/C
Y-site incompatibilities: Amiodarone, hetastarch, hydromorphone, idarubicin, vinorelbine tartrate
Additive compatibilities: Aztreonam, clindamycin, famotidine, fluconazole, metronidazole, verapamil
Additive incompatibilities: Amikacin, amobarbital, bleomycin, calcium gluceptate, calcium gluconate, colistimethate, erythromy-

cin, kanamycin, oxytetracycline, pentobarbital, polymyxin B, tetracycline

cephalexin
Implementation
- Do not break, crush, or chew caps
- Give in even doses around the clock; if GI upset occurs, give with food; product must be taken for 10-14 days to ensure organism death and prevent superinfection
- Shake susp, refrigerate, discard after 2 wk

cephradine
Implementation
PO route
- May be given with food for GI symptoms
- When giving susp, shake well; refrigerate unused portion

IM route
- Reconstitute 250 mg/1.2 ml, 500 mg/ml, 1 g/4 ml sterile or bacteriostatic water for inj; give deep in large muscle mass, massage

IV route
- Check for irritation, extravasation, phlebitis daily; change site q72hr
- For direct **IV** route, reconstitute 250-500 mg/5 ml sterile water, 0.9% NaCl, D₅W, or 1 g/10 ml, 2 g/20 ml; give over 3-5 min
- For intermittent inf, dilute 1 g/10 ml or more sterile water for inj, D₅W, D₁₀W, or D₅/0.9% NaCl; give over 30-60 min
- Store refrigerated 96 hr, room temperature 24 hr

Additive incompatibilities: Other antibiotics, calcium salts, D₅W, epinephrine, lidocaine, Ringer's or LR sol, NormosolR, 0.9% NaCl, TPN #61, tetracycline

Patient/family education
- Teach patient to report sore throat, bruising, bleeding, joint pain; may indicate blood dyscrasias (rare)
- Advise patient to contact prescriber if vaginal itching, loose foul-smelling stools, furry tongue occur; may indicate superinfection
- Instruct patient to take all medication prescribed for the length of time ordered
- Advise patient to notify prescriber of diarrhea with blood, pus, mucus, which may indicate pseudomembranous colitis

Evaluation
Positive therapeutic outcome
- Absence of signs/symptoms of infection (WBC <10,000/mm³, temp WNL, absence of red draining wounds, earache)
- Reported improvement in symptoms of infection
- Negative C&S

Treatment of anaphylaxis: Epinephrine, antihistamines, resuscitate if needed

---

CEPHALOSPORINS— 2ND GENERATION

C

cefaclor (Rx)
(sef'a-klor)
Ceclor, Raniclor

cefotetan (Rx)
(sef'oh-tee-tan)
Cefotan

cefoxitin (Rx)
(se-fox'i-tin)
Mefoxin

cefprozil (Rx)
(sef-proe'zill)
Cefzil

cefuroxime (Rx)
(sef-yoor-ox'eem)
Ceftin, Cefuroxime, Zinacef

loracarbef (Rx)
(lor-a-kar'beff)
Lorabid
Func. class.: Antiinfective
Chem. class.: Cephalosporin (2nd generation)

Pregnancy category D

Do not confuse:
cefaclor/cephalexin, Cefotan/Ceftin, cefprozil/cefazolin/cefuroxime, Cefzil/Ceftin/Kefzol

Action: Inhibits bacterial cell wall synthesis, rendering cell wall osmotically unstable, leading to cell death by binding to cell wall membrane

cefaclor
Therapeutic outcome: Bactericidal effects for the following: gram-negative bacilli *Haemophilus influenzae, Escherichia coli, Proteus mirabilis, Klebsiella;* gram-positive organisms *Streptococcus pneumoniae, Streptococcus pyogenes, Staphylococcus aureus*

Uses: Upper and lower respiratory tract, urinary tract, skin infections; otitis media; bone, joint infections

cefotetan
Therapeutic outcome: Bactericidal effects for the following: gram-negative organisms *Citrobacter, Haemophilus influenzae, Escherichia coli, Enterobacter aerogenes, Proteus mirabilis, Klebsiella, Salmonella,*

Shigella, Acinetobacter, Bacteroides fragilis, Neisseria, Serratia; gram-positive organisms *Streptococcus pneumoniae, Streptococcus pyogenes, Staphylococcus aureus*

Uses: Serious upper or lower respiratory tract, urinary tract, gynecologic, skin, bone, joint, gonococcal, intraabdominal infections

cefoxitin
Therapeutic outcome: Bactericidal effects for the following: gram-negative bacilli *Bacteroides fragilis, Haemophilus influenzae, Escherichia coli, Proteus, Klebsiella, Neisseria gonorrhoeae;* gram-positive organisms *Streptococcus pneumoniae, Streptococcus pyogenes, Staphylococcus aureus;* anaerobes including *Clostridium*

Uses: Lower respiratory tract, urinary tract, skin, bone, gynecologic, gonococcal infections; septicemia, peritonitis

cefprozil
Therapeutic outcome: Bactericidal effects for the following: gram-negative bacilli *Haemophilus influenzae, Escherichia coli;* gram-positive organisms *Streptococcus pneumoniae, Streptococcus pyogenes, Staphylococcus aureus*

Uses: Pharyngitis/tonsillitis, otitis media, secondary bacterial infection of acute bronchitis, and acute bacterial exacerbation of chronic bronchitis and uncomplicated skin and skin structure infections; acute sinusitis

cefuroxime
Therapeutic outcome: Bactericidal effects for the following: gram-negative bacilli *Haemophilus influenzae, Escherichia coli, Neisseria, Proteus mirabilis, Klebsiella;* gram-positive organisms: *Streptococcus pneumoniae, Streptococcus pyogenes, Staphylococcus aureus*

Uses: Serious lower respiratory tract, urinary tract, skin, bone, joint, gonococcal infections; septicemia, meningitis

loracarbef
Therapeutic outcome: Bactericidal effects for the following: gram-negative organisms *Haemophilus influenzae, Escherichia coli, Proteus mirabilis, Klebsiella;* gram-positive organisms *Streptococcus pneumoniae, Streptococcus pyogenes, Staphylococcus aureus*

Uses: Upper and lower respiratory tract, urinary tract, skin infections; otitis media, pharyngitis, tonsillitis

Dosage and routes
cefaclor
Adult: PO 250-500 mg q8hr, max 4 g/day
Child >1 mo: PO 20-40 mg/kg daily in divided doses q8hr, or total daily dose may be divided and given q12hr, max 1 g/day

Available forms: Caps 250, 500 mg; oral susp 125, 187, 250, 375 mg/5 ml; chew tabs (Raniclor) 250, 375 mg

cefotetan
Adult: **IV**/IM 1-2 g q12hr × 5-10 days

Renal dose
Adult: IM/**IV** CCr 10-30 ml/min q24hr or ½ dose q12hr; CCr <10 ml/min q48hr or ½ dose q24hr

Perioperative prophylaxis
Adult: **IV** 1-2 g ½-1 hr before surgery

Available forms: Inj 1, 2, 10 g

cefoxitin
Adult: IM/**IV** 1-2 g q6-8hr

Uncomplicated gonorrhea (outpatient)
Adult/adolescent/child ≥45 kg: IM 2 g as single dose with 1 g PO probenecid at same time

Renal dose
Adult: IM/**IV** after loading dose CCr 30-50 ml/min 1-2 g q8-12hr; CCr 10-29 ml/min 1-2 g q12-24hr; CCr <10 ml/min 0.5-1 g q12-24hr

Severe infections
Adult: IM/**IV** 2 g q4hr
Child ≥3 mo: IM/**IV** 80-160 mg/kg/day divided q4-6hr; max 12 g/day

Available forms: Powder for inj 1, 2, 10 g

cefprozil
Renal dose
CCr <30 ml/min 50% of dose

Upper respiratory infections
Adult: PO 500 mg q24hr × 10 days

Otitis media
Child 6 mo-12 yr: PO 15 mg/kg q12hr × 10 days

Lower respiratory infections
Adult: PO 500 mg q12hr × 10 days

Skin/skin structure infections
Adult: PO 250-500 mg q12hr × 10 days

Available forms: Tabs 250, 500 mg; susp 125, 250 mg/5 ml

C

cefuroxime
Adult and child: PO 250 mg q12hr; may increase to 500 mg of q12hr in serious infections
Adult: IM/**IV** 750 mg-1.5 g q8hr for 5-10 days

Urinary tract infections
Adult: PO 125 mg q12hr; may increase to 250 mg q12hr if needed

Otitis media
Child <2 yr: PO 125 mg bid
Child >2 yr: PO 250 mg bid

Surgical prophylaxis
Adult: **IV** 1.5 g ½-1 hr preop

Severe infections
Adult: IM/**IV** 1.5 g q6hr; may give up to 3 g q8hr for bacterial meningitis
Child >3 mo: IM/**IV** 50-100 mg/kg/day; may give up to 200-240 mg/kg/day **IV** in divided doses for bacterial meningitis (not recommended)
• Dosage reduction indicated in severe renal impairment (CCr <20 ml/min)

Uncomplicated gonorrhea
Adult: 1.5 g IM as single dose with oral probenecid in 2 separate sites

Available forms: Tabs 125, 250, 500 mg; inj 150, 750 mg, 1.5, 7.5 g; inj 750 mg; 1.5 g powder, susp 125, 250 mg/5 ml

loracarbef
Adult and child >13 yr: PO 200-400 mg q12hr
Child to 12 yr: PO 15-30 mg/kg/day in 2 divided doses q12hr

Renal dose
CCr 10-49 ml/min 50% of dose; CCr <10 ml/min q3-5 days

Available forms: Caps 200, 400 mg; oral susp 100, 200 mg/5 ml

Side effects/adverse reactions
CNS: Dizziness, headache, fatigue, paresthesia, fever, chills, confusion
GI: Diarrhea, nausea, vomiting, anorexia, dysgeusia, glossitis, bleeding; increased AST, ALT, bilirubin, LDH, alkaline phosphatase; abdominal pain, loose stools, flatulence, heartburn, stomach cramps, colitis, jaundice, **pseudomembranous colitis**
GU: Vaginitis, pruritus, candidiasis, increased BUN, **nephrotoxicity, renal failure,** pyuria, dysuria, reversible interstitial nephritis
HEMA: **Leukopenia, thrombocytopenia, agranulocytosis,** anemia, **neutropenia, lymphocytosis, eosinophilia, pancytope-** **nia, hemolytic anemia, leukocytosis, granulocytopenia**
INTEG: Rash, urticaria, dermatitis, **Stevens-Johnson syndrome**
RESP: Dyspnea
SYST: **Anaphylaxis, serum sickness,** superinfection

Contraindications: Hypersensitivity to cephalosporins or related antibiotics, seizures

Precautions: Pregnancy **B,** breastfeeding, children, renal/GI disease

cefaclor

Pharmacokinetics	
Absorption	Well absorbed
Distribution	Widely distributed; crosses placenta
Metabolism	Not metabolized
Excretion	Unchanged by kidneys (60%-80%); enters breast milk
Half-life	36-54 min; increased in renal disease

Pharmacodynamics	
Onset	15 min
Peak	½-1 hr
Duration	Unknown

cefotetan

Pharmacokinetics	
Absorption	Well absorbed (IM)
Distribution	Widely distributed; crosses placenta
Metabolism	Not metabolized
Excretion	Kidneys, unchanged; enters breast milk
Half-life	5 hr; increased in renal disease

Pharmacodynamics		
	IM	IV
Onset	Rapid	Immediate
Peak	1-3 hr	Infusion's end
Duration	Unknown	Unknown

cefoxitin

Pharmacokinetics	
Absorption	Well absorbed (IM)
Distribution	Widely distributed; crosses placenta
Metabolism	Not metabolized
Excretion	Kidneys, unchanged; enters breast milk
Half-life	½-1 hr; increased in renal disease

Adverse effects: *italic* = common, **bold** = life-threatening

Pharmacodynamics

	IM	IV
Onset	Rapid	Immediate
Peak	½ hr	Infusion's end
Duration	Unknown	Unknown

cefprozil

Pharmacokinetics

Absorption	Well absorbed
Distribution	Widely distributed; crosses placenta
Metabolism	Not metabolized
Excretion	Kidneys, unchanged; enters breast milk
Half-life	1-1½ hr; increased in renal disease

Pharmacodynamics

Unknown

loracarbef

Pharmacokinetics

Absorption	Well absorbed
Distribution	Widely distributed; crosses placenta
Metabolism	Not metabolized
Excretion	Kidneys, unchanged; enters breast milk
Half-life	1 hr; increased in renal disease

Pharmacodynamics

Onset	Rapid
Peak	1 hr
Duration	Unknown

Interactions
Individual drugs
Antacids: decreased absorption of cephalosporins
Furosemide: increased effect/toxicity
Plicamycin, valproic acid: increased bleeding
Probenecid: decreased excretion of product and increased blood levels/toxicity
Drug classifications
Aminoglycosides: increased effect/toxicity
Anticoagulants, antiplatelets, NSAIDs, thrombolytics: increased bleeding (cefotetan)
H₂-blockers: decreased effects of cephalosporins
Drug/herb
Acidophilus: do not use with antiinfectives; separate by several hours
Angelica, anise, arnica, bogbean, boldo, celery, chamomile, clove, fenugreek, feverfew,

garlic, ginger, ginkgo, ginseng *(Panax)*, horse chestnut, horseradish, licorice, meadowsweet, onion, papain, passion flower, poplar, prickly ash, red clover, turmeric, willow: increased bleeding risk (cefotetan)
Drug/lab test
False: increased creatinine (serum urine), urinary 17-KS
False positive: urinary protein, direct Coombs' test, urine glucose (Clinitest)
Interference: cross-matching

NURSING CONSIDERATIONS
Assessment
• Assess patient for previous sensitivity reaction to penicillins or other cephalosporins; cross-sensitivity between penicillins and cephalosporins is common
• Assess patient for signs and symptoms of infection including characteristics of wounds, sputum, urine, stool, WBC >10,000/mm³, earache, fever; obtain baseline information and during treatment
• Obtain C&S before beginning product therapy to identify if correct treatment has been initiated
• Assess for anaphylaxis: rash, urticaria, pruritus, dyspnea, chills, fever, joint pain; angioedema may occur a few days after therapy begins; epinephrine and resuscitation equipment should be available for anaphylactic reaction
• Identify urine output; if decreasing, notify prescriber (may indicate nephrotoxicity); also check for increased BUN, creatinine
• Monitor blood studies: AST, ALT, CBC, Hct, bilirubin, LDH, alkaline phosphatase, Coombs' test monthly if patient is on long-term therapy
• Monitor electrolytes: potassium, sodium, chloride monthly if patient is on long-term therapy
• Assess bowel pattern daily; if severe diarrhea occurs, product should be discontinued; may indicate pseudomembranous colitis
• Monitor for bleeding: ecchymosis, bleeding gums, hematuria, stool guaiac daily if on long-term therapy
• Assess for overgrowth of infection: perineal itching, fever, malaise, redness, pain, swelling, drainage, rash, diarrhea, change in cough, sputum

Nursing diagnoses
• Diarrhea (side effects)
• Fluid volume, risk for, deficient (side effects)
• Infection, risk for (uses)
• Injury, risk for (side effects)

- Knowledge, deficient (teaching)
- Noncompliance (teaching)

Implementation
cefaclor
- Do not break, crush, chew, or cut ext rel tabs
- Give in even doses around the clock; if GI upset occurs, give with food; product must be given for 10-14 days to ensure organism death and prevent superinfection
- Shake susp, refrigerate, discard after 2 wk

cefotetan
IM route
- Reconstitute 1 g/2 ml or 2 g/3 ml of sterile or bacteriostatic water for inj; may be diluted with 0.5% of 1% lidocaine to prevent pain; give deep in large muscle mass, massage

IV route
- May be stored 96 hr refrigerated or 24 hr room temperature
- Check for irritation, extravasation, phlebitis daily; change site q72hr
- For direct **IV** dilute in 1 g/10 ml or more and give over 5 min
- For intermittent inf further dilute in 50-100 ml of 0.9% NaCl or D₅W; give over 3-5 min; discontinue primary line while running intermittent inf

Syringe incompatibilities: Doxapram
Y-site compatibilities: Allopurinol, amifostine, aztreonam, diltiazem, famotidine, filgrastim, fluconazole, fludarabine, heparin, regular insulin, melphalan, meperidine, morphine, paclitaxel, sargramostim, tacrolimus, teniposide, theophylline, thiotepa
Additive incompatibilities: Aminoglycosides, tetracyclines, heparin

cefoxitin
IM route
- Reconstitute 1 g/2 ml of sterile water for inj; may be diluted with 0.5% or 1% lidocaine to prevent pain; give deep in large muscle mass, massage

IV route
- Check for irritation, extravasation, phlebitis daily; change site q72hr
- For direct **IV**, dilute 1 g/10 ml or 2 g/20 ml of sterile water for inj; shake, let stand until clear; give over 3-5 min
- For intermittent inf further dilute with 50-100 ml of D₅W, D₁₀W, D₅/0.25% NaCl, D₅/0.45% NaCl, D₅/0.9% NaCl, 0.9% NaCl D₅/LR, D₅/0.02%, sodium bicarbonate, Ringer's, or LR; give over 15-30 min; may store 96 hr refrigerated or 24 hr room temperature
- For cont inf dilute in 500-1000 ml; give over prescribed rate

Syringe compatibilities: Heparin, insulin
Y-site compatibilities: Acyclovir, amifostine, aztreonam, cyclophosphamide, diltiazem, famotidine, fluconazole, foscarnet, hydromorphone, magnesium sulfate, meperidine, morphine, ondansetron, perphenazine, temiposide, thiotepa
Y-site incompatibilities: Hetastarch
Additive compatibilities: Amikacin, cimetidine, clindamycin, gentamicin, kanamycin, multivitamins, sodium bicarbonate, tobramycin, verapamil, vit B/C
Additive incompatibilities: Aztreonam

cefprozil
IM route
- Reconstitute with 1 g/2 ml or 2 g/3 ml of sterile or bacteriostatic water for inj; may be diluted with 0.5% or 1% lidocaine to prevent pain; give deep in large muscle mass, massage

IV route
- Check for irritation, extravasation, phlebitis daily; change site q72hr
- For direct **IV**, dilute 1 g/10 ml or more and give over 5 min
- For intermittent inf further dilute with 50-100 ml of 0.9% NaCl or D₅W; give over 3-5 min; discontinue primary line while running intermittent inf

Syringe incompatibilities: Doxapram
Y-site compatibilities: Famotidine, fluconazole, fludarabine, regular insulin, meperidine, morphine, sargramostim
Additive incompatibilities: Aminoglycosides, tetracyclines, heparin

loracarbef
◆ Do not break, crush, or chew caps
- Give on an empty stomach, 1 hr before or 2 hr after a meal
- Oral susp should be shaken before administration; store for 2 wk at room temperature, discard after 2 wk

Patient/family education
- Teach patient to report sore throat, bruising, bleeding, joint pain; may indicate blood dyscrasias (rare)
- Advise patient to contact prescriber if vaginal itching, loose foul-smelling stools, furry tongue occur; may indicate superinfection
- Instruct patient to take all medication prescribed for the length of time ordered; to use yogurt or buttermilk to maintain intestinal flora, decrease diarrhea
- Advise patient to notify prescriber of diarrhea with blood or pus, which may indicate pseudomembranous colitis

Adverse effects: *italic* = common, **bold** = life-threatening

Evaluation
Positive therapeutic outcome
- Absence of signs/symptoms of infection (WBC <10,000/mm³, temp WNL, absence of red draining wounds, earache)
- Reported improvement in symptoms of infection
- Negative C&S

Treatment of anaphylaxis: Epinephrine, antihistamines, resuscitate if needed

---

CEPHALOSPORINS— 3RD GENERATION

cefdinir (Rx)
(sef'dih-ner)
Omnicef
cefditoren pivoxil (Rx)
(sef-dit'oh-ren pih-vox'il)
Spectracef
cefepime (Rx)
(sef'e-peem)
Maxipime
cefixime (Rx)
(sef-iks'ime)
Cefixime, Suprax
cefotaxime (Rx)
(sef-oh-taks'eem)
Claforan
cefpodoxime (Rx)
(sef-poe-docks'eem)
Vantin
ceftazidime (Rx)
(sef'tay-zi-deem)
Ceptaz, Fortaz, Tazicef, Tazidime
ceftibuten (Rx)
(sef-ti-byoo'tin)
Cedax
ceftizoxime (Rx)
(sef-ti-zox'eem)
Cefizox
ceftriaxone (Rx)
(sef-try-ax'one)
Rocephin
Func. class.: Broad-spectrum antibiotic
Chem. class.: Cephalosporin (3rd generation)

Pregnancy category B

Do not confuse:
ceftazidime/**ceftizoxime**, Vantin/**Ventolin**

Action: Inhibits bacterial cell wall synthesis, rendering cell wall osmotically unstable, leading to cell death

cefdinir
Therapeutic outcome: Bactericidal effects for the following: gram-negative organisms *Haemophilus influenzae, Haemophilus parainfluenzae, Moraxella catarrhalis;* gram-positive organisms *Streptococcus pneumoniae, Streptococcus pyogenes, Staphylococcus aureus*

Uses: Uncomplicated skin and skin structure infections, community-acquired pneumonia, acute exacerbations of chronic bronchitis, acute maxillary sinusitis, pharyngitis, tonsillitis, otitis media

cefditoren pivoxil
Therapeutic outcome: Bactericidal effects for the following organisms: *Haemophilus influenzae, Haemophilus parainfluenzae, Streptococcus pneumoniae, Moraxella catarrhalis, Streptococcus pyogenes, Staphylococcus aureus*

Uses: Acute bacterial exacerbation of chronic bronchitis, pharyngitis/tonsillitis; uncomplicated skin, skin structure infections

cefepime
Therapeutic outcome: Bactericidal effects for the following: gram-negative bacilli *Escherichia coli, Proteus, Klebsiella;* gram-positive organisms *Streptococcus pneumoniae, Streptococcus pyogenes, Staphylococcus aureus*

Uses: Lower respiratory tract, urinary tract, skin, bone, febrile neutropenia, intraabdominal infection

cefixime
Therapeutic outcome: Bactericidal effects for the following organisms: *Escherichia coli, Proteus mirabilis, Streptococcus pyogenes, Haemophilus influenzae, Moraxella catarrhalis, Streptococcus pneumoniae*

Uses: Uncomplicated UTI, pharyngitis/tonsillitis, otitis media, acute bronchitis, exacerbations of chronic bronchitis, uncomplicated gonorrhea

cefotaxime
Therapeutic outcome: Bactericidal effects for the following: gram-negative organisms *Haemophilus influenzae, Haemophilus parainfluenzae, Escherichia coli, Enterococcus faecalis, Neisseria gonorrhoeae, Neisseria meningitidis, Proteus mirabilis, Klebsiella, Citrobacter, Serratia, Salmonella,*

 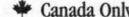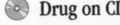

C

Shigella Pseudomonas; gram-positive organisms *Streptococcus pneumoniae, Streptococcus pyogenes, Staphylococcus aureus*

Uses: Lower serious respiratory tract, urinary tract, skin, bone, gonococcal infections; bacteremia, septicemia, meningitis, skin, skin structure infections, CNS infections, perioperative prophylaxis

cefpodoxime
Therapeutic outcome: Bactericidal effects for the following: gram-negative organisms *Neisseria gonorrhoeae, Haemophilus influenzae, Escherichia coli, Proteus mirabilis, Klebsiella;* gram-positive organisms *Streptococcus pneumoniae, Streptococcus pyogenes, Staphylococcus aureus*

Uses: Upper and lower respiratory tract, urinary tract, skin infections; otitis media, STDs

ceftazidime
Therapeutic outcome: Bactericidal effects for the following: gram-negative organisms *Haemophilus influenzae, Escherichia coli, Enterobacter aerogenes, Proteus mirabilis, Klebsiella, Citrobacter, Enterobacter, Salmonella, Serratia, Pseudomonas aeruginosa, Shigella, Acinetobacter, Bacteroides fragilis, Neisseria;* gram-positive organisms *Streptococcus pneumoniae, Streptococcus pyogenes, Staphylococcus aureus*

Uses: Serious upper or lower respiratory tract, urinary tract, skin, gynecologic, bone, joint, intraabdominal infections; septicemia, meningitis

ceftibuten
Therapeutic outcome: Bactericidal effects for the following: gram-negative bacilli *Haemophilus influenzae, Escherichia coli;* gram-positive organisms *Streptococcus pneumoniae, Streptococcus pyogenes, Staphylococcus aureus*

Uses: Pharyngitis, tonsilitis, otitis media, secondary bacterial infection of acute bronchitis

ceftizoxime
Therapeutic outcome: Bactericidal effects for the following: gram-negative organisms *Haemophilus influenzae, Escherichia coli, Enterobacter aerogenes, Proteus mirabilis, Klebsiella, Enterobacter;* gram-positive organisms *Streptococcus pneumoniae, Streptococcus pyogenes, Staphylococcus aureus, Neisseria gonorrhoeae*

Uses: Serious lower respiratory tract, urinary tract, skin, intraabdominal infections; septicemia, meningitis; bone, joint infections

ceftriaxone
Therapeutic outcome: Bactericidal effects on the following: gram-negative organisms *Haemophilus influenzae, Escherichia coli, Enterobacter aerogenes, Proteus mirabilis, Klebsiella, Citrobacter, Enterobacter, Salmonella, Shigella, Acinetobacter, Bacteroides fragilis, Neisseria, Serratia;* gram-positive organisms *Streptococcus pneumoniae, Streptococcus pyogenes, Staphylococcus aureus*

Uses: Serious lower respiratory tract, urinary tract, skin, gonococcal, intraabdominal infections; septicemia, meningitis; bone, joint infections, otitis media, PID

Dosage and routes
cefdinir
Uncomplicated skin and skin structure infections/community-acquired pneumonia
Adult and child ≥13 yr: PO 300 mg q12hr × 10 days
Child 6 mo-12 yr: PO 7 mg/kg q12hr or 14 mg/kg q24hr × 10 days

Acute exacerbations of chronic bronchitis/acute maxillary sinusitis
Adult and child ≥13 yr: PO 300 mg q12hr or 600 mg q24hr × 10 days or 300 mg bid × 5 days in some infections

Pharyngitis/tonsillitis
Adult and child ≥13 yr: PO 300 mg q12hr or 600 mg q24hr × 10 days
Child 6 mo-12 yr: PO 7 mg/kg q12hr × 5-10 days or 14 mg/kg q24hr × 10 days

Renal dose
CCr <30 ml/min 300 mg daily (adult); 7 mg/kg daily (child)

Available forms: Caps 300 mg, oral susp 125 mg/5 ml

cefditoren pivoxil
Adult: PO 200-400 mg bid

Renal dose
Adult: PO CCr 30-50 ml/min, max 200 mg bid; CCr <30 ml/min, max 200 mg daily

Available forms: Tabs 200 mg

cefepime
Febrile neutropenia
Adult: **IV** 2 g q3hr × 7 days or until neutropenia resolves

Adverse effects: *italic* = common, **bold** = life-threatening

Urinary tract infections (mild to moderate)
Adult: **IV**/IM 0.5-1 g q12hr × 7-10 days

Urinary tract infections (severe)
Adult: **IV** 2 g q12hr × 10 days

Pneumonia (moderate to severe)
Adult: **IV** 1-2 g q12hr × 10 days
Dosage reduction indicated in renal impairment (CCr <50 ml/min)

Uncomplicated gonorrhea
Adult: IM 2 g as a single dose with 1 g PO probenecid at the same time

Available forms: Powder for inj 500 mg, 1, 2 g

cefixime
Adult: PO 400 mg/day as a single dose or 200 mg q12hr
Child >50 kg or >12 yr: PO use adult dosage
Child <50 kg or <12 yr: PO 8 mg/kg/day as a single dose or 4 mg/kg q12hr

Renal dose
CCr 21-60 ml/min give 75% of dose; CCr <20 ml/min give 50% of dose

Available forms: Tabs 400 mg; powder for oral susp 100 mg/5 ml

cefotaxime
Adult: IM/**IV** 1-2 g q12hr
Child 1 mo-12 yr: IM/**IV** 50-180 mg/kg/day divided q6hr

Severe infections
Adult: IM/**IV** 2 g q4hr, max 12 g/day
Child 1 mo-12 yr: IM/**IV** 50-180 mg/kg in 4-6 divided doses

Uncomplicated gonorrhea
Adult: IM 1 g; dosage reduction indicated for severe renal impairment (CCr <30 ml/min)

Available forms: Powder for inj 500 mg, 1, 2, 10 g; 1, 2 g premixed frozen

cefpodoxime
Pneumonia
Adult >13 yr: PO 200 mg q12hr for 14 days

Uncomplicated gonorrhea
Adult >13 yr: PO 200 mg single dose

Skin and skin structure
Adult >13 yr: PO 400 mg q12hr for 7-14 days

Pharyngitis and tonsillitis
Adult >13 yr: PO 100 mg q12hr for 10 days

Child 5 mo-12 yr: PO 5 mg/kg q12hr (max 100 mg/dose or 200 mg/day) × 5-10 days

Uncomplicated UTI
Adult >13 yr: PO 100 mg q12hr for 7 days; dosing interval increased in presence of severe renal impairment

Acute otitis media
Child 5 mo-12 yr: PO 5 mg/kg q12hr for 10 days

Available forms: Tabs 100, 200 mg; granules for susp 50, 100 mg/5 ml

ceftazidime
Adult: **IV**/IM 1-2 g q8-12hr × 5-10 days
Child: **IV** 30-50 mg/kg q8hr, max 6 g/day
Neonate: **IV** 30-50 mg/kg q12hr

Renal dose
Adult: **IV** CCr <50 ml/min q12hr; CCr 10-30 ml/min q24hr; CCr <10 ml/min q48hr, CCr <10 ml/min give q48-72hr

Available forms: Inj 250, 500 mg, 1, 2, 6 g

ceftibuten
Adult: PO 400 mg daily × 10 days
Child 6 mo-12 yr: PO 9 mg/kg daily × 10 days

Renal dose
Adult: PO CCr 30-49 ml/min 200 mg q24hr; CCr 5-29 ml/min 100 mg q24hr

Available forms: Caps 400 mg; susp 90, 180 mg/5 ml

ceftizoxime
Adult: IM/**IV** 1-2 g q8-12hr, may give up to 4 g q8hr in life-threatening infections
Child >6 mo: IM/**IV** 50 mg/kg q6-8hr

Renal dose
Adult: IM/**IV** CCr 50-80 ml/min 500-1500 mg q8hr; CCr 5-49 ml/min 250-1000 mg q12hr

PID
Adult: **IV** 2 g q8hr, may increase to 4 g q8hr in severe infections

Available forms: Powder for inj 500 mg, 1, 2, 10 g; premixed 1 g, 2 g/50 ml

ceftriaxone
Adult: IM/**IV** 1-2 g daily, max 2 g q12-24hr
Child: IM/**IV** 50-75 mg/kg/day in equal doses q12hr

Uncomplicated gonorrhea
Adult: 250 mg IM as single dose
Reduce dosage in severe renal impairment (CCr <10 ml/min)

Meningitis
Adult and child: IM/**IV** 100 mg/kg/day in equal doses q12hr, max 4 g/day

Surgical prophylaxis
Adult: **IV** 1 g ½-2 hr preop

Available forms: Inj 250, 500 mg, 1, 2, 10 g

Adverse effects
CNS: Headache, dizziness, weakness, paresthesia, fever, chills, **seizures**, dyskinesia (cefdinir)
CV: **Heart failure**, syncope (cefdinir)
GI: Nausea, vomiting, diarrhea, anorexia, pain, glossitis, **bleeding**; increased AST, ALT, bilirubin, LDH, alkaline phosphatase; abdominal pain, **pseudomembranous colitis**, cholestasis (cefotaxime)
GU: **Proteinuria**, vaginitis, pruritus, candidiasis, increased BUN, **nephrotoxicity, renal failure**
HEMA: **Leukopenia, thrombocytopenia, agranulocytosis**, anemia, **neutropenia**, lymphocytosis, **eosinophilia, pancytopenia, hemolytic anemia**
INTEG: Rash, urticaria, dermatitis
RESP: Dyspnea
SYST: **Anaphylaxis, serum sickness, Stevens-Johnson syndrome, toxic epidermal necrolysis**

Contraindications: Hypersensitivity to cephalosporins, infants <1 mo

Precautions: Pregnancy **B,** breastfeeding, children, hypersensitivity to penicillins, renal/GI disease

cefdinir

Pharmacokinetics

Absorption	Well absorbed
Distribution	Widely distributed; crosses placenta
Metabolism	Not metabolized
Excretion	Kidneys, unchanged; enters breast milk
Half-life	Unknown

Pharmacodynamics

Unknown

cefditoren pivoxil

Pharmacokinetics

Absorption	Well absorbed after it is broken down (prodrug)
Distribution	Widely
Metabolism	Unknown
Excretion	Unknown
Half-life	100 mins

Pharmacodynamics

Onset	Rapid
Peak	0.5-3 hr
Duration	12 hrs

cefepime

Pharmacokinetics

Absorption	Well absorbed (IM)
Distribution	Widely distributed; crosses placenta
Metabolism	Not metabolized
Excretion	Kidneys, unchanged; enters breast milk
Half-life	2 hr; increased in renal disease

Pharmacodynamics

	IM	IV
Onset	Rapid	Immediate
Peak	79 min	Infusion's end
Duration	Unknown	Unknown

cefixime

Pharmacokinetics

Absorption	Unknown
Distribution	Protein binding 65%-70%
Metabolism	Unknown
Excretion	Urine, bile
Half-life	3-4 hr

Pharmacodynamics

Onset	Unknown
Peak	2-6 hr
Duration	Unknown

cefotaxime

Pharmacokinetics

Absorption	Widely distributed
Distribution	Breast milk, small amounts
Metabolism	Liver, active metabolites
Excretion	40%-65% unchanged, kidney
Half-life	1 hr

Pharmacodynamics

	IV	IM
Onset	5 min	30 min
Peak	Unknown	Unknown
Duration	Unknown	Unknown

cefpodoxime

Pharmacokinetics

Absorption	Well absorbed
Distribution	Widely distributed; crosses placenta
Metabolism	Not metabolized
Excretion	Kidneys, unchanged; enters breast milk
Half-life	2-3 hr, increased in renal disease

Pharmacodynamics

Unknown

ceftazidime

Pharmacokinetics

Absorption	Well absorbed (IM)
Distribution	Widely distributed; crosses placenta
Metabolism	Not metabolized
Excretion	Kidneys, unchanged; enters breast milk
Half-life	½-1 hr; increased in renal disease

Pharmacodynamics

	IM	IV
Onset	Rapid	Immediate
Peak	1 hr	Infusion's end

ceftibuten

Pharmacokinetics

Absorption	Well absorbed
Distribution	Widely distributed; crosses placenta
Metabolism	Not metabolized
Excretion	Kidneys, unchanged; enters breast milk
Half-life	1-1½ hr; increased in renal disease

Pharmacodynamics

Unknown

ceftizoxime

Pharmacokinetics

Absorption	Well absorbed (IM)
Distribution	Widely distributed; crosses placenta
Metabolism	Not metabolized
Excretion	Kidneys, unchanged; enters breast milk
Half-life	1½-2 hr; increased in renal disease

Pharmacodynamics

	IM	IV
Onset	Rapid	Immediate
Peak	1 hr	Infusion's end

ceftriaxone

Pharmacokinetics

Absorption	Well absorbed
Distribution	Widely distributed; crosses placenta; enters CSF
Metabolism	Liver
Excretion	Kidneys, partly
Half-life	5-8 hr

Pharmacodynamics

	IM	IV
Onset	Rapid	Immediate
Peak	1 hr	Infusion's end

Interactions
Individual drugs
Furosemide, probenecid: increased toxicity
Iron: decreased absorption of cefdinir
Plicamycin, valproic acid: increased bleeding
Drug classifications
Aminoglycosides: increased toxicity
Anticoagulants, NSAIDs, thrombolytics: increased bleeding
Drug/herb
Acidophilus: do not use with antiinfectives; separate by several hours
Angelica, anise, arnica, bogbean, boldo, celery, chamomile, clove, fenugreek, feverfew, garlic, ginger, ginkgo, ginseng *(Panax)*, horse chestnut, horseradish, licorice, meadowsweet, onion, papain, passion flower, poplar, prickly ash, red clover, turmeric, willow: increased risk of bleeding when used with cefoperazone
Drug/food
Iron-rich cereal, infants' formula: decreased absorption

Drug/lab test
Increased: ALT, AST, alkaline phosphatase,
LDH, bilirubin, BUN, creatinine
False increase: creatinine (serum urine),
urinary 17-KS
False positive: urinary protein, direct Coombs'
test, urine glucose
Interference: cross-matching

NURSING CONSIDERATIONS
Assessment
- Assess patient for previous sensitivity reaction to penicillins or other cephalosporins; cross-sensitivity between penicillins and cephalosporins is common
- Assess patient for signs and symptoms of infection including characteristics of wounds, sputum, urine, stool, WBC >10,000/mm^3, fever; obtain baseline information and during treatment
- Obtain C&S before beginning product therapy to identify if correct treatment has been initiated
- Assess for anaphylaxis: rash, urticaria, pruritus, chills, fever, joint pain; angioedema may occur a few days after therapy begins; epinephrine and resuscitation equipment should be available for anaphylactic reaction
- Identify urine output; if decreasing, notify prescriber (may indicate nephrotoxicity); also check for increased BUN, creatinine
- Monitor blood studies: AST, ALT, CBC, Hct, bilirubin, LDH, alkaline phosphatase, Coombs' test monthly if patient is on long-term therapy
- Monitor electrolytes: potassium, sodium, chloride monthly if patient is on long-term therapy
- Assess bowel pattern daily; if severe diarrhea occurs, product should be discontinued; may indicate pseudomembranous colitis
- Monitor for bleeding: ecchymosis, bleeding gums, hematuria, stool guaiac daily if on long-term therapy
- Assess for overgrowth of infection: perineal itching, fever, malaise, redness, pain, swelling, drainage, rash, diarrhea, change in cough, sputum

Nursing diagnoses
- Diarrhea (side effects)
- Infection, risk for (uses)
- Injury, risk for (side effects)
- Knowledge, deficient (teaching)

Implementation
cefdinir
PO route
- Give oral susp after adding 39 ml water to the 60 ml bottle; 65 ml water to the 12.0 ml bottle; discard unused portion after 10 days

cefditoren pivoxil
- Give for 10 days to ensure organism death, prevent superinfection
- Give with food if needed for GI symptoms
- Give after C&S is completed

cefepime
IM route
- Reconstitute 1 g/2 ml of sterile water for inj; may be diluted with 0.5% or 1% lidocaine to prevent pain; give deep in large muscle mass, massage
IV route
- Check for irritation, extravasation, phlebitis daily; change site q72hr
- For intermittent inf dilute with 50-100 ml of D$_5$W, give over 30 min
Solution compatibilities: 0.9% NaCl, D$_5$, 0.5, 1.0% lidocaine, bacteriostatic water for inj with parabens/benzyl alcohol

cefixime
- Do not break, crush, or chew tab
- Give for 10-14 days to ensure organism death, prevent superinfection

cefotaxime
IV route
- Dilute 1 g/10 ml D$_5$W, NS, sterile H$_2$O for inj and give over 3-5 min by Y-tube or 3-way stopcock; may be diluted further with 50-100 ml of 0.9% NaCl or D$_5$W; run over ½-1 hr; discontinue primary inf during administration; or may be diluted in larger volume of sol and given as a cont inf over 6-24 hr
- Give for 10-14 days to ensure organism death, prevent superinfection
- Thaw frozen container at room temperature or refrigeration, do not force thaw by immersion or microwave; visually inspect container for leaks
Syringe compatibilities: Heparin, oflaxacin
Y-site compatibilities: Acyclovir, amifostine, aztreonam, cyclophosphamide, diltiazem, famotidine, fludarabine, hydromorphone, lorazepam, magnesium sulfate, melphalan, meperidine, midazolam, morphine, ondansetron, perphenazine, sargramostim, teniposide, thiotepa, tolazoline, vinorelbine
Additive compatibilities: Clindamycin, metronidazole, verapamil

Adverse effects: *italic* = common, **bold** = life-threatening

cefpodoxime
IM route
- Reconstitute 1 g/2 ml or 2 g/3 ml of sterile or bacteriostatic water for inj; may be diluted with 0.5% of 1% lidocaine to prevent pain; give deep in large muscle mass, massage

IV route
- Check for irritation, extravasation, phlebitis daily; change site q72hr
- For direct **IV** dilute in 1 g/10 ml or more and give over 5 min
- For intermittent inf further dilute in 50-100 ml of 0.9% NaCl or D₅W; give over 3-5 min; discontinue primary line while running intermittent inf

Syringe incompatibilities: Doxapram
Y-site compatibilities: Famotidine, fluconazole, fludarabine, regular insulin, meperidine, morphine, sargramostim
Additive incompatibilities:
Aminoglycosides, heparin, tetracyclines

ceftazidime
IM route
- Reconstitute 500 mg/1.5 ml or 1 g/3 ml of sterile or bacteriostatic water for inj; may be diluted with 0.5% or 1% lidocaine to prevent pain; give deep in large muscle mass, massage

IV route
- Check for irritation, extravasation, phlebitis daily; change site q72hr
- For direct **IV** dilute 500 mg/5 ml or 1 g/10 ml sterile water for inj; give over 3-5 min; do not use sol with benzyl alcohol for neonates
- For intermittent inf further dilute 1 g/10 ml or more 0.9% NaCl, D₅W, D₁₀W, D₅/0.25% NaCl, D₅/0.45% NaCl, D₅/0.9% NaCl, or LR; give over 30-60 min
- Store for 96 hr refrigerated, 24 hr room temperature

Y-site compatibilities: Acyclovir, allopurinol, amifostine, aztreonam, ciprofloxacin, diltiazem, enalaprilat, esmolol, famotidine, filgrastim, fludarabine, foscarnet, granisetron, heparin, hydromorphone, labetalol, melphalan, meperidine, morphine, ondansetron, paclitaxel, rantidine, tacrolimus, teniposide, theophylline, thiotepa, vinorelbine tartrate, zidovudine
Y-site incompatibilities: Amsacrine, fluconazole, idarubicin, sargramostim
Additive compatibilities: Ciprofloxacin, clindamycin, fluconazole, metronidazole, ofloxacin
Additive incompatibilities: Aminoglycosides, sodium bicarbonate

ceftibuten
- Administer for 10 days to ensure organism death, prevent superinfection
- Administer after C&S

ceftizoxime
IM route
- Reconstitute 250 mg/0.9 ml, 500 mg/1.8 ml, 1 g/3.6 ml, 2 g/7.2 ml; may be diluted with 0.5% or 1% lidocaine to prevent pain; give deep in large muscle mass, massage

IV route
- Check for irritation, extravasation, phlebitis daily; change site q72hr
- For intermittent inf reconstitute 250 mg/2.4 ml, 500 mg/4.8 ml, 1 g/9.6 ml/2 g/19.2 ml sterile water for inj, D₅W, or 0.9% NaCl; do not use sol with benzyl alcohol for neonates; may be further diluted in 50-100 ml of D₅W, D₁₀W, 0.9% NaCl, or LR; give over 30-60 min
- May store 96 hr refrigerated, 24 hr room temperature

Y-site compatibilities: Acyclovir, allopurinol, amifostine, aztreonam, enalaprilat, esmolol, famotidine, fludarabine, foscarnet, hydromorphone, labetalol, melphalan, meperidine, morphine, ondansetron, sargramostim, teniposide, thiotepa, vinorelbine
Additive compatibilities: Clindamycin, metronidazole
Additive incompatibilities: Aminoglycosides

ceftriaxone
- Give IM inj deep in large muscle mass
- Give for 10-14 days to ensure organism death, prevent superinfection

IV route
- Give **IV** after diluting 250 mg/2.4 ml of D₅W, H₂O for inj, 0.9% NaCl; may be further diluted with 50-100 ml of 0.9% NaCl, D₅W, D₁₀W, shake; run over ½-1 hr
- Do not mix with calcium salts

Y-site compatibilities: Acyclovir, allopurinol, aztreonam, cisatracurium, diltiazem, DOXOrubicin liposome, fludarabine, foscarnet, heparin, melphalan, meperidine, methotrexate, morphine, paclitaxel, remifentanil, sargramostim, tacrolimus, teniposide, theophylline, vinorelbine, warfarin, zidovudine
Additive compatibilities: Amino acids or sodium bicarbonate, metronidazole

Patient/family education
- Teach patient to report sore throat, bruising, bleeding, joint pain; may indicate blood dyscrasias (rare)
- Advise patient to contact prescriber if vaginal itching, loose foul-smelling stools, furry tongue occur; may indicate superinfection

- Advise patient to notify prescriber of diarrhea with blood or pus, may indicate pseudomembranous colitis
- Cefditoren can be taken with oral contraceptives

Evaluation
Positive therapeutic outcome
- Absence of signs/symptoms of infection (WBC <10,000/mm³, temp WNL, absence of red draining wounds, earache)
- Reported improvement in symptoms of infection
- Negative C&S

Treatment of anaphylaxis: Epinephrine, antihistamines, resuscitate if needed

---

cephradine
See cephalosporins—1st generation

---

certolizumab (Rx)
(ser'tue-liz'oo-mab)
Cimzia
Func. class.: Biologic response modifier
Chem. class.: Anti-TNF (tissue necrosis factor) agent
Pregnancy category B

Action: Monoclonal antibody that neutralizes the activity of tumor necrosis factor alpha (TNF α) found in Crohn's disease; decreased infiltration of inflammatory cells

Therapeutic outcome: Absence of fever, mucus in stools

Uses: Crohn's disease, rheumatoid arthritis (moderate-severe)

Dosage and routes
Crohn's disease (moderate-severe)
Adult: SUBCUT 400 mg given as 2 inj at wk 0, 2, 4; if clinical response occurs, give 400 mg q4wk

Rheumatoid arthritis (moderate-severe)
Adult: SUBCUT 400 mg q2wk × 3 doses, then 200 mg q2wk; given with methotrexate

Available forms: Powder for inj 400 mg kit

Adverse effects
CNS: Dizziness, syncope, peripheral neuropathy, fever, **seizures, demyelinating disease of CNS**
CV: Hypotension, **heart failure, MI, cardiac dysrhythmia**

EENT: Optic neuritis, retinal hemorrhage, uveitis
GI: Increased LFTs, **hepatitis, bowel obstruction**
GU: UTI, renal disease
HEMA: Anemia, **aplastic anemia, pancytopenia, thrombocytopenia**
INTEG: Rash, urticaria, **angioedema**
RESP: Dyspnea, URI
SYST: **Anaphylaxis, malignancies, serum sickness,** bleeding, antibody formation, infection, lupus-like symptoms, lymphadenopathy, arthralgia, **suicidal ideation**

Contraindications: Influenzae, **IV** administration, sepsis, hypersensitivity

Black Box Warning: Infection

Precautions: Pregnancy **B**, breastfeeding, children, geriatric patients, AIDS, coagulopathy, diabetes, fungal infection, heart failure, hepatitis, human anti-chimeric antibody, immunosuppression, leukopenia, MS, cancer, neurologic disease, surgery, thrombocytopenia, TB, vaccinations, renal disease

Pharmacokinetics
Absorption	Unknown
Distribution	Unknown
Metabolism	Unknown
Excretion	Unknown
Half-life	Terminal 14 days

Pharmacodynamics
Onset	Unknown
Peak	54-171 hr
Duration	Unknown

Interactions
Individual drugs
Abatacept, adalimumab, anakinra, etanercept, infliximab, rilonacept: increased possible infections
Adalimumab, etanercept, infliximab: increased possible malignancies
Drug classifications
Immunosuppressive agents: increased possible infections
Live vaccines, toxoids: do not administer concurrently

NURSING CONSIDERATIONS
Assessment
- Monitor antibody test (ANA), hepatitis B serology, CBC
- Assess for rheumatoid arthritis, ROM, pain
- Assess GI symptoms: nausea, vomiting, abdominal pain, hepatitis, increased LFTs

Adverse effects: *italic* = common, **bold** = life-threatening

- Monitor periodic blood counts (CBC)
- Assess CV status: B/P, pulse, chest pain
- ⬥ Assess for allergic reaction, anaphylaxis: rash, dermatitis, urticaria, dyspnea, hypotension, fever, chills; discontinue if severe, administer epinephrine, corticosteroids, antihistamines; assess for allergies to murine proteins before starting therapy
- Assess infections: discontinue if infection occurs; do not administer to patients with active infections
- Identify TB, risk for HBV before beginning treatment; a TB test should be obtained; if present, TB should be treated prior to receiving infliximab

Nursing diagnoses
- Diarrhea (uses)
- Knowledge, deficient (teaching)
- Mobility, impaired physical (uses)

Implementation
- Store in refrigerator; do not freeze

SUBCUT route
- Give by SUBCUT only
- Allow reconstitution to warm to room temp; add 1 ml sterile water for inj to each vial; two vials will be needed for Crohn's disease
- Gently swirl; do not shake; full reconstitution may take up to 30 min; reconstituted product may remain at room temp for up to 2 hr or refrigerated up to 24 hr
- Warm to room temperature if reconstituted product has been refrigerated
- Use 2 syringes and 2 20-G needles
- Withdraw reconstituted sol from each vial into separate syringes; each will contain 200 mg; switch 20-G to 23-G needle; inject into 2 separate sites in abdomen or thigh

Patient/family education
- Instruct patient not to breastfeed while taking this product
- Advise patient to notify prescriber of GI symptoms, hypersensitivity reactions
- Caution patient not to operate machinery, drive if dizziness, vertigo occur

Evaluation
Positive therapeutic outcome
- Absence of fever, mucus in stools

---

cetirizine (Rx)
(se-tear'i-zeen)
Zyrtec
Func. class.: Antihistamine, peripherally selective (2nd generation)
Chem. class.: Piperazine, H₁ histamine antagonist

Pregnancy category B

Do not confuse:
Zyrtec/Xanax/Zantac

Action: Acts on blood vessels, GI, respiratory system by competing with histamine for H₁-receptor site; decreases allergic response by blocking pharmacologic effects of histamine; minimal anticholinergic/sedative action

Therapeutic outcome: Absence of allergy symptoms, rhinitis, and chronic idiopathic urticaria

Uses: Rhinitis, allergy symptoms, and chronic idiopathic urticaria

Dosage and routes
Adult and child ≥6 yr: PO 5-10 mg daily
Child 2-5 yr: PO 2.5 mg daily, may increase to 5 mg daily or 2.5 mg bid
Child 1-2 yr: PO 2.5 mg daily, may increase to 2.5 mg q12hr
Child 6-11 mo: PO 2.5 mg daily
Geriatric: PO 5 mg daily, may increase to 10 mg/day

Self-treatment of hay fever/other respiratory allergies
Adult/adolescent/child ≥6 yr: PO 10 mg/day, oral SOL 5-10 mg/day

Renal dose
Adult: PO CCr 11-31 ml/min 5 mg daily

Hemodialysis
Adult: PO 5 mg/day

Hepatic dose
Adult: PO 5 mg daily

Available forms: Tabs 5, 10 mg; syr 5 mg/5 ml

Adverse effects
CNS: Headache, stimulation, *drowsiness,* sedation, *fatigue,* confusion, blurred vision, tinnitus, restlessness, tremors, parodoxical excitation in children or geriatric
GI: Dry mouth, increased liver function tests, constipation
INTEG: Rash, eczema, photosensitivity, urticaria
RESP: Thickening of bronchial secretions; dry nose, throat

Contraindications: Hypersensitivity to this product or hydrOXYzine, breastfeeding, newborn or premature infants, severe hepatic disease

Precautions: Pregnancy B, children, geriatric, respiratory disease, closed-angle glaucoma, prostatic hypertrophy, bladder neck obstruction, asthma

Pharmacokinetics

Absorption	Well absorbed, rapid
Distribution	Protein binding 93%
Metabolism	Liver
Excretion	Kidneys
Half-life	8.3 hr, decreased in children, increased in renal/hepatic disease

Pharmacodynamics

Onset	½ hr
Peak	1-2 hr
Duration	24 hr

Interactions
Individual drugs
Alcohol: increased CNS depression
Drug classifications
CNS depressants, opioids, sedative/hypnotics: increased CNS depression
MAOIs: increased anticholinergic effect
Drug/herb
Corkwood: increased anticholinergic effect
Hops, Jamaican dogwood, kava, senna, valerian: increased effects
Drug/food
Prolongs absorption by 1.7 hr
Drug/lab test
False negative: skin allergy tests (discontinue antihistamine 3 days before testing)

NURSING CONSIDERATIONS
Assessment
• Assess respiratory status: rate, rhythm; increase in bronchial secretions, wheezing, chest tightness; provide fluids to 2 L/day to decrease secretion thickness
• Assess for allergy symptoms: pruritus, urticaria, watering eyes, baseline, during treatment

Nursing diagnoses
• Airway clearance, ineffective (uses)
• Injury, risk for (side effects)
• Knowledge, deficient (teaching)
• Noncompliance (teaching overuse)

Implementation
• Give without regard to meals
• Store in tight, light-resistant container

Patient/family education
• Teach all aspects of product uses; to notify prescriber if confusion, sedation, hypotension occur; to avoid driving or other hazardous activity if drowsiness occurs; to avoid alcohol or other CNS depressants that may potentiate effect
• Instruct patient to take without regard to meals
• Instruct patient not to exceed recommended dose; dysrhythmias may occur
• Advise patient to avoid using if breastfeeding
• Advise patient to avoid exposure to sunlight; burns may occur
• Advise patient to use sugarless gum, candy, frequent sips of water to minimize dry mouth
• Advise patient to avoid alcohol, OTC antihistamines, other CNS depressants

Evaluation
Positive therapeutic outcome
• Absence of runny or congested nose, rashes

Treatment of overdose:
Lavage, diazepam, vasopressors, phenytoin IV

---

cetrorelix (Rx)
(set-roe-ree'lix)
Cetrotide
Func. class.: Gonadotropin-releasing hormone antagonist
Chem. class.: Synthetic decapeptide
Pregnancy category X

Action: Inhibitor of pituitary gonadotropin secretion; initially increases LH and FSH, induces a rapid suppression of gonadotropin secretion

Therapeutic outcome: Pregnancy

Uses: For inhibition of premature LH surges in women undergoing controlled ovarian hyperstimulation

Dosage and routes
Single-dose regimen
Adult: SUBCUT 3 mg when serum estradiol level is at appropriate stimulation response, usually on stimulation day 7; if hCG has not been given within 4 days after inj of 3 mg cetrorelix, give 0.25 mg daily until day of hCG administration

Multiple-dose regimen
Adult: SUBCUT 0.25 mg is given on stimulation day 5 (either morning or evening) or 6 (morning) and continued daily until day hCG is given

Available forms: Inj 0.25, 3 mg

Adverse effects: *italic* = common, **bold** = life-threatening

Adverse effects
CNS: Headache
CV: Edema
ENDO: Ovarian hyperstimulation syndrome, abdominal pain (gyn)
GI: Nausea, vomiting, diarrhea
INTEG: Pain on inj; local site reactions, bruising, pruritus
OTHER: Rapid weight gain
RESP: Shortness of breath
SYST: **Fetal death, anaphylaxis**

Contraindications: Pregnancy **X**, breast-feeding, hypersensitivity, latex allergy, renal disease

Precautions: Geriatric

Pharmacokinetics	
Absorption	Unknown
Distribution	Protein binding 86%
Metabolism	Liver to metabolites
Excretion	Feces/urine
Half-life	Depends on dosage

Pharmacodynamics
Unknown

NURSING CONSIDERATIONS
Assessment
• Assess for suspected pregnancy; product should not be used
• Assess for latex allergy; product should not be used
• Monitor ALT, AST, GGT, alkaline phosphatase, serum progesterone, LH; ovarian ultrasound days 7-14

Nursing diagnoses
• Knowledge, deficient (teaching)

Implementation
• Give SUBCUT using abdomen, 1 inch away from navel, or upper thigh; swab inj area with disinfectant, clean a 2-in circle and allow to dry, pinch up area between thumb and finger, insert needle at 45-90 degrees to surface; if blood is drawn into the syringe, reposition needle without removing it; rotate inj sites
• Do not administer if patient is pregnant
• Protect from light

Patient/family education
• Instruct to report abdominal pain, vaginal bleeding, nausea, vomiting, diarrhea, shortness of breath, peripheral edema
• Teach self-administration technique if needed

Evaluation
Positive therapeutic outcome
• Pregnancy

cetuximab (Rx)
(se-tux′i-mab)
Erbitux
Func. class.: Antineoplastic—miscellaneous, monoclonal antibody
Chem. class.: Epidermal growth factor receptor inhibitor
Pregnancy category C

Action: Not fully understood; binds to epidermal growth factor receptors (EGFR); inhibits phosphorylation and activation of receptor-associated kinase resulting in inhibition of cell growth

Therapeutic outcome: Decrease in tumor size

Uses: Alone or in combination with irinotecan for EGFR expressing metastatic colorectal carcinoma, head/neck cancer

Dosage and routes
Adult: **IV** INF 400 mg/m² loading dose given over 120 min, max INF rate 5 ml/min, weekly maintenance dose (all other infusions) is 250 mg/m² given over 60 min, max INF rate 5 ml/min; premedicate with an H₁ antagonist (diphenhydrAMINE 50 mg **IV**); dosage adjustments are made for INF reactions or dermatologic toxicity

Available forms: Inj 50 ml, single-use vial with 100 mg of cetuximab (2 mg/ml)

Adverse effects
CNS: Headache, insomnia, depression
GI: Nausea, diarrhea, vomiting, anorexia, mouth ulceration, dehydration, constipation, abdominal pain
HEMA: **Leukepenia, anemia**
INTEG: Rash, pruritus, acne, dry skin, **toxic epidermal neurolysis, angioedema,** *blepharitis, cheilitis, cellulitis, cysts, alopecia, skin/nail disorder,* **acute infusion reactions, other skin toxicities**
MISC: Conjunctivitis, asthma, malaise, fever, **renal failure,** *hypomagnesemia*
MS: Back pain
RESP: **Interstitial lung disease,** *cough, dyspnea,* **pulmonary embolus,** *peripheral edema*
SYST: **Anaphylaxis, sepsis, infection**

Contraindications: Hypersensitivity to this product or murine proteins

Precautions: Pregnancy C, breastfeeding, child, geriatric, renal/hepatic disease, ocular, pulmonary disorders

Black Box Warning: Arrhythmias, CAD, infusion-related reactions, radiation

Pharmacokinetics

Absorption	Unknown
Distribution	Unknown
Metabolism	Unknown
Excretion	Unknown
Half-life	114 hrs

Pharmacodynamics

Onset	Unknown
Peak	168-235 g/ml, trough 41-85 g/ml
Duration	Steady state by 3rd weekly infusion

Drug/lab test
Increase: LFTs

NURSING CONSIDERATIONS
Assessment
◆ Monitor pulmonary changes: lung sounds, cough, dyspnea; interstitial lung disease may occur, may be fatal; discontinue therapy if confirmed
◆ Assess for toxic epidermal necrosis, angioedema, anaphylaxis
• Assess GI symptoms: frequency of stools, dehydration, abdominal pain, stomatitis
• Obtain K-RAS mutation in metastatic colorectal carcinoma; if K-RAS mutation in codon 12 or 13 is detected, then patient should not receive anti-EGFR antibody therapy

Nursing diagnoses
• Body image, disturbed (adverse reactions)
• Infection, risk for (adverse reactions)
• Injury, risk for (adverse reactions)
• Knowledge, deficient (teaching)

Implementation
IV infusion route
• Administer by **IV** infusion only, do not give by **IV** push or bolus
• Do not shake or dilute
• Infusion pump: draw up volume of a vial using appropriate syringe/needle (a vented spike or other appropriate transfer device); fill Erbitux into sterile evacuated container/bag, repeat until calculated volume has been put into the container. Use a new needle for each vial; give through in-line filter (low protein binding 0.22-micrometer); affix inf line and prime before starting inf, max rate 5 ml/min; flush line at end of inf with 0.9% NaCl

• Syringe pump: Draw up volume of a vial using appropriate syringe/needle (a vented spike); place syringe into syringe driver of a syringe pump and set rate; use an in-line filter 0.22 micrometer (low protein binding); connect inf line and start inf after priming; repeat until calculated volume has been given
• Use a new needle and filter for each vial, max 5 ml/min rate; use 0.9% NaCl to flush line after inf
• Do not piggyback to patient inf line
• Observe patient for adverse reactions for 1 hr after inf
• Inf reactions: if mild (Grade 1 or 2) reduce all doses by 50%; if severe (Grade 3 or 4) permanently discontinue
• Store refrigerated 36°-46° F, discard unused portions

Patient/family education
• Instruct patient to report adverse reactions immediately: SOB, severe abdominal pain, skin eruptions
• Explain reason for treatment, expected results
• Instruct patient to use contraception during treatment
• Advise patient to wear sunscreen and hats to limit sun exposure; sun exposure can exacerbate any skin reactions

Evaluation
Positive therapeutic outcome
• Decrease growth, spread of EGFR expressing metastatic colorectal carcinoma

---

charcoal, activated (OTC)
Actidose-Aqua, Actidose with Sorbitol, CharcoAid, Charcoal Plus, Charcocaps, Liqui-Char
Func. class.: Antiflatulent/antidote

Pregnancy category D

Action: Binds poisons, toxins, irritants; increases adsorption in GI tract; inactivates toxins and binds until excreted

Therapeutic outcome: Prevention of toxicity and death resulting from absorption of products

Uses: Poisoning, overdose

Unlabeled uses: Diarrhea, flatulence

Dosage and routes
Poisoning
Children should not get more than 1 dose of products with sorbitol

---

Adverse effects: *italic* = common, **bold** = life-threatening

Adult and child: PO 30-100 g or 1 g/kg, minimum dosage 30 g/250 ml of water; may give 20-40 g q6hr for 1-2 days in severe poisoning; take plenty of water

Available forms: Powder 15, 25 ♣, 30, 40, 120, 125, 240 g/container; oral susp 12.5 g/60 ml, 15 g/72 ml, 15 g/120 ml, 25 g/120 ml, 30 g/120 ml, 50 g/240 ml; ♣ 15 g/120 ml, 25 g/125 ml, 50 g/225 ml, 50 g/250 ml; tabs/caps should not be used in poisonings

Adverse effects

GI: Nausea, black stools, vomiting, constipation, diarrhea, abdominal pain

OTHER: **Pulmonary aspiration**

Contraindications: Pregnancy **D,** hypersensitivity to this product, unconsciousness, semiconsciousness, poisoning of cyanide, mineral acids, alkalis, gag reflex, depression, ethanol intoxication, intestinal obstruction, absent bowel sounds

Precautions: Pregnancy **(C),** hypersensitivity to quinidine, quinine

Pharmacokinetics	
Absorption	None
Distribution	None
Metabolism	None
Excretion	Feces (unchanged)
Half-life	Unknown

Pharmacodynamics	
Onset	1 min
Peak	Unknown
Duration	4-12 hr

Interactions

Individual drugs

Acetylcysteine: inactivation

Acarbose, carbamazepine, digoxin, ipecac, phenytoin: decreased effects

NURSING CONSIDERATIONS

Assessment

• Assess neurologic status including LOC, pupil reactivity, cough reflex, gag reflex, and swallowing ability before administration; do not give if neurologic status is impaired; aspiration may occur unless a protected airway is present

• Assess toxin, poison ingested, time of ingestion, and amount

• Monitor respiration, pulse, B/P to determine charcoal effectiveness if taken for barbiturate/opioid poisoning, serum electrolytes

Nursing diagnoses

• Injury, risk for (uses)

• Knowledge, deficient (teaching)

• Poisoning, risk for (uses)

Implementation

• Give after inducing vomiting unless vomiting contraindicated (i.e., cyanide or alkalis); mix with 8 oz of water or fruit juice to form thick syrup; do not use dairy products to mix charcoal; repeat dose if vomiting occurs soon after dose

• Space at least 2 hr before or after other products, or absorption will be decreased; use a laxative to promote elimination; constipation occurs often

• If patient unable to swallow, dilute to a less thick sol; keep container tightly closed to prevent absorption of gases

• Give through a nasogastric tube if patient unable to swallow

Patient/family education

• Tell patient stools will be black

• Teach patient about overdose/poison prevention and about keeping poison control chart available

Evaluation

Positive therapeutic outcome

• Alert, PERL (poisoning)

• Absence of distention

• Absence of odor in wounds

chloral hydrate (Rx)

(klor'al hye'drate)

Aquachloral, chloral hydrate, Novo-Chlorhydrate ♣, PMS-Chloral Hydrate, Somnote

Func. class.: Sedative/hypnotic, non-barbiturate

Chem. class.: Chloral derivative

Pregnancy category C

Controlled substance schedule IV (USA), schedule F (Canada)

Action: Reduced to product trichloroethanol, which produces mild cerebral depression, causing sleep; generalized CNS depression

Therapeutic outcome: Ability to sleep, sedation

Uses: Sedation, short-term treatment of insomnia, alcohol withdrawal, anxiety

Dosage and routes
Sedation
Adult: PO/RECT 250 mg tid after meals; max 2 g/day
Child: PO 25-50 mg/kg tid, max 500 mg tid
Alcohol withdrawal
Adult: PO/RECT 500 mg-1 g q6hr, max 2 g/day
Postop pain adjunct
Adult: PO 250 mg tid, after meals, max 2 g/day
Procedure sedation
Child: PO/RECT 25-50 mg/kg, max 100 mg/kg or 2 g
Insomnia
Adult: PO/RECT 500 mg-1 g 30 min before bedtime; max 2 g/day
Child: PO/RECT 50-75 mg/kg (one dose)
Renal disease
Adult: PO/RECT CCr <50 ml/min avoid use

Available forms: Caps 500 mg; SYR 250, 500 mg/5 ml; SUPP 325, 650 mg

Adverse effects
CNS: Drowsiness, dizziness, stimulation, nightmares, ataxia, hangover (rare), light-headedness, headache, paranoia, hallucinations
CV: Hypotension, **dysrhythmias**
GI: Nausea, vomiting, flatulence, diarrhea, unpleasant taste, **gastric necrosis,** abdominal pain
HEMA: **Eosinophilia, leukopenia**
INTEG: Rash, urticaria, **angioedema,** fever, purpura, eczema
RESP: **Depression**

Contraindications: Hypersensitivity to this product or triclofos, severe renal/hepatic disease, GI disorders (oral forms), gastritis

Precautions: Pregnancy **C,** breastfeeding, geriatric, severe cardiac disease, depression, suicidal individuals, asthma, intermittent porphyria, esophagitis, gastric/duodenal ulcers, gastritis

Pharmacokinetics
Absorption	Well absorbed (PO, RECT)
Distribution	Widely distributed; crosses placenta
Metabolism	Liver to trichloroethanol
Excretion	Kidneys (inactive metabolite), feces, breast milk
Half-life	8-10 hr; active metabolite

Pharmacodynamics
	PO	RECT
Onset	½-1 hr	Slow
Peak	Unknown	Unknown
Duration	4-8 hr	4-8 hr

Interactions
Individual drugs
Alcohol: increased action of both products
Furosemide: increased action of furosemide
Phenytoin: decreased effect of phenytoin
Drug classifications
Anticoagulants (oral): increased action of anticoagulants
CNS depressants: increased action of both products
Drug/herb
Black cohosh: increased hypotension
Catnip, chamomile, clary, cowslip, hops, kava, lavender, mistletoe, nettle, pokeweed, poppy, Queen Anne's lace, senega, valerian: increased sedative effect
Drug/lab test
Interferences: urine catecholamines, urinary 17-OHCS

NURSING CONSIDERATIONS
Assessment
• Assess patient's sleep pattern and note physical (sleep apnea, obstructed airway, pain/discomfort, urinary frequency) and psychologic (fear, anxiety) circumstances that interrupt sleep
• Assess patient's bedtime routine, presleep cues/props
• Assess potential for abuse; this product may lead to physical and psychologic dependency; amount of product should be limited
• Monitor blood studies: Hct, Hgb, RBCs, serum folate (if on long-term therapy), pro-time in patients receiving anticoagulants since action of anticoagulant may be increased
• Monitor mental status: mood, sensorium, affect, memory (long, short)
• Monitor physical dependency: more frequent requests for medication, shakes, anxiety, pinpoint pupils
• Monitor respiratory dysfunction: respiratory depression, character, rate, rhythm; hold product if respirations are <10/min or if pupils are dilated (rare)
• Assess for blood dyscrasias: fever, sore throat, bruising, rash, jaundice, epistaxis (rare)
• Assess previous history of substance abuse, cardiac disease, or gastritis

Adverse effects: *italic* = common, **bold** = life-threatening

Nursing diagnoses
- Anxiety (uses)
- Knowledge, deficient (teaching)
- Noncompliance (teaching)
- Sleep deprivation (uses)

Implementation
- Regulate environmental stimuli (light, noise, temperature), remove foods and fluids that interfere with sleep
- Place side rails up after giving medication for hypnotic; remove cigarettes/matches from patient's environment to prevent fires

PO route
- Do not break, crush, or chew caps
- Give ½-1 hr before bedtime for sleeplessness; give on empty stomach with full glass of water or juice for best absorption and to decrease corrosion (do not chew); after meals to decrease GI symptoms if used for sedation; dilute syr in 4 oz water or juice
⬥ Check dose of syrup carefully, fatal overdoses have occurred

Rectal route
- Store supp in dark container, in refrigerator; remove outer wrapper before insertion

Patient/family education
- Caution patient to avoid driving and other activities requiring alertness; to avoid alcohol ingestion or CNS depressants; serious CNS depression may result plus tachycardia, flushing, headache, hypotension
- Instruct patient not to discontinue medication quickly after long-term use; product should be tapered over 1-2 wk, delirium may occur; that benefits may take 2 nights to be noticed; withdrawal symptoms include tremors, anxiety, hallucinations, delirium
- Teach patient alternative measures to improve sleep (reading, exercise several hours before bedtime, warm bath, warm milk, TV, self-hypnosis, deep breathing)
- Instruct the patient about factors that contribute to sleep pattern disturbances (lifestyle, shift work, long work hours, environmental factors, frequent napping)
- Teach patient to take product as prescribed, not to double doses
- Avoid breastfeeding

Evaluation
Positive therapeutic outcome
- Ability to sleep at night
- Decreased amount of early morning awakening if taking product for insomnia
- Sedation

Treatment of overdose: Lavage, activated charcoal; monitor electrolytes, VS

chlorambucil (Rx)
(klor-am'byoo-sil)
Leukeran
Func. class.: Antineoplastic alkylating agent
Chem. class.: Nitrogen mustard
Pregnancy category D

Do not confuse:
Leukeran/leucovorin/Leukine

Action: Alkylates DNA, RNA; inhibits enzymes that allow synthesis of amino acids in proteins; activity is not cell cycle phase specific

Therapeutic outcome: Prevention of rapidly growing malignant cells

Uses: Chronic lymphocytic leukemia, non-Hodgkin's/Hodgkin's disease, other lymphomas

Unlabeled uses: Macroglobulinemia, ovarian, testicular carcinoma, non-Hodgkin's lymphoma, Behçet's syndrome

Dosage and routes
Adult: PO 0.1-0.2 mg/kg/day × 3-6 wk initially, then 4-10 mg/day maintenance
Geriatric: PO initially ≤2-4 mg/day
Child: PO 0.1-0.2 mg/kg/day (4.5 mg/m²/day) in divided doses or 4.5 mg/m²/day as 1 dose or in divided doses × 3-6 wk

Nephrotic syndrome
Child: PO 0.1-0.2 mg/kg daily with predniSONE × 8-12 wk

Available forms: Tabs 2 mg

Adverse effects
CNS: **Seizures,** tremors, confusion, agitation, ataxia, hallucinations
GI: Nausea, vomiting, diarrhea, weight loss, **hepatotoxicity,** *jaundice*
GU: Hyperuremia
HEMA: **Thrombocytopenia, leukopenia, pancytopenia** (prolonged use), **permanent bone marrow suppression**
INTEG: Alopecia (rare), dermatitis, rash, **Stevens-Johnson syndrome**
RESP: **Fibrosis, pneumonitis**

Contraindications: Breastfeeding, radiation therapy within 1 mo, chemotherapy within 1 mo, thrombocytopenia, recent smallpox vaccination

Black Box Warning: Pregnancy **D**

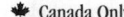

Precautions: *Pneumococcus* vaccination, children, tumor lysis syndrome

Black Box Warning: Bone marrow suppression, infertility, secondary malignancy

Pharmacokinetics	
Absorption	Rapidly, completely absorbed
Distribution	Crosses placenta
Metabolism	Liver, extensively
Excretion	Kidneys
Half-life	2 hr

Pharmacodynamics
Unknown

Interactions
Individual drugs
Filgrastim, sargramostim: contraindicated 24 hr prior to or after chemotherapy
Nalidixic acid: do not use in combination
Radiation: increased toxicity, bone marrow suppression
Drug classifications
Anticoagulants, salicylates: increased risk of bleeding
Antineoplastics: increased bone marrow suppression; increased toxicity

NURSING CONSIDERATIONS
Assessment
• Monitor CBC, differential, platelet count weekly; withhold product if WBC is <2000/mm^3 or granulocyte count <1000/mm^3; notify prescriber of results if WBC <20,000/mm^3, platelets <50,000/mm^3
• Monitor pulmonary function tests, chest x-ray films before, during therapy; chest film should be obtained q2wk during treatment; check for dyspnea, crackles, unproductive cough, chest pain, tachypnea
• Assess for increased uric acid levels, swelling, joint pain primarily in extremities; patient should be well hydrated to prevent urate deposits
• Monitor renal function studies: BUN, serum uric acid, urine CCr before, during therapy; I&O ratio; report fall in urine output of 30 ml/hr; monitor for decreased hyperuricemia
• Assess for jaundice of skin, sclera, dark urine, clay-colored stools, itchy skin, abdominal pain, fever, diarrhea
• Monitor for cold, fever, sore throat (may indicate beginning infection); identify edema in feet, joint, stomach pain, shaking; prescriber should be notified

• Assess for bleeding: hematuria, guaiac, bruising or petechiae, mucosa or orifices q8hr, no rectal temp

Nursing diagnoses
• Body image, disturbed (adverse reactions)
• Infection, risk for (adverse reactions)
• Injury, risk for (adverse reactions)
• Knowledge, deficient (teaching)

Implementation
• Give 1 hr before or 2 hr after meals to lessen nausea and vomiting or antacid before oral agent, give product after evening meal, before bedtime or 1 hr before breakfast; antiemetic 30-60 min before giving product to prevent vomiting
• Give allopurinol to maintain uric acid levels, alkalinization of urine; increase fluid intake to 2-3 L/day to prevent urate deposits, calculus formation
• Antibiotics for prophylaxis of infection may be prescribed, since infection potential is high
• Give all products PO if possible, avoid IM inj when platelets <100,000/mm^3
• Store in tight container

Patient/family education
• Teach patient to avoid use of products containing aspirin or ibuprofen, razors, commercial mouthwash, since bleeding may occur; to report symptoms of bleeding (hematuria, tarry stools)
• Instruct patient to report signs of anemia (fatigue, headache, irritability, faintness, shortness of breath)
• Instruct patient to report any changes in breathing or coughing even several mo after treatment; to avoid crowds and persons with respiratory tract or other infections
• Advise patient hair loss is common; discuss the use of wigs or hairpieces
• Instruct patient to drink 2-3 L of fluid daily unless contraindicated
• Caution patient not to have any vaccinations without the advice of the prescriber; serious reactions can occur
• Advise patient contraception is needed during treatment and for several months after the completion of therapy; may cause irreversible gonadal suppression

Evaluation
Positive therapeutic outcome
• Decreased size of tumor
• Decreased spread of malignancy
• Improved blood values
• Absence of sweating at night
• Increased appetite, increased weight

Adverse effects: *italic* = common, **bold** = life-threatening

chloramphenicol (Rx)

(klor-am-fen'i-kole)

chloramphenicol, Chloromycetin, Pentamycetin ♥

Func. class.: Antiinfective—miscellaneous

Chem. class.: Dichloroacetic acid derivative

Pregnancy category C

Action: Binds to 50S ribosomal subunit, which interferes with or inhibits protein synthesis

Therapeutic outcome: Bactericidal for *Haemophilus influenzae, Salmonella typhi, Rickettsia, Neisseria, Staphylococcus, Streptococcus, Escherichia coli* mycoplasma

Uses: Meningitis, bacteremia, abdominal, skin, soft tissue infections; not to be used if less toxic products can be used

Dosage and routes

Adult and child: PO/**IV** 50-75 mg/kg/day in divided doses q6hr; 100 mg/kg/day (for meningitis only); max 4 g/day

Premature infant and neonate: **IV** 25 mg/kg/day in divided doses q12-24hr

Available forms: Inj **IV** 1 g; caps 250 mg

Adverse effects

CNS: Headache, *depression*, confusion, peripheral neuritis

CV: **Gray syndrome in newborns: failure to feed, pallor, cyanosis, abdominal distention, irregular respiration, vasomotor collapse**

EENT: Optic neuritis, blindness

GI: *Nausea, vomiting, diarrhea,* abdominal pain, xerostomia, glossitis, colitis, pruritus ani

HEMA: **Anemia, thrombocytopenia, aplastic anemia, granulocytopenia, leukopenia, acute generalized exanthematous pustulosis (AGEP)** (rare)

INTEG: Itching, urticaria, contact dermatitis, rash

Contraindications: Hypersensitivity, severe renal/hepatic disease, minor infections, labor

Precautions: Pregnancy **C**, breastfeeding, infants, children, renal/hepatic disease, ulcerative colitis, pseudomembraneous colitis influenza, tympanic membrane perforation

Black Box Warning: Bone marrow depression (product-induced)

Pharmacokinetics

Absorption	Well absorbed (PO), completely absorbed (**IV**)
Distribution	Wide
Metabolism	Liver
Excretion	Kidneys, unchanged
Half-life	1½-4 hr

Pharmacodynamics

	PO	IV
Onset	15 min	Rapid
Peak	1-2 hr	Inf end
Duration	Unknown	Unknown

Interactions

Individual drugs

Folic acid: decreased action of folic acid

Hydantoins: increased action of hydantoins

Iron: increased action of iron

Rifampin: decreased action of rifampin

Vitamin B_{12}: decreased action of vit B_{12}

Drug classifications

Anticoagulants: increased PTT

Antidiabetics: increased action of antidiabetics

Barbiturates: increased levels of barbiturates

Penicillins: decreased action of penicillins

Drug/herb

Acidophilus: do not use with antiinfectives; separate by several hours

NURSING CONSIDERATIONS

Assessment

- Assess patient for previous sensitivity reaction to other antiinfectives; cross-sensitivity between penicillins and cephalosporins is common
- Assess patient for signs and symptoms of infection including characteristics of wounds, sputum, urine, stool, WBC >10,000/mm³, fever; obtain baseline information and during treatment
- Perform C&S testing before starting product therapy to identify if correct treatment has been initiated
- Monitor product level in impaired renal/hepatic systems; peak 15-20 mg/ml 3 hr after dose, trough 5-10 mg/ml before next dose
- Monitor blood studies: platelets q2day, CBC
- Assess bowel pattern daily; if severe diarrhea occurs, product should be discontinued
- Monitor for bleeding: ecchymosis, bleeding gums, hematuria, stool guaiac daily if on long-term therapy
- Assess for overgrowth of infection: perineal itching, fever, malaise, redness, pain, swelling, drainage, rash, diarrhea, change in cough, sputum

Nursing diagnoses
• Diarrhea (adverse reaction)
• Infection, risk for (uses)
• Injury, risk for (side effects)
• Knowledge, deficient (teaching)
• Noncompliance (teaching)

Implementation
PO route
⚠ Do not break, crush, or chew caps
• Give oral form on empty stomach with full glass of water
• Store cap in airtight container at room temperature
IV route
• Give after diluting 1 g/10 ml of sterile H_2O for inj or D_5W (10% sol); give >1 min
• May be further diluted in 50-100 ml of D_5W; give through Y-tube, 3-way stopcock, or additive inf set; run over ½-1 hr; store reconstituted sol at room temperature for up to 30 days
Syringe compatibilities: Ampicillin, cloxacillin, heparin, methicillin, penicillin G sodium
Y-site compatibilities: Acyclovir, cyclophosphamide, enalaprilat, esmolol, foscarnet, hydromorphone, labetalol, magnesium sulfate, meperidine, morphine, perphenazine, tacrolimus
Y-site incompatibilities: Fluconazole
Additive compatibilities: Amikacin, aminophylline, ascorbic acid, calcium chloride/gluconate, cephalothin, cephapirin, colistimethate, corticotropin, cyanocobalamin, dimenhyDRINATE, DOPamine, ephedrine, heparin, hydrocortisone, kanamycin, lidocaine, magnesium sulfate, metaraminol, methicillin, methyldopate, methylPREDNISolone, metronidazole, nafcillin, oxacillin, oxytocin, penicillin G potassium, penicillin G sodium, pentobarbital, phenylephrine, phytonadione, plasma protein fraction, potassium chloride, promazine, ranitidine, sodium bicarbonate, thiopental, verapamil, vit B

Patient/family education
• Teach patient all aspects of product therapy; need to complete entire course of medication to ensure organism death (10-14 days); culture may be taken after complete course of medication
• Advise patient to report sore throat, fever, fatigue, unusual bleeding, or bruising; could indicate bone marrow depression (may occur weeks or months after termination of product)
• Tell patient that product must be taken at regular intervals around the clock to maintain blood levels

Evaluation
Positive therapeutic outcome
• Decreased symptoms of infection

chloramphenicol ophthalmic
See Appendix B

chloramphenicol otic
See Appendix B

chlordiazepoxide (Rx)
(klor-dye-az-e-pox'ide)
Apo-Chlordiazepoxide ✦, Librium, Novopoxide ✦
Func. class.: Antianxiety
Chem. class.: Benzodiazepine, long-acting

Pregnancy category D
Controlled substance schedule IV

Do not confuse:
Librium/Librax

Action: Potentiates the actions of GABA, an inhibitory neurotransmitter, especially in the limbic system reticular formation, which depresses the CNS

Therapeutic outcome: Decreased anxiety, successful alcohol withdrawal, relaxation

Uses: Short-term management of anxiety, acute alcohol withdrawal, preoperative relaxation

Dosage and routes
Mild anxiety
Adult: PO 5-10 mg tid-qid
Geriatric: PO 5 mg bid initially, increase as needed
Child >6 yr: PO 5 mg bid-qid, max 10 mg bid-tid

Severe anxiety
Adult: PO 20-25 mg tid-qid

Preoperatively
Adult: PO 5-10 mg tid-qid on day before surgery; IM 50-100 mg 1 hr before surgery

Alcohol withdrawal
Adult: PO 50-100 mg q4-6hr prn, max 300 mg/day

Renal disease
Adult: PO CCr <10 ml/min give 50% dose

Liver disease
Adult: PO 5 mg bid-qid

Available forms: Caps 5, 25 mg

Adverse effects
CNS: *Dizziness, drowsiness,* confusion, headache, anxiety, tremors, stimulation, fatigue, depression, insomnia, hallucinations
CV: *Orthostatic hypotension,* **ECG changes, tachycardia,** hypotension, edema
EENT: *Blurred vision,* tinnitus, mydriasis
GI: Constipation, dry mouth, nausea, vomiting, anorexia, diarrhea
GU: Irregular periods, decreased libido
HEMA: **Agranulocytosis**
INTEG: Rash, dermatitis, itching

Contraindications: Pregnancy **D,** child <6 yr, hypersensitivity to benzodiazepines, closed-angle glaucoma, psychosis

Precautions: Geriatric, debilitated, renal/hepatic disease, suicidal ideation, abrupt discontinuation

Pharmacokinetics	
Absorption	Well absorbed (PO); slow, erratic (IM)
Distribution	Widely distributed; crosses placenta, blood-brain barrier
Metabolism	Liver extensively
Excretion	Kidneys, breast milk
Half-life	5-30 hr (increased in geriatric)

Pharmacodynamics			
	PO	IM	IV
Onset	30 min	15-30 min	1-5 min
Peak	Within 2 hr	Unknown	Unknown
Duration	4-6 hr	Unknown	Up to 1 hr

Interactions
Individual drugs
Alcohol: increased CNS depression
Cimetidine, disulfiram, fluoxetine, isoniazid, ketoconazole, metoprolol, propranolol, valproic acid: increased action of chlordiazepoxide
Levodopa: decreased action of levodopa

Drug classifications
CNS depressants: increased CNS depression
Contraceptives (oral): increased effect of chlordiazepoxide
CYP3A4 inhibitors (barbiturates, protease inhibitors, rifamycins): decreased effect of chlordiazepoxide
Drug/herb
Cowslip, kava, Queen Anne's lace, St. John's wort, valerian: decreased effect
Drug/lab test
False increase: 17-OHCS
False positive: pregnancy test (some methods)

NURSING CONSIDERATIONS
Assessment
• Assess anxiety reaction: inability to sleep, apprehension, dread, foreboding, or uneasiness related to unidentified source of danger
• Assess for previous product dependence or tolerance; if product dependent or tolerant, amount of medication should be restricted
• Monitor B/P (with patient lying, standing), pulse; if systolic B/P drops 20 mm Hg, hold product, notify prescriber
• Monitor blood studies: CBC during long-term therapy; blood dyscrasias have occurred rarely
• Monitor hepatic studies: AST, ALT, bilirubin, creatinine, LDH, alkaline phosphatase during long-term therapy
• Monitor mental status: mood, sensorium, affect, sleeping patterns, drowsiness, dizziness, suicidal tendencies

Nursing diagnoses
• Anxiety (uses)
• Knowledge, deficient (teaching)
• Noncompliance (teaching)

Implementation
PO route
• Give with food or milk for GI symptoms, crushed if patient unable to swallow medication whole; do not open capsules; provide sugarless gum, hard candy, frequent sips of water for dry mouth

Patient/family education
• Instruct patient that product may be taken with food; if dose is missed take as soon as remembered; do not double doses
• Tell patient to avoid OTC preparations unless approved by prescriber; to avoid alcohol ingestion or other psychotropic medications unless directed by a prescriber

- Caution patient to avoid driving and activities requiring alertness, since drowsiness may occur; until medication response is known, tell patient that drowsiness may worsen at beginning of treatment
- Instruct patient not to discontinue medication abruptly after long-term use; product should be tapered over 1 wk
- Caution patient to rise slowly or fainting may occur, especially in geriatric
- Advise patient that product should be avoided during pregnancy

Evaluation
Positive therapeutic outcome
- Increased well being
- Decreased anxiety, restlessness, sleeplessness, dread
- Successful alcohol withdrawal

Treatment of overdose: Lavage, VS, supportive care

---

chloroquine  (Rx)
(klor'oh-kwin)
Aralen HCl, Aralen Phosphate, chloroquine phosphate
Func. class.: Antimalarial
Chem. class.: Synthetic 4-aminoquinoline derivative

Pregnancy category C

Action: Inhibits parasite replications, transcription of DNA to RNA by forming complexes with DNA of parasite

Therapeutic outcome: Decreased symptoms of malaria, amebiasis

Uses: Malaria caused by *Plasmodium vivax, Plasmodium malariae, Plasmodium ovale, Plasmodium falciparum* (some strains), amebiasis

Dosage and routes
Malaria suppression
Adult and child: PO 5 mg base/kg/wk (child) or 500 mg (300 mg base)/wk (adult) on same day of week, max 300 mg base; treatment should begin 1-2 wk before exposure and for 8 wk after leaving endemic area; if treatment begins after exposure, 600 mg base for adult and 10 mg base/kg for children in 2 divided doses 6 hr apart

Extraintestinal amebiasis
Adult: PO 250 mg (150 mg base) qid × 2 days, then 250 mg (150 mg base) bid × 2-3 wk

Child: PO 10 mg/kg daily × 2-3 wk, max 300 mg/day

Available forms: Tabs 250 mg (150 mg base), 500 mg (300 mg base) phosphate; inj 50 mg (40 mg base)/ml HCl

Adverse effects
CNS: Headache, stimulation, fatigue, **seizure,** psychosis
CV: Hypotension, **heart block, asystole with syncope,** ECG changes
EENT: Blurred vision, corneal changes, retinal changes, difficulty focusing, tinnitus, vertigo, deafness, photophobia, corneal edema
GI: Nausea, vomiting, anorexia, diarrhea, cramps
HEMA: **Thrombocytopenia, agranulocytosis, hemolytic anemia, leukopenia**
INTEG: Pruritus, pigmentary changes, skin eruptions, lichen planus–like eruptions, eczema, **exfoliative dermatitis**

Contraindications: Hypersensitivity, retinal field changes

Precautions: Pregnancy C, breastfeeding, children, blood dyscrasias, severe GI disease, neurologic disease, alcoholism, hepatic disease, G6PD deficiency, psoriasis, eczema, seizures, preexisting auditory damage, infection

Pharmacokinetics
Absorption	Well absorbed
Distribution	Widely
Metabolism	Liver
Excretion	Kidneys, feces
Half-life	3-5 days

Pharmacodynamics
	PO	IM
Onset	Rapid	Rapid
Peak	1-3 hr	30 min
Duration	6-8 hr	Unknown

Interactions
Individual drugs
Cimetidine: decreased oral clearance, metabolism
Kaolin: decreased absorption
Magnesium: decreased action of chloroquine
Drug classifications
2D6 inhibitors (amiodarone, chlorpheniramine, fluoxetine, haloperidol, ritonavir, paroxetine, terbinafine, ticlopidine), CYP3A4

---

inhibitors (clarithromycin, diltiazem, doxy-cycline, erythromycin, itraconazole, ketoco-nazole, verapamil): decreased effects
Antacids (aluminum): decreased absorption

NURSING CONSIDERATIONS
Assessment
- Monitor liver studies weekly: ALT, AST, bilirubin; renal status: before exposure, monthly thereafter: BUN, creatinine, urine output, specific gravity, urinalysis
- Assess mental status often: affect, mood, behavioral changes; psychosis may occur
- Assess hepatic status: decreased appetite, jaundice, dark urine, fatigue
- Assess for toxicity: blurring vision, difficulty focusing, headache, dizziness, decreased knee and ankle reflexes, product should be discontinued immediately

Nursing diagnoses
- Diarrhea (side effects)
- Infection, risk for (uses)
- Injury, risk for (side effects)
- Knowledge, deficient (teaching)
- Noncompliance (teaching)

Implementation
PO route
- Give with meals to decrease GI symptoms; better to take on empty stomach 1 hr before or 2 hr after meals
- Give antiemetic if vomiting occurs
- Give after C&S is completed; monthly to detect resistance

IM route
- Give IM after aspirating to prevent inj into bloodstream

Additive compatibility: Promethazine

Patient/family education
- Advise patient that compliance with dosage schedule, duration is necessary
- Instruct patient that scheduled appointments must be kept or relapse may occur
- Caution patient to avoid alcohol while taking product
- Instruct diabetic to use blood glucose monitor to obtain correct result
- Teach patient to report weakness, fatigue, loss of appetite, nausea, vomiting, yellowing of skin or eyes, tingling/numbness of hands/feet
- Advise patient that urine may turn rust brown color
- Instruct patient to use sunglasses in bright sunlight to prevent photophobia

Evaluation
Positive therapeutic outcome
- Decreased symptoms of malaria

Treatment of overdose: Induce vomiting, gastric lavage, administer barbiturate (ultrashort-acting), vasopressor; tracheostomy may be necessary

---

chlorothiazide (Rx)
(klor-oh-thye′a-zide)
Diuril
Func. class.: Diuretic, antihypertensive
Chem. class.: Thiazide; sulfonamide deriva-tive

Pregnancy category B

Do not confuse:
chlorothiazide/chlorproMAZINE/chlorproPAMIDE/chlorthalidone

Action: Acts on the distal tubule and thick ascending limb of the loop of Henle in the kidney, increasing excretion of sodium, water, chloride, magnesium, potassium, and bicarbonate

Therapeutic outcome: Decreased BP, decreased edema in tissues peripherally, diuresis

Uses: Hypertension, diuresis, CHF, edema

Dosage and routes
Hypertension
Adult: PO/**IV** 500 mg-2 g daily; may divide bid

Edema
Adult: **IV** 250 mg q6-12hr
Child >6 mo: PO 10-20 mg/kg/day may divide bid
Child <6 mo: PO up to 40 mg/kg/day in 2 doses

Available forms: Tabs 250, 500 mg; oral susp 250 mg/5 ml; powder for inj 500 mg

Adverse effects
CNS: Paresthesia, headache, *dizziness, fatigue*
CV: Irregular pulse, orthostatic hypotension, volume depletion
EENT: Blurred vision
ELECT: Hypokalemia, hypercalcemia, hypo-natremia, hypochloremia
GI: Nausea, vomiting, anorexia, constipation, diarrhea, pancreatitis, GI irritation, ***hepatitis***
GU: Frequency, polyuria, incontinence
HEMA: **Aplastic anemia, hemolytic ane-mia, leukopenia, agranulocytosis, throm-bocytopenia, neutropenia**
INTEG: Rash, urticaria, purpura, photosensi-tivity, alopecia

META: Hyperglycemia, *hyperuricemia,* increased creatinine, BUN
SYST: **Anaphylaxis**

Contraindications: Hypersensitivity to thiazides or sulfonamides, anuria, renal decompensation, breastfeeding, hepatic coma

Precautions: Pregnancy **B**, geriatric, hypokalemia, renal/hepatic disease, gout, COPD, LE, diabetes mellitus, hyperlipidemia

Pharmacokinetics

	PO
Absorption	GI tract (10%-20%)
Distribution	Extracellular spaces; crosses placenta
Metabolism	Liver
Excretion	Urine, unchanged; breast milk
Half-life	1-2 hr

Pharmacodynamics

	PO	IV
Onset	2 hr	15 min
Peak	4 hr	½ hr
Duration	6-12 hr	2 hr

Interactions
Individual drugs
Alcohol: increased hypotension
Allopurinol, digoxin, lithium: increased toxicity
Amphotericin, mezlocillin, piperacillin, ticarcillin: increased hypokalemia
Cholestyramine, colestipol: decreased absorption of thiazides
Drug classifications
Antihypertensives: increased antihypertensive effect
Glucocorticoids: increased hypokalemia
Nitrates: increased hypotension
NSAIDs: decreased diuretic action
Nondepolarizing skeletal muscle relaxants: increased toxicity
Drug/herb
Aloe, buckthorn, cascara sagrada, Chinese rhubarb, gossypol, licorice, nettle, senna: increased hypokalemia (chronic use)
Aloe, cucumber, dandelion, horsetail, pumpkin, Queen Anne's lace: increased diuretic effect
St. John's wort: increased severe photosensitivity
Drug/lab test
Increased: calcium, amylase, parathyroid test, CPK
Decreased: PBI

False negative: phentolamine and tyramine tests
Interference: urine steroid tests

NURSING CONSIDERATIONS
Assessment
- Assess glucose in urine if patient is diabetic
- Monitor improvement in CVP q8hr
- Check for rashes, temp elevation daily
- Assess for confusion, especially in geriatric; take safety precautions if needed
- Monitor manifestations of hypokalemia; *RENAL:* acidic urine, reduced urine osmolality, nocturia; *CV:* hypotension, broad T wave, U wave, ectopy, tachycardia, weak pulse; *NEURO:* muscle weakness, altered LOC, drowsiness, apathy, lethargy, confusion, depression; *GI:* anorexia, nausea, cramps, constipation, distention, paralytic ileus; *RESP:* hypoventilation, respiratory muscle weakness
- Monitor for manifestations of hypomagnesemia; *CNS:* agitation, muscle twitching, paresthesias, hyperactive reflexes, positive Babinski's reflex, dysphagia, nystagmus, seizures, tetany; *GI:* nausea, vomiting, diarrhea, anorexia, abdominal distention; *CV:* ectopy, tachycardia, broad, flat, or inverted T waves, depressed ST segment, prolonged QT interval, decreased cardiac output, hypotension
- Monitor for manifestations of hyponatremia: *CV:* increased B/P, cold, clammy skin, hypovolemia or hypervolemia; *GI:* anorexia, nausea, vomiting, diarrhea, abdominal cramps; *NEURO:* lethargy, increased ICP, confusion, headache, seizures, coma, fatigue, tremors, hyperreflexia
- Monitor for manifestations of hyperchloremia: *NEURO:* weakness, lethargy, coma; *RESP:* coma, deep rapid breathing
- Assess fluid volume status: I&O ratios and record, count or weigh diapers as appropriate, weight, distended red veins, crackles in lung, color, quality, and specific gravity of urine, skin turgor, adequacy of pulses, moist mucous membranes, bilateral lung sounds, peripheral pitting edema; dehydration symptoms of decreasing output, thirst, hypotension, dry mouth and mucous membranes should be reported
- Monitor electrolytes: potassium, sodium, calcium, magnesium; also include BUN, blood pH, ABGs, uric acid, CBC, blood glucose
- Assess B/P before, during therapy with patient lying, standing, and sitting as appropriate; orthostatic hypotension can occur rapidly

Adverse effects: *italic* = common, **bold** = life-threatening

Nursing diagnoses
- Fluid volume, deficient
- Fluid volume, excess (uses)
- Knowledge, deficient (teaching)
- Urinary elimination, impaired (adverse reactions)

Implementation
- Give in AM to avoid interference with sleep
- Potassium replacement if potassium level is 3.0 mg/dl
- Give whole, or use oral sol; product may be crushed if patient is unable to swallow

PO route
- Give with food; if nausea occurs, absorption may be increased

IV route
- Do not use sol that is yellow, has a precipitate or crystals
- Administer **IV** after diluting 0.5 g/18 ml or more of sterile water for inj; may be diluted further with dextrose or NaCl: give over 5 min; sol is stable at room temperature for 24 hr

Additive compatibilities: Cimetidine, lidocaine, nafcillin, sodium bicarbonate
Additive incompatibilities: Amikacin, blood, blood products, chlorproMAZINE, codeine, hydrALAZINE, insulin, levorphanol, methadone, morphine, multivitamins, norepinephrine, polymyxin B, procaine, prochlorperazine, promazine, promethazine, streptomycin, tetracycline, triflupromazine, vancomycin

Patient/family education
- Teach patient to take medication early in the day to prevent nocturia
- Instruct patient to take with food or milk if GI symptoms of nausea and anorexia occur
- Teach patient to maintain a weekly record of weight and notify prescriber of weight loss >5 lb
- Caution patient that this product causes a loss of potassium, so food rich in potassium should be added to the diet; refer to a dietitian for assistance in planning
- Caution patient not to exercise in hot weather or stand for prolonged periods, since orthostatic hypotension will be enhanced; to use sunscreen to prevent burning
- Teach patient not to use alcohol or any OTC medications without prescriber's approval; serious product reactions may occur
- Emphasize the need to contact prescriber immediately if muscle cramps, weakness, nausea, dizziness, or numbness occur
- Teach patient to take own B/P and pulse and record

- Caution patient that orthostatic hypotension may occur; patient should rise slowly from sitting or reclining positions and lie down if dizziness occurs
- Teach patient to continue taking medication even if feeling better; this product controls symptoms but does not cure the condition
- Advise the patient with hypertension to continue other medical treatment (exercise, weight loss, relaxation techniques, cessation of smoking)

Evaluation
Positive therapeutic outcome
- Decreased edema
- Decreased B/P
- Increased diuresis

Treatment of overdose: Lavage if taken orally, monitor electrolytes; administer dextrose in saline; monitor hydration, CV, renal status

---

chlorpheniramine (OTC, Rx)
(klor-fen-ir′a-meen)
Aller-Chlor, Allergy, Chlo-Amine, Chlorate, chlorpheniramine maleate, Chlor-Trimeton, Chlor-Tripolon ✦, Novo-Pheniram ✦, PediaCare Allergy Formula, Phenetron, Telachor, Teldrin
Func. class.: Antihistamine (1st generation, nonselective)
Chem. class.: Alkylamine, H_1-receptor antagonist
Pregnancy category B

Do not confuse:
Teldrin/Tedral

Action: Acts on blood vessels, GI, respiratory system by competing with histamine for H_1-receptor site; decreases allergic response by blocking histamine

Therapeutic outcome: Absence of allergy symptoms and rhinitis

Uses: Allergy symptoms, rhinitis, conjunctivitis (allergic)

Dosage and routes
Adult/child ≥12 yr: PO 2-4 mg tid-qid, max 24 mg/day; TIME REL 8-12 mg bid-tid, max 24 mg/day; IM/SUBCUT/**IV** 5-40 mg/day, max 40 mg/day
Child 6-12 yr: PO 2 mg q4-6hr, max 12 mg/day; SUS REL 8 mg at bedtime or daily; SUS REL not recommended for child <6 yr; SUBCUT 87.5 mcg/kg or 2.5 mg/m² q6hr

Child 2-5 yr: PO 1 mg q4-6hr, max 4 mg/day

For self-treatment of hay fever or other upper respiratory allergies
Adult/adolescent/child ≥12 yr: PO 4 mg q4-6hr, max 24 mg/24 hr
Child 6-11 yr: PO 2 mg q4-6hr, max 12 mg/24 hr

Available forms: Chewable tabs 2 mg; tabs 4, 8, 12 mg; ext rel tabs 8, 12 mg; ext rel caps 8, 12 mg; syr 1, 2, 2.5 mg/5 ml; inj 10, 100 mg/ml

Adverse effects
CNS: Dizziness, drowsiness, poor coordination, fatigue, anxiety, euphoria, confusion, paresthesia, neuritis
EENT: Blurred vision, dilated pupils, tinnitus, nasal stuffiness, dry nose, throat, mouth
GI: Nausea, anorexia, diarrhea
GU: Retention, dysuria, frequency
HEMA: **Thrombocytopenia, agranulocytosis, hemolytic anemia**
INTEG: Photosensitivity
RESP: Increased thick secretions, wheezing, chest tightness

Contraindications: Newborns/neonates

Precautions: Pregnancy **B,** breastfeeding, geriatric, increased intraocular pressure, renal/cardiac disease, hypertension, bronchial asthma, seizure disorder, hyperthyroidism, prostatic hypertrophy, GI obstruction, peptic ulcer disease, emphysema, hypersensitivity to H_1-receptor antagonists, lower respiratory tract disease, stenosed peptic ulcers, bladder neck obstruction, closed-angle glaucoma

Pharmacokinetics

Absorption	Well absorbed (PO, SUBCUT, IM, **IV**)
Distribution	Widely distributed; crosses blood-brain barrier
Metabolism	Liver, mostly
Excretion	Kidneys, metabolite; breast milk (minimal)
Half-life	12-15 hr

Pharmacodynamics

	PO	PO-ER	SUBCUT	IM	IV
Onset	15-30 min	Unknown	Unknown	Unknown	Immediate
Peak	1-2 hr	Unknown	Unknown	Unknown	Unknown
Duration	4-12 hr	8-24 hr	4-12 hr	4-12 hr	4-12 hr

Interactions
Individual drugs
Alcohol: increased CNS depression
Atropine, haloperidol, quinidine: increased anticholinergic reactions
Drug classifications
Barbiturates, CNS depressants, opiates, sedative/hypnotics, tricyclics: increased CNS depression
MAOIs: increased effect of chlorpheniramine
Phenothiazines: increased anticholinergic reactions
Drug/herb
Corkwood, henbane leaf: increased anticholinergic effect
Hops, Jamaican dogwood, kava, khat, senega: increased sedative effect
Drug/lab test
False negative: skin allergy tests (discontinue antihistamines 3 days before testing)

NURSING CONSIDERATIONS
Assessment
• Assess respiratory status: rate, rhythm, increase in bronchial secretions, wheezing, chest tightness; provide fluids to 2 L/day to decrease secretion thickness
• Monitor I&O ratio: be alert for urinary retention, frequency, dysuria, especially geriatric; product should be discontinued if these occur
• **IV** administration may result in rapid drop in B/P, sweating, dizziness, especially in geriatric

Nursing diagnoses
• Airway clearance, ineffective (uses)
• Injury, risk for (side effects)
• Knowledge, deficient (teaching)
• Noncompliance (teaching, overuse)

Implementation
PO route
• Swallow time rel tabs and caps whole
• Do not break, crush, chew, or open time rel tabs
• Chewable tabs should be chewed and not swallowed whole
• May give with food to decrease GI upset
• Store in tight, light-resistant container
IM/SUBCUT route
• Use only 20 and 100 mg/ml strengths; does not need to be reconstituted or diluted
IV route
Give undiluted by direct **IV** (10 mg/ml strength only); administer 10 mg over 1 min or more

Additive incompatibilities: Calcium chloride, kanamycin, norepinephrine, pentobarbital

Patient/family education
• Teach all aspects of product use; to notify prescriber if confusion, sedation, hypotension, or difficulty voiding occurs; to avoid driving and other hazardous activity if drowsiness occurs; to avoid alcohol and other CNS depressants that may potentiate effect
• Teach patient not to exceed recommended dosage; dysrhythmias may occur
• Advise patient hard candy, gum, frequent rinsing of mouth may be used for dryness

Evaluation
Positive therapeutic outcome
• Absence of running or congested nose, rashes, conjunctivitis

Treatment of overdose: Administer lavage, diazepam, vasopressors, phenytoin IV

---

*chlorproMAZINE 💿 (Rx)
(klor-proe′ma-zeen)
chlorproMAZINE HCl, Chlorpromanyl ♣, Largactil ♣, Novo-Chlorpromazine ♣, Thorazine, Thor-Prom
Func. class.: Antipsychotic/neuroleptic/antiemetic
Chem. class.: Phenothiazine, aliphatic
Pregnancy category C

Do not confuse:
chlorproMAZINE/chlorothiazide/chlorproPAMIDE/chlorthalidone/prochlorperazine

Action: Depresses cerebral cortex, hypothalamus, limbic system, which control activity, aggression; blocks neurotransmission produced by dopamine at synapse; exhibits a strong α-adrenergic, anticholinergic blocking action; mechanism for antipsychotic effects is unclear

Therapeutic outcome: Decreased signs and symptoms of psychosis; control of nausea, vomiting, intractable hiccups, decreased anxiety preoperatively

Uses: Psychotic disorders, Tourette's syndrome, mania, schizophrenia, anxiety, intractable hiccups (adults), nausea, vomiting, preoperative relaxation, acute intermittent porphyria, behavioral problems in children, nonpsychotic patients with dementia

Unlabeled uses: Vascular headache

Dosage and routes
Psychosis
Adult: PO 10-50 mg q1-4hr initially, then increase up to 2 g/day if necessary; IM 10-50 mg q1-4hr, usual dose 300-800 mg/day
Geriatric: PO 10-25 mg daily-bid, increased by 10-25 mg/day q4-7day, max 800 mg/day
Child >6 mo: PO 0.5 mg/kg q4-6hr; IM 0.5 mg/kg q6-8hr; RECT 1 mg/kg q6-8hr

Nausea and vomiting
Adult: PO 10-25 mg q4-6hr prn; IM 25-50 mg q3hr prn; RECT 50-100 mg q6-8hr prn, max 400 mg/day; **IV** 25-50 mg daily-qid
Child ≥6 mo: PO 0.55 mg/kg q4-6hr; IM q6-8hr; RECT 1.1 mg/kg q6-8hr, max IM ≤5 yr or ≤22.7 kg 40 mg; max IM 5-10 yr or 22.7-45.5 kg 75 mg

Intractable hiccups
Adult: PO 25-50 mg tid-qid; IM 25-50 mg (used only if PO dose does not work); **IV** 25-50 mg in 500-1000 ml saline (only for severe hiccups)

Available forms: Tabs 10, 25, 50, 100, 200 mg; sus rel caps 30, 75, 150, 200, 300 mg; syr 10, 25, 100 mg/5 ml; conc 30, 40, 100 mg/ml; supp 25, 100 mg; inj 25 mg/ml

Adverse effects
CNS: **Neuroleptic malignant syndrome,** dizziness, *extrapyramidal symptoms: pseudoparkinsonism, akathisia, dystonia, tardive dyskinesia,* **seizures,** *headache*
CV: Orthostatic hypotension, hypertension, **cardiac arrest,** ECG changes, **tachycardia**
EENT: Blurred vision, glaucoma, dry eyes
GI: Dry mouth, nausea, vomiting, anorexia, constipation, diarrhea, cholestatic jaundice, weight gain
GU: Urinary retention, enuresis, impotence, amenorrhea, gynecomastia, breast engorgement
HEMA: Anemia, **leukopenia, leukocytosis, agranulocytosis**
INTEG: Rash, photosensitivity, dermatitis
RESP: **Laryngospasm,** dyspnea, **respiratory depression**

Contraindications: Hypersensitivity, circulatory collapse, liver damage, cerebral arteriosclerosis, coronary disease, severe hypo/hypertension, blood dyscrasias, coma, child <6 mo, brain damage, bone marrow depression, alcohol and barbiturate withdrawal, closed-angle glaucoma

Precautions: Pregnancy C, breastfeeding, geriatric, seizure disorders, hypertension, hepatic/cardiac disease, prostate enlargement, pulmonary/Parkinson's disease

---

◆ Alert   ♣ Canada Only   💿 Drug on CD   * "Tall Man" lettering (See Preface)

Black Box Warning: Dementia

Pharmacokinetics

Absorption	Variable (PO); well absorbed (IM)
Distribution	Widely distributed; crosses placenta
Metabolism	Liver, GI mucosa extensively
Excretion	Kidneys
Half-life	30 hr

Pharmacodynamics

	PO	RECT	IM	IV
Onset	½-1 hr	12 hr	Unknown	Rapid
Peak	Unknown	Unknown	Unknown	Unknown
Duration	4-6 hr*	3-4 hr	4-8 hr	Unknown

*Duration PO ext rel is 10-12 hr.

Interactions
Individual drugs
Alcohol: increased effects of both products, oversedation

Aluminum hydroxide, magnesium hydroxide: decreased absorption

Bromocriptine, levodopa: decreased antiparkinsonian activity

Epinephrine: increased toxicity

Lithium: decreased chlorproMAZINE levels

Valproic acid: increased valproic acid level

Warfarin: decreased anticoagulant effect

Drug classifications
Antacids: decreased absorption

Anticholinergics, antidepressants, antiparkinsonian agents: increased anticholinergic effects

Anticonvulsants: decreased seizure threshold

Antidepressants, antihistamines, barbiturate anesthetics, opioids, sedative/hypnotics: increased CNS depression

Antithyroid agents: increased agranulocytosis

Barbiturates: decreased serum chlorproMAZINE

β-Adrenergic blockers: increased effect of both products

Drug/herb
Betel palm, kava: increased EPS

Cola tree, hops, nettle, nutmeg: increased action

Henbane leaf: increased anticholinergic effect

Drug/lab test
Increased: liver function tests, cardiac enzymes, cholesterol, blood glucose, prolactin, bilirubin, PBI, cholinesterase, alkaline phosphatase, leukocytes, granulocytes, platelets, [131]I

Decreased: hormones (blood and urine)

False positive: pregnancy tests, PKU, urine

False negative: urinary steroids, 17-OHCS

NURSING CONSIDERATIONS
Assessment
• Assess mental status: orientation, mood, behavior, presence of hallucinations, and type before initial administration and monthly; this product should significantly reduce psychotic behavior

• Assess any potentially reversible cause of behavior problems in geriatric before, during therapy

• Check for swallowing of PO medication; check for hoarding or giving of medication to other patients

• Monitor I&O ratio; palpate bladder if low urinary output occurs, especially in geriatric; urinalysis recommended before, during prolonged therapy

• Monitor bilirubin, CBC, liver function studies monthly

• Assess affect, orientation, LOC, reflexes, gait, coordination, sleep pattern disturbances

• Monitor B/P with patient sitting, standing, lying; take pulse and respirations q4hr during initial treatment; establish baseline before starting treatment; report drops of 30 mm Hg; obtain baseline ECG, Q wave, and T wave changes

• Check for dizziness, faintness, palpitations, tachycardia on rising; severe orthostatic hypotension is common

⚠ Identify for neuroleptic malignant syndrome: hyperpyrexia, muscle rigidity, increased CPK, altered mental status; product should be discontinued

• Assess for EPS including akathisia (inability to sit still, no pattern to movements), tardive dyskinesia (bizarre movements of the jaw, mouth, tongue, extremities), pseudoparkinsonism (rigidity, tremors, pill rolling, shuffling gate); an antiparkinsonian product should be prescribed

• Assess for constipation, urinary retention daily; if these occur, increase bulk, water in diet

Nursing diagnoses
• Coping, ineffective (uses)
• Knowledge, deficient (teaching)
• Noncompliance (teaching)
• Thought processes, disturbed (uses)

Implementation
PO route
⚠ Do not break, crush, or chew time rel caps
• Give product in liquid form mixed in glass of juice or cola if hoarding is suspected

- Periodically attempt dosage reduction in patients with behavioral problems
- Give with full glass of water, milk; or give with food to decrease GI upset
- Store in tight, light-resistant container, oral sol in amber bottle

IM route

- Inject in deep muscle mass; do not give SUBCUT; may be diluted with 0.9% NaCl, 2% procaine as prescribed; do not administer sol with a precipitate
- Remain lying down after IM inj for at least 30 min

Rectal route

- Give after placing in refrigerator for 30 min if too soft to insert; this route is used for nausea, vomiting, hiccups

IV route

- Give by direct **IV** by diluting with 0.9% NaCl to a concentration of 1 mg/1 ml; administer at a rate of 1 mg/2 min
- Give by cont inf after diluting 50 mg/500-1000 ml of D_5W, $D_{10}W$, 0.9% NaCl, 0.45% NaCl, LR, Ringer's or combinations (used for intractable hiccups)

Syringe compatibilities:
Atropine, benztropine, butorphanol, diphenhydrAMINE, doxapram, droperidol, fentanyl, glycopyrrolate, hydromorphone, hydrOXYzine, meperidine, metoclopramide, midazolam, morphine, pentazocine, perphenazine, prochlorperazine, promazine, promethazine, scopolamine

Syringe incompatibilities:
Cimetidine, dimenhyDRINATE, heparin, pentobarbital, thiopental

Y-site compatibilities:
Amsacrine, cisatracurium, cisplatin, cladribine, cyclophosphamide, cytarabine, DOXOrubicin, DOXOrubicin liposome, famotidine, filgrastim, fluconazole, granisetron, heparin, hydrocortisone, ondansetron, potassium chloride, propofol, teniposide, thiotepa, vinorelbine

Additive compatibilities:
Ascorbic acid, ethacrynate, netilmicin, theophylline, vit B/C

Additive incompatibilities:
Aminophylline, amphotericin B, ampicillin, chloramphenicol, chlorothiazide, methicillin, methohexital, penicillin G, phenobarbital

Patient/family education

- Teach patient to use good oral hygiene; frequent rinsing of mouth, sugarless gum, candy, or ice chips for dry mouth
- Caution patient to avoid hazardous activities until product response is determined; dizziness, blurred vision may occur
- Inform patient that orthostatic hypotension occurs often and to rise from sitting or lying position gradually, to remain lying down after IM inj for at least 30 min; tell patient to avoid hot tubs, hot showers, tub baths, since hypotension may occur; tell patient that in hot weather heat stroke may occur; take extra precautions to stay cool
- Advise patient to avoid abrupt withdrawal of this product, or extrapyramidal symptoms may result; product should be withdrawn slowly
- Teach patient to avoid OTC preparations (cough, hay fever, cold) unless approved by prescriber, since serious product interactions may occur; avoid use with alcohol, CNS depressants, since increased drowsiness may occur
- Caution patient to use sunscreen and sunglasses to prevent burns
- Teach patient about extrapyramidal symptoms and necessity of meticulous oral hygiene, since oral candidiasis may occur
- Instruct patient to take antacids 2 hr before or after taking this product
- Instruct patient to report sore throat, malaise, fever, bleeding, mouth sores; if these occur, CBC should be drawn and product discontinued
- Teach that urine may turn pink or reddish-brown
- Teach patient to use contraceptive measures

Evaluation

Positive therapeutic outcome

- Decrease in emotional excitement, hallucinations, delusions, paranoia
- Reorganization of patterns of thought, speech
- Increase in target behaviors

Treatment of overdose: Lavage if orally ingested; provide airway, *do not induce vomiting or use epinephrine*

chlorthalidone (Rx)
(klor-tha'li-doan)

Apo-Chlorthalidone ✤, chlorthalidone, Hygroton, Thalitone, Uridon ✤

Func. class.: Diuretic, antihypertensive
Chem. class.: Thiazide-like phthalimidine derivative

Pregnancy category B

Do not confuse:
chlorthalidone/chlorothiazide/chlorproMAZINE/chlorproPAMIDE, Hygroton/Regroton, Uridon ✤/Vicodin

Action: Acts on the distal tubule and thick ascending limb of the loop of Henle in the kidney, increasing excretion of sodium, water, chloride, magnesium, potassium, and bicarbonate; possible arteriolar dilatation

Therapeutic outcome: Decreased B/P, decreased edema in lung tissues and peripherally, diuresis

Uses: Edema in congestive heart failure, nephrotic syndrome; may be used alone or as adjunct with antihypertensives; also for edema in corticosteroid, estrogen therapy

Dosage and routes
Hypertension
Adult: PO 25-200 mg/day or 100 mg 3 × wk
Edema
Adult: PO 50-100 mg/day or 100 mg on alternate days, max 200 mg/day
Geriatric: PO 12.5 mg daily or every other day

Available forms: Tabs 25, 50, 100 mg

Adverse effects
CNS: Paresthesia, headache, *dizziness, fatigue, weakness,* fever
CV: Hypertension, orthostatic hypotension, palpitations, volume depletion
EENT: Blurred vision
ELECT: Hypokalemia, hypercalcemia, hyponatremia, hypochloremia, hypomagnesemia
GI: Nausea, vomiting, anorexia, constipation, diarrhea, cramps, pancreatitis, GI irritation, jaundice
GU: Frequency, polyuria, **uremia,** glucosuria, impotence
HEMA: **Aplastic anemia, hemolytic anemia, leukopenia, agranulocytosis, thrombocytopenia, neutropenia**
INTEG: Rash, urticaria, purpura, photosensitivity
META: Hyperglycemia, hyperuricemia, increased creatinine, BUN, gout

Contraindications: Hypersensitivity to thiazides or sulfonamides, anuria, renal decompensation, breastfeeding

Precautions: Pregnancy **B,** geriatric, hypokalemia, renal/hepatic disease, gout, diabetes mellitus, hyperlipidemia, SLE, hypotension, CCr <25 ml/min

Pharmacokinetics
Absorption	Well absorbed
Distribution	Extracellular spaces; crosses placenta
Metabolism	Liver
Excretion	Urine, unchanged (30%-60%)
Half-life	40 hr

Pharmacodynamics
Onset	2 hr
Peak	6 hr
Duration	24-72 hr

Interactions
Individual drugs
Alcohol: increased hypotensive effect
Allopurinol, lithium: increased toxicity
Amphotericin B: increased hypokalemia
Cholestyramine, colestipol: decreased absorption of thiazides
Diazoxide: increased hyperglycemia, hypotension
Drug classifications
Glucocorticoids: increased hypokalemia
Nondepolarizing skeletal muscle relaxants: increased toxicity
Drug/herb
Buckthorn, cascara sagrada, Chinese rhubarb, gossypol, licorice, nettle, senna: increased hypokalemia (chronic use)
Cucumber, dandelion, horsetail, khella, pumpkin, Queen Anne's lace: increased hypotension
St. John's wort: severe photosensitivity
Drug/lab test
Increased: triglycerides, calcium, amylase, cholesterol, bilirubin, creatinine, low-density lipoproteins, serum/urine glucose (diabetics), uric acid
Decreased: PBI, parathyroid test, magnesium, potassium, sodium, urinary calcium

NURSING CONSIDERATIONS
Assessment
• Monitor manifestations of hypokalemia; *CV:* hypotension, broad T wave, U wave, ectopy, tachycardia, weak pulse; *GI:* anorexia, nausea, cramps, constipation, distention, paralytic ileus; *NEURO:* muscle weakness, altered LOC,

Adverse effects: *italic* = common, **bold** = life-threatening

drowsiness, apathy, lethargy, confusion, depression; *RENAL:* acidic urine, reduced urine, osmolality, nocturia; *RESP:* hypoventilation, respiratory muscle weakness
• Monitor for manifestations of hypomagnesemia; *CNS:* agitation, muscle twitching, paresthesias, hyperactive reflexes, positive Babinski's reflex, dysphagia, nystagmus, seizures, tetany; *CV:* ectopy, tachycardia, broad, flat or inverted T waves, depressed ST segment, prolonged QT, decreased cardiac output, hypotension; *GI:* nausea, vomiting, diarrhea, anorexia, abdominal distention
• Monitor for manifestations of hyponatremia; *CV:* increased B/P, cold, clammy skin, hypovolemia or hypervolemia; *GI:* anorexia, nausea, vomiting, diarrhea, abdominal cramps; *NEURO:* lethargy, increased ICP, confusion, headache, seizures, coma, fatigue, tremors, hyperreflexia
• Monitor for manifestations of hyperchloremia; *NEURO:* weakness, lethargy, coma; *RESP:* coma, deep rapid breathing
• Assess fluid volume status: I&O ratios and record, count or weigh diapers as appropriate, weight, distended red veins, crackles in lung, color, quality, and specific gravity of urine, skin turgor, adequacy of pulses, moist mucous membranes, bilateral lung sounds, peripheral pitting edema; dehydration symptoms of decreasing output, thirst, hypotension, dry mouth, and mucous membranes should be reported
• Monitor electrolytes: potassium, sodium, calcium, magnesium; also include BUN, blood pH, ABGs, uric acid, CBC, blood glucose
• Assess B/P before and during therapy with patient lying, standing, and sitting as appropriate; orthostatic hypotension can occur rapidly

Nursing diagnoses
• Fluid volume, deficient (adverse reactions)
• Fluid volume, excess (uses)
• Knowledge, deficient (teaching)
• Urinary elimination, impaired (side effect)

Implementation
• Brand names Thalitone/Hygroton should not be used interchangeably
• Give in AM to avoid interference with sleep
• Provide potassium replacement if potassium level is 3.0 mg/dl; give whole, or use oral solutions lightly; product may be crushed if patient is unable to swallow
• Give with food if nausea occurs; may crush tab and mix with fluids or applesauce for swallowing

Patient/family education
• Teach patient to take the medication early in the day to prevent nocturia
• Instruct patient to take with food or milk if GI symptoms of nausea and anorexia occur
• Teach patient to maintain weekly record of weight and notify prescriber of weight loss >5 lb
• Caution patient that this product causes a loss of potassium, so foods rich in potassium should be added to the diet; refer to a dietitian for assistance in planning
• Caution the patient not to exercise in hot weather or stand for prolonged periods, since orthostatic hypotension will be enhanced; to use sunscreen to prevent burns
• Teach patient not to use alcohol, or any OTC medications without prescriber's approval; serious product reactions may occur
• Emphasize the need to contact prescriber immediately if muscle cramps, weakness, nausea, dizziness, or numbness occur
• Teach patient to take own B/P and pulse and record
• Caution patient that orthostatic hypotension may occur; patient should rise slowly from sitting or reclining positions and lie down if dizziness occurs
• Teach patient to continue taking medication even if feeling better; this product controls symptoms but does not cure the condition
• Advise patient with hypertension to continue other medical treatment (exercise, weight loss, relaxation techniques, cessation of smoking)

Evaluation
Positive therapeutic outcome
• Decreased edema
• Decreased B/P
• Increased diuresis

Treatment of overdose: Lavage if taken orally, monitor electrolytes; administer dextrose in saline; monitor hydration, CV, renal status

cholecalciferol
See vitamin D

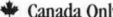

cholestyramine (Rx)

(koe-less-tear'a-meen)

LoCHOLEST, LoCHOLEST Light, Prevalite,
Questran, Questran Light

Func. class.: Antilipemic

Chem. class.: Bile acid sequestrant

Pregnancy category C

Action: Absorbs, combines with bile acids to form an insoluble complex that is excreted through feces; loss of bile acids lowers cholesterol levels

Therapeutic outcome: Decreasing cholesterol levels and low-density lipoproteins, decreased pruritus

Uses: Primary hypercholesterolemia, pruritus associated with biliary obstruction

Unlabeled uses: Diarrhea caused by excess bile acid

Dosage and routes
Adult: PO 4 g daily-bid, max 24 g/day
Child: PO 240 mg/kg/day in 3 divided doses; administer with food or drink, max 8 g/day, titrated up over several weeks to decrease GI effects

Available forms: Powder for susp 4 g/ cholestyramine/packet or scoop; tab 1 g

Adverse effects
CNS: Headache, dizziness, drowsiness, vertigo, tinnitus, anxiety
GI: Constipation, abdominal pain, nausea, fecal impaction, hemorrhoids, flatulence, vomiting, steatorrhea, peptic ulcer
HEMA: **Bleeding,** increased pro-time
INTEG: Rash, irritation of perianal area, tongue, skin
META: Decreased vit A, D, K, red cell folate content, **hyperchloremic acidosis**
MS: Muscle, joint pain

Contraindications: Hypersensitivity; biliary obstruction; hyperlipidemia III, IV, V

Precautions: Pregnancy **C,** breastfeeding, children

Pharmacokinetics

Absorption	Not absorbed
Distribution	Not distributed
Metabolism	Not metabolized; LDL lowered in 4-7 days, serum cholesterol lowered in 1 mo
Excretion	Binds with bile acids, feces
Half-life	Unknown

Pharmacodynamics

Onset	24-48 hr
Peak	1-3 wk
Duration	2-4 wk

Interactions
Individual drugs
Acetaminophen, amiodarone, clindamycin, clofibrate, gemfibrozil, glipizide, iron, penicillin G, phenytoin, propranolol, thyroid hormones, warfarin: decreased absorption of each specific product

Drug classifications
Cardiac glycosides, corticosteroids, tetracyclines, thiazides, vit A, D, E, K: decreased absorption

Drug/herb
Glucomannan: increased effect
Gotu kola: decreased effect

Drug/lab test
Increased: AST, ALT, alkaline phosphatase
Decreased: Na, K
Interference: cholecystography

NURSING CONSIDERATIONS
Assessment
• Assess nutrition: fat, protein, carbohydrates, nutritional analysis should be completed by dietitian
• Assess skin integrity after patient has been receiving product; itching, pruritus often occur from bile deposits on skin
• Monitor cardiac glycoside level if both products are being administered; cardiac glycoside levels will be decreased
• Monitor for signs of vit A, D, E, K deficiency; fasting LDL, HDL, total cholesterol, triglyceride levels, electrolytes if on extended therapy
• Monitor bowel pattern daily; increase bulk, water in diet if constipation develops

Nursing diagnoses
• Constipation (adverse reactions)
• Knowledge, deficient (teaching)
• Noncompliance (teaching)

Implementation
• Give product daily-bid, at bedtime; give all other medications 1 hr before cholestyramine or 4-6 hr after cholestyramine to avoid poor absorption; do not take dry; mix product with applesauce or stir into beverage (2-6 oz); let stand for 2 min; do not mix with carbonated beverages; avoid inhaling powder
• Provide supplemental doses of vit A, D, E, K if levels are low

Patient/family education
◆ Teach patient symptoms of hypoprothrombinemia: bleeding mucous membranes, dark

Adverse effects: *italic* = common, **bold** = life-threatening

tarry stools, hematuria, petechiae; report immediately
- Teach patient importance of compliance
- Teach patient that risk factors should be decreased: high-fat diet, smoking, alcohol consumption, absence of exercise
- Have patient mix product with 6 oz of milk, water, fruit juice; do not mix with carbonated beverages; rinse glass to make sure all medication is taken or may mix product in applesauce; allow to stand for 2 min before mixing

Evaluation

Positive therapeutic outcome
- Decreased cholesterol level (hyperlipidemia)
- Decreased diarrhea, pruritus (excess bile acids)

---

choline salicylate (Rx)
(koe'leen sa-lis'ih-late)
Arthropan
choline/magnesium salicylates (Rx)
CMT, Tricosal, Trilisate
Func. class.: Nonopioid analgesic
Chem. class.: Salicylate

Pregnancy category C

Action: Blocks pain impulses in CNS that occur in response to inhibition of prostaglandin synthesis; antipyretic action results from inhibition of hypothalamic heat-regulating center to produce vasodilatation to allow heat dissipation

Therapeutic outcome: Decreased pain, inflammation, fever

Uses: Mild to moderate pain or fever including arthritis, juvenile rheumatoid arthritis

Dosage and routes
435 mg of choline salicylate = 325 mg of aspirin

Choline salicylate
Adult and child >12 yr: PO 870-1740 mg qid; max 6 ×/day

Pain/fever
Adult: PO 435-870 mg q3-4hr prn

Choline/magnesium salicylates
Adult: PO 1500 mg bid
Child >37 kg: PO 2.2 g of salicylate/day divided bid
Child <37 kg: PO 50 mg of salicylate/kg/day divided bid

Available forms: Choline salicylate liquid 870 mg/5 ml; choline/magnesium salicylate tabs 500, 750, 1000 mg; liquid 500 mg/5 ml

Adverse effects
CNS: Stimulation, drowsiness, dizziness, confusion, **seizure**, headache, flushing, hallucinations, **coma**
CV: Rapid pulse, pulmonary edema
EENT: Tinnitus, hearing loss
ENDO: Hypoglycemia, hyponatremia, hypokalemia
GI: Nausea, vomiting, GI bleeding, diarrhea, heartburn, anorexia, **hepatitis, hepatotoxicity**
HEMA: **Thrombocytopenia, agranulocytosis, leukopenia, neutropenia, hemolytic anemia,** increased pro-time
INTEG: Rash, urticaria, bruising, sweating
RESP: Wheezing, hyperpnea, hyperventilation

Contraindications: Hypersensitivity to salicylates, GI bleeding, bleeding disorders, children <3 yr, vit K deficiency, children with flulike symptoms, Reye's syndrome

Precautions: Pregnancy C, breastfeeding, anemia, renal/hepatic disease, Hodgkin's disease

Pharmacokinetics

Absorption	Well absorbed
Distribution	Widely distributed; crosses placenta
Metabolism	Liver, extensively
Excretion	Kidney, active metabolites; breast milk
Half-life	2-3 hr (low doses); 9-17 hr (high doses)

Pharmacodynamics

Onset	15-30 min
Peak	1-3 hr
Duration	3-6 hr

Interactions
Individual drugs
Alcohol, aspirin, heparin, plicamycin: increased bleeding
Ammonium chloride, nizatidine: increased salicylate levels
Insulin, methotrexate, penicillins, phenytoin, valproic acid: increased effects
Probenecid, spironolactone, sulfinpyrazone: decreased effects
Drug classifications
Antacids (high doses), corticosteroids, steroids, urinary alkalizers: decreased effects of choline salicylate

---

Anticoagulants, hypoglycemics (oral), sulfonamides, thrombolytics: increased effects

Antiinflammatories, NSAIDs, steroids: increased gastric ulcers

β-Blockers, NSAIDs, sulfonamides: decreased effects

Urinary acidifiers: increased salicylate levels

Drug/herb

Bilberry, bogbean, chondroitin, horse chestnut, Irish moss, kelpware, pansy: increased bleeding risk

Drug/lab test

Increased: coagulation studies, liver function studies, serum uric acid, amylase, CO_2, urinary protein

Decreased: serum potassium, cholesterol

Interference: VMA, TSH, 5-HIAA

NURSING CONSIDERATIONS
Assessment
- Monitor pain: location, duration, type, intensity, before dose and 1 hr after
- Monitor musculoskeletal status: ROM before dose
- Identify fever, length of time and related symptoms
- Monitor liver function studies: AST, ALT, bilirubin, creatinine if patient is on long-term therapy
- Monitor renal function studies: BUN, urine creatinine if patient is on long-term therapy; check I&O ratio; decreasing output may indicate renal failure
- Monitor blood studies: CBC, Hct, Hgb, protime if patient is on long-term therapy
- ❶ Assess hepatotoxicity: dark urine, clay-colored stools, yellowing of the skin and sclera, itching, abdominal pain, fever, diarrhea if patient is on long-term therapy
- Assess for allergic reactions: rash, urticaria; if these occur, product may have to be discontinued
- Assess for ototoxicity: tinnitus, ringing, roaring in ears; audiometric testing needed before, after long-term therapy
- Check edema in feet, ankles, legs
- Identify prior product history; there are many product interactions

Nursing diagnoses
- Injury, risk for (side effects)
- Knowledge, deficient (teaching)
- Mobility, impaired physical (uses)
- Pain, acute (uses)
- Pain, chronic (uses)

Implementation
- Administer to patient crushed or whole
- Give with food or milk to decrease gastric symptoms; give 30 min before or 2 hr after meals; absorption may be slowed; sit upright for 30 min after dose
- Give antacids 1-2 hr after enteric products

Patient/family education
- Teach patient to report any symptoms of hepatotoxicity, renal toxicity, visual changes, ototoxicity, allergic reactions, bleeding (long-term therapy)
- Advise patient to take with 8 oz of water
- Caution patient not to exceed recommended dosage; acute poisoning may result
- Caution patient to read label on other OTC products; many contain aspirin products
- Inform patient that the therapeutic response takes 2 wk (arthritis)
- Teach patient to report tinnitus, confusion, diarrhea, sweating, hyperventilation
- Caution patient to avoid alcohol ingestion; GI bleeding may occur
- Teach patient that patients who have allergies may develop allergic reactions
- Caution patient to avoid buffered or effervescent products
- Teach patient not to give to children; Reye's syndrome may develop

Evaluation
Positive therapeutic outcome
- Decreased pain
- Decreased inflammation
- Decreased fever
- Increased mobility

Treatment of overdose: Lavage, activated charcoal, monitor electrolytes, VS

---

cidofovir (Rx)
(si-doh-foh'veer)
Vistide
Func. class.: Antiviral
Chem. class.: Nucleotide analog

Pregnancy category C

Action: Suppresses cytomegalovirus (CMV) replication by selective inhibition of viral DNA synthesis

Therapeutic outcome: Decreased symptoms of CMV

Uses: CMV retinitis in patients with HIV, used with probenecid

Dosage and routes
Adult: **IV** 5 mg/kg qwk × 2 wk; then 3 mg/kg q2wk, give with probenecid

Adverse effects: *italic* = common, **bold** = life-threatening

Renal dose
Adult: IV CCr ≤55 ml/min, do not use; SCr increase of 0.3-0.4 mg/dl above baseline, decrease dose to 3 mg/kg; SCr increase of ≥0.5 mg/dl above baseline or ≥2+ proteinuria, discontinue

Available forms: Inj 75 mg/ml

Adverse effects
CNS: *Fever, chills,* **coma,** confusion, abnormal thought, *dizziness,* bizarre dreams, *headache,* psychosis, tremors, somnolence, paresthesia, *amnesia, anxiety, insomnia,* **seizures**
CV: **Dysrhythmias,** hypo/hypertension
EENT: Retinal detachment in CMV retinitis
GI: Abnormal liver function tests, *nausea, vomiting, anorexia, diarrhea,* abdominal pain, **hemorrhage**
GU: **Hematuria,** increased creatinine, BUN, **nephrotoxicity**
HEMA: **Granulocytopenia, thrombocytopenia, irreversible neutropenia, anemia, eosinophilia**
INTEG: *Rash, alopecia, pruritus, acne,* urticaria, pain at inj site, phlebitis
RESP: Dyspnea

Contraindications: Hypersensitivity to this product or probenecid; sulfa products

Black Box Warning: Proteinuria, renal disease/failure

Precautions: Pregnancy **C,** breastfeeding, children <6 mo, geriatric, preexisting cytopenias, renal function impairment, platelet count <25,000/mm^3

Black Box Warning: Neutropenia, infertility, secondary malignancy

Pharmacokinetics
Absorption	Unknown
Distribution	Unknown
Metabolism	Unknown
Excretion	Unknown
Half-life	Terminal 2.6 hr

Pharmacodynamics
Unknown

Interactions
Individual drugs
Amphotericin B, foscarnet, pentamidine **IV:** increased nephrotoxicity; wait 7 days after use to begin cidofovir

Drug classifications
Aminoglycosides, NSAIDs, salicylates: increased nephrotoxicity; wait 7 days after use to begin cidofovir

NURSING CONSIDERATIONS
Assessment
• Obtain culture before treatment is initiated; cultures of blood, urine, and throat may all be taken; CMV is not confirmed by this method; the diagnosis is made by an ophthalmic exam
• Monitor renal, liver function, increased hematopoietic studies and BUN; serum creatinine, AST, ALT, creatinine, CCr, A-G ratio, baseline and drip treatment, blood counts should be done q2wk; watch for decreasing granulocytes, Hgb; if low, therapy may have to be discontinued and restarted after hematologic recovery; blood transfusions may be required
• Assess for GI symptoms: severe nausea, vomiting, diarrhea; severe symptoms may necessitate discontinuing product
• Assess electrolytes and minerals: calcium, phosphorous, magnesium, sodium, potassium; watch closely for tetany during first administration
• Assess for symptoms of blood dyscrasias (anemia, granulocytopenia); bruising, fatigue, bleeding, poor healing
• Assess allergic reactions: flushing, rash, urticaria, pruritus
• Assess for leukopenia, neutropenia, thrombocytopenia: WBCs, platelets q2day during 2 ×/day dosing and qwk thereafter; check for leukopenias, with daily WBC count in patients with prior leukopenia, with other nucleoside analogs, or for whom leukopenia counts are <1000 cells/mm^3 at start of treatment
• Monitor serum creatinine or CCr at least q2wk; give only to those with creatinine levels ≤1.5 mg/dl, CCr >55 ml/dl, urine protein <100 mg/dl

Nursing diagnoses
• Infection, risk for (uses)

Implementation
• Dilute in 100 ml 0.9% NaCl sol before administration; probenecid must be given PO 2 g 3 hr before the cidofovir INF and 1 g at 2 and 8 hr after ending the cidofovir INF; give 1 L of 0.9% NaCl sol **IV** with each INF of cidofovir, give saline INF over 1-2 hr period immediately before cidofovir; patient should be given a second L if the patient can tolerate the fluid load (second L given at time of cidofovir or immediately afterward and should be given over a 1-3 hr period)

 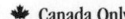

- Mix under strict aseptic conditions using gloves, gown, and mask, and using precautions for antineoplastics
- Administer after diluting in 100 ml of 0.9% NaCl
- Give slowly; do not give by BOL **IV, IV,** SUBCUT inj
- Use diluted sol within 12 hr, do not refrigerate or freeze; do not use sol with particulate matter or discoloration
- Refrigerate up to 24 hr; allow to warm to room temperature before using

Patient/family education
- Advise to notify prescriber if sore throat, swollen lymph nodes, malaise, fever occur; may indicate other infections
- Advise to report perioral tingling, numbness in extremities, and paresthesias; report rash immediately
- Teach that serious product interactions may occur if OTC products are ingested; check first with prescriber
- Teach that product is not a cure, but will control symptoms
- Advise that regular ophthalmic exams must be continued
- Advise that major toxicities may necessitate discontinuing product
- Advise to use contraception during treatment and that infertility may occur; men should use barrier contraception for 90 days after treatment

Evaluation
Positive therapeutic outcome
- Decreased symptoms of CMV

Treatment of overdose: Discontinue product; use hemodialysis, and increase hydration

---

cilastatin
See imipenem/cilastatin

---

cilostazol (Rx)
(sih-los′tah-zol)
Pletal
Func. class.: Platelet aggregation inhibitor
Chem. class.: Quinolinone derivative
Pregnancy category C

Do not confuse:
Pletal/Plendil

Action: Reversibly inhibits cellular phosphodiesterase; inhibits platelet aggrega-

tion induced by thrombin, ADP, collagen, arachidonic acid, epinephrine, stress

Therapeutic outcome: Increased walking distance

Uses: Intermittent claudication

Dosage and routes
Adult: PO 100 mg bid taken ≥30 min before or 2 hr after breakfast and dinner or 50 mg bid, if using products that inhibit CYP3A4 and CYP2C19; 12 wk of treatment may be needed for beneficial effect

Available forms: Tabs 50, 100 mg

Adverse effects
CNS: Dizziness, headache
CV: Palpitations, tachycardia, **nodal dysrhythmia,** postural hypotension
EENT: Blindness, diplopia, ear pain, tinnitus, retinal hemorrhage
GI: Nausea, vomiting, diarrhea, GI disorder, colitis, cholelithiasis, ulcer, esophagitis, gastritis, anorexia, *flatulence, dyspepsia*
GU: Cystitis, frequency, vaginitis, **vaginal hemorrhage,** hematuria
HEMA: **Bleeding (epistaxis, hematuria, retinal hemorrhage, GI bleeding), thrombocytopenia,** anemia, polycythemia; **aplastic anemia**
INTEG: Rash, urticaria, dry skin, **Stevens-Johnson syndrome**
MISC: Back pain, headache, *infection, myalgia, peripheral edema,* chills, fever, malaise, diabetes mellitus
RESP: Cough, pharyngitis, rhinitis, asthma, pneumonia

Contraindications: Hypersensitivity, acute MI, active bleeding conditions, hemostatic conditions

Black Box Warning: CHF

Precautions: Pregnancy **C,** breastfeeding, children, geriatric, past liver disease, renal/cardiac disease, increased bleeding risk, low platelet count, platelet dysfunction

Pharmacokinetics	
Absorption	Unknown
Distribution	95%-98% protein binding
Metabolism	Hepatic extensively by CYP450 enzymes
Excretion	Urine (74%), feces (20%)
Half-life	11-13 hr

Pharmacodynamics
Unknown

Interactions
Individual drugs
Abciximab, eptifibatide, ticlopidine, tirofiban: increased bleeding tendencies

Clarithromycin, CYP3A4 inhibitors, CYP2C19 inhibitors, diltiazem, erythromycin, omeprazole, verapamil: increased cilostazol levels

CYP3A4 inducers: decreased cilostazol

Fluconazole, fluoxetine, fluvoxamine, gemfibrozil, isoniazid, itraconazole, ketoconazole, omeprazole, voriconazole: may increase cilostazol levels; exercise caution when coadministering and reduce dose to 50 mg bid

Drug classifications
Anticoagulants, NSAIDs, thrombolytics: may increase bleeding tendencies

Protease inhibitors: increased cilostazol levels

Drug/herb
Agrimony, alfalfa, angelica, anise, bilberry, black haw, bogbean, buchu, chondroitin, dong quai, fenugreek, feverfew, garlic, ginger, ginkgo, ginseng, green tea, horse chestnut, Irish moss, kelp, kelpware, khella, lovage, lungwort, meadowsweet, motherwort, mugwort, nettle, papaya, parsley (large amounts), pau d'arco, pineapple, poplar, prickly ash, safflower, saw palmetto, senega, tonka bean, turmeric, white willow, wintergreen, yarrow: increased risk of bleeding

Chamomile, coenzyme Q10, flax, glucomannan, goldenseal, St. John's wort: decreased anticoagulant effect

Drug/food
Grapefruit juice: do not use; toxicity may occur

NURSING CONSIDERATIONS
Assessment
• Assess for underlying CV disease since cardiovascular risk is great; for severe headache, signs of toxicity
• Assess for CV lesions with repeated oral administration
• Assess for CHF
• Monitor blood studies: CBC, Hct, Hgb, pro-time if patient is on long-term therapy; thrombocytopenia, neutropenia may occur

Nursing diagnoses
• Injury, risk for (uses)
• Knowledge, deficient (teaching)

Implementation
• Give bid ≥1 hr before or 2 hr after meals; do not give with grapefruit juice

Patient/family education
• Advise patient to report any unusual bleeding to prescriber

• Caution patient to report side effects such as diarrhea, skin rashes, subcutaneous bleeding
• Teach patient that effects may take 2-4 wk, treatment of up to 12 wk may be required for necessary effect
• Teach patients with CHF about potential risks
• Advise patient to take ≥1 hr before or 2 hr after meals
• Advise patient that reading patient package insert is necessary
• Advise patient to discontinue tobacco use
• Advise that there are many drug and herb interactions; obtain approval by prescriber before use

Evaluation
Positive therapeutic outcome
• Increased walking distance and duration
• Decreased pain

---

cimetidine ⊚ (OTC, Rx)
(sye-met'i-deen)
Apo-Cimetidine ✤, cimetidine, Major Acid Reducer, Novocimetine ✤, Peptol ✤, Tagamet, Tagamet HB
Func. class.: H₂-receptor antagonist
Chem. class.: Imidazole derivative

Pregnancy category B

Action: Inhibits histamine at H₂-receptor site in the gastric parietal cells, which inhibits gastric acid secretion

Therapeutic outcome: Healing of duodenal or gastric ulcers; prevention of duodenal ulcers; decreases symptoms of gastroesophageal reflux disease (GERD) and Zollinger-Ellison syndrome

Uses: Short-term treatment of duodenal and gastric ulcers and maintenance; management of GERD, Zollinger-Ellison syndrome; prevention of upper GI bleeding; prevent, relieve heartburn, acid indigestion, upper GI bleeding

Unlabeled uses: Prevention of aspiration pneumonitis, stress ulcers

Dosage and routes
Treatment of active ulcers
Adult and child: PO 300 mg qid with meals, at bedtime × 8 wk or 400 mg bid, 800 mg at bedtime; after 8 wk give at bedtime dose only; **IV** BOL 300 mg/20 ml 0.9% NaCl over 1-2 min q6hr; **IV** INF 300 mg/50 ml D₅W over 15-20 min; IM 300 mg q6hr, max 2400 mg
Child: PO 20-40 mg/kg/day; IM/**IV** 5-10 mg/kg q6-8hr

Prophylaxis of duodenal ulcer
Adult and child >16 yr: 400 mg at
bedtime

GERD
Adult: PO 800-1600 mg/day in divided doses

Hypersecretory conditions
(Zollinger-Ellison syndrome)
Adult: PO/IM/**IV** 300-600 mg q6hr; may
increase to 12 g/day if needed; OTC use up to
200 mg daily or bid, max 2 ×/wk

Upper GI bleeding prophylaxis
Adult: **IV** 50 mg/hr; lowered in renal
disease

Aspiration pneumonitis
prophylaxis (unlabeled)
Adult: IM/**IV** 300 mg IM 1 hr before anesthesia, then 300 mg **IV** q4hr until patient is
alert, max 2400 mg/day

Renal dose
Adult: PO/**IV** CCr <30 ml/min 300 mg
q12hr

Available forms: Tabs 100, 200, 300,
400, 800 mg; liquid 200, 300 mg/5 ml; inj 300
mg/2 ml, 300 mg/50 ml 0.9% NaCl

Adverse effects
CNS: Confusion, headache, depression,
dizziness, anxiety, weakness, psychosis, tremors, **seizures**
CV: Bradycardia, tachycardia, **dysrhythmias**
GI: Diarrhea, abdominal cramps, **paralytic
ileus,** *jaundice*
GU: Gynecomastia, galactorrhea, impotence,
increase in BUN, creatinine
HEMA: **Agranulocytosis, thrombocytopenia, neutropenia, aplastic anemia, increase in pro-time**
INTEG: Urticaria, rash, alopecia, sweating,
flushing, **exfoliative dermatitis**
RESP: **Pneumonia**

Contraindications: Hypersensitivity

Precautions: Pregnancy **B,** breastfeeding,
child <16 yr, geriatric, organic brain syndrome, renal/hepatic disease

Pharmacokinetics

Absorption	Well absorbed (PO, IM); completely absorbed (**IV**)
Distribution	Widely distributed; crosses placenta
Metabolism	Liver (30%)
Excretion	Kidneys, unchanged (70%); breast milk
Half-life	1½-2 hr; increased in renal disease

Pharmacodynamics

	PO	IM/IV
Onset	½ hr	10 min
Peak	45-90 min	½ hr
Duration	4-5 hr	4-5 hr

Interactions
Individual drugs
Carbamazepine, chloroquine, lidocaine,
metronidazole, moricizine, phenytoin,
quinidine, quinine, valproic acid, warfarin:
increased toxicity (CYP450 pathway)
Itraconazole: decreased absorption of itra-
conazole
Ketoconazole: decreased absorption of ketoco-
nazole
Sucralfate: decreased cimetidine absorption
Drug classifications
Antacids: decreased absorption of cimetidine
Antidepressants (tricyclic), benzodiazepines,
β-adrenergic blockers, calcium channel
blockers, phenytoins, sulfonylureas,
theophyllines: increased toxicity (CYP450
pathway)
Drug/lab test
Increased: alkaline phosphatase, AST, creati-
nine, prolactin
False positive: Hemoccult, Gastroccult tests
False negative: TB skin tests

NURSING CONSIDERATIONS
Assessment
• Assess patient with ulcers or suspected
ulcers: epigastric or abdominal pain, hematemesis, occult blood in stools, blood in
gastric aspirate before and/or throughout
treatment; monitor gastric pH (≥5 should be
maintained)
• Monitor I&O ratio, BUN, creatinine, CBC
with differential periodically

Nursing diagnoses
• Knowledge, deficient (teaching)
• Pain, acute (uses)

Implementation
PO route
• Give with meals for lengthened product
effect; antacids 1 hr before or 1 hr after
cimetidine
IV route
• Give by direct **IV** after diluting 300 mg/20 ml
of 0.9% NaCl for inj; give over 5 min or more
• Give intermittent **IV** by diluting 300 mg/50
ml of D₅W; run over 15-20 min
• Give by cont inf after using total daily dose
(900 mg) diluted in 100-1000 ml D₅W given
over 24 hr

Adverse effects: *italic* = common, **bold** = life-threatening

• Store diluted sol at room temperature up to 48 hr

Syringe compatibilities: Atropine, butorphanol, cephalothin, diazepam, diphenhydrAMINE, doxapram, droperidol, fentanyl, glycopyrrolate, heparin, hydromorphone, hydrOXYzine, lorazepam, meperidine, midazolam, morphine, nafcillin, nalbuphine, penicillin G sodium, pentazocine, perphenazine, prochlorperazine, promazine, promethazine, scopolamine

Syringe incompatibilities: Cefamandole, cefazolin, chlorproMAZINE, pentobarbital, secobarbital

Y-site compatibilities: Acyclovir, amifostine, aminophylline, atracurium, aztreonam, cisatracurium, cisplatin, cladribine, cyclosphosphamide, cytarabine, diltiazem, DOXOrubicin, DOXOrubicin liposome, enalaprilat, esmolol, filgrastim, fluconazole, fludarabine, foscarnet, gallium, granisetron, haloperidol, heparin, hetastarch, idarubicin, inamrinone, labetalol, melphalan, meropenem, methotrexate, midazolam, ondansetron, paclitaxel, pancuronium, piperacillin/tazobactam, propofol, sargramostim, tacrolimus, teniposide, theophylline, thiotepa, tolazoline, vecuronium, vinorelbine, zidovudine

Y-site incompatibilities: Amsacrine

Additive compatibilities: Acetazolamide, amikacin, aminophylline, atracurium, cefoperazone, cefoxitin, chlorothiazide, clindamycin, colistimethate, dexamethasone, digoxin, epinephrine, erythromycin, ethacrynate, floxacillin, flumazenil, furosemide, gentamicin, insulin, isoproterenol, lidocaine, lincomycin, meropenem, metaraminol, methylPREDNISolone, norepinephrine, penicillin G potassium, phytonadione, polymyxin B, potassium chloride, protamine, quinidine, tacrolimus, tetracycline, vancomycin, verapamil, vit B complex, vit B/C

Additive incompatibilities: Amphotericin B

Patient/family education
• Advise patient that any gynecomastia or impotence that develops is reversible after treatment is discontinued
• Caution patient to avoid driving, other hazardous activities until stabilized on this medication; drowsiness or dizziness may occur
• Advise patient to avoid black pepper, caffeine, alcohol, harsh spices, extremes in temperature of food; tell patient to avoid OTC preparations: aspirin, cough, cold preparations; condition may worsen

• Advise patient that smoking decreases the effectiveness of the product; smoking cessation should be considered
• Teach patient that product must be continued for prescribed time to be effective and taken exactly as prescribed; doses are not to be doubled; to take missed dose when remembered up to 1 hr before next dose
• Instruct patient to report bruising, fatigue, malaise; blood dyscrasias may occur
• Have patient report to prescriber immediately any diarrhea, black tarry stools, sore throat, dizziness, confusion, or delirium

Evaluation
Positive therapeutic outcome
• Decreased pain in abdomen
• Healing of ulcers
• Absence of gastroesophageal reflux
• Gastric pH of ≥5

cinacalcet (Rx)
(sin-a-kal'set)
Sensipar
Func. class.: Calcium receptor agonist
Chem. class.: Polypeptide hormone

Pregnancy category C

Action: Directly lowers PTH levels by increasing sensitivity of calcium sensing receptors to extracellular calcium

Therapeutic outcome: Decreased symptoms of hypercalcemia

Uses: Hypercalcemia in parathyroid carcinoma, secondary hyperparathyroidism in chronic kidney disease on dialysis, primary hyperparathyroidism

Dosage and routes
Parathyroid carcinoma
Adult: PO 30 mg bid, titrate q2-4wk, with sequential doses of 30 mg bid, 60 mg bid, 90 mg bid, 90 mg tid-qid to normalize calcium levels

Secondary hyperparathyroidism
Adult: PO 30 mg daily, titrate no more frequently than 2-4 wks with sequential doses of 30, 60, 90, 120, 180 mg daily

Available forms: Tabs 30, 60, 90 mg

Adverse effects
CNS: Dizziness, asthenia, **seizures,** tetany, hallucinations, depression
CV: Hypertension, dysrhythmia exacerbation
GI: Nausea, diarrhea, vomiting, anorexia

MISC: Access infection, noncardiac chest pain, hypocalcemia
MS: Myalgia

Contraindications: Hypersensitivity

Precautions: Pregnancy **C**, breastfeeding, children, seizure disorders, hepatic disease, hypocalcemia

Pharmacokinetics

Absorption	93%-97% bound to plasma
Distribution	Unknown
Metabolism	Proteins metabolized by CYP3A4, 2D6, 1A2
Excretion	Renal (80% renal, 15% feces)
Half-life	30-40 hr

Pharmacodynamics

Unknown

Interactions
Individual drugs
Ketoconazole, erythromycin, itraconazole (products metabolized by CYP3A4); flecainide, vinBLAStine, thioridazine: adjustments may be necessary
Drug classifications
Tricyclics (metabolized by CYP2D6): adjustments may be necessary
Drug/food
High-fat meal: increased action

NURSING CONSIDERATIONS
Assessment
• Assess for hypocalcemia: cramping, seizures, tetany, myalgia, paresthesia
• Monitor calcium, phosphorous within 1 wk and iPTH 1-4 wk after initiation or dosage adjustment when maintenance is established; measure calcium, phosphorus monthly; iPTH q1-3mo, target range 150-300 pg/ml for iPTH level; biochemical markers of bone formation/resorption, radiologic evidence of fracture
• If calcium <8.4 mg/dl, do not start therapy

Nursing diagnoses
• Injury, risk for (uses)
• Knowledge, deficient (teaching)

Implementation
• Swallow tabs whole; do not break, crush, chew, or divide tabs
• Can be used alone or in combination with vit D sterols and/or phosphate binders
• Take with food or shortly after meal
Secondary hyperthyroidism
• Titrate q2-4wk to target iPTH consistent with National Kidney Foundation-Kidney Disease

Outcomes Quality Initiative (NKF-K/DOQI) for chronic kidney disease patient on dialysis of 150-300 pg/ml; if iPTH drops below 150-300 pg/ml, reduce dose of cinacalcet and/or vit D sterols or discontinue treatment
• Store at <77° F (25° C)

Patient/family education
• Instruct patient to take with food or shortly after a meal
• Instruct patient to immediately report cramping, seizures, muscle pain, tingling, tetany

Evaluation
Positive therapeutic outcome
• Calcium levels 9-10 mg/dl, decreasing symptoms of hypercalcemia

ciprofloxacin (Rx)
(sip-ro-floks'a-sin)
Cipro, Cipro XR, ProQuin XR
Func. class.: Urinary antiinfectives, broad-spectrum
Chem. class.: Fluoroquinolone
Pregnancy category C

Do not confuse:
ciprofloxacin/cephalexin

Action: Interferes with conversion of intermediate DNA fragments into high-molecular-weight DNA in bacteria; DNA gyrase inhibitor

Therapeutic outcome: Bactericidal action against the following: gram-positive organisms *Staphylococcus epidermidis,* methicillin-resistant strains of *Staphylococcus aureus;* gram-negative organisms *Escherichia coli, Klebsiella* species, *Enterobacter, Salmonella, Proteus vulgaris, Pseudomonas aeruginosa, Serratia, Campylobacter jejuni*

Uses: Adult urinary tract infections (including complicated); chronic bacterial prostatitis; acute sinusitis; infectious diarrhea; typhoid fever; complicated intraabdominal infections; nosocomial pneumonia; exposure to inhalation anthrax; conjunctivitis, corneal ulcers (ophthalmic)

Dosage and routes
Uncomplicated urinary tract infections
Adult: PO 250 mg q12hr × 3 days or 500 mg q24hr × 3 days

Complicated/severe urinary tract infections
Adult: PO 500 mg q12hr or 1000 mg q24hr × 7-14 days; **IV** 400 mg q12hr

Adverse effects: *italic* = common, **bold** = life-threatening

Respiratory, bone, skin, joint infections
Adult: PO 500-750 mg q12hr × 7-14 days; **IV** 400 mg q12hr

Corneal ulcers, conjunctivitis
Adult: Ophth 1-2 gtt q15-30min until infection is controlled, then 1-2 gtt 4-6 ×/day

Nosocomial pneumonia
Adult: IV 400 mg q8hr × 10-14 days

Intraabdominal infections, complicated
Adult: PO 500 mg q12hr × 7-14 days, **IV** 400 mg q12hr × 7-14 days, usually given with metronidazole

Acute sinusitis, mild/moderate
Adult: PO 500 mg q12hr × 10 days; **IV** 400 mg q12hr × 10 days

Inhalational anthrax (postexposure)
Adult: PO 500 mg q12hr × 60 days; **IV** 400 mg q12hr × 60 days
Child: PO 15 mg/kg/dose, max 500 mg/dose; **IV** max 400 mg/dose × 60 days

Infectious diarrhea
Adult: PO 500 mg q12hr × 5-7 days

Chronic bacterial prostatitis
Adult: PO 500 mg q12hr × 28 days; **IV** 400 mg q12hr × 28 days

Pyelonephritis, acute uncomplicated
Adult: PO 1000 mg q24hr × 7-14 days

Renal dose
Adult: PO CCr 30-50 ml/min PO 250-500 mg q12hr; CCr 5-29 ml/min PO 250-500 mg q18hr; **IV** 200-400 mg q18-24hr

Available forms: Tabs 100, 250, 500, 750 mg; ext rel tabs (XR) 500, 1000 mg; inj 200 mg/20 ml, 400 mg/40 ml, 200 mg/100 ml D$_5$, 400 mg/200 ml D$_5$; oral susp 250, 500 mg/5 ml

Adverse effects
CNS: *Headache,* dizziness, fatigue, insomnia, depression, *restlessness,* **seizures,** confusion
GI: *Nausea,* increased ALT, AST, flatulence, heartburn, *vomiting, diarrhea,* oral candidiasis, dysphagia, **pseudomembranous colitis,** dry mouth
HEMA: **Bone marrow depression**
INTEG: *Rash,* pruritus, urticaria, photosensitivity, flushing, fever, chills, **toxic epidermal necrolysis**

MISC: **Anaphylaxis, Stevens-Johnson syndrome,** visual impairment, QT prolongation
MS: Tremor, arthralgia, tendon rupture

Contraindications: Hypersensitivity to quinolones

Precautions: Pregnancy **C,** breastfeeding, children, geriatric, renal disease, epilepsy, QT prolongation, hypokalemia

Black Box Warning: Tendon pain/rupture, tendonitis

Pharmacokinetics

Absorption	Well absorbed (75%) (PO)
Distribution	Widely distributed
Metabolism	Liver (15%)
Excretion	Kidneys (40%-50%)
Half-life	3-4 hr; increased in renal disease

Pharmacodynamics

	PO	IV
Onset	Rapid	Immediate
Peak	1 hr	Infusion's end

Interactions
Individual drugs
Alfuzosin, arsenic trioxide, astemizole, bepridil, chloroquine, clopazine, cyclobenzapine, dasatinib, dolasetron, droperidol, flecainide, halofantrine, haloperidol, lapatinib, levomethadyl, methadone, octreotide, ondansetron, paliperidone, palonosetron, pentamidine, probucol, propafenone, ranolazine, risperidone, sertindole, sunitinib, tacrolimus, terfenadine, vardenafil, vorinostat, ziprasidone: increased QT prolongation
Calcium, enteral feeding, iron, sucralfate, zinc sulfate: decreased ciprofloxacin absorption
CycloSPORINE: increased nephrotoxicity
Probenecid: increased blood levels of ciprofloxacin, increased toxicity
Theophylline: increased theophylline levels, monitor blood levels
Warfarin: increased warfarin effect, monitor blood levels
Drug classifications
Antacids (containing magnesium, aluminum), iron salts: decreased absorption of ciprofloxacin
β-agonists, class IA/III antidysrhythmics, halogenated anesthetics, local anesthetics, macrolides, phenothiazines, tricyclics: increased QT prolongation

Drug/herb
Acidophilus: do not use with antiinfectives;
separate by several hours
Caffeine: increased caffeine levels
Fennel: decreased antiinfective effect
Yerba maté: increased toxicity
Drug/food
Dairy products, food: decreased absorption
Drug/lab test
Increased: AST, ALT, bilirubin, BUN, creatinine,
alkaline phosphatase, LDH, glucose, protein-
uria, albuminuria
Decreased: WBC, glucose

NURSING CONSIDERATIONS
Assessment
• Assess patient for previous sensitivity reaction
• Assess patient for signs and symptoms of
infection including characteristics of wounds,
sputum, urine, stool, WBC >10,000/mm³,
fever; obtain baseline information before,
during treatment
• Obtain C&S before beginning product
therapy to identify if correct treatment has
been initiated
• Assess for anaphylaxis: rash, urticaria,
dyspnea, pruritus, chills, fever, joint pain; may
occur a few days after therapy begins; epinephrine and resuscitation equipment should be
available for anaphylactic reaction
• Identify urine output; if decreasing, notify
prescriber (may indicate nephrotoxicity); also
check for increased BUN, creatinine
• Monitor blood studies: AST, ALT, CBC, Hct,
bilirubin, LDH, alkaline phosphatase, Coombs'
test monthly if patient is on long-term therapy
• Monitor electrolytes: potassium, sodium,
chloride monthly if patient is on long-term
therapy
• Assess bowel pattern daily; if severe diarrhea occurs, product should be discontinued
• Monitor for bleeding: ecchymosis, bleeding
gums, hematuria, stool guaiac daily if on
long-term therapy
• Assess for overgrowth of infection: perineal
itching, fever, malaise, redness, pain, swelling,
drainage, rash, diarrhea, change in cough,
sputum

Nursing diagnoses
• Diarrhea (side effects)
• Infection, risk for (uses)
• Injury, risk for (side effects)
• Knowledge, deficient (teaching)
• Noncompliance (teaching)

Implementation
PO route
• Give around the clock to maintain proper
blood levels
• Administer 2 hr before or 2 hr after antacids, zinc, iron, calcium
IV route
• Check for irritation, extravasation, phlebitis
daily
• For intermittent inf, dilute to 1-2 mg/ml of
D₅W, 0.9% NaCl; give over 60 min; it will
remain stable under refrigeration for 2 wk
Y-site compatibilities: Amifostine,
amino acids, aztreonam, calcium gluconate,
ceftazidime, cisatracurium, digoxin, diltiazem,
diphenhydrAMINE, DOBUTamine, DOPamine,
DOXOrubicin liposome, gallium, gentamicin,
granisetron, hydrOXYzine, lidocaine, lorazepam, metoclopramide, midazolam, midodrine,
piperacillin, potassium acetate, potassium
chloride, potassium phosphates, predniso-
LONE, promethazine, propofol, ranitidine,
remifentanil, Ringer's, sodium chloride,
tacrolimus, teniposide, thiotepa, tobramycin,
verapamil
Y-site incompatibilities: Heparin,
mezlocillin
Additive compatibilities: Amikacin,
aztreonam, ceftazidime, cycloSPORINE, gentamicin, metronidazole, netilmicin, piperacillin,
potassium acetate, potassium chloride, potassium phosphates, prednisoLONE, promethazine, propofol, ranitidine, Ringer's, sodium
chloride, tobramycin, vit B/C
Additive incompatibilities: Aminophylline, amoxicillin, clindamycin, floxacillin,
mezlocillin

Patient/family education
• Teach patient to report sore throat, bruising,
bleeding, joint pain; may indicate blood
dyscrasias (rare)
• Teach patient to contact prescriber if
adverse reaction occurs or if inflammation or
pain in tendon occurs
• Advise patient to contact prescriber if
vaginal itching, loose foul-smelling stools,
furry tongue occur; may indicate
superinfection; report itching, rash, pruritus,
urticaria
• Instruct patient to take all medication
prescribed for the length of time ordered;
product must be taken around the clock to
maintain blood levels; do not give medication
to others
• Advise patient to notify prescriber of diarrhea with blood or pus

---

Adverse effects: *italic* = common, **bold** = life-threatening

- Advise patient to rinse mouth frequently, use sugarless candy or gum for dry mouth

Evaluation
Positive therapeutic outcome
- Absence of signs/symptoms of infection (WBC <10,000/mm^3, temp WNL, absence of red draining wounds)
- Reported improvement in symptoms of infection

---

ciprofloxacin ophthalmic
See Appendix B

---

cisatracurium (Rx)
(sis-a-tra-cyoor'ee-um)
Nimbex
Func. class.: Neuromuscular blocker (nondepolarizing)

Pregnancy category B

Action: Inhibits transmission of nerve impulses by binding with cholinergic receptor sites, antagonizing action of acetylcholine

Therapeutic outcome: Paralysis of body for administration of anesthesia

Uses: Facilitation of endotracheal intubation, skeletal muscle relaxation during mechanical ventilation surgery, or general anesthesia

Dosage and routes
Adult: **IV** 0.15 and 0.2 mg/kg depending on desired time to intubate and length of surgery: use peripheral nerve stimulation to evaluate dosage
Child 2-12 yr: **IV** 0.1 mg/kg over 5-10 sec with halothane or opioid anesthesia

Available forms: Inj 2, 10 mg/ml

Adverse effects
CV: Bradycardia, tachycardia; increased, decreased B/P
EENT: Increased secretions
INTEG: Rash, flushing, pruritus, urticaria
RESP: **Prolonged apnea, bronchospasm, cyanosis, respiratory depression**

Contraindications: Hypersensitivity

Precautions: Pregnancy **B**, breastfeeding, children <2 yr, electrolyte imbalances, dehydration, cardiac/neuromuscular/respiratory disease

Pharmacokinetics	
Unknown	

Pharmacodynamics	
Onset	1-3 min
Peak	2-5 min
Duration	30-40 min

Interactions
Individual drugs
Carbamazepine, phenytoin: decreased duration of neuromuscular blockade
Isoflurane, lithium: increased neuromuscular blockade
Succinylcholine: decreased neuromuscular blockade
Drug classifications
Aminoglycosides, antibiotics (polymix), β-adrenergic blockers, opioids: increased neuromuscular blockade

NURSING CONSIDERATIONS
Assessment
- Assess for electrolyte imbalances (K, Mg), may lead to increased action of this product
- Assess vital signs (B/P, pulse, respirations, airway) until fully recovered; rate, depth, pattern of respirations; strength of handgrip
- Assess I&O ratio: check for urinary retention, frequency, hesitancy
- Assess recovery: decreased paralysis of face, diaphragm, legs, arms, rest of body
- Assess allergic reactions: rash, fever, respiratory distress, pruritus; product should be discontinued

Nursing diagnoses
- Breathing pattern, ineffective (uses)
- Communication, impaired verbal (adverse reactions)
- Knowledge, deficient (teaching)

Implementation
IV route
- Use nerve stimulator by anesthesiologist to determine neuromuscular blockade
- Give anticholinesterase to reverse neuromuscular blockade
- Give by slow **IV** only by qualified person; do not administer IM
- Store in light-resistant area
- Reassure if communication is difficult during recovery from neuromuscular blockage

Evaluation
Positive therapeutic outcome
- Paralysis of jaw, eyelid, head, neck, rest of body

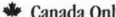

Treatment of overdose: Edrophonium or neostigmine, atropine, monitor VS; mechanical ventilation

---

⚠ HIGH ALERT

cisplatin (Rx)
(sis'pla-tin)
Platinol, Platinol-AQ
Func. class.: Antineoplastic alkylating agent
Chem. class.: Inorganic heavy metal

Pregnancy category D

Do not confuse:
cisplatin/carboplatin, Platinol/Paraplatin

Action: Alkylates DNA, RNA; inhibits enzymes that allow synthesis of amino acids in proteins; activity is not cell cycle phase specific

Therapeutic outcome: Prevention of rapidly growing malignant cells

Uses: Advanced bladder cancer; adjunctive in metastatic testicular cancer and metastatic ovarian cancer; osteosarcoma; soft tissue sarcomas; head, neck, esophageal, prostatic, lung, and cervical cancer; lymphoma

Dosage and routes
Dosage protocols may vary

Metastatic testicular cancer
Adult: IV 20 mg/m² daily × 5 days, repeat q3wk for 2 cycles or more, depending on response

Advanced bladder cancer
Adult: IV 50-70 mg/m² q3-4wk

Metastatic ovarian cancer
Adult: IV 100 mg/m² q4wk or 75-100 mg/m² q3wk with cyclophosphamide therapy; mix with 2 L of NaCl and 37.5 g mannitol over 6 hr

Available forms: Inj 0.5 mg/ml ✿, 1 mg/ml

Adverse effects
CNS: **Seizures,** peripheral neuropathy
CV: Cardiac abnormalities
EENT: Tinnitus, hearing loss, vestibular toxicity, blurred vision, altered color perception
GI: Severe nausea, vomiting, diarrhea, weight loss
GU: **Renal tubular damage,** renal insufficiency, impotence, sterility, amenorrhea, gynecomastia, hyperuremia
HEMA: **Thrombocytopenia, leukopenia, pancytopenia**
INTEG: Alopecia, dermatitis

META: Hypomagnesemia, hypocalcemia, hypokalemia, hypophosphatemia
RESP: **Fibrosis**
SYST: **Anaphylaxis**

Contraindications: Pregnancy **D**, breastfeeding, radiation therapy within 1 mo, chemotherapy within 1 mo, thrombocytopenia, recent smallpox vaccination, aluminum products used to prepare or administer cisplatin

Black Box Warning: Bone marrow suppression, platinum compound hypersensitivity, renal disease/failure, preexisting hearing impairment

Precautions: Geriatric patients, pneumococcal vaccination

Pharmacokinetics

Absorption	Complete
Distribution	Widely distributed, accumulates in body tissues for several months
Metabolism	Liver
Excretion	Kidneys
Half-life	30-100 hr

Pharmacodynamics
Unknown

Interactions
Individual drugs
Alcohol, aspirin: increased risk of bleeding
Bumetanide, ethacrynic acid, furosemide: ototoxicity
Phenytoin: decreased phenytoin effect
Drug classifications
Aminoglycosides, diuretics (loop) salicylates: increased nephrotoxicity
Myelosuppressive agents, radiation: increased myelosuppression
NSAIDs: increased risk of bleeding
Vaccines, live virus: decreased antibody response
Drug/lab test
Increased: uric acid, BUN, creatinine
Decreased: CCr, calcium, phosphate, potassium, magnesium
Positive: Coombs' test

NURSING CONSIDERATIONS
Assessment
• Monitor for bone marrow depression: CBC, differential, platelet count weekly; withhold product if WBC count is <4000/mm³ or platelet count is <100,000/mm³; notify prescriber of results if WBC <20,000/mm³, platelets <150,000/mm³
• Monitor renal function studies: BUN, creatinine, serum uric acid, urine CCr before,

Adverse effects: *italic* = common, **bold** = life-threatening

during therapy; I&O ratio; report fall in urine output to <30 ml/hr; dose should not be given if BUN <25 mg/dl; creatinine <1.5 mg/dl
- Assess for anaphylaxis: wheezing, tachycardia, facial swelling, fainting; discontinue product and report to prescriber; resuscitation equipment should be nearby
- Monitor temp q4hr (may indicate beginning of infection)
- Monitor liver function tests before, during therapy (bilirubin, AST, ALT, LDH) as needed or monthly; note yellowing of skin or sclera, dark urine, clay-colored stools, itchy skin, abdominal pain, fever, diarrhea
- Assess for increased uric acid levels, swelling, joint pain primarily in extremities; patient should be well hydrated to prevent urate deposits
- Assess for bleeding: hematuria, stool guaiac, bruising or petechiae, mucosa or orifices q8hr; note inflammation of mucosa, breaks in skin
- Identify dyspnea, crackles, nonproductive cough, chest pain, tachypnea
- Identify effects of alopecia on body image; discuss feelings about body changes
- Identify edema in feet, joint pain, stomach pain, shaking; prescriber should be notified

Nursing diagnoses
- Body image, disturbed (adverse reactions)
- Infection, risk for (adverse reactions)
- Injury, risk for (adverse reactions)
- Knowledge, deficient (teaching)

Implementation
- Hydrate patient with 0.9% NaCl over 8-12 hr before treatment
- Give all medications PO, if possible; avoid IM inj when platelets <100,000/mm³
- Give epinephrine, antihistamines, corticosteroids for hypersensitivity reaction; antiemetic 30-60 min before giving product to prevent vomiting, and prn; allopurinol or sodium bicarbonate to maintain uric acid level, alkalinization of urine; antibiotics for prophylaxis of infection; diuretic (furosemide 40 mg **IV**) or mannitol after infusion
- After diluting 10 mg/10 ml or 50 mg/50 ml sterile water for inj; withdraw prescribed dose, dilute ½ dose with 1000 ml D₅ 0.2 NaCl or D₅ 0.45 NaCl with 37.5 g mannitol; **IV** inf is given over 3-4 hr; use a 0.45 μm filter; total dose 2000 ml over 6-8 hr; check site for irritation, phlebitis; do not use equipment containing aluminum
- Prepare in biologic cabinet using gown, gloves, mask; do not allow product to come in contact with skin; use soap and water if contact occurs

Syringe compatibilities: Bleomycin, cyclophosphamide, doxapram, DOXOrubicin, droperidol, fluorouracil, furosemide, heparin, leucovorin, methotrexate, metoclopramide, mitomycin, vinBLAStine, vinCRIStine

Y-site compatibilities: Allopurinol, aztreonam, bleomycin, chlorproMAZINE, cimetidine, cladribine, cyclophosphamide, dexamethasone, diphenhydrAMINE, doxapram, DOXOrubicin, DOXOrubicin liposome, droperidol, famotidine, filgrastim, fludarabine, fluorouracil, furosemide, ganciclovir, granisetron, heparin, hydromorphone, leucovorin, lorazepam, melphalan, methotrexate, methylPREDNISolone, metoclopramide, mitomycin, morphine, ondansetron, paclitaxel, prochlorperazine, promethazine, propofol, ranitidine, sargramostim, teniposide, vinBLAStine, vinCRIStine, vinorelbine

Additive compatibilities: Carboplatin, cyclophosphamide with etoposide, etoposide, etoposide with floxuridine, floxuridine, floxuridine with leucovorin, hydrOXYzine, ifosfamide, ifosfamide with etoposide, leucovorin, magnesium sulfate, mannitol, ondansetron

Additive incompatibilities: Fluorouracil, mesna, thiotepa

Solution compatibilities: D₅/0.225% NaCl, D₅/0.45% NaCl, D₅/0.9% NaCl, D₅/0.45% NaCl with mannitol 1.875%, D₅/0.33% NaCl with mannitol 1.875%, D₅/0.33% NaCl with KCl 20 mEq and mannitol 1.875%, 0.9% NaCl, 0.45% NaCl, 0.3% NaCl, 0.225% NaCl, water

Solution incompatibilities: Sodium bicarbonate 5%, 0.1% NaCl, water

Patient/family education
- Teach patient to avoid use of products containing aspirin or ibuprofen, NSAIDs, alcohol (may cause GI bleeding), razors, commercial mouthwash; to report symptoms of bleeding (hematuria, tarry stools, bruising, petechiae)
- Advise patient to report numbness, tingling in face or extremities, poor hearing or joint pain, swelling
- Instruct patient to report signs of anemia (fatigue, headache, irritability, faintness, shortness of breath)
- Instruct patient to report any changes in breathing or coughing even several months after treatment; to avoid crowds and persons with respiratory tract or other infections
- Advise patient that hair may be lost during treatment; a wig or hairpiece may make patient

feel better; new hair may be different in color, texture
• Tell patient not to have any vaccinations without the advice of the prescriber; serious reactions can occur
• Caution patient contraception is needed during treatment and for several months after the completion of therapy

Evaluation
Positive therapeutic outcome
• Prevention of rapid division of malignant cells

---

citalopram (Rx)
(sigh-tal'oh-pram)
Celexa
Func. class.: Antidepressant
Chem class.: Selective serotonin reuptake inhibitor (SSRI)

Pregnancy category C

Do not confuse:
Celexa/Celebrex/Cerebyx/Cerebra

Action: Inhibits CNS neuron uptake of serotonin but not of norepinephrine; weak inhibitor of CYP450 enzyme system, making it more appealing than other products

Therapeutic outcome: Decreased symptoms of depression after 2-3 wk

Uses: Major depressive disorder

Unlabeled uses: Premenstrual disorders, panic disorder, social phobia, impulsive aggression in children, obsessive-compulsive disorder in adolescents, treatment of psychotic symptoms in nondepressed, demented patients, anxiety, hot flashes, menopause, adjunct in schizophrenia, PTSD

Dosage and routes
Depression
Adult: PO 20 mg daily AM or PM, may increase if needed to 40 mg/day after 1 wk; maintenance: after 6-8 wk of initial treatment, continue for 24 wk (32 wk total), reevaluate long-term usefulness (max 60 mg/day)

Hepatic dose/geriatric
Adult: PO 20 mg/day, may increase to 40 mg/day if no response

Panic disorder (unlabeled)
Adult: PO 20-60 mg/day

Premenstrual dysphoria, social phobia
Adult: PO 20-40 mg/day used intermittently in premenstrual dysphoria

Available forms: Tabs 10, 20, 40 mg; oral SOL 10 mg/5 ml

Adverse effects
CNS: Headache, nervousness, insomnia, drowsiness, anxiety, tremor, dizziness, fatigue, sedation, poor concentration, abnormal dreams, agitation, **seizures,** apathy, euphoria, hallucinations, delusions, psychosis, **suicidal attempts, malignant neuroleptic-like syndrome reactions**
CV: Hot flashes, palpitations, angina pectoris, **hemorrhage,** hypertension, 1st-degree tachycardia, 1st-degree AV block, bradycardia, MI, thrombophlebitis
GI: Nausea, diarrhea, dry mouth, anorexia, dyspepsia, constipation, cramps, vomiting, taste changes, flatulence, decreased appetite
GU: Dysmenorrhea, decreased libido, urinary frequency, urinary tract infection, amenorrhea, cystitis, impotence, urine retention
INTEG: Sweating, rash, pruritus, acne, alopecia, urticaria
MS: Pain, arthritis, twitching
RESP: Infection, pharyngitis, nasal congestion, sinus headache, sinusitis, cough, dyspnea, bronchitis, asthma, hyperventilation, pneumonia
SYST: Asthenia, viral infection, fever, allergy, chills, hyponatremia (geriatric patients)

Contraindications: Hypersensitivity

Precautions: Pregnancy C, breastfeeding, geriatric, renal/hepatic disease, seizure disorder

Black Box Warning: Children, suicidal ideation

Pharmacokinetics
Absorption	Well absorbed
Distribution	Unknown
Metabolism	Liver, by CYP1A2, CYP2D6
Excretion	Kidneys, steady state 28-35 days
Half-life	Unknown

Pharmacodynamics
Unknown

Interactions
Individual drugs
Alcohol: increased CNS depression
Carbamazepine, clonidine: decreased citalopram levels
Lithium, trazodone: increased serotonergic effects

Adverse effects: *italic* = common, **bold** = life-threatening

Pimoside, ziprasidone: increased QTc interval; do not use together

Drug classifications

Anticoagulants, NSAIDs, salicylates, thrombolytics: increased risk of bleeding

Antidepressants (tricyclics): increased effect, use cautiously

Antifungals (azole), macrolides: increased citalopram levels

β-Adrenergic blockers: increased plasma levels of β-blockers

Barbiturates, benzodiazepines, CNS depressants, sedatives/hypnotics: increased CNS depression

MAOIs: hypertensive crisis, seizures, fatal reactions; do not use together

Quinolones: increased QTc interval; do not use together

Serotonin receptor agonists, SNRIs, SSRIs: increased serotonin syndrome

Drug/herb

SAM-e, St. John's wort: serotonin syndrome; do not use with citalopram; fatal reaction may occur

Yohimbe: increased CNS stimulation

Drug/lab test

Increased: serum bilirubin, blood glucose, alkaline phosphatase

Decreased: VMA, 5-HIAA

False increase: increased urinary catecholamines

NURSING CONSIDERATIONS
Assessment

• Monitor B/P (lying, standing), pulse q4hr; if systolic B/P drops 20 mm Hg, hold product and notify prescriber; take vital signs q4hr in patients with cardiovascular disease

• Monitor blood studies: CBC, leukocytes, differential, cardiac enzymes if patient is receiving long-term therapy; check platelets; bleeding can occur

• Monitor hepatic studies: AST, ALT, bilirubin

• Check weight qwk; appetite may increase with product

• Assess ECG for flattening of T wave, bundle branch block, AV block, dysrhythmias in cardiac patients

• Assess EPS primarily in geriatric: rigidity, dystonia, akathisia

• Assess mental status: mood, sensorium, affect, suicidal tendencies; increase in psychiatric symptoms: depression, panic

• Monitor urinary retention, constipation; constipation is more likely to occur in children or geriatric

 Assess for withdrawal symptoms: headache, nausea, vomiting, muscle pain, weakness; usually do not occur unless product is discontinued abruptly

• Identify patient's alcohol consumption; if alcohol is consumed, hold dose until AM

Nursing diagnoses

• Coping, ineffective (uses)
• Injury, risk for (side effects)
• Knowledge, deficient (teaching)
• Noncompliance (teaching)

Implementation

• Give with food or milk for GI symptoms
• Give dosage at bedtime if oversedation occurs during day
• Leave orally disintegrating tabs on tongue and allow to dissolve before swallowing
• Store at room temperature; do not freeze

Patient/family education

• Teach patient that therapeutic effects may take 4-6 wk

• Instruct patient to use caution in driving or other activities requiring alertness because of drowsiness, dizziness, blurred vision; to avoid rising quickly from sitting to standing, especially geriatric patients

• Advise that suicidal ideas, behavior may occur in children or young adults

• Caution patient to avoid alcohol ingestion, other CNS depressants

• Advise patient not to discontinue medication quickly after long-term use: may cause nausea, headache, malaise

• Instruct patient to increase fluids, bulk in diet if constipation, urinary retention occur, especially geriatric

• Advise patient to take gum, hard sugarless candy, or frequent sips of water for dry mouth

• Teach patient how to use orally disintegrating tabs

Evaluation

Positive therapeutic outcome
• Decreased in depression
• Absence of suicidal thoughts

---

clarithromycin (Rx)

(clare-i-thro-mye'sin)

Biaxin, Biaxin XL

Func. class.: Antiinfective

Chem. class.: Macrolide

Pregnancy category C

Action: Binds to 50S ribosomal subunits of susceptible bacteria and suppresses protein synthesis

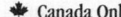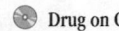

Therapeutic outcome: Bactericidal action against the following: *Streptococcus pneumoniae, Streptococcus pyogenes, Mycoplasma pneumoniae, Corynebacterium diphtheriae, Bordetella pertussis, Listeria monocytogenes, Haemophilus influenzae, Staphylococcus aureus, Mycobacterium avium (MAC), Legionella pneumophila, Moxarella catarrhalis, Neisseria gonorrhoeae,* complex infections in AIDS patients, *Helicobacter pylori* in combination with omeprazole

Uses: Mild to moderate infections of the upper respiratory tract, lower respiratory tract; uncomplicated skin and skin structure infections

Dosage and routes
Acute exacerbation of chronic bronchitis
Adult: PO 250-500 mg q12hr × 7-14 days or 1000 mg/day × 7 days (XL)

Pharyngitis/tonsillitis
Adult: PO 250 mg q12hr × 10 days

Community-acquired pneumonia
Adult: PO 250 mg q12hr × 7-14 days or 1000 mg/day × 7 days (XL)

Endocarditis prophylaxis
Adult: PO 500 mg 1 hr before procedure

MAC prophylaxis/treatment
Adult: PO 500 mg bid, will require an additional antiinfective for active infection

H. pylori *infection*
Adult: PO 500 mg/bid plus omeprazole 2 × 20 mg qAM (days 1-14), then omeprazole 20 mg qAM (days 15-28)

Acute maxillary sinusitis
Adult: PO 500 mg q12hr × 14 days

Most infections
Child: PO 7.5 mg/kg q12hr × 10 days, max 500 mg/dose for MAC

Renal dose
Adult: PO CCr <30 ml/min reduce dose by 50%

Available forms: Tabs 250, 500 mg; oral susp 125, 250 mg/5 ml; ext rel tab (XL) 500 mg

Adverse effects
CV: **Ventricular dysrhythmias, QT prolongation**
GI: Nausea, vomiting, diarrhea, **hepatotoxicity,** abdominal pain, stomatitis, heartburn, anorexia, abnormal taste, **pseudomembranous colitis**
GU: Vaginitis, moniliasis

HEMA: Leukopenia, thrombocytopenia, increased INR
INTEG: Rash, urticaria, pruritus, **Stevens-Johnson syndrome, toxic epidermal necrolysis**
MISC: Headache, hearing loss

Contraindications: Hypersensitivity to this product or other macrolides

Precautions: Pregnancy **C,** breastfeeding, geriatric, renal/hepatic disease, QT prolongation

Pharmacokinetics
Absorption	50%
Distribution	Widely distributed
Metabolism	Liver
Excretion	Kidneys, unchanged (20%-30%)
Half-life	4-6 hr

Pharmacodynamics
Onset	Unknown
Peak	2 hr
Duration	Unknown

Interactions
Individual drugs
Alprazolam, busPIRone, carbamazepine, cycloSPORINE, digoxin, disopyramide, felodipine, fluconazole, omeprazole, tacrolimus, theophylline: increased levels, increased toxicity

Carbamazepine: increased toxicity, from increased levels of carbamazepine, increased oral anticoagulants effect

Cisapride, pimozide: increased effect, increased dysrhythmias

Digoxin: increased blood levels of digoxin, increased digoxin effects, increased oral anticoagulants effect

Midazolam, tacrolimus: increased effects

Rifabutin, rifampin: decreased levels

Theophylline: increased toxicity from increased levels of theophylline, increased oral anticoagulants effect

Zidovudine: increased or decreased action

Drug classifications
All products metabolized by CYP3A enzyme system: increased action, risk of toxicity

Calcium channel blockers, benzodiazepines: increased effects

Class IA, III antidysrhythmics: increased QT prolongation

Ergots: increased levels, increased toxicity

HMG-CoA reductase inhibitors: increased levels

Adverse effects: *italic* = common, **bold** = life-threatening

Oral anticoagulants: increased effects of oral anticoagulants

Drug/herb

Acidophilus: do not use with antiinfectives; separate by several hours

Drug/lab test

Increased: 17-OHCS/17-KS, AST, ALT, BUN, creatinine, LDH, total bilirubin

Decreased: folate assay, WBC

NURSING CONSIDERATIONS

Assessment

- Assess patient for signs and symptoms of infection including characteristics of wounds, sputum, urine, stool, WBC >10,000/mm³, earache, fever; obtain baseline information before, during treatment
- Obtain C&S before beginning product therapy to identify if correct treatment has been initiated
- Monitor blood studies: AST, ALT, CBC, Hct, bilirubin, LDH, alkaline phosphatase, Coombs' test monthly if patient is on long-term therapy
- Assess bowel pattern daily; if severe diarrhea occurs, product should be discontinued
- Assess for overgrowth of infection: perineal itching, fever, malaise, redness, pain, swelling, drainage, rash, diarrhea, change in cough, sputum

Nursing diagnoses

- Diarrhea (side effects)
- Infection, risk for (uses)
- Knowledge, deficient (teaching)
- Noncompliance (teaching)

Implementation

- Do not break, crush, or chew ext rel tab
- Ensure adequate fluid intake (2 L) during diarrhea episodes
- Give q12hr to maintain serum level

Patient/family education

- Advise patient to contact physician if vaginal itching, loose foul-smelling stools, furry tongue occur; may indicate superinfection
- Instruct patient to take all medication prescribed for the length of time ordered
- Advise prescriber if pregnancy is planned or suspected

Evaluation

Positive therapeutic outcome

- Absence of signs/symptoms of infection: WBC <10,000/mm³, temp WNL, absence of red draining wounds
- Reported improvement in symptoms of infection

clavulanate

See amoxicillin/clavulanate, ticarcillin/clavulanate

clevidipine (Rx)

(klev-id′i-peen)

Cleviprex

Func. class.: Calcium channel blocker (L-type)

Chem. class.: Dihydropyridine

Pregnancy category C

Action: L-type calcium channels mediate the influx of calcium during depolarization in arterial smooth muscle; reduces mean arterial B/P by decreasing systemic vascular resistance

Therapeutic outcome: Decreased B/P

Uses: Treatment of hypertension when oral therapy is not feasible

Dosage and routes

Adult: CONT **IV** 1-2 mg/hr; dose may be doubled q90sec initially; as B/P reaches goal, adjust dose less frequently (5-10 min) with smaller increases in dose; most patients require 4-6 mg/hr, max 32 mg/hr; no more than 1000 ml should be infused per 24 hr period due to lipid load restrictions

Available forms: Single dose vial 50, 100 ml (0.5 mg/ml), intravenous emulsion

Adverse effects

CNS: Headache

CV: Hypotension, **MI, sinus tachycardia,** syncope, **reflex tachycardia, atrial fibrillation**

GI: Nausea, vomiting

GU: Renal failure

Contraindications: Hypersensitivity to this product, eggs, or soya lecithin; defective lipid metabolism; severe aortic stenosis; pancreatitis

Precautions: Pregnancy **C**, breastfeeding, children <18 yr, geriatric patients, heart failure, hyperlipidemia, hypertension, labor, phenochromocytoma

Pharmacokinetics

Absorption	Unknown
Distribution	Protein binding >99%
Metabolism	By esterases in blood, extravascular tissues
Excretion	Urine 63%-74%, feces 7%-22%
Half-life	Initially 1 min; terminal 15 min; increased in hepatic disease

Pharmacodynamics	
Onset	2-4 min
Peak	6-12 hr
Duration	Unknown

NURSING CONSIDERATIONS
Assessment
• Assess cardiac status: B/P, pulse, respiration, ECG; some patients have developed severe angina, acute MI after calcium channel blockers if obstructive CAD is severe; if not transitioned to other antihypertensive therapies following clevidipine infusion, patients should be monitored ≥8 hr for rebound hypertension; monitor for rebound hypertension following drug stoppage
• Monitor I&O ratio, weight daily; peripheral edema, dyspnea, jugular vein distention, crackles

Nursing diagnoses
• Knowledge, deficient (teaching)
• Noncompliance (teaching)

Implementation
• Do not give through same line as other medications
• Gently invert several times before use; do not use if discolored or particulate matter is present
• Give through central or peripheral line
• Use infusion device
• Store vials in refrigerator, do not freeze; leave vials in carton until use; product is photosensitive, however protection from light during administration is not required

Patient/family education
• Instruct patient to notify prescriber immediately if neurological symptoms, visual changes, or symptoms of CHF occur
• Instruct patient to continue follow up for hypertension

Evaluation
Positive therapeutic outcome
• Decreased B/P

---

clindamycin HCl (Rx)
(klin-dah-my'sin)
Cleocin HCl
clindamycin palmitate (Rx)
Cleocin Pediatric, Dalacin C Palmitate
clindamycin phosphate (Rx)
Cleocin Phosphate, Dalacin C, Dalacin C Phosphate
Func. class.: Antiinfective—miscellaneous
Chem. class.: Lincomycin derivative

Pregnancy category B

Action: Binds to 50S subunit of bacterial ribosomes; suppresses protein synthesis

Therapeutic outcome: Absence of infection

Uses: Infections caused by staphylococci, streptococci, *Rickettsia, Fusobacterium, Actinomyces, Peptococcus, Bacteroides, Pneumocystis jiroveci*

Dosage and routes
Adults: PO 150-450 mg q6hr, max 1.8 g/day; IM/**IV** 1.2-1.8 g/day in 2-4 divided doses q6-12hr, max 4800 mg/day
Child >1 mo: PO 8-25 mg/kg/day in divided doses q6-8hr; IM/**IV** 20-40 mg/kg/day in divided doses q6-8hr in 3-4 equal doses
Child <1 mo: 15-20 mg/kg/day divided q6-8hr

PID
Adult: **IV** 900 mg q8hr plus gentamicin

Bacterial endocarditis prophylaxis
Adult: 600 mg 1 hr before procedure

P. jiroveci pneumonia (unlabeled)
Adult: PO 1200-1800 mg/day in divided doses with 15-30 mg primaquine/day

Available forms: Phosphate: inj 150, 300, 600 mg base/4 ml; 900 mg base/ml; inj inf in D₅ 300, 600, 900 mg; HCl: caps 75, 150, 300 mg; palmitate: oral sol 75 mg/5 ml

Adverse effects
GI: Nausea, vomiting, abdominal pain, diarrhea, **pseudomembranous colitis,** *anorexia, weight loss,* increased AST, ALT, bilirubin, alkaline phosphatase, jaundice
GU: Vaginitis, urinary frequency
HEMA: **Leukopenia, eosinophilia, agranulocytosis, thrombocytopenia, polyarthritis**
INTEG: Rash, urticaria, pruritus, erythema, pain, abscess at inj site
SYST: **Stevens-Johnson syndrome, exfoliative dermatitis**

Adverse effects: *italic* = common, **bold** = life-threatening

Contraindications: Hypersensitivity to this product or lincomycin, tartrazine dye, ulcerative colitis/enteritis

Black Box Warning: Pseudomembranous colitis

Precautions: Pregnancy **B**, breastfeeding, geriatric, renal/liver/GI disease, asthma, allergy

Black Box Warning: Diarrhea

Pharmacokinetics

Absorption	Well absorbed (PO, IM), minimal (TOP)
Distribution	Widely distributed; crosses placenta
Metabolism	Liver, extensively
Excretion	Kidneys, breast milk
Half-life	2½ hr

Pharmacodynamics

	PO	IM	IV
Onset	Rapid	Rapid	Rapid
Peak	½-1 hr	1½ hr	Infusion's end

Interactions
Individual drugs
Erythromycin, chloramphenicol: decreased action of clindamycin
Kaolin: decreased absorption
Drug classifications
Neuromuscular blockers: increased neuromuscular blockade
Drug/herb
Acidophilus: do not use with antiinfectives; separate by several hours
Drug/lab test
Increased: alkaline phosphatase, bilirubin, CPK, AST, ALT

NURSING CONSIDERATIONS
Assessment
• Assess any patient with compromised renal system; product is excreted slowly in poor renal system function; toxicity may occur rapidly
• Assess patient for signs and symptoms of infection including characteristics of wounds, sputum, urine, stool, WBC >10,000/mm^3, fever; obtain baseline information before, during treatment
• Complete C&S testing before beginning product therapy; this will identify if correct treatment has been initiated
• Assess for allergic reactions: rash, urticaria, pruritus, chills, fever, joint pain; may occur a few days after therapy begins; epinephrine and resuscitation equipment should be available in case of an anaphylactic reaction
• Identify urine output; if decreasing, notify prescriber (may indicate nephrotoxicity); also look for increased BUN and creatinine levels
• Monitor blood studies: AST, ALT, CBC, Hct, bilirubin, LDH, alkaline phosphatase, Coombs' test monthly if patient is on long-term therapy
• Monitor electrolytes: potassium, sodium, chloride monthly if patient is on long-term therapy
• Assess bowel pattern daily; if severe diarrhea occurs, product should be discontinued; may indicate pseudomembranous colitis
• Monitor for bleeding: ecchymosis, bleeding gums, hematuria, stool guaiac daily if on long-term therapy
• Assess for overgrowth of infection: perineal itching, fever, malaise, redness, pain, swelling, drainage, rash, diarrhea, change in cough, sputum

Nursing diagnoses
• Diarrhea (adverse reactions)
• Infection, risk for (uses)
• Injury, risk for (adverse reaction)
• Knowledge, deficient (teaching)
• Noncompliance (teaching)

Implementation
PO route
• Do not break, crush, or chew caps
• Give with 8 oz of water; give with meals for GI symptoms
• Shake liquids well
• Do not refrigerate oral preparations; stable at room temperature for 2 wk
IM route
• If more than 600 mg must be given, divide into 2 inj
• Give deeply in large muscle mass; rotate sites
IV route
• Give by inf only; do not administer BOL dose; dilute 300 mg or more/50 ml or more of D$_5$W, 0.9% NaCl
• May be further diluted in greater amounts of D$_5$W, 0.9% NaCl and given as a cont inf in acute PID; give first dose 10 mg/min over ½ hr, then 0.75 mg/min; increased rates may be used to keep serum blood levels higher; run over >10 min; no more than 1200 mg in a 1 hr inf
Syringe compatibilities: Amikacin, aztreonam, gentamicin, heparin
Syringe incompatibilities: Tobramycin

Y-site compatibilities: Amifostine, amiodarone, amphotericin B cholesteryl, amsacrine, aztreonam, cisatracurium, cyclophosphamide, diltiazem, DOXOrubicin liposome, enalaprilat, esmolol, fludarabine, foscarnet, granisetron, heparin, hydromorphone, labetolol, magnesium sulfate, melphalan, meperidine, midazolam, morphine, multivitamins, odansetron, perphenazine, piperacillin/tazobactam, propofol, remifentanil, sargramostim, tacrolimus, teniposide, theophylline, thiotepa, vinorelbine, vit B/C, zidovudine

Y-site incompatibilities: Idarubicin

Additive compatibilities: Amikacin, ampicillin, aztreonam, cefamandole, cefazolin, cefepine, cefonicid, cefoperazone, cefotaxime, cefoxitin, ceftazidime, ceftizoxime, cefuroxime, cephalothin, cimetidine, fluconazole, heparin, hydrocortisone, kanamycin, methylPREDNISolone, metoclopramide, metronidazole, netilmicin, ofloxacin, penicillin G, pipercillin, potassium chloride, sodium bicarbonate, tobramycin, verapamil, vit B/C

Additive incompatibilities: Ciprofloxacin

Patient/family education
- Tell patient to take oral product with full glass of water; may take with food if GI symptoms occur; antiperistaltic products may worsen diarrhea
- Teach patient aspects of product therapy: need to complete entire course of medication to ensure organism death (10-14 days); culture may be taken after medication course has been completed
- Advise patient to report sore throat, fever, fatigue; may indicate superimposed infection
- Advise patient that product must be taken at equal intervals around clock to maintain blood levels

Evaluation
Positive therapeutic outcome
- Decreased temp, negative C&S

Treatment of hypersensitivity:
Withdraw product; maintain airway; administer epinephrine, aminophylline, O₂, **IV** corticosteroids

clindamycin topical
See Appendix B

clobetasol topical
See Appendix B

*clomiPHENE (Rx)
(kloe'mi-feen)
Clomid, clomiPHENE citrate, Serophene
Func. class.: Ovulation stimulant
Chem. class.: Nonsteroidal antiestrogenic

Pregnancy category X

Do not confuse:
clomiPHENE/clomiPRAMINE

Action: Increases LH, FSH release from the pituitary, which increases maturation of ovarian follicle, ovulation, development of corpus luteum

Therapeutic outcome: Pregnancy

Uses: Female infertility (ovulatory failure)

Dosage and routes
Adult: PO 50-100 mg daily × 5 days or 50-100 mg daily beginning on day 5 of cycle; may be repeated until conception occurs or 3 cycles of therapy have been completed

Available forms: Tabs 50 mg

Adverse effects
CNS: Headache, depression, restlessness, anxiety, nervousness, fatigue, insomnia, dizziness, flushing
CV: Vasomotor flushing, phlebitis, **deep vein thrombosis**
EENT: Blurred vision, diplopia, photophobia
GI: Nausea, vomiting, constipation, abdominal pain, bloating
GU: Polyuria, frequency of urination, **birth defects, spontaneous abortions,** multiple ovulation, breast pain, oliguria, abnormal uterine bleeding, ovarian cyst, hypertrophy of ovary
INTEG: Rash, dermatitis, urticaria, alopecia

Contraindications: Pregnancy X, hypersensitivity, hepatic disease, undiagnosed uterine bleeding, uncontrolled thyroid or adrenal dysfunction, intracranial lesion, ovarian cysts, endometrial carcinoma

Precautions: Hypertension, depression, seizures, diabetes mellitus, abnormal ovarian enlargement, ovarian hyperstimulation

Pharmacokinetics	
Absorption	Well distributed
Distribution	Unknown
Metabolism	Liver, extensively
Excretion	Feces
Half-life	5 days

Adverse effects: *italic* = common, **bold** = life-threatening

Pharmacodynamics
Unknown

Interactions
Drug/lab test
Increased: FSH/LH, BSP, thyroxine, TBG

NURSING CONSIDERATIONS
Assessment
• Determine liver function tests before therapy: AST, ALT, alkaline phosphatase
• Monitor serum progesterone, urinary excretion of pregnanediol to identify occurrence of ovulation
• Pelvic examination should be done to determine ovarian size, cervical condition
• Endometrial biopsy may be done in women over 35 to rule out endometrial carcinoma

Nursing diagnoses
• Knowledge, deficient (teaching)
• Sexual dysfunction (uses)

Implementation
• Give after discontinuing estrogen therapy
• Give at same time daily to maintain product level; begin on 5th day of menstrual cycle

Patient/family education
• Advise patient that multiple births are common after product is taken
• Instruct patient to notify prescriber immediately if low abdominal pain occurs; may indicate ovarian cyst, cyst rupture
• Advise patient to notify prescriber of photophobia, blurred vision, diplopia, abnormal bleeding, hot flashes, nausea, vomiting, headache
• Teach patient if dose is missed, double at next time; if more than one dose is missed, call prescriber
• Instruct patient that response usually occurs 4-10 days after last day of treatment
• Teach patient method for taking, recording basal body temp to determine whether ovulation has occurred; if ovulation can be determined (there is a slight decrease in temp, then a sharp increase for ovulation), to attempt coitus 3 days before and every other day until after ovulation
• Teach patient if pregnancy is suspected, to notify prescriber immediately

Evaluation
Positive therapeutic outcome
• Fertility

*clomiPRAMINE (Rx)
(klom-ip'ra-meen)
Anafranil
Func. class.: Tricyclic antidepressant
Chem. class.: Tertiary amine
Pregnancy category C

Do not confuse:
clomiPRAMINE/clomiPHENE/desipramine/Norpramin

Action: Potentiates serotonin and norepinephrine uptake; also increases dopamine metabolism, moderate anticholinergic effect

Therapeutic outcome: Decreased signs and symptoms of obsessive-compulsive disorder, decreased depression

Uses: Obsessive-compulsive disorder

Unlabeled uses: Dysphoria, anxiety, agoraphobia and other phobias

Dosage and routes
Obsessive-compulsive disorder
Adult: PO 25 mg at bedtime; increase gradually over 4 wk to a dosage of 75-250 mg/day in divided doses
Child 10-18 yr: PO 25-50 mg/day gradually increased or 3 mg/kg/day, whichever is smaller; max 200 mg/day

Available forms: Caps 25, 50, 75 mg

Adverse effects
CNS: Dizziness, tremors, mania, **seizures,** aggressiveness, drowsiness, headache, EPS, **neuroleptic malignant syndrome**
CV: Hypotension, tachycardia, **cardiac arrest**
EENT: Blurred vision
ENDO: Galactorrhea, hyperprolactinemia
GI: Constipation, dry mouth, nausea, dyspepsia, weight gain, **hepatic toxicity**
GU: Delayed ejaculation, anorgasmia, retention, decreased libido
HEMA: **Agranulocytosis, neutropenia, pancytopenia**
INTEG: Diaphoresis, photosensitivity
META: Hyponatremia
SYST: **Suicide in children/adolescents**

Contraindications: Hypersensitivity, immediately after MI

Precautions: Pregnancy C, breastfeeding, geriatric, seizures, suicidal patients, cardiac disease, glaucoma

Black Box Warning: Suicidal ideation, children

C

Pharmacokinetics

Absorption	Well absorbed
Distribution	Widely distributed
Metabolism	Liver, extensively
Excretion	Kidneys, breast milk
Half-life	19-37 hr; steady state 1-2 wk

Pharmacodynamics

Onset	≥2 wk
Peak	2-6 hr
Duration	Unknown

Interactions
Individual drugs
Alcohol: increased CNS depression

Carbamazepine: decreased clomiPRAMINE action

Cimetidine, fluoxetine, fluvoxamine, sertraline: increased clomiPRAMINE level; do not use together

Clonidine, epinephrine, norepinephrine: severe hypertension; avoid use

Clonidine, haloperidol, levodopa: decreased effect of these products

Phenytoin: decreased clomiPRAMINE action

Drug classifications
Barbiturates: decreased clomiPRAMINE levels

CNS depressants, general anesthetics: increased effects; do not use together

CYP1A2, CYP2D6: increased clomiPRAMINE level

MAOIs: hypertensive crisis, seizures; do not use together

Other tricyclics, phenothiazines, quinolones: QT prolongation

Skeletal muscle relaxants, opiates: decreased action of these products

Drug/herb
SAM-e, St. John's wort: serotonin syndrome, do not use together

Belladonna, corkwood, henbane leaf, jimsonweed: increased anticholinergic effect

Hops, kava, lavender: increased sedative effect

Scopolia: increased clomiPRAMINE effect

Drug/lab test
Increased: prolactin, TBG, AST, ALT

Decreased: serum thyroid hormone (T_3, T_4)

NURSING CONSIDERATIONS
Assessment
• Monitor B/P (with patient lying, standing), pulse q4hr; if systolic B/P drops 20 mm Hg hold product, notify prescriber; take VS q4hr in patients with cardiovascular disease

• Monitor blood studies: CBC, leukocytes, differential, cardiac enzymes if patient is receiving long-term therapy

• Monitor hepatic studies: AST, ALT, bilirubin

• Check weight weekly; appetite may increase with product

• Assess ECG for flattening of T wave, QTc prolongation bundle branch block, AV block, dysrhythmias in cardiac patients

• Assess for EPS primarily in geriatric: rigidity, dystonia, akathisia

• Assess mental status: mood, sensorium, affect, suicidal tendencies; increase in psychiatric symptoms: depression, panic, frequency of obsessive-compulsive behaviors

• Monitor urinary retention, constipation; constipation is more likely to occur in children or geriatric

• Assess for withdrawal symptoms: headache, nausea, vomiting, muscle pain, weakness; do not usually occur unless product was discontinued abruptly

• Identify alcohol consumption; if alcohol is consumed, hold dose until morning

Nursing diagnoses
• Coping, ineffective (uses)
• Injury, risk for physical (side effects)
• Knowledge, deficient (teaching)
• Noncompliance (teaching)

Implementation
• Do not break, crush, or chew caps
• Give with food or milk for GI symptoms
• Store at room temperature; do not freeze

Patient/family education
• Teach patient that therapeutic effects may take 4-6 wk

• Teach patient to use caution in driving or other activities requiring alertness because of drowsiness, dizziness, blurred vision; to avoid rising quickly from sitting to standing, especially geriatric

• Teach patient to avoid alcohol ingestion, other CNS depressants

• Teach patient not to discontinue medication quickly after long-term use: may cause nausea, headache, malaise

• Teach patient to wear sunscreen or large hat, since photosensitivity occurs

• Teach patient to increase fluids, bulk in diet if constipation, urinary retention occur, especially geriatric

• Teach patient to take gum, hard sugarless candy, or frequent sips of water for dry mouth

• Advise patient to notify prescriber if pregnancy is planned or suspected

• Teach patient that suicidal ideas, behavior may occur in children/young adults

Adverse effects: *italic* = common, **bold** = life-threatening

Evaluation
Positive therapeutic outcome
- Decrease in depression
- Absence of suicidal thoughts

Treatment of overdose: ECG monitoring, induce emesis, lavage, activated charcoal, administer anticonvulsant

---

clonazepam (Rx)
(kloe-na'zi-pam)
Apo-Clonazepam ✦, Gen-Clonazepam ✦, Klonopin, Klonopin wafers, Novo-Clonazepam ✦, Nu-Clonazepam ✦, PMS-Clonazepam, Rivotril
Func. class.: Anticonvulsant
Chem. class.: Benzodiazepine derivative

Pregnancy category D

Controlled substance schedule IV

Do not confuse:
clonazepam/lorazepam/clorazepate, Klonopin/clonidine

Action: Inhibits spike, wave formation in absence seizures (petit mal), decreases amplitude, frequency, duration, spread of discharge in minor motor seizures

Therapeutic outcome: Decreased frequency, severity of seizures

Uses: Absence, atypical absence, akinetic, myoclonic seizures, Lennox-Gastaut syndrome, panic disorder

Dosage and routes
Adult: PO max 1.5 mg/day in 3 divided doses; may be increased 0.5-1 mg q3day until desired response; max 20 mg/day; RECT 0.02 mg/kg
Child <10 yr or <30 kg: PO 0.01-0.03 mg/kg/day in divided doses q8hr, max 0.05 mg/kg/day; may be increased 0.25-0.5 mg q3day until desired response; max 0.1-0.2 mg/kg/day; RECT 0.05-0.1 mg/kg
Geriatric: PO 0.25 daily bid initially, increase by 0.25 daily q7-14day as needed

Available forms: Tabs 0.5, 1, 2 mg; orally disintegrating tabs 0.125, 0.25, 0.5, 1, 2 mg, wafer 0.125, 0.25, 0.5, 1, 2 mg

Adverse effects
CNS: Drowsiness, dizziness, confusion, behavioral changes, tremors, insomnia, headache, **suicidal tendencies,** slurred speech, anterograde amnesia
CV: Palpitations, bradycardia, tachycardia

EENT: Increased salivation, nystagmus, diplopia, abnormal eye movements
GI: Nausea, constipation, polyphagia, anorexia, xerostomia, diarrhea, gastritis, sore gums
GU: Dysuria, enuresis, nocturia, retention, libido changes
HEMA: **Thrombocytopenia, leukocytosis, eosinophilia**
INTEG: Rash, alopecia, hirsutism
RESP: **Respiratory depression,** dyspnea, congestion

Contraindications: Pregnancy **D,** hypersensitivity to benzodiazepines, acute closed-angle glaucoma, psychosis, severe liver disease

Precautions: Open-angle glaucoma, chronic respiratory disease, renal/hepatic disease, breastfeeding, geriatric

Pharmacokinetics
Absorption	Well absorbed
Distribution	Crosses blood-brain barrier, placenta
Metabolism	Liver, protein binding 85%
Excretion	Kidneys
Half-life	18-50 hr

Pharmacodynamics
Onset	½-1 hr
Peak	1-2 hr
Duration	6-12 hr

Interactions
Individual drugs
Alcohol: increased CNS depression
Carbamazepine: decreased clonazepam effect
Cimetidine, clarithromycin, diltiazem, erythromycin, fluoxetine: increased clonazepam effect
Phenobarbitol: decreased clonazepam effect
Phenytoin: decreased clonazepam levels
Drug classifications
Anticonvulsants, antidepressants, barbiturates, general anesthetics, opiates, sedative/hypnotics: increased CNS depression
Azoles, oral contraceptives: increased clonazepam effect
CYP3A4 inducers: decreased clonazepam effect
Drug/herb
Ginkgo, melatonin: increased clonazepam effect
Ginseng, santonica, St. John's wort: decreased clonazepam effect
Kava: increased sedative effect
Drug/lab test
Increased: AST, alkaline phosphatase

NURSING CONSIDERATIONS
Assessment
🔷 Assess mental status: mood, sensorium, affect, memory (long, short), especially geriatric; behavioral changes, suicidal thoughts/behaviors
• Assess for blood dyscrasias: fever, sore throat, bruising, rash, jaundice, epistaxis (long-term treatment only)
• Assess seizure activity including type, location, duration, and character; provide seizure precaution
• Assess renal studies: urinalysis, BUN, urine creatinine
• Monitor blood studies: RBCs, Hct, Hgb, reticulocyte counts weekly for 4 wk, then monthly
• Monitor hepatic studies: ALT, AST, bilirubin, creatinine
• Monitor product levels during initial treatment
• Assess for signs of physical withdrawal if medication suddenly discontinued
• Assess eye problems: need for ophthalmic examinations before, during, after treatment (slit lamp, fundoscopy, tonometry)
• Assess allergic reaction: red raised rash; if this occurs, product should be discontinued
• Monitor for toxicity: bone marrow depression, nausea, vomiting, ataxia, diplopia, cardiovascular collapse

Nursing diagnoses
• Injury, risk for (side effects)
• Knowledge, deficient (teaching)

Implementation
PO route
• Give on empty stomach for best absorption
Rectal route
• **IV** sol may be used rectally, 1 ml syringe inserted 3 cm into rectum
• Oral susp may be used rectally (1 mg/ml of product with 1 ml of water), use plastic tube (volume 2.2-3.3 ml)

Patient/family education
• Teach patient to carry/wear emergency ID card stating patient's name, products taken, condition, physician's name, phone number
• Caution patient to avoid driving, other activities that require alertness
• Caution patient to avoid alcohol ingestion or CNS depressants; increased sedation may occur
• Teach patient not to discontinue medication quickly after long-term use; taper off over several weeks

Evaluation
Positive therapeutic outcome
• Decreased seizure activity

Treatment of overdose: Lavage, activated charcoal, VS, flumazenil, monitor electrolytes

---

clonidine 🔄 (Rx)
(klon'i-deen)
Apo-Clonidine ✦, Catapres, Catapres-TTS, clonidine HCl, Dixarit ✦, Duraclon, Novo-Clonidine ✦, Nu-Clonidine ✦
Func. class.: Antihypertensive, centrally acting analgesic
Chem. class.: Centrally acting α-adrenergic agonist

Pregnancy category C

Do not confuse:
clonidine/Klonopin/clonazepam, Catapres/Cataflam/catarase

Action: Inhibits sympathetic vasomotor center in CNS, which reduces impulses in sympathetic nervous system; B/P, pulse rate, cardiac output decreased; prevents pain signal transmission in CNS by α-adrenergic receptor stimulation of the spinal cord

Therapeutic outcome: Decreased B/P in hypertension

Uses: Mild to moderate hypertension, used alone or in combination; severe pain in cancer patients (epidural)

Unlabeled uses: Opioid withdrawal, prevention of vascular headaches, treatment of menopausal symptoms, dysmenorrhea, attention deficit hyperactivity disorder (ADHD), autism, cycloSPORINE nephrotoxicity prophylaxis, diabetic neuropathy, ethanol withdrawal, Tourette's syndrome, hypertensive emergency

Dosage and routes
Hypertension
Adult: PO/TD 0.1 mg bid, then increase by 0.1-0.2 mg/day at weekly intervals, until desired response; range 0.2-0.6 mg/day in divided doses
Geriatric: PO 0.1 mg at bedtime, may increase gradually
Child: PO 5-10 mcg/kg/day in divided doses q8-12hr, max 0.9 mg/day

Opioid withdrawal (unlabeled)
Adult: PO 0.3-1.2 mg/day; may decrease by 50% × 3 days, then decrease by 0.1-0.2 mg/day or discontinue

Adverse effects: *italic* = common, **bold** = life-threatening

Severe pain
Adult: CONT EPIDURAL INF 30 mcg/hr
Child: CONT EPIDURAL INF 0.5 mcg/kg/hr,
then titrate to response

Menopausal symptoms (unlabeled)
Adult: TD 0.1 mg patch q1wk; PO 0.05-0.4 mg daily

ADHD/tic disorders in children/ autism (unlabeled)
Child: PO 0.05 mg/kg/day in 3-4 divided doses × 8 wk, max 0.3 mg/day

Tourette's syndrome (unlabeled)
Adult: PO 0.15-0.2 mg/day

Available forms: Tabs 0.025 ♣, 0.1, 0.2, 0.3 mg; transdermal sys 2.5, 5, 7.5 mg delivering 0.1, 0.2, 0.3 mg/24 hr, respectively; inj 100, 500 mcg/ml

Adverse effects
CNS: Drowsiness, sedation, headache, fatigue, nightmares, insomnia, mental changes, anxiety, depression, hallucinations, delirium
CV: Orthostatic hypotension, palpitations,
CHF: ECG abnormalities
EENT: Taste change, parotid pain
ENDO: Hyperglycemia
GI: Nausea, vomiting, malaise, constipation, *dry mouth*
GU: Impotence, dysuria, *nocturia,* gynecomastia
INTEG: Rash, alopecia, facial pallor, pruritus, hives, edema, burning papules, excoriation (TD patches)
MISC: Withdrawal symptoms
MS: Muscle, joint pain, leg cramps

Contraindications: Hypersensitivity; (epidural) bleeding disorders, anticoagulants

Precautions: Pregnancy **C**, breastfeeding, child <12 yr (transdermal), geriatric, MI (recent), diabetes mellitus, chronic renal failure, Raynaud's disease, thyroid disease, depression, COPD, asthma, noncompliant patients

Black Box Warning: Labor

Pharmacokinetics	
Absorption	Well absorbed (PO, TD)
Distribution	Widely distributed; crosses blood-brain barrier
Metabolism	Liver, extensively
Excretion	Kidneys, unchanged (30%)
Half-life	12-21 hr

Pharmacodynamics		
	PO	TD
Onset	½-1 hr	3 days
Peak	2-4 hr	Unknown
Duration	8-12 hr	8 hr (after removal)

Interactions
Individual drugs
Alcohol: increased CNS depression
Levodopa: decreased levodopa effect
Prazosin: decreased hypotensive effects
Verapamil: AV block
Drug classifications
Amphetamines, appetite suppressants, MAOIs, tricyclics: decreased hypotensive effects
Anesthetics, opiates, sedatives/hypnotics: increased CNS depression
Antidepressants (tricyclic), β-adrenergic blockers: life-threatening increase in B/P
Diuretics, nitrates: increased hypotensive effects
Drug/herb
Aconite: increased toxicity, death
Astragalus, capsicum peppers, cola tree, coltsfoot, guarana, khat, licorice: decreased antihypertensive effect
Barberry, betony, black catechu, black cohosh, bloodroot, broom, burdock, cat's claw, dandelion, goldenseal, hawthorn, Irish moss, Jamaican dogwood, kelp, khella, mistletoe, parsley, Queen Anne's lace, rue: increased antihypertensive effect
Drug/lab test
Increased: blood glucose
Decreased: VMA, urinary catecholamines, aldosterone

NURSING CONSIDERATIONS
Assessment
• Assess pain: location, intensity, character, alleviating, aggravation factors, baseline and frequency
• Perform blood studies: neutrophils, decreased platelets
• Perform renal studies: protein, BUN, creatinine; watch for increased levels that may indicate nephrotic syndrome: polyuria, oliguria, frequency
• Monitor baselines for renal/liver function tests before therapy begins; check potassium levels, although hyperkalemia rarely occurs
• Monitor B/P, pulse if the product is being used for hypertension; notify prescriber of changes
• Assess for opiate withdrawal in patients receiving the product for opioid withdrawal, including fever, diarrhea, nausea, vomiting,

cramps, insomnia, shivering, dilated pupils, weakness
• Check for edema in feet, legs daily; monitor I&O; check for decreasing output
• Note allergic reaction: rash, fever, pruritus, urticaria; product should be discontinued if antihistamines fail to help
• Note allergic reaction from patches: rash, urticaria, angioedema; should not continue to use
• Assess for symptoms of CHF: edema; dyspnea, wet crackles, B/P, weight gain, report significant changes

Nursing diagnoses
• Injury, risk for physical (side effects)
• Knowledge, deficient (teaching)
• Noncompliance (teaching)

Implementation
PO route
• Give last dose at bedtime
Transdermal route
• Apply patch weekly; remove old patch and wash off residue; apply to site without hair; best absorption over chest or upper arm; rotate sites with each application; clean site before application; apply firmly, especially around edges
• Store patches in cool environment, tabs in tight container

Patient/family education
• Instruct patient not to discontinue product abruptly, or withdrawal symptoms may occur: anxiety, increased B/P, headache, insomnia, increased pulse, tremors, nausea, sweating
• Caution patient not to use OTC (cough, cold, or allergy) products unless directed by prescriber
• Teach patient to comply with dosage schedule even if feeling better; product controls symptoms, does not cure
• Caution patient to change position slowly, to rise slowly to sitting or standing position to minimize orthostatic hypotension, especially geriatric
• Instruct patient to notify physician of mouth sores, sore throat, fever, swelling of hands or feet, irregular heartbeat, chest pain, signs of angioedema, increased weight
• Teach patient about excessive perspiration, dehydration, vomiting; diarrhea may lead to fall in B/P; consult prescriber if these occur
• Tell patient that product may cause dizziness, fainting; light-headedness may occur during first few days of therapy; use hard candy, saliva product, or frequent rinsing of mouth for dry mouth

• Advise patient that compliance is necessary; not to skip or stop product unless directed by prescriber
• Teach patient that product may cause skin rash or impaired perspiration
• Teach patient that response may take 2-3 days if product is given TD; instruct on administration of patch; return demonstration
• Teach patient to avoid hazardous activities, since product may cause drowsiness, dizziness
• Teach patient to administer 1 hr before meals

Evaluation
Positive therapeutic outcome
• Decrease in B/P in hypertension
• Decrease in withdrawal symptoms
• Decrease in pain
• Decrease in vascular headaches
• Decrease in dysmenorrhea
• Decrease in menopausal symptoms

Treatment of overdose: Supportive treatment; administer tolazoline, atropine, DOPamine prn

---

clopidogrel (Rx)
(klo-pid'oh-grel)
Plavix
Func. class.: Platelet aggregation inhibitor
Chem. class.: Thienopyridine derivative
Pregnancy category B

Action: Inhibits first and second phases of ADP-induced effects in platelet aggregation

Therapeutic outcome: Decreased possibility of stroke, MI by decreasing platelet aggregation

Uses: Reducing the risk of stroke, MI, peripheral arterial disease in high-risk patients, acute coronary syndrome, transient ischemic attack (TIA), unstable angina

Dosage and routes
Recent MI, stroke, peripheral arterial disease
Adult: PO 75 mg daily with or without aspirin

Acute coronary syndrome
Adult: PO loading dose 300 mg then 75 mg daily with aspirin

Available forms: Tabs 75 mg

Adverse effects
CNS: Headache, dizziness, depression, syncope, hyperesthesia, neuralgia
CV: Edema, hypertension, chest pain

Adverse effects: *italic* = common, **bold** = life-threatening

GI: Nausea, vomiting, diarrhea, GI discomfort, **GI bleeding, pancreatitis**
GU: **Glomerulonephritis**
HEMA: *Epistaxis,* purpura, **bleeding, neutropenia, aplastic anemia**
INTEG: Rash, pruritus
MISC: UTI, hypercholesterolemia, chest pain, fatigue, **intracranial hemorrhage, toxic epidermal necrolysis, Stevens-Johnson syndrome,** flu-like syndrome
MS: Arthralgia, back pain
RESP: Upper respiratory tract infection, dyspnea, rhinitis, bronchitis, cough, **bronchospasm**

Contraindications: Hypersensitivity, active bleeding

Precautions: Pregnancy **B,** breastfeeding, children, past liver disease, increased bleeding risk, neutropenia, agranulocytosis, renal disease, Asian/Black/Caucasian patients

Pharmacokinetics	
Absorption	Rapidly absorbed
Distribution	Unknown
Metabolism	Liver, extensively, protein binding 95%
Excretion	Kidneys, unchanged product
Half-life	8 hr

Pharmacodynamics	
Onset	Unknown
Peak	1-3 hr
Duration	Unknown

Interactions
Individual drugs
Abciximab, aspirin, eptifibatide, rifampin, ticlopidine, tirofiban, treprostinil: increased bleeding tendencies
Fluvastatin, phenytoin, tamoxifen, TOLBUTamide, torsemide, warfarin: increased action of each specific product
Drug classifications
Anticoagulants, NSAIDs, SSRIs, thrombolytics: increased bleeding tendencies
CYP3A4 inhibitors/substrates (atorvastatin, cerivistatin, simvistatin): decreased effects
CYP2C19 inhibitors: avoid use
NSAIDs: increased action of some NSAIDs
Drug/herb
Arginine: increased gastric irritation
Bilberry, saw palmetto: decreased clopidogrel effect
Bogbean, dong quai, feverfew, garlic, ginger, ginkgo biloba, green tea, horse chestnut: increased clopidogrel effect

Drug/lab test
Increased: AST, ALT, bilirubin, uric acid, total cholesterol, nonprotein nitrogen (NPN)

NURSING CONSIDERATIONS
Assessment
• Assess for symptoms of stroke, MI during treatment
• Monitor liver function tests: AST, ALT, bilirubin, creatinine if patient is on long-term therapy (4 mo or more)
• Monitor blood studies: CBC, Hct, Hgb, protime, cholesterol if patient is on long-term therapy; thrombocytopenia, neutropenia may occur

Nursing diagnoses
• Injury, risk for (uses)
• Knowledge, deficient (teaching)

Implementation
• Give with food to decrease gastric symptoms

Patient/family education
• Advise patient that blood work will be necessary during treatment
• Advise patient to report any unusual bleeding to prescriber, that it may take longer to stop bleeding
• Instruct patient to take with food or just after eating to minimize GI discomfort
• Caution patient to report diarrhea, skin rashes, subcutaneous bleeding, chills, fever, sore throat
• Teach patient to tell all health care providers that clopidogrel is used

Evaluation
Positive therapeutic outcome
• Absence of stroke

---

clorazepate (Rx)
(klor-az′e-pate)
APO-Clorazepate ✦, clorazepate, Novo-Clopate ✦, Gen-XENE, Tranxene, Tranxene-SD, Tranxene-SD Half Strength, Tranxene T-tab
Func. class.: Antianxiety, anticonvulsant, sedative/hypnotic
Chem. class.: Benzodiazepine, long-acting

Pregnancy category D
Controlled substance schedule IV

Do not confuse:
clorazepate/clonazepam

Action: Potentiates the actions of GABA; especially in limbic system, reticular formation has anticonvulsant effects

 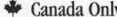

Therapeutic outcome: Decreased anxiety, restlessness, insomnia

Uses: Anxiety, acute alcohol withdrawal, adjunct in seizure disorders

Unlabeled uses: Insomnia

Dosage and routes
Anxiety
Adult: PO 15-60 mg/day in divided doses or 7.5 mg tid; EXT REL 11.25-22.5 mg at bedtime, do not use EXT REL to initiate therapy
Geriatric: PO 7.5 mg daily bid

Alcohol withdrawal
Adult: Day 1, PO 30 mg then 30-60 mg in divided doses; day 2, 45-90 mg in divided doses; day 3, 22.5-45 mg in divided doses; day 4, 15-30 mg in divided doses; then gradually reduce daily dose to 7.5-15 mg

Seizure disorders
Adult and child >12 yr: PO 7.5 mg tid; may increase by 7.5 mg/wk or less, max 90 mg/day
Child 9-12 yr: PO 3.75-7.5 mg bid; may increase by 3.75 mg/wk or less, max 60 mg/day

Insomnia (unlabeled)
Adult: PO 7.5-15 mg at bedtime
Geriatric: PO 3.75-7.5 mg at bedtime, max 15 mg at bedtime

Available forms: Tabs 3.75, 7.5, 15 mg; ext rel tab (Tranxene SD Half Strength) 11.25 mg, (Tranxene SD) 22.5 mg

Adverse effects
CNS: Dizziness, drowsiness, confusion, headache, anxiety, tremors, stimulation, fatigue, depression, insomnia, hallucinations, lethargy
CV: Orthostatic hypotension, **ECG changes, tachycardia,** hypotension, chest pain
EENT: Blurred vision, tinnitus, mydriasis
GI: Constipation, dry mouth, nausea, vomiting, anorexia, diarrhea
INTEG: Rash, dermatitis, itching

Contraindications: Pregnancy **D,** breastfeeding, children <9 yr, hypersensitivity to benzodiazepines, closed-angle glaucoma, psychosis

Precautions: Geriatric, debilitated, renal/hepatic disease, suicidal ideation, dependency problems

Pharmacokinetics	
Absorption	Well absorbed
Distribution	Widely distributed, crosses placenta, 97% protein binding
Metabolism	Liver
Excretion	Kidneys, breast milk
Half-life	30-200 hr

Pharmacodynamics	
Onset	1 hr
Peak	1-2 hr
Duration	Up to 24 hr

Interactions
Individual drugs
Alcohol: increased CNS depression
Cimetidine, disulfiram, fluoxetine, isoniazid, ketoconazole, propoxyphene, valproic acid: increased effects of clorazepate
Rifampin: decreased action of clorazepate
Drug classifications
Antidepressants, β-blockers (some), CYP3A4 inhibitors, MAOIs, oral contraceptives: increased clorazepate action
Barbiturates: decreased clorazepate effect
CNS depressants: increased CNS depression
Drug/herb
Catnip, chamomile, clary, cowslip, kava, mistletoe, nettle, pokeweed, poppy, Queen Anne's lace, senega, St. John's wort, valerian: increased CNS depression
Black cohosh: increased hypotension
Drug/lab test
Increased: AST/ALT
Decreased: HCT

NURSING CONSIDERATIONS
Assessment
• Assess seizures: duration, location, intensity, aura
• Monitor B/P (with patient lying, standing), pulse; if systolic B/P drops 20 mm Hg, hold product, notify prescriber
• Monitor blood studies: CBC during long-term therapy; blood dyscrasias have occurred rarely
• Monitor hepatic studies: AST, ALT, bilirubin, creatinine, LDH, alkaline phosphatase
• Monitor I&O; may indicate renal dysfunction
• Monitor mental status: mood, sensorium, affect, sleeping pattern, drowsiness, dizziness, physical dependency; withdrawal symptoms: headache, nausea, vomiting, muscle pain, weakness after long-term use; suicidal tendencies

Adverse effects: *italic* = common, **bold** = life-threatening

Nursing diagnoses
- Coping, ineffective (uses)
- Knowledge, deficient (teaching)
- Noncompliance (teaching)

Implementation
- Give with food or milk for GI symptoms
- Give crushed if patient cannot swallow whole (tab only)
- Do not use Tranxene SD to start treatment
- Use sugarless gum, hard candy, frequent sips of water for dry mouth
- Check to see PO medication has been swallowed

Patient/family education
- Teach patient that product may be taken with food
- Teach patient not to use for everyday stress or longer than 4 mo, unless directed by a prescriber; not to take more than prescribed amount; may be habit forming
- Caution patient to avoid OTC preparations unless approved by a prescriber
- Caution patient to avoid driving, activities that require alertness; drowsiness may occur, especially in geriatric
- Advise patient to avoid alcohol ingestion or other psychotropic medications, unless prescribed
- Advise patient not to discontinue medication abruptly after long-term use; restlessness, insomnia, irritability may occur
- Advise patient to rise slowly; fainting may occur
- Teach patient that drowsiness may worsen at beginning of treatment

Evaluation
Positive therapeutic outcome
- Decreased anxiety, restlessness
- Decreased seizure activity

Treatment of overdose: Lavage, VS, supportive care, flumazenil

---

clotrimazole topical
See Appendix B

---

clotrimazole vaginal antifungal
See Appendix B

---

clozapine (Rx)
(kloz'a-peen)
clozapine, Clozaril, Fazaclo
Func. class.: Antipsychotic
Chem. class.: Tricyclic dibenzodiazepine derivative

Pregnancy category B

Do not confuse:
Clozaril/Clinoril/Colazal

Action: Interferes with dopamine receptor binding with lack of EPS and tardive dyskinesia; also acts as an adrenergic, cholinergic, histaminergic, serotonergic antagonist

Therapeutic outcome: Decreased psychotic behavior

Uses: Management of psychotic symptoms in schizophrenic patients for whom other antipsychotics have failed, recurrent suicidal behavior; orally disintegrating tabs are not used for recurrent suicidal behavior

Unlabeled uses: Agitation, bipolar disorder, dementia, tremor in Parkinson's disease

Dosage and routes
Adult: PO 12.5 mg daily or bid; may increase by 25-50 mg/day; normal range 300-450 mg/day after 2 wk; do not increase dosage more than 2 times/wk; max 900 mg/day; use lowest dosage to control symptoms

Tremor in Parkinson's disease (unlabeled)
Adult: PO 40 mg at bedtime

Dementia with multiple behavioral disturbances (unlabeled)
Geriatric: PO 12.5 mg qd at bedtime, may increase by 12.5 mg every other day; max 50 mg/day

Available forms: Tabs 12.5, 25, 50, 100, 200 mg; orally disintegrating tabs 25, 100 mg

Adverse effects
CNS: Sedation, salivation, dizziness, headache, tremors, sleep problems, akinesia, fever, **seizures,** *sweating, akathisia, confusion, fatigue, insomnia, depression, slurred speech, anxiety,* **neuroleptic malignant syndrome,** agitation
CV: Tachycardia, hypo/hypertension, chest pain, ECG changes, orthostatic hypotension
EENT: Blurred vision
GI: Drooling or excessive salivation, constipation, nausea, abdominal discomfort, vomiting, diarrhea, anorexia, weight gain, dry

mouth, heartburn, dyspepsia, gastroesophageal reflux
GU: Urinary abnormalities, incontinence, ejaculation dysfunction, frequency, urgency, retention, dysuria
HEMA: Leukopenia, neutropenia, agranulocytosis, eosinophilia
MS: Weakness; pain in back, neck, legs; spasm; rigidity
RESP: Dyspnea, nasal congestion
OTHER: Diaphoresis

Contraindications: Hypersensitivity, severe granulocytopenia (WBC <3500/mm^3 before therapy), coma

Black Box Warning: Myeloproliferative disorders, CNS depression, uncontrolled epilepsy

Precautions: Pregnancy **B**, breastfeeding, children <16 yr, geriatric, renal/hepatic/cardiac/CV/pulmonary disease, seizures, prostatic enlargement, closed-angle glaucoma

Pharmacokinetics

Absorption	Well absorbed
Distribution	Widely distributed; crosses blood-brain barrier, placenta; 95% protein binding
Metabolism	Liver, CYP1A2, 2D6, 3A4
Excretion	Kidneys (50%), feces (30%) (metabolites)
Half-life	8-12 hr

Pharmacodynamics

Onset	Unknown
Peak	Unknown
Duration	8-12 hr

Interactions
Individual drugs
Alcohol: increased CNS depression
Caffeine, citalopram, erythromycin, fluoxetine, fluvoxamine, ketoconazole, risperidone, ritonavir, sertraline: increased clozapine levels
Carbamazepine, omeprazole, phenobarbital, rifampin: decreased clozapine level
Digoxin: increased plasma concentration of digoxin
Warfarin: increased plasma concentrations
Drug classifications
Benzodiazepines: increased hypotension, respiratory, cardiac arrest, collapse
CNS depressants, psychoactives: increased CNS depression
CYP1A2 inducers: decreased clozapine levels
CYP1A2 inhibitors, CYP3A4 inhibitors: increased clozapine level

Highly protein-bound products: increased plasma concentrations
Drug/herb
Betel palm, kava: increased EPS
Cola tree, hops, nettle, nutmeg: increased clozapine action
Kava, St. John's wort: increased CNS depression
Drug/food
Caffeine: increased clozapine levels
Drug/lab test
Increased: liver function tests, cardiac enzymes, cholesterol, blood glucose, bilirubin, PBI, cholinesterase, ^{131}I
False positive: pregnancy tests, PKU
False negative: urinary steroids, 17-OHCS

NURSING CONSIDERATIONS
Assessment
• Assess mental status: orientation, mood, behavior, presence of hallucinations, and type before initial administration and monthly; this product should significantly reduce psychotic behavior
• Check for swallowing of PO medication; check for hoarding or giving of medication to other patients
• Monitor I&O ratio; palpate bladder if low urinary output occurs, especially in geriatric; urinalysis recommended before, during prolonged therapy
• Monitor bilirubin, CBC, liver function test monthly; discontinue treatment if WBC <3000/mm^3 or if ANC <1500/mm^3; test qwk; may resume when normal; if WBC <2000/mm^3 or ANC <1000/mm^3, discontinue
• Assess affect, orientation, LOC, reflexes, gait, coordination, sleep pattern disturbances
• Monitor B/P with patient sitting, standing, and lying; take pulse and respirations q4hr during initial treatment; establish baseline before starting treatment; report drops of 30 mm Hg
• Check for dizziness, faintness, palpitations, tachycardia on rising
• Assess for neuroleptic malignant syndrome: hyperpyrexia, muscle rigidity, increased CPK, altered mental status; product should be discontinued
• Assess for EPS including akathisia (inability to sit still, no pattern to movements), tardive dyskinesia (bizarre movements of the jaw, mouth, tongue, extremities), pseudoparkinsonism (rigidity, tremors, pill rolling, shuffling gate)
• Assess for constipation, urinary retention daily; if these occur, increase bulk, water in diet

Adverse effects: *italic* = common, **bold** = life-threatening

Nursing diagnoses
- Coping, ineffective (uses)
- Knowledge, deficient (teaching)
- Noncompliance (teaching)
- Thought processes, disturbed (uses)

Implementation
- Decrease dosage in geriatric since metabolism is slowed
- Give with full glass of water, milk; or give with food to decrease GI upset
- Store in tight, light-resistant container; oral sol in amber bottle
- Patient-specific registration is required before administration; if WBC <3500 cells/mm³ or ANC <2000 cells/mm², therapy should not be started

Patient/family education
- Teach patient to use good oral hygiene; frequent rinsing of mouth, sugarless gum for dry mouth
- Caution patient to avoid hazardous activities until product response is determined
- Inform patient that orthostatic hypotension occurs often and to rise from sitting or lying position gradually
- Caution patient to avoid hot tubs, hot showers, tub baths, since hypotension may occur
- Teach patient to avoid OTC preparations (cough, hay fever, cold) unless approved by prescriber, since serious product interactions may occur; avoid use with alcohol, CNS depressants; increased drowsiness may occur
- Teach patient about EPS and necessity of meticulous oral hygiene, since oral candidiasis may occur
- Teach patient to report sore throat, malaise, fever, bleeding, mouth sores; if these occur, CBC should be performed and product discontinued
- Advise patient that in hot weather, heat stroke may occur; take extra precautions to stay cool
- Teach patient symptoms of agranulocytosis and need for blood test qwk for 6 mo, then q2wk; report flulike symptoms

Evaluation
Positive therapeutic outcome
- Decrease in emotional excitement, hallucinations, delusions, paranoia
- Reorganization of patterns of thought, speech

Treatment of anaphylaxis: Withdraw product, maintain airway; if diabetic, check blood glucose levels

---

codeine (Rx)
(koe'deen)
Paveral ✦
Func. class.: Opiate, phenanthrene derivative

Pregnancy category C

Controlled substance schedule II, III, IV, V (depends on content)

Do not confuse:
codeine/Lodine/Iodine/Cardene

Action: Depresses pain impulse transmission at the spinal cord level by interacting with opioid receptors; decreases cough reflex, GI motility

Therapeutic outcome: Pain relief, decreased cough, decreased diarrhea depending on route

Uses: Moderate to severe pain

Unlabeled uses: Diarrhea, nonproductive cough

Dosage and routes
Pain
Adult: PO IM/SUBCUT 15-60 mg q4hr prn
Child: PO 6-17 yr 3 mg/kg/day in divided doses q4hr prn

Cough
Adult: PO 10-20 mg q4-6hr, max 120 mg/day

Renal dose
Adult: PO CCr 10-50 ml/min 75% of dose; CCr <10 ml/min 50% of dose

Diarrhea (unlabeled)
Adult: PO 30 mg; may repeat qid prn

Available forms: Inj tab 30, 60 mg; tabs 15, 30, 60 mg; inj 15, 30 mg/ml

Adverse effects
CNS: Drowsiness, sedation, dizziness, agitation, dependency, lethargy, restlessness, euphoria, **seizures,** hallucinations, headache, confusion
CV: Bradycardia, palpitations, orthostatic hypotension, tachycardia, **circulatory collapse**
GI: Nausea, vomiting, anorexia, constipation, dry mouth
GU: Urinary retention
INTEG: Flushing, rash, urticaria, pruritus
RESP: **Respiratory depression, respiratory paralysis,** dyspnea
SYST: Anaphylaxis

Contraindications: Hypersensitivity to opiates, respiratory depression, increased

---

 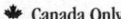

intracranial pressure, seizure disorders, severe respiratory disorders, breastfeeding

Precautions: Pregnancy **C**, geriatric, cardiac dysrhythmias, prostatic hypertrophy, bowel impacton

Pharmacokinetics

Absorption	Bioavailability 60%-90%
Distribution	Widely distributed; crosses placenta, protein binding 7%
Metabolism	Liver, extensively by CYP3A4; altered in ethnic groups
Excretion	Kidneys (up to 15%), breast milk
Half-life	3-4 hr

Pharmacodynamics

	PO	IM	SUBCUT
Onset	30-60 min	30-60 min	15-30 min
Peak	1-2 hr	30-60 min	Unknown
Duration	4 hr	4 hr	4 hr

Interactions
Individual drugs
Alcohol: increased CNS depression
Drug classifications
Antipsychotics, CYP2D6, hypnotics, opiates, sedative/skeletal muscle relaxants: increased CNS depression
MAOIs: increased toxicity; use cautiously
Drug/herb
Corkwood: increased anticholinergic effects
Gotu kola, Jamaican dogwood, kava, lavender, mistletoe, nettle, pokeweed, poppy, senega, valerian: increased CNS depression
St. John's wort: decreased codeine level
Drug/lab test
Increased: amylase, lipase

NURSING CONSIDERATIONS
Assessment
- Assess pain: intensity, type, alleviating factors
- Assess GI function: nausea, vomiting, constipation
- Assess cough: type, duration, ability to raise secretion for productive cough; do not use to suppress a productive cough
- Monitor VS after parenteral route; note muscle rigidity, product history, renal/hepatic function tests, respiratory dysfunction: respiratory depression, character, rate, rhythm; notify prescriber if respirations are <10/min
- Monitor CNS changes: dizziness, drowsiness, hallucinations, euphoria, LOC, pupil reaction
- Monitor allergic reactions: rash, urticaria

Nursing diagnoses
- Breathing pattern, ineffective (adverse reactions)
- Knowledge, deficient (teaching)
- Pain, acute (uses)
- Sensory perception, disturbed (adverse reactions)

Implementation
- Give with antiemetic if nausea, vomiting occur
- Administer when pain is beginning to return, determine dosage interval by patient response; continuous dosing of medication is more effective given prn; explain analgesic effect
- Medication should be slowly withdrawn after long-term use to prevent withdrawal symptoms
- Store in light-resistant container at room temp
PO route
- May be given with food or milk to lessen GI upset
IM/SUBCUT route
- Do not give if cloudy, or a precipitate has formed
IV route
- Give slowly by direct inj
Syringe compatibilities: Dimenhydrinate, glycopyrrolate, hydrOXYzine
Y-site compatibilities: Cefmetazole
Additive incompatibilities: Aminophylline, amobarbital, chlorothiazide, heparin, methicillin, pentobarbital, phenobarbital, phenytoin, secobarbital, thiopental

Patient/family education
- Teach patient to report any symptoms of CNS changes, allergic reactions; to avoid CNS depressants: alcohol, sedative/hypnotics for at least 24 hr after taking this product
- Discuss with patient that dizziness, drowsiness, and confusion are common
- Advise patient to avoid getting up without assistance
- Discuss in detail with patient all aspects of the product
- Advise patient not to breastfeed

Evaluation
Positive therapeutic outcome
- Decreased pain
- Decreased cough
- Decreased diarrhea

Treatment of overdose: Naloxone 0.4 ampule diluted in 10 ml 0.9% NaCl and given by direct **IV** push 0.02 mg q2min (adult)

Adverse effects: *italic* = common, **bold** = life-threatening

colchicine (Rx)
(kol'chi-seen)
Colcrys, Colsalide
Func. class.: Antigout agent
Chem. class.: Colchicum autumnale
alkaloid

Pregnancy category C

Action: Inhibits microtubule formation of lactic acid in leukocytes, which decreases phagocytosis and inflammation in joints

Therapeutic outcome: Decreased pain, inflammation of joints

Uses: Gout, gouty arthritis (prevention, treatment); to arrest progression of neurologic disability in multiple sclerosis

Unlabeled uses: Hepatic cirrhosis, familial Mediterranean fever, pericarditis, amyloidosis, Behçet's syndrome, biliary cirrhosis, dermatitis herpetiformis, idiopathic thrombocytopenic purpura, Paget's disease, pseudogout, pulmonary fibrosis

Dosage and routes
Gout prevention
Adult: PO 0.6-1.8 mg daily depending on severity

Gout treatment
Adult: PO 0.6-1.2 mg, then 0.5-1.2 mg q1hr, until pain decreases or side effects occur

Renal dose
Adult: PO CCr <30 ml/min for acute gout, do not repeat course for 2 wk, familial Mediterranean fever 0.3 mg daily, increase cautiously

Available forms: Tabs 0.5, 0.6, 1 mg ✦

Adverse effects
GI: Nausea, vomiting, anorexia, malaise, metallic taste, cramps, peptic ulcer, diarrhea
GU: Hematuria, **oliguria, renal damage**
HEMA: **Agranulocytosis, thrombocytopenia, aplastic anemia, pancytopenia**
INTEG: Chills, dermatitis, pruritus, purpura, erythema
MISC: Myopathy, alopecia, reversible azoospermia, peripheral neuritis

Contraindications: Hypersensitivity; serious GI disorders, severe renal/hepatic/cardiac disorders

Precautions: Pregnancy C, breastfeeding, children, geriatric, blood dyscrasias, hepatic disease

Pharmacokinetics

Absorption	Well absorbed
Distribution	WBCs
Metabolism	Deacetylates in liver
Excretion	Feces (metabolites/active product)
Half-life	4.4 hr

Pharmacodynamics

	PO
Onset	Unknown
Peak	½-2 hr
Duration	Unknown

Interactions
Individual drugs
CycloSPORINE, radiation: increased bone marrow depression
Clarithromycin, cycloSPORINE, erythromycin: toxicity
Ethanol: increased GI effects
Vitamin B_{12}: decreased action of vit B_{12}; may cause reversible malabsorption
Drug classifications
Bone marrow depressants: increased bone marrow depression
NSAIDs: increased GI effects
Drug/lab test
Increased: alkaline phosphatase, AST
False positive: urine, RBC, Hgb
Interference: urinary 17-hydroxycorticosteroids

NURSING CONSIDERATIONS
Assessment
• Assess pain and mobility of joints, uric acid levels returning to normal
• Monitor I&O ratio; observe for decrease in urinary output; CBC, platelets, reticulocytes before, during therapy (q3mo); may cause aplastic anemia, agranulocytosis, decreased platelets
• Assess for toxicity: weakness, abdominal pain, nausea, vomiting, diarrhea

Nursing diagnoses
• Knowledge, deficient (teaching)
• Mobility, impaired physical (uses)
• Pain, chronic (uses)

Implementation
PO route
• Give with food for GI symptoms

Patient/family education
• Caution patient to avoid alcohol, OTC preparations that contain alcohol
• Instruct patient to report any pain, redness, or hard area, usually in legs; rash, sore throat,

fever, bleeding, bruising, weakness, numbness, tingling
• Teach patient importance of complying with medical regimen (diet, weight loss, product therapy); bone marrow depression may occur

Evaluation
Positive therapeutic outcome
• Decreased stone formation on x-ray
• Decreased pain in kidney region
• Absence of hematuria
• Decreased pain in joints

Treatment of overdose: D/C medication, may need opioids to treat diarrhea

colesevelam (Rx)
(coal-see-vel'am)
Welchol
Func. class.: Antilipemic
Chem. class.: Bile acid sequestrant
Pregnancy category C

Action: Absorbs, combines with bile acids to form insoluble complex that is excreted through feces; loss of bile acids lowers cholesterol levels

Therapeutic outcome: Decreasing LDL cholesterol

Uses: Elevated LDL cholesterol, alone or in combination with HMG-CoA reductase inhibitor; type 2 diabetes (adjunct)

Dosage and routes
Monotherapy
Adult: PO 3 625 mg tabs bid with meals or 6 tabs daily with a meal; may increase to 7 tabs if needed

Combination therapy
Adult: PO 3 tabs bid with meals or 6 tabs daily with a meal given with an HMG-CoA reductase inhibitor

Type 2 diabetes, adjunct (to improve glycemic control)
Adult and geriatric: PO approx 3.8 g (6 tabs)/day or approx 1.9 g (3 tabs) bid

Available forms: Tabs 625 mg

Adverse effects
CNS: Headache, dizziness, drowsiness, vertigo, tinnitus
GI: Constipation, abdominal pain, nausea, fecal impaction, hemorrhoids, flatulence, vomiting, steatorrhea, peptic ulcer, GI obstruction

HEMA: Decreased red cell folate content; **bleeding,** decreased pro-time
INTEG: Rash, irritation of perianal area, tongue, skin
META: Decreased vit A, D, K, **hyperchloremic acidosis**
MS: Muscle, joint pain

Contraindications: Hypersensitivity, biliary obstruction; dysphagia, bowel disease, primary biliary cirrhosis, triglycerides >300 mg/dl, fat-soluble vitamin deficiency

Precautions: Pregnancy C, breastfeeding, children

Pharmacokinetics
Absorption	Unknown
Distribution	Unknown
Metabolism	Unknown
Excretion	Feces
Half-life	Unknown

Pharmacodynamics
LDL decreased in 4-7 days

Interactions
Individual drugs
Clindamycin, digoxin, diltiazem, gemfibrozil, glipiZIDE, iron, mycophenolate, penicillin G, phenytoin, propanolol, warfarin: decreased absorption of each specific product
Thyroid hormones: decreased absorption of thyroid
Drug classifications
Corticosteroids: decreased corticosteroid action
Tetracyclines: decreased absorption of tetracyclines
Thiazides: decreased absorption of thiazides
Vitamins (fat-soluble): decreased absorption of fat-soluble vitamins
Drug/herb
Glucomannan: increased effect
Gotu kola: decreased effect
Drug/lab test
Increased: liver function tests

NURSING CONSIDERATIONS
Assessment
• Assess cardiac glycoside level if both products are being administered
• Assess for signs of vit A, D, K deficiency
• Monitor fasting LDL, HDL, total cholesterol, triglyceride levels, electrolytes if on extended therapy
• Monitor bowel pattern daily; increase bulk, H_2O in diet for constipation

Adverse effects: *italic* = common, **bold** = life-threatening

Nursing diagnoses
- Constipation (adverse reactions)
- Knowledge, deficient (teaching)
- Noncompliance (teaching)

Implementation
- Give product daily, bid with meals; give all other medications 1 hr before colesevelam or 4 hr after colesevelam to avoid poor absorption; take with liquid
- Give supplemental doses of vit A, D, K if levels are low

Patient/family education
◆Teach the symptoms of hypoprothrombinemia: bleeding mucous membranes, dark tarry stools, hematuria, petechiae; report immediately
- Teach the importance of compliance; toxicity may result if doses missed
- Teach that risk factors should be decreased: high-fat diet, smoking, alcohol consumption, absence of exercise
- Advise not to discontinue suddenly

Evaluation
Positive therapeutic outcome
- Decreased cholesterol level (hyperlipidemia); diarrhea, pruritus (excess bile acids)

---

colestipol (Rx)
(koe-les′ti-pole)
Colestid
Func. class.: Antilipemic
Chem. class.: Bile acid sequestrant

Pregnancy category B

Action: Absorbs, combines with bile acids to form an insoluble complex that is excreted through feces; loss of bile acids lowers cholesterol levels

Therapeutic outcome: Decreasing cholesterol levels and low-density lipoproteins, decreased pruritus

Uses: Primary hypercholesterolemia, xanthomas

Unlabeled uses: Digoxin toxicity/overdose, pruritus, diarrhea due to increased bile acids after surgery

Dosage and routes
Adult: PO tabs 2 g daily-bid, may increase by 1 g/mo, max 16 g/day; powder 5-30 g mixed with liquid daily or in divided doses

Available forms: Powder/packet/scoop 5 g; tabs 1 g

Adverse effects
GI: Constipation, abdominal pain, nausea, fecal impaction, hemorrhoids, flatulence, vomiting, steatorrhea, peptic ulcer
HEMA: **Bleeding, increased pro-time**
INTEG: Rash, irritation of perianal area, tongue, skin
META: Decreased vit A, D, E, K, red folate content; **hyperchloremic acidosis**

Contraindications: Hypersensitivity, biliary obstruction

Precautions: Pregnancy **B**, breastfeeding, children, bleeding disorders

Pharmacokinetics
Absorption	Not absorbed
Distribution	Not distributed
Metabolism	Not metabolized
Excretion	Binds with bile acids, feces
Half-life	Unknown

Pharmacodynamics
Onset	24-48 hr
Peak	30 days
Duration	30 days

Interactions
Individual drugs
Clindamycin, digoxin, gemfibrozil, glipiZIDE, iron, penicillin G, propranolol, tetracycline, thyroid agents, warfarin: decreased action of each specific product
Phenytoin, TOLBUTamide: decreased effect of each specific product
Drug classifications
Corticosteroids: decreased corticosteroid action
Diuretics (thiazide): decreased absorption
Vitamins A, D, E, K: decreased absorption
Drug/herb
Glucomannan: increased effect
Gotu kola: decreased effect
Drug/lab test
Increased: Cl, PO_4, AST, ALT, alkaline phosphatase
Decreased: Na, K, Ca

NURSING CONSIDERATIONS
Assessment
- Assess nutrition: fat, protein, carbohydrates; nutritional analysis should be completed by dietitian
- Assess skin integrity after patient has been receiving product; itching, pruritus often occur from bile deposits on skin

---

 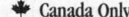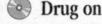

C

• Monitor cardiac glycoside level, if both products are being administered; cardiac glycoside levels will be decreased
• Monitor for signs of vit A, D, E, K deficiency; check serum cholesterol, triglyceride levels, electrolytes if on extended therapy
• Monitor bowel pattern daily; increase bulk, water in diet if constipation develops

Nursing diagnoses
• Constipation (adverse reactions)
• Knowledge, deficient (teaching)
• Noncompliance (teaching)

Implementation
• Swallow tabs whole; do not break, crush, or chew
• Give product daily or bid; give all other medications 1 hr before or 4 hr after colestipol to avoid poor absorption; give product mixed with applesauce or stirred into beverage (2-6 oz), let stand for 2 min; rinse glass to make sure all medication is taken; do not take dry
• Provide supplemental doses of vit A, D, E, K if levels are low

Patient/family education
◆ Teach patient symptoms of hypoprothrombinemia: bleeding mucous membranes, dark, tarry stools, hematuria, petechiae; report immediately
• Teach patient importance of compliance, not to miss or double doses
• Teach patient that risk factors should be decreased: high-fat diet, smoking, alcohol consumption, absence of exercise
• Tell patient to mix product with 6 oz of milk, water, fruit juice; may be mixed with carbonated beverages; rinse glass to make sure all medication is taken or may mix product in applesauce; allow to stand for 2 min before mixing

Evaluation
Positive therapeutic outcome
• Decreased cholesterol level (hyperlipidemia)

---

conivaptan (Rx)
(kon-ih-vap'-tan)
Vaprisol
Func. class.: Vasopressin receptor antagonist

Pregnancy category C

Action: Dual arginine vasopressin (AVP) antagonist with affinity for V_{1A}, V_2 receptors; level of circulating AVP in circulating blood is critical for regulation of water, electrolyte balance and is usually elevated in euvolemic/hypervolemic hyponatremia

Therapeutic outcome: Correct serum sodium levels

Uses: Euvolemia hyponatremia in those hospitalized, not indicated for CHF, hypervolemia, hyponatremia

Dosage and routes
Adult: **IV** INF loading dose 20 mg given over 30 min, then CONT **IV** over 24 hr; after 1 day, give for an additional 1-3 days as a CONT INF of 20 mg/day total, can be titrated up to 40 mg/day if serum sodium is not rising at the desired rate; max time 4 days

Available forms: 5 mg/ml (20 mg/4 ml) in single-use ampule; 20 mg/100 ml in D_5 for injection

Adverse effects
CNS: Headache, confusion, insomnia
CV: **Atrial fibrillation,** hypo/hypertension, orthostatic hypotension, phlebitis
GI: Nausea, vomiting, constipation, dry mouth
GU: Hematuria, polyuria, UTI, pollakiuria
HEMA: Anemia
INTEG: Erythemia, inj site reaction
META: Dehydration, hypo/hyperglycemia, hypokalemia, hypomagnesia, hyponatremia
MISC: Oral candidiasis, pain, peripheral edema, pneumonia

Contraindications: Hypersensitivity, hypovolemia

Precautions: Pregnancy **C**, breastfeeding, orthostatic/renal disease

Pharmacokinetics
Absorption	Unknown
Distribution	Protein binding 99%
Metabolism	By CYP3A4
Excretion	Unknown
Half-life	Terminal 5 hr

Pharmacodynamics
Unknown

Interactions
Individual drugs
Digoxin: decreased plasma concentration of conivaptan
Drug classifications
CYP3A4 inhibitors: increased plasma concentrations of conivaptan

---

Adverse effects: *italic* = common, **bold** = life-threatening

NURSING CONSIDERATIONS
Assessment
- Monitor renal/hepatic function
- Assess frequent sodium volume status; overly rapid correction of sodium concentration (>12 mEq/L per 24 hr) may result in osmotic demyelination syndrome
- Assess neurologic status: confusion, headache
- Assess CV status: atrial fibrillation, hyper/hypotension, orthostatic hypotension; monitor B/P, pulse
- Monitor other electrolytes (magnesium and potassium)

Nursing diagnoses
- Injury, risk for (uses)
- Knowledge, deficient (teaching)

Implementation
IV route
- Withdraw 4 ml (20 mg) of conivaptan, add to 100 ml D_5W, gently invert several times to mix, give over 30 min

Continuous IV infusion route
- Withdraw 4 ml (20 mg) of conivaptan, add to 250 ml D_5W, gently invert several times to mix, give over 24 hr; or 40 mg in 250 ml D_5W, gently invert several times to mix, give over 24 hr

Patient/family education
- Advise patient to avoid pregnancy, breastfeeding while taking this product
- Advise patient to report neurologic changes: headache, insomnia, confusion
- Teach patient administration procedure and expected result
- Advise patient to report inj site pain, redness, swelling

Evaluation
Positive therapeutic outcome
- Correction of serum sodium levels

CONTRACEPTIVES, HORMONAL

MONOPHASIC, ORAL
ethinyl estradiol/ desogestrel (Rx)
Apri, Cesia, Desogen, Kariva, Mircette, Ortho-Cept, Reclipsen, Solia, Velivet

ethinyl estradiol/ drospirenone (Rx)
Yasmin, Yaz 28

ethinyl estradiol/ ethynodiol (Rx)
Kelnor 1/35, Zovia

ethinyl estradiol/ levonorgestrel (Rx)
Alesse, Aviane-28, Enpresse, Jolessa, Lessina, Levlen, Levlite, Levora, Lutera, Nordette, Portia, Quasense, Seasonique, Sronyx

ethinyl estradiol/ norethindrone (Rx)
Brevicon, Genora 0.5/35, Genora 1/35, Junel 21 1/20, Junel 21 1.5/20, Loestrin 21 1.5/30, Loestrin 21 1/20, Microgestin, Modicon, N.E.E 1/35, Nelova 0.5/35E, Nelova 1/35E, Norcept-E 1/35, Norethin 1/35E, Norinyl 1+35, Norlestrin 1/50, Norlestrin 2.5/50, Nortrel

ethinyl estradiol/ norgestimate (Rx)
MonoNessa, Ortho-Cyclen, Previfem, Sprintec

ethinyl estradiol/ norgestrel (Rx)
Cryselle, Lo/Ovral, Low-Ogestrel, Ogestrel, Ovral

mestranol/ norethindrone (Rx)
Genora 1/50, Nelova 1/50m, Norethin 1/50m, Norinyl 1+50, Ortho-Novum 1/50

BIPHASIC, ORAL
ethinyl estradiol/ norethindrone (Rx)
Nelova 10/11, Ortho-Novum 10/11

TRIPHASIC, ORAL
ethinyl estradiol/ desogestrel (Rx)
Cyclessa

◆ Alert   ✤ Canada Only   ◐ Drug on CD   * "Tall Man" lettering (See Preface)

**ethinyl estradiol/
norethindrone** (Rx)
Necor 7/7/7, Nortrel 7/7/7, Ortho-Novum
7/7/7, Tri-Norinyl
**ethinyl estradiol/
norgestimate** (Rx)
Ortho Tri-Cyclen, Ortho Tri-Cyclen Lo
**ethinyl estradiol/
levonorgestrel** (Rx)
Enpresse, Tri-Levlen, Triphasil

EXTENDED CYCLE, ORAL
**ethinyl estradiol/
levonorgestrel** (Rx)
Seasonale

PROGESTIN, ORAL
norethindrone (Rx)
Errin, Ortho Micronor, Camila, Jolivette,
Nor-Q D

PROGRESSIVE ESTROGEN, ORAL
**ethinyl estradiol/
norethindrone acetate** (Rx)
Estrostep, Estrostep Fe

EMERGENCY
**levonorgestrel/ethinyl
estradiol** (Rx)
Preven
levonorgestrel (Rx)
Plan B
medroxyprogesterone (Rx)
Depo-Provera

INTRAUTERINE
levonorgestrel (Rx)
Mirena

IMPLANT
etonogestrel (Rx)
Implanon

VAGINAL RING
**ethinyl estradiol/
etonogestrel** (Rx)
Nuva Ring

TRANSDERMAL
**ethinyl estradiol/
norelgestromin** (Rx)
Ortho Evra

Action: Prevents ovulation by suppressing FSH, LH; *monophasic:* estrogen/progestin (fixed dose) used during a 21-day cycle; ovulation is inhibited by suppression of FSH and LH; thickness of cervical mucus and endometrial lining prevents pregnancy; *biphasic:* ovulation is inhibited by suppression of FSH and LH; alteration of cervical mucus, endometrial lining prevents pregnancy; *triphasic:* ovulation is inhibited by suppression of FSH and LH; change of cervical mucus, endometrial lining prevents pregnancy; variable doses of estrogen/progestin combinations may be similar to natural hormonal fluctuations; *extended cycle:* estrogen/progestin continuous for 84 days, off for 7 days, result 4 menstrual periods/yr; *progressive estrogen:* constant progestin with 3 progressive doses of estrogen; *progestin-only pill, implant, intrauterine:* change of cervical mucus and endometrial lining prevents pregnancy; ovulation may be suppressed

Therapeutic outcome: Prevention of pregnancy, decreased severity of endometriosis, hypermenorrhea

Uses: To prevent pregnancy, regulation of menstrual cycle, treatment of acne in women over 14 yr that other treatment has failed, emergency contraception; *injection:* inhibits gonadotropin secretion, ovulation, follicular maturation; *emergency:* inhibits ovulation and fertilization, decreases transport of sperm and egg from fallopian tube to uterus; *vaginal ring, transdermal:* inhibits ovulation, prevents sperm entry into uterus; *antiacne:* may decrease sex hormone binding globulin, results in decreased testosterone

Dosage and routes
Monophasic
Adult: PO take first tab on Sunday after start of menses × 21 days; skip 7 days; then repeat cycle; start on 1st day of menses × 21 days; skip 7 days, then repeat cycle; may contain 7 placebo tabs, where 1 tab is taken daily

Biphasic
Adult: PO Take 10 days of small progestin, then large progestin; estrogen is the same during cycle; skip 7 days, then repeat cycle; may contain 7 placebo tabs, where 1 tab is taken daily

Triphasic
Adult: PO estrogen dose remains constant, progestin changes throughout 21 day cycle, some products contain 28 tabs per month

Adverse effects: *italic* = common, **bold** = life-threatening

Extended cycle
Adult: PO start taking on first day of menses; continue for 84 days of active tab, then 7 days of placebo; repeat cycle

Progestin
Adult: PO start on 1st day of menses, then daily and continuously

Progressive estrogen
Adult: PO progestin dose remains constant, estrogen increases q7days throughout 21-day cycle, may include 7 placebo tabs for 28-day cycle

Emergency
Adult and adolescent: Give within 72 hr of intercourse, repeat 12 hr later; Plan B 1 tab, then 1 tab 12 hr later; Preven 2 tab, then 2 tab 12 hr later; Ovral (unlabeled) 2 white tabs; Lo/Ovral (unlabeled) 4 white tabs; Levlen (unlabeled), Nordette (unlabeled) 4 orange tabs; Triphasil (unlabeled), Tri-Levlen (unlabeled) 4 yellow tabs

Injectable
Adult: IM (Depo-Provera) 150 mg within 5 days of start of menses, or within 5 days postpartum (must not be breastfeeding); if breastfeeding, give 6 wk postpartum, repeat q3mo

Intrauterine
Adult: To be inserted using the levonorgestrel-releasing intrauterine system (LRIS) by those trained in procedure; inserted into uterine cavity within 7 days of the onset of menstruation; use should not exceed 5 years per implant

Vaginal ring
Adult: VAG insert 1 ring on or prior to day 5 of cycle, leave in place 3 wk; remove for 1 wk, then repeat

Transdermal
Adult: Transdermal apply patch within 7 days of menses, change weekly × 3 wk; no patch wk 4, repeat cycle

Implant
Adult: Subdermal in inner side of upper arm on days 1-5 of menses, replace q3yr

Acne
Adult: PO (Ortho Tri-Cyclen) take daily × 21 days, off 7 days

Adverse effects
CNS: Depression, fatigue, dizziness, nervousness, anxiety, headache
CV: Increased B/P, **cerebral hemorrhage, thrombosis, pulmonary embolism,** fluid retention, edema

EENT: Optic neuritis, retinal thrombosis, cataracts
ENDO: Decreased glucose tolerance, increased TBG, PBI, T_4, T_3
GI: Nausea, vomiting, cramps, diarrhea, bloating, constipation, change in appetite, **cholestatic jaundice**
GU: Breakthrough bleeding, amenorrhea, spotting, dysmenorrhea, galactorrhea, endocervical hyperplasia, vaginitis, cystitis-like syndrome, breast change
HEMA: Increased fibrinogen, clotting factor
INTEG: Chloasma, melasma, acne, rash, urticaria, erythema, pruritus, hirsutism, alopecia, photosensitivity

Contraindications: Pregnancy **X,** breastfeeding, women 40 yr and over, reproductive cancer, thrombophlebitis, MI, hepatic tumors, hepatic disease, CAD, CVA

Precautions: Depression, hypertension, renal disease, seizure disorders, lupus erythematosus, rheumatic disease, migraine headache, amenorrhea, irregular menses, breast cancer (fibrocystic), gallbladder disease, diabetes mellitus, heavy smoking, acute mononucleosis, sickle cell disease

Pharmacokinetics
Absorption	Unknown
Distribution	Unknown
Metabolism	Unknown
Excretion	Breast milk
Half-life	Unknown

Pharmacodynamics
Unknown

Interactions
Individual drugs
Griseofulvin, rifampin: decreased effectiveness of oral contraceptive
Drug classifications
Analgesics, antibiotics, anticonvulsants, antihistamines: decreased action of oral contraceptives
Anticoagulants (oral): decreased action of oral anticoagulants
Drug/herb
Alfalfa, black cohosh, chaste tree: altered action
Saw palmetto, St. John's wort: decreased oral contraceptive effect
Drug/food
Grapefruit juice: increased peak level

Drug/lab test
Increased: pro-time; clotting factors VII, VIII, IX, X; TBG, PBI, T₄, platelet aggregation, BSP, triglycerides, bilirubin, AST, ALT
Decreased: T₃, antithrombin III, folate, metyrapone test, GTT, 17-OHCS

NURSING CONSIDERATIONS
Assessment
• Assess for reproductive changes: change in breasts, tumors, positive Pap smear; product should be discontinued if changes occur
• Monitor glucose, thyroid function, liver function tests, B/P

Nursing diagnoses
• Body image, disturbed (adverse reactions)
• Injury, risk for (adverse reactions)
• Knowledge, deficient (teaching)
• Noncompliance (teaching)

Implementation
PO route
• If GI symptoms occur, medication may be taken with food; take at same time each day
Implant route
• Inject 6 cap subdermally
• Implant is effective for 5 yr, should be removed after that
IM route
• Administer inj deep in large muscle mass after shaking susp well; ensure pregnancy has not occurred if inj are 2 wk or more apart

Patient/family education
• Teach patient about detection of clots using Homans' sign; teach monitoring technique for heat, redness, pain, swelling
• Teach patient to use sunscreen or to avoid sunlight; photosensitivity can occur
• Teach patient to take at same time each day to ensure equal product level, to take another tab as soon as possible if one is missed
• Teach patient that after product is discontinued, pregnancy may not occur for several mo
• Instruct patient to report GI symptoms that occur after 4 mo
• Advise patient to use another birth control method during first 3 wk of oral contraceptive use
• Teach patient to report abdominal pain, change in vision, shortness of breath, change in menstrual flow, spotting, breakthrough bleeding, breast lumps, swelling, headache, severe leg pain, mental changes; that continuing medical care is needed: Pap smear and gynecologic exam q6mo

• Teach patient to notify physicians and dentist of oral contraceptive use

Evaluation
Positive therapeutic outcome
• Absence of pregnancy
• Decreased severity of endometriosis
• Decreased severity of hypermenorrhea

---

cortisone ⊛ (Rx)
(kor'ti-sone)
Cortone ✦, cortone acetate
Func. class.: Corticosteroid, synthetic
Chem. class.: Short-acting glucocorticoid
Pregnancy category D

Action: Decreases inflammation by suppression of migration of polymorphonuclear leukocytes and fibroblasts, reversal of increased capillary permeability, and lysosomal stabilization; suppresses adrenal function with long-term use

Therapeutic outcome: Replacement of cortisol in adrenal insufficiency

Uses: Inflammation, severe allergy, adrenal insufficiency; collagen, respiratory, dermatologic, rheumatic disorders

Dosage and routes
Adult: PO 25-300 mg daily or q2day, titrated to patient response
Child: PO 0.7-10 mg/kg/day

Available forms: Tabs 25 mg

Adverse effects
CNS: Depression, flushing, sweating, headache, mood changes
CV: Hypertension, **circulatory collapse, thrombophlebitis, embolism,** tachycardia, **necrotizing angiitis, CHF,** edema
EENT: Fungal infections, increased intraocular pressure, blurred vision, cataracts, glaucoma
GI: Diarrhea, nausea, abdominal distention, **GI hemorrhage,** increased appetite, **pancreatitis,** ulcerative esophagitis
HEMA: **Thrombocytopenia**
INTEG: Acne, poor wound healing, ecchymosis, bruising, petechiae, hirsutism
META: Sodium fluid retention; potassium loss, diabetes
MS: Fractures, osteoporosis, weakness, loss of muscle mass

Contraindications: Pregnancy **D,** child <2 yr, psychosis, hypersensitivity, idiopathic thrombocytopenia, acute glomerulonephritis, amebiasis, fungal infections, nonasthmatic bronchial disease, AIDS, TB, measles, varicella

Adverse effects: *italic* = common, **bold** = life-threatening

Precautions: Breastfeeding, diabetes mellitus, glaucoma, osteoporosis, seizure disorders, ulcerative colitis, CHF, myasthenia gravis, renal/hepatic disease, esophagitis, peptic ulcer

Pharmacokinetics
Absorption	Slowly (IM)
Distribution	Widely, crosses placenta
Metabolism	Liver
Excretion	Unknown
Half-life	8-12 hr

Pharmacodynamics
	PO
Onset	Unknown
Peak	2 hr
Duration	1½ days

Interactions
Individual drugs
Alcohol: increased side effects
Indomethacin: increased GI symptoms, increased side effects, increased action of cortisone
Ketoconazole: increased cortisone action
Phenobarbital, phenytoin: decreased effectiveness of cortisone
Rifampin, theophylline: decreased cortisone action
Drug classifications
Acetylcholinesterases, barbiturates: decreased cortisone action
Anticoagulants: decreased anticoagulant effect
Antidiabetics: decreased antidiabetic effect
Antiinfectives (macrolide), estrogens: increased cortisone action
Contraceptives (oral): increased action of cortisone
Diuretics (potassium-wasting), salicylates: increased side effects
NSAIDs: increased GI symptoms
Salicylates: increased GI symptoms, increased cortisone effects, increased side effects; decreased salicylate effect
Toxoids: decreased toxoid effect
Vaccines: decreased vaccine effect
Drug/herb
Aloe, buckthorn bark/berry, cascara sagrada bark, Chinese rhubarb, rhubarb root, senna leaf/fruits: increased potassium deficiency
Aloe, licorice, perilla: increased steroid effect
Drug/lab test
Increased: cholesterol, sodium, blood glucose, uric acid, calcium, urine glucose
Decreased: calcium, potassium, T_4, T_3, thyroid ^{131}I uptake test, urine 17-OHCS, 17-KS
False negative: skin allergy tests

NURSING CONSIDERATIONS
Assessment
• Assess for adrenal insufficiency symptoms: weakness, nausea, vomiting, confusion, anxiety, restlessness, decreased B/P, weight loss; check before, during treatment
• Monitor potassium, blood glucose for patient on long-term therapy; hypokalemia and hyperglycemia can occur
• Check B/P, pulse q4hr; notify prescriber if chest pain occurs
• Monitor I&O ratio and weight daily; be alert for decreasing urinary output and increasing edema with bilateral crackles, dyspnea, weight gain
• Monitor plasma cortisol levels during long-term therapy (normal level: 138-635 nmol/L if checked at 8 AM)
• Assess for symptoms of infection: increased temp, WBC even after withdrawal of medication; product masks symptoms of infection
• Monitor for potassium depletion: paresthesias, fatigue, nausea, vomiting, depression, polyuria, dysrhythmias, weakness, edema, hypertension, cardiac symptoms, weight daily; notify prescriber of weekly gain >5 lb
• Assess for mental changes: affect, mood, behavioral changes, aggression; depression, psychosis may occur
Nursing diagnoses
• Infection, risk for (adverse reactions)
• Injury, risk for (adverse reactions)
• Knowledge, deficient (teaching)
Implementation
PO route
• Administer in AM with food or milk to decrease GI symptoms
Patient/family education
• Advise patient to carry/wear emergency ID as corticosteroid user at all times
• Instruct patient to notify prescriber if therapeutic response decreases; dosage adjustment may be needed; teach not to discontinue this medication abruptly or adrenal crisis can result; teach all aspects of product usage, including cushingoid symptoms
• Caution patient to avoid all OTC products: salicylates, potassium, alcohol in cough products, cold preparations unless directed by prescriber; avoid high-sodium foods
• Teach patient symptoms of adrenal insufficiency: nausea, anorexia, fatigue, dizzi-

ness, dyspnea, weakness, joint pain, tarry stools, bruising, blurred vision
• Advise patient to avoid persons with known infections; report probable infection rapidly; product masks infection
• Caution patient that diet modification is necessary if on long-term treatment: increased calcium, potassium, and protein; also low sodium and carbohydrates
• Advise the patient to avoid exposure to chickenpox, measles
• Advise the patient to take PO dose in AM with food or fluid (milk)

Evaluation
Positive therapeutic outcome
• Decreased inflammation

---

cotrimoxazole
See trimethoprim/sulfamethoxazole

---

cyclobenzaprine (Rx)
(sye-kloe-ben′za-preen)
Amrix, cyclobenzaprine HCl, Cycloflex, Fexmid, Flexeril
Func. class.: Skeletal muscle relaxant, central acting
Chem. class.: Tricyclic amine salt
Pregnancy category B

Do not confuse:
cyclobenzaprine/cyproheptadine

Action: Reduction of tonic muscle activity at the brain stem; may be related to antidepressant effects

Therapeutic outcome: Relaxation of skeletal muscle

Uses: Adjunct for relief of muscle spasm and pain in musculoskeletal conditions

Unlabeled uses: Fibromyalgia

Dosage and routes
Musculoskeletal disorders
Adult: PO 5 mg tid × 1 wk, max 30 mg/day × 3 wk

Geriatric: PO 5 mg tid

Fibromyalgia (unlabeled)
Adult: PO 10 mg at bedtime, titrated up

Available forms: Tabs 5, 10 mg; ext rel tab 15, 30 mg

Adverse effects
CNS: Dizziness, weakness, drowsiness, headache, tremor, depression, insomnia, confusion, paresthesia, nervousness
CV: Postural hypotension, tachycardia, **dysrhythmias**
EENT: Diplopia, temporary loss of vision
GI: Nausea, vomiting, hiccups, dry mouth, constipation, hepatitis
GU: Urinary retention, frequency, change in libido
INTEG: Rash, pruritus, fever, facial flushing, sweating

Contraindications: Acute recovery phase of MI, dysrhythmias, heart block, CHF, hypersensitivity, child <12 yr, intermittent porphyria, thyroid disease

Precautions: Pregnancy **B**, breastfeeding, geriatric, renal/hepatic disease, addictive personality

Pharmacokinetics
Distribution	Well
Metabolism	Liver, partially
Excretion	Kidney (unchanged)
Half-life	1-3 days

Pharmacodynamics
Onset	1 hr
Peak	3-8 hr
Duration	12-24 hr

Interactions
Individual drugs
Alcohol: increased CNS depression
Erythromycin, levaquin: increased QT interval
Tramadol: do not use within 14 days
Drug classifications
Antidepressants (tricyclic), barbiturates, opiates, sedative/hypnotics: increased CNS depression
MAOIs: do not use within 14 days
Drug/herb
Kava: increased CNS depression

NURSING CONSIDERATIONS
Assessment
• Assess pain periodically: location, duration, mobility, stiffness, baseline
• Monitor ECG in epileptic patients; poor seizure control has occurred in patients taking this product
• Check for allergic reactions: rash, fever, respiratory distress
• Check for severe weakness, numbness, in extremities

Adverse effects: *italic* = common, **bold** = life-threatening

- Assess for CNS depression: dizziness, drowsiness, psychiatric symptoms

Nursing diagnoses
- Injury, risk for (adverse reactions)
- Knowledge, deficient (teaching)
- Mobility, impaired physical (uses)

Implementation
- Give without regard to meals
- Store in airtight container at room temperature

Patient/family education
- Teach patient not to discontinue medication quickly; insomnia, nausea, headache, spasticity, tachycardia will occur; product should be tapered off over 1-2 wk
- Caution patient not to take with alcohol, other CNS depressants
- Advise to avoid altering activities while taking this product
- Caution patient to avoid hazardous activities if drowsiness/dizziness occurs
- Caution patient to avoid using OTC medication: cough preparations, antihistamines, unless directed by prescriber
- Teach patient to use gum, frequent sips of water for dry mouth

Evaluation
Positive therapeutic outcome
- Decreased pain, spasticity; muscle spasms of acute, painful musculoskeletal conditions are generally short term; long-term therapy is seldom warranted

Treatment of overdose: Empty stomach with emesis, gastric lavage, then administer activated charcoal; use anticonvulsants if indicated; monitor cardiac function

---

cyclopentolate ophthalmic
See Appendix B

⚠ HIGH ALERT

cyclophosphamide 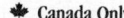 **(Rx)**
(sye-kloe-foss'fa-mide)
Cytoxan, Procytox ✦
Func. class.: Antineoplastic alkylating agent
Chem. class.: Nitrogen mustard

Pregnancy category D

Do not confuse:
cyclophosphamide/cycloSPORINE, Cytoxan/Cytosar/Cytotec/centoxin/Cytarabine

Action: Alkylates DNA; responsible for cross-linking DNA strands; activity is not cell cycle phase specific

Therapeutic outcome: Prevention of rapidly growing malignant cells

Uses: Hodgkin's disease, lymphomas, leukemia, multiple myeloma, neuroblastoma, retinoblastoma, Ewing's sarcoma, cancer of female reproductive tract, breast, lung, prostate; disseminated neuroblastoma

Dosage and routes
Adult: PO initially 1-5 mg/kg over 2-5 days; maintenance 1-5 mg/kg; **IV** initially 40-50 mg/kg in divided doses over 2-5 days; maintenance 10-15 mg/kg q7-10day, or 3-5 mg/kg q3day
Child: PO/IV 2-8 mg/kg or 60-250 mg/m² in divided doses × 6 or more days; maintenance **IV** 10-15 mg/kg q7-10 days or 30 mg/kg q3-4wk; dose should be reduced by half when bone marrow suppression occurs

Neuroblastoma
Child and infant: PO 150 mg/m²/day, days 1-7 with DOXOrubicin (**IV** 35 mg/m² on day 5) q21day × 5 cycles
Child: **IV** 70 mg/kg/day with hydration on days 1 and 2 with DOXOrubicin and vinCRIStine q21day for courses 1, 2, 4, 6, alternating with cisplatin and etoposide q21day for courses 3, 5, 7

Breast cancer
Adult: PO 100-200 mg/m²/day or 2 mg/kg/day × 4-14 days; **IV** 500-1000 mg/m² on day 1 in combination with fluorouracil and methotrexate or DOXOrubicin, or DOXOrubicin alone; also cyclophosphamide 600 mg/m², may be given dose-dense on day 1 of q14day with DOXOrubicin (60 mg/m²) with growth factor support

Operable node-positive breast cancer
IV (TAC regimen) Adult: 500 mg/m² with DOXOrubicin (50 mg/m² **IV**) then docetaxel (75 mg/m²) **IV** given 1 hr later × 6 cycles q3wk

Available forms: Inj **IV** 100, 200, 500 mg, 1, 2 g; tabs 25, 50 mg

Adverse effects
CNS: Headache, dizziness
CV: **Cardiotoxicity (high doses), myocardial fibrosis**
ENDO: Syndrome of inappropriate antidiuretic hormone (SIADH), gonadal suppression
GI: Nausea, vomiting, diarrhea, weight loss, colitis, **hepatotoxicity**
GU: **Hemorrhagic cystitis,** hematuria, neoplasms, amenorrhea, azoospermia, sterility, ovarian fibrosis

---

HEMA: **Thrombocytopenia, leukopenia, pancytopenia, myelosuppression**
INTEG: *Alopecia,* dermatitis
META: Hyperuricemia
MISC: Secondary neoplasms, **anaphylaxis**
RESP: **Pulmonary fibrosis, interstitial pneumonia**

Contraindications: Pregnancy **D,** breast-feeding, severely depressed bone marrow function, hypersensitivity

Precautions: Radiation therapy, cardiac disease

Pharmacokinetics

Absorption	Well absorbed (PO)
Distribution	Widely distributed; crosses placenta, blood-brain barrier (50%)
Metabolism	Liver to active product
Excretion	Kidneys, unchanged (30%)
Half-life	4-6½ hr

Pharmacodynamics
Unknown

Interactions
Individual drugs
Allopurinol: increased bone marrow suppression
Chloramphenicol: decreased cyclophosphamide effect
Digoxin: decreased digoxin levels
Insulin: increased hypoglycemia
Succinylcholine: increased neuromuscular blockade
Warfarin: increased warfarin action
Drug classifications
Diuretics (thiazides): increased bone marrow suppression
Barbiturates: increased toxicity of cyclophosphamide
Corticosteroids: decreased cyclophosphamide effect
Live virus vaccines: decreased antibody reaction

Drug/herb
St. John's wort: increased toxicity
Drug/lab test
Increased: uric acid
Decreased: pseudocholinesterase
False positive: Pap smear
False negative: PPD, mumps trichophytin, *Candida, Trichophyton,* Pap smear

NURSING CONSIDERATIONS
Assessment
◆ Assess symptoms indicating severe allergic reaction: rash, pruritus, urticaria, purpuric skin lesions, itching, flushing
• Assess for tachypnea, ECG changes, dyspnea, edema, fatigue
• Monitor CBC, differential, platelet count weekly; withhold product if WBC count is <2500/mm³ or platelet count is <75,000/mm³; notify prescriber of results
• Assess for hemorrhagic cystitis: renal function studies including BUN, creatinine, serum uric acid, urine CCr before, during therapy; I&O ratio; report fall in urine output to <30 ml/hr
• Monitor temp q4hr (elevated temp may indicate beginning of infection)
• Monitor liver function tests before, during therapy (bilirubin, AST, ALT, LDH) as needed or monthly; note jaundice of skin or sclera, dark urine, clay-colored stools, itchy skin, abdominal pain, fever, diarrhea
• Assess for bleeding: hematuria, stool guaiac, bruising or petechiae, mucosa or orifices q8hr
• Identify dyspnea, crackles, unproductive cough, chest pain, tachypnea
• Identify effects of alopecia on body image; discuss feelings about body changes

Nursing diagnoses
• Body image, disturbed (adverse reactions)
• Infection, risk for (adverse reactions)
• Injury, risk for (adverse reactions)
• Knowledge, deficient (teaching)

Implementation
• Give fluids **IV** or PO before chemotherapy to hydrate patient
• Give antacid before oral agent, after PM meals, before bedtime; antiemetic 30-60 min before giving product to prevent vomiting and prn; antibiotics for prophylaxis of infection
• Give top or syst analgesics for pain; give in AM so product can be eliminated before bedtime
IV route
• Give **IV** after diluting 100 mg/5 ml of sterile or bacteriostatic water; shake; let stand until clear; may be further diluted in up to 250 ml D₅ 0.9% NaCl, 0.45% NaCl, LR, Ringer's; give 100 mg or less/min through 3-way stopcock of glucose or saline inf
• Use 21-, 23-, or 25-G needle; check site for irritation, phlebitis
Syringe compatibilities: Bleomycin, cisplatin, doxapram, DOXOrubicin, droperidol, fluorouracil, furosemide, heparin, leucovorin, methotrexate, metoclopramide, mitomycin, mitoxantrone, vinBLAStine, vinCRIStine

Adverse effects: *italic* = common, **bold** = life-threatening

Y-site compatibilities: Amifostine, amikacin, ampicillin, azlocillin, aztreonam, bleomycin, cefamandole, cefazolin, cefepime, cefoperazone, cefotaxime, cefoxitin, cefuroxime, cephalothin, cephapirin, chloramphenicol, chlorproMAZINE, cimetidine, cisplatin, cladribine, clindamycin, dexamethasone, diphenhydrAMINE, DOXOrubicin, doxycycline, droperidol, erythromycin, famotidine, filgrastim, fludarabine, fluorouracil, furosemide, gallium, ganciclovir, gentamicin, granisetron, heparin, hydromorphone, idarubicin, kanamycin, leucovorin, lorazepam, melphalan, methotrexate, methylPREDNISolone, metoclopramide, metronidazole, mezlocillin, minocycline, mitomycin, moxalactam, nafcillin, ondansetron, oxacillin, paclitaxel, penicillin G potassium, piperacillin, piperacillin/tazobactam, prochlorperazine, promethazine, propofol, ranitidine, sargramostim, sodium bicarbonate, teniposide, tetracycline, thiotepa, ticarcillin, ticarcillin-clavulanate, tobramycin, trimethoprim-sulfamethoxazole, vancomycin, vinBLAStine, vinCRIStine, vinorelbine

Additive compatibilities: Cisplatin with etoposide, hydrOXYzine, methotrexate, methotrexate with fluorouracil, mitoxantrone, ondansetron

Solution compatibilities: Amino acids 4.25%/D_{25}, D_5/0.9% NaCl, D_5W, 0.9% NaCl

Patient/family education

• Teach patient to avoid use of products containing aspirin or ibuprofen, razors, commercial mouthwash, since bleeding may occur; to report symptoms of bleeding (hematuria, tarry stools, bruising)

• Instruct patient to report signs of anemia (fatigue, headache, irritability, faintness, shortness of breath)

• Teach patient to report any changes in breathing or coughing even several months after treatment

• Advise patient that hair may be lost during treatment; a wig or hairpiece may make patient feel better; new hair may be different in color, texture

• Teach patient not to have any vaccinations without the advice of the prescriber; serious reactions can occur

• Advise patient contraception is needed during treatment and for several months after the completion of therapy

Evaluation

Positive therapeutic outcome

• Prevention of rapid division of malignant cells

• Increased appetite, increased weight

---

*cycloSPORINE (Rx)
(sye-kloe-spor'een)
Gengraf, Neoral, Pulminiq, Sandimmune
Func. class.: Immunosuppressant
Chem. class.: Fungus-derived peptide

Pregnancy category C

Do not confuse:
cycloSPORINE/CycloSERINE/cyclophosphamide

Action: Produces immunosuppression by inhibiting T lymphocytes

Therapeutic outcome: Absence of transplant rejection

Uses: Organ transplants (liver, kidney, heart) to prevent rejection, rheumatoid arthritis, psoriasis

Unlabeled uses: Recalcitrant ulcerative colitis, aplastic anemia, Crohn's disease, GVHD, thrombocytopenia purpura, lupus, nephritis, myasthenia gravis, psoriatic arthritis

Dosage and routes
Prevention of transplant rejection
Adult and child: PO 15 mg/kg several hr before surgery, daily for 2 wk, reduce dosage by 2.5 mg/kg/wk to 5-10 mg/kg/day; **IV** 5-6 mg/kg several hr before surgery, daily, switch to PO form as soon as possible

Rheumatoid arthritis (Neoral/Gengraf)
Adult: PO 2.5 mg/kg/day divided bid, may increase 0.5-0.75 mg/kg/day after 8-12 wk, max 4 mg/kg/day

Psoriasis (Neoral/Gengraf)
Adult: PO 2.5 mg/kg/day divided bid × 4 wk, then increase by 0.5 mg/kg/day q2wk, max 4 mg/kg/day

Idiopathic thrombocytopenia purpura (unlabeled)
Adult: PO 1.25-2.5 mg/kg bid

Severe aplastic anemia (unlabeled)
Adult and child: PO 12 mg/kg/day or 15 mg/kg/day (child) with antithymocyte globulin (ATG)

Available forms: Oral sol (Neoral) 100 mg/ml; soft gel cap 25, 50, 100 mg; inj 50 mg/ml; inh sol 300 mg/4.8 ml

Adverse effects
CNS: Tremors, *headache*, **seizures**, confusion
GI: Nausea, vomiting, diarrhea, *oral candida*, *gum hyperplasia*, **hepatotoxicity**, pancreatitis

---

GU: **Albuminuria, hematuria, proteinuria, renal failure**
INTEG: Rash, acne, *hirsutism,* pruritus
META: Hyperkalemia, hypomagnesemia, hyperlipidemia, hyperuricemia
MISC: Infection

Contraindications: Hypersensitivity to polyxyethylated castor oil (inj only), psoriasis or rheumatoid arthrits in renal disease (Neoral/Gengraf), Gengraf/Neoral used with PUVA/UVB; methotrexate, coal tar, breastfeeding, ocular infections

Black Box Warning: Neoplastic disease, sunlight (UV) exposure, renal disease/failure, uncontrolled, malignant hypertension; radiation in psoriasis

Precautions: Pregnancy **C**, geriatric, severe renal/hepatic disease

Pharmacokinetics

Absorption	Poorly absorbed (PO)
Distribution	Crosses placenta
Metabolism	Liver to mercaptopurine
Excretion	Kidney, minimal
Half-life	Biphasic 1.2 hr, 25 hr

Pharmacodynamics

	PO
Onset	Unknown
Peak	4 hr
Duration	Unknown

Interactions
Individual drugs
Allopurinol, amiodarone, amphotericin B, bromocriptine, carvedilol, cimetidine, colchicine, foscarnet, imipenem-cilastatin, melphalan, metoclopramide: increased action, cycloSPORINE toxicity
Digoxin: increased digoxin level
Etoposide: increased etoposide level
Methotrexate: increased methotrexate level
Nafcillin, orlistat, phenobarbital, phenytoin, probucol terbinafine, ticlodipine, trimethoprim/sulfamethoxazole: decreased cycloSPORINE action
Sirolimus: increased sirolimus level
Tacrolimus: increased tacrolimus level
Drug classifications:
Androgens, antifungals (azole), β-blockers, calcium channel blockers, contraceptives (oral), corticosteroids, fluoroquinolones, macrolides, NSAIDs, selective serotonin reuptake inhibitors: increased cycloSPORINE levels, toxicity

Anticonvulsants, rifamycins: decreased cycloSPORINE levels
HMG-CoA reductase inhibitors, diuretics (potassium-sparing): increased effects of each product
Live virus vaccines: decreased antibody reaction
Drug/herb
Ginseng, maitake, mistletoe, schisandra, St. John's wort, turmeric: decreased effect
Safflower: increased effect
Drug/food
Grapefruit juice, food: increased slowed metabolism of product

NURSING CONSIDERATIONS
Assessment
• Monitor renal studies: BUN, creatinine at least monthly during treatment, 3 mo after treatment
• Monitor liver function studies: alkaline phosphatase, AST, ALT, bilirubin
• Monitor product blood levels during treatment
• Assess for hepatotoxicity: dark urine, jaundice, itching, light-colored stools; product should be discontinued
• Assess for nephrotoxicity: 6 wk postop, CyA trough level >200 ng/ml, intracapsular pressure <40 mm Hg, rise in creatinine 0.15 mg/dl/day

Nursing diagnoses
• Infection, risk for (uses)
• Knowledge, deficient (teaching)
• Mobility, impaired physical (uses)

Implementation
PO route
• Do not break, crush, or chew caps
• Use pipette provided to draw up oral sol; may mix with milk or juice, wipe pipette, do not wash
• Give for several days before transplant surgery with corticosteroids
• Microemulsion products (Neoral) and other products are not interchangeable
• Give with meals for GI upset or place product in chocolate milk
• Give with oral antifungal for *Candida* infections
IV route
• Give **IV** after diluting each 50 mg/20-100 ml of 0.9% NaCl or D$_5$W; run over 2-6 hr; use an inf pump, glass inf bottles only; may give as cont inf over 24 hr
Additive compatibilities: Ciprofloxacin

C

Y-site compatibility: Cefmetazole, propofol, sargramostim
Solution compatibilities: D$_5$W, NaCl 0.9%

• Give for several days before transplant surgery
• Give with corticosteroids

Patient/family education
• Advise patient to report fever, rash, severe diarrhea, chills, sore throat, fatigue, since serious infections may occur; also to report clay-colored stools, cramping (may indicate hepatotoxicity); tremors, bleeding gums, increased B/P
• Advise patient to limit UV exposure
• Caution patient to use contraceptive measures during treatment and for 12 wk after ending therapy; product is teratogenic
• Caution patient to avoid crowds and persons with known infections to reduce risk of infection

Evaluation
Positive therapeutic outcome
• Absence of graft rejection

---

cyproheptadine (Rx)
(si-proe-hep′ta-deen)
cyproheptadine HCl, PMS-Cyproheptadine
Func. class.: Antihistamine, H$_1$-receptor antagonist
Chem. class.: Piperidine
Pregnancy category B

Do not confuse:
cyproheptadine/cyclobenzaprine

Action: Acts on blood vessels, GI, respiratory system by competing with histamine for H$_1$-receptor site; decreases allergic response by blocking histamine; blocks serotonin to increase appetite and relieve vascular headaches

Therapeutic outcome: Absence of allergy symptoms and rhinitis

Uses: Allergy symptoms, rhinitis, pruritus, common cold, urticaria

Unlabeled uses: Appetite stimulant, management of vascular headache, nightmares, posttraumatic stress disorder

Dosage and routes
Adult: PO 4 mg tid-qid, max 0.5 mg/kg/day
Geriatric: PO 4 mg bid, may increase if needed
Child 6-14 yr: PO 4 mg bid-tid, max 16 mg/day

Child 2-6 yr: PO 2 mg bid-tid, max 12 mg/day

Nightmares, posttraumatic stress disorder (unlabeled)
Adult: PO 4-12 mg nightly, max 32 mg

Available forms: Tabs 4 mg; syr 2 mg/5 ml

Adverse effects
CNS: Dizziness, drowsiness, poor coordination, fatigue, anxiety, euphoria, confusion, paresthesia, neuritis
CV: Hypotension, palpitations, tachycardia
EENT: Blurred vision, dilated pupils; tinnitus; nasal stuffiness; dry nose, throat, mouth
GI: Constipation, dry mouth, nausea, vomiting, anorexia, diarrhea, weight gain, increased appetite
GU: Urinary retention, dysuria, urinary frequency
HEMA: **Hemolytic anemia, leukopenia, thrombocytosis, agranulocytosis**
INTEG: Rash, urticaria, photosensitivity
MISC: **Anaphylaxis**
RESP: Increased thick secretions, wheezing, chest tightness

Contraindications: Breastfeeding, geriatric patients, hypersensitivity to H$_1$-receptor antagonist, closed-angle glaucoma, neonates/infants

Precautions: Pregnancy **B**, cardiac disease, asthma, peptic ulcers, ileus, urinary retention, COPD, bladder neck obstruction, prostatic hypertrophy

Pharmacokinetics
Absorption	Well absorbed
Distribution	Unknown
Metabolism	Liver, complete
Excretion	Kidneys, (65%-75%); feces (25%-35%)
Half-life	Unknown

Pharmacodynamics
Onset	15-60 min
Peak	1-2 hr
Duration	8 hr

Interactions
Individual drugs
Alcohol: increased CNS depression
Drug classifications
Antidepressants (tricyclics), barbiturates, CNS depressants, opiates, sedative/hypnotics: increased CNS depression
MAOIs: increased anticholinergic effect

Drug/herb
Corkwood, henbane leaf: increased anticholinergic effect
Hops, Jamaican dogwood, kava, khat, senega: increased CNS depression

Drug/lab test
False negative: skin allergy tests (discontinue antihistamine 3 days before testing)

NURSING CONSIDERATIONS
Assessment
• Assess respiratory status: rate, rhythm, increase in bronchial secretions, wheezing, chest tightness; provide fluids to 2 L/day to decrease secretion thickness
• Monitor I&O ratio: be alert for urinary retention, frequency, dysuria, especially geriatric; product should be discontinued if these occur; monitor food intake, weight if using as an appetite stimulant

Nursing diagnoses
• Airway clearance, ineffective (uses)
• Injury, risk for (side effects)
• Knowledge, deficient (teaching)
• Noncompliance (teaching, overuse)

Implementation
• May give with food to decrease GI upset
• Syrup may be used for patients with difficulty swallowing or children
• Store in tight, light-resistant container

Patient/family education
• Teach all aspects of product uses; tell patient to notify prescriber if confusion, sedation, hypotension occur; to avoid driving and other hazardous activity if drowsiness occurs; to avoid alcohol and other CNS depressants that may potentiate effect
• Caution patient not to exceed recommended dosage; dysrhythmias may occur
• Teach patient hard candy, gum, frequent rinsing of mouth may be used for dryness
• Advise patient to avoid breastfeeding

Evaluation
Positive therapeutic outcome
• Absence of runny or congested nose, rashes

Treatment of overdose: Administer lavage, diazepam, vasopressors, phenytoin IV

! HIGH ALERT

cytarabine (Rx)
(sye-tare′a-been)
Ara-C, Cytosar ✤, Cytosar-U, cytosine arabinoside
cytarabine liposomal (Rx)
Depo Cyt
Func. class.: Antineoplastic, antimetabolite
Chem. class.: Pyrimidine nucleoside

Pregnancy category D

Do not confuse:
Cytosar ✤/Cytovene/Cytoxan

Action: Competes with physiologic substrate of DNA synthesis, thus interfering with cell replication in the S phase of the cell cycle (before mitosis)

Therapeutic outcome: Prevention of rapidly growing malignant cells

Uses: Acute myelocytic leukemia, acute lymphocytic leukemia, chronic myelocytic leukemia, lymphomatous meningitis (IT)

Unlabeled uses: Hodgkin's, non-Hodgkin's lymphoma

Dosage and routes
Acute nonlymphocytic/lymphocytic
Adult: **IV** INF 200 mg/m²/day × 5 days q2wk as single agent or 2-6 mg/kg/day (100-200 mg/m²/day) as single dose or 2-3 divided doses for 5-10 days until remission, used in combination; maintenance 70-200 mg/m²/day for 2-5 days qmo; SUBCUT maintenance 1 mg/kg 1-2 ×/wk

Meningeal leukemia
Adult and child: IT 5-75 mg/m² variable daily × 4 days to q2-7day

Refractory acute Hodgkin's/refractory non-Hodgkin's lymphoma (unlabeled)
Adult: **IV** 2 g/m²/day; on day 5 q21day, with etoposide, methylPREDNISolone, and cisplatin

Available forms: Powder for inj 100, 500 mg, 1, 2 g; sus rel (Depo Cyt) liposomal for IT use 10 mg/ml

Adverse effects
CNS: Neuritis, dizziness, headache, cerebellar syndrome, personality changes, ataxia, mechanical dysphasia, **coma; chemical arachnoiditis** (IT)
CV: Chest pain, **cardiopathy**
CYTARABINE SYNDROME: Fever, myalgia, bone pain, chest pain, rash, conjunctivitis, malaise (6-12 hr after administration)

Adverse effects: *italic* = common, **bold** = life-threatening

EENT: Sore throat, conjunctivitis
GI: *Nausea, vomiting, anorexia, diarrhea, stomatitis,* **hepatotoxicity,** abdominal pain, hematemesis, **GI hemorrhage**
GU: Urinary retention, **renal failure, hyperuricemia**
HEMA: Thrombophlebitis, bleeding, thrombocytopenia, leukopenia, myelosuppression, anemia
INTEG: *Rash, fever,* freckling, cellulitis
META: Hyperuricemia
RESP: Pneumonia, dyspnea, **pulmonary edema** (high doses)
SYST: Anaphylaxis

Contraindications: Pregnancy **D,** hypersensitivity

Precautions: Renal/hepatic disease, breastfeeding, children, tumor lysis syndrome, infection, hyperkalemia, hyperphosphatemia, hyperuricemia, hypocalcemia

Black Box Warning: Bone marrow suppression

Pharmacokinetics

Absorption	Complete
Distribution	Widely distributed; crosses blood-brain barrier, placenta
Metabolism	Liver, extensively
Excretion	Kidneys
Half-life	1-3 hr; IT 100-236 hr

Pharmacodynamics
Unknown

Interactions
Individual drugs
Digoxin oral: decreased digoxin effects
Filgrastim, G-CSF, GM-CSF, sargramostim: do not use within 24 hr
Flucytosine, methotrexate: increased toxicity, immunosuppression
Gentamicin: decreased effects
Radiation: increased toxicity, bone marrow suppression
Drug classifications
Anticoagulants, NSAIDs, platelet inhibitors, salicylates, thrombolytics: increased bleeding risk
Antineoplastics: increased toxicity, bone marrow suppression
Live virus vaccines: do not use together

NURSING CONSIDERATIONS
Assessment
• Assess buccal cavity q8hr for dryness, sores or ulceration, white patches, pain, bleeding,
dysphagia; obtain prescription for viscous lidocaine (Xylocaine)
• Assess symptoms indicating anaphylaxis: rash, pruritus, urticaria, purpuric skin lesions, itching, flushing; resuscitation equipment should be nearby
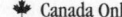 Assess for chemical arachnoiditis (IT): headache, nausea, vomiting, fever; neck rigidity/pain, meningism, CSF pleocytosis; may be decreased by dexamethasone
• Assess tachypnea, dyspnea, edema, fatigue; identify dyspnea, crackles, unproductive cough, chest pain, tachypnea; pulmonary edema may be fatal (rare)
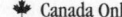 Assess for cytarabine syndrome 6-12 hr after infusion: fever, myalgia, bone pain, chest pain, rash, conjunctivitis, malaise; corticosteroid may be ordered
• Monitor CBC, differential, platelet count weekly; withhold product if WBC count is <1000/mm^3 or platelet count is <50,000/mm^3
• Assess for increased uric acid levels, swelling, joint pain primarily in extremities; patient should be well hydrated to prevent urate deposits
• Monitor renal function studies: BUN, creatinine, serum uric acid, urine CCr before and during therapy; I&O ratio; report fall in urine output to <30 ml/hr
• Monitor temp q4hr (may indicate beginning of infection)
• Monitor liver function tests before and during therapy (bilirubin, AST, ALT, LDH) as needed or monthly; note yellowing of skin or sclera, dark urine, clay-colored stools, pruritus, abdominal pain, fever, diarrhea; an antispasmodic may be used for GI symptoms
• Assess for bleeding: hematuria, stool guaiac, bruising or petechiae, mucosa or orifices q8hr; identify inflammation of mucosa, breaks in skin

Nursing diagnoses
• Body image, disturbed (adverse reactions)
• Infection, risk for (adverse reactions)
• Injury, risk for (adverse reactions)
• Knowledge, deficient (teaching)

Implementation
• Avoid contact with skin; very irritating; wash completely to remove
• Give fluids **IV** or PO before chemotherapy to hydrate patient
• Give antiemetic 30-60 min before giving product to prevent vomiting, and prn; antibiotics for prophylaxis of infection
• Increase fluids to 3 L/day
• Give top or syst analgesics for pain

- Give in AM so product can be eliminated before bedtime
- Give **IV** direct after diluting 100 mg/5 ml of sterile water for inj; give by direct **IV** over 1-3 min through free-flowing tubing

IM/SUBCUT route
- Reconstitute 100 mg/5 ml or 500 mg/10 ml with bacteriostatic water for inj with benzyl alcohol 0.9%; do not use sol with precipitate; stable for 48 hr

Intrathecal route
- Liposomal: withdraw product immediately before use; use within 4 hr, do not save unused portions, or use in-line filter; give directly into CSF by intraventricular reservoir or by direct inj into lumbar site
- Give slowly over 1-5 min; follow with lumbar puncture; instruct patient to lie flat; give dexamethasone 4 mg bid PO or **IV** × 5 days beginning on day of liposomal inj

IV infusion route
- May be further diluted in 50-100 ml 0.9% NaCl or D₅W and given over 30 min to 24 hr depending on dosage; may be given by cont inf also

Syringe compatibilities: Metoclopramide

Y-site compatibilities: Amifostine, amsacrine, aztreonam, cefepime, chlorproMAZINE, cimetidine, cladribine, dexamethasone, diphenhydrAMINE, droperidol, famotidine, filgrastim, fludarabine, gentamicin, granisetron, heparin, hydrocortisone, hydromorphone, idarubicin, lorazepam, melphalan, methotrexate, methylPREDNISolone, metoclopramide, morphine, ondansetron, paclitaxel, piperacillin/tazobactam, prochlorperazine, promethazine, propofol, ranitidine, sargramostim, sodium bicarbonate, teniposide, thiotepa, vinorelbine

Additive compatibilities: Corticotropin, DAUNOrubicin with etoposide, etoposide, hydrOXYzine, lincomycin, mitoxantrone, potassium chloride, prednisoLONE, ondansetron, sodium bicarbonate, vinCRIStine

Additive incompatibilities: Carbenicillin, fluorouracil, heparin, regular insulin, nafcillin, oxacillin, penicillin G sodium

Solution compatibilities: Amino acids, 4.25%/D₂₅, D₅/LR, D₅/0.2% NaCl, D₅/0.9% NaCl, D₁₀/0.9% NaCl, D₅W, invert glucose 10% in electrolyte #1, Ringer's LR, 0.9% NaCl, sodium lactate 1/6 mol/L, TPN #57

Patient/family education
- Advise patient that contraceptive measures are recommended during and 4 mo after therapy

- Teach patient to avoid use of products containing aspirin or ibuprofen, NSAIDs, razors, commercial mouthwash, since bleeding may occur; to report symptoms of bleeding (hematuria, tarry stools)
- Advise that fever, headache, nausea, vomiting are likely to occur, but to continue using dexamethasone with IT administration
- Provide liquid diet: carbonated beverages; gelatin may be added if patient is not nauseated or vomiting
- Provide rinsing of mouth tid-qid with water, club soda; brushing of teeth bid-qid with soft brush or cotton-tipped applicators for stomatitis; use unwaxed dental floss
- Advise patient to report signs of anemia (fatigue, headache, irritability, faintness, shortness of breath)
- Advise patient to avoid foods with citric acid, hot flavor, or rough texture if stomatitis is present, to use sponge brush and rinse with water after each meal; to report stomatitis: any bleeding, white spots, ulcerations in mouth; tell patient to examine mouth daily, report any symptoms
- Instruct patient to report any changes in breathing or coughing even several months after treatment; to avoid crowds and persons with respiratory tract or other infections; neurotoxicity
- Caution patient not to have any vaccinations without the advice of the prescriber; serious reactions can occur
- Advise patient to take 3 L/day fluids to prevent renal damage

Evaluation
Positive therapeutic outcome
- Prevention of rapid division of malignant cells

❗ HIGH ALERT

dacarbazine (Rx)
(da-kar′ba-zeen)
dacarbazine, DTIC ✦, DTIC-Dome
Func. class.: Antineoplastic—miscellaneous agent
Chem. class.: Imidazole

Pregnancy category C

Action: Alkylates DNA, RNA; inhibits enzymes that allow synthesis of amino acids in proteins; also responsible for breakage, cross-linking DNA strands; activity is not cell cycle phase specific

Therapeutic outcome: Prevention of rapidly growing malignant cells

Uses: Hodgkin's disease, malignant melanoma

Unlabeled uses: Malignant pheochromocytoma in combination with cyclophosphamide and vinCRIStine, metastatic soft tissue sarcoma in combination with other agents, carcinoma meningitis, neuroblastoma

Dosage and routes
Metastatic malignant melanoma
Adult: IV 2-4.5 mg/kg daily × 10 days or 100-250 mg/m² daily × 5 days; repeat q3wk depending on response

Hodgkin's disease
Adult: IV 150 mg/m² daily × 5 days with other agents, repeat q4wk or 375 mg/m² on day 1 when given in combination, repeat q28day

Osteogenic sarcoma (unlabeled)
Adult and child: IV 250 mg/m²/day as a cont INF × 4 days q28day

Soft tissue sarcoma (unlabeled)
Adult and child: IV 250-300 mg/m²/day as a cont INF × 3 days q21-28day

Carcinoma meningitis (unlabeled)
Adult: Intrathecal 5-30 mg in a fixed dose 2-3 × wk until disease controlled

Available forms: Powder for inj 10, 100, 200 mg

Adverse effects
CNS: Facial paresthesia, flushing, fever, malaise, confusion, headache, **seizures, cerebral hemorrhage,** blurred vision (high doses)
GI: Nausea, anorexia, vomiting, **hepatotoxicity** (rare)
HEMA: **Thrombocytopenia, leukopenia,** anemia
INTEG: Alopecia, dermatitis, pain at inj site, photosensitivity, severe sun reactions (high doses)
MISC: Flulike symptoms, malaise, fever, myalgia, hypotension
SYST: **Anaphylaxis**

Contraindications: Hypersensitivity, breastfeeding

Precautions: Renal disease

Black Box Warning: Pregnancy C (1st trimester), radiation therapy, hepatic disease, bone marrow suppression, secondary malignancy

Pharmacokinetics
Absorption	Complete bioavailability (**IV**)
Distribution	Widely distributed; concentrates in liver
Metabolism	Liver (50%, 5% protein bound)
Excretion	Kidneys, unchanged (50%)
Half-life	Initial 35 min, terminal 5 hr

Pharmacodynamics
Unknown

Interactions
Individual drugs
Phenobarbital, phenytoin: increased metabolism; decreased dacarbazine effect
Radiation: bone marrow suppression, toxicity
Drug classifications
Aminoglycosides: increased nephrotoxicity
Anticoagulants, salicylates: increased risk of bleeding
Antineoplastics, bone marrow–suppressing products: increased toxicity, bone marrow suppression
Diuretics, loop: increased ototoxicity
Live virus vaccines: increased adverse reactions; decreased antibody reaction

NURSING CONSIDERATIONS
Assessment
• Assess symptoms indicating severe allergic reaction: rash, pruritus, urticaria, purpuric skin lesions, itching, flushing; product should be discontinued
• Monitor CBC, differential, platelet count weekly; withhold product if WBC is <4000/mm³ or platelet count is <100,000/mm³
• Monitor renal function tests: BUN, creatinine, urine CCr before, during therapy; I&O ratio; report fall in urine output to <30 ml/hr
• Monitor temp q4hr (may indicate beginning of infection)
• Monitor liver function tests before, during therapy (bilirubin, AST, ALT, LDH) as needed or monthly; note jaundice of skin or sclera, dark urine, clay-colored stools, itchy skin, abdominal pain, fever, diarrhea; hepatotoxicity can be serious and fatal
• Assess for bleeding: hematuria, stool guaiac, bruising or petechiae, mucosa or orifices q8hr; check for inflammation of mucosa, breaks in skin
• Identify effects of alopecia on body image; discuss feelings about body changes

Nursing diagnoses
- Body image, disturbed (adverse reactions)
- Infection, risk for (adverse reactions)
- Injury, risk for (adverse reactions)
- Knowledge, deficient (teaching)

Implementation
- Give fluids **IV** or PO before chemotherapy to hydrate patient
- Give antiemetic 30-60 min before giving product to prevent vomiting, and prn; antibiotics for prophylaxis of infection
- Provide liquid diet: carbonated beverages; gelatin may be added if patient is not nauseated or vomiting
- After diluting 100 mg/9.9 ml of sterile water for inj (10 mg/ml), give by direct **IV** over 1 min through Y-tube or 3-way stopcock
- May be further diluted in 50-250 ml of D$_5$W or normal saline for inj and given over 30 min
- Watch for extravasation; give 3-5 ml of mixture of 4 ml sodium thiosulfate 10% plus 5 ml of sterile water SUBCUT as prescribed

Y-site compatibilities:
Amifostine, aztreonam, filgrastim, fludarabine, granisetron, melphalan, ondansetron, paclitaxel, sargramostim, teniposide, thiotepa, vinorelbine

Additive compatibilities:
Bleomycin, carmustine, cyclophosphamide, cytarabine, dactinomycin, DOXOrubicin, fluorouracil, mercaptopurine, methotrexate, ondansetron, vinBLAStine

Additive incompatibilities:
Hydrocortisone sodium succinate, cysteine

Patient/family education
- Teach patient to avoid use of products containing aspirin or ibuprofen, razors, commercial mouthwash, since bleeding may occur; to report symptoms of bleeding (hematuria, tarry stools)
- Instruct patient to report signs of anemia (fatigue, headache, irritability, faintness, shortness of breath)
- Advise patient that hair may be lost during treatment; a wig or hairpiece may make patient feel better; new hair may be different in color, texture
- Caution patient not to have any vaccinations without the advice of prescriber; serious reactions can occur
- Advise patient contraception is needed during treatment and for several months after the completion of therapy; product has teratogenic properties

Evaluation
Positive therapeutic outcome
- Prevention of rapid division of malignant cells

❗HIGH ALERT

D

daclizumab (Rx)
(dah-kliz'uh-mab)
Zenapax
Func. class.: Immunosuppressant
Chem class.: Humanized IgGl monoclonal antibody

Pregnancy category C

Action: Binds to the IL-2 receptor antagonist

Therapeutic outcome: Prevention of graft rejection

Uses: Acute allograft rejection in renal transplant patients

Dosage and routes
Adult: **IV** begin 24 hr prior to transplant, then 1 mg/kg as part of a regimen that includes cycloSPORINE and corticosteroids, mix calculated vol with 50 ml of 0.9% NaCl and give via peripheral/central vein over 15 min; do not admix; give q14day for a total of 5 doses

Available forms: Inj 5 mg/ml

Adverse effects
CNS: Chills, tremors, dizziness, insomnia, headache, prickly sensation, fatigue
CV: Hypo/hypertension, **tachycardia, thrombosis, bleeding,** chest pain
GI: Vomiting, nausea, diarrhea, constipation, abdominal pain, pyrosis
GU: Oliguria, dysuria, **renal tubular necrosis, renal damage, hydronephrosis**
INTEG: Impaired wound healing, acne
MISC: Edema, peripheral edema, allergic reaction, **anaphylaxis, bleeding, thrombosis**
RESP: Dyspnea, wheezing, **pulmonary edema,** coughing, atelectasis, congestion, hypoxia

Contraindications: Hypersensitivity to this product or murine protein

Precautions: Pregnancy C, breastfeeding, child <11 mo, geriatric, severe liver disease

Black Box Warning: Infection

Adverse effects: *italic* = common, **bold** = life-threatening

Pharmacokinetics
Unknown

Pharmacodynamics
Unknown

Interactions
Drug/herb
Ginseng, maitake, mistletoe, schisandra, St. John's wort, turmeric: decreased immunosuppressant effect
Safflower: increased immunosuppressant effect

NURSING CONSIDERATIONS
Assessment
- Monitor blood studies: Hgb, WBC, platelets during treatment qmo; if leukocytes are <3000/mm³, product should be discontinued
- Monitor liver function tests: alkaline phosphatase, AST, ALT, bilirubin
- Assess for hepatotoxicity: dark urine, jaundice, itching, light-colored stools; product should be discontinued
- Assess for anaphylaxis: have corticosteroids, epinephrine available

Nursing diagnoses
- Injury, risk for (uses)
- Knowledge, deficient (teaching)

Implementation
- Give all other medications PO if possible; avoid IM inj, since infection may occur

IV route
- Solution compatibilities 0.9% NaCl
- Protect undiluted sol from direct light; should be used with product for immunosuppression

Patient/family education
- Teach patient to report fever, chills, sore throat, fatigue, since serious infection may occur
- Instruct patient to use contraception (women) before, during, and for 4 mo after treatment
- Advise patient to avoid vaccinations during treatment
- Advise patient to drink fluids during treatment

Evaluation
Positive therapeutic outcome
- Absence of graft rejection

! HIGH ALERT

dactinomycin (Rx)
(dak-ti-noe-mye'sin)
Cosmegen
Func. class.: Antineoplastic, antibiotic

Pregnancy category D

Do not confuse:
dactinomycin/daptomycin

Action: Inhibits DNA, RNA, protein synthesis; derived from *Streptomyces parvulus;* replication is decreased by binding to DNA, which causes strand splitting; cell cycle nonspecific; a vesicant

Therapeutic outcome: Prevention of rapidly growing malignant cells, immunosuppression

Uses: Sarcomas, trophoblastic tumors in women, testicular cancer, Wilms' tumor, rhabdomyosarcoma

Unlabeled uses: Kaposi's sarcoma, malignant melanoma, osteogenic sarcoma, ovarian cancer, soft tissue sarcoma

Dosage and routes
Adult: **IV** 500 mcg/m²/day × 5 days; stop product for 2-4 wk, then repeat cycle
Child: **IV** 15 mcg/kg/day × 5 days, max 500 mcg/day; stop product until bone marrow recovery, then repeat cycle

Choriocarcinoma/hydatidiform mole
Adult: **IV** 1250 mcg/m² q14days × 4 cycles

Wilms' tumor/childhood rhabdomyosarcoma/Ewing's sarcoma
Adult and child: **IV** 15 mcg/kg/day × 5 days

Germ cell testicular cancer
Adult and child: **IV** 1000 mcg/m² as a single dose on day 1

Available forms: Inj 0.5 mg/vial

Adverse effects
CNS: Malaise, fatigue, lethargy, fever
EENT: Cheilitis, dysphagia, esophagitis
GI: Nausea, vomiting, anorexia, stomatitis, **hepatotoxicity,** abdominal pain, diarrhea
HEMA: **Thrombocytopenia, leukopenia, aplastic anemia**
INTEG: Rash, alopecia, pain at inj site, folliculitis, acne, desquamation, **extravasation**
MS: Myalgia

Contraindications: Hypersensitivity, herpes infections, child <6 mo

---

 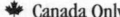

Black Box Warning: Pregnancy **D**

Precautions: Breastfeeding, renal/hepatic disease, bone marrow suppression, tumor lysis syndrome, infection

Black Box Warning: Accidental exposure, extravasation, secondary malignancy

Pharmacokinetics

Absorption	Complete bioavailability
Distribution	Widely distributed; crosses placenta
Metabolism	Unknown
Excretion	Bile; feces, unchanged (50%); kidneys (10%)
Half-life	36 hr

Pharmacodynamics

Unknown

Interactions
Individual drugs
Radiation: increased toxicity
Drug classifications
Antineoplastics: increased toxicity
Drug/lab test
Increased: uric acid

NURSING CONSIDERATIONS
Assessment
• Assess buccal cavity q8hr for dryness, sores or ulceration, white patches, pain, bleeding, dysphagia; obtain prescription for viscous lidocaine (Xylocaine)
◆ Assess symptoms indicating severe allergic reaction: rash, pruritus, urticaria, purpuric skin lesions, itching, flushing; product should be discontinued
• Monitor CBC, differential, platelet count weekly; withhold product if WBC is <4000/mm^3 or platelet count is <100,000/mm^3; notify prescriber of results if WBC <20,000/mm^3, platelets <150,000/mm^3
• Monitor renal function studies: BUN, creatinine, serum uric acid, urine CCr before, during therapy; I&O ratio; report fall in urine output to <30 ml/hr
• Monitor temp q4hr (may indicate beginning of infection)
• Monitor liver function tests before and during therapy (bilirubin, AST, ALT, LDH) as needed or monthly; note jaundice of skin or sclera, dark urine, clay-colored stools, itchy skin, abdominal pain, fever, diarrhea
• Assess for bleeding: hematuria, stool guaiac, bruising or petechiae, mucosa or orifices q8hr; check for inflammation of mucosa, breaks in skin

• Identify effects of alopecia on body image; discuss feelings about body changes

Nursing diagnoses
• Body image, disturbed (adverse reactions)
• Infection, risk for (adverse reactions)
• Injury, risk for (adverse reactions)
• Knowledge, deficient (teaching)
• Oral mucous membranes, impaired (adverse reactions)

Implementation
• Provide antacid before oral agent; give product after meals PM, before bedtime; antiemetic 30-60 min before giving product to prevent vomiting, and prn; antibiotics for prophylaxis of infection
• Provide liquid diet: carbonated beverages; gelatin may be added if patient is not nauseated or vomiting
• Help patient rinse mouth tid-qid with water, club soda, brush teeth bid-qid with soft brush or cotton-tipped applicators for stomatitis, use unwaxed dental floss
• Drug should be prepared by experienced personnel using proper precautions
• Give after diluting 0.5 mg/1.1 ml of sterile water for inj without preservative; use 2.2 ml (0.25 mg/ml), give by direct **IV** at 0.5 mg or less/min through Y-tube or 3-way stopcock of inf in progress
• Increase fluids to 3 L/day
Intermittent IV infusion route
• May be further diluted in 50 ml of D$_5$W or 0.9% NaCl for inf; run over 10-15 min
• Give hydrocortisone, sodium thiosulfate to infiltration area, and ice compress after stopping inf
• Store in darkness in cool environment
Y-site compatibilities: Allopurinol, amifostine, aztreonam, cefepime, fludarabine, granisetron, melphalan, ondansetron, sargramostim, teniposide, thiotepa, vinorelbine

Patient/family education
• Teach patient to avoid use of products containing aspirin or ibuprofen, razors, commercial mouthwash, since bleeding may occur; to report symptoms of bleeding (hematuria, tarry stools)
• Instruct patient to report signs of anemia (fatigue, headache, irritability, faintness, shortness of breath)
• Advise patient that hair may be lost during treatment; a wig or hairpiece may make patient feel better; new hair may be different in color, texture
• Caution patient not to have any vaccinations without the advice of the prescriber, serious reactions can occur

Adverse effects: *italic* = common, **bold** = life-threatening

- Advise patient that contraception is needed during treatment and for several months after the completion of therapy
- Advise patient to increase fluids to 3 L/day

Evaluation
Positive therapeutic outcome
- Prevention of rapid division of malignant cells

! HIGH ALERT

dalteparin (Rx)
(dahl′ta-pear-in)
Fragmin
Func. class.: Anticoagulant
Chem. class.: Low-molecular-weight heparin

Pregnancy category B

Action: Inhibits factor Xa/IIa (thrombin), resulting in anticoagulation

Therapeutic outcome: Absence of deep vein thrombosis

Uses: Unstable angina/non-Q-wave MI; prevention of deep vein thrombosis in abdominal surgery, hip replacement patients or those with restricted mobility during acute illness; pulmonary embolism

Unlabeled uses: Antiphospholipid antibody, arterial thromboembolism (after heart valve surgery), cerebral thromboembolism

Dosage and routes
Hip replacement surgery/
DVT prophylaxis
Adult: SUBCUT 2500 international units 2 hr before surgery and 2nd dose in the evening the day of surgery (4-8 hr postop), then 5000 international units SUBCUT 1st postop day and daily 5-10 days

Unstable angina/
non-Q-wave MI
Adult: SUBCUT 120 international units/kg q12hr × 5-8 days; max 10,000 international units q12hr × 5-8 days with concurrent aspirin, continue until stable

Deep vein thrombosis,
prophylaxis for abdominal
surgery
Adult: SUBCUT 2500 international units daily, evening prior to abdominal surgery and repeat daily × 5-10 days; in high-risk patients 5000 international units should be used

Available forms: Prefilled syringes, 2500, 5000 international units/0.2 ml; 7500 interna-

tional units/0.3 ml, 10,000 international units/ml

Adverse effects
CNS: **Intracranial bleeding**
HEMA: **Thrombocytopenia**
INTEG: Pruritus, superficial wound infection
SYST: Hypersensitivity, **hemorrhage, anaphylaxis** possible

Contraindications: Hypersensitivity to this product, heparin, pork products, benzyl alcohol; active major bleeding, hemophilia, leukemia with bleeding, thrombocytopenic purpura, cerebrovascular hemorrhage, cerebral aneurysm, those undergoing regional anesthesia for unstable angina, non-Q-wave MI, dalteparin-induced thrombocytopenia

Precautions: Pregnancy **B**, recent childbirth, breastfeeding, child, geriatric, hepatic disease, severe renal/cardiac disease, blood dyscrasias, bacterial endocarditis, acute nephritis, peptic ulcer disease, pericarditis, pericardial effusion, recent lumbar puncture, vasculitis, other diseases where bleeding is possible, uncontrolled hypertension; recent brain, spine, eye surgery; congenital or acquired disorders, hemorrhagic stroke, history of HIT

Black Box Warning: Epidural anesthesia

Pharmacokinetics	
Absorption	87%
Distribution	Unknown
Metabolism	Liver
Excretion	Kidney
Half-life	3-5 hr elimination

Pharmacodynamics	
Onset	Unknown
Peak	4 hr
Duration	Unknown

Interactions
Individual drugs
Aspirin: increased bleeding risk
Drug classifications
Anticoagulants, NSAIDs, platelet inhibitors, salicylates, thrombolytics: increased risk of bleeding
Drug/herb
Agrimony, alfalfa, angelica, anise, bilberry, black haw, bogbean, bromelain, buchu, chondroitin, cinchona bark, dong quai, fenugreek, feverfew, garlic, ginger, ginkgo, ginseng, horse chestnut, Irish moss, kelp, kelpware, khella, lovage, lungwort, meadowsweet, motherwort, mugwort, nettle, papaya,

---

parsley (large amounts), pau d'arco, pineapple, poplar, prickly ash, safflower, saw palmetto, senega, tonka bean, turmeric, wintergreen, yarrow: increased risk of bleeding

Chamomile, coenzyme Q10, flax, glucomannan, goldenseal, guar gum: decreased anticoagulant effect

NURSING CONSIDERATIONS
Assessment
• Assess for bleeding (Hct, occult blood in stools) during treatment since bleeding can occur

⬩ Assess for bleeding gums, petechiae, ecchymosis, black tarry stools, hematuria, epistaxis, decrease in Hct, B/P; may indicate bleeding, possible hemorrhage; notify prescriber immediately; product should be discontinued
• Assess for hypersensitivity: fever, skin rash, urticaria; notify prescriber immediately
• Assess for needed dosage change q1-2wk; dose may need to be decreased if bleeding occurs

Nursing diagnoses
• Injury, risk for (uses, adverse reactions)
• Knowledge, deficient (teaching)
• Tissue perfusion, ineffective (uses)

Implementation
SUBCUT route
• Cannot be used interchangeably (unit for unit with unfractionated heparin or LMWHs)
• Do not give IM or **IV** product route; approved in SUBCUT only; do not mix with other inj or sol
• Give by SUBCUT only; have patient sit or lie down; SUBCUT inj may be 2 in from umbilicus in a U-shape, upper outer side of thigh, around navel, or upper outer quadrangle of the buttocks; rotate inj sites
• Changing needles is not recommended; change inj site daily, use at same time of day

Patient/family education
• Advise patient to avoid OTC preparations that contain aspirin, other anticoagulants; serious product interaction may occur
• Advise patient to use soft-bristle toothbrush to avoid bleeding gums, avoid contact sports, use electric razor, avoid IM inj
• Instruct patient to report any signs of bleeding: gums, under skin, urine, stools; unusual bruising

Evaluation
Positive therapeutic outcome
• Absence of deep vein thrombosis

Treatment of overdose: Protamine sulfate 1% given **IV**; 1 mg protamine/100 anti-Xa international units of dalteparin given

dantrolene (Rx)
(dan'troe-leen)
Dantrium
Func. class.: Skeletal muscle relaxant, direct acting
Chem. class.: Hydantoin
Pregnancy category C

Do not confuse:
Dantrium/danazol

Action: Interferes with intracellular release from the sarcoplasmic reticulum of calcium necessary to initiate contraction; slows catabolism in malignant hyperthermia

Therapeutic outcome: Decreased muscle spasticity; absence of malignant hyperthermia

Uses: Spasticity in multiple sclerosis, stroke, spinal cord injury, cerebral palsy, prevention and treatment of malignant hyperthermia

Unlabeled uses: Neuroleptic malignant syndrome

Dosage and routes
Spasticity
Adult: PO 25 mg/day; may increase to 25-100 mg bid-qid, max 400 mg/day
Child: PO 0.5 mg/kg/day given in divided doses bid; may increase gradually; max 400 mg daily

Malignant hyperthermia
Adult and child: **IV** 1 mg/kg; may repeat to total dose of 10 mg/kg; PO 4-8 mg/kg/day in 4 divided doses × 3 days to prevent further hyperthermia; postcrisis follow-up 4-8 mg/kg/day for 1-3 days

Prevention of malignant hyperthermia
Adult and child: PO 4-8 mg/kg/day in 3-4 divided doses × 1-2 days before procedures; give last dose 4 hr preoperatively; **IV** 2.5 mg/kg prior to anesthesia

Neuroleptic malignant syndrome (unlabeled)
Adult: PO 100-300 mg/day in divided doses, **IV** 1.25-1.5 mg/kg

Available forms: Caps 25, 50, 100 mg; powder for inj 20 mg/vial

D

Adverse effects: *italic* = common, **bold** = life-threatening

Adverse effects

CNS: Dizziness, weakness, fatigue, drowsiness, headache, disorientation, insomnia, paresthesias, tremors, **seizures**
CV: Hypotension, chest pain, palpitations
EENT: Nasal congestion, blurred vision, mydriasis
*GI: **Hepatic injury,** nausea,* constipation, vomiting, increased AST and alkaline phosphatase, abdominal pain, dry mouth, anorexia, hepatitis, dyspepsia
GU: Urinary frequency, nocturia, impotence, crystalluria
HEMA: **Eosinophilia, aplastic anemia, leukopenia**
INTEG: Rash, pruritus, photosensitivity, extravasation tissue necrosis
RESP: Pleural effusion

Contraindications: Hypersensitivity, compromised pulmonary function, active hepatic disease, impaired myocardial function

Precautions: Pregnancy **C**, breastfeeding, geriatric, peptic ulcer disease, renal/cardiac, stroke, seizure disorder, diabetes mellitus, ALS, COPD, MS, mannitol/gelatin hypersensitivity, labor, lactase deficiency, extravasation

Black Box Warning: Active hepatic disease, females

Pharmacokinetics

Absorption	PO (30%-35%), poor
Distribution	Unknown
Metabolism	Liver, extensively
Excretion	Kidney
Half-life	9 hr

Pharmacodynamics

	PO	IV
Onset	Unknown	Immediate
Peak	5 hr	5 hr
Duration	Dose related	Dose related

Interactions

- Considered incompatible in sol or syringe; compatibility unknown
Individual drugs
Alcohol: increased CNS depression
Verapamil: increased dysrhythmias
Drug classifications
Antidepressants (tricyclic), antihistamines, barbiturates, opiates, sedative/hypnotics: increased CNS depression
Estrogens, hepatotoxic agents: increased hepatotoxicity

NURSING CONSIDERATIONS
Assessment
- Monitor I&O ratio; check for urinary retention, frequency, hesitancy, especially geriatric
- Monitor ECG in epileptic patients; poor seizure control has occurred with patients taking this product; assess for increased seizure activity in epilepsy patient
- Monitor hepatic function by frequent determination of AST, ALT, bilirubin, alkaline phosphatase, GGTP, renal function studies, CBC
- Assess for allergic reactions: rash, fever, respiratory distress
- Monitor for severe weakness, numbness in extremities
- Assess for CNS depression: dizziness, drowsiness, psychiatric symptoms
 Assess for signs of hepatotoxicity: jaundice, yellow sclera, pain in abdomen, nausea, fever; product should be discontinued if these signs and symptoms occur

Nursing diagnoses
- Injury, risk for (adverse reactions)
- Knowledge, deficient (teaching)
- Mobility, impaired physical (uses)
- Pain, chronic (uses)

Implementation
PO route
- Do not crush or chew caps; caps may be opened and mixed with juice and swallowed; drink immediately after mixing
- Give with meals for GI symptoms
- Store in airtight container at room temperature
IV route
- Administer **IV** after reconstituting 20 mg/60 ml sterile water for inj without bacteriostatic agent (333 mcg/ml); shake until clear; give by rapid **IV** push through Y-tube or 3-way stopcock; follow by prescribed doses immediately; may also give by intermittent inf over 1 hr before anesthesia; assess site for extravasation, phlebitis
- Protect diluted sol from light; use reconstituted sol within 6 hr
- Considered incompatible in sol or syringe, compatibility unknown

Patient/family education
- Notify prescriber of abdominal pain, jaundiced sclera, clay-colored stools, change in color of urine, rash, itching
- Caution patient not to take with alcohol, other CNS depressants; severe CNS depression can occur; avoid using OTC medication (cough preparations, antihistamines, alcohol, other

 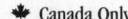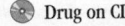

CNS depressants), unless directed by prescriber
- Tell patient that if improvement does not occur within 6 wk, prescriber may discontinue
- Caution patient to avoid hazardous activities if drowsiness, dizziness, blurred vision occurs; wait several days to identify patient response to medication
- Teach patient to use sunscreen, protective clothing for photosensitivity
- Instruct patient to take medication as prescribed; do not double doses; take missed dose within 1 hr of scheduled time

Evaluation
Positive therapeutic outcome
- Decreased pain, spasticity
- Absence or decreased symptoms of malignant hyperthermia

Treatment of overdose: Activated charcoal, supportive care

---

dapiprazole ophthalmic
See Appendix B

---

daptomycin (Rx)
(dap'toe-mye-sin)
Cubicin
Func. class.: Antiinfective—miscellaneous
Chem. class.: Lipopeptides
Pregnancy category B

Action: New class of antiinfective; binds to the bacterial membrane and results in a rapid depolarization of the membrane potential, leading to inhibition of DNA, RNA, and protein synthesis

Therapeutic outcome: Absence of infections

Uses: Complicated skin, skin structure infections caused by *Staphylococcus aureus*, including methicillin-resistant strains, *Streptococcus pyogenes, S. agalactiae, S. dysgalactiae, Enterococcus faecalis* (vancomycin-susceptible strains only)

Dosage and routes
Adult: **IV** INF 4 mg/kg over ½ hr diluted in 0.9% NaCl, give q24hr × 7-14 days
Adolescent/child/infant ≥5 mo (unlabeled): **IV** 4-6 mg/kg/day

Renal dose
Adult: **IV** CCr <30 ml/min; hemodialysis, CAPD 4 mg/kg q48hr

Available forms: Lyophilized powder for inj 500 mg

Adverse effects
CNS: Headache, insomnia, dizziness, confusion, anxiety, fatigue, fever
CV: Hypo/hypertension, **heart failure,** chest pain
GI: Nausea, constipation, diarrhea, vomiting, dyspepsia, **pseudomembranous colitis,** abdominal pain
GU: **Nephrotoxicity: increased BUN, creatinine, albumin**
HEMA: **Leukocytosis, anemia, thrombocytopenia**
INTEG: Rash, pruritus
MISC: Fungal infections, UTI, anemia
MS: Muscle pain or weakness, arthralgia, pain, **rhabdomyolysis**
RESP: Cough
SYST: **Anaphylaxis**

Contraindications: Hypersensitivity

Precautions: Pregnancy **B,** breastfeeding, children, geriatrics, GI/renal disease, myopathy, ulcerative/pseudomembranous colitis, rhabdomyolysis

Pharmacokinetics
Absorption	Unknown
Distribution	Protein binding 92%
Metabolism	Unknown
Excretion	Unknown
Half-life	Unknown

Pharmacodynamics
Unknown

Interactions
Drug classifications
HMG-CoA reductase inhibitors: myopathy
Drug/lab test
Increase: CPK, AST, ALT, BUN, creatinine, albumin

NURSING CONSIDERATIONS
Assessment
- Monitor I&O ratio: report hematuria, oliguria; nephrotoxicity may occur
◆ Monitor any patient with compromised renal system: BUN, creatinine; toxicity may occur
- Monitor blood tests: CBC
- Monitor C&S, product may be given as soon as culture is taken
- Monitor B/P during administration; hypo/hypertension may occur
- Assess signs of infection

Adverse effects: *italic* = common, **bold** = life-threatening

- Assess respiratory status: rate, character, wheezing
- Identify allergies before treatment, reaction of each medication

Nursing diagnoses
- Infection, risk for (uses)
- Knowledge, deficient (teaching)

Implementation
IV route
- Give after reconstitution with 5 ml 0.9% NaCl (250 mg/5 ml) or 10 ml 0.9% NaCl (500 mg/10 ml), further dilution is needed with 0.9% NaCl; infuse over ½ hr

Solution compatibilities: 0.9% NaCl, LR

Patient/family education
- Teach all aspects of product therapy
- Advise to report sore throat, fever, fatigue; could indicate superinfection

Evaluation
Positive therapeutic outcome
- Negative culture

---

darbepoetin (Rx)
(dar'bee-poh'-eh-tin)
Aranesp
Func. class.: Hematopoietic agent
Chem. class.: Recombinant human erythropoietin

Pregnancy category C

Action: Stimulates erythropoiesis by the same mechanism as endogenous erythropoietin; in response to hypoxia, erythropoietin is produced in the kidney and released into the bloodstream, where it interacts with progenitor stem cells to increase red cell production

Therapeutic outcome: Decreased anemia with increased RBCs

Uses: Anemia associated with chronic renal failure in patients on and not on dialysis and anemic in nonmyeloid malignancies receiving coadministered chemotherapy

Dosage and routes
Correction of anemia in chronic renal failure
Adult: SUBCUT/**IV** 0.45 mcg/kg as a single inj, titrate max target Hgb of 12 g/dl

Chemotherapy treatment
Adult: SUBCUT 2.5 mcg/kg/wk or 500 mcg q3wk

Epoetin alfa to darbepoetin conversion
Adult: SUBCUT/**IV** (epoetin alfa <2500 units/wk) 6.25 mcg/wk; (epoetin alfa 2500-4999 units/wk) 12.5 mcg/wk; (epoetin alfa 5000-10,999 units/wk) 25 mcg/wk; (epoetin alfa 11,000-17,999 units/wk) 40 mcg/wk; (epoetin alfa 18,000-33,999 units/wk) 60 mcg/wk; (epoetin alfa 34,000-89,999 units/wk) 100 mcg/wk; (epoetin alfa >90,000 units/wk) 200 mcg/wk

Available forms: Sol for inj 25, 40, 60, 100, 150, 200, 300, 500 mcg/ml

Adverse effects
CNS: **Seizures,** sweating, headache, dizziness, **stroke**
CV: *Hypo/hypertension,* **cardiac arrest,** *angina pectoris,* **thrombosis, CHF, acute MI, dysrhythmias,** chest pain, transient ischemic attacks, edema
GI: *Diarrhea, vomiting, nausea, abdominal pain, constipation*
HEMA: **Red cell aplasia**
MISC: *Infection, fatigue, fever,* **death,** *fluid overload,* **vascular access hemorrhage,** dehydration, sepsis
MS: *Bone pain, myalgia, limb pain, back pain*
RESP: *Upper respiratory infection, dyspnea, cough, bronchitis,* **pulmonary embolism**
SYST: *Allergic reactions,* **anaphylaxis**

Contraindications: Hypersensitivity to mammalian cell–derived products or human albumin, uncontrolled hypertension, red cell aplasia

Precautions: Pregnancy **C,** breastfeeding, children, seizure disorder, porphyria, hypertension, sickle cell disease, vit B_{12} folate deficiency, chronic renal failure, dialysis, latex hypersensitivity, CABG, angina, anemia

Black Box Warning: Hgb >12 g/dl, surgery

Pharmacokinetics	
Absorption	Slow, rate-limiting (SUBCUT)
Distribution	Vascular space
Metabolism	Metabolized in body (**IV**), extent unknown
Excretion	Unknown
Half-life	49 hr

Pharmacodynamics	
Onset	Onset of increased reticulocyte count 1-6 wk
Peak	34 hr
Duration	Unknown

Interactions
Individual drugs
◆ Do not use epoetin alfa with this product
Drug classifications
Androgens: increased darbepoetin alfa effect
Drug/lab test
Increased: WBC, platelets
Decreased: bleeding time

NURSING CONSIDERATIONS
Assessment
* Assess for serious allergic reactions: rash, urticaria; if anaphylaxis occurs, stop product, administer emergency treatment (rare)
* Assess blood studies: ferritin, transferrin monthly; transferrin sat ≥20%, ferritin ≥100 ng/ml; Hgb 2 ×/wk until stabilized in target range (30%-33%), then at regular intervals; those with endogenous erythropoietin levels of <500 units/L respond to this agent
* Assess renal studies: urinalysis, protein, blood, BUN, creatinine
* Assess B/P, Hct; check for rising B/P as Hct rises; antihypertensives may be needed
◆ Assess CV status: hypertension may occur rapidly, leading to hypertensive encephalopathy; Hgb >12 g/dl may lead to death
* Assess I&O ratio; report drop in output to <50 ml/hr
* Assess for seizures if Hgb is increased within 2 wk by 4 pts
* Assess CNS symptoms: cold sensation, sweating, pain in long bones
* Assess dialysis patients for thrill, bruit of shunts; monitor for circulation impairment

Nursing diagnoses
* Activity intolerance (uses)
* Fatigue (uses)
* Knowledge, deficient (teaching)

Implementation
IV/SUBCUT
* Do not shake, do not dilute, do not mix with other products or solutions
* Check for discoloration, particulate matter; do not use if present; discard unused portion; do not pool unused portion

Patient/family education
* Caution patient to avoid driving or hazardous activity during beginning of treatment
* Advise patient to monitor B/P
* Advise patient to take iron supplements, vit B₁₂, folic acid as directed
* Advise patient to report side effects to prescriber, to comply with treatment regimen
* Teach home administration and review information for patients and caregivers if home administration is deemed appropriate

Evaluation
Positive therapeutic outcome
* Increased reticulocyte count, Hgb/Hct
* Increased appetite
* Enhanced sense of well-being

Treatment of overdose: If polycythemia occurs, discontinue product temporarily; perform phlebotomy if clinically indicated

D

darunavir (Rx)
(dar-ue′na-vir)
Prezista
Func. class.: Antiretroviral
Chem. class.: Protease inhibitor

Pregnancy category B

Action: Inhibits human immunodeficiency virus (HIV-1) protease; this prevents maturation of virus

Therapeutic outcome: Decreased viral load, increase in CD4 counts

Uses: HIV-1 in combination with ritonavir and other antiretrovirals

Dosage and routes
Treatment-naive patients
Adult: PO 800 mg with ritonavir 100 mg qd
Child ≥6 yr/adolescents ≥30 kg, <40 kg: PO 450 mg bid with ritonavir 60 mg bid

Treatment-experienced patients
Adult: PO 600 mg with ritonavir 100 mg qd
Child ≥6 yr/adolescent ≥20 kg, <30 kg: PO 375 mg with ritonavir 50 mg bid

Available forms: Tabs 75, 150, 300, 400, 600 mg

Adverse effects
CNS: Headache, insomnia, dizziness, somnolence
GI: Diarrhea, abdominal pain, nausea, vomiting, anorexia, dry mouth
GU: Nephrolithiasis
INTEG: Rash
MS: Pain
OTHER: Asthenia, **insulin-resistant hyperglycemia,** hyperlipidemia, **ketoacidosis,** lipodystrophy

Contraindications: Hypersensitivity

Precautions: Pregnancy **B,** breastfeeding, children, renal/hepatic disease, history of renal stones, diabetes, hypercholesterolemia, sulfonamide hypersensitivity, antimicrobial resistance, bleeding, elderly, immune reconstitution syndrome, pancreatitis

Pharmacokinetics

Absorption	Unknown
Distribution	Protein binding 95%
Metabolism	By CYP3A
Excretion	Feces 79.5%, urine 13.9%
Half-life	Terminal 15 hr

Pharmacodynamics

Onset	Unknown
Peak	2.5-4 hr
Duration	Unknown

Interactions
Individual drugs

Atorvastatin, lovastatin, simvastatin: increased myopathy

Clarithromycin, zidovudine: increased levels of both products

Delavirdine, itraconazole, ketoconazole: increased darunavir levels

Efavirenz, fluconazole, nevirapine: decreased darunavir levels

Isoniazid: increased levels of isoniazid

◆Midazolam, pimozide, rifampin, triazolam: life-threatening dysrhythmias
Drug classifications

Anticonvulsants: decreased levels of both products

◆Ergots: life-threatening dysrhythmias; do not use concurrently

Oral contraceptives: increased levels of oral contraceptives

Rifamycins: decreased darunavir levels
Drug/herb

St. John's wort: decreased darunavir levels; avoid concurrent use
Drug/food

Darunavir: increased absorption

NURSING CONSIDERATIONS
Assessment
- Assess for complaints of lower back, flank pain; indicates kidney stones
- Assess for signs of infection, anemia, the presence of other STDs
- Monitor liver function tests: ALT, AST, bilirubin, amylase; all may be elevated
- Monitor viral load, CD4 during treatment; viral load should be decreasing, CD4 increasing
- Assess bowel pattern before, during treatment; if severe abdominal pain with bleeding occurs, product should be discontinued; monitor hydration
- Assess skin eruptions: rash, urticaria, itching
- Assess allergies before treatment, reaction of each medication; place allergies on chart

Nursing diagnoses
- Infection, risk for (uses)
- Knowledge, deficient (teaching)
- Noncompliance (teaching)

Implementation
- Give with food and ritonavir
- Give water to 1.5 L/day minimum to prevent nephrolithiasis

Patient/family education
- Instruct patient to take as prescribed; if dose is missed, take as soon as remembered up to 1 hr before next dose; do not double dose
- Advise patient that product must be taken in equal intervals around the clock to maintain blood levels for duration of therapy
◆ Advise patient that hyperglycemia may occur; watch for increased thirst, weight loss, hunger, dry, itchy skin; notify prescriber
- Teach patient to increase fluids to prevent kidney stones; if stone formation occurs, treatment may need to be interrupted
- Teach patient that product does not cure AIDS, only controls symptoms; do not donate blood

Evaluation
Positive therapeutic outcome
- Decreased viral load, increased CD4 counts

---

dasatinib (Rx)
(da-si'ti-nib)
Sprycel
Func. class.: Miscellaneous antineoplastic
Chem. class.: Protein-tyrosine kinase inhibitor

Pregnancy category D

Action: Inhibits BCR-ABL, SRC, LCK, YES, FYN, C-KIT, EPHA$_2$, and PDGFR-β tyrosine kinase created in chronic myeloid leukemia (CML)

Therapeutic outcome: Decrease in number of leukemic cells or size of tumor

Uses: Treatment of accelerated, chronic blast phase CML or acute lymphoblastic leukemia (ALL); chronic phase CML with resistance or intolerance to prior therapy

Dosage and routes
Accelerated or myeloid/lymphoid blast phase CML with resistance/ intolerance to prior therapy
Adult: PO 140 mg daily, titrated up to 180 mg bid in those resistant to therapy

Chronic phase CML with resistance/intolerance to prior therapy
Adult: PO 100 mg daily either AM or PM

Dosage reduction for those taking a strong CYP3A4 inhibitor
Adult: 20 mg daily

Available forms: Tabs 20, 50, 70, 100 mg

Adverse effects
CNS: **CNS hemorrhage,** headache, dizziness, insomnia, neuropathy, asthenia
CV: Dsyrhythmias, chest pain, CHF, pericardial effusion
GI: Nausea, **vomiting,** *anorexia, abdominal pain,* constipation, diarrhea, GI bleeding, muscositis, stomatitis
HEMA: **Neutropenia, thrombocytopenia, bleeding**
INTEG: Rash, pruritus
META: Fluid retention, edema, hypocalcemia, hypophosphatemia
MISC: Increased/decreased weight
MS: Pain, arthralgia, myalgia
RESP: Cough, dyspnea, pulmonary edema/hypertension, pneumonia, URI, **pleural effusion**

Contraindications: Pregnancy **D,** hypersensitivity

Precautions: Breastfeeding, children, geriatric

Pharmacokinetics	
Absorption	Unknown
Distribution	Protein binding 96%
Metabolism	By CYP3A4
Excretion	Feces 85%, urine 4%
Half-life	Terminal 1.3-5 hr

Pharmacodynamics	
Onset	0.5-6 hr
Peak	Unknown
Duration	Unknown

Interactions
Individual drugs
Clarithromycin, erythromycin, itraconazole, ketoconazole, nefazodine, telithromycin: increased dasatinib concentrations
Drug classifications
CYP3A4 inducers (dexamethasone, phenytoin, carbamazepine, rifampin, phenobarbital), H₂ blockers (famotidine), proton pump inhibitors (omeprazole): decreased dasatinib concentrations

CYP3A4 substrates (alfentanil, cycloSPORINE, ergots, fentanyl, pimozide, quinidine, sirolimus, tacrolimus): altered action
Protease inhibitors: increased dasatinib concentrations
Simvastatin: increased concentrations of this product
Drug/herb
St. John's wort: decreased dasatinib concentration

NURSING CONSIDERATIONS
Assessment
• Monitor ANC and platelets; in chronic phase if ANC <1 × 10⁹/L and/or platelets <50 ×10⁹/L, stop until ANC >1.5 × 10⁹/L and platelets >75 × 10⁹/L; in accelerated phase/blast crisis if ANC <0.5 × 10⁹/L and/or platelets <10 × 10⁹/L, determine whether cytopenia is related to biopsy/aspirate, if not, reduce dose by 200 mg, if cytopenia continues, reduce dose by another 100 mg; if cytopenia continues for 4 wk, stop product until ANC ≥1 × 10⁹/L
• Assess for renal toxicity: if bilirubin >3 × IULN, withhold until bilirubin levels return to <1.5 × IULN
• Assess for hepatotoxicity: monitor liver function tests, before treatment and qmo; if liver transaminases >5 × IULN, withhold until transaminase levels return to <2.5 × IULN
• Monitor CBC, differential, platelet count weekly; withhold product if WBC is <3500/mm³, or platelet count <100,000/mm³; notify prescriber of these results; product should be discontinued
• Monitor for signs of fluid retention, edema: weigh, monitor lung sounds, assess for edema, some fluid retention is dose dependent

Nursing diagnoses
• Infection, risk for (adverse reactions)
• Knowledge, deficient (teaching)
• Nutrition: less than body requirements, imbalanced (adverse reactions)

Implementation
• Do not break, crush, or chew tab
• Give after meal and with large glass of water
• Give nutritious diet with iron, vitamin supplement
• Store at 25° C (77° F)

Patient/family education
• Instruct patient to report adverse reactions immediately: SOB, swelling of extremities, bleeding
• Teach patient reason for treatment, expected result

Evaluation
Positive therapeutic outcome
• Decrease in number of leukemic cells

Adverse effects: *italic* = common, **bold** = life-threatening

! HIGH ALERT

*DAUNOrubicin (Rx)
(daw-noe-roo'bi-sin)
Cerubidine
*DAUNOrubicin citrate liposome (Rx)
DaunoXome
Func. class.: Antineoplastic, antibiotic
Chem. class.: Anthracycline glycoside

Pregnancy category D

Do not confuse:
DAUNOrubicin/DOXOrubicin

Action: Inhibits DNA synthesis, primarily; derived from *Streptomyces coeruleorubidus;* replication is decreased by binding to DNA, which causes strand splitting; cell cycle specific (S phase); a vesicant

Therapeutic outcome: Prevention of rapidly growing malignant cells; immunosuppression

Uses: Acute lymphocytic leukemia (ALL), acute myelogenous leukemia (AML); liposomal Kaposi's sarcoma

Dosage and routes
Use decreased dose for those >60 yr

DAUNOrubicin
In combination
Adult: IV 45-60 mg/m²/day × 3 days, then 2 days of subsequent courses in combination
Child: IV 25-60 mg/m² depending on cycle

DAUNOrubicin citrate liposome
Adult: IV 40 mg/m² q2wk

Renal dose
Adult: IV serum Cr >3 mg/dl reduce dose by 50%

Hepatic dose
Adult: IV serum bilirubin 1.2-3 mg/dl reduce dose by 25%; bilirubin >3 mg/dl reduce dose by 50%

Available forms: Inj 20 mg powder/vial, sol for inj 5 mg/ml (DaunoXome); liposome: dispersion for inj 2 mg/ml

Adverse effects
DAUNOrubicin
CNS: Fever, chills
CV: **Dysrhythmias, CHF, pericarditis, myocarditis,** peripheral edema
GI: *Nausea, vomiting, anorexia, mucositis,* **hepatotoxicity**
GU: Impotence, sterility, amenorrhea, gynecomastia, hyperuricemia

HEMA: **Thrombocytopenia, leukopenia, anemia**
INTEG: *Rash, extravasation,* dermatitis, reversible alopecia, cellulitis, thrombophlebitis at inj site
MISC: **Anaphylaxis**

DAUNOrubicin citrate liposome
CNS: Fatigue, headache, depression, insomnia, dizziness, malaise, neuropathy
CV: Chest pain, edema
GI: Abdominal pain, nausea, vomiting, *diarrhea,* constipation, stomatitis
INTEG: *Alopecia, sweating, pruritus*
MISC: *Allergic reactions, chest pain, fever,* edema, flulike symptoms
MS: *Rigors,* arthralgia, back pain
RESP: *Cough, dyspnea, rhinitis, sinusitis*

Contraindications: Pregnancy **D**, breastfeeding, hypersensitivity, systemic infections, cardiac disease, bone marrow depression

Precautions: Renal/hepatic disease, gout, tumor lysis syndrome, MI, infection, thrombocytopenia

Black Box Warning: Bone marrow suppression, cardiac disease, extravasation, renal failure

Pharmacokinetics

Absorption	Complete
Distribution	Widely distributed; crosses placenta
Metabolism	Liver, extensively
Excretion	Biliary (40%-50%)
Half-life	18½ hr, liposome 55½ hr

Pharmacodynamics
Unknown

Interactions
Individual drugs
Cyclophosphamide, radiation: increased toxicity
Drug classifications
Antineoplastics: increased toxicity
Live virus vaccines: decreased antibody reaction
NSAIDs, salicylates: increased risk of bleeding
Drug/lab test
Increased: uric acid

NURSING CONSIDERATIONS
Assessment
• Assess buccal cavity q8hr for dryness, sores or ulceration, white patches, pain, bleeding, dysphagia; obtain prescription for viscous lidocaine (Xylocaine)

 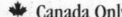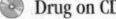

- Assess symptoms indicating severe allergic reaction: rash, pruritus, urticaria, purpuric skin lesions, itching, flushing; product should be discontinued
- Assess chest x-ray, echocardiography, radionuclide angiography, ECG; watch for ST-T wave changes, low QRS and T, possible dysrhythmias (sinus tachycardia, heart block, PVCs); watch for CHF (jugular vein distention, weight gain, edema, crackles), may occur after 2-6 mo of treatment
- Monitor CBC, differential, platelet count weekly, leukocyte nadir within 2 wk after administration, recovery within 3 wk; do not administer if absolute granulocyte count is <750/mm^3 (liposome)
- Assess for increased uric acid levels, swelling, joint pain primarily in extremities; patient should be well hydrated to prevent urate deposits
- Monitor renal function tests: BUN, creatinine, serum uric acid, urine CCr baseline and before each dose; I&O ratio; report fall in urine output to <30 ml/hr
- Monitor temp q4hr (may indicate beginning of infection)
- Monitor liver function tests baseline and before each dose (bilirubin, AST, ALT, LDH) as needed or monthly; note jaundice of skin or sclera, dark urine, clay-colored stools, itchy skin, abdominal pain, fever, diarrhea; hepatotoxicity can be severe
- Assess for bleeding: hematuria, stool guaiac, bruising or petechiae, mucosa or orifices q8hr; check for inflammation of mucosa, breaks in skin
- Identify effects of alopecia on body image; discuss feelings about body changes

Nursing diagnoses

- Body image, disturbed (adverse reactions)
- Cardiac output, decreased (adverse reactions)
- Infection, risk for (adverse reactions)
- Injury, risk for (adverse reactions)
- Knowledge, deficient (teaching)

Implementation

- Avoid contact with skin; very irritating; wash completely to remove
- Give fluids **IV** or PO before chemotherapy to hydrate patient; give antiemetic 30-60 min before giving product to prevent vomiting, and prn; antibiotics for prophylaxis of infection
- Provide liquid diet: carbonated beverages; gelatin may be added if patient is not nauseated or vomiting
- Help patient rinse mouth tid-qid with water, club soda, brush teeth bid-qid with soft brush or cotton-tipped applicators for stomatitis, use unwaxed dental floss
- Product should be prepared by experienced personnel using proper precautions

Cerubidine
IV route
- Give after diluting 20 mg/4 ml sterile water for inj (5 mg/ml); rotate; further dilute in 10-15 ml 0.9% NaCl; give over 3-5 min by direct **IV** through Y-tube or 3-way stopcock of inf of D$_5$W or 0.9% NaCl
Intermittent IV infusion route
- Dilute further in 50-100 ml 0.9% NaCl, LR, D$_5$W; give over 15 min (50 ml), 30 min (100 ml)

Y-site compatibilities: Amifostine, filgrastim, granisetron, melphalan, methotrexate, ondansetron, sodium bicarbonate, teniposide, thiotepa, vinorelbine
Y-site incompatibilities: Fludarabine
Additive compatibilities: Cytarabine with etoposide, hydrocortisone; not recommended for admixing
Additive incompatibilities: Dexamethasone, heparin
Solution compatibilities: D$_{3.3}$/0.3% NaCl, D$_5$W, Normosol-R, Ringer's, 0.9% NaCl

DaunoXome
IV route
- Dilute with D$_5$W (1 mg/ml); give over 60 min, do not use in-line filter, reconstituted sol may be stored ≤6 hr refrigerated; do not admix

Patient/family education

- Teach patient to avoid use of products containing aspirin or ibuprofen, razors, commercial mouthwash, since bleeding may occur; to report symptoms of bleeding (hematuria, tarry stools)
- Instruct patient to report signs of anemia (fatigue, headache, irritability, faintness, shortness of breath); signs of infection; bleeding, bruising, shortness of breath, swelling, change in heart rate; to avoid crowds, those with known infections
- Advise patient that hair may be lost during treatment; a wig or hairpiece may make patient feel better; new hair may be different in color, texture
- Caution patient not to have any vaccinations without the advice of the prescriber; serious reactions can occur
- Advise patient that contraception is needed during treatment and for 4 mo after the completion of therapy
- Advise patient to avoid alcohol, aspirin, NSAIDs

Evaluation
Positive therapeutic outcome
• Prevention of rapid division of malignant cells

---

decitabine (Rx)
(de-sit'-a-been)
Dacogen
Func. class.: DNA demethylation agent
Chem. class.: Cytosine analog
Pregnancy category D

Action: Incorporated into DNA and inhibits DNA methylation, halting growth of rapid proliferation of blasts

Therapeutic outcome: Decreasing blast count

Uses: Treatment of naïve and experienced myelodysplasic syndrome

Dosage and routes
Adult: CONT **IV** first treatment cycle: 15 mg/m^2 over 3 hr, q8hr × 3 days; subsequent treatment cycles: repeat above cycle q6wk for at least 4 cycles; a partial or complete response may take more than 4 cycles

Available forms: Powder for injection, lyophilized 50 mg, in single dose vial

Adverse effects
CNS: Headache, anxiety, dizziness, hypoesthesia, insomnia, confusion
CV: Edema, murmur, hypotension
GI: Nausea, anorexia, vomiting, diarrhea, constipation, stomatitis, abdominal pain, dyspepsia
HEMA: Neutropenia, thrombocytopenia, leukopenia, anemia
INTEG: Alopecia, ecchymosis, erythema, pallor, petechiae, pruritus, rash, swelling face, urticaria, hematoma, cellulitis
META: Decreased potassium, sodium, magnesium, albumin; increased bilirubin, increased/decreased glucose
MS: Myalgia, arthralgia, back pain, chest wall pain, pain in limbs
RESP: Cough, crackles, hypoxia, pharyngitis, pneumonia, pulmonary edema

Contraindications: Pregnancy **D**, breastfeeding, children, hypersensitivity to this product, severe neurotoxicity, severe blood dyscrasias

Precautions: Severe renal/hepatic disease, men (men should not father a child while receiving treatments or for 2 months after treatment ends), dental work, infections, thrombocytopenia

Pharmacokinetics
Absorption	Unknown
Distribution	Protein binding <1%
Metabolism	Liver, granulocytes, intestinal epithelium, whole blood
Excretion	Unknown
Half-life	Terminal 0.2-0.8 hr

Pharmacodynamics
Unknown

Interactions
Drug classifications
Do not use with live virus vaccines

NURSING CONSIDERATIONS
Assessment
• Monitor CBC (RBC, Hct, Hgb), differential, platelet count weekly; withhold product if WBC <4000/mm^3, platelets <75,000/mm^3, or RBC, Hct, Hgb is low; notify prescriber of results
• Monitor renal studies: BUN, serum uric acid, urine CCr, electrolytes before, during therapy
• Monitor temp q4hr; fever may indicate beginning infection; no rectal temps
• Monitor hepatic studies before, during treatment: bilirubin, AST, ALT, alkaline phosphatase, as needed or monthly
• Assess for bleeding: hematuria, hemepositive stools, bruising or petechiae, mucosa or orifices daily; blood dyscrasias can occur
• Assess for dyspnea, crackles, unproductive cough, chest pain, tachypnea, fatigue, increased pulse, pallor, lethargy, personality changes
• Assess buccal cavity daily for dryness, ulceration, white patches, oral pain, bleeding, dysphagia
• Assess GI symptoms: frequency of stools, cramping; if severe diarrhea occurs, electrolytes may need to be given

Nursing diagnoses
• Injury, risk for (uses)
• Knowledge, deficient (teaching)

Implementation
• Use procedures for handling and disposal of products
• Rinse mouth tid-qid with water or club soda; brush teeth tid with soft toothbrush or cotton-tipped applicator for stomatitis; use unwaxed dental floss
• Store at room temperature, away from light

Patient/family education

- Advise patient to report bleeding; not to use commercial mouthwashes, razors
- Teach patient to report signs of infection: increased temp, sore throat, flulike symptoms
- Teach patient to report signs of anemia: fatigue, headache, faintness, shortness of breath, irritability
- Advise patient to avoid citric acid, rough-textured foods, if stomatitis is present
- Teach patient to notify prescriber if pregnancy is suspected or planned; use contraception while taking this product
- Teach patient to avoid breastfeeding while taking this product
- Instruct patient not to operate machinery or perform other hazardous activities while taking this product
- Teach patient that men should not father a child while taking this product, pregnancy category **D**
- Teach patient to inform prescriber of kidney or liver disease
- Teach patient not to receive vaccinations while taking this product
- Advise to drink 2-3 L of fluids/day unless contraindicated

Evaluation
Positive therapeutic outcome
- Decreased blast count

---

delavirdine (Rx)
(de-la-veer'deen)
Rescriptor
Func. class.: Antiretroviral
Chem. class.: Nonnucleoside reverse transcriptase inhibitor (NNRTI)

Pregnancy category C

Action: Binds directly to reverse transcriptase and blocks RNA, DNA polymerase causing a disruption of the enzyme's site

Therapeutic outcome: Improvement of HIV-1 infection

Uses: HIV-1 in combination with other antiretrovirals

Dosage and routes
Adult and child ≥16 yr: PO 400 mg tid; max 1200 mg/day

Available forms: Tabs 100, 200 mg

Adverse effects
CNS: Headache, fatigue, anxiety, insomnia, fever

GI: Diarrhea, anorexia, abdominal pain, nausea, vomiting, dyspepsia, **hepatotoxicity**
GU: **Nephrotoxicity**
HEMA: **Neutropenia, leukopenia, thrombocytopenia, anemia, granulocytopenia**
INTEG: Rash, pruritus
MISC: Cough
MS: Pain, myalgia
SYST: **Stevens-Johnson syndrome**

Contraindications: Hypersensitivity

Precautions: Pregnancy **C**, breastfeeding, children, hepatic disease, exfoliative dermatitis, hepatitis, immune reconstitution syndrome, achlorhydria, antimicrobial resistance

Pharmacokinetics

Absorption	Well
Distribution	98% protein bound
Metabolism	Liver, extensively by CYP3A4
Excretion	Kidneys, feces
Half-life	2-11 hr

Pharmacodynamics

Onset	Unknown
Peak	1 hr
Duration	8 hr

Interactions
Individual drugs
Alprazolam, amprenavir, atorvastatin, clarithromycin, dapsone, felodipine, indinavir, lovastatin, midazolam, NIFEdipine, saquinavir, simvastatin: increased level of each specific product
Alprazolam, astemizole, cisapride, midazolam, pimozide, sildenafil, terfenadine, triazolam: life-threatening reactions; do not combine
Clarithromycin, quinidine, warfarin: increased level of both products
Didanosine: decreased delavirdine levels, decreased action of didanosine
Fluoxetine, ketoconazole: increased level of delavirdine
Drug classifications
Amphetamines, antidysrhythmics, benzodiazepines, calcium channel blockers, ergots, sedative/hypnotics, and other 3A4, 2D6 inhibitors: increased serious life-threatening adverse reaction
Antacids, anticonvulsants, protease inhibitors, rifamycins: decreased delavirdine levels
Antidysrhythmics, sedative/hypnotics: life-threatening reactions; do not combine

Adverse effects: *italic* = common, **bold** = life-threatening

Contraceptives (oral): decreased action of oral contraceptives

Ergots: increased levels of ergots

Drug/herb

St. John's wort: decreased delavirdine level

NURSING CONSIDERATIONS
Assessment
- Assess signs of infection, anemia
- Assess liver function tests: ALT, AST; renal studies
- Assess C&S before product therapy; product may be taken as soon as culture is taken; repeat C&S after treatment; determine the presence of other STDs
- Assess bowel pattern before, during treatment; if severe abdominal pain with bleeding occurs, product should be discontinued; monitor hydration
- Assess skin eruptions; rash, urticaria, itching
- Assess allergies before treatment, reaction to each medication; place allergies on chart
- Assess plasma delavirdine concentrations (trough 10 µm)
- Assess CBC, blood chemistry, plasma HIV RNA, absolute CD4$^+$/CD8$^+$/cell counts/%, serum β$_2$ microglobulin, serum ICD+24 antigen levels
- Assess for signs of delavirdine toxicity: severe nausea, vomiting, maculopapular rash

Nursing diagnoses
- Diarrhea (side effects)
- Infection, risk for (uses)
- Knowledge, deficient (teaching)

Implementation
- Add 4 tabs/3-4 oz of water, let stand, stir, swallow, rinse glass, swallow; use only 100 mg tabs for dispersion
- Do not give within 1 hr of antacids or didanosine
- Take in equal intervals around the clock

Patient/family education
- Advise patient to take as prescribed; if dose is missed, take as soon as remembered up to 1 hr before next dose; do not double dose
- Advise patient that product must be taken in equal intervals around the clock to maintain blood levels for duration of therapy
- Advise patient that tabs may be dissolved; drink right away, rinse cup with water, and drink that to get all medication
- Instruct patient to make sure health care provider knows of all the medications being taken
- Advise patient that if severe rash, mouth sores, swelling, aching muscles/joints, or eye redness occur, stop taking and notify health care provider
- Advise patient not to breastfeed if taking this product
- Teach patient that this product is not a cure, only controls symptoms

Evaluation
Positive therapeutic outcome
- Increased CD4$^+$ cell count
- Decreased viral load
- Improvement in symptoms of HIV

demecarium ophthalmic
See Appendix B

denileukin diftitox (Rx)
(den-ih-loo'kin dif'tih-tox)
Ontak
Func. class.: Antineoplastic—miscellaneous agent

Pregnancy category C

Action: A recombinant DNA-derived cytotoxic protein that interacts with high-affinity IL-2 receptors on the cell surface and inhibits cellular protein synthesis

Therapeutic outcome: Prevention of rapidly growing malignant cells

Uses: Cutaneous T-cell lymphoma that expresses CD25 component of the IL-2 receptor

Unlabeled uses: Non-Hodgkin's lymphoma, psoriasis

Dosage and routes
Adult: IV 9-18 mcg/kg/day given for 5 days q21day, give over ≥15 min

Available forms: sol for inj, frozen 150 mcg/ml

Adverse effects
CNS: Dizziness, paresthesia, nervousness, confusion, insomnia
CV: Hypo/hypertension, vasodilatation, tachycardia, thrombosis, dysrhythmia, hypertension, **capillary leak syndrome**
EENT: Persistent visual impairment
GI: Nausea, anorexia, vomiting, diarrhea, constipation, dyspepsia, dysphagia
GU: Hematuria, albuminuria, pyuria, creatinine increase
HEMA: **Thrombocytopenia, leukopenia,** *anemia*
INTEG: Rash, pruritus, sweating

META: Hypoalbuminemia, edema, hypocalcemia, weight decrease, dehydration, hypokalemia

MISC: Fever, chills, asthenia, infection, pain, headache, chest pain, flulike symptoms, **serious infection,** capillary leak syndrome

MS: Myalgia, arthralgia

RESP: Dyspnea, cough, pharyngitis, rhinitis

Contraindications: Hypersensitivity to denileukin, diphtheria toxin, interleukin-2

Precautions: Pregnancy C, breastfeeding, children, geriatric, CAD, *E. coli,* protein hypersensitivity, immunosuppression, peripheral vascular disease

Black Box Warning: Capillary leak syndrome, infection-related reactions, visual disturbances

---

Pharmacokinetics

Absorption	Complete bioavailability (**IV**)
Distribution	Widely distributed; concentrates in liver/kidneys
Metabolism	Proteolytic degradation
Excretion	Unknown
Half-life	Unknown

Pharmacodynamics

Unknown

Interactions
Drug classifications

Antineoplastics, bone marrow suppressing products, radiation: increased bone marrow suppression

Live virus vaccines: increased adverse reactions; decreased antibody reaction

NURSING CONSIDERATIONS
Assessment

• Assess symptoms indicating severe allergic reaction: rash, pruritus, urticaria, purpuric skin lesions, itching, flushing; product should be discontinued

• Assess for vascular leak syndrome after 2 wk of treatment: hypotension, edema, hypoalbuminemia; monitor weight, B/P, serum albumin, edema

• Obtain CD25 expression on skin biopsy samples

• Monitor CBC, differential, platelet count weekly; withhold product if WBC count is <4000/mm^3 or platelet count is <100,000/mm^3

• Monitor renal function studies: BUN, creatinine, urine CCr before, during therapy; I&O ratio; report fall in urine output to <30 ml/hr

• Monitor temp q4hr (may indicate beginning of infection)

• Monitor liver function tests before, during therapy (bilirubin, AST, ALT, LDH) as needed or monthly; note jaundiced skin or sclera, dark urine, clay-colored stools, itchy skin, abdominal pain, fever, diarrhea; hepatotoxicity can be serious and fatal

• Assess for bleeding: hematuria, stool guaiac, bruising or petechiae, mucosa or orifices q8hr; check for inflammation of mucosa, breaks in skin

Nursing diagnoses
• Body image, disturbed (adverse reactions)
• Infection, risk for (adverse reactions)
• Injury, risk for (adverse reactions)
• Knowledge, deficient (teaching)

Implementation
• Give fluids **IV** or PO before chemotherapy to hydrate patient

• Give antiemetic 30-60 min before giving product to prevent vomiting, and prn; antibiotics for prophylaxis of infection

• Provide liquid diet: carbonated beverages; gelatin may be added if patient is not nauseated or vomiting

• Prepare and hold sol in plastic syringes or soft plastic **IV** bags only

• Draw calculated dose from vial, inject into empty **IV** infusion bag; for each 1 ml of product removed from vial, no more than 9 ml of sterile saline without preservative should be added to **IV** bag; infuse over ≥15 min; do not give by BOL; do not admix with other products; do not use a filter

• Use within 6 hr, discard unused portions

• Watch for extravasation; give 3-5 ml of mixture of 4 ml sodium thiosulfate 10% plus 5 ml sterile water SUBCUT as prescribed

Patient/family education
• Teach patient to avoid use of products containing aspirin or NSAIDs, razors, commercial mouthwash, since bleeding may occur; to report symptoms of bleeding (hematuria, tarry stools)

• Instruct patient to report signs of anemia (fatigue, headache, irritability, faintness, shortness of breath)

• Caution patient not to have any vaccinations without the advice of prescriber; serious reactions can occur

• Advise patient contraception is needed during treatment and for several months after the completion of therapy; product has teratogenic properties

---

Adverse effects: *italic* = common, **bold** = life-threatening

Evaluation
Positive therapeutic outcome
- Prevention of rapid division of malignant cells

---

desipramine (Rx)
(dess-ip'ra-meen)
Apo-Desipramine ♣, desipramine HCl, Norpramin, Pertofrane ♣
Func. class.: Antidepressant, tricyclic
Chem. class.: Dibenzazepine, secondary amine

Pregnancy category C

Action: Blocks reuptake of norepinephrine, serotonin into nerve endings, increasing action of norepinephrine, serotonin in nerve cells

Therapeutic outcome: Decreased depression

Uses: Depression

Unlabeled uses: Chronic pain, ADHD, bulimia, diabetic neuropathy, panic disorder, social phobia

Dosage and routes
Major depression
Adult: PO 50-75 mg/day in 1-4 divided doses; titrate by 25-50 mg qwk up to 300 mg/day in single or divided doses
Geriatric: PO 25 mg/day at bedtime, titrate qwk; may increase to 150 mg/day
Child >12 yr: PO 25-50 mg/day in divided doses, max 150 mg/day
Child 6-12 yr: PO 1-3 mg/kg/day in divided doses, give >3 mg/kg/day with close medical monitoring; max 5 mg/kg/day

Available forms: Tabs 10, 25, 50, 75, 100, 150 mg

Adverse effects
CNS: Dizziness, drowsiness, confusion, headache, anxiety, tremors, stimulation, weakness, insomnia, nightmares, EPS (geriatric), increased psychiatric symptoms, paresthenia, suicidal ideation
CV: Orthostatic hypo/hypertension, ECG changes, tachycardia, palpitations
EENT: Blurred vision, tinnitus, mydriasis, ophthalmoplegia
GI: Diarrhea, dry mouth, nausea, vomiting, **paralytic ileus,** increased appetite, cramps, epigastric distress, jaundice, **hepatitis,** stomatitis, constipation, weight gain
GU: Retention, **acute renal failure**
HEMA: **Agranulocytosis, thrombocytopenia, eosinophilia, leukopenia**

INTEG: Rash, urticaria, sweating, pruritus, photosensitivity

Contraindications: Hypersensitivity to tricyclics, closed-angle glaucoma, acute MI

Precautions: Pregnancy **C**, breastfeeding, geriatric, severe depression, increased intraocular pressure, seizure disorder, CV disease, prostatic hypertrophy, thyroid disease

Black Box Warning: Suicidal patients, children <18 yr

Pharmacokinetics
Absorption	Well
Distribution	Widely, protein binding 92%
Metabolism	Extensively, liver
Excretion	Unknown
Half-life	12-24 hr

Pharmacodynamics
Unknown

Interactions
Individual drugs
Alcohol: increased CNS depression
Cimetidine, diltiazem, fluvoxamine, fluoxetine, paroxetine, sertraline, verapamil: increased desipramine level
Clonidine: increased life-threatening B/P elevations, do not use concurrently
Epinephrine, norepinephrine: increased hypertension
Drug classifications
Barbiturates, opioids, CNS depressants: increased CNS depression
MAOIs: increased hyperpyrexia, seizures, excitation; do not use within 14 days of MAOIs
Tricyclic antidepressants: increased QT interval
Drug/herb
Evening primrose oil: may lower seizure threshold; do not use concurrently
Chamomile, hops, kavan, valerian: increased CNS depression
St. John's wort, SAM-e: may increase serotonin syndrome; avoid concurrent use
Drug/lab test
Increase: serum bilirubin, blood glucose, alkaline phosphatase

NURSING CONSIDERATIONS
Assessment
- Monitor B/P (lying, standing), pulse q4hr; if systolic B/P drops 20 mm Hg, hold product, notify prescriber; take vital signs q4hr in patients with CV disease

---

🔷 Alert   ♣ Canada Only   🔘 Drug on CD   ＊ "Tall Man" lettering (See Preface)

- Monitor blood studies: CBC, leukocytes, differential, cardiac enzymes if patient is receiving long-term therapy
- Monitor hepatic studies: AST, ALT, bilirubin
- Check weight qwk; appetite may increase with this product
- Monitor ECG for flattening T wave, bundle branch block, AV block, dysrhythmias in cardiac patients
- Assess for EPS primarily in geriatric: rigidity, dystonia, akathisia
- Assess for seizure activity in those with a history of seizures
- Assess mental status: mood, sensorium, affect, suicidal tendencies, increase in psychiatric symptoms: depression, panic
- Assess for urinary retention, constipation; constipation most likely in children
- Assess for withdrawal symptoms: headache, nausea, vomiting, muscle pain, weakness; not usual unless product discontinued abruptly
- Assess for alcohol consumption; if consumed, hold dose until morning

Nursing diagnoses
- Coping, ineffective (uses)
- Knowledge, deficient (teaching)
- Noncompliance (teaching)

Implementation
- Increase fluids, bulk in diet for constipation, especially in geriatric
- Take with food or milk for GI symptoms
- Crush if patient is unable to swallow medication whole
- Give dosage at bedtime if oversedation occurs during day; may take entire dose at bedtime; geriatric may not tolerate once a day dosing
- Give gum, hard candy, frequent sips of water for dry mouth
- Store at room temperature
- Provide assistance with ambulation during beginning of therapy for drowsiness/dizziness
- Provide safety measures, primarily in the geriatric
- Check to see that PO medication is swallowed

Patient/family education
- Advise patient that therapeutic effects may take 2-3 wk
- Teach patient that suicidal thoughts and behavior may occur
- Advise patient to use caution in driving, other activities requiring alertness because of drowsiness, dizziness, blurred vision
- Teach patient to avoid alcohol ingestion, other CNS depressants
- Teach patient not to discontinue medication quickly after long-term use; may cause nausea, headache, malaise
- Teach patient to wear sunscreen or large hat, since photosensitivity occurs

Evaluation
Positive therapeutic outcome
- Decreased depression

Treatment of overdose: ECG monitoring; induce emesis; lavage, activated charcoal; administer anticonvulsant

---

desloratadine (Rx)
(des-lor-at'ah-deen)
Clarinex, Clarinex RediTabs
Func. class.: Antihistamine, 2nd generation
Chem. class.: Selective histamine (H_1) receptor antagonist

Pregnancy category C

Action: Binds to peripheral histamine receptors, providing antihistamine action without sedation

Therapeutic outcome: Decreased nasal stuffiness, itching, swollen eyes

Uses: Seasonal/perennial allergic rhinitis, chronic idiopathic urticaria

Dosage and routes
Adult and child ≥12 yr: PO 5 mg daily
Child 6-11 yr: PO 2.5 mg daily
Child 1-5 yr: PO 1.25 mg daily
Child 6-11 mo: PO 1 mg daily

Renal/hepatic dose
Adult: PO 5 mg every other day

Available forms: Tabs 5 mg; orally disintegrating (Reditabs) 2.5, 5 mg; syr 0.5 mg/ml

Adverse effects
CNS: Sedation (more common with increased doses), headache, psychomotor hyperactivity, **seizures,** fatigue
GI: **Hepatitis,** nausea, dry mouth
MISC: Flulike symptoms

Contraindications: Hypersensitivity, infants/neonates

Precautions: Pregnancy C, bronchial asthma, renal/hepatic impairment, child, breastfeeding

---

Pharmacokinetics

Absorption	Unknown
Distribution	Bound to plasma proteins (82%-87%)
Metabolism	Liver (active metabolites)
Excretion	Urine, feces (metabolites)
Half-life	8½-28 hr

Pharmacodynamics

Onset	1 hr, relief in 1 day
Peak	1½ hr
Duration	24 hr

Interactions
Drug/food
Food may prolong time to peak with orally disintegrating tabs

NURSING CONSIDERATIONS
Assessment
• Assess for allergy: hives, rash, rhinitis; monitor respiratory status; test interaction, antigen skin test

Nursing diagnoses
• Airway clearance, ineffective (uses)
• Knowledge, deficient (teaching)
• Noncompliance (teaching, overuse)

Implementation
• May administer without regard to meals
• Store in airtight container at room temperature

Patient/family education
• Advise patient to avoid driving, other hazardous activities if drowsiness occurs; to observe caution until product's effects are known
• Advise patient that product may cause photosensitivity; use sunscreen or stay out of the sun to prevent burns
• Caution patient to avoid use of other CNS depressants
• Teach not to remove Reditabs from blister until ready to use; to place Reditabs directly on tongue; may take with or without water

Evaluation
Positive therapeutic outcome
• Absence of running or congested nose, other allergy symptoms

desmopressin (Rx)
(des-moe-press'in)
DDAVP, Minirin, Octostim ✤, Stimate
Func. class.: Pituitary hormone
Chem. class.: Synthetic antidiuretic hormone
Pregnancy category B

Action: Promotes reabsorption of water by action on renal tubular epithelium in the kidney; causes smooth muscle constriction and increase in plasma factor VIII levels, which increases platelet aggregation resulting in vasopressor effect; similar to vasopressin

Therapeutic outcome: Prevention of nocturnal enuresis, decreased bleeding in hemophilia A, von Willebrand's disease type 1, control and stabilization of water in diabetes insipidus

Uses: Hemophilia A, von Willebrand's disease type 1, nonnephrogenic diabetes insipidus, symptoms of polyuria/polydipsia caused by pituitary dysfunction, nocturnal enuresis

Dosage and routes
Primary nocturnal enuresis
Adult and child ≥6 yr: INTRANASAL 20 mcg (10 mcg in each nostril) at bedtime, may increase to 40 mcg; PO 0.2 mg at bedtime, may be increased to max 0.6 mg at bedtime

Diabetes insipidus
Adult: Intranasal 0.1-0.4 ml daily in divided doses (1-4 sprays with pump); SUBCUT/**IV** 0.5-1 ml daily in divided doses
Child 3 mo-12 yr: Intranasal 0.05-0.3 ml daily in divided doses

Hemophilia/von Willebrand's disease
Adult and child >3 mo: IV 0.3 mcg/kg in NaCl over 15-30 min; may repeat if needed

Antihemorrhagic
Adult and child >3 mo: **IV** 0.3 mcg/kg
Adult and child <50 kg: Intranasal 1 spray in one nostril
Adult and child >50 kg: 1 spray each nostril

Available forms: Inj 4, 15 mcg/ml, Rhinal Tube del 2.5 mg/vial (0.1 mg/ml); tabs 0.1, 0.2 mg; nasal spray pump 10 mcg/spray (0.1 mg/ml); nasal sol 1.5 mg/ml (150 mcg/dose)

Adverse effects
CNS: Drowsiness, headache, lethargy, flushing
CV: Increased B/P, palpitations, tachycardia
EENT: Nasal irritation, congestion, rhinitis

GI: Nausea, heartburn, cramps
GU: *Vulval pain*
META: Hyponatremia, hypernatremia
SYST: Anaphylaxis **(IV)**

Contraindications: Hypersensitivity, nephrogenic diabetes insipidus, severe renal disease

Precautions: Pregnancy **B,** breastfeeding, CAD, hypertension, cystic fibrosis, thrombus

Pharmacokinetics

Absorption	Nasal (up to 20%)
Distribution	Unknown
Metabolism	Unknown
Excretion	Unknown; breast milk
Half-life	8 min (initial), 76 min (terminal)

Pharmacodynamics

	PO	INTRANASAL	SUBCUT/IV
Onset	1 hr	1 hr	Rapid
Peak	4-7 hr	1-4 hr	15-30 min
Duration	Unknown	8-20 hr	3 hr

Interactions
Individual drugs
Alcohol, demeclocycline, epinephrine (large doses), heparin, lithium: decreased antidiuretic action
Carbamazepine, chlorpropamide, clofibrate: increased antidiuretic action

NURSING CONSIDERATIONS
Assessment
• Monitor I&O ratio, urine osmolality, specific gravity, weight daily; check for edema in extremities; if water retention is severe, diuretic may be prescribed; check pulse, B/P when giving product **IV** or SUBCUT
• Assess for water intoxication: lethargy, behavioral changes, disorientation, neuromuscular excitability, dehydration, poor skin turgor, severe thirst, dry skin, tachycardia
• Assess intranasal use: nausea, congestion, cramps, headache; usually decreased with decreased dosage
• Monitor for enuresis during treatment (nocturnal enuresis)
• Assess for allergic reaction, including anaphylaxis (**IV** route)
• Assess for nasal mucosa changes: congestion, edema, discharge, scarring (nasal route)
• Monitor urine volume osmolality and plasma osmolality (diabetes insipidus)
• Monitor factor VIII coagulant activity before using for hemostasis

Nursing diagnoses
• Fluid volume, deficient (uses)
• Fluid volume, excess (side effects)
• Knowledge, deficient (teaching)

Implementation
• Draw medication into tube, insert tube into nostril to instill product and blow on other end to deliver sol into nasal cavity; rinse after use
• Store in refrigerator or cool environment
IV, direct route
• Give undiluted over 1 min in diabetes insipidus or **IV** for hemophilia
Intermittent IV infusion route
• Give single dose diluted in 50 ml of 0.9% NaCl (adult and child >10 kg); a single dose/10 ml as an **IV** inf over 15-30 min in von Willebrand's disease or hemophilia A

Patient/family education
• Use demonstration, return demonstration to teach technique for nasal instillation
• Teach patient to notify prescriber of dyspnea, vomiting, cramping, drowsiness, headache, nasal congestion
• Caution patient to avoid OTC products (cough, hay fever), since these preparations may contain epinephrine and decrease product response; do not use with alcohol
• Advise patient to carry/wear emergency ID or other identification specifying disease and medication used
• Advise patient if dose is missed, take when remembered, up to 1 hr before next dose; do not double doses, avoid fluids from 1 hr to up to 8 hr after PO dose
• Teach patient to report upper respiratory infection, nasal congestion

Evaluation
Positive therapeutic outcome
• Absence of severe thirst
• Decreased urine output, osmolality
• Absence of bleeding (hemophilia)

---

desonide topical
See Appendix B

---

desoximetasone topical
See Appendix B

---

desoxyephedrine nasal agent
See Appendix B

---

desoxyribonuclease
See fibrinolysin/desoxyribonuclease

dexamethasone (Rx)
(dex-ah-meth'ah-sone)
Decadron, Deronil ✦, Dexasone ✦, Dexon, Hexadrol, Mymethasone
dexamethasone acetate (Rx)
Dalalone DP, Dalalone LA, Decadron-LA, Decaject-LA, Dexacen LA-8, Dexasone-LA, Dexone LA, Solurex-LA
dexamethasone sodium phosphate (Rx)
Dalalone, Decadron Phosphate, Decaject, Dexacen-4, Dexone, Hexadrol Phosphate, Solurex
Func. class.: Corticosteroid, synthetic
Chem. class.: Glucocorticoid, long-acting

Pregnancy category C

Do not confuse:
Decadron/Percodan

Action: Decreases inflammation by suppression of migration of polymorphonuclear leukocytes, fibroblasts, reversal of increased capillary permeability and lysosomal stabilization

Uses: Inflammation, allergies, neoplasms, cerebral edema, septic shock, collagen disorders

Dosage and routes
Inflammation
Adult: PO 0.75-9 mg/day, in divided doses q6-12hr; or phosphate IM 0.5-9 mg/day divided q6-12hr; or acetate IM 4-16 mg q1-3wk
Child: PO 0.024-0.34 mg/kg/day in divided doses q6-12hr

Shock
Adult: **IV** (phosphate) single dose 1-6 mg/kg or **IV** 40 mg q2-6hr as needed up to 72 hr

Cerebral edema
Adult: **IV** (phosphate) 10 mg, then 4-6 mg IM q6hr × 2-4 days, then taper over 1 wk
Child: PO/IM/**IV** loading dose 1-2 mg/kg, then 1-1.5 mg/kg/day, max 16 mg/day divided q4-6hr for 2-4 days, then taper down qwk

Adrenocortical insufficiency
Adult: PO 0.5-9 mg/day in divided doses
Child: PO 0.03-0.3 mg/kg/day divided in 2-4 doses

Suppression test
Adult: PO 1 mg at 11 PM or 0.5 mg q6hr × 48 hr

Croup (unlabeled)
Child: PO 0.024-0.34 mg/kg/day or 0.66-10 mg/m^2/day in 2-4 divided doses; a single dose of 0.6 mg/kg has been used for mild to moderate croup; IM/**IV** 0.06-0.3 mg/kg/day or 1.2-10 mg/m^2/day in divided doses q6-12hr; a single dose of 0.6 mg/kg IM has been used for severe croup

Available forms: Dexamethasone: tabs 0.25, 0.5, 0.75, 1, 1.5, 2, 4, 6 mg; elix 0.5 mg/5 ml; oral sol 0.5 mg/5 ml, 1 mg/ml; inj acetate 8, 16 mg/ml; inj phosphate 4, 10, 20, 24 mg/ml

Adverse effects
CNS: Depression, flushing, sweating, headache, mood changes, euphoria, psychosis, **seizures,** insomnia
CV: Hypertension, **circulatory collapse, thrombophlebitis, embolism,** tachycardia, edema, cardiomyopathy
EENT: Fungal infections, increased intraocular pressure, blurred vision, cataracts, glaucoma
ENDO: Hypothalmic-pituitary-adrenal axis suppression, hyperglycemia, sodium, fluid retention
GI: Diarrhea, nausea, abdominal distention, **GI hemorrhage,** *increased appetite,* **pancreatitis**
HEMA: **Thrombocytopenia,** transient leukocytosis
INTEG: Acne, poor wound healing, ecchymosis, petechiae, hirsutism
META: Hypokalemia
MS: Fractures, osteoporosis, weakness, arthralgia, myopathy

Contraindications: Psychosis, hypersensitivity to corticosteroids or benzyl alcohol, idiopathic thrombocytopenia, acute glomerulonephritis, amebiasis, fungal infections, nonasthmatic bronchial disease, child <2 yr, AIDS, TB, glaucoma, ocular infection

Precautions: Pregnancy **C**, breastfeeding, diabetes mellitus, osteoporosis, seizure disorders, ulcerative colitis, CHF, myasthenia gravis, renal disease, peptic ulcer, esophagitis

Pharmacokinetics	
Absorption	Unknown
Distribution	Unknown
Metabolism	Liver
Excretion	Kidneys
Half-life	36-54 hr

◆ Alert　　✦ Canada Only　　🔘 Drug on CD　　* "Tall Man" lettering (See Preface)

Pharmacodynamics		
	PO	IM
Onset	1 hr	Unknown
Peak	1-2 hr	8 hr
Duration	2½ days	6 days-3 wk

Interactions
Individual drugs
Alcohol, amphotericin B, cycloSPORINE, digoxin, indomethacin: increased side effects

Ambenonium, isoniazid, neostigmine, sometrem: decreased effects of each specific product

Cholestyramine, colestipol, ephedrine, phenytoin, rifampin, theophylline: decreased action of dexamethasone

Indomethacin, ketoconazole: increased action of dexamethasone

Drug classifications
Antacids, barbiturates: decreased action of dexamethasone

Antibiotics (macrolide), contraceptives (oral), estrogens, salicylates: increased action of dexamethasone

Anticholinesterases, anticoagulants, anticonvulsants, antidiabetics, salicylates, toxoids/vaccines: decreased effects of each specific product

Diuretics, salicylates: increased side effects

Drug/herb
Aloe, buckthorn bark/berry, cascara sagrada, Chinese rhubarb, senna pod/leaf: increased hypokalemia

Aloe, licorice, perilla: increased corticosteroid effect

Drug/lab test
Increased: cholesterol, Na, blood glucose, uric acid, Ca, urine glucose

Decreased: Ca, K, T_4, T_3, thyroid ^{131}I uptake test, urine 17-OHCS, 17-KS, PBI

False negative: skin allergy tests

NURSING CONSIDERATIONS
Assessment
• Monitor K, blood, urine glucose while on long-term therapy; hypokalemia and hyperglycemia

• Monitor weight daily; notify prescriber of weekly gain >5 lb

• Monitor B/P q4hr, pulse; notify prescriber of chest pain

• Monitor I&O ratio; be alert for decreasing urinary output, increasing edema

• Monitor plasma cortisol levels during long-term therapy (normal: 138-635 nmol/L SI units when assessed at 8 AM), prolonged use can cause cushingoid symptoms

• Assess infection: fever, WBC even after withdrawal of medication; product masks infection

• Assess potassium depletion: paresthesias, fatigue, nausea, vomiting, depression, polyuria, dysrhythmias, weakness

• Assess edema, hypertension, cardiac symptoms

• Assess mental status: affect, mood, behavioral changes, aggression

Nursing diagnoses
• Infection, risk for (adverse reaction)
• Knowledge, deficient (teaching)
• Mobility, impaired physical (uses)

Implementation
PO route
• Give with food or milk to decrease GI symptoms

• Provide assistance with ambulation in patient with bone tissue disease to prevent fractures

IM route
• IM inj deep in large muscle mass; rotate sites; avoid deltoid; use 21-G needle

• In one dose in AM to prevent adrenal suppression; avoid SUBCUT administration, may damage tissue

IV route
• IV undiluted direct over 1 min or less or diluted with 0.9% NaCl or D_5W and give as an IV inf at prescribed rate

• After shaking susp (parenteral); do not give susp IV

• Titrated dose; use lowest effective dose

Dexamethasone sodium phosphate
Syringe compatibilities: Granisetron, metoclopramide, ranitidine, sufentanil

Y-site compatibilities: Acyclovir, allopurinol, amifostine, amikacin, amphotericin B cholesteryl, amsacrine, aztreonam, cefepime, cisatracurium, cisplatin, cladribine, cyclophosphamide, cytarabine, DOXOrubicin, DOXOrubicin liposome, famotidine, filgrastim, fluconazole, fludarabine, foscarnet, heparin, melphalan, meperidine, meropenem, morphine, ondansetron, paclitaxel, piperacillin/tazobactam, potassium chloride, propofol, remifentanil, sargramostim, sodium bicarbonate, sufentanil, tacrolimus, teniposide, theophylline, vinorelbine, vit B/C, zidovudine

Additive compatibilities: Aminophylline, bleomycin, cimetidine, floxacillin, furosemide, lidocaine, meropenem, nafcillin, netilmicin, ondansetron, prochlorperazine, ranitidine, verapamil

Adverse effects: *italic* = common, **bold** = life-threatening

Patient/family education

- Advise that emergency ID as corticosteroid user should be carried or worn
- Teach to notify prescriber if therapeutic response decreases; dosage adjustment may be needed
- Teach not to discontinue abruptly or adrenal crisis can result
- Teach to avoid OTC products: salicylates, alcohol in cough products, cold preparations unless directed by prescriber
- Instruct patient to contact prescriber if surgery, trauma, stress occurs, dose may need to be adjusted
- Teach patient all aspects of product usage, including cushingoid symptoms
- Instruct patient to notify prescriber of infection
- Teach symptoms of adrenal insufficiency: nausea, anorexia, fatigue, dizziness, dyspnea, weakness, joint pain
- Advise patient to avoid exposure to chickenpox or measles, persons with infections

Evaluation

Positive therapeutic outcome
Decreased inflammation

---

dexamethasone ophthalmic
See Appendix B

---

dexamethasone topical
See Appendix B

---

dexlansoprazole (Rx)
dex-lan-so-prey′zole
Kapidex
Func. class.: Anti-ulcer–proton pump inhibitor
Chem. class.: Benzimidazole

Pregnancy category B

Action: Suppresses gastric secretion by inhibiting hydrogen/potassium ATPase enzyme system in gastric parietal cell; characterized as gastric acid pump inhibitor, since it blocks final step of acid production

Therapeutic outcome: Reduction in gastric pain, swelling, fullness

Uses: Gastroesophageal reflux disease (GERD), severe erosive esophagitis, heartburn

Dosage and routes
Erosive esophagitis
Adult: **PO** 60 mg qd for up to 8 wk; maintenance: PO 30 mg qd for up to 6 mo

GERD
Adult: **PO:** 30 mg qd × 4 wk

Available forms: Del rel caps 30, 60 mg

Adverse effects

CNS: Headache, dizziness, confusion, agitation, amnesia, depression, **anxiety**, **seizures**, insomnia
CV: Chest pain, angina, bradycardia, palpitations, **CVA**, hypertension, **MI**
EENT: Tinnitus
GI: Diarrhea, abdominal pain, vomiting, nausea, constipation, flatulence, colitis
HEMA: Anemia, **neutropenia, thrombocytopenia, pernicious anemia, thrombosis**
INTEG: Rash, urticaria, pruritus
META: Gout
MS: Arthralgia, myalgia
RESP: Upper respiratory infections, cough, epistaxis, dyspnea, **pneumonia**
SYST: Anaphylaxis

Contraindications: Hypersensitivity

Precautions: Pregnancy **B**, breastfeeding, children, proton-pump hypersensitivity, gastric cancer, hepatic disease, vit B_{12} deficiency

Pharmacokinetics

Absorption	57%-64%
Distribution	Protein binding 97%
Metabolism	Liver extensively
Excretion	Urine, feces; clearance decreased in geriatric, renal/hepatic disease
Half-life	Plasma 1-2 hr, 4-5 hr

Pharmacodynamics
Unknown

Interactions
Individual drugs
Calcium carbonate, indinavir, iron, itraconazole, ketoconazole: decreased absorption of each specific product

Drug classifications
CYP2C19, 3A4 (fluvoxamine, voriconazole): increased dexlansoprazole effect
Sucralfate: delayed absorption of dexlansoprazole

NURSING CONSIDERATIONS
Assessment
- Assess GI system: bowel sounds q8hr, abdomen for pain, swelling, anorexia

---

- Monitor liver enzymes (AST, ALT, alkaline phosphatase) during treatment

Nursing diagnoses
- Knowledge, deficient (teaching)
- Pain, chronic (uses)

Implementation
- Swallow del rel cap whole; do not break, crush, chew, or open

Patient/family education
- Instruct patient to report severe diarrhea; product may have to be discontinued
- Inform diabetic patient that hypoglycemia may occur
- Encourage patient to avoid hazardous activities; dizziness may occur
- Tell patient to avoid alcohol, salicylates, ibuprofen; may cause GI irritation

Evaluation
Positive therapeutic outcome
- Absence of gastric pain, swelling, fullness

---

dexmedetomidine (Rx)
(deks-med-ee-tome′a-dine)
Precedex
Func. class.: Sedative, α_2-adrenoceptor agonist

Pregnancy category C

Action: Produces α_2-agonist activity as seen at low and moderate doses; also, α_1 at high doses

Uses: Sedation in mechanically ventilated, intubated patients in ICU

Dosage and routes
Adult: **IV** loading dose of 1 mcg/kg over 10 min, then 0.2-0.7 mcg/kg/hr, do not use for more than 24 hr

Available forms: Inj 100 mcg/ml

Adverse effects
CV: Bradycardia, hypo/hypertension, **atrial fibrillation, infarction, cardiac arrest**
GI: Nausea, thirst
GU: Oliguria
HEMA: Leukocytosis, anemia
MISC: Hyperkalemia
RESP: **Pulmonary edema, pleural effusion, hypoxia,** respiratory acidosis

Contraindications: Hypersensitivity, chronic hypertension

Precautions: Pregnancy **C**, breastfeeding, children, geriatric, respiratory depression, severe respiratory disorders, cardiac dysrhyth-mias, hypovolemia, diabetes, CV/renal/hepatic disease

Pharmacokinetics
Absorption	Unknown
Distribution	Unknown
Metabolism	Unknown
Excretion	Unknown
Half-life	8 min

Pharmacodynamics
Unknown

Interactions
Individual drugs
Alcohol: increased CNS depression
Drug classifications
Anesthetics (inhalational), antipsychotics, opiates, sedative/hypnotics, skeletal muscle relaxants: increased CNS depression
Antihypertensives: increased hypotension

NURSING CONSIDERATIONS
Assessment
- Assess inj site: phlebitis, burning, stinging
- Monitor ECG for changes: atrial fibrillation; monitor geriatric more closely
- Assess CNS changes: movement, jerking, tremors, dizziness, LOC, pupil reaction
- Assess respiratory dysfunction: respiratory depression, character, rate, rhythm; notify prescriber if respirations are <10/min
- Assess cardiac status: B/P, heart rate

Nursing diagnoses
- Injury, risk for (uses)

Implementation
IV route
- Give after diluting with D_5W, 0.9% NaCl; withdraw 2 ml of product and add to 48 ml of 0.9% NaCl to a total of 50 ml; shake to mix well; use controlled infusion device
- Give only with resuscitative equipment available
- Give only by qualified persons trained in management of ICU sedation
Solution compatibilities: LR, D_5W, 0.9% NaCl, 20% mannitol
Additive compatibilities: Atracurium, atropine, etomidate, fentanyl, glycopyrrolate, midazolam, mivacurium, morphine, pancuronium, phenylephrine, succinylcholine, thiopental, vecuronium
- Provide safety measures: side rails, night-light, call bell within easy reach

Evaluation
Positive therapeutic outcome
- Induction of sedation

Adverse effects: *italic* = common, **bold** = life-threatening

dexmethylphenidate (Rx)
(dex'meth-ul-fen'ih-dayt)
Focalin, Focalin XR
Func. class.: Central nervous system (CNS) stimulant, psychostimulant

Pregnancy category C

Controlled substance schedule II

Action: Increases release of norepinephrine and dopamine into the extraneuronal space, also blocks reuptake of norepinephrine and dopamine into the presynaptic neuron; mode of action in treating attention deficit hyperactivity disorder (ADHD) is unknown

Therapeutic outcome: Increased alertness, decreased fatigue, ability to stay awake (narcolepsy), increased attention span, decreased hyperactivity (ADHD)

Uses: ADHD, adjunctive treatment

Dosage and routes
Adult: PO EXT REL 10 mg/day, may adjust to 20 mg/day in 10 mg increments
Child >6 yr: PO 2.5 mg bid with doses at least 4 hr apart, gradually increase to a max of 20 mg/day (10 mg bid); for those taking methylphenidate, use ½ of methylphenidate dose initially, then increase as needed to max 20 mg/day; EXT REL 5 mg/day, may adjust to 20 mg/day in 5 mg increments

Available forms: Tabs 2.5, 5, 10 mg; ext rel caps (Focalin XR) 5, 10, 20 mg

Adverse effects
CNS: Dizziness, headache, drowsiness, nervousness, insomnia, **toxic psychosis, neuroleptic malignant syndrome (rare)**, Gilles de la Tourette's syndrome
CV: Palpitations, B/P changes, angina, **dysrhythmias, tachycardia**
GI: *Nausea, anorexia,* abnormal liver function, **hepatic coma,** *abdominal pain*
HEMA: Leukopenia, anemia, thrombocytopenic purpura
INTEG: **Exfoliative dermatitis,** urticaria, rash, erythema multiforme
MISC: *Fever,* arthralgia, scalp hair loss

Contraindications: Hypersensitivity to methylphenidate, anxiety, history of Gilles de la Tourette's syndrome; children <6 yr, glaucoma, concurrent treatment with MAOIs or within 14 days of discontinuing treatment with MAOIs, breastfeeding, tics, psychosis

Precautions: Pregnancy **C,** hypertension, depression, seizures, CV disorders, alcoholism

Black Box Warning: Substance abuse

Pharmacokinetics
Absorption	Readily absorbed
Distribution	Unknown
Metabolism	Liver
Excretion	Kidneys
Half-life	2.2 hr

Pharmacodynamics
	PO	EXT REL
Onset	½-1 hr	Unknown
Peak	1-1 ½ hr	4 hr
Duration	4 hr	8 hr

Interactions
Drug classifications
Anticoagulants (coumarin) (e.g., warfarin), anticonvulsants, selective serotonin reuptake inhibitors, tricyclics: increased effects
Antihypertensives: decreased effects
Decongestants, vasoconstrictors: increased sympathomimetic effect
MAOIs: hypertensive crisis if coadministered or given within 14 days
Vasopressors: hypertensive crisis
Drug/herb
Horsetail, yohimbe: increased stimulant effect
Melatonin: increased synergistic effect

NURSING CONSIDERATIONS
Assessment
- Assess VS, B/P; may reverse antihypertensives; check patients with cardiac disease more often for increased B/P
- Assess CBC, differential, platelet counts during long-term therapy, urinalysis; in diabetes: blood/urine glucose; insulin changes may have to be made, since eating will decrease
- Assess height, growth rate q3mo in children; growth rate may be decreased
- Assess mental status: mood, sensorium, affect, stimulation, insomnia, aggressiveness
- Assess withdrawal symptoms: headache, nausea, vomiting, muscle pain, weakness
- Assess appetite, sleep, speech patterns
- Assess for attention span, decreased hyperactivity in persons with ADHD

Nursing diagnoses
- Coping, disabled family (uses)
- Coping, ineffective (uses)
- Knowledge, deficient (teaching)
- Thought processes, disturbed (uses, adverse reactions)

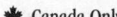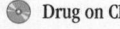

Implementation
- Do not break, crush, or chew ext rel caps
- Twice daily at least 4 hr apart; ext rel once a day
- Without regard to meals

Patient/family education
- Advise patient to decrease caffeine consumption (coffee, tea, cola, chocolate); may increase irritability, stimulation
- Advise patient to avoid OTC preparations unless approved by prescriber
- Caution patient to taper off product over several wk to avoid depression, increased sleeping, lethargy
- Caution patient to avoid alcohol ingestion
- Caution patient to avoid hazardous activities until stabilized on medication
- Advise patient to get needed rest; patients will feel more tired at end of day
- Notify all health providers including school nurse of medication and schedule
- Discuss information instructions provided in patient information section

Evaluation
Positive therapeutic outcome
- Decreased hyperactivity or ability to stay awake

Treatment of overdose: Administer fluids; hemodialysis or peritoneal dialysis; antihypertensive for increased B/P; administer short-acting barbiturate before lavage

---

dextroamphetamine (Rx)
(dex-troe-am-fet'a-meen)
Dextroamphetamine, Dexedrine
Func. class.: Cerebral stimulant
Chem. class.: Amphetamine

Pregnancy category C
Controlled substance schedule II

Action: Increases release of norepinephrine, dopamine in cerebral cortex to reticular activating system

Therapeutic outcome: Increased alertness, decreased fatigue, ability to stay awake (narcolepsy); increased attention span, decreased hyperactivity (ADHD)

Uses: Narcolepsy, attention deficit disorder with hyperactivity

Unlabeled use: Obesity

Dosage and routes
Narcolepsy
Adult: PO 5 mg bid, titrate daily dose by no more than 10 mg/wk, max 60 mg/day

Child 6-12 yr: PO 5 mg daily increasing by no more than 5 mg/day at weekly intervals
ADHD
Adult: PO 5-60 mg/day in divided doses
Child 6-12 yr: PO 5 mg daily-bid increasing by 5 mg/day at weekly intervals
Child 3-5 yr: PO 2.5 mg daily increasing by 2.5 mg/day at weekly intervals (max 40 mg/day)

Available forms: Tabs 5, 10 mg, oral sol 5 mg/5 ml

Adverse effects
CNS: Hyperactivity, insomnia, restlessness, talkativeness, dizziness, headache, chills, stimulation, dysphoria, irritability, aggressiveness, tremor, dependence, addiction
CV: Palpitations, **tachycardia,** hypertension, decrease in heart rate, **dysrhythmias**
GI: Anorexia, dry mouth, diarrhea, constipation, weight loss, metallic taste
GU: Impotence, change in libido
INTEG: Urticaria

Contraindications: Hypersensitivity to sympathomimetic amines, hyperthyroidism, hypertension, glaucoma, severe arteriosclerosis, drug abuse, anxiety, anorexia nervosa, tartrazine dye hypersensitivity

Black Box Warning: CV disease, substance abuse

Precautions: Pregnancy C, breastfeeding, child <3 yr, Gilles de la Tourette's disorder, depression

Pharmacokinetics
Absorption	Well absorbed
Distribution	Widely distributed; crosses placenta
Metabolism	Liver
Excretion	Kidneys, pH dependent: increased pH, increased reabsorption
Half-life	10-30 hr; increased when urine is alkaline

Pharmacodynamics
Onset	½ hr
Peak	1-3 hr
Duration	4-10 hr

Interactions
Individual drugs
AcetaZOLAMIDE, sodium bicarbonate: increased effect of dextroamphetamine
Ammonium chloride, ascorbic acid: decreased effect of dextroamphetamine

---

Adverse effects: *italic* = common, **bold** = life-threatening

Haloperidol: increased CNS effect

Phenytoin: decreased absorption of phenytoin

Drug classifications

Adrenergic blockers: decreased adrenergic blocking effect

Antacids: increased effect of dextroamphetamine

Antidepressants (tricyclic), phenothiazines: increased CNS effect

Antidiabetics: decreased antidiabetic effect

Barbiturates: decreased absorption of barbiturate

MAOIs: hypertensive crisis if used within 14 days

Drug/herb

Eucalyptus: decreased stimulant effect

Khat: increased stimulant effect

St. John's wort: increased serotonin syndrome

Drug/food

Caffeine: increased amine effect

NURSING CONSIDERATIONS
Assessment

• Monitor VS, B/P, since this product may reverse antihypertensives; check patients with cardiac disease more often for increased B/P

• Monitor CBC, urinalysis; for diabetic patients monitor blood, urine glucose; insulin changes may be required, since eating will decrease

• Monitor height and weight q3mo since growth rate in children may be decreased; appetite is suppressed so weight loss is common during the first few months of treatment

• Monitor mental status: mood, sensorium, affect, stimulation, insomnia; aggressiveness may occur; depression with crying spells may occur after product has worn off

• Assess for physical dependency; should not be used for extended time except in ADHD; dosage should be decreased gradually to prevent withdrawal symptoms

• Assess for narcoleptic symptoms before medication and after; ability to stay awake should increase significantly

• In children or adults with ADHD, monitor for improved organizational skills, attention span, attending to tasks, impulse control, socialization, and ability to get along better with others

• Assess for withdrawal symptoms: headache, nausea, vomiting, muscle pain, weakness; product tolerance develops after long-term use; dosage should not be increased if tolerance develops; this medication has a high abuse potential

Nursing diagnoses

• Coping, compromised family (uses)

• Coping, ineffective (uses)

• Knowledge, deficient (teaching)

• Thought processes, disturbed (uses, adverse reactions)

Implementation

• Give at least 6 hr before bedtime to avoid sleeplessness; titrate to patient's response; lowest dosage should be used to control symptoms

• Give gum, hard candy, frequent sips of water for dry mouth at beginning of treatment; these symptoms tend to lessen with time

Patient/family education

• Advise patient to decrease caffeine consumption (coffee, tea, cola, chocolate), which may increase irritability and stimulation; to avoid OTC preparations unless approved by prescriber; to avoid alcohol ingestion; these may cause serious drug interactions

• Advise patient to take before meals (obesity)

• Caution patient to taper off product over several weeks, or depression, increased sleeping, lethargy may occur

• Caution patient to avoid hazardous activities until patient is stabilized on medication

• Instruct patient not to double doses if medication is missed; prescriber may suggest product holidays (ADHD) during the school year to assess progress and determine continued product necessity

• Instruct patient/family to notify prescriber if significant side effects occur: tremors, insomnia, palpitations, restlessness, product changes may be needed

• Inform patient that if dry mouth occurs, to use frequent sips of water, sugarless gum, hard candy during beginning therapy; dry mouth lessens with continued treatment

• Advise patient to get needed rest; patients will feel more tired at end of day; to give last dose at least 6 hr before bedtime to avoid insomnia

Evaluation
Positive therapeutic outcome

• Decreased activity in ADHD

• Absence of sleeping during day in narcolepsy

Treatment of overdose: Administer fluids, hemodialysis, peritoneal dialysis, antihypertensives for increased B/P; ammonium chloride for increased excretion

dextromethorphan (OTC)
(dex-troe-meth-or'fan)
Buckley's DM, Creo-Terpin, Delsym,
dextromethorphan, ElixSure Cough,
Hold DM, PediaCare Children's Long-
Acting Cough, Robafan, Robitussin Cough
with Honey, Robitussin Cough Long Acting,
Scot-Tussin DM Cough Chasers, Sucrets
Cough Control, Suppress, Triaminic Long-
Acting Cough, Tylenol Children's Simply
Cough, Vicks Formula 44 Cough Relief,
Wal-Tussin, Zicam Cough Mist Max
Func. class.: Antitussive, nonopioid
Chem. class.: Levorphanol derivative

Pregnancy category C

Action: Depresses cough center in medulla
by direct effect related to levorphanol

Therapeutic outcome: Absence of
cough

Uses: Nonproductive cough carried by minor
respiratory tract infections or irritants that
might be inhaled

Dosage and routes
Adult and child ≥12 yr: PO 10-20 mg
q4hr, or 30 mg q6-8hr, max 120 mg/day; SUS
REL LIQUID 60 mg q12hr, max 120 mg/day
Child 6-12 yr: PO 5-10 mg q4hr; SUS REL
LIQUID 30 mg bid, max 60 mg/day; LOZENGE
5-10 mg q1-4hr, max 60 mg/day
Child 4-6 yr: PO 2.5-7.5 mg q4-8hr, max
30 mg/day, SUS REL LIQ 15 ml bid
Child <4 yr: PO: not recommended

Available forms: Loz 5 mg; liquid 7.5,
15 mg/5 ml; syr 15 mg/15 ml, 10 mg/5 ml;
15 mg/5 ml, 30 mg/15 ml; caps 15 mg; gel
caps 15 mg; spray mist 6 mg/actuation

Adverse effects
CNS: Dizziness, sedation, confusion, ataxia,
fatigue
GI: Nausea

Contraindications: Hypersensitivity

Precautions: Pregnancy **C**, fever, hepatic
disease, asthma/emphysema, chronic cough

Pharmacokinetics
Absorption	Rapid (PO); slow (SUS REL)
Distribution	Unknown
Metabolism	Liver
Excretion	Kidneys
Half-life	Terminal 11 hr

Pharmacodynamics
	PO	PO-SUS
Onset	15-30 min	Unknown
Peak	Unknown	Unknown
Duration	3-6 hr	12 hr

Interactions
Individual drugs
Alcohol: increased CNS depression
Amiodarone, fluoxetine, quinidine,
    sibutramine: increased adverse reactions
Furazolidone, linezolide, procarbazine:
    increased hypotension, hyperpyrexia; do not
    give within 2 wk (MAOI activity)
Drug classifications
Antihistamines, antidepressants, opiates,
    sedative/hypnotics: increased CNS depres-
    sion
MAOIs: increased hypotension, hyperpyrexia,
    do not give within 2 wk of MAOIs
Serotonin receptor agonists, SSRIs: increased
    adverse reactions

NURSING CONSIDERATIONS
Assessment
• Assess cough: type, frequency, character
including sputum; provide adequate hydration
to 2 L/day to decrease viscosity of secretions

Nursing diagnoses
• Airway clearance, ineffective (uses)
• Knowledge, deficient (teaching)

Implementation
• Administer decreased dosage to geriatric
patients; their metabolism may be slowed; do
not provide water within 30 min of administration because it dilutes product
• Shake susp before administration

Patient/family education
• Caution patient to avoid driving or other
hazardous activities until stabilized on this
medication; may cause drowsiness, dizziness
in some individuals
• Advise patient to avoid smoking, smoke-
filled rooms, perfumes, dust, environmental
pollutants, cleaners, which increase cough;
may use gum, hard candy to prevent dry mouth
• Advise patient to avoid alcohol or other CNS
depressants while taking this medication;
drowsiness will be increased
• Caution patient that any cough lasting over a
few days should be assessed by prescriber

Evaluation
Positive therapeutic outcome
• Absence of dry, irritating cough

D

dextrose (D-glucose) (Rx)
Glucose, Glutose, Insta-Glucose
Func. class.: Caloric agent

Action: Needed for adequate utilization of amino acids; decreases protein, nitrogen loss; prevents ketosis

Therapeutic outcome: Provides calories, prevents severe hypoglycemia

Uses: Increases intake of calories; increases fluids in patients unable to take adequate fluids, calories orally; acute hypoglycemia

Dosage and routes
Adult and child: **IV**, depends on individual requirements

Hypoglycemia
Adult: PO/**IV** 10-25 mg

Available forms: Inj IV 2.5%, 5%, 10%, 20%, 25% 30%, 38.5%, 40%, 50%, 60%, 70%; oral gel 40%; chewable tabs 5 g

Adverse effects
CNS: Confusion, **loss of consciousness,** dizziness
CV: Hypertension, **CHF, pulmonary edema, intracranial hemorrhage**
ENDO: Hyperglycemia, rebound hypoglycemia, hyperosmolar syndrome, hyperglycemic nonketolytic syndrome, aluminum toxicity, hypokalemia, hypomagnesium
GI: Nausea
GU: Glycosuria, osmotic diuresis
INTEG: Chills, flushing, warm feeling, rash, urticaria, extravasation necrosis
RESP: Pulmonary edema

Contraindications: Hyperglycemia, delirium tremens, hemorrhage (cranial/spinal), CHF, anuria, allergy to corn products

Precautions: Renal/liver/cardiac disease, diabetes mellitus, carbohydrate intolerance

Pharmacokinetics
Absorption	Well absorbed (PO); completely absorbed (**IV**)
Distribution	Widely distributed
Metabolism	Unknown
Excretion	Unknown
Half-life	Unknown

Pharmacodynamics
	PO	IV
Onset	Rapid	Immediate
Peak	Rapid	Immediate
Duration	Rapid	Immediate

Interactions
Drug classifications
Corticosteroids: increased fluid retention/electrolyte excretion

NURSING CONSIDERATIONS
Assessment
• Assess I&O, skin turgor, edema, electrolytes (potassium, sodium, calcium, chloride, magnesium), blood glucose, ammonia, phosphate
• Monitor inj site for extravasation: redness along vein, edema at site, necrosis, pain, hard tender area; site should be changed immediately
• Monitor temp q4hr for increased fever, indicating infection; if infection suspected, inf is discontinued and tubing, bottle, catheter tip cultured
• Monitor serum glucose in patients receiving hypertonic glucose 5% and over
• Assess nutritional status: calorie count by dietitian; GI system function

Nursing diagnoses
• Fluid volume, excess (adverse reactions)
• Knowledge, deficient (teaching)
• Nutrition, less than body requirements, imbalanced (uses)

Implementation
PO route
• Oral glucose preparations (gel, chewable tabs) are to be used for conscious patients only; serum blood glucose should be monitored after first oral dose; if glucose has not increased by 20 mg/100 ml in 20-30 min, dose should be repeated and serum glucose checked again
IV route
• Give only protein (4%) and dextrose (up to 12.5%) via peripheral vein; stronger sol requires central **IV** administration
• May be given undiluted via prepared sol; give 10% sol (5 ml/15 sec), 20% sol (1000 ml/3 hr or more), 50% sol (500 ml/30-60 min); too rapid **IV** administration may cause fluid overload and hyperglycemia
• After changing **IV** catheter, change dressing q24hr with aseptic technique

Patient/family education
• Teach patient reason for dextrose infusion
• Provide literature and information on when and how to use oral products for hypoglycemia
• Review hypo/hyperglycemia symptoms
• Review blood glucose monitoring procedure

 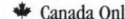

Evaluation
Positive therapeutic outcome
- Increased weight
- Blood glucose level at normal limits for patient
- Adequate hydration

---

diazepam 😊 (Rx)
(dye-az'e-pam)
Apo-Diazepam ✦, Diastat, diazepam, Diazepam Intensol, Diazemuls ✦, Novo-Diapam ✦, PMS-Diazepam ✦, Valium, Vivol ✦

Func. class.: Antianxiety, anticonvulsant, skeletal muscle relaxant, central acting
Chem. class.: Benzodiazepine, long-acting

Pregnancy category D

Controlled substance schedule IV

Do not confuse:
diazepam/Ditropan/lorazepam

Action: Potentiates the actions of GABA, especially in limbic system, reticular formation; enhances presympathetic inhibition, inhibits spinal polysynaptic afferent paths

Therapeutic outcome: Decreased anxiety, restlessness, insomnia

Uses: Anxiety, acute alcohol withdrawal, adjunct in seizure disorders; preoperative skeletal muscle relaxation; rectally for acute repetitive seizures

Dosage and routes
Anxiety/convulsive disorders
Adult: PO 2-10 mg bid-qid; IM/IV 2-10 mg q3-4hr
Geriatric: PO 1-2 mg daily-bid, increase slowly as needed
Child >6 mo: IM/IV 0.04-0.3 mg/kg/dose q2-4hr, max 0.6 mg/kg in an 8-hr period

Precardioversion
Adult: IV 5-15 mg 5-10 min precardioversion

Preendoscopy
Adult: IV 2.5-20 mg, IM 5-10 mg ½ hr preendoscopy

Muscle relaxation
Adult: PO 2-10 mg tid-qid or EXT REL 15-30 mg daily; IM/IV 5-10 mg repeat in 2-4 hr
Geriatric: PO 2-5 mg bid-qid; IM/IV 2-5 mg, may repeat in 2-4 hr

Tetanic muscle spasms
Child >5 yr: IM/IV 5-10 mg q3-4hr prn

Infants >30 days: IM/IV 1-2 mg q3-4hr prn

Status epilepticus
Adult: IM/IV 5-10 mg, 2 mg/min, may repeat q10-15min; max 30 mg; may repeat in 2-4 hr if seizures reappear
Child >5 yr: IV 1 mg slowly; IM 1 mg q2-5min
Child 1 mo-5 yr: IV 0.2-0.5 mg slowly; IM 0.2-0.5 mg slowly q2-5min up to 5 mg; may repeat in 2-4 hr prn

Seizures other than status epilepticus
Adult: RECT 0.2 mg/kg, may repeat 4-12 hr later
Child 6-11 yr: RECT 0.3 mg/kg, may repeat 4-12 hr later
Child 2-5 yr: RECT 0.5 mg/kg, may repeat 4-12 hr later

Alcohol withdrawal
Adult: IV 10 mg initially, then 5-10 mg q3-4hr prn

Available forms: Tabs 2, 5, 10 mg; inj 5 mg/ml; oral sol 5 mg/5 ml, 5 mg/ml; gel, rectal delivery system 10 mg, twin packs; ext rel cap 15 mg

Adverse effects
CNS: Dizziness, drowsiness, confusion, headache, anxiety, tremors, stimulation, fatigue, depression, insomnia, hallucinations, ataxia, fatigue
CV: Orthostatic hypotension, **ECG changes, tachycardia,** hypotension
EENT: Blurred vision, tinnitus, mydriasis, nystagmus
GI: Constipation, dry mouth, nausea, vomiting, anorexia, diarrhea
HEMA: **Neutropenia**
INTEG: Rash, dermatitis, itching
RESP: **Respiratory depression**

Contraindications: Pregnancy **D,** hypersensitivity to benzodiazepines, closed-angle glaucoma, coma, respiratory depression, untreated open-angle glaucoma, renal/hepatic disease, sleep apnea

Precautions: Breastfeeding, geriatric, debilitated, addiction, child <6 mo, asthma, bipolar disorder, COPD, CNS depression, labor, Parkinson's disease, neutropenia, psychosis, seizures, substance abuse, smoking

---

Adverse effects: *italic* = common, **bold** = life-threatening

Pharmacokinetics

Absorption	Rapid (PO); erratic (IM)
Distribution	Widely distributed; crosses blood-brain barrier, placenta; protein binding 99%
Metabolism	Liver, extensively, CYP2C19, CYP3A4
Excretion	Kidneys, breast milk
Half-life	20-80 hr

Pharmacodynamics

	PO	IM	IV
Onset	½ hr	15 min	Immediate
Peak	1-2 hr	½-1½ hr	15 min
Duration	2-3 hr	1-1½ hr	15 min-1 hr

Interactions
Individual drugs
Alcohol: increased CNS depression
Cimetidine, valproic acid: increased toxicity
CYP3A4 inducers (carbamazepine, ethetoin, fosphenytoin, phenytoins, rifampin): decreased diazepam effect
Disulfiram, isoniazid, propranolol, valproic acid: decreased metabolism of diazepam
Drug classifications
Barbiturates, CNS depressants, CYP3A4 inhibitors, selective serotonin reuptake inhibitors: increased toxicity
CNS depressants: increased CNS depression
CYP3A4 inducers (barbiturates): decreased diazepam effect
Oral contraceptives: decreased metabolism of diazepam
Drug/herb
Cola tree, St. John's wort: decreased diazepam effect
Cowslip, goldenseal, kava, melatonin, mistletoe, pokeweed, poppy, Queen Anne's lace, valerian: increased diazepam effect
Drug/lab test
Increased: AST/ALT, serum bilirubin
Decreased: radioactive iodine uptake
False increase: 17-OHCS

NURSING CONSIDERATIONS
Assessment
• Assess degree of anxiety; what precipitates anxiety and whether product controls symptoms; other signs of anxiety: dilated pupils, inability to sleep, restlessness, inability to focus
• Assess for alcohol withdrawal symptoms, including hallucinations (visual, auditory), delirium, irritability, agitation, fine to coarse tremors
• Monitor B/P (with patient lying, standing), pulse, respiratory rate; if systolic B/P drops 20 mm Hg, hold product, notify prescriber; monitor respirations q5-15min if given **IV**
• Monitor blood studies: CBC during long-term therapy; blood dyscrasias have occurred (rarely); hepatic studies: ALT, AST
• Monitor for seizure control; type, duration, and intensity of seizures; what precipitates seizures
• Monitor hepatic studies: AST, ALT, bilirubin, creatinine, LDH, alkaline phosphatase
• Assess mental status: mood, sensorium, affect, sleeping pattern, drowsiness, dizziness, suicidal tendencies, and ability of product to control these symptoms; check for tolerance, withdrawal symptoms: headache, nausea, vomiting, muscle pain, weakness after long-term use
• Assess for muscle spasms, pain relief

Nursing diagnoses
• Anxiety (uses)
• Coping, ineffective (uses)
• Injury, risk for (uses, adverse reactions)
• Knowledge, deficient (teaching)
• Noncompliance (teaching)

Implementation
PO route
• Give with food or milk for GI symptoms
• Crush tab if patient is unable to swallow medication whole
• Use sugarless gum, hard candy, frequent sips of water for dry mouth
• Reduce opioid dosage by one third if given concomitantly with diazepam
• Check to see if PO medication has been swallowed
• Concentrate: use calibrated dropper only; mix with water, juice, pudding, applesauce; consume immediately
Rectal route
• Do not use more than 5 ×/mo or for an episode q5day
IV route
• Administer **IV** into large vein; do not dilute or mix with any other product; give **IV** 5 mg or less/min or total dose over 3 min or more (children, infants); cont inf is not recommended; inject closest vein insertion as possible; do not dilute or mix with other products
• Check **IV** site for thrombosis or phlebitis, which may occur rapidly
Sterile emulsion for injection route
• Use **IV** only, within 6 hr, flush line after use and after 6 hr
Syringe compatibilities: Cimetidine

Syringe incompatibilities: Benzquinamide, doxapram, glycopyrrolate, heparin, nalbuphine

Y-site compatibilities: Cefmetazole, DOBUTamine, nafcillin, quinidine, sufentanil

Y-site incompatibilities: Hydromorphone, fluconazole, foscarnet, heparin, pancuronium, potassium chloride, vecuronium, vit B with C

Additive compatibilities: Netilmicin, verapamil

Patient/family education

• Advise patient that product may be taken with food; that product is not to be used for everyday stress or used longer than 4 mo unless directed by prescriber; take no more than prescribed amount; may be habit forming
• Caution patient to avoid OTC preparations unless approved by a prescriber; to avoid alcohol, other psychotropic medications unless prescribed; that smoking may decrease diazepam effect by increasing diazepam metabolism; not to discontinue medication abruptly after long-term use, gradually taper
• Inform patient to avoid driving, activities that require alertness; drowsiness may occur; to rise slowly or fainting may occur, especially in geriatric
• Advise patient not to become pregnant while using this product
• Inform patient that drowsiness may worsen at beginning of treatment

Evaluation
Positive therapeutic outcome
• Decreased anxiety, restlessness, insomnia

Treatment of overdose: Lavage, VS, supportive care, flumazenil

---

diazoxide (Rx)
(dye-az-ox′ide)
Diazoxide parenteral, Proglycem
Func. class.: Antihypertensive
Chem. class.: Vasodilator

Pregnancy category C

Action: Vasodilates arteriolar smooth muscle by direct relaxation; a reduction in blood pressure with concomitant increases in heart rate, cardiac output; reduces release of insulin from the pancreas

Therapeutic outcome: Decreased B/P, increased blood glucose

Uses: Hypertensive crisis when urgent decrease of diastolic pressure required (**IV**); increase blood glucose levels in hyperinsulinism

Dosage and routes
Hypoglycemia
Adult and child: PO 3-8 mg/kg/day in 2-3 divided doses q8-12hr
Infant and neonate: PO 8-15 mg/kg/day in 2-3 divided doses 8-12 hr

Hypertension
Adult: **IV** BOL 1-3 mg/kg rapidly up to a max of 150 mg in a single inj; dose may be repeated at 5-15 min intervals until desired response is achieved; give **IV** in 30 sec or less
Child: **IV** BOL 1-2 mg/kg rapidly: administration same as adult; max 150 mg

Available forms: Caps 50 mg; oral susp 50 mg/ml; inj 15 mg/ml, 300 mg/20 ml

Adverse effects
CNS: Headache, weakness, anxiety, dizziness, **seizures, cerebral ischemia, paralysis,** sleepiness, euphoria, anxiety, EPS, confusion, tinnitus, blurred vision
CV: Palpitations, hypotension, **shock, MI,** T-wave changes, angina pectoris, **supraventricular tachycardia, edema,** rebound hypertension
ENDO: Hyperglycemia in diabetics, transient hyperglycemia in nondiabetics, increased uric acid
GI: Nausea, vomiting, dry mouth
GU: Breast tenderness, increased BUN, fluid, electrolyte imbalances, Na, water retention
HEMA: **Thrombocytopenia,** decreased Hgb, Hct
INTEG: Rash

Contraindications: Hypersensitivity to this product or thiazides, sulfonamides, hypertension of aortic coarctation or AV shunt, pheochromocytoma, dissecting aortic aneurysm, hypoglycemia

Precautions: Pregnancy **C,** breastfeeding, children, tachycardia, fluid/electrolyte imbalances, impaired cerebral or circula tion

Pharmacokinetics

Absorption	Well absorbed (PO); completely absorbed (**IV**)
Distribution	Crosses blood-brain barrier, placenta, protein binding >90%
Metabolism	Liver (50%)
Excretion	Kidneys, unchanged (50%)
Half-life	20-36 hr

Pharmacodynamics		
	PO	IV
Onset	1 hr	1-2 min
Peak	8-12 hr	5 min
Duration	8 hr	3-12 hr

Interactions
Drug classifications
Antihypertensives: severe hypotension
Diuretics (thiazides): increased hyperurice-
mic, antihypertensive effects of diazoxide
Hydantoins: decreased anticonvulsant effect
NSAIDs, salicylates: decreased antihypertensive
effect
Sulfonylureas: increased hyperglycemia
Drug/herb
Aconite: increased toxicity, death

NURSING CONSIDERATIONS
Assessment
- Assess for allergies to sulfonamide; cross-
sensitivity may occur
- Assess B/P q5min until stabilized
- Monitor electrolytes, blood studies: potassium, sodium, chloride, carbon dioxide, CBC,
serum glucose
- Monitor weight daily, I&O; edema in feet,
legs daily; check skin turgor, dryness of
mucous membranes for hydration status
- Assess for crackles, dyspnea, orthopnea;
peripheral edema, fatigue, weight gain, jugular
vein distention (CHF)
- Assess for signs of hyperglycemia: acetone
breath, increased urinary output, severe thirst,
lethargy, dizziness

Nursing diagnoses
- Cardiac output, decreased (adverse reac-
tions)
- Injury, risk for (side effects)
- Knowledge, deficient (teaching)

Implementation
PO route
- Shake susp before using
- Store protected from light and heat
IV route
- Give by direct **IV** over 30 sec or less; may
repeat q5-15min until desired response; do
not administer dark solution
- Give to patient in recumbent position; keep
in that position for 1 hr after
Syringe compatibility: Heparin
Y-site incompatibilities: Hydralazine,
propranolol

Evaluation
Positive therapeutic outcome
- Decreased B/P in hypertension

Treatment of overdose: Administer
levarterenol, DOPamine, or norepinephrine
for hypotension, dialysis

---

dibucaine topical
See Appendix B

---

diclofenac ophthalmic
See Appendix B

---

diclofenac epolamine (Rx)
(dye-kloe'fen-ak)
Flector
diclofenac potassium (Rx)
Cataflam, Voltaren Rapide ✤
diclofenac sodium (Rx)
Apo-Dilo ✤, Cambia, Novo-Difenac ✤,
Solaraze Topical Gel, Voltram Topical Gel,
Voltaren, Voltaren XR, Zipsor
Func. class.: Nonsteroidal antiinflammatory
(NSAIDs), nonopioid analgesic
Chem. class.: Phenylacetic acid

Pregnancy category C

Do not confuse:
Cataflam/Catapres

Action: Inhibits prostaglandin synthesis by
decreasing enzyme needed for biosynthesis;
analgesic, antiinflammatory, antipyretic properties

Therapeutic outcome: Decreased pain,
inflammation

Uses: Acute, chronic rheumatoid arthritis,
osteoarthritis, ankylosing spondylitis, analgesia, primary dysmenorrhea; patch, mild-
moderate pain

Dosage and routes
Osteoarthritis
Adult: PO (Cataflam) 50 mg bid-tid, max
150 mg/day; DEL REL (Voltaren) 50 mg bid-tid
or 75 mg bid, max 150 mg/day; EXT REL
(Voltaren-XR) 100 mg qd, max 150 mg/day;
TOP gel 1% (Voltaren gel) 4 g for each lower
extremity qid, max 16 g/day; 2 g for each
upper extremity qid, max 8 g/day

Rheumatoid arthritis
Adult: PO (Cataflam) 50 mg tid-qid, max
225 mg/day; DEL REL (Voltaren) 50 mg tid-qid
or 75 mg bid, max 225 mg/day; EXT REL
(Voltaren-XR) 100 mg qd, may increase to 200
mg/day, max 225 mg/day

Ankylosing spondylitis
Adult: PO DEL REL (Voltaren) 25 mg qid and 25 mg at bedtime, max 125 mg/day

Acute migraine with/without aura
Adult: PO (powder for oral SOL) (Cambia) 50 mg as a single dose; mix contents of packet in 1-2 oz water

Mild to moderate pain
Adult: PO (Zipsor) 25 mg qid

Dysmenorrhea or nonrheumatic inflammatory conditions
Adult: PO (Cataflam) 50 mg tid or 100 mg initially, then 50 mg tid, max 200 mg 1st day, then 150 mg/day

Pain of strains/sprains
Adult: TOP Patch (Flector) apply patch to area bid

Actinic keratosis
Adult: TOP Gel (Solaraze) apply to area bid

Renal dose
Avoid use of Voltaren gel in advanced renal disease

Available forms: Epolamine: topical patch 1.3%; potassium: tabs 50 mg, sodium: del rel tabs (enteric-coated) 25, 50, 75, 100 mg; tabs liquid filled 25 mg; oral sol

Adverse effects
CNS: Dizziness, headache, drowsiness, fatigue, tremors, confusion, insomnia, anxiety, depression, nervousness, paresthesia, muscle weakness
CV: **CHF,** tachycardia, peripheral edema, palpitations, dysrhythmias, hypo/hypertension, fluid retention, **MI, stroke**
EENT: Tinnitus, hearing loss, blurred vision, **laryngeal edema**
GI: Nausea, anorexia, vomiting, diarrhea, jaundice, **cholestatic hepatitis,** constipation, flatulence, cramps, dry mouth, peptic ulcer, GI bleeding, **hepatotoxicity**
GU: **Nephrotoxicity: dysuria, hematuria, oliguria, azotemia, cystitis, UTI**
HEMA: **Blood dyscrasias,** epistaxis, bruising
INTEG: Purpura, rash, pruritus, sweating, erythema, petechiae, photosensitivity, alopecia
RESP: Dyspnea, hemoptysis, pharyngitis, **bronchospasm,** rhinitis, shortness of breath
SYST: **Anaphylaxis**

Contraindications: Hypersensitivity to aspirin, iodides, other NSAIDs; asthma, serious CV disease

Black Box Warning: Treatment of perioperative pain (CABG) surgery

Precautions: Pregnancy **C** (1st trimester), not recommended in 2nd half of pregnancy, breastfeeding, children, bleeding disorders, GI/cardiac disorders, hypersensitivity to other antiinflammatory agents, CCr <30 ml/min

Black Box Warning: GI bleeding, MI, stroke

D

Pharmacokinetics
Absorption	Well absorbed (PO, ophth)
Distribution	Crosses placenta; 99% bound to plasma proteins
Metabolism	Liver (50%)
Excretion	Breast milk
Half-life	2.5 hr

Pharmacodynamics
	PO	OPHTH	TOP (PATCH)
Onset	Unknown	Unknown	Unknown
Peak	2-3 hr	Unknown	12 hr
Duration	Unknown	Unknown	Unknown

Interactions
Individual drugs
Aspirin: increased GI side effects
CycloSPORINE, lithium, methotrexate, phenytoin: increased toxicity
Drug classifications
ACE inhibitors, β-blockers, diuretics: decreased antihypertensive effect
Anticoagulants, NSAIDs, platelet inhibitors, salicylates, SSRIs, thrombolytics: increased risk of bleeding
Antidiabetics: increased need for dosage adjustment
Biphosphonates, corticosteroids, diuretics (potassium-sparing): hyperkalemia
NSAIDs: increased GI side effects
Drug/herb
Arginine, gossypol: increased gastric irritation
Bearberry, bilberry: increased NSAIDs effect
Bogbean, chondroitin, garlic, ginger, gingko, saw palmetto, turmeric: increased bleeding risk
St. John's wort: increased severe photosensitivity

NURSING CONSIDERATIONS
Assessment
• Assess for pain of rheumatoid arthritis, osteoarthritis, ankylosing spondylitis; check ROM, inflammation of joints, characteristics of pain
• Assess ophthalmic patients for pain, inflammation, redness, swelling
◆ Monitor blood counts during therapy; watch for decreasing platelets; if low, therapy may

Adverse effects: *italic* = common, **bold** = life-threatening

need to be discontinued, restarted after hematologic recovery
- Assess for asthma, aspirin hypersensitivity, nasal polyps; may develop hypersensitivity
- Monitor liver function tests (may be elevated) and uric acid (may be decreased—serum; increased—urine) periodically; also BUN, creatinine, electrolytes (may be elevated)
- ⚠ Monitor for blood dyscrasias (thrombocytopenia): bruising, fatigue, bleeding, poor healing

Nursing diagnoses
- Injury, risk for (side effects)
- Knowledge, deficient (teaching)
- Mobility, impaired physical (uses)
- Pain, chronic (uses)

Implementation
PO route
- Do not break, crush, chew, or dissolve enteric-coated or ext rel tabs
- Administer with food or milk to decrease gastric symptoms
- Remain upright for ½ hr

Topical route (patch) (Flector)
- Wash hands before handling patch
- Remove and release liner before administration
- Use only on normal, intact skin
- Remove before bath, shower, swimming
- Discard removed patch in trash away from children, pets

Topical route (gel)
- Apply to intact skin
- Use only for osteoarthritis: mild-moderate pain

Ophthalmic route
- Administer with patient recumbent or tilting head back; pull down on lower lid; when conjunctival sac is exposed, instill 1 drop; wait a few minutes before instilling other drops

Patient/family education
- Teach patient that product must be continued for prescribed time to be effective; to avoid aspirin, NSAIDs, acetaminophen, or other OTC medications unless approved by prescriber, alcoholic beverages; to contact prescriber before surgery regarding when to discontinue this product
- Caution patient to report bleeding, bruising, fatigue, malaise, since blood dyscrasias do occur
- Advise patient to report hepatotoxicity: flulike symptoms, nausea, vomiting, jaundice, pruritus, lethargy
- Instruct patient to use sunscreen to prevent photosensitivity

- Teach patient to avoid use in 3rd trimester of pregnancy
- Instruct patient to use caution when driving; drowsiness, dizziness may occur
- Teach patient to take with a full glass of water to enhance absorption; remain upright for ½ hr; if dose is missed, take as soon as remembered within 2 hr if taking 1-2 ×/day; do not double doses
- Teach to report respiratory difficulty; trouble swallowing
- Advise to notify all providers that product is being used

Evaluation
Positive therapeutic outcome
- Decreased pain in arthritic conditions
- Decreased inflammation in arthritic conditions
- Decreased ocular irritation

---

didanosine (Rx)
(dye-dan'oh-seen)
ddI, dideoxyinosine, Pediatric Videx, Videx EC
Func. class.: Antiretroviral
Chem. class.: Synthetic purine nucleoside reverse transcriptase inhibitor (NRTI)
Pregnancy category B

Action: Nucleoside analog incorporating into cellular DNA by viral reverse transcriptase, thereby terminating the cellular DNA chain that prevents viral replication

Therapeutic outcome: Antiviral against the retroviruses, primarily HIV-1

Uses: HIV-1 infection in combination with other antiretrovirals

Dosage and routes
Adult: PO >60 kg, DEL REL caps 400 mg daily; <60 kg, DEL REL caps 250 mg daily
Child: PO (child BSA 1.1-1.4 m²); reconstituted pediatric powder 125 mg q8-12hr; PO (child BSA 0.8-1 m²); reconstituted pediatric powder 94 mg q8-12hr; PO (child BSA 0.5-0.7 m²); reconstituted pediatric powder 62 mg q8-12hr; PO (child BSA <0.4 m²); reconstituted pediatric powder 31 mg q8-12hr

Videx EC cap
Renal dose
Adult >60 kg: PO CCr 30-59 ml/min 200 mg/day; CCr 10-29 ml/min 125 mg/day; CCr <10 ml/min 125 mg/day
Adult <60 kg: PO CCr 30-59 ml/min 125 mg/day; CCr 10-29 ml/min 125 mg/day; CCr <10 ml/min, avoid use

---

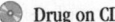

Available forms: Powder for oral sol 10 mg/ml; del rel caps 125, 200, 250, 400

Adverse effects
CNS: Peripheral neuropathy, seizures, confusion, *anxiety,* hypertonia, abnormal thinking, asthenia, *insomnia, CNS depression,* pain, dizziness, chills, fever
CV: Hypertension, vasodilatation, **dysrhythmia,** syncope, **CHF,** palpitations
EENT: Ear pain, otitis, photophobia, visual impairment, retinal depigmentation
GI: Pancreatitis, *diarrhea, nausea,* vomiting, *abdominal pain,* constipation, stomatitis, dyspepsia, liver abnormalities, flatulence, taste perversion, dry mouth, oral thrush, melena, increased ALT, AST, alkaline phosphatase, amylase, **hepatic failure**
GU: Increased bilirubin, uric acid
HEMA: Leukopenia, granulocytopenia, thrombocytopenia, anemia
INTEG: *Rash, pruritus,* alopecia, ecchymosis, hemorrhage, petechiae, sweating
MS: Myalgia, arthritis, myopathy, muscular atrophy
RESP: Cough, pneumonia, dyspnea, asthma, epistaxis, hypoventilation, sinusitis
SYST: Lactic acidosis, anaphylaxis

Contraindications: Hypersensitivity, lactic acidosis, pancreatitis, phenylketonuria

Precautions: Pregnancy **B,** breastfeeding, children, renal disease, sodium-restricted diets, elevated amylase, preexistent peripheral neuropathy, hyperuricemia, gout, CHF

Black Box Warning: Hepatic disease, lactic acidosis, pancreatitis

Pharmacokinetics
Absorption	Rapidly absorbed (up to 40%)
Distribution	Unknown
Metabolism	Not metabolized
Excretion	Kidneys (55%)/feces
Half-life	0.8-1.6 hr, shorter in children

Pharmacodynamics
Onset	Unknown
Peak	Up to 1 hr, del rel 2 hr
Duration	Unknown

Interactions
Individual drugs
Allopurinol, tenofovir: increased didanosine level; adjust dose as needed
Dapsone, ketoconazole: decreased absorption of each specific product
Itraconazole: decreased concentrations
Methadone: decreased didanosine level

Drug classifications
Aluminum, antacids, magnesium: increased side effects
Antiretrovirals, other: decreased concentration
Fluoroquinolones, tetracyclines: decreased concentrations of each specific product
Drug/food
Do not use with acidic juices
Decreased: absorption 50%

NURSING CONSIDERATIONS
Assessment
• Assess for peripheral neuropathy: tingling or pain in hands and feet, distal numbness; onset usually occurs 2-6 mo after beginning treatment, if these occur during therapy, product may be decreased or discontinued
• Assess for pancreatitis: abdominal pain, nausea, vomiting, elevated liver enzymes; product should be discontinued, since condition can be fatal
• Assess children by dilated retinal examination q6mo to rule out retinal depigmentation
• Monitor CBC, differential, platelet count monthly; withhold product if WBC is <4000/mm^3 or platelet count is <75,000 mm^3, viral load, CD4$^+$ count; notify prescriber of results
• Monitor renal function studies: BUN, serum uric acid, urine CCr before, during therapy; these may be elevated throughout treatment
• Assess for anaphylaxis, lactic acidosis
• Monitor temp q4hr; may indicate beginning of infection
• Monitor liver function tests before, during therapy (bilirubin, AST, ALT, amylase, alkaline phosphatase) as needed or monthly

Nursing diagnoses
• Infection, risk for (uses)
• Injury, risk for (adverse reactions)
• Knowledge, deficient (teaching)

Implementation
• Give on empty stomach 1 hr before or 2 hr after meals q12hr; food decreases effectiveness of product; adjust dose in renal impairment
• Pediatric powder for oral sol should be prepared in the pharmacy; shake before using
• Packets for oral sol must be mixed with ½ glass of water, not fruit juice; stir until dissolved; drink immediately
• Store caps in tightly closed bottle at room temperature; store oral sol after dissolving at room temperature ≤4 hr
• Do not take dapsone at same time as ddI

Patient/family education
• Advise patient to take on empty stomach; not to mix powder with fruit juice; to drink powder

immediately after mixing; to use exactly as prescribed
• Instruct patient to report signs of infection: increased temp, sore throat, flulike symptoms; to avoid crowds and those with known infections
• Instruct patient to report signs of anemia: fatigue, headache, faintness, shortness of breath, irritability
• Advise patient to report numbness/tingling in extremities
• Instruct patient to report bleeding; avoid use of razors and commercial mouthwash
• Advise patient that hair may be lost during therapy; a wig or hairpiece may make patient feel better
• Caution patient to avoid OTC products and other medications without approval of prescriber; to avoid alcohol
• Teach patient not to have any sexual contact without use of a condom; needles should not be shared; blood from infected individual should not come in contact with another's mucous membranes

Evaluation
Positive therapeutic outcome
• Absence of opportunistic infection, symptoms of HIV

---

difenoxin with atropine
See diphenoxylate with atropine

❗ HIGH ALERT

digoxin 💿 (Rx)
(di-jox'in)
digoxin, Lanoxicaps, Lanoxin
Func. class.: Inotropic antidysrhythmic, cardiac glycoside
Chem. class.: Digitalis preparation

Pregnancy category C

Do not confuse:
Lanoxin/Lasix/Lonox/Lomotil/Xanax/Levoxine

Action: Inhibits sodium-potassium ATPase, which makes more calcium available for contractile proteins, resulting in increased cardiac output; increases force of contraction (positive inotropic effect); decreases heart rate (chronotropic effect); decreases AV conduction speed

Therapeutic outcome: Decreased edema, pulse, respiration, crackles

Uses: Rapid digitalization in acute and chronic CHF, atrial fibrillation, atrial flutter, atrial tachycardia; cardiogenic shock, paroxysmal atrial tachycardia

Dosage and routes
Adult: **IV** *digitalizing dose* 0.6-1.0 mg given as 50% of the dose initially, additional fractions given at 4-8 hr intervals; PO *digitalizing dose* 0.75-1.25 mg given as 50% of the dose initially, additional fractions given at 4-8 hr intervals; *maintenance* 0.125-0.5 mg/day (tabs), or 0.350-0.5 mg/day (gelatin cap)
Child >10 yr: **IV** *digitalizing dose* 8-12 mcg/kg given as 50% of the dose initially, additional fractions given at 4-8 hr intervals; PO *digitalizing dose* 0.01-0.015 mg/kg given as 50% of the dose initially, additional fractions given at 6-8 hr intervals; maintenance 25%-35% of the loading dose daily as a single dose
Child 5-10 yr: **IV** *digitalizing dose* 0.015-0.03 mg/kg given as 50% of the dose initially, additional fractions given at 4-8 hr intervals; PO *digitalizing dose* 0.02-0.035 mg/kg given as 50% of the dose initially, additional fractions given at 6-8 hr intervals; *maintenance* 25%-35% of the loading dose daily in 2 divided doses
Child 2-5 yr: **IV** *digitalizing dose* 0.025-0.035 mg/kg given as 50% of the dose initially, additional fractions given at 4-8 hr intervals; PO *digitalizing dose* 0.03-0.04 mg/kg given as 50% of the dose initially, additional fractions given at 6-8 hr intervals; *maintenance* 25%-35% of the loading dose daily in 2 divided doses
Child 1-2 yr: **IV** *digitalizing dose* 0.03-0.05 mg/kg given as 50% of the dose initially, additional fractions given at 4-8 hr intervals; PO *digitalizing dose* 0.035-0.06 mg/kg given as 50% of the dose initially, additional fractions given at 4-8 hr intervals; *maintenance* 25%-35% of the loading dose daily in 2 divided doses
Infant: **IV** *digitalizing dose* 0.02-0.03 mg/kg given as 50% of the dose initially, additional fractions given at 4-8 hr intervals; PO *digitalizing dose* 0.025-0.035 mg/kg given as 50% of the dose initially, additional fractions given at 6-8 hr intervals; *maintenance* 25%-35% of the loading dose daily in 2 divided doses
Premature infant: **IV** *digitalizing dose* 0.015-0.025 mg/kg given as 50% of the dose initially, additional fractions given at 4-8 hr intervals; PO *digitalizing dose* 0.02-0.03 mg/kg given as 50% of the dose initially, additional fractions given at 6-8 hr intervals;

---

maintenance 20%-30% of the loading dose daily in 2 divided doses

Available forms: Caps 0.05, 0.1, 0.2 mg; elix 0.05 mg/ml; tabs 0.125, 0.25, 0.5 mg; inj 0.5 ❧, 0.25 mg/ml; pediatric inj 0.1 mg/ml

Adverse effects
CNS: Headache, drowsiness, apathy, confusion, disorientation, fatigue, depression, hallucinations
CV: **Dysrhythmias,** hypotension, bradycardia, **AV block**
EENT: Blurred vision, yellow-green halos, photophobia, diplopia
GI: Nausea, vomiting, anorexia, abdominal pain, diarrhea

Contraindications: Hypersensitivity to digoxin, ventricular fibrillation, ventricular tachycardia, carotid sinus syndrome, 2nd- or 3rd-degree heart block

Precautions: Pregnancy **C,** breastfeeding, geriatric, renal disease, acute MI, AV block, severe respiratory disease, hypothyroidism, sinus nodal disease, hypokalemia

Pharmacokinetics

Absorption	Unknown
Distribution	Widely distributed; 20%-25% protein bound
Metabolism	Liver, small amount; also intestinal bacteria
Excretion	Urine
Half-life	1½ days

Pharmacodynamics

	PO	IV
Onset	½-1½ hr	5-30 min
Peak	2-6 hr	1-5 hr
Duration	After steady state	6-8 days

Interactions
Individual drugs
Amiodarone, diltiazem, NIFEdipine, propantheline, quinidine, verapamil: increased digoxin levels
Amphotericin B, carbenicillin, ticarcillin: increased hypokalemia, increased toxicity
Calcium IV: increased hypercalcemia, hypomagnesemia, digoxin toxicity
Cholestyramine, colestipol, metoclopramide, thyroid hormones: decreased digoxin levels
Kaolin/pectin: decreased absorption
Drug classifications
Antacids: decreased digoxin absorption
Anticholinergics: increased digoxin blood levels

Antidysrhythmics, β-adrenergic blockers: increased bradycardia
Diuretics (thiazide) corticosteroids: increased hypokalemia, hypercalcemia, hypomagnesemia, digoxin toxicity
Sympathomimetics: increased cardiac dysrhythmia risk
Drug/herb
Aconite, hawthorn, horsetail: increased toxicity
Aloe, betel palm, broom, buckthorn, cascara sagrada castor, Chinese rhubarb, figwort, fumitory, hawthorn, khat, kudzu, licorice, lily of the valley, Mayapple, mistletoe, motherwort, night blooming cereus, oleander, pheasant's eye, purple foxglove, Queen Anne's lace, rhubarb, rue, senna, Siberian ginseng, squill, yellow dock: increased digoxin action
Bethroot, goldenseal, St. John's wort: decreased digoxin effect
Blackroot: forms insoluble complex
Cocoa, coffee, cola, guarana, horsetail, licorice, yerba maté: increased hypokalemia
Indian snakeroot: increased bradycardia
Psyllium: decreased digoxin absorption
Drug/lab test
Increased: CPK

NURSING CONSIDERATIONS
Assessment
• Assess and document apical pulse for 1 min before giving product; if pulse <60 in adult or <90 in an infant or is significantly different, take again in 1 hr; if <60 in adult, call prescriber; note rate, rhythm, character
• Monitor electrolytes: potassium, sodium, chloride, magnesium, calcium; renal function studies: BUN, creatinine; other blood studies: ALT, AST, bilirubin, Hct, Hgb, product levels (therapeutic level 0.5-2 ng/ml) before initiating treatment and periodically thereafter
• Monitor I&O ratio, daily weights; monitor turgor, lung sounds, edema
• Monitor cardiac status: apical pulse, character, rate, rhythm; resolution of atrial dysrhythmias by ECG; if tachydysrhythmia develops, hold product; delay cardioversion while product levels are determined
• Monitor ECG continuously during parenteral loading doses and for patients with suspected toxicity; provide hemodynamic monitoring for patients with heart failure or administer multiple cardiac products

Nursing diagnoses
• Cardiac output, decreased (uses)
• Gas exchange, impaired (adverse reactions)
• Knowledge, deficient (teaching)

Adverse effects: *italic* = common, **bold** = life-threatening

Implementation
• Do not give at same time as antacids or other products that decrease absorption
PO route
• Give PO with or without food; may crush tabs
• Take medication at same time each day
• Give potassium supplements if ordered for potassium levels <3, or give foods high in potassium: bananas, orange juice
IV route
• Give **IV** undiluted or 1 ml of product/4 ml sterile water, D₅, or 0.9% NaCl; give over >5 min through Y-tube or 3-way stopcock; during digitalization, close monitoring is necessary
• Store protected from light
Syringe compatibilities: Heparin, milrinone
Syringe incompatibility: Doxapram
Y-site compatibilities: Amrinone, cefmetazole, ciprofloxacin, cisatracurium, diltiazem, famotidine, meperidine, meropenem, midazolam, milrinone, morphine, potassium chloride, propofol, remifentanil, tacrolimus, vit B/C
Y-site incompatibilities: Fluconazole, foscarnet
Additive compatibilities: Bretylium, cimetidine, floxacillin, furosemide, lidocaine, ranitidine, verapamil
Additive incompatibility: DOBUTamine

Patient/family education
• Caution patient to avoid OTC medications including cough, cold, allergy preparations, antacids, since many adverse product interactions may occur; do not take antacid at same time
• Instruct patient to notify prescriber of any loss of appetite, lower stomach pain, diarrhea, weakness, drowsiness, headache, blurred or yellow-green vision, rash, depression; teach toxic symptoms of this product and when to notify prescriber
• Advise patient to maintain a sodium-restricted diet as ordered; to take potassium supplements as ordered to prevent toxicity
• Instruct patient to report shortness of breath, difficulty breathing, weight gain, edema, persistent cough
• Teach patient purpose of product is to regulate the heart's functioning
• Teach patient as outpatient to check and record pulse for 1 min before taking dose; if there is a change of >15 bpm from usual pulse, prescriber should be notified
• Teach patient to take medication at the same time each day, take missed doses within 12 hr; do not double doses; notify prescriber if doses are missed for 2 days or more; how to monitor heart rate
• Advise patient to carry/wear emergency ID describing dosage and reason for digoxin

Evaluation
Positive therapeutic outcome
• Decreased weight, edema, pulse, respiration, crackles
• Increased urine output
• Serum digoxin level 0.5-2 ng/ml

Treatment of overdose: Discontinue product, administer potassium, monitor ECG, administer an adrenergic blocking agent, digoxin immune FAB

digoxin immune FAB (ovine) ⊛ (Rx)
(di-jox'in)
Digibind, DigiFab
Func. class.: Antidote, digoxin specific
Pregnancy category C

Action: Antibody fragments bind to free digoxin or to reverse toxicity by not allowing digoxin or digitoxin to bind to sites of action

Therapeutic outcome: Correction of digoxin toxicity

Uses: Reversal of life-threatening digoxin or digitoxin toxicity, including severe bradycardia, ventricular tachycardia/fibrillation, severe hypertension

Dosage and routes
1 (38 mg) vial binds 0.5 mg digoxin
Digoxin toxicity (known amount) (tabs, oral sol, IM)
Adult and child: **IV** dose (mg) = dose ingested (mg) × 0.8/1000 × 38 or 40 mg/vial
Toxicity (known amount) (cap, **IV***)*
Adult and child: **IV** dose = dose ingested (mg)/0.5 × 38 or 40 mg/vial
Toxicity (known amount) by serum digoxin concentrations (SDCs)
Adult and child: **IV** SDC (nanograms/ml) × kg of weight/100 × 38 or 40 mg/vial
Digoxin toxicity (unknown amount)
Adult and child >20 kg: **IV** 228 mg (6 vials)

Infant and child <20 kg: **IV** 38 mg (1 vial)

Acute ingestion
Adult: **IV** 10 vials (380 mg)

Life-threatening ingestion
Adult: **IV** 20 vials (760 mg)

Skin test
Adult: ID 9.5 mcg

Available forms: Inj 38 mg/vial (binds 0.5 mg of digoxin), 40 mg/vial (binds 0.5 mg digoxin)

Adverse effects
CV: **CHF,** *ventricular rate increase,* **atrial fibrillation,** *low cardiac output,* hypotension
INTEG: *Hypersensitivity,* allergic reactions, facial swelling, redness, phlebitis
META: *Hypokalemia*
MISC: **Anaphylaxis** (rare)
RESP: **Impaired respiratory function, rapid respiratory rate**

Contraindications: Mild digoxin toxicity, hypersensitivity to this product, papain, or ovine protein

Precautions: Pregnancy **C,** breastfeeding, children, geriatric, cardiac/renal disease, hypocalcemia, heart failure, allergy to ovine proteins

Pharmacokinetics	
Absorption	Complete
Distribution	Widely distributed into plasma, interstitial fluids
Metabolism	Unknown
Excretion	Kidneys
Half-life	Biphasic (14-20 hr); increased in renal disease

Pharmacodynamics	
Onset	30 min (variable)
Peak	Unknown
Duration	Unknown

Interactions
Individual drugs
Considered incompatible with all products in syringe or sol
Drug/lab test
Interference: immunoassay (digoxin)

NURSING CONSIDERATIONS
Assessment
• Assess for hypokalemia: ST depression, flat T waves, presence of U wave, ventricular dysrhythmias

• Obtain information on previous allergies: previous exposure to sheep (ovine) proteins; scratch test may be performed before use of this product; hypersensitive reactions are more common in persons with previous exposure
• Monitor VS before, during, and after infusion
• Monitor heart rate, B/P q10min during inf and after completion until stabilized; hemodynamic monitoring is used for unstable or hypotensive patients; check potassium levels until toxicity is resolved
• Assess for oxygen or perfusion deficit: hypotension, chest pain, dizziness, loss of consciousness
• Assess respiratory status: auscultate lung fields for bibasilar crackles in patients with advanced CHF, B/P, volume overload

Nursing diagnoses
• Injury, risk for (uses)
• Knowledge, deficient (teaching)

Implementation
• Test doses have proven to be ineffective in the general population; only use test dose in those with known allergies or those previously treated with digoxin immune FAB
• For test dose dilute 0.1 ml or reconstituted product (9.5 mg/ml) in 9.9 ml sterile isotonic saline, inj 0.1 ml (1:100 dilution) ID and observe for wheal with erythema; read in 20 min
• For scratch test, place 1 drop of sol on skin and make a scratch through the drop with a sterile needle; read in 20 min
• Give after diluting 40 mg/4 ml of sterile water (10 mg/ml), mix gently; may be further diluted with 0.9% NaCl; sol should be clear, colorless
• Give by BOL if cardiac arrest is imminent or **IV** over 30 min using a 0.22-µm filter
• Store reconstituted sol for up to 4 hr in refrigerator; do not freeze DigiFab

Patient/family education
• Teach that purpose of medication is to bind excess digoxin and reduce high blood levels
• Instruct patients to report fever, chills, itching, sweating, dyspnea, delayed hypersensitivity
• Advise other prescribers that this medication has been used previously

Evaluation
Positive therapeutic outcome
• Correction of digoxin toxicity
• Digoxin blood level 0.5-2 ng/ml
• Digitoxin blood level 9-25 ng/ml

dihydroergotamine
See ergotamine

dihydrotachysterol (Rx)
(dye-hye-droh-tak-iss'ter-ole)
DHT Intensol ✤, Hytakerol
Func. class.: Parathyroid agent (calcium regulator)
Chem. class.: Vitamin D analog

Pregnancy category C

Action: Increases intestinal absorption of calcium, increases renal tubular absorption of phosphorus; is able to regulate calcium levels by regulation of calcitonin, parathyroid hormone

Therapeutic outcome: Prevention of continued calcium loss in bones

Uses: Hypoparathyroidism, pseudohypoparathyroidism, postoperative tetany

Dosage and routes
*Hypoparathyroidism/
pseudohypoparathyroidism*
Adult: PO 0.75-2.5 mg daily × 4 days, maintenance 0.2-1 mg daily regulated by serum calcium levels
Neonate: PO 0.05-0.1 mg/day
Child/infant: PO 1-5 mg qd × 4 days then 0.5-1.5 mg qd

Rickets (vit D resistant)
Child: PO 0.25-1 mg/day

Available forms: Tabs 0.125, 0.2, 0.4 mg; caps 0.125 mg; oral sol 0.2, 0.25 mg/5 ml, 0.2 mg/ml ✤ (Intensol)

Adverse effects
CNS: Drowsiness, headache, vertigo, fever, lethargy, depression
CV: **Dysrhythmias,** hypertension
EENT: Tinnitus
GI: Nausea, diarrhea, vomiting, jaundice, anorexia, dry mouth, constipation, cramps, metallic taste, thirst
GU: **Polyuria,** hypercalciuria, hyperphosphatemia, **hematuria,** nocturia, renal calculi
MS: Myalgia, arthralgia, decreased bone development, weakness, ataxia

Contraindications: Hypersensitivity, renal disease, hyperphosphatemia, hypercalcemia, hypervitaminosis D

Precautions: Pregnancy **C,** breastfeeding, renal calculi, CV disease

Pharmacokinetics
Absorption	Well absorbed from small intestine
Distribution	Liver, fat
Metabolism	Liver
Excretion	Feces (inactive, active metabolites)
Half-life	Unknown

Pharmacodynamics
Onset	2 wk
Peak	2 wk
Duration	2-9 wk

Interactions
Individual drugs
Cholestyramine, colestipol, mineral oil: decreased absorption of dihydrotachysterol
Phenytoin: decreased effect of dihydrotachysterol
Verapamil: increased dysrhythmias
Drug classifications
Barbiturates, corticosteroids: decreased effect of dihydrotachysterol
Calcium supplements, diuretics (thiazide): increased hypercalcemia
Cardiac glycosides: increased dysrhythmias
Drug/lab test
False increase: cholesterol

NURSING CONSIDERATIONS
Assessment
• Monitor BUN, urinary calcium, AST, ALT, cholesterol, alkaline phosphatase, creatinine, uric acid, chloride, magnesium, electrolytes, urine pH, phosphate; may increase calcium; should be kept at 9-10 mg/dl; keep vit D at 50-135 international units/dl, phosphate at 70 mg/dl; these tests should be checked before and throughout treatment
• Monitor for increased blood level, since toxic reaction may occur rapidly
• Monitor for dry mouth, metallic taste, polyuria, bone pain, muscle weakness, headache, fatigue, tinnitus, change in LOC, irregular pulse, dysrhythmias, increased respirations, anorexia, nausea, vomiting, cramps, diarrhea, constipation; may indicate hypercalcemia; if these occur, discontinue product, give laxatives, low-calcium diet
• Monitor renal status: decreased urinary output (oliguria, anuria), edema in extremities, weight gain >5 lb, periorbital edema
• Assess nutritional status; check diet for sources of vit D (milk, some seafood), calcium (dairy products, dark green vegetables); phosphates (dairy products) must be avoided

Nursing diagnoses
- Knowledge, deficient (teaching)
- Nutrition: less than body requirements, imbalanced (uses)

Implementation
- Do not break, crush, or chew caps
- May be increased q4wk depending on blood level; give with meals for GI symptoms
- Store in tight, light-resistant containers at room temperature
- Restrict sodium, potassium if required
- Restriction of fluids may be required for chronic renal failure

Patient/family education
- Teach symptoms of hypercalcemia and when to report symptoms to prescriber
- Teach patient about foods rich in calcium, vit D; provide list of calcium-rich foods; renal failure patients are given a renal diet
- Caution patient not to double doses, take exactly as prescribed

Evaluation
Positive therapeutic outcome
- Prevention of bone deficiencies
- Calcium, phosphorus at normal levels

⚠ HIGH ALERT

diltiazem (Rx)
(dil-tye´a-zem)
Apo-Diltiaz ✤, Cardizem, Cardizem CD, Cardizem LA, Cartia XT, Dilacor-XR, Diltia XR, diltiazem, Novo-Diltiazem ✤, Nu-Diltiaz, Ratio-Diltiazem CD, Syn-Diltiazem ✤, Taztia XT, Tiamate, Tiazac, Tiazem
Func. class.: Calcium channel blocker, antianginal, antiarrhythmic class IV, antihypertensive
Chem. class.: Benzothiazepine

Pregnancy category C

Do not confuse:
Cardizem/Cardene

Action: Inhibits calcium ion influx across cell membrane during cardiac depolarization, produces relaxation of coronary vascular smooth muscle, dilates coronary arteries, slows SA/AV node conduction times, dilates peripheral arteries

Therapeutic outcome: Decreased angina pectoris, dysrhythmias, B/P

Uses
Oral: Angina pectoris due to hypertension, coronary artery spasm

Parenteral: Atrial fibrillation, flutter; paroxysmal supraventricular tachycardia

Dosage and routes
Hypertension
Adult: PO 60-120 mg bid (SUS REL) (Cardizem SR), max 540 mg/day, or 180-240 mg (EXT REL) daily

Prinzmetal's or variant angina, chronic stable angina
Adult: PO 30 mg qid, increasing dose gradually to 180-360 mg/day in divided doses or (SR) 60-120 mg bid; may increase to 240-360 mg/day or 120 or 180 mg EXT REL (LA, CD, XT, XR products) PO daily

Atrial fibrillation, flutter, paroxysmal supraventricular tachycardia
Adult: IV 0.25 mg/kg as BOL over 2 min initially, then 0.35 mg/kg may be given after 15 min; if no response, may give CONT INF 5-15 mg/hr for up to 24 hr

Available forms: Tabs 30, 60, 90, 120 mg; ext rel tab 120, 180, 240, 300, 360, 420 mg; ext rel caps 60, 90, 120, 180, 240, 300, 360, 420 mg; inj 5 mg/ml (5, 10 ml)

Adverse effects
CNS: Headache, fatigue, drowsiness, dizziness, depression, weakness, insomnia, tremor, paresthesia
CV: **Dysrhythmia,** *edema,* **CHF,** bradycardia, hypotension, palpitations, **heart block**
GI: Nausea, vomiting, diarrhea, gastric upset, *constipation,* increased liver function tests
GU: Nocturia, polyuria, **acute renal failure**
INTEG: Rash, pruritus at inj site, flushing, photosensitivity, burning
RESP: Rhinitis, dyspnea, pharyngitis

Contraindications: Sick sinus syndrome, 2nd- or 3rd-degree heart block, hypotension less than 90 mm Hg systolic, acute MI, pulmonary congestion, cardiogenic shock

Precautions: Pregnancy **C,** breastfeeding, children, CHF, aortic stenosis bradycardia, GERD, hepatic disease, hiatal hernia, ventricular dysfunction, elderly

Pharmacokinetics	
Absorption	Well absorbed
Distribution	Not known
Metabolism	Liver, extensively
Excretion	Metabolites (96%)
Half-life	3½-9 hr

Adverse effects: *italic* = common, **bold** = life-threatening

Pharmacodynamics

	PO	PO–SUS REL	IV
Onset	½ hr	Unknown	Unknown
Peak	2-3 hr	Unknown	Unknown
Duration	6-8 hr	12 hr	Unknown

Interactions
Individual drugs
Carbamazepine, lithium, lovastatin, methylPREDNISolone: increased effects of each specific product
Cimetidine: increased effects of diltiazem
CycloSPORINE: increased cycloSPORINE effect
Digoxin: increased digoxin effect
Theophylline: increased effect, toxicity

Drug classifications
Anesthetics: increased effects of anesthetics
β-Adrenergic blockers: increased bradycardia, CHF, increased β-blocker effect
Benzodiazepines: increased effect of benzodiazepines
HMG-CoA reductase inhibitors: increased effects

Drug/herb
Barberry, betel palm, burdock, goldenseal, khat, khella, lily of the valley, plantain: increased diltiazem effect
Yohimbe: decreased diltiazem effect

Drug/food
Grapefruit juice: increased hypotension

NURSING CONSIDERATIONS
Assessment
• Assess fluid volume status: I&O ratio and record, weight, distended red veins, crackles in lung, color, quality, and specific gravity of urine, skin turgor, adequacy of pulses, moist mucous membranes, bilateral lung sounds, peripheral pitting edema; dehydration symptoms of decreasing output, thirst, hypotension, dry mouth and mucous membranes should be reported
• Monitor B/P and pulse, respiration, ECG and intervals (PR, QRS, QT); PCWP, CVP often during infusion; if B/P drops 30 mm Hg, stop infusion and call prescriber
• Monitor ALT, AST, bilirubin daily; if these are elevated, hepatotoxicity is suspected
• If platelets are <150,000/mm^3, product is usually discontinued and another product started
• Assess for extravasation: change site q48hr

Nursing diagnoses
• Cardiac output, decreased (uses)
• Knowledge, deficient (teaching)

Implementation
PO route
• Cardizem LA ext rel tab 24 hr: give qd, either AM or PM, without regard to meals
• Dilacor XR/Diltia XT ext rel cap 24 hr give qd, take on empty stomach, swallow whole, do not cut, crush, chew, open
• Tiazac, Tiztia XT: give qd without regard to meals
• Conventional regular-rel tab: give before meals and at bedtime
• Cardizem CD or equivalent (Cartia XT) generic ext rel cap 24 hr: give qd, without regard to meals
• Give with meals for GI symptoms; may sprinkle (reg tab) on applesauce after crushing
• Store in airtight container at room temperature

Oral suspension (unlabeled)
• Grind 16, 90 mg diltiazem reg rel tab into fine powder
• In separate container, mix 60 ml Ora-Sweet and 60 ml Ora-Plus
• Add small amount of sol to powder to form paste, add geometric amounts of base to achieve desired vol, place in amber container

IV route
• Give direct **IV** undiluted over 2 min
• For continuous inf dilute 125 mg/100 ml (1.25 mg/ml) or 250 mg/250 ml (1 mg/ml) or 250 mg/500 ml (0.5 mg/ml) of D$_5$W, 0.9% NaCl, D$_5$/0.45% NaCl; give 10 mg/hr; may increase by 5 mg/hr to 15 mg/hr; may continue inf up to 24 hr

Y-site compatibilities: Albumin, amikacin, amphotericin B, aztreonam, bretylium, bumetanide, cefazolin, cefotaxime, cefotetan, cefoxitin, ceftazidime, ceftriaxone, cefuroxime, cimetidine, ciprofloxacin, clindamycin, digoxin, DOBUTamine, DOPamine, doxycycline, epinephrine, erythromycin, esmolol, fentanyl, fluconazole, gentamicin, hetastarch, hydromorphone, imipenem-cilastatin, labetalol, lidocaine, lorazepam, meperidine, metoclopramide, metronidazole, midazolam, milrinone, morphine, multivitamins, niCARdipine, nitroglycerin, norepinephrine, oxacillin, penicillin G potassium, pentamidine, piperacillin, potassium chloride, potassium phosphates, ranitidine, sodium nitroprusside, theophylline, ticarcillin, ticarcillin/clavulanate, tobramycin, trimethoprim-sulfamethoxazole, vancomycin, vecuronium

Patient/family education
- Caution patient to avoid hazardous activities until stabilized on product and dizziness is no longer a problem
- Instruct patient to limit caffeine consumption; to avoid grapefruit juice; to avoid alcohol and OTC products unless directed by prescriber
◆ Tell patient to comply in all areas of medical regimen; diet, exercise, stress reduction, product therapy; to notify prescriber of irregular heartbeat, shortness of breath, swelling of feet and hands, pronounced dizziness, constipation, nausea, hypotension
- Teach patient to use as directed even if feeling better; may be taken with other cardiovascular products (nitrates, β-blockers); how to take pulse, B/P before taking product; to change position slowly

Evaluation
Positive therapeutic outcome
- Decreased anginal pain
- Decreased B/P
- Absence of dysrhythmias

Treatment of overdose: Atropine for AV block, vasopressor for hypotension

---

*dimenhyDRINATE (OTC, Rx)
(dye-men-hye′dri-nate)
Apo-Dimenhydrate ✦, Calm-X, Children's Dramamine, dimenhyDRINATE, Dimetabs, Dramamine, Dramanate, Dymenate, Gravol ✦, Gravol L/A ✦, Nauseatol ✦, Novo-Dimenate ✦, PMS-Dimenhydrinate ✦, Travamine ✦
Func. class.: Antiemetic, antihistamine, anticholinergic
Chem. class.: H₁-receptor antagonist, ethanolamine derivative

Pregnancy category B

Do not confuse:
dimenhyDRINATE/diphenhydrAMINE

Action: Vestibular stimulator is decreased; anticholinergic, antiemetic, antihistamine response; competes with histamine for H₁ receptors in GI tract, blood vessels, respiratory tract; central anticholinergic activity, which results in decreased vestibular stimulation and blockade of chemorecepter trigger zone

Therapeutic outcome: Absence of motion sickness

Uses: Motion sickness, nausea, vomiting, vertigo

Dosage and routes
Adult: PO 50-100 mg q4hr; IM/IV 50 mg q4hr as needed ✦
Child 6-12 yr: PO 25-50 mg q6-8hr prn, max 150 mg/day
Child 2-5 yr: PO 12.5-25 mg q6-8hr, max 75 mg/day

Available forms: Tab 50 mg; inj 50 mg/ml ✦; elix 15 mg/5 ml ✦; chew tab 50 mg

Adverse effects
CNS: Drowsiness, restlessness, headache, dizziness, insomnia, confusion, nervousness, tingling, vertigo
CV: Hypertension, *hypotension,* palpitations
EENT: Dry mouth, blurred vision, diplopia, nasal congestion, photosensitivity
GI: Nausea, anorexia, vomiting, *constipation*
INTEG: Rash, urticaria, fever, chills, flushing
MISC: **Anaphylaxis**

Contraindications: Hypersensitivity

Precautions: Pregnancy **B,** breastfeeding, children, geriatric, cardiac dysrhythmias, asthma, prostatic hypertrophy, bladder neck obstruction, closed-angle glaucoma, stenosing peptic ulcer, pyloroduodenal obstruction

Pharmacokinetics
Absorption	Well absorbed (PO, IM)
Distribution	Unknown; crosses placenta
Metabolism	Liver
Excretion	Kidneys, breast milk
Half-life	Unknown

Pharmacodynamics
	PO	IM	IV
Onset	15-60 min	30 min	Immediate
Peak	1-2 hr	1-2 hr	Unknown
Duration	4-6 hr	4-6 hr	4-6 hr

Interactions
Individual drugs
Alcohol: increased effect
Drug classifications
CNS depressants, anticholinergics, tricyclics, opiates, sedative/hypnotics, MAOIs: increased effects
Drug/herb
Corkwood, henbane leaf, jimsonweed, scopolia: increased anticholinergic effect
Hops, Jamaican dogwood, khat, senega: increased effect
Drug/lab test
False negative: skin allergy tests (discontinue antihistamines 3 days before testing)

Adverse effects: *italic* = common, **bold** = life-threatening

NURSING CONSIDERATIONS
Assessment

- Assess for signs of toxicity to other products or masking of symptoms of disease (brain tumor, intestinal obstruction); monitor GI symptoms including nausea, vomiting, abdominal pain, increased bowel sounds
- Monitor VS, B/P; check patients with cardiac disease more often
- Monitor I&O; check for dehydration (poor skin turgor, increased specific gravity, tachycardia, severe thirst) especially in the geriatric

Nursing diagnoses

- Injury, risk for (side effects)
- Knowledge, deficient (teaching)

Implementation

PO route
- Tabs may be swallowed whole, chewed, or allowed to dissolve; give 1-2 hr before activity that may cause motion sickness; use measuring device for liquid for correct dosing

IM route
- Give IM inj in large muscle mass; aspirate to avoid **IV** administration; massage

IV route
- Give **IV** directly after diluting 50 mg/10 ml or NaCl inj; give 50 mg or less over 2 min

Syringe compatibilities: Atropine, diphenhydrAMINE, droperidol, fentanyl, heparin, hydromorphone, meperidine, metoclopramide, morphine, pentazocine, perphenazine, ranitidine, scopolamine

Syringe incompatibilities: Butorphanol, chlorproMAZINE, glycopyrrolate, hydrOXYzine, midazolam, pentobarbital, prochlorperazine, promazine, promethazine, thiopental

Y-site compatibilities: Acyclovir

Y-site incompatibilities: Aminophylline, heparin, hydrocortisone sodium succinate, hydrOXYzine, phenobarbital, phenytoin, prednisoLONE, prochlorperazine, promazine, promethazine

Additive compatibilities: Amikacin, calcium gluconate, chloramphenicol, corticotropin, erythromycin, heparin, hydrOXYzine, methicillin, norepinephrine, penicillin G potassium, pentobarbital, phenobarbital, potassium chloride, prochlorperazine, vancomycin, vit B/C

Additive incompatibilities: Tetracycline, thiopental

Patient/family education

- Teach all aspects of product uses; to notify prescriber if confusion, sedation, hypotension occur; to avoid driving and other hazardous activity if drowsiness occurs; to avoid alcohol and other CNS depressants that may potentiate effect
- Tell patient not to exceed recommended dosage
- Inform patient hard candy, gum, frequent rinsing of mouth may be used for dryness
- Advise patient that a false negative result may occur with skin testing; these procedures should not be scheduled until 4 days after discontinuing use
- Caution patient to avoid hazardous activities, activities requiring alertness; dizziness may occur; instruct patient to request assistance with ambulation

Evaluation

Positive therapeutic outcome
- Absence of motion sickness
- Absence of nausea, vomiting

---

dinoprostone (Rx)
(dye-noe-prost'one)
Cervidil Vaginal Insert, Prepidil, Endocervical Gel, Prostin E Vaginal Suppository
Func. class.: Oxytocic, abortifacient
Chem. class.: Prostaglandin E_2

Pregnancy category C

Do not confuse:
Prepidil/bepridil

Action: Stimulates uterine contractions similar to labor by myometrium stimulation, causing abortion; acts within 30 hr for complete abortion

Therapeutic outcome: Beginning of labor, fetal expulsion

Uses: Abortion during 2nd trimester, benign hydatidiform mole, expulsion of uterine contents in fetal deaths to 28 wk, missed abortion, cervical effacement and dilatation in term pregnancy when they have not occurred spontaneously

Dosage and routes
Abortifacient/2nd trimester/ missed abortion/benign hydatidiform mole/intrauterine fetal death
Adult: VAG SUPP 20 mg; repeat q3-5hr until abortion occurs; max dose 240 mg

Cervical ripening
Adult: GEL warm to room temperature; choose correct length shielded catheter (10 or 20 mm); fill catheter by pushing plunger; have

patient recumbent for 15-30 min; insert one 10 mg insert

Available forms: Vag supp 20 mg; gel 0.5 mg/3 g (prefilled syringe); vag insert 10 mg

Adverse effects
CNS: Headache, dizziness, chills, fever
CV: Hypotension, **dysrhythmias**
EENT: Blurred vision
GI: Nausea, vomiting, diarrhea
GU: Vaginitis, vaginal pain, vulvitis, vaginismus
INTEG: Rash, skin color changes
MS: Leg cramps, joint swelling, weakness
Insert: Uterine hyperstimulation, fever, nausea, vomiting, diarrhea, abdominal pain
Gel: Uterine contractile abnormality, GI side effects, back pain, fever
Fetal: Bradycardia (i.e., deceleration)
Suppository: Uterine rupture, anaphylaxis

Contraindications: Hypersensitivity, C-section, surgery

Precautions: Pregnancy **C**, renal/hepatic/cardiac disease, asthma, anemia, jaundice, diabetes mellitus, seizure disorders, hypertension, glaucoma, uterine fibrosis, cervical stenosis, pelvic surgery, PID, respiratory disease

Black Box Warning: Hypotension, diarrhea, fever, vomiting

Pharmacokinetics

Absorption	Rapidly absorbed
Distribution	Unknown
Metabolism	Enzymes
Excretion	Kidneys
Half-life	Unknown

Pharmacodynamics

	GEL	SUPP
Onset	Rapid	10 min
Peak	30-45 min	Unknown
Duration	Unknown	2-3 hr

Interactions
Individual drugs
Alcohol: decreased oxytoxic effect
Drug classifications
Other oxytocics: increased effect

NURSING CONSIDERATIONS
Assessment
• Assess dilatation and effacement of the cervix, uterine contractions, fetal heart tones; watch for contractions lasting over 1 min, hypertonus, fetal distress; product should be slowed or discontinued

• Assess for fever that occurs approximately 30 min after supp insertion (abortion)
• Monitor for nausea, vomiting, diarrhea; these may require medication
• Assess for hypersensitivity reaction: dyspnea, rash, chest discomfort
• Assess respiratory rate, rhythm, depth; notify prescriber of abnormalities, in pulse, B/P
• Check vaginal discharge; itching, irritation indicates vaginal infection

Nursing diagnoses
• Injury, risk for (side effects)
• Knowledge, deficient (teaching)

Implementation
Suppository route
• Warm supp by running warm water over package; insert high in vagina, wear gloves to prevent absorption; have patient recumbent for at least 10 min

Gel route
• Do not allow to come in contact with skin; use soap and water to wash after use
• Gel should be at room temperature
• Place patient in dorsal or lithotomy position to insert gel into cervical canal; remove catheter; discard all items after use, keep supine 15-30 min

Patient/family education
• Teach patient all aspects of treatment including purpose of medication and expected results
• Tell patient that gel may produce warmth in her vagina
• Caution patient that if contractions are longer than 1 min to notify nurse or prescriber
• Advise patient to notify prescriber of cramping, pain, increased bleeding, chills, increased temp, or foul-smelling discharge; these symptoms may indicate uterine infection
• Advise patient to remain supine 10-15 min after insertion of suppository, 2 hr after insert, 15-30 min after gel

Evaluation
Positive therapeutic outcome
• Progression of labor
• Abortion

D

*diphenhydrAMINE
(OTC, Rx)
(dye-fen-hye'dra-meen)
Allerdryl ♣, AllerMax, Allermed,
Banophen, Benadryl, Benadryl 25, Benadryl
Kapseals, Benahist 10, Benahist 50, Ben-
Allergin-50, Benoject-10, Benoject-50,
Benylin Cough, Bydramine, Compoz,
Diphenadryl, Diphen Cough, Diphenhist,
diphenhydrAMINE HCl, Dormin, Genahist,
Hydramine, Hydramyn, Hydril, Hyrexin-50,
Insomnal ♣, Nidryl, Nighttime Sleep Aid,
Nordryl, Nordryl Cough, Nytol, Phendry,
Siladril, Sleep-Eze 3, Sominex 2, Tusstat,
Twilite, Uni-Bent Cough, Wehdryl
Func. class.: Antihistamine (1st generation,
nonselective), antitussive
Chem. class.: Ethanolamine derivative,
H₁-receptor antagonist

Pregnancy category B

Do not confuse:
diphenhydrAMINE/dicyclomine/
dimenhyDRINATE

Action: Acts on blood vessels, GI, respiratory system by competing with histamine for
H₁-receptor site; decreases allergic response
by blocking histamine

Therapeutic outcome: Absence of
allergy symptoms and rhinitis, decreased
dystonic symptoms, absence of motion sickness, absence of cough, ability to sleep

Uses: Allergy symptoms, rhinitis, motion
sickness, antiparkinsonism, nighttime sedation, infant colic, nonproductive cough,
insomnia in children

Dosage and routes
Adult and child >12 yr: PO 25-50 mg
q4-6hr, max 300 mg/day; IM/**IV** 10-50 mg,
max 300 mg/day
Child 6-12 yr: PO/IM/**IV** 5 mg/kg/day in 4
divided doses, max 150 mg/day

Nighttime sleep aid
Adult and child ≥12 yr: PO 25-50 mg at
bedtime

Antitussive (syrup only)
Adult and child ≥12 yr: 25 mg q4hr,
max 150 mg/24 hr
Child 6-12 yr: 12.5 mg q4hr, max 75
mg/24 hr

Renal dose
Adult: PO CCr >50 ml/min give dose q6hr;
CCr 10-50 ml/min dose q6-12hr; CCr <10
ml/min dose q12-18hr

Available forms: Caps 25, 50 mg; tabs
25, 50 mg; chew tabs 12.5 mg; elix 12.5 mg/5
ml; syr 12.5 mg/5 ml; inj 10, 50 mg/ml; orally
disintegrating tabs 12.5, 25 mg

Adverse effects
CNS: Dizziness, drowsiness, poor coordina-
tion, fatigue, anxiety, euphoria, confusion,
paresthesia, neuritis, **seizures**
CV: Hypotension, palpitations
EENT: Blurred vision, dilated pupils, tinnitus,
nasal stuffiness, dry nose, throat, mouth
GI: Nausea, anorexia, diarrhea
GU: Retention, dysuria, frequency
HEMA: **Thrombocytopenia, agranulocyto-
sis, hemolytic anemia**
INTEG: Photosensitivity
MISC: **Anaphylaxis**
RESP: Increased thick secretions, wheezing,
chest tightness

Contraindications: Hypersensitivity to
H₁-receptor antagonist, acute asthma attack,
lower respiratory tract disease, neonates

Precautions: Pregnancy **B**, breastfeeding,
children <2 yr, increased intraocular pressure,
renal/cardiac disease, hypertension, bronchial
asthma, seizure disorder, stenosed peptic
ulcers, hyperthyroidism, prostatic hypertrophy,
bladder neck obstruction

Pharmacokinetics

Absorption	Well absorbed (PO, IM); com-
pletely absorbed (**IV**)
Distribution	Widely distributed; crosses
placenta
Metabolism	Liver (95%)
Excretion	Kidneys, breast milk
Half-life	2½-7 hr

Pharmacodynamics

	PO	IM	IV
Onset	15-60 min	30 min	Immediate
Peak	1-4 hr	1-4 hr	Unknown
Duration	4-8 hr	4-8 hr	4-8 hr

Interactions
Individual drugs
Alcohol: increased CNS depression
Drug classifications
Antidepressants (tricyclic), barbiturates, CNS
depressants, opiates, sedative/hypnotics:
increased CNS depression
MAOIs: increased effect of diphenhydrAMINE
Drug/herb
Corkwood, henbane leaf: increased anticholin-
ergic effect

 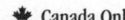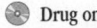

Hops, Jamaican dogwood, khat, senega: increased effect

Drug/lab test

False negative: skin allergy tests (discontinue antihistamines 3 days before testing)

NURSING CONSIDERATIONS
Assessment
- Assess respiratory status: rate, rhythm, increase in bronchial secretions, wheezing, chest tightness; provide fluids to 2 L/day to decrease secretion thickness
- Monitor I&O ratio: be alert for urinary retention, frequency, dysuria, especially geriatric; product should be discontinued if these occur
- Monitor CBC during long-term therapy; blood dyscrasias may occur but are rare
- If giving for dystonic reactions, assess type of involuntary movements and evaluate response to this medication
- Assess cough characteristics including type, frequency, thickness of secretions; evaluate response to this medication if using for cough

Nursing diagnoses
- Injury, risk for (side effects)
- Knowledge, deficient (teaching)
- Sleep deprivation (uses)

Implementation
- Give 20 min before bedtime if using for sleep aid

PO route
- Give with meals if GI symptoms occur; absorption rate may be slightly decreased; cap may be opened and product mixed with food/fluids for patients with swallowing difficulties

IM route
- Give IM inj in large muscle mass; aspirate to avoid **IV** administration; rotate sites

IV route
- Give **IV** undiluted 25 mg/min; may be diluted with 0.9% NaCl, D_5W, $D_{10}W$, 0.45% NaCl, D_5/0.9% NaCl, D_5/0.45% NaCl, D_5/0.25% NaCl, LR, Ringer's; give 25 mg/min or less

Syringe compatibilities: Atropine, butorphanol, chlorproMAZINE, cimetidine, cisatracurium, dimenhyDRINATE, DOXOrubicin liposome, droperidol, fentanyl, fluphenazine, glycopyrrolate, hydromorphone, hydrOXYzine, meperidine, metoclopramide, midazolam, morphine, nalbuphine, pentazocine, perphenazine, prochlorperazine, promazine, promethazine, ranitidine, remifentanil, scopolamine, sufentanil

Syringe incompatibilities: Pentobarbital, phenytoin, thiopental

Y-site compatibilities: Abciximab, aldesleukin, amifostine, amsacrine, ciprofloxacin, cisplatin, cladribine, cyclophosphamide, cytarabine, DOXOrubicin, famotidine, filgrastim, fluconazole, fludarabine, gallium, granisetron, heparin, hydrocortisone, idarubicin, melphalan, meperidine, meropenem, methotrexate, ondansetron, paclitaxel, piperacillin/tazobactam, potassium chloride, propofol, sargramostim, sufentanil, tacrolimus, teniposide, thiotepa, vinorelbine, vit B/C

Y-site incompatibilities: Foscarnet

Additive compatibilities: Amikacin, aminophylline, ascorbic acid, bleomycin, cephapirin, erythromycin, hydrocortisone, lidocaine, methyldopate, nafcillin, netilmicin, penicillin G potassium, penicillin G sodium, polymyxin B, vit B/C

Additive incompatibilities: Amobarbital, cephalothin, thiopental

Patient/family education
- Tell patient that a false-negative result may occur with skin testing; these procedures should not be scheduled until 3 days after discontinuing use
- Caution patient to avoid hazardous activities and activities requiring alertness, since dizziness may occur; instruct patient to request assistance with ambulation
- Teach patient to use sunscreen to prevent photosensitivity
- Advise patient to avoid alcohol, other depressants; may potentiate effect; CNS depression may occur
- Teach all aspects of product uses; to notify prescriber if confusion, sedation, hypotension occur; to avoid driving and other hazardous activity if drowsiness occurs; to avoid alcohol or other CNS depressants that may potentiate effect
- Teach patient to avoid breastfeeding

Evaluation
Positive therapeutic outcome
- Absence of motion sickness
- Absence of nausea, vomiting
- Ability to sleep
- Absence of cough
- Decrease in involuntary movements

Treatment of overdose:
- Administer lavage, diazepam, vasopressors, phenytoin IV

diphenoxylate with atropine (Rx)
(dye-fen-ox'i-late)
Lomotil, Lonox
difenoxin/atropine (Rx)
(dye-fen-ox'in/a'troe-peen)
Motofen
Func. class.: Antidiarrheal
Chem. class.: Phenylpiperidine derivative, opiate agonist

Pregnancy category C

Controlled substance schedule V
diphenoxylate/atropine; **IV**
difenoxin/atropine (US)

Do not confuse:
Lomotil/Lamictal/Lamasil/Lanoxin/Lasix/
Ludomil

Action: Inhibits gastric motility by acting on mucosal receptors responsible for peristalsis; related to opioid analgesics as adjunct

Therapeutic outcome: Decreased loose stools

Uses: Acute nonspecific and acute exacerbations of chronic functional diarrhea

Dosage and routes
diphenoxylate/atropine
Adult: PO 5 mg qid, titrated to patient response, max 8 tabs/24 hr
Child 2-12 yr: PO (liquid only) 0.3-0.4 mg/kg/day in 4 divided doses

difenoxin/atropine
Adult: PO initially 2 tabs, then 1 tab after each loose stool or q3-4hr prn, max 8 tabs/day

Available forms: diphenoxylate/atropine: tab 2.5 mg diphenoxylate/0.025 mg atropine; liq 2.5 mg diphenoxylate/0.025 mg atropine/5 ml; difenoxin/atropine: tabs 1 mg difenoxin/0.025 atropine

Adverse effects
CNS: Dizziness, drowsiness, light-headedness, headache, fatigue, nervousness, insomnia, confusion
EENT: Blurred vision, burning eyes
GI: Nausea, vomiting, dry mouth, epigastric distress, constipation, **paralytic ileus, toxic megacolon**
MISC: **Anaphylaxis, angioedema**
RESP: **Respiratory depression**

Contraindications: Hypersensitivity, pseudomembranous colitis, child <2 yr, severe electrolyte imbalances, diarrhea associated with organisms that penetrate intestinal mucosa

Precautions: Pregnancy **C**, breastfeeding, hepatic disease, ulcerative colitis, severe hepatic disease, substance abuse, dehydration

Pharmacokinetics	
Absorption	Well absorbed
Distribution	Unknown
Metabolism	Liver, active metabolite
Excretion	Kidneys
Half-life	2½ hr

Pharmacodynamics	
Onset	45-60 min
Peak	2 hr
Duration	3-4 hr

Interactions
Individual drugs
Alcohol: increased action of alcohol
Amantadine, amoxapine, diphenhydramine, clemastine, clozapine, cyclobenzaprine, disopyramide, loperamide, maprotiline, olanzapine: decreased GI motility, possible toxic megacolon
Drug classifications
Anticholinergics: increased anticholinergic effect
Antimuscarinics, phenothiazines, tricyclics: decreased GI motility, possible toxic megacolon
Barbiturates: increased action of barbiturates
CNS depressants: increased action of CNS depressants
MAOIs: hypertensive crisis; do not use together
Opiates: increased action of opioids
Drug/herb
Nutmeg: increased antidiarrheal effect

NURSING CONSIDERATIONS
Assessment
• Monitor electrolytes (potassium, sodium, chloride) if on long-term therapy; fluid status, skin turgor
• Assess bowel pattern before, during treatment; check for rebound constipation after termination of medication; check bowel sounds
• Check response after 48 hr; if no response, product should be discontinued and other treatment initiated
• Assess for abdominal distention and toxic megacolon, which may occur in ulcerative colitis
• Assess hepatic function if on long-term therapy

 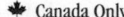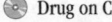

Nursing diagnoses
• Constipation (adverse reactions)
• Diarrhea (uses)
• Knowledge, deficient (teaching)
• Noncompliance (teaching)

Implementation
• Give for 48 hr only; tabs may be given with food, crushed and mixed with fluids; liquid should be measured accurately

Patient/family education
• Advise patient to avoid alcohol and OTC products unless directed by prescriber; may cause increased CNS depression
• Caution patient not to exceed recommended dosage; that product may be habit forming
• Advise patient that product may cause drowsiness; to avoid hazardous activities until response to product is determined
• Teach patient that dry mouth can be decreased by frequent sips of water, hard candy, sugarless gum

Evaluation
Positive therapeutic outcome
• Decreased diarrhea

---

dipivefrin ophthalmic
See Appendix B

---

dipyridamole (Rx)
(dye-peer-id'a-mole)
Apo-Dipyridamole ✦, dipyridamole, Novo-Dipiradol ✦, Persantine, Persantine IV
Func. class.: Coronary vasodilator, antiplatelet agent
Chem. class.: Nonnitrate

Pregnancy category B

Action: Inhibits adenosine uptake, which produces coronary vasodilatation; increases oxygen saturation in coronary tissues, coronary blood flow; acts on small vessels with little effect on vascular resistance; may increase development of collateral circulation; decreased platelet aggregation by the inhibition of phosphodiesterases (enzymes)

Therapeutic outcome: Inhibition of platelet aggregation; absence of ischemic attacks, reinfarction

Uses: Prevention of transient ischemic attacks, inhibition of platelet adhesion to prevent myocardial reinfarction, thromboembolism, with warfarin in prosthetic heart valves, prevention of coronary bypass graft occlusion with aspirin; **IV** form used to evaluate coronary artery disease; used as alternative to exercise in thallium myocardial perfusion imaging to evaluate coronary artery disease

Dosage and routes
Transient ischemic attacks
Adult: PO 50 mg tid, 1 hr before meals, max 400 mg daily

Inhibition of platelet adhesion
Adult: PO 75-100 mg qid in combination with aspirin or warfarin

Thallium myocardial perfusion imaging
Adult: **IV** 570 mcg/kg

Available forms: Tabs 25, 50, 75 mg; inj 10 mg/2 ml

Adverse effects
CNS: Headache, dizziness, weakness, fainting, syncope; **IV**: transient cerebral ischemia, weakness
CV: Postural hypotension; **IV**: **MI**
GI: Nausea, vomiting, anorexia, diarrhea
INTEG: Rash, flushing
RESP: **IV**: **Bronchospasm**

Contraindications: Hypersensitivity

Precautions: Pregnancy **B**, breastfeeding, hypotension

Pharmacokinetics
Absorption	30%-50% (PO)
Distribution	Widely distributed; crosses placenta
Metabolism	Liver
Excretion	Bile, undergoes enterohepatic recirculation; enters breast milk
Half-life	10 hr

Pharmacodynamics
	PO	IV
Onset	Unknown	Unknown
Peak	1.25 hr	6 min
Duration	6 hr	½ hr
Therapeutic effect	Several mo	

Interactions
Individual drugs
Aspirin, cefamandole, cefotetan, cefoperazone, plicamycin, sulfinpyrazone, valproic acid: increased risk of bleeding
Digoxin: increased digoxin effect
Theophylline: prevention of coronary vasodilation

Adverse effects: *italic* = common, **bold** = life-threatening

Drug classifications
Anticoagulants, NSAIDs, salicylates, thrombolytics: increased risk of bleeding
Drug/herb
Arginine: increased gastric irritation
Bilberry, saw palmetto: decreased antiplatelet effect
Bogbean, dong quai, feverfew, garlic, ginger, ginkgo, grapeseed, primrose: increased antiplatelet effect

NURSING CONSIDERATIONS
Assessment
• Monitor B/P, pulse baseline and during treatment until stable; take B/P with patient lying, standing; orthostatic hypotension is common
• Assess cardiac status: chest pain, what aggravates or ameliorates condition
• If using by **IV** route, monitor VS before, during, and after infusion; monitor for chest pain, bronchospasm; use ECG for identifying dysrhythmias; use aminophylline up to 250 mg **IV** for bronchospasm and chest pain; if chest pain is unrelieved with the 250 mg dose of aminophylline, give SL dose of nitroglycerin

Nursing diagnoses
• Cardiac output, decreased (uses)
• Knowledge, deficient (teaching)
• Pain, acute (uses)

Implementation
PO route
• Give with 8 oz of water; to improve absorption give on an empty stomach; if GI symptoms occur may give with meals
• Tabs may be crushed, mixed with food or fluids for swallowing difficulty or swallowed whole
• Store at room temperature
Intermittent IV infusion route
• Give by **IV** after diluting to at least 1:2 ratio using D₅W, 0.45% NaCl, or 0.9% NaCl; 20-50 ml should be given; give over 4 min; do not give undiluted

Patient/family education
• Teach patient that this medication is not a cure; that product may have to be taken continuously in evenly spaced doses only as directed; if a dose is missed, take one when remembered up to 4 hr; do not double doses
• Advise patient to rise slowly from sitting or lying down to prevent orthostatic hypotension
• Caution patient not to use alcohol or OTC medication unless approved by prescriber
• Caution patient to avoid hazardous activities until stabilized on medication; dizziness may occur

Evaluation
Positive therapeutic outcome
• Absence of reinfarction, ischemic attacks

Treatment of overdose: Administer **IV** phenylephrine

---

disopyramide (Rx)
(dye-soe-peer′a-mide)
disopyramide, Norpace, Norpace CR, Rhythmodan ✦, Rythmodan-LA ✦
Func. class.: Antidysrhythmic (class IA)
Chem. class.: Nonnitrate
Pregnancy category C

Action: Prolongs action potential duration and effective refractory period; reduces disparity in refractory period between normal and infarcted myocardium; prevents increased myocardial excitability and conduction contractility

Therapeutic outcome: Suppression of supraventricular dysrhythmias

Uses: PVCs, ventricular tachycardia, supraventricular tachycardia

Unlabeled uses: Atrial flutter, fibrillation

Dosage and routes
Adult: PO 100-200 mg q6hr; SUS REL cap 200-400 mg q12hr
Child 12-18 yr: PO 6-15 mg/kg/day, in divided doses q6hr
Child 5-12 yr: PO 10-15 mg/kg/day in divided doses q6hr
Child 1-4 yr: PO 10-20 mg/kg/day in divided doses q6hr
Child <1 yr: PO 10-30 mg/kg/day, in divided doses q6hr

Renal dose
Adult: PO CCr >40 ml/min 100 mg q6hr; CCr 30-40 ml/min dose q8hr; CCr 15-30 ml/min dose q12hr; CCr <15 ml/min dose q24hr

Available forms: Caps 100, 150 mg; cont rel caps 100, 150 mg; sus rel tabs 150 mg ✦

Adverse effects
CNS: Headache, dizziness, psychosis, fatigue, depression, paresthesias, insomnia
CV: Hypotension, bradycardia, angina, PVCs, tachycardia, increases in QRS and QT segments, **cardiac arrest,** edema, weight gain, AV block, **CHF,** syncope, chest pain
EENT: Blurred vision, dry nose, throat, eyes, closed-angle glaucoma
GI: Dry mouth, constipation, nausea, anorexia, flatulence, diarrhea, vomiting

---

GU: Retention, hesitancy, impotence
HEMA: **Thrombocytopenia, agranulocytosis,** anemia (rare), decreased Hgb, Hct
INTEG: Rash, pruritus, urticaria
META: Hypoglycemia, hypokalemia
MS: Weakness, pain in extremities

Contraindications: Hypersensitivity, 2nd- or 3rd-degree heart block, cardiogenic shock, CHF (uncompensated), sick sinus syndrome

Black Box Warning: QT prolongation

Precautions: Pregnancy C, breastfeeding, children, geriatric patients, diabetes mellitus, renal/hepatic disease, myasthenia gravis, closed-angle glaucoma, cardiomyopathy, conduction abnormalities, potassium imbalance

Black Box Warning: Arrhythmias, MI, torsades de pointes

Pharmacokinetics

Absorption	Well absorbed
Distribution	Widely distributed
Metabolism	Liver
Excretion	Kidneys
Half-life	4-10 hr

Pharmacodynamics

	PO	PO–SUS REL
Onset	½-3½ hr	Unknown
Peak	2 hr	Unknown
Duration	1½-8 hr	12 hr

Interactions
Individual drugs
Atenolol, erythromycin, lidocaine, procainamide, propranolol, quinidine: increased effects of disopyramide
Phenobarbital, phenytoin, rifampin: decreased effects of disopyramide
Drug classifications
Anticholinergics: increased side effects, urinary retention
Antidysrhythmics: increased disopyramide effect
Drug/herb
Aconite: increased toxicity, death
Aloe, broom, buckthorn (chronic use), cascara sagrada (chronic use), Chinese rhubarb, figwort, fumitory, goldenseal, kudzu, licorice, senna: increased effect
Coltsfoot: decreased effect
Horehound: increased serotonin effect
Drug/lab test
Increased: liver enzymes, lipids, BUN, creatinine
Decreased: Hgb/Hct, blood glucose

NURSING CONSIDERATIONS
Assessment
- Assess respiratory status: auscultate lung fields for bibasilar crackles in patients with advanced CHF
- Monitor I&O ratio and electrolytes: potassium, sodium, chloride; watch for decreasing urinary output, possible retention
- Monitor liver function tests: AST, ALT, bilirubin, alkaline phosphatase
- Monitor ECG to determine product effectiveness, measure PR, QRS, QT intervals; check for PVCs, other dysrhythmias; monitor B/P for hypotension; check for prolonged widening QT intervals, QRS complex; if QT or QRS increase by 50% or more, withhold next dose, notify prescriber
- Monitor for dehydration or hypovolemia
- Monitor for CNS symptoms: psychosis, numbness, depression; if these occur, product should be discontinued

Nursing diagnoses
- Cardiac output, decreased (uses)
- Knowledge, deficient (teaching)

Implementation
- Do not break, crush, or chew sus rel tabs
- Give 1 hr before or 2 hr after meals
- If changing from regular release to sus rel cap, give sus rel 6 hr after last dose of regular release

Patient/family education
- Teach patient to report side effects immediately to prescriber; to take exactly as prescribed; if dose is missed take when remembered if within 3-4 hr of next dose; do not double doses
- Teach patient to complete follow-up appointment with prescriber including pulmonary function tests, chest x-ray
- Instruct patient that dry mouth may be relieved by frequent sips of water, hard candy, sugarless gum
- Caution patient to make position changes from lying to standing slowly to prevent orthostatic hypotension

Evaluation
Positive therapeutic outcome
- Decreased PVCs, ventricular tachycardia

Treatment of overdose: Administer O_2, artificial ventilation, ECG; administer DOPamine for circulatory depression; administer diazepam or thiopental for seizures, isoproterenol

Adverse effects: *italic* = common, **bold** = life-threatening

divalproex sodium
See valproate

---

*DOBUTamine (Rx)
(doe-byoo'ta-meen)
DOBUTamine
Func. class.: Adrenergic direct-acting β₁-agonist, inotropic agent, cardiac stimulant
Chem. class.: Catecholamine

Pregnancy category B

Do not confuse:
DOBUTamine/DOPamine, Dobutrex/Diamox

Action: Causes increased contractility, increased cardiac output without marked increase in heart rate by acting on β₁-receptors in heart; minor α/β₂ effects

Therapeutic outcome: Cardiac output increased with decreased fatigue and dyspnea

Uses: Cardiac decompensation due to organic heart disease or cardiac surgery

Unlabeled uses: Cardiogenic shock in children, congenital heart disease in children undergoing cardiac catherization

Dosage and routes
Adult and child: **IV** INF 2-20 mcg/kg/min; may increase to 40 mcg/kg/min if needed

Available forms: Inj 12.5 mg/ml

Adverse effects
CNS: *Anxiety,* headache, dizziness, fatigue
CV: Palpitations, tachycardia, hypo/hypertension, PVCs, angina
ENDO: Hypokalemia
GI: Heartburn, nausea, vomiting
MS: Muscle cramps (leg)
RESP: Dyspnea

Contraindications: Hypersensitivity, idiopathic hypertrophic subaortic stenosis

Precautions: Pregnancy **B**, breastfeeding, children, hypertension, CAD, MI, hypovolemia, dysrhythmias

Pharmacokinetics	
Absorption	Complete
Distribution	Unknown
Metabolism	Liver
Excretion	Kidneys
Half-life	2 min

Pharmacodynamics	
Onset	1-5 min
Peak	10 min
Duration	<10 min

Interactions
Individual drugs
Atomoxetine: increased pressor effect, dysrhythmias
Bretylium, oxytocin: increased dysrhythmias
Guanethidine: increased severe hypertension
Oxytocin: increased pressor effects
Drug classifications
Anesthetics: increased dysrhythmias
Antidepressants (tricyclic), COMT inhibitors, MAOIs, oxytocics: increased pressor response, dysrhythmias
β-Blockers: decreased action of DOBUTamine

NURSING CONSIDERATIONS
Assessment
• Assess for hypovolemia; if present, correct before beginning treatment with DOBUTamine; avoid use in patients with atrial fibrillation before digitalization
• Monitor ECG for dysrhythmias, ischemia during treatment; some patients may not need continuous ECG monitoring; also monitor PCWP, CVP, CO₂, urinary output; notify prescriber if <30 ml/hr
• Assess for heart failure: bibasilar crackles, S₃ gallop, dyspnea, neck vein distention in patients with cardiomyopathy or CHF
• Assess for oxygenation or perfusion deficit: decreased B/P, chest pain, dizziness, loss of consciousness
• Monitor B/P and pulse q5min during infusion; if B/P drops 30 mm Hg, stop infusion and call prescriber
• Monitor ALT, AST, bilirubin daily
• Monitor for sulfite sensitivity, which may be life threatening

Nursing diagnoses
• Cardiac output, decreased (uses)
• Knowledge, deficient (teaching)

Implementation
IV route
• Reconstitute 250 mg/10 ml of D₅W or sterile water for inj; may add another 10 ml to dissolve completely if needed, then dilute in 50 ml or more of D₅W, 0.9% NaCl, 0.45% NaCl, D₅/0.45% NaCl, D₅/0.9% NaCl, D₅/LR, LR; titrate to patient response; use infusion pump for correct dose
• Use a CVP catheter or large peripheral vein, use infusion pump, titrate to patient response
• Change **IV** site q48hr

Syringe compatibilities: Heparin, ranitidine

Syringe incompatibility: Doxapram

Y-site compatibilities: Amifostine, inamrinone, atracurium, aztreonam, bretylium, calcium chloride, calcium gluconate, ciprofloxacin, cladribine, diazepam, diltiazem, DOPamine, enalaprilat, epinephrine, famotidine, fentanyl, fluconazole, granisetron, haloperidol, hydromorphone, regular insulin, labetalol, lidocaine, lorazepam, magnesium sulfate, meperidine, milrinone, morphine, niCARdipine, nitroglycerin, norepinephrine, pancuronium, potassium chloride, propofol, ranitidine, sodium nitroprusside, streptokinase, tacrolimus, theophylline, thiotepa, tolazoline, vecuronium, verapamil, zidovudine

Y-site incompatibilities: Acyclovir, alteplase, aminophylline, foscarnet, phytonadione

Additive compatibilities: Amiodarone, atracurium, atropine, DOPamine, enalaprilat, epinephrine, flumazenil, hydrALAZINE, isoproterenol, lidocaine, meperidine, meropenem, metaraminol, morphine, nitroglycerin, norepinephrine, phentolamine, phenylephrine, procainamide, propranolol, ranitidine, verapamil

Additive incompatibilities: Acyclovir, aminophylline, bumetanide, calcium gluconate, diazepam, digoxin, furosemide, insulin, magnesium sulfate, phenytoin, potassium phosphate, sodium bicarbonate

Patient/family education
• Teach patient reason for medication and expected results, reason for all monitoring and procedures
• Advise patient to report dyspnea, headache, **IV** site discomfort, chest pain, numbness of extremities

Evaluation
Positive therapeutic outcome
• Increased cardiac output
• Decreased PCWP, adequate CVP
• Decreased dyspnea, fatigue, edema, ECG
• Increased urine output

Treatment of overdose: Discontinue product, support circulation

docetaxel (Rx)
(doe-se-tax′el)
Taxotere
Func. class.: Antineoplastic—miscellaneous
Pregnancy category D

D

Do not confuse:
Taxotere/Taxol

Action: Inhibits the reorganization of the microtubule network needed for interphase and mitotic cellular functions; also causes abnormal bundles of microtubules during cell cycle and multiple esters of microtubules during mitosis

Therapeutic outcome: Prevention of rapidly growing malignant cells

Uses: Locally advanced or metastatic breast cancer, non–small-cell lung cancer, androgen independent metastatic prostate cancer, postsurgery operable node-positive breast cancer, induction treatment of locally advanced squamous cell cancer of the head/neck, adjuvant treatment of breast cancer with carboplatin and trastuzumab

Dosage and routes
• Other regimens are used

Locally advanced or metastatic breast cancer after failure of other chemotherapy
Adult: **IV** 60-100 mg/m^2 given over 1 hr q3wk; if neutrophil count is <500/mm^3 for >1 wk, reduce dose by 25%

Operable node positive breast cancer
Adult: **IV** (TAC regimen) 75 mg/m^2 1 hr after DOXOrubicin 50 mg/m^2 and cyclophosphamide 500 mg/m^2 q3wk for 6 cycles

Adjuvant treatment of operable stage I-III invasive breast cancer in combination with cyclophosphamide
Adult: **IV** (TC) regimen docetaxel 75 mg/m^2 with cyclophosphamide 600 mg/m^2 q21day × 4 cycles

Locally advanced or metastatic non–small-cell lung cancer after failure of cisplatin chemotherapy
Adult: **IV** 75 mg/m^2 over 1 hr q3wk; if neutrophil count is <500/mm^3 for >1 wk, reduce dose to 55 mg/m^2; if patient develops grade 3 peripheral neuropathy, stop product

Unresectable, locally advanced or metastatic non–small-cell lung cancer previously treated with chemotherapy
Adult: **IV** 75 mg/m^2 over 1 hr, then cisplatin 75 mg/m^2 **IV** given over 30-60 min q3wk; reduce dose to 65 mg/m^2 in those with hematologic or nonhematologic toxicities

Androgen-independent metastatic prostate cancer
Adult: **IV** 75 mg/m^2 given over 1 hr q3wk, with 5 mg predniSONE PO bid continuously; give dexamethasone 8 mg PO at 12 hr, 3 hr, and 1 hr prior to docetaxel; if neutrophil count is <500 cells/mm^3 for more than 1 wk or other toxicities occur, reduce dose to 60 mg/m^2

Adjuvant postsurgery treatment of operable node-positive breast cancer
Adult: **IV** 75 mg/m^2 over 1 hr, given 1 hr after DOXOrubicin 50 mg/m^2, cyclophosphamide 500 mg/m^2 q3wk × 6 cycles

Squamous cell cancer of head/neck
Adult: **IV** 75 mg/m^2 over 1 hr, then cisplatin 75 mg/m^2 over 1 hr on day 1, then 5-FU 750 mg/m^2/day CONT INF × 5 days, repeat cycle q3wk

Available forms: Inj 20, 80 mg in single dose vials

Adverse effects
CNS: **Seizures**
CV: Hypotension, fluid retention, peripheral edema, flushing, MI, sinus tachycardia
GI: Nausea, vomiting, diarrhea, **hepatotoxicity,** stomatitis, colitis
HEMA: **Neutropenia, leukopenia, thrombocytopenia, anemia,** bleeding, infections, **myelosuppression**
INTEG: Alopecia, nail pain, rash, skin eruptions
MISC: Amenorrhea, fever of unknown origin, **secondary malignancy, Stevens-Johnson syndrome**
MS: Arthralgia, myalgia, back pain
NEURO: Peripheral neuropathy
RESP: Dyspnea, **pulmonary edema, fibrosis, embolism**
SYST: Hypersensitivity reactions, AML, **death**

Contraindications: Pregnancy **D,** breastfeeding, hypersensitivity to this product, severe hepatic disease, bilirubin exceeding upper normal limit, or severely elevated ALT, AST, alkaline phosphatase

Black Box Warning: Hypersensitivity to other products with polysorbate 80, neutropenia (neutrophils <1500/mm^3)

Precautions: Children, CV disease, pulmonary disorders, bone marrow depression, herpes zoster, pleural effusion

Black Box Warning: Edema, hepatic disease, lung cancer, taxane hypersensitivity

Pharmacokinetics	
Absorption	Completely absorbed
Distribution	Unknown
Metabolism	Liver, extensively
Excretion	Fecal
Half-life	11.1 hr

Pharmacodynamics	
Onset	Rapid
Peak	Unknown
Duration	Unknown

Interactions
Individual drugs
CycloSPORINE, erythromycin, ketoconazole, troleadomycin: altered metabolism of docetaxel
Drug classifications
Antineoplastics, radiation: increased myelosuppression
Live virus vaccines: decreased immune response

NURSING CONSIDERATIONS
Assessment
• Assess CNS changes: confusion, paresthesias, dysethenia, pain, weakness: if severe, product should be discontinued
• Check buccal cavity q8hr for dryness, sores or ulceration, white patches, oral pain, bleeding, dysphagia; obtain prescription for viscous lidocaine (Xylocaine) to use in mouth
• Assess symptoms indicating severe allergic reaction, anaphylaxis: rash, pruritus, urticaria, purpuric skin lesions, itching, flushing
• Monitor CBC, differential, platelet count weekly; withhold product if WBC is <1500/mm^3 or platelet count is <100,000/mm^3, notify prescriber of results
• Monitor renal function tests: BUN, creatinine, serum uric acid, urine CCr before, during therapy; check I&O ratio; report fall in urine output to <30 ml/hr
• Monitor temp q4hr (may indicate beginning of infection)
• Monitor liver function tests before, during therapy (bilirubin, AST, ALT, LDH) as needed

or monthly; check for jaundice of skin and sclera, dark urine, clay-colored stools, itchy skin, abdominal pain, fever, diarrhea
• Assess for bleeding: hematuria, stool guaiac, bruising or petechiae, mucosa or orifices q8hr; check for inflammation of mucosa, breaks in skin
• Assess effects of alopecia on body image; discuss feelings about body changes

Nursing diagnoses
• Body image, disturbed (adverse reactions)
• Infection, risk for (adverse reactions)
• Injury, risk for (adverse reactions)
• Knowledge, deficient (teaching)

Implementation
• Give top or systemic analgesics for pain to lessen effects of stomatitis
• Give liquid diet: carbonated beverages; gelatin may be added if patient is not nauseated or vomiting
IV route
• Use gloves and cytotoxic handling precautions
• Allow vials to warm to room temperature, withdraw all diluent and inject in vial of docetaxel, rotate gently to mix, allow to stand to decrease foaming, then withdraw the required amount (10 mg/ml) and inject in 250 ml of 0.9% NaCl or D_5W, mix gently, give over 1 hr
Y-site compatibilities: Acyclovir, amikacin, aminophylline, ampicillin/sulbactam, butorphanol, calcium gluconate, cefepime, cefotetan, ceftazidime, ceftriaxone, cimetidine, diphenhydrAMINE, droperidol, famotidine, fluconazole, furosemide, ganciclovir, gentamicin, granisetron, haloperidol, heparin, hydrocortisone, hydromorphone, lorazepam, magnesium sulfate, mannitol, meperidine, mesna, metoclopramide, morphine, ondansetron, potassium chloride, prochlorperazine, ranitidine, sodium bicarbonate, vancomycin, zidovudine

Patient/family education
• Inform patient that nonhormonal contraceptive measures are recommended during therapy and >4 mo after; teratogenic effects are possible
• Teach patient to avoid use of products containing aspirin or ibuprofen, razors, commercial mouthwash, since bleeding may occur; to report symptoms of bleeding (hematuria, tarry stools)
• Instruct patient to report signs of anemia (fatigue, headache, irritability, faintness, shortness of breath) and CNS reactions (con-

fusion, psychosis, nightmares, seizures, severe headaches)
• Inform patient that hair may be lost during treatment; a wig or hairpiece may make patient feel better; new hair may be different in color and texture
• Inform patient that receiving vaccinations during therapy may cause serious reactions
• Instruct patient to rinse mouth tid-qid with water, club soda; brush teeth bid-qid with soft brush or cotton-tipped applicators for stomatitis; use unwaxed dental floss

Evaluation
Positive therapeutic outcome
• Prevention of rapid division of malignant cells

---

docosanol topical
See Appendix B

---

docusate calcium (OTC)
(dok′yoo-sate)
DC Softgels, Dioctocal, Pro-Cal-Sof, Sulfalax, Surfak
docusate sodium (OTC)
Colace, Correctol Extra Gentle, Diocto, Docu, DOK, DOS, DSS, Dulcolax Stool Softener, Ex-Lax, Fleet Sof-Lax, Modane, Regulex ✦, Silace, Therevac SB
Func. class.: Laxative, emollient
Chem. class.: Anionic surfactant

Pregnancy category C

Action: Increases water, fat penetration in intestine; allows for easier passage of stool; increases electrolyte, water secretion in colon

Therapeutic outcome: Passage of softened stool, absence of constipation

Uses: To soften stools, prevent constipation, soften fecal impaction (rectal route)

Dosage and routes
Adult: PO 50-300 mg/day (docusate sodium) or 240 mg (docusate calcium or docusate potassium) prn Enema 4 ml (docusate sodium)
Child >12 yr: Enema 2 ml (docusate sodium)
Child 6-12 yr: PO 40-150 mg/day (docusate sodium) in divided doses
Child 3-6 yr: PO 20-60 mg/day (docusate sodium) in divided doses
Child <3 yr: PO 10-40 mg/day (docusate sodium) in divided doses

Available forms: Docusate calcium: caps 240 mg; docusate sodium: caps 50, 100, 250 mg; tabs 100 mg; syr 20 mg/5 ml, 50 mg/15 ml, 100 mg/30 ml, 150 mg/15 ml; oral sol 10, 50 mg/ml; enema 283 mg/3.9 g cap

Adverse effects
EENT: Bitter taste, throat irritation
GI: Nausea, anorexia, cramps, diarrhea
INTEG: Rash

Contraindications: Hypersensitivity, obstruction, fecal impaction, nausea/vomiting
Precautions: Pregnancy **C**, breastfeeding

Pharmacokinetics

Absorption	Minimal (PO)
Distribution	Unknown
Metabolism	Not metabolized
Excretion	Bile
Half-life	Unknown

Pharmacodynamics

	PO	RECT
Onset	24-72 hr	4-6 hr
Peak	Unknown	Unknown
Duration	Unknown	Unknown

Interactions
Individual drugs
Mineral oil: toxicity
Drug/herb
Flax, senna: increased laxative action

NURSING CONSIDERATIONS
Assessment
• Assess cramping, rectal bleeding, nausea, vomiting; if these symptoms occur, product should be discontinued; identify cause of constipation; identify whether fluids, bulk, or exercise is missing from lifestyle

Nursing diagnoses
• Constipation (uses)
• Diarrhea (side effects)
• Knowledge, deficient (teaching)
• Noncompliance (teaching)

Implementation
PO route
• Dilute oral sol in juice or other fluid to disguise taste
• Give tabs or caps with 8 oz of liquid; give on empty stomach for increased absorption, results

Patient/family education
• Discuss with patient that adequate fluid consumption is as necessary as bulk, exercise for adequate bowel function
• Teach patient that normal bowel movements do not always occur daily
• Advise patient not to use in presence of abdominal pain, nausea, vomiting; tell patient to notify prescriber if unrelieved constipation or if symptoms of electrolyte imbalance occur: muscle cramps, pain, weakness, dizziness, excessive thirst
• Advise patient that product may take up to 3 days to soften stools
• Instruct patient to take oral preparation with a full glass of water and increase fluid intake unless on fluid restrictions
• Caution patients with heart disease to avoid using the Valsalva maneuver to expedite evacuation

Evaluation
Positive therapeutic outcome
• Decreased constipation within 3 days

dofetilide
(doff-ee-till'-lide)
Tikosyn
Func. class.: Antidysrhythmic (Class III)
Pregnancy category C

Action: Blocks cardiac ion channel carrying the rapid component of delayed potassium current, no effect on sodium channels

Therapeutic outcome: Absence of atrial fibrillation

Uses: Atrial fibrillation, flutter, maintenance of normal sinus rhythm

Dosage and routes
Adult: PO 125-500 mcg bid depending on CCr; may be adjusted q2-3hr to get appropriate increase in QTc

Renal dose: PO initial dose for CCr >60 mg/ml 500 mcg bid; CCr 40-60 mg/min 250 mcg bid; CCr 20-39 mg/min 125 mcg bid; CCr <20 mg/min do not use

Available forms: Caps 125, 250, 500 mcg

Adverse effects
CNS: Syncope, dizziness, headache
CV: Hypotension, postural hypotension, bradycardia, angina, PVCs, substernal pressure, precipitation of angina, transient hypertension
GI: Nausea, vomiting, severe diarrhea, anorexia
RESP: Dyspnea, respiratory infections

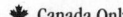

Contraindications: Hypersensitivity, digoxin toxicity, aortic stenosis, pulmonary hypertension, children, severe renal disease

Black Box Warning: QT prolongation, torsades de pointes

Precautions: Pregnancy **C**, breastfeeding, AV block, bradycardia, electrolyte imbalance

Black Box Warning: Renal disease, arrhythmias

Pharmacokinetics
Absorption	>90%
Distribution	Steady state 2-3 days
Metabolism	Not metabolized
Excretion	Kidneys 80%
Half-life	10 hr

Pharmacodynamics
Unknown

Interactions
Individual drugs
Amiloride, cimetidine, ketoconazole, megestrol, metformin, prochlorperazine, triamterene, trimethoprim/sulfamethoxazole, verapamil: do not use together
Drug classifications
Diuretics, potassium depletion: increased hypokalemia
Drug/herb
♦Aconite: toxicity, death
Aloe, broom, buckthorn (chronic use), cascara sagrada (chronic use), Chinese rhubarb, figwort, fumitory, goldenseal, kudzu, licorice: increased effect
Coltsfoot: decreased effect
Horehound: increased serotonin effect

NURSING CONSIDERATIONS
Assessment
• Monitor ECG continuously to determine product effectiveness; measure PR, QRS, QT intervals; check for PVCs, other dysrhythmias; monitor B/P continuously; this product is available only to facilities that have been educated in its administration; patient must be hospitalized
• Before administration, QTc must be determined using an average of 5-10 beats; if the QTc >440 msec or 500 msec in ventricular conduction abnormalities, do not use; do not use if heart rate <60 bpm
• Before dosing, identify CCr, using CCr to determine dosing

Nursing diagnoses
• Cardiac output, decreased (uses)
• Gas exchange, impaired (adverse reactions)
• Knowledge, deficient (teaching)

Implementation
• Give for 3 days with patient hospitalized
• Give dofetilide after withholding class I or III antidysrhythmic for 3 half-lives of dofetilide before starting dofetilide

Patient/family education
• Notify prescriber if fast heartbeats with fainting or dizziness occur
• Notify all prescribers of all medications and supplements taken
• Teach patient that if a dose is missed, do not double, take next dose at usual time

Evaluation
Positive therapeutic outcome
• Increased control in atrial fibrillation

dolasetron (Rx)
(do-la′se-tron)
Anzemet
Func. class.: Antiemetic
Chem. class.: 5-HT receptor antagonist
Pregnancy category B

Action: Prevents nausea, vomiting by blocking serotonin peripherally, centrally, and in the small intestine

Therapeutic outcome: Control of nausea, vomiting

Uses: Prevention of nausea, vomiting associated with cancer chemotherapy and prevention of postoperative nausea, vomiting

Unlabeled uses: Radiotherapy-induced nausea/vomiting

Dosage and routes
Prevention of nausea/vomiting associated with cancer chemotherapy
Adult and child 2-16 yr: **IV** 1.8 mg/kg as a single dose ½ hr before chemotherapy
Adult: PO 100 mg 1 hr before chemotherapy
Child 2-16 yr: PO 1.8 mg/kg 1 hr before chemotherapy, max 100 mg

Prevention of postoperative nausea/vomiting

Adult: IV 12.5 mg as a single dose 15 min before cessation of anesthesia; PO 100 mg 2 hr before surgery (prevention only)

Child 2-16 yr: IV 0.35 mg/kg as a single dose 15 min before cessation of anesthesia; PO 1.2 mg/kg within 2 hr before surgery (prevention only)

Available forms: Tabs 50, 100 mg; inj 20 mg/ml (12.5 mg/0.625 ml)

Adverse effects

CNS: Headache, dizziness, fatigue, drowsiness
CV: **Dysrhythmias,** ECG changes, hypo/hypertension, tachycardia, bradycardia
GI: Diarrhea, constipation, increased AST, ALT, abdominal pain, anorexia
GU: Urinary retention, oliguria
MISC: Rash, **bronchospasm**

Contraindications: Hypersensitivity

Precautions: Pregnancy **B**, breastfeeding, children, geriatric, hypokalemia, electrolyte imbalances, granisetron, ondansetron, palonosetron hypersensitivity, QT prolongation

Pharmacokinetics

Absorption	Completely absorbed
Distribution	Unknown
Metabolism	Liver, extensively
Excretion	Kidneys
Half-life	Unknown

Pharmacodynamics
Unknown

Interactions
Individual drugs
Cimetidine: increased dolasetron levels
Rifampin: decreased dolasetron levels
Drug classifications
Antidysrhythmics: increased dysrhythmias
Loop diuretics, thiazide: increased QT prolongation

NURSING CONSIDERATIONS
Assessment
• Assess for absence of nausea, vomiting during chemotherapy
• Assess for hypersensitivity reaction: rash, bronchospasm
• Assess for cardiac conditions; electrolyte imbalances or dysrhythmias

Nursing diagnoses
• Knowledge, deficient (teaching)
• Noncompliance (teaching)

Implementation
IV route
• Administer by inj 100 mg/30 sec or less or diluted in 50 ml of compatible sol; give over 15 sec
• Store at room temperature for 24 hr after dilution

Patient/family education
• Instruct patient to report diarrhea, constipation, rash, or changes in respirations; may cause headache; use analgesic
• Teach patient reason for medication and expected results

Evaluation
Positive therapeutic outcome
• Absence of nausea, vomiting during cancer chemotherapy

donepezil (Rx)
(don-ep-ee′zill)
Aricept, Aricept ODT
Func. class.: Anti-Alzheimer agent
Chem. class.: Reversible cholinesterase inhibitor

Pregnancy category C

Action: Elevates acetylcholine concentrations (cerebral cortex) by slowing degradation of acetylcholine released in cholinergic neurons; does not alter underlying dementia

Therapeutic outcome: Decreased symptoms of Alzheimer's disease

Uses: Treatment of mild to severe dementia in Alzheimer's disease

Unlabeled uses: Subcortical vascular dementia, dementia with Lewy bodies, Pick's disease

Dosage and routes
Adult: PO 5 mg/day at bedtime; may increase to 10 mg/day after 4-6 wk

Available forms: Tabs 5, 10 mg; oral sol 1 mg/ml; orally disintegrating tabs 5, 10 mg (Aricept ODT)

Adverse effects
CNS: Dizziness, insomnia, somnolence, headache, fatigue, abnormal dreams, syncope, **seizures,** drowsiness, agitation, depression
CV: **Atrial fibrillation,** hypo/hypertension, **sinus bradycardia, AV block**
GI: Nausea, vomiting, anorexia, *diarrhea,* abdominal pain, weight loss, **GI bleeding**
GU: Frequency, UTI, incontinence

 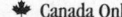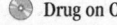

INTEG: Rash, flushing, diaphoresis, bruising
MS: Cramps, arthritis, arthralgia
RESP: Rhinitis, URI, cough, pharyngitis

Contraindications: Hypersensitivity to this product or piperidine derivatives

Precautions: Pregnancy **C,** breastfeeding, children, sick sinus syndrome, history of ulcers, GI bleeding, hepatic disease, bladder obstruction, asthma, seizures, COPD

Pharmacokinetics

Absorption	Well
Distribution	Unknown
Metabolism	Liver to metabolities
Excretion	Unknown
Half-life	10 hr (single dose)

Pharmacodynamics
Unknown

Interactions
Individual drugs
Carbamazepine, dexamethasone, phenobarbital, phenytoin, rifampin: decreased donepezil effect
Succinylcholine: synergistic effects
Drug classification
Anticholinergics: decreased activity
Cholinergic agonists, cholinesterase inhibitors: synergistic effects
NSAIDs: increased gastric acid secretions
CYP2D6, CYP3A4 inducers: decreased donepezil effects
CYP2D6, CYP3A4 inhibitors: increased donepezil effects
Drug/herb
St. John's wort: decreased donepezil effect

NURSING CONSIDERATIONS
Assessment
• Monitor B/P, heart rate: hypo/hypertension
• Assess mental status: affect, mood, behavioral changes, depression, complete suicide assessment
• Assess GI status: nausea, vomiting, anorexia, diarrhea
• Assess GU status: urinary frequency, incontinence

Nursing diagnoses
• Confusion, chronic (uses)
• Memory, impaired (uses)

Implementation
• Give between meals; may be given with meals for GI symptoms
• Administer dosage adjusted to response no more than q4-6wk

• Provide assistance with ambulation during beginning therapy; dizziness, ataxia may occur
• Oral sol: measure with calibrated oral syringe or other calibrated device
• Orally disintegrating tabs: allow to dissolve on tongue before swallowing

Patient/family education
• Advise patient to report side effects: twitching, nausea, vomiting, sweating, dizziness; indicates overdose
• Advise patient to use product exactly as prescribed
• Advise patient to notify prescriber of nausea, vomiting, diarrhea (dose increase or beginning treatment), or rash
• Advise patient not to increase or abruptly decrease dose, serious consequences may result
• Instruct patient that product is not a cure

Evaluation
Positive therapeutic outcome
• Decrease in confusion; improved mood

⚠ HIGH ALERT

*DOPamine (Rx)
(doe'pa-meen)
DOPamine HCl, Revimine ✦
Func. class.: Agonist, vasopressor, inotropic agent
Chem. class.: Catecholamine

Pregnancy category C

Do not confuse:
DOPamine/DOBUTamine

Action: Causes increased cardiac output; acts on β_1- and α-receptors, causing vasoconstriction in blood vessels; when low doses are administered, causes renal and mesenteric vasodilatation; β_1 stimulation produces inotropic effects with increased cardiac output

Therapeutic outcome: Increased B/P, cardiac output

Uses: Shock; to increase perfusion; hypotension, cardiogenic/septic shock

Dosage and routes
Shock
Adult: **IV** INF 1-20 mcg/kg/min, max 50 mcg/kg/min; titrate to patient's response
Child: **IV** 1-20 mcg/kg/min adjust depending on response

COPD
Adult: **IV** 4 mcg/kg/min

Adverse effects: *italic* = common, **bold** = life-threatening

CHF
Adult: IV 3-10 mcg/kg/min

RDS
Infant: IV 5 mcg/kg/min

Available forms: Inj 40, 80, 160 mg/ml; conc for **IV** inf 0.8, 1.6, 3.2 mg/ml in 250, 500 ml D₅W

Adverse effects
CNS: Headache, anxiety
CV: Palpitations, **tachycardia,** *hypertension,* **ectopic beats,** *angina,* **wide QRS complex,** peripheral vasoconstriction, hypotension
GI: Nausea, vomiting, diarrhea
INTEG: Necrosis, tissue sloughing with extravasation, **gangrene**
RESP: Dyspnea

Contraindications: Hypersensitivity, ventricular fibrillation, tachydysrhythmias, pheochromocytoma, hypovolemia

Precautions: Pregnancy **C,** breastfeeding, geriatric, arterial embolism, peripheral vascular disease, sulfite hypersensitivity, acute MI

Black Box Warning: Extravasation

Pharmacokinetics	
Absorption	Complete
Distribution	Widely
Metabolism	Liver
Excretion	Kidney, plasma
Half-life	2 min

Pharmacodynamics	
Onset	2-5 min
Peak	Unknown
Duration	<10 min

Interactions
Individual drugs
Phenytoin: bradycardia, hypotension
Drug classifications
α-Adrenergic blockers, β-adrenergic blockers: decreased action of DOPamine
Anesthetics (general): increased dysrhythmias
Antidepressants (tricyclic): increased pressor response
Ergots: severe hypertension
MAOIs: increased hypertension (severe), do not use within 2 wk; increased pressor effect; hypertensive crisis may result
Oxytocics: increased B/P
Drug/lab test
Increased: urinary catecholamine, serum glucose

NURSING CONSIDERATIONS
Assessment
• Monitor ECG for dysrhythmias, ischemia during treatment; some patients may not need continuous ECG monitoring; also monitor PCWP, CVP, CO₂, urinary output; notify prescriber if <30 ml/hr
• Assess for heart failure: bibasilar crackles, S₃ gallop, dyspnea, neck vein distention in patients with cardiomyopathy or CHF
• Assess for oxygenation or perfusion deficit: decreased B/P, chest pain, dizziness, loss of consciousness
• Monitor B/P and pulse q5min during inf; if B/P drops 30 mm Hg, stop inf and call prescriber
• Check for extravasation: change site q48hr

Nursing diagnoses
• Cardiac output, decreased (uses)
• Fluid volume, excess (uses)
• Knowledge, deficient (teaching)
• Tissue perfusion, ineffective (uses)

Implementation
Continuous infusion route
• Dilute 200-400 mg/250-500 ml of D₅W, 0.9% NaCl, D₅/LR, D₅/0.45% NaCl, D₅/0.9% NaCl, LR; do not use discolored sol; sol is stable for 24 hr; give 0.5-5 mcg/kg/min; may increase by 1-4 mcg/kg/min q15-30min until desired patient response; use infusion pump
Syringe compatibilities: Doxapram, heparin, ranitidine
Y-site compatibilities: Aldesleukin, amifostine, amiodarone, inamrinone, atracurium, aztreonam, cefmetazole, cefpirome, ciprofloxacin, cladribine, diltiazem, DOBUTamine, enalaprilat, epinephrine, esmolol, famotidine, fentanyl, fluconazole, foscarnet, granisetron, haloperidol, heparin, hydrocortisone, hydromorphone, labetalol, lidocaine, lorazepam, meperidine, methylPREDNISolone, metronidazole, midazolam, milrinone, morphine, niCARdipine, nitroglycerin, norepinephrine, ondansetron, pancuronium, piperacillin/tazobactam, potassium chloride, propofol, ranitidine, sargramostim, sodium nitroprusside, streptokinase, tacrolimus, theophylline, thiotepa, tolazoline, vecuronium, verapamil, vit B/C, warfarin, zidovudine
Additive compatibilities: Aminophylline, atracurium, bretylium, calcium chloride, cephalothin, chloramphenicol, DOBUTamine, enalaprilat, flumazenil, heparin, hydrocortisone, kanamycin, lidocaine, meropenem, methylPREDNISolone, nitroglycerin, oxacillin, potassium chloride, ranitidine, verapamil

Patient/family education
- Teach patient reason for medication, expected results, reason for all monitoring, and procedures
- Advise patient to report all side effects

Evaluation
Positive therapeutic outcome
- Increased cardiac output

Treatment of overdose: Discontinue product, support circulation; give a short-acting α-blocker

---

doripenem (Rx)
(dore-i-pen'em)
Doribax
Func. class.: Antiinfective—miscellaneous
Chem. class.: Carbapenem

Pregnancy category B

Action: Bactericidal, interferes with cell wall replication of susceptible organisms; osmotically unstable cell wall swells, bursts from osmotic pressure

Therapeutic outcome: Negative C&S; decreasing symptoms and signs of infection

Uses: Serious infections caused by *Acinetobacter baumannii, Bacteroides caccae, Bacteroides fragilis, Bacteroides thetaiotaomicron, Bacteroides uniformis, Bacteroides vulgatus, Escherichia coli, Klebsiella pneumoniae, Peptostreptococcus micros, Proteus mirabilis, Pseudomonas aeruginosa, Streptococcus contellatus, Streptococcus intermedius;* complicated urinary tract infections, pyelonephritis, complicated intraabdominal infections

Dosage and routes
Adult: **IV** 500 mg every 8 hr × 5-14 days; if improvement occurs after 3 days, switch to an appropriate oral product

Available forms: Powder for inj 500 mg

Adverse effects
CNS: **Seizures,** headache
GI: Diarrhea, nausea, vomiting, **pseudomembranous colitis, hepatitis**
HEMA: **Neutropenia, leukopenia**
INTEG: *Rash,* urticaria, phlebitis, erythema at inj site, **Stevens-Johnson syndrome, toxic epidermal necrolysis,** pruritus
SYST: **Anaphylaxis**

Contraindications: Hypersensitivity to carbapenems (meropenem, doripenem, imipenem), penicillin, β-lactam; viral infection

Precautions: Pregnancy **B,** breastfeeding, geriatric, renal disease, seizure disorder, pseudomembranous colitis

Pharmacokinetics
Absorption	Unknown
Distribution	To most body fluids/tissue
Metabolism	Unknown
Excretion	Mainly unchanged in urine, 70% recovered in 48 hr
Half-life	1 hr, extended in renal disease

Pharmacodynamics
Unknown

Interactions
Individual drugs
Probenecid: increased doripenem plasma levels
Divalproex sodium, valproic acid: decreased effects
Drug/herb
Acidophilus: do not use with antiinfectives; separate by several hours
Drug/lab test
Increased: AST, ALT, LDH, BUN, alkaline phosphatase, bilirubin, creatinine
False positive: direct Coombs' test

NURSING CONSIDERATIONS
Assessment
- Assess sensitivity to carbapenem antibiotics, penicillins
- Monitor renal disease: lower dose may be required
- Monitor bowel pattern daily; if severe diarrhea occurs, product should be discontinued; may indicate pseudomembranous colitis
- Monitor for infection: temp, sputum, characteristics of wound, before, during, and after treatment
- ◆ Monitor for allergic reactions, anaphylaxis: rash, urticaria, pruritus; may occur few days after therapy begins
- Monitor overgrowth of infection: perineal itching, fever, malaise, redness, pain, swelling, drainage, rash, diarrhea, change in cough, sputum

Nursing diagnoses
- Infection, risk for (uses)
- Knowledge, deficient (teaching)

Implementation
- Give after C&S is taken
- When giving 500-mg dose: constitute vial with 10 ml of sterile water for inj or NaCl 0.9%; gently shake; (50 mg/ml); sol must be

D

Adverse effects: *italic* = common, **bold** = life-threatening

further diluted using a 21-G needle; withdraw susp and add to 100-ml infusion bag of D_5W; gently shake until clear

• When giving 250-mg dose: constitute vial with 10 ml of sterile water for inj or NaCl 0.9%; gently shake; (50 mg/ml); sol must be further diluted using a 21-G needle; withdraw susp and add to 100-ml infusion bag of D_5W; gently shake; remove 55 ml of solution; discard; the remaining sol contains 250 mg doripenem (4.5 mg/ml)

Solution compatibilities: D_5W, 0.9% NaCl, sterile water for inj

Patient/family education

• Instruct patient to report severe diarrhea; may indicate pseudomembranous colitis
• Instruct patient to report sore throat, bruising, bleeding, joint pain; may indicate blood dyscrasias (rare)
• Instruct patient to report overgrowth of infection: black, furry tongue; vaginal itching; foul-smelling stools
• Advise patient to avoid breastfeeding; product is excreted in breast milk

Evaluation

Positive therapeutic outcome
• Negative C&S
• Absence of symptoms and signs of infection

Treatment of hypersensitivity:

Epinephrine, antihistamines; resuscitate if needed (anaphylaxis)

---

dorzolamide ophthalmic
See Appendix B

---

doxapram (Rx)
(dox'a-pram)
Dopram
Func. class.: Analeptic (respiratory/cerebral stimulant)

Pregnancy category B

Action: Respiratory stimulation through activation of peripheral carotid chemoreceptor in low dosages; with higher dosages medullary respiratory centers are stimulated, with progressive general CNS stimulation

Therapeutic outcome: Ease of breathing, ABGs at normal limits

Uses: COPD, postanesthesia CNS and respiratory depression, prevention of acute hypercapnia, product-induced CNS depression

Unlabeled uses: Treatment of apnea in premature infants when methylxanthines have failed

Dosage and routes
Postanesthesia stimulation
Adult: **IV** inj 0.5-1 mg/kg, max 1.5 mg/kg total as a single inj; **IV** INF 250 mg in 250 ml SOL, max 4 mg/kg; run at 1-3 mg/min

Drug-induced CNS depression
Adult: **IV** priming dose of 2 mg/kg, repeated in 5 min; repeat q1-2hr until patient awakens; **IV** INF priming dose 2 mg/kg at 1-3 mg/min, max 3 g/day

COPD (hypercapnia)
Adult: **IV** INF 1-2 mg/min, max 3 mg/min for no longer than 2 hr

Apnea of premature infant (unlabeled)
Infant: **IV** 1-1.5 mg/kg/hr loading dose followed by INF of 0.5-2.5 mg/kg/hr

Available forms: Inj **IV** 20 mg/ml

Adverse effects

CNS: **Seizures** (clonus/generalized), *headache,* restlessness, dizziness, confusion, paresthesias, flushing, sweating, bilateral Babinski's sign, rigidity, depression
CV: *Chest pain, hypertension, change in heart rate,* lowered T waves, tachycardia, dysrhythmias
EENT: Pupil dilation, sneezing
GI: Nausea, vomiting, diarrhea, desire to defecate
GU: Retention, incontinence, elevation of BUN, albuminuria
INTEG: Pruritus, irritation at inj site
RESP: **Laryngospasm, bronchospasm,** rebound hypoventilation, dyspnea, cough, tachypnea, hiccups

Contraindications: Hypersensitivity, seizure disorders, severe hypertension, severe bronchial asthma, severe dyspnea, severe cardiac disorders, flail chest, pneumothorax, pulmonary embolism, severe respiratory disease

Precautions: Pregnancy **B,** breastfeeding, children, bronchial asthma, pheochromocytoma, severe tachycardia, dysrhythmias, hypertension, hyperthyroidism

Pharmacokinetics

Absorption	Complete
Distribution	Unknown
Metabolism	Liver
Excretion	Kidneys, metabolites
Half-life	2.5-4 hr

Pharmacodynamics

Onset	20-40 sec
Peak	1-2 min
Duration	5-10 min

Interactions
Individual drugs
Cyclopropane, enflurane, halothane: increased dysrhythmias; delay use of doxapram for 10 min after inh anesthetics
Drug classifications
MAOIs, sympathomimetics: synergistic pressor effect

NURSING CONSIDERATIONS
Assessment
• Monitor B/P, heart rate, deep tendon reflexes, level of consciousness, ABGs before administration q30min; check for Po_2, Pco_2, O_2 saturation during treatment
• Monitor ECG; watch for hypertension, increased pulse, increased pulmonary artery pressures
• Monitor for hypertension: dysrhythmias, tachycardia, dyspnea, skeletal muscle hyperactivity; may indicate overdosage; discontinue if these occur
• Assess for respiratory stimulation: increased respiratory rate, depth, abnormal rhythm; check for patent airway; elevate head of bed to 45 degrees or higher, position patient on side
• Check for extravasation: redness, inflammation, pain; may cause phlebitis; change **IV** site q48hr

Nursing diagnoses
• Breathing pattern, ineffective (uses)
• Gas exchange, impaired (uses)
• Knowledge, deficient (teaching)

Implementation
• May give **IV** diluted with equal parts of sterile water for inj; may be diluted 250 mg/250 ml (1 mg/ml) of D_5W, $D_{10}W$ (dilute 400 mg/180 ml of compatible **IV** sol [2 mg/ml] and run as inf over 2 hr)
• Give **IV** undiluted over 5 min; **IV** inf at 1-3 mg/min; adjust for desired respiratory response, using infusion pump **IV**; if an inf is used after initial dose, start at 1-3 mg/min; adjust for desired respiratory response, using infusion pump **IV**; if an inf is used after initial dose, start at 1-3 mg/min depending on patient response; discontinue after 2 hr; wait 1-2 hr and repeat
• Give only after adequate airway is established; ensure O_2, **IV** barbiturates, resuscitative equipment available

• Discontinue inf if side effects occur; narrow margin of safety
Syringe compatibilities: Amikacin, bumetadine, chlorproMAZINE, cimetidine, cisplatin, cyclophosphamide, DOPamine, doxycycline, epinephrine, hydrOXYzine, imipramine, isoniazid, lincomycin, methotrexate, netilmicin, phytonadione, pyridoxine, terbutaline, thiamine, tobramycin, vinCRIStine
Syringe incompatibilities: Aminophylline, ascorbic acid, cefoperazone, cefotaxime, cefotetan, cefuroxime, dexamethasone, diazepam, digoxin, DOBUTamine, folic acid, furosemide, hydrocortisone, ketamine, methylPREDNISolone, minocycline, thiopental, ticarcillin

Patient/family education
• Teach all aspects of product, purpose, expected reactions
• Caution patient if difficulty breathing or shortness of breath occurs to notify nurse or prescriber

Evaluation
Positive therapeutic outcome
• Increased breathing capacity
• ABGs WNL for patient

---

doxazosin (Rx)
(dox-ay'zoe-sin)
Cardura, Cardura XL
Func. class.: Peripheral α adrenergic blocker, antihypertensive
Chem. class.: Quinazoline

Pregnancy category C

Do not confuse:
Cardura/Coumadin/Cardene/Ridaura

Action: Peripheral blood vessels are dilated, peripheral resistance lowered; reduction in B/P results from peripheral α-adrenergic receptors being blocked

Therapeutic outcome: Decreased B/P, decreased symptoms of benign prostatic hypertrophy (BPH)

Uses: Hypertension alone or as an adjunct, urinary outflow obstruction, symptoms of benign prostatic hyperplasia

Unlabeled uses: BPH with finesteride

Dosage and routes
BPH
Adult: PO 1 mg/day, increase in stepwise manner to 2, 4, 8 mg/day as needed at 1-2 wk intervals, max 8 mg

---

Adverse effects: *italic* = common, **bold** = life-threatening

Hypertension
Adult: PO 1 mg/day, increasing up to 16 mg daily if required; usual range 4-16 mg/day
Geriatric: PO 0.5 mg nightly, gradually increase

Available forms: Tabs 1, 2, 4, 8 mg; ext rel tabs 4, 8 mg

Adverse effects
CNS: *Dizziness,* headache, drowsiness, anxiety, depression, vertigo, weakness, fatigue, asthenia
CV: Palpitations, *orthostatic hypotension,* **tachycardia,** edema, **dysrhythmias,** chest pain
EENT: Epistaxis, tinnitus, dry mouth, red sclera, pharyngitis, rhinitis
GI: Nausea, vomiting, diarrhea, constipation, abdominal pain
GU: Incontinence, polyuria, priapism

Contraindications: Hypersensitivity to quinazolines

Precautions: Pregnancy **C**, breastfeeding, children, hepatic disease

Pharmacokinetics

Absorption	Well absorbed
Distribution	Not known; 98% plasma protein bound
Metabolism	Liver, extensively (<63%)
Excretion	Kidneys
Half-life	22 hr

Pharmacodynamics

Onset	2 hr
Peak	2-6 hr
Duration	6-12 hr

Interactions
Individual drugs
Alcohol, sildenafil, vardenafil: increased hypotensive effects
Clonidine: decreased antihypertensive effect
Drug classifications
Other antihypertensives, nitrates: increased hypotensive effects
Drug/herb
Angelica, hawthorn: increased doxazosin effect
Butcher's broom, capsicum peppers: decreased doxazosin effect
Yohimbe: increased toxicity

NURSING CONSIDERATIONS
Assessment
• Monitor B/P (lying, standing) and pulse, syncope; check for edema in feet, legs daily; I&O; monitor for weight daily; notify prescriber of changes
• Assess skin turgor, dryness of mucous membranes for hydration status
• Assess for orthostatic hypotension; tell patient to rise slowly from sitting or lying position; assess pulse, jugular venous distention q4hr, crackles, dyspnea, orthopnea with B/P

Nursing diagnoses
• Cardiac output, decreased (uses)
• Injury, risk for (side effects)
• Knowledge, deficient (teaching)
• Noncompliance (teaching)

Implementation
• Store in tight container at 86° F (30° C) or less
• May be used in combination with other antihypertensives
• May be given with food to prevent GI symptoms

Patient/family education
• Teach patient not to discontinue product abruptly; emphasize the importance of complying with dosage schedule, even if feeling better; if dose is missed take as soon as remembered; take at same time each day
• Instruct patient to take 1st dose at bedtime to decrease orthostatic B/P changes
• Teach patient not to use OTC products (cough, cold, allergy) unless directed by prescriber; also to avoid large amounts of caffeine
• Emphasize the need to rise slowly to sitting or standing position to minimize orthostatic hypotension
• Teach patient to notify prescriber of mouth sores, sore throat, fever, swelling of hands or feet, irregular heartbeat, chest pain
• Caution patient to report excessive perspiration, dehydration, vomiting, diarrhea; may lead to fall in B/P
• Caution patient that product may cause dizziness, fainting, light-headedness; may occur during 1st few days of therapy; to avoid hazardous activities
• Teach patient how to take B/P, and normal readings for age-group; to take B/P q7days

Evaluation
Positive therapeutic outcome
• Decreased B/P in hypertension
• Decreased symptoms of BPH

Treatment of overdose: Administer volume expanders or vasopressors; discontinue product; place in supine position

doxepin (Rx)

(dox'e-pin)

doxepin HCl, Novo-Doxepin ✦, Prudoxin Cream, Triadapin ✦, Zonolon Topical Cream

Func. class.: Antidepressant, tricyclic; antianxiety

Chem. class.: Dibenzoxepin, tertiary amine

Pregnancy category
B (Topical)
C (PO)

Action: Blocks reuptake of norepinephrine, serotonin into nerve endings, increasing action of norepinephrine, serotonin in nerve cells; has anticholinergic effects

Therapeutic outcome: Decreased symptoms of depression after 2-3 wk

Uses: Major depression, anxiety, topical: lichen simplex, atopic dermatitis, eczema

Unlabeled uses: Insomnia, migraine prophylaxis; topical: pruritus

Dosage and routes
Depression/anxiety

Adult: PO 25-75 mg/day, may increase to 300 mg/day for severely ill, give in divided doses if >150 mg/day

Geriatric: PO 10-25 mg at bedtime, increase qwk by 10-25 mg to desired dose, max 150 mg/day

Pruritus

Adult: PO 10 mg at bedtime, may increase to 25 mg at bedtime; TOP apply a thin film qid ≥3 hr apart

Available forms: Caps 10, 25, 50, 75, 100, 150 mg; oral conc 10 mg/ml; cream 5%

Adverse effects

CNS: Dizziness, drowsiness, confusion, headache, anxiety, tremors, stimulation, weakness, insomnia, nightmares, EPS (geriatric), increased psychiatric symptoms, paresthesia, **suicidal ideation**

CV: Orthostatic hypotension, ECG changes, **tachycardia,** *hypertension,* palpitations, **dysrhythmias**

EENT: Blurred vision, tinnitus, mydriasis, ophthalmoplegia, glossitis

GI: Diarrhea, dry mouth, nausea, vomiting, **paralytic ileus,** increased appetite, cramps, epigastric distress, jaundice, **hepatitis,** stomatitis, constipation

GU: Retention, **acute renal failure**

HEMA: **Agranulocytosis, thrombocytopenia, eosinophilia, leukopenia,** pancytopenia, purpuric disorder

INTEG: Rash, urticaria, sweating, pruritus, photosensitivity

Contraindications: Hypersensitivity to tricyclics, urinary retention, closed-angle glaucoma, prostatic hypertrophy

Precautions: Pregnancy **C** (PO), **B** (topical), breastfeeding, geriatric, seizures

Black Box Warning: Suicidal patients, children

Pharmacokinetics

Absorption	Well absorbed
Distribution	Widely distributed; crosses placenta
Metabolism	Liver, extensively
Excretion	Kidneys, breast milk
Half-life	8-24 hr

Pharmacodynamics
Unknown

Interactions
Individual drugs

Alcohol: increased CNS depression

Cimetidine, fluoxetine, fluvoxamine, paroxetine, sertraline: increased doxepin effect

Clonidine: increased hypertensive crisis; do not use together

Epinephrine, norepinephrine: increased hypertensive action

Drug classifications

Antiarrhythmics, 1C (propafenone, flecainide), quinolones: increased QT interval

Barbiturates, benzodiazepines, CNS depressants, sedative/hypnotics: increased CNS depression

MAOIs: hypertensive crisis, seizures, hyperpyretic crisis

SSRIs: increased toxicity

Drug/herb

Belladonna, corkwood, henbane, jimsonweed: increased anticholinergic effect

Evening primrose oil, hops, kava, lavender, scopolia: increased action of doxepin

SAM-e, St. John's wort: increased serotonin syndrome

Yohimbe: increased hypertension

Drug/lab test

Increased: serum bilirubin, blood glucose, alkaline phosphatase, LFTs

NURSING CONSIDERATIONS
Assessment
• Monitor B/P (with patient lying, standing), pulse q4hr; if systolic B/P drops 20 mm Hg, hold product, notify prescriber; take VS q4hr in patients with CV disease
• Monitor blood studies: CBC, leukocytes, differential, cardiac enzymes if patient is receiving long-term therapy
• Monitor liver function tests: AST, ALT, bilirubin
• Check weight weekly; appetite may increase with product
• Assess ECG for flattening of T wave, bundle branch block, AV block, dysrhythmias in cardiac patients; product should be discontinued gradually several days before surgery
• Assess for EPS primarily in geriatric: rigidity, dystonia, akathisia
• Assess mental status: mood, sensorium, affect, suicidal tendencies; increase in psychiatric symptoms: depression, panic
• Monitor urinary retention, constipation; constipation is more likely to occur in children or geriatric
• Assess for withdrawal symptoms: headache, nausea, vomiting, muscle pain, weakness; do not usually occur unless product was discontinued abruptly
• Identify alcohol consumption; if alcohol is consumed, hold dose until AM

Nursing diagnoses
• Coping, ineffective (uses)
• Injury, risk for (side effects)
• Knowledge, deficient (teaching)

Implementation
• Oral conc should be diluted with 120 ml of water, milk, or orange, grapefruit, tomato, prune, pineapple juice; do not mix with grape juice
• Give with food or milk for GI symptoms; do not give with carbonated beverages
• Give dosage at bedtime if oversedation occurs during day; may take entire dose at bedtime; geriatric may not tolerate once/day dosing
• Store at room temperature; do not freeze
• Provide safety measures, primarily for geriatric

Patient/family education
• Tell patient that therapeutic effects of decreased depression may take 2-3 wk, antianxiety effects sooner; to use caution in driving and other activities requiring alertness because of drowsiness, dizziness, blurred vision
• Advise patient to avoid rising quickly from sitting to standing, especially geriatric
• Teach patient to avoid alcohol ingestion, other CNS depressants: may potentiate effects; not to discontinue medication quickly after long-term use: may cause nausea, headache, malaise
• Teach patient to wear sunscreen or large hat, since photosensitivity occurs
• Teach patient that clinical worsening and suicidal ideation may occur
• Teach patient to increase fluids, bulk in diet if constipation occurs, especially geriatric; to take gum, hard sugarless candy, or frequent sips of water for dry mouth
• Teach patient to report urinary retention immediately

Evaluation
Positive therapeutic outcome
• Decrease in depression
• Absence of suicidal thoughts

Treatment of overdose: ECG monitoring, induce emesis, lavage, activated charcoal, administer anticonvulsant

---

doxercalciferol (Rx)
(dox-er-kal′-cif-er-ol)
Hectorol
Func. class.: Parathyroid agent (calcium regulator)
Chem. class.: Vitamin D hormone
Pregnancy category C

Action: Synthetic vit D analog, reduces parathyroid hormone

Therapeutic outcome: Calcium at normal level

Uses: To lower high parathyroid hormone levels in patients undergoing chronic kidney dialysis and those in stages 3 or 4 of chronic renal disease prior to dialysis

Dosage and routes
Adult: PO iPTH level >400 pg/ml 10 mcg 3 ×/wk at dialysis; dose titration iPTH level decreased by <50% and >300 pg/ml increase by 2.5 mcg at 8 wk intervals as necessary; iPTH level 150-300 pg/ml maintain; iPTH levels <100 pg/ml suspend for 1 wk, then resume at a dose that is at least 2.5 mcg lower
Adult: IV BOL initial iPTH level >400 pg/ml 4 mcg 3 ×/wk at the end of dialysis, or approximately every other day; dose titration iPTH level decreased by <50% and >300 pg/ml increase by 1-2 mcg at 8 wk intervals; iPTH

level 150-300 pg/ml maintain; iPTH level <100 pg/ml suspend for 1 wk, then resume at a dose that is at least 1 mcg lower

Available forms: Caps 2.5 mcg; inj 2 mcg/ml

Adverse effects
CNS: Drowsiness, headache, lethargy
GI: Nausea, diarrhea, vomiting, anorexia, dry mouth, constipation, cramps, metallic taste
GU: Polyuria, hypercalciuria, hyperphosphatemia, hematuria
MS: Myalgia, arthralgia, decreased bone development
RESP: Shortness of breath

Contraindications: Hypersensitivity, hyperphosphatemia, hypercalcemia, vit D toxicity

Precautions: Pregnancy **C**, breastfeeding, renal calculi, CV disease, hepatic disease

Pharmacokinetics

Absorption	Unknown
Distribution	Unknown
Metabolism	Liver
Excretion	Unknown
Half-life	32-37 hr, terminal

Pharmacodynamics

Peak	11-12 hr

Interactions
Individual drugs
Cholestyramine, magnesium antacids, mineral oil: decreased doxercalciferol levels, do not use together

NURSING CONSIDERATIONS
Assessment
• Assess GI symptoms, polyuria, flushing, head swelling, tingling, headache; may indicate hypercalcemia
• Identify nutritional status; check diet for sources of vit D (milk, some seafood), calcium (dairy products, dark green vegetables), phosphates
• Monitor BUN, creatinine, uric acid, chloride electrolytes, urine pH, urinary calcium, magnesium, phosphate, urinalysis (calcium should be kept at 9-10 mg/dl; vit D 50-135 international units/dl), alkaline phosphatase baseline and q3-6mo
◆ Assess for increased product level, since toxic reactions occur rapidly; have calcium chloride on hand if calcium level drops too low; check for tetany

Nursing diagnoses
• Injury, risk for (adverse reactions)
• Knowledge, deficient (teaching)
• Pain, chronic (uses)

Implementation
• Do not break, crush, or chew caps
• Give with meals for GI symptoms

Patient/family education
• Teach patient the symptoms of hypercalcemia and about foods rich in calcium
• Advise patient to avoid products with sodium: cured meats, dairy products, cold cuts, olives, beets, pickles, soups, meat tenderizers in chronic renal failure
• Advise patient to avoid products with potassium: oranges, bananas, dried fruit, peas, dark green leafy vegetables, milk, melons, beans in chronic renal failure
• Advise patient to avoid OTC products containing calcium, potassium, sodium, or antacids in chronic renal failure
• Instruct patient to avoid all preparations containing vit D
• Instruct patient to monitor weight weekly

Evaluation
Positive therapeutic outcome
• Calcium levels 9-10 mg/dl

/ HIGH ALERT

*DOXOrubicin (Rx)
(dox-oh-roo'bi-sin)
Adriamycin PFS, Adriamycin RDF, Rubex
*DOXOrubicin liposome (Rx)
Doxil
Func. class.: Antineoplastic, antibiotic
Chem. class.: Anthracycline glycoside

Pregnancy category D

Do not confuse:
DOXOrubicin/DAUNOrubicin/idarubicin/idamycin, Adriamycin/Aredia/Idamycin

Action: Inhibits DNA synthesis primarily; derived from *Streptomyces peucetius;* replication is decreased by binding to DNA, which causes strand splitting; active throughout entire cell cycle; a vesicant

Therapeutic outcome: Prevention of rapidly growing malignant cells

Uses: Wilms' tumor; bladder, breast, liver, lung, ovarian, stomach, testicular, thyroid cancer; Hodgkin's disease; acute lymphoblastic leukemia; myeloblastic leukemia; neuroblastomas; lymphomas; sarcomas; *Doxil:*

Adverse effects: *italic* = common, **bold** = life-threatening

AIDS-related Kaposi's sarcoma, metastatic ovarian carcinoma

Dosage and routes
DOXOrubicin
Adult: **IV** 60-75 mg/m² q3wk, or 30 mg/m² on days 1-3 of 4-wk cycle, max 550 mg/m² cumulative dose
Child: **IV** 30 mg/m²/day × 3 days, may repeat q4wk

Hepatic dose
Adult: **IV** bilirubin 1.2-3 mg/dl give 50% of dose, bilirubin 3.1-5 mg/dl give 25% of dose

DOXOrubicin liposome
Kaposi's sarcoma
Adult: **IV** 20 mg/m² q3wk

Ovarian cancer (DOXOrubicin liposomal)
Adult: **IV** 50 mg/m² (doxorubicin equivalent) given 1 mg/min if no adverse reactions, may increase to finish INF in 1 hr

Available forms: Inj 10, 20, 50, 100, 150 mg; liposomal dispersion for inj (Doxil) 20 mg/ml, 50 mg/30 ml

Adverse effects
CV: Increased B/P, **sinus tachycardia, PVCs,** chest pain, **bradycardia, extrasystole**
GI: Nausea, vomiting, anorexia, mucositis, **hepatotoxicity**
GU: Impotence, sterility, amenorrhea, gynecomastia, hyperuricemia
HEMA: **Thrombocytopenia, leukopenia, anemia**
INTEG: Rash, *necrosis at inj site,* dermatitis, reversible alopecia, cellulitis, thrombophlebitis at inj site

Contraindications: Pregnancy **D** (1st trimester), breastfeeding, hypersensitivity, systemic infections, cardiac disorders

Precautions: Renal/cardiac disease, gout

Black Box Warning: Hepatic disease, bone marrow suppression (severe), extravasation, heart failure, secondary malignancy

Pharmacokinetics
Absorption	Complete bioavailability
Distribution	Widely distributed; crosses placenta
Metabolism	Liver, extensively
Excretion	Bile (40%-50%)
Half-life	12 min; 3½ hr; 29⅔ hr

Pharmacodynamics
Unknown

Interactions
Individual drugs
Cyclophosphamide: increased cardiotoxicity, increased hemorrhagic cystitis risk
Mercaptopurine, radiation: increased toxicity, hypersensitivity
Radiation: increased toxicity
Drug classifications
Antineoplastics: increased toxicity, bone marrow suppression
Live virus vaccines: decreased antibody response
Drug/lab test
Increased: uric acid

NURSING CONSIDERATIONS
Assessment
• Monitor ECG; watch for ST-T wave changes, low QRS and T; possible dysrhythmias (sinus tachycardia, heart block, PVCs); signs of irreversible cardiomyopathy
• Assess buccal cavity q8hr for dryness, sores or ulceration, white patches, pain, bleeding, dysphagia; obtain prescription for viscous lidocaine (Xylocaine)
• Assess symptoms indicating severe allergic reaction: rash, pruritus, urticaria, purpuric skin lesions, itching, flushing; product should be discontinued
• Assess tachypnea, ECG changes, dyspnea, edema, fatigue
• Monitor CBC, differential, platelet count weekly; withhold product if WBC is <4000/mm³ or platelet count is <100,000/mm³; notify prescriber of results if WBC <20,000/mm³, platelets <150,000/mm³
• Assess for increased uric acid levels, swelling, joint pain, primarily extremities; patient should be well hydrated to prevent urate deposits
• Monitor renal function studies: BUN, creatinine, serum uric acid, urine CCr before, during therapy; I&O ratio; report fall in urine output to <30 ml/hr
• Monitor temp q4hr (may indicate beginning of infection)
• Monitor liver function tests before, during therapy (bilirubin, AST, ALT, LDH) as needed or monthly; note jaundice of skin or sclera, dark urine, clay-colored stools, itchy skin, abdominal pain, fever, diarrhea
• Assess for bleeding: hematuria, stool guaiac, bruising or petechiae, mucosa or orifices q8hr; inflammation of mucosa, breaks in skin
• Identify effects of alopecia on body image; discuss feelings about body changes

 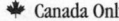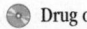

Nursing diagnoses
- Body image, disturbed (adverse reactions)
- Infection, risk for (adverse reactions)
- Injury, risk for (adverse reactions)
- Knowledge, deficient (teaching)

Implementation
- Avoid contact with skin; very irritating; wash completely to remove; give fluids **IV** or PO before chemotherapy to hydrate patient
- Give antiemetic 30-60 min before giving product to prevent vomiting and prn; give antibiotics for prophylaxis of infection
- Provide liquid diet: carbonated beverages; gelatin may be added if patient is not nauseated or vomiting
- Product should be prepared by experienced personnel using proper precautions
- Do not interchange DOXOrubicin with DOXOrubicin liposome
- Give **IV** after diluting 10 mg/5 ml of NaCl for inj; another 5 ml of diluent/10 mg is recommended; shake; give over 3-5 min; give through Y-tube or 3-way stopcock through free-flowing D₅ inf or 0.9% NaCl
- **IV** liposome inj (Doxil): dilute dose up to 90 mg/250 ml of D₅W, give over ½ hr; do not admix with other solution medications
- Use hydrocortisone, dexamethasone, or sodium bicarbonate (1 mEq/1 ml) for extravasation: apply ice compress
- Dose modifications for HFS: Toxicity Grade 1, redose unless patient has experienced previous grade 3 or 4; Grade 2, delay dosing up to 2 wk, or until resolved to grades 0 or 1; Grade 3 delay dosing up to 2 wk or until resolved to grades 0 or 1; resume dose at 25% decrease, return to original dosing after interval; Grade 4 delay dosing up to 2 wk or until grades 0 or 1; resume dose at 25% decrease, then return to original dose; if after 2 wk there is no resolution, discontinue

Syringe compatibilities: Bleomycin, cisplatin, cyclophosphamide, droperidol, fluorouracil, leucovorin, methotrexate, metoclopramide, mitomycin, vinCRIStine

Syringe incompatibilities: Furosemide, heparin

Y-site compatibilities: Amifostine, aztreonam, bleomycin, chlorproMAZINE, cimetidine, cisplatin, cladribine, cyclophosphamide, dexamethasone, diphenhydrAMINE, droperidol, famotidine, filgrastim, fludarabine, fluorouracil, granisetron, hydromorphone, leucovorin calcium, lorazepam, melphalan, methotrexate, methylPREDNISolone, metoclopramide, mitomycin, morphine, ondansetron, paclitaxel, prochlorperazine, promethazine,

propofol, ranitidine, sargramostim, sodium bicarbonate, teniposide, thiotepa, vinBLAStine, vinCRIStine, vinorelbine

Y-site incompatibilities: Furosemide, heparin

Additive compatibilities: Ondansetron

Additive incompatibilities: Aminophylline, cephalothin, dexamethasone, diazepam, fluorouracil, hydrocortisone

Patient/family education
- Help patient to rinse mouth tid-qid with water or club soda, brush teeth bid-qid with soft brush or cotton-tipped applicators for stomatitis, use unwaxed dental floss
- Advise patient to add 2-3 L of fluids unless contraindicated prior to and for 24-48 hr after, to decrease possible hemorrhagic cystitis
- Tell patient that urine and other body fluids may be red-orange for 48 hr; contraceptive measures are recommended during and 4 mo after therapy; product is teratogenic to fetus
- Advise patient to avoid use of products containing aspirin or ibuprofen, razors, commercial mouthwash, since bleeding may occur; to report symptoms of bleeding (hematuria, tarry stools)
- Instruct patient to report signs of anemia (fatigue, headache, irritability, faintness, shortness of breath)
- Inform patient that hair may be lost during treatment; a wig or hairpiece may make patient feel better; new hair may be different in color, texture
- Caution patient not to have any vaccinations without the advice of the prescriber; serious reactions can occur

Evaluation
Positive therapeutic outcome
- Prevention of rapid division of malignant cells

---

doxycycline (Rx)
(dox-i-sye′kleen)
Adoxa, Apo-Doxy ✢, Doryx, Doxy, Doxycaps, Doxycin ✢, doxycycline, Monodox, Novodoxyclin ✢, Periostat, Vibramycin, Vibra-Tabs
Func. class.: Antiinfective
Chem. class.: Tetracycline

Pregnancy category D

Do not confuse:
doxycycline/doxepin

Action: Inhibits protein synthesis, phosphorylation in microorganisms by binding to 30S

Adverse effects: *italic* = common, **bold** = life-threatening

ribosomal subunits, reversibly binding to 50S ribosomal subunits; bacteriostatic

Therapeutic outcome: Bactericidal action against the following: gram-positive pathogens *Bacillus anthracis, Clostridium perfringens, Clostridium tetani, Listeria monocytogenes, Nocardia, Propionibacterium acnes, Actinomyces israelii;* gram-negative pathogens *Haemophilus influenzae, Legionella pneumophila, Yersinia enterocolitica, Yersinia pestis, Neisseria gonorrhoeae, Neisseria meningitidis, Mycoplasma, Chlamydia*

Uses: Syphilis, gonorrhea, *Chlamydia, Rickettsia,* lymphogranuloma venereum, uncommon gram-negative or gram-positive organisms, malaria prophylaxis, acne, anthrax, chronic periodontitis, Lyme disease

Unlabeled uses: Traveler's diarrhea, prevention of chronic bronchitis

Dosage and routes
Most infections
Adult: PO/**IV** 100 mg q12hr on day 1, then 100 mg/day; **IV** 200 mg in 1-2 INF on day 1, then 100-200 mg/day
Child >8 yr (>45 kg): PO/**IV** 2.2-4.4 mg/kg/day in divided doses q12hr

Gonorrhea (uncomplicated) (patients allergic to penicillin)
Adult: PO 100 mg q12hr × 7 days, or 300 mg followed 1 hr later by another 300 mg

Malaria prophylaxis
Adult: 100 mg/day 1-2 days prior to travel, daily during travel, and 4 wk after return

Chlamydia trachomatis
Adult: PO 100 mg bid × 7days

Syphilis
Adult: PO 100 mg bid × 14 days

Anthrax
Adult and child >8 yr: **IV** 100 mg q12hr, change to PO when able × 60 days
Child ≤8 yr: PO 2.2 mg/kg q12h × 60 days; **IV** 100 mg q12hr, change to PO when able × 60 days

Lyme disease
Adult: PO 100 mg bid × 14-21 days

Periodontitis
Adult: 20 mg bid after sealing and root planing for ≤9 mo; give close to meal AM or PM

Available forms: Tabs 100 mg; caps 50, 100 mg; syr 50 mg/5 ml; powder for inj 100, 200 mg; powder for oral susp 25 mg/5 ml; mouth products: tabs 20 mg; inj 42.5 mg

Adverse effects
CNS: Fever
CV: Pericarditis
EENT: Dysphagia, glossitis, decreased calcification of deciduous teeth, oral candidiasis, tooth discoloration
GI: *Nausea, abdominal pain, vomiting, diarrhea,* anorexia, enterocolitis, **hepatotoxicity,** flatulence, abdominal cramps, gastric burning, stomatitis
GU: *Increased BUN*
HEMA: **Eosinophilia, neutropenia, thrombocytopenia, hemolytic anemia**
INTEG: Rash, urticaria, photosensitivity, increased pigmentation, **exfoliative dermatitis,** pruritus
SYST: **Stevens-Johnson syndrome, angioedema**

Contraindications: Pregnancy **D,** children <8 yr, esophageal ulceration, hypersensitivity to tetracyclines

Precautions: Hepatic disease, breastfeeding, pseudomembranous ulcerative colitis

Pharmacokinetics
Absorption	Well absorbed
Distribution	Widely distributed, crosses placenta
Metabolism	Some hepatic recycling
Excretion	Bile, feces; kidneys unchanged (20%-40%), enters breast milk
Half-life	14-17 hr; increased in severe renal disease

Pharmacodynamics
	PO	IV
Onset	1½-4 hr	Immediate
Peak	1½-4 hr	Infusion's end

Interactions
Individual drugs
Bismuth, carbamazepine, cimetidine, cholestyramine, colestipol, kaolin/pectin, NaHCO$_3$, phenytoin, rifampin, sucralfate: decreased effect of doxycycline
Digoxin: decreased effect of digoxin
Iron: forms chelates, decreased absorption
Penicillins: decreased effects of penicillins
Warfarin: increased effect of warfarin
Drug classifications
Alkali products, antacids, barbiturates: decreased effect of doxycycline
Anticoagulants (oral): increased effect of anticoagulants
Contraceptives (oral): decreased effect of oral contraceptive

 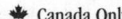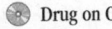

Drug/herb
Acidophilus: do not use with antiinfectives; separate by several hours
Bromelain: increased action
Drug/food
Decreased: absorption with dairy products
Drug/lab test
Increased: BUN, alkaline phosphatase, bilirubin, amylase, ALT, AST
False increase: urinary catecholamines, ALT, AST

NURSING CONSIDERATIONS
Assessment
• Assess patient for previous sensitivity reaction
• Assess patient for signs and symptoms of infection including characteristics of wounds, sputum, urine, stool, WBC >10,000/mm³, fever; obtain baseline information before, during treatment
• Obtain C&S before beginning product therapy to identify if correct treatment has been initiated
• Assess for allergic reactions: rash, urticaria, pruritus, chills, fever, joint pain; angioedema may occur a few days after therapy begins
• Assess bowel pattern daily; if severe diarrhea occurs, product should be discontinued
• Monitor for bleeding: ecchymosis, bleeding gums, hematuria, stool guaiac daily if on long-term therapy; blood dyscrasias may occur
• Assess for overgrowth of infection: perineal itching, fever, malaise, redness, pain, swelling, drainage, rash, diarrhea, change in cough, sputum

Nursing diagnoses
• Diarrhea (side effects)
• Infection, risk for (uses)
• Injury, risk for (side effects)
• Knowledge, deficient (teaching)
• Noncompliance (teaching)

Implementation
PO route
• Do not break, crush, or chew caps
• Give around the clock to maintain proper blood levels; give with food to increase absorption of product; do not give within 3 hr of other agents; product reactions may occur
• Give with 8 oz of water, 1 hr before bedtime to prevent ulceration
• Shake liquid preparation well before giving; use calibrated device for proper dosing
• Do not give with iron, calcium, magnesium products or antacids, which decrease absorption and form insoluble chelate

IV route
• Check for irritation, extravasation, phlebitis daily; change site q72hr
• For intermittent inf, dilute each 100 mg/10 ml of 0.9% NaCl, sterile water for inj; further dilute in at least 100 ml of 0.9% NaCl, D₅W, Ringer's, LR, D₅/LR; protect from direct light; keep at room temperature; give over 1-4 hr; IV sol stable for 12 hr at room temperature, 72 hr refrigerated, discard if precipitate forms
Syringe compatibilities: Doxapram
Y-site compatibilities: Acyclovir, amifostine, amiodarone, aztreonam, cyclophosphamide, diltiazem, filgrastim, fludarabine, granisetron, hydromorphone, magnesium sulfate, melphalan, meperidine, morphine, ondansetron, perphenazine, propofol, sargramostim, tacrolimus, teniposide, theophylline, thiotepa, vinorelbine
Y-site incompatibilities: Hetastarch
Additive compatibilities: Ranitidine

Patient/family education
• Teach patient to report sore throat, bruising, bleeding, joint pain; may indicate blood dyscrasias (rare)
• Advise patient to contact prescriber if vaginal itching, loose foul-smelling stools, furry tongue occur; may indicate superinfection; report itching, rash, pruritus, urticaria
• Instruct patient to take all medication prescribed for the length of time ordered; product must be taken around the clock to maintain blood levels; do not give medication to others
• Advise patient to notify prescriber of diarrhea with blood or pus

Evaluation
Positive therapeutic outcome
• Absence of signs/symptoms of infection (WBC <10,000/mm³, temp WNL, absence of red draining wounds)
• Reported improvement in symptoms of infection

⚠ HIGH ALERT

dronedarone (Rx)
(drone-da-rone)
Multaq
Func. class.: Antidysrhythmic (Class III)
Chem. class.: Iodinated benzofuran derivative

Pregnancy category X

Action: Prolongs action potential duration and effective refractory period, noncompetitive

Adverse effects: *italic* = common, **bold** = life-threatening

α- and β-adrenergic inhibition; increases PR and QT intervals, decreases sinus rate, decreases peripheral vascular resistance

Therapeutic outcome: Decreased amount and severity of ventricular dysrhythmias

Uses: Atrial fibrillation, atrial flutter

Dosage and routes
Adult: PO 400 mg bid; discontinue class I, III antidysrhythmias or strong CYP3A4 inhibitors prior to beginning treatment; max 800 mg/day

Available forms: Tabs 400 mg

Adverse effects
CV: Bradycardia, **Heart Failure, QT prolongation, torsades de pointes**
ENDO: Hypo/hyperthyroidism
GI: Nausea, vomiting, diarrhea, abdominal pain
INTEG: Rash, photosensitivity

Contraindications: Pregnancy **X,** breastfeeding, severe sinus node dysfunction, 2nd- or 3rd-degree AV block; bradycardia, hypersensitivity, heart failure, hepatic disease, QT prolongation

Precautions: Children, electrolyte imbalances, elderly, Asian patients, females

Pharmacokinetics

Absorption	Slow, variable (PO) up to 65%
Distribution	Body tissues; crosses placenta
Metabolism	Liver
Excretion	Bile, kidney (minimal)
Half-life	15-100 day

Pharmacodynamics

	PO
Onset	1-3 wk
Peak	Unknown
Duration	Up to months

Interactions
Individual drugs
CycloSPORINE, dextromethorphan, digoxin, disopyramide, flecainide, methotrexate, phenytoin, procainamide, quinidine, theophylline: increased blood levels, increased toxicity
Warfarin: increased bleeding

Drug classifications
β-Adrenergic blockers, calcium channel blockers: increased bradycardia

Drug/herb
Aconite: increased toxicity, death
Aloe, broom, buckthorn (chronic use), cascara sagrada (chronic use), Chinese rhubarb, figwort, fumitory, goldenseal, kudzu, licorice, senna: increased effect
Coltsfoot: decreased effect
Horehound: increased serotonin effect

Drug/food
Grapefruit juice: toxicity

Drug/lab test
Increased: T4

NURSING CONSIDERATIONS
Assessment
• Monitor I&O ratio; monitor electrolytes: potassium, creatinine, magnesium
• Monitor liver function studies: AST, ALT, bilirubin, alkaline phosphatase
• Monitor ECG to determine product effectiveness; measure PR, QRS, QT intervals; check for PVCs, other dysrhythmias; monitor B/P continuously for hypo/hypertension; check for rebound hypertension after 1-2 hr
• Monitor serum creatine, potassium, magnesium
• Monitor for dehydration or hypovolemia
• Assess for hypothyroidism: lethargy, dizziness, constipation, enlarged thyroid gland, edema of extremities, cool, pale skin
• Monitor hyperthyroidism: restlessness, tachycardia, eyelid puffiness, weight loss, frequent urination, menstrual irregularities, dyspnea, warm, moist skin
• Monitor cardiac rate, respiration: rate, rhythm, character, chest pain, ventricular tachycardia, supraventricular tachycardia or fibrillation
• Assess sight and vision before treatment and throughout therapy; microdeposits on the cornea may cause blurred vision, halos, and photophobia

Nursing diagnoses
• Cardiac output, decreased (uses)
• Gas exchange, impaired (adverse reactions)
• Knowledge, deficient (teaching)

Implementation
• Start with patient hospitalized and monitored
PO route
• Give reduced dosage slowly with ECG monitoring only
• Give loading dose with food to decrease nausea
Intermittent IV infusion route
• Give 1000 mg/24 hr during loading/maintenance

- Initial loading: add 3 ml (150 mg) 100 ml D₅W (1.5 mg/ml); give over 10 min
- Loading inf: add 18 ml (900 mg) 500 ml D₅W (1.8 mg/ml); give over 6 hr
- Maintenance inf: Give remainder of loading inf 540 mg over 18 hr (0.5 mg/min)

Continuous infusion route
- After 24 hr, give 1-6 mg/ml at 0.5 mg/ml, max 30 mg/min

Y-site compatibilities: Amikacin, bretylium, clindamycin, DOBUTamine, DOPamine, doxycycline, erythromycin, esmolol, gentamicin, insulin (regular), isoproterenol, labetalol, lidocaine, metaraminol, metronidazole, midazolam, morphine, nitroglycerin, norepinephrine, penicillin G potassium, phentolamine, phenylephrine, potassium chloride, procainamide, tobramycin, vancomycin

Additive compatibilities: DOBUTamine, lidocaine, potassium chloride, procainamide, verapamil

Solution compatibilities: D₅W, 0.9% NaCl

Patient/family education
- Instruct patient to report side effects immediately to prescriber
- Instruct patient that skin discoloration is usually reversible, but skin may turn bluish on neck, face, arms when used for long periods
- Advise patient that dark glasses may be needed for photophobia
- Instruct patient to use sunscreen and protective clothing to prevent burning associated with photosensitivity
- Instruct patient to take medication as prescribed, not to double doses
- Instruct patient to complete follow-up appointment with health care provider, including pulmonary function studies, chest x-ray

Evaluation
Positive therapeutic outcome
- Decreased dysrhythmias

Treatment of overdose: Administer O₂, artificial ventilation, ECG, DOPamine for circulatory depression, diazepam or thiopental for seizures, isoproterenol

---

❗HIGH ALERT

droperidol (Rx)
(droe-per′i-dole)
droperidol, Inapsine
Func. class.: Neuroleptic, tranquilizer, antiemetic
Chem. class.: Butyrophenone derivative

Pregnancy category C

D

Action: Acts on CNS at subcortical levels, producing tranquilization, sleep; antiemetic; mild α-blockade

Therapeutic outcome: Maintenance of anesthesia

Uses: Premedication for surgery; induction, maintenance in general anesthesia; postoperatively for nausea and vomiting

Dosage and routes
Induction, adjunct
Adult: **IV**/IM 1.25-2.5 mg, may give additional 1.25 mg
Child 2-12 yr: **IV** 0.05-0.1 mg/kg titrate to response

Premedication
Adult: IM 2.5 mg ½-1 hr before surgery, may give 1.25-2.5 mg additionally
Child 2-12 yr: IM 0.05-0.1 mg/kg

Available forms: Inj 2.5 mg/ml

Adverse effects
CNS: EPS: Dystonia, akathisia, flexion of arms, fine tremors; *dizziness, anxiety, drowsiness, restlessness,* hallucinations, depression, **seizures, neuroleptic malignant syndrome**
CV: **Tachycardia,** *hypotension,* **prolonged QT prolongation, torsades de pointes**
EENT: Upward rotation of eyes, oculogyric crisis
INTEG: Chills, *facial sweating, shivering*
RESP: **Laryngospasm, bronchospasm**

Contraindications: Hypersensitivity, breastfeeding, child <2 yr

Precautions: Pregnancy **C**, geriatric, CV disease (hypotension, bradydysrhythmias), renal/hepatic disease, Parkinson's disease, pheochromocytoma, CHF, hypokalemia, hypomagnesemia, cardiac hypertrophy

Black Box Warning: QT prolongation, torsades de pointes

Pharmacokinetics

Absorption	Well absorbed (IM)
Distribution	Crosses blood-brain barrier, placenta
Metabolism	Liver
Excretion	Kidneys, unchanged (10%)
Half-life	2-3 hr

Pharmacodynamics

	IM/IV
Onset	3-10 min
Peak	30 min
Duration	3-6 hr

Interactions
Individual drugs
Alcohol: increased CNS depression
Lithium: increased side effects of lithium
Drug classifications
Antihistamines, antipsychotics, barbiturates, CNS depressants, opiates: increased CNS depression
Antihypertensives, nitrates: increased hypotension
Class IA/III antiarrhythmics, some phenothiazines, some quinolones, tricyclics, others: QT prolongation
Drug/herb
Kava: increased action

NURSING CONSIDERATIONS
Assessment
◆ Check VS q10min during **IV** administration, q30min after IM dose; for increasing heart rate or decreasing B/P, notify prescriber at once; do not place patient in Trendelenburg's position, sympathetic blockade may occur, causing respiratory arrest
• Assess extrapyramidal reactions: dystonia, akathisia, extended neck, restlessness, tremors; if these occur, an anticholinergic should be given
• If given for nausea or vomiting, monitor for significant loss of fluids, bowel sounds before, during administration
• ECG prior to and 2-3 hr after administration for serious arrhythmias

Nursing diagnoses
• Injury, risk for (adverse reactions)
• Knowledge, deficient (teaching)

Implementation
• Protect from light
IM route
• Give deeply in large muscle mass

IV route
• Give direct **IV** undiluted; give through Y-tube or 3-way stopcock at 10 mg or less/min; titrate to patient response
• Intermittent inf may be given by adding dose to 250 ml of LR, D₅W, 0.9% NaCl; give slowly, titrate to patient response
• Give anticholinergics (benztropine, diphenhydrAMINE) for extrapyramidal reaction
• Give only with resuscitative equipment nearby
Syringe compatibilities: Atropine, bleomycin, butorphanol, chlorproMAZINE, cimetidine, cisplatin, cyclophosphamide, dimenhyDRINATE, diphenhydrAMINE, DOXOrubicin, fentanyl, glycopyrrolate, hydrOXYzine, meperidine, metoclopramide, midazolam, mitomycin, morphine, nalbuphine, pentazocine, perphenazine, prochlorperazine, promazine, promethazine, scopolamine, vinBLAStine, vinCRIStine
Syringe incompatibilities: Fluorouracil, furosemide, heparin, leucovorin, methotrexate, pentobarbital
Y-site compatibilities: Amifostine, aztrenonam, bleomycin, cisatracurium, cisplatin, cladribine, cyclophosphamide, cytarabine, DOXOrubicin, DOXOrubicin liposome, famotidine, filgrastim, fluconazole, fludarabine, granisetron, hydrocortisone sodium succinate, idarubicin, melphalen, meperidine, metoclopramide, mitomycin, ondansetron, paclitaxel, potassium chloride, propofol, remifentanil, sargramostim, teniposide, thiotepa, vinBLAStine, vinCRIStine, vinorelbine, vit B/C
Y-site incompatibilities: Fluorouracil, foscarnet, furosemide, leucovorin, methotrexate, nafcillin
Additive incompatibilities: Barbiturates

Patient/family education
• Advise patient that orthostatic hypotension is common; to rise from lying or sitting position slowly; to avoid ambulation without assistance
• Caution patient that drowsiness may occur; to call for assistance for ambulation

Evaluation
Positive therapeutic outcome
• Decreased anxiety
• Absence of vomiting during and after surgery

 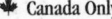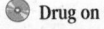

drotrecogin alfa (Rx)

(droh'treh-koh-jin al'fah)

Xigris

Func. class.: Thrombolytic agent

Chem. class.: Recombinant human activated protein C

Pregnancy category C

Action: Activated protein C exerts an anti-thrombotic effect by inhibiting factor Va/VIIIa

Therapeutic outcome: Reduction of mortality in adult patients with severe sepsis who have a high risk of death

Uses: Severe sepsis (sepsis associated with acute organ dysfunction)

Dosage and routes

Adult: **IV** INF 24 mcg/kg/hr × 96 hr; based on actual body weight

Available forms: Powder for inj, lyophilized, 5 mg, 20 mg

Adverse effects

HEMA: Decreased Hct, **bleeding**

SYST: GI, GU, **intracranial, intraabdominal, intrathoracic, retroperitoneal bleeding; surface bleeding**

Contraindications: Hypersensitivity, internal active bleeding, intraspinal surgery, CNS neoplasms, ulcerative colitis, enteritis, hepatic disease, hypocoagulation, within 3 mo of hemorrhagic stroke, epidural catheter in place, cerebral embolism/thrombosis/hemorrhage, within 2 mo of major surgery, trauma

Precautions: Pregnancy **C**, breastfeeding, children, within 6 wk of GI bleeding, prothrombin time INR >3, use >96 hr, hepatic disease, within 3 mo of ischemic stroke

Pharmacokinetics

Absorption	Rapid
Distribution	Plasma
Metabolism	Unknown
Excretion	Unknown
Half-life	Unknown

Pharmacodynamics

Onset	Within 2 hr of beginning infusion
Peak	96 hr
Duration	2 hr postinfusion

Interactions

Individual drugs

Asprin, cilostazol, clopidogrel, dipyridamole, indomethacin, phenylbutazone, ticlopidine: increased bleeding risk

Drug classifications

Anticoagulants, glycoprotein IIb/IIIa inhibitors, thrombolytics, other NSAIDs: increased bleeding risk

D

NURSING CONSIDERATIONS

Assessment

🔴 Assess for bleeding during treatment; hematuria, hematemesis, bleeding from mucous membranes, epistaxis, ecchymosis; may require transfusion (rare), continue to assess for bleeding

- Assess blood studies (Hct, platelets, PTT, pro-time, TT, APTT) before starting therapy; pro-time or APTT must be less than 2 × control before starting therapy; PTT or pro-time q3-4hr during treatment
- Assess VS, B/P, pulse, respirations, neurologic signs, temp at least q4hr; temp >104° F (40° C) indicates internal bleeding; systolic pressure increase >25 mm Hg should be reported to prescriber

🔴 Assess for neurologic changes that may indicate intracranial bleeding

🔴 Assess for retroperitoneal bleeding: back pain, leg weakness, diminished pulses

Nursing diagnoses

- Knowledge, deficient (teaching)

Implementation

- Store in refrigerator at 2°-8° C (36°-46° F); do not freeze
- Protect unreconstituted vials from light; keep in carton until time of use

IV route

- Reconstitute 5 mg vial/2.5 ml; 20 mg vial/10 ml sterile water for inj to a concentration of 2 mg/ml; slowly add sterile water for inj; do not shake or invert; gently swirl until dissolved
- Further dilute with 0.9% NaCl, slowly withdraw prescribed amount and add to bag of 0.9% NaCl, direct stream to side of bag, gently invert bag; do not transport infusion bag between locations using mechanical delivery systems
- Use immediately after reconstituting; may be held for only 3 hr at controlled room temperature 59°-86° F, must complete inf within 12 hr after preparation
- Do not use if discolored or if particulate is present
- If using an infusion pump, usual concentration is 100-200 mcg/ml; if using a syringe

pump, usual concentration is 100-1000 mcg/ml

- Use a dedicated **IV** line, or dedicated lumen of central venous catheter, may use only 0.9% NaCl, LR, dextrose, or dextrose/saline mixtures through same line
- Do not expose to heat or direct sunlight
- Discontinue 2 hr prior to invasive surgery or procedures introducing risk of bleeding

Evaluation
Positive therapeutic outcome
- Decreasing symptoms of sepsis, lack of mortality

---

duloxetine (Rx)
(du-lox'uh-teen)
Cymbalta
Func. class.: Antidepressant—miscellaneous
Chem. class: Serotonin, norepinephrine reuptake inhibitor (SNRI)

Pregnancy category C

Action: Unknown, may potentiate serotonergic, noradrenergic activity in the CNS. In studies duloxetine is a potent inhibitor of neuronal serotonin and norepinephrine reuptake

Therapeutic outcome: Decreased depression, decreased neuropathic pain

Uses: Major depressive disorder (MDD), neuropathic pain associated with diabetic neuropathy, generalized anxiety disorder, fibromyalgia

Dosage and routes
Depression
Adult: PO 40-60 mg/day as a single dose or 2 divided doses

Diabetic neuropathy
Adult: PO 60 mg qday

Generalized anxiety disorder
Adult: PO 60 mg/day, may start with 30 mg/day × 1 wk, then increase to 60 mg/day

Fibromyalgia
Adult: PO 30 mg/day × 1 wk, then 60 mg/day

Renal dose
Adult: PO Start with 20 mg, gradually increase; avoid use in severe renal disease

Available forms: Caps 20, 30, 60 mg

Adverse effects
CNS: Insomnia, anxiety, dizziness, tremor, somnolence, fatigue, decreased appetite, decreased weight, agitation, diaphoresis, hallucinations, **neuroleptic malignant syndrome–like reaction,** aggression, **seizures**
CV: **Thrombophlebitis,** peripheral edema, palpitations, hypertension, **supraventricular dysrhythmia**
EENT: Abnormal vision
ENDO: Hypoglycemia
GI: Constipation, diarrhea, dysphagia, *nausea,* vomiting, anorexia, dry mouth, colitis, gastritis, abdominal pain, **hepatic failure**
GU: Abnormal ejaculation, urinary hesitation, ejaculation delayed, erectile dysfunction, urinary frequency/retention, gyn bleeding
INTEG: Photosensitivity, bruising, sweating, **Stevens-Johnson syndrome**
MS: Gait disturbances, muscle spasm, restless leg syndrome
SYST: **Anaphylaxis, angioedema**

Contraindications: Hypersensitivity, closed-angle glaucoma, alcohol intoxication, alcoholism, hepatic disease, hepatitis, jaundice

Precautions: Pregnancy C, breastfeeding, geriatric, mania, hypertension, cardiac/renal/hepatic disease, seizures, hepatotoxicity, increased intraocular pressure, anorexia nervosa, bleeding, dehydration, diabetes, hyponatremia, hypotension, hypovolemia, orthostatic hypotension, abrupt drug withdrawal

Black Box Warning: Children, suicidal ideation

Pharmacokinetics
Absorption	Well absorbed
Distribution	90% protein binding
Metabolism	Extensively metabolized (CYP2D6, CYP1A2) in the liver to an active metabolite
Excretion	70% of product recovered in urine, 20% in feces
Half-life	12 hr

Pharmacodynamics
Unknown

Interactions
Individual drugs
Alcohol: increased ALT, bilirubin
Drug classifications
◆ MAOIs: coadministration (or within 14 days of MAOIs use) is contraindicated: hyperthermia, rigidity, rapid fluctuations of VS, mental status changes, neuroleptic malignant syndrome

---

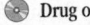

Opioids, antihistamines, sedative/hypnotics: increased CNS depression

CYP1A2 inhibitors (fluvoxamine, quinolone antiinfectives); CYP2D6 inhibitors (fluoxetine, quinidine, paroxetine): increased action of duloxetine

CYP2D6 extensively metabolized products (flecainide, phenothiazines, propafenone, tricyclics, thioridazine): narrow therapeutic index

SSRIs: increased serotonin syndrome

Drug/herb

Chamomile, hops, kava, lavender, skullcap, valerian: increased CNS depression

Corkwood, jimsonweed: increased anticholinergic effect

SAM-e, St. John's wort: serotonin syndrome

Yohimbe: increased hypertension

NURSING CONSIDERATIONS
Assessment
• Assess B/P lying, standing; pulse q4hr; if systolic B/P drops 20 mm Hg, hold product, notify prescriber; take VS q4hr in patients with CV disease

• Monitor hepatic studies: AST, ALT, bilirubin

• Monitor weight qwk; weight loss or gain; appetite may increase; peripheral edema may occur

• Offer sugarless gum, hard candy, frequent sips of water for dry mouth

• Assess mental status: mood, sensorium, affect, suicidal tendencies, increase in psychiatric symptoms; depression, panic

• Assess for withdrawal symptoms: headache, nausea, vomiting, muscle pain, weakness; not usual unless product is discontinued abruptly

◆ Assess for neuroleptic malignant syndrome–like reaction

Nursing diagnoses
• Injury, risk for (uses)
• Knowledge, deficient (teaching)
• Noncompliance (teaching)

Implementation
• Swallow caps whole; do not break, crush, or chew; do not sprinkle on food or mix with liquid

• Give without regard to food

• Store in tight container at room temperature; do not freeze

• Provide assistance with ambulation during beginning therapy, since drowsiness, dizziness occur

• Check to see if PO medication was swallowed

Patient/family education
• Advise that product is dispensed in small amounts because of suicide potential, especially in the beginning of therapy

• Teach patient/family to use caution when driving or other activities requiring alertness because of drowsiness, dizziness, blurred vision

• Advise patient to avoid alcohol ingestion, MAOIs, other CNS depressants

• Advise patient not to discontinue medication quickly after long-term use; may cause nausea, headache, malaise

• Advise patient to wear sunscreen or large hat, since photosensitivity may occur

• Advise patient to notify prescriber if pregnancy is planned or suspected, or if breastfeeding

• Tell patient that improvement may occur in 4-8 wk

• Advise that clinical worsening and suicide risk may occur

Evaluation
Positive therapeutic outcome
• Decreased depression

dutasteride (Rx)
(doo-tass′ter-ide)
Avodart
Func. class.: Sex hormone, 5α-reductase inhibitor
Chem. class.: Synthetic 4-azasteroid compound

Pregnancy category X

Action: Inhibits both types 1 and 2 forms of a steroid enzyme that converts testosterone to 5 µ-dihydrotestosterone (DHT), which is responsible for the initial growth of prostatic tissue

Therapeutic outcome: Decreased symptoms of benign prostatic hyperplasia (BPH)

Uses: Treatment of symptomatic BPH in men with an enlarged prostate gland, or may be used in combination with tamsulosis

Unlabeled uses: Alopecia

Dosage and routes
Adult: PO 0.5 mg/day

Alopecia (unlabeled)
Adult: PO 0.5-2.5 mg/day

Available forms: Caps 0.5 mg

Adverse effects: *italic* = common, **bold** = life-threatening

Adverse effects
GU: Decreased libido, impotence, gynecomastia, ejaculation disorders (rare), mastalgia, teratogenesis
INTEG: **Serious skin infections**

Contraindications: Pregnancy **X**, breastfeeding, children, women, hypersensitivity

Precautions: Hepatic disease

Pharmacokinetics	
Absorption	Absolute bioavailability ~60%
Distribution	Protein binding 99%
Metabolism	Liver (CYP3A4)
Excretion	Feces
Half-life	5 wk at steady state

Pharmacodynamics	
Onset	Rapid
Peak	2-3 hr
Duration	Levels detectable 4-6 mo posttreatment

Interactions
Individual drugs
Cimetidine, ciprofloxacin, diltiazem, ketoconazole, ritonavir, verapamil: increased dutasteride concentrations
Drug classifications
Antiretroviral protease inhibitors or other CYP3A4-metabolized products: increased dutasteride concentrations
Drug/lab test
Increased: TSH
Decreased: PSA

NURSING CONSIDERATIONS
Assessment
• Assess for decreasing symptoms in BPH: decreasing urinary retention, frequency, urgency, nocturia
• Assess PSA levels, digital rectal exam, urinary obstruction; determine the absence of urinary cancer before starting treatment
• Assess liver function tests: ALT, AST, bilirubin; blood studies: CBC with differential, serum creatitine, serum electrolytes

Nursing diagnoses
• Body image, disturbed (adverse reactions)
• Knowledge, deficient (teaching)

Implementation
• Swallow caps whole: do not break, crush, chew, or open
• May be given without regard to meals

Patient/family education
• Advise patient to notify prescriber if therapeutic response decreases, if edema occurs

• Caution patient not to discontinue product abruptly
• Inform patient about changes in sex characteristics
• Caution patient not to donate blood for at least 6 mo after last dose to prevent possible blood administration to pregnant female
• Advise patient and family that caps should not be handled by pregnant women since this product can be absorbed through the skin
• Inform patient that ejaculate volume may decrease during treatment, that product rarely interferes with sexual function
• Advise patient to read patient information leaflet before starting therapy and reread it upon prescription renewal

Evaluation
Positive therapeutic outcome
• Decreased levels of DHT (5 α-dihydrotestosterone)
• Decreased urinary frequency
• Decreased urinary retention
• Decreased urinary urgency
• Decreased nocturia

---

dyphylline (Rx)
(dye'fi-lin)
Dylix, dyphylline, Lufyllin, Neothylline
Func. class.: Bronchodilator, phosphodiesterase inhibitor
Chem. class.: Xanthine, theophylline derivative

Pregnancy category C

Action: Relaxes smooth muscle of respiratory system by blocking phosphodiesterase, which increases cyclic AMP; cyclic AMP results in positive inotropic, chronotropic effects, bronchodilatation, stimulation of CNS

Therapeutic outcome: Bronchodilatation with ease of breathing

Uses: Bronchial asthma, bronchospasm in chronic bronchitis and emphysema, COPD

Dosage and routes
Adult and child >6 yr: PO up to 15 mg/kg/dose, max 60 mg/kg/day
Renal dose
Adult: PO CCr 50-80 ml/min 75% of original dose; CCr 10-50 mg/ml 50% of original dose; CCr <10 ml/min 25% of original dose

Available forms: Tabs 200, 400 mg; elix 33.3, 53.3 mg/5 ml

Adverse effects
CNS: Anxiety, restlessness, insomnia, dizziness, **seizures,** headache, light-headedness, muscle twitching
CV: Palpitations, sinus tachycardia, hypotension, flushing, **dysrhythmias, circulatory failure**
GI: Nausea, diarrhea, *vomiting, anorexia,* dyspepsia, epigastric pain, rectal irritation, bleeding, reflux
INTEG: Flushing, urticaria
OTHER: Fever, dehydration, **albuminuria,** hyperglycemia, increased diuresis
RESP: Tachypnea, **respiratory arrest**

Contraindications: Hypersensitivity to xanthines

Precautions: Pregnancy C, breastfeeding, children, geriatric, CHF, cor pulmonale, diabetes mellitus, hypertension, renal/hepatic disease, glaucoma, hyperthyroidism, peptic ulcer, seizure disorder

Pharmacokinetics
Absorption	Well absorbed (PO)
Distribution	Unknown
Metabolism	Liver
Excretion	Kidneys (85%), breast milk
Half-life	2 hr; increased in renal disease

Pharmacodynamics
	PO	IM
Onset	Unknown	Unknown
Peak	1 hr	Unknown
Duration	6 hr	Unknown

Interactions
Individual drugs
Cimetidine, erythromycin, propranolol, probenecid: increased action of dyphylline
Phenytoin: decreased levels of phenytoin, increased metabolism of dyphylline
Drug classifications
Barbiturates: increased metabolism of dyphylline
β-Adrenergic blockers: increased cardiotoxicity
Uricosurics: decreased elimination of dyphylline

NURSING CONSIDERATIONS
Assessment
• Monitor dyphylline blood levels (therapeutic level is <20 mcg/ml); toxicity (dysrhythmias, seizures, diuresis, flushing, headache) may occur with small increase above 20 mcg/ml, especially geriatric; determine whether theophylline was given recently (24 hr)
• Monitor I&O; an increase in diuresis occurs; dehydration may result in geriatric or children
• Assess respiratory rate, rhythm, depth; before, during treatment auscultate lung fields bilaterally; notify prescriber of abnormalities
• Assess for allergic reactions: rash, urticaria; if these occur, product should be discontinued
• Assess for product toxicity: nausea, vomiting, anorexia, cramping, diarrhea, confusion

Nursing diagnoses
• Activity intolerance (uses)
• Airway clearance, ineffective (uses)
• Injury, risk for (uses, adverse reactions)
• Knowledge, deficient (teaching)

Implementation
PO route
• Give around the clock to maintain blood levels, daily dose each AM
• Give 1 hr before or 2 hr after meals to increase absorption; elix should be measured accurately
• Take with 8 oz of water and food if GI upset occurs
• Increase fluids to 2 L/day
IM route
• Inject slowly; do not give by **IV** route; do not administer if cloudy or a precipitate occurs, avoid this route, do not give **IV**

Patient/family education
• Teach patient to take doses as prescribed, not to skip doses or double dose; patient should check OTC medications and current prescription medications for ephedrine, which increases CNS stimulation; tell patient not to drink alcohol or caffeine products (tea, coffee, chocolate, colas) or CV effects may occur, not to change brands
• Advise patient to avoid hazardous activities; dizziness may occur
• Caution patient if GI upset occurs, to take product with 8 oz of water and food
• Teach patient to notify prescriber of change in smoking habit; a change in dosage may be required
• Instruct patient to report nausea, vomiting, insomnia, tachycardia, dysrhythmias, seizures, or restlessness; can indicate toxicity
• Teach patient to increase fluids to 2 L/day to decrease viscosity of secretions
• Advise patient to obtain product level q6-12mo

Evaluation
Positive therapeutic outcome
• Decreased dyspnea
• Clear lung fields bilaterally

econazole topical
See Appendix B

ecothiophate ophthalmic
See Appendix B

efavirenz (Rx)
(ef-ah-veer′enz)
Sustiva
Func. class.: Antiretroviral
Chem. class.: Nonnucleoside reverse transcriptase inhibitor (NNRTI)

Pregnancy category D

Action: Binds directly to reverse transcriptase and blocks RNA, DNA, polymerase, causing a disruption of the enzyme's site

Therapeutic outcome: Improvement of HIV-1 infection

Uses: HIV-1 in combination with other antiretrovirals

Dosage and routes
Given in combination with protease inhibitor or nucleoside analog reverse transcriptase inhibitors (NRTIs)
Adult and child >40 kg: PO 600 mg/day at bedtime
Child:
10-15 kg: PO 200 mg/day at bedtime
15-20 kg: PO 250 mg/day at bedtime
20-25 kg: PO 300 mg/day at bedtime
25-32.5 kg: PO 350 mg/day at bedtime
32.5-40 kg: PO 400 mg/day at bedtime

Available forms: Caps 50, 100, 200 mg; tabs 600 mg

Adverse effects
CNS: Headache, dizziness, fatigue, impaired cognition, insomnia, abnormal dreams, depression, anxiety, drowsiness
GI: Diarrhea, abdominal pain, *nausea,* hyperlipidemia, constipation, increased liver function tests
GU: Hematuria, kidney stones
INTEG: Rash, **erythema multiforme, Stevens-Johnson syndrome, toxic epidermal necrosis**

Contraindications: Pregnancy **D**, hypersensitivity

Precautions: Liver disease, breastfeeding, children <3 yr, renal disease, myelosuppression, depression, seizures

Pharmacokinetics
Absorption	Well
Distribution	Highly protein bound (99%)
Metabolism	Liver
Excretion	Kidneys, feces
Half-life	Terminal 52-76 hr

Pharmacodynamics
Onset	Unknown
Peak	3-5 hr
Duration	Unknown

Interactions
Individual drugs
Alcohol: increased CNS depression
Carbamazepine: decreased efavirenz levels
Cisapride, midazolam, triazolam: do not give together
Clarithromycin, indinavir, methadone, saquinavir: decreased level of each specific product
Midazolam, triazolam, warfarin: increased level of each specific product
Ritonavir: increased levels of both products
Drug classifications
Anticonvulsants, ergots, statins (except pravastatin, fluvastatin): increased levels of each specific product
Antidepressants, antihistamines, opioids: increased CNS depression
Benzodiazepines, ergots: do not give together
CYP3A4 inhibitors (conivaptan, ambrisentan, sorafenib): decreased efavirenz metabolism
CYP3A4 inducers (carbamazepine, rifamycins): decreased efavirenz effect
Estrogens: increased level of both products
Rifamycins: decreased efavirenz action
Drug/herb
St. John's wort: decreased efavirenz level; do not use together
Drug/food
Increased: absorption of high-fat foods
Drug/lab test
Increased: ALT
False positive: cannabinoids

NURSING CONSIDERATIONS
Assessment
- Assess signs of infection, anemia
- Assess liver studies: ALT, AST; renal tests
- Assess bowel pattern before, during treatment; if severe abdominal pain with bleeding occurs, product should be discontinued; monitor hydration
- Assess skin eruptions; rash, urticaria, itching
- Assess allergies before treatment, reaction to each medication

 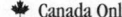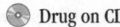

- Assess CBC, blood chemistry, plasma HIV RNA, absolute $CD4^+$/$CD8^+$/cell counts/%, serum β_2 microglobulin, serum ICD+24 antigen levels, cholesterol, hepatic enzymes
- Assess for signs of toxicity: severe nausea/vomiting, maculopapular rash

Nursing diagnoses
- Diarrhea (side effects)
- Infection, risk for (uses)
- Knowledge, deficient (teaching)

Implementation
- Give at bedtime to decrease CNS side effects, give on empty stomach

Patient/family education
- Inform patient that product does not cure disease but controls symptoms; HIV still can be transmitted to others
- Advise patient to take as prescribed; if dose is missed, take as soon as remembered; do not double dose; take on empty stomach with water/juice
- Instruct patient to make sure health care provider knows of all the medications being taken, supplements, herbs, OTC products
- Advise patient that if severe rash occurs, stop taking and notify health care provider
- Advise patient not to breastfeed or become pregnant (serious birth defects have occurred) if taking this product
- Advise patient that adverse reactions (rash, dizziness, abnormal dreams, insomnia), lessen after a month
- Teach patient to avoid hazardous activities if dizziness, drowsiness occurs

Evaluation
Positive therapeutic outcome
- Increased CD4, cell counts
- Decreased viral load
- Improvement in symptoms and progression of HIV-1 infection

---

eletriptan (Rx)
(el-ee-trip'tan)
Relpax
Func. class.: Antimigraine agent

Pregnancy category C

Action: Binds selectively to the vascular $5\text{-}HT_1$-receptor subtype, exerts antimigraine effect; causes vasoconstriction in cranial arteries

Therapeutic outcome: Decreased severity of migraine

Uses: Acute treatment of migraine with or without aura

Dosage and routes
Adult: **PO** 20 mg, may increase if needed, max 40 mg (single dose); may repeat in 2 hr if headache improves but returns, max 80 mg/24 hr

Available forms: Tabs 20, 40 mg

Adverse effects
CNS: Dizziness, headache, anxiety, paresthesia, asthenia, somnolence, flushing, fatigue, hot/cold sensation, chills, vertigo, hypertonia
CV: Chest pain, palpitations, hypertension
GI: Nausea, dry mouth
MS: Weakness, back pain
RESP: Chest tightness, pressure

Contraindications: Concurrent use of ergotamine-containing preparations, uncontrolled hypertension, hypersensitivity, basilar or hemiplegic migraine, ischemic bowel disease, severe renal/hepatic disease, coronary artery vasospasm, peripheral vascular disease, heart disease

Precautions: Pregnancy **C**, breastfeeding, children, geriatric, postmenopausal women, men >40 yr, risk factors of CAD, MI, or other cardiac disease, hypercholesterolemia, obesity, diabetes, impaired renal/hepatic function

Pharmacokinetics	
Absorption	Unknown
Distribution	Unknown
Metabolism	Liver
Excretion	Urine, feces
Half-life	Unknown

Pharmacodynamics	
Onset	Of pain relief 2 hr
Peak	Unknown
Duration	Unknown

Interactions
Individual drugs
Clarithromycin, erythromycin, itraconazole, ketoconazole, nelfinavir, propanolol, ritonavir: increased plasma concentration of eletriptan
Drug classifications
CYP3A4 inhibitors: increased concentration of eletriptan
Drug/herb
Butterbur: increased effect

Adverse effects: *italic* = common, **bold** = life-threatening

NURSING CONSIDERATIONS
Assessment
• Monitor B/P; signs/symptoms of coronary vasospasms
• Assess for tingling, hot sensation, burning, feeling of pressure, numbness, flushing
• Assess stress level, activity, recreation, coping mechanisms
• Assess neurologic status: LOC, blurring vision, nausea, vomiting, tingling in extremities preceding headache
• Identify ingestion of tyramine foods (pickled products, beer, wine, aged cheese), food additives, preservatives, colorings, artificial sweeteners, chocolate, caffeine, which may precipitate these types of headaches

Nursing diagnoses
• Knowledge, deficient (teaching)
• Pain, acute (uses)

Implementation
• Swallow tabs whole; do not break, crush, or chew
• Provide quiet, calm environment with decreased stimulation from noise, bright light, excessive talking

Patient/family education
• Have patient report any side effects to prescriber
• Teach patient to use contraception while taking product
• Teach patient to have dark, quiet environment
• Teach patient that product does not prevent or reduce number of migraine attacks

Evaluation
Positive therapeutic outcome
• Decreased severity of migraine

---

eltrombopag
Promacta
See Appendix A, Selected New Drugs

---

emedastine ophthalmic
See Appendix B

---

emtricitabine (Rx)
(em-tri-sit'uh-bean)
Emtriva
Func. class.: Antiretroviral
Chem. class.: Nucleoside reverse transcriptase inhibitor (NRTI)

Pregnancy category B

Action: Synthetic nucleoside analog of cytosine; inhibits replication of HIV virus by competing with the natural substrate and then becoming incorporated into cellular DNA by viral reverse transcriptase, thereby terminating cellular DNA chain

Therapeutic outcome: Decreasing symptoms of HIV

Uses: HIV-1 infection with other antiretrovirals

Unlabeled uses: HBV (hepatitis B virus) infection

Dosage and routes
Oral cap and sol are not interchangeable
Adult: PO (caps) 200 mg/day; oral SOL 240 mg (24 ml) daily
Child 3 mo-17 yr: PO (caps) 200 mg/day; oral SOL 6 mg/kg/day, max 240 mg (24 ml)

Renal dose
Adult: PO CCr 30-49 ml/min 200 mg q48hr, SOL 120 mg q24hr; CCr 15-29 ml/min 200 mg q72hr, SOL 80 mg q24hr; CCr <15 ml/min 200 mg q96hr, SOL 60 mg q24hr

Available forms: Caps 200 mg; oral sol 10 mg/ml; oral cap and sol are not interchangeable

Adverse effects
CNS: Headache, abnormal dreams, depression, dizziness, insomnia, neuropathy, paresthesia, *asthenia*
GI: Nausea, vomiting, diarrhea, anorexia, abdominal pain, dyspepsia, **hepatomegaly with stenosis (may be fatal)**
INTEG: Rash, skin discoloration
MS: Arthralgia, myalgia
RESP: Cough
SYST: Change in body fat distribution, **lactic acidosis**

Contraindications: Hypersensitivity

Black Box Warning: Lactic acidosis

Precautions: Pregnancy **B**, breastfeeding, children, geriatric, renal disease

Black Box Warning: Hepatic insufficiency, chronic hepatitis B virus (HBV) infection

---

Pharmacokinetics

Absorption	Rapidly, extensively absorbed
Distribution	Protein binding <4%
Metabolism	Unknown
Excretion	Excreted unchanged in urine (86%), feces (14%)
Half-life	10 hr

Pharmacodynamics

Onset	Unknown
Peak	1-2 hr
Duration	Unknown

NURSING CONSIDERATIONS
Assessment
- Monitor liver, renal function tests: AST, ALT, bilirubin, amylase, lipase, triglycerides periodically during treatment
- ⚠ Assess for lactic acidosis, severe hepatomegaly with steatosis; if lab reports confirm these conditions, discontinue treatment

Nursing diagnoses
- Infection, risk for (uses)
- Injury, risk for (adverse reactions)
- Knowledge, deficient (teaching)

Implementation
- Give without regard to meals
- Store at 25° C (77° F)
- Take at same time every day
- Oral cap and solution are not interchangeable

Patient/family education
- Teach that GI complaints resolve after 3-4 wk of treatment
- Advise not to breastfeed while taking this product
- Instruct that product must be taken at same time of day to maintain blood level
- Advise that product will control symptoms, but is not a cure for HIV; patient is still infectious, may pass HIV virus on to others
- Instruct that other products may be necessary to prevent other infections
- Advise that changes in body fat distribution may occur

Evaluation
Positive therapeutic outcome
- Decrease in signs/symptoms of HIV

enalapril/enalaprilat (Rx)
(e-nal'a-pril/e-nal'a-pril-at)
Vasotec
Func. class.: Antihypertensive
Chem. class.: Angiotensin-converting enzyme (ACE) inhibitor

Pregnancy category D

E

Do not confuse:
enalapril/Eldepryl/ramipril/Anafranil

Action: Selectively suppresses renin-angiotensin-aldosterone system; inhibits ACE; prevents conversion of angiotensin I to angiotensin II, resulting in dilatation of arterial and venous vessels

Therapeutic outcome: Decreased B/P in hypertension; decreased preload, afterload in CHF

Uses: Hypertension, CHF, left ventricular dysfunction

Dosage and routes
Hypertension
Adult: PO 2.5-5 mg/day, may increase or decrease to desired response, range 10-40 mg/day; **IV** 0.625-1.25 mg q6hr over 5 min
Child: PO 0.08 mg/kg/day in 1-2 divided doses, max 0.58 mg/kg/day; **IV** 5-10 mcg/kg/dose q8-24hr

Patients on diuretics
Adult: **IV** 0.625 mg over 5 min, may give additional doses of 1.25 mg q6hr

CHF
Adult: PO 2.5-20 mg/day in 2 divided doses, max 40 mg/day in divided doses

Renal dose
Adult: PO CCr <30 ml/min 2.5 mg/day, increase gradually; **IV** CCr >30 ml/min 1.25 mg q6hr; CCr <30 ml/min 0.625 mg as one-time dose, increase as per B/P

Available forms: Enalapril: tabs 2.5, 5, 10, 20 mg; enalaprilat: inj 1.25 mg/ml

Adverse effects
CNS: Insomnia, dizziness, paresthesias, headache, fatigue, anxiety
CV: Hypotension, chest pain, tachycardia, **dysrhythmias,** syncope, angina, **MI,** orthostatic hypotension
EENT: Tinnitus, visual changes, sore throat, double vision, dry burning eyes
GI: Nausea, vomiting, colitis, cramps, diarrhea, constipation, flatulence, dry mouth, loss of taste
GU: **Proteinuria, renal failure,** increased frequency of polyuria or oliguria

Adverse effects: *italic* = common, **bold** = life-threatening

HEMA: **Agranulocytosis, neutropenia**
INTEG: Rash, purpura, alopecia, hyperhidrosis, photosensitivity
META: Hyperkalemia
RESP: Dyspnea, dry cough, crackles, **angioedema**

Contraindications: Hypersensitivity, history of angioedema

Black Box Warning: Pregnancy **D**

Precautions: Breastfeeding, renal disease, hyperkalemia, hepatic failure, dehydration, bilateral renal artery stenosis

Pharmacokinetics

Absorption	Well absorbed (PO), complete (**IV**)
Distribution	Unknown
Metabolism	Liver (active metabolite—enalaprilat)
Excretion	Kidneys (60%—enalaprilat, 20%—enalapril)
Half-life	Enalaprilat 11 hr, increased in renal disease

Pharmacodynamics

	PO	IV
Onset	1 hr	15 min
Peak	4-6 hr	1-4 hr
Duration	24 hr	6 hr

Interactions
Individual drugs
Alcohol: increased hypotension (large amounts)
Allopurinol: increased hypersensitivity
CycloSPORINE, indomethacin: increased potassium levels
Digoxin, lithium: increased serum levels
Rifampin: decreased effects of enalapril
Drug classifications
Antacids: decreased effects of enalapril
Diuretics, general anesthesia, nitrates, other antihypertensives, phenothiazines: increased hypotension
Diuretics (potassium-sparing), potassium supplements, salt substitutes: increased potassium levels
Drug/herb
Arginine: fatal hypokalemia
Pill-bearing spurge: increased effect
Pineapple, yohimbe: decreased effect
St. John's wort: severe photosensitivity
Drug/lab test
Increased: ALT, AST, bilirubin, alkaline phosphatase, glucose, uric acid
False positive: ANA titer

NURSING CONSIDERATIONS
Assessment
• Monitor blood studies: neutrophils, decreased platelets with differential baseline and q3mo; if neutrophils <1000/mm³, discontinue treatment
• Monitor B/P, orthostatic hypotension, syncope; if changes occur, dosage change may be required; obtain peak/trough levels
• Monitor electrolytes: K, Na, Cl during 1st 2 wk of therapy
• Monitor renal studies: protein, BUN, creatinine; increased levels may indicate nephrotic syndrome and renal failure
• Monitor renal symptoms: polyuria, oliguria, frequency, dysuria
• Establish baselines in renal, liver function tests before therapy begins and 1 wk into therapy
• Check potassium levels throughout treatment, although hyperkalemia rarely occurs
• Check for edema in feet, legs daily
• Assess for allergic reactions: rash, fever, pruritus, urticaria; product should be discontinued if antihistamines fail to help

Nursing diagnoses
• Cardiac output, decreased (uses)
• Injury, risk for (adverse reactions)
• Knowledge, deficient (teaching)
• Noncompliance (teaching)

Implementation
PO route
• Store in air-tight container at 86° F (30° C) or less
• Severe hypotension may occur after 1st dose of this medication; decreased hypotension may be prevented by reducing or discontinuing diuretic therapy 3 days before beginning benazepril therapy
• Give by **IV** inf of 0.9% NaCl (as ordered) to expand fluid volume if severe hypotension occurs
IV route
• Give **IV** direct over 5 min
• Dilute in 50 ml of 0.9% NaCl, D₅W, D₅/0.9% NaCl, D₅/LR; diluted solution may be used for 24 hr
Y-site compatibilities: Allopurinol, amifostine, amikacin, aminophylline, ampicillin, ampicillin/sulbactam, aztreonam, butorphanol, calcium gluconate, cefazolin, cefoperazone, ceftazidime, ceftizoxime, chloramphenicol, cimetidine, cladribine, clindamycin, dextran 40, DOBUTamine, DOPamine, erythromycin lactobionate, esmolol, famotidine, fentanyl, filgrastim, ganciclovir, gentamicin, granisetron, heparin, hetastarch,

hydrocortisone, labetalol, lidocaine, magnesium sulfate, melphalan, meropenem, methylPREDNISolone, metronidazole, morphine, nafcillin, niCARDipine, penicillin G potassium, phenobarbital, piperacillin, piperacillin/tazobactam, potassium chloride, potassium phosphate, propofol, ranitidine, teniposide, thiotepa, tobramycin, trimethoprim/sulfamethoxazole, vancomycin, vinorelbine

Y-site incompatibilities: Amphotericin B, phenytoin

Additive compatibilities: DOBUTamine, DOPamine, heparin, meropenem, nitroglycerin, nitroprusside, potassium chloride

Patient/family education
• Advise patient not to discontinue product abruptly; advise patient to tell all persons associated with health care that product is being taken
• Teach patient not to use OTC products (cough, cold, allergy medications) unless directed by physician, to avoid potassium, salt substitutes; serious side effects can occur; xanthines, such as coffee, tea, chocolate, cola, can prevent action of product
• Instruct patient on the importance of complying with dosage schedule, even if feeling better; to continue with medical regimen to decrease B/P: exercise, cessation of smoking, decreasing stress, diet modifications
• Emphasize the need to rise slowly to sitting or standing position to minimize orthostatic hypotension; not to exercise in hot weather, which can cause increased hypotension
• Advise patient to notify prescriber of mouth sores, sore throat, fever, swelling of hands or feet, irregular heartbeat, chest pain, coughing, shortness of breath
• Caution patient to report excessive perspiration, dehydration, vomiting, diarrhea; may lead to fall in B/P
• Caution patient that product may cause skin rash or impaired perspiration; that angioedema may occur and to discontinue if it occurs
• Caution patient that product may cause dizziness, fainting, light-headedness; may occur during 1st few days of therapy; to avoid activities that may be hazardous
• Teach patient how to take B/P, and normal readings for age-group

Evaluation
Positive therapeutic outcome
• Decreased B/P in hypertension

Treatment of overdose: Lavage, **IV** atropine for bradycardia; **IV** theophylline for bronchospasm, digoxin, O_2; diuretic for cardiac failure, hemodialysis

---

enfuvirtide (Rx)
(en-fyoo′vir-tide)
Fuzeon
Func. class.: Antiretroviral
Chem. class.: Fusion inhibitor

Pregnancy category B

Action: Inhibitor of the fusion of HIV-1 with CD4+ cells

Therapeutic outcome: Decreasing symptoms of HIV

Uses: Treatment of HIV-1 infection in combination with other antiretrovirals

Dosage and routes
Adult: SUBCUT 90 mg (1 ml) bid
Child 6-16 yr and <42.6 kg: SUBCUT 2 mg/kg bid, max 90 mg bid; 11-15.5 kg 27 mg/0.3 ml bid; 15.6-20 kg 36 ml/0.4 ml bid; 20.1-24.5 kg 45 mg/0.5 ml bid; 24.6-29 kg 54 mg/0.6 ml bid; 29.1-33.5 kg 63 mg/0.7 ml bid; 33.6-38 kg 72 mg/0.8 ml bid; 38.1-42.5 kg 81 mg/0.9 ml bid

Available forms: Powder for inj, lyophilized 108 mg (90 mg/ml when reconstituted)

Adverse effects
CNS: Anxiety, peripheral neuropathy, taste disturbance, **Guillain-Barré syndrome,** insomnia, depression
GI: Abdominal pain, anorexia, constipation, pancreatitis
GU: **Glomerulonephritis, renal failure**
HEMA: **Thrombocytopenia, neutropenia**
INTEG: Inj site reactions
MISC: Influenza, cough, conjunctivitis, lymphadenopathy, myalgias, hyperglycemia, pneumonia, rhinitis, fatigue

Contraindications: Breastfeeding, hypersensitivity

Precautions: Pregnancy **B,** children <6 yr, liver disease, myelosuppression, infections

Pharmacokinetics
Absorption	Well
Distribution	92% protein binding
Metabolism	Undergoes catabolism
Excretion	Unknown
Half-life	Terminal 3.8 hr

Adverse effects: *italic* = common, **bold** = life-threatening

Pharmacodynamics

Onset	Unknown
Peak	8 hrs
Duration	Unknown

NURSING CONSIDERATIONS
Assessment
• Assess for signs of infection, inj site reactions
• Monitor renal studies: BUN, creatinine, renal failure may occur
• Monitor bowel pattern before, during treatment; if severe abdominal pain or constipation occurs, notify prescriber; monitor hydration
• Assess skin eruptions, rash, urticaria, itching
• Identify allergies before treatment, reaction to each medication
• CBC, blood chemistry, plasma HIV RNA, absolute CD4+/CD8+ cell counts/%, serum β_2 microglobulin, serum ICD+24 antigen levels, cholesterol

Nursing diagnoses
• Infection, risk for (uses)
• Injury, risk for (adverse reactions)
• Knowledge, deficient (teaching)

Implementation
• Give SUBCUT, bid; rotate sites; preferred sites are upper arm, anterior thigh, abdomen

Patient/family education
• Instruct to notify prescriber if pregnancy is suspected, or if breastfeeding
• Advise that pneumonia may occur, to contact prescriber if cough, fever occur
• Teach that hypersensitive reactions may occur: rash, pruritus; stop product, contact prescriber
• Teach that this product is not a cure for HIV-1 infection but controls symptoms; HIV-1 can still be transmitted to others
• Teach that this product is to be used in combination only with other antiretrovirals

Evaluation
Positive therapeutic outcome
• Increased CD4 cell counts; decreased viral load; slowing progression of HIV-1 infection

⚠ HIGH ALERT

enoxaparin (Rx)
(ee-nox′a-par-in)
Lovenox
Func. class.: Anticoagulant, antithrombotic
Chem. class.: Unfractionated porcine heparin (low-molecular-weight heparin)
Pregnancy category B

Do not confuse:
enoxaparin/enoxacin, Lovenox/Lotronex

Action: Prevents conversion of fibrinogen to fibrin and prothrombin to thrombin by enhancing inhibitory effects of antithrombin III; produces higher ratio of anti-factor Xa to anti-factor IIa

Therapeutic outcome: Prevention of deep vein thrombosis

Uses: Prevention of DVT, pulmonary emboli in hip and knee replacement, abdominal surgery at risk for thrombosis; unstable angina/non–Q-wave MI

Dosage and routes
DVT prevention before hip/knee surgery
Adult: SUBCUT 30 mg bid given 12-24 hr postoperatively for 7-10 days until DVT risk is diminished

DVT prevention before hip replacement
Adult: SUBCUT 40 mg/day started 9-15 hr preop or 30 mg bid started 12-24 hr postop, continued until DVT risk is diminished or is adequately an anticoagulant

DVT prophylaxis before abdominal surgery
Adult: SUBCUT 40 mg/day × 7-10 days to prevent thromboembolic complications, start 24 hr before surgery

Treatment of DVT/PE
Adult: SUBCUT (outpatient without PE) 1 mg/kg q12hr or 1.5 mg/kg/day (outpatient/inpatient); warfarin should be started within 72 hr and continued until INR is 2-3 (usually 7 days)

Prevention of ischemic complications in unstable angina/non–Q-wave MI with aspirin
Adult: SUBCUT/**IV** 1 mg/kg q12hr until stable with aspirin 100-325 mg/day × ≥2 days

Available forms: Prefilled syringes/inj 30 mg/0.3 ml, 40 mg/0.4 ml, 60 mg/0.6 ml, 80 mg/0.8 ml, 100 mg/1 ml, 120 mg/0.8 ml, 150 mg/ml; multidose vials 100 mg/ml (3 ml)

Adverse effects
CNS: Fever, confusion
GI: Nausea
HEMA: **Hemorrhage, hypochromic anemia, thrombocytopenia,** bleeding
INTEG: Ecchymosis, inj site hematoma
META: Hyperkalemia in renal failure
SYST: Edema, peripheral edema

Contraindications: Hypersensitivity to this product, benzyl alcohol, heparin, or pork; hemophilia; leukemia with bleeding; peptic ulcer disease; thrombocytopenic purpura, heparin-induced thrombocytopenia, active major bleeding

Precautions: Pregnancy **B,** breastfeeding, children, geriatric, severe renal/hepatic disease, blood dyscrasias, severe hypertension, subacute bacterial endocarditis, acute nephritis, recent burn, spinal surgery, indwelling catheters, low weight (men <57 kg, women <45 kg)

Black Box Warning: Lumbar puncture, epidural/spinal anesthesia

Pharmacokinetics
Absorption	Well absorbed (90%)
Distribution	Unknown
Metabolism	Unknown
Excretion	Kidneys
Half-life	4½ hr

Pharmacodynamics
Onset	Unknown
Peak	3-5 hr
Duration	Unknown

Interactions
Drug classifications
Anticoagulants, antiplatelets, NSAIDs, salicylates, thrombolytics: increased bleeding
Drug/herb
Agrimony, alfalfa, angelica, anise, basil, bay, bilberry, black currant, black haw, bogbean, bromelain, buchu, cat's claw, chondroitin, cinchona bark, dong quai, evening primrose, fenugreek, feverfew, fish oils, garlic, ginger, ginkgo, ginseng, horse chestnut, Irish moss, kava, kelp, kelpware, khella, licorice, lovage, lungwort, meadowsweet, motherwort, mugwort, nettle, papaya, parsley (large amounts), pau d'arco, pineapple, poplar, prickly ash, red clover, safflower, saw palmetto, skullcap, tonka bean, turmeric, wintergreen, yarrow: increased risk of bleeding

Chamomile, coenzyme Q10, flax, glucomannan, goldenseal, guar gum: decreased anticoagulant effect
Drug/lab test
Increased: AST/ALT
Decreased: platelets

NURSING CONSIDERATIONS
Assessment
• Monitor blood studies (Hct, CBC, coagulation studies, occult blood in stools), anti-Xa levels q3mo; platelet count q2-3day; thrombocytopenia may occur
• Assess patient for bleeding gums, petechiae, ecchymosis, black tarry stools, hematuria, epistaxis, decrease in B/P; indicate bleeding and possible hemorrhage; notify prescriber immediately
• Assess for neurosymptoms in patients who have received spinal anesthesia

Nursing diagnoses
• Injury, risk for (uses, adverse reactions)
• Knowledge, deficient (teaching)
• Tissue perfusion, ineffective (uses)

Implementation
• Give at same time each day to maintain steady blood levels
SUBCUT route
• Administer SUBCUT deeply; do not give IM, begin 1 hr before surgery, do not aspirate, do not expel bubble from syringe before administration; sol is clear to yellow; do not use sol with precipitate; apply gentle pressure for 1 min
• Give to recumbent patient, rotate sites (left/right anterolateral, left/right posterolateral abdominal wall)
• Leave vascular access sheath in place for 6 hr after dose, then give next dose, 6 hr after sheath removed
IV route
• Use multidose vial for **IV** administration; use TB syringe or other graduated syringe to measure dose; give **IV** BOL through IV line; flush after
• If withdrawing from multidose vial, use TB syringe for proper measurement
• Prefilled syringes (30, 40 mg) are not graduated; do not use for partial doses
• Do not mix with other products or infusion fluids
◆ Give only this product when ordered; not interchangeable with heparin or LMWHs

Patient/family education
• Warn patient to avoid OTC preparations unless directed by prescriber because they could cause serious product interactions

---

Adverse effects: *italic* = common, **bold** = life-threatening

• Instruct patient to use soft-bristled toothbrush to avoid bleeding gums; to avoid contact sports; to use electric razor; to avoid IM inj
• Advise patient to report any signs of bleeding, bruising: gums, under skin, urine, stools

Evaluation
Positive therapeutic outcome
• Absence of DVT

---

entacapone (Rx)
(en-ta'-ka-pone)
Comtan
Func. class.: Antiparkinsonian agent
Chem. class.: COMT

Pregnancy category C

Action: Inhibits COMT (catechol *O*-methyltransferase) and alters the plasma pharmacokinetics of levodopa; given with levodopa/carbidopa

Therapeutic outcome: Decreased symptoms of Parkinson's disease (involuntary movements)

Uses: Parkinsonism in those experiencing end of dose, decreased effect as an adjunct to levodopa/carbidopa

Dosage and routes
Adult: PO 200 mg given with carbidopa/levodopa, max 1600 mg/day

Available forms: Tabs 200 mg film coated

Adverse effects
CNS: Involuntary choreiform movements, dyskinesia, hypokinesia, hyperkinesia, hand tremors, fatigue, headache, anxiety, twitching, numbness, weakness, confusion, agitation, nightmares, psychosis, hallucinations, hypomania, severe depression, dizziness, **neuroleptic malignant syndrome**
CV: Orthostatic hypotension
GI: Nausea, vomiting, anorexia, abdominal distress, dry mouth, flatulence, dyspepsia, gastritis, *GI disorder, diarrhea, constipation,* bitter taste
INTEG: Rash, sweating, alopecia
MISC: Dark urine and other body fluids, back pain, dyspnea, purpura, fatigue, asthenia, infection-bacterial, **rhabdomyolysis**

Contraindications: Hypersensitivity

Precautions: Pregnancy C, breastfeeding, children, renal/hepatic disease, affective disorders, psychosis

Pharmacokinetics
Absorption	Well absorbed
Distribution	Protein binding 98%
Metabolism	Liver extensively
Excretion	Kidneys, feces; breast milk
Half-life	0.5 hr initial, 2.5 hr second

Pharmacodynamics
Onset	Unknown
Peak	Unknown
Duration	≤8 hr

Interactions
Individual drugs
Ampicillin, chloramphenicol, erythromycin, probenecid, rifampin: decreased excretion of entacapone
Bitolterol, DOBUTamine, DOPamine, epinephrine, isoetharine, methyldopa, norepinephrine: increased CV reactions; avoid use
Drug classifications
MAOIs: prevent catecholamine metabolism; do not use together
Drug/herb
Kava: decreased effect
Ma huang: increased B/P

NURSING CONSIDERATIONS
Assessment
• Assess for neuroleptic malignant syndrome: high temp, increased CPK, rigidity, change in consciousness
• Monitor B/P, respiration during initial treatment; hypotension should be reported
• Assess mental status: affect, mood, behavioral changes, depression; complete suicide assessment
• Monitor liver function enzymes: AST, ALT, alkaline phosphatase; also check LDH, bilirubin, CBC
• Assess for involuntary movements in parkinsonism: akinesia, tremors, staggering gait, muscle rigidity, drooling; these symptoms should improve with therapy when given with levodopa/carbidopa

Nursing diagnoses
• Injury, risk for (uses)
• Knowledge, deficient (teaching)
• Mobility, impaired physical (uses)
• Noncompliance (teaching)

Implementation
• Adjust dosage to patient response
• Give with meals to decrease GI upset; limit protein taken with product
• Give only after MAOIs have been discontinued for 2 wk

◆ Alert ♣ Canada Only 🔵 Drug on CD * "Tall Man" lettering (See Preface)

Patient/family education
- Advise patient that hallucinations, mental changes, nausea, dyskinesia can occur
- Caution patient to change positions slowly to prevent orthostatic hypotension; not to drive or operate machinery until stabilized on medication and mental performance is not affected
- Instruct patient to use product exactly as prescribed
- Inform patient that urine, sweat may darken
- Inform patient to notify prescriber if pregnancy is suspected; if breastfeeding, product is excreted in breast milk

Evaluation
Positive therapeutic outcome
- Decreased akathisia, other involuntary movements when used with levodopa/carbidopa
- Increased mood when used with levodopa/carbidopa

---

entecavir (Rx)
(en-te'ka-veer)
Baraclude
Func. class.: Antiviral
Chem. class.: Guanosine nucleoside analog

Pregnancy category C

Action: Inhibits hepatitis B virus DNA polymerase by competing with natural substrates and by causing DNA termination after its incorporation into viral DNA; causes viral DNA death

Therapeutic outcome: Improved liver function tests in chronic hepatitis B (HBV)

Uses: Chronic hepatitis B (HBV)

Dosage and routes
Chronic hepatitis B (nucleoside treatment-naive)
Adult and adolescent ≥16 yr: PO 0.5 mg/day

Chronic hepatitis B while receiving lamivudine or known lamivudine resistance mutations
Adult and adolescent ≥16 yr: PO 1 mg/day

Renal dose
Adult: PO CCr ≥50 ml/min 0.5 mg/day; CCr 30-49 ml/min 0.25 mg daily, 0.5 mg/day for lamivudine refractory patient; CCr 10-29 ml/min 0.15 mg/day, 0.3 for lamivudine refractory patient; CCr <10 ml/min 0.05 mg PO/day, 0.1 mg for lamivudine refractory patient

Available forms: Tabs, film coated 0.5, 1 mg; oral sol 0.05 mg/ml

Adverse effects
CNS: *Headache*, fatigue, dizziness, insomnia
ENDO: Hyperglycemia
GI: *Dyspepsia*, nausea, vomiting, diarrhea, elevated liver function enzymes
INTEG: Alopecia, rash
SYST: **Lactic acidosis, severe hepatomegaly with stenosis**

Contraindications: Hypersensitivity

Precautions: Pregnancy **C**, breastfeeding, child, geriatric, severe renal disease

Black Box Warning: Hepatic disease, hepatitis, lactic acidosis

Pharmacokinetics	
Absorption	100%
Distribution	Extensively to tissues, protein binding 13%
Metabolism	Unknown
Excretion	Unchanged 62%-73% via kidneys
Half-life	Terminal 128-149 hr

Pharmacodynamics	
Onset	Unknown
Peak	0.5-1.5 hr
Duration	Unknown

Interactions
Drug/food
High-fat meal: decreased absorption
Drug/lab test
Increased: ALT, AST, total bilirubin, amylase, lipase, creatinine, blood glucose, urine glucose
Decreased: platelets, albumin

NURSING CONSIDERATIONS
Assessment
- Assess for nephrotoxicity: increasing CCr, BUN
- Assess for HIV before beginning treatment because HIV resistance may occur in patients with chronic hepatitis B infection
- Assess for lactic acidosis, severe hepatomegaly with stenosis
- Monitor geriatric patients more carefully; may develop renal, cardiac symptoms more rapidly
- Assess for exacerbations of hepatitis after discontinuing treatment; monitor liver function tests

Nursing diagnoses
- Infection, risk for (uses)
- Injury, risk for (uses, adverse reactions)

Adverse effects: *italic* = common, **bold** = life-threatening

Implementation
- Give by mouth on empty stomach 2 hr before or after food
- Store in cool environment; protect from light

Patient/family education
- Teach patient not to take with food
- Teach patient to take exactly as prescribed
- Advise patient not to stop medication without approval of prescriber
- Advise that optimal duration of treatment is unknown
- Teach patient to avoid use with other medications unless approved by prescriber
- Teach patient to notify prescriber of decreased urinary output, blood in urine
- Teach patient symptoms of lactic acidosis: muscle pain, severe tiredness, weakness, trouble breathing, stomach pain with nausea/vomiting, coldness in arms/legs, fast/irregular heartbeat, dizziness
- Teach patient symptoms of hepatotoxicity: eyes/skin turns yellow, dark urine, light bowel movements, no appetite for days, nausea, stomach pain
- Advise patient that product does not cure, but lowers the amount of HBV in body
- Teach patient that product does not stop the spreading of HBV to others by sex, sharing needles, or being exposed to blood

Evaluation
Positive therapeutic outcome
- Decreased symptoms of chronic hepatitis B, improving liver function tests

---

⚠ HIGH ALERT

ephedrine (Rx, OTC)
(e-fed′rin)

ephedrine sulfate, Pretz-D
Func. class.: Bronchodilator, nonselective, adrenergic, mixed direct and indirect effects; bronchodilator, nasal decongestant, vasopressor
Chem. class.: Phenylisopropylamine

Pregnancy category C

Do not confuse:
ephedrine/epinephrine

Action: Increases contractility and heart rate by acting on β-receptors in the heart; also acts on α-receptors, causing vasoconstriction in blood vessels

Therapeutic outcome: Decreased nasal congestion, bronchodilatation, stimulation, increased B/P

Uses: Shock; increased perfusion; hypotension, bronchodilatation; nasal congestion; depression

Dosage and routes
Bronchodilator
Adult and child >12 yr: PO 12.5-50 mg q3-4hr prn, max 150 mg/24 hr; NASAL 2-3 sprays in each nostril q4hr
Child 2-12 yr: PO 2-3 mg/kg or 100 mg/m²/day in 4-6 divided doses

Nasal decongestant
Adult: Fill dropper to the level marked, then use in each nostril q4hr or less

Hypotension
Adult: PO 25 mg daily-qid; IM/SUBCUT 25-50 mg; **IV** 10-25 mg max 150 mg/24 hr
Child: SUBCUT/**IV** 25-100 mg/m²/day in 4-6 divided doses

Available forms: Inj 25, 30, 50 mg/ml; caps 25, 50 mg

Adverse effects
CNS: Tremors, anxiety, insomnia, sweating, headache, dizziness, confusion, hallucinations, **seizures, CNS depression, cerebral hemorrhage,** weakness, drowsiness
CV: Palpitations, tachycardia, hypertension, chest pain, **dysrhythmias**
GI: Anorexia, nausea, vomiting
GU: Dysuria, urinary retention
RESP: Dyspnea

Contraindications: Hypersensitivity to sympathomimetics, closed-angle glaucoma, nonanaphylactic shock during general anesthesia, diabetes mellitus, hypertension

Precautions: Pregnancy **C,** breastfeeding, cardiac disorders, hyperthyroidism, prostatic hypertrophy, angina, diabetes mellitus

Pharmacokinetics
Absorption	Well absorbed (PO/IM/SUBCUT), complete (**IV**)
Distribution	Unknown
Metabolism	Liver
Excretion	Kidneys—unchanged
Half-life	3-5 hr

Pharmacodynamics
	PO	SUBCUT	IM	IV	NASAL
Onset	¼-1 hr	Unkn	15-30 min	5 min	Unkn
Peak	Unkn	Unkn	Unkn	Unkn	Unkn
Duration	2-4 hr	1 hr	1 hr	2 hr	6 hr

Interactions
Individual drugs
Guanethidine: decreased effect of guanethedine

Levodopa: increased dysrhythmias

Methyldopa: decreased effect of ephedrine

Drug classifications
α-Adrenergic blockers, antidepressants (tricyclic), diuretics, rauwolfia alkaloids, urinary acidifiers: decreased effect of ephedrine

Anesthetics (halothane), cardiac glycosides: increased dysrhythmias

Ergots: hypertensive crisis

MAOIs: increased chance of hypertensive crisis; do not use together

Oxytoxics: increased severe hypertension

Sympathomimetics: increased adrenergic side effects

Urinary alkalizers: increased effect of ephedrine

NURSING CONSIDERATIONS
Assessment
• Monitor respiratory function: vital capacity, forced expiratory volume, ABGs, lung sounds, heart rate, baseline rhythm (bronchodilator)

• Monitor for evidence of allergic reactions, paradoxical bronchospasm; withhold dose; notify prescriber

• Monitor ECG, B/P, pulse q5min when using **IV** route (shock)

• Assess for paresthesias and coldness of extremities; peripheral blood flow may decrease; long-term use may produce pseudo anxiety state requiring sedatives, increased lactic acid with severe metabolic acidosis

• Assess nasal congestion to identify factors contributing to ongoing congestion (nasal use)

• Assess mental status and sleeping patterns: mood, sensorium, ability to stay awake

Nursing diagnoses
• Airway clearance, ineffective (uses)

• Gas exchange, impaired (uses)

• Knowledge, deficient (teaching)

• Sleep deprivation (uses)

Implementation
PO route
• Administer several hr (up to 6 hr) before bedtime to prevent sleeplessness

IV route
• Give **IV** directly undiluted using 3-way stopcock or Y-site; give 10-25 mg slowly; may repeat in 5-10 min

• Use clear sol without precipitate; unused sol should be discarded; protect from light

Syringe compatibilities: Pentobarbital

Y-site compatibilities: Etomidate, propofol

Additive compatibilities: Chloramphenicol, lidocaine, metaraminol, nafcillin, penicillin G potassium

Solution compatibilities: 0.9% NaCl, 0.45% NaCl, D_5W, $D_{10}W$, Ringer's, LR

Patient/family education
• Advise patient to avoid use of OTC medications: extra stimulation may occur; not to use alcohol

Evaluation
Positive therapeutic outcome
• Increased B/P (vasopressor)

• Ability to stay awake (absence of narcolepsy) or improved mood (absence of depression)

• Absence of bronchospasm

• Decreased nasal congestion

---

ephedrine nasal agent
See Appendix B

---

epinastine ophthalmic
See Appendix B

⚠ HIGH ALERT

epinephrine (Rx, OTC)
(ep-i-nef'rin)
Adrenalin, Ana-Guard, AsthmaHaler Mist, AsthmaNefrin (racepinephrine), Bronitin Mist, Bronkaid Mist, epinephrine, Epinal, Epitrate, Eppy/N, Epinephrine Pediatric, EpiPen, EpiPen Jr., Medihaler, microNefrin, Nephron, Primatene Mist, S-2, Sus-Phrine, Vaponefrin (racepinephrine)
Func. class.: Bronchodilator, nonselective adrenergic agonist, cardiac stimulant, vasopressor
Chem. class.: Catecholamine

Pregnancy category C

Do not confuse:
epinephrine/ephedrine

Action: β_1- and β_2-agonist causing increased levels of cyclic AMP producing bronchodilatation, cardiac and CNS stimulation; large doses cause vasoconstriction via α-receptors; small doses can cause vasodilation via β_2-vascular receptors

---

Adverse effects: *italic* = common, **bold** = life-threatening

Therapeutic outcome: Vasoconstrictor, cardiac stimulator, bronchodilator, decreased aqueous humor

Uses: Acute asthmatic attacks, hemostasis, bronchospasm, anaphylaxis, allergic reactions, cardiac arrest, adjunct in anesthesia, shock

Dosage and routes
Asthma
Adult and child: INH 1-2 puffs of 1:100 or 2.25% racemic q15min

Bronchodilator
Adult: SUBCUT/IM 0.3-0.5 mg (1:1000 SOL) q10-15min-4hr, max 1 mg/dose

Anaphylactic reaction/asthma
Adult: SUBCUT/IM 0.3-0.5 mg, repeat q10-15min, max 1 mg/dose; epinephrine susp 0.5 mg SUBCUT, may repeat 0.5-1.5 mg q6hr
Child: SUBCUT 0.01 mg/kg, repeat q15min × 2 doses, then q4hr as needed, up to 0.5 mg/dose; epinephrine susp 0.025 mg/kg SUBCUT, may repeat q6hr, max 0.75 mg in child ≤30 kg

Cardiac arrest (ACLS)
Adult: **IV** 1 mg q3-5min; Endotracheal 2-25 mg; IC 0.3-0.5 mg

Symptomatic bradycardia/pulseless arrest (PALS)
Child: **IV** 0.01 mg/kg, may repeat q3-5min; Endotracheal give 2-10 × **IV** dose diluted to a volume of 3-5 mg of 0.9% NaCl, followed by positive pressure ventilation

Available forms: Aerosol 0.16, 0.2, 0.25 mg/spray, inj 1:1000 (1 mg/ml), 1:200 (5 mg/ml), 0.01 mg/ml (1:100,000), 0.1 mg/ml (1:10,000), 0.5 mg/ml (1:2000); sol for nebulization 1:100, 1.25% 2.25% (base)

Adverse effects
CNS: Tremors, anxiety, insomnia, headache, dizziness, weakness, drowsiness, confusion, hallucinations, **cerebral hemorrhage**
CV: Palpitations, tachycardia, hypertension, *dysrhythmias,* increased T-wave
GI: Anorexia, nausea, vomiting
MISC: Sweating, dry eyes
RESP: Dyspnea

Contraindications: Hypersensitivity to sympathomimetics, closed-angle glaucoma, nonanaphylactic shock during general anesthesia

Precautions: Pregnancy **C**, breastfeeding, cardiac disorders, hyperthyroidism, diabetes mellitus, prostatic hypertrophy, hypertension, organic brain syndrome, local anesthesia of certain areas, labor, cardiac dilatation, coronary insufficiency, cerebral arteriosclerosis, organic heart disease

Pharmacokinetics
Absorption	Well absorbed (PO), complete (**IV**)
Distribution	Unknown, crosses placenta
Metabolism	Liver
Excretion	Breast milk
Half-life	Unknown

Pharmacodynamics
	SUBCUT	IM	IV	INH
Onset	3-5 min	5-10 min	Immediate	1 min
Peak	Unknown	Unknown	Unknown	Unknown
Duration	1-4 hr	1-4 hr	Unknown	1-4 hr

Interactions
Drug classifications
α-Adrenergic blockers: decreased hypertensive effects

Antidepressants (tricyclics): increased chance of hypertensive crisis; do not use together

MAOIs: increased chance of hypertensive crisis, do not use together

Other sympathomimetics: toxicity

NURSING CONSIDERATIONS
Assessment
• Monitor respiratory function: vital capacity, forced expiratory volume, ABGs, lung sounds, heart rate, rhythm (baseline); amount, color of sputum
• Monitor ECG during administration continuously; if B/P increases, product should be decreased; check B/P, pulse q5min after parenteral route; CVP, PCWP, SVR; inadvertent high arterial B/P can result in angina, aortic rupture, cerebral hemorrhage
• Check inj site for tissue sloughing; if this occurs, administer phentolamine mixed with 0.9% NaCl
• Monitor for evidence of allergic reactions, paradoxical bronchospasm: withhold dose, notify prescriber; sulfite sensitivity, which may be life threatening

Nursing diagnoses
• Airway clearance, ineffective (uses)
• Cardiac output, decreased (uses)
• Gas exchange, impaired (uses)
• Knowledge, deficient (teaching)
• Sensory perception, disturbed, visual (uses) (ophth)

 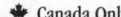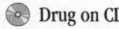

Implementation
- Check for correct concentration, route, dosage before administration
- Use this medication before other medications and allow at least 5 min between each to prevent overstimulation

IM/SUBCUT route
- Rotate inj sites, massage well, do not use gluteal (IM) site
- Shake susp before using

Inhalation route
- Use 2.25% sol diluted in nebulizer/respirator
- Rinse mouth after inh
- 10 gtt of a 1% sol should be placed in nebulizer
- Dilute racepinephrine 2.25% sol

Endotracheal route
- Only used in intubated patient; use **IV** dose that should be injected by endotracheal tube into bronchi

IV route
- Give after diluting 1 mg of 1:1000 sol/10 ml or more; 0.9% NaCl yields 1:10,000 sol, give 1 mg/min
- Give by continuous inf after further diluting in 0.9% NaCl, D_5W, $D_{10}W$, D_5/LR, LR via 3-way stopcock; for Y-site, use infusion pump, protect from light; increase dose of insulin in diabetic patients

Syringe compatibilities: Doxapram, heparin, milrinone

Y-site compatibilities: Amrinone, atracurium, calcium chloride, calcium gluconate, diltiazem, DOBUTamine, DOPamine, famotidine, fentanyl, furosemide, heparin, hydrocortisone sodium succinate, hydromorphone, labetalol, lorazepam, midazolam, milrinone, morphine, niCARdipine, nitroglycerin, norepinephrine, pancuronium, phytonadione, potassium chloride, propofol, ranitidine, vecuronium, vit B/C

Y-site incompatibilities: Ampicillin

Additive compatibilities: Amikacin, cimetidine, DOBUTamine, floxacillin, furosemide, metaraminol, ranitidine, verapamil

Additive incompatibilities: Aminophylline, mephentermine, sodium bicarbonate, warfarin

Patient/family education
- Tell patient not to use OTC medications; extra stimulation may occur; to use this medication before other medications and allow at least 5 min between each, to prevent overstimulation
- Teach patient that paradoxical bronchospasm may occur and to stop product immediately and notify prescriber; to limit caffeine products such as chocolate, coffee, tea, and colas
- Patient should rinse mouth after inh
- Patient should report blurred vision, irritation with ophth preparations

Evaluation
Positive therapeutic outcome
- Absence of dyspnea, wheezing
- Improved airway exchange, improved ABGs
- Decreased aqueous humor
- Stabilization of heart rate and cardiac output

Treatment of overdose: Administer a β_2-adrenergic blocker, vasodilators, α-blocker

---

epinephrine/epinephryl borate ophthalmic
See Appendix B

---

epinephrine nasal agent
See Appendix B

❗ HIGH ALERT

epirubicin (Rx)
(ep-i-roo'-bi-sin)
Ellence
Func. class.: Antineoplastic, antibiotic
Chem. class.: Anthracycline

Pregnancy category D

Action: Inhibits DNA synthesis primarily; replication is decreased by binding to DNA, which causes strand splitting; maximum cytotoxic effects at S and G_2 phases; a vesicant

Therapeutic outcome: Prevention of rapidly growing malignant cells

Uses: Breast cancer as an adjuvant therapy, with axillary node involvement, after resection

Unlabeled uses: Used in combination for treatment of advanced forms of cancer

Dosage and routes
Adult: **IV** INF 100-120 mg/m² initially given with other antineoplastics (cyclophosphamide, 5-fluorouracil); given in repeated 3-4 wk cycles

Epirubicin dosage adjustments
Adult: **IV** 100 mg/m² on day 1 of each cycle; toxicity nadir platelet counts <50,000 mm³, ANC 250 mm³, neutropenic fever or grade 3 or 4 nonhematologic toxicity; next cycle give 75% of day 1 dose; delay next cycle

until platelets are ≥100,000 mm³, ANC >1500 mm³, and nonhematologic toxicities have recovered to < grade 1

Hepatic dose
Adult: **IV** Bilirubin 1.2-3 mg/dl or AST 2-4 × normal upper limit, 50% of starting dose; bilirubin >3 mg/dl or AST >4 × normal upper limit, 25% of starting dose

Available forms: Inj (2 mg/ml) 10 mg/5 ml, 50 mg/25 ml, 150 mg/75 ml, 200 mg/100 ml

Adverse effects
CV: Increased B/P, **sinus tachycardia, PVCs,** chest pain, **bradycardia, extrasystole**
GI: Nausea, vomiting, diarrhea, anorexia, mucositis
GU: Hot flashes, amenorrhea, hyperuricemia
HEMA: Thrombocytopenia, leukopenia, anemia, neutropenia, secondary AML
INTEG: Rash, necrosis, pain at inj site, reversible alopecia
MISC: Hot flashes, febrile neutropenia, lethargy, fever, conjunctivitis, tumor lysis syndrome

Contraindications: Pregnancy **D,** breastfeeding, hypersensitivity to this product, anthracyclines, anthracenediones, systemic infections, baseline neutrophil count <1500 cell/mm³, severe myocardial insufficiency, recent MI

Black Box Warning: Severe hepatic disease

Precautions: Children, geriatric, renal/hepatic/cardiac disease, gout, previous anthracycline use

Black Box Warning: Bone marrow suppression (severe), heart failure, extravasation, secondary malignancy

Pharmacokinetics
Absorption	Complete bioavailability
Distribution	Widely distributed, crosses placenta
Metabolism	Liver, extensively
Excretion	Bile (60%)
Half-life	3 min; 2.5 hr; 33 hr

Pharmacodynamics
Unknown

Interactions
Individual drugs
Cimetidine, radiation: increased toxicity
Drug classifications
Antineoplastics: increased toxicity
Live virus vaccines: decreased antibody response

NURSING CONSIDERATIONS
Assessment
• Monitor left ventricular ejection fraction, multigated acquisition scan or echocardiogram, ECG; watch for ST-T wave changes, low QRS and T; possible dysrhythmias (sinus tachycardia, heart block, PVCs) may occur; assess tachypnea, ECG changes, dyspnea, edema, fatigue; cardiac status: B/P, pulse, character, rhythm, rate, ABGs
• Assess for bone marrow depression, infection
• Assess symptoms indicating severe allergic reaction: rash, pruritus, urticaria, purpuric skin lesions, itching, flushing; product should be discontinued
• Monitor CBC, differential, platelet count weekly; withhold product if baseline neutrophil count is <1500/mm³; notify prescriber of results if WBC <20,000/mm³, platelets <150,000/mm³; leukocyte nadir occurs 10-14 days after administration; recovery by 21st day
• Assess for increased uric acid levels, swelling, joint pain, primarily extremities; patient should be well hydrated to prevent urate deposits
• Monitor renal function studies: BUN, creatinine, serum uric acid, urine CCr before, during therapy; I&O ratio; report fall in urine output to <30 ml/hr; dosage adjustment is needed if serum creatinine >5 mg/dl
• Monitor liver function tests before, during therapy (bilirubin, AST, ALT, LDH) as needed or monthly; note jaundice of skin or sclera, dark urine, clay-colored stools, itchy skin, abdominal pain, fever, diarrhea
• Assess for bleeding: hematuria, stool guaiac, bruising or petechiae, mucosa or orifices q8hr; inflammation of mucosa, breaks in skin
• Identify effects of alopecia on body image; discuss feeling about body changes

Nursing diagnoses
• Body image, disturbed (adverse reactions)
• Infection, risk for (adverse reactions)
• Injury, risk for (adverse reactions)
• Knowledge, deficient (teaching)

Implementation
• Avoid contact with skin; very irritating; wash completely to remove; give fluids **IV** or PO before chemotherapy to hydrate patient
• Give antiemetic 30-60 min before giving product to prevent vomiting and prn
• Administer prophylactic antibiotic with a fluoroquinolone or trimethoprim/sulfamethoxazole if dose of epirubicin is 120 mg/m²

 Alert   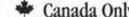 Canada Only   Drug on CD   * "Tall Man" lettering (See Preface)

- Provide liquid diet: carbonated beverages; gelatin may be added if patient is not nauseated or vomiting
- Product should be prepared by experienced personnel using proper precautions
- Give into tubing of free-flowing **IV** inf 0.9% NaCl or D₅ over 3-5 min; do not admix with other products in syringe
- Use hydrocortisone, dexamethasone, or sodium bicarbonate (1 mEq/1 ml) for extravasation: apply ice compress

Patient/family education

- Advise patient to avoid use of products containing aspirin or NSAIDs, razors, commercial mouthwash, since bleeding may occur; to report symptoms of bleeding (hematuria, tarry stools)
- Instruct patient to report signs of anemia (fatigue, headache, irritability, faintness, shortness of breath)
- Inform patient that hair may be lost during treatment; a wig or hairpiece may make patient feel better; new hair may be different in color, texture
- Caution patient not to have any vaccinations without the advice of the prescriber; serious reactions can occur
- Advise patient to use contraception during treatment and 4 mo afterward
- Advise patient that urine may appear red for 2 days
- Instruct patient to avoid crowds, persons with known infection
- Caution patient to avoid OTC medications, supplements unless approved by prescriber

Evaluation

Positive therapeutic outcome
- Prevention of rapid division of malignant cells

---

eplerenone (Rx)
(ep-ler-ee′known)
Inspra
Func. class.: Antihypertensive

Pregnancy category B

Action: Binds to mineralocorticoid receptor and blocks the binding of aldosterone, a component of the renin-angiotensin-aldosterone system (RAAS)

Therapeutic outcome: Absence of hypertension

Uses: Hypertension, alone or in combination with thiazide diuretics, CHF, post-MI

Dosage and routes
Adult: **PO** 50 mg/day initially, may increase to 50 mg bid after 4 wk; start dose at 25 mg/day if patient is taking CYP3A4 inhibitors

CHF/post-MI
Adult: PO 25 mg/day initially, may increase to 50 mg/day max

Available forms: Tabs 25, 50, 100 mg

Adverse effects
CNS: Headache, dizziness, fatigue
CV: Angina, **MI**
GI: Increased GGT diarrhea, abdominal pain, increased ALT
GU: Increased BUN, creatinine, gynecomastia, mastodynia (males), abnormal vaginal bleeding
META: Hyperkalemia, hyponatremia, hypercholesteremia, hypertriglyceridemia, increased uric acid
RESP: Cough

Contraindications: Breastfeeding, children, hypersensitivity, increased serum creatinine >2 mg/dl (male) or >1.8 mg/dl (female), potassium >5.5 mEq/L, type 2 diabetes with microalbuminuria, hepatic disease, CCr <30 ml/min, CCr <50 ml/min in hypertension

Precautions: Pregnancy **B**, breastfeeding, geriatric, impaired renal/hepatic function, hyperkalemia

Pharmacokinetics
Absorption	Unknown
Distribution	Protein binding 50%
Metabolism	Liver (CYP3A4 inhibitor)
Excretion	Urine
Half-life	4-6 hr

Pharmacodynamics
Onset	Unknown
Peak	1½ hr
Duration	Unknown

Interactions
Individual drugs
Erythromycin, fluconazole, itraconazole, ketoconazole, saquinavir, verapamil: increased levels of eplerenone; reduce dose of eplerenone
Lithium: increased serum lithium levels
Drug classifications
ACE inhibitors, angiotensin II antagonists, diuretics (potassium-sparing), NSAIDs, potassium supplements: increased hyperkalemia

Adverse effects: *italic* = common, **bold** = life-threatening

CYP3A4 inhibitors: increased levels of eplerenone; reduce dose of eplerenone
NSAIDs: decreased antihypertensive effect

Drug/herb
Aconite: increased toxicity, death
Astragalus, cola tree: increased or decreased antihypertensive effect
Barberry, betony, black catechu, black cohosh, bloodroot, broom, burdock, cat's claw, dandelion, goldenseal, hawthorn, Irish moss, Jamaican dogwood, kelp, khella, mistletoe, parsley: increased antihypertensive effect
Coltsfoot, guarana, khat, licorice, yohimbe: decreased antihypertensive effect
St. John's wort: decreased levels of eplerenone

Drug/food
Grapefruit juice: increased product level by 25%

NURSING CONSIDERATIONS
Assessment
• Monitor B/P at peak/trough level of product, orthostatic hypotension, syncope when used with diuretic
• Monitor renal studies: protein, BUN, creatinine; increased liver function tests; uric acid may be increased
• Monitor potassium levels, hyperkalemia may occur

Nursing diagnoses
• Cardiac output, decreased (uses)
• Diarrhea (side effects)
• Knowledge, deficient (teaching)
• Noncompliance (teaching)
• Tissue perfusion, ineffective (uses)

Implementation
• Store in tight container at 86° F (30° C) or less

Patient/family education
• Advise not to discontinue product abruptly
• Advise not to use OTC products (cough, cold, allergy) unless directed by prescriber; do not use salt substitutes containing potassium without consulting prescriber
• Teach the importance of complying with dosage schedule, even if feeling better
• Teach that product may cause dizziness, fainting, light-headedness; may occur during first few days of therapy
• Teach how to take B/P, and normal readings for age-group

Evaluation
Positive therapeutic outcome
• Decreased in B/P

epoetin (Rx)
(ee-poe'e-tin)
Epogen, EPO, Eprex ✿, Procrit
Func. class.: Antianemic, biologic modifier, hormone
Chem. class.: Amino acid polypeptide
Pregnancy category C

Action: Erythropoietin is one factor controlling rate of red cell production; product is developed by recombinant DNA technology

Therapeutic outcome: Decreased anemia with increased RBCs

Uses: Anemia caused by reduced endogenous erythropoietin production, primarily end-stage renal disease; to correct hemostatic defect in uremia; anemia caused by AZT (zidovudine) treatment in HIV-positive patients; anemia caused by chemotherapy; reduction of allogeneic blood transfusion in surgery patients

Unlabeled uses: Anemia in premature preterm infants

Dosage and routes
Anemia secondary to chemotherapy
Adult: SUBCUT 150 units/kg 3 ×/wk, may increase after 2 mo up to 300 units/kg 3 ×/wk

Anemia in chronic renal failure
Adult: SUBCUT/**IV** 50-100 units/kg 3 ×/wk, then adjust to maintain the target Hct of 30%-36%
Child: **IV**/SUBCUT 50 units/kg 3 ×/wk

Anemia secondary to zidovudine treatment
Adult: SUBCUT/**IV** 100 units/kg 3 ×/wk × 2 mo; may increase by 50-100 units/kg q1-2mo, up to 300 units/kg 3 ×/wk

Surgery
Adult: SUBCUT 300 units/kg/day × 10 days before surgery, the day of surgery, and for 4 days postsurgery or 600 units/kg 3, 2, 1 wk before and on day of surgery

Available forms: Inj 2000, 3000, 4000, 10,000, 20,000, 40,000 units/ml

Adverse effects
CNS: **Seizures,** coldness, sweating, headache
CV: Hypertension, **hypertensive encephalopathy, CHF,** edema, **DVT**
INTEG: Pruritus, rash, inj site reaction
MISC: Iron deficiency
MS: Bone pain
RESP: Cough

Contraindications: Hypersensitivity to mammalian cell-derived products or human albumin; uncontrolled hypertension

Precautions: Pregnancy **C,** breastfeeding, children <1 mo, seizure disorder, porphyria, CV disease, hemodialysis, latex allergy, hypertension, history of CABG; multidose preserved formulation contains benzyl alcohol and should not be used in premature infants

Black Box Warning: Hgb >12 g/dl, surgery

Pharmacokinetics

Absorption	Well absorbed (SUBCUT), completely absorbed (**IV**)
Distribution	Increased RBC count 2-6 wk
Metabolism	Unknown
Excretion	Unknown
Half-life	5-14 hr

Pharmacodynamics

	SUBCUT/IV
Onset	Unknown
Peak	Immediate
Duration	Unknown

Interactions
Drug classifications
Anticoagulants: need for increased heparin during hemodialysis

NURSING CONSIDERATIONS
Assessment
• Monitor renal studies: urinalysis, protein, blood, BUN, creatinine; I&O; report drop in output to <50 ml/hr
◆ Monitor blood studies: ferritin, transferrin monthly, transferrin sat ≥20%; ferritin ≥100 ng/ml; Hct 2 ×/wk until stabilized in target range (30%-36%), then at regular intervals; those with endogenous erythropoietin levels of <500 units/L respond to this agent; check for symptoms of anemia: fatigue, pallor, dyspnea; monitor Hct 2 ×/wk in chronic renal failure; those being treated with zidovudine or cancer patients should be monitored weekly, then periodically after stabilization; death may occur in Hgb >12 g/dl
• Assess for CNS symptoms: coldness, sweating, pain in long bones
• Assess CV status: B/P before, during treatment; hypertension may occur rapidly, leading to hypertension encephalopathy; antihypertensives may be needed
• Assess patient during hemodialysis for bruits, thrills, or shunts; product prevents severe anemia in chronic renal failure; clotting may need to be treated with increased anticoagulant
• Assess for seizures if Hct is increased within 2 wk by 4 pts
• Monitor serum iron levels, ferritin, transferrin levels; iron therapy may be needed to prevent recurring anemia
• Monitor B/P, check for rising B/P as Hct rises
• Monitor blood studies: BUN, creatinine, uric acid, platelets, WBC, phosphorus, potassium, bleeding time; Hct, Hgb, RBCs, reticulocytes should be checked in chronic renal failure
• For hypersensitivity reactions: Skin rashes, urticaria (rare), antibody development does not occur
◆ For pure cell aplasia (PRCA) in absence of other causes, evaluate by testing sera for recombinant erythropoietin antibodies; any loss of response to epoetin should be evaluated

Nursing diagnoses
• Activity intolerance (uses)
• Fatigue (uses)
• Knowledge, deficient (teaching)

Implementation
SUBCUT route
• Before injecting, preservative-free, single-dose formulation may be admixed by using 0.9% NaCl, USP, with benzyl alcohol 0.9% at a 1:1 ratio to reduce injection site discomfort
IV route
• Administer by direct route at end of dialysis by venous line, do not shake vial
• If Hct increases by 4% in 2 wk, decrease dose by 25 units/kg; increase dose if Hct does not increase by 5-6 pts after 8 wk of therapy; suggested target Hct range 30%-36%
• Give additional heparin to lower chance of clots
Solution compatibilities: Do not dilute or administer with other solutions

Patient/family education
• Teach patient how to take B/P
• Advise patients to take iron supplements, vit B₁₂, folic acid as directed
• Teach patient to avoid driving or hazardous activity during treatment
• Teach patients with renal disease to include high-iron and low-potassium foods in their diets (meat, dark green leafy vegetables, eggs, enriched breads)
• Teach patient the reason for treatment, expected results
• Advise patient to use contraception

E

Adverse effects: *italic* = common, **bold** = life-threatening

Evaluation
Positive therapeutic outcome
- Increased appetite
- Enhanced sense of well-being
- Increase in reticulocyte count in 2-6 wk, Hgb, Hct

---

eprosartan (Rx)
(ep-roh-sar'tan)
Teveten
Func. class.: Antihypertensive
Chem. class.: Angiotensin II receptor antagonist (Subtype AT_1)

Pregnancy category
C (1st trimester),
D (2nd/3rd trimesters)

Action: Blocks the vasoconstrictor and aldosterone-secreting effects of angiotensin II; selectively blocks the binding of angiotensin II to the AT_1 receptor found in tissues

Therapeutic outcome: Decreased B/P

Uses: Hypertension, alone or in combination with other antihypertensives

Dosage and routes
Adult: PO 600 mg/day; dose may be divided and given bid with total daily doses ranging from 400-800 mg

Available forms: Tabs 400, 600 mg

Adverse effects
CNS: Dizziness, depression, fatigue, headache
CV: Chest pain
EENT: Sinusitis
GI: Diarrhea, dyspepsia, abdominal pain
GU: UTI
META: Hypertriglyceridemia
MS: Myalgia, arthralgia
RESP: Cough, upper respiratory infection, rhinitis, pharyngitis, viral infection
SYST: Anaphylaxis

Contraindications: Hypersensitivity

Black Box Warning: Pregnancy **D** (2nd/3rd trimesters)

Precautions: Pregnancy **C** (1st trimester), breastfeeding, children, geriatric, hypersensitivity to ACE inhibitors, renal/hepatic disease, angioedema

Pharmacokinetics
Absorption	Absolute bioavailability ~13%; food delays absorption
Distribution	Protein binding 98%
Metabolism	Moderate renal impairment increases product levels by 30%, hepatic impairment increases levels by 40%
Excretion	Urine, feces
Half-life	5-9 hr

Pharmacodynamics
Onset	Unknown
Peak	1-2 hr
Duration	Unknown

Interactions
Drug classifications
NSAIDs, salicylates: decreased antihypertensive effect
Drug/herb
Aconite: increased toxicity, death
Astragalus, cola tree: increased or decreased antihypertensive effect
Barberry, betony, black catechu, black cohosh, bloodroot, broom, burdock, cat's claw, dandelion, goldenseal, hawthorn, Irish moss, Jamaican dogwood, kelp, khella, mistletoe, parsley: increased antihypertensive effect
Coltsfoot, guarana, khat, licorice, yohimbe: decreased antihypertensive effect
Drug/lab test
Increased: ALT, AST, alkaline phosphatase
Decreased: Hgb

NURSING CONSIDERATIONS
Assessment
- Assess B/P with position changes, pulse q4hr; note rate, rhythm, quality
- Assess electrolytes: K, Na, Cl
- Assess baselines in renal, liver function tests before therapy begins
- Assess for edema in feet, legs daily
- Assess skin turgor, dryness of mucous membranes for hydration status

Nursing diagnoses
- Fluid volume, deficient (adverse reactions)
- Injury, risk for (adverse reactions)
- Knowledge, deficient (teaching)
- Noncompliance (teaching)

Implementation
- May be given without regard to meals

Patient/family education
- Advise patient to comply with dosage schedule, even if feeling better

---

 	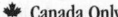	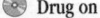

- Advise patient to notify prescriber of fever, swelling of hands or feet, chest pain
- Inform patient that excessive perspiration, dehydration, diarrhea may lead to fall in blood pressure; consult prescriber if these occur
- Inform patient that product may cause dizziness; advise to avoid hazardous activities until effect is known
- Advise patient not to take this medication if pregnant or breastfeeding, or if allergic reaction to this product has occurred
- Advise patient to take missed dose as soon as possible, unless within 1 hr of next dose

Evaluation
Positive therapeutic outcome
- Decreased B/P

! HIGH ALERT

eptifibatide (Rx)
(ep-tih-fib'ah-tide)
Integrilin
Func. class.: Antiplatelet agent
Chem. class.: Glycoprotein IIb/IIIa inhibitor

Pregnancy category B

Action: Platelet glycoprotein antagonist; reversibly prevents fibrinogen, von Willebrand's factor from binding to the glycoprotein IIb/IIIa receptor, inhibiting platelet aggregation

Therapeutic outcome: Decreased platelets

Uses: Acute coronary syndrome, including those undergoing percutaneous coronary intervention (PCI)

Dosage and routes
Acute coronary syndrome
Adult: **IV** BOL 180 mcg/kg as soon as diagnosed, max 22.6 mg; then **IV** CONT INF 2 mcg/kg/min until discharge or coronary artery bypass graft (CABG) up to 72 hr, max 15 mg/hr

PCI in patients without acute coronary syndrome
Adult: **IV** BOL 180 mcg/kg given immediately before PCI; then 2 mcg/kg/min × 18 hr and a second 180 mcg/kg BOL, 10 min after 1st BOL; continue INF for up to 18-24 hr at a rate of 1 mcg/kg/min

Renal dose
Adult: **IV** BOL CCr <50 ml/min 2-4 mg/dl same loading dose, then ½ usual INF dose

Available forms: Sol for inj 2 mg/ml (10 ml), 0.75 mg/ml (100 ml)

Adverse effects
CV: **Stroke,** hypotension
GU: Hematuria
***HEMA:* Thrombocytopenia**
SYST: **Bleeding, anaphylaxis**

Contraindications: Hypersensitivity, active internal bleeding, history of bleeding, stroke within 2 yr, major surgery with severe trauma, severe hypertension, history of intracranial bleeding, current or planned use of another parenteral GPIIb/IIIa inhibitor, dependence on renal dialysis, coagulopathy, AV malformation, aneurysm

Precautions: Pregnancy **B,** breastfeeding, children, geriatric, bleeding, renal function impairment

Pharmacokinetics	
Absorption	Unknown
Distribution	Protein binding 25%
Metabolism	Limited
Excretion	Kidneys
Half-life	1.5-2 hr

Pharmacodynamics	
Onset	Within 1 hr

Interactions
Individual drugs
Abciximab, aspirin, clopidogrel, dipyridamole, heparin, ticlopidine, valproate: increased bleeding
Drug classifications
Anticoagulants, NSAIDs, thrombolytics: increased bleeding
Platelet receptor inhibitors IIb, IIIa: do not give together
Drug/herb
Arnica, chamomile, clove, dong quai, feverfew, garlic, ginger, ginkgo, Panax ginseng

NURSING CONSIDERATIONS
Assessment
- Monitor platelets, Hgb, Hct, creatinine, pro-time/APTT baseline, INR, within 6 hr of loading dose and daily thereafter; patients undergoing PCI should have ACT monitored; maintain APTT 50-70 sec unless PCI is to be performed; during PCI, ACT should be 200-300 sec; if platelets drop <100,000/mm³, obtain additional platelet counts; if thrombocytopenia is confirmed, discontinue product; also draw Hct, Hgb, serum creatinine

- Assess for bleeding: gums, bruising, ecchymosis, petechiae; from GI, GU tract, cardiac catheter sites, IM inj sites

Nursing diagnoses
- Knowledge, deficient (teaching)
- Tissue perfusion, ineffective (uses)

Implementation
- Aspirin and heparin may be given with this product; check for bleeding
- Discontinue heparin before removing femoral artery sheath after PCI

IV route
- After withdrawing the BOL dose from 10-ml vial, give **IV** push over 1-2 min; follow BOL dose with cont inf using infusion pump, give product undiluted directly from the 100-ml vial, spike the 100-ml vial with a vented infusion set; use caution when centering the spike on the circle of the stopper top
- Do not use discolored sol or those with particulate

Y-site compatibilities: Alteplase, atropine, DOBUTamine, heparin, lidocaine, meperidine, metoprolol, midazolam, morphine, nitroglycerin, verapamil

Solution compatibilities: 0.9% NaCl, D₅/0.9% NaCl
- Discontinuing product before CABG
- Give all medications PO if possible, avoid IM inj and catheters

Patient/family education
- Teach patient to report bruising, bleeding, chest pain immediately
- Inform patient of reason for medication and expected results

Evaluation
Positive therapeutic outcome
- Decreased platelets

---

ergocalciferol
See vitamin D

---

ergonovine (Rx)
(er-goe-noe′veen)
Ergometrine, ergotrate
Func. class.: Oxytocic
Chem. class.: Ergot alkaloid

Pregnancy category Unknown

Action: Stimulates uterine and vascular smooth muscle contractions, decreases bleeding

Therapeutic outcome: Uterine contraction, decreases bleeding

Uses: Treatment of postpartum or postabortion hemorrhage

Unlabeled uses: Variant angina diagnosis

Dosage and routes
Oxytoxic
Adult: PO/SL 0.2-0.4 mg q6-12hr; IM 0.2 mg q2-4hr, max 5 doses; **IV** 0.2 mg given over 1 min

Variant angina diagnosis (unlabeled)
Adult: **IV** 50 mg q5min up to 400 mcg or until chest pain occurs

Available forms: Inj 0.2, 0.25 ✤ mg/ml; tab 0.2 mg

Adverse effects
CNS: Headache, dizziness, fainting
CV: Hypertension, chest pain
EENT: Tinnitus
GI: Nausea, vomiting, diarrhea
GU: Cramping
INTEG: Sweating
RESP: Dyspnea

Contraindications: Hypersensitivity to ergot medication, augmentation of labor, before delivery of placenta, spontaneous abortion (threatened), PID

Precautions: Renal/cardiac/hepatic disease, asthma, anemia, seizure disorders, hypertension, glaucoma, obliterative vascular disease

Pharmacokinetics

Absorption	Well absorbed (IM), completely absorbed (**IV**)
Distribution	Unknown
Metabolism	Liver
Excretion	Kidneys
Half-life	Unknown

Pharmacodynamics

	IM	IV
Onset	2-5 min	Immediate
Peak	Unknown	Unknown
Duration	3 hr	45 min

Interactions
Drug classifications
Ergots, sympathomimetics: increased hypertension
Drug/herb
Horehound: increased serotonin effect

 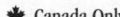

NURSING CONSIDERATIONS
Assessment
- Monitor B/P, pulse; watch for change that may indicate hemorrhage; check respiratory rate, rhythm, depth; notify prescriber of abnormalities
- Assess fundal tone, nonphasic contractions; check for relaxation or severe cramping
- Assess for ergotism or overdose: nausea, vomiting, weakness, muscular pain, insensitivity to cold, paresthesia of extremities; product should be decreased or infusion discontinued
- Before administering ergonovine, calcium levels should be checked; if hypocalcemia is present, correction should be made to increase effectiveness of this product
- Monitor prolactin levels and decreased breast milk production

Nursing diagnoses
- Injury, risk for (adverse reactions)
- Knowledge, deficient (teaching)
- Tissue perfusion, ineffective (uses)

Implementation
IM route
- Contractions begin in 2-5 min, product is given q2-4hr for contractions to continue; give deeply in large muscle mass; rotate inj sites if additional doses are given
IV route
- Give **IV** directly after dilution with 5 ml of 0.9% NaCl, give over >1 min through Y-site of free-running **IV** of 0.9% NaCl or D$_5$W
Additive compatibilities: Amikacin, cephapirin, sodium bicarbonate

Patient/family education
- Advise patient to report increased blood loss, increased temp, or foul-smelling lochia; about the need for pad count
- Inform patient that cramping is normal; pad count should be done to determine amount of bleeding
- Tell patient not to smoke during treatment to prevent excessive vasoconstriction

Evaluation
Positive therapeutic outcome
- Absence of severe bleeding

Treatment of overdose: Stop product; give vasodilators, heparin, dextran

---

ergotamine (Rx)
(er-got'a-meen)
Ergostat, Ergomar, Gynergen
dihydroergotamine
(dy-hy'droh-er-got'ah-meen)
DHE 45, Dihydroergotamine Sandoz ✤, Migranal
Func. class.: α-Adrenergic blocker, vascular headache suppressant
Chem. class.: Ergot alkaloid–amino acid

Pregnancy category X

Action: Constricts smooth muscle in peripheral, cranial blood vessels; relaxes uterine muscle; blocks serotonin release

Therapeutic outcome: Absence of headache

Uses: Vascular headache (migraine, histamine, cluster)

Dosage and routes
ergotamine
Adult: SL 1 tab (2 mg), may use q30min, max 3 tabs (6 mg)/24 hr or 10 mg/wk
dihydroergotamine
Adult: SUBCUT/IM 1 mg, may repeat in 1 hr to 3 mg, max 3 mg/day or 6 mg/wk; **IV** 0.5-1 mg, may repeat in 1 hr, max 2 mg/day or 6 mg/wk; Intranasal 1 spray in each nostril, repeat in 15 min, max 3 mg/24 hr, 4 mg/wk
Child >6 yr: SUBCUT/IM 0.5 mg, may repeat in 1 hr; **IV** 0.25 mg, may repeat in 1 hr

Severe acute migraine
Child 12-16 yr: **IV** 0.25-0.5 mg, may repeat q20min for 1-2 doses

Available forms: Ergotamine: SL tab 2 mg; tabs 1 mg; dihydroergotamine: inj 1 mg/ml; nasal spray 4 mg/ml

Adverse effects
CNS: Numbness in fingers, toes, headache, weakness
CV: Transient tachycardia, chest pain, bradycardia, edema, claudication, increase or decrease in B/P, **MI**, peripheral vascular ischemia
GI: Nausea, vomiting, diarrhea, abdominal cramps
MS: Muscle pain

Contraindications: Pregnancy **X**, hypersensitivity to ergot preparations, occlusion (peripheral, vascular), renal/hepatic disease, peptic ulcer, intermittent claudication, glaucoma, CVA

Adverse effects: *italic* = common, **bold** = life-threatening

Black Box Warning: CAD, hypertension, Raynaud's disease, peripheral vascular disease, angina

Precautions: Breastfeeding, children, geriatric, anemia, basilar/hemiplagic migraine

Black Box Warning: MI, stroke, Buerger's disease, cardiac disease

Pharmacokinetics

Absorption	Erratic (PO), poor (SL), rapidly (SUBCUT, IM)
Distribution	Crosses blood-brain barrier
Metabolism	Liver—extensively
Excretion	Kidneys (metabolites)
Half-life	Biphasic 2.7 hr, 21 hr

Pharmacodynamics

	PO	SL	IM/SUBCUT	IV
Onset	1-2 hr	Unknown	Unknown	Unknown
Peak	½-3 hr	Unknown	Unknown	¼-2 hr
Duration	Unknown	Unknown	8 hr	8 hr

Interactions
Individual drugs
Nicotine: increased vasoconstriction
Drug classifications
β-Blockers, contraceptives (oral), vasoconstrictors, other migraine agents: increased vasoconstriction
CYP450384 inhibitors (protease inhibitors, some macrolides, azole antifungals): increased ergot toxicity; do not use together
Drug/herb
Horehound: increased serotonin effect

NURSING CONSIDERATIONS
Assessment
• Assess characteristics of pain: duration, intensity, location, frequency, alleviating factors; also identify if halos, nausea, vomiting, blurred vision occur with headache; assess before, during treatment
• Assess for ergotism or overdose: nausea, vomiting, weakness, muscular pain, insensitivity to cold, paresthesia of extremities; product should be decreased or infusion discontinued
• Check for hypertension: B/P, pulse, monitor all peripheral pulses; if hypertension occurs, notify prescriber; also check for tachycardia or bradycardia

Nursing diagnoses
• Injury, risk for (adverse reactions)
• Knowledge, deficient (teaching)
• Pain, acute (uses)

Implementation
SL route
• Do not break, crush, chew, or swallow SL tab
• Place tab under tongue, do not drink, eat, or smoke until tab has dissolved
Inhalation route
• Teach patient how to use inhaler, protect ampules from heat/light
IV route
• Give dihydroergotamine undiluted over 1 min

Patient/family education
• Caution patient not to smoke during treatment to prevent excessive vasoconstriction
• Advise patient to avoid alcohol or OTC medications unless approved by prescriber
• Tell patient to inform prescriber if pregnancy occurs

Evaluation
Positive therapeutic outcome
• Decreasing headache

Treatment of overdose: Stop product, give vasodilators, heparin, dextran

---

erlotinib (Rx)
(er-loe'tye-nib)
Tarceva
Func. class.: Misc. antineoplastic
Chem. class.: Epidermal growth factor receptor inhibitor

Pregnancy category D

Action: Not fully understood. Inhibits intracellular phosphorylation of cell surface receptors associated with epidermal growth factor receptors.

Therapeutic outcome: Decrease in tumor size

Uses: Non–small cell lung cancer (NSCLC), pancreatic cancer

Unlabeled uses: Squamous cell, head and neck cancer

Dosage and routes
CYP3A4 inducers concurrently (such as rifampin or phenytoin)
Dosage increase is advised

 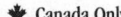

CYP3A4 inhibitors (atazanavir, clarithromycin, indinavir, itraconazole, ketoconazole, telithromycin, ritonavir, saquinavir, troleandomycin, nelfinavir)
Dosage reduction may be needed.

Non–small cell lung cancer (NSCLC)
Adult: PO 150 mg/day

Pancreatic cancer
Adult: PO 100 mg/day in combination with gemcitabine

Available forms: Tabs 25, 100, 150 mg

Adverse effects
CNS: **CVA,** anxiety, depression, headache, rigors
CV: **MI/ischemia**
EENT: Ocular changes, *conjunctivitis, eye pain*
GI: Nausea, diarrhea, vomiting, anorexia, mouth ulceration, **hepatic failure, GI perforation**
GU: **Renal impairment/failure**
HEMA: **DVT**
INTEG: **Rash, Stevens-Johnson–like skin reactions, toxic epidermal necrolysis**
MISC: Fatigue, infection
RESP: **Interstitial lung disease,** *cough, dyspnea,* **ARDs, pulmonary fibrosis**
SYST: **Hepatorenal syndrome**

Contraindications: Pregnancy **D,** breastfeeding, hypersensitivity

Precautions: Renal, hepatic; ocular, pulmonary disorders; children; geriatric

Pharmacokinetics	
Absorption	Slowly absorbed
Distribution	Unknown
Metabolism	Metabolized by CYP3A4
Excretion	Feces (86%), urine (<4%)
Half-life	36 hr

Pharmacodynamics	
Onset	Unknown
Peak	3-7 hr
Duration	Unknown

Interactions
Individual drugs
Metoprolol, warfarin: increased plasma concentrations

Drug classifications
CYP3A4 inducers (phenytoin, rifampin, carbamazepine, phenobarbital): decreased erlotinib levels
CYP3A4 inhibitors (clarithromycin, erythromycin, itraconazole, ketoconazole, telithromycin): increased erlotinib concentrations
Drug/herb
St. John's wort: decreased erlotinib levels

NURSING CONSIDERATIONS
Assessment
⬥ Assess for MI/ischemia, CVA in pancreatic cancer
⬥ Assess for pulmonary changes: lung sounds, cough, dyspnea; interstitial lung disease may occur, may be fatal; discontinue therapy if confirmed
• Assess for ocular changes: eye irritation, corneal erosion/ulcer, aberrant eyelash growth
• Assess for GI symptoms: frequency of stools; if diarrhea is poorly tolerated, therapy may be discontinued for up to 14 days
• Monitor blood studies: INR, LFTs, PT

Nursing diagnoses
• Body image, disturbed (adverse reactions)
• Infection, risk for (adverse reactions)
• Injury, risk for (adverse reactions)
• Knowledge, deficient (teaching)

Implementation
• Administer 1 hr before or 2 hr after food

Patient/family education
⬥ Teach patient to report adverse reactions immediately: SOB, severe abdominal pain, persistent diarrhea or vomiting, ocular changes, skin eruptions
• Explain reason for treatment, expected results
• Advise patient to use contraception during treatment

Evaluation
Positive therapeutic outcome
• Decrease non–small cell lung cancer cells

ertapenem (Rx)
(er-tah-pen'em)
Invanz
Func. class.: Antiinfective—miscellaneous
Chem. class.: Carbapenem
Pregnancy category B

Do not confuse:
Invanz/Aninza

E

Adverse effects: *italic* = common, **bold** = life-threatening

Action: Interferes with cell wall replication of susceptible organisms; osmotically unstable cell wall swells, bursts from osmotic pressure

Therapeutic outcome: Bactericidal action against the following organisms: *Bacteroides fragilis, Bacteroides distasonis, Bacteroides ovatus, Bacteroides thetaiotaomicron, Bacteroides uniformis; Clostridium clostridioforme, Escherichia coli, Eubacterium lentum, Haemophilus influenzae* (β lactamase–negative), *Klebsiella pneumoniae, Moraxella catarrhalis, Peptostreptococcus* sp., *Porphyromonas asaccharolytica, Prevotella bivia, Staphylococcus aureus* (methicillin-susceptible); *Streptococcus agalactiae, Streptococcus pneumoniae* (penicillin-susceptible), *Streptococcus pyogenes*

Uses: Adult patients with moderate to severe intraabdominal infections, complicated skin/skin structure infections, community-acquired pneumonia, complicated UTI, acute pelvic infections; infection prophylaxis prior to elective colorectal surgery

Dosage and routes
Complicated intraabdominal infections
Adult: IM/**IV** 1 g/day × 5-14 days
Child 3 mo-12 yr: IM/**IV** 15 mg/kg bid × 5-14 days

Complicated skin/skin structure infections
Adult: IM/**IV** 1 g/day × 7-14 days
Child 3 mo-12 yr: IM/**IV** 15 mg/kg bid × 7-14 days

Community-acquired pneumonia
Adult: IM/**IV** 1 g/day × 10-14 days
Child 3 mo-12 yr: IM/**IV** 15 mg/kg bid × 10-14 days

Complicated UTI
Adult: IM/**IV** 1 g/day × 10-14 days
Child 3 mo-12 yr: IM/**IV** 15 mg/kg bid × 10-14 days

Acute pelvic infections
Adult: IM/**IV** 1 g/day × 3-10 days
Child 3 mo-12 yr: IM/**IV** 15 mg/kg bid × 3-10 days

Surgical infection prophylaxis
Adult: **IV** 1 g as a single dose 1 hr prior to surgical incision

Available forms: Powder, lyophilized, 1 g

Adverse effects
CNS: Insomnia, **seizures**, dizziness, *headache*
CV: **Tachycardia**

GI: Diarrhea, nausea, vomiting, **pseudomembranous colitis**
GU: Vaginitis
INTEG: Rash, urticaria, *pruritus,* pain at inj site, *infused vein complication, phlebitis/thrombophlebitis,* erythema at inj site
RESP: Dyspnea, cough, pharyngitis, crackles, respiratory distress
SYST: **Anaphylaxis**

Contraindications: Hypersensitivity to this product or its components, to amide-type local anesthetics (IM only); anaphylactic reactions to β-lactams

Precautions: Pregnancy **B,** breastfeeding, children, geriatric, renal/hepatic/GI disease

Pharmacokinetics
Absorption	Almost completely absorbed (IM); completely (**IV**)
Distribution	85%-95% plasma protein bound
Metabolism	Liver (IM, **IV**)
Excretion	Urine (80%), feces (10%), breast milk (IM, **IV**)
Half-life	4 hr (**IV**)

Pharmacodynamics
	IM	IV
Onset	Unknown	Immediate
Peak	2.3 hr	Dose-dependent
Duration	Unknown	Unknown

Interactions
Individual drugs
Probenecid: increased ertapenem plasma levels; do not coadminister
Drug/herb
Acidophilus: do not use with antiinfectives; separate by several hours
Drug/lab test
Increased: hepatic enzymes

NURSING CONSIDERATIONS
Assessment
• Assess for sensitivity to carbapenem antibiotics, other β-lactam antibiotics, penicillins
• Assess for renal disease: lower dose may be required
• Assess bowel pattern daily: if severe diarrhea occurs, product should be discontinued; may indicate pseudomembranous colitis
• Assess for infection: temp, sputum, characteristics of wound before, during, after treatment
⬥ Assess for allergic reactions, anaphylaxis: rash, urticaria, pruritus; may occur a few days after therapy begins

- Assess for overgrowth of infection: perineal itching, fever, malaise, redness, pain, swelling, drainage, rash, diarrhea, change in cough or sputum

Nursing diagnoses
- Diarrhea (adverse reaction)
- Infection, risk for (uses)
- Injury, risk for (adverse reactions)
- Knowledge, deficient (teaching)
- Noncompliance (teaching)

Implementation
- Administer by **IV** or IM
- Give after C&S is taken

IM route
- Reconstitute 1 g vial of ertapenem with 3.2 ml of 1% lidocaine HCl without epinephrine, shake well
- Withdraw contents, administer deep IM in large muscle mass, use within 1 hr

IV route
- Do not co-infuse or mix with other medications; do not use diluents containing dextrose
- Reconstitute 1 g vial of ertapenem with either 10 ml of water for inj, 0.9% NaCl, or bacteriostatic water for inj
- Shake well to dissolve, transfer contents of reconstituted vial to 50 ml 0.9% NaCl inj
- Complete inf within 6 hr

Patient/family education
- Advise patient to report severe diarrhea; may indicate pseudomembranous colitis
- Advise patient to report overgrowth of infection: black, furry tongue, vaginal itching, foul-smelling stools
- Caution patient to avoid breastfeeding; product is excreted in breast milk

Evaluation
Positive therapeutic outcome
- Negative C&S, absence of signs and symptoms of infection

Treatment of overdose: Administer epinephrine, antihistamines; resuscitate if needed (anaphylaxis)

erythromycin base (Rx)
(eh-rith-roh-my'sin)
Apo Erythro ✦, E-base, E-Mycin, Eramycin, Erybid ✦, Eryc, Ery-Tab, Erythromid ✦, Erythromycin Base Filmtab, Erythromycin Delayed-Release, Novo-Rythro Encap ✦, PCE
erythromycin estolate (Rx)
Ilosone, Novo-Rythro ✦
erythromycin ethylsuccinate (Rx)
Apo-Erythro-ES ✦, EES, Ery Ped, Novo-Rythro ✦
erythromycin gluceptate (Rx)
erythromycin lactobionate (Rx)
Erythrocin
erythromycin stearate (Rx)
Apo-Erythro-S ✦, Novo-Rythro ✦
Func. class.: Antiinfective
Chem. class.: Macrolide

Pregnancy category B

Do not confuse:
erythromycin/azithromycin

Action: Binds to 50S ribosomal subunits of susceptible bacteria and suppresses protein synthesis

Therapeutic outcome: Bactericidal action against the following organisms: *Neisseria gonorrhoeae, Streptococcus pneumoniae, Mycoplasma pneumoniae, Corynebacterium diphtheriae, Bordetella pertussis, Borrelia burgdorferi, Listeria monocytogenes, Treponema pallidum;* streptococci, staphylococci; gram-negative pathogens: *Neisseria, Haemophilus influenzae* (when used with sulfonamides), *Legionella pneumophila, Chlamydia trachomatis, Entamoeba histolytica*

Uses: Mild to moderate respiratory tract, skin, soft tissue infections, Legionnaire's disease, syphilis

Dosage and routes
Soft tissue infections
Adult: PO 250-500 mg q6hr (base, estolate, stearate); PO 400-800 mg q6hr (ethylsuccinate); **IV** INF 15-20 mg/kg/day (lactobionate) divided q6hr
Child: PO 30-50 mg/kg/day in divided doses q6hr (salts); **IV** 20-40 mg/kg/day in divided doses q6hr (lactobionate), max adult dose

Adverse effects: *italic* = common, **bold** = life-threatening

N. gonorrhoeae/*PID*
Adult: **IV** 500 mg q6hr × 3 days (gluceptate, lactobionate), then PO 250 mg (base, estolate, stearate) or 400 mg (ethylsuccinate) q6hr × 1 wk

Syphilis
Adult: PO 500 mg qid × 14 days

Chlamydia
Adult: PO 500 mg q6hr × 1 wk or 250 mg qid × 2 wk
Infant: PO 50 mg/kg/day in 4 divided doses × 3 wk or more
Newborn: PO 50 mg/kg/day in 4 divided doses × 2 wk or more

Intestinal amebiasis
Adult: PO 250 mg q6hr × 10-14 days (base, estolate, stearate)
Child: PO 30-50 mg/kg/day in divided doses q6hr × 10-14 days (base, estolate, stearate)

Available forms: Base: enteric-coated tab 250, 333, 500 mg; film-coated tab 250, 500 mg; enteric-coated caps, 250, 333 mg; estolate: tabs 500 mg; caps 125, 250 mg; drops 100 mg/ml; susp 125, 250 mg/5 ml; stearate: film-coated tabs, 250 mg; ethylsuccinate: chewable tabs 200 mg; susp 100 mg/2.5 ml, 200, 400 mg/5 ml; powder for inj 500 mg, 1 g (lactobionate); 1 g (as gluceptate)

Adverse effects
CNS: **Seizures**
CV: **Dysrhythmias, QT prolongation**
EENT: Hearing loss, tinnitus
GI: Nausea, vomiting, diarrhea, **hepatotoxicity,** abdominal pain, stomatitis, heartburn, anorexia, pruritus ani, **pseudomembranous colitis**
GU: Vaginitis, moniliasis
INTEG: Rash, urticaria, pruritus, thrombophlebitis (**IV** site)
SYST: **Anaphylaxis**

Contraindications: Hypersensitivity, preexisting liver disease (estolate)

Precautions: Pregnancy **B**, breastfeeding, geriatric, hepatic/GI disease, QT prolongation, seizure disorder, myasthenia gravis

Pharmacokinetics	
Absorption	Well absorbed (PO)
Distribution	Widely distributed; minimally distributed (CSF); crosses placenta
Metabolism	Liver, partially
Excretion	Bile, unchanged; kidneys (minimal), unchanged
Half-life	1-3 hr

Pharmacodynamics		
	PO	IV
Onset	1 hr	Rapid
Peak	4 hr	Infusion's end
Duration	Unknown	Unknown

Interactions
Individual drugs
Alfentanil, alprazolam, bromocriptine, busPIRone, carbamazepine, cilostazol, clindamycin, clopazine, cycloSPORINE, diazepam, digoxin, disopyramide, felodipine, methylPREDNISolone, midazolam, quinidine, rifabutin, sildenafil, tacrolimus, tadalafil, theophylline, triazolam, vardenafil, vinBLAStine, warfarin: increased toxicity, increased action
Diltiazem, itraconazole, ketoconazole, nefazodone, pimozide, sparfloxacin, verapamil: increased serious dysrhythmias, do not use together

Drug classifications
Ergots: increased action, toxicity
HMG-CoA reductase inhibitors: increased action, toxicity
Protease inhibitors: serious dysrhythmias
Drug/herb
Acidophilus: do not use with antiinfectives
Drug/lab test
Increased: AST/ALT
Decreased: folate assay
False increase: 17-OHCS/17-KS

NURSING CONSIDERATIONS
Assessment
• Assess patient for previous sensitivity reaction
• Assess patient for signs and symptoms of infection including characteristics of wounds, sputum, urine, stool, WBC >10,000/mm^3, earache, fever; obtain baseline information before, during treatment
• Obtain C&S test results before beginning product therapy to identify if correct treatment has been initiated
• Assess for allergic reactions: rash, urticaria may occur a few days after therapy begins
• Identify urine output; if decreasing, notify prescriber (may indicate nephrotoxicity); also monitor increases in BUN, creatinine
• Monitor blood studies: AST, ALT, CBC, Hct, bilirubin, LDH, alkaline phosphatase, Coombs' test monthly if patient is on long-term therapy
• Monitor electrolytes: potassium, sodium, chloride monthly if patient is on long-term therapy

- Assess bowel pattern daily; if severe diarrhea occurs, product should be discontinued
- Assess for overgrowth of infection: perineal itching, fever, malaise, redness, pain, swelling, drainage, rash, diarrhea, change in cough, sputum

Nursing diagnoses
- Diarrhea (adverse reactions)
- Infection, risk for (uses)
- Injury, risk for (adverse reactions)
- Knowledge, deficient (teaching)
- Noncompliance (teaching)

Implementation
PO route
- Give around the clock on an empty stomach, at least 1 hr before or 2 hr after meals; may be taken with food if GI upset occurs; do not take with juices; take dose with a full glass of water; use calibrated measuring device for drops or susp; shake well
- Store susp in refrigerator
- Chewable tab may be crushed or chewed, not swallowed whole
- Do not crush or chew enteric-coated tab

IV route
- Add 10 ml of sterile water for inj without preservatives to 250- or 500-mg vials and 20 ml to 1-g vial; sol is stable for 1 wk after reconstitution if refrigerated

Intermittent IV infusion
- Dilute further in 100-250 ml of 0.9% NaCl or D₅W
- Give over 20-60 min to avoid phlebitis; assess for pain along vein; slow inf if pain occurs; apply ice to site and notify prescriber if unable to relieve pain

Continuous infusion
- May also be administered as an inf in a dilution of 1 g/L of 0.9% NaCl, D₅W, over 4 hr

Syringe incompatibilities: Heparin

Additive compatibilities: Calcium gluconate, hydrocortisone, lidocaine, methicillin, penicillin G potassium, potassium chloride, sodium bicarbonate

Additive incompatibilities: Aminophylline, cephapirin, pentobarbital, secobarbital, streptomycin, tetracycline

Erythromycin lactobionate
Syringe compatibilities: Methicillin

Syringe incompatibilities: Ampicillin, heparin

Y-site compatibilities: Acyclovir, amiodarone, cyclophosphamide, enalaprilat, esmolol, famotidine, foscarnet, hydromorphone, idarubicin, labetalol, lorazepam, magnesium sulfate, meperidine, midazolam, morphine, multivitamins, perphenazine, vit B/C, zidovudine

Y-site incompatibilities: Fluconazole

Additive compatibilities: Aminophylline, ampicillin, cimetidine, diphenhydrAMINE, hydrocortisone, lidocaine, methicillin, penicillin G potassium, penicillin G sodium, pentobarbital, polymyxin B, potassium chloride, prednisoLONE, prochlorperazine, promazine, ranitidine, sodium bicarbonate, verapamil

Additive incompatibilities: Cephalothin, colistimethate, floxacillin, furosemide, heparin, metaraminol, metoclopramide, tetracycline, vit B/C

Patient/family education
- Teach patient to report sore throat, bruising, bleeding, joint pain; may indicate blood dyscrasias (rare)
- Advise patient to contact prescriber if vaginal itching, loose foul-smelling stools, furry tongue occur; may indicate super infection
- Instruct patient to take all medication prescribed for the length of time ordered

Evaluation
Positive therapeutic outcome
- Absence of signs/symptoms of infection (WBC <10,000/mm³, temp WNL, absence of red, draining wounds, earache)
- Reported improvement in symptoms of infection

Treatment of overdose: Withdraw product, maintain airway, administer epinephrine, aminophylline, O₂, **IV** corticosteroids

erythromycin ophthalmic
See Appendix B

erythromycin topical
See Appendix B

escitalopram (Rx)
(es-sit-tal'oh-pram)
Lexapro
Func. class.: Antidepressant, selective serotonin reuptake inhibitor

Pregnancy category C

Action: Inhibits CNS neuron uptake of serotonin but not of norepinephrine

Therapeutic outcome: Decreased symptoms of depression

Uses: General anxiety disorder; major depressive disorder in adults/adolescents

Unlabeled uses: Panic disorder, social phobia

Dosage and routes

Adult: PO 10 mg/day in AM or PM; after 1 wk if no clinical improvement is noted, dose may be increased to 20 mg/day PM; maintenance 10-20 mg/day; reassess to determine need for treatment

Geriatric/hepatic dose: PO 10 mg/day

Available forms: Tabs 5, 10, 20 mg; oral sol 5 mg (as base)/5 ml (contains sorbitol)

Adverse effects

CNS: Headache, nervousness, insomnia, drowsiness, anxiety, tremor, dizziness, fatigue, sedation, poor concentration, abnormal dreams, agitation, **seizures,** apathy, euphoria, hallucinations, delusions, psychosis, **neuroleptic malignant syndrome–like reactions**

CV: Hot flashes, palpitations, angina pectoris, **hemorrhage,** hypertension, **tachycardia,** 1st-degree AV block, **bradycardia, MI, thrombophlebitis,** postural hypotension

EENT: Visual changes, ear/eye pain, photophobia, tinnitus

GI: Nausea, diarrhea, dry mouth, anorexia, dyspepsia, constipation, cramps, vomiting, taste changes, flatulence, decreased appetite

GU: Dysmenorrhea, decreased libido, urinary frequency, UTI, amenorrhea, cystitis, impotence, urine retention

INTEG: Sweating, rash, pruritus, acne, alopecia, urticaria, photosensitivity

MS: Pain, arthritis, twitching

RESP: Infection, pharyngitis, nasal congestion, sinus headache, sinusitis, cough, dyspnea, bronchitis, asthma, hyperventilation, pneumonia

SYST: Asthenia, viral infection, fever, allergy, chills

Contraindications: Hypersensitivity

Precautions: Pregnancy **C,** breastfeeding, geriatric, renal/hepatic disease, history of seizures

Black Box Warning: Children ≤12 yr/ adolescents, suicidal ideation

Pharmacokinetics

Absorption	Unknown
Distribution	Unknown
Metabolism	Liver
Excretion	Urine
Half-life	Unknown

Pharmacodynamics

Unknown

Interactions

Individual drugs

Alcohol: increased CNS depression

Amantadine, bromocriptine, busPIRone, lithium, tryptophan: increased serotonin syndrome

BusPIRone: increased symptoms of OCD

Carbamazepine, lithium, phenytoin, warfarin: increased levels or toxicity of each specific product

Cyproheptadine: decreased escitalopram effect

Diazepam: increased half-life of diazepam

Haloperidol: increased effect of haloperidol

Drug classifications

Antidepressants, amphetamines: increased serotonin syndrome

Antidepressants, opioids, sedatives: increased CNS depression

Antidysrhythmics, antipsychotics: increased levels, toxicity

Highly protein-bound products: increased side effects of escitalopram

MAOIs: do not use with or 14 days before escitalopram

NSAIDs, salicylates: increased bleeding risk

Phenothiazines: increased levels of phenothiazines

Tricyclics: increased levels of tricyclics

Drug/herb

Corkwood, jimsonweed: increased anticholinergic effect

Hops, kava, lavender: increased CNS effect

SAM-e, St. John's wort: do not use together

Yohimbe: increased hypertension

Drug/lab test

Increased: serum bilirubin, blood glucose, alkaline phosphatase

Decreased: VMA, 5-HIAA

False increase: urinary catecholamines

NURSING CONSIDERATIONS
Assessment

- Assess mental status: mood, sensorium, affect, suicidal tendencies, increase in psychiatric symptoms, depression, panic
- Assess appetite in bulimia nervosa, weight

 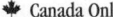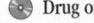

daily, increase nutritious foods in diet, watch for bingeing and vomiting
- Assess allergic reactions: itching, rash, urticaria; product should be discontinued; may need to give antihistamine
- Monitor B/P (lying/standing), pulse q4hr; if systolic B/P drops 20 mm Hg, hold product, notify prescriber; take VS q4hr in patients with cardiovascular disease
- Monitor blood studies: CBC, leukocytes, differential, cardiac enzymes if patient is receiving long-term therapy; check platelets; bleeding can occur
- Monitor liver function tests: AST, ALT, bilirubin, creatinine; thyroid function studies
- Monitor weight qwk; appetite may decrease with product
- Monitor ECG for flattening of T wave, bundle branch, AV block, dysrhythmias in cardiac patients
- Monitor alcohol consumption; if alcohol is consumed, hold dose until AM

Nursing diagnoses
- Coping, ineffective (uses)
- Injury, risk for (uses/adverse reactions)
- Knowledge, deficient (teaching)

Implementation
- Give with food or milk for GI symptoms; give with full glass of water
- Give crushed if patient is unable to swallow medication whole
- Give dosage at bedtime if oversedation occurs during the day
- Give gum, hard candy, frequent sips of water for dry mouth
- Oral sol: measure with calibrated device
- Store at room temperature; do not freeze
- Provide assistance with ambulation during therapy, because drowsiness, dizziness occur
- Provide safety measures primarily in geriatric
- Check to see if PO medication swallowed

Patient/family education
- Teach that therapeutic effect may take 1-4 wk
- Advise to use caution in driving, other activities requiring alertness because of drowsiness, dizziness, blurred vision
- Advise to use sunscreen to prevent photosensitivity
- Advise to avoid alcohol ingestion, other CNS depressants
- Advise patient to notify prescriber if pregnant or plan to become pregnant or breastfeed
- Advise patient to change positions slowly; orthostatic hypotension may occur
- Teach to avoid all OTC products unless approved by prescriber
- Teach patient to report immediately signs of urinary retention
- Teach patient that clinical worsening and suicide risk may occur
- Teach using MedGuide provided
- Teach about drug interactions

Evaluation
Positive therapeutic outcome
- Decreased depression

Treatment of overdose: Activated charcoal, supportive care

esmolol (Rx)
(ez'moe-lole)
Brevibloc
Func. class.: β-Adrenergic blocker (antidysrhythmic II)

Pregnancy category C

Do not confuse:
esmolol/Osmitrol, Brevibloc/Brevital

Action: Competitively blocks stimulation of β_1-adrenergic receptors in the myocardium; produces negative chronotropic, inotropic activity (decreases rate of SA node discharge, increases recovery time), slows conduction of AV node, decreases heart rate, decreases O_2 consumption in myocardium; also decreases renin-aldosterone-angiotensin system at high doses; inhibits β_2-receptors in bronchial system at higher doses

Therapeutic outcome: Decreased supraventricular tachycardia

Uses: Supraventricular tachycardias, non-compensatory sinus tachycardia, hypertensive crisis, intraoperative and postoperative tachycardia and hypertension

Dosage and routes
Adult: **IV** Loading dose 500 mcg/kg/min over 1 min; maintenance 50 mcg/kg/min for 4 min; if no response in 5 min, give 2nd loading dose; then increase INF to 100 mcg/kg/min for 4 min; if no response, repeat loading dose, then increase maintenance INF by 50 mcg/kg/min (max of 200 mcg/kg/min); titrate to patient response
Child: **IV** A total loading dose of 600 mcg/kg over 2 min, maintenance **IV** INF 200 mcg/kg/min, titrate upwards by 50-100 mcg/kg/min q5-10min until B/P, heart rate reduced by >10%

Available forms: Inj 10 mg, 250 mg/ml

Adverse effects: *italic* = common, **bold** = life-threatening

Adverse effects

CNS: Confusion, light-headedness, paresthesia, somnolence, fever, dizziness, fatigue, headache, depression, anxiety, **seizures**

CV: Hypotension, bradycardia, chest pain, peripheral ischemia, shortness of breath, CHF, conduction disturbances 1st-, 2nd-, 3rd-degree heart block

GI: *Nausea,* vomiting, anorexia, gastric pain, flatulence, constipation, heartburn, bloating

GU: Urinary retention, impotence, dysuria

INTEG: *Induration, inflammation at inj site,* discoloration, edema, erythema, burning, pallor, flushing, rash, pruritus, dry skin, alopecia

RESP: **Bronchospasm,** dyspnea, cough, wheezing, nasal stuffiness, **pulmonary edema**

Contraindications: Heart block (2nd- or 3rd-degree), cardiogenic shock, CHF, cardiac failure, hypersensitivity, severe bradycardia

Precautions: Pregnancy **C**, breastfeeding, geriatric patients, hypotension, peripheral vascular disease, diabetes, hypoglycemia, thyrotoxicosis, renal disease, atrial fibrillation, bronchospasms, hyperthyroidism

Black Box Warning: Abrupt discontinuation

Pharmacokinetics

Absorption	Complete
Distribution	Unknown
Metabolism	Liver
Excretion	Kidneys
Half-life	9 min

Pharmacodynamics

Onset	Rapid
Peak	Unknown
Duration	1-2 min

Interactions
Individual drugs

Amphetamine, ephedrine, epinephrine, norepinephrine, phenylephrine, pseudoephedrine: increased α-adrenergic stimulation

Digoxin: increased digoxin levels

Thyroid hormones: decreased effect of esmolol, decreased action of thyroid hormone

Drug classifications

MAOIs: avoid use

Drug/herb

Aloe, buckthorn, cascara sagrada, senna: increased hypokalemia

Betel palm, butterbur, cola tree, figwort, fumitory, guarana, hawthorn, lily of the valley, motherwort, plantain: increased β-blocking effect

Coenzyme Q10, yohimbe: decreased β-blocking effect

Jamborandi tree: increased CV reactions

Drug/lab test

Interference: glucose/insulin tolerance test

NURSING CONSIDERATIONS
Assessment
- Monitor B/P during beginning treatment, periodically thereafter; pulse q4hr; note rate, rhythm, quality; apical/radial pulse before administration; notify prescriber of any significant changes (pulse <50 bpm)
- Check for baselines in renal, liver function tests before therapy begins
- Assess for edema in feet, legs daily, monitor I&O, daily weight; check for jugular vein distention, crackles bilaterally, dyspnea (CHF)
- Monitor skin turgor, dryness of mucous membranes for hydration status, especially geriatric

Nursing diagnoses
- Cardiac output, decreased (uses)
- Injury, risk for (adverse reactions)
- Knowledge, deficient (teaching)
- Noncompliance (teaching)

Implementation
- Give by intermittent inf after diluting 5 g/500 ml of D_5W, 0.9% NaCl, D_5/0.45% NaCl, D_5/LR, D_5/0.9% NaCl, 0.45% NaCl, LR (10 mg/ml)
- Give loading dose over 1 min, then maintenance dose over 4 min, may repeat loading dose q5min with increased maintenance dose; maintenance dose max 200 mcg/kg/min administered up to 48 hr; dosage should be tapered at a rate of 25 mcg/kg/min
- Store at room temperature for 24 hr; sol should be clear

Y-site compatibilities: Amikacin, aminophylline, ampicillin, amiodarone, atracurium, butorphanol, calcium chloride, cefazolin, cefmetazole, cefoperazone, ceftazidime, ceftizoxime, chloramphenicol, cimetidine, cisatracurium, clindamycin, diltiazem, DOPamine, enalaprilat, erythromycin, famotidine, fentanyl, gentamicin, heparin, hydrocortisone, regular insulin, labetalol, magnesium sulfate, methyldopate, metronidazole, midazolam, morphine, nafcillin, nitroglycerin, norepinephrine, nitroprusside, pancuronium, penicillin G potassium, phenytoin, piperacillin, polymyxin B, potassium chloride, potassium phosphate, propofol, ranitidine, remifentanil, streptomycin, tacrolimus, tobramycin,

trimethoprim/sulfamethoxazole, vancomycin, vecuronium
Y-site incompatibilities: Furosemide
Additive compatibilities: Aminophylline, atracurium, bretylium, heparin
Additive incompatibilities: Diazepam, procainamide, sodium bicarbonate, thiopental

Patient/family education
- Teach patient need for medication and expected results
- Caution patient to rise slowly to prevent orthostatic hypotension
- Advise patient to notify if pain, swelling occurs at **IV** site

Evaluation
Positive therapeutic outcome
- Absence of dysrhythmias

Treatment of overdose: Defibrillation, vasopressor for hypotension

---

esomeprazole (Rx)
(es'oh-mep'rah-zohl)
Nexium
Func. class.: Anti-ulcer, proton pump inhibitor
Chem. class.: Benzimidazole
Pregnancy category B

Action: Suppresses gastric secretion by inhibiting hydrogen/potassium ATPase enzyme system in the gastric parietal cell; characterized as gastric acid pump inhibitor, since it blocks final step of acid production

Therapeutic outcome: Absence of duodenal ulcers; decreased gastroesophageal reflux

Uses: Gastroesophageal reflux disease (GERD), severe erosive esophagitis; treatment of active duodenal ulcers in combination with antiinfectives for *Helicobacter pylori* infection; long-term use in hypersecretory conditions

Dosage and routes
Active duodenal ulcers associated with H. pylori
Adult: PO 40 mg/day × 10 days in combination with clarithromycin 500 mg bid × 10 days and amoxicillin 1000 mg bid × 10 days

Hepatic dose
Adult: PO/**IV** max 20 mg/day (severe hepatic disease)

GERD/erosive gastritis
Adult: PO 20 or 40 mg/day × 4-8 wk; no adjustment needed in renal, liver failure, geriatric; **IV** 20 or 40 mg/day up to 10 days

Child and adolescent 12-17 yr: PO 20-40 mg/day 1 hr before meals up to 8 wk
Child 1-11 yr: PO 10 mg/day 1 hr before meals for up to 8 wk

Available forms: Del rel caps 20, 40 mg; powder for **IV** inj 20, 40 mg/vial; del rel powder for oral susp 20, 40 mg

Adverse effects
CNS: Headache, dizziness
GI: Diarrhea, flatulence, abdominal pain, constipation, dry mouth, **hepatic failure, hepatitis**
INTEG: Rash, dry skin
MISC: **Heart failure**
RESP: Cough, **pneumonia**
SYST: **Stevens-Johnson syndrome, toxic epidermal necrolysis, exfoliative dermatitis**

Contraindications: Hypersensitivity

Precautions: Pregnancy **B**, breastfeeding, children, geriatric

Pharmacokinetics
Absorption	Unknown
Distribution	97% plasma protein bound
Metabolism	Liver (metabolites)
Excretion	Urine (metabolites), feces (metabolites); in geriatric, elimination rate decreased, bioavailability increased
Half-life	1-1½ hr

Pharmacodynamics
Onset	Unknown
Peak	1½ hr
Duration	Unknown

Interactions
Individual drugs
Calcium carbonate, dapsone, indinavir, iron, itraconazole, ketoconazole, vitamin B_{12}: decreased effect
Diazepam, digoxin, penicillins: increased effect, toxicity

NURSING CONSIDERATIONS
Assessment
- Assess GI system: bowel sounds q8hr, abdomen for pain, swelling, anorexia
- Assess hepatic enzymes: AST, ALT, alkaline phosphatase during treatment

Nursing diagnoses
- Knowledge, deficient (teaching)
- Pain, acute (uses)
- Pain, chronic (uses)

Adverse effects: *italic* = common, **bold** = life-threatening

Implementation
- Swallow caps whole; do not break, crush, or chew
- Administer at least 1 hr before eating

Patient/family education
- Instruct patient to report severe diarrhea; product may have to be discontinued
- Advise diabetic patients that hypoglycemia may occur
- Advise patient to avoid hazardous activities; dizziness may occur
- Advise patient to avoid alcohol, salicylates, ibuprofen; may cause GI irritation

Evaluation
Positive therapeutic outcome
- Absence of epigastric pain, swelling, fullness

---

estradiol (Rx)
(ess-tra-dye'ole)
Estrace
estradiol cypionate (Rx)
depGynogen, Depo-Estradiol, Depogen, Dura-Estrin, E-Cypionate, Estragyn LAS, Estro-Cyp, Estrofem, Estroject-LA, Estro-L.A.
estradiol topical emulsion (Rx)
Estrasorb
estradiol valerate (Rx)
Clinagen LA, Delestrogen, Dioval, Duragan, Estra-L, Estro-span, Femogex ♣, Gynogen LA, Menaval, Valergen
estradiol transdermal system (Rx)
Alora, Climara, Esclim, Estraderm, FemPatch, Vivelle
estradiol vaginal tablet (Rx)
Vagifem
estradiol vaginal ring (Rx)
Estring
estradiol gel (Rx)
Divigel, Elestrin
estradiol spray (Rx)
Evamist
Func. class.: Estrogen, progestin
Chem. class.: Nonsteroidal synthetic estrogen

Pregnancy category X

Action: Needed for adequate functioning of female reproductive system; affects release of pituitary gonadatropins, inhibits ovulation, promotes adequate calcium use in bone structure

Therapeutic outcome: Decreased tumor size in prostatic cancer; increased estrogen levels in menopause, female hypogonadism

Uses: Vasomotor symptoms associated with menopause, inoperable breast cancer (selected cases), prostatic cancer, atrophic vaginitis, kraurosis vulvae, hypogonadism, primary ovarian failure, prevention of osteoporosis, castration

Dosage and routes
Hormone replacement/menopause symptoms
Adult: Transdermal 0.05-0.1 mg/24 hr apply 2 ×/wk; GEL apply entire unit dose packet to 5 × 7-inch area of upper thigh daily, alternate thighs; Spray 1 spray to inner surface of forearm daily in AM

Menopause/hypogonadism/castration/ovarian failure
Adult: PO 1-2 mg/day 3 wk on, 1 wk off or 5 days on, 2 days off; IM 1-5 mg q3-4wk (cypionate), 10-20 mg q4wk (valerate); TOP Estraderm 0.05 mg/24 hr applied 2 ×/wk, Climara 0.05 mg/hr applied 1 ×/wk in a cyclic regimen; women with hysterectomy may use continuously

Prostatic cancer
Adult: IM 30 mg q1-2wk (valerate); PO 1-2 mg tid (oral estradiol)

Breast cancer
Adult: PO 10 mg tid × 3 mo or longer

Atropic vaginitis/kraurosis vulvae
Adult: VAG cream 2-4 g/day × 1-2 wk, then 1 g 1-3 ×/wk cycled; VAG tab 1/day × 2 wk, maintenance 1 tab 2 ×/wk; VAG ring inserted and left in place continuously for 3 mo

Vasomotor symptoms
Adult: TOP after cleaning and drying skin on left thigh, calf, rub in contents of pouch using both hands until completely absorbed; wash hands

Available forms: Estradiol: tabs 0.5, 1, 2 mg; valerate: inj 10, 20, 40 mg/ml; transdermal 0.025, 0.0375, 0.05, 0.075, 0.1 mg/24-hr release rate; vag cream 100 mcg/g; vag ring 2 mg/90 days; vag tab 25 mcg; topical emulsion: 2.5 mg; gel 0.1% (Divigel); spray (Evamist) 1.53 mg/acuation

Adverse effects
CNS: Dizziness, headache, migraine, depression, **seizures**

CV: Hypertension, thrombophlebitis, edema, **thromboembolism, stroke, pulmonary embolism, MI,** chest pain
EENT: Contact lens intolerance, increased myopia, astigmatism, throat swelling, eyelid edema
GI: Nausea, vomiting, diarrhea, anorexia, pancreatitis, cramps, constipation, increased appetite, increased weight, **cholestatic jaundice, hepatic adenoma**
GU: Amenorrhea, cervical erosion, breakthrough bleeding, dysmenorrhea, vaginal candidiasis, breast changes, *gynecomastia, testicular atrophy, impotence,* **increased risk of breast, endometrial cancer,** changes in libido; **toxic shock, vaginal wall ulceration/erosion (vag ring)**
INTEG: Rash, urticaria, acne, hirsutism, alopecia, oily skin, seborrhea, purpura, melasma
META: Folic acid deficiency, hypercalcemia, hyperglycemia

Contraindications: Pregnancy **X,** breastfeeding, reproductive cancer, genital bleeding (abnormal, undiagnosed)

Black Box Warning: Breast/endometrial cancer, thromboembolic disorders, MI, stroke

Precautions: Hypertension, asthma, blood dyscrasias, gallbladder disease, CHF, diabetes mellitus, bone disease, depression, migraine headache, seizure disorders, renal/hepatic disease, family history of cancer of breast or reproductive tract, smoking, uterine fibroids, vaginal irritation/infection

Black Box Warning: Cardiac disease, dementia

Pharmacokinetics

Absorption	Well absorbed
Distribution	Widely distributed, crosses placenta
Metabolism	Unknown
Excretion	Unknown
Half-life	Unknown

Pharmacodynamics

	PO	IM	IV
Onset	Rapid	Slow	Rapid
Peak	Unknown	Unknown	Unknown
Duration	Unknown	Unknown	Unknown

Interactions
Individual drugs
Calcium, phenylbutazone, rifampin: decreased estradiol action

CycloSPORINE, dantrolene: increased toxicity
Tamoxifen: decreased tamoxifen action
Drug classifications
Anticoagulants: decreased action of anticoagulants
Anticonvulsants, barbiturates: decreased estradiol action
Corticosteroids: increased action of corticosteroids
Hypoglycemics (oral): decreased action of hypoglycemics
Drug/herb
Alfalfa, hops: increased estrogen effect
Black cohosh, DHEA: altered estrogen effect
Saw palmetto, St. John's wort: decreased estrogen effect
Drug/food
Grapefruit juice: increased estrogen level
Drug/lab test
Increased: BSP retention test; PBI; T_4; serum sodium; platelet aggregation; thyroxine-binding globulin (TBS); prothrombin; factors VII, VIII, IX, X; triglycerides
Decreased: serum folate, serum triglyceride, T_3 resin uptake test, glucose tolerance test, antithrombin III, pregnanediol, metyrapone test
False positive: LE prep, ANA titer

NURSING CONSIDERATIONS
Assessment
• Monitor blood glucose in patient with diabetes; hyperglycemia may occur
• Monitor B/P q4hr; watch for increase caused by water and sodium retention
• Monitor I&O ratio; be alert for decreasing urinary output and increasing edema; monitor weight daily; notify prescriber if weekly weight gain is >5 lb; if increased, diuretic may be ordered
• Obtain liver function tests baseline, periodically, including AST, ALT, bilirubin, alkaline phosphatase, periodic folic acid level
• Assess edema, hypertension, cardiac symptoms, jaundice
• Assess mental status: affect, mood, behavioral changes, aggression; depression may occur, product may need to be discontinued
• Assess female patient for intact uterus; if so, progesterone should be added to estrogen therapy to decrease risk of endometrial cancer

Nursing diagnoses
• Injury, risk for (adverse reactions)
• Sexual dysfunction (uses)

Implementation
PO route
- Give titrated dose, use lowest effective dose
- Give with food or milk to decrease GI symptoms

IM route
- Administer deeply in large muscle mass; product is painful
- Rotate syringe to mix oil and medication

Transdermal route
- Apply to area free of hair to ensure adhesion on trunk of body 2 ×/wk; press firmly and hold in place for 10 sec to ensure good contact
- Start transdermal dose 7 days before last PO dose if routes are to be changed

Topical route spray (Evamist)
- Use daily; spray to inner upper arm; may increase to 2-3 ×/day based on response; let dry for 2 min

Vaginal route
- Place cream in applicator by attaching tube to applicator; squeeze cream into tube to mark; insert with patient reclining
- Applicator should be washed after each use

Patient/family education
- Tell patient to take exactly as prescribed; do not double doses
- ◆ Advise patient that increased weight gain and symptoms of fluid retention should be reported to prescriber: edema of feet, ankles, sacral area; abnormal vaginal bleeding; breast lumps; hepatic disease (dark urine, clay-colored stools, jaundice of skin, sclera, pruritus); to report dermal rash with transdermal patch
- ◆ Caution patient that thromboembolic symptoms should be reported: tenderness in legs, chest pain, dyspnea, headaches, blurred vision
- Inform patient to use sunscreen and protective clothing because sunburns may occur
- Advise patient to stop smoking; smokers have a greater chance of thromboembolic disorder
- Tell patient to use nonhormonal birth control and to notify prescriber if pregnancy is suspected

Evaluation
Positive therapeutic outcome
- Reversal of menopausal symptoms
- Decrease in tumor size in prostatic or breast cancer
- Decrease in itching, inflammation of vagina
- Absence of symptoms of osteoporosis

---

estrogens, conjugated
☺ (Rx)
Cenestin, C.E.S ✦, Congest, Premarin, Premphase

estrogens, conjugated synthetic B (Rx)
Enjuvia

Pregnancy category X

Do not confuse:
Premarin/Provera

Action: Needed for adequate functioning of female reproductive system; affects release of pituitary gonadotropins; inhibits ovulation; promotes adequate calcium use in bone structures

Therapeutic outcome: Decreased tumor size in prostatic cancer; increased estrogen levels in menopause, female hypogonadism

Uses: Symptoms associated with menopause, inoperable breast cancer, prostatic cancer, abnormal uterine bleeding, hypogonadism, primary ovarian failure, prevention of osteoporosis

Dosage and routes
Estrogens, conjugated
Menopause
Adult: PO 0.3-1.25 mg/day 3 wk on, 1 wk off

Prevention of osteoporosis
Adult: PO 0.625 mg/day or in a cycle

Atrophic vaginitis
Adult: VAG cream 2-4 g/day × 21 days, off 7 days, repeat

Prostatic cancer
Adult: PO 1.25-2.5 mg tid

Advanced inoperable breast cancer
Adult: PO 10 mg tid × 3 mo or longer

Abnormal uterine bleeding
Adult: **IV**/IM 25 mg, repeat in 6-12 hr

Primary ovarian failure
Adult: PO 1.25 mg/day 3 wk on, 1 wk off

Hypogonadism
Adult: PO 2.5-7.5 mg/day × 20 days/mo

Estrogens, conjugated synthetic B
Menopause
Adult: PO 0.625 mg/day initially, may increase based on response

Available forms: Tabs 0.3, 0.45, 0.625, 0.9, 1.25, 2.5 mg; inj 25 mg/vial; vag cream 0.625 mg/g; synthetic B: tabs 0.625, 1.25 mg

---

Adverse effects

CNS: Dizziness, headache, migraine, depression, **seizures,** mood disturbances

CV: Hypertension, thrombophlebitis, edema, **thromboembolism, stroke, pulmonary embolism, MI,** chest pain

EENT: Contact lens intolerance, increased myopia, astigmatism

GI: *Nausea,* vomiting, diarrhea, anorexia, pancreatitis, cramps, constipation, increased appetite, **cholestatic jaundice, hepatic adenoma,** weight gain/loss

GU: Amenorrhea, cervical erosion, breakthrough bleeding, dysmenorrhea, vaginal candidiasis, breast changes, *gynecomastia, testicular atrophy, impotence,* **increased risk of breast, endometrial cancer,** libido changes

INTEG: Rash, urticaria, acne, hirsutism, alopecia, oily skin, seborrhea, purpura, melasma

META: Folic acid deficiency, hypercalcemia, hyperglycemia

Contraindications: Pregnancy **X,** breastfeeding, thromboembolic disorders, reproductive cancer, genital bleeding (abnormal, undiagnosed), hypersensitivity

Black Box Warning: Endometrial cancer

Precautions: Hypertension, asthma, blood dyscrasias, gallbladder disease, CHF, diabetes mellitus, bone disease, depression, migraine headache, seizure disorders, renal/hepatic disease, family history of cancer of breast or reproductive tract, smoking, dementia, hypothyroidism, obesity, SLE

Black Box Warning: Cardiac disease, dementia

Pharmacokinetics

Absorption	Well absorbed (PO), completely absorbed **(IV)**
Distribution	Widely distributed, crosses placenta
Metabolism	Liver—exclusively; hepatic recirculation
Excretion	Kidney
Half-life	Unknown

Pharmacodynamics

	PO	IM	IV
Onset	Rapid	Slow	Immediate
Peak	Unknown	Unknown	Unknown
Duration	Unknown	Unknown	Unknown

Interactions

Individual drugs

CycloSPORINE, dantrolene: increased toxicity

Phenylbutazone, rifampin: decreased action of estrogens

Tamoxifen: decreased tamoxifen action

Drug classifications

Anticoagulants: decreased action of anticoagulants

Anticonvulsants, barbiturates: decreased action of estrogens

Corticosteroids: increased action of corticosteroids

Oral hypoglycemics: decreased action of hypoglycemics

Drug/herb

Alfalfa, hops: increased estrogen level

Black cohosh, DHEA: altered estrogen effect

Saw palmetto, St. John's wort: decreased estrogen level

Drug/food

Grapefruit juice: increased estrogen level

Drug/lab test

Increased: BSP retention test; PBI, T_4; serum sodium; platelet aggregation; thyroxine-binding globulin (TBG); prothrombin; factors VII, VIII, IX, X; triglycerides

Decreased: serum folate, serum triglyceride, T_3 resin uptake test, glucose tolerance test, antithrombin III, pregnanediol, metyrapone test

False positive: LE prep, ANA titer

NURSING CONSIDERATIONS

Assessment

• Monitor blood glucose in patient with diabetes; hyperglycemia may occur

• Monitor B/P q4hr; watch for increase caused by water and sodium retention

• Monitor I&O ratio; be alert for decreasing urinary output and increasing edema; monitor weight daily; notify prescriber if weekly weight gain is >5 lb; if increased, diuretic may be ordered

• Obtain liver function tests, including AST, ALT, bilirubin, alkaline phosphatase

• Assess edema, hypertension, cardiac symptoms, jaundice

• Assess mental status: affect, mood, behavioral changes, aggression; depression may occur; product may need to be discontinued

• Assess female patient for intact uterus; if so, progesterone should be added to estrogen therapy to decrease risk of endometrial cancer; abnormal uterine bleeding, breast exam

E

Nursing diagnoses
- Injury, risk for (adverse reactions)
- Sexual dysfunction (uses)

Implementation
PO route
- Give titrated dose, use lowest effective dose
- Give in 1 dose in AM for prostatic cancer, vaginitis, hypogonadism
- Give with food or milk to decrease GI symptoms

IM route
- Reconstitute after withdrawing at least 5 ml of air from container and inject sterile diluent on vial side, rotate to dissolve
- Give IM inj deeply in large muscle

Vaginal route
- Place cream in applicator by attaching tube to applicator, squeeze cream into tube to mark, insert with patient recumbent
- Applicator should be washed after each use

IV, direct route
- Reconstitute as for IM, inject into distal port of running **IV** line of D₅W, 0.9% NaCl, LR, at a rate of 5 mg/min or less

Y-site compatibilities: Heparin/hydrocortisone, potassium chloride, vit B/C

Patient/family education
- Caution patient to take exactly as prescribed and not to double doses
- ◆ Advise patient that increased weight gain and symptoms of fluid retention should be reported to prescriber: edema of feet, ankles, sacral area; abnormal vaginal bleeding; breast lumps; hepatic disease (dark urine, clay-colored stools, jaundice of skin, sclera, pruritus)
- ◆ Caution patient that thromboembolic symptoms should be reported: pain, redness, tenderness in legs; chest pain, dyspnea, headaches, blurred vision
- Inform patient that sunburns may occur and to use sunscreen and protective clothing
- Advise patient to stop smoking; smokers have a greater chance of thromboembolic disorder
- Tell patient to use nonhormonal birth control, and to notify prescriber if pregnancy is suspected
- Tell patient that vasomotor symptoms improve in 2 wk, max relief 8 wk

Evaluation
Positive therapeutic outcome
- Reversal of menopause symptoms
- Decrease in tumor size in prostatic, breast cancer
- Decrease in itching, inflammation of vagina
- Absence of symptoms of osteoporosis

---

eszopiclone (Rx)
(es-zop'i-klone)
Lunesta
Func. class.: Sedative/hypnotic, non-benzodiazepine
Chem. class.: Cyclopyrrolone

Pregnancy category C

Controlled substance schedule IV

Action: Interacts with GABA receptors

Therapeutic outcome: Ability to sleep and stay asleep throughout the night

Uses: Insomnia

Dosage and routes
Adult: PO 2 mg immediately before bed, may increase to 3 mg if needed

Hepatic dose/CYP3A4 inhibitors
Adult: PO 1 mg immediately before bed in severe hepatic disease

Available forms: Tabs 1, 2, 3 mg

Adverse effects
CNS: Worsening depression, hallucinations, headache, daytime drowsiness, **suicidal thoughts/actions**, migraine, restlessness, anxiety, sleep driving, sleep walking
CV: Peripheral edema, chest pain
GI: Dry mouth, bitter taste (dysgeusia)
GU: Gynecomastia, dysmenorrhea
INTEG: Rash, **angioedema**

Contraindications: Hypersensitivity, ethanol intoxication

Precautions: Pregnancy C, breastfeeding, children, geriatric, severe hepatic disease

Pharmacokinetics
Absorption	Unknown
Distribution	Unknown
Metabolism	Extensively in the liver by CYP3A4, CYP2E1, protein binding 52%-59%
Excretion	Via kidneys
Half-life	6 hr, geriatric 9 hr

Pharmacodynamics
Onset	Rapid
Peak	1 hr
Duration	6 hr

Interactions
Drug classifications
CNS depressants: increased CNS depression
CYP3A4 inhibitors (clarithromycin, itraconazole, ketoconazole, nefazodone, nelfinavir,

ritonavir, troleandomycin): increased toxicity due to decreased eszopiclone elimination
Drug/food
High-fat meal: decreased product action

NURSING CONSIDERATIONS
Assessment
- Assess sleep pattern: ability to go to sleep, stay asleep; early morning awakenings; conservative methods used
- Monitor for abuse of this or other products

Nursing diagnoses
- Injury, risk for (adverse reactions)
- Knowledge, deficient (teaching)
- Sleep deprivation (uses)

Implementation
- Do not break, crush, or chew tab
- Give immediately before bedtime
- Avoid use with a high fat meal

Patient/family education
- Caution patient that daytime drowsiness may occur; not to engage in hazardous activities until effect is known
- Advise patient that all other medications and supplements should be avoided unless approved by prescriber
- Advise patient to notify prescriber if pregnancy is suspected or planned

Evaluation
Positive therapeutic outcome
- Ability to sleep and stay asleep throughout the night

---

etanercept (Rx)
(eh-tan'er-sept)
Enbrel
Func. class.: Antirheumatic agent (disease-modifying)

Pregnancy category B

Action: Binds to tumor necrosis factor (TNF), which decreases inflammation and immune response

Therapeutic outcome: Decreased pain, inflammation

Uses: Acute, chronic rheumatoid arthritis that has not responded to other disease-modifying agents; polyarticular course juvenile rheumatoid arthritis (JRA), ankylosing spondylitis, plaque psoriasis, psoriatic arthritis

Unlabeled uses: Crohn's disease

Dosage and routes
Rheumatoid/psoriatic arthritis, ankylosing spondylitis
Adult: SUBCUT 50 mg qwk
Child 2-17 yr: SUBCUT 0.8 mg/kg/wk, max 50 mg/wk

Plaque psoriasis
Adult: SUBCUT 50 mg 2 ×/wk × 3 mo
Adolescent and child 4-17 yr (unlabeled): SUBCUT 0.8 mg/kg/wk, max 50 mg/wk

Juvenile rheumatoid arthritis (JRA)
Adolescent and child 2-17 yr:
SUBCUT 0.8 mg/kg/wk, max 50 mg/wk

Available forms: Powder for inj 25 mg; inj 50 mg/ml; auto injector, single use

Adverse effects
CNS: Headache, asthenia, dizziness
GI: Abdominal pain, dyspepsia, vomiting
HEMA: Pancytopenia, **anemia, thrombocytopenia, leukopenia, neutropenia**
INTEG: Rash, *inj site reaction,* keratoderma blenorrhagicum
RESP: Pharyngitis, rhinitis, *cough, URI,* non-URI sinusitis
SYST: **Serious infections, sepsis, death, malignancies**

Contraindications: Sepsis, active infections

Black Box Warning: Hypersensitivity to this product, latex, benzyl alcohol

Precautions: Pregnancy **B**, breastfeeding, children <4 yr, geriatric, malignancies, CHF

Black Box Warning: Infection

Pharmacokinetics

Absorption	Rapidly (60%)
Distribution	Unknown
Metabolism	Unknown
Excretion	Unknown
Half-life	115 hr

Pharmacodynamics
Unknown

Interactions
Individual drugs
Anakinra, cyclophosphamide: avoid use
Drug classifications
Immunizations: should be brought up to date before treatment
Immunizations, vaccines: do not give concurrently

Adverse effects: *italic* = common, **bold** = life-threatening

NURSING CONSIDERATIONS
Assessment
- Assess for pain of rheumatoid arthritis; check ROM, inflammation of joints, characteristics of pain
- Assess inj site for pain, swelling; usually occurs after 2 inj (4-5 days)

Nursing diagnoses
- Injury, risk for (side effects)
- Knowledge, deficient (teaching)
- Mobility, impaired physical (uses)
- Pain, chronic (uses)

Implementation
- Administer after reconstituting 1 ml of supplied diluent, slowly inject diluent into vial; swirl contents, do not shake; sol should be clear/colorless, do not use if cloudy or discolored
- Do not admix with other sol or medications; do not use filter
- May be injected SUBCUT into upper arm, abdomen, thigh; rotate inj sites

Patient/family education
- Teach patient that product must be continued for prescribed time to be effective; to avoid aspirin, alcoholic beverages
- Instruct patient to use caution when driving; dizziness may occur
- Teach patient about self-administration, if appropriate: inj should be made in thigh, abdomen, upper arm; rotate sites at least 1 in from old site

Evaluation
Positive therapeutic outcome
- Decreased pain in arthritic conditions
- Decreased inflammation in arthritic conditions

---

ethambutol (Rx)
(e-tham'byoo-tole)
Etibi ✤, Myambutol
Func. class.: Antitubercular
Chem. class.: Diisopropylethylene diamide derivative

Pregnancy category B

Do not confuse:
ethambutol/Ethmozine

Action: Inhibits RNA synthesis, decreases tubercle bacilli replication

Therapeutic outcome: Resolution of TB infection

Uses: Pulmonary TB, as an adjunct, other mycobacterial infections

Dosage and routes
Adult and child >13 yr: PO 15-25 mg/kg/day as a single dose or 50 mg/kg 2 ×/wk or 25-30 mg/kg 3 ×/wk

Renal dose
Adult: PO CCr 10-50 ml/min dose q24-36hr; CCr <10 ml/min dose q48hr

Retreatment
Adult: PO 25 mg/kg/day as single dose × 2 mo with at least 1 other product, then decrease to 15 mg/kg/day as single dose, max 2.5 g/day
Child: PO 15 mg/kg/day

Available forms: Tabs 100, 400 mg

Adverse effects
CNS: *Headache, confusion,* fever, malaise, dizziness, *disorientation,* hallucinations
EENT: Blurred vision, optic neuritis, photophobia, decreased visual acuity
GI: *Abdominal distress, anorexia, nausea, vomiting*
INTEG: Dermatitis, pruritus, **toxic epidermal necrolysis,** erythema multiforme
META: *Elevated uric acid, acute gout,* liver function impairment
MISC: **Thrombocytopenia,** joint pain, bloody sputum, **anaphylaxis**

Contraindications: Hypersensitivity, optic neuritis, child <13 yr

Precautions: Pregnancy **B,** breastfeeding, renal disease, diabetic retinopathy, cataracts, ocular defects, hepatic and hematopoietic disorders

Pharmacokinetics
Absorption	Rapidly absorbed
Distribution	Widely distributed, crosses blood-brain barrier, placenta
Metabolism	Liver
Excretion	Kidneys—unchanged
Half-life	3 hr, increased in liver, kidney disease

Pharmacodynamics
Onset	Rapid
Peak	2-4 hr
Duration	Unknown

Interactions
Individual drugs
Ethionamide: increased adverse reactions
Drug classifications
Aluminum, antacids: decreased absorption
Neurotoxic agents, other: increased neurotoxicity

 Alert   ✤ Canada Only   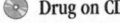 Drug on CD   * "Tall Man" lettering (See Preface)

NURSING CONSIDERATIONS
Assessment
- Obtain C&S tests including sputum tests before initiating treatment; monitor qmo to detect resistance
- Monitor liver function tests qwk × 2 wk, then q2mo: ALT, AST, bilirubin; renal studies: before, qmo: BUN, creatinine, output, specific gravity, urinalysis, uric acid
- Assess patient's mental status often: affect, mood, behavioral changes; psychosis may occur with hallucinations, confusion
- Assess patient's hepatic status: decreased appetite, jaundice, dark urine, fatigue
- Assess patient for visual disturbance that may indicate optic neuritis: blurred vision, change in color perception; may lead to blindness

Nursing diagnoses
- Diarrhea (adverse reactions)
- Infection, risk for (uses)
- Knowledge, deficient (teaching)
- Noncompliance (teaching)
- Sensory perception, disturbed (adverse reactions)

Implementation
- Give with meals to decrease GI symptoms, at same time each day to maintain blood level
- Give 2 hr before antacids
- Give antiemetic if vomiting occurs

Patient/family education
- Advise patient that compliance with dosage schedule and duration is necessary to eradicate disease; to keep scheduled appointments including ophthalmic appointments or relapse may occur
- Caution patient to report weakness, fatigue, loss of appetite, nausea, vomiting, yellowing of skin or eyes, tingling/numbness of hands/feet, weight gain, or decreased urine output
- Instruct patient to report any visual changes; rash; hot, swollen, painful joints; numbness or tingling of extremities to physician
- Caution patient to inform prescriber if pregnancy is suspected

Evaluation
Positive therapeutic outcome
- Decreased symptoms of TB
- Decrease in acid-fast bacteria

etidronate (Rx)
(eh-tih-droe′nate)
Didronel
Func. class.: Bone resorption inhibitor
Chem. class.: Bisphosphonate

Pregnancy category C

Do not confuse:
etidronate/etomidate/etretinate

Action: Decreases bone resorption and new bone development (accretion)

Therapeutic outcome: Decreased bone reabsorption, calcium levels WNL

Uses: Paget's disease, heterotopic ossification, hypercalcemia of malignancy

Dosage and routes
Paget's disease
Adult: PO 5-10 mg/kg/day, 2 hr before meals with water, max 20 mg/kg/day, max 6 mo or 11-20 mg/kg/day for max of 3 mo

Heterotopic ossification
Adult: PO 20 mg/kg/day × 2 wk, then 10 mg/kg/day for 10 wk, total 12 wk

Hypercalcemia
Adult: **IV** 7.5 mg/kg/day × 3 days, then 20 mg/kg/day (PO)

Heterotopic ossification/hip replacement
Adult: PO 20 mg/kg/day × 4 wk before and 3 mo after surgery (4 months total)

Available forms: Tabs 200, 400 mg

Adverse effects
CNS: Headache
CV: **Atrial fibrillation**
GI: Nausea, constipation, gastritis, esophagitis
GU: **Nephrotoxicity**
MISC: Dyspnea; low magnesium, phosphorus, alopecia, **Stevens-Johnson syndrome, angioedema**
MS: Bone pain, hypocalcemia, decreased mineralization of nonaffected bones, **osteonecrosis of the jaw,** arthralgia, leg cramps

Contraindications: Clinically overt osteomalacia

Precautions: Pregnancy **C,** breastfeeding, children, renal disease, restricted vit D, calcium, colitis, vitamin D deficiency, anemia, esophagitis, pathologic fractures, asthma, coagulopathy, dental disease, GERD, hiatal hernia, hyperparathyroidism, infection, phosphate hypersensitivity, severe renal disease with creatinine >5 mg/dl, poor dentition

E

Adverse effects: *italic* = common, **bold** = life-threatening

Pharmacokinetics

Absorption	Poorly absorbed (PO), completely absorbed (**IV**)
Distribution	50% bond to crystals in osteogenesis
Metabolism	None
Excretion	Feces (unabsorbed), kidney (unchanged)
Half-life	5-7 hr; in bone >3 mo

Pharmacodynamics

	PO	IV
Onset	4 wk	24 hr
Peak	Unknown	3-4 days
Duration	Up to 1 yr	10-12 days

Interactions
Individual drugs
Warfarin: increased protime
Drug classifications
Aluminum, antacids, calcium, iron products, or mineral supplements with magnesium: decreased absorption of etidronate
Drug/food
Dairy products: decreased absorption of etidronate

NURSING CONSIDERATIONS
Assessment
• Assess for GI symptoms, polyuria, flushing, head swelling, tingling, headache; may indicate hypercalcemia; nervousness, irritability, twitching, seizures, spasm, paresthesia: indicates hypocalcemia at start of treatment
• Identify nutritional status; evaluate diet for sources of vit D (milk, some seafood), calcium (dairy products, dark green vegetables), phosphates
• Monitor BUN, creatinine, alk phos, calcium, phosphate, urinalysis (calcium: should be kept at 9-10 mg/dl), albumin, alkaline phosphatase baseline and q3-6mo; check urine sediment for casts throughout treatment
• Assess for bone pain, weakness during treatment
• Assess for increased product level; toxic reactions occur rapidly; have calcium chloride or gluconate on hand if calcium level drops too low; check for tetany
• Assess for dental health

Nursing diagnoses
• Injury, risk for (adverse reactions)
• Knowledge, deficient (teaching)
• Pain, chronic (uses)

Implementation
PO route
• Administer on empty stomach to improve absorption (2 hr before meals); avoid simultaneous vitamins/minerals, antacids with calcium, iron, magnesium, or aluminum
IV route
• Used in hypercalcemias; give by intermittent inf after diluting 300 mg/250 ml or more 0.9% NaCl; run over 2-3 hr, therapy should not last >6 mo

Patient/family education
• Teach method of inj if patient will be responsible for self-medication
• Caution patient to notify prescriber if hypercalcemia recurs: renal calculi, nausea, vomiting, thirst, lethargy, deep bone or flank pain, heat over bone, restricted mobility
• Teach patient that warmth and flushing occur and last 1 hr
• Teach patient to follow a low-calcium diet as prescribed (Paget's disease, hypercalcemia)
• Advise patient to notify prescriber of diarrhea, nausea; dose may be divided to lessen these symptoms
• Inform patient that metallic taste may occur with **IV** dosing
• Advise patient to continue with good hygiene

Evaluation
Positive therapeutic outcome
• Calcium levels 9-10 mg/dl
• Decreasing symptoms of Paget's disease including pain
• Decreased bone loss in osteoporosis

---

etodolac (Rx)
(ee-toe-doe'lak)
Lodine, Lodine XL
Func. class.: Nonsteroidal antiinflammatory, nonopioid analgesic

Pregnancy category C

Do not confuse:
Lodine/codeine/iodine

Action: Inhibits prostaglandin synthesis by decreasing enzyme needed for biosynthesis; analgesic, antiinflammatory properties

Therapeutic outcome: Decreased pain, inflammation

Uses: Mild to moderate pain, osteoarthritis

Dosage and routes
Osteoarthritis
Adult: PO 800-1200 mg/day in divided doses q6-8hr initially, then adjust to 600-1200

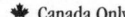

mg/day in divided doses; max 1200 mg/day; patients <60 kg max 20 mg/kg

Analgesia
Adult: PO 200-400 mg q6-8hr prn for acute pain; max 1200 mg/day; patients <60 kg max 20 mg/kg

Available forms: Caps 200, 300 mg; tabs 400, 500 mg; ext rel tabs 400, 600 mg

Adverse effects
CNS: Dizziness, headache, drowsiness, fatigue, tremors, confusion, insomnia, anxiety, depression, light-headedness, vertigo
CV: Tachycardia, peripheral edema, fluid retention, palpitations, dysrhythmias, CHF
EENT: Tinnitus, hearing loss, blurred vision, photophobia
GI: Nausea, anorexia, vomiting, diarrhea, jaundice, **cholestatic hepatitis,** constipation, flatulence, cramps, dry mouth, peptic ulcer, dyspepsia, **GI bleeding**
GU: **Nephrotoxicity, dysuria, hematuria, oliguria, azotemia, cystitis, UTI**
HEMA: **Blood dyscrasias**
INTEG: Erythema, urticaria, purpura, rash, pruritus, sweating, **Stevens-Johnson syndrome**
SYST: **Angioedema, anaphylaxis**

Contraindications: Hypersensitivity; patients in whom aspirin, iodides, or other NSAIDs have produced asthma, rhinitis, urticaria, nasal polyps, angioedema, bronchospasm; avoid in 2nd half of pregnancy

Precautions: Pregnancy **C,** breastfeeding, children, geriatric, bleeding, GI/cardiac/renal/hepatic disorders

Pharmacokinetics	
Absorption	Well absorbed
Distribution	Highly bound to plasma protein
Metabolism	Unknown
Excretion	Unknown
Half-life	7 hr

Pharmacodynamics	
Onset	½ hr
Peak	1-2 hr
Duration	4-12 hr

Interactions
Individual drugs
Aspirin: may increase GI toxicity
CycloSPORINE, digoxin, lithium, methotrexate, phenytoin: increased toxicity

Drug classifications
Antacids: delayed etodolac effect
β-Adrenergic blockers: decreased effect
Diuretics: decreased effectiveness of diuretics
Drug/herb
Arginine, gossypol: increased gastric irritation
Bearberry, bilberry: increased NSAIDs action
Bogbean, chondroitin, saw palmetto, turmeric: increased bleeding risk
St. John's wort: severe photosensitivity

NURSING CONSIDERATIONS
Assessment
• Assess pain: location, frequency, characteristics; relief after medication
• Assess for GI bleeding: black stools, hematemesis
• Assess for asthma, aspirin hypersensitivity, nasal polyps that may be hypersensitive to etodolac
• Monitor blood counts during therapy; watch for decreasing platelets; if low, therapy may need to be discontinued, then restarted after hematologic recovery; watch for blood dyscrasia (thrombocytopenia): bruising, fatigue, bleeding, poor healing

Nursing diagnoses
• Injury, risk for (adverse reactions)
• Knowledge, deficient (teaching)
• Mobility, impaired physical (uses)
• Pain, acute (uses)
• Pain, chronic (uses)

Implementation
• Do not break, crush, or chew ext rel tabs
• Administer with full glass of water to enhance absorption
• Administer with food or milk to decrease gastric symptoms; food will slow absorption slightly, will not decrease absorption

Patient/family education
• Inform patient that product must be continued for prescribed time to be effective; to avoid aspirin, alcoholic beverages, NSAIDs
• Caution patient to report bleeding, bruising, fatigue, malaise because blood dyscrasias can occur
• Instruct patient to use caution when driving; drowsiness, dizziness may occur
• Teach patient to take with a full glass of water to enhance absorption

Evaluation
Positive therapeutic outcome
• Decreased pain
• Decreased inflammation
• Increased mobility

⚠ HIGH ALERT

etoposide (Rx)
(e-toe′poe-side)
Toposar, VP-16
etoposide phosphate (Rx)
Etopophos
Func. class.: Antineoplastic—miscellaneous
Chem. class.: Semisynthetic podophyllotoxin

Pregnancy category D

Action: Inhibits mitotic activity through metaphase to mitosis; also inhibits cells from entering mitosis, depresses DNA, RNA synthesis, cell cycle specific S and G_2, binds to a complex of DNA and topoisomerase II

Therapeutic outcome: Prevention of rapid growth of malignant cells

Uses: Leukemias, small cell carcinoma of the lung, testicular cancer

Unlabeled uses: Lymphomas

Dosage and routes
Testicular cancer
Adult: IV 50-100 mg/m²/day × 5 days given q3-5wk or 200-250 mg/m²/wk, or 125-140 mg/m²/day 3 × wk, q5wk

Small cell carcinoma of the lung
Adult: PO 70 mg/m²/day × 4 days, repeated q3-4wk; **IV** 35 mg/m²/day × 4 days, up to 50 mg/m²/day × 5 day q3-4wk

Available forms: Inj 20 mg/ml, caps 50 mg

Adverse effects
CNS: Headache, *fever,* peripheral neuropathy, paresthesia, confusion
CV: Hypotension, **MI,** dysrhythmia
GI: Nausea, vomiting, anorexia, **hepatotoxicity,** dyspepsia, diarrhea, constipation
GU: Nephrotoxicity
HEMA: **Thrombocytopenia, leukopenia, myelosuppression, anemia**
INTEG: Rash, alopecia, phlebitis at **IV** site, radiation recall, **Stevens-Johnson syndrome**
RESP: **Bronchospasm,** pleural effusion
SYST: **Anaphylaxis**

Contraindications: Pregnancy **D,** breastfeeding, hypersensitivity, severe renal/hepatic disease

Precautions: Children, renal/hepatic disease, gout

Black Box Warning: Bone marrow depression, infection, bleeding

Pharmacokinetics
Absorption	Variably absorbed
Distribution	Rapidly absorbed, 97% protein binding, crosses placenta
Metabolism	Liver—some
Excretion	Kidneys, unchanged 50%, breast milk
Half-life	3 hr initially, 15 hr terminally

Pharmacodynamics
Unknown

Interactions
Individual drugs
Radiation: increased bone marrow depression
Drug classifications
Antineoplastics: increased bone marrow depression
Live virus vaccines: increased adverse reactions

NURSING CONSIDERATIONS
Assessment
• Monitor B/P (baseline and q15min) during administration
• Monitor CBC, differential, platelet count weekly; withhold product if WBC is <4000/mm³ or platelet count is <75,000/mm³; notify prescriber of results; recovery will take 3 wk
• Monitor renal function tests: BUN, urine CCr before, during therapy; I&O ratio; report fall in urine output of 30 ml/hr; for decreased hyperuricemia
• Monitor for cold, fever, sore throat (may indicate beginning of infection); notify prescriber if these occur
• Assess for bleeding: hematuria, guaiac, bruising or petechiae, mucosa or orifices q8hr; no rectal temp; avoid IM inj; use pressure to venipuncture sites
• Identify nutritional status: an antiemetic may need to be prescribed
◆ Assess for symptoms indicating severe allergic reactions: rash, pruritus, urticaria, itching, flushing, bronchospasm, hypotension; epinephrine and crash cart should be nearby

Nursing diagnoses
• Body image, disturbed (adverse reactions)
• Infection, risk for (adverse reactions)
• Injury, risk for (adverse reactions)
• Knowledge, deficient (teaching)

Implementation
PO route
• Caps need to be refrigerated

IV route
- Give by intermittent inf
- Sol should be prepared by qualified personnel and only under controlled conditions
- Use Luer-Lok tubing to prevent leakage; do not let sol come in contact with skin; if contact occurs, wash well with soap and water
- Give after diluting 100 mg/250 ml or more D₅W or NaCl to a concentration of 0.2-0.4 mg/ml; infuse over 30-60 min; phosphate may be given over 5 min-3½ hr; may dilute further to 0.1 mg/ml in 0.9% NaCl, D₅W
- Give hyaluronidase 150 units/ml to 1 ml NaCl to infiltration area; ice compress for treatment of vesicant activity

Y-site compatibilities: Allopurinol, amifostine, aztreonam, cladribine, fludarabine, granisetron, melphalan, ondansetron, paclitaxel, piperacillin/tazobactam, sargramostim, sodium bicarbonate, teniposide, thiotepa, vinorelbine

Y-site incompatibility: Idarubicin

Additive compatibilities: Carboplatin, cisplatin, cytarabine, floxuridine, fluorouracil, hydrOXYzine, ifosfamide, ondansetron

Patient/family education
- Teach patient to avoid use of products containing aspirin or ibuprofen, razors, commercial mouthwash because bleeding may occur; to report symptoms of bleeding (hematuria, tarry stools)
- Instruct patient to report signs of anemia (fatigue, headache, irritability, faintness, shortness of breath)
- Teach patient to report any changes in breathing or coughing even several months after treatment
- Advise patient that contraception will be necessary during treatment because teratogenesis may occur
- Caution patient that hair loss may occur during treatment; a wig or hairpiece may make patient feel better; new hair will be different in color, texture
- Advise patient to avoid vaccinations during treatment because serious reactions may occur
- Teach patient to report signs/symptoms of infection: fever, chills, sore throat; patient should avoid crowds and persons with known infections

Evaluation
Positive therapeutic outcome
- Decreased spread of malignant, leukemic cells

etravirine (Rx)
(e-tra'veer-een)
Intelence
Func. class.: Antiretroviral
Chem. class.: Non-nucleoside reverse transcriptase inhibitor (NNRTI)

Pregnancy category B

Action: Binds directly to reverse transcriptase, blocking the RNA- and DNA-dependent DNA polymerase action, causing a disruption of the enzyme's catalytic site

Therapeutic outcome: Increased CD4 count, decrease viral load

Uses: In combination with other antiretroviral agents for HIV infection in treatment-experienced patients with evidence of HIV replication despite ongoing antiretroviral therapy

Dosages and routes
Adult: PO 200 mg bid after a meal, max 400 mg/day; not established in treatment-naïve patients

Available forms: Tabs 100 mg

Adverse effects
CNS: Headache, insomnia, amnesia, anxiety, confusion, fatigue, nightmares, peripheral neuropathy, **seizures, stroke,** tremor
CV: **Atrial fibrillation,** hypertension, MI
EENT: Blurred vision
GI: Nausea, vomiting, diarrhea, anorexia, abdominal pain, increased AST/ALT, constipation, flatulence, gastritis, GERD, **hematemesis, hepatitis,** hepatomegaly, **pancreatitis**
GU: **Renal failure**
HEMA: **Hemolytic anemia, neutropenia, thrombocytopenia, anemia**
INTEG: Rash, erythema multiforme, **angioedema, Stevens-Johnson syndrome**
OTHER: Diabetes mellitus, gynecomastia, hyperamylasemia, hypercholesterolemia, hyperglycemia, hyperlipidemia
RESP: Dyspnea, **bronchospasm**

Contraindications: Hypersensitivity, breastfeeding

Precautions: Pregnancy **B,** impaired hepatic function, children, antimicrobial resistance, geriatric patients, hepatitis, hypercholesterolemia, hypertriglycerides, immune reconstitution syndrome

Pharmacokinetics

Absorption	Unknown
Distribution	Plasma protein binding 99.9%
Metabolism	By CYP3A4, 2C9, 2C19
Excretion	Feces
Half-life	21-61 hr

Pharmacodynamics
Unknown

Interactions
Individual drugs
Amiodarone, atazanavir, clarithromycin, flecainide, fosamprenavir, lidocaine, mexiletine, propafenone, quinidine, sildenafil, tadalafil, vardenafil: decreased levels

Atazanavir, carbamazepine, delavirdine, fosamprenavir, fosphenytoin, phenytoin, phenobarbital, rifapentine, rifampin, tipranavir: do not use concurrently

Bepridil, darunavir, dexamethasone, disopyramide, efavirenz, nevirapine, ritonavir, saquinavir, tipranavir: decreased etravirine levels

CycloSPORINE, sirolimus, tacrolimus: altered effect

Diazepam, rifampin, voriconazole, warfarin: increased levels

Fluconazole, itraconazole, ketoconazole, lopinavir, posaconazole, ritonavir, voriconazole: increased etravirine levels

Methadone: increased withdrawal symptoms

Drug classifications
HMG-CoA reductase inhibitors: increased myopathy, rhabdomyolysis

Drug/herb
St. John's wort: decreased etravirine

NURSING CONSIDERATIONS
Assessment
• Assess symptoms of HIV and for possible infections; increased temp

🔷 Monitor for fatal hypersensitivity reactions: fever, rash, nausea, vomiting, fatigue, cough, dyspnea, diarrhea, abdominal discomfort; treatment should be discontinued and not restarted

• Assess blood dyscrasias (anemia, granulocytopenia): bruising, fatigue, bleeding, poor healing

• Monitor renal studies: BUN, serum uric acid, CCr before, during therapy; these may be elevated throughout treatment

• Monitor hepatic studies before, during therapy: bilirubin, AST, ALT, amylase, alk phos, creatine phosphokinase, creatinine, qmo

• Monitor blood counts q2wk; monitor viral load and CD4 counts during treatment; watch for decreasing granulocytes, Hgb; if low, therapy may have to be discontinued and restarted after hematologic recovery; blood transfusions may be required

• Monitor cholesterol/lipid profile during treatment

Nursing diagnoses
• Infection, risk for (uses)
• Knowledge, deficient (teaching)

Implementation
• Give in combination with other antiretrovirals with food

• Store in cool environment; protect from light

Patient/family education
• Inform patient that product is not a cure but will control symptoms; patient is still infective, may pass AIDS virus on to others

• Instruct patient to notify prescriber of sore throat, swollen lymph nodes, malaise, fever; other infections may occur; to stop product and notify prescriber immediately if skin rash, fever, cough, shortness of breath, GI symptoms occur; advise all health care providers that allergic reaction has occurred with etravirine

• Advise patient that follow-up visits must be continued since serious toxicity may occur; blood counts must be done

• Instruct patient to use contraception during treatment; still able to transmit disease

• Give patient Medication Guide and Warning Card, discuss points on guide

• Inform patient that other products may be necessary to prevent other infections

• Advise patient to take medication following a meal

Evaluation
Positive therapeutic outcome
• Increased CD4 count, decrease viral load

---

everolimus (Rx)
(e-ve-ro′-li-mus)
Affinitor
Func. class.: Antineoplastic (miscellaneous)
Chem. class.: Immunosuppressant, macrolide

Pregnancy category D

Action: Proliferation signal inhibitor that inhibits mammalian target of rapamycin (mTOR); this pathway is dysregulated in cancer

---

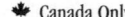

Uses: Renal cell cancer in those with failed treatment with suritinib or sorafenib

Therapeutic outcome: Decreasing tumor size, spread of malignancy

Dosage and routes
Adult: PO 10 mg qd as long as clinically beneficial; with strong 3A4 inducers 10 mg qd, may increase by 5-mg increments to 20 mg qd

Hepatic dose
Adult: PO (Child-Pugh B) 5 mg qd; not to be used in Child-Pugh C

Available forms: Tabs 5, 10 mg

Adverse effects
CNS: Headache, insomnia, paresthesia, chills, fever
CV: Hypertension, *CHF,* peripheral edema
EENT: Blurred vision, photophobia
GI: Nausea, vomiting, diarrhea
GU: **Renal failure**
HEMA: **Anemia, leukopenia, thrombocytopenia**
INTEG: Rash, acne
META: Hyperglycemia, increased creatinine, *hyperlipemia,* hyperphosphatemia, weight loss
RESP: **Pleural effusion,** *dyspnea*

Contraindications: Breastfeeding; hypersensitivity to this product, rapamine, and torisel

Precautions: Pregnancy **D,** children <13 yr, renal/hepatic disease, diabetes mellitus, infection, hyperlipidemia, plural effusion

Pharmacokinetics	
Absorption	Rapid
Distribution	Protein binding 74%
Metabolism	Extensively by CYP3A4
Excretion	Unknown
Half-life	30 hr, reduced by high fat meal

Pharmacodynamics	
Onset	Unknown
Peak	1-2 hr
Duration	Unknown

Interactions
Individual drugs
Cimetidine, cyclosporine, danazol, erythromycin: increased blood levels of these products
Carbamazepine, phenobarbital, phenytoin, rifamycin, rifapentine: decreased blood levels of everolimus

Drug classifications
Antifungals, calcium channel blockers, HIV-protease inhibitors: increased blood levels of these products
Vaccines: decreased effect
Drug/herb
St. John's wort: may decrease the effect of everolimus
Drug/food
Alters bioavailability; use consistently with or without food; do not use with grapefruit juice

NURSING CONSIDERATIONS
Assessment
• Monitor lipid profile: cholesterol, triglycerides, a lipid-lowering agent may be needed; blood glucose
⬥ Monitor blood studies: Hgb, WBC, platelets during treatment qmo; if leukocytes <3000/mm^3 or platelets <100,000/mm^3, product should be discontinued or reduced; decreased hemoglobulin level may indicate bone marrow suppression
• Monitor hepatic studies: alk phos, AST, ALT, amylase, bilirubin, and for hepatotoxicity: dark urine, jaundice, itching, light-colored stools; product should be discontinued

Nursing Diagnoses
• Injury, risk for (adverse reactions)
• Infection, risk for (adverse reactions)
• Knowledge, deficient (teaching)

Implementation
• Swallow tabs whole with a full glass of water; do not chew, crush, or break
• Take at same time of day
• Follow procedure for proper handling of antineoplastics
• Give all medications PO if possible, avoiding IM inj; bleeding may occur
• Store protected from light, at room temperature

Patient/family education
• Advise to report fever, rash, severe diarrhea, chills, sore throat, fatigue; serious infections may occur; clay-colored stools, cramping (hepatotoxicity)
• Advise to avoid crowds, persons with known infections to reduce risk of infection
• Teach to use contraception before, during, and 12 wk after product has been discontinued; avoid breastfeeding
• Advise not to use with grapefruit juice
• Inform to avoid vaccines
• Advise to take up to 6 hr after normally scheduled time if dose is missed

E

Adverse effects: italic = common, **bold** *= life-threatening*

- Advise that product may decrease male/female fertility
- Teach that drinking alcohol is not recommended

Evaluation
Positive therapeutic outcome
- Decreasing size of tumor, spread of malignancy

---

exemestane (Rx)
(x-ee-mes´-tane)
Aromasin
Func. class.: Antineoplastic
Chem. class.: Aromatase inhibitor
Pregnancy category D

Action: Lowers serum estradiol concentrations; many breast cancers have strong estrogen receptors

Therapeutic outcome: Prevention of rapidly growing malignant cells

Uses: Advanced breast carcinoma that has not responded to other therapy in estrogen receptor–positive patients (postmenopausal)

Dosage and routes
Adult: PO 25 mg/day after meals; may need 50 mg/day if taken with a potent CYP3A4 inhibitor

Available forms: Tabs 25 mg

Adverse effects
CNS: Headache, fatigue, depression, insomnia, anxiety
CV: Hypertension
GI: Nausea, vomiting, increased appetite, diarrhea, constipation, abdominal pain, hot flashes
HEMA: Lymphopenia
MS: Fracture, bone loss
RESP: Cough, dyspnea

Contraindications: Pregnancy **D**, breastfeeding, hypersensitivity, premenopausal women

Precautions: Children, geriatric, renal/hepatic disease

Pharmacokinetics
Absorption	Rapidly absorbed
Distribution	Unknown
Metabolism	Liver
Excretion	Feces, urine
Half-life	24 hr

Pharmacodynamics
Unknown

Interactions
Drug classifications
CYP3A4 inducers, estrogens: decreased exemestane action

NURSING CONSIDERATIONS
Assessment
- Assess B/P; hypertension may occur

Nursing diagnoses
- Injury, risk for (adverse reactions)
- Knowledge, deficient (teaching)

Implementation
- Give with food or fluids for GI upset
- Store in light-resistant container at room temperature

Patient/family education
- Instruct patient to report any complaints, side effects to prescriber; if dose is missed, do not double next dose
- Advise patient that hot flashes can occur and are reversible after discontinuing treatment
- Inform patient about who should be told about therapy

Evaluation
Positive therapeutic outcome
- Decreased spread of malignant cells in breast cancer

---

exenatide (Rx)
(ex-en´a-tide)
Byetta
Func. class.: Antidiabetic
Chem. class.: Incretin mimetic
Pregnancy category C

Action: Binds and activates known human GLP-1 receptor, mimics natural physiology for self-regulating glycemic control

Therapeutic outcome: Decreased polyuria, polydipsia, polyphagia; improved A1c

Uses: Type 2 diabetes mellitus given in combination with metformin, sulfonylurea, or a thiazolidinedione

Dosage and routes
Adult: SUBCUT 5 mcg bid 1 hr before morning and evening meal; may increase to 10 mcg bid after 1 mo of therapy

Available forms: Inj 5, 10 mcg

Adverse effects
CNS: Headache, dizziness, jittery feeling, restlessness, weakness
ENDO: **Hypoglycemia**
GI: Nausea, vomiting, diarrhea, dyspepsia, anorexia, gastroesophageal reflux, weight loss

Contraindications: Hypersensitivity

Precautions: Pregnancy **C,** geriatric, severe renal/hepatic/GI disease

Pharmacokinetics

Absorption	Unknown
Distribution	Unknown
Metabolism	Unknown
Excretion	Glomerular filtration
Half-life	Unknown

Pharmacodynamics

Onset	Unknown
Peak	2.1 hr
Duration	Unknown

Interactions
Individual drugs
Acetaminophen: may increase the effect of acetaminophen
Acetaminophen (elixir), digoxin, lovastatin: decreased action of these products
Alcohol, disopyramide: increased hypoglycemia
Dextrothyroxine, niacin, triamterene: decreased hypoglycemia
Erythromycin, metoclopramide: do not use with exenatide
Drug classifications
ACE inhibitors, anabolic steroids, androgens, corticosteroids, fibric acid derivatives, sulfonylureas: increased hypoglycemia
Estrogens, MAOIs, oral contraceptives, progestins, thiazide diuretics: decreased hypoglycemia
Phenothiazines: increased hyperglycemia

NURSING CONSIDERATIONS
Assessment
• Monitor fasting blood, glucose, A1c levels, postprandial glucose during treatment to determine diabetes control
• Assess for hypo/hyperglycemic reaction that can occur soon after meals; for severe hypoglycemia give **IV** D$_{50}$W, then **IV** dextrose solution
• Assess for nausea, vomiting, ability to tolerate product

Nursing diagnoses
• Injury, risk for (uses)
• Knowledge, deficient (teaching)
• Noncompliance (teaching)

Implementation
• Give SUBCUT only, do not give **IV**/IM
• Pen needles must be purchased separately and be compatible
• Prime prior to use
• Inject into thigh, abdomen, upper arm
• Give 1 hr before meals; if patient is NPO, may need to hold dose to prevent hypoglycemia
• Store in refrigerator; unopened pen, may be stored at room temperature after opening for up to 30 days

Patient/family education
• Teach patient symptoms of hypo/hyperglycemia, what to do about each; to have glucagon emergency kit available; to carry a glucose source (candy, sugar cube) to treat hypoglycemia
• Advise patient that product must be continued on daily basis; explain consequences of discontinuing product abruptly
• Teach patient that diabetes is a lifelong illness; product will not cure disease
• Advise that all food in diet plan must be eaten to prevent hypoglycemia
• Advise patient to carry emergency ID with prescriber and medications
• Advise patient to continue weight control, dietary restrictions, exercise, hygiene
• Inform patient that regular blood glucose monitoring and A1c testing is needed
• Advise patient to notify prescriber if pregnant or intend to become pregnant
• Advise patient to read "Information for the Patient" and "Pen User Manual"; provide education on self-injection

Evaluation
Positive therapeutic outcome
• Decrease in polyuria, polydipsia, polyphagia, clear sensorium; improved A1c, weight; absence of dizziness, stable gait

---

ezetimibe (Rx)
(ehz-eh-tim'bee)
Zetia
Func. class.: Antilipemic
Pregnancy category C

Action: Inhibits absorption of cholesterol by the small intestine

Adverse effects: *italic* = common, **bold** = life-threatening

Therapeutic outcome: Decreased cholesterol levels

Uses: Hypercholesterolemia, homozygous familial hypercholesterolemia (HoFH), homozygous sitosterolemia

Dosage and routes
Adult: PO 10 mg/day; may be given with HMG-CoA reductase inhibitor at same time; may be given with bile acid sequestrant; give ezetimibe 2 hr before or 4 hr after the bile acid sequestrant

Available forms: Tabs 10 mg

Adverse effects
CNS: Fatigue, dizziness, headache
GI: Diarrhea, abdominal pain
MISC: Chest pain, jittery
MS: Myalgias, arthralgias, back pain
RESP: Pharyngitis, sinusitis, cough, URI

Contraindications: Hypersensitivity, severe hepatic disease

Precautions: Pregnancy C, breastfeeding, children, hepatic disease

Pharmacokinetics	
Absorption	Unknown
Distribution	Unknown
Metabolism	Small intestine, liver
Excretion	Urine (11%), feces (78%)
Half-life	Unknown

Pharmacodynamics
Unknown

Interactions
Individual drugs
Cholestyramine: decreased ezetimibe action
CycloSPORINE: increased action of ezetimibe
Drug classifications
Antacids: decreased action of ezetimibe
Fibric acid derivatives: increased ezetimibe action
Drug/herb
Glucomannan: increased effect
Gotu kola: decreased effect

NURSING CONSIDERATIONS
Assessment
• Monitor lipid levels, liver function tests baseline, periodically during treatment

Nursing diagnoses
• Knowledge, deficient (teaching)
• Noncompliance (teaching)

Implementation
• Give without regard to meals

Patient/family education
• Teach patient that compliance is needed
• Advise that risk factors should be decreased: high-fat diet, smoking, alcohol consumption, absence of exercise
• Advise patient to notify prescriber if pregnancy is suspected or planned

Evaluation
Positive therapeutic outcome
• Decreased cholesterol

❗HIGH ALERT

factor VIIa, recombinant (Rx)
Niastase ✽, NovoSeven, NovoSeven RT
Func. class.: Antihemophilic

Pregnancy category C

Action: Promotes hemostasis by activating the intrinsic pathway of coagulation

Therapeutic outcome: Prevention of hemorrhage

Uses: Bleeding in hemophilia A or B, with inhibitors to factor VIII or IX, acquired hemophilia, factor VII deficiency

Unlabeled uses: Coumarin toxicity

Dosage and routes
Bleeding prophylaxis or hemophilic with inhibitors to factor VIII/IX
Adult: IV BOL 90 mcg/kg q2hr until hemostasis occurs, or until therapy is deemed to be inadequate; posthemostatic doses q3-6hr may be required

Bleeding prophylaxis factor VII deficiency
Adult: IV BOL 15-30 mcg/kg over 2-5 min q4-6hr

Acquired hemophilia
Adult/adolescent/child: IV BOL 70-90 mcg/kg q2-3hr

Available forms: Lyophilized powder 1.2 mg/vial (1200 mcg/vial), 2.4 mg/vial (2400 mcg/vial), 4.8 mg/vial (4800 mcg/vial) recombinant human coagulation factor VIIa (rFVIIa); NovoSeven RT: 1 mg, 2 mg, 5 mg powder for injection

Adverse effects
CNS: Fever, headache, **cerebral artery occlusion**
CV: **Ischemic heart disease, MI,** hypertension

 Alert   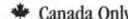 **Canada Only**   🕲 **Drug on CD**   * "Tall Man" lettering (See Preface)

INTEG: Pain, redness at inj site, pruritus, purpura, rash

SYST: **Hemorrhage not otherwise specified, hemarthrosis, fibrinogen plasma decrease,** hypertension, bradycardia, **DIC, coagulation disorder, thrombosis, acute renal failure**

Contraindications: Hypersensitivity to this product or mouse, hamster, or bovine products

Precautions: Pregnancy **C**, breastfeeding, children, DIC, septicemia, intracranial hemorrhage

Pharmacokinetics

Absorption	Unknown
Distribution	Unknown
Metabolism	Unknown
Excretion	Unknown
Half-life	2-3 hr

Pharmacodynamics
Unknown

Interactions
Individual drugs
Activated prothrombin complex concentrate, prothrombin complex concentrate: do not use together

NURSING CONSIDERATIONS
Assessment
• Assess VS, B/P, pulse, respirations, neurologic signs, temp at least q4hr, temp 104° F (40° C) or indicators of internal bleeding, cardiac rhythm
• Monitor pro-time, APTT, plasma FVII clotting
• Monitor for thrombosis; dose should be reduced or stopped

Nursing diagnoses
• Injury, risk for (uses, adverse reactions)
• Tissue perfusion, ineffective (uses)

Implementation
IV route
• Bring to room temperature; for 1.2 mg vial/2.2 ml sterile water for inj; 4.8 mg vial/8.5 ml sterile water for inj; remove caps from stopper, cleanse stopper with alcohol, allow to dry, draw back plunger of sterile syringe and allow air into syringe, insert needle of syringe into sterile water for inj, inject the air and withdraw amount required, insert syringe needle with diluent into product vial, aim to side so liquid runs down vial wall, gently swirl until dissolved; use within 3 hr; give by BOL over 3-5 min

• Do not admix; keep refrigerated until ready to use; avoid sunlight

Evaluation
Positive therapeutic outcome
• Therapeutic response: hemostasis

⚠ HIGH ALERT

factor IX complex (human)
Alpha Nine SD, BeneFIX, Konyne 80, Mononine, Profilnine/Alpha Nine, Proplex T, Proplex SX-T
Func. class.: Hemostatic
Chem. class.: Factors II, VII, IX, X

Pregnancy category C

Action: Causes an increase in blood levels of clotting factors II, VII, IX, X; factor IX (human) has IX activity only

Therapeutic outcome: Replacement of factors II, VII, IX, X

Uses: Hemophilia B (Christmas disease), factor IX deficiency, anticoagulant reversal, control of bleeding in patients with factor VIII inhibitors; reversal of overdose of anticoagulants in emergencies

Dosage and routes
Bleeding in hemophilia A and inhibitors of factor VIII (Proplex T, Konyne 80)
Adult and child: 75 units/kg, repeat in 12 hr

Factor IX complex (human) bleeding in hemophilia B
Adult and child: **IV** Establish 25% of normal factor IX activity or 60-75 units/kg then 10-20 units/kg/day × 1-2 wk

Prophylaxis of bleeding in hemophilia B
Adult and child: **IV** 10-20 units/kg 1-2 ×/wk

Reversal of oral anticoagulant
Adult and child: 15 units/kg

Factor VII deficiency (use Proplex T only)
Adult and child: 0.5 units/kg × body weight (kg) × desired factor IX increase (in % of normal); repeat q4-6hr if needed

Factor IX (human) minor to moderate hemorrhage
Use only Alpha Nine, Alpha Nine SD
Adult and child: **IV** Dose to increase plasma factor IX level to 20%-30% in one dose

---

Adverse effects: *italic* = common, **bold** = life-threatening

Serious hemorrhage
Adult and child: IV Dose to increase plasma factor IX level to 30%-50% given as daily INF

Minor hemorrhage (Mononine only)
Adult and child: IV dose to increase plasma factor IX level to 15%-25% (20-30 units/kg), may repeat in 24 hr if needed

Major hemorrhage
Adult and child: IV dose to increase plasma factor IX level to 25%-50% (75 units/kg) q18-30hr for up to 10 days

Available forms: Inj (number of units noted on label)

Adverse effects
CNS: *Headache, dizziness,* malaise, paresthesia, *lethargy, chills, fever, flushing*
CV: *Hypotension,* tachycardia, **MI, venous thrombosis, pulmonary embolism**
GI: Nausea, vomiting, abdominal cramps, jaundice, **viral hepatitis**
HEMA: **Thrombosis, hemolysis, AIDS, DIC**
INTEG: Rash, flushing, *urticaria*
RESP: Bronchospasm

Contraindications: Hypersensitivity to mouse/hamster protein, hepatic disease, DIC, elective surgery, mild factor IX deficiency

Precautions: Pregnancy **C**, neonates, infants

Pharmacokinetics	
Absorption	40% (PO), complete (**IV**)
Distribution	Unknown
Metabolism	Rapidly cleared from plasma, liver 30%
Excretion	Kidneys—70% unchanged
Half-life	24 hr

Pharmacodynamics
Unknown

Interactions
Individual drugs
Aminocaproic acid: increased risk of thrombosis; do not use together
Warfarin: decreased effect of warfarin
Drug classifications
Incompatible with protein products

NURSING CONSIDERATIONS
Assesment
• Monitor blood studies (coagulation factor assays by % normal: 5% prevents spontaneous hemorrhage, 30%-50% for surgery, 80%-100% for severe hemorrhage); check for bleeding q15-30min, immobilize and apply ice to affected joints
• Monitor for increased B/P, pulse
• Monitor I&O; if urine becomes orange or red, notify prescriber
• Assess for allergic or pyrogenic reaction: fever, chills, rash, itching; slow inf rate if not severe
◆ Assess for DIC: bleeding, ecchymosis, hypersensitivity, changes in coagulation tests

Nursing diagnoses
• Injury, risk for (uses)
• Knowledge, deficient (teaching)
• Tissue perfusion, ineffective (uses)

Implementation
IV route
• Give hepatitis B vaccine before administration
• Give **IV** after warming to room temperature 3 ml/min or less, with plastic syringe only; do not admix
• Give after dilution with provided diluent, 50 or 25 units/ml; max 10 ml/min; decrease rate if fever, headache, flushing, tingling occur
• Give after crossmatch is completed if patient has blood type A, B, AB, to determine incompatibility with factor
• Store reconstituted sol for 3 hr at room temperature or up to 2 yr if refrigerated (powder); check expiration date
• Incompatible with protein products
BeneFIX
• Allow vials of concentrate/diluent to warm to room temperature
• After removing flip-top cap from vial, wipe top of vial with alcohol swab; let dry
• Peel back cover from vial adapter package; do not remove
• Place vial adapter over vial; press firmly until snaps; attach plunger rod to diluent syringe and break plastic tip cap from diluent syringe
• Lift the package away from the adapter and connect diluent syringe; depress plunger; swirl contents

Patient/family education
• Advise patient to report any signs of bleeding: gums, under skin, urine, stools, emesis
• Caution patient about risk of viral hepatitis, AIDS; that immunization for hepatitis B may be given first; to be tested q2-3mo for HIV, even though the risk is low
• Tell patient to carry/wear emergency ID identifying disease and treatment; avoid salicylates, NSAIDs; inform other health professionals about condition

Evaluation
Positive therapeutic outcome
- Prevention of hemorrhage

famciclovir (Rx)
(fam-sye-klo'vir)
Famvir
Func. class.: Antiviral
Chem. class.: Guanosine nucleoside

Pregnancy category B

Action: Inhibits DNA polymerase and viral DNA synthesis by the conversion of this guanosine nucleoside to penciclovir

Therapeutic outcome: Decreasing size and number of lesions

Uses: Treatment of acute herpes zoster (shingles), genital herpes, recurrent mucocutaneous herpes simplex virus (HSV) in HIV patients, initial episodes of herpes genitalis, herpes labialis in the immunocompromised

Dosage and routes
Herpes zoster
Adult: PO 500 mg q8hr × 7 days

Renal dose
Adult: PO CCr ≥ 60 ml/min 500 mg q8hr; 40-59 ml/min 500 mg q12hr; 20-39 ml/min 500 mg q24hr; CCr <20 ml/min 250 mg q24hr

Recurrent HSV
Adult: PO 125 mg q12hr × 5 days

Renal dose
Adult: PO CCr <39 ml/min 125 mg q24hr × 5 days

Suppression of recurrent HSV
Adult: PO 250 mg q12hr up to 1 yr

Renal dose
Adult: PO CCr 20-39 ml/min 125 mg q12hr × 5 days; CCr <20 ml/min 125 mg q24hr × 5 days

Genital herpes/herpes labialis (recurrent)
Adult: PO 125 mg bid × 5 days or 1000 mg bid for 1 day; begin treatment at first sign of recurrence

Suppression of recurrent genital herpes
Adult: PO 250 mg bid for up to a year

Herpes genitalis initial episodes
Adult: PO 250 mg tid × 7-10 days

Available forms: Tabs 125, 250, 500 mg

Adverse effects
CNS: Headache, fatigue, dizziness, paresthesia, somnolence, fever
GI: Nausea, vomiting, diarrhea, constipation, abdominal pain, anorexia
GU: Decreased sperm count
INTEG: Pruritus
MS: Back pain, arthralgia
RESP: Pharyngitis, sinusitis

Contraindications: Hypersensitivity to this product, penciclovir, acyclovir, ganciclovir, valacyclovir, or valganciclovir

Precautions: Pregnancy **B,** breastfeeding, renal disease

Pharmacokinetics
Absorption	Well absorbed, 77%
Distribution	Protein binding 20%
Metabolism	Intestinal tissue, blood, liver
Excretion	Breast milk, kidney, bile
Half-life	Terminal 2-3 hr

Pharmacodynamics
Onset	Unknown
Peak	1 hr
Duration	8 hr

Interactions
Individual drugs
Cimetidine: decreased metabolism
Digoxin, probenecid, theophylline: decreased renal excretion

NURSING CONSIDERATIONS
Assessment
- Assess amount and distribution of lesions; also burning, itching, or pain (early symptoms of herpes infection); neuralgia during, after treatment
- Monitor renal function tests: urine CCr, BUN before, during treatment if patient has decreased renal function; dose may need to be lowered
- Monitor bowel pattern before, during treatment; diarrhea may occur

Nursing diagnoses
- Infection, risk for (uses)
- Knowledge, deficient (teaching)

Implementation
- Give with or without meals; absorption does not appear to be lowered when taken with food
- Give within 72 hr of the appearance of rash in herpes zoster

F

Patient/family education

- Teach patient how to recognize signs of beginning of infection
- Teach patient how to prevent the spread of infection to others
- Teach patient reason for medication and expected results
- Advise patient that this medication does not prevent spread of disease to others, that condoms should be used
- Advise women with genital herpes to have yearly Pap smears; cervical cancer is more likely

Evaluation
Positive therapeutic outcome
- Decreased size and spread of lesions

---

famotidine (Rx, OTC)
(fa-moe'ti-deen)
Maximum Strength Pepcid, Mylanta AR, Pepcid, Pepcid AC, Pepcid AC Acid Controller, Pepcid RPD ✤
Func. class.: H₂-histamine receptor antagonist, antiulcer agent

Pregnancy category B

Action: Inhibits histamine at H_2-receptor site in gastric parietal cells, which inhibits gastric acid secretion while pepsin remains at a stable level

Therapeutic outcome: Healing of duodenal ulcers or gastric ulcers; prevention of duodenal ulcers; decreases symptoms of gastroesophageal reflux disease or Zollinger-Ellison syndrome, heartburn

Uses: Short-term treatment of active duodenal ulcer, maintenance therapy for duodenal ulcer, Zollinger-Ellison syndrome, multiple endocrine adenomas, gastric ulcers, heartburn, gastroesophageal reflux disease

Unlabeled uses: GI disorders in those taking NSAIDs, urticaria, prevention of stress ulcers, aspiration pneumonitis, inactivation of oral pancreatic enzymes in pancreatic disorders, prevention of paclitaxel hypersensitivity reactions

Dosage and routes
Active ulcer
Adult: PO 40 mg/day at bedtime × 4-8 wk, then 20 mg/day at bedtime if needed (maintenance); **IV** 20 mg q12hr if unable to take PO
Child 1-16 yr: PO 0.5 mg/kg/day at bedtime or divided bid, max 40 mg/day

Hypersecretory conditions
Adult: PO 20 mg q6hr; may give 160 mg q6hr if needed; **IV** 20 mg q12hr if unable to take PO
Child 1-16 yr: PO 1 mg/kg/day divided bid, max 40 mg bid

Paclitaxel hypersensitivity reactions
Adult: **IV** 20 mg ½ hr before INF

Heartburn relief/prevention
Adult: PO 10 mg with water, 15 min-1 hr before eating

Renal dose
Adult: PO CCr <50 ml/min; give 50% of dose or extend interval to q36-48hr

Available forms: Tabs 10, 20, 40 mg; powder for oral susp 40 mg/5 ml; inj 10 mg/ml, 20 mg/50 ml 0.9% NaCl; orally disintegrating tabs (RPD) 20, 40 mg; chew tabs 10 mg; gel cap 10 mg

Adverse effects
CNS: Headache, dizziness, paresthesia, depression, anxiety, somnolence, insomnia, fever, **seizures in renal disease**
CV: **Dysrhythmias**
EENT: Taste change, tinnitus, orbital edema
GI: Constipation, nausea, vomiting, anorexia, cramps, abnormal liver enzymes, diarrhea
HEMA: **Thrombocytopenia, aplastic anemia**
INTEG: Rash, **toxic epidermal necrolysis, Stevens-Johnson syndrome**
MS: Myalgia, arthralgia
RESP: **Pneumonia**

Contraindications: Hypersensitivity

Precautions: Pregnancy **B**, breastfeeding, children <12 yr, geriatric, severe renal/hepatic disease

Pharmacokinetics

Absorption	50% absorbed (PO)
Distribution	Plasma, protein binding (15%-20%)
Metabolism	Liver (30% active metabolizing)
Excretion	Kidneys (70%)
Half-life	2½-3½ hr

Pharmacodynamics

	PO	IV
Onset	30-60 min	Immediate
Peak	1-3 hr	½-3 hr
Duration	6-12 hr	8-15 hr

Interactions
Individual drugs
Ketoconazole: decreased absorption of ketoconazole
Drug classifications
Antacids: decreased absorption of famotidine

NURSING CONSIDERATIONS
Assessment
• Assess patient with ulcers or suspected ulcers: epigastric, abdominal pain, hematemesis, occult blood in stools, blood in gastric aspirate before treatment; throughout treatment, monitor gastric pH (5 should be maintained)
• Monitor I&O ratio, BUN, creatinine, CBC with differential monthly
Nursing diagnoses
• Knowledge, deficient (teaching)
• Pain, acute (uses)
Implementation
PO route
• Give antacids 1 hr before or 2 hr after famotidine; may be given with foods or liquid
• Administer oral susp after shaking well; discard unused sol after 1 mo
IV route
• Give **IV** direct after diluting 2 ml of product (10 mg/ml) in 0.9% NaCl to total volume of 5-10 ml; inject over 2 min to prevent hypotension
• Administer **IV** intermittent inf after diluting 20 mg of product in 100 ml of LR, 0.9% NaCl, D_5W, $D_{10}W$; run over 15-30 min
• Store in cool environment (oral); **IV** sol is stable for 48 hr at room temperature; do not use discolored sol
Y-site compatibilities: Acyclovir, allopurinol, amifostine, aminophylline, amphotericin, ampicillin, ampicillin/sulbactam, inamrinone, amsacrine, atropine, aztreonam, bretylium, calcium gluconate, cefazolin, cefoperazone, cefotaxime, cefotetan, cefoxitin, ceftazidime, ceftizoxime, ceftriaxone, cefuroxime, cephalothin, cephapirin, chlorproMAZINE, cisplatin, cladribine, cyclophosphamide, cytarabine, dexamethasone, dextran 40, digoxin, diphenhydrAMINE, DOBUTamine, DOPamine, DOXOrubicin, droperidol, enalaprilat, epinephrine, erythromycin lactobionate, esmolol, filgrastim, fluconazole, fludarabine, folic acid, gentamicin, granisetron, haloperidol, heparin, hydrocortisone, hydromorphone, hydrOXYzine, imipenem/cilastatin, regular insulin, isoproterenol, labetalol, lidocaine, lorazepam, magnesium sulfate, melphalan, meperidine, methotrexate, methylPREDNISolone, metoclopramide, mezlocillin, midazolam, morphine, nafcillin, nitroglycerin, nitroprusside, norepinephrine, ondansetron, oxacillin, paclitaxel, perphenazine, phenylephrine, phenytoin, phytonadione, piperacillin, potassium chloride, potassium phosphate, procainamide, propofol, sargramostim, sodium bicarbonate, teniposide, theophylline, thiamine, thiotepa, ticarcillin, ticarcillin/clavulanate, verapamil, vinorelbine
Additive compatibilities: Cefazolin, cefmetazole, flumazenil

Patient/family education
• Caution patient to avoid driving, other hazardous activities until stabilized on this medication; dizziness may occur
• Advise patient to avoid black pepper, caffeine, alcohol, harsh spices, extremes in temperature of food; tell patient to avoid OTC preparations: aspirin, cough, cold preparations; condition may worsen
• Advise patient to avoid taking OTC and prescription preparations of this product concurrently
• Tell patient that smoking decreases the effectiveness of the product; that smoking cessation should be considered
• Instruct patient that product must be continued for prescribed time to be effective and taken exactly as prescribed; doses are not to be doubled; take missed dose when remembered up to 1 hr before next dose
• Tell patient to report bruising, fatigue, malaise; blood dyscrasias may occur
• Tell patient to report diarrhea, black tarry stools, sore throat, rash, dizziness, confusion, or delirium to prescriber immediately

Evaluation
Positive therapeutic outcome
• Decreased pain in abdomen
• Healing of ulcers

fat emulsions (Rx)
(fat ee-mul'shuns)
Intralipid 10%, Intralipid 20%, Liposyn II 10%, Liposyn II 20%, Liposyn III 10%, Liposyn III 20%, Soyacal 20%
Func. class.: Caloric
Chem. class.: Fatty acid, long chain
Pregnancy category C

Action: Needed for energy, heat production; consists of neutral triglycerides, primarily unsaturated fatty acids

Therapeutic outcome: Increased available calories and fatty acids

Uses: Increase calorie intake, prevent fatty acid deficiency

Dosage and routes
Deficiency
Adult and child: **IV** 8%-10% of required calorie intake (intralipid)

Adjunct to TPN
Adult: **IV** 1 ml/min over 15-30 min (10%) or 0.5 ml/min over 15-30 min (20%); may increase to 500 ml over 4-8 hr if no adverse reactions occur; max 2.5 g/kg
Child: **IV** 0.1 ml/min over 10-15 min (10%) or 0.05 ml/ min over 10-15 min (20%); may increase to 1 g/kg over 4 hr if no adverse reactions occur; max 4 g/kg

Prevention of deficiency
Adult: **IV** 500 ml 2 ×/wk (10%), given 1 ml/min for 30 min, max 500 ml over 6 hr
Child: **IV** 5-10 ml/kg/day (10%), given 0.1 ml/min for 30 min, max 100 ml/hr

Available forms: Inj 10% (50, 100, 200, 250, 500 ml), 20% (50, 100, 200, 250, 500 ml)

Adverse effects
CNS: Dizziness, headache, drowsiness, **focal seizures**
CV: **Shock**
GI: Nausea, vomiting, **hepatomegaly**
HEMA: **Hyperlipemia, hypercoagulation, thrombocytopenia, leukopenia, leukocytosis**
RESP: Dyspnea, **fat in lung tissue**

Contraindications: Hypersensitivity to this product, eggs, soybeans, or legumes; hyperlipemia; lipid necrosis; acute pancreatitis accompanied by hyperlipemia; hyperbilirubinemia of the newborn; renal insufficiency; hepatic damage

Precautions: Pregnancy **C**, term newborns, severe liver disease, diabetes mellitus, thrombocytopenia, gastric ulcers, premature, sepsis

Pharmacokinetics	
Absorption	Completely absorbed
Distribution	Intravascular space
Metabolism	Conversion to triglycerides, then to free fatty acids
Excretion	Unknown
Half-life	Unknown

Pharmacodynamics
Unknown

NURSING CONSIDERATIONS
Assessment
• Monitor triglycerides, free fatty acid levels, platelet counts daily to prevent fat overload, thrombocytopenia
• Monitor liver function tests: AST, ALT, Hct, Hgb; notify prescriber if abnormal
• Assess nutritional status: calorie count by dietitian; monitor weight daily

Nursing diagnoses
• Knowledge, deficient (teaching)
• Nutrition: less than body requirements, imbalanced (uses)

Implementation
• Administer using infusion pump at prescribed rate; do not use in-line filter sized for lipid emulsion; clogging will occur
• Do not use mixed sol that looks oily or is not separated; discard unused sol
• Change **IV** tubing at each inf: infection may occur with old tubing
• Give by intermittent inf at a rate of 10% sol (1 ml/min); 20% sol (0.5 ml/min) initially for 15-30 min; may be increased to 10% sol (120 ml/hr) or 20% sol (62.5 ml/hr) if no adverse reactions occur; max 500 ml during the first day; children should be given 10% (0.1 mg/ml) or 20% (0.05 ml/min) initially for 15-30 min, may be increased 1 g/kg/4 hr, max 10% (100 ml/hr) or 20% (50 ml/hr)

Y-site compatibilities:
Ampicillin, cefamandole, cefazolin, cefoxitin, cephapirin, clindamycin, digoxin, DOPamine, erythromycin, furosemide, gentamicin, IL-2, isoproterenol, lidocaine, kanamycin, norepinephrine, oxacillin, penicillin G potassium, ticarcillin, tobramycin

Y-site incompatibilities:
Amikacin, tetracycline

Additive compatibilities:
Cefamandole, chloramphenicol, cimetidine, cycloSPORINE, diphenhydrAMINE, famotidine, heparin, hydrocortisone, multivitamins, nizatidine, penicillin G potassium

Patient/family education
• Teach patient reason for use of lipids and expected results

Evaluation
Positive therapeutic outcome
• Increased weight
• Fatty acids at adequate levels

 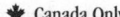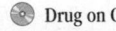

febuxostat (Rx)

(feb-ux'oh-stat)

Uloric

Func. class.: Antigout drug, antihyperuricemic

Chem. class.: Xanthene oxidase inhibitor

Pregnancy category C

Action: Inhibits the enzyme xanthine oxidase, reducing uric acid synthesis; more selective for xanthine oxidase than allopurinol

Therapeutic outcome: Decreased signs/symptoms of gout, hyperuricemia

Uses: Chronic gout, hyperuricemia

Dosage and routes

Adult: PO 40 mg qd, may increase to 80 mg qd if uric acid levels are >6 mg/dl after 2 wk of therapy

Available forms: Tabs 40, 80 mg

Adverse effects

CNS: Weakness, flushing

CV: **MI, atrial fibrillation, atrial flutter, AV block,** bradycardia, hyper/hypotension, palpitations, **sinus tachycardia, stroke,** angina

EENT: Retinopathy, cataracts, epistaxis

GI: Nausea, vomiting, anorexia, constipation, diarrhea, dyspepsia, hematemesis, hepatitis, hepatomegaly, weight gain/loss, cholecystitis, cholelithiasis, melena

GU: Renal failure, urinary urgency/frequency/ incontinence, nephrolithiasis, hemateria

HEMA: **Thrombocytopenia, anemia, pancytopenia, leukopenia, bone marrow suppression**

INTEG: Rash

MISC: Arthralgia, gout flare

Contraindications: Hypersensitivity

Precautions: Pregnancy C, breastfeeding, children, renal/hepatic/cardiac/neoplastic disease, stroke, MI, organ transplant, Lesch-Nyhan syndrome

Pharmacokinetics

Absorption	Unknown
Distribution	Protein binding 99.2%
Metabolism	Unknown
Excretion	Feces, urine
Half-life	5-8 hr

Pharmacodynamics

Onset	Unknown
Peak	1-1.5 hr
Duration	Unknown

Interactions

Individual drugs

Azathioprine: increased toxicity

Rasburicase: increased xanthine nephropathy, calculi

Mercaptopurine, theophylline: increased myelosuppression

Drug classifications

Antineoplastics: increased xanthine nephropathy, calculi

NURSING CONSIDERATIONS

Assessment

* Monitor uric acid levels q2wk; uric acid levels should be 6 mg/dl or less
* Monitor CBC, AST, BUN, creatinine before starting treatment, periodically
* Monitor I&O ratio; increase fluids to 2 L/day to prevent stone formation and toxicity
* Assess for rash, hypersensitivity reactions; discontinue
* Assess for gout: joint pain, swelling; may use with NSAIDs for acute gouty attacks and gout flare

Nursing diagnoses

* Pain, chronic (uses)
* Noncompliance (teaching)
* Knowledge, deficient (teaching)

Implementation

PO route

* Give with meals to prevent GI symptoms; may crush and add to foods or fluids
* Give a few days before antineoplastic therapy

Patient/family education

* Inform that tabs may be crushed
* Teach to take as prescribed; if dose is missed, take as soon as remembered; do not double dose
* Teach to increase fluid intake to 2 L/day unless contraindicated
* Advise to avoid alcohol, caffeine; will increase uric acid levels
* Advise to report cardiovascular events to prescriber

Evaluation

Positive therapeutic outcome

* Decreased pain in joints, decreased stone formation in kidneys, decreased uric acid levels

F

Adverse effects: *italic* = common, **bold** = life-threatening

felodipine (Rx)

(feh-loh'dih-peen)

Renedil ✦

Func. class.: Calcium-channel blocker, antihypertensive, antianginal

Chem. class.: Dihydropyridine

Pregnancy category C

Action: Inhibits calcium ion influx across cell membrane, resulting in inhibition of excitation/contraction

Therapeutic outcome: Decreased B/P in hypertension

Uses: Essential hypertension, alone or with other antihypertensives, angina pectoris, Prinzmetal's angina (vasospastic)

Dosage and routes
Adult: PO 5 mg/day initially, usual range 2.5-10 mg/day; max 10 mg/day; do not adjust dosage at intervals of <2 wk
Geriatric: PO 2.5 mg/day

Hepatic dose
Adult: PO 2.5-5 mg/day, max 10 mg/day

Available forms: Ext rel tabs 2.5, 5, 10 mg

Adverse effects
CNS: Headache, fatigue, drowsiness, dizziness, anxiety, depression, nervousness, insomnia, light-headedness, paresthesia, tinnitus, psychosis, somnolence
CV: **Dysrhythmias,** edema, **CHF,** hypotension, palpitations, **MI, pulmonary edema,** tachycardia, syncope, AV block, angina
GI: Nausea, vomiting, diarrhea, gastric upset, constipation, increased liver function studies, dry mouth
GU: Nocturia, polyuria
HEMA: Anemia
INTEG: Rash, pruritus
MISC: Flushing, sexual difficulties, cough, nasal congestion, shortness of breath, wheezing, epistaxis, respiratory infection, chest pain, **Stevens-Johnson syndrome,** gingival hyperplasia

Contraindications: Hypersensitivity, sick sinus syndrome, 2nd- or 3rd-degree heart block, hypotension <90 mm Hg systolic

Precautions: Pregnancy C, breastfeeding, children, geriatric, CHF, hepatic injury, renal disease

Pharmacokinetics
Absorption	Well absorbed
Distribution	Unknown; protein binding >99%
Metabolism	Liver, extensively
Excretion	Kidneys
Half-life	11-16 hr

Pharmacodynamics
Onset	2-3 hr
Peak	2½-5 hr
Duration	<24 hr

Interactions
Individual drugs
Alcohol, fentanyl, quinidine: increased hypotension
Digoxin, disopyramide, phenytoin: increased bradycardia, increased CHF
Erythromycin, ketoconazole, itraconazole, propanolol: increased toxicity
Drug classifications
β-Adrenergic blockers: increased bradycardia, CHF
Nitrates: increased hypotension
NSAIDs: decreased antihypertensive effects
Drug/herb
Aconite: increased toxicity, death
Astragalus, cola tree: increased or decreased antihypertensive effect
Barberry, betony, black catechu, black cohosh, bloodroot, broom, burdock, cat's claw, dandelion, ginkgo, ginseng, goldenseal, Irish moss, Jamaican dogwood, kelp, khella, mistletoe, parsley: increased antihypertensive effect
Coltsfoot, guarana, khat, licorice, St. John's wort, yohimbe: decreased antihypertensive effect
Drug/food
Grapefruit juice: increased felodipine level

NURSING CONSIDERATIONS
Assessment
• Assess fluid volume status: I&O ratio and record; weight; skin turgor; adequacy of pulses; moist mucous membranes; bilateral lung sounds; peripheral pitting edema; dehydration symptoms of decreasing output, thirst, hypotension, dry mouth, and mucous membranes should be reported; for CHF: weight gain, crackles, dyspnea, edema, jugular venous distention
• Monitor ALT, AST, bilirubin daily if these are elevated
• Monitor cardiac status: B/P, pulse, respiration, ECG, periodically

 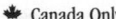

- Assess for anginal pain: duration; intensity; ameliorating, aggravating factors

Nursing diagnoses
- Cardiac output, decreased (uses)
- Knowledge, deficient (teaching)

Implementation
- Do not break, crush, or chew ext rel tabs
- Give once a day with food for GI symptoms

Patient/family education
- Caution patient to avoid hazardous activities until stabilized on product and dizziness is no longer a problem
- Instruct patient to limit caffeine consumption; to avoid alcohol and OTC products unless directed by prescriber
- Urge patient to comply in all areas of medical regimen: diet, exercise, stress reduction, product therapy; to notify prescriber of irregular heartbeat, shortness of breath, swelling of feet and hands, pronounced dizziness, constipation, nausea, hypotension
- Advise patient to use protective clothing, sunscreen to prevent photosensitivity
- Teach patient to change positions slowly to prevent orthostatic hypotension
- Advise patient to obtain correct pulse; to contact prescriber if pulse is <50 bpm
- Teach patient to use as directed even if feeling better; may be taken with other CV products (nitrates, β-blockers); that capsules may appear in stools but are insignificant

Evaluation
Positive therapeutic outcome
- Decreased B/P
- Decreased anginal attacks
- Increase in activity tolerance

---

fenofibrate (Rx)
(fen-oh-fee'brate)
Antara, Lipofem, Lofibra, Tricor, Triglide
Func. class.: Antilipemic
Chem. class.: Fibric acid derivative

Pregnancy category C

Action: Increases lipolysis and elimination of triglyceride-rich particles from plasma by activating lipoprotein lipase, resulting in triglyceride change in size and composition of LDL, leading to rapid breakdown of LDL; mobilizes triglycerides from tissue; increases excretion of neutral sterols

Therapeutic outcome: Decreasing cholesterol levels and low-density lipoproteins, decreased pruritus

Uses: Patients with types IV, V hyperlipidemia who do not respond to other treatment and who are at risk for pancreatitis Fredrickson type IIa, IIb, hypertriglyceridemia

Unlabeled uses: Polymetabolic syndrome X

Dosage and routes
Hypertriglyceridemia
Adult: PO (Antara) 43-130 mg/day; (Lofibra) 67-200 mg/day; (Tricor) 48-145 mg/day; (Triglide) 50-160 mg/day

Primary hypercholesterolemia/ mixed hyperlipidemia
Adult: PO (Antara) 130 mg/day; (Lofibra) 200 mg/day; (Tricor) 145 mg/day; (Triglide) 160 mg/day

Renal dose (geriatric)
Adult: PO (Tricor) CCr 30-80 ml/min 48 mg/day; CCr <30 ml/min contraindicated
Adult: PO (Triglide, Lipofem) CCr 11-49 ml/min 50 mg/day; (Antara) 43 mg/day; (Lofibra) 67 mg/day; (Antara, Lipofem, Lofibra, Triglide) CCr <10 ml/min, contraindicated

Available forms: Tabs (Triglide) 50, 160 mg; (Tricor) 48, 145 mg; micronized cap (Antara) 45, 87, 130 mg; (Lofibra) 67, 134, 200 mg; cap (Lipofem) 50, 150 mg

Adverse effects
CNS: Fatigue, weakness, drowsiness, dizziness, insomnia, depression, vertigo
CV: Angina, **dysrhythmias,** hypertension
GI: Nausea, vomiting, dyspepsia, increased liver enzymes, flatulence, hepatomegaly, gastritis
GU: Dysuria, proteinuria, oliguria, urinary frequency
HEMA: Anemia, **leukopenia,** ecchymosis, **thrombosis, pulmonary embolism**
INTEG: Rash, urticaria, pruritus
MISC: Polyphagia, weight gain
MS: Myalgias, arthralgias, myopathy
RESP: Pharyngitis, bronchitis, cough

Contraindications: Hypersensitivity, severe renal/hepatic disease, primary biliary cirrhosis, preexisting gallbladder disease

Precautions: Pregnancy C, breastfeeding, geriatric, peptic ulcer, pancreatitis, renal/ hepatic disease

F

Pharmacokinetics	
Absorption	Unknown
Distribution	Protein binding 99%
Metabolism	Liver
Excretion	Urine 60%
Half-life	20 hr

Pharmacodynamics	
Onset	Unknown
Peak	6-8 hr
Duration	Unknown

Interactions
Drug classifications
Anticoagulants (oral): increased effect of anticoagulants
Bile acid sequestrants: decreased absorption
CycloSPORINE: increased nephrotoxicity
HMG-CoA reductase inhibitors: do not use together, rhabdomyolysis may occur
Drug/herb
Glucomannan: increased effect
Gotu kola: decreased effect
Drug/food
Increased absorption

NURSING CONSIDERATIONS
Assessment
• Assess lipid levels, liver function tests, baseline and periodically during treatment; CPK if muscle pain occurs, CBC, Hct, Hgh, pro-time with anticoagulant therapy
• Assess for pancreatitis, cholelithiasis, renal failure, rhabdomyolysis (when combined with HMG-CoA reductase inhibitors), myositis; product should be discontinued
• Assess nutrition: fat, protein, carbohydrates, nutritional analysis should be completed by dietitian
• Assess skin integrity after patient has been receiving product; itching, pruritus often occur from bile deposits on skin
• Monitor cardiac glycoside level if both products are being administered; cardiac glycoside levels should be decreased
• Monitor for signs of vit A, D, K deficiency; serum cholesterol, triglyceride levels, electrolytes if on extended therapy
• Monitor bowel pattern daily; increase bulk, water in diet if constipation develops

Nursing diagnoses
• Knowledge, deficient (teaching)
• Noncompliance (teaching)

Implementation
• Do not break, crush, or chew tabs
• Give with evening meal; if dose is increased, take with breakfast and evening meal

• Store in cool environment in tight, light-resistant container

Patient/family education
• Inform patient that compliance is needed
• Teach patient that risk factors—high-fat diet, smoking, alcohol consumption, absence of exercise—should be decreased
• Caution patient to notify prescriber if pregnancy is planned or suspected
• Teach patient to notify prescriber if the GI symptoms of diarrhea, abdominal or epigastric pain, nausea, or vomiting occur
• Instruct patient to report GU symptoms: dysuria, proteinuria, oliguria, decreased libido, impotence
• Advise patient to notify prescriber of muscle pain, weakness, fever, fatigue, epigastric pain

Evaluation
Positive therapeutic outcome
• Decrease in cholesterol to desired level after 8 wk

---

fenofibric acid (Rx)
(fen-oh-fye-brick)
TriLipix, Fibricor
Func. class.: Antilipemic
Chem. class.: Fibric acid derivative
Pregnancy category C

Action: An active metabolite of fenofibrate; increases lipolysis and elimination of triglyceride-rich particles from plasma by activating lipoprotein lipase, resulting in triglyceride change in size and composition of LDL, leading to rapid breakdown of LDL; mobilizes triglycerides from tissue; increases excretion of neutral sterols

Therapeutic outcome: Triglyceride level returning to normal

Uses: Hyperlipoproteinemia; hypertriglyceridemia

Dosage and routes
Combination with HMG-CoA reductase inhibitors to reduce triglycerides and increase HDL-C in those with mixed dyslipidemia or coronary heart disease
Adult: DEL REL cap PO 135 mg qd
Severe hypertriglyceridemia
Adult: DEL REL cap PO 45-135 qd; tabs 35-105 mg qd

Available forms: Tabs 35, 105 mg; cap, gastro-resistant pellet 45, 135 mg

Adverse effects

CNS: Fatigue, weakness, drowsiness, dizziness, insomnia, depression, vertigo, asthenia, headache
CV: Hypertension
EENT: Blurred vision
GI: Nausea, vomiting, dyspepsia, increased liver enzymes, abdominal pain, cholecystitis, cholelithiasis, constipation, diarrhea, hepatitis, jaundice, pancreatitis
GU: Impotence, decreased libido
HEMA: Anemia, leukopenia, **thrombosis/pulmonary embolism, agranulocytosis, eosinophilia**
INTEG: Rash, urticaria, pruritus, **Stevens-Johnson syndrome**
MISC: Infection
MS: Myalgias, arthralgias, myopathy, back pain, MS pain
RESP: Pharyngitis, cough

Contraindications: Hypersensitivity, severe renal/hepatic disease, primary biliary cirrhosis, preexisting gallbladder disease, breastfeeding

Precautions: Pregnancy **C**, geriatric patients, pancreatitis, thromboembolic disease

Pharmacokinetics

Absorption	QA64
Distribution	Protein binding 99%
Metabolism	Liver, converted to fenofibric acid
Excretion	Urine 60%
Half-life	20 hr

Pharmacodynamics

Onset	Unknown
Peak	4-5 hr (del rel cap), 2.5 hr (tab)
Duration	Unknown

Interactions
Individual drugs

CycloSPORINE: increased nephrotoxicity
Drug classifications

Monitor use with HMG-CoA reductase inhibitors; rhabdomyolysis may occur
Bile acid sequestrants: decreased absorption of fenofibrate
Oral anticoagulants: increased anticoagulant effect
Drug/herb

Glucomannan: increased effect
Gotu cola: decreased effect
Drug/food

Increase: absorption

NURSING CONSIDERATIONS
Assessment

- Monitor lipid levels, LFTs baseline, periodically during treatment, CBC with differential, CPK, serum bilirubin (direct/indirect)
- Assess for pancreatitis, cholelithiasis renal failure, rhabdomyolysis (when combined with HMG CoA reductase inhibitors), myositis; product should be discontinued

Nursing diagnosis

- Risk of injury (uses)
- Noncompliance (teaching)
- Knowledge, deficient (teaching)

Implementation

- Give product with meals; may increase q4-8wk

Patient/family education

- Teach patient that compliance is needed
- Advise that risk factors should be decreased: high-fat diet, smoking, alcohol consumption, absence of exercise
- Inform to notify prescriber if pregnancy is suspected or planned
- Teach patient to report GU symptoms: decreased libido, impotence
- Advise to notify prescriber of muscle pain, weakness, fever, fatigue; epigastric pain

Evaluation:

Positive therapeutic outcome
- Decreased triglycerides

---

fenoldopam (Rx)
(fen-nahl'doh-pam)
Corlopam
Func. class.: Antihypertensive, vasodilator
Pregnancy category B

Action: Agonist at D_1-like dopamine receptors; binds to α_2-adrenoreceptors; increases renal blood flow

Therapeutic outcome: B/P, decreased

Uses: Hypertensive crisis, malignant hypertension

Unlabeled uses: Prevention of contrast agent-associated nephrotoxicity

Dosage and routes
Adult: **IV** 0.1-1.6 mcg/kg/min
Child: CONT IV 0.2 mcg/kg/min with effects within 5 min; may increase dose to 0.3-0.5 mcg/kg/min q20-30min depending on response

Available forms: Inj conc 10 mg/ml in single-use ampules; inj 10 mg/ml

Adverse effects

CNS: Headache, anxiety, dizziness, insomnia
CV: Hypotension, ST-T-wave changes, angina
pectoris, palpitations, **MI, ischemic heart
disease,** *flushing*
GI: Nausea, vomiting, constipation, diarrhea
HEMA: Leukocytosis, bleeding
INTEG: Sweating
META: Increased BUN, glucose, LDH, creatinine, hypokalemia

Contraindications: Hypersensitivity, sulfite sensitivity

Precautions: Pregnancy **B,** breastfeeding, children, tachycardia, intraocular pressure, hypokalemia

Pharmacokinetics

Absorption	Unknown
Distribution	Steady state 20 min
Metabolism	Unknown
Excretion	Unknown
Half-life	5 min (elimination)

Pharmacodynamics

Unknown

Interactions
Drug classifications

β-Adrenergic blockers: increased hypotension
Drug/herb

Aconite: increased toxicity, death
Astragalus, cola tree: increased or decreased antihypertensive effect
Barberry, betony, black catechu, black cohosh, bloodroot, broom, burdock, cat's claw, dandelion, goldenseal, Irish moss, Jamaican dogwood, kelp, khella, mistletoe, parsley: increased antihypertensive effect
Coltsfoot, guarana, khat, licorice: decreased antihypertensive effect

NURSING CONSIDERATIONS
Assessment

• Monitor B/P q5min until stabilized, then q1hr × 2 hr, then q4hr; pulse, jugular venous distention q4hr
• Monitor electrolytes, blood studies: K, Na, Cl, CO_2, CBC, serum glucose
• Assess skin turgor, dryness of mucous membranes for hydration status
• Assess **IV** site for extravasation, rate

Nursing diagnoses

• Knowledge, deficient (teaching)
• Noncompliance (teaching)
• Tissue perfusion, ineffective (uses)

Implementation
IV route

• Administer after diluting contents of ampules in 0.9% NaCl, or 5% dextrose inj (40 mcg/ml); then add 4 ml of conc (40 mg of product/1000 ml); 2 ml of conc (20 mg of product/500 ml); 1 ml of conc (10 mg of product/250 ml); do not admix
• Give to patient in recumbent position; keep in that position for 1 hr after administration
• Diluted sol is stable in normal light/temperature for 24 hr

Patient/family education

• Teach patient reason for medication and expected results
• Instruct patient to report dyspnea, chest pain, bleeding

Evaluation
Positive therapeutic outcome

• Decreased B/P

⚠ HIGH ALERT

fentanyl (Rx)
(fen′ta-nill)
Actiq, fentanyl, Fentanyl Fentora, Onsolis, Sublimaze
fentanyl transdermal (Rx)
Duragesic
Func. class.: Opioid analgesic
Chem. class.: Synthetic phenylpiperidine derivative

Pregnancy category C
Controlled substance schedule II

Do not confuse:
fentanyl/Sufenta

Action: Inhibits ascending pain pathways in CNS, increases pain threshold, alters pain perception by binding to opiate receptors

Therapeutic outcome: Relief of pain, supplement to anesthesia

Uses: Controls moderate to severe pain; preoperatively, postoperatively; adjunct to general anesthetic, adjunct to regional anesthesia; *Fentanyl:* for anesthesia as pre-medication, conscious sedation; *Actiq:* for breakthrough cancer pain

Dosage and routes
Fentanyl
Anesthetic
Adult: **IV** 25-100 mcg (0.7-2 mcg/kg) q2-3min prn

Anesthesia supplement
Adult and child >12 yr: IM/IV 2-20 mcg/kg IV INF 0.025-0.25 mcg/kg/min

Induction and maintenance
Adult: IV BOL 5-40 mcg/kg
Child 2-12 yr: IV 2-3 mcg/kg

Preoperatively
Adult and child >12 yr: IM/IV 0.05-0.1 mg q30-60min before surgery

Postoperatively
Adult and child >12 yr: IM/IV 0.05-0.1 mg q1-2hr prn

Sedation/analgesia
Adult and child >12 yr: IV 0.5-1 mcg/kg/dose; may repeat after 30-60 min
Child 1-12 yr: IV BOL 1-2 mcg/kg/dose; may repeat after 30-60 min intervals; CONT IV 1-5 mcg/kg/hr after IV BOL dose
Neonate: IV BOL 0.5-3 mcg/kg/dose; CONT IV 0.5-2 mcg/kg/hr after IV BOL

Actiq
Adult: Transmucosal 200 mcg, redose if needed 15 min after completion of 1st dose, max 2 doses during titration period

Fentora
Adult: BUCCAL 100 mcg placed above rear molar between upper cheek and gum

Fentanyl transdermal
Adult: 25 mcg/hr; may increase until pain relief occurs; apply patch to flat surface on upper torso and wear for 72 hr; apply new patch to different site for continued relief

Available forms: Inj 0.05 mg/ml; lozenges 100, 200, 300, 400 mcg; lozenges on a stick 200, 400, 600, 800, 1200, 1600 mcg; buccal tab 100, 200, 400, 600, 800 mcg; oral dissolving film (Onsolis) 120, 200, 400, 600, 800 mcg; transdermal patch 12, 25, 50, 75, 100 mcg/hr

Adverse effects
CNS: Dizziness, delirium, euphoria, sedation
CV: **Bradycardia, cardiac arrest,** hypo/hypertension
EENT: Blurred vision, miosis
GI: Nausea, vomiting, constipation
GU: Urinary retention
INTEG: Rash, diaphoresis
MS: Muscle rigidity
RESP: **Respiratory depression, arrest, laryngospasm**

Contraindications: Hypersensitivity to opiates, myasthenia gravis

Precautions: Pregnancy C, breastfeeding, geriatric, respiratory depression, increased ICP, seizure disorders, cardiac dysrhythmias

Black Box Warning: Children, accidental exposure, ambient temperature increase, fever, opioid-naive patients, skin abrasion (TD patch), substance abuse, severe respiratory disorders

Pharmacokinetics
Absorption	Well absorbed (IM), completely absorbed (**IV**)
Distribution	Unknown, crosses placenta
Metabolism	Extensively—liver, 80% bound to plasma proteins
Excretion	Kidneys—up to 25% unchanged, breast milk
Half-life	1½-6 hr; 17 hr after removal of patch (TD)

Pharmacodynamics
	IM	IV	TD
Onset	7-8 min	Rapid	6 hr
Peak	30 min	3-5 min	12-24 hr
Duration	1-2 hr	½-1 hr	72 hr

Interactions
Individual drugs
Alcohol: Increased respiratory depression, hypotension, increased sedation
Drug classifications
Antipsychotics, opioids, skeletal muscle relaxants: effects increased
CNS depressants, sedative/hypnotics: increased respiratory depression, hypotension
CYP3A4 inducers (carbamazepine, phenobarbital, phenytoin, rifampin): decreased fentanyl effect
Drug/herb
Corkwood: increased anticholinergic effect
Gotu kola, Jamaican dogwood, kava, lavender, mistletoe, nettle, pokeweed, poppy, senega, St. John's wort, valerian: increased fentanyl action
Drug/lab test
Increased: amylase, lipase

NURSING CONSIDERATIONS
Assessment
• Monitor VS after parenteral route (B/P, pulse, respiration); note muscle rigidity; take drug history before administering product; check renal/liver function tests; assess for respiratory dysfunction: respiratory depression, character, rate, rhythm; notify prescriber if respirations are <10/min
• Monitor CNS changes: dizziness, drowsiness, hallucinations, euphoria, LOC, pupil reaction

Adverse effects: *italic* = common, **bold** = life-threatening

- Monitor allergic reactions: rash, urticaria; product should be discontinued
- Assess for pain: intensity, location, duration, type, before and 15 min after IM route or 3-5 min after **IV** route

Nursing diagnoses
- Breathing pattern, ineffective (adverse reactions)
- Knowledge, deficient (teaching)
- Pain, acute (uses)
- Sensory perception, disturbed: visual, auditory (adverse reactions)

Implementation
- Give by inj (IM, **IV**), only with resuscitative equipment available; give slowly to prevent rigidity
- Store in light-resistant area at room temperature

Transmucosal route
- Remove foil just before administration; instruct patient to place between cheek and lower gum, moving it back and forth and suck, not chew (Actiq); place above rear molar (Fentora); place film on the inside of the cheek (Onsolis); all products not used or partially used should be flushed down the toilet

Transdermal route
- Apply patch to chest on a flat area with skin intact; for skin preparation, use clear water with no soap; clip hair, skin should be dry before applying patch; apply immediately after removing from package and press firmly in place with palm of hand; flush old patch down toilet immediately upon removal

Use pain dosing
- Dosage is titrated based on patient's report of pain; dosage is determined by calculating the previous 24-hr requirement and converting to equianalgesic morphine dose
- To convert to another opioid analgesic, remove transdermal patch and begin treatment with half the equal pain-controlling dose of the new analgesic in 12-18 hr

IV route
- Give **IV** undiluted by anesthesiologist or diluted with 5 ml or more sterile water or 0.9% NaCl given through Y-tube or 3-way stopcock given at 0.1 mg or less/1.2 min

Syringe compatibilities: Alprostadil, atracurium, atropine, bupivacaine/ketamine, butorphanol, chlorproMAZINE, cimetidine, clonidine/lidocaine, dimenhyDRINATE, diphenhydrAMINE, droperidol, heparin, hydromorphone, hydrOXYzine, meperidine, metoclopramide, midazolam, morphine, pentazocine, perphenazine, prochlorperazine, promazine, promethazine, ranitidine, scopolamine

Syringe incompatibilities: Pentobarbital

Y-site compatibilities: Amphotericin B cholesteryl, atracurium, cisatracurium, diltiazem, dobutamine, DOPamine, enalaprilat, epinephrine, esmolol, etomidate, furosemide, heparin, hydrocortisone, hydromorphone, labetalol, lorazepam, midazolam, milrinone, morphine, nafcillin, niCARdipine, nitroglycerin, norepinephrine, pancuronium, potassium chloride, propofol, ranitidine, remifentanil, sargramostim, thiopental, vecuronium, vit B/C

Additive compatibilities: Bupivacaine, caffeine citrate, clonidine, droperidol, epinephrine, ketamine, lidocaine, ziconotide

Additive incompatibilities: Methohexital, pentobarbital, thiopental

Solution compatibilities: D_5W, 0.9% NaCl

Patient/family education
- Advise patient to report any symptoms of CNS changes, allergic reactions
- Instruct patient to avoid CNS depressants: alcohol, sedative/hypnotics for at least 24 hr after taking this product
- Teach patient that dizziness, drowsiness, confusion are common, and to avoid getting up without assistance
- Discuss in detail with patient all aspects of the product
- Teach patient CNS changes: physical dependence; not to use with alcohol, other CNS depressants

Transdermal route
- Discuss with patient that excessive heat may increase absorption; excessive perspiration may alter adhesiveness
- Discuss with patient that hair may need to be clipped before applying
- Teach patient how to dispose of patch: place sticky sides together and flush in toilet

Evaluation
Positive therapeutic outcome
- Maintenance of anesthesia
- Decreased breakthrough cancer pain
- General pain relief

Treatment of overdose: Naloxone 0.2-0.8 **IV**, O_2, **IV** fluids, vasopressors

ferrous fumarate (Rx, OTC)
(fer'us fyu'-muh-rāt)
Femiron, Feostat, Feostat Drops,
Hemocyte, Ircon, Nephro-Fer,
Novofumar ✦, Palafer ✦, Span-FF

ferrous gluconate (Rx, OTC)
Fergon, Fertinic ✦, Novoferrogluc ✦

**ferric gluconate
complex** (Rx, OTC)
Ferrlecit

ferrous sulfate (Rx, OTC)
Apo-Ferrous Sulfate ✦, ED-INSOL, Feosol,
Fer-gen-sol, Fer-Iron Drops, Fero-Grad,
Mol-Iron

ferrous sulfate, dried
(Rx, OTC)
Fe⁵⁰, Feosol, Feratab, Novoferrosulfa ✦,
PMS-Ferrous Sulfate, Slow Fe

iron, carbonyl (OTC)
(kar'boh-nil)
Feosol

iron polysaccharide (OTC)
(pah-lee-sack'ah-ride)
Hytinic, Niferex, Nu-Iron, Nu-Iron 150
Func. class.: Hematinic
Chem. class.: Iron preparation

Pregnancy category B, C

Action: Replaces iron stores needed for red blood cell development, energy and O_2 transport, utilization; fumarate contains 33% elemental iron; gluconate, 12%; sulfate, 20%; iron, 30%; ferrous sulfate exsiccated

Therapeutic outcome: Prevention and correction of iron deficiency

Uses: Iron deficiency anemia, prophylaxis for iron deficiency in pregnancy, nutritional supplementation

Dosage and routes
Fumarate
Adult: PO 50-100 mg tid
Child: PO 3 mg/kg/day (elemental iron) tid-qid

Gluconate
Adult: PO 200-600 mg daily-tid
Child 6-12 yr: PO 300-900 mg/day
Child <6 yr: PO 100-300 mg/day

Sulfate
Adult: PO 0.750-1.5 g/day in divided doses tid
Child 6-12 yr: 600 mg/day in divided doses

Pregnancy
Adult: PO 300-600 mg/day in divided doses

Complex
Adult: **IV** INF (125 mg) 10 ml/100 ml of NaCl for inj given over 1 hr

Iron polysaccharide
Adult: 100-200 mg tid
Child: PO 4-6 mg/kg/day in 3 divided doses

Available forms: *Fumarate:* tabs 63, 195, 200, 324, 325 mg; chewable tabs 100 mg; controlled-release tabs 300 mg; oral susp 100 mg/5 ml, 45 mg/0.6 ml; *gluconate:* tabs 300, 320, 325 mg; caps 86, 325, 435 mg; film-coated tabs 300 mg; elix 300 mg/5 ml; *sulfate:* tabs 195, 300, 325 mg; enteric-coated tabs 325 mg; ext rel tabs, time-rel caps 525 mg; dried: tabs 200 mg; ext rel tabs 160 mg; ext rel caps 160 mg; complex: inj 62.5 mg/5 ml (12.5 mg/ml); *iron polysaccharide:* tabs 50 mg; caps 150 mg; sol 100 mg/5 ml

Adverse effects
GI: Nausea, constipation, epigastric pain, black and red tarry stools, vomiting, diarrhea
INTEG: Temporarily discolored tooth enamel and eyes
SYST: **Hypersensitivity reactions (Ferrlecit)**

Contraindications: Hypersensitivity, ulcerative colitis/regional enteritis, hemosiderosis/hemochromatosis, peptic ulcer disease, hemolytic anemia, cirrhosis

Precautions: Pregnancy **B** (ferric gluconate complex), **C** (iron dextran, oral products); anemia (long-term)

Black Box Warning: Accidental exposure

Pharmacokinetics	
Absorption	Up to 30%
Distribution	Bound to transferrin, crosses placenta
Metabolism	Recycled
Excretion	Feces, urine, skin, breast milk
Half-life	Unknown

Pharmacodynamics
Unknown

Interactions
Individual drugs
Chloramphenicol, vit C: increased absorption of iron products

Adverse effects: *italic* = common, **bold** = life-threatening

Cholestyramine: decreased absorption of iron
L-Thyroxine: decreased L-thyroxine absorption
Levodopa: decreased absorption of levodopa
Methyldopa: decreased absorption of methyldopa
Penicillamine: decreased absorption of penicillamine
Tetracycline: decreased absorption of tetracycline
Vit E: decreased absorption of iron preparations

Drug classifications
Antacids, H₂ antagonists, proton pump inhibitors: decreased absorption of iron preparations
Fluoroquinolones: decreased absorption of fluoroquinolone

Drug/herb
Allspice, bilberry, condurango, elderberry, eye bright (PO), gentian, ground ivy, marshmallow, meadowsweet, mistletoe, motherwort, nettle, raspberry, valerian, tea made with artichoke, hawthorn, horse chestnut, lady mantle, lemon balm, oak bark, plantain, poplar, prickly ash, sage: decreased iron absorption
Anise: increased iron effect
Black catechu: forms insoluble complex

Drug/food
Caffeine, dairy products, eggs: decreased absorption

Drug/lab test
False positive: occult blood

NURSING CONSIDERATIONS
Assessment
• Monitor blood studies: Hct, Hgb, reticulocytes, bilirubin before treatment, at least monthly; iron studies (Fe, TIBC, ferritin)
• Assess for toxicity: nausea, vomiting, diarrhea (green, then tarry stools,) hematemesis, pallor, cyanosis, shock, coma
• Assess bowel elimination; if constipation occurs, increase water, bulk, activity before laxatives are required
• Assess nutrition: amount of iron in diet (meat, dark green leafy vegetables, dried beans, dried fruits, eggs); provide referral to dietitian if indicated
• Identify cause of iron loss or anemia, including salicylates, sulfonamides, antimalarials, quinidine

Nursing diagnoses
• Fatigue (uses)
• Knowledge, deficient (teaching)
• Nutrition, less than body requirements, imbalanced (uses)

Implementation
• Swallow all tabs whole; do not break, crush, or chew
• Give between meals for best absorption; may give with juice; do not give with antacids or milk, delay at least 1 hr; if GI symptoms occur, give after meals even if absorption is decreased; eggs, milk products, chocolate, caffeine interfere with absorption; ferrous gluconate is less GI irritating than ferrous sulfate
• Give liquid preparations through plastic straw to avoid discoloration of tooth enamel; dilute thoroughly
• Give at least 1 hr before bedtime because corrosion may occur in stomach
• Give for <6 mo for anemia
• Store in airtight, light-resistant container

Patient/family education
• Advise patient that iron will make stools black or dark green; that iron poisoning may occur if increased beyond recommended level
• Keep out of reach of children
• Caution patient not to substitute one iron salt for another; elemental iron content differs (e.g., 300 mg ferrous fumarate contains about 100 mg elemental iron, whereas 300 mg ferrous gluconate contains only about 30 mg elemental iron)
• Caution patient to avoid reclining position for 15-30 min after taking product to avoid esophageal corrosion; to follow diet high in iron
• Caution patient to avoid taking iron, dairy products, calcium supplements, vit C together; they compete for absorption

Evaluation
Positive therapeutic outcome
• Decreased fatigue, weakness
• Improvement in Hct, Hgb, reticulocytes

Treatment of overdose: Induce vomiting; give eggs, milk until lavage can be done

---

ferumoxytol (Rx)
(fer′ue-mox′i-tol)
Feraheme
Func. class.: Hematinic

Pregnancy category B

Action: Iron is carried by transferrin to the bone marrow, where it is incorporated into hemoglobin

Uses: Iron deficiency anemia in chronic kidney disease

 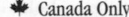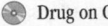

Therapeutic outcome: Resolution of iron deficiency anemia in chronic kidney disease

Unlabeled uses: MRI

Dosage and routes
Adult: **IV** 510 mg of elemental iron followed by a second dose 3-8 days later; if giving during dialysis, give after B/P is stable and after 1 hr of hemodialysis

Available forms: 510 mg/17 ml solution for injection

Adverse effects
CNS: Headache, dizziness
CV: Chest pain, hypo/hypertension, hypervolemia, edema
GI: Nausea, vomiting, abdominal pain, constipation, diarrhea
INTEG: Rash, pruritus, urticaria, fever
MISC: **Anaphylaxis**
MS: Back pain
RESP: Dyspnea, cough

Contraindications: Hypersensitivity, hemochromatosis

Precautions: Pregnancy **B**, breastfeeding, children, geriatric patients, all anemias excluding iron deficiency anemia, iron overload, dialysis, hepatic disease, hypotension, MRI, sideroblastic anemia, thalassemia

Pharmacokinetics	
Absorption	Unknown
Distribution	Unknown
Metabolism	Unknown
Excretion	Unknown
Half-life	15 hr

Pharmacodynamics
Unknown

Interactions
Oral iron; do not use: iron toxicity

NURSING CONSIDERATIONS
Assessment
• Monitor blood studies: Hct, Hgb, reticulocytes, transferrin, plasma iron concentrations, ferritin, total iron-binding, bilirubin before treatment, at least monthly
• Assess for allergy: anaphylaxis, rash, pruritus, fever, wheezing; notify prescriber immediately, keep emergency equipment available
• Assess cardiac status: hypo/hypertension, hypervolemia
• Assess for toxicity: nausea, vomiting, diarrhea, fever, abdominal pain (early symptoms),

cyanotic-looking lips, nailbeds, seizures, CV collapse (late symptoms)

Nursing diagnoses
• Activity intolerance (uses)
• Knowledge deficient (teaching)

Implementation
• Use only with epinephrine, Solu-Medrol available in case of anaphylactic reaction during dose
IV route
• Give directly in dialysis line by slow inj or inf, give by slow inj at 1 ml/min (5 min/vial); inf, dilute each vial exclusively in a max of 100 ml of 0.9% NaCl, give at rate of 100 mg of iron/15 min, discard unused portions

Perform/provide
• Store at room temperature in cool environment, do not freeze

Patient/family education
• Teach to report itching, rash, chest pain, headache, vertigo, nausea, vomiting, abdominal pain, joint/muscle pain, numbness, tingling
• Teach that iron poisoning may occur if increased beyond recommended level; not to take oral iron preparation
• May alter MRI studies

Evaluation
Positive therapeutic outcome
• Increased serum iron levels, Hct, Hgb

Treatment of overdose: Discontinue product, treat allergic reaction, give diphenhydrAMINE or epinephrine as needed, give iron-chelating product in acute poisoning

fesoterodine (Rx)
(fess'oh-ter-oh-deen)
Toviaz
Func. class.: Overactive bladder product
Chem. class.: Muscarinic receptor antagonist

Pregnancy category C

Action: Relaxes smooth muscles in urinary tract by inhibiting acetylcholine at postganglionic sites

Therapeutic outcome: Absence of urinary frequency, urgency, incontinence

Uses: Overactive bladder (urinary frequency, urgency), urinary incontinence

Dosage and routes
Adult and geriatric: PO EXT REL 4 mg/day, may increase to 8 mg/day based on

F

response, max 4 mg/day in those taking potent CYP3A4 inhibitors

Renal dose
Adult: PO EXT REL max 4 mg/day in severe renal impairment

Available forms: Ext rel tabs 4, 8 mg

Adverse effects
CV: Chest pain, angina, QT prolongation
EENT: Xerophthalmia
GI: Nausea, vomiting, abdominal pain, constipation, dry mouth
GU: Dysuria, urinary retention
INTEG: Rash
MISC: Peripheral edema
MS: Back pain
RESP: Cough
SYST: Infection

Contraindications: GI obstruction, ileus, pyloric stenosis, urinary retention, gastric retention, hypersensitivity

Precautions: Pregnancy **C**, breastfeeding, children, renal/hepatic disease, closed-angle glaucoma, urinary tract obstruction, ambient temperature increase, autonomic neuropathy, constipation, contact lenses, hazardous activity, GERD, gastroparesis, myasthenia gravis, prostatic hypertrophy, toxic megacolon, ulcerative colitis

Pharmacokinetics	
Absorption	Rapidly
Distribution	Protein binding 50%
Metabolism	Unknown
Excretion	Urine/feces
Half-life	7 hr

Pharmacodynamics
Unknown

Interactions
Drug classifications
Anticholinergics, antimuscarinics: increased anticholinergic effect
Antiretroviral protease inhibitors, azole antifungals, macrolide antiinfectives: increased action of fesoterodine
Diuretics: increased urinary frequency
Drug/herb
Caffeine, green tea, guarana: decreased fesoterodine
Drug/food
Grapefruit juice: increased fesoterodine level
Cola, coffee, tea: decreased fesoterodine level
Drug/lab test
Increased: LFTs

NURSING CONSIDERATIONS
Assessment
• Assess urinary patterns: distention, nocturia, frequency, urgency, incontinence
• Assess for allergic reactions: rash; if this occurs, product should be discontinued

Nursing diagnoses
• Knowledge, deficient (teaching)
• Incontinence, urge urinary (uses)
• Urinary elimination, impaired (uses)

Implementation
• Do not break, crush, or chew ext rel product
• Give without regard to meals
• Store at room temperature; protect from moisture

Patient/family education
• Advise patient not to drink liquids before bedtime
• Instruct the patient on the importance of bladder maintenance

Evaluation
Positive therapeutic outcome
• Absence of urinary frequency, urgency, incontinence

fexofenadine (Rx)
(fex-oh-fin'a-deen)
Allegra
Func. class.: Histamine antagonist, 2nd generation
Chem. class.: Piperidine, peripherally selective
Pregnancy category C

Do not confuse:
Allegra/Viagra

Action: Acts on blood vessels, GI, respiratory system by competing with histamine for H_1-receptor site; decreases allergic response by blocking pharmacologic effects of histamine; less sedation rate than with other antihistamines; causes increased heart rate, vasodilatation, increased secretions

Therapeutic outcome: Absence of allergy symptoms and rhinitis

Uses: Rhinitis, allergy symptoms, chronic idiopathic urticaria

Dosage and routes
Adult and child >12 yr: PO 60 mg bid or 180 mg/day
Child 6-11 yr: PO 30 mg bid; Orally

disintegrating tab 30 mg bid dissolved on tongue

Renal dose
Adult and child ≥12 yr: PO CCr <80 ml/min 60 mg/day

Available forms: Caps 60 mg; tabs 30, 60, 180 mg; oral susp 6 mg/ml; orally disintegrating tab 30 mg

Adverse effects
CNS: Headache, stimulation, drowsiness, sedation, fatigue, confusion, blurred vision, tinnitus, restlessness, tremors, paradoxical excitation in children or geriatric
CV: Hypotension, palpitations, bradycardia, tachycardia, **dysrhythmias (rare)**
GI: Nausea, diarrhea, abdominal pain, vomiting, constipation
GU: Frequency, dysuria, urinary retention, impotence
HEMA: **Hemolytic anemia, thrombocytopenia, leukopenia, agranulocytosis, pancytopenia**
INTEG: Rash, eczema, photosensitivity, urticaria
RESP: Thickening of bronchial secretions; dry nose, throat

Contraindications: Breastfeeding, newborn or premature infants, hypersensitivity, severe hepatic disease

Precautions: Pregnancy C, children, geriatric, respiratory disease, closed-angle glaucoma, prostatic hypertrophy, bladder neck obstruction, asthma

Pharmacokinetics	
Absorption	Well absorbed
Distribution	Unknown
Metabolism	Liver
Excretion	Kidneys
Half-life	Unknown

Pharmacodynamics	
Onset	1 hr
Peak	2-3 hr
Duration	12-24 hr

Interactions
Drug classifications
Aluminum, antacids, magnesium: decreased fexofenadine effect
Drug/herb
Corkwood, henbane leaf: increased anticholinergic effect
Hops, Jamaican dogwood, khat, senega, St. John's wort: increased sedation

Drug/food
Apple, orange, grapefruit, pomegranate juice: decreased absorption
Drug/lab test
False negative: skin allergy tests (discontinue antihistamine 3 days before testing)

NURSING CONSIDERATIONS
Assessment
• Assess respiratory status: rate, rhythm, increase in bronchial secretions, wheezing, chest tightness; provide fluids to 2 L/day to decrease secretion thickness
• Monitor I&O ratio: be alert for urinary retention, frequency, dysuria, especially geriatric; product should be discontinued if these occur

Nursing diagnoses
• Airway clearance, ineffective (uses)
• Injury, risk for (side effects)
• Knowledge, deficient (teaching)
• Noncompliance (teaching, overuse)

Implementation
• Give on an empty stomach 1 hr before or 2 hr after meals to facilitate absorption, with food or milk for GI symptoms, do not take with juice
• Orally disintegrating tab: allow to dissolve, swallow
• Store in tight, light-resistant container

Patient/family education
• Teach all aspects of product uses; to notify prescriber if confusion, sedation, hypotension occur; to avoid driving or other hazardous activity if drowsiness occurs; to avoid alcohol or other CNS depressants that may potentiate effect
• Instruct patient to take 1 hr before or 2 hr after meals to facilitate absorption
• Instruct patient not to exceed recommended dose; dysrhythmias may occur
• Teach patient that hard candy, gum, frequent rinsing of mouth may be used for dryness

Evaluation
Positive therapeutic outcome
• Absence of running or congested nose, rashes

Treatment of overdose:
Administer lavage, diazepam, vasopressors, **IV** phenytoin

F

Adverse effects: *italic* = common, **bold** = life-threatening

fibrinogen, concentrate, human
Ria STAP
See Appendix A, Selected New Drugs

filgrastim (Rx)
(fill-gras′stim)
G-CSF, granulocyte colony stimulator, Neupogen
Func. class.: Biologic modifier
Chem. class.: Granulocyte colony-stimulating factor

Pregnancy category C

Action: Stimulates proliferation and differentiation of neutrophils; a glycoprotein

Therapeutic outcome: Absence of infection

Uses: To decrease infection in patients receiving antineoplastics that are myelosuppressive; to increase WBC in patients with product-induced neutropenia; bone marrow depression

Unlabeled uses: Neutropenia in HIV infection, aplastic anemia, ganciclovir-induced neutropenia, zidovudine-induced neutropenia

Dosage and routes
After myelosuppressive chemotherapy
Adult and child: **IV**/SUBCUT 5 mcg/kg/day in a single dose × 14 days; may increase by 5 mcg/kg in each chemotherapy cycle

After bone marrow transplantation
Adult: **IV**/SUBCUT 10 mcg/kg as an INF (**IV**) over 4 or 24 hr, begin 24 hr after chemotherapy and 24 hr after bone marrow transplantation

Peripheral blood progenitor cell collection/therapy
Adult: 10 mcg/kg/day as a BOL or CONT INF × 4 days or more before leukapheresis, continue to last leukapheresis, may alter dose if WBC >100,000/mm³

Severe neutropenia (chronic), idiopathic/cyclical
Adult: SUBCUT 5 mcg/kg daily

Available forms: Inj 300 mcg/ml, 480 mcg/1.6 ml, 480 mcg/0.8 ml, 3000 mcg/0.5 ml

Adverse effects
CNS: Fever, headache
GI: Nausea, vomiting, diarrhea, mucositis, anorexia
HEMA: **Thrombocytopenia,** excessive leukocytosis
INTEG: Alopecia, exacerbation of skin conditions, urticaria, vasculitis
MS: Osteoporosis, skeletal pain
OTHER: Chest pain, hypotension
RESP: **Acute respiratory distress syndrome,** wheezing, alveolar hemorrhage

Contraindications: Hypersensitivity to proteins of *Escherichia coli*

Precautions: Pregnancy **C**, breastfeeding, children, cardiac conditions, myeloid malignancies, radiation therapy, sepsis, sickle cell disease, chemotherapy, respiratory disease

Pharmacokinetics	
Absorption	Well absorbed (SUBCUT), completely absorbed (**IV**)
Distribution	Unknown
Metabolism	Unknown
Excretion	Unknown
Half-life	Unknown

Pharmacodynamics		
	IV	SUBCUT
Onset	5-60 min	5-60 min
Peak	24 hr	2-8 hr
Duration	up to 1 wk	up to 1 wk

Interactions
Individual drugs
Lithium: do not use concurrently
Drug classifications
Antineoplastics: increased neutrophils, do not use together 24 hr before or after antineoplastics
Drug/lab test
Increased: uric acid, lactate dehydrogenase, alkaline phosphatase

NURSING CONSIDERATIONS
Assessment
• Monitor blood studies: CBC, platelet count before treatment and twice weekly; neutrophil counts (ANC) may be increased for 2 days after therapy, but treatment should continue until ANC >10,000/mm³
• Assess for bone pain: frequency, intensity, duration; analgesics may be given; opiates should not be used
• Check B/P, heart rate, respiration; baseline, during treatment

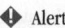 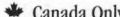

Nursing diagnoses
- Infection, risk for (uses)
- Knowledge, deficient (teaching)
- Pain, acute (adverse reaction)

Implementation
IV route
- Give 300 mcg/ml or 480 mcg/1.6 ml; allow to warm to room temperature; give single dose over 1 min or less through Y-tube or medport
- Dilute in D_5W to a conc of 5-15 mcg/ml, vial is for one-time use; give over 15-30 min (chemotherapy); over 4-24 hr (bone marrow transplantation); do not use 0.9% NaCl to dilute product
- Use single-use vials; after dose is withdrawn, do not reenter vial
- Do not shake; discard any product left out for >24 hr
- Do not use earlier than 24 hr after antineoplastics, bone marrow infusion
- Give for 2 wk or until ANC = 10,000/mm³ after the expected chemotherapy neutrophil nadir
- Store in refrigerator; do not freeze; may store at room temperature for up to 24 hr

Y-site compatibilities: Acyclovir,
allopurinol, amikacin, aminophylline, ampicillin, ampicillin/sulbactam, aztreonam, bleomycin, bumetanide, buprenorphine, butorphanol, calcium gluconate, carboplatin, carmustine, cefazolin, cefotetan, ceftazidime, chlorproMAZINE, cimetidine, cisplatin, cyclophosphamide, cytarabine, dacarbazine, DAUNOrubicin, dexamethasone, diphenhydrAMINE, DOXOrubicin, doxycycline, droperidol, enalaprilat, famotidine, floxuridine, fluconazole, fludarabine, gallium, ganciclovir, granisetron, haloperidol, hydrocortisone, hydromorphone, hydrOXYzine, idarubicin, ifosfamide, leucovorin, lorazepam, mechlorethamine, melphalan, meperidine, mesna, methotrexate, metoclopramide, miconazole, minocycline, mitoxantrone, morphine, nalbuphine, netilmicin, ondansetron, plicamycin, potassium chloride, promethazine, ranitidine, sodium bicarbonate, streptozocin, ticarcillin, ticarcillin/clavulanate, tobramycin, trimethoprim-sulfamethoxazole, vancomycin, vinBLAStine, vinCRIStine, vinorelbine, zidovudine

Patient/family education
- Teach patient technique for self-administration: dose, side effects, disposal of containers and needles; provide instruction sheet

Evaluation
Positive therapeutic outcome
- Absence of infection

---

finasteride (Rx)
(fin-ass'te-ride)
Propecia, Proscar
Func. class.: Androgen hormone inhibitor, hair stimulant
Chem. class.: 5-α-Reductase inhibitor

Pregnancy category X

Do not confuse:
Proscar/ProSom/Prozac
finasteride/furosemide

Action: Inhibits 5-α-reductase and reduction in dihydrotestosterone (DHT); DHT induces androgenic effects by binding to androgen receptors in the cell nuclei of the prostate gland, liver, skin; prevents development of benign prostatic hypertrophy (BPH)

Therapeutic outcome: Reduced prostate size

Uses: Symptomatic BPH; male-pattern baldness (Propecia)

Dosage and routes
BPH
Adult: PO 5 mg/day × 6-12 mo

Male pattern baldness
Adult: PO 1 mg/day for 3 mo or more for results

Available forms: Tabs (Propecia) 1 mg, (Proscar) 5 mg

Adverse effects
GU: Impotence, decreased libido, decreased volume of ejaculate
INTEG: Rash
MISC: Breast tenderness

Contraindications: Pregnancy **X**, breastfeeding, children, women who are pregnant or may become pregnant should not handle tabs, hypersensitivity

Precautions: Large residual urinary volume, severely diminished urinary flow, liver function abnormalities

---

Pharmacokinetics

Absorption	63%, readily
Distribution	Plasma protein binding, crosses blood-brain barrier
Metabolism	Liver
Excretion	Kidneys—metabolites (39%), feces (57%)
Half-life	6-15 hr

Adverse effects: *italic* = common, **bold** = life-threatening

Pharmacodynamics	
Onset	Immediate
Peak	1-2 hr
Duration	14 days

Interactions
Drug classifications
Anticholinergics, bronchodilators (adrenergic), theophylline: decreased effect of finasteride
Drug/lab test
Decreased: PSA levels (finasteride)

NURSING CONSIDERATIONS
Assessment
• Assess urinary patterns, residual urinary volume, severely diminished urinary flow; PSA levels and digital rectal exam results before initiating therapy and periodically thereafter
• Monitor liver function tests before initiating treatment; extensively metabolized in liver

Nursing diagnoses
• Knowledge, deficient (teaching)
• Urinary elimination, impaired (uses)

Implementation
• Administer without regard to meals; give for a minimum of 6 mo; not all patients will respond
• Store at temp <86° F (30° C); protect from light; keep container tightly closed

Patient/family education
• Advise patient that pregnant women or women who may become pregnant should not touch crushed tab or come into contact with semen of a patient taking this product; may adversely affect development of male fetus
• Inform patient that volume of ejaculate may be decreased during treatment; impotence and decreased libido may also occur
• Inform patient that Propecia results may not occur for 3 mo
• Inform patient that Proscar results may not occur for 6-12 mo

Evaluation
Positive therapeutic outcome
• Decreased postvoiding dribbling, frequency, nocturia
• Increased urinary flow
• Regression of prostate size
• Hair growth within 3-6 mo

flavocoxid (Rx)
(flav-uh-kox'id)
Limbrel
Func. class.: Oral nutritional supplement

Pregnancy category Unknown

Action: Exhibits anti-inflammatory, analgesic properties, thought to be due to inhibition of prostaglandin synthesis via inhibition of cyclooxygenase

Therapeutic outcome: Decreased pain, inflammation in osteoarthritis

Uses: For dietary management of osteoarthritis

Dosage and routes
Adult: PO 250 or 500 mg q12hr

Available forms: Caps 250 mg

Adverse effects
MISC: Hypertension, increase in varicose veins, psoriasis
MS: Fluid accumulation in the knees

Contraindications: Hypersensitivity

Precautions: Pregnancy **Unknown,** breastfeeding, children <18 yr, history of stomach ulcers

Pharmacokinetics	
Absorption	Unknown
Distribution	Unknown
Metabolism	Primarily via glucuronidation and sulfation
Excretion	Unknown
Half-life	Unknown

Pharmacodynamics
Unknown

NURSING CONSIDERATIONS
Assessment
• Assess for pain of rheumatoid arthritis, osteoarthritis; check ROM, inflammation of joints, characteristics of pain

Nursing diagnoses
• Injury, risk for (uses)
• Knowledge, deficient (teaching)

Implementation
• Administer 1 hr before or after meals, food increases absorption

Patient/family education
• Teach patient that product does not take the place of other products, including corticosteroids for osteoarthritis

- Advise patient to notify prescriber if pregnancy is planned or suspected

Evaluation
Positive therapeutic outcome
- Decreased pain, inflammation in arthritic conditions

---

flecainide (Rx)
(flek'a-nide)
Tambocor
Func. class.: Antidysrhythmic (Class IC)

Pregnancy category C

Action: Decreases conduction in all parts of the heart, with greatest effect on the His-Purkinje system, which stabilizes the cardiac membrane

Therapeutic outcome: Absence of dysrhythmias

Uses: Life-threatening ventricular dysrhythmias, sustained ventricular tachycardia; supraventricular tachydysrhythmias, paroxysmal atrial fibrillation/flutter associated with disabling symptoms

Unlabeled uses: Atrial fibrillation, single dose

Dosage and routes
PSVTT/PAT
Adult: PO 50-100 mg q12hr; may increase every 4 days by 50 mg q12hr to desired response; max 300 mg/day

Life-threatening ventricular dysrhythmias
Adult: PO 100 mg q12hr, may increase by 50 mg q12hr q4days; max 400 mg/day

Renal dose
Adult: PO CCr <35 ml/min dose 50%-75%

Available forms: Tabs 50, 100, 150 mg

Adverse effects
CNS: *Headache, dizziness,* involuntary movement, confusion, psychosis, restlessness, irritability, paresthesias, ataxia, flushing, somnolence, depression, anxiety, malaise, fatigue, asthenia, tremors
CV: *Hypotension,* **bradycardia,** angina, PVCs, **heart block, cardiovascular collapse, arrest, dysrhythmias, CHF, fatal ventricular tachycardia**
EENT: Tinnitus, *blurred vision,* hearing loss, corneal deposits, dry eyes
GI: Nausea, vomiting, anorexia, constipation, abdominal pain, flatulence, change in taste, diarrhea
GU: Impotence, decreased libido, polyuria, urinary retention
HEMA: **Leukopenia, thrombocytopenia**
INTEG: Rash, urticaria, edema, swelling
RESP: Dyspnea, **respiratory depression**

Contraindications: Hypersensitivity, severe heart block, cardiogenic shock, nonsustained ventricular dysrhythmias, frequent PVCs, non–life-threatening dysrhythmias

Precautions: Pregnancy **C**, breastfeeding, children, renal/hepatic disease, CHF, respiratory depression, myasthenia gravis, geriatric, electrolyte abnormalities

Black Box Warning: MI, cardiac arrhythmias

Pharmacokinetics
Absorption	Well absorbed
Distribution	Widely distributed
Metabolism	Liver
Excretion	30% kidneys, unchanged
Half-life	14 hr

Pharmacodynamics
Onset	Unknown
Peak	3 hr
Duration	Unknown

Interactions
Individual drugs
Amiodarone, cimetidine, ritonavir: increased level of flecainide
Digoxin: increased digoxin levels
Disopyramide, verapamil: increased CV depressant action
Propanolol: increased both products
Drug classifications
Acidifying agents, alkalizing agents: increased or decreased effect
β-Adrenergic blockers: increased CV depressant action
Drug/herb
Aconite: increased toxicity, death
Aloe, broom, buckthorn (chronic use), cascara sagrada (chronic use), Chinese rhubarb, figwort, fumitory, goldenseal, kudzu, licorice: increased effect
Coltsfoot: decreased effect
Horehound: increased serotonin effect
Drug/lab test
Increased: CPK

NURSING CONSIDERATIONS
Assessment
- Monitor ECG continuously to determine product effectiveness; measure PR, QRS,

---

Adverse effects: *italic* = common, **bold** = life-threatening

QT intervals; check for PVCs, other dysrhythmias; monitor B/P continuously for hypo/hypertension and rebound hypertension (after 1-2 hr); check for dehydration or hypovolemia
- Monitor I&O ratio; electrolytes: K (potassium), Na (sodium), Cl (chloride); check weight daily and for signs of CHF or pulmonary toxicity: dyspnea, fatigue, cough, fever, chest pain, jugular vein distention, crackles; if these occur, product should be discontinued
- Monitor liver function studies: AST, ALT, bilirubin, alkaline phosphatase
- Assess patient for CNS symptoms: confusion, psychosis, numbness, depression, involuntary movements; if these occur, product should be discontinued
- Monitor cardiac rate, respiration: rate, rhythm, character, chest pain; watch for ventricular tachycardia, supraventricular tachycardia, or fibrillation

Nursing diagnoses
- Cardiac output, decreased (uses)
- Knowledge, deficient (teaching)

Implementation
- Give reduced dosage slowly with ECG monitoring; do not increase dose fewer than 4 days apart
- Give with meals if GI upset occurs

Patient/family education
- Instruct patient to report side effects immediately to prescriber
- Instruct patient to complete follow-up appointment with health care provider, including pulmonary function tests, chest x-ray
- Teach patient to change position slowly from lying or sitting to standing to minimize orthostatic hypotension
- Advise patient not to skip or double doses
- Advise patient to carry/wear emergency ID with disorder, medications taken
- Advise patient to avoid hazardous activities that require alertness until response is known

Evaluation
Positive therapeutic outcome
- Absence of dysrhythmias

fluconazole (Rx)
(floo-kon'a-zole)
Diflucan
Func. class.: Antifungal
Pregnancy category C

Do not confuse:
Diflucan/Diprivan

Action: Inhibits ergosterol biosynthesis, causes direct damage to membrane phospholipids in the cell wall of fungi

Therapeutic outcome: Fungistatic fungicidal against the following susceptible organisms: *Candida, Cryptococcus neoformans*

Uses: Oropharyngeal candidiasis; chronic mucocutaneous candidiasis; systemic, vaginal, urinary candidiasis; cryptococcal meningitis; prevention of candidiasis in bone marrow transplant in those who receive chemotherapy and/or radiation therapy

Dosage and routes
Vaginal candidiasis
Adult: PO 150 mg as a single dose

Serious fungal infections
Adult: PO/**IV** 50-400 mg initially, then 200 mg once daily for 4 wk
Child: 6-12 mg/kg/day

Oropharyngeal candidiasis
Adult: PO/**IV** 200 mg initially, then 100 mg/day for at least 2 wk
Child: PO/**IV** 6 mg/kg initially, then 3 mg/kg/day for ≥2 wk

Prevention of candidiasis in bone marrow transplant
Adult: PO/**IV** 400 mg/day

Renal dose
Adult: PO CCr <50 ml/min dose 50%

Available forms: Tabs 50, 100, 150, 200 mg; inj 2 mg/ml; powder for oral susp 50, 200 mg/ml

Adverse effects
CNS: Headache
GI: Nausea, vomiting, diarrhea, cramping, flatus, increased AST, ALT, **hepatotoxicity**
INTEG: **Stevens-Johnson syndrome**

Contraindications: Hypersensitivity to this product or azoles

Precautions: Pregnancy C, breastfeeding, renal/hepatic disease

Pharmacokinetics

Absorption	Well absorbed (PO)
Distribution	Widely distributed (peritoneum, CSF)
Metabolism	<10%—liver
Excretion	80% kidneys (unchanged)
Half-life	30 hr, increased in renal disease

Pharmacodynamics

	PO	IV
Onset	Unknown	Immediate
Peak	2-4 hr	Infusion's end
Duration	Unknown	Unknown

Interactions
Individual drugs
CycloSPORINE, phenytoin, rifabutin, tacrolimus, theophylline: increased plasma concentrations
Warfarin: increased anticoagulation
Zidovudine: increased effect
Drug classification
Contraceptives (oral): decreased effect
Oral antidiabetics: hypoglycemia
Drug/herb
Gossypol: increased nephrotoxicity

NURSING CONSIDERATIONS
Assessment
• Assess for signs and symptoms of infection: clearing of CSF culture during treatment, obtain C&S baseline and during treatment, product may be started as soon as culture is taken
• Monitor for hepatotoxicity: increased AST, ALT, alkaline phosphatase, bilirubin; product will be discontinued if hepatotoxicity occurs

Nursing diagnoses
• Infection, risk for (uses)
• Injury, risk for (adverse reactions)
• Knowledge, deficient (teaching)

Implementation
• Take with food to reduce GI effects
PO route
• Shake oral susp before each use
IV route
• Give after diluting according to package directions; run at 200 mg/hr or less; do not use plastic containers in connections
• Do not admix
• Administer **IV** using an in-line filter, using distal veins; check for extravasation and necrosis q2hr
• Give product only after C&S confirms organism, product needed to treat condition
• Store protected from moisture and light, diluted sol is stable for 24 hr

Y-site compatibilities: Acyclovir, aldesleukin, allopurinol, amifostine, amikacin, aminophylline, ampicillin/sulbactam, aztreonam, benztropine, cefazolin, cefepime, cefotetan, cefoxitin, chlorproMAZINE, cimetidine, dexamethasone, diphenhydrAMINE, DOBUTamine, DOPamine, droperidol, famotidine, filgrastim, fludarabine, foscarnet, gallium, ganciclovir, gentamicin, granisetron, heparin, hydrocortisone, immune globulin, leucovorin, lorazepam, melphalan, meperidine, meropenem, metoclopramide, metronidazole, midazolam, morphine, nafcillin, nitroglycerin, ondansetron, oxacillin, paclitaxel, pancuronium, penicillin G, potassium, phenytoin, piperacillin/tazobactam, prochlorperazine, promethazine, propofol, ranitidine, sargramostim, sulfamethoxazole, tacrolimus, teniposide, theophylline, thiotepa, ticarcillin/clavulanate, tobramycin, vancomycin, vecuronium, vinorelbine, zidovudine

Y-site incompatibilities: Amphotericin B, ampicillin, calcium gluconate, cefotaxime, ceftriaxone, ceftazidime, cefuroxime, chloramphenicol, clindamycin, diazepam, digoxin, erythromycin lactobionate, furosemide, haloperidol, hydrOXYzine, imipenem/cilastatin, pentamidine, ticarcillin, trimethoprim/sulfamethoxazole

Additive compatibilities: Acyclovir, amikacin, amphotericin B, cefazolin, ceftazidime, clindamycin, gentamicin, heparin, meropenem, metronidazole, morphine, piperacillin, potassium chloride, theophylline

Patient/family education
• Caution patient that long-term therapy may be needed to clear infection; to take entire course of medication; take in equal intervals (PO)
• Teach patient the signs and symptoms of hepatotoxicity: nausea, vomiting, clay-colored stools, dark urine, anorexia, fatigue, jaundice; prescriber should be notified immediately
• Inform patient that medication may be taken with food to reduce GI effects
• Advise patient to consider using alternative contraception if using oral contraceptives

Evaluation
Positive therapeutic outcome
• Decreasing oral candidiasis, fever, malaise, rash
• Negative C&S for infecting organism

Adverse effects: *italic* = common, **bold** = life-threatening

fludrocortisone (Rx)
(floo-droe-kor'ti-sone)
Func. class.: Corticosteroid, synthetic
Chem. class.: Mineralocorticoid
Pregnancy category C

Action: Promotes increased reabsorption of sodium and loss of potassium, water, hydrogen from the distal renal tubules

Therapeutic outcome: Treatment of adrenal insufficiency symptoms

Uses: Adrenal insufficiency, salt-losing adrenogenital syndrome, Addison's disease

Unlabeled uses: Renal tubular acidosis (type IV), idiopathic orthostatic hypertension

Dosage and routes
Adult: PO 100-200 mcg/day
Child: PO 50-100 mcg/day

Idiopathic hypotension (unlabeled)
Adult: PO 50-100 mcg/day

Available forms: Tabs 100 mcg (0.1 mg)

Adverse effects
CNS: Flushing, sweating, headache, paralysis, dizziness, **seizures**
CV: Hypertension, **circulatory collapse, thrombophlebitis, embolism,** tachycardia, **CHF,** edema
ENDO: Weight gain, adrenal suppression, hyperglycemia
META: Hypokalemia
MISC: Hypersensitivity, cataracts, GI ulcers, **anaphylaxis**
MS: Fractures, osteoporosis, weakness

Contraindications: Hypersensitivity, acute glomerulonephritis, amebiasis, psychoses, Cushing's syndrome, fungal infections, child <2 yr

Precautions: Pregnancy **C**, breastfeeding, child >2 yr, osteoporosis, CHF, hypertension, diabetes

Pharmacokinetics
Absorption	Well absorbed
Distribution	Widely
Metabolism	Liver
Excretion	Kidneys, breast milk
Half-life	3½ hr

Pharmacodynamics
Onset	Unknown
Peak	1.5 hr
Duration	Unknown

Interactions
Individual drugs
Amphotericin B, mezlocillin, piperacillin: increased hypokalemia
Phenytoin: decreased action of fludrocortisone
Rifampin: decreased effect of fludrocortisone
Drug classifications
Barbiturates: decreased action of fludrocortisone
Diuretics (loop), thiazides, potassium-wasting products: decreased potassium levels
Drug/herb
Aloe, buckthorn, cascara sagrada, Chinese rhubarb, senna: increased hypokalemia
Aloe, licorice, perilla: increased corticosteroid effect
Drug/food
Increased salt/sodium ingestion: increased B/P
Drug/lab test
Increased: potassium, sodium
Decreased: hematocrit

NURSING CONSIDERATIONS
Assessment
• Monitor patient for fluid retention: weigh daily, notify prescriber of weekly gain >5 lb; B/P q4hr, pulse; notify prescriber if chest pain occurs; I&O ratio; be alert for decreasing urinary output and increasing edema
• Check for potassium depletion: paresthesias, fatigue, nausea, vomiting, depression, polyuria, dysrhythmias, weakness; also sodium, chloride

Nursing diagnoses
• Fluid volume, deficient (uses)
• Fluid volume, excess (adverse reactions)
• Knowledge, deficient (teaching)

Implementation
• Administer titrated dose; use lowest effective dose; scored tab may be broken if lower dose is necessary
• Give with food or milk to decrease GI symptoms

Patient/family education
• Advise patient to carry/wear emergency ID as steroid user at all times during diagnosis and treatment
• Caution patient not to discontinue this medication abruptly; Addisonian crisis may occur
• Counsel patient to follow dietary regimen recommended by prescriber; should include high potassium and, possibly, low sodium
• Advise patient to report weight gain >5 lb; edema in legs, hands; abdominal cramping; muscle cramps; nausea; vomiting; anorexia;

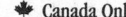 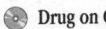

dizziness or weakness, infection, trauma, stress
- Advise patient not to breastfeed
- Tell patient to avoid exposure to disease, trauma

Evaluation
Positive therapeutic outcome
- Correction of adrenal insufficiency
- Electrolytes and fluids in normal range

flumazenil (Rx)
(flu-maz'e-nil)
Anexate ✤, Romazicon
Func. class.: Benzodiazepine receptor antagonist
Chem. class.: Imidazobenzodiazepine derivative

Pregnancy category C

Action: Antagonizes the actions of benzodiazepines on the CNS, competitively inhibits the activity at the benzodiazepine receptor complex

Therapeutic outcome: Reversed benzodiazepine toxic effects

Uses: Reversal of the sedative effects of benzodiazepines

Dosage and routes
Reversal of conscious sedation or in general anesthesia
Adult: **IV** 0.2 mg (2 ml) given over 15 sec; wait 45 sec, then give 0.2 mg (2 ml) if consciousness does not occur; may be repeated at 60-sec intervals as needed (max 3 mg/hr) or 1 mg/5 min
Child: **IV** 10 mcg (0.01 mg)/kg; cumulative dose of 1 mg or less

Management of suspected benzodiazepine overdose
Adult: **IV** 0.2 mg (2 ml) given over 30 sec; wait 30 sec, then give 0.3 mg (3 ml) over 30 sec if consciousness does not occur; further doses of 0.5 mg (5 ml) can be given over 30 sec at intervals of 1 min up to cumulative dose of 3 mg
Child: **IV** 10 mcg (0.01 mg/kg); cumulative dose of less than 1 mg

Available forms: Inj 0.1 mg/ml

Adverse effects
CNS: Dizziness, agitation, emotional lability, confusion, **seizures,** somnolence, panic attacks

CV: Hypertension, palpitations, cutaneous vasodilatation, **dysrhythmias,** bradycardia, tachycardia, chest pain
EENT: Abnormal vision, blurred vision, tinnitus
GI: Nausea, vomiting, hiccups
SYST: Headache, inj site pain, increased sweating, fatigue, rigors

Contraindications: Hypersensitivity to this product or benzodiazepines, serous tricyclic overdose, patients given benzodiazepine for control of life-threatening condition

Precautions: Pregnancy C, breastfeeding, children, geriatric, ambulatory patients, renal/hepatic disease, status epilepticus, head injury, labor and delivery, hypoventilation, panic disorder, drug/alcohol dependency

Black Box Warning: Benzodiazepine dependence, seizures

Pharmacokinetics
Absorption	Complete
Distribution	Unknown
Metabolism	Liver
Excretion	Unknown
Half-life	41-79 min

Pharmacodynamics
Onset	1-2 min
Peak	10 min
Duration	Unknown

Interactions
Individual drugs
Zaleplon, zolpidem: antagonize action
Drug classifications
Benzodiazepines: antagonize action
Toxicity: mixed product overdosage

NURSING CONSIDERATIONS
Assessment
- Assess cardiac status using continuous monitoring
- Assess for seizures, protect patient from injury; most likely in those who usually experience withdrawal from sedatives
- Assess for GI symptoms: nausea, vomiting; place in side-lying position to prevent aspiration
- Assess for allergic reactions: flushing, rash, urticaria, pruritus

Nursing diagnoses
- Injury, risk for (uses)
- Poisoning, risk for (uses)

F

Implementation
• Give directly undiluted or diluted in 0.9% NaCl, D₅W, or LR; give over 15 sec into running **IV**
• Use large vein
• Check airway and **IV** access before administration
• Stable for 24 hr if drawn into a syringe or mixed with other solutions
Additive compatibilities: Aminophylline, cimetidine, DOBUTamine, DOPamine, famotidine, heparin, lidocaine, procainamide, ranitidine

Patient/family education
• Caution patient that amnesia may continue
• Instruct patient to avoid any hazardous activities for 18-24 hr after discharge
• Inform patient not to take any alcohol or nonprescription products for 18-24 hr; serious reactions may occur

Evaluation
Positive therapeutic outcome
• Decreased sedation, respiratory depression
• Absence of toxicity

---

flunisolide nasal agent
See Appendix B

---

fluocinolone topical
See Appendix B

---

fluorometholone ophthalmic
See Appendix B

⚠ HIGH ALERT

fluorouracil (Rx)
(flure-oh-yoor'a-sil)
5-FU, Adrucil, Carac, Efudex, Fluoroplex
Func. class.: Antineoplastic, antimetabolite
Chem. class.: Pyrimidine antagonist

Pregnancy category X

Do not confuse:
fluorouracil/flucytosine

Action: Inhibits DNA, RNA synthesis; interferes with cell replication by competitively inhibiting thymidylate synthesis; cell cycle–specific (S phase); a vesicant

Therapeutic outcome: Prevention of rapidly growing malignant cells

Uses: *Systemic:* cancer of breast, colon, rectum, stomach, pancreas; *Topical:* superficial basal cell carcinoma; multiple actinic keratoses

Dosage and routes
Doses vary widely

Advanced colorectal cancer
Adult: IV 370 mg/m² given after leucovorin or 425 mg/m² given after leucovorin daily × 5 days; repeat q4-5wk

Other cancer
Adult: IV 12 mg/kg/day × 4 days, max 800 mg/day; may repeat with 6 mg/kg on day 6, 8, 10, 12; maintenance is 10-15 mg/kg/wk as a single dose, max 1 g/wk

Actinic/solar keratoses
Adult: TOP 1% cream/SOL 1-2 ×/day or 2%-5% SOL for hands

Superficial basal cell carcinoma
Adult: TOP 5% cream/SOL 2 ×/day × 3-12 wk

Available forms: Inj 50 mg/ml; cream 1, 5%; SOL 1, 2, 5%

Adverse effects
Systemic use
CNS: Lethargy, malaise, weakness, acute cerebellar dysfunction
CV: Myocardial ischemia, angina
EENT: Epistaxis, light intolerance, lacrimation
GI: Anorexia, stomatitis, diarrhea, nausea, vomiting, **hemorrhage,** enteritis, glossitis
HEMA: **Thrombocytopenia, leukopenia, myelosuppression, anemia, agranulocytosis**
INTEG: Rash, fever, photosensitivity

Contraindications: Pregnancy **X,** breastfeeding, hypersensitivity, poor nutritional status, serious infections, major surgery within 1 mo

Black Box Warning: Myelosuppression

Precautions: Children, renal/hepatic disease, angina

Black Box Warning: GI bleeding

Pharmacokinetics	
Absorption	Completely bioavailable (**IV**), minimal (topical)
Distribution	Widely distributed, concentration in tumor
Metabolism	Liver—converted to active metabolite
Excretion	Lungs (60%-80%), kidneys (up to 15%)
Half-life	20 hr terminal

 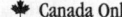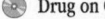

Pharmacodynamics
Unknown

Interactions
Individual drugs
Radiation: increased toxicity, bone marrow
  suppression
Drug classifications
Antineoplastics: increased toxicity, bone
  marrow depression
Live virus vaccines: decreased antibody re-
  sponse
Drug/lab test
Increased: AST, ALT, LDH, serum bilirubin, Hct,
  Hgb, WBC, platelets, 5-HIAA
Decreased: albumin

NURSING CONSIDERATIONS
Assessment
- Monitor ECG; watch for ST-T wave changes,
  low QRS and T, possible dysrhythmias (sinus
  tachycardia, heart block, PVCs)
- Assess buccal cavity q8hr for dryness, sores
  or ulceration, white patches, oral pain, bleeding, dysphagia; obtain prescription for viscous
  lidocaine (Xylocaine)
- Assess tachypnea, ECG changes, dyspnea,
  edema, fatigue; identify dyspnea, crackles,
  unproductive cough, chest pain, tachypnea
- Monitor CBC, differential, platelet count
  daily (**IV**); withhold product if WBC is <4000/
  mm³ or platelet count is <100,000/mm³;
  notify prescriber of results if WBC <20,000/
  mm³, platelets <50,000/mm³; nadir of leukopenia within 2 wk, recovery 1 mo
- Monitor renal function studies: BUN, creatinine, serum uric acid, urine CCr before,
  during therapy; I&O ratio; report fall in urine
  output to <30 ml/hr
- Monitor temp q4hr (may indicate beginning
  of infection)
- Monitor liver function tests before, during
  therapy (bilirubin, AST, ALT, LDH) as needed
  or monthly; jaundice of skin, sclera, dark
  urine, clay-colored stools, itchy skin, abdominal pain, fever, diarrhea
- Assess for bleeding: hematuria, stool guaiac,
  bruising or petechiae, mucosa or orifices
  q8hr; inflammation of mucosa, breaks in skin

Nursing diagnoses
- Body image, disturbed (adverse reactions)
- Infection, risk for (adverse reactions)
- Injury, risk for (adverse reactions)
- Knowledge, deficient (teaching)

Implementation
- Avoid contact with skin (very irritating);
  wash completely to remove

- Give fluids **IV** or PO before chemotherapy
  to hydrate patient
- Give antiemetic 30-60 min before giving
  product to prevent vomiting, and prn for
  several days thereafter; antibiotics for prophylaxis of infection
- Provide liquid diet: carbonated beverages;
  gelatin may be added if patient is not nauseated or vomiting
- Provide rinsing of mouth tid-qid with water,
  club soda; brushing of teeth bid-qid with soft
  brush or cotton-tipped applicators for
  stomatitis; use unwaxed dental floss
Topical route
- Wear gloves when applying; may use with a
  loose dressing, use a plastic or wooden
  applicator
IV route
- Prepare in biologic cabinet using gloves,
  gown, mask
- **IV** undiluted; may inject through Y-tube or
  3-way stopcock; give over 1-3 min
- May be diluted in 0.9% NaCl, D₅W, given
  over 2-8 hr as an **IV** inf
Syringe compatibilities: Bleomycin,
cisplatin, cyclophosphamide, furosemide,
heparin, leucovorin, methotrexate, metoclopramide, mitomycin, vinBLAStine, vinCRIStine
Syringe incompatibilities: Droperidol
Y-site compatibilities: Allopurinol,
amifostine, aztreonam, bleomycin, cefepime,
cisplatin, cyclophosphamide, DOXOrubicin,
fludarabine, furosemide, granisetron, heparin,
hydrocortisone, leucovorin, mannitol, melphalan, methotrexate, metoclopramide, mitomycin, paclitaxel, piperacillin/tazobactam,
potassium chloride, propofol, sargramostin,
thiotepa, thiposide, vinBLAStine, vinCRIStine,
vit B/C
Y-site incompatibilities: Droperidol,
vinorelbine
Additive compatibilities: Bleomycin,
cephalothin, cyclophosphamide, etoposides,
floxuridine, hydromorphone, ifosfamide,
leucovorin, methotrexate, mitoxantrone,
prednisoLONE, vinCRIStine
Additive incompatibilities: Carboplatin, cisplatin, cytarabine, diazepam, DOXO-
rubicin
Solution compatibilities: Amino acids
4.25%/D₂₅, D₅/LR, D₃.₃/0.3% NaCl, D₅W, 0.9%
NaCl, TPN #23

Patient/family education
- Caution patient that contraceptive measures
  are recommended during therapy
- Teach patient to avoid using aspirin, NSAIDs,
  or ibuprofen-containing products, razors,

Adverse effects: *italic* = common, **bold** = life-threatening

commercial mouthwash because bleeding may occur; to report symptoms of bleeding (hematuria, tarry stools)
- Instruct patient to report signs of anemia (fatigue, headache, irritability, faintness, SOB)
- Instruct patient to report signs of stomatitis (bleeding, white spots, ulcerations in the mouth); tell patient to examine mouth daily, to report symptoms; viscous lidocaine (Xylocaine) may be used
- Teach patient to avoid crowds, persons with known infections
- Advise patient to avoid vaccinations during therapy, to use sunscreen or stay out of the sun to prevent burns; about hair loss; explore use of wigs or other products until hair regrowth occurs

Evaluation
Positive therapeutic outcome
- Prevention of rapid division of malignant cells

---

fluoxetine (Rx)
(floo-ox'uh-teen)
Prozac, Prozac Weekly, Sarafem
Func. class.: Antidepressant, selective serotonin reuptake inhibitor
Pregnancy category C

Do not confuse:
Prozac/Proscar/Prilosec/Prosom, Sarafem/Serophene

Action: Inhibits CNS neuron uptake of serotonin, but not of norepinephrine

Therapeutic outcome: Decreased symptoms of depression after 2-3 wk

Uses: Major depressive disorder, obsessive-compulsive disorder (OCD), bulimia nervosa; *Sarafem:* premenstrual dysphoric disorder (PMDD), panic disorder

Unlabeled uses: Alcoholism, anorexia nervosa, attention deficit hyperactivity disorder, bipolar II affective disorder, borderline personality disorder, cataplexy, narcolepsy, kleptomania, migraine, obesity, posttraumatic stress disorder, schizophrenia, Gilles de la Tourette's syndrome, trichotillomania, levodopa-induced dyskinesia, social phobia

Dosage and routes
Depression/OCD
Adult: PO 20 mg/day AM; after 4 wk if no clinical improvement is noted, dose may be increased to 20 mg bid in AM, afternoon; max 80 mg/day; PO 90 mg weekly

Geriatric: PO 5-10 mg/day, increase as needed
Child 5-18 yr: PO 5-10 mg/day, max 20 mg/day

Bulimia nervosa
Adult: PO 60 mg/day in AM

ADHD (unlabeled)
Adult: PO 20-60 mg/day

Alcoholism (unlabeled)
Adult: PO 20-80 mg/day

Anorexia nervosa (unlabeled)
Adult: PO 10 mg every other day-20 mg/day

Bipolar II affective disorder (unlabeled)
Adult: PO 10 mg every other day-20 mg/day

Borderline personality disorder (unlabeled)
Adult: PO 20 mg/day

Kleptomania (unlabeled)
Adult: PO 60-80 mg/day

Migraine, chronic daily headaches (unlabeled)
Adult: PO 10-80 mg/day

Narcolepsy (unlabeled)
Adult: PO 20-40 mg/day

Posttraumatic stress disorder (unlabeled)
Adult: PO 10-80 mg/day

Premenstrual dysphoric disorder (Sarafem)
Adult: PO 20 mg/day, may be taken daily 14 days before menses

Schizophrenia (unlabeled)
Adult: PO 20-60 mg/day

Available forms: Caps 10, 20, 40 mg; tabs 10, 20 mg; oral sol 20 mg/5 ml; del rel caps (Prozac Weekly) 90 mg

Adverse effects
CNS: Headache, nervousness, insomnia, drowsiness, anxiety, tremor, dizziness, fatigue, sedation, poor concentration, abnormal dreams, agitation, **seizures,** apathy, euphoria, hallucinations, delusions, psychosis, **suicidal ideation, neuroleptic malignant syndrome–like reactions**
CV: Hot flashes, palpitations, angina pectoris, **hemorrhage,** hypertension, **tachycardia,** 1st-degree AV block, **bradycardia, MI, thrombophlebitis**
EENT: Visual changes, ear/eye pain, photophobia, tinnitus

GI: Nausea, diarrhea, dry mouth, anorexia, dyspepsia, constipation, cramps, vomiting, taste changes, flatulence, decreased appetite
GU: Dysmenorrhea, decreased libido, urinary frequency, urinary tract infection, amenorrhea, cystitis, impotence, urine retention
INTEG: Sweating, rash, pruritus, acne, alopecia, urticaria
MS: Pain, arthritis, twitching
RESP: Infection, pharyngitis, nasal congestion, sinus headache, sinusitis, cough, dyspnea, bronchitis, asthma, hyperventilation, pneumonia
SYST: Asthenia, viral infection, fever, allergy, chills, hyponatremia

Contraindications: Hypersensitivity

Precautions: Pregnancy **C,** breastfeeding, geriatric, diabetes mellitus

Black Box Warning: Children, suicidal ideation

Pharmacokinetics

Absorption	Well absorbed
Distribution	Crosses blood-brain barrier
Metabolism	Liver, extensively to norfluoxetine
Excretion	Kidneys, unchanged (12%), metabolite (7%); steady state 28-35 days, protein binding 94%
Half-life	1-3 days metabolite up to 1 wk

Pharmacodynamics

Onset	Unknown
Peak	6-8 hr
Duration	Unknown

Interactions
Individual drugs
Alcohol: increased CNS depression
BusPIRone: increased worsening of OCD
Carbamazepine, digoxin, lithium, phenytoin, warfarin: increased toxicity
Cyproheptadine: decreased fluoxetine effect
Diazepam: increased half-life of diazepam
Haloperidol: increased haloperidol effect
Thioridazine: do not use, or use within 5 wk of discontinuing fluoxetine
Drug classifications
Antidepressants, opioids, sedative/hypnotics: increased CNS depression
Highly protein-bound products: increased side effects
MAOIs: hypertensive crisis, seizures; do not use with or 14 days prior to fluoxetine

Phenothiazines, tricyclics: increased levels
Serotonin precursors (tryptophan): do not use together
Drug/herb
Corkwood, jimsonweed: increased anticholinergic effect
Hops, kava, lavender: increased CNS effect
St. John's wort, SAM-e: do not use together; increased risk of serotonin syndrome
Drug/lab test
Increased: serum bilirubin, blood glucose, alkaline phosphatase
Decreased: VMA, 5-HIAA
False increase: urinary catecholamines

NURSING CONSIDERATIONS
Assessment
• Monitor B/P (lying, standing), pulse q4hr; if systolic B/P drops 20 mm hg, hold product and notify prescriber; take VS q4hr in patients with CV disease
• Monitor blood studies: CBC, leukocytes, differential, cardiac enzymes if patient is receiving long-term therapy, check platelets, bleeding can occur
• Monitor hepatic studies: AST, ALT, bilirubin
• Check weight qwk; appetite may increase with product
• Assess ECG for flattening of T wave, bundle branch block, AV block, dysrhythmias in cardiac patients
• Assess mental status: mood, sensorium, affect, suicidal tendencies; increase in psychiatric symptoms: depression, panic; monitor for seizures; seizure potential is increased
• Monitor urinary retention, constipation; constipation is more likely to occur in children or geriatric
• Identify patient's alcohol consumption; if alcohol is consumed, hold dose until AM
• Assess appetite in bulimia nervosa, weight daily, increase nutritious foods in diet, watch for bingeing and vomiting
• Assess allergic reactions: itching, rash, urticaria, product should be discontinued; may need to give antihistamine

Nursing diagnoses
• Coping, ineffective (uses)
• Injury, risk for (side effects)
• Knowledge, deficient (teaching)
• Noncompliance (teaching)

Implementation
• Give with food or milk for GI symptoms
• Give dosage at bedtime if oversedation occurs during day; may take entire dose at bedtime; geriatric may not tolerate once/day

dosing, crush if patient unable to swallow whole (tabs only)
- Prozac weekly: Give on same day each week
- Store at room temperature; do not freeze

Patient/family education
- Teach patient that therapeutic effects may take 1-4 wk
- Instruct patient to use caution in driving or other activities requiring alertness because of drowsiness, dizziness, blurred vision; to avoid rising quickly from sitting to standing, especially geriatric; to use sunscreen to prevent photosensitivity
- Caution patient to avoid alcohol ingestion, other CNS depressants
- Advise patient not to discontinue medication quickly after long-term use: may cause nausea, headache, malaise
- Instruct patient to increase fluids, bulk in diet if constipation, urinary retention occur, especially geriatric
- Advise patient to take gum, hard sugarless candy, or frequent sips of water for dry mouth
- Teach patient to avoid all OTC products unless approved by prescriber
- Advise patient to change positions slowly, orthostatic hypotension may occur
- Teach that suicidal thoughts, behavior may occur in young adults, children

Evaluation
Positive therapeutic outcome
- Decrease in depression
- Absence of suicidal thoughts
- Decreased symptoms of OCD

Treatment of overdose: Activated charcoal, supportive care

---

fluoxymesterone (Rx)
(floo-oks-i-mes'te-rone)
Androxy
Func. class.: Hormone-androgen
Chem. class.: Alkylated derivative of testosterone

Pregnancy category X
Controlled substance schedule C-III

Action: Androgens are responsible for sexual maturation, suppression of gonadotropin-releasing hormones, LH, FSH, by a negative feedback mechanism

Therapeutic outcome: Decreased advance of inoperable female breast cancer, male puberty

Uses: Inoperable female breast cancer, male hypogonadism, delayed male puberty

Dosage and routes
Androgen replacement in male hypogonadism
Adult: PO 5 mg 1-4 ×/day, may increase dose, max 40 mg/day

Delayed male puberty
Adult and adolescent: PO 2.5-10 mg/day × 4-6 mo, max 20 mg/day

Inoperable female breast cancer
Adult: PO 10-40 mg/day in divided doses, continue for ≥2-3 mo

Available forms: Tabs 10 mg

Adverse effects
CV: **Heart failure**
GI: **Hepatitis**
GU: Amenorrhea, feminization, virilization, prostatic hypertrophy, priapism, oligospermia, oligomenorrhea, gynecomastia
HEMA: Coagulation disorders (clotting factors II, V, VII, X)
INTEG: Alopecia, acne, hirsutism, seborrhea
MISC: Edema, hypercalcemia

Contraindications: Pregnancy **X,** breastfeeding, prostate cancer, male breast cancer

Precautions: Diabetes mellitus, CV/hepatic/renal disease, elderly, hypercalcemia, hypothyroidism

Pharmacokinetics	
Absorption	Unknown
Distribution	Unknown, crosses placenta
Metabolism	Liver
Excretion	Urine, breast milk
Half-life	9.2 hr

Pharmacodynamics
Unknown

Interactions
Individual drugs
CycloSPORINE: increased nephrotoxicity
Darbepoetin, epoetin: increased erythropoiesis; avoid concurrent administration
Insulin: decreased glucose levels may alter need for insulin
Warfarin: increased PT
Drug classifications
5-α-reductase inhibitors (dutasteride, finasteride): decreased androgen effect
Antidiabetics (oral): decreased glucose levels may alter need for oral antidiabetics

 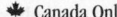

Corticosteroids: edema
Hepatotoxic agents (other): increased hepatotoxicity
Drug/herb
Saw palmetto: decreased fluoxymesterone effect
Drug/food
Soy: decreased fluoxymesterone effect

NURSING CONSIDERATIONS
Assessment
• Monitor weight daily; notify prescriber if weekly weight gain is >5 lb
• Monitor I&O ratio; be alert for decreasing urinary output, increasing edema
• Assess growth rate in children; growth rate may be uneven (linear/bone growth) with extended use
• Monitor electrolytes: K, Na, Cl, Ca; cholesterol
• Monitor hepatic studies: ALT, AST, bilirubin
• Assess edema, hypertension, cardiac symptoms
• Assess signs of masculinization in female: increased libido, deepening of voice, decreased breast tissue, enlarged clitoris, menstrual irregularities; male: gynecomastia, impotence, testicular atrophy
• Assess hypercalcemia: lethargy, polyuria, polydipsia, nausea, vomiting, constipation; product may have to be decreased
• Assess hypoglycemia in diabetics; oral antidiabetic action is increased

Nursing diagnoses
• Injury, risk for (adverse reactions)
• Knowledge, deficient (teaching)

Implementation
• Give as a single dose or up to 4 ×/day
• Store at controlled room temperature (68°-77° F)

Patient/family education
• Instruct patient to notify prescriber if therapeutic response decreases; if edema occurs
• Teach patient about changes in sex characteristics
• Instruct women to report menstrual irregularities, voice changes, acne, facial hair growth
• Advise patient to notify prescriber if pregnancy is planned or suspected; use contraception while taking product
• Inform patient that 2-3–mo course is necessary to determine objective treatment in breast cancer
• Advise patient to report signs/symptoms of hepatic disorder

Evaluation
Positive therapeutic outcome
• Decreased advance of inoperable female breast cancer, male puberty

---

fluphenazine decanoate (Rx)
(floo-fen'ah-zeen)
Modecate ✦, Modecate Concentrate, Prolixin Decanoate
fluphenazine enanthate (Rx)
Moditen Enanthate ✦, Prolixin Enanthate
fluphenazine hydrochloride (Rx)
Apo-Fluphenazine ✦, Moditen HCL ✦, Moditen HCl-H.P. ✦, Permitil ✦, Prolixin
Func. class.: Antipsychotic/neuroleptic
Chem. class.: Phenothiazine, piperazine

Pregnancy category C

Do not confuse:
Prolixin/Proloid

Action: Depresses cerebral cortex, hypothalamus, limbic system, which control activity and aggression; blocks neurotransmission produced by dopamine at synapse; exhibits strong α-adrenergic and anticholinergic blocking action; mechanism for antipsychotic effects is unclear

Therapeutic outcome: Decreased signs and symptoms of psychosis

Uses: Psychotic disorders, schizophrenia

Dosage and routes
Decanoate
Adult and child >16 yr: IM/SUBCUT 12.5-25 mg q1-3wk, may increase slowly
Child 12-16 yr: IM/SUBCUT 6.25-18.75 mg, then repeat q1-3wk, then increase slowly, max 25 mg
Child 5-12 yr: IM/SUBCUT 3.125-12.5 mg, then repeat q1-3wk, increase slowly
Enanthate
Adult: IM/SUBCUT 25 mg q1-3wk, max 100 mg/dose
HCl
Adult: PO 2.5-10 mg, in divided doses q6-8hr, max 40 mg/day; IM initially 1.25 mg then 2.5-10 mg in divided doses q6-8hr
Child: PO 0.25-3.5 mg/day in divided doses q4-6hr, max 10 mg/day

Available forms: HCl: tabs 1, 2.5, 5, 10 mg; elix 2.5 mg/5 ml; inj 2.5 mg/ml;

Adverse effects: *italic* = common, **bold** = life-threatening

decanoate: inj 25 mg/ml; enanthate: inj 25 mg/ml

Adverse effects

CNS: EPS, pseudoparkinsonism, akathisia, dystonia, tardive dyskinesia, drowsiness, headache, **seizures, neuroleptic malignant syndrome**
CV: Orthostatic hypotension, hypertension, **cardiac arrest,** ECG changes, **tachycardia**
EENT: Blurred vision, glaucoma, dry eyes
GI: Dry mouth, nausea, vomiting, anorexia, constipation, diarrhea, jaundice, weight gain, **paralytic ileus, hepatitis,** cholecystic jaundice
GU: Urinary retention, urinary frequency, enuresis, impotence, amenorrhea, gynecomastia
HEMA: Anemia, **leukopenia, leukocytosis, agranulocytosis, aplastic anemia, thrombocytopenia**
INTEG: Rash, photosensitivity, dermatitis
RESP: Laryngospasm, dyspnea, **respiratory depression**

Contraindications: Hypersensitivity,
circulatory collapse, liver damage, cerebral arteriosclerosis, coronary disease, severe hypo/hypertension, blood dyscrasias, coma, brain damage, bone marrow depression, alcohol and barbiturate withdrawal, closed-angle glaucoma

Precautions: Pregnancy **C,** breastfeeding,
children <12 yr, geriatric, seizure disorders, hypertension, hepatic/cardiac disease

Black Box Warning: Dementia

Pharmacokinetics

Absorption	Well absorbed (PO, IM)
Distribution	Widely absorbed, crosses blood-brain barrier, placenta
Metabolism	Liver, extensively, not dialyzable
Excretion	Kidneys (metabolites)
Half-life	HCl-4.7-15.3 hr, enanthate 3½-4 days, decanoate 6.8-14.3 days

Pharmacodynamics

	PO/IM	IM	IM
	HCl	Enanthate	Decanoate
Onset	1 hr	1-2 days	1-3 days
Peak	1½-2 hr	2-3 days	1-2 days
Duration	6-8 hr	1-3 wk	>4 wk

Interactions
Individual drugs

Alcohol: increased effects of both products, oversedation

Epinephrine: increased toxicity
Levodopa: decreased antiparkinson activity
Lithium: decreased effects of lithium

Drug classifications

Anticholinergics: increased anticholinergic effects
Barbiturates: decreased effect of fluphenazine, oversedation
CNS depressants: oversedation
Smoking: decreased effects of fluphenazine

Drug/herb

Betel palm, kava: increased EPS
Cola tree, hops, kava, nettle, nutmeg: possible increased action
Henbane leaf: increased anticholinergic effect

Drug/lab test

Increased: liver function tests, cardiac enzymes, cholesterol, blood glucose, prolactin, bilirubin, cholinesterase
Decreased: hormones (blood and urine)
False positive: pregnancy tests, PKU, urinary steroids, 17-OHCS

NURSING CONSIDERATIONS
Assessment

• Assess mental status: orientation, mood, behavior, presence of hallucinations, and type before initial administration and monthly; this product should significantly reduce psychotic behavior
• Check for swallowing of PO medication; check for hoarding or giving of medication to other patients
• Monitor I&O ratio, palpate bladder if low urinary output occurs, especially in geriatric; urinalysis recommended before, during prolonged therapy
• Monitor bilirubin, CBC, liver function tests monthly
• Assess affect, orientation, LOC, reflexes, gait, coordination, sleep pattern disturbances
• Monitor B/P with patient sitting, standing, and lying down; take pulse and respirations q4hr during initial treatment; establish baseline before starting treatment; report drops of 30 mm Hg; obtain baseline ECG, Q-wave and T-wave changes
• Check for dizziness, faintness, palpitations, tachycardia on rising; severe orthostatic hypotension is common
◆ Assess for neuroleptic malignant syndrome: hyperpyrexia, muscle rigidity, increased CPK, altered mental status; product should be discontinued
• Assess for EPS including akathisia (inability to sit still, no pattern to movements), tardive dyskinesia (bizarre movements of the jaw, mouth, tongue, extremities), pseudoparkin-

sonism (rigidity, tremors, pill rolling, shuffling gait); an antiparkinson product should be prescribed
• Assess for constipation, urinary retention daily; if these occur, increase bulk, water in diet

Nursing diagnoses
• Coping, ineffective (uses)
• Knowledge, deficient (teaching)
• Noncompliance (teaching)
• Thought processes, disturbed (uses)

Implementation
PO route
• Give product in liquid form mixed in glass of juice or cola if hoarding is suspected; do not mix in caffeine drinks, tannics, or pectinates; decrease dose in geriatric
• Give PO with full glass of water, milk; or give with food to decrease GI upset
• Take antacids 2 hr before or after this product
• Store in tight, light-resistant container; oral sol in amber bottle
SUBCUT route
• May be given by this route; however, it is painful
IM route
• Inject in deep muscle mass, use a 21-G needle into dorsal gluteal site, keep patient recumbent for 30 min to prevent orthostatic hypotension
Syringe compatibilities: Benztropine, diphenhydrAMINE, hydrOXYzine

Patient/family education
• Teach patient to use good oral hygiene; frequent rinsing of mouth, sugarless gum for dry mouth
• Caution patient to avoid hazardous activities until product response is determined; dizziness, blurred vision may occur
• Inform patient that orthostatic hypotension occurs often and to rise from sitting or lying position gradually; tell patient to avoid hot tubs, hot showers, tub baths because hypotension may occur; tell patient that in hot weather, heat stroke may occur; extra precautions are necessary to stay cool
• Instruct patient to avoid abrupt withdrawal of this product, or EPS may result; product should be withdrawn slowly
• Teach patient to avoid OTC preparations (cough, hay fever, cold) unless approved by physician because serious product interactions may occur; avoid use with alcohol, CNS depressants; increased drowsiness may occur
• Instruct patient to use a sunscreen and sunglasses to prevent burns

• Teach patient about EPS and necessity of meticulous oral hygiene because oral candidiasis may occur
• Instruct patient to take antacids 2 hr before or after this product
• Advise patient to report sore throat, malaise, fever, bleeding, mouth sores; if these occur, CBC should be performed and product discontinued

Evaluation
Positive therapeutic outcome
• Decrease in emotional excitement, hallucinations, delusions, paranoia
• Reorganization of patterns of thought, speech

Treatment of overdose: Lavage if orally ingested; provide airway; *do not induce vomiting or use epinephrine*

---

flurandrenolide topical
See Appendix B

---

flurazepam (Rx)
(flure-az'e-pam)
Apo-flurazepam ✚, flurazepam, Novoflupam ✚, Somnol ✚
Func. class.: Sedative-hypnotic
Chem. class.: Benzodiazepine, long-acting

Pregnancy category X

Controlled substance schedule IV (USA), Targeted (CDSA IV) (Canada)

Do not confuse:
flurazepam/temazepam

Action: Produces CNS depression at the limbic, thalamic, hypothalamic levels of CNS; may be mediated by neurotransmitter γ-aminobutyric acid (GABA); results are sedation, hypnosis, skeletal muscle relaxation, anticonvulsant activity, anxiolytic action

Therapeutic outcome: Ability to sleep, relaxation

Uses: Insomnia, short term

Dosage and routes
Adult: PO 15-30 mg at bedtime; may repeat dose once if needed
Geriatric: PO 15 mg at bedtime; may increase if needed
Hepatic dose
Adult: PO 5 mg at bedtime
Available forms: Caps 15, 30 mg

Adverse effects: *italic* = common, **bold** = life-threatening

Adverse effects

CNS: Lethargy, drowsiness, daytime sedation, dizziness, confusion, light-headedness, headache, anxiety, irritability, complex sleep-related reactions (sleep driving, sleep eating) *CV:* Chest pain, pulse changes, palpitations *GI:* Nausea, vomiting, diarrhea, heartburn, abdominal pain, constipation **HEMA: Leukopenia, granulocytopenia (rare)** *MISC:* Physical, psychologic dependence, blurred vision, **apnea**

Contraindications: Pregnancy **X**, breastfeeding, intermittent porphyria, uncontrolled pain, sleep apnea, hypersensitivity to this product or benzodiazepines

Precautions: Anemia, renal/hepatic disease, suicidal individuals, drug abuse, geriatric, psychosis, children <15 yr, angioedema, pulmonary disease

Pharmacokinetics

Absorption	Well absorbed
Distribution	Widely absorbed, crosses blood-brain barrier, crosses placenta, protein binding 97%
Metabolism	Liver to active, inactive metabolites
Excretion	Kidneys, breast milk
Half-life	2½ hr, 30-200 hr active metabolites

Pharmacodynamics

Onset	15-30 min
Peak	½-1 hr
Duration	7-8 hr

Interactions
Individual drugs

Alcohol: increased CNS depression
Cimetidine, disulfiram, fluoxetine, isoniazid, ketoconazole, propranolol, valproic acid: increased action of flurazepam
Probenecid: increased effects of flurazepam
Rifampin: decreased action of flurazepam
Theophylline: decreased effect of flurazepam
Drug classifications
Barbiturates: decreased effect of flurazepam
CNS depressants: increased CNS depression
CYP3A4 inhibitors, oral contraceptives: increased effect of flurazepam
Drug/herb
Black cohosh: increased hypotension
Catnip, chamomile, clary, cowslip, kava, lavender, mistletoe, nettle, pokeweed, poppy, Queen Anne's lace, senega, valerian: increased effect
St. John's wort: decreased flurazepam effect

Drug/lab test
Increased: AST, ALT, serum bilirubin
Decreased: radioactive iodine uptake
False increase: urinary 17-OHCS

NURSING CONSIDERATIONS
Assessment

• Assess anxiety reaction: inability to sleep, apprehension, dread, foreboding, or uneasiness related to unidentified source of danger
• Assess for previous product dependence or tolerance; if product dependent or tolerant, amount of medication should be restricted
• Monitor B/P (lying, standing), pulse; if systolic B/P drops 20 mm Hg, hold product, notify prescriber; I&O, may indicate renal dysfunction
• Monitor blood studies: CBC during long-term therapy; blood dyscrasias have occurred rarely
• Monitor hepatic studies: AST, ALT, bilirubin, creatinine, LDH, alkaline phosphatase
• Monitor patient's mental status: mood, sensorium, affect, sleeping patterns, drowsiness, dizziness, suicidal tendencies
• Assess for withdrawal signs if discontinued abruptly
• Assess for excessive sedation, impaired coordination, especially in the geriatric

Nursing diagnoses
• Knowledge, deficient (teaching)
• Noncompliance (teaching)
• Sleep pattern, disturbed (uses)

Implementation

Give ½-1 hr before bedtime for sleeplessness; caps may be opened and mixed with food; give after meals to decrease GI symptoms if used for sedation
• Best to avoid in geriatric patients; long half-life
• Provide assistance with ambulation after receiving dose
• Provide safety measures: nightlight, call bell within easy reach
• Check to see if PO medication has been swallowed
• Store in tight container in cool environment

Patient/family education
• Inform patient that product may be taken with food; if dose is missed take as soon as remembered; do not double doses
• Advise patient to avoid OTC preparations unless approved by a physician, to avoid alcohol ingestion or other psychotropic

 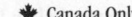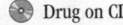

medications unless approved by prescriber, that 1-2 wk of therapy may be required before therapeutic effects occur
• Caution patient to avoid driving, activities requiring alertness; drowsiness may occur; until medication response is known, tell patient that drowsiness may worsen at beginning of treatment
• Instruct patient not to discontinue medication abruptly after long-term use
• Caution patient to rise slowly or fainting may occur, especially in geriatric
• Inform patient that hangover is common in geriatric
• Teach patients to use contraceptives; pregnancy category **X**

Evaluation

Positive therapeutic outcome
• Increased well-being
• Decreased anxiety, restlessness, sleeplessness, dread

Treatment of overdose: Lavage, activated charcoal; monitor electrolytes, VS

---

flurbiprofen ophthalmic
See Appendix B

---

flutamide (Rx)
(floo′ta-mide)
Apo-Flutamide ✤, Novo-Flutamide ✤
Func. class.: Antineoplastic hormone
Chem. class.: Antiandrogen

Pregnancy category D

Action: Interferes with androgen uptake in the nucleus or androgen activity in target tissues; arrests tumor growth in androgen-sensitive tissue (i.e., prostate gland)

Therapeutic outcome: Prevention of rapidly growing malignant cells

Uses: Metastatic prostatic carcinoma, stage D_2 in combination with LHRH agonistic analogs (leuprolide), B_2-C in combination with goserelin and radiation

Dosage and routes
Adult: PO 250 mg q8hr tid, for a daily dosage of 750 mg

Available forms: Caps 125, 250 ✤ mg

Adverse effects
CNS: Hot flashes, drowsiness, confusion, depression, anxiety, paresthesia

GI: Diarrhea, nausea, vomiting, increased liver function studies, **hepatitis,** anorexia, **hepatotoxicity**
GU: Decreased libido, impotence, gynecomastia
HEMA: Leukopenia, thrombocytopenia, hemolytic anemia
INTEG: Irritation at site, rash, photosensitivity
MISC: Edema, neuromuscular and pulmonary symptoms, hypertension

Contraindications: Pregnancy **D**, hypersensitivity

Black Box Warning: Severe hepatic disease

Precautions: G6PD deficiency, hemoglobinopathy, lactase deficiency, polycystic ovary syndrome, tobacco smoking

Pharmacokinetics

Absorption	Well absorbed
Distribution	Unknown
Metabolism	Liver
Excretion	Unknown
Half-life	6 hr

Pharmacodynamics
Unknown

Interactions
Individual drugs
Leuprolide: decreased flutamide action
Warfarin: increased PT

NURSING CONSIDERATIONS
Assessment
• Monitor CBC, bilirubin, creatinine, AST, ALT, alkaline phosphatase, which may be elevated; product may need to be discontinued
• Identify CNS symptoms: drowsiness, confusion, depression, anxiety

Nursing diagnoses
• Body image, disturbed (adverse reactions)
• Infection, risk for (adverse reactions)
• Injury, risk for (adverse reactions)
• Knowledge, deficient (teaching)
• Sexual dysfunction (adverse reactions)

Implementation
• Used in combination with LHRH agonist (leuprolide)
• May be given with food or fluids

Patient/family education
• Tell the patient to report side effects: decreased libido, impotence, breast enlargement,

F

Adverse effects: *italic* = common, **bold** = life-threatening

hot flashes, diarrhea, which occur when the two products are given together; also nausea, vomiting; jaundice in eyes, skin; dark urine, clay-colored stools, hepatotoxicity may occur
• Inform patient that this product is taken with leuprolide for medical castration; do not change dosing

Evaluation
Positive therapeutic outcome
• Prevention of rapid division of malignant cells

---

fluticasone (Rx)
(floo-tic′a-sone)
Flovent HFA, Flovent Diskus ✽
Func. class.: Corticosteroids, inhalation; antiasthmatic

Pregnancy category C

Action: Decreases inflammation by inhibiting mast cells, macrophages, and leukotrienes; antiinflammatory and vasoconstrictor properties

Therapeutic outcome: Decreased severity of asthma

Uses: Prevention of chronic asthma during maintenance treatment in those requiring oral corticosteroids; nasal symptoms of seasonal/perennial and allergic/nonallergic rhinitis

Dosage and routes
Prevention of chronic asthma during maintenance treatment in those requiring oral corticosteroids
Flovent HFA
Adult and child ≥12 yr: INH 88-660 mcg bid (in those previously taking bronchodilators alone); INH 88-220 mcg bid, max 440 mcg bid (in those previously taking inhaled corticosteroids); INH 440 mcg bid, max 880 mcg bid (in those previously taking oral corticosteroids)
Flovent Diskus ✽
Adult and child ≥12 yr: INH 100 mcg bid, max 500 mcg (in those previously taking bronchodilators alone); INH 100-250 mcg bid, max 500 mcg bid (in those previously taking inhaled corticosteroids); INH 500-1000 mcg bid, max 1000 mcg bid (in those previously taking oral corticosteroids)
Child 4-11 yr: INH initially 50 mcg bid, max 100 mcg bid (in those previously taking bronchodilators alone or inhaled corticosteroids)

Nasal symptoms of seasonal/perennial rhinitis
Flonase
Adult: Nasal spray 2 sprays (100 mcg) in each nostril daily or 1 spray (50 mcg) in each nostril bid; when symptoms are controlled, decrease to 1 spray (50 mcg) in each nostril every day
Adolescent and child ≥4 yr: Nasal spray 1 spray (50 mcg) in each nostril daily; may increase to 2 sprays (100 mcg) in each nostril daily; max 2 sprays in each nostril daily

Available forms: Nasal spray 50 mcg/metered spray; oral inh aerosol 44, 110, 220 mcg; oral inh powder 50, 100, 250 mcg

Adverse effects
CNS: Fever, headache, nervousness, dizziness, migraines, numbness in fingers
EENT: Pharyngitis, sinusitis, rhinitis, laryngitis, hoarseness, dry eyes, cataracts, nasal discharge, epistaxis
GI: Diarrhea, abdominal pain, nausea, vomiting, *oral candidiasis,* gastroenteritis
GU: UTI
INTEG: Urticaria, dermatitis
META: Hyperglycemia, growth retardation in children, cushingoid features
MISC: Influenza, **eosinophilic conditions, angioedema, Churg-Strauss syndrome,** adrenal insufficiency (high doses)
MS: Osteoporosis, muscle soreness, joint pain
RESP: Upper respiratory infection, dyspnea, cough, bronchitis, **bronchospasm**

Contraindications: Hypersensitivity, primary treatment in status asthmaticus

Precautions: Pregnancy **C,** breastfeeding, active infections, glaucoma, diabetes, immunocompromised patients

Pharmacokinetics	
Absorption	30% aerosol, 13.5% powder
Distribution	Protein binding 91%
Metabolism	In liver after absorption in lung
Excretion	<5% in urine and feces
Half-life	7.8 hr

Pharmacodynamics		
	NASAL INH	ORAL INH
Onset	12 hr	24 hr
Peak	Several days	Several days
Duration	1-2 wk	1-2 wk

Interactions
Drug classifications
CYP450 3A4 inhibitors (ketoconazole): increased fluticasone levels

---

 Alert   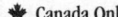 Canada Only   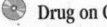 Drug on CD   * "Tall Man" lettering (See Preface)

Drug/lab test
Increased: urine/serum glucose

NURSING CONSIDERATIONS
Assessment
• Assess respiratory status: lung sounds, pulmonary function tests during and several months after change from systemic to inhalation corticosteroids
• Assess for withdrawal symptoms from oral corticosteroids: depression, pain in joints, fatigue
⚠ Monitor adrenal insufficiency: nausea, weakness, fatigue, hypotension, hypoglycemia, anorexia; may occur when changing from systemic to inhalation corticosteroids; may be life-threatening
• Monitor growth rate in children
• Monitor adrenal function tests periodically: hypothalamic–pituitary-adrenal axis suppression in long-term treatment

Nursing diagnoses
• Airway clearance, ineffective (uses)
• Noncompliance (teaching)

Implementation
• Give at 1 min intervals
• Decrease dose to lowest effective dose after desired effect; decrease dose at 2- to 4-wk intervals

Patient/family education
• Advise patient to use bronchodilator first before using inhalation, if taking both
• Caution patient not to use for acute asthmatic attack; for acute asthma, may require oral corticosteroids
• Advise patient to avoid smoking, smoke-filled rooms, those with URIs, those not immunized against chickenpox or measles

Evaluation
Positive therapeutic outcome
• Decreased severity of asthma

---

fluticasone nasal agent
See Appendix B

---

fluticasone topical
See Appendix B

---

fluvastatin (Rx)
(flu'vah-stay-tin)
Lescol, Lescol XL
Func. class.: Antilipidemic
Chem. class.: HMG-CoA reductase inhibitor
Pregnancy category X

Action: Inhibits HMG-CoA reductase enzyme, which reduces cholesterol synthesis

Therapeutic outcome: Decreased cholesterol levels and LDLs, increased HDLs

Uses: As an adjunct in primary hypercholesterolemia (types Ia, Ib), coronary atherosclerosis in CAD; to reduce the risk of undergoing coronary revascularization in patients with CAD

Dosage and routes
Adult: PO 20-40 mg/day in PM initially, usual range 20-80, max 80 mg; may be given in 2 doses (40 mg AM, 40 mg PM); dosage adjustments may be made in 4-wk intervals or more

Available forms: Caps 20, 40 mg; ext rel tab 80 mg

Adverse effects
CNS: Headache, dizziness, insomnia, **ALS (Lou Gehrig's disease)**
EENT: Lens opacities
GI: Nausea, constipation, diarrhea, abdominal pain, cramps, dyspepsia, flatus, liver dysfunction, pancreatitis
HEMA: **Thrombocytopenia, hemolytic anemia, leukopenia**
INTEG: Rash, pruritus
MISC: Fatigue, influenza, photosensitivity
MS: Myalgia, *arthritis, arthralgia,* myositis, **rhabdomyolysis**
RESP: Upper respiratory infection, rhinitis, cough, pharyngitis, sinusitis

Contraindications: Pregnancy X, breast-feeding, hypersensitivity, active liver disease

Precautions: Past liver disease, alcoholism, severe acute infections, trauma, hypotension, uncontrolled seizure disorders, severe metabolic disorders, electrolyte imbalance

Pharmacokinetics
Absorption	Unknown
Distribution	Steady state 4-5 wk
Metabolism	Liver
Excretion	Feces, kidneys
Half-life	1-6 days

Pharmacodynamics
Unknown

Adverse effects: *italic* = common, **bold** = life-threatening

Interactions
Individual drugs

Alcohol, cimetidine, lithium, ranitidine, omeprazole, saquinavir: increased fluvastatin effect

Clofibrate, cycloSPORINE, erythromycin, gemfibrozil, niacin: increased myalgia, myositis

Clozapine, methadone, propranolol, theophylline: increased levels of these products

Digoxin, warfarin: increased action

Pimozide, thioridazine: increased QTc interval

Tramadol: increased serotonin syndrome

Drug classifications:

Azole antiinfectives given with clofibrate: increased myalgia, increased myositis

MAOIs: increased serotonin syndrome

Tricyclics: increased levels of tricyclics

Drug/herb

Glucomannan: increased effect

Gotu kola, St. John's wort: decreased effect

Drug/food

Grapefruit juice: possible increased fluvastatin toxicity

Oat bran, high fat: decreased absorption

NURSING CONSIDERATIONS
Assessment

• Assess nutrition: fat, protein, carbohydrates; nutritional analysis should be completed by dietitian before treatment

• Monitor bowel pattern daily; diarrhea may be a problem

• Assess fasting lipid profile (cholesterol, LDL, HDL, triglycerides) q8wk, then q3-6mo when stable

• Monitor liver function studies q1-2mo during the first 1½ yr of treatment; AST, ALT, liver function test results may be increased

• Monitor renal studies in patients with compromised renal system: BUN, I&O ratio, creatinine

• Obtain ophth exam before, 1 mo after treatment begins, annually; lens opacities may occur

Nursing diagnoses

• Diarrhea (adverse reactions)

• Knowledge, deficient (teaching)

• Noncompliance (teaching)

Implementation

• Give with evening meal; if dosage is increased, take with breakfast and evening meal

• Store in cool environment in airtight, light-resistant container

Patient/family education

• Inform patient that compliance is needed for positive results to occur, not to double doses

• Advise patient to notify prescriber if GI symptoms of diarrhea, abdominal or epigastric pain, nausea, vomiting, or if chills, fever, sore throat occur; also muscle pain, weakness, tenderness

• Advise patient that treatment is chronic

• Advise patient that blood studies and eye exam will be necessary during treatment

• Instruct patient to report suspected pregnancy, not to use during pregnancy

• Advise patient that previously prescribed regimen will continue, including diet, exercise, smoking cessation

• Advise patient to use sunscreen or stay out of the sun to prevent burns

• Instruct patient to notify all health care providers of products taken

Evaluation
Positive therapeutic outcome

• Decreased LDL, VLDL, total cholesterol levels

• Improved ratio of HDLs

---

folic acid (vitamin B₉) (PO, OTC; IM/IV, Ph)
(foe-lik a′sid)

Apo-Folic ✦, Folate, Folvite, Novofolacid ✦, Vitamin B₉

Func. class.: Vitamin B-complex group, water-soluble vitamin

Chem. class.: Supplement

Pregnancy category A

Action: Needed for erythropoiesis; increases RBC, WBC, and platelet formation in megaloblastic anemias

Therapeutic outcome: Absence of macrocytic, megaloblastic anemias

Uses: Megaloblastic or macrocytic anemia caused by folic acid deficiency; liver disease; alcoholism; hemolysis; intestinal obstruction; pregnancy; to reduce risk of neural tube defect

Dosage and routes
RDA

Adult (pregnant/breastfeeding): PO 600 mcg/day

Adult and child ≥14 yr: PO 400 mcg
Child 9-13 yr: PO 300 mcg
Child 4-8 yr: PO 200 mcg
Child 1-3 yr: PO 150 mcg
Infant 6 mo-1 yr: PO 80 mcg
Neonate and infant <6 mo: PO 65 mcg

Megaloblastic/macrocytic anemia due to folic acid or nutritional deficiency
Pregnant/lactating: PO 800-1000 mcg

Therapeutic dose
Adult and child: PO/IM/SUBCUT/**IV** up to 1 mg/day

Maintenance dose
Adult and child >4 yr: PO/IM/**IV**/SUBCUT 0.4 mg/day
Child <4 yr: PO/IM/**IV**/SUBCUT up to 0.3 mg/day
Infant: PO/IM/**IV**/SUBCUT up to 0.1 mg/day
Pregnant/lactating: PO/IM/**IV**/SUBCUT 0.8-1 mg/day

Prevention of neural tube defects during pregnancy
Adult: PO 0.6 mg/day

Prevention of megaloblastic anemia during pregnancy
Adult: PO/IM/SUBCUT up to 1 mg/day during pregnancy

Tropical sprue
Adult: PO 3-15 mg/day

Available forms: Tabs 0.1, 0.4, 0.8, 1, 5 mg; inj 5, 10 mg/ml

Adverse effects
INTEG: Flushing
RESP: **Bronchospasm**

Contraindications: Hypersensitivity, anemias other than megaloblastic/macrocytic anemia, vit B_{12} deficiency anemia, uncorrected pernicious anemia

Precautions: Pregnancy **A**

Pharmacokinetics	
Absorption	Well absorbed
Distribution	Liver, crosses placenta
Metabolism	Liver (converted to active metabolite)
Excretion	Kidneys (unchanged)
Half-life	Unknown

Pharmacodynamics	
Onset	Unknown
Peak	½-1 hr
Duration	Unknown

Interactions
Individual drugs
Carbamazepine: increased need for folic acid
Fosphenytoin: decreased fosphenytoin levels, may increase seizures
Methotrexate, sulfasalazine, trimethoprim: decreased action of folic acid
Phenytoin: decreased phenytoin levels, may increase seizures
Drug classifications
Estrogens, glucocorticoids, hydantoins: increased need for folic acid
Sulfonamides: decreased action of folic acid

NURSING CONSIDERATIONS
Assessment
• Assess patient for fatigue, dyspnea, weakness, shortness of breath, activity intolerance (signs of megaloblastic anemia)
• Monitor Hgb, Hct, and reticulocyte count; folate levels: 6-15 mcg/ml baseline, throughout treatment
• Assess nutritional status: bran, yeast, dried beans, nuts, fruits, fresh vegetables, asparagus; if high folic acid foods are missing from the diet, a referral to a dietitian may be indicated
• Identify products currently taken: alcohol, oral contraceptives, estrogens, glucocorticoids, carbamazepine, hydantoins, trimethoprim; these products may cause increased folic acid use by the body and contribute to deficiency if taking other neurotoxic products

Nursing diagnoses
• Activity intolerance (uses)
• Fatigue (uses)
• Knowledge, deficient (teaching)
• Nutrition: less than body requirements, imbalanced (uses)

Implementation
IV route
• Give **IV** directly, undiluted 5 mg or less over 1 min or more, or may be added to most **IV** sol or TPN
• Store in light-resistant container
Y-site compatibilities: Famotidine
Solution compatibilities: $D_{20}W$
Solution incompatibilities: $D_{40}W$, $D_{50}W$, calcium gluconate

Patient/family education
• Advise patient to take product exactly as prescribed; not to double doses, toxicity may occur
• Instruct patient to notify prescriber of side effects; rash or fever may indicate hypersensitivity

Adverse effects: *italic* = common, **bold** = life-threatening

- Advise patient that urine may become more yellow
- Instruct patient to increase intake of foods rich in folic acid in diet as recommended by dietitian or health care provider
- Teach patient to avoid breastfeeding

Evaluation
Positive therapeutic outcome
- Absence of fatigue, weakness, dyspnea
- Absence of symptoms of megaloblastic anemia
- Increase in reticulocyte count within 5 days
- Absence of neural tube defect

❗ HIGH ALERT

fondaparinux (Rx)
(fon-dah-pair'ih-nux)
Arixtra
Func. class.: Anticoagulant, antithrombotic
Chem. class.: Synthetic, selective factor Xa inhibitor

Pregnancy category B

Do not confuse:
Arixtra/Anti-Xa

Action: Acts by antithrombin III (ATIII)-mediated selective inhibition of factor Xa; neutralization of factor Xa interrupts blood coagulation and inhibits thrombin formation; does not inactivate thrombin (activated factor II) or affect platelets

Therapeutic outcome: Prevention of deep vein thrombosis

Uses: Prevention/treatment of deep vein thrombosis, pulmonary emboli in hip and knee replacement, hip fracture or abdominal surgery

Dosage and routes
Deep vein thrombosis/PE
Adult <50 kg: SUBCUT 5 mg/day × 5 days or more until INR is 2-3; may give warfarin within 72 hr of fondaparinux
Adult 50-100 kg: SUBCUT 7.5 mg/day × 5 days or more until INR is 2-3; may give warfarin within 72 hr of fondaparinux
Adult >100 kg: SUBCUT 10 mg/day × 5 days or more until INR is 2-3; may give warfarin within 72 hr of fondaparinux

Prevention of deep vein thrombosis
Adult: SUBCUT 2.5 mg/day, given 6 hr after surgery; continue for 5-9 days; hip surgery up to 32 days; abdominal surgery up to 24 days

Available forms: Inj 2.5 mg/0.5 ml, 5 mg/0.4 ml, 7.5 mg/0.6 ml, 10 mg/0.8 ml prefilled syringes

Adverse effects
CNS: Fever, confusion, headache, dizziness, *insomnia*
GI: Nausea, vomiting, diarrhea, dyspepsia, *constipation,* increased AST, ALT
GU: UTI, urinary retention
HEMA: Anemia, minor bleeding, purpura, hematoma, **thrombocytopenia, major bleeding (intracranial, cerebral, retroperitoneal hemorrhage), postoperative hemorrhage,** heparin-induced thrombocytopenia
INTEG: Local reaction—*rash,* pruritus, inj site bleeding, increased wound drainage, bullous eruption
META: Hypokalemia
MISC: Hypotension, pain, *edema*

Contraindications: Hypersensitivity to this product; hemophilia, leukemia with bleeding, peptic ulcer disease, hemorrhagic stroke, surgery, thrombocytopenic purpura, weight <50 kg, severe renal disease (CCr <30 ml/min), active major bleeding, bacterial endocarditis

Precautions: Pregnancy **B**, breastfeeding, children, geriatric, alcoholism, hepatic disease (severe), blood dyscrasias, heparin-induced thrombocytopenia, uncontrolled severe hypertension, subacute bacterial endocarditis, acute nephritis, mild-moderate renal disease

Black Box Warning: Spinal/epidural anesthesia, lumbar puncture

Pharmacokinetics	
Absorption	Rapidly, completely absorbed
Distribution	Blood; does not bind to plasma proteins except 94% to ATIII
Metabolism	Unknown
Excretion	Eliminated unchanged in 72 hr in normal renal function
Half-life	17-21 hr

Pharmacodynamics	
Onset	Unknown
Peak	3 hr
Duration	Unknown

Interactions
Before starting fondaparinux, discontinue use of other products that may increase the risk of hemorrhage; monitor closely if coadministration is essential

---

Individual drugs
Abciximab, clopidogrel, dipyridamole, eptifibatide, quinidine, tirofiban, valproic acid:
increased risk of bleeding
Drug classifications
NSAIDs, salicylates: increased risk of bleeding
Drug/herb
Agrimony, alfalfa, angelica, anise, basil, bay,
bilberry, black haw, bogbean, bromelain,
buchu, chondroitin, cinchona bark, dong
quai, fenugreek, feverfew, garlic, ginger,
ginkgo, ginseng, horse chestnut, Irish moss,
kelp, kelpware, khella, lovage, lungwort,
meadowsweet, motherwort, mugwort, nettle,
papaya, parsley (large amounts), pau
D'arco, pineapple, poplar, prickly ash,
safflower, saw palmetto, tonka bean, turmeric, wintergreen, yarrow: increased risk
of bleeding
Chamomile, coenzyme Q10, flax, glucomannan, goldenseal, guar gum: decreased
anticoagulant effect

NURSING CONSIDERATIONS
Assessment
• Assess blood studies (Hct, CBC, coagulation
studies, platelets, occult blood in stools),
anti-Xa; thrombocytopenia may occur
• Assess for bleeding: gums, petechiae,
ecchymosis, black tarry stools, hematuria;
notify prescriber
• Assess for neurologic symptoms in patients
who have received spinal anesthesia

Nursing diagnoses
• Injury, risk for (uses, adverse reactions)
• Knowledge, deficient (teaching)
• Tissue perfusion, ineffective (uses)

Implementation
• Do not mix with other products or
solutions; cannot be used interchangeably
(unit to unit) with other anticoagulants
• Administer for 5-9 days
• Give only after screening patient for bleed-
ing disorders
• Administer SUBCUT only; do not give IM
• Store at 77° F (25° C); do not freeze
SUBCUT route
• Check for discolored sol or sol with
particulate; if present, do not give
• Begin 2 hr prior to surgery
• Administer to recumbent patient, rotate inj
sites (left/right anterolateral, left/right postero-
lateral abdominal wall)
• Wipe surface of inj site with alcohol swab,
twist plunger cap and remove, remove rigid
needle guard by pulling straight off needle, do

not aspirate, do not expel air bubble from
surface
• Insert whole length of needle into skin fold
held with thumb and forefinger
• When product is injected, a soft click may
be felt or heard
• Give at same time each day to maintain
steady blood levels
• Avoid all IM inj that may cause bleeding
◆ Administer only this product when ordered;
not interchangeable with heparin

Patient/family education
• Advise patient to use soft-bristle toothbrush
to avoid bleeding gums, to use electric razor
• Advise patient to report any signs of
bleeding: gums, under skin, urine, stools
• Caution patient to avoid OTC products
containing aspirin

Evaluation
Positive therapeutic outcome
• Absence of deep vein thrombosis

---

formoterol (Rx)
(for-moh'ter-ahl)
Foradil Aerolizer, Perforomist
Func. class.: β-Adrenergic agonist
Chem. class.: Sympathomimetic catechol-
amine
Pregnancy category C

Do not confuse:
Foradil/Toradol

Action: Has β_1 and β_2 action; relaxes
bronchial smooth muscle and dilates the
trachea and main bronchi by increasing levels
of cAMP, which relaxes smooth muscles;
causes increased contractility and heart rate by
acting on β-receptors in the heart

Therapeutic outcome: Bronchodilatation, increased heart rate and cardiac output
from action on β-receptors in heart

Uses: Maintenance, treatment of asthma,
COPD, prevention of exercise-induced bronchospasm

Dosage and routes
*Maintenance, treatment of
asthma*
Adult and child ≥5 yr: INH AM and PM
long-term, 1 cap (12 mcg) q12hr using
aerolizer inhaler
Maintenance of COPD
Adult: INH 12 mcg q12hr

F

Prevention of exercise-induced bronchospasm
Adult and child ≥12 yr: INH prn occasionally 1 cap (12 mcg) at least 15 min before exercise

Available forms: INH powder in cap 12 mcg

Adverse effects
CNS: Tremors, *anxiety*, insomnia, headache, dizziness, stimulation
CV: Palpitations, tachycardia, hypertension
GI: Nausea, vomiting, xerostomia
RESP: Bronchial irritation, dryness of oropharynx, **bronchospasms (overuse);** infection, inflammatory reactions (child)

Contraindications: Hypersensitivity to sympathomimetics, closed-angle glaucoma

Precautions: Pregnancy **C**, geriatric, cardiac disorders, hyperthyroidism, diabetes mellitus, prostatic hypertrophy, hypertension

Black Box Warning: Respiratory insufficiency

Pharmacokinetics

Absorption	Rapid (INH)
Distribution	Plasma protein binding 61%-64% at concentrations of 0.1-100 ng/mL; 31%-38% at concentrations of 5-500 ng/mL
Metabolism	Liver, lungs, GI tract
Excretion	Urine, feces
Half-life	10 hr mean terminal elimination half-life

Pharmacodynamics

Onset	Unknown
Peak	5 min (INH)
Duration	Unknown

Interactions
Drug classifications
β-Blockers: decreased action of formoterol
MAOIs, antidepressants (tricyclics): serious dysrhythmias
Sympathomimetics: increased action of both products

NURSING CONSIDERATIONS
Assessment
• Assess respiratory function: B/P, pulse, lung sounds
• Assess I&O ratio; check for urinary retention, frequency, hesitancy
• Assess for paresthesias and coldness of extremities; peripheral blood flow may decrease

Nursing diagnoses
• Airway clearance, ineffective (uses)
• Gas exchange, impaired (uses)
• Knowledge, deficient (teaching)

Implementation
• Store at room temperature, protect from heat, moisture
• Do not use discolored sol
• Rinse mouth after use

Patient/family education
• Review package insert with patient and inform about all aspects of product
• Teach correct use of inhaler
• Teach use of spacer device in children or geriatric
• Advise patient to avoid getting aerosol in eyes
• Instruct patient to rinse mouth after use
• Advise patient to wash inhaler in warm water and dry daily
• Advise patient to avoid smoking, smoke-filled rooms, persons with respiratory infections

Evaluation
Positive therapeutic outcome
• Absence of dyspnea, wheezing
• Improved airway exchange
• Improved ABGs

Treatment of overdose: Administer β-blocker

fosamprenavir (Rx)
(fos-am-pren′a-veer)
Lexiva
Func. class.: Antiretroviral
Chem. class.: Protease inhibitor

Pregnancy category C

Action: Prodrug of amprenavir; inhibits human immunodeficiency virus (HIV) protease, which prevents maturation of the infectious virus

Therapeutic outcome: Decreasing symptoms of HIV

Uses: HIV-1 infection in combination with antiretrovirals

Dosage and routes
Therapy-naïve patients
Adult: PO 1400 mg bid without ritonavir, or fosamprenavir 1400 mg/day and ritonavir 200 mg/day, or fosamprenavir 700 mg bid and ritonavir 100 mg bid

Protease-experienced patients (PI)
Adult: PO 700 mg bid and ritonavir 100 mg bid

Combination with efavirenz
Adult: PO add another 100 mg/day of ritonavir for a total of 300 mg/day when all three products are given

Hepatic dose
Adult: PO (Child-Pugh 5-6) 700 mg bid without ritonavir (treatment-naive patients) or 700 mg bid with ritonavir 100 mg qd (treatment-naive or experienced patients); (Child-Pugh 7-9) 700 mg bid without ritonavir (treatment-naive patients) or 450 mg bid with ritonavir 100 mg qd (treatment-naive or experienced patients); (Child-Pugh 10-15) 350 mg bid without ritonavir (treatment-naive patients) or 300 mg bid with ritonavir 100 mg qd (treatment-naive or experienced patients)

Available forms: Tabs 700 mg (equivalent to 600 mg amprenavir)

Adverse effects
CNS: Headache, fatigue, depression, oral paresthesia
GI: Nausea, diarrhea, vomiting, abdominal pain
INTEG: Rash, pruritus
MISC: Redistribution or accumulation of body fat, hyperglycemia, **Stevens-Johnson syndrome**

Contraindications: Hypersensitivity to protease inhibitors

Precautions: Pregnancy C, breastfeeding, geriatric, liver disease, hemolytic anemia, diabetes, sulfa sensitivity

Pharmacokinetics	
Absorption	Unknown
Distribution	90% protein binding
Metabolism	In the liver by CYP4503AY (CYP3A4)
Excretion	Excretion of unchanged product is minimal
Half-life	Unknown

Pharmacodynamics	
Onset	Unknown
Peak	1½-4 hr
Duration	Unknown

Interactions
Individual drugs
🔷Amiodarone, flecainide, lidocaine, midazolam, pimozide, propafenone, triazolam: serious life-threatening reactions

Carbamazepine, delavirdine, phenobarbital, phenytoin, rifampin: avoid use; may lose virologic response and possibly lead to resistance to fosamprenavir
Carbamazepine, efavirenz, lopinavir/ritonavir, nevirapine, phenytoin, ranitidine, saquinavir: decreased fosamprenavir levels
Itraconazole, ketoconazole, rifbutin, sildenafil, vardenafil: increased effect
Methadone: decreased effect
Warfarin: may affect coagulation
Drug classifications
Antacids: decreased fosamprenavir levels
🔷Barbiturates, calcium channel blockers, ergots, H₂ receptor antagonists, proton pump inhibitors: serious life-threatening reactions
Contraceptives (oral): decreased effect
Estrogens, H₂ receptor antagonists, oral contraceptives, proton pump inhibitors: avoid use; may lose virologic response and possibly lead to resistance of fosamprenavir
HMG-CoA reductase inhibitors: increased toxicity
Drug/herb
Avoid use with St. John's wort because may lose virologic response and possibly lead to resistance of fosamprenavir
Drug/lab test
Increased: serum glucose, AST, ALT, triglycerides

NURSING CONSIDERATIONS
Assessment
• Assess bowel pattern before, during treatment; monitor hydration
• Assess skin eruptions, rash, urticaria, itching
• Monitor viral load, CD4 cell counts baseline, throughout treatment

Nursing diagnoses
• Infection, risk for (uses)
• Injury, risk for (adverse reactions)
• Knowledge, deficient (teaching)

Implementation
• Administer without regard to food
• Patients receiving phosphodiesterase type 5 inhibitors may be at increased risk for PDE5 inhibitor adverse effects

Patient/family education
• Advise to avoid taking with other medications unless directed by provider
• Teach that product does not cure, but does manage symptoms; that product does not prevent transmission of HIV to others
• Advise to use nonhormonal form of birth control while taking this product

Adverse effects: *italic* = common, **bold** = life-threatening

Adverse effects: *italic* = common, **bold** = life-threatening

- Instruct if dose is missed, take as soon as remembered up to 1 hr before next dose; do not double dose
- Instruct not to alter dose or stop therapy without talking to physician
- Advise physician if patient has a sulfa allergy
- Advise to report all medications, including herbal supplements, to physician

Evaluation
Positive therapeutic outcome
- Decreasing symptoms of HIV

fosaprepitant (Rx)
(phos-a-prep'ih-tant)
Emend
Func. class.: Antiemetic
Chem. class.: Miscellaneous

Pregnancy category B

Action: A selective antagonist of human substance P/neurokinin 1 (NK$_1$) receptors decreasing emetic reflex, prodrug of aprepitant

Therapeutic outcome: Absence of nausea, vomiting during cancer chemotherapy

Uses: Prevention of nausea/vomiting associated with cancer chemotherapy (highly emetogenic/moderately emetogenic) including high-dose cisplatin, used in combination with other antiemetics; postoperative nausea/vomiting

Dosage and routes
Adult: **IV** INF 115 mg over 15 min, 30 min prior to chemotherapy as an alternate to the 1st dose of aprepitant on day 1 of the aprepitant-CINV regimen

Available forms: Powder for inj 115 mg

Adverse effects
CNS: Headache, *dizziness,* insomnia, anxiety, depression, confusion, peripheral neuropathy
CV: Bradycardia, tachycardia, DVT, hypo/hypertension
GI: Diarrhea, constipation, abdominal pain, anorexia, gastritis, increased AST/ALT, *nausea,* vomiting, heartburn
GU: Increased BUN, serum creatine, proteinuria, dysuria
HEMA: Anemia, **thrombocytopenia, neutropenia**
INTEG: Pruritus, rash, urticaria, **anaphylaxis**
MISC: Asthenia, fatigue, dehydration, fever, hiccups, tinnitus, **Stevens-Johnson syndrome**

Contraindications: Hypersensitivity to this product or polysorbate 80

Precautions: Pregnancy **B,** breastfeeding, children, hepatic disease, geriatric patients; continuous use for nausea and vomiting not recommended

Pharmacokinetics

Absorption	Unknown
Distribution	Protein binding 95%
Metabolism	In liver by CYP3A4 enzymes to an active metabolite; rapidly converted to aprepitant (within 30 mins)
Excretion	Unknown
Half-life	13 hr

Pharmacodynamics
Unknown

Interactions
Individual drugs
Paroxetine: increased action of both products
Drug classifications
CYP2C9 substrates (warfarin, tolbutamide, phenytoin), oral contraceptives: decreased action
CYP3A4 inducers (rifampin, carbamazepine, phenytoin): decreased aprepitant action
CYP3A4 inhibitors (ketoconazole, itraconazole, nefazodone, troleandomycin, clarithromycin, ritonavir, nelfinavir, diltiazem): increased aprepitant action
CYP3A4 substrates (pimozide, cisapride, dexamethasone, terfenadine, astemizole, methylPREDNISolone, midazolam, alprazolam, triazolam, docetaxel, paclitaxel, etoposide, irinotecan, imatinib, ifosfamide, vinorelbine, vinBLAStine, vinCRIStine): increased action
Drug/food
Grapefruit juice: decreased effect

NURSING CONSIDERATIONS
Assessment
- Assess CV status: hyper/hypotension, bradycardia, tachycardia, DVT
- Assess for absence of nausea, vomiting during chemotherapy
- Monitor LFTs

Nursing diagnoses
- Knowledge, deficient (teaching)
- Nausea (uses)

Implementation
IV INF route
- Give **IV** route
- Approved only as a substitute for the 1st dose of aprepitant in 3-day regimen
- Use aseptic technique for reconstitution; inject 5 ml of 0.9% NaCl into the vial, directing stream to wall of vial to prevent foam; swirl; do not shake
- Prepare inf bag with 110 ml of NS; do not dilute or reconstitute with any divalent cations such as calcium, magnesium, including LR, Hartmann's sol
- Withdraw the entire volume from vial and transfer to inf bag; total volume 115 ml (1 mg/ 1 ml)
- Gently invert bag 2-3 times; reconstituted sol is stable for 24 hr at lower room temp or <25° C
- Visually inspect for particulates and discoloration
- Infuse over 15 min

Patient/family education
- Instruct patient to report diarrhea, constipation
- Instruct patient to report all medications and herbals to prescriber prior to taking this medication
- Advise patient to use nonhormonal form of contraception while taking this agent; oral contraceptive effect may be decreased
- Advise patient on warfarin to have clotting monitored closely during 2-wk period following administration of aprepitant
- Instruct patient to avoid breastfeeding

Evaluation
Positive therapeutic outcome
- Absence of nausea, vomiting during cancer chemotherapy

foscarnet (Rx)
(foss-kar'net)
Foscavir
Func. class.: Antiviral
Chem. class.: Inorganic pyrophosphate organic analog
Pregnancy category C

Action: Antiviral activity is produced by selective inhibition at the pyrophosphate binding site on virus-specific DNA polymerases and reverse transcriptases at concentrations that do not affect cellular DNA polymerases

Therapeutic outcome: Virostatic agents against CMV retinitis

Uses: Treatment of CMV, retinitis, herpes simplex virus (HSV) infections; used with ganciclovir for relapsing patients

Dosage and routes
CMV retinitis
Adult: **IV** INF 60 mg/kg given over at least 1 hr, q8hr × 2-3 wk initially, or 90 mg/kg q12hr, usually given with at least 750-1000 ml of 0.9% NaCl daily
HSV
Adult: **IV** 40 mg/kg q8-12hr × 2-3 wk
Renal dose
Adult: **IV**
Male:
$$\frac{140 - \text{age}}{72 \times \text{serum creatinine (mg/dl)}} = CCr$$

Female: 0.85 × above value; dose based on table provided in package insert

Available forms: Inj 6000 mg/250 ml, 12,000 mg/500 ml (24 mg/ml)

Adverse effects
CNS: Fever, dizziness, *headache,* **seizures,** *fatigue,* neuropathy, tremor, ataxia, dementia, stupor, EEG abnormalities, vertigo, **coma,** abnormal gait, hypertonia, extrapyramidal disorders, hemiparesis, **paralysis,** hyperreflexia, paraplegia, **tetany,** hyporeflexia, neuralgia, neuritis, **cerebral edema,** *paresthesia,* depression, *confusion, anxiety,* insomnia, somnolence, amnesia, hallucinations, agitation
CV: Hypertension, palpitations, ECG abnormalities, 1st-degree AV block, nonspecific ST-T segment changes, hypotension, cerebrovascular disorder, cardiomyopathy, **cardiac arrest,** bradycardia, **dysrhythmias**
EENT: Visual field defects, vocal cord paralysis, speech disorders, taste perversion, eye pain, conjunctivitis, tinnitus, otitis
GI: Nausea, vomiting, diarrhea, anorexia, abdominal pain, constipation, dysphagia, rectal hemorrhage, dry mouth, melena, flatulence, ulcerative stomatitis, pancreatitis, enteritis, enterocolitis, glossitis, proctitis, stomatitis, increased amylases, gastroenteritis, **pseudomembranous colitis,** duodenal ulcer, **paralytic ileus, esophageal ulceration,** abnormal A-G ratio, increased AST, ALT, cholecystitis, **hepatitis,** dyspepsia, tenesmus, hepatosplenomegaly, jaundice
GU: **Acute renal failure,** decreased CCr and increased serum creatinine, **glomerulonephritis,** toxic nephropathy, **nephrosis, renal tubular disorders, pyelonephritis, uremia, hematuria, albuminuria,** dysuria, polyuria

Adverse effects: *italic* = common, **bold** = life-threatening

HEMA: Anemia, **granulocytopenia, leukopenia, thrombocytopenia, platelet abnormalities, thrombosis, pulmonary embolism, coagulation disorders, decreased prothrombin, hypochromic anemia, pancytopenia, hemolysis, leukocytosis,** lymphadenopathy, epistaxis, lymphopenia
INTEG: *Rash,* sweating, pruritus, skin ulceration, seborrhea, skin discoloration, alopecia, acne, dermatitis, pain/inflammation at injection site, facial edema, dry skin, urticaria
MS: Arthralgia, myalgia
RESP: *Coughing, dyspnea,* pneumonia, sinusitis, pharyngitis, **pulmonary infiltration,** stridor, **pneumothorax, hemoptysis, bronchospasm,** bronchitis, **respiratory depression, pleural effusion, pulmonary hemorrhage,** rhinitis
SYST: *Hypokalemia, hypocalcemia, hypomagnesemia,* increased alkaline phosphatase, LDH, BUN, acidosis, hypophosphatemia, hyperphosphatemia, dehydration, glycosuria, increased creatine phosphokinase, hypervolemia, infection, **sepsis, death, ascites,** hyponatremia, hypochloremia, hypercalcemia

Contraindications: Hypersensitivity, CCr <0.4 ml/min/kg

Precautions: Pregnancy **C,** breastfeeding, children, geriatric, seizure disorders, severe anemia

Black Box Warning: Renal disease, electrolyte/mineral imbalances

Pharmacokinetics

Absorption	Complete (**IV**)
Distribution	14%-17% plasma protein binding
Metabolism	Not metabolized
Excretion	Kidneys (79%-92%) unchanged, breast milk
Half-life	18-88 hr; increased in renal disease

Pharmacodynamics

Onset	48 hr
Peak	2 wk
Duration	Unknown

Interactions
Individual drugs
Amphotericin B, cycloSPORINE, lithium: increased nephrotoxicity
Pentamidine: increased hypocalcemia
Drug classifications
Aminoglycosides, NSAIDs: increased nephrotoxicity

NURSING CONSIDERATIONS
Assessment
- Culture should be done before treatment with foscarnet is begun; cultures of blood, urine, and throat may all be taken; CMV is not confirmed by this method; the diagnosis is made by an ophth exam
- Assess kidney and liver function; increased hemopoietic studies: BUN, serum creatinine, creatinine clearance, if CCr <0.4 ml/min/kg, discontinue product; AST, ALT, A-G ratio, baseline, during treatment; blood counts should be done q2wk; watch for decreasing granulocytes, Hgb; if low, therapy may have to be discontinued and restarted after hematologic recovery; blood transfusions may be required
- Assess for GI symptoms: severe nausea, vomiting, diarrhea; severe symptoms may necessitate discontinuing product
- Monitor electrolytes and minerals: calcium, phosphorous, magnesium, sodium, potassium; watch closely for tetany during first administration
◆ Assess for symptoms of blood dyscrasias (anemia, granulocytopenia); bruising, fatigue, bleeding, poor healing
- Assess for symptoms of allergic reactions: flushing, rash, urticaria, pruritus

Nursing diagnoses
- Infection, risk for (uses)
- Injury, risk for (adverse reactions)
- Knowledge, deficient (teaching)

Implementation
IV route
- Administer increased fluids before, during product administration to induce diuresis and minimize renal toxicity
- Administer via inf pump, at no more than 1 mg/kg/min; do not give by rapid or bolus **IV;** give by central venous line or peripheral vein; standard 24 mg/ml sol may be used without dilution if using by central line; dilute the 24 mg/ml sol to 12 mg/ml with D_5W or 0.9% NaCl if using peripheral vein
- Monitor patient closely during therapy; if tingling, numbness, paresthesias occur, stop inf and obtain lab sample for electrolytes
Y-site compatibilities: Aldesleukin, aminophylline, amikacin, ampicillin, aztreonam, benzquinamide, cefazolin, cefoperazone, cefoxitin, ceftazidime, ceftizoxime, ceftriaxone, cefuroxime, chloramphenicol, cimetidine, clindamycin, dexamethasone, DOPamine, erythromycin, fluconazole, flucytosine, furosemide, gentamicin, heparin, hydrocortisone, hydromorphone, hydrOXYzine,

imipenem-cilastatin, metoclopramide, metronidazole, miconazole, morphine, nafcillin, oxacillin, penicillin G potassium, phenytoin, piperacillin, ranitidine, ticarcillin/clavulanate, tobramycin

Y-site incompatibilities: Acyclovir, amphotericin B, calcium, cotrimoxazole, diazepam, digoxin, gancyclovir, haloperidol, leucovorin, midazolam, pentamidine, phenytoin, prochlorperazine, vancomycin

Patient/family education

• Advise patient to notify prescriber if sore throat, swollen lymph nodes, malaise, fever occur, may indicate presence of other infections

• Advise patient to report perioral tingling, numbness in extremities, and paresthesias; inf should be stopped and electrolytes should be requested

• Caution patient that serious product interactions may occur if OTC products are ingested; check first with prescriber

• Inform patient that product is not a cure, but will control symptoms

• Advise patient that ophth exams must be continued

Evaluation

Positive therapeutic outcome

• Improvement in CMV retinitis

---

fosinopril (Rx)

(foss-in-o′pril)

Monopril

Func. class.: Antihypertensive

Chem. class.: Angiotensin-converting enzyme (ACE) inhibitor

Pregnancy category D

Do not confuse:

Monopril/minoxidil/Accupril/Monoket

Action: Selectively suppresses renin-angiotensin-aldosterone system; inhibits ACE; prevents conversion of angiotensin I to angiotensin II; results in dilatation of arterial, venous vessels

Therapeutic outcome: Decreased B/P in hypertension

Uses: Hypertension, alone or in combination with thiazide diuretics, systolic CHF

Dosage and routes

Hypertension

Adult: PO 10 mg/day initially, then 20-40 mg/day divided bid or daily, max 80 mg/day

CHF

Adult: PO 10 mg/day, then up to 40 mg/day, increased over several weeks; use lower dose in those undergoing diuresis before fosinopril

Available forms: Tabs 10, 20, 40 mg

Adverse effects

CNS: Insomnia, paresthesia, headache, dizziness, fatigue, memory disturbance, tremor, mood change

CV: Hypotension, chest pain, palpitations, angina, orthostatic hypotension, dysrhythmias, tachycardia

GI: Nausea, constipation, vomiting, diarrhea

GU: **Proteinuria,** increased BUN, creatinine, decreased libido

HEMA: Decreased Hct, Hgb, **eosinophilia, leukopenia, neutropenia**

INTEG: **Angioedema,** rash, flushing, sweating, photosensitivity, pruritus

META: Hyperkalemia

MS: Arthralgia, myalgia

RESP: Cough, sinusitis, dyspnea, **bronchospasm**

Contraindications: Breastfeeding, children, hypersensitivity to ACE inhibitors

Black Box Warning: Pregnancy D

Precautions: Geriatric, impaired liver function, hypovolemia, blood dyscrasias, CHF, COPD, asthma, angioedema, hyperkalemia, renal artery stenosis, renal disease

Pharmacokinetics	
Absorption	30%
Distribution	Crosses placenta
Metabolism	Liver—converted to fosinoprilat
Excretion	50% kidneys (metabolites), 50% feces
Half-life	12 hr—fosinoprilat

Pharmacodynamics	
Onset	1 hr
Peak	2-6 hr
Duration	24 hr

Interactions

Individual drugs

Alcohol (acute ingestion): increased hypotension (large amounts)

Allopurinol: increased hypersensitivity

Digoxin, hydralazine, lithium, prazosin: increased toxicity

Indomethacin: decreased antihypertensive effect

F

Drug classifications

Adrenergic blockers, antihypertensives, diuretics, ganglionic blockers, nitrates, phenothiazines: increased hypotension

Antacids: decreased absorption

Diuretics (potassium-sparing), sympathomimetics, vasodilators: increased toxicity

NSAIDs, salicylates: decreased antihypertensive effect

Drug/herb

⚠Arginine: fatal hypokalemia

Hawthorn, pill-bearing spurge: increased antihypertensive effect

Pineapple, yohimbe: decreased antihypertensive effect

St. John's wort: severe photosensitivity

Drug/lab test

Increased: AST, ALT, alkaline phosphatase, glucose, bilirubin, uric acid

Positive: ANA titer

False positive: urine acetone

NURSING CONSIDERATIONS
Assessment

• Monitor blood studies: neutrophils, decreased platelets; obtain WBC with differential baseline and qmo × 6 mo, then q2-3mo × 1 yr; if neutrophils <1000/mm³, discontinue

• Monitor B/P, check for orthostatic hypotension, syncope; if changes occur, dosage change may be required

• Monitor renal studies: protein, BUN, creatinine; watch for increased levels that may indicate nephrotic syndrome and renal failure; monitor urine daily for protein; monitor renal symptoms: polyuria, oliguria, frequency, dysuria

• Establish baselines in renal, liver function tests before therapy begins

• Check potassium levels throughout treatment although hyperkalemia rarely occurs

• Check for edema in feet, legs daily, monitor weight daily

• Assess for allergic reactions: rash, fever, pruritus, urticaria; product should be discontinued if antihistamines fail to help

Nursing diagnoses

• Cardiac output, decreased (uses)
• Injury, risk for (side effects)
• Knowledge, deficient (teaching)
• Noncompliance (teaching)

Implementation

• Store in airtight container at 86° F (30° C) or less

• Severe hypotension may occur after 1st dose of this medication; hypotension may be prevented by reducing or discontinuing diuretic therapy 3 days before beginning benzapril therapy

Patient/family education

• Advise patient not to discontinue product abruptly; warn patient to tell all persons associated with his or her care

• Teach patient not to use OTC products (cough, cold, allergy) unless directed by prescriber because serious side effects can occur; xanthines such as coffee, tea, chocolate, cola can prevent action of product

• Teach patient the importance of complying with dosage schedule, even if feeling better; to continue with medical regimen to decrease B/P: exercise, smoking cessation, decreasing stress, diet modifications

• Emphasize the need to rise slowly to sitting or standing position to minimize orthostatic hypotension; not to exercise in hot weather or increased hypotension can occur

• Teach patient to notify prescriber of mouth sores, sore throat, fever, swelling of hands or feet, irregular heartbeat, chest pain, coughing, shortness of breath

• Instruct patient to report excessive perspiration, dehydration, vomiting, diarrhea; may lead to fall in B/P

• Caution patient that product may cause dizziness, fainting, light-headedness; may occur during 1st few days of therapy; to avoid activities that may be hazardous

• Teach patient how to take B/P, and normal readings for age-group

• Advise patient to notify prescriber if pregnancy is planned or suspected

Evaluation
Positive therapeutic outcome

• Decreased B/P in hypertension

Treatment of overdose: 0.9% NaCl **IV** inf, hemodialysis

---

fosphenytoin (Rx)
(foss-fen'i-toy-in)
Cerebyx
Func. class.: Anticonvulsant
Chem. class.: Hydantoin, phosphate phenytoin ester

Pregnancy category D

Action: Inhibits spread of seizure activity in motor cortex by altering ion transport; increases AV conduction; prodrug of phenytoin

Therapeutic outcome: Decreased seizures, absence of dysrhythmias

Uses: Generalized tonic-clonic seizures, status epilepticus, partial seizures

Dosage and routes
All doses in PE (phenytoin sodium equivalent)

Status epilepticus
Adult and adolescent: **IV** 15-20 mg PE/kg

Nonemergency/maintenance dosing
Adult and adolescent >16 yr: IM/IV 10-20 mg PE/kg 10 mg dose; 4-6 mg PE/kg/day (maintenance); start maintenance 12 hr after loading dose; give in 2-3 divided doses

Available forms: Inj 150 mg (100 mg PE), 750 mg (500 mg PE), 50 mg/ml vials

Adverse effects
CNS: Drowsiness, dizziness, insomnia, paresthesias, depression, **suicidal tendencies,** aggression, headache, confusion, paresthesia
CV: Hypotension, **ventricular fibrillation,** hypertension, **CHF, shock**
EENT: Nystagmus, diplopia, blurred vision
GI: Nausea, vomiting, diarrhea, constipation, anorexia, weight loss, **hepatitis,** jaundice, gingival hyperplasia
HEMA: **Agranulocytosis, leukopenia, aplastic anemia, thrombocytopenia, megaloblastic anemia**
INTEG: Rash, lupus erythematosus, **Stevens-Johnson syndrome,** hirsutism, hypersensitivity, pruritus
SYST: Hyperglycemia, hypokalemia, **toxic epidermal necrolysis (Asian patients positive for HLA-B 1502)**

Contraindications: Pregnancy **D,** hypersensitivity, psychiatric conditions, bradycardia, SA and AV block, Stokes-Adams syndrome, absence seizures

Precautions: Breastfeeding, allergies, renal/hepatic disease, myocardial insufficiency, hypoalbuminemia, hypothyroidism, Asian patients positive for HLA-B 1502

Pharmacokinetics
Absorption	Unknown
Distribution	Protein binding 99%
Metabolism	Liver: converted to phenytoin
Excretion	Kidneys
Half-life	Unknown

Pharmacodynamics
Unknown

Interactions
Individual drugs
Alcohol: decreased effects of fosphenytoin (chronic use)
Amiodarone, chloramphenicol, cimetidine: increased fosphenytoin level
Carbamazepine, folic acid, rifampin, theophylline, tramadol: decreased effects of fosphenytoin
Drug classifications
Antacids, antihistamines, antineoplastics, CYP1A2 inducers: decreased effects of fosphenytoin
Antidepressants (tricyclics), CYP1A2 inhibitors, estrogens, H$_2$-receptor antagonists, phenothiazines, salicylates, sulfonamides: increased fosphenytoin level
Drug/herb
Ginseng, santonica, valerian: decreased anticonvulsant effect
Ginkgo: increased anticonvulsant effect
Drug/lab test
Increased: glucose, alkaline phosphatase
Decreased: dexamethasone, metyrapone test serum, PBI, urinary steroids

NURSING CONSIDERATIONS
Assessment
• Assess product level: toxic level 30-50 mcg/ml, wait at least 2 hr after dose before testing, 4 hr after IM dose
• Assess seizure activity including type, location, duration, and character; provide seizure precaution
• Assess renal studies: urinalysis, BUN, urine creatinine
• Monitor hepatic studies: ALT, AST, bilirubin, creatinine
• Assess allergic reaction: red raised rash; if this occurs, product should be discontinued
• Monitor for toxicity: bone marrow depression, nausea, vomiting, ataxia, diplopia, cardiovascular collapse, slurred speech, confusion
• Assess product level: toxic level 30-50 mcg/ml
⬥Assess for rash, discontinue as soon as rash develops, serious adverse reactions such as Stevens-Johnson syndrome can occur
⬥ Assess mental status: mood, sensorium, affect, memory (long, short), especially geriatric; suicidal thoughts/behaviors
• Assess for blood dyscrasias: fever, sore throat, bruising, rash, jaundice, epistaxis (long-term treatment only)
• Monitor blood studies: RBC, Hct, Hgb, reticulocyte counts weekly for 4 wk then

F

monthly; also check thyroid function tests, serum calcium, albumin, phosphorus

Nursing diagnoses
- Injury, risk for (uses, adverse reactions)
- Knowledge, deficient (teaching)
- Noncompliance (teaching)

Implementation
IV route
- Administer by direct **IV** after diluting with D₅ or 0.9% NaCl to 1.5-25 mg PE/ml
Solution compatibilities: D₅W, D₁₀W, amino acid inj 10%, D₅LR, D₅/0.9% NaCl, Plasmalyte A, LR
Additive compatibilities: Potassium chloride

Patient/family education
- Teach patient the reason for and expected outcome of treatment
- Instruct patient not to use machinery or engage in hazardous activity; drowsiness, dizziness may occur
- Advise patient to carry/wear emergency ID identifying product used, name of prescriber
- Advise patient to notify prescriber of rash, bleeding, bruising, slurred speech, jaundice of skin or eyes, joint pain, nausea, vomiting, severe headache
- Advise patient to keep all medical appointments, including lab work, physical assessment
- Advise patient to notify prescriber if pregnancy is planned or suspected; to use contraception with this product

Evaluation
Positive therapeutic outcome
- Decreased seizure activity

---

fospropofol
Lusedra
See Appendix A, Selected New Drugs

---

frovatriptan (Rx)
(froh-vah-trip'tan)
Frova
Func. class.: Antimigraine agent
Chem. class.: 5-HT₁ receptor agonist

Pregnancy category C

Action: Binds selectively to the vascular 5-HT₁B, 5-HT₁D receptor subtypes, exerts antimigraine effect; binds to benzodiazepine receptor sites, causes vasoconstriction in cranium

Therapeutic outcome: Absence of migraines

Uses: Acute treatment of migraine with or without aura

Dosage and routes
Adult: PO 2.5 mg; a 2nd dose may be taken after ≥2 hr; max 3 tabs/day (7.5 mg)

Available forms: Tabs 2.5 mg

Adverse effects
CNS: Hot sensation, paresthesia, *dizziness,* headache, fatigue, cold sensation, insomnia, anxiety, somnolence, **seizures**
CV: Flushing, chest pain, palpitation
GI: Dry mouth, dyspepsia, abdominal pain, diarrhea, vomiting, nausea
MS: Skeletal pain

Contraindications: Angina pectoris, history of MI, documented silent ischemia, Prinzmetal's angina, ischemic heart disease, concurrent ergotamine-containing preparations, uncontrolled hypertension, hypersensitivity, basilar or hemiplegic migraine; ischemic bowel disease; peripheral vascular disease, severe hepatic disease, prophylactic migraine treatment

Precautions: Pregnancy **C**, breastfeeding, children, geriatric, postmenopausal women, men >40 yr, risk factors for CAD, hypercholesterolemia, obesity, diabetes, impaired hepatic function, seizure disorder

Pharmacokinetics

Absorption	Absolute bioavailability of PO dose ~20% in males, 30% in females
Distribution	Protein binding 15%; reversibly bound to blood cells at equilibrium 60%
Metabolism	Liver
Excretion	Urine (32%), feces (62%)
Half-life	25-29 hr

Pharmacodynamics

Onset	10 min-2 hr
Peak	2-4 hr
Duration	Unknown

Interactions
Individual drugs
Estrogen, propranolol: increased effects of frovatriptan
Drug classifications
CYP1A2 inhibitors (cimetidine, ciprofloxacin, erythromycin), oral contraceptives: increased frovatriptan levels

 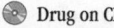

Selective serotonin reuptake inhibitors, other serotonin agonists (dextromethorphan, tramadol, antidepressants): increased toxicity

Drug/herb
Butterbur: increased effect

NURSING CONSIDERATIONS
Assessment
- Assess B/P; signs/symptoms of coronary vasospasms
- Assess for stress level, activity, recreation, coping mechanisms
- Assess neurologic status: LOC, paresthesia, hot/cold sensations, dizziness, headache, fatigue
- Assess for ingestion of tyramine-containing foods (pickled products, beer, wine, aged cheese), food additives, preservatives, colorings, artificial sweeteners, chocolate, caffeine, which may precipitate these types of headaches

Nursing diagnoses
- Knowledge, deficient (teaching)
- Pain, acute (uses)

Implementation
- Ensure that tablets are swallowed whole
- Provide quiet, calm environment with decreased stimulation from noise, bright light, excessive talking

Patient/family education
- Instruct patient to report any side effects to prescriber
- Advise patient to use contraception while taking product
- Advise patient that photosensitivity may occur, to use sunscreen and wear protective clothing when outdoors
- Advise patient to have dark, quiet environment available

Evaluation
Positive therapeutic outcome
- Decrease in frequency, severity of migraine

Treatment of overdose: No specific antidote; monitor patient closely for ≥48 hr, treat any symptoms as necessary

fulvestrant (Rx)
(full-ves'trant)
Faslodex
Func. class.: Antineoplastic
Pregnancy category D

Action: Inhibits cell division by binding to cytoplasmic estrogen receptors; resembles normal cell complex but inhibits DNA synthesis and estrogen response of target tissue

Therapeutic outcome: Decreased tumor size, spread of malignancy

Uses: Advanced breast carcinoma in estrogen-receptor–positive patients (usually postmenopausal)

Dosage and routes
Adult: IM 250 mg qmo

Available forms: Inj 50 mg/ml

Adverse effects
CNS: Headache, depression, dizziness, insomnia, paresthesia, anxiety
GI: Nausea, vomiting, anorexia, constipation, diarrhea, abdominal pain
HEMA: **Anemia**
INTEG: Rash, sweating, hot flashes, inj site pain
MS: Bone pain, arthritis, back pain
RESP: Pharyngitis, dyspnea, cough
SYST: **Angioedema**

Contraindications: Pregnancy **D**, breastfeeding, children, hypersensitivity

Precautions: Hepatic disease

Pharmacokinetics	
Absorption	Unknown
Distribution	Unknown
Metabolism	CYP3A4
Excretion	Feces 90%
Half-life	40 days

Pharmacodynamics
Unknown

NURSING CONSIDERATIONS
Assessment
- Monitor for side effects, report to prescriber

Nursing diagnoses
- Infection, risk for (adverse reactions)
- Knowledge, deficient (teaching)
- Nutrition: less than body requirements, imbalanced (adverse reactions)

F

Adverse effects: *italic* = common, **bold** = life-threatening

Implementation

- Give IM 5 ml as a single inj or 2, 2.5 ml inj; give slowly in buttock
- Give antacid before oral agent; give product after evening meal, before bedtime
- Give antiemetic 30-60 min before giving product to prevent vomiting
- Provide liquid diet, if needed, including cola, Jell-O; dry toast or crackers may be added if patient is not nauseated or vomiting
- Provide nutritious diet with iron, vitamin supplements as ordered
- Increase fluids to 2 L/day unless contraindicated
- Store in refrigerator

Patient/family education

- Advise patient to report any complaints, side effects to prescriber
- Teach patient to increase fluids to 2 L/day unless contraindicated
- Advise patient to report vaginal bleeding immediately
- Teach patient that tumor flare—increase in size of tumor, increased bone pain—may occur and will subside rapidly; may take analgesics for pain
- Teach that premenopausal women must use mechanical birth control because ovulation may be induced

Evaluation

Positive therapeutic outcome

- Decreased tumor size, spread of malignancy

---

furosemide 🔘 (Rx)
(fur-oh'se-mide)

Apo-Furosemide ✦, Furoside ✦, Lasix, Lasix Special ✦, Myrosemide, Novosemide ✦, Uritol ✦
Func. class.: Loop diuretic
Chem. class.: Sulfonamide derivative

Pregnancy category C

Do not confuse:
furosemide/torsemide, Lasix/Lanoxin/Lomotil/Luvox

Action: Acts on the ascending loop of Henle in the kidney, inhibiting reabsorption of electrolytes sodium and chloride, causing excretion of sodium, calcium, magnesium, chloride, water, and some potassium; decreases reabsorption of sodium and chloride and increases excretion of potassium in the distal tubule of the kidney; responsible for slight antihypertensive effect and peripheral vasodilatation

Therapeutic outcome: Decreased edema in lung tissue, peripherally; decreased B/P

Uses: Pulmonary edema, edema in CHF, nephrotic syndrome, ascites, hepatic disease, hypertension

Unlabeled uses: Hypercalcemia in malignancy

Dosage and routes
Adult: PO 20-80 mg/day in AM, may give another dose in 6 hr, up to 600 mg/day; IM/**IV** 20-40 mg, increased by 20 mg q2hr until desired response
Child: PO/IM/**IV** 2 mg/kg, may increase by 1-2 mg/kg/q6-8hr up to 6 mg/kg

Acute pulmonary edema
Adult: **IV** 40 mg given over several min, repeated in 1 hr; increase to 80 mg if needed

Hypertensive crisis/acute renal failure
Adult: **IV** 100-200 mg over 1-2 min

Antihypercalcemia
Adult: IM/**IV** 80-100 mg q1-4hr or PO 120 mg/day or divided bid
Child: IM/**IV** 25-50 mg, repeat q4hr if needed

Available forms: Tabs 20, 40, 80 mg; oral sol 8 mg/ml, 10 mg/ml; inj IM, **IV** 10 mg/ml

Adverse effects
CNS: Headache, fatigue, weakness, vertigo, paresthesias
CV: Orthostatic hypotension, chest pain, ECG changes, **circulatory collapse**
EENT: Loss of hearing, ear pain, tinnitus, blurred vision
ELECT: Hypokalemia, hypochloremic alkalosis, hypomagnesemia, hyperuricemia, hypocalcemia, hyponatremia, metabolic alkalosis
ENDO: Hyperglycemia
GI: Nausea, diarrhea, dry mouth, vomiting, anorexia, cramps, oral or gastric irritations, pancreatitis
GU: Polyuria, **renal failure,** *glycosuria*
HEMA: **Thrombocytopenia, agranulocytosis, leukopenia, neutropenia, anemia**
INTEG: Rash, pruritus, purpura, **Stevens-Johnson syndrome,** sweating, photosensitivity, urticaria
MS: Cramps, stiffness

Contraindications: Hypersensitivity to sulfonamides; anuria, hypovolemia, breastfeeding, infants, electrolyte depletion

---

Precautions: Pregnancy **C**, diabetes mellitus, dehydration, severe renal disease, cirrhosis, ascites

Pharmacokinetics

	PO
Absorption	GI tract (60%-70%)
	PO/IM/IV
Distribution	Crosses placenta
Metabolism	Liver (30%-40%)
Excretion	Breast milk, urine, feces
Half-life	½-1 hr

Pharmacodynamics

	PO	IM	IV
Onset	1 hr	½ hr	5 min
Peak	1-2 hr	Unknown	½ hr
Duration	6-8 hr	4-8 hr	2 hr

Interactions
Individual drugs
Cisplatin, vancomycin: increased risk of ototoxicity

Digoxin: increased toxicity

Lithium: decreased renal clearance, causing increased toxicity

Drug classifications
Aminoglycosides: increased ototoxicity

Anticoagulants, salicylates: increased effects

Antihypertensives: increased antihypertensive effect

Nitrates: increased hypotensive action

Nondepolarizing skeletal muscle relaxants: increased toxicity

Drug/herb
Aloe, cucumber, dandelion, horsetail, khella, pumpkin, Queen Anne's lace: increased diuretic effect

St. John's wort: severe photosensitivity

Drug/lab test
Interference: GTT

Increase: LDL

NURSING CONSIDERATIONS
Assessment
• Assess patient for tinnitus, hearing loss, ear pain; periodic testing of hearing is needed when high doses of this product are given by **IV** route

• Monitor for renal, cardiac, neurologic, GI, pulmonary manifestations of hypokalemia: acidic urine, reduced urine osmolality, nocturia, polyuria and polydipsia; hypotension, broad T-wave, U-wave, ectopy, tachycardia, weak pulse; muscle weakness, altered LOC, drowsiness, apathy, lethargy, confusion, depression; anorexia, nausea, cramps, constipation, distention, paralytic ileus; hypoventilation, respiratory muscle weakness

• Monitor for CNS, GI, cardiovascular, integumentary, neurologic manifestations of hypocalcemia: personality changes, anxiety, disturbances, depression and psychosis; nausea, vomiting, constipation, abdominal pain from muscle spasm; decreased contractility, decreased cardiac output, hypotension, lengthened ST segment, prolonged QT interval; scaling eczema, alopecia, hyperpigmentation; tetany, muscle twitching, cramping, grimacing, seizure, altered deep tendon reflexes, spasm

• Monitor for CNS, neuromuscular, GI, cardiac manifestations of hypomagnesemia, agitation; muscle twitching, paresthesias, hyperactive reflexes, positive Babinski reflex, dysphagia, nystagmus, seizures, tetany; nausea, vomiting, diarrhea, anorexia, abdominal distention; ectopy, tachycardia, broad, flat or inverted T-waves, depressed ST segment, prolonged QT, decreased cardiac output, hypotension

• Monitor for CV, GI, neurologic manifestations of hyponatremia: increased B/P, cold, clammy skin, hypovolemia or hypervolemia; anorexia, nausea, vomiting, diarrhea, abdominal cramps; lethargy, increased ICP, confusion, headache, seizures, coma, fatigue, tremors, hyperreflexia

• Monitor for neurologic, respiratory manifestations of hyperchloremia: weakness, lethargy, coma; deep rapid breathing

• Assess fluid volume status: I&O ratios and record, count or weigh diapers as appropriate, weight, distended red veins, crackles in lung, color, quality, and specific gravity of urine, skin turgor, adequacy of pulses, moist mucous membranes, bilateral lung sounds, peripheral pitting edema; dehydration symptoms of decreasing output, thirst, hypotension, dry mouth and mucous membranes should be reported

• Monitor electrolytes: potassium, sodium, calcium, magnesium; also include BUN, blood pH, ABGs, uric acid, CBC, blood glucose

• Assess B/P before and during therapy lying, standing, and sitting as appropriate; orthostatic hypotension can occur rapidly

Nursing diagnoses
• Fluid volume, deficient (side effects)
• Fluid volume, excess (uses)
• Knowledge, deficient (teaching)

Implementation
• Give in AM to avoid interference with sleep
• Potassium replacement if potassium level is <3.0 mg/dl, or use oral sol slightly; product may be crushed if patient is unable to swallow

---

Adverse effects: *italic* = common, **bold** = life-threatening

PO route

• With food or milk if nausea occurs; absorption may be reduced

IV route

• Do not use sol that is yellow, has a precipitate or crystals

IV, direct route

• Give undiluted through Y-tube on 3-way stopcock; give 20 mg or less/min

Intermittent IV inf route

• May be added to 0.9% NaCl, D_5W, $D_{10}W$, $D_{20}W$; invert sugar 10% in electrolyte #1, LR, use within 24 hr to ensure compatibility; give through Y-tube or 3-way stopcock; give at 4 mg/min or less, use inf pump

Syringe compatibilities: Bleomycin, cisplatin, cyclophosphamide, fluorouracil, heparin, leucovorin, methotrexate, mitomycin

Syringe incompatibilities: Doxapram, DOXOrubicin, droperidol, metaclopramide, milrinone

Y-site compatibilities: Allopurinol, amifostine, amikacin, aztreonam, bleomycin, cefepime, cefmetazole, cisplatin, cladribine, cyclophosphamide, cytarabine, dexamethasone, epinephrine, fentanyl, fludarabine, fluorouracil, foscarnet, gallium, granisetron, heparin, hydrocortisone, hydromorphone, indomethacin, kanamycin, leucovorin, lorazepam, melphalan, meropenem, methotrexate, mitomycin, morphine, nitroglycerin, norepinephrine, paclitaxel, piperacillin/tazobactam, potassium chloride, propofol, ranitidine, sargramostim, tacrolimus, teniposide, thiotepa, tobramycin, tolazoline, vit B complex with C

Y-site incompatibilities: Amsacrine, bleomycin, DOXOrubicin, droperidol, esmolol, fluconazole, gentamicin, idarubicin, metoclopramide, milrinone, netilmicin, ondansetron, quinidine, vinBLAStine, vinCRIStine

Additive compatibilities: Amikacin, aminophylline, ampicillin, atropine, bumetanide, calcium gluconate, cefamandole, cefoperazone, cefuroxime, cimetidine, cloxacillin, dexamethasone, diamorphine, digoxin, epinephrine, heparin, isosorbide, kanamycin, lidocaine, meropenem, morphine, nitroglycerin, penicillin G, potassium chloride, ranitidine, scopolamine, sodium bicarbonate, theophylline, tobramycin, verapamil

Additive incompatibilities: Bleomycin, DOBUTamine, gentamicin, chlorproMAZINE, diazepam, erythromycin, isoproterenol, meperidine, metoclopramide, netilmicin, opium alkaloids, prochlorperazine, tetracycline

Patient/family education

• Teach patient to take the medication early in the day to prevent nocturia

• Instruct the patient to take with food or milk if GI symptoms of nausea and anorexia occur

• Teach patient to maintain a record of weight on a weekly basis and notify physician of weight loss of >5 lb

• Caution the patient that this product causes a loss of potassium, that food rich in potassium should be added to the diet; refer to a dietitian for assistance in planning

• Caution the patient to rise slowly from sitting or reclining positions, not to exercise in hot weather or stand for prolonged periods of time because orthostatic hypotension will be enhanced; lie down if dizziness occurs

• Advise patient to wear protective clothing and sunscreen to prevent photosensitivity

• Teach patient not to use alcohol or any OTC medications without physician's approval; serious product reactions may occur

• Emphasize the need to contact physician immediately if muscle cramps, weakness, nausea, dizziness, or numbness occurs

• Teach patient to take and record own B/P and pulse

• Teach patient to continue taking medication even if feeling better; this product controls symptoms but does not cure the condition

• Advise the patient with hypertension to continue other medical treatment (exercise, weight loss, relaxation techniques, cessation of smoking)

Evaluation

Positive therapeutic outcome

• Decreased edema
• Decreased B/P
• Lowered calcium level in malignancy
• Increased diuresis

gabapentin (Rx)
(gab'a-pen-tin)
Neurontin
Func. class.: Anticonvulsant
Pregnancy category C

Do not confuse:
Neurontin/Noroxin/Neoral

Action: Mechanism unknown; may increase seizure threshold; structurally similar to GABA; gabapentin binding sites in neocortex, hippocampus

Therapeutic outcome: Decreased seizure activity

Uses: Adjunct treatment of partial seizures, with or without generalization in patients >12 yr; adjunct in partial seizures in children 3-12 yr, postherpetic neuralgia

Unlabeled uses: Tremors in multiple sclerosis, neuropathic pain, bipolar disorder, migraine prophylaxis, diabetic neuropathy

Dosage and routes
Adult and child >12 yr: PO 900-1800 mg/day in 3 divided doses; may titrate by giving 300 mg on the first day, 300 mg bid on second day, 300 mg tid on third day; may increase to 1800 mg/day by adding 300 mg on subsequent days
Child 5-12 yr: PO 10-15 mg/kg/day in 3 divided doses, initially titrate dose upward over approximately 3 days; 25-35 mg/kg/day; all given in 3 divided doses
Child 3-4 yr: PO 10-15 mg/kg/day in 3 divided doses, initially titrate dose upward over approximately 3 days, 40 mg/kg/day; all given in 3 divided doses

Postherpetic neuralgia
Adult: PO 300 mg on day 1, 600 mg/day divided bid on day 2, 900 mg/day divided tid, may titrate to 1800-3600 mg divided tid if needed

Renal dose
Adult and child >12 yr: CCr 30-60 ml/min 400-1400 mg divided; CCr 15-30 ml/min 200-700 mg/day; CCr <15 ml/min 100-300 mg/day

Available forms: Caps 100, 300, 400 mg; tabs 600, 800 mg; oral sol 250 mg/5 ml

Adverse effects
CNS: Drowsiness, confusion, dizziness, fatigue, anxiety, somnolence, ataxia, amnesia, abnormal thinking, unsteady gait, depression; 3-12 yr old, emotional lability, aggression, thought disorder, hyperkinesia, hostility, **seizures, suicidal ideation**
CV: Vasodilatation, peripheral edema, hypotension
EENT: Dry mouth, blurred vision, diplopia, nystagmus
GI: Constipation, increased appetite, dental abnormalities, nausea, vomiting
GU: Impotence, bleeding, *UTI*
HEMA: **Leukopenia,** decreased WBC
INTEG: Pruritus, abrasion, **Stevens-Johnson syndrome**
MS: Myalgia
RESP: Rhinitis, pharyngitis, coughing

Contraindications: Hypersensitivity to this product

Precautions: Pregnancy **C**, breastfeeding, children <12 yr, geriatric, renal disease, hemodialysis

Pharmacokinetics
Absorption	Unknown
Distribution	Unknown
Metabolism	None
Excretion	Urine unchanged
Half-life	5-7 hr, 130 hr in ESRD

Pharmacodynamics
Unknown

Interactions
Individual drugs
Alcohol: increased CNS depression
Ketorolac, sevelamer: decreased gabapentin levels
Drug classifications
Antacids: decreased gabapentin levels
Antihistamines, sedatives, all other CNS depressants: increased CNS depression
Drug/herb
Chamomille, hops, kava, skullcap, valerian: increased CNS depression
Drug/lab test
False positive: urinary protein using Ames N-multistix SG

NURSING CONSIDERATIONS
Assessment
- Assess seizures: aura, location, duration, activity at onset
- Assess renal studies: urinalysis, BUN, urine creatinine q3mo
- Assess mental status: mood, sensorium, affect, behavioral changes, suicidal thoughts/behaviors; if mental status changes, notify prescriber
- Assess eye problems, need for ophth exam before, during, after treatment (slit lamp, fundoscopy, tonometry)

Nursing diagnoses
- Knowledge, deficient (teaching)
- Noncompliance (teaching)

Implementation
- Do not break, crush, or chew caps
- Give at least 2 hr after meals with antacids; give without regard to meals
- Store at room temperature away from heat and light
- Provide assistance with ambulation during early part of treatment; dizziness occurs
- Provide seizure precautions: padded side rails, move objects that may harm patient

Patient/family education

- Advise patient to carry/wear emergency ID stating patient's name, products taken, condition, prescriber's name and phone number
- Teach patient to avoid driving, other activities that require alertness
- Teach patient not to discontinue medication quickly after long-term use, withdrawal-precipitated seizures may occur, not to double dose; if dose is missed, take if 2 hr or more before next dose
- Teach patient to gradually withdraw over 7 days; abrupt withdrawal may precipitate seizures
- Teach patient to use hard candy, gum, and frequent rinsing of mouth for dry mouth
- Teach patient to increase fluids, bulk in diet for constipation
- Advise patient to notify prescriber if pregnancy is planned or suspected, avoid breastfeeding

Evaluation

Positive therapeutic outcome

- Decreased seizure activity; document on patient's chart

Treatment of overdose: Lavage, VS

galantamine (Rx)

(gah-lan'tah-meen)
Razadyne, Razadyne ER
Func. class.: Anti-Alzheimer's agent, cholinesterase inhibitor

Pregnancy category B

Action: Enhances cholinergic functioning by increasing acetylcholine

Therapeutic outcome: Decreased signs and symptoms of Alzheimer's dementia

Uses: Mild to moderate dementia of Alzheimer's disease, vascular dementia

Dosage and routes

Adult: PO 4 mg bid with morning and evening meals; after 4 wk or more may increase to 8 mg bid; after another 4 wk may increase to 12 mg bid; usual dose 16-24 mg/day in 2 divided doses; EXT REL 8 mg/day in AM; may increase to 16 mg/day after 4 wk, and 24 mg/day after another 4 wk

Hepatic dose
Adult: (Child-Pugh 7-9) PO max 16 mg/day
Adult: (Child-Pugh 10-15) PO avoid use

Renal dose
Adult: PO CCr 10-70 ml/min; max 16 mg/day

CCr <9 ml/min: PO avoid use

Available forms: Tabs 4, 8, 12 mg; ext rel tabs 8, 16, 24 mg; oral sol 4 mg/ml

Adverse effects

CNS: Tremors, insomnia, depression, dizziness, headache, somnolence, fatigue
CV: Bradycardia, chest pain
GI: Nausea, vomiting, anorexia, abdominal distress, flatulence, diarrhea
GU: Urinary incontinence, bladder outflow obstruction, hematuria
HEMA: Anemia
META: Weight decrease
MS: Asthenia
RESP: URI, rhinitis

Contraindications: Hypersensitivity to this product, breastfeeding, children, GI bleeding, jaundice, renal failure, renal/hepatic/cardiac disease

Precautions: Pregnancy **B,** respiratory disease, seizure disorder, peptic ulcer, asthma, bradycardia, heart block, geriatric patients, surgery, urinary tract obstruction

Pharmacokinetics

Absorption	Rapidly and completely absorbed
Distribution	18% protein binding
Metabolism	P450 enzyme
Excretion	Kidneys; clearance decreased in geriatric, hepatic disease, females (20% lower)
Half-life	Elimination 7 hr

Pharmacodynamics

Unknown

Interactions

Individual drugs
Amitriptyline, cimetidine, erythromycin, fluvoxamine, ketoconazole, paroxetine, quinidine: increased galantamine bioavailability

Drug classifications
Cholinesterase inhibitors, cholinomimetics: synergistic effect
CYP3A4 inducers (bosentan, carbamazepine, fosphenytoin, nevirapine, oxcarbazepine, phenytoin, rifabutin, rifampin, rifapentine, troglitazone): decreased galantamine effect
CYP3A4 inhibitors (antiretroviral protease inhibitors, clarithromycin, conivaptan, delavirdine, diltiazem, efavirenz, erythromycin, fluconazole, fluvoxamine, imatinib, itraconazole, ketoconazole, nefazodone, nicardipine, troleandomycin, verapamil,

voriconazole, zafirlukast): increased galan-
tamine effect
NSAIDs: increased GI effects
Drug/herb
Jimsonweed, scopolia: cholinergic antagonism
Pill-bearing spurge: increased effect

NURSING CONSIDERATIONS
Assessment
• Assess liver function enzymes: AST, ALT,
alkaline phosphatase, LDH, bilirubin, CBC
• Assess for severe GI effects: nausea, vomiting, anorexia, weight loss
• Assess B/P, heart rate, respiration during
initial treatment
• Assess mental status: affect, mood, behavioral changes, depression

Nursing diagnoses
• Knowledge, deficient (teaching)
• Thought processes, disturbed

Implementation
• Give with meals, morning and evening, ext
rel product can be opened and sprinkled on
food; do not crush/chew
• Dose increase after minimum of 4 wk at
prior dose; if dose is interrupted for several
days, restart at lower dose, titrate to current
dose
• Provide assistance with ambulation during
beginning therapy
• Perform complete suicide assessment

Patient/family education
• Teach patient or caregiver correct procedure for giving oral sol, using instruction sheet
provided
• Instruct patient or caregiver to notify prescriber of severe GI effects
• Instruct patient or caregiver to report
hypo/hypertension, slow heart rate

Evaluation
Positive therapeutic outcome
• Decreased symptoms of dementia
• Increased coherence
• Improved cognitive performance (memory,
orientation, attention, reasoning, language,
praxis)

Treatment of overdose: Administer
IV atropine titrated to effect at an initial dose
of 0.5-1 mg, with subsequent doses based on
clinical response; provide general supportive
measures

ganciclovir (Rx)
(gan-sye'kloe-vir)
Cytovene, Vitrasert
Func. class.: Antiviral
Chem. class.: Synthetic nucleoside analog

Pregnancy category C

Do not confuse:
Cytovene/Cytosar

Action: Inhibits replication of herpes viruses
in vitro; competitively inhibits human cytomegalovirus (CMV) DNA polymerase and is incorporated, resulting in termination of DNA
elongation

Therapeutic outcome: Decreased
proliferation of virus responsible for CMV
retinitis

Uses: CMV retinitis in immunocompromised
persons, including those with AIDS, after
indirect ophthalmoscopy confirms diagnosis;
prophylaxis of CMV in transplantation

Unlabeled uses: CMV pneumonia in
organ transplant patients, CMV gastroenteritis
in patients with irritable bowel syndrome, CMV
pneumonitis

Dosage and routes
Induction treatment
Adult: IV 5 mg/kg/dose given over 1 hr
q12hr × 2-3 wk

Maintenance treatment
Adult: IV INF 5 mg/kg/day given over 1 hr,
daily × 7 days/wk; or 6 mg/kg/day × 5 days/
wk; PO 1000 mg tid with food or 500 mg q3hr
while awake; Intravitreal 4.5-mg implant

Prevention of CMV infection
Adult: IV 5 mg/kg/dose over 1 hr q12hr ×
1-2 wk, then 5 mg/kg/day × 7 days/wk, then 6
mg/kg/day × 5 days/wk; PO 1000 mg tid,
starting 10 days post-transplant × 14 wks

Renal dose
CCr <70 ml/min reduce dose

Available forms: Powder for inj 500
mg/vial, caps 250, 500 mg; implant, intravitreal 4.5 mg

Adverse effects
CNS: *Fever,* chills, **coma,** *confusion,* abnormal thoughts, dizziness, bizarre dreams,
headache, psychosis, tremors, somnolence,
paresthesia, weakness, **seizures,** peripheral
neuropathy
CV: Dysrhythmia, hypo/hypertension
EENT: Retinal detachment in CMV retinitis,
cataracts, ocular hypertension, ocular pain,
conjunctival scarring

Adverse effects: *italic* = common, **bold** = life-threatening

GI: *Abnormal liver function tests, nausea, vomiting, anorexia, diarrhea, abdominal pain,* **hemorrhage, perforation, pancreatitis**
GU: **Hematuria,** *increased creatinine,* BUN
HEMA: **Granulocytopenia, thrombocytopenia, irreversible neutropenia, anemia, eosinophilia, pancytopenia**
INTEG: *Rash,* alopecia, *pruritus,* urticaria, pain at inj site, phlebitis, **Stevens-Johnson syndrome**
RESP: Dyspnea

Contraindications: Hypersensitivity to acyclovir, famciclovir, penciclovir, valacyclovir, valganciclovir, or ganciclovir

Black Box Warning: ANC <500/mm³, platelet count <25,000/mm³ (intravitreal)

Precautions: Pregnancy **C,** breastfeeding, children <6 mo, geriatric, preexisting cytopenias, renal function impairment, radiation therapy

Black Box Warning: Secondary malignancy, bone marrow suppression, anemia, infertility, neutropenia

Pharmacokinetics

Absorption	Completely absorbed, increased bioavailability with fatty foods
Distribution	Crosses blood-brain barrier, CSF
Metabolism	Not metabolized
Excretion	Kidneys (90%) unchanged, breast milk
Half-life	3 hr

Pharmacodynamics
Unknown

Interactions
Individual drugs
Adriamycin, amphotericin B, cycloSPORINE, dapsone, DOXOrubicin, flucytosine, mycophenolate, pentamidine, probenecid, trimethoprim/sulfa combinations, vinBLAStine, vinCRIStine: increased ganciclovir toxicity
Didanosine: decreased effect
Imipenem with cilastatin: increased chance of seizures
Probenecid: decreased renal clearance of ganciclovir
Radiation, zidovudine: severe granulocytopenia; do not give together
Tenofovir: increased effect

Drug classifications
Antineoplastics: severe granulocytopenia; do not give together
Nucleoside analogs: increased toxicity

NURSING CONSIDERATIONS
Assessment
• Culture should be done before treatment with ganciclovir is initiated; cultures of blood, urine, and throat may all be taken; CMV is not confirmed by this method; the diagnosis is made by an ophthalmic exam
• Assess kidney, liver function; increases in hemopoietic studies: BUN, serum creatinine, AST creatinine clearance, ALT, A-G ratio, baseline, and drip treatment; blood counts should be done q2wk; watch for decreasing granulocytes, Hgb; if low, therapy may have to be discontinued and restarted after hematologic recovery; blood transfusions may be required
• Assess for GI symptoms: severe nausea, vomiting, diarrhea; severe symptoms may necessitate discontinuing product
• Monitor electrolytes and minerals: calcium, phosphorus, magnesium, sodium, potassium; watch closely for tetany during 1st administration
• Assess for symptoms of blood dyscrasias (anemia, granulocytopenia): bruising, fatigue, bleeding, poor healing
• Assess for symptoms of allergic reactions: flushing, rash, urticaria, pruritus
• Monitor for leukopenia/neutropenia/thrombocytopenia: WBCs, platelets q2day during 2 ×/day dosing and qwk thereafter; check for leukopenia with daily WBC count in patients with prior leukopenia with other nucleoside analogs or for whom leukopenia counts are <1000 cells/mm³ at start of treatment
• Monitor serum creatinine or creatinine clearance at least q2wk
• Assess for seizures, dysrhythmias

Nursing diagnoses
• Infection, risk for (uses)
• Injury, risk for (uses, adverse reactions)
• Knowledge, deficient (teaching)

Implementation
PO route
• Give with food
IV route
• Medicine should be mixed under strict aseptic conditions using gloves, gown, and mask, and using precautions for antineoplastics

 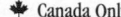

Intermittent IV inf route
• Administer **IV** after diluting 500 mg/10 ml of sterile water for inj (50 mg/ml); shake; further dilute in 100 ml of D₅W, 0.9% NaCl, LR, Ringer's and run over 1 hr; use inf pump, in-line filter
• Give slowly; do not give by BOL **IV**, IM, SUBCUT inj
• Use reconstituted sol within 12 hr, do not refrigerate or freeze; inf sol is stable for 14 days when refrigerated; do not use sol with particulate matter or discoloration, fludarabine, sargramostim
Y-site compatibilities: Allopurinol, cisplatin, cyclophosphamide, enalaprilat, etoposide, filgrastim, fluconazole, gatifloxacin, granisetron, linezolid, melphalan, methotrexate, paclitaxel, propofol, tacrolimus, teniposide, thiotepa
Y-site incompatibilities: Amsacrine, fludarabine, foscarnet, ondansetron, sargramostim, vinorelbine

Patient/family education
• Advise patient to notify prescriber if sore throat, swollen lymph nodes, malaise, fever occur; may indicate other infections
• Advise patient to report perioral tingling, numbness in extremities, and paresthesias
• Caution patient that serious product interactions may occur if OTC products are ingested; check first with prescriber
• Inform patient that product is not a cure, but will control symptoms
• Advise patient that regular blood tests, ophth exams must be continued
• Inform patient that major toxicities may necessitate discontinuing product
• Instruct patient to use contraception during treatment and that infertility may occur; men should use barrier contraception for 90 days after treatment
• Teach patient to take PO with food
• Teach patient to report infection: fever, chills, sore throat; blood dyscrasias: bruising, bleeding, petechiae
• Tell patient to avoid crowds, persons with respiratory infection
• Advise patient to use sunscreen to prevent burns

Evaluation
Positive therapeutic outcome
• Decreased symptoms of CMV infection

ganciclovir ophthalmic
See Appendix B

ganirelix (Rx)
(gan-i-rell'-ex)
Orgalutran ✦
Func. class.: Gonadotropin-releasing hormone antagonist
Chem. class.: Synthetic decapeptide
Pregnancy category X

Action: Inhibitor of pituitary gonadotropin secretion; initially increases LH and FSH, induces a rapid suppression of gonadotropin secretion

Therapeutic outcome: Pregnancy

Uses: For inhibition of premature LH surges in women undergoing controlled ovarian hyperstimulation

Dosage and routes
Adult: SUBCUT 250 mcg/day during early to midfollicular phase; continue until day of hCG administration

Available forms: Inj 250 mcg/0.5 ml

Adverse effects:
CNS: Headache
ENDO: Ovarian hyperstimulation syndrome, abdominal pain (gynecologic)
GI: Nausea
GU: Spotting, breakthrough bleeding, decreased urine, **fetal death**
INTEG: Pain on inj
SYST: **Fetal death**

Contraindications: Pregnancy **X**, breastfeeding, hypersensitivity, latex allergy

Pharmacokinetics
Absorption	Unknown
Distribution	Unknown
Metabolism	To metabolites
Excretion	Unknown
Half-life	13-16 hr

Pharmacodynamics
Onset	Unknown
Peak	Unknown
Duration	Treatment length

NURSING CONSIDERATIONS
Assessment
• Monitor reproductive tests: serum progesterone, LH, estradiol, ovarian ultrasound, pelvic exam, baseline, during treatment

G

- Assess for suspected pregnancy; product should not be used
- Assess for latex allergy; product should not be used

Nursing diagnoses
- Knowledge, deficient (teaching)
- Sexual dysfunction (uses)

Implementation
- Administer SUBCUT using abdomen, around navel, or upper thigh, swab inj area with disinfectant, clean a 2-in circle and allow to dry, pinch up area between thumb and finger, insert needle at 45-90 degrees to surface; if positioned correctly, no blood will be drawn back into syringe; if blood is drawn into syringe, reposition needle without removing it, inject slowly
- Protect from light

Patient/family education
- Teach patient to report abdominal pain, vaginal bleeding

Evaluation
Positive therapeutic outcome
- Pregnancy

---

gatifloxacin ophthalmic
See Appendix B

---

gefitinib (Rx)
(ge-fi′tye-nib)
Iressa
Func. class.: Antineoplastic—miscellaneous
Chem. class.: Epidermal growth factor receptor inhibitor

Pregnancy category D

Action: Not fully understood; inhibits intracellular phosphorylation of cell surface receptors associated with epidermal growth factor receptors

Therapeutic outcome: Decreased growth and spread of malignant cells

Uses: Advanced/metastatic non–small cell lung cancer (NSCLC) in those who have not responded to platinum or docetaxel products

Dosage and routes
Adult: PO 250 mg/day
CYP3A4 inducers concurrently (such as rifampin or phenytoin)
Adult: PO 500 mg/day

Available forms: Tabs 250 mg

Adverse effects
EENT: Amblyopia, conjunctivitis, eye pain, corneal erosion/ulcer
GI: Nausea, diarrhea, vomiting, anorexia, **pancreatitis,** mouth ulceration, **hepatotoxicity**
INTEG: Rash, pruritus, acne, dry skin, **toxic epidermal neurolysis, angioedema**
MISC: Peripheral edema, hemorrhage
RESP: **Interstitial lung disease,** cough, dyspnea, pneumonia

Contraindications: Pregnancy **D**, breastfeeding, children, hypersensitivity

Precautions: Renal/hepatic/ocular/pulmonary disorders, geriatric

Pharmacokinetics
Absorption	Slowly
Distribution	Unknown
Metabolism	Unknown
Excretion	In feces (86%), urine (<4%)
Half-life	Unknown

Pharmacodynamics
Onset	Unknown
Peak	3-7 hr
Duration	Unknown

Interactions
Individual drugs
Cimetidine, phenytoin, ranitidine, rifampin, sodium bicarbonate: decreased levels
Clarithromycin, erythromycin, itraconazole, ketoconazole: increased concentration
Clozapine: increased bone marrow suppression
Metoprolol, warfarin: increased plasma concentration
Drug/herb
St. John's wort: decreased gefitinib levels

NURSING CONSIDERATIONS
Assessment
◆ Assess pulmonary changes: lung sounds, cough, dyspnea; interstitial lung disease may occur, may be fatal; discontinue therapy if confirmed
- Assess ocular changes: eye irritation, corneal erosion/ulcer, aberrant eyelash growth
◆ Assess for pancreatitis: abdominal pain, levels of amylase, lipase
◆ Assess for toxic epidermal necrosis, angioedema
- Monitor GI symptoms: frequency of stools; if diarrhea is poorly tolerated, therapy may be discontinued for up to 14 days

Nursing diagnoses
- Body image, disturbed (adverse reactions)
- Infection, risk for (adverse reactions)
- Injury, risk for (adverse reactions)
- Knowledge, deficient (teaching)

Implementation
- Give without regard to food

Patient/family education
- Teach to report adverse reactions immediately: SOB, severe abdominal pain, occular changes, skin eruptions
- Advise of reason for treatment, expected results
- Advise to use contraception during treatment

Evaluation
Positive therapeutic outcome
- Decreased non–small cell lung cancer cells

---

gemcitabine (Rx)
(gem-sit′a-been)
Gemzar
Func. class.: Antineoplastic—miscellaneous
Chem. class.: Nucleoside analog
Pregnancy category D

Do not confuse:
Gemzar/**Zinecard**

Action: Exhibits antitumor activity by killing cells undergoing DNA synthesis (S phase) and blocking G_1/S-phase boundary

Therapeutic outcome: Prevention of growth of tumor

Uses: Adenocarcinoma of the pancreas (nonresectable stage II, III, or metastatic stage IV); in combination with cisplatin for inoperable, advanced, or metastatic non–small cell lung cancer; advanced breast cancer in combination with paclitaxel; with carboplatin for ovarian cancer, biliary tract cancer

Dosage and routes
Pancreatic carcinoma (nonresectable stage II, III, IV)
Adult: **IV** 1000 mg/m^2 given over ½ hr qwk × 7 wk, then 1 wk rest period; subsequent cycles should be infused once qwk × 3 wk out of every 4 wk

Non–small cell lung cancer
4 wk schedule
Adult: **IV** 1000 mg/m^2 given over ½ hr on days 1, 8, 15 of each 28-day cycle; give cisplatin **IV** 100 mg/m^2 on day 1 after gemcitabine

3 wk schedule
Adult: **IV** 1250 mg/m^2 given over ½ hr on days 1, 8 of each 21-day cycle; give cisplatin 100 mg/m^2 after the INF of gemcitabine on day 1

Advanced breast cancer
Adult: **IV** 1250 mg/m^2 over ½ hr on days 1 and 8 of a 21-day cycle; give paclitaxel on day 1, 175 mg/m^2 over 3 hr prior to gemcitabine

Available forms: Lyophilized powder for inj 20 mg/ml

Adverse effects
GI: Diarrhea, nausea, vomiting, anorexia, constipation, stomatitis
GU: Proteinuria, hematuria
HEMA: Leukopenia, anemia, neutropenia, thrombocytopenia
INTEG: Irritation at site, rash, alopecia
MISC: Dyspnea, fever, **hemorrhage,** infection, flulike syndrome, paresthesia, peripheral edema

Contraindications: Pregnancy **D**, breastfeeding, hypersensitivity

Precautions: Children, geriatric, myelosuppression, irradiation, renal/hepatic disease

Pharmacokinetics	
Absorption	Unknown
Distribution	Crosses placenta
Metabolism	Unknown
Excretion	Unknown
Half-life	42-379 min

Pharmacodynamics
Unknown

Interactions
Individual drug
Alcohol: increased bleeding
Drug classifications
Anticoagulants, NSAIDs, salicylates: increased bleeding
Antineoplastics, radiation: increased myelosuppression, diarrhea
Live virus vaccines: decreased antibody response
Drug/lab test
Increased: BUN, AST, ALT, alkaline phosphatase, bilirubin, creatinine

NURSING CONSIDERATIONS
Assessment
- Monitor CBC, differential, platelet count before each dose; absolute granulocyte count >1000/mm^3, platelets >100,000/mm^3, give complete dose; absolute granulocyte count

G

Adverse effects: *italic* = common, **bold** = life-threatening

500-1000/mm^3, platelets 50,000-100,000/mm^3, give 75%; absolute granulocyte count <500/mm^3, platelets <50,000/mm^3, do not give
- Assess for blood dyscrasias: bruising, bleeding, petechiae
- Monitor I&O, nutritional intake
- Monitor renal/hepatic studies before, during treatment; may increase AST, ALT, alkaline phosphatase, bilirubin, BUN, creatinine
- Assess food preferences: list likes, dislikes
- Assess buccal cavity for dryness, sores or ulceration, white patches, oral pain, bleeding, dysphagia
- Assess GI symptoms: frequency of stools; cramping
- Assess signs of dehydration: rapid respirations, poor skin turgor, decreased urine output, dry skin, restlessness, weakness

Nursing diagnoses
- Infection, risk for (adverse reactions)
- Nutrition: less than body requirements, imbalanced (adverse reaction)

Implementation
- Give increased fluid intake to 2-3 L/day to prevent dehydration, unless contraindicated
- Provide antiemetic agents before and after treatment

IV route
- Prepare in biologic cabinet using gown, mask, gloves
- After reconstituting with 0.9% NaCl 5 ml/200 mg vial of product or 25 ml/1 g of product, shake (40 mg/ml); may be further diluted with 0.9% NaCl to concentrate as low as 0.1 mg/ml; discard unused portion, give over ½ hr, do not admix

Patient/family education
- Teach patient to rinse mouth tid-qid with water, club soda; brush teeth bid-tid with soft brush or cotton-tipped applicator for stomatitis; use unwaxed dental floss
- Advise patient to avoid foods with citric acid or hot or rough texture if stomatitis is present; to drink adequate fluids
- Advise patient to report stomatitis; any bleeding, white spots, ulcerations in mouth; tell patient to examine mouth daily, report symptoms
- Advise patient to report signs of anemia: fatigue, headache, faintness, shortness of breath, irritability; hematuria, dysuria
- Advise patient to use contraception during therapy and for 4 mo after
- Instruct patient to avoid use with NSAIDs, salicylates, alcohol; not to receive vaccinations during treatment

- Teach about possible hair loss and what can be done
- Advise to report flu-like symptoms, swelling of feet/legs, bruising; bleeding of gums, blood in urine, stools, emesis
- Teach to avoid crowds, persons with known upper respiratory infections
- Advise to use soft bristle toothbrush, electric razor

Evaluation
Positive therapeutic outcome
- Decrease in tumor size, decrease in spread of cancer, symptom relief

Treatment of overdose:
Induce vomiting, provide supportive care

---

gemfibrozil (Rx)
(gem-fye′broe-zil)
gemfibrozil, Lopid
Func. class.: Antilipemic
Chem. class.: Fibric acid derivative

Pregnancy category C

Do not confuse:
Lopid/Levbid/Slo-bid

Action: Inhibits biosynthesis of VLDL, decreases triglycerides, increases HDLs

Therapeutic outcome: Decreased hepatic triglyceride production, VLDL; accelerates removal of cholesterol from liver

Uses: Type IIb, IV, V hyperlipidemia as adjunct with diet therapy

Dosage and routes
Adult: PO 1200 mg in divided doses bid 30 min before meals

Available forms: Tabs 600 mg; caps 300 mg ❦

Adverse effects
CNS: Fatigue, vertigo, headache, paresthesia, dizziness, somnolence
GI: Nausea, vomiting, *dyspepsia, diarrhea, abdominal pain*
HEMA: **Leukopenia, anemia, eosinophilia, thrombocytopenia**
INTEG: Rash, urticaria, pruritus
MISC: Task perversion

Contraindications: Severe renal/hepatic disease, preexisting gallbladder disease, primary biliary cirrhosis, hypersensitivity

Precautions: Pregnancy C, breastfeeding, monitor hematologic and hepatic function

 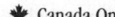

Pharmacokinetics

Absorption	Well absorbed
Distribution	Unknown, plasma protein binding >90%
Metabolism	Liver—minimal
Excretion	Kidney—unchanged (70%), feces (6%)
Half-life	1½ hr

Pharmacodynamics

Onset	1-2 hr
Peak	1-2 hr
Duration	2-4 months

Interactions
Individual drugs
CycloSPORINE: decreased cycloSPORINE effect
Drug classifications
Anticoagulants (oral): increased effect of anticoagulants
HMG-CoA reductase inhibitors: increased risk of myositis, myalgia
Sulfonylureas: increased hypoglycemic effect
Drug/herb
Glucomannan: increased effect
Gotu kola: decreased effect
Drug/lab test
Increased: liver function tests, CPK, BSP, thymol turbidity, glucose
Decreased: Hgb, Hct, WBC

NURSING CONSIDERATIONS
Assessment
- Assess nutrition: fat, protein, carbohydrates; nutritional analysis should be performed by dietitian before treatment is initiated
- Assess renal, liver function tests, CBC, blood glucose if patient is on long-term therapy; if liver function test results increase, product should be discontinued
- Monitor bowel pattern daily; diarrhea may be a problem
- Monitor triglycerides, cholesterol, lipids baseline, during treatment; LDL and VLDL should be watched closely and if increased, product should be discontinued

Nursing diagnoses
- Diarrhea (adverse reactions)
- Knowledge, deficient (teaching)
- Noncompliance (teaching)

Implementation
- Give 30 min before AM and PM meals

Patient/family education
- Inform patient that compliance is needed for positive results to occur; not to double

doses; that product may be discontinued if no improvement in 3 mo
- Caution patient to decrease risk factors: high-fat diet, smoking, alcohol consumption, lack of exercise
- Advise patient to notify prescriber if GI symptoms of diarrhea, abdominal or epigastric pain, nausea, vomiting occur; or if chills, fever, sore throat occur; also occurrence of muscle cramps, abdominal cramps, severe flatulence

Evaluation
Positive therapeutic outcome
- Decreased cholesterol levels, serum triglyceride and improved ratio with HDLs

G

gemifloxacin (Rx)
(gem-ah-flox'a-sin)
Factive
Func. class.: Antiinfective
Chem. class.: Fluoroquinolone

Pregnancy category C

Action: Inhibits DNA gyrase, which is an enzyme involved in replication, transcription, and repair of bacterial DNA

Therapeutic outcome: Negative C&S, decreasing symptoms of infection

Uses: Acute bacterial exacerbation of chronic bronchitis caused by *Streptococcus pneumoniae, Haemophilus influenzae, H. parainfluenzae, Moraxella catarrhalis;* community-acquired pneumonia caused by *Streptococcus pneumoniae* including multiproduct-resistant strains, *H. influenzae, M. catarrhalis, Mycoplasma pneumoniae, Chlamydia pneumoniae, Klebsiella pneumoniae*

Dosage and routes
Adult: PO 320 mg/day × 5-10 days depending on type of infection

Renal dose
Adult: PO CCr ≤40 ml/min 160 mg q24hr

Available forms: Tabs 320 mg

Adverse effects
CNS: *Dizziness, headache,* somnolence, depression, insomnia, nervousness, confusion, agitation, **seizures**
CV: QT prolongation, vasodilatation
EENT: Visual disturbances
GI: Diarrhea, *nausea,* vomiting, anorexia, flatulence, heartburn, dry mouth; increased AST, ALT; constipation, abdominal pain, oral thrush, glossitis, stomatitis, **pseudomembranous colitis**
HEMA: **Thrombocytopenia, neutropenia**

Adverse effects: *italic* = common, **bold** = life-threatening

INTEG: Rash, pruritus, urticaria, *photosensitivity*

SYST: **Anaphylaxis, Stevens-Johnson syndrome**

Contraindications: Hypersensitivity to quinolones

Precautions: Pregnancy C, breastfeeding, children, geriatric, hypokalemia, hypomagnesemia, renal disease, seizure disorders, excessive exposure to sunlight, psychosis, increased intracranial pressure, history of QT interval prolongation, dysrhythmias

Black Box Warning: Tendon pain/rupture, tendinitis

Pharmacokinetics

Absorption	Rapidly, bioavailability 71%
Distribution	Unknown
Metabolism	Unknown
Excretion	In urine as active product, metabolites
Half-life	4-12 hr

Pharmacodynamics

Onset	Unknown
Peak	1-2 hr
Duration	Unknown

Interactions
Individual drugs
Probenecid: may increase toxicity
Drug classifications
Antacids containing aluminum, iron, magnesium, sucralfate, zinc: decreased absorption; give 2 hr before or 3 hr after meals
Antiarrhythmics (amiodarone, disopyramide, procainamide, quinidine, sotalol), antidepressants (tricyclics): may decrease effect, resulting in life-threatening dysrhythmias, QT prolongation
Drugs that increase QT prolongation: increased QT prolongation
Drug/herb
Do not use acidophilus with antiinfectives; separate by several hours

NURSING CONSIDERATIONS
Assessment
• Monitor renal, liver function tests: BUN, creatinine, AST, ALT
• Monitor I&O ratio; urine pH, <5.5 is ideal
• Assess CNS symptoms: insomnia, vertigo, headache, agitation, confusion
◆ Assess allergic reactions and anaphylaxis: rash, flushing, urticaria, pruritus, chills, fever, joint pain; may occur a few days after therapy begins; epinephrine and resuscitation equip-

ment should be available for anaphylactic reaction
• Monitor bowel pattern daily; if severe diarrhea occurs, product should be discontinued
• Assess for overgrowth of infection: perineal itching, fever, malaise, redness, pain, swelling, drainage, rash, diarrhea, change in cough, sputum

Nursing diagnoses
• Infection, risk for (uses)
• Knowledge, deficient (teaching)
• Noncompliance (teaching)

Implementation
• Give with or without food
• Theophylline should not be used with this product; toxicity may result
• Administer 2 hr before or 3 hr after antacids, iron, zinc, or buffered products; 2 hr before sucralfate

Patient/family education
• Advise that fluids must be increased to 2 L/day to avoid crystallization in kidneys
• Instruct that if dizziness or light-headedness occurs, to ambulate, perform activities with assistance
• Instruct to complete full course of product therapy
• Teach to contact prescriber if adverse reactions occur
• Teach to avoid iron- or mineral-containing supplements or aluminum/magnesium antacids within 2 hr before or 3 hr after dosing
• Advise that photosensitivity may occur and sunscreen should be used
• Advise to use frequent rinsing of mouth, sugarless candy or gum for dry mouth
• Teach to avoid other medication unless approved by prescriber

Evaluation
Positive therapeutic outcome
• Negative C&S, absence of signs/symptoms of infection

! HIGH ALERT

gemtuzumab (Rx)
(gem-tue-zue′mab)
Mylotarg
Func. class.: Antineoplastic—miscellaneous
Chem. class.: Monoclonal antibody

Pregnancy category D

Action: Composed of recombinant humanized IgG$_4$ κ antibody, binds to CD33 antigen that is released in myeloid cells

Therapeutic outcome: Decreasing signs/symptoms of leukemia

Uses: Acute myeloid leukemia (AML) in patients with first relapse who are 60 yr or older

Dosage and routes
Adult: **IV** 9 m/m^2 as a 2 hr INF; before giving INF, give diphenhydrAMINE 50 mg PO, acetaminophen 650-1000 mg PO 1 hr; then use acetaminophen 650-1000 mg q4hr for additional 2 doses prn

Available forms: Powder for inj, lyophilized 5 mg

Adverse effects
CNS: Dizziness, insomnia, depression, headache
CV: Hypertension, **hemorrhage,** tachycardia, hypotension
HEMA: **Prolonged neutropenia, thrombocytopenia**
INTEG: Rash, herpes simplex, local reaction, petechiae, pruritus
GI: Anorexia, diarrhea, constipation, nausea, stomatitis, vomiting, **fatal liver toxicity**
GU: Hematuria, **vaginal hemorrhage**
META: Hypokalemia, hypomagnesemia
MISC: Fever, myalgias, headache, chills, peripheral edema
RESP: Cough, pneumonia, epistaxis, rhinitis, dyspnea

Contraindications: Pregnancy **D,** breastfeeding

Black Box Warning: Hypersensitivity to this product or murine protein, severe myelosuppression

Precautions: Children, severe renal disease

Black Box Warning: Hepatic disease, pulmonary disease, infusion-related reactions

Pharmacokinetics
Absorption	Unknown
Distribution	Unknown
Metabolism	Unknown
Excretion	Unknown
Half-life	45, 100 hr, respectively

Pharmacodynamics
Unknown

Interactions
Drug classifications
Antineoplastics, other, radiation: increased bone marrow suppression

NURSING CONSIDERATIONS
Assessment
- Assess for pulmonary symptoms: cough, dyspnea
- Monitor blood studies: BUN, creatinine, AST, ALT, electrolytes, bilirubin, CBC, uric acid
- Assess for symptoms of infection; chills, fever, headache may be masked by product
- Assess CNS reaction: LOC, mental status, dizziness, confusion
- Assess cardiac status: lung sounds; ECG before, during treatment, especially in those with cardiac disease
- Assess bone marrow depression: bruising, bleeding, blood in stools, urine, sputum, emesis

Nursing diagnoses
- Infection, risk for (adverse reactions)
- Nutrition: less than body requirements, imbalanced (adverse reactions)
- Oral mucous membrane, impaired (adverse reactions)

Implementation
- Do not give **IV** push or bolus
- Protect from light, use biologic safety hood, allow to come to room temperature
- Reconstitute each vial with 5 ml of sterile water for inj using sterile syringes, swirl each vial, check for discoloration or particulate matter, give over 2 hr, use a separate line with 1.2-micron terminal filter
- May be premedicated with methylPREDNISolone and antiemetics
- Store reconstituted sol for ≤8 hr in refrigerator

Patient/family education
- Advise patient to take acetaminophen for fever
- Instruct patient to avoid hazardous tasks, since confusion, dizziness may occur; avoid prolonged sunlight, use sunscreen
- Instruct patient to report signs of infection: sore throat, fever, diarrhea, vomiting
- Teach patient to avoid immunizations, crowds, people with known infections
- Teach patient that product is very toxic

Evaluation
Positive therapeutic outcome
- Improvement in blood counts

G

gentamicin (Rx)
(jen-ta-mye'sin)
Cidomycin ✳, G-mycin, Garamycin,
Gentamicin Sulfate, Jenamicin
Func. class.: Antiinfective
Chem. class.: Aminoglycoside

Pregnancy category C

Do not confuse:
Garamycin/kanamycin

Action: Interferes with protein synthesis in bacterial cell by binding to ribosomal subunit, causing misreading of genetic code; inaccurate peptide sequence forms in protein chain, causing bacterial death

Therapeutic outcome: Bactericidal effects for the following organisms: *Pseudomonas aeruginosa, Proteus, Klebsiella, Serratia, Escherichia coli, Enterobacter, Citrobacter, Staphylococcus, Shigella, Salmonella, Acinetobacter, Bacillus anthracis*

Uses: Severe systemic infections of CNS; respiratory, GI, and urinary tracts; bone; skin; soft tissues; acute PID caused by susceptible strains

Dosage and routes
Severe systemic infections
Adult: **IV** INF 3-6 mg/kg/day in 3 divided doses q8hr; dilute in 50-200 ml 0.9% NaCl or D₅W given over 30 min-1 hr; IM 3 mg/kg/day in divided doses q8hr
Child: **IV**/IM 2-2.5 mg/ kg q8hr
Neonate and infant: **IV**/IM 2.5 mg/kg q8-12hr
Neonate <1 wk: 2.5 mg/kg q12-24hr

Renal dose
Adult: IM/**IV** 1-1.7 mg/kg initially, then adjust according to CCr levels

Available forms: Inj 10, 40 mg/ml; premixed inj 40, 60, 70, 80, 100 mg/50 ml; 40, 60, 80, 90, 100, 120, 160, 180 mg/ml

Adverse effects
CNS: Confusion, depression, numbness, tremors, **seizures,** muscle twitching, **neurotoxicity,** dizziness, vertigo
CV: Hypotension, hypertension, palpitations, edema
EENT: Ototoxicity, deafness, visual disturbances, tinnitus
GI: Nausea, vomiting, anorexia, increased ALT, AST, bilirubin, hepatomegaly, **hepatic necrosis,** splenomegaly
GU: Oliguria, hematuria, **renal damage, azotemia, renal failure, nephrotoxicity,** proteinuria

HEMA: **Agranulocytosis, thrombocytopenia, leukopenia, eosinophilia,** anemia
INTEG: Rash, burning, urticaria, dermatitis, alopecia, photosensitivity

Contraindications: Hypersensitivity to this or other aminoglycosides, fungal/viral/mycobacterial infection

Black Box Warning: Severe renal disease

Precautions: Breastfeeding, geriatric, neonates

Black Box Warning: Pregnancy **D,** mild renal disease, hearing deficits, myasthenia gravis, Parkinson's disease

Pharmacokinetics
Absorption	Well absorbed (IM)
Distribution	Distributed in extracellular fluids, poorly distributed in CSF; crosses placenta
Metabolism	Liver, minimal
Excretion	Mostly unchanged (79%) kidneys
Half-life	1-2 hr; infants 6-7 hr; increased in renal disease

Pharmacodynamics
	IM	IV
Onset	Rapid	Rapid
Peak	½-1½ hr	Infusion's end
Duration	Unknown	Unknown

Interactions
Individual drugs
Acyclovir, amphotericin B, cidofovir, cisplatin, ethacrynic acid, furosemide, mannitol, methoxyflurane, polymyxin, vancomycin: increased ototoxicity, neurotoxicity, nephrotoxicity
Drug classifications
Aminoglycosides, cephalosporins, penicillins: increased otoxicity, neurotoxicity, nephrotoxicity
Nondepolarizing neuromuscular blockers: increased neuromuscular blockade, respiratory depression
Drug/herb
Do not use acidophilus with antiinfectives; separate by several hours

NURSING CONSIDERATIONS
Assessment
• Assess patient for previous sensitivity reaction
• Assess patient for signs and symptoms of infection including characteristics of wounds, sputum, urine, stool, WBC >10,000/mm³, fever; obtain baseline, during treatment

 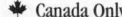

- Complete C&S before beginning product therapy; this will ensure that correct treatment has been initiated
- Assess for allergic reactions: rash, urticaria, pruritus, chills, fever, joint pain may occur a few days after therapy begins
- Identify urine output; if decreasing, notify prescriber (may indicate nephrotoxicity); also, increased BUN, creatinine, urine CCr <80 ml/min
- Monitor blood studies: AST, ALT, CBC, Hct, bilirubin, LDH, alkaline phosphatase, Coombs' test monthly if patient is on long-term therapy
- Monitor electrolytes: potassium, sodium, chloride, magnesium monthly if patient is on long-term therapy
- Monitor for bleeding: ecchymosis, bleeding gums, hematuria; assess stool guaiac daily if on long-term therapy
- Assess for overgrowth of infection: perineal itching, fever, malaise, redness, pain, swelling, drainage, rash, diarrhea, change in cough, sputum
- Obtain weight before treatment; calculation of dosage is usually based on ideal body weight but may be calculated on actual body weight
- Monitor I&O ratio; urinalysis daily for proteinuria, cells, casts; report sudden change in urine output
- Monitor VS during inf, watch for hypotension, change in pulse
- Assess **IV** site for thrombophlebitis including pain, redness, swelling q30min, change site if needed; apply warm compresses to discontinued site
- Obtain serum peak, measured at 30-60 min after **IV** inf or 60 min after IM inj, trough level measured just before next dose; blood level should be 2-4 times bacteriostatic level
- Assess urine pH if product is used for UTI; urine should be kept alkaline
- Assess for deafness by audiometric testing, ringing, roaring in ears, vertigo; assess hearing before, during, after treatment
- Assess for dehydration: high specific gravity, decrease in skin turgor, dry mucous membranes, dark urine

Nursing diagnoses
- Diarrhea (side effects)
- Infection, risk for (uses)
- Injury, risk for (side effects)
- Knowledge, deficient (teaching)
- Noncompliance (teaching)

Implementation
IM route
- Give inj deeply in large muscle mass; rotate sites

Topical route
- Wash hands, wear gloves, clean skin before applying
IV route
- Give in even doses around the clock; product must be given for 10-14 days to ensure organism death and prevent superinfection
- Give by intermittent inf over ½-1 hr, flush with 0.9% NaCl or D_5W after inf
- Separate aminoglycosides and penicillins by ≥1 hr
- Store in tight container

Syringe compatibilities: Clindamycin, methicillin, penicillin G sodium

Y-site compatibilities: Acyclovir, amifostine, amiodarone, amsacrine, atracurium, aztreonam, cefpirome, ciprofloxacin, cyclophosphamide, cytarabine, diltiazem, enalaprilat, esmolol, famotidine, fluconazole, fludarabine, foscarnet, granisetron, hydromorphone, IL-2, insulin, labetalol, lorazepam, magnesium sulfate, melphalan, meperidine, meropenem, midazolam, morphine, multivitamins, ondansetron, paclitaxel, pancuronium, perphenazine, sargramostim, tacrolimus, teniposide, theophylline, thiotepa, tolazine, vecuronium, vinorelbine, vit B with C, zidovudine

Y-site incompatibilities: Idarubicin, indomethacin, zidovudine

Additive compatibilities: Atracurium, aztreonam, bleomycin, cefoxitin, cimetidine, ciprofloxacin, fluconazole, meropenem, methicillin, metronidazole, ofloxacin, penicillin G sodium, ranitidine, verapamil

Patient/family education
- Teach patient to report sore throat, bruising, bleeding, joint pain; may indicate blood dyscrasias (rare)
- Advise patient to contact prescriber if vaginal itching, loose foul-smelling stools, furry tongue occur; may indicate superimposed infection

Evaluation
Positive therapeutic outcome
- Absence of signs/symptoms of infection (WBC <10,000/mm^3, temp WNL, absence of red, draining wounds)
- Reported improvement in symptoms of infection

Treatment of overdose: Withdraw product, hemodialysis

G

Adverse effects: *italic* = common, **bold** = life-threatening

gentamicin ophthalmic
See Appendix B

gentamicin topical
See Appendix B

glatiramer (Rx)
(glah-teer′a-mer)
Copaxone
Func. class.: Multiple sclerosis agent

Pregnancy category B

Action: Unknown; may modify the immune responses responsible for multiple sclerosis (MS)

Therapeutic outcome: Decreased symptoms of MS

Uses: Reduction of the frequency of relapses in patients with relapsing-remitting MS after first clinical episode with MRI results consistent with MS

Dosage and routes
Adult: SUBCUT 20 mg/day

Available forms: Inj premixed 20 mg/ml

Adverse effects
CNS: Anxiety, hypertonia, tremor, vertigo, speech disorder, agitation, confusion
CV: Migraine, palpitations, syncope, tachycardia, vasodilatation, chest pain, hypertension
EENT: Ear pain, blurred vision
GI: Nausea, vomiting, diarrhea, anorexia, gastroenteritis
GU: Urgency, dysmenorrhea, vaginal moniliasis
HEMA: Ecchymosis, lymphadenopathy
INTEG: Pruritus, rash, sweating, urticaria, erythema, injection site reaction
META: Edema, weight gain
MS: Arthralgia, back pain, neck pain, increased muscle tone
RESP: Bronchitis, dyspnea, laryngismus, rhinitis

Contraindications: Hypersensitivity to this product or mannitol

Precautions: Pregnancy **B**, breastfeeding, children <18 yr, immune disorders, renal disease

Pharmacokinetics
Unknown

Pharmacodynamics
Unknown

NURSING CONSIDERATIONS
Assessment
• Monitor blood, renal, liver function tests before treatment
• Assess for CNS symptoms: anxiety, confusion, vertigo
• Assess GI status: diarrhea, vomiting, abdominal pain, gastroenteritis
• Assess cardiac status: tachycardia, palpitations, vasodilatation, chest pain

Nursing diagnoses
• Knowledge, deficient (teaching)
• Noncompliance (teaching)

Implementation
SUBCUT route
• Use a sterile syringe/needle to transfer the supplied diluent into the vial, rotate vial gently, do not shake; withdraw medication using a syringe with 27-G needle; administer SUBCUT into hip, thigh, arm; discard unused portion
• Use SUBCUT route only; do not give IM or **IV**
• Do not use sol that contains precipitate or is discolored

Patient/family education
• Give written, detailed instructions about the product; provide initial and return demonstrations on inj procedure; give information on use and disposal of product
• Advise patient that blurred vision, sweating may occur
• Advise patient that irregular menses, dysmenorrhea, or metorrhagia as well as breast pain may occur; use contraception during treatment
• Advise patient that if pregnancy is suspected or if nursing to notify prescriber
• Advise patient not to change dosing or to stop taking product without advice of prescriber

Evaluation
Positive therapeutic outcome
• Decreased symptoms of multiple sclerosis

glimepiride (Rx)
(gly-meh′pih-ride)
Amaryl
*__glipiZIDE__ (Rx)
(glip-i′zide)
Glucotrol, Glucotrol XL
Func. class.: Antidiabetic
Chem. class.: Sulfonylurea (2nd generation)
Pregnancy category C

Do not confuse:
glipiZIDE/glucotrol/glyBURIDE

Action: Causes functioning β-cells in pancreas to release insulin, leading to drop in blood glucose levels; may improve insulin binding to insulin receptors or increase the number of insulin receptors with prolonged administration; may also reduce basal hepatic glucose secretion; not effective if patient lacks functioning β-cells

Therapeutic outcome: Decrease in polyuria, polydipsia, polyphagia, clear sensorium, absence of dizziness, stable gait

Uses: Type 2 diabetes mellitus

Dosage and routes
Glimepiride
Adult: PO 1-2 mg/day with breakfast, then increase q1-2wk, max 8 mg/day
Geriatric: PO 1 mg/day, may increase if needed

Renal dose
Adult: CCr <20 ml/min; PO 1 mg/day with breakfast, may titrate upward as needed

GlipiZIDE
Adult: PO 5 mg initially before breakfast, then increase to desired response; max 40 mg/day in divided doses or 15 mg/dose; (XL) PO 5 mg/day with breakfast, may increase to 10 mg/day; max 20 mg/day
Geriatric: PO 2.5 mg/day, may increase if needed

Hepatic dose
Adult: PO 2.5 mg initially, then increase to desired response; max 40 mg/day in divided doses or 15 mg/dose

Available forms: Glimepiride: tabs 1, 2, 4 mg; glipiZIDE: tabs 5, 10 mg scored; EXT REL tabs 2.5, 5, 10 mg

Adverse effects
CNS: Headache, weakness, dizziness, drowsiness, tinnitus, fatigue, vertigo
ENDO: Hypoglycemia
GI: Hepatotoxicity, cholestatic jaundice, nausea, vomiting, diarrhea, heartburn

HEMA: Leukopenia, thrombocytopenia, agranulocytosis, aplastic anemia, increased AST, ALT, alkaline phosphatase, pancytopenia, hemolytic anemia
INTEG: Rash, allergic reactions, pruritus, urticaria, eczema, photosensitivity, erythema, allergic vasculitis

Contraindications: Hypersensitivity to sulfonylureas, type 1 diabetes, diabetic ketoacidosis

Precautions: Pregnancy C, geriatric, cardiac disease, severe renal/hepatic disease, G6PD deficiency

Pharmacokinetics

Absorption	Completely absorbed GI tract
Distribution	Unknown
Metabolism	Liver
Excretion	Via kidneys
Half-life	2-4 hr

Pharmacodynamics

Onset	1-1½ hr
Peak	1-3 hr
Duration	10-24 hr

Interactions
Individual drugs
Charcoal, cholestyramine, diazoxide, isoniazid, rifampin: possible decreased action of glipiZIDE
Chloramphenicol, cimetidine, clofibrate, fenfluramine, fluconazole, gemfibrozil, guanethidine, insulin, methyldopa, phenylbutazone, probenecid, sulfinpyrizine: increased hypoglycemia
Digoxin: increased action of digoxin
Drug classifications
Androgens, anticoagulants, H₂-antagonists, magnesium salts, MAOIs, NSAIDs, salicylates, sulfonamides, tricyclics, urinary acidifiers: increased hypoglycemia
β-Blockers: may mask symptoms of hypoglycemia
Diuretics (thiazide), hydantoins, urinary alkalinizers: possible decreased action of glipiZIDE
Glycosides: increased action of glycosides
Drug/herb
Alfalfa, aloe, basil, bay, bilberry, bitter melon, black catechu, buchu, burdock, coriander, dandelion, eyebright (po), garlic, glucomannan, glucosamine, goat's rue, gymnema, horehound, horse chestnut, jambul, myrrh, myrtle: increased antidiabetic effect

Adverse effects: *italic* = common, **bold** = life-threatening

Bee pollen, blue cohosh, broom, chromium, elecampane, eucalyptus, gotu kola: decreased antidiabetic effect

Broom, buchu, dandelion, glucosamine, juniper: decreased hypoglycemic effect

Chromium, coenzyme Q10, fenugreek, ginseng: increased or decreased hypoglycemic effect

Karela: increased glucose tolerance

Drug/lab test
Increase: AST, ALT, LDH, BUN, creatinine

NURSING CONSIDERATIONS
Assessment
• Assess for hypoglycemic/hyperglycemic reactions that can occur soon after meals; hypoglycemic reactions (sweating, weakness, dizziness, anxiety, tremors, hunger); hyperglycemic reactions
• Monitor CBC, A1c (baseline, q3mo) during treatment; check liver function tests periodically: AST, LDH; renal tests: BUN, creatinine during treatment

Nursing diagnoses
• Injury, risk for (adverse reactions)
• Knowledge, deficient (teaching)
• Noncompliance (teaching)
• Nutrition: less than body requirements, imbalanced (adverse reactions)
• Nutrition: more than body requirements, imbalanced (uses)

Implementation
• Do not break, crush, or chew ext rel tabs
• Convert from other oral hypoglycemic agents or insulin dosage of <40 units/day; change may be made without gradual dosage change.
• Patients taking >40 units/day of insulin convert gradually by receiving oral hypoglycemic agents and 50% of previous insulin dosage for 3-5 days
• Monitor serum or urine glucose and ketones 3 ×/day during conversion
• Give product 30 min before breakfast; if large dose is required, may be divided into 2 doses; give with meals to decrease GI upset and provide best absorption; if patient is NPO, may need to hold dose to prevent hypoglycemia
• Give tab crushed and mixed with meal or fluids for patients with difficulty swallowing
• For severe hypoglycemia give **IV** D$_{50}$W, then **IV** dextrose solution
• Store in tight container in cool environment

Patient/family education
• Teach patient to check for symptoms of cholestatic jaundice: dark urine, pruritus, yellow sclera; if these occur, prescriber should be notified
• Teach patient to use capillary blood glucose test
• Teach patient symptoms of hypo/hyperglycemia, what to do about each
• Instruct patient that product must be continued on daily basis; explain consequence of discontinuing product abruptly
• Teach patient to take product in AM to prevent hypoglycemic reactions at night
• Caution patient to avoid OTC medications unless approved by a prescriber
• Teach patient that diabetes is a lifelong illness; that this product is not a cure
• Teach patient to avoid alcohol; inform about disulfiram reaction (nausea, headache, cramps, flushing, hypoglycemia)
• Instruct patient that all food included in diet plan must be eaten to prevent hypoglycemia
• Advise patient to use sunscreen or stay out of the sun to prevent burns
• Advise patient to carry/wear emergency ID and carry a glucagon emergency kit for emergency purposes; also prescriber name, phone number, and medications taken
• Teach patient ext rel tab may appear in stool

Evaluation
Positive therapeutic outcome
• Decrease in polyuria, polydipsia, polyphagia; clear sensorium; absence of dizziness; stable gait
• Improved serum glucose, A1c

---

*glyBURIDE (Rx)
(glye′byoor-ide)
Apo-Glyburide ✦, DiaBeta ✦, Euglucon ✦, Gen-Glybe ✦, Glynase PresTab, Micronase, Novo-Glyburide ✦, Nu-Glyburide ✦
Func. class.: Antidiabetic
Chem. class.: Sulfonylurea (2nd generation)
Pregnancy category C

Do not confuse:
glyBURIDE/Glucotrol/glipiZIDE, DiaBeta/Zebeta

Action: Causes functioning β-cells in pancreas to release insulin, leading to drop in blood glucose levels; may improve insulin binding to insulin receptors and increase number of insulin receptors with prolonged administration; may also reduce basal hepatic glucose secretion; not effective if patient lacks functioning β-cells

Therapeutic outcome: Decrease in polyuria, polydipsia, polyphagia, clear sensorium, absence of dizziness, stable gait

Uses: Type 2 diabetes mellitus

Dosage and routes
DiaBeta/Micronase
Adult: PO 1.25-5 mg initially, then increased to desired response at weekly intervals up to 20 mg/day; may be given as a single or divided dose
Geriatric: PO 1.25 mg initially, then increased to desired response; max 20 mg/day, maintenance 1.25-20 mg/day

Glynase PresTab (micronized)
Adult: PO 1.5-3 mg/day initially, may increase by 1.5 mg/wk, max 12 mg/day
Geriatric: PO 0.75-3 mg/day, may increase by 1.5 mg/wk

Available forms: Tabs (DiaBeta) 1.25, 2.5, 5 mg; tabs micronized (Glynase PresTab) 1.5, 3, 6 mg

Adverse effects
CNS: *Headache, weakness,* paresthesia, tinnitus, fatigue, vertigo
ENDO: **Hypoglycemia**
GI: Nausea, fullness, heartburn, **hepatoxicity, cholestatic jaundice,** vomiting, diarrhea
HEMA: **Leukopenia, thrombocytopenia, agranulocytosis, aplastic anemia,** increased AST, ALT, alkaline phosphatase
INTEG: Rash, allergic reactions, pruritus, urticaria, eczema, photosensitivity, erythema
MS: Joint pains

Contraindications: Hypersensitivity to sulfonylureas, type 1 diabetes, diabetic ketoacidosis, renal failure

Precautions: Pregnancy **C,** geriatric, cardiac/thyroid disease, severe renal/hepatic disease, severe hypoglycemic reactions

Pharmacokinetics
Absorption	Completely absorbed GI tract
Distribution	99% plasma protein binding
Metabolism	Liver
Excretion	Urine, feces (metabolites), crosses placenta
Half-life	10 hr

Pharmacodynamics
Onset	2-4 hr
Peak	4 hr
Duration	24 hr

Interactions
Individual drugs
Charcoal, cholestyramine, isoniazid, rifampin: decreased action of glyBURIDE
Chloramphenicol, fenfluramine, fluconazole, gemfibrozil, guanethidine, insulin, methyldopa, phenylbutazone, probenecid, sulfinpyrazone: increased hypoglycemia
Diazoxide: both products may have action decreased
Digoxin: increased level

Drug classifications
Androgens, anticoagulants, antidepressants (tricyclics), H_2-antagonists, magnesium salts, MAOIs, NSAIDs, salicylates, sulfonamides, urinary acidifiers: increased hypoglycemia
β-Adrenergic blockers: increased masking of symptoms of hypoglycemia
Diuretics (thiazide), hydantoins, urinary alkalinizers: decreased action of glyBURIDE

Drug/herb
Alfalfa, aloe, basil, bay, bilberry, bitter melon, black catechu, buchu, burdock, coriander, dandelion, eyebright (po), garlic, glucomannan, glucosamine, goat's rue, gymnema, horehound, horse chestnut, jambul, myrrh, myrtle: increased antidiabetic effect
Bee pollen, blue cohosh, broom, chromium, elecampane, eucalyptus, gotu kola: decreased antidiabetic effect
Broom, buchu, dandelion, glucosamine, juniper: decreased hypoglycemic effect
Chromium, coenzyme Q10, fenugreek, ginseng: increased or decreased hypoglycemic effect
Karela: increased glucose tolerance

Drug/lab test
Increased: AST, ALT, LDH, BUN, creatinine

NURSING CONSIDERATIONS
Assessment
• Assess for hypo/hyperglycemic reactions that can occur soon after meals; hypoglycemic reactions (sweating, weakness, dizziness, anxiety, tremors, hunger); hyperglycemic reactions
• Monitor CBC, A1c (baseline, q3mo) during treatment; check liver function tests periodically, AST, LDH, and renal studies: BUN, creatinine during treatment

Nursing diagnoses
• Injury, risk for (adverse reactions)
• Knowledge, deficient (teaching)
• Noncompliance (teaching)
• Nutrition: less than body requirements, imbalanced (adverse reactions)

*Adverse effects: *italic* = common, **bold** = life-threatening*

- Nutrition: more than body requirements, imbalanced (uses)

Implementation
- Conversion from other oral hypoglycemic agents or insulin dosage of <40 units/day; change may be made without gradual dosage change
- Patients taking >40 units/day of insulin convert gradually by receiving oral hypoglycemic agents and 50% of previous insulin dosage for 3-5 days
- Monitor serum or urine glucose and ketones 3 ×/day during conversion
- Give product 30 min before breakfast; if large dose is required, may be divided into two; give with meals to decrease GI upset and provide best absorption; if patient is NPO, may need to hold dose to avoid hypoglycemia
- Give tab crushed and mixed with meal or fluids for patients with difficulty swallowing
- For severe hypoglycemia, give **IV** $D_{50}W$, then **IV** dextrose sol
- Store in tight container in cool environment

Patient/family education
- Teach patient to check for symptoms of cholestatic jaundice: dark urine, pruritus, yellow sclera; if these occur, prescriber should be notified
- Teach patient to use capillary blood glucose test
- Teach patient symptoms of hypo/hyperglycemia, what to do about each
- Instruct patient that product must be continued on daily basis; explain consequence of discontinuing product abruptly
- Teach patient to take product in AM to prevent hypoglycemic reactions at night
- Caution patient to avoid OTC medications unless approved by a prescriber
- Teach patient that diabetes is a lifelong illness; that this product is not a cure
- Instruct patient that all food included in diet plan must be eaten to prevent hypoglycemia
- Advise patient to carry/wear emergency ID and carry a glucagon emergency kit for emergency purposes: have sugar packets available; also prescriber name, phone number, and medications
- Advise patient to use sunscreen or stay out of the sun to prevent burns

Evaluation
Positive therapeutic outcome
- Decrease in polyuria, polydipsia, polyphagia; clear sensorium; absence of dizziness; stable gait
- Improved serum glucose, A1c

glycopyrrolate (Rx)
(glye-koe-pye′roe-late)
glycopyrrolate, Robinul, Robinul-Forte
Func. class.: Cholinergic blocker, antispasmodic
Chem. class.: Quaternary ammonium compound

Pregnancy category B

Action: Inhibits action of acetylcholine at receptor sites in autonomic nervous system, which controls secretions, free acids in stomach

Therapeutic outcome: Decreased secretions in the respiratory tract, GI system

Uses: Decreased secretions before surgery, reversal of neuromuscular blockade, peptic ulcer disease, irritable bowel syndrome, bradycardia, drooling

Dosage and routes
Preoperatively
Adult: IM 4.4 mcg/kg ½-1 hr before surgery, max 0.1 mg
Child >2 yr (unlabeled): IM 4 mcg/kg 30-60 min before surgery
Child <2 yr (unlabeled): IM 4-9 mcg/kg

Intraoperative
Adult: IV 0.1 mg; may repeat 2-3 min prn
Child: IM/IV 4 mcg/kg q2-3min prn; max 0.1 mg/dose

Reversal of neuromuscular blockage
Adult and child: IV 200 mcg for each 1 mg of neostigmine or 5 mg IV of pyridostigmine simultaneously

GI disorders
Adult: PO 1-2 mg bid-tid; max 6 mg/day; IM/IV 100-200 mcg tid-qid, titrated to patient response

Antidysrhythmic
Adult: IV 100 mcg, may repeat q2min
Child: IV 4.4 mcg/kg, may repeat q2min, max 100 mcg

Secretion control
Child: PO 40-100 mcg/kg/dose tid-qid; IM/IV 4-10 mcg/kg/dose q3-4hr; max 0.2 mg/dose or 0.8 mg/24hr

Available forms: Tabs 1, 2 mg; inj 200 mcg 0.2 mg/ml

Adverse effects
CNS: Confusion, anxiety, restlessness, irritability, delusions, hallucinations, headache, sedation, depression, incoherence, dizziness, lethargy, flushing, weakness, **seizures**

CV: Palpitations, tachycardia, postural hypotension, paradoxical bradycardia
EENT: Blurred vision, photophobia, dilated pupils, difficulty swallowing, increased intraocular pressure, mydriasis, cycloplegia
GI: *Dryness of mouth, constipation,* nausea, vomiting, abdominal distress, paralytic ileus, altered taste perception
GU: Hesitancy, retention, impotence
INTEG: Urticaria, allergic reactions
MISC: Suppression of breastfeeding, nasal congestion, decreased sweating, **malignant hyperthermia**
SYST: Anaphylaxis

Contraindications: Children <3 yr, hypersensitivity, closed-angle glaucoma, myasthenia gravis, GI/GU obstruction, tachycardia, myocardial ischemia, hepatic disease, ulcerative colitis, toxic megacolon, prostatic hypertrophy

Precautions: Pregnancy **B**, breastfeeding, geriatric, pulmonary/renal disease, CHF, hyperthyroidism, CAD, Down-syndrome, hiatal hernia, hypertension

Pharmacokinetics

Absorption	Well absorbed (PO, SUBCUT, IM)
Distribution	Unknown
Metabolism	Not metabolized
Excretion	Unchanged feces
Half-life	2 hr

Pharmacodynamics

	PO	IM	IV
Onset	Unknown	15-30 min	Immediate
Peak	1 hr	30-45 min	10-15 min
Duration	8-12 hr	2-7 hr	2-7 hr

Interactions
Individual drugs
Alcohol, amantadine: increased anticholinergic effect
Drug classifications
Antacids: decreased absorption of glycopyrrolate
Antidepressants (tricyclic), antihistamines, phenothiazines: increased anticholinergic effect
Antidiarrheals: decreased absorption of glycopyrrolate

NURSING CONSIDERATIONS
Assessment
• Monitor I&O ratio; retention commonly causes decreased urinary output; check for urinary hesitation; palpate bladder if retention occurs

• Monitor ECG for ectopic ventricular beats, PVC, tachycardia
• Monitor for bowel sounds; check for constipation; increase fluids, bulk, exercise if constipation occurs
• Assess mental status: affect, mood, CNS depression, worsening of psychiatric symptoms during early therapy

Nursing diagnoses
• Knowledge, deficient (teaching)

Implementation
PO route
• Give PO with or after meals to prevent GI upset; may give with fluids other than water
IM route
• Give IM inj deeply in large muscle mass
IV route
• Administer **IV** undiluted, give at a rate of 0.2 mg or less over 5-15 min through Y-tube or 3-way stopcock; do not add to **IV** sol
• Administer parenteral dose with patient recumbent to prevent postural hypotension
Syringe compatibilities: Atropine, benzquinamide, chlorproMAZINE, cimetidine, codeine, diphenhydrAMINE, droperidol, droperidol/fentanyl, hydromorphone, hydrOXYzine, levorphanol, lidocaine, meperidine, meperidine/promethazine, midazolam, morphine, nalbuphine, neostigmine, oxymorphone, procaine, prochlorperazine, promazine, promethazine, pyridostigmine, ranitidine, scopolamine, triflupromazine, trimethobenzamide
Y-site compatibilities: Propofol
Solution compatibilities: D$_5$W, 0.9% NaCl, Ringer's D$_5$/0.45% NaCl

Patient/family education
• Caution patient not to operate machinery or engage in hazardous activities if drowsiness, blurred vision occurs
• Advise patient not to take OTC products, cough, cold preparations with alcohol, antihistamines without approval of prescriber
• Teach patient to avoid hot temperature; since sweating is decreased, heat stroke is possible
• Advise patient to notify prescriber of eye pain, blurred vision, light sensitivity
• Caution patient not to discontinue this product abruptly; tapering should be done over 1 wk

Evaluation
Positive therapeutic outcome
• Decreased secretions, bronchial, GI
• Decreased pain in GI disorders
• Reversal of neuromuscular blockade

Adverse effects: *italic* = common, **bold** = life-threatening

golimumab
Simponi
See Appendix A, Selected New Drugs

goserelin (Rx)
(goe'se-rel-lin)
Zoladex
Func. class.: Gonadotropin-releasing hormone, antineoplastic
Chem. class.: Synthetic decapeptide analog of LHRH

Pregnancy category D, X

Action: Inhibitor of pituitary gonadotropin secretion; initially increases LH and FSH, with increases in testosterone, reduction in sex steroid levels (substitute serum testosterone levels)

Therapeutic outcome: Decrease in tumor size and spread of malignant cells

Uses: Advanced prostate cancer Stage B2-C (10.8 mg); endometriosis, advanced breast cancer, endometrial thinning (3.6 mg)

Dosage and routes
Adult: SUBCUT 3.6 mg q4wk (implant) or 10.8 mg q12wk

Endometrial thinning
Adult: SUBCUT 1-2 depot inj; usually 1 depot, surgery performed at 4 wk; if 2 depots, surgery performed 2-4 wk after 2nd depot

Available forms: Depot inj 3.6, 10.8 mg

Adverse effects
CNS: Headaches, **spinal cord compression,** anxiety, depression, dizziness, insomnia, lethargy, hot flashes, emotional lability
CV: **Dysrhythmia, cerebrovascular accident,** hypertension, **MI,** chest pain, CHF
ENDO: Gynecomastia, breast tenderness, hot flashes
GI: Nausea, vomiting, constipation, diarrhea, ulcer
GU: *Spotting, breakthrough bleeding, decreased libido,* renal insufficiency, urinary obstruction, urinary tract infection, impotence
INTEG: Rash, pain on inj, diaphoresis
MS: Osteoneuralgia
RESP: COPD, URI

Contraindications: Pregnancy **D** (breast cancer), **X** (endometriosis), breastfeeding, nondiagnosed vaginal bleeding, children, 10.8 mg dose in women, hypersensitivity to LHRH, LHRH-agonist analogs

Precautions: Spinal cord decompression, renal disease, bone mineral density loss

Pharmacokinetics
Absorption	Well absorbed
Distribution	Unknown
Metabolism	Unknown
Excretion	Unknown
Half-life	4½ hr

Pharmacodynamics
Onset	Unknown
Peak	14-28 days
Duration	Treatment length

Interactions
Drug/lab test
Increased: alkaline phosphatase, estradiol, FSH, LH, testosterone levels
Decreased: testosterone levels, progesterone

NURSING CONSIDERATIONS
Assessment
• Assess for relief of bone pain (back pain), change in motor function
• Monitor I&O ratios, palpate bladder for distention (urinary obstruction) at beginning of treatment; renal insufficiency and obstruction may occur
• Monitor acid phosphatase, PSA baseline and periodically
• Obtain pregnancy test prior to therapy

Nursing diagnoses
• Knowledge, deficient (teaching)
• Sexual dysfunction (uses)

Implementation
• Administer via implant inserted by qualified persons into upper subcutaneous tissue in abdominal wall q28day or q12wk (10.8 mg); do not attempt to remove air bubbles from syringe

Patient/family education
• Caution patient that gynecomastia and postmenopausal symptoms may occur but will decrease after treatment is discontinued; that bone pain may increase, then decrease
• Teach patient to contact prescriber if difficulty urinating, hot flashes occur during treatment
• Advise patient not to breastfeed while taking product; use effective nonhormonal contraception

Evaluation
Positive therapeutic outcome
• More normal levels of PSA, acid phosphatase, alkaline phosphatase; testosterone level of <25 mg/dl

 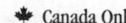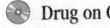

granisetron (Rx)
(grane-iss'e-tron)
Kytril
Func. class.: Antiemetic
Chem. class.: 5-HT₃ receptor antagonist

Pregnancy category B

Action: Prevents nausea, vomiting by blocking serotonin peripherally, centrally, and in the small intestine

Therapeutic outcome: Absence of nausea and vomiting

Uses: Prevention of nausea, vomiting associated with cancer chemotherapy including high-dose cisplatin, radiation

Unlabeled uses: Acute nausea, vomiting after surgery

Dosage and routes
Nausea, vomiting in chemotherapy
Adult and child ≥2 yr: IV 10 mcg/kg over 5 min, 30 min before the start of cancer chemotherapy, TD apply 1 patch (3.1 mg/24 hr) to upper arm 24-48 hr before chemotherapy
Adult: PO 1 mg bid, give 1st dose 1 hr before chemotherapy and next dose 12 hr after 1st

Nausea, vomiting in radiation therapy
Adult: PO 2 mg/day 1 hr prior to radiation

Available forms: Inj 1 mg/ml; tabs 1 mg, oral sol 2 mg/10 ml; patch TD 3.1 mg/24 hr

Adverse effects
CNS: Headache, asthenia, anxiety, dizziness
CV: Hypertension
GI: Diarrhea, *constipation,* increased AST, ALT, *nausea*
HEMA: Leukopenia, anemia, **thrombocytopenia**
MISC: Rash, **bronchospasm**

Contraindications: Hypersensitivity

Precautions: Pregnancy **B**, breastfeeding, children, geriatric, ondansetron hypersensitivity

Pharmacokinetics

Absorption	Unknown
Distribution	Unknown
Metabolism	Liver
Excretion	Unknown
Half-life	10-12 hr

Pharmacodynamics
Unknown

Interactions
Drug classifications
Antipsychotics: increased EPS

NURSING CONSIDERATIONS
Assessment
- Assess patient for absence of nausea, vomiting during chemotherapy
- Assess patient for hypersensitive reaction: rash, bronchospasm

Nursing diagnoses
- Fluid volume, deficient (uses)
- Knowledge, deficient (teaching)

Implementation
- Administer **IV**
- Dilute in 0.9% NaCl for inj or D₅W (20-50 ml), give over 5-15 min
- Store at room temp for 24-hr dilution

Y-site compatibilities: Acyclovir, allopurinol, amifostine, amikacin, aminophylline, amphotericin B cholesteryl, ampicillin, ampicillin/sulbactam, amsacrine, aztreonam, bleomycin, bumetanide, buprenorphine, butorphanol, calcium gluconate, carboplatin, carmustine, cefazolin, cefepime, cefonicid, cefoperazone, cefotaxime, cefotetan, cefoxitin, ceftazidime, ceftizoxime, ceftriaxone, cefuroxime, chlorproMAZINE, cimetidine, ciprofloxacin, cisplatin, cladribine, clindamycin, cyclophosphamide, cytarabine, dacarbazine, dactinomycin, DAUNOrubicin, dexamethasone, diphenhydrAMINE, DOBUTamine, DOPamine, DOXOrubicin, DOXOrubicin liposome, doxycycline, droperidol, enalaprilat, etoposide, famotidine, filgrastim, floxuridine, fluconazole, fluorouracil, fludarabine, furosemide, gallium, ganciclovir, gentamicin, haloperidol, heparin, hydrocortisone, hydromorphone, hydrOXYzine, idarubicin, ifosfamide, imipenem-cilastatin, leucovorin, lorazepam, magnesium sulfate, melphalan, meperidine, mesna, methotrexate, methylPREDNISolone, metoclopramide, metronidazole, mezlocillin, miconazole, minocycline, mitomycin, mitoxantrone, morphine, nalbuphine, netilmicin, ofloxacin, paclitaxel, piperacillin, piperacillin/tazobactam, plicamycin, potassium chloride, prochlorperazine, promethazine, propofol, ranitidine, sargramostim, sodium bicarbonate, streptozocin, teniposide, thiotepa, ticarcillin, ticarcillin/clavulanate, tobramycin, trimethoprim/sulfamethoxazole, vancomycin, vinBLAStine, vinCRIStine, vinorelbine, zidovudine

G

Adverse effects: *italic* = common, **bold** = life-threatening

Y-site incompatibilities: Fluorouracil, furosemide, sodium bicarbonate
Additive compatibilities: Dexamethasone, methylPREDNISolone
Solution compatibilities: D₅W, 0.9% NaCl

Patient/family education
• Advise patient to report diarrhea, constipation, rash, or changes in respirations

Evaluation
Positive therapeutic outcome
• Absence of nausea, vomiting during cancer chemotherapy

---

guaifenesin (Rx, OTC)
(gwye-fen'e-sin)
All Fen Jr., Altarussin, Benylin-E ✦, Diabetic Tussin Expectorant, Ganidin NR, guaifenesin, Guaifenesin NR, Guiatuss, Humibid, Mucinex, Naldecon Senior EX, Organidin NR, Refenesen, Robitussin Chest Congestion, Scot-Tussin Expectorant, Siltussin DAS, Siltussin SA
Func. class.: Expectorant

Pregnancy category C

Action: Increases the volume and reduces the viscosity of secretions in the trachea and bronchi to facilitate secretion removal

Therapeutic outcome: Decreased cough

Uses: Productive and nonproductive cough

Dosage and routes
Adult and child ≥12 yr: PO 200-400 mg q4hr, or EXT REL 600-1200 mg q12hr; max 2.4 g/day
Child 6-12 yr: PO 100-200 mg q4hr or EXT REL 600 mg q12hr; max 1.2 g/day
Child 2-5 yr: PO: 50-100 mg q4hr; max 600 mg/day

Available forms: Tabs 200, 400 mg; ext rel tabs 600, 1200 mg; syr 100 mg/5 ml; oral sol 100 mg/5 ml; oral granules 50, 100 mg/packet

Adverse effects
CNS: Drowsiness, headache, dizziness
GI: Nausea, anorexia, vomiting

Contraindications: Hypersensitivity, chronic persistent cough

Precautions: Pregnancy **C**, breastfeeding, CHF, asthma, emphysema, fever

Pharmacokinetics
Absorption	Well absorbed
Distribution	Unknown
Metabolism	Unknown
Excretion	Unknown
Half-life	1 hr

Pharmacodynamics
	PO	PO–EXT REL
Onset	½ hr	Unknown
Peak	Unknown	Unknown
Duration	4-6 hr	12 hr

NURSING CONSIDERATIONS
Assessment
• Assess cough: type, frequency, character, including characteristics of sputum; lung sounds bilaterally; fluids should be increased to 2 L/day to decrease secretion viscosity (thickness)

Nursing diagnoses
• Airway clearance, ineffective (uses)
• Knowledge, deficient (teaching)

Implementation
• Store at room temperature; provide room humidification to assist with liquefying secretions
• Avoid fluids for ½ hr after administration

Patient/family education
• Caution patient to avoid driving, other hazardous activities if drowsiness occurs (rare)
• Advise patient to avoid smoking, smoke-filled rooms, perfumes, dust, environmental pollutants, cleansers
• Instruct patient to notify prescriber if dry, nonproductive cough lasts over 7 days

Evaluation
Positive therapeutic outcome
• Absence of dry cough
• Thinner, more productive cough that raises secretions

---

halcinonide topical
See Appendix B

---

haloperidol (Rx)
(hal-oh-pehr'ih-dol)
Apo-Haloperidol ✤, Haldol, Novo-Peridol ✤, Peridol ✤
haloperidol decanoate (Rx)
Haldol Decanoate, Haldol LA ✤
haloperidol lactate (Rx)
Haldol, Haldol Concentrate, Haloperidol Intensol
Func. class.: Antipsychotic/neuroleptic
Chem. class.: Butyrophenone

Pregnancy category C

Do not confuse:
haloperidol/Halotestin, Haldol/Stadol

Action: Depresses cerebral cortex, hypothalamus, limbic system, which control activity and aggression; blocks neurotransmission produced by dopamine at synapse; exhibits strong α-adrenergic, anticholinergic blocking action; mechanism for antipsychotic effects unclear

Therapeutic outcome: Decreased signs and symptoms of psychosis

Uses: Psychotic disorders, control of tics, vocal utterances in Gilles de la Tourette syndrome, short-term treatment of hyperactive children showing excessive motor activity, prolonged parenteral therapy in chronic schizophrenia, organic mental syndrome with psychotic features, hiccups (short-term), emergency sedation of severely agitated or delirious patients

Unlabeled uses: Nausea, vomiting in surgery, autism, migraine headache

Dosage and routes
Psychosis
Adult: PO 0.5-5 mg bid or tid initially depending on severity of condition; increase to desired dosage, max 100 mg/day; IM (lactate) 2-5 mg q4-8hr or bid-tid; initial dose IM (decanoate) is 10-15 mg × daily oral dose at 4-wk interval; do not administer **IV**; max 100 mg
Geriatric: PO/IM 0.25-0.5 mg daily-bid, titrate q3-4day by 0.25-0.5 mg/dose
Child 3-12 yr: PO/IM (lactate) 0.05-0.15 mg/kg/day

Chronic schizophrenia
Adult: IM 50-100 mg q4wk (decanoate)
Child 3-12 yr: PO/IM 0.05-0.15 mg/kg/day

Tics/vocal utterances
Adult: PO 0.5-5 mg bid or tid, increased until desired response occurs
Child 3-12 yr: PO 0.05-0.075 mg/kg/day

Hyperactive children
Child 3-12 yr: PO 0.05-0.075 mg/kg/day

Available forms: Tabs 0.5, 1, 2, 5, 10, 20 mg; lactate: conc 2 mg/ml; inj 5 mg/ml; decanoate: 50, 100 mg/ml

Adverse effects
CNS: EPS, pseudoparkinsonism, akathisia, dystonia, tardive dyskinesia, drowsiness, headache, **seizures, neuroleptic malignant syndrome,** confusion
CV: Orthostatic hypotension, hypertension, **cardiac arrest,** ECG changes, **tachycardia, QT prolongation, sudden death**
EENT: Blurred vision, glaucoma, dry eyes
GI: Dry mouth, nausea, vomiting, anorexia, constipation, diarrhea, jaundice, weight gain, **ileus, hepatitis**
GU: Urinary retention, urinary frequency, dysuria, enuresis, impotence, amenorrhea, gynecomastia
INTEG: Rash, photosensitivity, dermatitis
RESP: **Laryngospasm,** dyspnea, **respiratory depression**
SYST: **Risk of death (dementia)**

Contraindications: Children <3 yr, hypersensitivity, blood dyscrasias, coma, brain damage, bone marrow depression, alcohol and barbiturate withdrawal states, Parkinson's disease, angina, epilepsy, urinary retention, closed-angle glaucoma

Precautions: Pregnancy **C,** breastfeeding, geriatric, seizure disorders, hypertension, hepatic/cardiac/pulmonary disease

Black Box Warning: Dementia

Pharmacokinetics
Absorption	Well absorbed (PO, IM); decanoate (IM) absorbed slowly
Distribution	High concentrations in liver, crosses placenta, protein binding 92%
Metabolism	Liver, extensively
Excretion	Kidneys, breast milk
Half-life	Terminal half-life 12-36 hr (metabolized)

Pharmacodynamics
	PO	IM	IM (decanoate)
Onset	Erratic	½ hr	3-9 days
Peak	2-6 hr	30-45 min	4-11 days
Duration	8-12 hr	4-8 hr	3 wk

Adverse effects: *italic* = common, **bold** = life-threatening

Interactions
Individual drugs
Alcohol: increased effects of both products, oversedation
Carbamazepine: decreased effects of haloperidol
Epinephrine: increased toxicity
Levodopa: decreased effects of levodopa
Lithium: increased toxicity; decreased effects of lithium
Phenobarbital: decreased effects of haloperidol

Drug classifications
Anticholinergics: increased anticholinergic effects
Barbiturate anesthetics: oversedation
β-Adrenergic blockers: increased effects of both products
CNS depressants: oversedation

Drug/herb
Chamomile, cola tree, hops, kava, nettle, nutmeg, skullcap, valerian: increased action
Betel palm, kava: increased EPS
Jimsonweed, scopolia: antagonist action

Drug/lab test
Increased: liver function tests, cardiac enzymes, cholesterol, blood glucose, prolactin, bilirubin, PBI, cholinesterase, alkaline phosphatase
Decreased: hormones (blood and urine), protime
False positive: pregnancy tests, PKU
False negative: urinary steroids

NURSING CONSIDERATIONS
Assessment
• Assess mental status: orientation, mood, behavior, presence and type of hallucinations before initial administration and monthly; this product should significantly reduce psychotic behavior
• Check for swallowing of PO medication; check for hoarding or giving of medication to other patients
• Monitor I&O ratio; palpate bladder if low urinary output occurs, especially in geriatric; urinalysis is recommended before, during prolonged therapy
• Monitor bilirubin, CBC, liver function tests monthly
• Assess affect, orientation, LOC, reflexes, gait, coordination, sleep pattern disturbances
• Monitor B/P with patient sitting, standing, and lying; take pulse and respirations q4hr during initial treatment; establish baseline before starting treatment; report drops of 30 mm Hg; obtain baseline ECG, Q-wave and T-wave changes

• Check for dizziness, faintness, palpitations, tachycardia on rising; severe orthostatic hypotension is common
• Assess for neuroleptic malignant syndrome: hyperpyrexia, muscle rigidity, increased CPK, altered mental status; product should be discontinued immediately; if seizures, hypo/hypertension, tachycardia occur, notify prescriber immediately
• Assess for EPS including akathisia (inability to sit still, no pattern to movements), tardive dyskinesia (bizarre movements of the jaw, mouth, tongue, extremities), pseudoparkinsonism (ragged tremors, pill rolling, shuffling gate); an antiparkinsonian product should be prescribed
• Assess for constipation and urinary retention daily; if these occur, increase bulk, water in diet

Nursing diagnoses
• Coping, ineffective (uses)
• Knowledge, deficient (teaching)
• Noncompliance (teaching)
• Thought processes, disturbed (uses)

Implementation
PO route
• Give product in liquid form mixed in glass of juice or caffeine-free cola if hoarding is suspected; do not mix in caffeine drinks, tannics, pectins
• Give decreased dosage in geriatric because of slower metabolism
• Give PO with full glass of water, milk; or give with food to decrease GI upset
• Give antacids 2 hr before or after this product
• Store in tight, light-resistant container; oral sol in amber bottle
IM route
• Inject in deep muscle mass, do not give SUBCUT; use 21-gauge 2-in needle; do not administer sol with a precipitate; give <3 ml per inj site; give slowly, may be painful
• Patient should remain lying down after IM inj for at least 30 min
IV route
• Give undiluted for psychotic episode at 5 mg/min
• Give by intermittent inf after dilution in 30-50 ml of D_5W, run over ½ hr
Syringe compatibilities: Hydromorphone, sufentanil
Y-site compatibilities: Amifostine, amsacrine, aztreonam, cimetidine, cisatracurium, cladribine, DOBUTamine, DOPamine, DOXOrubicin liposome, famotidine, filgrastim, fludarabine, granisetron, lidocaine, lorazepam,

melphalan, midazolam, nitroglycerin, norepinephrine, ondansetron, paclitaxel, phenylephrine, propofol, remifentanil, sufentanil, tacrolimus, teniposide, theophylline, thiotepa,
vinorelbine

Y-site incompatibilities: Fluconazole,
foscarnet, heparin, sargramostim

Patient/family education

• Teach patient to use good oral hygiene; use
frequent rinsing of mouth, sugarless gum for
dry mouth; oral candidiasis may occur

• Advise patient to avoid hazardous activities
until product response is determined; dizziness, blurred vision are common

• Inform patient that orthostatic hypotension
occurs often and to rise from sitting or lying
position gradually; tell patient to avoid hot
tubs, hot showers, tub baths, since hypotension may occur; tell patient that in hot weather
heat stroke may occur; take extra precautions
to stay cool

• Instruct patient to avoid abrupt withdrawal
of this product, or EPS may result; product
should be withdrawn slowly

• Caution patient to avoid OTC preparations
(cough, hay fever, cold) unless approved by
prescriber, since serious product interactions
may occur; avoid use with alcohol, CNS depressants since increased drowsiness may
occur

• Advise patient to use a sunscreen and
sunglasses to prevent burns

• Instruct patient to take antacids 2 hr before
or after this product

• Tell patient to report sore throat, malaise,
fever, bleeding, mouth sores; if these occur,
CBC should be obtained and product discontinued

Evaluation
Positive therapeutic outcome

• Decrease in emotional excitement, hallucinations, delusions, paranoia, reorganization of
patterns of thought, speech; improvement in
specific behaviors

Treatment of overdose: Lavage if
orally ingested; provide airway; *do not induce
vomiting*

❗HIGH ALERT

heparin 🔵 **(Rx)**
(hep′a-rin)
Calcilean 🍁, Calciparine, Hepalean 🍁,
heparin sodium, Heparin Leo 🍁, Hep-
Lock, Hep-Lock U/P
Func. class.: Anticoagulant, antithrombotic

Pregnancy category C

Do not confuse:
heparin/Hespan

Action: Prevents conversion of fibrinogen to
fibrin and prothrombin to thrombin by enhancing inhibitory effects of antithrombin III

Therapeutic outcome: Prevention of
thrombi

Uses: Prevention of deep vein thrombosis
(DVT) and pulmonary emboli (PE) (treatment
and prevention), MI, open heart surgery,
disseminated intravascular clotting syndrome,
atrial fibrillation with embolization; as an
anticoagulant in transfusion and dialysis
procedures; prevention of DVT/PE; to maintain
patency of indwelling venipuncture devices,
diagnosis, treatment of disseminated intravascular coagulation (DIC)

Dosage and routes
Deep vein thrombosis/MI
Adult: **IV** BOL 5000-7000 units q4hr then
titrated to PTT or ACT level; **IV** INF after BOL
dose, then 1000 units/hr titrated to PTT or ACT
level
Child: **IV** INF 50 units/kg, maintenance 100
units/kg q4hr or 20,000 units/m^2 daily

Anticoagulation
Adult: SUBCUT 5000 units **IV** then 10,000-
20,000 units, then 8,000-10,000 units q8hr or
15,000-20,000 units q12hr; intermittent **IV**
BOL 10,000 units, then 5000-10,000 units
q4-6hr; CONT **IV** INF 5000 units (35-70
units/kg), then 20,000-40,000 units given over
24 hr
Child >1 yr: Intermittent **IV** BOL 50-100
units/kg, then 50-100 units/kg q4hr; CONT INF
75 units/kg, then 20 units/kg/hr, adjust to
maintain aPTT at 60-85 sec
Neonates, infants <1 yr: CONT **IV** INF
75 units/kg, then 28 units/kg/hr, adjust to
maintain aPTT at 60-85 sec

Cardiovascular surgery
Adult: **IV** INF 150-300 units/kg
Child, infants, neonates: IA 100
units/kg in artery prior to cardiac catheter

Prophylaxis for DVT/PE
Adult: SUBCUT 5000 units q8-12hr

Heparin flush
Adult and child: **IV** 10-100 units/ml

Arterial line patency
Neonates: IA 0.5-2 units/ml

Available forms: Sol for inj 10, 100, 1000, 5000, 7500, 10,000, 20,000, 40,000 units/ml; premixed 1000 units/500 ml, 2000 units/1000 ml, 12,500 units/250 ml, 25,000 units/250 ml, 25,000 units/500 ml; lock flush preparations 10 units/ml

Adverse effects
CNS: Fever, chills, headache
GU: Hematuria
HEMA: **Hemorrhage, thrombocytopenia, anemia**
INTEG: Rash, dermatitis, urticaria, pruritus, delayed transient alopecia, hematoma, cutaneous necrosis (SUBCUT)
SYST: **Anaphylaxis**

Contraindications: Hypersensitivity, hemophilia, leukemia with bleeding, peptic ulcer disease, severe thrombocytopenic purpura, renal/hepatic disease (severe), blood dyscrasias, severe hypertension, subacute bacterial endocarditis, acute nephritis

Precautions: Pregnancy **C,** children, geriatric, alcoholism, hyperlipidemia, diabetes, renal disease

Pharmacokinetics

Absorption	Well absorbed (SUBCUT)
Distribution	Unknown
Metabolism	Partially in kidney, liver
Excretion	Lymph, spleen, in urine (<50% unchanged)
Half-life	1½ hr

Pharmacodynamics

	SUBCUT	IV
Onset	½-1 hr	5 min
Peak	2 hr	10 min
Duration	8-12 hr	2-6 hr

Interactions
Individual drugs
Dextran, dipyridole, ticlopidine: increased action of heparin
Diazepam: increased action of diazepam
Digoxin: decreased action of heparin
Streptokinase: resistance to heparin

Drug classifications
Anticoagulants (oral), cephalosporins, NSAIDs, penicillins, platelet inhibitors, salicylates: increased action of heparin
Antihistamines, tetracyclines: decreased action of heparin
Corticosteroids: decreased action of corticosteroids
Drug/herb
Agrimony, alfalfa, angelica, anise, basil, bay, bilberry, black haw, bogbean, bromelain, buchu, chamomile, chondroitin, cinchona bark, dong quai, fenugreek, feverfew, garlic, ginger, ginkgo, ginseng, horse chestnut, Irish moss, kelp, kelpware, khella, lovage, lungwort, meadowsweet, motherwort, mugwort, nettle, papaya, parsley (large amounts), pau d'arco, pineapple, poplar, prickly ash, safflower, saw palmetto, tonka bean, turmeric, wintergreen, yarrow: increased risk of bleeding
Coenzyme Q10, flax, glucomannan, goldenseal, guar gum: decreased anticoagulant effect
Drug/lab test
Increased: ALT, AST, INR, pro-time, PTT, potassium
Decreased: platelets, triglycerides, cholesterol, plasma free fatty acids

NURSING CONSIDERATIONS
Assessment
• Assess for blood studies (Hct, occult blood in stools) q3mo if patient is on long-term therapy
• Monitor PPT, which should be 1½-2 × control, PTT; often done daily, APTT, ACT
• Monitor platelet count q2-3day; thrombocytopenia may occur on fourth day of treatment and resolve, or continue to eighth day of treatment
◆ Assess for bleeding gums, petechiae, ecchymosis, black tarry stools, hematuria, epistaxis, decrease in Hct, B/P; may indicate bleeding and possible hemorrhage; notify prescriber immediately; HIT may occur after product discontinuation
• Monitor for hypersensitivity: fever, skin rash, urticaria; notify prescriber immediately

Nursing diagnoses
• Injury, risk for (uses, adverse reactions)
• Knowledge, deficient (teaching)
• Tissue perfusion, ineffective (uses)

Implementation
SUBCUT route
• Give SUBCUT with at least 25-G ⅜-in needle; do not massage area or aspirate fluid when giving SUBCUT inj; give in abdomen between

pelvic bones, rotate sites; do not pull back on plunger, leave in for 10 sec; apply gentle pressure for 1 min
• Give at same time each day to maintain steady blood levels
• Changing needles is not recommended
Heparin lock route
• Do not mistake heparin sodium injection 10,000 units/ml and Hep-Lock U/P 10 units/ml; they have similar blue labeling
• Inject 10-100 units/0.5-1 ml after each inf or q8-12hr
IV route
• Cannot be used interchangeably (unit for unit) with LMWHs or heparinoids
• Give directly; **IV** loading dose over 1 min
• Give **IV** diluted in 0.9% NaCl, dextrose, Ringer's and by intermittent or cont inf; inf may run from 4-24 hr; use infusion pump
• When product is added to inf sol for cont **IV**, invert container at least 6 × to ensure adequate mixing

Syringe compatibilities: Aminophylline, amphotericin B, ampicillin, atropine, azlocillin, bleomycin, cefamandole, cefazolin, cefoperazone, cefotaxime, cefoxitin, chloramphenicol, cimetidine, cisplatin, clindamycin, cyclophosphamide, diazoxide, digoxin, dimenhyDRINATE, DOBUTamine, DOPamine, epinephrine, fentanyl, fluorouracil, furosemide, leucovorin, lidocaine, lincomycin, methotrexate, metoclopramide, mezlocillin, mitomycin, moxalactam, nafcillin, naloxone, neostigmine, nitroglycerin, norepinephrine, pancuronium, penicillin G, phenobarbital, piperacillin, sodium nitroprusside, succinylcholine, trimethoprim-sulfamethoxazole, verapamil, vinCRIStine

Y-site compatibilities: Acyclovir, aldesleukin, allopurinol, amifostine, aminophylline, ampicillin, ampicillin/sulbactam, atracurium, atropine, aztreonam, betamethasone, bleomycin, calcium gluconate, cefazolin, cefotetan, ceftazidime, ceftriaxone, cephalothin, cephapirin, chlordiazepoxide, chlorproMAZINE, cimetidine, cisplatin, cladribine, clindamycin, conjugated estrogens, cyanocobalamin, cyclophosphamide, cytarabine, dexamethasone, digoxin, diphenhydrAMINE, DOPamine, DOXOrubicin liposome, edrophonium, enalaprilat, epinephrine, erythromycin, esmolol, ethacrynate, famotidine, fentanyl, fluconazole, fludarabine, fluorouracil, foscarnet, furosemide, gallium, granisetron, hydrALAZINE, hydrocortisone, hydromorphone, regular insulin, isoproterenol, kanamycin, leucovorin, lidocaine, lorazepam, magnesium sulfate, melphalan, menadiol sodium, meperi-

dine, meropenem, methicillin, methotrexate, methoxamine, methyldopa, methylergonovine, metoclopramide, metronidazole, midazolam, milrinone, minocycline, mitomycin, morphine, nafcillin, neostigmine, nitroglycerin, nitroprusside, norepinephrine, ondansetron, oxacillin, oxytocin, paclitaxel, pancuronium, penicillin G potassium, pentazocine, phytonadione, piperacillin, piperacillin/tazobactam, propofol, potassium chloride, prednisoLONE, procainamide, prochlorperazine, propofol, propranolol, pyridostigmine, ranitidine, remifentanil, sargramostim, scopolamine, sodium bicarbonate, streptokinase, succinylcholine, tacrolimus, teniposide, theophylline, thiopental, thiotepa, ticarcillin, ticarcillin/clavulanate, trimethobenzamide, vecuronium, vinBLAStine, vinorelbine, warfarin, zidovudine

Y-site incompatibilities: Alteplase, ciprofloxacin, dacarbazine, diazepam, DOBUTamine, DOXOrubicin, ergotamine, gentamicin, haloperidol, idarubicin, methotrimeprazine, phenytoin, promethazine, tobramycin, trifluupromazine

Additive compatibilities: Aminophylline, amphotericin, ascorbic acid, bleomycin, calcium gluconate, cefepime, cephapirin, chloramphenicol, clindamycin, colistimethate, dimenhyDRINATE, doxacillin, DOPamine, enalaprilat, erythromycin, esmolol, floxacillin, fluconazole, flumazenil, furosemide, hydrocortisone, isoproterenol, lidocaine, lincomycin, magnesium sulfate, meropenem, methyldopa, methylPREDNISolone, metronidazole/sodium bicarbonate, nafcillin, norepinephrine, octreotide, penicillin G, potassium chloride, prednisoLONE, promazine, ranitidine, sodium bicarbonate, verapamil, vit B complex, vit B complex with C

Additive incompatibilities: Amikacin, erythromycin lactobionate, gentamicin, kanamycin, meperidine, methadone, morphine, polymyxin B, streptomycin

Patient/family education
• Advise patient to avoid OTC preparations that may cause serious product interactions unless directed by prescriber; may contain aspirin or other anticoagulants
• Tell patient that product may be held during active bleeding (menstruation), depending on condition
• Caution patient to use soft-bristle toothbrush to avoid bleeding gums; avoid contact sports; use electric razor; avoid IM inj

- Instruct patient to carry/wear emergency ID or other identification identifying product taken and condition treated
- Advise patient to report any signs of bleeding: gums, under skin, urine, stools; or unusual bruising even after discontinuing product

Evaluation
Positive therapeutic outcome
- Decrease of DVT
- PTT of 1.5-2.5 × control
- Free-flowing **IV**

Treatment of overdose: Withdraw product, give protamine sulfate 1 mg protamine/100 units heparin

---

hepatitis B immune globulin (Rx)
(hep-a-tite′iss)
BayHep B, Nabi-HB
Func. class.: Immune globulin

Pregnancy category C

Action: Provides passive immunity to hepatitis B

Therapeutic outcome: Passive immunity to hepatitis B

Uses: Prevention of hepatitis B virus in exposed patients, including passive immunity in neonates born to HBsAg-positive mothers

Dosage and routes
Adult and child: IM 0.06 ml/kg (usual 3-5 ml) within 7 days of exposure; repeat 28 days after exposure, if patient wishes not to receive the hepatitis B vaccine

Neonates born to hepatitis B surface antigen–positive persons
Neonate: IM 0.5 ml within 12 hr of birth

Available forms: Inj 1-, 4-, 5-ml vials; neonatal syringe 0.5 ml

Adverse effects
CNS: Headache, dizziness, fever
GI: Nausea, vomiting
INTEG: Soreness at inj site, urticaria, erythema, swelling
SYST: Induration, **anaphylaxis, angioedema**

Contraindications: Hypersensitivity to immune globulins, coagulation disorders

Precautions: Pregnancy C, breastfeeding, children, geriatric, hemophilia, active infection, IgA deficiency

Pharmacokinetics
Absorption	Slowly absorbed
Distribution	Unknown
Metabolism	Unknown
Excretion	Unknown
Half-life	3 wk

Pharmacodynamics
Onset	1-7 days
Peak	3-10 days
Duration	2-6 mo

Interactions
Drug classifications
MMR, rotavirus vaccines, varicella: do not use within 3 mo of hepatitis B immune globulin

NURSING CONSIDERATIONS
Assessment
- Assess for history of allergies, skin conditions (eczema, psoriasis, dermatitis), reactions to vaccinations
- Assess for skin reactions: rash, induration, urticaria
- Assess for sneezing, pruritus, angioedema, dysphagia, vomiting, abdominal pain
⬥ Assess for anaphylaxis: inability to breathe, bronchospasm, hypotension, wheezing, diaphoresis, fever, flushing; epinephrine and emergency equipment should be available

Nursing diagnoses
- Infection, risk for (uses)
- Knowledge, deficient (teaching)

Implementation
- Give after rotating vial; do not shake
- Give in deltoid (adult) or anterolateral thigh for better protection; give 2-ml dose in two different sites; do not give **IV**
- Refrigerate unused portion; sol should be clear, light amber, and thick

Patient/family education
- Teach patient purpose of medication and expected results
- Give patient a list of adverse reactions that need to be reported immediately: wheezing, vomiting, sneezing, abdominal pain, sweating, tightness in chest
- Advise patient that pain, rash, swelling at inj site can be expected
- Give patient written record of immunization

Evaluation
Positive therapeutic outcome
- Prevention of hepatitis B

---

homatropine ophthalmic
See Appendix B

---

*hydrALAZINE (Rx)
(hye-dral′a-zeen)
Apresoline, Novo-Hylazin ✦, hydrALAZINE HCl
Func. class.: Antihypertensive, direct-acting peripheral vasodilator
Chem. class.: Phthalazine
Pregnancy category C

Do not confuse:
hydrALAZINE/hydrOXYzine, Apresoline/allopurinol

Action: Vasodilates arterioles in smooth muscle by direct relaxation; reduces B/P with reflex increases in heart rate, stroke volume, cardiac output

Therapeutic outcome: Decreased B/P in hypertension, decreased afterload in CHF

Uses: Essential hypertension, severe essential hypertension

Unlabeled uses: CHF

Dosage and routes
Hypertension
Adult: PO 10 mg qid 2-4 days, then 25 mg for rest of 1st wk, then 50 mg qid individualized to desired response; max 300 mg/day
Child: PO 0.75-1 mg/kg/day in 4 divided doses; max 25 mg/dose

Hypertensive crisis
Adult: **IV** BOL 10-20 mg q4-6hr; administer PO as soon as possible; IM 10-50 mg q4-6hr
Child: **IV** BOL 0.1-0.6 mg/kg q4-6hr; IM 0.1-0.6 mg/kg q4-6hr

CHF
Adult: PO 10-25 mg bid, max 75 mg tid

Available forms: Inj 20 mg/ml; tabs 10, 25, 50, 100 mg

Adverse effects
CNS: Headache, tremors, dizziness, anxiety, peripheral neuritis, depression, fever, chills
CV: Palpitations, reflex tachycardia, angina, **shock,** rebound hypertension
GI: Nausea, vomiting, anorexia, diarrhea, constipation, paralytic ileus
GU: Urinary retention
HEMA: **Leukopenia, agranulocytosis,** anemia, **thrombocytopenia**
INTEG: Rash, pruritus, urticaria

MISC: Nasal congestion, muscle cramps, *lupuslike symptoms,* flushing, edema, dyspnea

Contraindications: Hypersensitivity to hydrALAZINEs, mitral valvular rheumatic heart disease, dissecting aortic aneurysm

Precautions: Pregnancy **C,** breastfeeding, geriatric, CVA, advanced renal disease, CAD, liver disease, SLE

Pharmacokinetics
Absorption	Rapidly absorbed (PO); well absorbed (IM); completely absorbed (**IV**)
Distribution	Widely distributed; crosses placenta
Metabolism	GI mucosa, liver extensively
Excretion	Kidneys, urine (12%-14%)
Half-life	2-8 hr

Pharmacodynamics
	PO	IM	IV
Onset	½ hr	10-30 min	5 20 min
Peak	1-2 hr	1 hr	10-80 min
Duration	6-12 hr	4-6 hr	4-6 hr

Interactions
Individual drugs
Alcohol: increased hypotension
Indomethacin: decreased effects of hydrALAZINE
Drug classifications
β-Adrenergic blockers: increased effects
MAOIs: severe hypotension
Other antihypertensives: increased hypotension
Sympathomimetics (epinephrine, norepinephrine): increased tachycardia, angina
Drug/herb
Aconite: increased toxicity, death
Astragalus, cola tree: increased or decreased antihypertensive effect
Barberry, betony, black catechu, black cohosh, bloodroot, broom, burdock, cat's claw, dandelion, goldenseal, hawthorn, Irish moss, Jamaican dogwood, kelp, khella, mistletoe, parsley: increased antihypertensive effect
Coltsfoot, guarana, khat, licorice, yohimbe: decreased antihypertensive effect

NURSING CONSIDERATIONS
Assessment
• Assess cardiac status: B/P q5min for 2 hr, then qhr for 2 hr, then q4hr; pulse, jugular venous distention q4hr

H

- Monitor electrolytes, blood studies: potassium, sodium, chloride, carbon dioxide, CBC, serum glucose; LE prep, ANA titer before starting treatment
- Monitor weight daily, I&O; edema in feet, legs daily; check skin turgor, dryness of mucous membranes for hydration status
- Assess for crackles, dyspnea, orthopnea; peripheral edema, fatigue, weight gain, jugular vein distention (CHF)
- For fever, joint pain, rash, sore throat (lupuslike symptoms), notify prescriber

Nursing diagnoses
- Cardiac output, decreased (adverse reactions)
- Injury, risk for (side effects)
- Knowledge, deficient (teaching)

Implementation
PO route
- Give with meals to enhance absorption
- Store protected from light and heat
IV route
- Give by IV undiluted through Y-tube or 3-way stopcock, give each 10 mg over 1 min or more
- Administer with patient in recumbent position; keep in that position for 1 hr after administration
Y-site compatibilities: Heparin, hydrocortisone, potassium chloride, verapamil, vit B/C
Y-site incompatibilities: Aminophylline, ampicillin, diazoxide, furosemide, paclitaxel
Additive incompatibilities: Aminophylline, ampicillin, chlorothiazide, edetate calcium disodium, ethacrynate, hydrocortisone, melphalan, mephentermine, methohexital, nitroglycerin, phenobarbital, verapamil, vinorelbine
Additive compatibilities: DOBUTamine

Patient/family education
- Teach patient to take with food to increase bioavailability (PO)
- Teach patient to avoid OTC preparations unless directed by prescriber
- Advise patient to notify prescriber if chest pain, severe fatigue, fever, muscle or joint pain occur
- Advise patient to rise slowly to prevent orthostatic hypertension
- Advise patient to notify prescriber if pregnancy is suspected

Evaluation
Positive therapeutic outcome
- Decreased B/P in hypertension

Treatment of overdose: Administer vasopressors, volume expanders for shock; if PO, lavage or give activated charcoal, digitalization

hydrochlorothiazide
(Rx)
(hye-droe-klor-oh-thye′a-zide)
Apo-Hydro ✿, Esidrix, HCTZ, Hydro-Chlor, hydrochlorothiazide, Hydro-D, HydroDIURIL, Microzide, Neo-Codema ✿, Novohydrazide ✿, Oretic, Urozide ✿
Func. class.: Diuretic, antihypertensive
Chem. class.: Thiazide, sulfonamide derivative

Pregnancy category B

Action: Acts on the distal tubule in the kidney, increasing excretion of sodium, water, chloride, and potassium

Therapeutic outcome: Decreased B/P, decreased edema in lung tissues peripherally

Uses: Edema, hypertension, diuresis, CHF; edema in corticosteroid, estrogen, NSAID therapy; idiopathic lower extremity edema

Dosage and routes
Adult: PO 12.5-100 mg/day
Geriatric: PO 12.5 mg/day, initially
Child >6 mo: PO 2 mg/kg/day in divided doses
Child <6 mo: PO 2-4 mg/kg/day in divided doses

Available forms: Tabs 25, 50, 100 mg; caps 12.5 mg; oral sol 10 mg/5 ml, 100 mg/ml

Adverse effects
CNS: Drowsiness, paresthesia, depression, headache, *dizziness, fatigue, weakness,* fever
CV: Irregular pulse, orthostatic hypotension, palpitations, volume depletion, allergic myocarditis
EENT: Blurred vision
ELECT: *Hypokalemia,* hypercalcemia, hyponatremia, hypochloremia, hypomagnesemia
GI: *Nausea, vomiting, anorexia,* constipation, diarrhea, cramps, pancreatitis, GI irritation, **hepatitis**
GU: *Frequency,* polyuria, **uremia,** glucosuria, hyperuricemia
HEMA: **Aplastic anemia, hemolytic anemia, leukopenia, agranulocytosis, thrombocytopenia, neutropenia**

INTEG: Rash, urticaria, purpura, photosensitivity, alopecia, erythema multiforme
META: Hyperglycemia, hyperuricemia, increased creatinine, BUN

Contraindications: Hypersensitivity to thiazides or sulfonamides, anuria, renal decompensation, hypomagnesemia

Precautions: Pregnancy **B**, breastfeeding, hypokalemia, renal/hepatic disease, gout, COPD, lupus erythematosus, diabetes mellitus, hyperlipidemia, CCr <25 ml/min

Pharmacokinetics

Absorption	Variable
Distribution	Extracellular spaces; crosses placenta
Metabolism	Excreted unchanged in urine
Excretion	Breast milk
Half-life	6-15 hr

Pharmacodynamics

Onset	2 hr
Peak	4 hr
Duration	6-12 hr

Interactions
Individual drugs
Amphotericin B: increased hypokalemia
Cholestyramine, colestipol: decreased absorption of hydrochlorothiazide
Diazoxide: increased hyperglycemia, hyperuricemia, hypotension
Lithium: increased toxicity
Drug classifications
Antidiabetics: decreased effect of antidiabetic agent
Cardiac glycosides, nondepolarizing skeletal muscle relaxants: increased toxicity
Diuretics (loop): increased effects of diuretic
Glucocorticoids: increased hypokalemia
NSAIDs: increased risk of renal failure
Drug/herb
Aloe, buckthorn, cascara sagrada, Chinese rhubarb, gossypol, licorice, nettle, senna: increased hypokalemia
Cucumber, dandelion, ginkgo, horsetail, khella, licorice, nettle, pumpkin, Queen Anne's lace: increased effect
St. John's wort: severe photosensitivity
Drug/lab test
Increased: BSP, retention, amylase, parathyroid test
Decreased: PBI, PSP

NURSING CONSIDERATIONS
Assessment
- Monitor glucose in urine if patient is diabetic
- Assess improvement in CVP q8hr
- Check for rashes, temp elevation daily
- Assess for confusion, especially in geriatric patients; take safety precautions if needed
- Monitor manifestations of hypokalemia: acidic urine, reduced urine, osmolality, nocturia; hypotension, broad T-wave, U-wave, ectopy, tachycardia, weak pulse; muscle weakness, altered LOC, drowsiness, apathy, lethargy, confusion, depression; anorexia, nausea, cramps, constipation, distention, paralytic ileus; hypoventilation, respiratory muscle weakness
- Monitor for manifestations of hypomagnesemia: agitation, muscle twitching, paresthesias, hyperactive reflexes, positive Babinski reflex, dysphagia, nystagmus, seizures, tetany; nausea, vomiting, diarrhea, anorexia, abdominal distention; ectopy, tachycardia, broad, flat, or inverted T-waves, depressed ST segment, prolonged QT interval, decreased cardiac output, hypotension
- Monitor for manifestations of hyponatremia: increased B/P, cold, clammy skin, hypovolemia or hypervolemia; anorexia, nausea, vomiting, diarrhea, abdominal cramps; lethargy, increased ICP, confusion, headache, seizures, coma, fatigue, tremors, hyperreflexia
- Monitor for manifestations of hyperchloremia: weakness, lethargy, coma, deep rapid breathing
- Assess fluid volume status: I&O ratios, record, count, or weigh diapers as appropriate; weight; distended red veins; crackles in lungs; color, quality, and specific gravity of urine; skin turgor; adequacy of pulses; moist mucous membranes; bilateral lung sounds; peripheral pitting edema; assess for dehydration: symptoms of decreasing output, thirst, hypotension; dry mouth and mucous membranes should be reported
- Monitor electrolytes: potassium, sodium, calcium, magnesium; also include BUN, blood pH, ABGs, uric acid, CBC, blood glucose, renal function
- Assess B/P before, during therapy with patient lying, standing, and sitting as appropriate; orthostatic hypotension can occur rapidly

Nursing diagnoses
- Fluid volume, deficient (side effects)
- Fluid volume, excess (uses)
- Knowledge, deficient (teaching)
- Urinary elimination, impaired (side effects)

H

Implementation

- Give in AM to avoid interference with sleep
- Provide potassium replacement if potassium level is ≤3.0 mg/dl; give whole tab or use oral sol lightly; product may be crushed if patient is unable to swallow
- Administer with food; if nausea occurs, absorption may be increased

Patient/family education

- Teach patient to take the medication early in the day to prevent nocturia
- Instruct patient to take with food or milk if GI symptoms of nausea and anorexia occur
- Teach patient to maintain a weekly record of weight and notify prescriber of weight loss >5 lb
- Caution patient that this product causes a loss of potassium and that food rich in potassium should be added to the diet; refer to a dietitian for assistance in planning
- Caution patient to rise slowly from sitting or reclining positions, not to exercise in hot weather or stand for prolonged periods since orthostatic hypotension will be enhanced; lie down if dizziness occurs
- Teach patient not to use alcohol or any OTC medications without prescriber's approval; serious product reactions may occur
- Emphasize the need to contact prescriber immediately if muscle cramps, weakness, nausea, dizziness, or numbness occurs
- Teach patient to take own B/P and pulse and record findings
- Teach patient to continue taking medication even if feeling better; this product controls symptoms but does not cure the condition
- Advise patient with hypertension to continue other medical treatment (exercise, weight loss, relaxation techniques, cessation of smoking)

Evaluation

Positive therapeutic outcome

- Decreased edema
- Decreased B/P
- Increased diuresis

Treatment of overdose: Lavage if taken orally, monitor electrolytes, administer dextrose in saline, monitor hydration, CV, renal status

hydrocodone (Rx)
(hye-droe-koe'done)
Hycodan ✳, Robidone ✳, Tussigon

hydrocodone/ acetaminophen (Rx)
Anexsia, Bancap HC, Ceta-Plus, Co-Gesic, Duocet, Hydrocet, Hydrogesic, Lorcet, Lortab, NorCo, Panlor, Polygesic, Stagesic, T-Gesic, Vanacet, Vicodin, Vicodin ES, Vicodin HP, Xodol, Zamicet, Zydone

hyprocodone/ibuprofen (Rx)
Ibudone, Reprexain, Vicoprofen
Func. class.: Antitussive opioid analgesic/ nonopioid analgesic

Pregnancy category C

Controlled substance schedule III

Do not confuse:
hydrocodone/hydrocortisone, Hycodan/ Vicodin

Action: Acts directly on cough center in medulla to suppress cough; binds to opiate receptors in the CNS to reduce pain

Therapeutic outcome: Pain relief, decreased cough, decreased diarrhea

Uses: Hyperactive and nonproductive cough, mild to moderate pain

Dosages and routes
Analgesic
Adult: PO 2.5-10 mg q3-6hr prn

Antitussive
Adult: PO 5 mg q4-6hr prn, max 30 mg/24 hr

Available forms: Hydrocodone: tabs 5 mg (Hycodan); syr 5 mg/ml (Hycodan, Robidone ✳; hydrocodone/acetaminophen: tabs 2.5 mg hydrocodone/500 mg acetaminophen (Lortabs 2.5/500), 5 mg hydrocodone/400 mg acetaminophen (Zydone), 5 mg hydrocodone/500 mg acetaminophen (Anexsia 5/500, Co-Gesic, Dolacet, Hydrocet, Hydrogesic, Hy-Phen, Lorcet, Lortab 5/500, Maragesic-H, Panacet 5/500, Stagesic, T-Gesic, Vicodin); 7.5 mg hydrocodone/400 mg acetaminophen (Zydone), 7.5 mg hydrocodone/500 mg acetaminophen (Lortab) 7.5/500, 7.5 mg hydrocodone/650 mg acetaminophen (Anexsia 7.5/650, Lorcet Plus), 7.5 mg hydrocodone/750 mg acetaminophen (Vicodin ES), 10 mg hydrocodone/325 mg acetaminophen (Norco), 10 mg hydrocodone/500 mg acetaminophen (Lortab 10/500), 10 mg hydrocodone/650 mg acetaminophen (Lorcet 10/650, Vicodin HP), 10 mg hydrocodone/660 acetaminophen (Anexia 10/660); caps 5 mg hydrocodone/500 mg acetaminophen (Bancap-HC, Dolacet, Hydrocet, Hydrogesic, Loracet-HD, Maragesic-H, Stragesic, T-Gesic, Zydone); elixir or oral sol 2.5 mg hydrocodone/167 mg acetaminophen/5 ml; hydrocodone/aspirin: tabs 5 mg hydrocodone/ 500 mg aspirin (Alor 5/500, Azdone, Damason-P, Lortab ASA, Panasal 5/500); hydrocodone/ibuprofen: tabs 7.5 mg hydrocodone/200 mg ibuprofen (Vicoprofen)

Adverse effects

CNS: Drowsiness, dizziness, light-headedness, confusion, headache, sedation, euphoria, dysphoria, weakness, hallucinations, disorientation, mood changes, dependence, **seizures**
CV: Palpitations, tachycardia, bradycardia, change in B/P, **circulatory depression,** syncope, **cardiac arrest (child)**
EENT: Tinnitus, blurred vision, miosis, diplopia
GI: Nausea, vomiting, anorexia, constipation, cramps, dry mouth, ulcers
GU: Increased urinary output, dysuria, urinary retention
INTEG: Rash, urticaria, flushing, pruritus
RESP: **Respiratory depression,** pulmonary edema, bronchopneumonia, **respiratory arrest (child)**

Contraindications: Acne rosacea/vulgaris, Cushing's, measles, perioral dermatitis, varicella, abrupt discontinuation, hypersensitivity to this product or benzyl

Precautions: Pregnancy **C,** breastfeeding, neonates, addictive personality, increased ICP, MI (acute), severe heart disease, respiratory depression, renal/hepatic disease, bowel impaction, urinary retention, viral infection, ulcerative colitis, seizures, sulfite hypersensitivity, psychosis, hypertension, hyperthyroidism

Pharmacokinetics

Absorption	Well absorbed
Distribution	Unknown; crosses placenta
Metabolism	Liver, extensively
Excretion	Kidneys
Half-life	3½-4½ hr

Pharmacodynamics

	PO (analgesic)	PO (antitussive)
Onset	10-20 min	Unknown
Peak	30-60 min	Unknown
Duration	4-6 hr	4-6 hr

Interactions
Individual drugs
Alcohol: increased CNS depression
Drug classifications
Antidepressants (tricyclics), CNS depressants, general anesthetics, opioids, phenothiazines, sedative/hypnotics, skeletal muscle relaxants: increased CNS depression
MAOIs: increased severe reactions
Drug/herb
Corkwood: increased anticholinergic effect
Jamacian dogwood, lavender, mistletoe, nettle, pokeweed, poppy, senega, valerian: increased CNS depression
Drug/lab test
Increased: amylase, lipase

NURSING CONSIDERATIONS
Assessment
- Assess pain: intensity, type, location, duration, precipitating factor
- Monitor VS after parenteral route; note muscle rigidity; product history; liver; renal function tests; cough; and respiratory dysfunction: respiratory depression, character, rate, rhythm; notify prescriber if respirations are <10/min
- Monitor CNS changes: dizziness, drowsiness, hallucinations, euphoria, LOC, pupil reaction
- Monitor allergic reactions: rash, urticaria
- Obtain history of ulcers if using ibuprofen combination product

Nursing diagnoses
- Breathing pattern, ineffective (adverse reactions)
- Knowledge, deficient (teaching)
- Pain, acute (uses)
- Sensory perception, disturbed: visual, auditory (adverse reactions)

Implementation
- Do not break, crush, or chew tabs; only scored tabs can be broken
- Give with antiemetic if nausea, vomiting occur
- Give when pain is beginning to return; determine dosage interval by patient response; continuous dosing of medication is more effective than given prn
- Medication should be slowly withdrawn after long-term use to prevent withdrawal symptoms
- Max 4 g acetaminophen with combination product
- Store in light-resistant container at room temperature
- May be given with food or milk to lessen GI upset

H

Adverse effects: *italic* = common, **bold** = life-threatening

Patient/family education
• Instruct patient to report any symptoms of CNS changes, allergic reactions; to avoid CNS depressants: alcohol, sedative/hypnotics for at least 24 hr after taking this product
• Teach patient that dizziness, drowsiness, and confusion are common and to avoid getting up without assistance, driving, or other hazardous activities
• Discuss in detail all aspects of the product

Evaluation
Positive therapeutic outcome
• Decreased pain
• Decreased cough

Treatment of overdose: Naloxone HCl (Narcan) 0.2-0.8 **IV**, O$_2$, **IV** fluids, vasopressors

---

hydrocortisone (Rx)
(hy-droh-kor'tih-sone)
Cortef, Cortenema, Hydrocortone
hydrocortisone acetate (Rx)
Cortifoam, Hydrocortone Acetate
hydrocortisone cypionate (Rx)
Cortef
hydrocortisone sodium phosphate (Rx)
Hydrocortone Phosphate
hydrocortisone sodium succinate (Rx)
A-hydroCort, Solu-Cortef
Func. class.: Short-acting glucocorticoid
Chem. class.: Natural nonfluorinated, group IV potency (valerate), group VI potency (acetate and plain)

Pregnancy category C

Do not confuse:
hydrocortisone/hydrocodone

Action: Decreases inflammation by suppressing migration of polymorphonuclear leukocytes and fibroblasts and reversing increased capillary permeability and lysosomal stabilization (systemic); antipruritic, antiinflammatory (topical)

Therapeutic outcome: Decreased inflammation

Uses: Severe inflammation, septic shock, adrenal insufficiency, ulcerative colitis, collagen disorders

Dosage and routes
Adrenal insufficiency/inflammation
Adult: PO 5-30 mg bid-qid; IM/**IV** 100-250 mg (succinate), then 50-100 mg IM as needed; IM/**IV** 15-240 mg q12hr (phosphate)

Shock prevention
Adult: IM/**IV** 500 mg-2 g q2-6hr (succinate)
Child: IM/**IV** 0.16-1 mg/kg bid-tid (succinate)

Colitis
Adult: PO 20-240 mg (base)/day in 2-4 divided doses; enema 100 mg nightly for 21 days
Child: PO 2-8 mg (base)/kg/day or 60-240 mg (base)/m^2/day in 3-4 divided doses

Topical route
Adult and child >2 yr: Apply to affected area daily-qid

Available forms: Tabs 5, 10, 20 mg; inj 25, 50 mg/ml; enema 100 mg/60 ml; acetate: inj 25 ✿, 50 mg/ml ✿, enema 10% aerosol foam, supp 25 mg; cypionate: oral susp 10 mg/5 ml; phosphate: inj 50 mg/ml; succinate: inj 100 mg ✿, 250 mg ✿, 500 mg ✿, 1000 mg/vial ✿

Adverse effects
CNS: Depression, flushing, sweating, headache, mood changes
CV: Hypertension, **circulatory collapse, thrombophlebitis, embolism,** tachycardia, edema
EENT: Fungal infections, increased intraocular pressure, blurred vision
GI: Diarrhea, nausea, abdominal distention, **GI hemorrhage,** increased appetite, **pancreatitis**
HEMA: **Thrombocytopenia**
INTEG: Acne, poor wound healing, ecchymosis, petechiae
MS: Fractures, osteoporosis, weakness

Contraindications: Children <2 yr, psychosis, hypersensitivity, idiopathic thrombocytopenia (IM), acute glomerulonephritis, amebiasis, fungal infections, nonasthmatic bronchial disease, AIDS, TB, recent MI (associated with left-ventricular rupture)

Precautions: Pregnancy **C,** breastfeeding, diabetes mellitus, glaucoma, osteoporosis, seizure disorders, ulcerative colitis, CHF, myasthenia gravis, renal disease, esophagitis, peptic ulcer, metastatic carcinoma

---

Pharmacokinetics

Absorption	Well absorbed (PO); systemic (topical)
Distribution	Crosses placenta
Metabolism	Liver, extensively
Excretion	Kidney
Half-life	3-5 hr, adrenal suppression 3-4 days

Pharmacodynamics

	PO	IM	IV	TOPICAL
Onset	1-2 hr	20 min	Rapid	Min to hr
Peak	1 hr	4-8 hr	Unkn	Hr to days
Duration	1½ days	1½ days	1½ days	Hr to days

Interactions
Individual drugs
Alcohol, amphotericin B, cycloSPORINE, digoxin: increased side effects

Cholestyramine, colestipol, ephedrine, phenytoin, rifampin, theophylline: decreased action of hydrocortisone

Drug classifications
Anticoagulants, calcium supplements, toxoids, vaccines: decreased action of each specific drug

Anticonvulsants: decreased effects of anticonvulsant

Antidiabetics: decreased effects of antidiabetics

Barbiturates: decreased action of hydrocortisone

Diuretics: increased side effects

NSAIDs, salicylates: increased risk of GI bleeding

Drug/herb
Aloe, buckthorn, cascara sagrada, cat's claw, Chinese rhubarb, echinacea, senna, St. John's wort: increased hypokalemia

Aloe, licorice, perilla: increased corticosteroid effect

Drug/lab test
Increased: cholesterol, sodium, blood glucose, uric acid, calcium, urine glucose

Decreased: calcium, potassium, T_4, T_3, thyroid ^{131}I uptake test, urine 17-OHCS, 17-KS

False negative: skin allergy tests

NURSING CONSIDERATIONS
Assessment
• Monitor potassium, blood glucose, urine glucose while patient is on long-term therapy; hypokalemia and hyperglycemia may occur

• Monitor I&O ratio; be alert for decreasing urinary output and increasing edema; weigh daily; notify prescriber of weekly gain >5 lb or edema, hypertension, cardiac symptoms

• Monitor plasma cortisol levels during long-term therapy (normal level is 138-635 nmol/L when obtained at 8 AM); check adrenal function periodically for hypothalamic-pituitary-adrenal axis suppression

• Assess for infection: increased temp, WBC even after withdrawal of medication; product masks infection symptoms; if fever develops, product should be discontinued

• Check for potassium depletion: paresthesias, fatigue, nausea, vomiting, depression, polyuria, dysrhythmias, weakness

• Assess mental status: affect, mood, behavioral changes, aggression

• Check nasal passages during long-term treatment for changes in mucus (nasal)

• Assess for systemic absorption: increased temp, inflammation, irritation (topical)

Nursing diagnoses
• Infection, risk for (adverse reactions)
• Knowledge, deficient (teaching)
• Noncompliance (teaching) (topical/nasal preparation)

Implementation
PO route
• Give with food or milk to decrease GI symptoms
Rectal route
• Use applicator provided
• Clean applicator after each use
Topical route
• Apply only to affected areas; do not get in eyes
• Cleanse and dry area before applying medication, then cover with occlusive dressing (only if prescribed); seal to normal skin; change q12hr; systemic absorption may occur; use only on dermatoses; do not use on weeping, denuded, or infected area
• Use for a few days after area has cleared
• Store at room temperature
Nasal route
• Patient should clear nasal passages before administration; use decongestant if needed; shake inhaler, invert, tilt head backward, insert nozzle into nostril, away from septum; hold other nostril closed and depress activator, inhale through nose, exhale through mouth
IV route
• Give only sodium phosphate product **IV**; reconstitute with sol provided; give 100 mg over >1 min
• May be given by intermittent inf in compatible sol
• Give titrated dose; use lowest effective dosage

Sodium phosphate preparations
Syringe compatibilities: Fluconazole, fludarabine, metoclopramide

Adverse effects: *italic* = common, **bold** = life-threatening

Additive compatibilities: Amikacin, amphotericin B, bleomycin, cephapirin, metaraminol, sodium bicarbonate, verapamil

Y-site compatibilities: Allopurinol, amifostine, aztreonam, cefepime, cladribine, famotidine, filgrastim, fluconazole, fludarabine, granisetron, melphalan, ondansetron, paclitaxel, piperacillin/tazobactam, teniposide, thiotepa, vinorelbine

Sodium succinate preparations
Syringe compatibilities: Metoclopramide, thiopental

Y-site compatibilities: Acyclovir, allopurinol, amifostine, aminophylline, ampicillin, amphotericin B cholesteryl, inamrinone, amsacrine, atracurium, atropine, aztreonam, betamethasone, calcium gluconate, cefepime, cefmetazole, cephalothin, cephapirin, chlordiazepoxide, chlorproMAZINE, cisatracurium, cladribine, cyanocobalamin, cytarabine, dexamethasone, digoxin, diphenhydrAMINE, DOPamine, DOXOrubicin liposome, droperidol, edrophonium, enalaprilat, epinephrine, esmolol, conjugated estrogens, ethacrynate, famotidine, fentanyl, fentanyl/droperidol, filgrastim, fludarabine, fluorouracil, foscarnet, furosemide, gallium, granisetron, heparin, hydrALAZINE, regular insulin, isoproterenol, kanamycin, lidocaine, lorazepam, magnesium sulfate, melphalan, menadiol, meperidine, methicillin, methoxamine, methylergonovine, minocycline, morphine, neostigmine, norepinephrine, ondansetron, oxacillin, oxytocin, paclitaxel, pancuronium, penicillin G potassium, pentazocine, phytonadione, piperacillin/tazobactam, prednisoLONE, procainamide, prochlorperazine, propofol, propranolol, pyridostigmine, remifentanil, scopolamine, sodium bicarbonate, succinylcholine, tacrolimus, teniposide, theophylline, thiotepa, trimethaphan, trimethobenzamide, vecuronium, vinorelbine

Y-site incompatibilities: Diazepam, ergotamine tartrate, idarubicin, phenytoin, sargramostim

Additive compatibilities: Amikacin, aminophylline, amphotericin B, calcium chloride, calcium gluconate, cephalothin, cephapirin, chloramphenicol, clindamycin, cloxacillin, corticotropin, DAUNOrubicin, diphenhydrAMINE, DOPamine, erythromycin, floxacillin, lidocaine, magnesium sulfate, mephentermine, metronidazole/sodium bicarbonate, mitomycin, mitoxantrone, netilmicin, netilmicin/potassium chloride, norepinephrine, penicillin G potassium/sodium, piperacillin, polymyxin B, potassium chloride, sodium bicarbonate, theophylline, thiopental, vancomycin, verapamil, vit B/C

Additive incompatibilities: Bleomycin, DOXOrubicin

Patient/family education
- Teach patient all aspects of product usage, including cushingoid symptoms
- Advise patient to carry/wear emergency ID as corticosteroid user; not to discontinue abruptly; adrenal crisis can result
- Instruct patient to notify prescriber if therapeutic response decreases; dosage adjustment may be needed
- Instruct patient to notify prescriber of signs of infection
- Teach patient that product can mask infections and cause hypoglycemia (diabetic)
- Teach patient to avoid live-virus vaccines if using steroids long term
- Caution patient to avoid OTC products unless directed by prescriber: salicylates, alcohol in cough products, cold preparations
- Teach patient symptoms of adrenal insufficiency: nausea, anorexia, fatigue, dizziness, dyspnea, weakness, joint pain; and when to notify prescriber
- Advise patient that long-term therapy may be needed to resolve infection (1-2 mo depending on type of infection)

Nasal route
- Instruct patient to clear nasal passages if sneezing attack occurs, then repeat dose; to continue using product even if mild nasal bleeding occurs; bleeding is usually transient
- Teach method of instillation after providing written instruction from manufacturer on instillation

Evaluation
Positive therapeutic outcome
- Decrease in runny nose (nasal)
- Decreased inflammation
- Absence of severe itching, patches on skin, flaking (top)
- Decreased GI symptoms

---

hydrocortisone topical
See Appendix B

⚠ HIGH ALERT

hydromorphone (Rx)
(hye-droe-mor′fone)
Dilaudid, Dilaudid-HP, Hydromorphone HCl, Hydrostat IR, PMS Hydromorphone
Func. class.: Antitussive, opioid analgesic agonist
Chem. class.: Phenanthrene derivative, guaifenesin

Pregnancy category C

Controlled substance schedule II

Do not confuse:
hydromorphone/meperidine/morphine, Dilaudid/Demerol

Action: Inhibits ascending pain pathways in CNS, increases pain threshold, alters pain perception

Therapeutic outcome: Decreased cough, decreased pain

Uses: As an antitussive to suppress cough; moderate to severe pain

Dosage and routes
Antitussive
Adult: PO 1 mg q3-4hr prn
Child 6-12 yr: PO 0.5 mg q3-4hr
Geriatric: PO 1-2 mg q4-6hr

Available forms: Inj 1, 2, 4, 10 mg/ml; tabs 2, 4, 8 mg; oral sol 5 mg/5 ml; supp 3 mg

Adverse effects
CNS: Dizziness, drowsiness, *sedation, confusion,* headache, euphoria, mood changes, **seizures**
CV: Hypotension, bradycardia, palpitations, change in B/P, tachycardia, peripheral vasodilatation
EENT: Miosis, diplopia, blurred vision, tinnitus
GI: Nausea, constipation, vomiting, anorexia, dry mouth, cramps, paralytic ileus
GU: Increased urinary output, dysuria, urinary retention
INTEG: Urticaria, rash, flushing, bruising, diaphoresis, pruritus
RESP: **Respiratory depression,** dyspnea

Contraindications: Hypersensitivity

Precautions: Pregnancy C, breastfeeding, children <18 yr, increased ICP, addictive personality, renal/hepatic disease, MI (acute), severe heart disease, bowel impaction, abrupt discontinuation, COPD

Black Box Warning: Respiratory depression, opioid-naive patients, substance abuse

Pharmacokinetics
Absorption	Well absorbed (PO), complete (**IV**)
Distribution	Unknown; crosses placenta
Metabolism	Liver, extensively
Excretion	Kidneys
Half-life	2-3 hr

Pharmacodynamics
	PO/IM/SUBCUT	IV	RECT
Onset	15-30 min	10-15 min	15-30 min
Peak	30-60 min	15-30 min	30-90 min
Duration	4-5 hr	2-3 hr	4-5 hr

H

Interactions
Individual drugs
Alcohol: increased respiratory depression, hypotension, sedation
Drug classifications
Antipsychotics, opiates, sedative/hypnotics, skeletal muscle relaxants: increased effects
MAOIs: increased severe reactions
Drug/herb
Chamomile, hops, Jamaican dogwood, kava, lavender, mistletoe, nettle, pokeweed, poppy, senega, skullcap, St. John's wort, valerian: increased action
Corkwood: increased anticholinergic effect
Drug/lab test
Increased: amylase

NURSING CONSIDERATIONS
Assessment
• Assess pain control, sedation by scoring on 0-10 scale; around-the-clock dosing is best for pain control
• Monitor VS after parenteral route; note muscle rigidity; product history, renal, liver function tests; respiratory dysfunction: respiratory depression, character, rate, rhythm; notify prescriber if respirations are <10/min
• Monitor CNS changes: dizziness, drowsiness, hallucinations, euphoria, LOC, pupil reaction
• Monitor allergic reactions: rash, urticaria; bowel function, constipation

Nursing diagnoses
• Breathing pattern, ineffective (adverse reactions)
• Knowledge, deficient (teaching)
• Pain, acute (uses)
• Sensory perception, disturbed: visual, auditory (adverse reactions)

Implementation

- Give with antiemetic if nausea, vomiting occur
- Give when pain is beginning to return; determine dosage interval by patient response; continuous dosing of medication is more effective given prn; explain analgesic effect
- Withdraw medication slowly after long-term use to prevent withdrawal symptoms
- Store in light-resistant container at room temperature

PO route

- May be given with food or milk to lessen GI upset

IM/SUBCUT route

- Do not give if sol is cloudy or a precipitate has formed; rotate inj sites

IV route

- Give by direct **IV** after diluting with 5 ml or more of sterile water or 0.9% NaCl for inj
- Give slowly at 2 mg over 3-5 min or less through Y-connector or 3-way stopcock

Syringe compatibilities: Atropine, bupivacaine, ceftazidime, chlorproMAZINE, cimetidine, dimenhyDRINATE, diphenhydrAMINE, fentanyl, glycopyrrolate, haloperidol, hydrOXYzine, lorazepam, midazolam, pentazocaine, pentobarbital, prochlorperazine, promethazine, ranitidine, scopolamine, tetracaine, thiethylperazine, trimethobenzamide

Y-site compatibilities: Acyclovir, allopurinol, amifostine, amikacin, amsacrine, aztreonam, cefamandole, cefepime, cefmetazole, cefoperazone, cefotaxime, cefoxitin, ceftazidime, ceftizoxime, cefuroxime, cephalothin, cephapirin, chloramphenicol, cisplatin, cladribine, clindamycin, cyclophosphamide, cytarabine, diltiazem, DOBUTamine, DOPamine, DOXOrubicin, doxycycline, epinephrine, erythromycin lactobionate, famotidine, fentanyl, filgrastim, fludarabine, foscarnet, furosemide, gentamicin, granisetron, heparin, kanamycin, labetalol, lorazepam, magnesium sulfate, melphalan, methotrexate, metronidazole, mezlocillin, midazolam, milrinone, morphine, moxalactam, nafcillin, niCARdipine, nitroglycerin, norepinephrine, ondansetron, oxacillin, paclitaxel, penicillin G potassium, piperacillin, piperacillin/tazobactam, propofol, ranitidine, teniposide, thiotepa, ticarcillin, tobramycin, trimethoprim/sulfamethoxazole, vancomycin, vecuronium, vinorelbine

Y-site incompatibilities: Ampicillin, diazepam, minocycline, phenobarbital, phenytoin, sargramostim

Additive compatibilities: Bupivacaine, clonidine, fluorouracil, heparin, midazolam, ondansetron, potassium chloride, promethazine, verapamil, ziconotide

Additive incompatibilities: Sodium bicarbonate, thiopental

Solution compatibilities: D$_5$W, D$_5$/0.45% NaCl, D$_5$/0.9% NaCl, D$_5$/LR, D$_5$/Ringer's, 0.45% NaCl, 0.9% NaCl, Ringer's and LR

Patient/family education

- Instruct patient to report any symptoms of CNS changes, allergic reactions; to avoid CNS depressants: alcohol, sedative/hypnotics for at least 24 hr after taking this product
- Advise patient that dizziness, drowsiness, and confusion are common and to avoid getting up without assistance, driving, or other hazardous activities
- Discuss in detail all aspects of the product

Evaluation

Positive therapeutic outcome

- Decreased pain
- Decreased cough

Treatment of overdose: Naloxone HCl (Narcan) 0.2-0.8 **IV**, O$_2$, **IV** fluids, vasopressors

---

hydroxychloroquine (Rx)

(hye-drox-ee-klor'oh-kwin)
Plaquenil, Quineprox
Func. class.: Antimalarial, antirheumatic (DMARDs)
Chem. class.: 4-Aminoquinoline derivative

Pregnancy category C

Action: Inhibits parasite replications, transcription of DNA to RNA by forming complexes with DNA in parasite

Therapeutic outcome: Resolution of infection

Uses: Malaria caused by *Plasmodium vivax, P. malariae, P. ovale, P. falciparum* (some strains); LE, rheumatoid arthritis

Dosage and routes
Malaria
Adult: PO suppression or prevention 200 mg qwk, begin 1-2 wk before travel, continue 4 wk after returning; treatment 400 mg, then 200 mg at 6, 24, 48 hr after 1st dose
Child: PO suppression or prevention 5 mg/kg qwk, begin 1-2 wk before travel, continue 4 wk after returning; treatment 10 mg/kg, then 5 mg/kg at 6, 24, 48 hr after 1st dose

Lupus erythematosus
Adult: PO 400 mg daily-bid; length depends on patient response; maintenance 200-400 mg/day

Rheumatoid arthritis
Adult: PO 400-600 mg/day for 4-12 wk; then 200-300 mg/day after good response
Child: PO 3-5 mg/kg/day max 400 mg/day

Available forms: Tabs 200 mg

Adverse effects
CNS: Headache, stimulation, fatigue, irritability, **seizures**, bad dreams, dizziness, confusion, psychosis, decreased reflexes
CV: Hypotension, heart block, **asystole with syncope**
EENT: Blurred vision, corneal changes, retinal changes, difficulty focusing, tinnitus, vertigo, deafness, photophobia, corneal edema
GI: Nausea, vomiting, anorexia, diarrhea, cramps
HEMA: **Thrombocytopenia, agranulocytosis, leukopenia, aplastic anemia**
INTEG: Pruritus, pigmentation changes, skin eruptions, lichen planus–like eruptions, eczema, **exfoliative dermatitis**, alopecia, **Stevens-Johnson syndrome**

Contraindications: Hypersensitivity, retinal field changes

Black Box Warning: Children (long-term), ocular disease

Precautions: Pregnancy **C**, breastfeeding, blood dyscrasias, severe GI disease, neurologic disease, alcoholism, hepatic disease, G6PD deficiency, psoriasis, eczema

Pharmacokinetics
Absorption	Well absorbed
Distribution	Widely distributed, crosses placenta
Metabolism	Liver
Excretion	Urine/feces
Half-life	3-5 day

Pharmacodynamics
Onset	Rapid
Peak	1-2 hr
Duration	Days-weeks

Interactions
Individual products
Magnesium, aluminum products: decreased malarial action
Digoxin: increased levels
Rabies vaccine: increased antibody titer

NURSING CONSIDERATIONS
Assessment
- Assess for lupus erythematosus, malaria symptoms
- Assess for rheumatoid arthritis: pain, swelling, ROM, temp of joints
- Assess ophthalmic exam baseline, q6mo if long-term treatment or product dosage >150 mg/day
- Assess hepatic studies qwk: AST, ALT, bilirubin
- Assess blood studies: CBC, platelets; WBC, RBC, platelets may be decreased; if severe, product should be discontinued
- Assess for decreased reflexes: knee, ankle
- Assess ECG during therapy
- Assess for depression of T-waves, widening of QRS complex
- Assess allergic reactions: pruritus, rash, urticaria
- Assess blood dyscrasias: malaise, fever, bruising, bleeding (rare)
- Assess for ototoxicity (tinnitus, vertigo, change in hearing); audiometric testing should be done before, after treatment
- ⬥ Assess for toxicity: blurring vision, difficulty focusing, headache, dizziness, knee, ankle reflexes; product should be discontinued immediately

Nursing diagnoses
- Infection, risk for (uses)
- Knowledge, deficient (teaching)
- Pain, chronic (uses)

Implementation
- Give before or after meals with milk, at same time each day to maintain product level
- Tabs may be crushed and mixed with food, fluids
- Malaria prophylaxis should be started 2 wk prior to exposure and 4-6 wk after leaving exposure area
- Store in tight, light-resistant container at room temperature

Patient/family education
- Teach patient to use sunglasses in bright sunlight to decrease photophobia
- Teach patient that urine may turn rust or brown
- Teach patient to report hearing, visual problems, fever, fatigue, bruising, bleeding, which may indicate blood dyscrasias

Evaluation
Positive therapeutic outcome
- Decreased symptoms of malaria, LE, rheumatoid arthritis

Adverse effects: *italic* = common, **bold** = life-threatening

Treatment of overdose: Induce vomiting; gastric lavage; administer barbiturate (ultra–short-acting), vasopressor, ammonium chloride; tracheostomy may be necessary

---

hydroxyurea (Rx)
(hye-drox-ee-yoo-ree′ah)
Droxia, Hydrea
Func. class.: Antineoplastic, antimetabolite
Chem. class.: Synthetic urea analog

Pregnancy category D

Action: Acts by inhibiting DNA synthesis without interfering with RNA or protein synthesis; incorporates thymidine into DNA, causing direct damage to DNA strands; cell cycle specific (S phase)

Therapeutic outcome: Prevention of rapidly growing malignant cells

Uses: Melanoma, chronic myelogenous leukemia, recurrent or metastatic ovarian cancer, squamous cell carcinoma of the head and neck, sickle cell anemia, psoriasis

Dosage and routes
Solid tumors
Adult: PO 80 mg/kg as a single dose q3day or 20-30 mg/kg as a single dose daily

In combination with radiation
Adult: PO 80 mg/kg as a single dose q3day; should be started 7 days before irradiation

Resistant chronic myelogenous leukemia
Adult: PO 10-30 mg/kg/day as a single daily dose

Sickle cell anemia
Adult: PO 15 mg/kg/day, may increase by 5 mg/kg/day q12wk; max 35 mg/kg/day

Renal dose
Adult: CCr 10-50 ml/min dose 50%; CCr <10 ml/min PO dose 20%

Available forms: Caps 200, 300, 400, 500 mg

Adverse effects
CNS: Headache, confusion, hallucinations, dizziness, **seizures**
CV: Angina, ischemia
GI: Nausea, vomiting, anorexia, diarrhea, stomatitis, constipation, **hepatotoxicity**
GU: Increased BUN, uric acid, creatinine, temporary renal function impairment
HEMA: **Leukopenia, anemia, thrombocytopenia, megaloblastic erythropoiesis**
INTEG: Rash, urticaria, pruritus, dry skin, facial erythema

MISC: Fever, chills, malaise, secondary cancers, tumor lysis syndrome
META: Hyperphosphatemia, hyperuricemia, hypocalcemia

Contraindications: Pregnancy **D**, breastfeeding, hypersensitivity

Black Box Warning: Leukopenia (<2500/mm³), thrombocytopenia (<100,000/mm³), anemia (severe)

Precautions: Renal disease (severe)

Pharmacokinetics

Absorption	Well absorbed
Distribution	Crosses blood-brain barrier
Metabolism	Liver (50%)
Excretion	Kidneys, unchanged (50%), eliminated as CO_2
Half-life	Terminal 3.5-4.5 hr

Pharmacodynamics

Onset	Unknown
Peak	1-4 hr
Duration	Unknown

Interactions
Individual drugs
Radiation: increased toxicity
Drug classifications
Anticoagulants, NSAIDs: increased bleeding
Antineoplastics: increased toxicity
Drug/lab test
Increased: renal function tests

NURSING CONSIDERATIONS
Assessment
• Assess buccal cavity q8hr for dryness, sores or ulceration, white patches, oral pain, bleeding, dysphagia; obtain prescription for viscous lidocaine (Xylocaine)
• Assess symptoms indicating severe allergic reaction: rash, pruritus, urticaria, purpuric skin lesions, itching, flushing
• Monitor CBC, differential, platelet count weekly; withhold product if WBC is <2500/mm³ or platelet count is <100,000/mm³; notify prescriber of results if WBC <20,000/mm³, platelets <150,000/mm³
• Assess for increased uric acid levels, swelling, joint pain primarily in extremities; patient should be well hydrated to prevent urate deposits
• Monitor renal function studies: BUN, creatinine, serum uric acid, urine CCr before, during therapy; I&O ratio; report fall in urine output to <30 ml/hr

---

 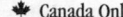

- Monitor temp (may indicate beginning of infection)
- Monitor liver function tests before, during therapy (bilirubin, AST, ALT, LDH) as needed or monthly
- Assess for bleeding: hematuria, stool guaiac, bruising or petechiae, mucosa or orifices q8hr; check for inflammation of mucosa, breaks in skin
⬥ Assess for tumor lysis syndrome

Nursing diagnoses
- Body image, disturbed (adverse reactions)
- Infection, risk for (adverse reactions)
- Injury, risk for (adverse reactions)
- Knowledge, deficient (teaching)

Implementation
- Do not crush or chew caps; for difficulty swallowing, caps can be opened and contents mixed with water
- Avoid contact with skin, very irritating; wash completely to remove
- Give fluids **IV** or PO before chemotherapy to hydrate patient
- Give antiemetic 30-60 min before giving product and prn to prevent vomiting; antibiotics for prophylaxis of infection
- Provide liquid diet: carbonated beverages; gelatin may be added if patient is not nauseated or vomiting

Patient/family education
- Advise patient that contraceptive measures are recommended during therapy
- Teach patient to avoid use of products containing aspirin or ibuprofen, razors, commercial mouthwash, since bleeding may occur; instruct patient to report symptoms of bleeding (hematuria, tarry stools)
- Teach patient to rinse mouth tid-qid with water, club soda; brush teeth bid-qid with soft brush or cotton-tipped applicators for stomatitis; use unwaxed dental floss
- Instruct patient to report signs of anemia (fatigue, headache, irritability, faintness, shortness of breath)
- Advise patient to report any changes in breathing or coughing even several mo after treatment; to avoid crowds and persons with respiratory tract or other infections
- Caution patient not to have any vaccinations without the advice of the prescriber, serious reactions can occur

Evaluation
Positive therapeutic outcome
- Prevention of rapid division of malignant cells

---

*hydrOXYzine (Rx)
(hye-drox'i-zeen)
ANX, Apo-hydroxyzine ✦, Atarax, hydroxyzine, Hyzine-50, Multi-pax ✦, Novohydroxyzine ✦, Vistaril
Func. class.: Antianxiety, sedative, hypnotic, antihistamine, antiemetic
Chem. class.: Piperazine derivative

Pregnancy category C

Do not confuse:
hydrOXYzine/hydrALAZINE, Atarax/amoxicillin/Ativan, Vistaril/Versed

Action: Depresses subcortical levels of CNS, including limbic system, reticular formation; anticholinergic, antiemetic, antihistaminic responses; competes with H_1-receptor sites

Therapeutic outcome: Absence of allergy symptoms, rhinitis, pruritus, absence of nausea/vomiting, sedation, absence of anxiety

Uses: Anxiety preoperatively; postoperatively to prevent nausea, vomiting; to potentiate opioid analgesics; sedation; pruritus; prevention of alcohol, product withdrawal

Dosage and routes
Anxiety
Adult: PO 25-100 mg tid qid, max 600 mg/day; IM 50-100 mg q4-6hr
Geriatric: PO max 50 mg/day
Child >6 yr: PO 50-100 mg/day in divided doses
Child <6 yr: PO 50 mg/day in divided doses

Alcohol withdrawal
Adult: IM 50-100 mg, then q4-6hr

Preoperatively/postoperatively
Adult: IM 25-100 mg q4-6hr
Child: IM 0.5-1.1 mg/kg q4-6hr

Pruritus
Adult: PO 25 mg tid-qid; IM 50-100 mg, then q4-6hr prn, switch to PO as soon as feasible
Geriatric: PO 10 mg tid-qid, max 50 mg/day
Child: PO 50-100 mg/day in divided doses; IM 0.5-1 mg/kg/dose q4-6hr prn, use PO when possible

Antiemetic
Adult: IM 25-100 mg/dose q4-6hr prn

Renal dose
Adult: PO CCr <50 ml/min reduce dose by 50%

Available forms: Tabs 10, 25, 50, 100 mg; caps 10, 25, 50, 100 mg; oral susp 5 mg/5 ml; inj 25, 50 mg/ml

Adverse effects: *italic* = common, **bold** = life-threatening

Adverse effects
CNS: *Dizziness, drowsiness,* confusion, headache, tremors, fatigue, depression, **seizures**
CV: Hypotension
GI: Dry mouth, nausea, diarrhea, increased appetite, weight gain

Contraindications: Pregnancy (1st trimester), breastfeeding, acute asthma, hypersensitivity to this product or cetirizine

Precautions: Pregnancy **C** (2nd/3rd trimesters), geriatric, debilitated patients, renal/hepatic disease, closed-angle glaucoma, COPD, prostatic hypertrophy, asthma

Pharmacokinetics

Absorption	Well absorbed
Distribution	Not known
Metabolism	Liver, completely
Excretion	Feces, urine, bile
Half-life	3 hr

Pharmacodynamics

	PO/IM
Onset	15-60 min
Peak	2-4 hr
Duration	4-6 hr

Interactions
Individual drugs
Alcohol: increased CNS depression
Atropine, disopyramide, haloperidol, quinidine: increased anticholinergic reactions
Drug classifications
Analgesics, barbiturates, CNS depressants, opiates, sedative/hypnotics: increased CNS depression
Antidepressants, antihistamines, MAOIs, phenothiazines: increased anticholinergic reactions
Drug/herb
Corkwood, henbane leaf, jimsonweed, scopolia: increased anticholinergic effect
Chamomile, cowslip, hops, Jamaican dogwood, khat, kava, Queen Anne's lace, senega, skullcap, valerian: increased sedative action

NURSING CONSIDERATIONS
Assessment
• Assess mental status: mood, sensorium, affect, behavior, increased sedation
• Assess respiratory status: rate, rhythm, increase in bronchial secretions, wheezing, chest tightness; provide fluids to 2 L/day to decrease secretion thickness

• Monitor I&O ratio: be alert for urinary retention, frequency, dysuria, especially in the geriatric; product should be discontinued if these occur
• Observe for drowsiness, dizziness
• Assess cough characteristics including type, frequency, thickness of secretions; evaluate response to this medication if using for cough

Nursing diagnoses
• Anxiety (uses)
• Injury, risk for (side effects)
• Knowledge, deficient (teaching)

Implementation
PO route
• Take 1 hr after or 2 hr before meals to facilitate absorption
• May crush tab if patient unable to swallow whole
• Give with meals if GI symptoms occur; absorption may be slightly decreased
• Caps may be opened and product mixed with food/fluids for patients with swallowing difficulties
IM route
• Give IM inj in large muscle mass; aspirate to prevent **IV** administration; use Z-track method; severe necrosis can result with improper technique; never give **IV**/SUBCUT
Syringe compatibilities: Atropine, atropine/meperidine, benzquinamide, bupivacaine, butorphanol, chlorproMAZINE, cimetidine, codeine, diphenhydrAMINE, doxapram, droperidol, fentanyl, fluphenazine, glycopyrrolate, hydromorphone, lidocaine, meperidine, meperidine/atropine, methotrimeprazine, metoclopramide, midazolam, morphine, nalbuphine, oxymorphone, pentazocine, perphenazine, procaine, prochlorperazine, promazine, promethazine, remifentanil, scopolamine, sufentanil, thiothixene
Syringe incompatibilities: Aminophylline, chloramphenicol, dimenhyDRINATE, heparin, penicillin G potassium, pentobarbital, phenobarbital, phenytoin
Additive compatibilities: Cisplatin, cyclophosphamide, cytarabine, dimenhyDRINATE, etoposide, lidocaine, mesna, methotrexate, nafcillin

Patient/family education
• Caution patient to avoid hazardous activities and activities requiring alertness, since dizziness may occur; instruct patient to request assistance with ambulation
• Advise patient to avoid alcohol, other CNS depressants including cough, cold preparations; CNS depression may occur

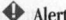 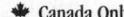

- Teach all aspects of product use; to notify prescriber if confusion, sedation, hypotension occur; to avoid driving and other hazardous activity if drowsiness occurs
- Caution patient not to exceed recommended dosage; dysrhythmias may occur
- Tell patient hard candy, gum, frequent rinsing of mouth may be used for dryness

Evaluation
Positive therapeutic outcome
- Absence of nausea, vomiting
- Decreased anxiety

Treatment of overdose: Lavage if orally ingested, VS, supportive care, **IV** norepinephrine for hypotension

---

Hylan G-F 20
Synvisc, Synvisc One
See Appendix A, Selected New Drugs

---

hyoscyamine (Rx)
(hye-oh-sye'a-meen)
Anaspaz, A-Spas S/L, Cystospaz, Donnamar, ED-SPAZ, Gastrosed, Levsin, Levsinex, NuLev Timecaps
Func. class.: Anticholinergic/antispasmodics
Chem. class.: Belladonna alkaloid

Pregnancy category C

Action: Inhibits muscarinic actions of acetylcholine at postganglionic parasympathetic neuroeffector sites, reduces rigidity, tremors, hyperhidrosis of parkinsonism

Therapeutic outcome: Absence of peptic ulcer after treatment

Uses: Treatment of peptic ulcer disease in combination with other products; other GI disorders, other spastic disorders, IBS, urinary incontinence

Dosage and routes
Adult: PO/SL 0.125-0.25 mg tid-qid before meals, at bedtime; TIME REL 0.375-0.75 mg q12hr; IM/SUBCUT/**IV** 0.25-0.5 mg q6hr
Geriatric: Max 1.5 mg/day in divided doses or max 4 biphasic tabs
Child 2-12 yr: PO individualized based on weight, max 0.75 mg/24 hr
Child <2 yr: PO individualized based on weight

Available forms: Tabs 0.125, 0.15 mg; time rel caps 0.375 mg; time rel tabs 0.375 ml; sol 0.125 mg/ml; elix 0.125 mg/ml; inj 0.5 mg/ml

Adverse effects
CNS: Confusion, stimulation in geriatric, headache, insomnia, dizziness, drowsiness, anxiety, weakness, hallucination
CV: Palpitations, tachycardia
EENT: Blurred vision, photophobia, mydriasis, cycloplegia, increased ocular tension
GI: Dry mouth, constipation, paralytic ileus, heartburn, nausea, vomiting, dysphagia, absence of taste
GU: Urinary hesitancy, retention, impotence
INTEG: Urticaria, rash, pruritus, anhidrosis, fever, allergic reactions

Contraindications: Hypersensitivity to anticholinergics, closed-angle glaucoma, GI obstruction, myasthenia gravis, paralytic ileus, GI atony, toxic megacolon, prostatic hypertrophy

Precautions: Pregnancy **C**, geriatric, hyperthyroidism, CAD, dysrhythmias, CHF, ulcerative colitis, hypertension, hiatal hernia, renal/hepatic disease, urinary retention

Pharmacokinetics	
Absorption	Well
Distribution	Cross blood-brain barrier, placenta
Metabolism	Liver
Excretion	Urine
Half-life	3½ hr

Pharmacodynamics		
	PO	IM/IV/SUBCUT
Onset	30 min	2-3 min
Peak	Unknown	Unknown
Duration	4-6 hr	4-6 hr

Interactions
Individual drugs
Amantidine: increased anticholinergic effect
Ketoconazole, levodopa: decreased effects
Drug classifications
Antacids: decreased hyoscyamine effect
Antidepressants (tricyclics), antihistamines, H₁, MAOIs: increased anticholinergic effect
Phenothiazines: decreased effect of phenothiazines
Drug/herb
Black catechu: increased constipation
Butterbur, jimsonweed: increased anticholinergic effect
Jaborandi tree, pill-bearing spurge: decreased anticholinergic effect

H

Adverse effects: *italic* = common, **bold** = life-threatening

NURSING CONSIDERATIONS
Assessment
- Monitor VS, cardiac status: checking for dysrhythmias, increased rate, palpitations
- Monitor I/O ratio; check for urinary retention or hesitancy
- Monitor GI complaints: pain, bleeding (frank or occult), nausea, vomiting, anorexia

Nursing diagnoses
- Constipation (adverse reactions)
- Injury, risk for (adverse reactions)
- Knowledge, deficient (teaching)

Implementation
- Do not break, crush, or chew time rel caps
- Give ½ hour before meals for better absorption
- Give decreased dose to geriatric patients; metabolism may be slowed
- Store in tight container protected from light

Patient/family education
- Teach patient to avoid driving, other hazardous activities until stabilized on medication
- Teach patient to avoid alcohol or other CNS depressants; will enhance sedating properties of this product
- Teach patient to avoid hot environments; heat stroke may occur; product suppresses perspiration
- Teach patient to use sunglasses when outside to prevent photophobia; may cause blurred vision
- Teach patient to use gum, hard candy, frequent rinsing of mouth for dryness of oral cavity
- Teach patient to increase fluids, bulk, exercise to decrease constipation

Evaluation
Positive therapeutic outcome
- Absence of epigastric pain, bleeding, nausea, vomiting

---

ibandronate (Rx)
(eye-ban′dro-nate)
Boniva
Func. class.: Bone-resorption inhibitor, electrolyte modifier
Chem. class.: Bisphosphonate
Pregnancy category C

Action: Inhibits bone resorption, apparently without inhibiting bone formation and mineralization; absorbs calcium phosphate crystals in bone and may directly block dissolution of hydroxyapatite crystals of bone; more potent than other products

Therapeutic outcome: Increased bone mineral density

Uses: Osteoporosis and prophylaxis

Unlabeled uses: Hypercalcemia, osteolytic metastases, Paget's disease

Dosage and routes
Postmenopausal osteoporosis
Adult: PO 2.5 mg/day or 150 mg qmo; **IV** BOL 3 mg q3mo

Prophylaxis
Adult: PO 2.5 mg/day or 150 mg qmo

Paget's disease (unlabeled)
Adult: **IV** 2 mg as a single dose

Osteolytic metastases (unlabeled)
Adult: **IV** 6 mg over 1 hr × 3 days, repeat q4wk

Hypercalcemia (unlabeled)
Adult: **IV** INF 2 mg over 2 hr

Renal dose
Adult: PO CCr <30 ml/min, avoid use

Available forms: Tabs 2.5, 150 mg; sol for inj 3 mg/ml

Adverse effects
CNS: Fever, insomnia, dizziness, headache
CV: Hypertension, **atrial fibrillation**
EENT: Ocular pain/inflammation, uveitis
GI: Constipation, nausea, vomiting, diarrhea, dyspepsia
INTEG: Rash, inj site reaction
META: Hypomagnesemia, hypophosphatemia, hypocalcemia, hypercholesterolemia
MS: Bone pain, myalgia, osteonecrosis of the jaw

Contraindications: Achalasia, esophageal stricture, hypocalcemia, intraarterial administration, renal failure, vitamin D deficiency, hypersensitivity to bisphosphonates

Precautions: Pregnancy **C**, breastfeeding, children, geriatric, anemia, chemotherapy, coagulopathy, dental disease, diabetes mellitus, dysphagia, GI/renal disease, GERD, hypertension, infection, multiple myeloma, phosphate hypersensitivity

Pharmacokinetics

Absorption	Poor
Distribution	Taken up primarily by bones, 86%-99% protein binding
Metabolism	Unknown
Excretion	Primarily by kidneys
Half-life	5-60 hr

 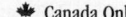

Pharmacodynamics

Onset	Unknown
Peak	0.5-2 hr
Duration	Up to 1 mo

Interactions
Individual drugs
Calcium, vitamin D: decreased ibandronate effect

CycloSPORINE, tacrolimus: possible increased neurotoxicity
Drug classifications
Aminoglycosides, NSAIDs, radiopaque contrast agents: possible increased neurotoxicity

Loop diuretics: increased hypocalcemia
Drug/food
• Do not take with food, calcium

NURSING CONSIDERATIONS
Assessment
• Assess for blood studies: electrolytes, Ca, P, Mg; creatinine/BUN
• Assess for atrial fibrillation
• Assess dental health; before dental extraction, give antiinfectives
• Assess for bone pain; use analgesics
• Monitor DEXA scan for bone mineral density

Nursing diagnoses
• Injury, risk for (uses)
• Knowledge, deficient (teaching)

Implementation
PO route
• Give early AM with a glass of water; if qmo, give on same day of each month
IV route
• Use single-dose prefilled syringe; discard unused portion, give over 15-30 sec
• Store at room temperature

Patient/family education
• Teach patient to report hypercalcemic relapse: nausea, vomiting, bone pain, thirst; unusual muscle twitching, muscle spasms, severe diarrhea, constipation
• Advise patient to continue with dietary recommendations, including calcium and vit D
• Instruct patient to obtain an analgesic from provider for bone pain
• Advise patient that if nausea/vomiting occur, small, frequent meals may help
• Teach patient to report vision symptoms: blurred vision, edema, inflammation; report to prescriber
• Teach to report if pregnancy is planned or suspected or if planning to breastfeed

• Encourage to exercise regularly, to stop smoking, and decrease alcohol
• Advise to take in AM at least 60 min before other meds, food, beverages
• Teach to sit upright ≥60 min after PO dose

Evaluation
Positive therapeutic outcome
• Increased bone mineral density

---

ibritumomab tiuxetan (Rx)
(ee-brit-u-moe′mab)
Zevalin
Func. class.: Radiopharmaceutical

Pregnancy category D

Action: High affinity for indium-111, yttrium-90; induces CD20$^+$ B-cell lines

Therapeutic outcome: Decrease in tumor size, spread of malignancy

Uses: Non-Hodgkin's lymphoma, B-cell NHL

Dosage and routes
Adult: Ritaximab 250 mg/m^2 given first; within 4 hr, give 5 mCi (1.6 mg total) over 10 min, then repeat 7-9 days later

Available forms: Inj 3.2 mg/2 ml

Adverse effects
CV: **Cardiac dysrhythmias**
GI: *Nausea, vomiting, anorexia,* abdominal pain, diarrhea
GU: **Renal failure**
HEMA: **Leukopenia, neutropenia, thrombocytopenia,** anemia
INTEG: *Irritation at site, rash,* **fatal mucocutaneous infections (rare)**
OTHER: Fever, chills, asthenia, headache, **angioedema,** hypotension, myalgia, **bronchospasm, hemorrhage,** infections, cough, dyspnea, dizziness, anxiety
SYST: **Stevens-Johnson syndrome, secondary malignancies (AML, MDS), fatal infections**

Contraindications: Pregnancy **D,** murine proteins, prior murine antibody exposure

Black Box Warning: Hypersensitivity to this agent, neutropenia, thrombocytopenia

Precautions: Breastfeeding, children, geriatric, cardiac conditions, immunizations after therapy

Black Box Warning: Altered biodistribution, infusion-related reaction

---

Adverse effects: *italic* = common, **bold** = life-threatening

Pharmacokinetics

Absorption	Unknown
Distribution	Unknown
Metabolism	Unknown
Excretion	Unknown
Half-life	30 hr

Pharmacodynamics
Unknown

NURSING CONSIDERATIONS
Assessment
• Assess for infection, murine antibody titers
 Assess for signs of fatal infusion reaction: hypoxia, pulmonary infiltrates, ARDS, MI, ventricular fibrillation, cardiogenic shock; most fatal infusion reactions occur with first infusion; potentially fatal
• Assess biodistribution: first image 2-24 hr, second image 48-72 hr, third image 90-120 hr (optimal)
• Assess for signs of severe mucocutaneous reactions: Stevens-Johnson syndrome, lichenoid dermatitis, toxic epidermal lysis; occur 1-13 wk after product was given
 Assess for tumor lysis syndrome: acute renal failure requiring hemodialysis, hyperkalemia, hypocalcemia, hyperuricemia, hyperphosphatemia
• Monitor CBC, differential, platelet count weekly; withhold product if WBC is <3500/mm^3 or platelet count <150,000/mm^3; notify prescriber of these results
• Monitor GI symptoms: frequency of stools
• Assess for signs of dehydration: rapid respirations, poor skin turgor, decreased urine output, dry skin, restlessness, weakness

Nursing diagnoses
• Infection, risk for (adverse reactions)
• Knowledge, deficient (teaching)
• Nutrition: less than body requirements, imbalanced (adverse reactions)

Implementation
• Do not use as BOL or **IV** direct
• Provide increased fluid intake to 2-3 L/day to prevent dehydration, unless contraindicated
IV infusion route
• See manufacturer's product labeling for preparation
• Have emergency equipment nearby with epinephrine, antihistamines, corticosteroids

Patient/family education
• Teach patient radiation safety precautions, disposal of body fluids
• Teach patient symptoms of infection
• Teach patient decreased blood count precautions
• Advise patient to report adverse reactions
• Advise patient to use contraception during and for 12 mo after therapy
• Teach patient neutropenia and bleeding precautions

Evaluation
Positive therapeutic outcome
• Improvement in blood counts
• Decreased evidence of disease

---

ibuprofen 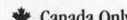 (OTC)
(eye-byoo-proe'fen)
Actiprofen 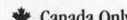, Advil, Advil Liqui-Gels, Advil Migraine, Apo-Ibuprofen 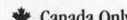, Bayer Select Ibuprofen Pain Relief, Caldolol, Children's Advil, Children's Motrin, Excedrin IB, Genpril, Haltran, ibuprofen, IBU-TAB, Infant's Motrin, Junior Strength Advil, Medipren, Menadol, Midol Maximum Strength Cramp Formula, Motrin, Motrin IB, Motrin Junior Strength, Motrin Migraine Pain, Novoprofen 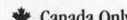, Nu-Ibuprofen, Nuprin, PediaCare Children's Fever, PediaCare Fever, Pediatric Advil Drops
Func. class.: Nonsteroidal antiinflammatory; nonopiate analgesic, antipyretic
Chem. class.: Propionic acid derivative

Pregnancy category B

Do not confuse:
Nuprin/Lupron

Action: Inhibits prostaglandin synthesis by decreasing enzyme needed for biosynthesis; analgesic, antiinflammatory, antipyretic

Therapeutic outcome: Decreased pain, inflammation, fever

Uses: Rheumatoid arthritis, osteoarthritis, primary dysmenorrhea, gout, dental pain, musculoskeletal disorders, fever, migraine

Dosage and routes
Self-treatment of minor aches/pain
Adult/adolescent: PO (OTC product) 200 mg q4-6hr, may increase to 400 mg q4-6hr; max 1200 mg/day

Analgesia
Adult: PO 200-400 mg q4-6hr; max 3.2 g/day; OTC use max 1200 mg/day
Child: PO 4-10 mg/kg/dose q6-8hr

 Alert   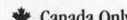 Canada Only   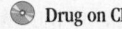 Drug on CD   * "Tall Man" lettering (See Preface)

Moderate-severe pain (hospitalized patients)
Adult: **IV** 400-800 mg q6hr as an adjunct to opiate agonist therapy

Dysmenorrhea
Adult: PO 400 mg q4hr; max 1200 mg/day

Antipyretic
Child 6 mo-12 yr: PO 5 mg/kg (temp <102.5° F or 39.2° C), 10 mg/kg (temp >102.5° F), may repeat q4-6hr; max 40 mg/kg/day

Antiinflammatory
Adult: PO 300-800 mg tid-qid; max 3.2 g/day
Child: PO 30-40 mg/kg/day in 3-4 divided doses; max 50 mg/kg/day

Patent ductus arteriosus (PDA) (Neoprofen)
Premature neonate ≤32 wk gestation who weighs 500-1500 g: **IV** 10 mg/kg initially, then if needed, 2 doses 5 mg/kg at 24 hr intervals; if oliguria occurs, hold dose

Available forms: Tabs 100, 200, 300, 400, 600, 800 mg; liqui-gel caps 200 mg; oral susp 100 mg/5 ml; liquid 100 mg/5 ml; chew tabs 50, 100 mg; drops 50 mg/1.25 ml; inj 10 mg/ml (NeoProfen); inj (Caldolor) 100 mg/ml

Adverse effects
CNS: Headache, dizziness, drowsiness, fatigue, tremors, confusion, insomnia, anxiety, depression
CV: Tachycardia, peripheral edema, palpitations, dysrhythmias, **CV thrombotic events, MI, stroke**
EENT: Tinnitus, hearing loss, blurred vision
GI: Nausea, anorexia, vomiting, diarrhea, jaundice, **hepatitis,** constipation, flatulence, cramps, dry mouth, peptic ulcer, **GI bleeding, ulceration, necrotizing enterocolitis, GI perforation**
GU: **Nephrotoxicity,** dysuria, hematuria, oliguria, azotemia
HEMA: **Blood dyscrasias,** increased bleeding time
INTEG: Purpura, rash, pruritus, sweating, urticaria, **necrotizing fasciitis**
SYST: **Anaphylaxis, Stevens-Johnson syndrome**

Contraindications: Avoid in 2nd/3rd trimester of pregnancy, hypersensitivity, asthma, severe renal/hepatic disease

Black Box Warning: Perioperative pain in CABG

Precautions: Pregnancy **B** (1st trimester), breastfeeding, children, geriatric, bleeding disorders, GI disorders, cardiac disorders, hypersensitivity to other antiinflammatory agents, CHF, CCr <25 ml/min

Black Box Warning: GI bleeding, MI, stroke

Pharmacokinetics
Absorption	Well absorbed
Distribution	Not known; crosses placenta
Metabolism	Liver, extensively
Excretion	Kidneys, unchanged (10%)
Half-life	1.8-2 hr

Pharmacodynamics
Onset	½ hr
Peak	1-2 hr
Duration	4-6 hr

Interactions
Individual drugs
Alcohol, aspirin: increased GI reactions
Aspirin: decreased ibuprofen action
Cefotetan, valproic acid, warfarin: increased risk of bleeding
CycloSPORINE, digoxin, lithium, methotrexate, probenecid: increased toxicity
Furosemide: decreased effect of furosemide
Insulin: increased hypoglycemia
Radiation: increased risk of blood dyscrasias
Drug classifications
Anticoagulants, antiplatelet agents, thrombolytics: increased risk of bleeding
Anticoagulants (oral): increased toxicity
Antidiabetics (oral): increased hypoglycemia
Antihypertensives: decreased effect of antihypertensives
Antineoplastics: increased risk of blood dyscrasias
Corticosteroids, NSAIDs: increased GI reactions
Diuretics: decreased effectiveness of diuretics (thiazides)
Drug/herb
Arginine, gossypol: increased gastric irritation
Arnica, bogbean, chamomile, chondroitin, clove, dong quai, fenugreek, feverfew, garlic, ginger, ginkgo, ginseng *(Panax):* increased risk of bleeding
Bearberry, bilberry: increased NSAIDs effect

NURSING CONSIDERATIONS
Assessment
- Assess for infection; may mask symptoms
- Assess pain: location, duration, type, intensity before dose, 1 hr after

Adverse effects: *italic* = common, **bold** = life-threatening

- Assess musculoskeletal status: ROM before dose, 1 hr after
- Monitor liver function tests: AST, ALT, bilirubin, creatinine if patient is on long-term therapy
- Monitor renal function tests: BUN, urine creatinine if patient is on long-term therapy
- Assess cardiac status: edema (peripheral), tachycardia, palpitations; monitor B/P, pulse for character, quality, rhythm
- Monitor blood studies: CBC, Hct, Hgb, pro-time if patient is on long-term therapy
- Check I&O ratio; decreasing output may indicate renal failure if patient is on long-term therapy
- Assess hepatotoxicity: dark urine, clay-colored stools, jaundice of skin and sclera, itching, abdominal pain, fever, diarrhea if patient is on long-term therapy
- Assess for history of peptic ulcer disorder; asthma, aspirin, hypersensitivity, check closely for hypersensitivity reactions
- Assess for allergic reactions: rash, urticaria; if these occur, product may have to be discontinued
- Assess for ototoxicity: tinnitus, ringing, roaring in ears; audiometric testing needed before, after long-term therapy
- Assess for visual changes: blurring, halos; may indicate corneal, retinal damage
- Identify prior product history; there are many product interactions
- Identify fever: length of time in evidence and related symptoms

Nursing diagnoses
- Injury, risk for (side effects)
- Knowledge, deficient (teaching)
- Mobility, impaired physical (uses)
- Pain, acute (uses)
- Pain, chronic (uses)

Implementation
PO route
- Administer to patient crushed or whole; 800-mg tab may be dissolved in water
- Give with food or milk to decrease gastric symptoms; give 2 hr before or 30 min after meals; absorption may be slowed
- Shake susp well before use

IV route
- Must be well hydrated prior to administration
- Dilute to ≤4 mg/ml (0.9% NaCl, LR, D₅); infuse over ≥30 min
- Discard unused portion

Patient/family education
- Teach patient to report any symptoms of hepatotoxicity, renal toxicity, visual changes, ototoxicity, allergic reactions, bleeding if patient is on long-term therapy
- Caution patient not to exceed recommended dosage; acute poisoning may result
- Advise patient to read label on other OTC products
- Inform patient that the therapeutic response takes 1 mo (arthritis)
- Caution patient to avoid alcohol ingestion, salicylates, NSAIDs; GI bleeding may occur
- Advise patient with allergies that allergic reactions may develop
- Advise patient to use sunscreen to prevent photosensitivity
- Advise to report use of this product to all health care providers

Evaluation
Positive therapeutic outcome
- Decreased pain
- Decreased inflammation
- Decreased fever
- Increased mobility

Treatment of overdose: Lavage, activated charcoal, induce diuresis

---

⚠ HIGH ALERT

ibutilide (Rx)
(eye-byoo'te-lide)
Corvert
Func. class.: Antidysrhythmic (Class III)

Pregnancy category C

Action: Prolongs duration of action potential and effective refractory period

Uses: For rapid conversion of atrial fibrillation/flutter occurring within 1 wk of coronary artery bypass or valve surgery

Dosage and routes
Atrial fibrillation/flutter
Adult: **IV** INF (≥60 kg) 1 vial (1 mg) given over 10 min, may repeat same dose in 10 min; **IV** INF (<60 kg) 0.01 mg/kg given over 10 min, may repeat same dose in 10 min

Atrial fibrillation/flutter after cardiac surgery
Adult ≥60 kg: **IV** INF 0.5 mg; may repeat 1 time
Adult <60 kg: **IV** INF 0.005 mg/kg; may repeat 1 time

Available forms: Inj 0.1 mg/ml

Adverse effects
CNS: Headache
CV: Hypotension, bradycardia, **sinus arrest, CHF, dysrhythmias,** hypertension, extrasystoles, ventricular tachycardia, bundle branch block, AV block, palpitations, supraventricular extrasystoles, syncope, **prolonged QT interval**
GI: Nausea

Contraindications: Hypersensitivity

Precautions: Pregnancy **C,** breastfeeding, children <18 yr, geriatric, sinus node dysfunction, 2nd- or 3rd-degree AV block, electrolyte imbalances, bradycardia, renal/hepatic disease, CHF

Black Box Warning: QT prolongation, torsades de pointes, ventricular arrhythmias, ventricular tachycardia

Pharmacokinetics
Absorption	Unknown
Distribution	Unknown
Metabolism	Liver
Excretion	Kidney
Half-life	6 hr

Pharmacodynamics
Unknown

Interactions
Individual drugs
Digoxin: masking of cardiotoxicity
Drug classifications
Antidepressants (tricyclics/tetracyclics): prodysrhythmia
Antihistamines, H₂-receptor antagonists, phenothiazines: increased prodysrhythmia
Class Ia antidysrhythmics (disopyramide, quinidine, procainamide), class III agents (amiodarone, sotalol): do not use within 5 hr of ibutilide
Drug/herb
Aconite: increased toxicity, death
Aloe, broom, buckthorn (chronic use), cascara sagrada (chronic use), Chinese rhubarb, figwort, fumitory, goldenseal, kudzu, licorice: increased effect
Coltsfoot: decreased effect
Horehound: increased serotonin effect

NURSING CONSIDERATIONS
Assessment
• Monitor I&O ratio; monitor electrolytes: potassium, sodium, chloride
• Monitor liver function tests: AST, ALT, bilirubin, alkaline phosphatase
• Monitor ECG continuously to determine product effectiveness; measure PR, QRS, QT intervals; check for PVCs, other dysrhythmias; monitor B/P continuously for hypo/hypertension; check for rebound hypertension after 1-2 hr; discontinue product when atrial fibrillation/flutter ceases
• Monitor for dehydration or hypovolemia
• Assess for CNS symptoms: confusion, psychosis, numbness, depression, involuntary movements; if these occur product should be discontinued
• Monitor cardiac rate, respiration; rate, rhythm, character, chest pain, ventricular tachycardia, supraventricular tachycardia or fibrillation

Nursing diagnoses
• Cardiac output, decreased (uses)
• Gas exchange, impaired (adverse reactions)
• Knowledge, deficient (teaching)

Implementation
IV route
• Give reduced dosage slowly with ECG monitoring only
• Give undiluted or diluted in 50 ml of 0.9% NaCl or D₅W (0.017 mg/ml), give over 10 min
• Solution is stable for 48 hr refrigerated or 24 hr at room temperature
• Do not admix with other solution, products

Patient/family education
• Instruct patient to report side effects immediately to prescriber

Evaluation
Positive therapeutic outcome
• Decrease in atrial fibrillation/flutter

❗ HIGH ALERT

idarubicin (Rx)
(eye-da-roo'bi-sin)
Idamycin, Idamycin PFS
Func. class.: Antineoplastic, antibiotic
Chem. class.: Anthracycline glycoside
Pregnancy category D

Do not confuse:
idarubicin/DOXOrubicin/DAUNOrubicin/epirubicin, Idamycin/Adriamycin

Action: Non–cell cycle specific; topoisomerase II inhibitor, a vesicant

Therapeutic outcome: Prevention of rapidly growing malignant cells

Uses: Used in combination with other antineoplastics for acute myelocytic leukemia in adults

Adverse effects: *italic* = common, **bold** = life-threatening

Unlabeled uses: Breast cancer, liquid tumors

Dosage and routes
Adult: **IV** 8-12 mg/m²/day × 3 days in combination with cytarabine (induction)

Renal/hepatic dose
Adult: **IV** if bilirubin is 2.6-5 mg/dl, give 50% of dose; if bilirubin >5 mg/dl, do not use; if CCr >2.5 mg/dl, give 50% of dose

Available forms: Inj 1 mg/ml

Adverse effects
CNS: Fever, chills, headache, **seizures**
CV: **Dysrhythmias, CHF, pericarditis, myocarditis,** peripheral edema, angina, **MI, myocardial toxicity**
GI: Nausea, vomiting, abdominal pain, mucositis, diarrhea, **hepatotoxicity**
GU: **Nephrotoxicity,** red urine
HEMA: **Thrombocytopenia, leukopenia, anemia**
INTEG: Rash, **extravasation,** dermatitis, reversible alopecia, urticaria, thrombophlebitis, tissue necrosis at inj site
SYST: **Infection,** tumor lysis syndrome

Contraindications: Pregnancy **D,** breastfeeding, hypersensitivity

Black Box Warning: Myelosuppression, bilirubin >5 mg/dl

Precautions: Children, gout, bone marrow depression, preexisting CV disease

Black Box Warning: Renal/hepatic disease, heart failure

Pharmacokinetics

Absorption	Complete bioavailability
Distribution	Rapidly distributed, protein binding 97%
Metabolism	Liver, extensively
Excretion	Bile
Half-life	22 hr

Pharmacodynamics
Unknown

Interactions
Individual drugs
Radiation: increased toxicity
Drug classifications
Antineoplastics: increased toxicity
Live virus vaccines: decreased antibody response
Drug/lab test
Increased: uric acid

NURSING CONSIDERATIONS
Assessment
• Assess for tumor lysis syndrome: hyperkalemia, hyperphosphatemia, hyperuricemia, hypocalcemia
• Assess symptoms indicating severe allergic reaction: rash, pruritus, urticaria, purpuric skin lesions, itching, flushing; product should be discontinued
• Assess for tachypnea, ECG changes, dyspnea, edema, fatigue
• Assess for cardiac toxicity: CHF, dysrhythmias, cardiomyopathy; cardiac studies should be done before and periodically during treatment; ECG, chest x-ray, MUGA
• Monitor CBC, differential, platelet count weekly; withhold product if WBC is <4000/mm³ or platelet count is <100,000/mm³; notify prescriber of results if WBC <20,000/mm³, platelets <150,000/mm³
• Monitor renal function studies: BUN, uric acid, urine CCr, electrolytes, before, during therapy
• Monitor temp (may indicate beginning of infection)
• Monitor liver function tests before, during therapy (bilirubin, AST, ALT, LDH) as needed or monthly; note jaundice of skin and sclera, dark urine, clay-colored stools, itchy skin, abdominal pain, fever, diarrhea; hepatoxicity can be severe
• Assess for bleeding: hematuria, stool guaiac, bruising or petechiae, mucosa or orifices, assess for inflammation of mucosa, breaks in skin
• Identify effects of alopecia on body image; discuss feelings about body changes
◆ Assess for local irritation, pain, burning at injection site, extravasation, a vesicant

Nursing diagnoses
• Body image, disturbed (adverse reactions)
• Cardiac output, decreased (adverse reactions)
• Infection, risk for (adverse reactions)
• Injury, risk for (adverse reactions)
• Knowledge, deficient (teaching)

Implementation
• Avoid contact with skin; very irritating; wash completely to remove
• Give fluids **IV** or PO before chemotherapy to hydrate patient
• Administer antiemetic 30-60 min before giving product and prn to prevent vomiting; administer antibiotics for prophylaxis of infection
• Give a liquid diet: carbonated beverages;

 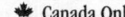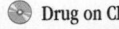

gelatin may be added if patient is not nauseated or vomiting

• Product should be prepared by experienced personnel using proper precautions (biologic cabinet, wearing gown, gloves, mask)

• Give after reconstituting 5-mg vial with 5 ml of 0.9% NaCl (1 mg/1 ml); give over 10-15 min through Y-tube or 3-way stopcock of inf of D₅ or 0.9% NaCl; discard unused portion

• Apply ice compress after stopping inf (extravasation)

• Store at room temperature for 3 days after reconstituting or 7 days refrigerated

Y-site compatibilities: Amifostine, amikacin, aztreonam, cimetidine, cladribine, cyclophosphamide, cytarabine, diphenhydrA-MINE, droperidol, erythromycin, filgrastim, granisetron, imipenem/cilastatin, magnesium sulfate, mannitol, melphalan, metoclopromide, potassium chloride, ranitidine, sargramostim, thiotepa, vinorelbine

Y-site incompatibilities: Acyclovir, ampicillin/sulbactam, cefazolin, ceftazidine, clindamycin, dexamethasone, etoposide, furosemide, gentamicin, hydrocortisone, lorazepam, meperidine, methotrexate, mezlocillin, sargramostim, sodium bicarbonate, vancomycin, vinCRIStine

Solution compatibilities: D₃.₃/0.3% NaCl, D₅/0.9% NaCl, D₅W, Ringer's, 0.9% NaCl, LR

Patient/family education

• Teach patient to avoid use of products containing aspirin or ibuprofen, razors, commercial mouthwash, since bleeding may occur; to report symptoms of bleeding (hematuria, tarry stools)

• Instruct patient to report signs of anemia (fatigue, headache, irritability, faintness, shortness of breath)

• Advise patient that hair may be lost during treatment; a wig or hairpiece may make patient feel better; new hair may be different in color, texture

• Teach patient to rinse mouth tid-qid with water, club soda; brush teeth bid-qid with soft brush or cotton-tipped applicators for stomatitis; use unwaxed dental floss

• Tell patient not to have any vaccinations without the advice of the prescriber; serious reactions can occur

• Advise patient that contraception is needed during treatment and for several mo after the completion of therapy

• Teach patient to report signs of CHF, cardiac toxicity, beginning infection

• Advise patient to avoid crowds, those with upper respiratory illness

• Advise that all body fluids change color

Evaluation

Positive therapeutic outcome

• Prevention of rapid division of malignant cells

⚠ HIGH ALERT

ifosfamide ⊛ (Rx)
(i-foss'fa-mide)

Ifex

Func. class.: Antineoplastic alkylating agent

Chem. class.: Nitrogen mustard

Pregnancy category D

Do not confuse:
ifosfamide/cyclophosphamide

Action: Alkylates DNA, RNA; inhibits enzymes that allow synthesis of amino acids in proteins; also responsible for cross-linking DNA strands; activity is not cell cycle stage specific

Therapeutic outcome: Prevention of rapidly growing malignant cells

Uses: Testicular cancer

Unlabeled uses: Soft-tissue sarcoma, Ewing's sarcoma, non Hodgkin's lymphoma, lung/pancreatic cancer, sarcoma

Dosage and routes

Adult: **IV** 1.2-2 g/m²/day × 5 days; repeat course q3wk; give with mesna

Renal dose

Adult: **IV** CCr 31-60 ml/min give 75% of dose; CCr 10-30 ml/min give 50% of dose; CCr <10 ml/min, do not give

Available forms: Inj 1, 3 g vials

Adverse effects

CNS: Facial paresthesia, fever, malaise, somnolence, confusion, depression, hallucinations, dizziness, disorientation, **seizures, coma,** cranial nerve dysfunction

GI: Nausea, vomiting, anorexia, **hepatotoxicity,** stomatitis, constipation, diarrhea

GU: **Hematuria, nephrotoxicity, hemorrhagic cystitis,** dysuria, urinary frequency

HEMA: **Thrombocytopenia, leukopenia, anemia**

INTEG: Dermatitis, alopecia, pain at inj site, hyperpigmentation

META: Metabolic acidosis

Adverse effects: *italic* = common, **bold** = life-threatening

Contraindications: Pregnancy **D**, hypersensitivity

Black Box Warning: Bone marrow suppression

Precautions: Renal/hepatic disease, breastfeeding, children

Black Box Warning: Coma, hemorrhagic cystitis

Pharmacokinetics

Absorption	Complete bioavailability
Distribution	Saturation at high dosages
Metabolism	Liver
Excretion	Breast milk
Half-life	15 hr, depends on dose

Pharmacodynamics

Unknown

Interactions
Individual drugs
Allopurinol: increased toxicity
Radiation: increased bone marrow suppression
Drug classifications
Anticoagulants, NSAIDs, salicylates, thrombolytics: increased bleeding risk
Antineoplastics: increased bone marrow suppression
CYP3A4 inducers, barbiturates: increased toxicity
CYP3A4 inhibitors: decreased ifosfamide effect
Live virus vaccines: decreased antibody response

NURSING CONSIDERATIONS
Assessment
 Monitor CBC, differential, platelet count weekly; withhold product if WBC is <2000 or platelet count is <50,000; notify prescriber of results if WBC <10,000/mm^3, platelets <100,000/mm^3, severe myelosuppression
• Monitor renal function studies: BUN, serum uric acid, urine CCr before, during therapy; I&O ratio; report fall in urine output of 30 ml/hr
• Monitor for cold, fever, sore throat (may indicate beginning of infection); identify edema in feet and joints, stomach pain, shaking; prescriber should be notified
• Assess for bleeding: hematuria, guaiac, bruising or petechiae, mucosa or orifices; no rec temp
• Monitor liver function tests before, during therapy (ALT, AST, LDH); jaundice of skin, sclera, dark urine, clay-colored stools, itching, abdominal pain, fever, diarrhea that may indicate liver involvement

Nursing diagnoses
• Body image, disturbed (adverse reactions)
• Infection, risk for (adverse reactions)
• Injury, risk for (adverse reactions)
• Knowledge, deficient (teaching)

Implementation
• Always give with mesna and increase fluids to 3 L/day to prevent ifosfamide-induced hemorrhagic cystitis
• Give ≥3 L/day fluids **IV** or PO before and after chemotherapy to hydrate patient to prevent hemorrhagic cystitis
• Give antiemetic 30-60 min before giving product and prn to prevent vomiting
• Provide liquid diet: carbonated beverages; gelatin may be added if patient is not nauseated or vomiting
• Give **IV** after diluting 1 g/20 ml of sterile or bacteriostatic water for inj with parabens or benzyl only; shake
• Give by intermittent inf after further diluting with D$_5$W, LR, 0.9% NaCl, sterile water for inj (1 g/20 ml = 50 mg/ml; 1 g/50 ml = 20 mg/ml; 1 g/200 ml = 5 mg/ml); give over ≥30 min; may also give as a cont inf over 72 hr
• Store powder at room temperature
Syringe compatibilities: Mesna
Y-site compatibilities: Allopurinol, amifostine, aztreonam, filgrastim, fludarabine, gallium, granisetron, melphalan, ondansetron, paclitaxel, piperacillin/tazobactam, propofol, sargramostim, teniposide, thiotepa, vinorelbine
Additive compatibilities: Carboplatin, cisplatin, etoposide, fluorouracil, mesna

Patient/family education
• Teach patient to avoid use of products containing aspirin or NSAIDs, razors, commercial mouthwash, since bleeding may occur; to report symptoms of bleeding (hematuria, tarry stools)
• Instruct patient to report signs of anemia (fatigue, headache, irritability, faintness, shortness of breath)
• Advise patient to report any changes in breathing or coughing even several mo after treatment; to avoid crowds and persons with respiratory tract or other infections
• Teach patient that hair loss is common; discuss the use of wigs or hairpieces; that hair may be a different texture when regrowth occurs
• Caution patient not to have any vaccinations without the advice of the prescriber; serious reactions can occur

 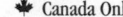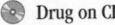

- Advise patient that contraception is needed during treatment and for several mo after completion of therapy
- Advise patient to report confusion, hallucinations, extreme drowsiness, numbness, tingling; avoid use of alcohol for ≥4 months after treatment

Evaluation
Positive therapeutic outcome
- Prevention of rapid division of malignant cells
- Absence of swelling at night
- Increased appetite, increased weight

---

iloperidone (Rx)
(ill-o-pehr'ih-dohn)
Fanapt
Func. class.: Antipsychotic
Chem. class.: Benzisoxazole derivative

Pregnancy category C

Action: Unknown; may be mediated through both dopamine type 2 (D2) and serotonin type 2 (5-HT2) antagonism

Therapeutic outcome: Decreased signs/symptoms of schizophrenia

Uses: Schizophrenia

Dosage and routes
Adult: PO 1 mg bid, day 1; 2 mg bid, day 2, 4 mg bid, day 3; 6 mg bid, day 4; 8 mg bid, day 5; 10 mg bid, day 6; 12 mg bid, day 7; max 24 mg/day in two divided doses

Available forms: Tabs 1, 2, 4, 6, 8, 10, 12 mg; titration pack

Adverse effects
CNS: EPS, pseudoparkinsonism, akathisia, dystonia, tardive dyskinesia; drowsiness, **seizures, neuroleptic malignant syndrome,** dizziness, delirium, depression, paranoia, fatigue, hostility, lethargy, restlessness, vertigo, tremor
CV: Orthostatic hypotension, **heart failure, AV block, QT prolongation,** tachycardia
EENT: Blurred vision, cataracts, nystagmus, tinnitus
GI: Nausea, vomiting, *anorexia, constipation,* jaundice, weight gain/loss, abdominal pain, stomatitis
GU: Hyperprolactinemia, urinary retention/incontinence, testicular pain, **renal failure**
MISC: **Renal artery occlusion**
HEMA: **Agranulocytosis, leukopenia, neutropenia**

Contraindications: Breastfeeding, hypersensitivity

Precautions: Pregnancy **C**, children, geriatric patients, renal/hepatic disease, breast cancer, Parkinson's disease, dementia with Lewy bodies, seizure disorder, QT prolongation, bundle branch block, acute MI, ambient temperature increase, AV block, stroke, substance abuse, suicidal ideation, tardive dyskinesia, torsades de pointes, blood dyscrasias

Pharmacokinetics
Absorption	Unknown
Distribution	Unknown
Metabolism	Extensively-liver (major metabolite) CYP2D6, CYP3A4
Excretion	Urine
Half-life	Terminal 18 hr extensive metabolizers; 33 hr poor metabolizers

Pharmacodynamics
Onset	Unknown
Peak	2-4 hr
Duration	Unknown

Interactions
Individual drugs
Alcohol: increased sedation
Bepridil, chloroquine, clarithromycin, droperidol, erythromycin, grepafloxacin, halofantrine, haloperidol, methadone, pentamidine, probucol, sparfloxacin: increased QT prolongation
Other CNS depressants: increased sedation
Drug classifications
CYP2D6, 3A4 inducers (carbamazepine, barbiturates, phenytoins, rifampin): decreased iloperidone action
CYP2D6, 3A4 inhibitors (SSRIs), other antipsychotics: increased EPS
Class IA/ III antidysrhythmics, some phenothiazines, β-agonists, local anesthetics, tricyclics: increased QT prolongation
Drug/herb
Betel palm, kava: increased EPS
Cola tree, hops, nettle, nutmeg: increased action
Kava: increased CNS depression
Drug/lab test
Increase: prolactin levels

NURSING CONSIDERATIONS
Assessment
- Assess mental status before initial administration

- Monitor swallowing of PO medication; check for hoarding or giving of medication to other patients
- Monitor I&O ratio; palpate bladder if urinary output is low
- Monitor bilirubin, CBC, hepatic studies qmo
- Monitor urinalysis before, during prolonged therapy
- Assess affect, orientation, LOC, reflexes, gait, coordination, sleep pattern disturbances
- Monitor B/P standing and lying; also pulse, respirations; take these q4hr during initial treatment; establish baseline before starting treatment; report drops of 30 mm Hg; watch for ECG changes; QT prolongation may occur
- Assess for dizziness, faintness, palpitations, tachycardia on rising
- Assess for EPS, including akathisia, tardive dyskinesia (bizarre movements of the jaw, mouth, tongue, extremities), pseudoparkinsonism (rigidity, tremors, pill rolling, shuffling gait)
- Assess for serious reactions in the geriatric patient: fatal pneumonia, heart failure, sudden death
- Assess for neuroleptic malignant syndrome: hyperthermia, increased CPK, altered mental status, muscle rigidity
- Assess skin turgor daily
- Assess for constipation, urinary retention daily; if these occur, increase bulk and water in diet
- Monitor weight gain, hyperglycemia, metabolic changes in diabetes

Nursing Diagnoses
- Thought processes, disturbed (uses)
- Coping, ineffective (uses)
- Noncompliance (teaching)
- Knowledge, deficient (teaching)

Implementation
- Give reduced dose in geriatric patients
- Give anticholinergic agent on order from prescriber, to be used for EPS
- Avoid use with CNS depressants
- Provide decreased stimulus by dimming lights, avoiding loud noises
- Provide supervised ambulation until patient is stabilized on medication; do not involve in strenuous exercise program because fainting is possible; patient should not stand still for a long time
- Give increased fluids to prevent constipation
- Provide sips of water, candy, gum for dry mouth
- Store in tight, light-resistant container (PO); unopened vials in refrigerator; protect from light; do not freeze

Patient/family education
- Teach that orthostatic hypotension may occur and to rise from sitting or lying position gradually
- Advise to avoid hot tubs, hot showers, tub baths; hypotension may occur
- Teach to avoid abrupt withdrawal of this product; EPS may result; product should be withdrawn slowly
- Teach to avoid OTC preparations (cough, hay fever, cold) unless approved by prescriber; serious product interactions may occur; avoid use of alcohol; increased drowsiness may occur
- Advise to avoid hazardous activities if drowsy or dizzy
- Teach compliance with product regimen
- Teach to report impaired vision, tremors, muscle twitching
- Teach that heat stroke may occur in hot weather; take extra precautions to stay cool
- Advise to use contraception; inform prescriber if pregnancy is planned or suspected

Evaluation
Positive therapeutic outcome
- Decrease in emotional excitement, hallucinations, delusions, paranoia; reorganization of patterns of thought, speech

Treatment of overdose: Lavage if orally ingested; provide airway; *do not induce vomiting*

---

imatinib (Rx)
(im-ah-tin'ib)
Gleevec
Func. class.: Antineoplastic—miscellaneous
Chem. class.: Protein-tyrosine kinase inhibitor
Pregnancy category D

Action: Inhibits Bcr-Abl tyrosine kinase created in chronic myeloid leukemia (CML)

Therapeutic outcome: Decreased tumor size, prevention of spread of cancer

Uses: Treatment of chronic myeloid leukemia (CML), Philadelphia chromosome positive in blast cell crisis or chronic failure after treatment failure with interferon alfa; gastrointestinal stromal tumors (GIST), positive for KIT; chronic eosinophilic leukemia, acute lymphocytic leukemia, dermatofibrosarcoma protuberans, myelodysplastic syndrome

Dosage and routes
CML, chronic phase
Adult: PO 400-600 mg/day
Child: PO 340 mg/m^2/day

CML, accelerated phase/blast crisis
Adult: PO 600-800 mg/day

GIST
Adult: PO 400 or 800 mg/day

Hepatic dose
Adult: PO total bilirubin 1.5-3 × ULN and any AST, decrease initial dose to 400 mg/day; total bilirubin >3 × ULN and any AST, decrease initial dose to 300 mg/day

Renal dose
Adult: PO CCr 40-59 ml/min, max 600 mg/day; CCr 20-39 ml/min decrease initial dose by 50%, max 400 mg/day; CCr <20 ml/min use with caution 100 mg/day

Available forms: Tabs 100, 400 mg

Adverse effects
CNS: **CNS hemorrhage,** headache, dizziness, insomnia
CV: **Hemorrhage, heart failure,** cardiac tamponade, hypereosinophilia, cardiac toxicity
EENT: Blurred vision, conjunctivitis
GI: *Nausea,* **hepatotoxicity,** *vomiting, dyspepsia,* **GI hemorrhage,** *anorexia,* abdominal pain, GI perforation, diarrhea
HEMA: **Neutropenia, thrombocytopenia, bleeding**
INTEG: *Rash, pruritus,* alopecia, photosensitivity
META: Edema, fluid retention, hypokalemia
MISC: Fatigue, epistaxis, pyrexia, night sweats, increased weight, flulike symptoms, hypothyroidism
MS: Cramps, pain, arthralgia, myalgia
RESP: Cough, dyspnea, nasopharyngitis, pneumonia, URI, pleural effusion, edema

Contraindications: Pregnancy **D,** hypersensitivity

Precautions: Breastfeeding, children, geriatric, cardiac/renal/hepatic disease

Pharmacokinetics
Absorption	Well absorbed, bound to plasma protein (98%)
Distribution	Unknown
Metabolism	Liver (metabolites)
Excretion	Feces, primarily (metabolites)
Half-life	18-40 hr

Pharmacodynamics
Onset	Unknown
Peak	2-4 hr
Duration	24 hr (imatinib), 40 hr (metabolite)

Interactions
Individual drugs
Acetaminophen: increased hepatotoxicity
CYP3A4 inducers (carbamazepine, dexamethasone, phenobarbital, phenytoin, rifampin): decreased imatinib concentrations
CYP3A4 inhibitors (clarithromycin, erythromycin, ketoconazole, itraconazole): increased imatinib concentrations
Simvastatin: increased plasma concentrations
Warfarin: increased plasma concentration of warfarin; avoid coadministration; use low-molecular-weight anticoagulants instead

Drug classifications
Calcium channel blockers, ergots: increased plasma concentrations

Drug/herb
St. John's wort: decreased imatinib concentration

NURSING CONSIDERATIONS
Assessment
• Assess ANC and platelets; in chronic phase if ANC <1 × 10^9/L and/or platelets <50 × 10^9/L, stop until ANC >1.5 × 10^9/L and platelets >75 × 10^9/L; in accelerated phase/blast crisis if ANC <0.5 × 10^9/L and/or platelets <10 × 10^9/L, determine whether cytopenia is related to biopsy/aspirate, if not, reduce dose by 200 mg, if cytopenia continues, reduce dose by another 100 mg; if cytopenia continues for 4 wk, stop product until ANC ≥1 × 10^9/L
• Assess for hepatotoxicity: monitor liver function tests before treatment, qmo
• Assess CBC, differential, platelet count weekly; withhold product if WBC is <3500/mm^3 or platelet count <100,000/mm^3; notify prescriber of these results
• Assess food preferences: list likes, dislikes
• Assess GI symptoms: frequency of stools
• Assess signs of fluid retention, edema: weigh, monitor lung sounds, assess for edema, 50-ml fluid retention is dose dependent

Nursing diagnoses
• Injury, risk for (side effects)
• Knowledge, deficient (teaching)

Implementation
• Give with meal and large glass of water to decrease GI symptoms
• Store at 25° C (77° F)

Adverse effects: *italic* = common, **bold** = life-threatening

Patient/family education
- Instruct patient to report adverse reactions immediately: shortness of breath, swelling of extremities, bleeding
- Teach patient reason for treatment, expected result
- Instruct patient to eat a nutritious diet with iron, vit supplement, low fiber, few dairy products

Evaluation
Positive therapeutic outcome
- Decrease in leukemic cells, size of tumors

---

imipenem/
cilastatin (Rx)
(i-me-pen'em sye-la-stat'in)
Primaxin IM, Primaxin IV
Func. class.: Antiinfective—miscellaneous penicillin
Chem. class.: Carbapenem

Pregnancy category   C

Do not confuse:
imipenem/Omnipen, Primaxin/Premarin

Action: Interferes with cell wall replication of susceptible organisms; osmotically unstable cell wall swells and bursts from osmotic pressure; addition of cilastatin prevents renal inactivation that occurs with high urinary concentrations of imipenem

Therapeutic outcome: Bactericidal action against the following: *Streptococcus pneumoniae,* group A β-hemolytic streptococci, *Staphylococcus aureus,* enterococcus; gram-negative organisms: *Klebsiella, Proteus, Escherichia coli, Acinetobacter, Serratia, Pseudomonas aeruginosa; Salmonella, Shigella, Haemophilus influenzae, Listeria* sp.

Uses: Serious infections caused by gram-positive or gram-negative organisms

Dosage and routes
Adult: **IV** 250-500 mg q6-8hr; severe infections may require 1 g q8hr; may give IM q12hr (total daily IM dose >1500 mg not recommended); mild to moderate infections
Child: **IV** 60-100 mg/kg/day in divided doses, max 4 g/day; IM 10-15 mg/kg q6hr

Renal dose
Adult: **IV** CCr 30-70 ml/min give 50% dose q6-8hr; CCr 20-30 ml/min give 40% of dose q8-12hr; CCr 5-20 ml/min give 25% of dose q12hr

Available forms: IV inj 250, 500; IM inj 500, 750 mg

Adverse effects
CNS: Fever, somnolence, **seizures,** confusion, dizziness, weakness, myoclonus
CV: Hypotension, palpitations, tachycardia
GI: Diarrhea, nausea, vomiting, **pseudomembranous colitis, hepatitis,** glossitis
GU: **Renal toxicity/failure**
HEMA: **Eosinophilia, neutropenia,** decreased Hgb, Hct
INTEG: Rash, urticaria, pruritus, pain at inj site, phlebitis, erythema at inj site
RESP: Chest discomfort, dyspnea, hyperventilation
SYST: **Anaphylaxis, Stevens-Johnson syndrome**

Contraindications: Hypersensitivity, IM hypersensitivity to local anesthetics of the amide type

Precautions: Pregnancy **C,** breastfeeding, children, geriatric, hypersensitivity to penicillins, seizure disorders, renal disease, head trauma

Pharmacokinetics

Absorption	Complete bioavailability (**IV**)
Distribution	Widely distributed; crosses placenta
Metabolism	Liver
Excretion	Kidneys, unchanged (70%-80%); breast milk
Half-life	1 hr; increased in renal disease

Pharmacodynamics

	IM	IV
Onset	Unknown	Rapid
Peak	Unknown	½-1 hr

Interactions
Individual drugs
Aminophylline, cycloSPORINE, ganciclovir, theophylline: increased risk of seizures
Probenecid: increased imipenem plasma levels
Valproic acid: decreased effect of valproic acid
Drug classifications
β-Lactam antibiotics: increased antagonistic effect
Drug/herb
Do not use acidophilus with antiinfectives; separate by several hours
Drug/lab test
Increased: AST, ALT, LDH, BUN, alkaline phosphatase, bilirubin, creatinine
False positive: direct Coombs' test

NURSING CONSIDERATIONS
Assessment
- Assess patient for previous penicillin sensitivity reaction, may have sensitivity to this product
- Assess patient for signs and symptoms of infection, including characteristics of wounds, sputum, urine, stool, WBC >10,000/mm³, fever; obtain baseline information before, during treatment
- Complete C&S tests before beginning product therapy to identify if correct treatment has been initiated
- Assess for allergic reactions, anaphylaxis: rash, urticaria, pruritus, chills, wheezing, laryngeal edema, fever, joint pain; angioedema may occur a few days after therapy begins; epiNEPHrine, resuscitation equipment should be available for anaphylactic reaction
- Identify urine output; if decreasing, notify prescriber (may indicate nephrotoxicity); also check for increased BUN, creatinine
- Monitor blood studies: AST, ALT, CBC, Hct, bilirubin, LDH, alkaline phosphatase, Coombs' test monthly if patient is on long-term therapy
- Monitor electrolytes: potassium, sodium, chloride monthly if patient is on long-term therapy
- Assess bowel pattern daily; if severe diarrhea occurs, product should be discontinued; may indicate pseudomembranous colitis
- Monitor for bleeding: ecchymosis, bleeding gums, hematuria, stool guaiac daily if patient is on long-term therapy
- Assess for overgrowth of infection: perineal itching, fever, malaise, redness, pain, swelling, drainage, rash, diarrhea, change in cough, sputum

Nursing diagnoses
- Diarrhea (adverse reactions)
- Infection, risk for (uses)
- Injury, risk for (adverse reactions)
- Knowledge, deficient (teaching)
- Noncompliance (teaching)

Implementation
IM route
- Reconstitute 500 mg/2 ml or 750 mg/3 ml lidocaine without epiNEPHrine; shake well, withdraw and administer entire vial; give inj deep in large muscle mass, massage
IV route
- Reconstitute each 250 or 500 mg/10 ml of compatible diluent; shake well; transfer the resulting susp to ≥100 ml of compatible diluent; add 10 ml to each previously reconstituted vial and shake to ensure all medication is used; transfer the remaining contents of the vial to the inf container; do not administer susp by direct inj; reconstitute 120-ml inf bottles/100 ml of a compatible diluent; shake until clear; may use 0.9% NaCl, D₅W, D₁₀W, D₅/0.2% sodium bicarbonate, D₅/0.9% NaCl, D₅/0.45% NaCl, D₅/0.225% NaCl, mannitol 2.5%, 5%, or 10%
- Give by intermittent inf: each 250- or 500-mg dose over 20-30 min, and each 1-g dose over 40-60 min; administer over 15-20 min for pediatric patients; do not administer direct **IV**; do not admix with other antibiotics

Y-site compatibilities: Acyclovir, amifostine, aztreonam, cefepime, diltiazem, famotidine, fludarabine, foscarnet, granisetron, idarubicin, regular insulin, melphalan, methotrexate, ondansetron, propofol, tacrolimus, teniposide, thiotepa, vinorelbine, zidovudine

Y-site incompatibilities: Fluconazole, meperidine, sargramostim

Additive incompatibilities: Fluconazole, meperidine, sargramostim

Patient/family education
- Teach patient to report sore throat, bruising, bleeding, joint pain; may indicate blood dyscrasias (rare)
- Advise patient to contact prescriber if vaginal itching, loose foul-smelling stools, furry tongue occur; may indicate superinfection
- Advise patient to notify prescriber of diarrhea with blood or pus; may indicate pseudomembranous colitis

Evaluation
Positive therapeutic outcome
- Absence of signs/symptoms of infection (WBC <10,000/mm³, temp WNL, absence of red, draining wounds)
- Reported improvement in symptoms of infection

Treatment of anaphylaxis: Epinephrine, antihistamines, resuscitate if needed

imipramine 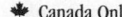 (Rx)
(im-ip'ra-meen)
Apo-Imipramine ✶, Imipramine HCl,
Impril ✶, Novo Pramine ✶, Tipramine,
Tofranil, Tofranil PM
Func. class.: Antidepressant, tricyclic
Chem. class.: Dibenzazepine, tertiary amine

Pregnancy category D

Do not confuse:
imipramine/desipramine

Action: Blocks reuptake of norepinephrine and serotonin into nerve endings, increasing action of norepinephrine and serotonin in nerve cells; has anticholinergic effects

Therapeutic outcome: Decreased symptoms of depression after 2-3 wk; decreased bedwetting in children

Uses: Depression, enuresis in children

Unlabeled uses: Chronic pain, migraine headaches, cluster headaches as adjunct, incontinence

Dosage and routes
Adult: PO 100 mg/day in divided doses; may increase by 25-50 mg up to 200 mg, max 300 mg/day; may give daily dose at bedtime
Geriatric: PO 25-50 mg at bedtime, may increase to 100 mg/day in divided doses
Child ≥6 yr (unlabeled): PO 1.5 mg/kg/day in divided doses; max 100 mg/day

Enuresis
Child 6-12 yr: PO 10-25 mg at bedtime, max 75 mg

Available forms: Tabs 10, 25, 50 mg; caps 75, 100, 125, 150 mg

Adverse effects
CNS: Dizziness, drowsiness, confusion, headache, anxiety, tremors, stimulation, weakness, insomnia, nightmares, EPS (geriatric), increased psychiatric symptoms, paresthesia, **seizures**
CV: Orthostatic hypotension, ECG changes, tachycardia, hypertension, palpitations, **dysrhythmias**
EENT: Blurred vision, tinnitus, mydriasis
GI: Diarrhea, dry mouth, nausea, vomiting, **paralytic ileus,** increased appetite, cramps, epigastric distress, jaundice, **hepatitis,** stomatitis, constipation, taste change
GU: Retention, **acute renal failure**
HEMA: **Agranulocytosis, thrombocytopenia, eosinophilia, leukopenia**
INTEG: Rash, urticaria, sweating, pruritus, photosensitivity, hyperpigmentation (rare)

Contraindications: Pregnancy **D**, hypersensitivity to tricyclics, recovery phase of MI, AV block, bundle-branch block, ileus, QT prolongation

Precautions: Suicidal patients, severe depression, increased intraocular pressure, closed-angle glaucoma, urinary retention, cardiac/hepatic disease, hyperthyroidism, electroshock therapy, elective surgery, breastfeeding, geriatric, seizure disorders, prostatic hypertrophy, MI

Black Box Warning: Children

Pharmacokinetics
Absorption	Well absorbed
Distribution	Widely distributed; crosses placenta
Metabolism	Liver, extensively
Excretion	Kidneys, breast milk
Half-life	6-20 hr

Pharmacodynamics
	PO	IM
Onset	1 hr	1 hr
Peak	Unknown	Unknown
Duration	Unknown	Unknown

Interactions
Individual drugs
Alcohol: increased effects
Clonidine: hyperpyretic crisis, seizures, hypertensive episode
Clonidine, guanethidine: decreased effects
Gatifloxacin, levofloxacin, moxifloxacin, ziprasidone: increased QT interval
Drug classifications
MAOIs: hyperpyretic crisis, hypertensive episode, seizures
Selective serotonin reuptake inhibitors: increased toxicity; avoid concurrent use
Sympathomimetics (direct acting [epinephrine]), barbiturates, benzodiazepines, CNS depressants: increased effects
Sympathomimetics (indirect acting [ephedrine]): decreased effects
Tricyclic antidepressants: increased QT interval
Drug/herb
Belladonna, corkwood, henbane, jimsonweed, scopolia: increased anticholinergic effect
Chamomile, hops, kava, lavender, skullcap, valerian: increased imipramine effect
SAM-e, St. John's wort: serotonin syndrome
Yohimbe: increased hypertension
Drug/lab test
Increased: serum bilirubin, blood glucose, alkaline phosphatase
Decreased: VMA, 5-HIAA, urinary catecholamines

NURSING CONSIDERATIONS
Assessment
- Monitor B/P (with patient lying, standing), pulse q4hr; if systolic B/P drops 20 mm Hg, hold product, notify prescriber; take vital signs q4hr in patients with CV disease
- Monitor blood studies: CBC, leukocytes, differential, cardiac enzymes if patient is receiving long-term therapy
- Monitor hepatic studies: AST, ALT, bilirubin
- Check weight weekly; appetite may increase with product
- Assess ECG for flattening of T wave, bundle branch block, AV block, dysrhythmias in cardiac patients
- Assess for EPS primarily in geriatric: rigidity, dystonia, akathisia
- Assess mental status: mood, sensorium, affect, suicidal tendencies; increase in psychiatric symptoms: depression, panic
- Monitor urinary retention, constipation; constipation is more likely to occur in children or geriatric
- ⭑ Assess for withdrawal symptoms: headache, nausea, vomiting, muscle pain, weakness, diarrhea, insomnia, restlessness; do not usually occur unless product was discontinued abruptly
- Identify alcohol consumption; if alcohol is consumed, hold dose until AM

Nursing diagnoses
- Coping, ineffective (uses)
- Injury, risk for (side effects)
- Knowledge, deficient (teaching)
- Noncompliance (teaching)

Implementation
PO route
- Do not break, crush, or chew caps
- Give with food or milk
- Store at room temperature; do not freeze

Syringe compatibilities: Doxapram
Y-site compatibilities: Cladribine

Patient/family education
- Teach patient that therapeutic effects may take 2-3 wk
- Teach patient to use caution in driving and other activities requiring alertness because of drowsiness, dizziness, blurred vision; to avoid rising quickly from sitting position, especially geriatric; orthostatic hypotension may occur
- Teach patient to avoid alcohol ingestion, other CNS depressants during treatment
- Teach patient not to discontinue medication quickly after long-term use: may cause nausea, headache, malaise
- Teach patient to wear sunscreen or large hat, since photosensitivity occurs

- Teach patient to increase fluids, bulk in diet if constipation, urinary retention occur, especially geriatric
- Teach patient to take gum, hard sugarless candy, or frequent sips of water for dry mouth

Evaluation
Positive therapeutic outcome
- Decreased depression
- Absence of suicidal thoughts
- Decreased enuresis in children
- Decreased pain

Treatment of overdose: ECG monitoring, lavage, activated charcoal, administer anticonvulsant

---

immune globulin IM (IMIG, IG1M) (Rx)
Bay Gam 15%, Flebogamma 5%, Flebogamma DIF 5%, Gammagard liquid 10%, Gamunex 10%, Privigen 10%, Vivaglobin

immune globulin IV (IGIV, IVIG) (Rx)
Carimune NF, Flebogamma 5%, Gamimune-N, Gammagard Liquid, Gammar-P IV, Gammagard S/D, Gammaplex, Gamune, Iveegram EN, Octagam, Panglobulin NF, Polygam S/D, Privigen

immune globulin SC (SCIG, IGSC) (Rx)
Bay Gam 15%, Flebogamma 5%, Flebogamma DIF, Gammagard Liquid 10%, Gamunex 10%, Privigen 10%, Vivaglobin
Func. class.: Immune serum
Chem. class.: IgG

Pregnancy category C

Do not confuse:
Iveegam/Invega

Action: Provides passive immunity to hepatitis A, measles, varicella, rubella, immune globulin deficiency; contains γ-globulin antibodies (IgG)

Therapeutic outcome: Absence of infection

Uses: Immunodeficiency syndrome, B-cell chronic lymphocytic leukemia, Kawasaki syndrome, bone marrow transplantation, pediatric HIV infection, agammaglobulinemia, hepatitis A, B exposure, measles exposure, measles vaccine complications, purpura, rubella exposure, chickenpox exposure, chronic inflammatory demyelinating polyneuropathy

Adverse effects: *italic* = common, **bold** = life-threatening

Unlabeled uses: IV posttransfusion purpura, Guillain-Barré syndrome

Dosage and routes
Immune globulin IM (IMIG, IGIM)
Hepatitis A prophylaxis
Adult, geriatric, adolescent, children, infant (unlabeled): IM 0.02 ml/kg for those who have not received Hepatitis A vaccine and have been exposed in the last 2 wk

Measles prophylaxis (exposed in last 6 days)
Adult: IM 0.25 ml/kg (immunocompetent)
Child (unlabeled): IM 0.5 ml/kg as a single dose, max 15 ml (immunocompromised)

Varicella prophylaxis
Adult: IM 0.6-1.2 ml/kg as soon as possible and if varicella-zoster immune globulin is not available

Rubella prophylaxis in exposed/ susceptible who will not consider a therapeutic abortion
Adult: Pregnant females IM 0.55 ml/kg

Immunoglobulin deficiency
Adult: 1.32 ml/kg, then 0.66 ml/kg (at least 100 mg/kg) q3-4wk

Immune globulin IV (IVIG, IGIV)
Primary immunodeficiency
Gammagard S/D
Adult/adolescent/child: **IV** 300-600 mg/kg q3-4wk

Polygam S/D
Adult/adolescent/child: **IV** 100 mg/kg qmo; initially 200-400 mg/kg may be used

Gammar-P IV
Adult: **IV** 200-400 mg/kg q3-4wk
Adolescent/child: **IV** 200 mg/kg q3-4wk

Gamunex
Adult/adolescent/child: **IV** INF 300-600 mg/kg (3-6 ml/kg) q3-4wk; initial infusion rate 1 mg/kg/min (max 8 mg/kg/min)

Iveegam EN
Adult/adolescent/child: **IV** 200 mg/kg qmo; max 800 mg/kg qmo

Panglobulin NF/Carimune NF
Adult/adolescent/child: **IV** 200 mg/kg qmo

Octagam/Gammagard Liquid/ Flebogamma 5%
Adult/adolescent/child: **IV** 300-600 mg/kg q3-4wk

Privigen
Adult/adolescent/child ≥3 yr: **IV** 200-800 mg q3-4wk

Idiopathic thrombocytopenic purpura (ITP)
Panglobulin NF/Carimune NF
Adult/child: **IV** 400 mg/kg qd × 2-5 days; in acute ITP of childhood, only 2 of the 5 days are needed if initial platelets are 30,000-50,000 mcl after 2 doses

Gammagard S/D/Polygam S/D
Adult/adolescent/child: **IV** 1000 mg/kg as a single dose; may give on alternate days for up to 3 doses

Gamunex
Adult/adolescent/child: **IV** INF total dose of 2000 mg/kg, divided as 1000 mg/kg (10 ml/kg) given on 2 consecutive days; initial rate is 1 mg/kg/min (max 8 mg/kg/min), if after 1st dose adequate platelets are observed after 24 hr, may withhold 2nd dose

Privigen
Adult/adolescent ≥15 yr: 1 g/kg/day × 2 days

Kawasaki disease
Iveegam EN
Child: **IV** 400 mg/kg qd × 4 consecutive days or a single dose of 2000 mg/kg over 10 hr; give with aspirin 100 mg/kg/day through 14th day of illness, then 3-5 mg/kg each day thereafter for 5 wk

Gammagard S/D/Polygam S/D
Infant/child: **IV** 1000 mg/kg (single dose) or 400 mg/kg/day × 4 days beginning within 7 days of fever onset, with aspirin 80-100 mg/kg/day × 4 divided doses

Immune globulin SC (SCIG/IGSC)
Adult/child >2 yr: SC infusion 100-200 mg/kg qwk; Vivaglobin brand of SGIG 160 mg IgG/ml, SC inj; max 15 ml for injection, given at max of 20 ml/hr

Available forms: IM (Bay Gam) inj 2, 10 ml vial; **IV** (Gamimune N, Venoglobulin-S) 5%, 10% sol; powder for inj (Carimune NF) 1-, 3-, 6-, 12-g vials; (Gammagard S/D) 50 mg protein/ml in 2.5-, 5-, 10-g vials; (Gammar-P IV) 1-, 2.5-, 5-, 10-g vials; (Iveegam) 500 mg, 1-, 2.5-, 5-g vials; (Panglobulin) 6-, 12-g vials; (Polygam S/D) 2.5-, 5-, 10-g vials; sol for inj (Gamunex) 1-, 2.5-, 5-, 10-, 20-g vials

Adverse effects
CNS: Headache, fatigue, malaise
GI: Abdominal pain
INTEG: Pain at inj site, rash, pruritus, chills
MS: Arthralgia, chest pain
SYST: Lymphadenopathy, **anaphylaxis**

Contraindications: Hypersensitivity
Precautions: Pregnancy **C**

Pharmacokinetics

Absorption	Well absorbed (IM); completely absorbed (**IV**)
Distribution	Rapidly
Metabolism	Liver, catabolism
Excretion	Kidneys
Half-life	3-4 wk

Pharmacodynamics

	IM	IV
Onset	Unknown	Rapid
Peak	Unknown	Unknown
Duration	Unknown	Unknown

Interactions
Drug classifications
Live virus vaccines: do not give within 3 mo
Drug/lab test
Interference: glucose testing system

NURSING CONSIDERATIONS
Assessment
• Assess for exposure date: this product should be given within 6 days of measles, 1 wk of hepatitis B, 14 days of hepatitis A; if the date of exposure is outside these limits, immune globulin will not be effective
• Monitor blood studies in leukemia, idiopathic thrombocytopenic purpura: WBCs (leukemia), platelets
• Identify the number of inj of this product patient has received; multiple inj may lead to sensitization (diaphoresis, fever, chills, malaise)
• Assess for anaphylaxis in patient receiving **IV** immune globulin: diaphoresis, flushing, nausea, vomiting, wheezing, difficulty breathing, hypotension, chest tightness, fever, weakness, sneezing, abdominal pain; VS should be monitored during inf and 1 hr after beginning inf; emergency equipment should be available with epinephrine and antihistamines to treat anaphylaxis

Nursing diagnoses
• Infection, risk for (uses)
• Knowledge, deficient (teaching)

Implementation
IM route
• Give IM (IGIM) inj in deltoid or anterolateral thigh in adults or anterolateral thigh in young children; if large amounts are given, several injections may be needed
• Do not give the IM preparation **IV**, SUBCUT, or intradermally

• Sol should be transparent and clear or slightly colored
IV route
• Warm to room temperature before administration (diluent, powder for inj)
• A transfer device is provided by manufacturer; this product should not be agitated or shaken
• Do not give the **IV** preparation SUBCUT, IM, or intradermally
• Check for adverse reaction during inf; stop inf if adverse reactions are present
Y-site compatibilities: Fluconazole, sargramostim
Gamimune N: Dilute **IV** with D₅; give 0.01 ml/kg/min; may increase to 0.02-0.04 ml/kg/min if no adverse reactions are present; may increase to 0.08 ml/kg/hr; sol should be refrigerated; do not freeze
Gammagard S/D: Reconstitute with sterile water for inj (50 mg protein/ml); give within 2 hr of reconstitution; give 0.5 ml/kg/hr; may increase to 4 ml/kg/hr if no adverse reactions occur; use inf set provided
Gammar-P IV: Give 0.01 ml/kg/min (50 mg/ml sol) over 15-30 min; may increase to 0.02 ml/kg/min; if adverse reactions are not present, may increase to 0.03-0.06 ml/kg/min; do not freeze; store at room temperature
Iveegam (5%): Give 1-2 ml/min; refrigerate, do not freeze
Sandoglobulin: IV diluted with provided diluent; give 0.5-1 ml/min over 15-30 min; may increase to 1.5-2.5 ml/min; other inf may be given 2-2.5 ml/min; store at room temperature
Venoglobulin I: Give 50 mg/ml sol 0.01-0.02 ml/kg/min over 30 min if no adverse reactions; increase 0.04 ml/kg/min; store at room temperature

Patient/family education
• Advise patient that passive immunity is temporary; explain reason for and expected results of this product
• Advise patient that pain and tenderness may occur at inj site

Evaluation
Positive therapeutic outcome
• Prevention of infection
• Increased platelets

Treatment of anaphylaxis: epinephrine, diphenhydrAMINE, O₂, vasopressors, corticosteroids

! HIGH ALERT

inamrinone ⊛ (Rx)
(in-am'rih-nohn)
Inocor
Func. class.: Inotropic agent
Chem. class.: Bipyrimidine derivative

Pregnancy category C

Do not confuse:
inamrinone/amiodarone

Action: Positive inotropic agent with vasodilator properties; reduces preload and afterload by direct relaxation of vascular smooth muscle; increases myocardial contractility

Therapeutic outcome: Increased inotropic effect resulting in increased cardiac output

Uses: Short-term management of CHF that has not responded to other medication (diuretics, other vasodilators); can be used with digoxin

Dosage and routes
Adult and child: **IV** BOL 0.75 mg/kg given over 2-3 min; start INF of 5-10 mcg/kg/min; may give another BOL 30 min after start of therapy, max 10 mg/kg total daily dose
Infants: **IV** 3-4.5 mg/kg in divided doses, then give by INF 10 mcg/kg/min
Neonates: **IV** 3-4.5 mg/kg in divided doses, then give by INF 3-5 mcg/kg/min

Renal dose
Adult: **IV** CCr >10 ml/min 100% of dose; CCr <10 ml/min 50%-75% of dose

Available forms: Inj 5 mg/ml

Adverse effects
CV: **Dysrhythmias,** *hypotension,* chest pain
GI: *Nausea, vomiting, anorexia,* abdominal pain, **hepatotoxicity (rare), ascites,** jaundice, hiccups
HEMA: **Thrombocytopenia**
INTEG: Allergic reactions, burning at inj site
RESP: Pleuritis, **pulmonary densities, hypoxemia**

Contraindications: Hypersensitivity to this product or bisulfites, severe aortic disease, severe pulmonic valvular disease, acute MI

Precautions: Pregnancy **C,** breastfeeding, children, geriatric, renal/hepatic disease, atrial flutter/fibrillation, asthma

Pharmacokinetics

Absorption	Complete bioavailability
Distribution	Unknown
Metabolism	Liver, 50%
Excretion	Kidney, metabolites (60%-90%)
Half-life	4-6 hr, increased in CHF

Pharmacodynamics

Onset	2-5 min
Peak	10 min
Duration	Variable

Interactions
Individual drugs
Disopyramide: excessive hypotension
Drug classifications
Antihypertensives: excessive hypotension
Cardiac glycosides: increased additive effect
Drug/herb
Aloe, buckthorn, cascara sagrada, senna: increased inamrinone action
Drug/lab test
Increased: hepatic enzymes
Decreased: potassium

NURSING CONSIDERATIONS
Assessment
• Monitor manifestations of hypokalemia: *RENAL:* acidic urine, reduced urine, osmolality, nocturia; *CV:* hypotension, broad T-wave, U-wave, ectopy, tachycardia, weak pulse; *NEURO:* muscle weakness, altered LOC, drowsiness, apathy, lethargy, confusion, depression; *GI:* anorexia, nausea, cramps, constipation, distention, paralytic ileus; *RESP:* hypoventilation, respiratory muscle weakness
• Assess fluid volume status: CVP in geriatric, I&O ratio and record, weight, distended red veins, crackles in lung, color, quality, and specific gravity of urine, skin turgor, adequacy of pulses, moist mucous membranes, bilateral lung sounds, peripheral pitting edema; dehydration symptoms of decreasing output, thirst, hypotension, dry mouth, and mucous membranes should be reported
• Monitor electrolytes: potassium, sodium, calcium, magnesium; also include BUN, blood pH, ABGs
• Monitor B/P and pulse, PCWP, CVP, index, often during inf; if B/P drops 30 mm Hg, stop inf and call prescriber
• Monitor ALT, AST, bilirubin daily; if these are elevated, hepatotoxicity is suspected
◆ If platelets are <150,000/mm³, product is usually discontinued and another product started
• Assess for extravasation: change site q48hr

Nursing diagnoses
- Cardiac output, decreased (uses)
- Fluid volume, excess (uses)
- Knowledge, deficient (teaching)

Implementation
- Patients with low potassium levels (hypokalemia) should receive potassium supplements before inamrinone administration
- Administer potassium supplements if ordered for potassium levels <3.0 mg/dl; correct before using inamrinone

IV route
- Do not mix directly with dextrose sol; chemical reaction occurs over 24 hr; precipitate forms if inamrinone and furosemide come in contact

IV, direct route
- May inject into running dextrose inf through Y-connector or directly into tubing; may give undiluted over 2-3 min or dilute with 0.9%, 0.45% NaCl to concentration of 1-3 mg/ml; run at prescribed rate by cont inf; another loading dose may be given in 30 min

Continous IV route
- Give after diluting with 0.9% or 0.45% NaCl (1-3 mg/ml); do not dilute with dextrose sol; decomposition of product will occur; use inf pump; use sol within 24 hr of dilution; titrate to patient response

Syringe compatibilities: Propranolol, verapamil

Y-site compatibilities: Aminophylline, atropine, bretylium, calcium chloride, cimetidine, cisatracurium, digoxin, DOBUTamine, DOPamine, epinephrine, famotidine, hydrocortisone, isoproterenol, lidocaine, metaraminol, methylPREDNISolone, nitroglycerin, nitroprusside, norepinephrine, phenylephrine, potassium chloride, procainamide, propranolol, remifentanil, verapamil

Y-site incompatibilities: Furosemide, inamrinone, sodium bicarbonate

Patient/family education
- Teach patient reason for medication and expected results
- Instruct patient to make position changes slowly; orthostatic hypotension may occur
- Teach patient signs and symptoms of hypersensitivity reactions and hypokalemia
- Advise patient that burning may occur at **IV** site

Evaluation
Positive therapeutic outcome
- Increased cardiac output
- Decreased PCWP, adequate CVP
- Decreased dyspnea, fatigue, edema, ECG

Treatment of overdose: Discontinue product, support circulation

---

indapamide (Rx)
(in-dap'a-mide)
indapamide, Lozide ✦
Func. class.: Diuretic, thiazide-like, antihypertensive
Chem. class.: Thiazide-like sulfonamide derivative

Pregnancy category B

Action: Acts on proximal section of distal renal tubule by inhibiting reabsorption of sodium, may act by direct vasodilatation caused by blocking of calcium channels

Therapeutic outcome: Decreased B/P, decreased edema in lung tissues, peripherally

Uses: Edema of CHF, hypertension, diuresis

Dosage and routes
Edema
Adult: PO 2.5 mg/day in AM; may be increased to 5 mg/day if needed

Antihypertensive
Adult: PO 1.25-5 mg/day; may increase to 5 mg/day over 8 wks

Available forms: Tabs 1.25, 2.5 mg

Adverse effects
CNS: Depression, *headache, dizziness, fatigue, weakness, nervousness, agitation,* extremity numbness
CV: Orthostatic hypotension, palpitations, volume depletion, PVCs, dysrhythmias, vasculitis
EENT: Blurred vision, nasal congestion, increased intraocular pressure
ELECT: Hypokalemia, hypercalcemia, hyponatremia, hypochloremic alkalosis, hypomagnesemia, hyperuricemia, hyperglycemia
GI: Nausea, vomiting, anorexia, constipation, diarrhea, cramps, abdominal pain, dry mouth
GU: Frequency, polyuria, nocturia, impotence
INTEG: Rash, *pruritus*
MS: Cramps

Contraindications: Hypersensitivity, anuria, hepatic coma

Precautions: Pregnancy **B,** breastfeeding, hypokalemia, severe renal disease, hepatic disease, ascites, dehydration, CCr <25 ml/min (not effective)

Pharmacokinetics	
Absorption	Well absorbed
Distribution	Widely distributed
Metabolism	Liver; 7%
Excretion	Unchanged (urine)
Half-life	14-18 hr

Pharmacodynamics	
Onset	1-2 hr
Peak	2 hr
Duration	Up to 36 hr

Interactions
Individual drugs
Amphotericin B: decreased potassium
Cholestyramine, colestipol: decreased absorption
Diazoxide: hyperglycemia
Digoxin, lithium: increased toxicity
Indomethacin: decreased hypotensive effect
Drug classifications
Anticoagulants, antidiabetics, antigout agents: decreased effects
Diuretics (other), steroids: decreased potassium
Muscle relaxants, steroids: increased toxicity
NSAIDs: decreased hypotensive effects
Drug/herb
Aloe, buckthorn, cascara sagrada, Chinese cucumber, licorice, senna: increased hypokalemia
Aloe, cucumber, dandelion, horsetail, pumpkin, Queen Anne's lace: increased diuretic effect
St. John's wort: severe photosensitivity
Drug/lab test
Increased: calcium, parathyroid test, glucose, uric acid

NURSING CONSIDERATIONS
Assessment
• Check for rashes, temp elevation daily
• Monitor patients that receive cardiac glycosides for increased hypokalemia, toxicity
• Monitor manifestations of hypokalemia: acidic or reduced urine, osmolality, nocturia; hypotension, broad T-wave, U-wave, ectopy, tachycardia, weak pulse; muscle weakness, altered LOC, drowsiness, apathy, lethargy, confusion, depression; anorexia, nausea, cramps, constipation, distention, paralytic ileus; hypoventilation, respiratory muscle weakness
• Monitor for manifestations of hypomagnesemia: agitation, muscle twitching, paresthesias, hyperactive reflexes, positive Babinski reflex, dysphagia, nystagmus, seizures, tetany; nausea, vomiting, diarrhea, anorexia, abdominal distention; ectopy, tachycardia, broad, flat- or inverted T-waves, depressed ST segment, prolonged QT interval, decreased cardiac output, hypotension
• Monitor for manifestations of hyponatremia: increased B/P, cold, clammy skin, hypo/hypervolemia; anorexia, nausea, vomiting, diarrhea, abdominal cramps; lethargy, increased ICP, confusion, headache, seizures, coma, fatigue, tremors, hyperreflexia
• Monitor for manifestations of hyperchloremia: weakness, lethargy, coma, deep rapid breathing
• Assess fluid volume status: I&O ratios and record, weight, distended red veins, crackles in lung, color, quality and specific gravity of urine, skin turgor, adequacy of pulses, moist mucous membranes, bilateral lung sounds, peripheral pitting edema; dehydration symptoms of decreasing output, thirst, hypotension, dry mouth and mucous membranes should be reported
• Monitor electrolytes: potassium, sodium, calcium, magnesium; also include BUN, blood pH, ABGs, uric acid, CBC, blood glucose
• Assess B/P before, during therapy with patient lying, standing, and sitting as appropriate; orthostatic hypotension can occur rapidly

Nursing diagnoses
• Fluid volume, deficient (side effects)
• Fluid volume, excess (uses)
• Knowledge, deficient (teaching)
• Urinary elimination, impaired (side effect)

Implementation
• Give in AM to avoid interference with sleep
• Provide potassium replacement if potassium level is <3.0 mg/dl; give whole
• Give with food and milk if nausea occurs, absorption may be increased

Patient/family education
• Teach patient to take the medication early in the day to prevent nocturia
• Instruct the patient to take with food or milk if GI symptoms of nausea and anorexia occur
• Teach patient to maintain weekly record of weight and notify prescriber of weight loss >5 lb
• Caution the patient that this product causes a loss of potassium, so food rich in potassium should be added to the diet; refer to a dietitian for assistance in planning
• Caution the patient to rise slowly from sitting or reclining positions, not to exercise in hot weather or stand for prolonged periods, since

orthostatic hypotension will be enhanced; lie down if dizziness occurs
• Teach patient not to use alcohol or any OTC medications without prescriber's approval; serious product reactions may occur
• Emphasize the need to contact prescriber immediately if muscle cramps, weakness, nausea, dizziness, or numbness occur
• Teach patient to take own B/P and pulse and record findings
• Teach patient to continue taking medication even if feeling better; this product controls symptoms but does not cure the condition
• Advise the patient with hypertension to continue other medical treatment (exercise, weight loss, relaxation techniques, cessation of smoking)

Evaluation
Positive therapeutic outcome
• Decreased edema
• Decreased B/P
• Increased diuresis

Treatment of overdose: Lavage, monitor electrolytes, administer **IV** fluids, monitor hydration, CV, renal status

indinavir (Rx)
(en-den'a-veer)
Crixivan
Func. class.: Antiretroviral
Chem. class.: Protease inhibitor
Pregnancy category C

Do not confuse:
idinavir/Denavir

Action: Inhibits HIV-1 protease; this prevents maturation of the infectious virus

Therapeutic outcome: Decreased signs/symptoms of HIV-1 infection

Uses: HIV-1 in combination with other antiretrovirals

Unlabeled uses: Prevention of HIV-1 after exposure

Dosage and routes
Adult: PO 800 mg q8hr; 400 mg bid with ritonavir 400 mg bid; or 800 mg bid with ritonavir 100-200 mg bid; decrease dose to 600 mg bid when given with lopinavir, ritonavir

Hepatic dose
Adult: PO 600 mg q8hr

Available forms: Caps 100, 200, 333, 400 mg

Adverse effects
CNS: Headache, insomnia, dizziness, somnolence
GI: Diarrhea, abdominal pain, nausea, vomiting, anorexia, dry mouth
GU: Nephrolithiasis
INTEG: Rash
MISC: Asthenia, **insulin-resistant hyperglycemia,** hyperlipidemia, **ketoacidosis,** lipodystrophy
MS: Pain

Contraindications: Hypersensitivity, breastfeeding

Precautions: Pregnancy **C,** children, renal/hepatic disease, history of renal stones, diabetes, hypercholesterolemia, hemophilia

Pharmacokinetics
Absorption	Unknown
Distribution	Unknown
Metabolism	60% protein binding; liver
Excretion	20% unchanged, urine
Half-life	Terminal 1-2 hr

Pharmacodynamics
Unknown

Interactions
Individual drugs
Clarithromycin, zidovudine: increased levels of both products
Isoniazid: increased isoniazid level
Midazolam, rifampin, triazolam: increased life-threatening dysrhythmias
Drug classifications
Anticonvulsants: decreased effect of both products
CYP3A4 inducers (barbiturates, carbamazepine, efavirenz, fluconazole, modafinil, nevirapine, non-nucleoside reverse transcriptase inhibitors, phenytoin, rifamycins): decreased indinavir levels
CYP3A4 inhibitors (aprepitant, azole antifungals, delavirdine, itraconazole, ketoconazole, nefazodone, protease inhibitors, verapamil); phosphotriesterases: increased indinavir levels
CYP3A4 substrates (azole antifungals, benzodiazepines, calcium channel blockers, immunosuppressants, macrolides, sildenafil, SSRIs, statins, tadalafil, vardenafil): decreased effect of these substrates
Ergots: increased life-threatening dysrhythmias
Oral contraceptives: increased levels of oral contraceptives
Statins (atorvastatin, lovastatin, simvastatin): increased myopathy

Adverse effects: *italic* = common, **bold** = life-threatening

Drug/herb
St. John's wort: decreased indinavir level, avoid use

Drug/food
High fat, high protein, grapefruit juice: decreased absorption

Drug/lab test
Increased: AST, ALT, amylase, total bilirubin

NURSING CONSIDERATIONS
Assessment
• Assess for lower back, flank pain, indicates kidney stones
• Monitor signs of infection, anemia
• Monitor liver studies: ALT, AST; total bilirubin, amylase; all may be elevated
• Determine the presence of other STDs
• Assess bowel pattern before, during treatment; if severe abdominal pain with bleeding occurs, product should be discontinued; monitor hydration
• Assess skin eruptions: rash, urticaria, itching
• Assess allergies before treatment, reaction of each medication; place allergies on chart
• Monitor viral load CD4 during treatment

Nursing diagnoses
• Infection, risk for (uses)
• Knowledge, deficient (teaching)

Implementation
• Do not break, crush, or chew caps
• Give with water, 1 hr before or 2 hr after meals; may be given with other liquids or small meal; do not give with high-fat, high-protein meals
• Give in equal intervals around the clock
• Dosage adjustment will need to be considered when given with efavirenz
• Give water to 1.5 L/day minimum, to prevent nephrolithiasis

Patient/family education
• Advise to take as prescribed; if dose is missed, take as soon as remembered up to 1 hr before next dose; do not double dose
• Advise that product must be taken in equal intervals around the clock to maintain blood levels for duration of therapy
• Instruct patient to increase fluids to prevent kidney stones; if stone formation occurs, treatment may need to be interrupted
• Inform patient that product does not cure AIDS, controls symptoms only; not to donate blood
• Advise patient that hyperglycemia may occur; watch for symptoms (thirst, hunger, dry, itchy skin); notify prescriber

Evaluation
Positive therapeutic outcome
• Decreased signs/symptoms of infection, HIV

---

indomethacin (Rx)
(in-doe-meth'a-sin)
Apo-Indomethacin ❧, Indameth ❧, Indocid ❧, Indocin, Indocin IV, Indocin PDA ❧, Indocin SR, indomethacin, Indomethacin Extended-Release, Indomethacin SR, Novomethacin ❧, Nu-Indo ❧
Func. class.: NSAID (nonsteroidal antiinflammatory), antirheumatic
Chem. class.: Propionic acid derivative

Pregnancy category
B (1st trimester),
D (2nd/3rd trimesters)

Action: Inhibits prostaglandin synthesis by decreasing enzyme needed for biosynthesis; analgesic, antiinflammatory, antipyretic

Therapeutic outcome: Decreased pain, inflammation; closure of patent ductus arteriosus (premature infants)

Uses: Rheumatoid arthritis, ankylosing spondylitis, osteoarthritis, bursitis, tendinitis, acute gouty arthritis; closure of patent ductus arteriosus in premature infants (**IV**)

Dosage and routes
Arthritis/antiinflammatory
Adult: PO 25-50 mg bid-qid, max 200 mg/day; SUS REL 75 mg daily; may increase to 75 mg bid

Acute gouty arthritis
Adult: PO 100 mg initially, then 50 mg tid; use only for acute attack, then reduce dosage

Patent ductus arteriosus
Longer or repeated treatment courses may be necessary for very premature infants
Infant <2 days: IV 0.2 mg/kg, then 0.1 mg/kg × 2 doses after 12, 24 hr
Infant 2-7 days: IV 0.2 mg/kg, then 0.2 mg/kg × 2 doses after 12, 24 hr
Infant >7 days: IV 0.2 mg/kg, then 0.25 mg/kg × 2 doses after 12, 24 hr

Available forms: Caps 25, 50 mg; sus rel caps 75 mg; oral susp 5 mg/ml; rectal supp 50 mg; inj 1-mg vials

Adverse effects
CNS: Dizziness, drowsiness, fatigue, tremors, confusion, insomnia, anxiety, depression, *headache*

CV: Tachycardia, peripheral edema, palpitations, dysrhythmias, hypertension, **CV thrombotic events, MI, stroke**

EENT: Tinnitus, hearing loss, blurred vision

GI: Nausea, anorexia, *vomiting,* diarrhea, jaundice, **cholestatic hepatitis,** *constipation,* flatulence, cramps, dry mouth, peptic ulcer, **ulceration, perforation, GI bleeding**

GU: **Nephrotoxicity (dysuria, hematuria, oliguria, azotemia)**

HEMA: **Blood dyscrasias,** prolonged bleeding

INTEG: Purpura, rash, pruritus, sweating

Contraindications: Pregnancy **D** (3rd trimester) hypersensitivity, asthma, ulcer disease, neonates, aortic coarctation, bleeding, salicylate/NSAID hypersensitivity

Black Box Warning: Perioperative pain in CABG

Precautions: Pregnancy **B** (1st trimester), breastfeeding, children, bleeding disorders, GI disorders, cardiac disorders, asthma, diabetes, acute bronchospasm, ulcerative colitis, seizures, Parkinson's disease, renal/hepatic disease, depression

Black Box Warning: Stroke, GI bleeding, MI

Pharmacokinetics

Absorption	Well absorbed (PO); erratic (RECT); complete (**IV**)
Distribution	Crosses blood-brain barrier; placenta, 99% plasma protein binding
Metabolism	Liver, extensively
Excretion	Breast milk
Half-life	4.5 hr

Pharmacodynamics

	PO	PO–EXT REL	IV
Onset	1-2 hr	½ hr	2 day
Peak	3 hr	Unknown	Unknown
Duration	4-6 hr	4-6 hr	Unknown

Interactions
Individual drugs

Abciximab, aspirin, cefamandole, cefoperazone, cefotetan, clopidogrel, eptifibatide, plicamycin, ticlodipine, tirofiban, valproic acid: increased bleeding risk

CycloSPORINE, lithium, methotrexate, probenecid, zidovudine: increased toxicity

Digoxin, penicillamine, phenyton: increased effect of each specific product

Drug classifications

Aminoglycosides: increased effects of aminoglycosides

Anticoagulants, SNRIs, SSRIs, thrombolytics: increased risk of bleeding

Antihypertensives: decreased effect of antihypertensives

Diuretics (potassium sparing): increased hyperkalemia

Drug/herb

Anise, arnica, bogbean, chamomile, chondroitin, clove, dong quai, feverfew, garlic, ginger, ginkgo, ginseng *(Panax):* increased bleeding risk

Arginine, gossypol: increased gastric irritation

Bearberry, bilberry: increased NSAIDs effect

NURSING CONSIDERATIONS
Assessment
- Assess for patent ductus arteriosus: respiratory rate, character, heart sounds
- Assess for joint pain (duration, intensity, ROM), baseline and during treatment
- Assess for confusion, mood changes, hallucinations, especially in geriatric
- Assess renal, liver, blood studies: BUN, creatinine, AST, ALT, Hgb before treatment, periodically thereafter; if renal function decreases, do not give subsequent doses
- Assess for cardiac disease, CV, thrombotic events (MI, stroke) prior to administration

Nursing diagnoses
- Knowledge, deficient (teaching)
- Mobility, impaired physical (uses)
- Pain, acute (uses)
- Pain, chronic (uses)

Implementation
PO route
- Swallow sus rel cap whole; do not break, crush, or chew sus rel cap
- Give with food or milk to decrease gastric symptoms and prevent ulceration
- Shake susp; do not mix with other liquids

Rectal route
- Have patient retain rect supp for 1 hr after insertion

IV route
- Give after diluting 1-2 mg/ml or more normal saline or sterile water for inj without preservative; give over 5-10 sec to avoid dramatic shift in cerebral blood flow; avoid extravasation

Y-site compatibilities: Furosemide, insulin (regular), potassium chloride, sodium bicarbonate, sodium nitroprusside

Patient/family education
- Advise patient to report change in vision, blurring, rash, tinnitus, black stools

Adverse effects: *italic* = common, **bold** = life-threatening

- Tell patient not to use for any other condition than prescribed
- Advise patient to avoid use with OTC medications for pain unless approved by prescriber, to report use to all providers
- Advise patient to avoid hazardous activities, since dizziness or drowsiness can occur
- Instruct patient to use sunscreen to prevent photosensitivity

Evaluation
Positive therapeutic outcome
- Decreased stiffness
- Increased joint mobility
- Decreased pain

---

infliximab (Rx)
(in-fliks'ih-mab)
Remicade
Func. class.: Monoclonal antibody

Pregnancy category B

Action: Monoclonal antibody that neutralizes the activity of tumor necrosis factor α (TNFα) that has been found in Crohn's disease; decreased infiltration of inflammatory cells

Therapeutic outcome: Decreased cramping and blood in stools

Uses: Crohn's disease, fistulizing, moderate-severe; rheumatoid arthritis given with methotrexate, plaque psoriasis, ankylosing spondylitis, ulcerative colitis, psoriatic arthritis, psoriasis

Unlabeled uses: Behçet syndrome, uveitis, juvenile arthritis

Dosage and routes
Crohn's disease (moderate-severe/fistulizing)
Adult: **IV** INF 5 mg/kg initially, then repeat dose 2, 6 wk, 8 wk thereafter, may increase to 10 mg/kg if needed

Rheumatoid arthritis
Adult: **IV** 3 mg/kg initially, and 2, 6 wk and q8wk thereafter, given with methotrexate

Available forms: Powder for inj 100 mg

Adverse effects
CNS: Headache, dizziness, depression, vertigo, fatigue, anxiety, fever, **seizures,** *chills, flulike symptoms,* demyelinating disease
CV: Chest pain, hypo/hypertension, tachycardia, **CHF, acute coronary syndrome**

GI: Nausea, vomiting, abdominal pain, stomatitis, constipation, dyspepsia, flatulence
GU: Dysuria, frequency
HEMA: **Anemia, leukopenia, thrombocytopenia, pancytopenia**
INTEG: Rash, dermatitis, urticaria, dry skin, sweating, flushing, hematoma, pruritus, keratoderma blennorrhagicum
MS: Myalgia, back pain, arthralgia
RESP: URI, pharyngitis, bronchitis, cough, dyspnea, sinusitis
SYST: **Anaphylaxis, fatal infections, sepsis, malignancies, immunogenicity, Stevens-Johnson syndrome, toxic epidermal necrolysis**

Contraindications: Hypersensitivity to murines, moderate to severe CHF (NYHA class III/IV)

Precautions: Pregnancy **B,** breastfeeding, children, geriatric, COPD, hepatotoxicity, hematologic abnormalities

Black Box Warning: Infection, neoplastic disease, TB

Pharmacokinetics
Absorption	Unknown
Distribution	Vascular compartment
Metabolism	Unknown
Excretion	Unknown
Half-life	9½ days

Pharmacodynamics
Unknown

Interactions
Drug classifications
Live virus vaccines: do not administer live vaccines concurrently

NURSING CONSIDERATIONS
Assessment
- Assess GI symptoms: nausea, vomiting, abdominal pain
- Take periodic blood counts: CBC
- Assess CV status: B/P, pulse, chest pain
◆ Assess for allergic reaction, anaphylaxis: rash, dermatitis, urticaria, fever, chills, dyspnea, hypotension; discontinue if severe; administer epinephrine, corticosteroids, antihistamines; assess for allergy to murine proteins before starting therapy
- Fatal infections: discontinue if infection occurs, do not administer to patients with active infections

• Identify TB before beginning treatment; a TB test should be obtained; if present, TB should be treated prior to receiving infliximab

Nursing diagnoses
• Diarrhea (uses)
• Injury, risk for (uses)
• Knowledge, deficient (teaching)

Implementation
IV inf route
• Administer immediately after reconstitution; reconstitute each vial with 10 ml of sterile water for inj, further dilute total dose/250 ml of 0.9% NaCl inj to a total conc of between 0.4 and 4 mg/ml; use 21-G or smaller needle for reconstitution, direct sterile water at glass wall of vial, gently swirl
• Give over ≥2 hr, use polyethylene-lined inf with in-line, sterile, low-protein-bind filter
• Do not admix
• Provide refrigerated storage, do not freeze

Patient/family education
• Teach patient not to breastfeed while taking this product
• Advise patient to notify prescriber of GI symptoms, hypersensitivity reactions
• Advise patient not to operate machinery or drive if dizziness, vertigo occurs

Evaluation
Positive therapeutic outcome
• Absence of blood in stool
• Reported improvement in comfort
• Weight gain

! HIGH ALERT

INSULINS

RAPID ACTING
insulin glulisine (Rx)
Apidra
insulin aspart (Rx)
Novolog, Novolog Flexpen, Novolog PenFill
insulin lispro (Rx)
Humalog

SHORT ACTING
insulin, regular 🕲 (OTC)
Humulin R ✣, Novolin R, Novolin R PenFill, Novolin R Prefilled
insulin, regular concentrated (Rx)
regular (concentrated)

INTERMEDIATE ACTING
insulin, isophane suspension (NPH) 🕲 (OTC)
Humulin N, Novolin N, Novolin N PenFill, Novolin N Prefilled

LONG ACTING
insulin detemir (Rx)
Levemir
insulin glargine (Rx)
Lantus

MIXTURES
insulin, isophane suspension and regular insulin (Rx)
Humulin 70/30, Humalin 30/70 ✣, Novolin 70/30, Novolin 70/30 PenFill, Novolin 70/30 Prefilled, Novolin ge 30/70 ✣
isophane insulin suspension (NPH) and insulin mixtures (Rx)
Humulin 50/50
insulin lispro mixture (Rx)
Humalog Mix 75/25
insulin aspart mixture (Rx)
Novolog 70/30
Func. class.: Antidiabetic, pancreatic hormone
Chem. class.: Modified structures of endogenous human insulin

Pregnancy category B, C

Do not confuse:
Lantus/lente, Novolin 70/30 PenFill/Novolin 70/30 Prefilled

Action: Decreases blood glucose; by transport of glucose into cells and the conversion of

---

Adverse effects: *italic* = common, **bold** = life-threatening

glucose to glycogen, indirectly increases blood pyruvate and lactate, decreases phosphate and potassium; insulin may be human (processed by recombinant DNA technologies)

Therapeutic outcome: Decreased blood glucose levels in diabetes mellitus

Uses: Type 1 diabetes mellitus, type 2 diabetes mellitus, gestational diabetes, insulin lispro may be used in combination with sulfonylureas in children >3 yr

Dosage and routes
Insulin glulisine
Adult/adolescent/child ≥4 yr: SUBCUT dosage individualized, give within 15 min before or 20 min after starting a meal
Adult: **IV** dilute to 1 unit/ml in INF systems with 0.9% NaCl, using PVC Viaflex INF bags and PVC tubing, use dedicated line

Insulin aspart
Adult/adolescent/child ≥6 yr: Intermittent SUBCUT total daily dose is given as 2-4 inj/day just prior to beginning of a meal; in general, 50%-70% of total daily insulin may be given as insulin aspart, the remainder should be intermediate or long-acting insulin; CONTINUOUS SUBCUT used with external insulin pump via cont SUBCUT insulin INF (CSII), the insulin dose should be based on the insulin dose from the previous regimen

Insulin lispro
Adult: SUBCUT 15 min before meals

Human regular
Adult: SUBCUT ½-1 hr before meals

Insulin, isophane suspension
Adult: SUBCUT dosage individualized by blood, urine glucose; usual dose 7-26 units; may increase by 2-10 units/day if needed

Insulin detemir
Adult: SUBCUT 1 or 2 times/day; if 1 time, give with evening meal

Insulin glargine
Adult and child ≥6 yr: SUBCUT 10 international units/day, range 2-100 international units/day

Regular insulin (ketoacidosis)
Adult: **IV** 5-10 units, then 5-10 units/hr until desired response, then switch to SUBCUT dose; **IV**/INF 2-12 units (50 units/500 ml of normal saline)
Child: **IV** 0.1 units/kg

Replacement
Adult and child: SUBCUT 0.5-1 units/kg/day qid given 30 min before meals
Adolescent: SUBCUT 0.8-1.2 mg/kg/day; this dosage is used during rapid growth

Available forms: NPH inj 100 units/ml; regular inj 100 units/ml, cartridges 100 units/ml; insulin analog inj 100 units/ml; isophane insulin inj 100 units/ml, cartridges 100 units/ml; insulin lispro 100 units/ml, 1.5-ml cartridges; insulin lispro Humalog Pen sol for inj 100 units/ml; insulin glulisine inj 100 units/ml; insulin glargine inj 100 units/ml; insulin detemir inj 100 units/ml in 10 vials, 3-ml cartridges; insulin aspart inj 100 mg/ml (Flexpen, PenFill)

Pharmacodynamics

Rapid acting	
Insulin glulisine	Onset 15-30 min, peak ½-1½ hr, duration 3-4 hr
Insulin aspart	Onset 10-20 min, peak 1-3 hr, duration 3-5 hr
Insulin lispro	Onset 15-30 min, peak ½-1½ hr, duration 3-4 hr
Short acting	
Insulin regular	Onset 30 min, peak 2.5-5 hr, duration up to 6 hr
Intermediate acting	
Insulin, isophane suspension (NPH)	Onset 1.5-4 hr, peak 4-12 hr, duration up to 24 hr
Long acting	
Insulin detemir	Onset 0.8-2 hr, peak unknown, duration up to 24 hr (concentration dependent)
Insulin glargine	Onset 1.5 hr, no peak identified, duration ≥24 hr
Mixtures	
Insulin, isophane suspension and regular insulin (70/30)	Onset 10-20 min, peak 2.4 hr, duration up to 24 hr
Isophane insulin suspension (NPH) and insulin mixtures (50/50)	Onset ½-1 hr, peak dual, duration 10-16 hr

Adverse effects
EENT: Blurred vision, dry mouth
INTEG: Flushing, rash, urticaria, warmth, *lipodystrophy,* lipohypertrophy, swelling, redness
META: Hypoglycemia, rebound hyperglycemia (Somogyi effect 12-72 hr or longer)
MISC: Peripheral edema
SYST: **Anaphylaxis; possible cancer risk (insulin glargine)**

Contraindications: Hypersensitivity to protamine; creosol (aspart)

Precautions: Pregnancy **B** (lispro, aspart), **C** (all others)

Pharmacokinetics	
Absorption	Rapidly absorbed (SUBCUT)
Distribution	Widely distributed
Metabolism	Liver, muscle, kidney
Excretion	Kidneys
Half-life	Regular 3-5 min; NPH 10 min

Interactions
Individual drugs
Alcohol: increased hypoglycemia
Dobutamine: increased insulin need
Epinephrine: decreased hypoglycemia
Fenfluramine, guanethedine, phenylbutazone, sulfinpyrazone, tetracycline: decreased insulin need
Drug classifications
Anabolic steroids, β-adrenergic blockers, hypoglycemics (oral), salicylates: increased hypoglycemia
Contraceptives (oral), corticosteroids, diuretics (thiazide), thyroid hormones: decreased hypoglycemia
Estrogens: increased insulin need
MAOIs: decreased insulin need
Drug/herb
Aceitilla, adiantam, agrimony, aloe gel, banana flowers/roots, banyan stem bark, bilberry, bitter melon, broom, bugleweed, burdock, carob, cumin, damiana, dandelion, eucalyptus, fenugreek, fo-ti, garlic, goat's rue, guar gum, horse chestnut, jambul, juniper, konjac, maitake, onion, psyllium, reishi: increased hypoglycemia
Alfalfa, aloe, basil, bay, bilberry, bitter melon, black catechu, buchu, burdock, coriander, dandelion, eyebright (po), fenugreek, garlic, ginseng, glucomannan, glucosamine, goat's rue, gymnema, horehound, horse chestnut, jambul, myrrh, myrtle: increased antidiabetic effect

Annato, cocoa seeds, coffee beans, cola seeds, guarana, ma huang, rosemary, yerba maté: decreased hypoglycemic effect
Bee pollen, blue cohosh, broom, chromium, elecampane, eucalyptus, gotu kola: decreased antidiabetic effect
Chromium: increased or decreased hypoglycemia
Karela: increased glucose tolerance

Drug/lab test
Increased: VMA
Decreased: potassium, calcium
Interference: liver, thyroid function tests

NURSING CONSIDERATIONS
Assessment
- Fasting blood glucose, also A1c may be drawn to identify treatment effectiveness q3mo
- Urine ketones during illness; insulin requirements may increase during stress, illness, surgery
- For hypoglycemic reaction that can occur during peak time (sweating, weakness, dizziness, chills, confusion, headache, nausea, rapid weak pulse, fatigue, tachycardia, memory lapses, slurred speech, staggering gait, anxiety, tremors, hunger)
- For hyperglycemia: acetone breath, polyuria, fatigue, polydipsia, flushed, dry skin, lethargy

Nursing diagnoses
- Injury, risk for (adverse reactions)
- Knowledge, deficient (teaching)
- Noncompliance (teaching)

Implementation
- Store at room temperature for <1 mo (some insulins); keep away from heat and sunlight; refrigerate all other supply; NPH, premixed insulins are cloudy; regular, rapid-acting analogs, long-acting analogs are clear; do not freeze—**IV** route, regular only
SUBCUT route
- Give after warming to room temperature by rotating in palms to prevent injecting cold insulin; use only insulin syringes with markings or syringe matching units/ml; rotate inj sites within one area: abdomen, upper back, thighs, upper arm, buttocks; keep record of sites
- Give increased dosages if tolerance occurs
- Premixed insulins and NPH are cloudy suspensions
- Regular human insulin, rapid-acting analogs, and long-acting analogs are clear; do not use if cloudy, thick, or discolored

CONT SUBCUT route (insulin infusion CSII)
• Do not mix with other insulins when using a pump
• Insulin lispro 3 ml cartridges are to be used in Disetronic H-TRON plus V100 pump using Disetronic rapid inf sets; the inf set and the cartridge adapter should be changed q3day; replace 3 ml cartridge q6days

IV route (insulin glulisine only)
• Dilute to 1 international unit/ml in infusion systems with 0.9% NaCl using PVC viaflex inf bags and PVC tubing; use dedicated line; do not admix

IV route (regular only)
◆ When regular insulin is administered IV, monitor glucose, potassium often to prevent fatal hypoglycemia, hypokalemia
• **IV** direct, undiluted via vein, Y-site, 3-way stopcock; give at 50 units/min or less
• Give by cont inf after diluting with **IV** sol and run at prescribed rate; use **IV** inf pump for correct dosing; give reduced dose at serum glucose level of 250 mg/100 ml

Additive compatibilities: Bretylium, cimetidine, lidocaine, meropenem, ranitidine, verapamil

Additive incompatibilities: Aminophylline, amobarbital, chlorothiazide, cytarabine, DOBUTamine, pentobarbital, phenobarbital, phenytoin, secobarbital, sodium bicarbonate, thiopental

Syringe compatibilities: Metoclopramide

Y-site compatibilities: Amiodarone, ampicillin, ampicillin/sulbactam, aztreonam, cefazolin, cefotetan, DOBUTamine, esmolol, famotidine, gentamicin, heparin, heparin/hydrocortisone, imipenem/cilastatin, indomethacin, magnesium sulfate, meperidine, meropenem, midazolam, morphine, nitroglycerin, oxytocin, pentobarbital, potassium chloride, propofol, ritodrine, sodium bicarbonate, sodium nitroprusside, tacrolimus, terbutaline, ticarcillin, ticarcillin/clavulanate, tobramycin, vancomycin, vit B/C

Y-site incompatibilities: Nafcillin

Patient/family education
• Advise patient that blurred vision occurs; not to change corrective lens until vision is stabilized 1-2 mo
• Advise patient to keep insulin, equipment available at all times; carry a glucagon kit, candy, or lump sugar to treat hypoglycemia
• Inform patient that product does not cure diabetes but controls symptoms

• Advise patient to carry emergency ID as diabetic
• Instruct patient to recognize hypoglycemia reaction: headache, tremors, fatigue, weakness
• Instruct patient to recognize hyperglycemia reaction: frequent urination, thirst, fatigue, hunger
• Teach patient the dosage, route, mixing instructions, any diet restrictions, disease process
• Teach patient the symptoms of ketoacidosis: nausea, thirst, polyuria, dry mouth, decreased B/P, dry, flushed skin, acetone breath, drowsiness, Kussmaul respirations
• Advise patient that a plan is necessary for diet, exercise; all food on diet should be eaten; exercise routine should not vary
• Teach patient about blood glucose testing; make sure patient is able to determine glucose level
• Advise patient to avoid OTC products unless directed by prescriber

Evaluation
Positive therapeutic outcome
• Decrease in polyuria, polydipsia, polyphagia; clear sensorium; absence of dizziness; stable gait
• Blood glucose level under control

Treatment of overdose: Glucose 25 g **IV,** via dextrose 50% sol, 50 ml, or glucagon 1 mg

---

interferon alfa-2a (recombinant) (Rx)
(in-ter-feer'on)
Roferon-A
interferon alfa-2b (recombinant) (Rx)
a-2-interferon, Intron-A
Func. class.: Antineoplastic—miscellaneous
Chem. class.: Protein product

Pregnancy category C

Do not confuse:
Roferon-A/Imferon

Action: Antiviral action inhibits viral replication by reprogramming virus; antitumor action suppresses cell proliferation; immunomodulating action phagocytizes target cells; may also inhibit virus replication in virus-infested cells

Therapeutic outcome: Prevention of rapid growth of malignant cells; treatment of hepatitis non-A, non-B (liver function improvement)

Uses: Hairy cell leukemia in persons >18 yr; condylomata acuminata (alfa 2b); chronic hepatitis C (alfa 2b); 2a only chronic myelogenous leukemia; 2b only hepatitis B, malignant melanoma

Unlabeled uses: Bladder tumors, carcinoid tumors, non-Hodgkin's lymphoma, essential thrombocytopenia, cytomegaloviruses, herpes simplex, human papilloma virus–associated diseases

Dosage and routes
Hairy cell leukemia (2a)
Adult: SUBCUT/IM 3 million international units/day × 16-24 wk, then 3 million international units 3 ×/wk maintenance

Condylomata acuminata (2a)
Adult: Intralesional 1 million international units/lesion 3 ×/wk × 3 wk

Alfa-2b hairy-cell leukemia
Adult: SUBCUT/IM 2 million international units/m^2 3 ×/wk × up to 6 mo

Condylomata acuminata
Adult: Intralesional 1 million international units (0.1 ml) injected into each lesion 3 ×/wk on alternating days for 3 wk; treat ≤5 warts per course

Chronic hepatitis B
Adult: SUBCUT/IM 30-35 million international units/wk × 16 wk given 5 million international units/day or 10 million international units 3 ×/wk

Available forms: Alfa-2a: inj 3, 6, 36 million international units/ml; alfa-2b: inj 3, 5, 10, 18, 25 million international units/vial; powder for inj 5, 10, 18, 25, 50 million international units/vial

Adverse effects
CNS: Dizziness, confusion, numbness, paresthesia, hallucinations, **seizures, coma,** amnesia, anxiety, mood changes, depression, somnolence, paranoia, irritability, hostility, encephalopathy
CV: Edema, hypotension, hypertension, chest pain, palpitations, dysrhythmias, **CHF, MI, CVA,** tachycardia, syncope
GI: Weight loss, taste changes, nausea, anorexia, diarrhea, xerostomia
GU: Impotence
HEMA: **Neutropenia, thrombocytopenia**
INTEG: Rash, dry skin, itching, alopecia, flushing, photosensitivity, **serious skin infection**
MISC: Flulike symptoms: fever, fatigue, myalgias, headache, chills, optic neuritis, **anaphylaxis, angioedema**

Contraindications: Hypersensitivity

Precautions: Pregnancy **C,** breastfeeding, children, severe hypotension, dysrhythmia, tachycardia, severe renal/hepatic disease, seizure disorder, optic neuritis, ocular disease, thyroid/pulmonary disease

Black Box Warning: Autoimmune disorders, cardiac disease, infection, depression

Pharmacokinetics
Absorption	80%-90% (SUBCUT/IM)
Distribution	Unknown
Metabolism	Renal tubular (degraded)
Excretion	Kidneys
Half-life	3.7-8.5 hr (2a); 2-7 hr (2b)

Pharmacodynamics
Onset	Unknown
Peak	3-8 hr
Duration	Unknown

Interactions
Individual drugs
Aminophylline: increased toxicity, blood levels
Clozapine, warfarin, zidovudine: increased neutropenia
Drug/lab test
Interference: AST, ALT, LDH, alkaline phosphatase, WBC, platelets, granulocytes, creatinine

NURSING CONSIDERATIONS
Assessment
• Assess cardiac status: lung sounds, ECG before, during treatment, especially in those with cardiac disease, hypo/hypertension, MI, CHF, CVA may occur
• Assess bone marrow depression: bruising, bleeding, blood in stools, urine, sputum, emesis
• Assess mental status: depression, suicidal thoughts, hallucinations, amnesia
• Assess for symptoms of infection; may be masked by drug fever; fever, chills, headache, sore throat may occur 6 hr after dose; give acetaminophen for symptoms
• Assess liver, thyroid function tests
• In AIDS patients with Kaposi's sarcoma, assess characteristics of lesions during therapy; symptoms should decrease
• Assess for bleeding: hematuria, stool guaiac, bruising or petechiae, mucosa or orifices q8hr; check for inflammation of mucosa, breaks in skin; avoid IM inj, rectal temp, or any other procedures that break the skin
• Assess for CNS reaction: LOC, mental status, dizziness, confusion, poor coordination,

difficulty speaking, behavior changes; notify prescriber (alfa-2b)

Nursing diagnoses
• Body image, disturbed (adverse reactions)
• Infection, risk for (adverse reactions)
• Injury, risk for (adverse reactions)
• Knowledge, deficient (teaching)

Implementation
• Sol should be prepared by qualified personnel only under controlled conditions in biologic cabinet using gown, gloves, and mask
• Use Luer-Lok tubing to prevent leakage; do not let sol come in contact with skin; if contact occurs, wash well with soap and water
• Give at bedtime to minimize side effects
• Give acetaminophen as ordered to alleviate fever and headache

Alfa-2a
• SUBCUT/IM after reconstituting 18 million units/3 ml of diluent provided (6 million units/ml)
• 36 million units/ml is used for Kaposi's sarcoma only
• Store reconstituted sol; must be used within 24 hr

Alfa-2b
• Give by IM/SUBCUT after reconstituting 3-5 million international units/1 ml, 10 million international units/2 ml, 25 million international units/5 ml, of diluent provided; mix gently, do not shake; each brand has different dilution directions; check patient insert

Intralesional route (2b)
• Give by intralesional route after reconstituting 10 million international units/1 ml of bacteriostatic water for inj; no more than 5 lesions can safely be treated at a time; using a 25-G needle inject 0.1 ml into base at center

Patient/family education
• Caution patient to avoid hazardous tasks, since confusion, dizziness may occur; fatigue is common; activity may have to be altered; to take at bedtime to minimize flulike symptoms; to take acetaminophen for fever; avoid prolonged sunlight
• Advise patient that brands of this product should not be changed; each form is different, with different dosages
• Caution patient not to become pregnant while taking product; possible mutagenic effects; impotence may occur during treatment but is temporary
• Advise patient to report signs of infection: sore throat, fever, diarrhea, vomiting; sores or white patches in mouth

◆ Advise patient that suicidal ideation is common; notify prescriber if severe or incapacitating

Evaluation
Positive therapeutic outcome
• Improved leukocytes, Hgb, platelets
• Decreased amount of genital warts

interferon alfacon-1 (Rx)
(in-ter-feer'on al'fa-kon)
Infergen
Func. class.: Recombinant type 1 interferon

Pregnancy category C

Action: Induces biologic responses and has antiviral, antiproliferative, and immunomodulatory effects

Therapeutic outcome: Decreased signs/symptoms of hepatitis C

Uses: Chronic hepatitis C infections in those 18 yr and older with compensated liver disease who have anti-HCV antibodies or HCV RNA

Unlabeled uses: Hairy cell leukemia when used with G-CSF

Dosage and routes
Adult: SUBCUT 9 mcg as a single inj 3 ×/wk × 24 wk; leave at least 48 hr between injections

Available forms: Inj 9 mg/0.3 ml, 15 mcg/0.5 ml, 30 mcg/ml

Adverse effects
CNS: Headache, fatigue, fever, rigors, insomnia, dizziness, agitation, nervousness, anxiety, lability, abnormal thinking, depression
CV: Hypertension, palpitation, tachycardia
EENT: Tinnitus, earache, conjunctivitis, eye pain
GI: Abdominal pain, nausea, diarrhea, anorexia, dyspepsia, vomiting, constipation, flatulence, hemorrhoids, decreased salivation
GU: Dysmenorrhea, vaginitis, menstrual disorders
HEMA: **Granulocytopenia, thrombocytopenia, leukopenia,** ecchymosis, **aplastic anemia**
INTEG: Alopecia, pruritus, rash, erythema, dry skin
MISC: **Anaphylaxis, angioedema,** flulike illness
MS: Back, limb, neck, skeletal pain, rigors
RESP: Pharyngitis, upper respiratory infection, cough, sinusitis, rhinitis, respiratory tract congestion, epistaxis, dyspnea, bronchitis

Contraindications: Hypersensitivity to α-interferons, or products from *Escherichia coli*

Precautions: Pregnancy **C**, breastfeeding, children <18 yr, thyroid disorders, myelosuppression, hepatic disease, alcoholism, geriatric patients, seizure disorder, hepatitis

Black Box Warning: Cardiac disease, autoimmune disorder, infection, depression

Pharmacokinetics
Unknown

Pharmacodynamics
Onset	Unknown
Peak	24-36 hr
Duration	Unknown

NURSING CONSIDERATIONS
Assessment
- Assess CBC, liver function tests, ECG, platelet counts, heme concentration, ANC, serum creatinine concentration, albumin, bilirubin, TSH, T₄
- Assess for myelosuppression, low dose if neutrophil count is <500 × 10-6/L or if platelets are <50 × 10-9/L
- Assess for hypersensitivity, discontinue immediately if hypersensitivity occurs

Nursing diagnoses
- Infection, risk for (uses)
- Knowledge, deficient (teaching)

Patient/family education
- Provide patient or family member with written, detailed instructions about the product
- Caution patient to use contraception during treatment

Evaluation
Positive therapeutic outcome
- Decreased hepatitis C signs/symptoms

---

interferon beta-1a (Rx)
(in-ter-feer'on)
Avonex, Rebif
interferon beta-1b (Rx)
Betaseron, Extavia
Func. class.: Multiple sclerosis agent, immune modifier
Chem. class.: Interferon, *Escherichia coli* derivative

Pregnancy category C

Action: Antiviral, immunoregulatory; action not clearly understood; biologic response-modifying properties mediated through specific receptors on cells, inducing expression of interferon-induced gene products

Therapeutic outcome: Decreased symptoms of multiple sclerosis

Uses: Ambulatory patients with relapsing or remitting multiple sclerosis

Unlabeled uses: May be useful in treatment of AIDS, AIDS-related Kaposi's sarcoma, malignant melanoma, metastatic renal cell carcinoma, cutaneous T cell lymphoma, acute non-A/non-B hepatitis

Dosage and routes
Interferon beta-1a
Remitting-relapsing multiple sclerosis
Adult: IM (Avonex) 30 mcg qwk; SUBCUT (Rebif) 22 or 44 mcg 3 ×/wk with each dose 48 hr apart

Interferon beta-1b
Relapsing/remitting multiple sclerosis
Adult: SUBCUT 0.0625 mg every other day for wk 1 and 2; then 0.125 mg every other day for wk 3 and 4; then 0.1875 mg every other day for wk 5 and 6; then 0.25 mg every other day thereafter; higher doses should not be used

Available forms: Beta-1a (Avonex): 33 mcg (6.6 million international units/vial); (Rebif) 22 mcg, 44 mcg/0.5 ml; beta-1b: powder for inj 0.3 mg (9.6 m international units)

Adverse effects
CNS: Headache, fever, pain, chills, mental changes, depression, hypertonia, **suicide attempts, seizures**
CV: Migraine, palpitations, hypertension, tachycardia, peripheral vascular disorders
EENT: Conjunctivitis, blurred vision

Adverse effects: *italic* = common, **bold** = life-threatening

GI: Diarrhea, constipation, vomiting, abdominal pain
GU: Dysmenorrhea, irregular menses, metrorrhagia, cystitis, breast pain
HEMA: Decreased lymphocytes, ANC, **WBC,** *lymphadenopathy,* anemia
INTEG: Sweating, inj site reaction
MS: Myalgia, **myasthenia**
RESP: Sinusitis, dyspnea

Contraindications: Hypersensitivity to natural or recombinant interferon-beta or human albumin, hamster protein, rotavirus vaccine

Precautions: Pregnancy C, breastfeeding, children <18 yr, chronic progressive multiple sclerosis, depression, mental disorders, seizure disorders, latex allergy, autoimmune disorders, bone marrow suppression, hepatotoxicity, cardiac disease, alcoholism, chickenpox, herpes zoster

Pharmacokinetics
Absorption	50% is absorbed
Distribution	Unknown
Metabolism	Unknown
Excretion	Unknown
Half-life	8 min–4½ hr (beta-1b), 8.6 hr (beta-1a)

Pharmacodynamics
	BETA-1A	BETA-1B
Onset	Up to 12 hr	Rapid
Peak	48 hr	2-8 hr
Duration	4 days	Unknown

Interactions
Individual drugs
Zidovudine: decreased clearance
Drug classifications
Antineoplastics: increased myelosuppression
Drug/herb
Astragalus, echinacea, melatonin: change in immunomodulation
Drug/lab test
Increased: liver function tests
Interference: vaccines, toxoids; avoid concurrent use

NURSING CONSIDERATIONS
Assessment
• Monitor blood, renal, liver function tests: CBC, differential, platelet counts, BUN, creatinine, ALT, urinalysis; if neutrophil count is <750/mm³, or if AST, ALT is 10 × greater than upper normal limit, or if bilirubin is 5 × greater than upper normal limit; when neutrophil count exceeds 750/mm³ and liver function

or renal studies return to normal, treatment may resume at 50% original dosage
• Assess for CNS symptoms: headache, fatigue, depression; if depression occurs and is severe, product should be discontinued
• Assess for multiple sclerosis symptoms
• Assess mental status: depression, depersonalization, suicidal thoughts, insomnia
• Monitor GI status: diarrhea or constipation, vomiting, abdominal pain
• Monitor cardiac status: increased B/P, tachycardia

Nursing diagnoses
• Knowledge, deficient (teaching)
• Mobility, impaired physical (uses)

Implementation
• Reconstitute 0.3 mg (9.6 million international units)/1.2 ml of supplied diluent (0.2 mg or 8 million international units concentration); rotate vial gently, do not shake; withdraw 1 ml using a syringe with 27G needle; administer SUBCUT only into hip, thigh, arm; discard unused portion
• Products are not interchangeable
Interferon beta-1a
• Reconstitute with 1.1 ml of diluent, swirl, give within 6 hr
Interferon beta-1b
• Reconstitute by injecting diluent provided (1.2 ml) into vial, swirl (8 milli-international units/ml), use 27-G needle for inj
• Give acetaminophen for fever, headache; use SUBCUT route only; do not give IM or **IV**
• Store reconstituted sol in refrigerator; do not freeze; do not use sol that contains precipitate or is discolored

Patient/family education
• Provide patient or family member with written, detailed instructions about the product; provide initial and return demonstrations on inj procedure; give information on use and disposal of product
• Inform patient that blurred vision, sweating may occur
• Advise women patients that irregular menses, dysmenorrhea, or metrorrhagia as well as breast pain may occur; use contraception during treatment; product may cause spontaneous abortion
• Teach patient to use sunscreen to prevent photosensitivity
• Instruct patient to notify prescriber if pregnancy is suspected
• Teach patient inj technique and care of equipment

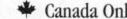 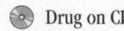

- Instruct patient to notify prescriber of increased temp, chills, muscle soreness, fatigue

Evaluation
Positive therapeutic outcome
- Decreased symptoms of multiple sclerosis

---

interferon gamma-1b (Rx)
(in-ter-feer'on)
Actimmune
Func. class.: Biologic response modifier
Chem. class.: Lymphokine, interleukin type

Pregnancy category C

Action: Species-specific protein synthesized in response to viruses; potent phagocyte-activating effects; capable of mediating the killing of *Staphylococcus aureus, Toxoplasma gondii, Leishmania donovani, Listeria monocytogenes, Mycobacterium avium-intracellulare;* enhances oxidative metabolism of macrophages; enhances antibody-dependent cellular cytotoxicity

Therapeutic outcome: Decreased signs/symptoms of infection (serious) in chronic granulomatous disease

Uses: Serious infections associated with chronic granulomatous disease, osteopetrosis

Unlabeled uses: Osteoporosis, *Mycobacterium avium* complex (MAC), ovarian cancer, pulmonary fibrosis

Dosage and routes
Adult: SUBCUT 50 mcg/m^2 (1.5 million units/m^2) for patients with a surface area of >0.5 m^2; 1.5 mcg/kg/dose for patient with a surface area of <0.5/m^2; give on Monday, Wednesday, Friday for 3 ×/wk dosing

Available forms: Inj 100 mcg (2 million units)/single-dose vial

Adverse effects
CNS: Headache, fatigue, depression, fever, chills
GI: Nausea, anorexia, abdominal pain, weight loss, diarrhea, vomiting
HEMA: **Leukopenia, thrombocytopenia**
INTEG: Rash, pain at inj site
MS: Myalgia, arthralgia

Contraindications: Hypersensitivity to interferon γ, *Escherichia coli*–derived products

Precautions: Pregnancy **C**, breastfeeding, children <1 yr, cardiac disease, seizure/CNS disorders, myelosuppression

Pharmacokinetics
Absorption	Slowly absorbed 89%
Distribution	Unknown
Metabolism	Unknown
Excretion	Unknown
Half-life	5.9 hr

Pharmacodynamics
Onset	Unknown
Peak	7 hr
Duration	Unknown

Interactions
Individual drugs
Aminophylline, theophylline: increased levels
Fosphenytoin, phenytoin, warfarin: increased interference
Drug classifications
Myelosuppressive agents: increased myelosuppression
Toxoids, vaccines: interference with antibody reaction

NURSING CONSIDERATIONS
Assessment
- Monitor blood, renal, hepatic studies: CBC with differential, platelet count, BUN, creatinine, ALT, urinalysis before, q3mo during treatment
- Assess for infection: headache, fever, chills, fatigue; these are common adverse reactions
- Monitor CNS symptoms: headache, fatigue, depression

Nursing diagnoses
- Infection, risk for (uses)
- Knowledge, deficient (teaching)

Implementation
- Give at bedtime to minimize adverse reactions; administer acetaminophen for fever, headache; use 50% of the dosage prescribed if severe reactions occur or discontinue treatment until reactions subside
- Give in right or left deltoid and anterior thigh; warm to room temperature before use; do not leave at room temperature over 12 hr (unopened vial); does not contain preservatives
- Store in refrigerator upon receipt; do not freeze; do not shake

Patient/family education
- Provide patient or family member with written, detailed instructions about the

product; provide initial and return demonstrations on inj procedure; give information on use and disposal of product
• Caution patient to use contraception during treatment

Evaluation
Positive therapeutic outcome
• Decreased serious infections
• Improvement in existing infections and inflammatory conditions

---

ipratropium (Rx)
(i-pra-troe'pee-um)
Atrovent HFA
Func. class.: Anticholinergic, bronchodilator
Chem. class.: Synthetic quaternary ammonium compound

Pregnancy category B

Do not confuse:
Atrovent/Alupent

Action: Inhibits interaction of acetylcholine at receptor sites on the bronchial smooth muscle, resulting in decreased cyclic guanosine monophosphate (cGMP) and bronchodilatation

Therapeutic outcome: Bronchodilatation

Uses: Bronchodilatation during bronchospasm for patients with COPD; rhinorrhea in children 6-11 yr (nasal spray)

Dosage and routes
Adult: 1-4 INH qid, max 24 puffs/24 hr; SOL 250-500 mcg (1 unit dose) given 3-4 ×/day
Child: INH 1-2 inhalations q6-8hr; NEB 125-250 mcg q4-6hr
Child 5-12 yr: NASAL 1 spray in each nostril

Available forms: Aerosol 18 mcg/actuation; nasal spray 0.03%, 0.06%; sol for inh 0.0125% ♣, 0.02%

Adverse effects
CNS: Anxiety, dizziness, headache, nervousness
CV: Palpitations
EENT: Dry mouth, blurred vision
GI: Nausea, vomiting, cramps
INTEG: Rash
RESP: Cough, worsening of symptoms, **bronchospasm**

Contraindications: Hypersensitivity to this product, atropine, soya lecithin

Precautions: Pregnancy **B**, breastfeeding, children <12 yr, closed-angle glaucoma, prostatic hypertrophy, bladder neck obstruction

Pharmacokinetics

Absorption	Minimal
Distribution	Does not cross blood-brain barrier
Metabolism	Liver, minimal
Excretion	Unknown
Half-life	2 hr

Pharmacodynamics

Onset	5-15 min
Peak	1-1½ hr
Duration	3-6 hr

Interactions
Individual drugs
Disopyramide: increased anticholinergic action
Drug classifications
Antihistamines, phenothiazines: increased anticholinergic action
Bronchodilators (other): increased toxicity
Drug/herb
Black catechu: increased constipation
Butterbur, jimsonweed: increased anticholinergic effect
Green tea (large amounts), guarana: increased bronchodilator effect
Jamborandi tree, pill-bearing spurge: decreased anticholinergic effect

NURSING CONSIDERATIONS
Assessment
• Monitor respiratory function: vital capacity, FEV, ABGs, lung sounds, heart rate, rhythm (baseline, during treatment); if severe bronchospasm is present, a more rapid medication is required
• Monitor for evidence of allergic reactions, paradoxic bronchospasm; withhold dose and notify prescriber; identify if patient is allergic to belladonna products or atropine; allergy to this product may occur

Nursing diagnoses
• Airway clearance, ineffective (uses)
• Gas exchange, impaired (uses)
• Knowledge, deficient (teaching)

Implementation
• Give after shaking container; have patient exhale, place mouthpiece in mouth, inhale slowly, hold breath, remove, exhale slowly; allow at least 1 min between inhalations

---

- Give this medication before other medications and allow at least 5 min between each
Nebulizer route
- Use solution in nebulizer with a mouthpiece rather than a face mask
Nasal route
- Prime pump, initially requires 7 actuations of the pump, priming again is not necessary if used regularly
- Store in light-resistant container; do not expose to temperature over 86° F (30° C)

Patient/family education
- Advise patient not to use OTC medications unless approved by prescriber; extra stimulation may occur; to use this medication before other medications and allow at least 5 min between each to prevent overstimulation
- Teach patient that compliance is necessary with number of inhalations/24 hr, or overdose may occur
- Instruct patient to use spacer device if geriatric
- Teach patient the proper use of the inhaler; review package insert with patient; to avoid getting aerosol in eyes: blurring may result; to wash inhaler in warm water daily and dry; to avoid smoking, smoke-filled rooms, persons with respiratory tract infections
- Teach patient if paradoxic bronchospasm occurs to stop product immediately and notify prescriber; to limit caffeine products such as chocolate, coffee, tea, and colas
- Instruct patient on administration of dose, not to use more than prescribed; serious side effects may occur; if dose is missed, take when remembered; space other doses on new time schedule; do not double doses

Evaluation
Positive therapeutic outcome
- Absence of dyspnea, wheezing after 1 hr
- Improved airway exchange
- Improved ABGs

---

irbesartan (Rx)
(er-be-sar′tan)
Avapro
Func. class.: Antihypertensive
Chem. class.: Angiotensin II receptor (Type AT_1)

Pregnancy category
C (1st trimester),
D (2nd/3rd trimesters)

Do not confuse:
Avapro/Anaprox

Action: Blocks the vasoconstrictor and aldosterone-secreting effects of angiotensin II; selectively blocks the binding of angiotensin II to the AT_1 receptor found in tissues

Therapeutic outcome: Decreased B/P

Uses: Hypertension, alone or in combination, nephropathy in type 2 diabetic patients

Unlabeled uses: Heart failure

Dosage and routes
Hypertension
Adult: PO 150 mg/day; may be increased to 300 mg/day

Nephropathy in type 2 diabetic patients
Adult: PO maintenance dose 300 mg/day, start 75 mg/day
Child 13-16 yr: PO 150 mg/day, may increase to 300 mg/day
Child 6-12 yr: PO 75 mg/day may increase to 150 mg/day

Volume and salt depleted patients
Adult: PO 75 mg/day

Available forms: Tabs 75, 150, 300 mg

Adverse effects
CNS: Dizziness, anxiety, headache, fatigue
CV: Hypotension
GI: Diarrhea, dyspepsia
MISC: Edema, chest pain, rash, tachycardia, UTI, **angioedema,** hyperkalemia
RESP: Cough, upper respiratory infection, rhinitis, pharyngitis, sinus disorder

Contraindications: Hypersensitivity

Black Box Warning: Pregnancy **D** (2nd/3rd trimesters)

Precautions: Pregnancy C (1st trimester), breastfeeding, children <6 yr, geriatric, renal/hepatic disease, renal artery stenosis, hypersensitivity to ACE inhibitors

Pharmacokinetics

Absorption	Well
Distribution	Bound to plasma proteins (90%)
Metabolism	Liver (minimal)
Excretion	Feces, urine
Half-life	11-15 hr

Pharmacodynamics

Unknown

Interactions
Drug classifications
CYP2C9 inhibitors: increased irbesartan level
Diuretics (potassium sparing), potassium salt substitutes: increased hyperkalemia
NSAIDs: decreased antihypertensive effect
Drug/herb
Aconite: increased toxicity, death
Astragalus, cola tree: increased or decreased antihypertensive effect
Barberry, betony, black catechu, black cohosh, bloodroot, broom, burdock, cat's claw, dandelion, goldenseal, hawthorn, Irish moss, Jamaican dogwood, kelp, khella, mistletoe, parsley: increased antihypertensive effect
Coltsfoot, guarana, khat, licorice, yohimbe: decreased antihypertensive effect

NURSING CONSIDERATIONS
Assessment
• Assess B/P, pulse q4hr; note rate, rhythm, quality
• Monitor electrolytes: potassium, sodium, chloride
• Obtain baselines for renal, liver function tests before therapy begins
• Monitor for edema in feet, legs daily
• Assess for skin turgor, dryness of mucous membranes for hydration status

Nursing diagnoses
• Fluid volume, deficient (side effects)
• Knowledge, deficient (teaching)
• Noncompliance (teaching)

Implementation
• Administer without regard to meals

Patient/family education
• Advise patient to comply with dosage schedule, even if feeling better
• Inform patient that product may cause dizziness, fainting, light-headedness
• Caution patient to rise slowly to sitting or standing position to minimize orthostatic hypotension
• Advise patient to notify prescriber if pregnancy is suspected

Evaluation
Positive therapeutic outcome
• Decreased B/P

---

irinotecan (Rx)
(ear-een-oh-tee'kan)
Camptosar
Func. class.: Antineoplastic hormone
Chem. class.: Topoisomerase inhibitor

Pregnancy category D

Action: Cytotoxic by producing damage to single-strand DNA during DNA synthesis, binds to topoisomerase I

Therapeutic outcome: Prevention in growth of tumor size

Uses: Metastatic carcinoma of colon or rectum, or 1st line treatment in combination with fluorouracil (5-FU) and leucovorin for metastatic carcinoma of colon or rectum

Dosage and routes
Single agent
Adult: **IV** 125 mg/m^2 given over 1½ hr qwk × 4 wk, then 2 wk rest period, may be repeated; 4 wk or 2 wk off

Combination dosage schedule
Regimen 1: Irinotecan 75-125 mg/m^2, leucovorin 20 mg/m^2, 5-FU 300-500 mg/m^2, depending on dosing levels

Regimen 2: Irinotecan 120-180 mg/m^2, leucovorin 200 mg/m^2, 5-FU-BOL 240-400 mg/m^2, 5-FU INF 360-600 mg/m^2

Hepatic dose
Adult: **IV** 100 mg/m^2 qwk × 4 wk, then 2 wk rest; may repeat cycle or 300 mg/m^2 q3wk as tolerated

Available forms: Inj 20 mg/ml

Adverse effects
CNS: Fever, headache, chills, dizziness
CV: Vasodilatation, edema, **thromboembolism**
GI: **Severe diarrhea,** *nausea, vomiting,* anorexia, constipation, cramps, flatus, stomatitis, dyspepsia, **hepatotoxicity**
HEMA: **Leukopenia,** anemia, **neutropenia**
INTEG: Irritation at site, rash, sweating, alopecia
MISC: Asthenia, weight loss, back pain
RESP: Dyspnea, increased cough, rhinitis

Contraindications: Pregnancy **D**, hypersensitivity

Precautions: Breastfeeding, children, geriatric, irradiation, hepatic disease

Black Box Warning: Myelosuppression, diarrhea

Pharmacokinetics

Absorption	Complete
Distribution	Widely, 30%-68% bound to plasma proteins, increased risk of toxicity in those homozygous for UGT1A128
Metabolism	Unknown
Excretion	Urine/bile
Half-life	6-12 hr

Pharmacodynamics

Unknown

Interactions

Individual products

Carbamazepine, phenobarbital, phenytoin: decreased irinotecan levels

Fluorouracil: increased toxicity

Radiation: increased myelosuppression, diarrhea

Drug classifications

Anticoagulants, NSAIDs: increased bleeding risk

Antineoplastics: increased myelosuppression, diarrhea

CYP3A4 inducers (dexamethasone): increased lymphocytopenia

CYP3A4 inhibitors (ketoconazole): increased irinotecan levels

Diuretics: increased dehydration

Drug/herb

St. John's wort: decreased product level; avoid concurrent use

Drug/lab test

Increased: ALK phos, AST

NURSING CONSIDERATIONS

Assessment

• Assess for CNS symptoms: fever, headache, chills, dizziness

• Assess CBC, differential, platelet count weekly; use colony-stimulating factor if WBC is <2000/mm^3, platelet count is <100,000/mm^3, Hgb ≤9 g/dl, neutrophils ≤1000/mm^3; notify prescriber of these results, product should be discontinued and colony-stimulating factor given

• Assess buccal cavity for dryness, sores or ulceration, white patches, oral pain, bleeding, dysphagia

• Assess GI symptoms: frequency of stools; cramping; severe life-threatening diarrhea may occur with fluid and electrolyte imbalances

• Assess early diarrhea and other cholinergic symptoms, treat with atropine; late diarrhea can be life threatening, must be treated promptly with loperimide

• Assess signs of dehydration: rapid respirations, poor skin turgor, decreased urine output; dry skin, restlessness, weakness

• Assess for bone marrow depression: bruising, bleeding, blood in stools, urine, sputum, emesis

Nursing diagnoses

• Infection, risk for (adverse reactions)

• Knowledge, deficient (teaching)

Implementation

• Give antiemetics and dexamethasone 10 mg at least ½ hr before antineoplastics

• Give after preparing in biologic cabinet using gloves, mask, gown

IV route

• Give by intermittent inf after diluting with 0.9% NaCl or D$_5$W (0.12-1.1 mg/ml); give over 1½ hr

• Do not admix with other solutions or medications

• Provide increased fluid intake to 2-3 L/day to prevent dehydration, unless contraindicated

• Provide rinsing of mouth tid-qid with water, club soda; brushing of teeth bid-tid with soft brush or cotton-tipped applicator for stomatitis; use unwaxed dental floss

• Provide nutritious diet with iron, low fiber, few dairy products; avoid raw fruits, vegetables, herbals

• Stable for 24 hr at room temperature, 48 hr if refrigerated

Patient/family education

• Advise patient to avoid foods with citric acid or hot or rough texture if stomatitis is present; to drink adequate fluids

• Advise patient to report stomatitis; any bleeding, white spots, ulcerations in mouth; tell patient to examine mouth daily, report symptoms

• Advise patient to report signs of anemia: fatigue, headache, faintness, shortness of breath, irritability

• Advise patient to use contraception during therapy

• Advise patient to avoid vaccinations while taking this product

• Instruct patient to report diarrhea that occurs 24 hr after administration; severe dehydration can occur rapidly

- Teach patient to avoid salicylates, NSAIDs, alcohol; bleeding may occur

Evaluation
Positive therapeutic outcome
- Decrease in tumor size, decrease in spread of cancer

Treatment of overdose: Induce vomiting, provide supportive care, prevent dehydration

---

iron, carbonyl
See ferrous fumarate

---

iron dextran (Rx)
DexFerrum, Imferon, InFed
Func. class.: Hematinic
Chem. class.: Ferric hydroxide complex with dextran

Pregnancy category C

Do not confuse:
Imferon/Imuran/Roferon-A/Interferon

Action: Iron is carried by transferrin to the bone marrow, where it is incorporated into hemoglobin

Therapeutic outcome: Prevention and resolution of iron-deficiency anemia

Uses: Iron-deficiency anemia in patients who cannot take oral preparations

Dosage and routes
Adult and child: IM 0.5 ml as a test dose by Z-track, then no more than the following per day:
Adult <50 kg: IM 100 mg
Adult >50 kg: IM 250 mg
Child 5-9 kg: IM 50 mg
Infant <5 kg: IM 25 mg
Adult: **IV** 0.5 ml (25 mg) test dose, then 100 mg/day after 2-3 days; give 25 mg test dose, wait 5 min, then INF over 6-12 hr or follow equation:

$$\frac{0.3 \times \text{weight (lb)} \times 100 \text{ Hgb (g/dl)} \times 100}{14.8} = \text{mg iron}$$

Patients <30 lb (66 kg) should be given 80% of above formula dose

Available forms: Inj IM/**IV** 50 mg/ml (2 ml, 10 ml vials)

Adverse effects
CNS: Headache, paresthesia, dizziness, shivering, weakness, **seizures**
CV: Chest pain, **shock,** hypotension, tachycardia
GI: Nausea, vomiting, metallic taste, abdominal pain
HEMA: **Leukocytosis**
INTEG: Rash, pruritus, urticaria, fever, sweating, chills, brown skin discoloration, pain at inj site, necrosis, sterile abscesses, phlebitis
MISC: **Anaphylaxis**
RESP: Dyspnea

Contraindications:
Black Box Warning: Hypersensitivity

Precautions: Pregnancy C, breastfeeding, infants <4 mo, children, acute renal disease, asthma, rheumatoid arthritis (**IV**), all anemias excluding iron-deficiency anemia, hepatic/cardiac/renal disease, neonates, ankylosing spondylitis, lupus, hypotension

Pharmacokinetics
Absorption	Well absorbed; lymphatics over wk or mo
Distribution	Crosses placenta
Metabolism	Slow; blood loss, desquamation
Excretion	Breast milk, feces, urine, bile
Half-life	6 hr

Pharmacodynamics
Unknown

Interactions
Individual drugs
Chloramphenicol: decreased reticulocyte response
Oral iron: do not use together, increased toxicity
Drug/lab test
False increase: serum bilirubin
False decrease: serum calcium
False positive: ^{99m}Tc diphosphate bone scan, iron test (large doses >2 ml)

NURSING CONSIDERATIONS
Assessment
- Observe for 1 hr after test dose
- Monitor blood studies: Hct, Hgb, reticulocytes, transferrin, plasma iron concentrations, ferritin, total iron-binding bilirubin before treatment, at least monthly

---

 Alert   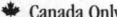 Canada Only   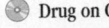 Drug on CD   * "Tall Man" lettering (See Preface)

- Assess for allergic reaction and anaphylaxis; rash, pruritus, fever, chills, wheezing; notify prescriber immediately, keep emergency equipment available
- Assess cardiac status: anginal pain, hypotension, tachycardia
- Assess for nutrition: amount of iron in diet (meat, dark green leafy vegetables, dried fruits, eggs); cause of iron loss or anemia, including salicylates, sulfonamides
- Monitor pulse, B/P during **IV** administration
- Assess for toxicity: nausea, vomiting, diarrhea, fever, abdominal pain (early symptoms); cyanotic lips, nailbeds, seizures, CV collapse (late symptoms)

Nursing diagnoses
- Activity intolerance (uses)
- Fatigue (uses)
- Knowledge, deficient (teaching)

Implementation
IM route
- Discontinue oral iron before parenteral; give only after test dose of 25 mg by preferred route; wait at least 1 hr before giving remaining portion
- Give IM inj deep in large muscle mass; use Z-track method and 19-G, 20-G 2-, 3-inch needle; ensure needle is long enough to place product deep in muscle; change needles after withdrawing medication and injecting to prevent skin and tissue staining
IV route
- Give **IV** after flushing tubing with 10 ml of 0.9% NaCl; give undiluted; give 1 ml (50 mg) or less over 1 min or more; flush line after use with 10 ml of 0.9% NaCl; patient should remain recumbent for 30-60 min to prevent orthostatic hypotension
- **IV** inj requires single-dose vial without preservative; verify on label **IV** use is approved
- Give by cont inf after diluting in 50-250 ml of 0.9% NaCl for inf; administer over 4-5 hr
- Give only with epinephrine available in case of anaphylactic reaction during dose
- Store at room temperature in cool environment

Additive compatibilities: Netilmicin

Patient/family education
- Caution patient that iron poisoning may occur if increased beyond recommended level; to not take oral iron preparation or vitamins containing iron unless approved by prescriber
- Advise patient that delayed reaction may occur 1-2 days after administration and last 3-4 days (**IV**) or 3-7 days (IM); report fever, chills, malaise, muscle/joint aches, nausea, vomiting, backache
- Advise patient to avoid breastfeeding
- Advise patient that stools may become dark

Evaluation
Positive therapeutic outcome
- Increased serum iron levels, Hct, Hgb

Treatment of overdose:
- Discontinue product, treat allergic reaction, give diphenhydrAMINE or epinephrine as needed for anaphylaxis; give iron-chelating product in acute poisoning

iron polysaccharide
See ferrous fumarate

iron sucrose (Rx)
Venofer
Func. class.: Hematinic
Chem. class.: Ferric hydroxide complex with dextran

Pregnancy category B

Action: Iron is carried by transferrin to the bone marrow, where it is incorporated into hemoglobin

Therapeutic outcome: Improved signs/symptoms of iron deficiency anemia; iron levels improved

Uses: Iron deficiency anemia

Unlabeled uses: Dystrophic epidermolysis bullosa (DEB)

Dosage and routes
Adult: **IV** 5 ml (100 mg of elemental iron) given during dialysis, most will need 1000 mg of elemental iron over 10 sequential dialysis sessions

Available forms: Inj 20 mg/ml

Adverse effects
CNS: Headache, dizziness
CV: Chest pain, hypo/hypertension, hypervolemia
GI: Nausea, vomiting, abdominal pain
INTEG: Rash, pruritus, urticaria, fever, sweating, chills
MISC: **Anaphylaxis**
RESP: Dyspnea, pneumonia, cough

Contraindications: Hypersensitivity, all anemias excluding iron deficiency anemia, iron overload

Precautions: Pregnancy **B,** breastfeeding (**IV**), children, geriatric, abdominal pain, anaphylactic shock, arthralgia, chest pain, cough, diarrhea, dizziness, dyspnea, edema, increased LFTs, fever, headache, heart failure, hyper/hypotension, infection, MS pain, nausea/vomiting, seizures, weakness

Pharmacokinetics

Absorption	Unknown
Distribution	Unknown
Metabolism	Unknown
Excretion	Urine
Half-life	6 hr

Pharmacodynamics
Unknown

Interactions
Individual drugs
Chloramphenicol: decreased iron sucrose
Dimercaprol, iron (oral): increased toxicity; do not use together

NURSING CONSIDERATIONS
Assessment
• Monitor blood studies: Hct, Hgb, reticulocytes, transferrin, plasma iron concentrations, ferritin, total iron binding, bilirubin before treatment, at least monthly
• Assess for allergy: anaphylaxis, rash, pruritus, fever, chills, wheezing; notify prescriber immediately, keep emergency equipment available
• Assess cardiac status: hypotension, hypertension, hypervolemia
• Assess for toxicity: nausea, vomiting, diarrhea, fever, abdominal pain (early symptoms), cyanotic-looking lips and nailbeds, seizures, CV collapse (late symptoms)

Nursing diagnoses
• Knowledge, deficient (teaching)
• Nutrition, less than body requirements, imbalanced (uses)

Implementation
◆ Give only with epinephrine, solu-medrol in case of anaphylactic reaction during dose
IV route
• Give directly in dialysis line by slow inj or inf; give by slow inj at 1 ml/min (5 min/vial); inf dilute each vial exclusively in a maximum of 100 ml of 0.9% NaCl, give at rate of 100 mg of iron/15 min, discard unused portions
• Store at room temperature in cool environment, do not freeze

Patient/family education
• Teach patient that iron poisoning may occur if increased beyond recommended level; not to take oral iron preparations
• Teach patient to report itching, rash, chest pain, headache, vertigo, nausea, vomiting, abdominal pain, joint/muscle pain, numbness, tingling

Evaluation
Positive therapeutic outcome
• Increased serum iron levels, Hct, Hgb

Treatment of overdose: Discontinue product, treat allergic reaction, give diphenhydrAMINE or epinephrine as needed, give iron-chelating product in acute poisoning

isoflurophate ophthalmic
See Appendix B

isoniazid (Rx)
(eye-soe-nye′a-zid)
INH, isoniazid, Isotamine ✳, Nydrazid, PMS-Isoniazid ✳
Func. class.: Antitubercular
Chem. class.: Isonicotinic acid hydrazide

Pregnancy category C

Action: Bactericidal interference with lipid, nucleic acid biosynthesis

Therapeutic outcome: Resolution of TB infection

Uses: Treatment, prevention of TB; other infections caused by mycobacteria

Dosage and routes
Treatment
Adult: PO/IM 5 mg/kg/day up to 300 mg/day, max 900 mg 2-3 ×/wk
Child and infant: PO/IM 10-20 mg/kg/day in 1-2 divided doses; max 300 mg/day or 20-40 mg/kg, max 900 mg 2-3 ×/wk

Available forms: Tabs 50, 100, 300 mg; inj 100 mg/ml; powder 50 mg/5 ml; syr 50 mg/5 ml

Adverse effects
Hypersensitivity: Fever, skin eruptions, lymphadenopathy, vasculitis
CNS: Peripheral neuropathy, dizziness, memory impairment, **toxic encephalopathy, seizures,** psychosis, slurred speech
EENT: Blurred vision, optic neuritis
GI: Nausea, vomiting, epigastric distress, **jaundice, fatal hepatitis**

HEMA: **Agranulocytosis, hemolytic ane-mia, aplastic anemia, thrombocytopenia, eosinophilia, methemoglobinemia**
MISC: Dyspnea, vit B$_6$ deficiency, pellagra, hyperglycemia, metabolic acidosis, gynecomastia, rheumatic syndrome, systemic lupus erythematosus–like syndrome

Contraindications: Hypersensitivity

Black Box Warning: Acute liver disease

Precautions: Pregnancy **C,** child <13 yr, diabetic retinopathy, cataracts, ocular defects, renal/hepatic disease, **IV** drug users, people >35 yr, postpartum period, HIV, neuropathy

Black Box Warning: Female (Hispanic), alcoholism

Pharmacokinetics	
Absorption	Well
Distribution	Widely
Metabolism	Liver
Excretion	Kidneys
Half-life	1-4 hr

Pharmacodynamics		
	PO	IM
Onset	Rapid	Rapid
Peak	1-2 hr	45-60 min
Duration	6-8 hr	6-8 hr

Interactions
Individual drugs
Alcohol, carbamazepine, cycloSERINE, ethion-amide, meperidine, phenytoin, rifampin, warfarin: increased toxicity
BCG vaccine, ketoconazole: decreased effectiveness
Drug classifications
Antacids, aluminum: decreased absorption
Benzodiazepines: increased toxicity
Drug/food
Tyramine foods: increased toxicity

NURSING CONSIDERATIONS
Assessment
• Obtain C&S tests, including sputum tests, before treatment; monitor every mo to detect resistance
• Monitor liver function tests weekly: ALT, AST, bilirubin, increased results may indicate hepatitis; renal studies during treatment, monthly: BUN, creatinine, output, specific gravity, urinalysis, uric acid
• Assess mental status often: affect, mood, behavioral changes; psychosis may occur with hallucinations, confusion

• Assess hepatic status: decreased appetite, jaundice, dark urine, fatigue
• Assess for visual disturbance that may indicate optic neuritis: blurred vision, change in color perception; may lead to blindness

Nursing diagnoses
• Diarrhea (adverse reactions)
• Infection, risk for (uses)
• Injury, risk for (adverse reactions)
• Knowledge, deficient (teaching)
• Noncompliance (teaching)

Implementation
• Give antiemetic for vomiting
• Provide a list of foods to avoid while taking this product
PO route
• Give with meals to decrease GI symptoms; absorption is better when taken on empty stomach, 1 hr before or 2 hr after meals
IM route
• Give inj deep in large muscle mass, massage; rotate inj sites, warm inj to room temperature to dissolve crystals

Patient/family education
• Instruct patient that compliance with dosage schedule for duration is necessary; not to skip or double doses; that scheduled appointments must be kept or relapse may occur
• Caution patient to avoid alcohol while taking product or hepatotoxicity may result; to avoid ingestion of aged cheeses, fish or hypertensive crisis may result; give patient written directions on which foods to avoid while taking this medication
• Tell patient to report peripheral neuritis: weakness, tingling/numbness of hands/feet, fatigue; hepatotoxicity: loss of appetite, nausea, vomiting, jaundice of skin or eyes

Evaluation
Positive therapeutic outcome
• Decreased symptoms of TB
• Culture negative for TB

Treatment of overdose:
Pyridoxine

isosorbide dinitrate (Rx)
(eye-soe-sor´bide)
Apo-ISDN ✤, Cedocard-SR ✤,
Coronex ✤, Dilatrate-SR, ISDN, Iso-Bid,
Isonate, Isorbid, Isordil, Isosorbide dinitrate,
Isotrate, Novosorbide ✤, Sorbitrate
isosorbide mononitrate (Rx)
Imdur, ISMO, Isotrate ER, Monoket
Func. class.: Antianginal, vasodilator
Chem. class.: Nitrate

Pregnancy category C

Do not confuse:
Imdur/Imuran/Inderal/K-Dur, Monoket/
Monopril

Action: Relaxation of vascular smooth
muscle, which leads to decreased preload,
afterload, thus decreasing left ventricular
end-diastolic pressure, systemic vascular
resistance, and reducing cardiac O_2 demand

Therapeutic outcome: Relief and
prevention of angina pectoris

Uses: Treatment, prevention of chronic stable
angina pectoris; diffuse esophageal spasm

Dosage and routes
Dinitrate
Adult: PO 5-40 mg qid; SL buccal tab 2.5-5
mg; may repeat q5-10min × 3 doses; chew tab
5-10 mg prn or q2-3hr as prophylaxis; SUS
REL cap 40-80 mg q8-12hr

Mononitrate
Adult: PO (ISMO, Monoket) 10-20 mg bid,
7 hr apart; (Imdur) initiate at 30-60 mg/day as
a single dose, increase q3day as needed; may
increase to 120 mg/day; max 240 mg/day

Available forms: Dinitrate: sus rel caps
40 mg; tabs 2.5, 5, 10, 20, 30 mg; SL tabs 2.5,
5, 10 mg; chew tabs 5, 10 mg; mononitrate:
tabs (Monoket, ISMO) 10, 20 mg; ext rel tabs
(Imdur, ER) 30, 60, 120 mg

Adverse effects
CNS: Vascular headache, flushing, dizziness,
weakness, faintness
CV: Postural hypotension, tachycardia,
collapse, syncope, palpitations
GI: Nausea, vomiting, diarrhea
INTEG: Pallor, sweating, rash
MISC: Twitching, hemolytic anemia, **methe-
moglobinemia**

Contraindications: Hypersensitivity to
this product or nitrates, severe anemia, increased ICP, cerebral hemorrhage, acute MI

Precautions: Pregnancy **C,** breastfeeding,
children, postural hypotension, MI, CHF,
severe renal/hepatic disease

Pharmacokinetics

Absorption	Well
Distribution	Unknown
Metabolism	Liver
Excretion	Urine, metabolites
Half-life	Dinitrate 1 hr, mononitrate 5 hr

Pharmacodynamics

	SUS REL	SL	PO
Onset	Up to 4 hr	2-5 min	15-30 min
Peak	Unknown	Unknown	Unknown
Duration	6-8 hr	1-4 hr	4-6 hr

Interactions
Individual drugs
Alcohol: increased hypotension
◆Sildenafil, tadalafil, vardenafil: fatal hypoten-
sion
Drug classifications
Antihypertensives, β-adrenergic blockers,
calcium channel blockers, diuretics,
phenothiazines: increased hypotension
Drug/herb
Blue cohosh: decreased antianginal effect

NURSING CONSIDERATIONS
Assessment
• Assess for pain: duration, time started,
activity being performed, character, intensity
• Monitor for orthostatic B/P, pulse at base-
line, during treatment

Nursing diagnoses
• Cardiac output, decreased (uses)
• Knowledge, deficient (teaching)
• Tissue perfusion, ineffective (uses)

Implementation
PO route
• Swallow sus rel cap and ext rel tab whole;
do not break, crush, or chew
• Do not swallow SL tab; tab should be
dissolved under tongue
• Chew tab should be chewed thoroughly
• Give 1 hr before or 2 hr after meals with 8
oz of water
SL route
• Hold SL tab under tongue until dissolved (a
few min); do not take anything PO when SL tab
is in place

Patient/family education
• Instruct patient to not skip or double doses;
if dose is missed take when remembered if 2
hr before next dose (dinitrate), 6 hr before

next dose (sus rel), or 8 hr before next dose (mononitrate)
- Caution patient to avoid alcohol and OTC medications unless approved by prescriber
- Inform patient that product may be taken before stressful activity: exercise, sexual activity
- Advise patient that SL tab may sting mucous membranes
- Caution patient to avoid driving and hazardous activities if dizziness occurs
- Advise patient to comply with complete medical regimen
- Caution patient to make position changes slowly to prevent orthostatic hypotension

Evaluation
Positive therapeutic outcome
- Decrease in, prevention of anginal pain

---

isradipine (Rx)
(is-ra'di-peen)
DynaCirc CR
Func. class.: Calcium channel blocker, antihypertensive, antianginal
Chem. class.: Dihydropyridine

Pregnancy category C

Do not confuse:
DynaCirc/Dynabac/Dynacin

Action: Inhibits calcium ion influx across cell membrane during cardiac depolarization; produces relaxation of coronary vascular smooth muscle and peripheral vascular smooth muscle; dilates coronary vascular arteries

Therapeutic outcome: Decreased B/P

Uses: Essential hypertension

Dosage and routes
Adult: PO 2.5 mg bid; increase at 2-4 wk intervals up to 10 mg bid or 5 mg/day; CONT REL may be increased q2-4wk, max 20 mg/day

Available forms: Caps 2.5, 5 mg; cont rel tabs 5, 10 mg

Adverse effects
CNS: Headache, fatigue, dizziness, fainting, sleep disturbances, weakness, depression, drowsiness
CV: Peripheral edema, tachycardia, hypotension, chest pain, **dysrhythmias,** syncope
GI: Nausea, vomiting, diarrhea, gastric upset, constipation, **hepatitis,** abdominal pain, distention, dry mouth
GU: Nocturia, urinary frequency
HEMA: **Leukopenia**

INTEG: Rash, pruritus, urticaria
MISC: Flushing

Contraindications: Sick sinus syndrome, 2nd- or 3rd-degree heart block, hypotension <90 mm Hg systolic, hypersensitivity

Precautions: Pregnancy **C**, breastfeeding, children, geriatric, CHF, hypotension, renal/hepatic disease

Pharmacokinetics

Absorption	Well absorbed
Distribution	High plasma protein binding (95%)
Metabolism	Liver, extensively and rapidly
Excretion	Kidney
Half-life	8 hr

Pharmacodynamics

Onset	1-2 hr
Peak	1.5 hr (immediate rel), 7-18 hr (cont rel)
Duration	12 hr

Interactions
Individual drugs
Disopyramide: increased bradycardia, conduction effects
Fentanyl: increased hypotension
Rifampin, ranitidine: increased serum concentration of isradipine
Cimetidine: decreased serum concentration of isradipine
Flovastatin: decreased flovastatin concentration
Lovastatin: decreased lovastatin concentration
Drug classifications
Antihypertensives, nitrates: increased hypotension
β-Adrenergic blockers: increased synergistic effect
CYP3A4 inducers: decreased serum concentration of isradipine
CYP3A4 inhibitors: decreased serum concentration of isradipine
NSAIDs, salicylates: decreased antihypertensive action
Drug/herb
Aconite: increased toxicity, death
Astragalus, cola tree: increased or decreased antihypertensive effect
Barberry, betony, black catechu, black cohosh, bloodroot, broom, burdock, cat's claw, dandelion, ginkgo, ginseng, goldenseal, hawthorn, Irish moss, Jamaica dogwood, kelp, khella, mistletoe, parsley: increased antihypertensive effect

Adverse effects: *italic* = common, **bold** = life-threatening

Coltsfoot, guarana, khat, licorice, St. John's wort, yohimbe: decreased antihypertensive effect

NURSING CONSIDERATIONS
Assessment
• Assess fluid volume status: I&O ratio and record, weight, distended red veins, crackles in lung, color, quality, and specific gravity of urine, skin turgor, adequacy of pulses, moist mucous membranes, bilateral lung sounds, peripheral pitting edema; dehydration symptoms of decreasing output, thirst, hypotension, dry mouth and mucous membranes should be reported
• Monitor ALT, AST, bilirubin; if these are elevated, hepatotoxicity is suspected
• Assess renal, hepatic status, electrolytes before, during treatment
• Monitor cardiac status: B/P, pulse, respiration, ECG; assess anginal pain, precipitating, ameliorating factors

Nursing diagnoses
• Cardiac output, decreased (uses)
• Knowledge, deficient (teaching)

Implementation
• Do not break, crush, or chew caps, cont rel tabs
• Give once a day with full glass of water; with food for GI symptoms

Patient/family education
• Instruct patient to avoid hazardous activities until stabilized on product and dizziness is no longer a problem
• Instruct patient to limit caffeine consumption; to avoid alcohol and OTC products unless directed by prescriber
• Advise patient to comply in all areas of medical regimen: diet, exercise, stress reduction, product therapy; to notify prescriber of irregular heartbeat, shortness of breath, swelling of feet and hands, pronounced dizziness, constipation, nausea, hypotension
• Teach patient to use as directed even if feeling better
• Teach patient to take with a full glass of water

Evaluation
Positive therapeutic outcome
• Decreased B/P

Treatment of overdose: Defibrillation, atropine for AV block, vasopressor for hypotension

itraconazole (Rx)
(it-tra-kon′a-zol)
Sporanox
Func. class.: Antifungal (systemic)
Chem. class.: Triazole derivative

Pregnancy category C

Action: Alters cell membranes and inhibits several fungal enzymes

Therapeutic outcome: Fungistatic against *Histoplasma capsulatum, Blastomyces dermatitis, Cryptococcus neoformans, Aspergillus fumigatus, Candida*

Uses: Systemic candidiasis, chronic mucocandidiasis, oral thrush, candiduria, histoplasmosis, chromomycosis, paracoccidioidomycosis, blastomycosis (pulmonary and extrapulmonary), aspergillosis onychomycosis

Unlabeled uses: Dermatomycosis, chromoblastomycosis, coccidioidomycosis, pityriasis versicolor, sebopsoriasis, vaginal candidiasis, cryptococcal, subcutaneous mycoses, dimorphic infections, leishmaniasis, fungal keratitis, alternariosis, zygomycosis

Dosage and routes
Dose varies with type of infection
Adult: PO 200 mg/day with food; may increase to 400 mg/day if needed; life-threatening infections may require a loading dose of 200 mg tid × 3 days; **IV** 200 mg bid × 4 doses, then 200 mg/day; give each dose over 1 hr, maintenance PO 200-400 mg/day
Child: PO 3-5 mg/kg/day

Available forms: Caps 100 mg; oral sol 10 mg/ml; inj 10 mg/ml

Adverse effects
CNS: Headache, dizziness, insomnia, somnolence, depression
CV: Hypertension
GI: Nausea, vomiting, anorexia, diarrhea, cramps, abdominal pain, flatulence, **GI bleeding, hepatotoxicity**
GU: Gynecomastia, impotence, decreased libido
INTEG: Pruritus, fever, rash, **toxic epidermal necrolysis**
MISC: Edema, fatigue, malaise, hypokalemia, tinnitus, **rhabdomyolysis**

Contraindications: Hypersensitivity, fungal meningitis, onychomycosis, or dermatomycosis in cardiac dysfunction, females

Black Box Warning: Heart failure, ventricular dysfunction, coadministration with other drugs

Precautions: Pregnancy **C**, breastfeeding, children, cardiac/hepatic disease, achlorhydria or hypochlorhydria (product-induced)

Pharmacokinetics

Absorption	Variable
Distribution	Tissue, plasma, CSF, highly protein bound
Metabolism	Liver, extensively, inhibits CYP4503A enzyme
Excretion	Feces, breast milk
Half-life	20-21 hr

Pharmacodynamics

Onset	Unknown
Peak	4 hr
Duration	Unknown

Interactions
Individual drugs
BusPIRone: increased busPIRone levels, toxicity

Busulfan, clarithromycin, cycloSPORINE, diazepam, digoxin, felodipine, fentanyl, indinavir, isradipine, niCARdipine, NIFEdipine, nimodipine, phenytoin, ritonavir, saquinavir, tacrolimus, warfarin: increased toxicity

Didanosine: decreased antifungal action

Dofetilide, pimozide, quinidine: life-threatening CV reaction

Midazolam (oral): increased sedation

Quinidine: increased tinnitus, hearing loss, increased toxicity

Rifamycins: decreased action of itraconazole

Triazolam: increased sedation

Drug classifications
Antacids, H_2-receptor antagonists: decreased action of itraconazole

Calcium channel blockers: increased edema

Contraceptives (oral): decreased effect

Hepatotoxic products: hepatotoxicity

Oral hypoglycemics: increased effects of oral hypoglycemics

Drug/herb
Gossypol: nephrotoxicity

Drug/food
Increased: absorption

NURSING CONSIDERATIONS
Assessment
• Assess for infection: WBC, sputum baseline, periodically, may start treatment before obtaining results

◆ Monitor for hepatotoxicity: increasing AST, ALT, alkaline phosphatase, bilirubin

• Monitor for allergic reaction: dermatitis, rash; product should be discontinued, antihistamines (mild reaction) or epinephrine (severe reaction) administered; check inj site for thrombophlebitis

• Monitor for hypokalemia, check potassium level: anorexia, drowsiness, weakness, decreased reflexes, dizziness, increased urinary output, increased thirst, paresthesias; if these occur, product should be decreased or discontinued and potassium administered

Nursing diagnoses
• Infection, risk for (uses)
• Injury, risk for (adverse reaction)
• Knowledge, deficient (teaching)

Implementation
PO route
• Swallow caps whole; do not break, crush, or chew
• Give caps after full meal to ensure absorption
• Give with food or milk to prevent nausea and vomiting
• Take 2 hr before administration of other products that increase gastric pH
• Store in tight container at room temperature
• Oral sol and caps are not interchangeable on a mg/mg basis
• Oral sol: patient should swish in mouth vigorously

IV route
• **IV** after adding full contents 25 ml to 50 ml of NaCl, mix gently, use flow control device, give over 1 hr; use separate line, flush after use

Patient/family education
• Advise patient that long-term therapy may be needed to clear infection (1 wk-6 mo depending on type of infection)
• Teach patient side effects and when to notify prescriber
• Instruct patient to avoid hazardous activities if dizziness occurs
• Instruct patient to take 2 hr before administration of other products that increase gastric pH (antacids, H_2-blockers, omeprazole, sucralfate, anticholinergics)
• Teach patient importance of compliance with product regimen
• Instruct patient to notify prescriber of GI symptoms, signs of liver dysfunction (fatigue, nausea, anorexia, vomiting, dark urine, pale stools)

Evaluation
Positive therapeutic outcome
• Decreased fever, malaise, rash
• Negative C&S for infectious organism

Adverse effects: *italic* = common, **bold** = life-threatening

ixabepilone (Rx)
(ix-ab-ep'i-lone)
Ixempra
Func. class.: Antineoplastic—miscellaneous
Chem. class.: Epothilone
Pregnancy category D

Action: Microtubule stabilizing agent; microtubles are needed for cell division

Therapeutic outcome: Decreased tumor size, spread of malignancy

Uses: Breast cancer

Dosage and routes
Breast cancer, metastatic or locally advanced given with capecitabine, and resistant to anthracycline, taxane
Adult: **IV** INF 40 mg/m² over 3 hr q3wk plus capecitabine PO 2000 mg/m²/day in 2 divided doses on days 1-14 q21day; in those with BSA >2.2 m², dose should be calculated for a BSA of 2.2 m²

Breast cancer, metastatic or locally advanced resistant/refractory to anthracyclines, taxanes, capecitabine
Adult: **IV** INF 40 mg/m² over 3 hr q3wk; in those with BSA >2.2 m², dose should be calculated for a BSA of 2.2 m²

Dosage reduction in those taking a strong CYP3A4 inhibitor
Adult: **IV** INF 20 mg/m² over 3 hr q3wk

Available forms: Powder for inj 15, 45 mg

Adverse effects
CNS: Peripheral neuropathy, chills, fatigue, fever, flushing, headache, insomnia, impaired cognition, asthenia
CV: Bradycardia, hypotension, abnormal ECG, angina, atrial flutter, cardiomyopathy, chest pain, edema, MI, vasculitis
GI: Nausea, vomiting, diarrhea, abdominal pain, anorexia, colitis, constipation, gastritis, jaundice, GERD, **hepatic failure,** trismus
GU: **Renal failure**
HEMA: **Neutropenia, thrombocytopenia, anemia,** infections, coagulopathy
INTEG: Alopecia, rash, hot flashes
META: Hypokalemia, metabolic acidosis
MS: Arthralgia, myalgia
RESP: Bronchospasm, cough, dyspnea
SYST: Hypersensitivity reactions, **anaphylaxis,** dehydration

Contraindications: Pregnancy **D**, hypersensitivity to products with polyoxyethylated castor oil, breastfeeding

Black Box Warning: Hepatic disease

Precautions: Children, geriatric, neutropenia of <1500/mm³, alcoholism, bone marrow suppression, cardiac dysrhythmias, cardiac/renal/hepatic disease, diabetes mellitus, peripheral neuropathy, thrombocytopenia, ventricular dysfunction

Pharmacokinetics
Absorption	Unknown
Distribution	Unknown
Metabolism	Liver by P45CYP3A4
Excretion	Feces 65%, urine 21%
Half-life	Terminal 52 hr

Pharmacodynamics
Unknown

Interactions
Drug classifications
CYP3A4 inducers (aminoglutethimide, barbiturates, bexarotene, bosentan, carbamazepine, dexamethasone, efavirenz, griseofulvin, modafinil, nafcillin, nevirapine, oxcarbazepine, phenytoin, rifamycin, topiramate): decreased ixabepilone levels
CYP3A4 inhibitors (amiodarone, amprenavir, aprepitant, atazanavir, chloramphenicol, clarithromycin, conivaptan, cycloSPORINE, danazol, darunavir, dalforpristan, delavirdine, diltiazem, erythromycin, estradiol, fluconazole, fluvoxamine, fosamprenavir, imatinib, indinavir, isoniazid, itraconazole, ketoconazole, lopinavir, miconazole, nefazodone, nelfinavir, propoxyphene, ritonavir, RU-486, saquinavir, tamoxifen, telithromycin, troleandomycin, verapamil, voriconazole, zafirlukast): increased ixabepilone level
Drug/herb
St. John's wort: avoid use
Drug/food
Grapefruit products: avoid use

NURSING CONSIDERATIONS
Assessment
• Monitor CBC, differential, platelet count prior to therapy, qwk; withhold product if WBC is <1500/mm³ or platelet count is <100,000/mm³, notify prescriber
• Monitor temp q4hr (may indicate beginning infection)
• Monitor liver function tests before, during therapy (bilirubin, AST, ALT, LDH) prn or qmo;

 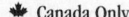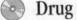

check for jaundiced skin and sclera, dark urine, clay-colored stool, itchy skin, abdominal pain, fever, diarrhea
- Monitor VS during 1st hr of inf; check IV site for signs of infiltration
⚠ Assess for hypersensitive reactions, anaphylaxis including hypotension, dyspnea, angioedema, generalized urticaria; discontinue inf immediately; keep emergency equipment available
- Assess effects of alopecia on body image; discuss feelings about body changes

Nursing diagnoses
- Injury, risk for (uses, adverse reactions)
- Knowledge, deficient (teaching)

Implementation
- Give antiemetic 30-60 min before giving product and prn
IV route
- Let kit stand at room temperature for 30 min; to reconstitute, withdraw supplied diluent (8 ml for 15 mg vials, 23.5 ml for 45 mg vials); slowly inject solution into vial; gently swirl and invert to mix, final conc 2 mg/ml; further dilute in LR in DEHP-free bags; final conc should be 0.2-0.6 mg/ml; after added, mix by manual rotation
- Diluted sol is stable for 6 hr at room temperature; inf must be completed within 6 hr
- Use in-line filter 0.2-1.2 micron
- Give over 3 hr

Patient/family education
- Teach patient to report signs of infection: fever, sore throat, flulike symptoms
- Teach patient to report signs of anemia: fatigue, headache, faintness, shortness of breath
- Teach patient to report any complaints or side effects to nurse or prescriber
- Caution patient that hair may be lost during treatment; a wig or hairpiece may make patient feel better; new hair may be different in color, texture
- Advise patient that pain in muscles and joints 2-5 days after inf is common
- Advise patient to use nonhormonal type of contraception
- Instruct patient to avoid receiving vaccinations while on this product

Evaluation
Positive therapeutic outcome
- Decreased tumor size, spread of malignancy

ketoconazole (Rx)
(kee-toe-koe′na-zole)
Func. class.: Antifungal
Chem. class.: Imidazole derivative
Pregnancy category C

Action: Alters cell membrane and inhibits several fungal enzymes leading to cell death

Therapeutic outcome: Fungistatic/fungicidal against susceptible organisms: *Blastomycoses, Candida, Coccidioides, Cryptococcus, Histoplasma;* topical route: tinea cruris, tinea corporis, tinea versicolor, *Pityrosporum ovale*

Uses: Systemic candidiasis, chronic mucocandidiasis, oral thrush, candiduria, coccidioidomycosis, histoplasmosis, chromomycosis, paracoccidioidomycosis, blastomycosis, tinea cruris, tinea corporis, tinea versicolor, *Pityrosporum ovale*

Unlabeled uses: Cushing's syndrome, advanced prostatic cancer

Dosage and routes
Adult: PO 200-400 mg once/day for 1-2 wk (candidiasis), 6 wk (other infections); 400 mg tid (prostate cancer, unlabeled)
Children >2 yr: 3.3-6.6 mg/kg/day as single daily dose

Available forms: Tabs 200 mg; oral susp ✱ 100 mg/5 ml topical (see Appendix B)

Adverse effects
CNS: Headache, dizziness, somnolence
GI: Nausea, vomiting, anorexia, diarrhea, abdominal pain, **hepatotoxicity**
GU: Gynecomastia, impotence
HEMA: **Thrombocytopenia, leukopenia, hemolytic anemia**
INTEG: Pruritus, fever, chills, photophobia, rash, dermatitis, purpura, urticaria
SYST: **Anaphylaxis**

Contraindications: Breastfeeding, hypersensitivity, fungal meningitis

Black Box Warning: Coadministration with other drugs

Precautions: Pregnancy **C**, children <2 yr, renal disease, achlorhydria (product induced)
Black Box Warning: Hepatic disease

K

Adverse effects: *italic* = common, **bold** = life-threatening

Pharmacokinetics

Absorption	pH dependent; decreased pH, increased absorption
Distribution	Widely distributed; crosses placenta
Metabolism	Liver, partially
Excretion	Feces, bile, breast milk
Half-life	Biphasic: 2 hr, 8 hr

Pharmacodynamics

Onset	Unknown
Peak	1-3 hr
Duration	Unknown

Interactions
Individual drugs
Alcohol: increased hepatotoxicity

Alfentanil, alprazolam, amprenavir, atorvastatin, carbamazepine, cerivastatin, clarithromycin, cyclophosphamide, cycloSPORINE, donepezil, erythromycin, fentanyl, ifosfamide, indinavir, lovastatin, midazolam, nelfinavir, nisoldipine, quinidine, ritonavir, saquinavir, sildenafil, simvastatin, sufentanil, tamoxifen, triazolam, vinBLAStine, vinCRIStine, zolpidem: increased toxicity, inhibition of CYP450 3A4 pathway

ddI, isoniazid, phenytoin, rifampin: decreased effect of ketoconazole

Paclitaxel: inhibited metabolism

Theophylline: decreased effectiveness

Warfarin: increased effects of warfarin

Drug classifications
Antacids, anticholinergics, gastric acid pump inhibitors, H$_2$-receptor agonists: decreased ketoconazole action

Anticoagulants (oral): increased effects of oral anticoagulants

Calcium channel blockers, corticosteroids, vinca alkaloids: increased toxicity, decreased CYP4503A4 pathway

Contraceptives (oral): decreased effect of oral contraceptives

Hepatotoxic agents: increased hepatotoxicity

Drug/herb
Gossypol: nephrotoxicity

Yew: decreased ketoconazole action

NURSING CONSIDERATIONS
Assessment
• Assess for signs and symptoms of infection: drainage, sore throat, urinary pain, hematuria, fever

• Obtain cultures for C&S before beginning treatment; therapy may be started after culture is taken

◆ Monitor for hepatotoxicity: increased AST, ALT, alkaline phosphatase, bilirubin; product is discontinued if hepatotoxicity occurs

Nursing diagnoses
• Infection, risk for (uses)
• Injury, risk for (adverse reactions)
• Knowledge, deficient (teaching)

Implementation
PO route
• Give in the presence of acid products only; do not use alkaline products, proton pump inhibitors, H$_2$-antagonists, or antacids within 2 hr of product; may give coffee, tea, acidic fruit juices, cola; give with food to decrease GI symptoms; dissolve tab/4 ml of aqueous sol 0.2 N HCl, use straw to avoid contact, rinse with water afterward and swallow

• Give with HCl if achlorhydria is present

• Store in tight container at room temperature

Topical route
• Use enough medication to cover fungally infected and surrounding area; rub in; do not use occlusive dressing; do not get in eyes

Shampoo
• Hair should be wet; apply shampoo, lather, rub gently into scalp and hair for 1 min; rinse; reapply × 3 min; continue treatment 2 ×/wk for 1 mo, no more than once q3day

Patient/family education
• Advise patient that long-term therapy may be needed to clear infection (1 wk-6 mo depending on infection)

• Advise patient to avoid hazardous activities if dizziness occurs

• Instruct patient to take 2 hr before administration of other products that increase gastric pH (antacids, H$_2$-blockers, omeprazole, sucralfate, anticholinergics)

• Stress the importance of compliance with product regimen

• Advise patient to notify prescriber of GI symptoms, signs of liver dysfunction (fatigue, nausea, anorexia, vomiting, dark urine, pale stools)

• Teach patient proper hygiene: hand washing, nail care, use of concomitant topical agents if prescribed

• Caution patient to avoid alcohol, since nausea, vomiting, hypertension may occur

• Advise patient to use sunscreen or avoid direct sunlight to prevent photosensitivity

• Advise patient to notify prescriber of sore throat, fever, skin rash, which may indicate superinfection

• Advise patient to use sunglasses to prevent photophobia

Evaluation
Positive therapeutic outcome
- Decreased oral candidiasis, fever, malaise, rash
- Negative C&S for infectious organism
- Absence of dandruff, scaling

---

ketoconazole topical
See Appendix B

---

ketoprofen (OTC, Rx)
(ke-to-proe'fen)
Apo-Keto ✤, Apo-Keto-E ✤, Ketoprofen, Orudis-E ✤, Orudis-SR ✤, Rhodis ✤
Func. class.: NSAID; nonopioid analgesic, antirheumatic
Chem. class.: Propionic acid derivative

Pregnancy category
B (1st trimester),
D (2nd/3rd trimesters)

Action: Inhibits prostaglandin synthesis by decreasing enzyme needed for biosynthesis; analgesic, antiinflammatory, antipyretic

Therapeutic outcome: Decreased pain, inflammation

Uses: Mild to moderate pain; osteoarthritis; rheumatoid arthritis; dysmenorrhea; OTC relief of minor aches, pains

Dosage and routes
Antiinflammatory
Adult: PO 150-300 mg in divided doses tid-qid, max 300 mg/day or EXT REL 200 mg/day

Analgesic
Adult: PO 25-50 mg q6-8hr, max 300 mg/day

Available forms: Caps 50, 75 mg; ext rel caps 200 mg

Adverse effects
CNS: Dizziness, drowsiness, fatigue, tremors, confusion, insomnia, anxiety, depression, headache
CV: Tachycardia, peripheral edema, palpitations, dysrhythmias, hypertension, **CV thrombotic events, MI, stroke**
EENT: Tinnitus, hearing loss, blurred vision
GI: Nausea, anorexia, vomiting, diarrhea, jaundice, **hepatitis,** constipation, flatulence, cramps, dry mouth, peptic ulcer, **GI bleeding**

GU: **Nephrotoxicity: dysuria, hematuria, oliguria, azotemia**
HEMA: **Blood dyscrasias**
INTEG: Purpura, rash, pruritus, sweating
SYST: **Anaphylaxis**

Contraindications: Pregnancy **D**, 2nd/3rd trimesters; hypersensitivity, asthma, severe renal/hepatic disease, ulcer disease

Black Box Warning: Perioperative pain in CABG

Precautions: Pregnancy **B** (1st trimester), breastfeeding, children, geriatric, bleeding/GI/cardiac disorders, hypersensitivity to other antiinflammatory agents

Black Box Warning: GI bleeding, MI, stroke

Pharmacokinetics
Absorption	Well absorbed
Distribution	Not known
Metabolism	Liver
Excretion	Kidneys
Half-life	2-4 hr; 5.4 hr (ext rel)

Pharmacodynamics
Onset	Unknown
Peak	1.2 hr; 6.8 hr (ext rel)
Duration	Unknown

Interactions
Individual drugs
Alcohol: increased adverse GI reactions, toxicity
Aspirin: increased ketoprofen levels, increased adverse GI reactions
Cefamandole, cefaperazone, cefotetan, clopidogrel, eptifibatide, plicamycin, ticlopidine, tirofiban, valproic acid: increased risk of bleeding
CycloSPORINE, digoxin, lithium, methotrexate, phenytoin: increased ketoprofen levels, increased toxicity
Insulin: increased hypoglycemia
Probenecid: increased ketoconazole levels
Radiation: increased risk of hematologic toxicity
Drug classifications
Anticoagulants, thrombolytics: increased risk of bleeding
Antihypertensives: decreased effect of antihypertensives
Antineoplastics: increased hematologic toxicity
Corticosteroids: increased adverse GI reactions

Adverse effects: *italic* = common, **bold** = life-threatening

Diuretics: decreased effectiveness of diuretics
NSAIDs: increased adverse GI reactions
Sulfonylureas: increased hypoglycemia
Drug/herb
Anise, arnica, bogbean, chamomile, chondroi-tin, clove, dong quai, feverfew, garlic, ginger, ginkgo, ginseng *(Panax):* increased risk of bleeding
Arginine, gossypol: increased gastric irritation
Bearberry, bilberry: increased NSAIDs effect
Drug/lab test
Increased: bleeding time, potassium, BUN, alkaline phosphatase, AST, ALT, creatinine, LDH
Decreased: blood glucose, Hct, Hgb, CCr, platelets, leukocytes
Interference: urine albumin, 17 KS, 17 hy-droxycorticosteroids, bilirubin

NURSING CONSIDERATIONS
Assessment
• Assess for pain: type, location, intensity; ROM before and 1-2 hr after treatment
• Monitor renal, liver function tests: AST, ALT, bilirubin, creatinine, BUN, urine creatinine, CBC Hct, Hgb, pro-time if patient is on long-term therapy
• Check I&O ratio; decreasing output may indicate renal failure (long-term therapy)
• Assess hepatotoxicity: dark urine, clay-colored stools, jaundice of skin and sclera, itching, abdominal pain, fever, diarrhea if patient is on long-term therapy
• Assess for allergic reactions: rash, urticaria; if these occur, product may have to be discontin-ued
• Assess for ototoxicity: tinnitus, ringing, roaring in ears; audiometric testing needed before, after long-term therapy
• Assess for visual changes: blurring, halos; may indicate corneal, retinal damage
• Assess for GI bleeding: blood in sputum, emesis, stools
• Check edema in feet, ankles, legs
• Identify prior product history; there are many product interactions
• Monitor pain: location, duration, type, intensity, before dose and 1 hr after; ROM before dose and after
• Assess for CV thrombotic events: MI, stroke

Nursing diagnoses
• Injury, risk for (adverse reactions)
• Knowledge, deficient (teaching)
• Mobility, physical impaired (uses)
• Pain, acute (uses)
• Pain, chronic (uses)

Implementation
• Swallow whole; do not break, crush, chew, or open ext rel cap
• Give with 8 oz of water and sit upright for 30 min after dose to prevent ulceration
• Give with food or milk to decrease gastric symptoms; give 30 min before or 2 hr after meals; absorption may be slowed

Patient/family education
• Teach patient to report any symptoms of hepatotoxicity, renal toxicity, visual changes, ototoxicity, allergic reactions, bleeding (long-term therapy)
• Advise patient to take with 8 oz of water and sit upright for 30 min after dose to prevent ulceration
• Caution patient not to exceed recommended dosage; acute poisoning may result; to take as prescribed; do not double dose
• Advise patient to read label on other OTC products; many contain other antiinflammato-ries
• Advise patient to use sunscreen to prevent photosensitivity
• Inform patient that the therapeutic response takes 2 wk (arthritis)
• Teach patient to report tinnitus, confusion, diarrhea, sweating, hyperventilation, blurred vision, fever, joint aches
• Caution patient to avoid alcohol ingestion; GI bleeding may occur
• Teach patient to report use to all providers

Evaluation
Positive therapeutic outcome
• Decreased pain
• Decreased inflammation
• Increased mobility
• Decreased fever

ketorolac (Rx)
(kee'toe-role-ak)
Acular
Func. class.: NSAID, nonopioid analgesic
Chem. class.: Acetic acid

Pregnancy category
C; D (third trimester)

Action: Inhibits prostaglandin synthesis by decreasing an enzyme needed for biosynthesis; analgesic, antiinflammatory, antipyretic effects

Therapeutic outcome: Decreased pain, inflammation, ocular itching

Uses: Mild to moderate pain (short term); decreased ocular itching in seasonal allergic conjunctivitis (ophthalmic)

Dosage and routes
Adult <65 yr: PO 20 mg, then 10 mg q4-6hr prn, max 40 mg/day; IM (single dose) 30-60 mg; **IV** 15-30 mg; IM (multiple dosing) 15 mg q6hr, max 60 mg/day × 5 days combined either PO/IM/**IV**

Adult >65 yr, renal disease, <50 kg: PO 10 mg q4-6hr prn, max 40 mg/day; IM (single dose) 30 mg; **IV** 15 mg; IM/**IV** (multiple dosing) 15 mg q6hr, max 60 mg/day × 5 days combined either PO/IM/**IV**

Ophthalmic route
Adult: 1 gtt (0.25 mg) qid × 7 days
Child: **IV** 1 mg/kg then 0.5 mg/kg q6hr

Available forms: Inj 15, 30 mg/ml (prefilled syringes); ophth 0.5% sol; tabs 10 mg

Adverse effects
CNS: Dizziness, *drowsiness,* tremors, **seizures**
CV: Hypertension, flushing, syncope, pallor, edema, vasodilatation, **CV thrombotic events, MI, stroke**
EENT: Tinnitus, hearing loss, blurred vision
GI: Nausea, anorexia, vomiting, diarrhea, constipation, flatulence, cramps, dry mouth, peptic ulcer, **GI bleeding, perforation,** taste change, **hepatitis, hepatic failure**
GU: Nephrotoxicity: **dysuria, hematuria, oliguria, azotemia**
HEMA: **Blood dyscrasias,** prolonged bleeding
INTEG: Purpura, rash, pruritus, sweating, **angioedema, Stevens-Johnson syndrome, toxic epidermal necrolysis**

Contraindications: Pregnancy **D** (3rd trimester), hypersensitivity, asthma, hepatic disease, peptic ulcer disease, CV bleeding

Black Box Warning: Breastfeeding, severe renal disease, labor and delivery, perioperative pain in CABG, prior to major surgery, epidural/intrathecal administration, GI bleeding, hypovolemia

Precautions: Pregnancy **C,** bleeding disorders, GI/cardiac disorders, hypersensitivity to other antiinflammatory agents, CCr <25 ml/min

Black Box Warning: Children, geriatric, MI, stroke

Pharmacokinetics
Absorption	Rapidly, completely absorbed
Distribution	Bound to plasma proteins (99%)
Metabolism	Liver (<50%)
Excretion	Kidney, metabolites (92%); breast milk (6%); feces
Half-life	6 hr (IM); increased in renal disease

Pharmacodynamics
	IM	OPHTH/PO
Onset	Up to 10 min	Unknown
Peak	50 min IM; 2-3 hr PO	Unknown
Duration	4-6 hr PO	Unknown

Interactions
Individual drugs
Alcohol, aspirin: increased GI effects
Aspirin: increased ketorolac levels, contraindicated
Cefamandole, cefoperazone, cefotetan, clopidogrel, eptifibatide, plicamycin, ticlopidine, tirofiban, valproic acid: increased risk of bleeding
CycloSPORINE, lithium, methotrexate, pentoxifylline, probenecid: increased toxicity
Drug classifications
ACE inhibitors: increased renal impairment
Anticoagulants: increased effects
Antihypertensives: decreased antihypertensive effect
Cephalosporins (some), salicylates, SNRIs, SSRIs, thrombolytics: increased risk of bleeding
Corticosteroids, NSAIDs, potassium products, steroids: increased GI effects
Diuretics: decreased diuretic effect
NSAIDs (other): increased ketorolac levels; contraindicated
Drug/herb
Anise, arnica, bogbean, chamomile, chondroitin, clove, dong quai, feverfew, garlic, ginger, ginkgo, ginseng *(Panax):* increased risk of bleeding
Arginine, gossypol: increased gastric irritation
Bearberry, bilberry: increased NSAIDs effect
Drug/lab test
Increased: AST, ALT, LDH, alkaline phosphatase, bleeding time, BUN, creatinine, potassium
Decreased: blood glucose, Hct/Hgb, platelets

NURSING CONSIDERATIONS
Assessment
◆ Monitor blood counts during therapy; watch for decreasing platelets; if low, therapy may need to be discontinued and restarted after

hematologic recovery; assess for blood dyscrasia (thrombocytopenia): bruising, fatigue, bleeding, poor healing
• Monitor for aspirin sensitivity, asthma; these patients may be more likely to develop hypersensitivity to NSAIDs
• Assess patient's eyes: redness, swelling, tearing, itching
• Monitor for pain: type, location, intensity, ROM before and 1 hr after treatment
• Assess for GI bleeding: blood in sputum, emesis, stools
• Assess for CV thrombotic events: MI, stroke

Nursing diagnoses
• Injury, risk for (adverse reactions)
• Knowledge, deficient (teaching)
• Mobility, impaired physical (uses)
• Pain, acute (uses)

Implementation
PO route
• Administer to patient crushed or whole
• Max 5 days
• Give with full glass of water; give with food or milk to decrease gastric symptoms; give 30 min before or 2 hr after meals; absorption may be slowed
IM/IV route
• **IV** give undiluted ≥15 sec
• Give IM inj deeply into large muscle mass
• Store at room temperature, protect from light
Y-site compatibilities: Cisatracurium, remifentanil, sufentanil
Syringe incompatibilities: Morphine, meperidine, promethazine, hydrOXYzine
Solution compatibilities: D_5W, 0.9% NaCl, LR, D_5, plasmalate

Patient/family education
• Teach patient that product must be continued for prescribed time to be effective; to avoid aspirin, alcoholic beverages, other NSAIDs, acetaminophen
• Caution patient to report bleeding, bruising, fatigue, malaise, since blood dyscrasias do occur
• Instruct patient to use caution when driving; drowsiness, dizziness may occur
• Teach patient to take with a full glass of water to enhance absorption
• Caution patient that this product may cause eye redness, burning if soft contact lenses are worn
• Advise to report use to all health care providers

Evaluation
Positive therapeutic outcome
• Decreased pain
• Decreased inflammatory response
• Increased mobility
• Decreased ocular itching

ketorolac ophthalmic
See Appendix B

ketotifen ophthalmic
See Appendix B

labetalol (Rx)
(la-bet'a-lole)
Trandate
Func. class.: Antihypertensive, antianginal
Chem. class.: α- and β-blocker
Pregnancy category C

Do not confuse:
Trandate/Tridate

Action: Produces decreases in B/P without reflex tachycardia or significant reduction in heart rate through mixture of α-blocking, β-blocking effects; elevated plasma resins are reduced

Therapeutic outcome: Decreased B/P

Uses: Mild to moderate hypertension; treatment of severe hypertension (**IV**)

Unlabeled uses: Hypertension in patients with pheochromocytoma, hypertension in clonidine withdrawal

Dosage and routes
Hypertension
Adult: PO 100 mg bid; may be given with a diuretic; may increase to 200 mg bid after 2 days; may continue to increase q1-3day; max 2400 mg/day in divided doses

Hypertensive crisis
Adult: IV INF 200 mg/160 ml D_5W, run at 2 mg/min or 1.6 ml/min; stop INF after desired response obtained; repeat q6-8hr as needed; IV BOL 20 mg over 2 min; may repeat 20-80 mg q10min, max 300 mg

Available forms: Tabs 100, 200, 300 mg; inj 5 mg/ml in 20-ml ampules

Adverse effects
CNS: Dizziness, mental changes, drowsiness, fatigue, headache, catatonia, depression, anxiety, nightmares, paresthesias, lethargy

CV: *Orthostatic hypotension,* **bradycardia, CHF,** chest pain, **ventricular dysrhythmias,** AV block, scalp tingling

EENT: *Tinnitus,* visual changes, sore throat, double vision, dry burning eyes

GI: *Nausea, vomiting, diarrhea,* dyspepsia, taste distortion

GU: Impotence, dysuria, ejaculatory failure

HEMA: Agranulocytosis, thrombocytopenia, purpura (rare)

INTEG: Rash, alopecia, urticaria, pruritus, fever

RESP: Bronchospasm, dyspnea, wheezing

Contraindications: Hypersensitivity to β-blockers, cardiogenic shock, heart block (2nd or 3rd degree), sinus bradycardia, CHF, bronchial asthma

Precautions: Pregnancy **C,** breastfeeding, geriatric, major surgery, diabetes mellitus, thyroid/renal/hepatic disease, COPD, well-compensated heart failure, CAD, nonallergic bronchospasm, peripheral vascular disease

Black Box Warning: Abrupt discontinuation

Pharmacokinetics

Absorption	Bioavailability 25% (PO); complete (**IV**)
Distribution	Crosses placenta, CNS
Metabolism	Liver, extensively
Excretion	Breast milk, kidneys, bile
Half-life	6-8 hr

Pharmacodynamics

	PO	IV
Onset	1-2 hr	5 min
Peak	2-4 hr	15 min
Duration	8-12 hr	2-4 hr

Interactions
Individual drugs
Alcohol (large amounts), cimetidine, nitroglycerin: increased hypotension

Glutethimide: decreased effect of labetalol

Indomethacin, lidocaine: decreased effect of each specific product

Verapamil: increased myocardial depression

Drug classifications
Antihypertensives: increased hypotension

β-Blockers, bronchodilators, sympathomimetics, xanthines: decreased effects

Diuretics: increased hypotension

General anesthetics, hydantoins: increased myocardial depression

MAOIs: do not use within 2 wk

NSAIDs, salicylates: decreased antihypertensive effect

Theophyllines: decreased bronchodilatation

Drug/herb
Aconite: increased toxicity, death

Astragalus, cola tree: increased or decreased antihypertensive effect

Barberry, betony, black catechu, black cohosh, bloodroot, broom, burdock, cat's claw, dandelion, goldenseal, hawthorn, Irish moss, Jamaican dogwood, kelp, khella, mistletoe, parsley: increased antihypertensive effect

Coltsfoot, guarana, khat, licorice, yohimbe: decreased antihypertensive effect

Drug/lab test
Increased: ANA titer, blood glucose, alkaline phosphatase, LDH, AST, ALT, BUN, potassium, triglycerides, uric acid

False increase: urinary catecholamines

NURSING CONSIDERATIONS
Assessment
• Monitor B/P at beginning of treatment, periodically thereafter; pulse q4hr; note rate, rhythm, quality: apical/radial pulse before administration, notify prescriber of any significant changes (pulse <50 bpm)

• Check for baselines in renal, liver function tests before therapy begins

• Assess for edema in feet, legs daily, monitor I&O, daily weight; check for jugular vein distention, crackles bilaterally, dyspnea (CHF)

• Monitor skin turgor, dryness of mucous membranes for hydration status, especially geriatric

Nursing diagnoses
• Cardiac output, decreased (uses)
• Injury, risk for (side effects)
• Knowledge, deficient (teaching)
• Noncompliance (teaching)

Implementation
PO route
• Given before meals, at bedtime; tab may be crushed or swallowed whole; give with food to prevent GI upset, increase absorption; reduce dosage in renal dysfunction

• Store protected from light, moisture; place in cool environment

IV route
• Give **IV** undiluted 20 mg/2 min; may increase q10min 40-80 mg until desired effect

• Give **IV** cont inf by diluting in LR, D₅W, D₅ in 0.2%, 0.9%, 0.33% NaCl or Ringer's; inf is titrated to patient response; 200 mg of product/160 ml sol (1 mg/ml); 300 mg of product/240 ml sol (1 mg/ml); 200 mg

of product/250 ml sol (2 mg/3ml); use inf pump
• Keep patient recumbent during and for 3 hr after inf, monitor VS q5-15min

Y-site compatibilities: Amikacin, aminophylline, amiodarone, ampicillin, butorphanol, calcium gluconate, cefazolin, ceftazidime, ceftizoxime, chloramphenicol, cimetidine, clindamycin, diltiazem, DOBUT-amine, DOPamine, enalaprilat, epinephrine, erythromycin, esmolol, famotidine, fentanyl, gentamicin, hydromorphone, lidocaine, lorazepam, magnesium sulfate, meperidine, metronidazole, midazolam, milrinone, mor-phine, niCARdipine, nitroglycerin, nitroprus-side, norepinephrine, oxacillin, penicillin G potassium, piperacillin, potassium chloride, potassium phosphate, propofol, ranitidine, sodium acetate, tobramycin, trimethoprim/sulfamethoxazole, vancomycin, vecuronium

Y-site incompatibilities: Cefoperazone, nafcillin

Solution compatibilities: D_5R, D_5LR, $D_{2\frac{1}{2}}$/0.45% NaCl, D_5/0.2% NaCl, D_5/0.33% NaCl, D_5/0.9% NaCl, D_5W, Ringer's, LR

Solution incompatibilities: Sodium bicarbonate 5%

Patient/family education
• Teach patient not to discontinue product abruptly, or precipitate angina might occur; taper over 2 wk
• Teach patient not to use OTC products containing α-adrenergic stimulants (such as nasal decongestants, cold preparations); to avoid alcohol, smoking; to limit sodium intake as prescribed
• Teach patient how to take pulse and B/P at home; advise when to notify prescriber
• Instruct patient to comply with weight control, dietary adjustments, modified exercise program
• Advise patient to carry/wear emergency ID to identify products being taken, allergies; that product controls symptoms but does not cure the condition
• Caution patient to avoid hazardous activities if dizziness, drowsiness are present
• Teach patient to report symptoms of CHF: difficulty breathing, especially on exertion or when lying down, night cough, swelling of extremities, bradycardia, dizziness, confusion, depression, fever
• Teach patient to take product as prescribed, not to double or skip doses; take any missed doses as soon as remembered if at least 4 hr until next dose

Evaluation
Positive therapeutic outcome
• Decreased B/P in hypertension (after 1-2 wk)
• Absence of dysrhythmias

Treatment of overdose: Lavage, **IV** atropine for bradycardia, **IV** theophylline for bronchospasm, digoxin, O_2, diuretic for cardiac failure, hemodialysis, **IV** glucose for hyperglycemia, **IV** diazepam (or phenytoin) for seizures

lacosamide (Rx)
(la-koe′sa-mide)
Vimpat
Func. class.: Anticonvulsant
Chem. class.: Functionalized amino acid

Pregnancy category C

Action: May act through action at sodium channels; exact action is unknown

Therapeutic outcome: Decrease in severity of seizures

Uses: Adjunctive therapy of partial seizures

Dosage and routes
Adult and child ≥17 yr: PO 50 mg bid, may increase qwk by 50 mg bid to 200-400 mg/day; **IV** 50 mg 2 ×/day, infuse over 30-60 min, may be increased 100 mg/day weekly, up to 200-400 mg/day maintenance

Available forms: Film coated tabs 50, 100, 150, 200 mg; **IV** 20 ml single use vials (200 mg/20 ml)

Adverse effects
CNS: Dizziness, syncope, tremor, vertigo, ataxia, drowsiness, fever, hypoesthesia, pares-thesias, depression, fatigue, headache, confu-sion, irritability, psychological dependence, **suicidal ideation**
CV: **Atrial fibrillation/flutter, AV block,** bradycardia, myocarditis, orthostatic hypoten-sion, palpitations, **QT prolongation**
EENT: Diplopia, blurred vision, nystagmus, tinnitus
GI: Nausea, constipation, vomiting, **hepatitis,** diarrhea, dyspepsia
HEMA: **Anemia, neutropenia**
INTEG: Rash, erythemia, inj site reaction, pruritus, xerostomia
MS: Asthenia, dysarthria

Contraindications: Hypersensitivity

Precautions: Pregnancy C, breastfeeding, allergies, renal/hepatic disease, geriatric patients, child <17 yr, acute MI, atrial fibrillation/flutter, AV block, bradycardia, cardiac disease, congenital heart disease, dehydration, depression, dialysis, hazardous activity, electrolyte imbalance, heart failure, labor, QT prolongation, sick sinus syndrome, substance abuse, suicidal ideation, syncope, torsades de pointes

Pharmacokinetics

Absorption	Unknown
Distribution	Protein binding <15%
Metabolism	Liver
Excretion	Kidneys (95% unchanged)
Half-life	13 hr (PO)

Pharmacodynamics

Onset	Unknown
Peak	1-4 hr (PO)
Duration	Unknown

Interactions
Individual drugs
⚑Bepridil, chloroquine, clarithromycin, droperidol, erythromycin, grepafloxacin, halofantrine, haloperidol, methadone, pentamidine, probucol, sparfloxacin: increased QT prolongation
Drug classifications
⚑Anesthetics (local), β-agonists, class 1A/III antidysrhythmics, some phenothiazines, tricyclic antidepressants: increased QT prolongation
Drug/lab test
Increased: LFTs

NURSING CONSIDERATIONS
Assessment
- Assess for seizures: duration, type, intensity, precipitating factors
- Monitor for renal function: albumin concentration
- Assess CV status: orthostatic hypotension, QT prolongation; monitor cardiac status throughout treatment
- Assess mental status: mood, sensorium, affect, memory (long, short), depression, suicidal ideation, psychological dependence
- Assess for rash, hypersensitivity reactions

Nursing diagnoses
- Injury, risk for (uses)
- Knowledge, deficient (teaching)

Implementation
- Store PO products/**IV** vials at room temperature; solution is stable for 24 hrs when mixed with compatible diluents in glass or PVC bags at room temperature

PO route
- Give without regard to meals
IV route
- May give undiluted or mixed in 0.9% NaCl, D₅, or LR
- Infuse over 30-60 min
- Do not use if discolored or particulates are present; discard unused portions

Patient/family education
- Caution patient not to discontinue product abruptly; seizures may occur
- Advise patient to avoid hazardous activities until stabilized on product
- Instruct patient to carry emergency ID stating product use
- Advise patient to notify prescriber of suicidal thoughts or actions, syncope, cardiac changes
- Instruct patient to notify prescriber if pregnancy is planned or suspected
- Teach patient that interactions with other medications may occur
- Give patient MediGuide for proper use and risks

Evaluation
Positive therapeutic outcome
- Decrease in severity of seizures

lactulose (Rx)
(lak´tyoo-lose)
Cephulac, Cholac, Chronulac, Constilac, Constulose, Duphalac, Enulose, Evalose, Heptalac, Kristalose, Lactulax ✦, Lactulose PSE, Portalac
Func. class.: Laxative (hyperosmotic/ammonia detoxicant)
Chem. class.: Lactose synthetic derivative

Pregnancy category B

Action: Increases osmotic pressure; draws fluid into colon; prevents absorption of ammonia in colon; increases water in stool

Therapeutic outcome: Decreased constipation, decreased blood ammonia level

Uses: Chronic constipation, portal-systemic encephalopathy in patients with hepatic disease

Dosage and routes
Constipation
Adult: PO 15-30 ml/day (10-20 g), may increase to 60 ml/day prn
Child (unlabeled): PO 7.5 ml/day

Encephalopathy
Adult: PO 30-45 ml tid or qid until stools are soft; retention enema 300 ml diluted

---

Adverse effects: *italic* = common, **bold** = life-threatening

Infant (unlabeled): PO 2.5-10 ml/day in divided doses
Child (unlabeled): PO 40-90 ml/day in divided doses given 2-4 ×/day

Available forms: Syr 10 g/15 ml, single-use packets (Kristalose) 10, 20 g

Adverse effects
GI: Nausea, vomiting, anorexia, abdominal cramps, diarrhea, flatulence, *distention, belching*
META: Hypernatremia

Contraindications: Hypersensitivity, low-galactose diet

Precautions: Pregnancy **B**, breastfeeding, geriatric and debilitated patient, diabetes mellitus

Pharmacokinetics	
Absorption	Poorly absorbed
Distribution	Not known
Metabolism	Colonic bacteria to acids
Excretion	Kidneys, unchanged
Half-life	Unknown

Pharmacodynamics
Unknown

Interactions
Individual drugs
Neomycin: decreased lactulose effect
Drug classifications
Antiinfectives (oral): decreased lactulose effect
Laxatives: do not use together
Drug/herb
Flax, senna: increased laxative effect

NURSING CONSIDERATIONS
Assessment
• Monitor glucose levels in diabetic patients (increases)
• Monitor blood, urine, electrolytes if used often by patient; may cause diarrhea, hypokalemia, hypernatremia; check I&O ratio to identify fluid loss
• Assess cramping, rectal bleeding, nausea, vomiting; if these symptoms occur, product should be discontinued; identify cause of constipation; identify whether fluids, bulk, or exercise is missing from lifestyle
• Monitor blood ammonia level (30-70 mg/100 ml); monitor for clearing of confusion, lethargy, restlessness, irritability (hepatic encephalopathy); may decrease ammonia level by 50%

Nursing diagnoses
• Constipation (uses)
• Diarrhea (adverse reactions)
• Knowledge, deficient (teaching)
• Noncompliance (teaching)

Implementation
PO route
• Give with full glass of fruit juice, water, milk to increase palatability of oral form; increase fluids by 2 L/day; do not give with other laxatives; if diarrhea occurs, reduce dosage
Rectal route
• Administer retention enema by diluting 300 ml of lactulose/700 ml of water or of 0.9% NaCl; administer by rec balloon catheter; retain for 30-60 min; repeat if evacuated too quickly

Patient/family education
• Discuss with patient that adequate fluid consumption is necessary
• Teach patient that normal bowel movements do not always occur daily
• Teach patient not to use in presence of abdominal pain, nausea, vomiting; tell patient to notify prescriber of unrelieved constipation or if symptoms of electrolyte imbalance occur: muscle cramps, pain, weakness, dizziness, excessive thirst
• Teach patient not to use laxatives for long-term therapy; bowel tone will be lost
• Do not give at bedtime as a laxative; may interfere with sleep
• Notify prescriber if diarrhea occurs; may indicate overdosage

Evaluation
Positive therapeutic outcome
• Decreased constipation
• Decreased blood ammonia level
• Clearing of mental state

lamivudine (Rx)
(lam-i'vue-dine)
Epivir, Epivir-HBV, 3TC
Func. class.: Antiretroviral
Chem. class.: Nucleoside reverse transcriptase inhibitor (NRTI)
Pregnancy category C

Do not confuse:
lamivudine/Lamotrigine

Action: Inhibits replication of HIV virus by incorporating into cellular DNA by viral reverse transcriptase, thereby terminating the cellular DNA chain

Therapeutic outcome: Improved symptoms of HIV infection

Uses: HIV infection in combination with other antiretrovirals; chronic hepatitis B (Epivir-HBV)

Unlabeled uses: Prophylaxis of HIV postexposure with indinavir and zidovudine

Dosage and routes
HIV infection
Adult and child >12 yr: PO 150 mg bid or 300 mg/day
Child 3 mo-12 yr: PO 4 mg/kg bid; max 150 mg bid

Renal dose
Adult: PO CCr 30-49 ml/min 150 mg/day; CCr 15-29 ml/min 150 mg (1st dose), then 100 mg/day; CCr 5-14 ml/min 150 mg/day (1st dose), then 50 mg/day; CCr <5 ml/min 50 mg (1st dose), then 25 mg/day

Chronic hepatitis B
Adult: PO 100 mg/day
Child/adolescent 2-17 yr: PO 3 mg/kg/day, max 100 mg

Available forms: Oral sol (Epivir) 10 mg/ml, tabs 100, 150, 300/mg; oral sol (Epivir-HBV) 5 mg/ml, tabs 100 mg

Adverse effects
CNS: Fever, headache, malaise, dizziness, insomnia, depression, fatigue, chills, **seizures**
EENT: Taste change, hearing loss, photophobia
GI: Nausea, vomiting, diarrhea, anorexia, cramps, dyspepsia, **hepatomegaly with steatosis, pancreatitis**
HEMA: **Neutropenia,** anemia, **thrombocytopenia**
INTEG: Rash
MS: Myalgia, arthralgia, pain
RESP: Cough
SYST: **Lactic acidosis, anaphylaxis, Stevens-Johnson syndrome**

Contraindications: Hypersensitivity

Black Box Warning: Lactic acidosis

Precautions: Pregnancy **C,** breastfeeding, children, geriatric, granulocyte count <1000/mm^3 or Hgb <9.5 g/dl, renal disease, pancreatitis, peripheral neuropathy

Black Box Warning: Severe hepatic dysfunction

Pharmacokinetics

Absorption	Rapidly absorbed
Distribution	Extravascular space
Metabolism	Protein binding <36%
Excretion	Unchanged in urine
Half-life	Terminal half-life 5-7 hr

Pharmacodynamics
Unknown

Interactions
Individual drugs
Trimethoprim/sulfamethoxazole: increased level of lamivudine
Zalcitabine: decreased both products
Zidovudine: increased level
Drug/lab test
Increased: ALT, bilirubin
Decreased: Hgb, neutrophil, platelet count

NURSING CONSIDERATIONS
Assessment
• Monitor blood counts q2wk; watch for neutropenia, thrombocytopenia, Hgb, CD4, viral load, lipase, triglycerides periodically during treatment; if low, therapy may have to be discontinued and restarted after hematologic recovery; blood transfusions may be required
• Monitor liver function tests: AST, ALT, bilirubin; amylase
• Monitor children for pancreatitis: abdominal pain, nausea, vomiting
• Assess for lactic acidosis, severe hepatomegaly with steatosis: obtain baseline liver function tests; if elevated, discontinue treatment; discontinue even if liver function tests are normal and symptoms of lactic acidosis, severe hepatomegaly develop

Nursing diagnoses
• Infection, risk for (uses)
• Injury, risk for (adverse reactions)
• Knowledge, deficient (teaching)

Implementation
• Administer PO daily, bid without regard to meals
• Give with other antiretrovirals only
• Store in cool environment; protect from light

Patient/family education
• Teach patient that GI complaints and insomnia resolve after 3-4 wk of treatment
• Tell patient that product is not a cure for AIDS but will control symptoms

---

Adverse effects: *italic* = common, **bold** = life-threatening

- Teach patient to notify prescriber of sore throat, swollen lymph nodes, malaise, fever; other infections may occur
- Teach patient that virus is still infective, may pass AIDS virus to others
- Encourage patient to continue follow-up visits since serious toxicity may occur; blood counts must be done q2wk
- Teach patient that product must be taken as prescribed, even if feeling better
- Tell patient that other products may be necessary to prevent other infections
- Teach patient that product may cause fainting or dizziness

Evaluation
Positive therapeutic outcome
- Absence of infection, symptoms of HIV infection

---

lamotrigine (Rx)
(lam-o-trye′geen)
Lamictal, Lamictal CD, Lamictal ODT, Lamictal XR
Func. class.: Anticonvulsant—miscellaneous
Chem. class.: Phenyltriazine
Pregnancy category C

Do not confuse:
lamotrigine/lamivudine, Lamictal/Lamisil/Lomotil

Action: Unknown; may inhibit voltage-sensitive sodium channels

Therapeutic outcome: Decrease in intensity and amount of seizures

Uses: Adjunct in the treatment of partial, tonic-clonic seizures, children with Lennox-Gastaut syndrome, bipolar disorder

Unlabeled uses: Absence seizures

Dosage and routes
Seizures: monotherapy
Adult: PO 50 mg/day for wk 1 and 2, then increase to 100 mg divided bid for wk 3 and 4; maintenance 300-500 mg/day; receiving enzyme inducing AEDs (carbamazepine, phenobarbital, phenytoin, primidone) but not valproic acid; EXT REL 50 mg/day × 1-2 wks, then 100 mg/day during wks 3-4, then 200 mg/day during wk 5, then 300 mg/day during wk 6, then 400 mg/day during wk 7; after wk 7 range is 400-600 mg/day
Child: PO 2 mg/kg/day in 2 divided doses × 2 wk, then 10 mg/kg/day, max 15 mg/kg/day or 400 mg/day

Seizures: multiple therapy with valproate
Adult: PO 25 mg every other day, then 25 mg/day wk 3-4, increase by 25-50 mg q1-2wk; maintenance 100-400 mg/day
Child: PO 0.1-0.2 mg/kg/day initially, then increase q2wk as needed to 2 mg/kg/day or 150 mg/day

Bipolar disorder
Adult: PO wk 1-2 25 mg/day; wk 3-4 50 mg/day; wk 5 100 mg/day; wk 6-7 200 mg/day; for patients taking valproic acid: wk 1-2 25 mg every other day; wk 3-4 25 mg/day; wk 5 50 mg/day; wk 6 100 mg/day; wk 7 100 mg/day

Hepatic dose
Adult (Child-Pugh grade B): PO reduce by 25%
Adult (Child-Pugh grade C): PO reduce by 50%

Available forms: Tabs 25, 100, 150, 200 mg; chew tabs 5, 25 mg; oral disintegrating tab 25, 50, 100, 200 mg; oral disintegrating 25-50, 50-100, 25-50-100 mg titration kit; PO ext rel 25-50-100, 50-100-200 mg titration kit; PO 25-100 mg starter kit

Adverse effects
CNS: Fever, insomnia, tremor, depression, anxiety, *dizziness,* ataxia, *headache,* **suicidal ideation**
EENT: Nystagmus, *diplopia, blurred vision*
GI: Nausea, *vomiting, anorexia,* abdominal pain, **hepatotoxicity**
GU: Dysmenorrhea
HEMA: Anemia, **DIC, leukopenia, thrombocytopenia**
INTEG: **Rash (potentially life-threatening),** alopecia, photosensitivity
SYST: **Stevens-Johnson syndrome, angioedema,** toxic epidermal necrolysis

Contraindications: Hypersensitivity

Precautions: Pregnancy **C** (cleft lip/palate in 1st trimester), breastfeeding, geriatric, renal/hepatic/cardiac disease, severe depression, suicidal, blood dyscrasias

Black Box Warning: Children <16 yr

Pharmacokinetics	
Absorption	Well absorbed, rapid
Distribution	Protein binding 55%
Metabolism	Glucuronic acid
Excretion	Crosses placenta, excreted in breast milk
Half-life	Terminal 24 hrs; 15 hrs with enzyme inducers

Pharmacodynamics	
Onset	Unknown
Peak	1.4-2.3 hr
Duration	Unknown

Interactions
Individual drugs
Acetaminophen, carbamazepine, oxcarbazepine, phenobarbital, phenytoin, primidone: decreased lamotrigine serum concentration

Valproic acid: decreased metabolic clearance of lamotrigine

Drug classifications
CYP3A4 inhibitors: decreased metabolic clearance of lamotrigine

Contraceptives (oral), estrogens, succinimides, rifamycins: decreased lamotrigine serum concentration

Drug/herb
Ginkgo: increased anticonvulsant effect

Ginseng, santonica: decreased anticonvulsant effect

NURSING CONSIDERATIONS
Assessment
⊕ Assess for rash (Stevens-Johnson syndrome or toxic epidermal necrolysis) in pediatric patients; product should be discontinued at first sign of rash
• Assess for seizure activity: duration, type, intensity, halo before seizure
• Assess for hypersensitive reactions
⊕ Assess mental status: suicidal thoughts/behaviors

Nursing diagnoses
• Injury, risk for (uses)
• Knowledge, deficient (teaching)

Implementation
• Give correct starter kit, errors have occurred
• Give in divided doses with or after meals to decrease adverse effects
• May be given with food or fluids
• Dispersible tabs should be swallowed whole, chewed, dispersed in water or diluted fruit juice; if chewed, a small amount of water should be taken

Patient/family education
• Caution patient not to discontinue product abruptly; seizures may occur
• Caution patient to avoid hazardous activities until stabilized on product
• Advise patient to notify prescriber of skin rash or increased seizure activity

• Instruct patient to report to prescriber if pregnancy is suspected or planned
• Teach patient to use sunscreen and protective clothing; photosensitivity occurs
• Advise patient to carry/wear emergency ID stating product use

Evaluation
Positive therapeutic outcome
• Decrease in severity of seizures

lansoprazole (Rx, OTC)
(lan-soe′prah-zole)
Prevacid, Prevacid 24 HR, Prevacid IV, Prevacid SoluTab
Func. class.: Anti-ulcer–proton pump inhibitor
Chem. class.: Benzimidazole

Pregnancy category B

Do not confuse:
Prevacid/Pravachol/Prinivil

Action: Suppresses gastric secretion by inhibiting hydrogen/potassium ATPase enzyme system in gastric parietal cell; characterized as gastric acid pump inhibitor since it blocks final step of acid production

Therapeutic outcome: Reduction in gastric pain, swelling, fullness

Uses: Gastroesophageal reflux disease (GERD), severe erosive esophagitis, poorly responsive systemic GERD, pathologic hypersecretory conditions (Zollinger-Ellison syndrome, systemic mastocytosis, multiple endocrine adenomas); possibly effective for treatment of duodenal, gastric ulcers, maintenance of healed duodenal ulcers

Dosage and routes
Frequent heartburn
Adult: PO 15 mg qd up to 14 days
NG tube
Adult: Use intact granules mixed in 40 ml of apple juice injected through NG tube, then flush with apple juice
Duodenal ulcer
Adult: PO 15 mg/day before meals for 4 wk, then 15 mg/day to maintain healing of ulcers; ulcers associated with *Helicobacter:* 30 mg lansoprazole, 500 mg clarithromycin, 1 g amoxicillin bid × 14 days or 30 mg lansoprazole, 1 g amoxicillin tid × 14 days

Erosive esophagitis
Adult: **IV** 30 mg over 30 min or for up to 7 days; switch to PO as soon as patient can tolerate, for 6-8 wk

Pathologic hypersecretory conditions
Adult: PO 60 mg/day, may give up to 90 mg bid, administer doses of >120 mg/day in divided doses

GERD/esophagitis
Adult/adolescent: PO 15-30 mg/day × 8 wk
Child 1-11 yr (>30 kg): PO 30 mg/day ≤12 wk
Child 1-11 yr (≤30 kg): 15 mg/day ≤12 wk

Available forms: del rel caps 15, 30 mg; granules for oral susp 15, 30 mg/packet; orally disintegrating tabs 15, 30 mg; lyophilized powder for IV inj 30 mg/vial

Adverse effects
CNS: Headache, dizziness, confusion, agitation, amnesia, depression
CV: Chest pain, angina, tachycardia, bradycardia, palpitations, **CVA**, hypo/hypertension, **MI, shock**, vasodilatation
EENT: Tinnitus, taste perversion, deafness, eye pain, otitis media
GI: Diarrhea, abdominal pain, vomiting, nausea, constipation, flatulence, acid regurgitation, anorexia, irritable colon, microscopic colitis
GU: **Hematuria,** glycosuria, impotence, kidney calculus, breast enlargement
HEMA: **Hemolysis,** anemia
INTEG: Rash, urticaria, pruritus, alopecia
META: Weight gain/loss, gout
RESP: Upper respiratory infections, cough, epistaxis, asthma, bronchitis, dyspnea, **pneumonia**

Contraindications: Hypersensitivity

Precautions: Pregnancy **B,** breastfeeding, children

Pharmacokinetics
Absorption	Rapid after granules leave stomach
Distribution	Protein binding 97%
Metabolism	Liver extensively
Excretion	Urine, feces; clearance decreased in geriatric, renal/hepatic disease
Half-life	Plasma 1.5 hr

Pharmacodynamics
Unknown

Interactions
Individual products
Calcium carbonate, indinavir, iron, itraconazole, ketoconazole: decreased absorption of each specific product
Sucralfate: delayed absorption of lansoprazole

NURSING CONSIDERATIONS
Assessment
• Assess GI system; bowel sounds q8hr, abdomen for pain, swelling, anorexia
• Monitor liver enzymes (AST, ALT, alkaline phosphatase) during treatment

Nursing diagnoses
• Knowledge, deficient (teaching)
• Pain, chronic (uses)

Implementation
• Swallow del rel cap whole; do not break, crush, chew, or open
• Administer before eating

Patient/family education
• Instruct patient to report severe diarrhea; product may have to be discontinued
• Inform diabetic patient that hypoglycemia may occur
• Encourage patient to avoid hazardous activities; dizziness may occur
• Tell patient to avoid alcohol, salicylates, ibuprofen; may cause GI irritation

Evaluation
Positive therapeutic outcome
• Absence of gastric pain, swelling, fullness

---

lapatinib (Rx)
(la-pa'tin-ib)
Tykerb
Func. class.: Antineoplastic—miscellaneous
Chem. class.: Biologic response modifier, signal transduction inhibitor (STIs)

Pregnancy category D

Action: Reverses tyrosine kinase of both the epidermal growth factor receptor (ERbB1) and human epidermal receptor type 2 (HER2) (ERbB2)

Therapeutic outcome: Decrease in breast cancer progression

Uses: Advanced, metastatic breast cancer patients with tumor that overexpresses HER2 protein and who has received previous chemotherapy

Dosage and routes
Adult: PO 1250 mg (5 tabs)/day 1 hr before or after food on days 1-21 plus capecitabine

---

 Alert   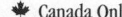 Canada Only   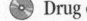 Drug on CD   * "Tall Man" lettering (See Preface)

2000 mg/m^2/day in 2 divided doses on days 1-14 in a repeating 21-day cycle; continue until therapeutic response or toxicity occurs

Hepatic dose
Adult (Child-Pugh C): PO 750 mg/day

Available forms: Tabs 250 mg

Adverse effects
CNS: Fatigue, insomnia, palmar-plantar erythrodysesthesia (hand/foot syndrome)
CV: **Heart failure,** palpitations, **QT prolongation**
GI: Anorexia, diarrhea, dyspepsia, mouth ulcerations, nausea, vomiting, xerosis
HEMA: **Anemia, neutropenia, thrombocytopenia**
INTEG: Rash
RESP: Dyspnea, pneumonitis

Contraindications: Pregnancy **D,** hypersensitivity, breastfeeding, torsades de pointes

Precautions: Geriatric, cardiac disease, bradycardia, hypertension, hypokalemia, hypomagnesemia, QT prolongation

Black Box Warning: Hepatic disease

Pharmacokinetics

Absorption	Incomplete
Distribution	Steady state 6-7 days
Metabolism	Liver, extensively, by P450 enzymes CYP3A4, CYP3A5; >99% protein bound
Excretion	Unknown
Half-life	Elimination 24 hr; increased in hepatic disease

Pharmacodynamics

Onset	Unknown
Peak	4 hr
Duration	Unknown

Interactions
Individual drugs
Arsenic trioxide, bepridil, chlorpromazine, chloroquine, grepafloxacin, halofantrine, haloperidol, levomethadyl, mesoridazine, pentamine, probucol, sparfloxacin, thioridazine: increased QT prolongation
Drug classifications
CYP3A4 inhibitors (amiodarone, amprenavir, aprepitant, atazanavir, chloramphenicol, clarithromycin, conivaptan, dalfopristin, danazol, darunavir, delavirdine, diltiazem, efavirenz, erythromycin, estradiol, fluconazole, fluvoxamine, imatinib, indinavir, isoniazid, itraconazole, ketoconazole, miconazole, mifepristone, nefazodone, nelfinavir, propoxyphene, quinupristin, ritonavir, RU-486, saquinavir, telithromycin, troleandomycin, verapamil, voriconazole, zafirlukast): increased effect of lapatinib; avoid concurrent use
CYP3A4 inhibitors (amiodarone, clarithromycin, erythromycin, telithromycin, troleandomycin), class IA, III antidysrhythmics: increased QT prolongation
CYP3A4 substrates (methadone, pimozide, quetiapine, quinidine, risperidone, terfenadine, ziprasidone): increased effect of these products, QT prolongation

NURSING CONSIDERATIONS
Assessment
• Assess cardiac status: EEG for QT prolongation, ejection fraction; chest pain, palpitations, dyspnea
• Assess hepatic status: liver function tests; jaundice of sclera, skin; dose should be reduced in hepatic disease
• Assess for skin toxicities NCI CTC grade 2 or greater; discontinue use in those with decreased left ventricular ejection fraction (LVEF) or for a LVEF that drops below the institution's lower limit of normal; the product may be restarted after 2 wk if the LVEF recovers to normal at 1000 mg/day; restart at 1250 mg/day when toxicity improves to grade 1 or better

Nursing diagnoses
• Injury, risk for (uses, adverse reactions)
• Knowledge, deficient (teaching)

Implementation
• Give once a day, with water, on an empty stomach, 1 hr before or after food
• Do not use with grapefruit products
• Store at room temperature, away from heat

Patient/family education
• Instruct patient to take with a full glass of water, once a day, 1 hr before or after food; do not take with food or grapefruit products
• Advise patient to take as directed only; if a dose is missed, take as soon as remembered; if it is close to the next dose, take only that dose; do not double
• Teach patient to report to prescriber: chest pain, difficulty breathing, fever, chills, sore throat, bleeding, bruising, yellow skin or eyes, severe fatigue, dizziness, palpitations
• Advise patient of other side effects that may occur, but do not need to be reported: nausea, diarrhea, heartburn, mouth sores, rash, numbness/pain in hands/feet

L

Adverse effects: *italic* = common, **bold** = life-threatening

- Advise patient to use adequate contraception, as the fetus could be damaged from this product

Evaluation
Positive therapeutic outcome
- Decrease in breast cancer progression

latanoprost ophthalmic
See Appendix B

leflunomide (Rx)
(leh-floo'noh-mide)
Arava
Func. class.: Antirheumatic (DMARDs)
Chem. class.: Immune modulator, pyrimidine synthesis inhibitor

Pregnancy category X

Action: Inhibits an enzyme involved in pyrimidine synthesis and has antiproliferative, antiinflammatory effect

Therapeutic outcome: Decreased pain, joint swelling, increased mobility

Uses: Rheumatoid arthritis, to reduce disease process as well as symptoms

Unlabeled uses: Juvenile rheumatoid arthritis

Dosage and routes
Adult: PO loading dose 100 mg/day × 3 days, maintenance 20 mg/day; may be decreased to 10 mg/day if not well tolerated

Juvenile rheumatoid arthritis (unlabeled)
Adolescent and child >40 kg: PO 20 mg
Adolescent and child 20-40 kg: PO 15 mg
Adolescent and child 10-19.9 kg: PO 10 mg

Available forms: Tabs 10, 20, 100 mg

Adverse effects
CNS: Dizziness, insomnia, depression, paresthesia, anxiety, migraine, neuralgia, headache
CV: Palpitations, hypertension, chest pain, angina pectoris, peripheral edema
EENT: Pharyngitis, oral candidiasis, stomatitis, dry mouth, blurred vision
GI: Nausea, anorexia, vomiting, constipation, flatulence, diarrhea, increased liver function tests, **hepatotoxicity**
HEMA: Anemia, ecchymosis, hyperlipidemia

INTEG: Rash, pruritus, alopecia, acne, hematoma, herpes infections
RESP: Pharyngitis, rhinitis, bronchitis, cough, respiratory infection, pneumonia, sinusitis
SYST: **Opportunistic/fatal infections**

Contraindications: Breastfeeding, hypersensitivity, jaundice, lactase deficiency, hepatic disease

Black Box Warning: Pregnancy **X**

Precautions: Children, renal disorders, vaccinations, infection, alcoholism, immunosuppression

Pharmacokinetics
Absorption	Unknown
Distribution	Unknown
Metabolism	Liver
Excretion	Kidneys
Half-life	Unknown

Pharmacodynamics
Unknown

Interactions
Individual drugs
Activated charcoal, cholestyramine: decreased effect of leflunomide
Methotrexate: increased leflunomide side effects
Rifampin: increased rifampin levels
Drug classifications
Hepatotoxic agents: increased side effects of leflunomide
Live virus vaccines: decreased antibody reaction
NSAIDs: increased NSAID effect

NURSING CONSIDERATIONS
Assessment
- Screen for latent TB before starting treatment
- Monitor liver function tests: if ALT elevations are >2 times baseline, reduce dose to 10 mg/day
- Obtain CBC with differential, pregnancy test, electrolytes
- Assess arthritic symptoms: ROM, mobility, swelling of joints, baseline, during treatment

Nursing diagnoses
- Knowledge, deficient (teaching)
- Mobility, impaired physical (uses)
- Pain, chronic (uses)

Implementation
- Give with full glass of water to enhance absorption

 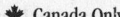

• Give PO with food, milk, or antacids for GI upset
• To eliminate product give cholestyramine 8 g tid × 11 days, check levels

Patient/family education
• Teach patient that product must be continued for prescribed time to be effective
• Instruct patient to take with food, milk, or antacids to avoid GI upset
• Advise patient to use caution when driving; drowsiness, dizziness may occur
• Advise patient to take with a full glass of water to enhance absorption
• Advise patient to avoid pregnancy while taking this product
• Inform patient that hair may be lost, review alternatives
• Advise patient to avoid live virus vaccinations during treatment

Evaluation
Positive therapeutic outcome
• Increased joint mobility without pain
• Decreased joint swelling

---

lenalidomide (Rx)
(len-a-lid'o-mide)
Revlimid
Func. class.: Antianemic, biologic response modifier, hormone
Chem. class.: Thalidomide derivative/TNF modifier

Pregnancy category X

Action: Decreases secretion of inflammatory cytokines and increases secretion of antiinflammatory cytokines, also COX-2 inhibition

Therapeutic outcome: Increase in reticulocyte count

Uses: Transfusion-dependent anemia due to low or intermediate-1–risk myelodysplastic syndrome (MDS); multiple myeloma in combination with dexamethasone

Dosage and routes
Transfusion-dependent anemia
Adult: PO 10 mg/day

Multiple myeloma
Adult: PO 25 mg/day on days 1-21, with dexamethasone 40 mg/day on days 1-4, 9-12, 17-20 of each 28-day cycle for first 4 therapy cycles; starting with cycle 5, leave lenalidomide the same, give dexamethasone 40 mg/day on days 1-4 of a 28-day cycle

Treatment of patients with transfusion-dependent anemia due to low- or intermediate-1–risk MDS associated with a deletion 5q cytogenetic abnormality with or without additional cytogenetic abnormalities
Adult: PO 10 mg/day; continue/adjust based on clinical toxicity/lab findings

Treatment of multiple myeloma in combination with dexamethasone in patients who have failed to respond to at least one prior therapy
Adult: PO 25 mg/day on days 1-21 along with dexamethasone 40 mg/day PO on days 1-4, 9-12, 17-20 of each 28-day cycle for the first 4 therapy cycles; starting with cycle 5, the lenalidomide dose stays the same, but only give dexamethasone 40 mg/day PO on days 1-4 q28day; continue/adjust dosing based on clinical and laboratory findings

Dosage adjustments of lenalidomide for hematologic toxicities associated with MDS Thrombocytopenia or neutropenia that develops within 4 wk of starting at 10 mg/day PO: Reduce dose from 10 mg/day PO to 5 mg/day PO; withhold lenalidomide if platelet count <50,000/mm³ from a baseline of at least 100,000/mm³, if platelet count falls to 50% of the baseline value, if the baseline is <100,000/mm³, if absolute neutrophil count (ANC) <750/mm³ from a baseline of at least 1000/mm³, or if <500/mm³ from a baseline of <1000/mm³; the new dose of 5 mg/day PO may begin once the platelet count is at least 50,000/mm³ (30,000/mm³ if the baseline <60,000/mm³), and the ANC returns to at least 1000/mm³ or 500/mm³ for patients with a baseline <1000/mm³
Thrombocytopenia or neutropenia that develops after 4 wk of starting at 10 mg/day PO: Reduce dose from 10 mg/day PO to 5 mg/day PO; withhold lenalidomide if platelet count <30,000/mm³, if platelet count <50,000/mm³ and a platelet transfusion, if neutrophils <500/mm³ for at least 7 days, or if <500/mm³ and a temp of at least 38.5° C are present; the new dose of 5 mg/day PO may begin once the platelet count is at least 30,000/mm³ without hemostatic failure, and the ANC is at least 500/mm³

Thrombocytopenia or neutropenia that develops while taking 5 mg/day PO: Reduce dose from 5 mg/day PO to 5 mg PO every other day; withhold lenalidomide if platelet count <30,000/mm³, platelet count <50,000/mm³ and a platelet transfusion, neutrophils <500/mm³ for at least 7 days, or if <500/mm³ and a temp of at least 38.5° C are present; the new dose of 5 mg PO every other day may begin once the platelet count is at least 30,000/mm³ without hemostatic failure, and the ANC is at least 500/mm³

Dosage adjustments of lenalidomide for toxicities associated with multiple myeloma
Thrombocytopenia: Reduce dose from 25 mg/day PO to 15 mg/day PO; withhold lenalidomide if platelet count <30,000/mm³; check CBC qwk; the new dose of 15 mg/day PO may begin once the platelet count is at least 30,000/mm³; withhold lenalidomide each time the platelet count is <30,000/mm³; a new dose of 5 mg less than the previous dose should be started once the platelet count is at least 30,000/mm³; do not dose below 5 mg/day PO
Neutropenia without other toxicity: Hold dose; withhold lenalidomide and add G-CSF if neutrophils <1000/mm³; check CBC weekly; resume lenalidomide at 25 mg/day PO once neutrophils are at least 1000/mm³, and neutropenia is the only toxicity
Neutropenia with other toxicity: Reduce dose from 25 mg/day PO to 15 mg/day PO; withhold lenalidomide and add G-CSF if neutrophils <1000/mm³; check CBC qwk; resume lenalidomide at 15 mg/day PO once neutrophils are at least 1000/mm³; withhold lenalidomide and add G-CSF each time the neutrophils are <1000/mm³; if other toxicity is present, a new dose of 5 mg less than the previous dose should be started once the neutrophils are at least 1000/mm³; do not dose below 5 mg/day PO
Other grade 3 or 4 toxicity judged to be related to lenalidomide: Reduce dose from 25 mg/day PO to 15 mg/day PO; withhold lenalidomide and resume lenalidomide at 15 mg/day PO once the toxicity has resolved to grade 2 or less; withhold lenalidomide each time a grade 3 or 4 toxicity occurs; a new dose of 5 mg less than the previous dose should be started once the toxicity has resolved to grade 2 or less; do not dose below 5 mg/day PO

Renal dose
Adult: PO CCr 30-59 ml/min, 5 mg q24hr (MDS), 10 mg q24hr (multiple myeloma); CCr <30 ml/min (not requiring dialysis), 5 mg q48hr (MDS), 15 mg q48hr (multiple myeloma)

Available forms: Caps 5, 10, 15, 25 mg
Adverse effects
CNS: Depression, dizziness, fatigue, fever, headache, sweating, peripheral enuropathy
CV: Chest pain, hypotension, palpitations
GI: Abdominal pain, anorexia, constipation, diarrhea, nausea/vomiting, dysgeusia, xerosis
HEMA: **Anemia, leukopenia, pancytopenia, thrombocytopenia, neutropenia**
META: Hypokalemia, hypomagnesemia
MS: Arthralgia, back pain, myalgia
RESP: Cough, dyspnea, **pulmonary embolism,** epistaxis, rhinitis
SYST: Angioedema

Contraindications: Breastfeeding, hypersensitivity

Black Box Warning: Pregnancy **X,** females

Precautions: Accidental exposure, bone marrow suppression, children, dental disease, uterine bleeding, geriatric, fungal/viral infections, smoking

Black Box Warning: Neutropenia/thrombocytopenia, thromboembolic disease

Pharmacokinetics	
Absorption	Rapid
Distribution	Unknown
Metabolism	Unknown
Excretion	Unknown
Half-life	Elimination 3 hr

Pharmacodynamics
Unknown

Interactions
Drug classifications
Anticoagulants, NSAIDs, platelet inhibitors, salicylates, thrombolytics: increased bleeding risk
Toxoids, vaccines: decreased immune response

NURSING CONSIDERATIONS
Assessment
• Monitor blood tests: HCT, Hgb, electrolytes
• Monitor B/P for hypotension
• Assess blood dyscrasias
• Assess for hypersensitivity reactions: skin rashes, urticaria (rare)

Nursing diagnoses
• Activity intolerance (uses)
• Knowledge, deficient (teaching)

 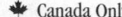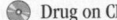

Implementation
- Give PO, with dexamethasone for multiple myeloma
- Do not crush or open caps
- All persons involved must comply with the condition of rev assist program

Patient/family education
- Advise patient to avoid driving or hazardous activity during beginning of treatment

Evaluation
Positive therapeutic outcome
- Increase in reticulocyte count

! HIGH ALERT

lepirudin 🔵 (Rx)
(lep-ih-roo'din)
Refludan
Func. class.: Anticoagulant
Chem. class.: Thrombin inhibitor, hirudin

Pregnancy category B

Action: Direct inhibitor of thrombin that is highly specific

Therapeutic outcome: Absence of thrombocytopenia, stroke, MI, or other thromboembolic conditions

Uses: Anticoagulation in those with heparin-induced thrombocytopenia (HIT) and other thromboembolic conditions

Unlabeled uses: Adjunct therapy in unstable angina, acute MI without ST elevation, prevention of DVT, PCI

Dosage and routes
Heparin-induced thrombocytopenia (not receiving thrombolytic therapy concurrently)
Adult: **IV** 0.4 mg/kg (≤110 kg) over 15-20 sec; then 0.15 mg/kg (≤110 kg/hr) as a CONT INF for 2-10 days or longer

Concomitant use with thrombolytic therapy
Adult: **IV** BOL 0.2 mg/kg initially, then CONT **IV** INF 0.1 mg/kg/hr

Renal dose
Adult: **IV** BOL 0.2 mg/kg over 15-20 sec; CCr 45-60 ml/min 0.075 mg/kg/hr; CCr 30-44 ml/min 0.045 mg/kg/hr; CCr 15-29 ml/min 0.0225 mg/kg/hr

Available forms: Powder for inj 50 mg

Adverse effects
CNS: Fever, **intracranial bleeding**
CV: **Heart failure, pericardial effusion, ventricular fibrillation**
GI: GI bleeding, abnormal liver function tests
GU: **Hematuria,** abnormal kidney function, vaginal bleeding
HEMA: **Hemorrhage, thrombocytopenia, anemia**
INTEG: Allergic skin reactions
RESP: Pneumonia, stridor, dyspnea, **bronchospasm**
SYST: **Multiorgan failure, sepsis, anaphylaxis**

Contraindications: Hypersensitivity to hirudins

Precautions: Pregnancy **B**, breastfeeding, children, women, geriatric, intracranial bleeding, hepatic disease, recent major surgery, hemorrhagic diathesis, bacterial endocarditis, severe uncontrolled hypertension, advanced renal disease, recent active peptic ulcer, recent CVA, stroke, intracerebral surgery

Pharmacokinetics
Absorption	Unknown
Distribution	Unknown
Metabolism	Possibly by the release of amino acids during catabolism
Excretion	50% unchanged in urine
Half-life	Unknown

Pharmacodynamics
Unknown

Interactions
Individual drugs
Aspirin, cefamandole, cefoperazone, cefotetan, clopidogrel, dipyridamole, eptifibatide, plicamycin, ticlopidine, tirofiban, valproic acid: increased bleeding risk
Drug classifications
NSAIDs, thrombolytics, warfarin derivatives: increased bleeding risk
Drug/herb
Agrimony, alfalfa, angelica, anise, basil, bay, bilberry, black haw, bogbean, bromelain, buchu, chondroitin, cinchona bark, dong quai, fenugreek, feverfew, garlic, ginger, ginkgo, ginseng, horse chestnut, Irish moss, kelp, kelpware, khella, lovage, lungwort, meadowsweet, motherwort, mugwort, nettle, papaya, parsley (large amounts), pau d'arco, pineapple, poplar, prickly ash, safflower, saw palmetto, tonka bean, turmeric, wintergreen, yarrow: increased risk of bleeding

L

Chamomile, coenzyme Q10, flax, glucomannan, goldenseal, guar gum: decreased
anticoagulant effect

NURSING CONSIDERATIONS
Assessment
• Obtain baseline APTT before treatment: do
not start treatment if APTT ratio is ≥2.5; then
APTT 4 hr after initiation of treatment and at
least daily thereafter; if APTT is above target,
stop infusion for 2 hr, then restart at 50%, take
APTT in 4 hr; if below target, increase inf rate
by 20%, take APTT in 4 hr, max inf rate 0.21
mg/kg/hr without checking for coagulation
abnormalities
• Monitor APTT, which should be 1.5-
2.5 × control
 Assess bleeding gums, petechiae, ecchymosis, black tarry stools, hematuria/epistaxis, B/P,
vaginal bleeding, puncture sites; may indicate
bleeding and possible hemorrhage
• Assess fever, skin rash, urticaria
• Monitor Hgb, Hct, platelets, serum creatinine, urinalysis, stool guaiac

Nursing diagnoses
• Injury, risk for (side effects)
• Knowledge, deficient (teaching)
• Tissue perfusion, ineffective (uses)

Implementation
• Administer after reconstitution and further
dilution under sterile conditions; use water for
inj or 0.9% NaCl; for further dilution 0.9%
NaCl or D_5; for rapid and complete reconstitution, inject 1 ml of diluent into vial and shake
gently, use immediately, warm to room temperature before use
• Avoid all IM inj that may cause bleeding
IV route
• Administer **IV** bol: use sol with conc of 5
mg/ml, reconstitute 5 mg (1 vial)/1 ml of
water for inj or 0.9% NaCl, use body weight for
correct weight calculation
• Administer **IV** inf: use sol with a conc of 0.2
or 0.4 mg/ml; reconstitute 100 mg (2 vials)
with 1 ml each (2 ml) water for inj or 0.9%
NaCl, transfer to inf bag with either 500 or 250
ml of 0.9% NaCl or D_5W

Patient/family education
• Teach patient to use soft-bristle toothbrush
to avoid bleeding gums, avoid contact sports,
use electric razor, avoid IM inj
• Teach patient to report any signs of
bleeding: gums, under skin, urine, stools

Evaluation
Positive therapeutic outcome
• Absence of thrombocytopenia without
significant bleeding

letrozole (Rx)
(let'tro-zohl)
Femara
Func. class.: Antineoplastic, nonsteroidal
aromatase inhibitor

Pregnancy category D

Action: Binds to the heme group of
aromatase; inhibits conversion of androgens to
estrogens to reduce plasma estrogen levels

Therapeutic outcome: Decreased
spread of malignancy

Uses: Early, advanced, or metastatic breast
cancer in postmenopausal women

Dosage and routes
Adult: PO 2.5 mg/day

Available forms: Tabs 2.5 mg

Adverse effects
CNS: Somnolence, dizziness, depression,
anxiety, *headache, lethargy*
CV: Angina, **MI, CVA, thromboembolic
events,** peripheral edema, hypertension
GI: Nausea, vomiting, anorexia, constipa-
tion, heartburn, diarrhea
GU: **Endometrial cancer, vaginal bleed-
ing, endometrial proliferation disorder**
INTEG: Rash, pruritus, alopecia, sweating
MISC: Hot flashes, night sweats, **second
malignancies, anaphylaxis, angioedema**
MS: Arthralgia, arthritis, bone fracture, myal-
gia, osteoporosis
RESP: Dyspnea, cough

Contraindications: Pregnancy **D,** hypersensitivity, premenopausal females

Precautions: Hepatic disease, respiratory
disease, osteoporosis

Pharmacokinetics
Absorption	Well absorbed
Distribution	Widely
Metabolism	Liver
Excretion	Kidneys
Half-life	Terminal 48 hr

Pharmacodynamics
Onset	Unknown
Peak	2-6 wk
Duration	Unknown

Interactions
Drug classifications
Estrogens, oral contraceptives: decreased
  letrozole effect

 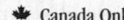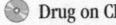

NURSING CONSIDERATIONS
Assessment
- Monitor temperature q4hr; may indicate beginning of infection
- Monitor liver function tests before, during therapy (bilirubin, AST, ALT, LDH) as needed or monthly

Nursing diagnoses
- Body image, disturbed (adverse reactions)
- Infection, risk for (adverse reactions)
- Injury, risk for (adverse reactions)
- Knowledge, deficient (teaching)

Implementation
- May administer biphosphates to increase bone density
- Give with food or fluids for GI upset
- Give in equal intervals q6hr

Patient/family education
- Advise patient to avoid use of alcohol, which potentiates this product
- Tell patient that product may be taken without regard to meals
- Teach patient to report vaginal bleeding, diarrhea, chest/bone pain
- Advise patient to use adequate contraception in perimenopausal, recently postmenopausal women

Evaluation
Positive therapeutic outcome
- Prevention of rapid division of malignant cells, postmenopausal cancer, prostate cancer

Treatment of overdose: Induce vomiting, provide supportive care

leucovorin (Rx)
(loo-koe-vor'in)
Citrovorum Factor, Folinic Acid, leucovorin calcium
Func. class.: Vitamin/folic acid antagonist antidote
Chem. class.: Tetrahydrofolic acid derivative

Pregnancy category C

Do not confuse:
leucovorin/Leukeran/Leukine
folinic acid/folic acid

Action: Needed for normal growth patterns; prevents toxicity during antineoplastic therapy by protecting normal cells

Therapeutic outcome: Reversal of severe toxic effects of folic acid antagonists

Uses: Megaloblastic or macrocytic anemia caused by folic acid deficiency, overdose of folic acid antagonist, methotrexate toxicity, toxicity caused by pyrimethamine/trimethoprim/trimetrexate, pneumocystosis, toxoplasmosis

Dosage and routes
Megaloblastic anemia caused by enzyme deficiency
Adult and child: PO/IM/**IV** up to 6 mg/day

Megaloblastic anemia caused by deficiency of folate
Adult and child: IM 1 mg or less/day until adequate response

Advanced colorectal cancer
Adult: **IV** 200 mg/m^2, then 5-fluorouracil 370 mg/m^2; or leucovorin 20 mg/m^2, then 5-fluorouracil 425 mg/m^2; give daily × 5 days q4-5wk

Methotrexate toxicity—leucovorin rescue
Adult and child: PO/IM/**IV** (normal elimination) given 6 hr after dose of methotrexate 10 mg/m^2 until methotrexate is $<5 \times 10^{-8}$ m, CCr has increased 50% above prior level, or methotrexate level is 5×10^{-8} m at 24 hr or at 48 hr level is $>9 \times 10^{-8}$ m; give leucovorin 100 mg/m^2 q3hr until level drops to $<10^{-8}$ m

Pyrimethamine/trimethoprim toxicity
Adult and child: PO/IM 5-15 mg/day

Available forms: Tabs 5, 10, 15, 25 mg; inj 3, 5 mg/ml; powder for inj 10 mg/ml

Adverse effects
HEMA: Thrombocytosis (intraarterial)
INTEG: Rash, pruritus, erythema, urticaria
RESP: Wheezing

Contraindications: Hypersensitivity to this product or folic acid, benzyl alcohol, anemias other than megaloblastic not associated with vit B$_{12}$ deficiency

Precautions: Pregnancy C, seizures, elderly, neonates, stomatitis, vomiting, breastfeeding

Pharmacokinetics
Absorption	Rapidly absorbed (PO); completely absorbed (**IV**)
Distribution	Widely distributed
Metabolism	Liver
Excretion	Kidney
Half-life	3½ hr

L

Pharmacodynamics

	PO/IM/IV
Onset	Up to 5 min
Peak	Unknown
Duration	4-6 hr

Interactions
Individual drugs
Chloramphenicol: decreased folate levels
Fluorouracil: increased toxicity
Phenobarbital: increased metabolism of
phenobarbital
Drug classifications
Hydantoins: increased metabolism of hydantoins

NURSING CONSIDERATIONS
Assessment
• Obtain CCr before leucovorin rescue and daily to detect nephrotoxicity, methotrexate level
• Monitor I&O, urine pH q6hr; maintain at >7 to prevent neurotoxicity; watch for nausea and vomiting; if vomiting occurs IM or **IV** route may be necessary
• Assess products currently taken: alcohol, hydantoins, trimethoprim may cause increased folic acid use by body
• Assess for allergic reactions: rash, dyspnea, wheezing
• Assess neurologic status (rescue), weakness, fatigue
• Monitor calcium levels
• Assess for megaloblastic anemia, plasma lactic acid, reticulocyte count, Hct, Hgb

Nursing diagnoses
• Injury, risk for (uses)
• Knowledge, deficient (teaching)
• Nutrition: less than body requirements, imbalanced (uses)

Implementation
• Instruct patient about leucovorin rescue; have patient drink 3 L of fluid each day of rescue
• Do not give concurrently with systemic methotrexate
PO route
• Use PO route only if patient is not vomiting
IM route
• Treatment of megaloblastic anemia uses IM dosing
• Give within 1 hr of folic acid antagonist, no reconstitution needed
• Give increased fluid intake if used to treat folic acid inhibitor overdose
• Provide protection from light and heat when storing ampules

IV route
• Reconstitute 50 mg/5 ml of bacteriostatic water or sterile water for inj (10 mg/ml) or 100 mg/10 ml; use immediately if sterile water for inj is used to reconstitute
• Give by direct **IV** over 160 mg/min or less (16 ml of 10 mg/ml sol/min)
• Give by intermittent inf after diluting in 100-500 ml of 0.9% NaCl, D_5W, $D_{10}W$, LR, Ringer's
Syringe compatibilities: Bleomycin, cisplatin, cyclophosphamide, DOXOrubicin, fluorouracil, furosemide, heparin, methotrexate, metoclopramide, mitomycin, vinBLAStine, vinCRIStine
Y-site compatibilities: Amifostine, aztreonam, bleomycin, cefepime, cisplatin, cladribine, cyclophosphamide, DOXOrubicin, filgrastim, fluconazole, fluorouracil, furosemide, granisetron, heparin, methotrexate, metoclopramide, mitomycin, piperacillin/tazobactam, tacrolimus, teniposide, thiotepa, vinBLAStine, vinCRIStine
Additive compatibilities: Cisplatin, cisplatin/floxuridine, floxuridine

Patient/family education
• Advise patient to take product exactly as prescribed; to notify prescriber of side effects immediately
• Advise patient to report signs of hypersensitivity reaction immediately
• Advise patient with folic acid deficiency to eat folic acid–rich foods: bran, yeast, dried beans, nuts, fruits, fresh green leafy vegetables, asparagus
• Advise patient to avoid breastfeeding

Evaluation
Positive therapeutic outcome
• Increased weight
• Improved orientation, well-being
• Absence of fatigue
• Reversal of toxicity: methotrexate, folic acid antagonist overdose

---

⬥ Alert   ♣ Canada Only   🔵 Drug on CD   * "Tall Man" lettering (See Preface)

! HIGH ALERT

leuprolide (Rx)
(loo-proe'lide)
Eligard, Lupron Depo, Lupron, Lupron Depot, Lupron Depot-3 month, Lupron Depot-4 month, Viadur
Func. class.: Antineoplastic hormone
Chem. class.: Gonadotropin-releasing hormone

Pregnancy category X

Do not confuse:
Lupron/Lopurin/Nuprin

Action: Causes initial increase in circulating levels of LH, FSH; continuous administration results in decreased LH, FSH; in men testosterone is reduced to castration levels; in premenopausal women estrogen is reduced to menopausal levels

Therapeutic outcome: Prevention of rapidly growing malignant cells in prostate cancer, decreased pain in endometriosis, resolution of central precocious puberty (CPP)

Uses: Metastatic prostate cancer (inj implant), management of endometriosis (depot), CPP, uterine leiomyomata (fibroids)

Dosage and routes
Prostate cancer
Adult: SUBCUT 1 mg/day; IM 7.5 mg/dose qmo; Viadur implant (72 mg) qyr; or IM 22.5 mg q3mo; or IM 30 mg q4mo

Endometriosis/fibroids
Adult: IM 3.75 mg qmo for 6 mo, 11.25 mg q3mo for 6 mo, or IM 30 mg q4mo

Central precocious puberty
Child: SUBCUT 50 mcg/kg/day; increase as needed by 10 mcg/kg/day
Child >37.5 kg: IM 15 mg q4wk
Child 25-37.5 kg: IM 11.25 mg q4wk
Child ≤25 kg: 7.5 mg q4wk

Available forms: Inj 5 mg/ml; powder for inj, lyophilized 7.5 mg; microspheres for inj, lyophilized 3.75, 7.5, 11.25, 15, 22.5, 30 mg; implant 72 mg; depot 7.5, 22.5, 30, 45 mg; depot 3.75, 11.25 mg; intradermal kit 65 mg

Adverse effects
CNS: Memory impairment, depression, **seizures**
CV: **MI, pulmonary emboli, dysrhythmias,** peripheral edema
GI: Anorexia, diarrhea, **GI bleeding,** nausea, vomiting

GU: Edema, hot flashes, impotence, decreased libido, amenorrhea, vaginal dryness, gynecomastia, **profuse vaginal bleeding**
INTEG: Alopecia
MS: Bone pain

Contraindications: Pregnancy **X**, breastfeeding, hypersensitivity to GnRH or analogs, thromboembolic disorders, undiagnosed vaginal bleeding; Viadur implant or Eligard should not be used in women or children

Precautions: Edema, hepatic disease, CVA, MI, seizures, hypertension, diabetes mellitus, CHF, depression, osteoporosis, spinal cord compression, urinary tract obstruction

Pharmacokinetics

Absorption	Rapidly absorbed (SUBCUT); slowly absorbed (IM depot)
Distribution	Unknown
Metabolism	Unknown
Excretion	Unknown
Half-life	3-4 hr

Pharmacodynamics
Unknown

Interactions
Individual drugs
Flutamide, megestrol: increased antineoplastic action

NURSING CONSIDERATIONS
Assessment
• Assess for symptoms of endometriosis/fibroids including lower abdominal pain, excessive vaginal bleeding, bloating if product is given for the diagnosis of endometriosis
• If giving this product for CPP, the diagnosis should have been confirmed by development of secondary sex characteristics in children <9 yr; also included to confirm the diagnosis of CPP is estradiol/testosterone, GnRH test, tomography of head, adrenal steroid, chorionic gonadotropin, wrist x-ray, height, weight; patients diagnosed with CPP display the signs of testicular growth, facial, body hair (males), breast development, menses (females)
• Monitor liver function tests before, during therapy (bilirubin, AST, ALT, LDH) as needed or monthly; prostate-specific antigen in prostate cancer
• Monitor PSA in prostate cancer; calcium, testosterone, bone mineral density
• Monitor pituitary gonadotropic and gonadal function during therapy and 4-8 wk after therapy is decreased; check LH, FSH, acid phosphate at beginning of treatment

Adverse effects: *italic* = common, **bold** = life-threatening

- Monitor worsening of signs and symptoms (normal during beginning therapy): fatigue, increased pulse, pallor, lethargy, edema in feet, joints, stomach pain, shaking
- Monitor renal status: I&O ratio, check for bladder distention daily during beginning therapy (renal obstruction)

Nursing diagnoses
- Injury, risk for (adverse reactions)
- Knowledge, deficient (teaching)
- Sexual dysfunction (adverse reactions)

Implementation
- Use syringe and product packaged together; give deep in large muscle mass; rotate sites
- Use depot only IM; never give SUBCUT
- Unused vials may be stored at room temperature
- Give monthly: reconstitute single-use vial with 1 ml of diluent; if multiple vials are used, withdraw 0.5 ml and inject into each vial (1 ml), withdraw all and inject
- Give 3 month: reconstitute microspheres using 1.5 ml of diluent and inject in vial, shake, withdraw and inject; 12-month: inserted into upper arm; at the end of 12 months, implant must be removed

Patient/family education
- Advise patient to notify prescriber if menstruation continues; menstruation should stop; to use a nonhormonal method of contraception during therapy
- Instruct patient to report any complaints, side effects to nurse or prescriber; hot flashes may occur; record weight, report gain of 2 lb/day
- Teach patient how to prepare, administer; to rotate sites for SUBCUT inj; to keep accurate records of dosing (prostate cancer)
- Instruct patient that tumor flare may occur: increase in size of tumor, increased bone pain; tell patient that bone pain disappears after 1 wk; may take analgesics for pain; premenopausal women must use mechanical birth control; ovulation may be induced
- Advise the patient not to breastfeed while taking this product
- Inform patient that voiding problems may increase in beginning of therapy, but will decrease in several weeks

Evaluation
Positive therapeutic outcome
- Decreased size, spread of malignancy
- Decreased pain in endometriosis, fibroids
- Decreased signs of CPP
- Increased follicle maturation

levalbuterol (Rx)
(lev-al-bute′er-ole)
Xopenex
Func. class.: Bronchodilator
Chem. class.: Adrenergic β_2-agonist

Pregnancy category C

Action: Causes bronchodilatation by action on β_2 (pulmonary) receptors by increasing levels of cyclic adenosine monophosphate (cAMP), which relaxes smooth muscle; produces bronchodilatation; CNS, cardiac stimulation, increased diuresis, and increased gastric acid secretion

Therapeutic outcome: Increased ability to breathe because of bronchodilatation

Uses: Treatment or prevention of bronchospasm (reversible obstructive airway disease)

Dosage and routes
Adult and child ≥12 yr: INH 0.63 mg tid, q6-8hr by nebulization; may increase to 1.25 mg q8hr
Child 6-11 yr: INH 0.31 mg tid via nebulization, max 0.63 mg tid

Available forms: Inh sol 0.63, 1.25 mg/3 ml

Adverse effects
CNS: Tremors, anxiety, insomnia, headache, dizziness, stimulation, *restlessness,* hallucinations, flushing, irritability
CV: Palpitations, tachycardia, hypertension, angina, hypotension, dysrhythmias, **QT prolongation**
EENT: Dry nose, irritation of nose and throat
GI: Heartburn, nausea, vomiting
INTEG: Rash
META: Hypokalemia, hyperglycemia
MS: Muscle cramps
RESP: Cough
SYST: **Anaphylaxis, angioedema**

Contraindications: Hypersensitivity to sympathomimetics, tachydysrhythmias, severe cardiac disease

Precautions: Pregnancy **C**, breastfeeding, cardiac disorders, hyperthyroidism, diabetes mellitus, hypertension, prostatic hypertrophy, closed-angle glaucoma, seizures, renal disease, QT prolongation

Pharmacokinetics

Absorption	Unknown
Distribution	Unknown
Metabolism	Liver extensively, tissues
Excretion	Unknown, breast milk
Half-life	Unknown

 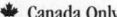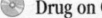

Pharmacodynamics	
	INH
Onset	5-15 min
Peak	1-1½ hr
Duration	6-8 hr

Interactions
Drug classifications
Adrenergics: increased levalbuterol action
Antidepressants (tricyclics): increased levalbuterol action
β-Adrenergic blockers: decreased levabuterol action
Bronchodilators (aerosol): increased action of bronchodilator
MAOIs: increased levalbuterol action
Drug/herb
Cola nut, guarana, tea (black/green), coffee, yerba maté: increased stimulation

NURSING CONSIDERATIONS
Assessment
- Assess cardiac status: palpitations, increased or decreased B/P, dysrhythmias, QT prolongation
- Assess respiratory function: vital capacity, forced expiratory volume, ABGs, lung sounds, heart rate, rhythm (baseline, during therapy); character of sputum; color, consistency, amount
- Determine that patient has not received theophylline therapy before giving dose, to prevent additive effect; client's ability to self-medicate
- Monitor for evidence of allergic reactions; paradoxic bronchospasm, anaphylaxis, angioedema; withhold dose; notify prescriber

Nursing diagnoses
- Airway clearance, ineffective (uses)
- Gas exchange, impaired (uses)
- Knowledge, deficient (teaching)

Implementation
- Give by nebulization q6-8hr; wait at least 1 min between inhalation of aerosols
- Use this medication before other medications and allow 5 min between each to prevent overstimulation

Patient/family education
- Tell patient not to use OTC medications before consulting prescriber; extra stimulation may occur; instruct patient to use this medication before other medications and allow at least 5 min between each to prevent overstimulation; to limit caffeine products such as chocolate, coffee, tea, and cola or herbs such as cola nut, guarana, yerba maté

🔸 Teach patient that if paradoxic bronchospasm occurs to stop product immediately and notify prescriber

Evaluation
Positive therapeutic outcome
- Absence of dyspnea and wheezing after 1 hr
- Improved airway exchange
- Improved ABGs

Treatment of overdose: Administer a β₁-adrenergic blocker

---

levetiracetam (Rx)
(lev-ee-tye′ra-see-tam)
Keppra, Keppra XR
Func. class.: Anticonvulsant

Pregnancy category C

Action: Unknown; may inhibit nerve impulses by limiting influx of sodium ions across cell membrane in motor cortex

Therapeutic outcome: Absence of seizures

Uses: Adjunctive therapy in partial onset seizures, primary generalized tonic-clonic seizures

Dosage and routes
Adjunctive treatment of partial seizures
Adult and adolescent ≥16 yr: IV
500 mg bid, may titrate by 1000 mg/day q2wk; max 3000 mg/day in divided doses; EXT REL 1000 mg/day, may increase q2wk, max 3000 mg/day

Myoclonic seizures/tonic-clonic seizures/partial seizures
Adult and adolescent >16 yr: PO/IV
500 mg bid, may increase by 1000 mg/day q2wk; max 3000 mg/day

Renal dose
Adult: PO CCr 50-80 ml/min, 500-1000 mg q12hr, EXT REL 1000-2000 q24hr, max 2000 mg/day; CCr 30-49 ml/min, 250-750 mg q12hr, EXT REL 500-1500 mg q24hr, max 1500 mg/day; CCr <30 ml/min 250-500 mg q12hr, EXT REL 500-1000 mg q24hr, max 1000 mg/day

Available forms: Tabs 500, 1000 mg; oral sol 100 mg/ml; SOL for inj 100 mg/ml, ext rel tab 500 mg

Adverse effects
CNS: Dizziness, somnolence, asthenia, psychosis, **suicidal ideation**

Adverse effects: *italic* = common, **bold** = life-threatening

HEMA: Decreased Hct, Hgb, RBC, infection
MISC: Abdominal pain, pharyngitis, infection

Contraindications: Hypersensitivity

Precautions: Pregnancy **C**, breastfeeding, children, geriatric, cardiac/renal disease, psychosis

Pharmacokinetics

Absorption	Rapidly absorbed
Distribution	Widely distributed, not protein bound
Metabolism	Small amount liver
Excretion	Kidneys (66%) unchanged
Half-life	6-8 hr longer in renal disease/geriatric

Pharmacodynamics
Unknown

Interactions
Individual drugs
Alcohol: avoid using
Carbamazepine: increased carbamazepine toxicity
Sevelamer: decreased levetiracetam absorption; separate by 1 hr before, 3 hr after sevelamer

NURSING CONSIDERATIONS
Assessment
• Monitor urine function tests (BUN, urine protein) periodically during treatments
🔶 Assess seizure activity including type, location, duration, and character; provide seizure precautions
• Assess blood studies: RBC, Hct, Hgb
🔶 Assess mental status: mood, sensorium, affect, behavioral changes, suicidal thoughts/behaviors

Nursing diagnoses
• Injury, risk for (side effects)
• Knowledge, deficient (teaching)

Implementation
PO route
• Give with food, milk to decrease GI symptoms (rare)
• Store at room temperature (PO); diluted preparation stable for 24 hr at room temperature in polyvinyl bags
IV route
• Single-use vials: dilute in 100 mg of 0.9% NaCl, D₅, LR; give over 15 min

Patient/family education
• Teach patient to carry/wear emergency ID stating patient's name, products taken, condition, prescriber's name, phone number

• Caution patient to avoid driving, other activities that require alertness until stabilized on medication
• Teach patient not to discontinue medication quickly after long-term use
• Teach patient to use a nonhormonal type of contraception to prevent harm to the fetus
• Teach patient to take exactly as prescribed, do not double or omit doses
• Advise not to breastfeed

Evaluation
Positive therapeutic outcome
• Decreased seizure activity

levobetaxolol ophthalmic
See Appendix B

levobunolol ophthalmic
See Appendix B

levocabastine ophthalmic
See Appendix B

levocetirizine (Rx)
(lee-voh-she-teer'ah-zeen)
Xyzal
Func. class.: Antihistamine, low sedating
Chem. class.: H₁-histamine blocker
Pregnancy category B

Action: Acts on blood vessels, GI, respiratory system by competing with histamine for H₁-receptor site; decreases allergic response by blocking pharmacologic effects of histamine; minimal anticholinergic action

Therapeutic outcome: Absence of running or congested nose or rashes

Uses: Perennial or seasonal rhinitis, allergy symptoms, chronic idiopathic urticaria

Dosage and routes
Adult and child ≥12 yr: PO 2.5-5 mg/day in the evening
Child 6-11 yr: PO (oral SOL) 2.5 mg/day in the evening
Child 2-5 yr: PO (oral SOL) 1.25 mg/day in the evening
Geriatric: PO 2.5-5 mg/day in the evening
Renal dose
Adult: PO CCr 50-80 ml/min 2.5 mg/day; CCr 30-50 ml/min 2.5 mg every other day; CCr

10-30 ml/min 2.5 mg 2 ×/wk; CCr <10 ml/min, do not use

Available forms: Tabs 5 mg; oral sol 2.5 mg/5 ml

Adverse effects
CNS: Drowsiness, fatigue, asthenia
GI: Dry mouth, increased liver function tests
INTEG: Rash, transient

Contraindications: Breastfeeding; end-stage renal disease; dialysis; child 6-11 yr with renal disease; hypersensitivity to this product, cetrizine, hydroxyzine

Precautions: Pregnancy **B**

Pharmacokinetics	
Absorption	Rapid
Distribution	Unknown
Metabolism	Protein binding 91%-92%
Excretion	Urine 85.4%, feces 12.9%
Half-life	8 hr

Pharmacodynamics	
Onset	Unknown
Peak	0.9 hr
Duration	Unknown

Interactions
Individual drugs
Alcohol: increased CNS depression
Ritonavir: increased half life; decreased clearance of levocetirizine
Drug classifications
MAOIs, phenothiazines, tricyclics: increased anticholinergic/sedative effect
Other CNS depressants: increased CNS depression
Drug/herb
Corkwood: increased anticholinergic effect
Hops, Jamaican dogwood, kava, senega, valerian: increased effect
Drug/lab test
False negative: skin allergy tests

NURSING CONSIDERATIONS
Assessment
• Allergy symptoms: pruritus, urticaria, watering eyes, baseline, during treatment
• Respiratory status: rate, rhythm, increase in bronchial secretions, wheezing, chest tightness
• Liver function tests, serum creatinine, BUN

Nursing diagnoses
• Knowledge, deficient (teaching)
• Noncompliance (teaching)

Implementation
• Give without regard to meals in the evening; tabs are scored and may be broken in half
• Store in tight, light-resistant container

Patient/family education
• Teach patient all aspects of product use; to notify prescriber if confusion, sedation, hypotension occur
• Advise patient to avoid driving, other hazardous activities if drowsiness occurs
• Advise patient to avoid alcohol, other CNS depressants
• Inform patient that product is not recommended during breastfeeding

Evaluation
Positive therapeutic outcome
• Absence of running or congested nose or rashes

Treatment of overdose: Administer diazepam, vasopressors, IV phenytoin

---

levofloxacin (Rx)
(lev-o-floks'a-sin)
Levaquin
Func. class.: Antiinfective
Chem. class.: Fluoroquinolone antibacterial

Pregnancy category C

Action: Interferes with conversion of intermediate DNA fragments into high molecular weight DNA in bacteria; DNA gyrase inhibitor; inhibits topoisomerase **IV**

Therapeutic outcome: Bacteriocidal action against the following: *Streptococcus pneumoniae, Haemophilus influenzae, Haemophilus parainfluenzae, Moraxella catarrhalis, Klebsiella pneumoniae, Mycoplasma pneumoniae, Escherichia coli, Serratia marcescens, Chlamydia pneumoniae, Legionella pneumophilia, Enterococcus faecalis, Staphylococcus epidermidis, Staphylococcus pyogenes*

Uses: Acute sinusitis, acute chronic bronchitis, community-acquired pneumonia, uncomplicated skin infections, complicated UTI, cellulitis, PID, prostatitis, inhalational anthrax (postexposure), acute pyelonephritis, inhalation anthrax in children

Unlabeled uses: Gonococcal infections, disseminated

Dosage and routes
Acute bacterial exacerbation of chronic bronchitis
Adult: PO/**IV** 500 mg q24hr × 7 days

Adverse effects: *italic* = common, **bold** = life-threatening

Acute bacterial sinusitis
Adult: PO 500 mg q24hr × 10-14 days or
750 mg q24hr × 5 days

Acute pyelonephritis
Adult: PO 250 mg q24hr × 10 days

Chronic bacterial prostatitis
Adult: PO 500 mg q24hr × 28 days

Postexposure inhalational anthrax
Adult/adolescent/child >50 kg:
PO/**IV** 500 mg q24hr × 60 days
Infant >6 mo and child <50 kg: **IV** 8
mg/kg q12hr, max 250 mg/dose, × 60 days

Pneumonia, community acquired
Adult: PO/**IV** 500 mg q24hr × 7-14 days or
750 mg q24hr × 5 days

Pneumonia, nosocomial
Adult: PO/**IV** 750 mg q24hr × 7-14 days

SSSI, complicated
Adult: PO/**IV** 750 mg q24hr × 7-14 days

SSSI, uncomplicated
Adult: PO 500 mg q24hr × 7-10 days

UTI, complicated
Adult: PO/**IV** 250 mg q24hr × 10 days

UTI, uncomplicated
Adult: PO 250 mg q24hr × 3 days

Gonococcal infection,
disseminated (unlabeled)
Adult: **IV** 250 mg q24hr × 24-48 hr, then
PO 500 mg/day x 7 days

PID
Adult: **IV** 500 mg q24hr × 14 days

Renal disease
Adult: PO/**IV** CCr 20-49 ml/min initial 500
mg, then 250 mg q24hr; CCr 10-19 ml/min
250 or 500 mg, depending on condition, then
250 mg q48hr

Available forms: Single-use vials (500,
750 mg), premixed flexible container; 250
mg/50 ml D_5W, 500 mg/100 ml D_5W, 750
mg/150 ml D_5W; tabs 250, 500, 750 mg

Adverse effects:
CNS: Headache, dizziness, *insomnia,* anxiety,
seizures, encephalopathy, paresthesia
CV: Chest pain, palpitations, vasodilatation, QT
prolongation
EENT: Dry mouth, visual impairment
GI: Nausea, flatulence, *vomiting,* diarrhea,
abdominal pain, **pseudomembranous
colitis, hepatotoxicity**
GU: Vaginitis, crystalluria
HEMA: Eosinophilia, **hemolytic anemia,**
lymphophemia

INTEG: Rash, pruritus, photosensitivity,
epidermal necrolysis
MISC: Hypoglycemia, hypersensitivity, tendon
rupture
RESP: Pneumonitis
SYST: **Anaphylaxis, multisystem organ
failure, Stevens-Johnson syndrome**

Contraindications: Hypersensitivity to
quinolones, photosensitivity

Precautions: Pregnancy **C,** breastfeeding,
children

Black Box Warning: Tendon pain/rupture,
tendonitis

Pharmacokinetics

Absorption	Unknown
Distribution	Unknown
Metabolism	Liver
Excretion	Kidneys unchanged
Half-life	6-8 hr

Pharmacodynamics

Onset	Immediate
Peak	Infusion's end
Duration	Unknown

Interactions
Individual drugs
Calcium, iron, sucralfate, zinc: decreased
absorption of levofloxacin
Foscarnet: increased CNS stimulation, seizures
Magnesium: decreased levofloxacin
absorption; do not use in same **IV** line
Probenecid: increased levofloxacin levels
Theophylline: decreased theophylline
clearance; toxicity may result
Warfarin: increased bleeding
Drug classifications
Antacids (magnesium, aluminum): decreased
absorption of levofloxacin
NSAIDs: increased CNS stimulation, seizures
QT prolonging agents: increased QT prolonga-
tion
Drug/herb
Acidophilus: do not use with antiinfectives;
separate by several hours
Cola tree: increased antiinfective effect
Drug/lab test
Decreased: glucose, lymphocytes

NURSING CONSIDERATIONS
Assessment
• Assess patient for previous sensitivity reac-
tion
• Assess patient for signs and symptoms of
infection, including characteristics of wounds,

 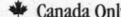

sputum, urine, stool, WBC >10,000/mm^3, fever; baseline, during treatment
• Obtain C&S before beginning product therapy to identify if correct treatment has been initiated
• Assess for allergic reactions and anaphylaxis: rash, urticaria, pruritus, chills, fever, joint pain; may occur a few days after therapy begins; epinephrine and resuscitation equipment should be available for anaphylactic reaction
• Determine urine output; if decreasing, notify prescriber (may indicate nephrotoxicity); also check for increased BUN, creatinine
• Monitor blood tests: AST, ALT, CBC, Hct, bilirubin, LDH, alkaline phosphatase, Coombs' test monthly if patient is on long-term therapy
• Monitor electrolytes: potassium, sodium, chloride monthly if patient is on long-term therapy
• Assess bowel pattern daily; if severe diarrhea occurs, product should be discontinued
• Monitor for bleeding: ecchymosis, bleeding gums, hematuria, stool guaiac daily if on long-term therapy
• Assess for overgrowth of infection: perineal itching, fever, malaise, redness, pain, swelling, drainage, rash, diarrhea, change in cough, sputum

Nursing diagnoses
• Diarrhea (side effects)
• Infection, risk for (uses)
• Injury, risk for (side effects)
• Knowledge, deficient (teaching)
• Noncompliance (teaching)

Implementation
• Give PO 4 hr before or 2 hr after antacids, iron, calcium, zinc
• Check for irritation, extravasation, phlebitis daily
• Give product around the clock to maintain blood levels
• Do not use theophylline with this product

Patient/family education
• Teach patient to report sore throat, bruising, bleeding, joint pain; may indicate blood dyscrasias (rare)
• Advise patient to contact prescriber if vaginal itching, loose foul-smelling stools, furry tongue occur, may indicate superinfection; report itching, rash, pruritus, urticaria
• Instruct patient to take all medication prescribed for the length of time ordered; product must be taken around the clock to maintain blood levels; do not give medication to others

• Advise patient to notify prescriber of diarrhea with blood or pus
• Instruct patient to take 4 hr before antacids, iron, calcium, zinc products
• Tell patient to complete full course of therapy; to increase fluid intake to 2 L/day to prevent crystalluria
• Advise patient to avoid hazardous activities until response to product is known
• Instruct patient to rinse mouth frequently and use sugarless candy or gum for dry mouth
• Instruct patient to avoid taking other medications unless approved by prescriber
• Advise patient to avoid sun exposure or use sunscreen to prevent phototoxicity

Evaluation
Positive therapeutic outcome
• Absence of signs/symptoms of infection (WBC <10,000/mm^3, temp WNL)
• Reported improvement in symptoms of infection

levofloxacin ophthalmic
See Appendix B

L

levoleucovorin (Rx)
(lee-voe-loo-koe-voe'rin)
Fusilev
Func. class.: Chemotherapy protectant
Chem. class.: Tetrahydrofolic acid derivative
Pregnancy category C

Action: Acts as a replacement to rescue cells from the effects of folate antagonists

Therapeutic outcome: Prevention of methotrexate toxicity

Uses: For methotrexate toxicity prophylaxis

Dosage and routes
For levoleucovorin rescue following high-dose methotrexate treatment for osteosarcoma
Adult and child >6 yr: **IV** 7.5 mg (approximately 5 mg/m^2) q6hr × 10 doses starting 24 hr after the beginning of methotrexate INF; max >16 ml (160 mg) of the reconstituted SOL/min

For inadvertent overdose of methotrexate
Adult and child >6 yr: **IV** 7.5 mg q6hr until serum methotrexate conc <0.01 micromolar; max >16 ml (160 mg) of the reconstituted SOL/min

Adverse effects: *italic* = common, **bold** = life-threatening

Available forms: Powder for inj 50 mg

Adverse effects
CNS: **Seizures,** syncope
GI: Nausea, vomiting, stomatitis
GU: Abnormal renal function
INTEG: *Rash, pruritus,* anaphylaxis, *urticaria*
RESP: Dyspnea

Contraindications: Hypersensitivity to this agent or folic acid, mannitol; intrathecal administration

Precautions: Pregnancy **C,** breastfeeding, children <6 yr, megaloblastic/pernicious anemia, seizure disorder, vitamin B$_{12}$ deficiency

Interactions
Individual drugs
Fluorouracil: increased toxicity
Methotrexate, pyrimethamine, trimethoprim, trimetrexate: decreased effect of these products
Drug classifications
Barbiturates, hydantoins: increased metabolism

NURSING CONSIDERATIONS
Assessment
• Monitor CCr, creatinine before levoleucovorin rescue and daily to detect methotrexate level
• Monitor CBC with differential
• Assess other products taken: hydantoins, trimethoprim may cause increased folic acid use by body
• Assess neurologic status (rescue): weakness, fatigue

Nursing diagnoses
• Injury, risk for (uses)
• Knowledge, deficient (teaching)

Implementation
• Give within 1 hr of folic acid antagonist
• Do not give concurrently with systemic methotrexate
• Increase fluid intake if used to treat folic acid inhibitor overdose
• Protect from light and heat
IV route
• For **IV** reconstitute 50 mg vial/5.3 ml of normal saline (10 mg/ml)
IV, direct route
• Give 160 mg/min or less (16 ml of 10 mg/ml sol/min)
Intermittent IV route
• Further dilute to a final concentration of 0.5 mg/ml-5 mg/ml

Patient/family education
• Teach patient to eat folic acid rich foods for folic acid deficiency: bran, yeast, dried beans, nuts, fresh, green leafy vegetables
• Advise patient to notify prescriber of side effects
• Instruct patient to report signs of hyposensitivity reaction immediately
• Inform patient to avoid breastfeeding

Evaluation
Positive therapeutic outcome
• Prevention of methotrexate toxicity

---

levothyroxine **(Rx)**
(lee-voe-thye-rox′een)
Eltroxin ✤, Levo-T, Levothroid, levothyroxine sodium, Levoxyl, PMS-Levothyroxine Sodium ✤, Synthroid, T$_4$, Unithroid
Func. class.: Thyroid hormone
Chem. class.: Levoisomer of thyroxine
Pregnancy category A

Do not confuse:
Synthroid/Symmetrel

Action: Controls protein synthesis; increases metabolic rate, cardiac output, renal blood flow, O$_2$ consumption, body temp, blood volume, growth, development at cellular level; exact mechanism unknown

Therapeutic outcome: Correction of lack of thyroid hormone

Uses: Hypothyroidism, myxedema coma, thyroid hormone replacement, thyrotoxicosis, congenital hypothyroidism, some types of thyroid cancer, pituitary TSH suppression

Dosage and routes
Severe hypothyroidism
Adult: PO 12.5-25 mcg/day, increase by 25 mcg q2-4wk, average dose 100-200 mcg/day, max 200 mcg/day; IM/**IV** 50-100 mcg/day as a single dose or 50% of usual oral dosage or (Adult >50 yr without heart disease or <50 yr with heart disease) PO 25-50 mcg/day, titrate q6-8wk or (Adult >50 yr with heart disease) PO 12.5-25 mcg/day, titrate by 12.5-25 mcg q6-8wk
Child >12 yr: PO 2-3 mcg/kg/day given as a single dose AM
Child 6-12 yr: PO 4-5 mcg/kg/day given as a single dose AM
Child 1-5 yr: PO 5-6 mcg/kg/day given as a single dose AM

Child 6-12 mo: PO 6-8 mcg/kg/day given as a single dose AM
Child <6 mo: PO 8-10 mcg/kg/day given as a single dose AM

Myxedema coma
Adult: IV 200-500 mcg; may increase by 100-300 mcg after 24 hr; give oral medication as soon as possible

Subclinical hypothyroidism
Adult: PO 1 mcg/kg/day may be sufficient

Available forms: Powder for inj 200, 500 mcg/vial; tabs 0.025, 0.05, 0.075, 0.088, 0.1, 0.112, 0.125, 0.137, 0.15, 0.175, 0.2, 0.3 mg

Adverse effects
CNS: Anxiety, insomnia, tremors, headache, **thyroid storm,** excitability
CV: Tachycardia, palpitations, angina, dysrhythmias, hypertension, **cardiac arrest**
GI: Nausea, diarrhea, increased or decreased appetite, cramps
MISC: Menstrual irregularities, weight loss, sweating, heat intolerance, fever, alopecia, decreased bone mineral density

Contraindications: Adrenal insufficiency, recent MI, thyrotoxicosis, hypersensitivity to beef, alcohol intolerance (inj only)

Black Box Warning: Obesity treatment

Precautions: Pregnancy A, breastfeeding, geriatric, angina pectoris, hypertension, ischemia, cardiac disease, diabetes

Pharmacokinetics
Absorption	Erratic (PO); complete (IV)
Distribution	Widely distributed
Metabolism	Liver; enterohepatic recirculation
Excretion	Feces via bile; breast milk (small amounts)
Half-life	6-7 days

Pharmacodynamics
	PO	IV
Onset	3-5 days	6-8 hr
Peak	12-48 hr	12-48 hr
Duration	Unknown	Unknown

Interactions
Individual drugs
Aluminum, calcium, iron, magnesium, sucralfate: decreased levothyroxine effects
Cholestyramine, colestipol, ferrous sulfate: decreased absorption of levothyroxine
Digoxin: decreased effect of digoxin
Insulin: increased requirement for insulin

Drug classifications
Antacids: decreased levothyroxine effects
Anticoagulants (oral): increased anticoagulant effect
Antidepressants (tricyclics): increased tricyclic effect
epinephrine products: increased cardiac insufficiency risk
Estrogens: decreased thyroid hormone effects
Hypoglycemics: decreased hypoglycemic effect
Selective serotonin reuptake inhibitors: decreased levothyroxine effects
Sympathomimetics: increased sympathomimetic effect
Drug/herb
Agar, bugleweed, carnitine, kelpware, soy, spirulina: decreased thyroid hormone effect
Drug/lab test
Increased: CPK, LDH, AST, blood glucose
Decreased: thyroid function tests

NURSING CONSIDERATIONS
Assessment
• Determine if the patient is taking anticoagulants, antidiabetic agents; document on chart
• Take B/P, pulse before each dose; monitor I&O ratio and weight every day in same clothing, using same scale, at same time of day
• Monitor height, weight, psychomotor development, and growth rate if given to a child
• Monitor T₃, T₄, which are decreased; radioimmunoassay of TSH, which is increased; radioactive iodine uptake (RAIU), which is increased if patient is on too low a dosage of medication
• Monitor pro-time (may require decreased anticoagulant); check for bleeding, bruising
• Assess for increased nervousness, excitability, irritability, which may indicate too high a dosage of medication, usually after 1-3 wk of treatment
• Assess cardiac status: angina, palpitations, chest pain, change in VS; the geriatric patient may have undetected cardiac problems and baseline ECG should be completed before treatment

Nursing diagnoses
• Knowledge, deficient (teaching)
• Noncompliance (teaching)

Implementation
PO route
• Give in AM if possible as a single dose to decrease sleeplessness; give at same time each day to maintain product level
• Give crushed and mixed with water, nonsoy formula, or breast milk for infants/children

- Give only for hormone imbalances; not to be used for obesity, male infertility, menstrual conditions, lethargy; give lowest dosage that relieves symptoms; lower dosage for the geriatric and in cardiac diseases
- Store in tight, light-resistant container
- Remove medication 4 wk before RAIU test

IV route
- Give **IV** after diluting with provided diluent (0.9% NaCl), 0.5 mg/5 ml; shake well; give through Y-tube or 3-way stopcock; give 0.1 mg or less over 1 min; do not add to **IV** inf; 0.1 mg = 1 ml; discard any unused portion

Patient/family education
- Teach patient that product is not a cure but controls symptoms and treatment is long term
- Instruct patient to report excitability, irritability, anxiety, sweating, heat intolerance, chest pain, palpitations, which indicate overdose
- Advise patient not to switch brands unless approved by prescriber; bioavailability may differ; do not take with food; absorption will be decreased
- Teach patient that product may be discontinued after giving birth; thyroid panel will be evaluated after 1-2 mo
- Teach patient or parent that hyperthyroid child will show almost immediate behavior/personality change; that hair loss will occur in child but is temporary
- Caution patient that product is not to be taken to reduce weight
- Caution patient to avoid OTC preparations with iodine; read labels; other medications should not be used unless approved by prescriber
- Teach patient to avoid iodine-rich food: iodized salt, soybeans, tofu, turnips, high iodine seafood, some bread

Evaluation
Positive therapeutic outcome
- Absence of depression
- Weight loss, increased diuresis, pulse, appetite
- Absence of constipation, peripheral edema, cold intolerance, pale, cool dry skin, brittle nails, alopecia, coarse hair, menorrhagia, night blindness, paresthesias, syncope, stupor, coma, rosy cheeks
- Improved levels of T_3, T_4 by laboratory tests
- Child: age-appropriate weight, height, and psychomotor development

Treatment of overdose: Withhold dose for up to 1 wk; acute overdose: gastric lavage or induced emesis, activated charcoal; provide supportive treatment to control symptoms

---

⚠ HIGH ALERT

lidocaine, parenteral
🌐 **(Rx)**
(lye′doe-kane)
LidoPen Auto-Injector, Xylocaine, Xylocard ✠, Zingo
Func. class.: Antidysrhythmic (class IB)
Chem. class.: Aminoacyl amide

Pregnancy category B

Action: Increases electrical stimulation threshold of ventricle and His-Purkinje system, which stabilizes cardiac membrane and decreases automaticity

Therapeutic outcome: Decreased ventricular dysrhythmia

Uses: Ventricular tachycardia, ventricular dysrhythmias during cardiac surgery, MI, digoxin toxicity, cardiac catheterization

Dosage and routes
Adult: **IV** BOL 50-100 mg (1-1.5 mg/kg) over 2-3 min; repeat q3-5min, max 300 mg in 1 hr; begin **IV** INF 20-50 mcg/kg/min; IM 200-300 mg (4.3 mg/kg) in deltoid muscle, may repeat in 1-1½ hr if needed
Child: ID (Zingo) 0.5 mg applied 1-3 min prior to needle insertion

CHF, reduced liver function
Geriatric: **IV** BOL ½ adult dose
Child: **IV** BOL 1 mg/kg, then **IV** INF 30 mcg/kg/min

Available forms: **IV** inf 0.2% (2 mg/ml), 0.4% (4 mg/ml), 0.8% (8 mg/ml); **IV** admixture 4% (40 mg/ml), 10% (100 mg/ml), 20% (200 mg/ml); **IV** direct 1% (10 mg/ml), 2% (20 mg/ml); IM 300 mg/3 ml; (Zingo) needle free (powder intradermal)

Adverse effects
CNS: Headache, dizziness, involuntary movement, confusion, tremor, *drowsiness,* euphoria, **seizures**
CV: Hypotension, bradycardia, **heart block, cardiovascular collapse, arrest**
EENT: Tinnitus, blurred vision
GI: Nausea, vomiting, anorexia
HEMA: **Methemoglobinemia**
INTEG: Rash, urticaria, edema, swelling
MISC: Febrile response, phlebitis at inj site
RESP: Dyspnea, **respiratory depression**

Contraindications: Hypersensitivity to amides, severe heart block, supraventricular dysrhythmias, Adams-Stokes syndrome, Wolff-Parkinson-White syndrome

---

Precautions: Pregnancy **B**, breastfeeding, children, geriatric, renal/hepatic disease, CHF, respiratory depression, malignant hyperthermia, myasthenia gravis, weight <50 kg

Pharmacokinetics

Absorption	Complete bioavailability (**IV**)
Distribution	Erythrocytes, cardiovascular endothelium
Metabolism	Liver
Excretion	Kidneys
Half-life	Biphasic 8 min, 1-2 hr

Pharmacodynamics

	IV	IM
Onset	2 min	5-15 min
Peak	Unknown	½ hr
Duration	20 min	1½ hr

Interactions
Individual drugs
Cimetidine, metoprolol, phenytoin, propranolol: increased lidocaine effects
Tubocurarine: increased neuromuscular blockade
Drug classifications
Barbiturates: decreased lidocaine effects
Neuromuscular blockers: increased neuromuscular blockade
Drug/herb
Aconite: increased toxicity, death
Aloe, broom, buckthorn (chronic use), cascara sagrada (chronic use), Chinese rhubarb, figwort, fumitory, goldenseal, kudzu, licorice, senna: increased effect
Coltsfoot: decreased effect
Horehound: increased serotonin effect
Drug/lab test
Increased: CPK

NURSING CONSIDERATIONS
Assessment
• Assess for oxygenation or perfusion deficit: decreased B/P, chest pain, dizziness, loss of consciousness
• Assess respiratory status: auscultate lung fields for bibasilar crackles in patients with advanced CHF
• Assess for urinary retention: check for pain, abdominal absorption, palpate bladder; check males with benign prostatic hypertrophy; anticholinergic reaction may cause retention
• Monitor I&O ratio, electrolytes (potassium, sodium, chloride); watch for decreasing urinary output, possible retention
• Monitor liver function tests: AST, ALT, bilirubin, alkaline phosphatase

• Monitor ECG continuously to determine product effectiveness, measure PR, QRS, QT intervals, check for PVCs, other dysrhythmias; monitor B/P continuously for hypo/hypertension; check for rebound hypertension after 1-2 hr, prolonged PR/QT intervals, QRS complex; if QT or QRS increases by 50% or more, withhold next dose, notify prescriber
• Monitor for CNS symptoms: confusion, numbness, depression, involuntary movements; if these occur, product should be discontinued
• Monitor blood levels (therapeutic level 1.5-5 mcg/ml), notify prescriber of abnormal results

Nursing diagnoses
• Cardiac output, decreased (uses)
• Gas exchange, impaired (adverse reactions)
• Knowledge, deficient (teaching)

Implementation
IM route
• Administer in deltoid, aspirate to prevent **IV** administration
• Check site daily for extravasation
IV route
• Give **IV** bolus undiluted (1%, 2% only); give 6 mg or less over 1 min; if using an **IV** line, use port near insertion site, flush with 0.9% NaCl (50 ml)
• Store at room temperature; sol should be clear
• Give by cont inf after adding 1 g/250-1000 ml of D₅W; give 1-4 mg/min; use infusion pump for correct dosage; pediatric inf is 120 mg of lidocaine/100 ml of D₅W; 1-2.5 ml/kg/hr = 20-50 mcg/kg/min; use only 1%, 2% sol
Solution compatibilities: D₅W, D₅/0.9% NaCl, D₅/0.45% NaCl, D₅/LR, LR, 0.9% NaCl, 0.45% NaCl
Syringe compatibilities: Cloxacillin, glycopyrrolate, heparin, hydrOXYzine, methicillin, metoclopramide, milrinone, moxalactam, nalbuphine
Syringe incompatibilities: Cefazolin
Y-site compatibilities: Alteplase, amiodarone, inamrinone, cefazolin, ciprofloxacin, diltiazem, DOBUTamine, DOPamine, enalaprilat, etomidate, famotidine, haloperidol, heparin, heparin with hydrocortisone, labetalol, meperidine, morphine, nitroglycerin, nitroprusside, potassium chloride, propofol, streptokinase, theophylline, vit B/C, warfarin
Additive compatibilities: Alteplase, aminophylline, amiodarone, atracurium, bretylium, calcium chloride, calcium gluceptate, calcium gluconate, chloramphenicol, chlorothiazide, cimetidine, dexamethasone,

digoxin, diphenhydrAMINE, DOBUTamine, DOPamine, ephedrine, erythromycin, floxacillin, flumazenil, furosemide, heparin, hydrocortisone, nafcillin, hydrOXYzine, regular insulin, mephentermine, metaraminol, nafcillin, nitroglycerin, penicillin G potassium, pentobarbital, phenylephrine, potassium chloride, procainamide, prochlorperazine, promazine, ranitidine, sodium bicarbonate, sodium lactate, theophylline, verapamil, vit B/C

Additive incompatibilities: Methohexital, phenytoin; do not admix with blood transfusions

Infiltration
Physician may order lidocaine with epinephrine to minimize systemic absorption and prolong local anesthesia

Patient/family education
• Teach patient or family reason for use of medication and expected results
◆ Instruct patient in at-home use of Lidopen Auto-Injector; patient should call prescriber before use if heart attack is imminent

Evaluation
Positive therapeutic outcome
• Decreased B/P, dysrhythmias
• Decreased heart rate
• Normal sinus rhythm

Treatment of overdose: Oxygen, artificial ventilation, ECG, administer DOPamine for circulatory depression, diazepam or thiopental for seizures; decreased product or discontinuation may be required

---

lidocaine topical
See Appendix B

---

lindane (OTC)
(lin-dane)
GBH, G-Well, Hexit ✤, Kwell, lindane, PMS-Lindane ✤
Func. class.: Scabicide/pediculicide
Chem. class.: Chlorinated hydrocarbon (synthetic)

Pregnancy category C

Action: Stimulates nervous system of arthropods, resulting in seizures, death of organism

Therapeutic outcome: Resolution of infestation

Uses: Scabies, lice (head/pubic/body), nits

Dosage and routes
Lice
Adult and child: TOP/Cream/Lotion wash area with soap and water, remove visible crusts; apply to skin surfaces; remove with soap, water 8-12 hr after application; may reapply in 1 wk if needed; shampoo using 30 ml work into lather, rub for 5 min, rinse, dry with towel; use fine-toothed comb to remove nits; most require 1 oz, max 2 oz

Scabies
Adult and child: TOP apply 1% cream/lotion to skin from neck to bottom of feet, toes; repeat in 1 wk if necessary; most require 1 oz, max 2 oz

Available forms: Lotion, shampoo, cream (1%)

Adverse effects
CNS: Tremors, **seizures,** stimulation, dizziness (chronic inhalation of vapors), anxiety, **CNS toxicity**
CV: **Ventricular fibrillation** (chronic inhalation of vapors)
GI: *Nausea, vomiting, diarrhea,* liver damage (inhalation of vapors)
GU: **Kidney damage** (chronic inhalation of vapors)
HEMA: **Aplastic anemia** (chronic inhalation of vapors), myelosuppression
INTEG: *Pruritus, rash, irritation, contact dermatitis*

Contraindications: Hypersensitivity; patients with known seizure disorders; Norwegian (crusted) scabies

Black Box Warning: Premature neonate; inflammation of skin, abrasions, or breaks in skin; seizure disorder

Precautions: Pregnancy **C,** breastfeeding, infants, children <10 yr; avoid contact with eyes

Pharmacokinetics
Absorption	20%
Distribution	Fat
Metabolism	Liver
Excretion	Kidneys
Half-life	18 hr

Pharmacodynamics
Onset	Rapid
Peak	Rapid
Duration	3 hr

Interactions
Oil-based hair dressing: increased absorption; wash, rinse, and dry hair before using lindane

NURSING CONSIDERATIONS
Assessment
• Assess head, hair for lice and nits before, after treatment; if scabies are present, check all skin surfaces
• Identify source of infection: school, family members, sexual contacts

Nursing diagnoses
• Knowledge, deficient (teaching)
• Skin integrity, impaired (uses)

Implementation
• Apply to body areas, scalp only; do not apply to face, lips, mouth, eyes, any mucous membrane, anus, or meatus
• Give topical corticosteroids as ordered to decrease contact dermatitis; provide antihistamines
• Apply menthol or phenol lotions to control itching
• Give topical antibiotics for infection
• Provide isolation until areas on skin, scalp have cleared and treatment is completed
• Remove nits by using a fine-toothed comb rinsed in vinegar after treatment, use gloves

Patient/family education
• Advise patient to wash all inhabitants' clothing, using insecticide; preventive treatment may be required for all persons living in same house, using lotion or shampoo to decrease spread of infection; use rubber gloves when applying product
• Instruct patient that itching may continue for 4-6 wk; that product must be reapplied if accidently washed off, or treatment will be ineffective; remove after specified time to prevent toxicity
• Advise patient not to apply to face; if accidental contact with eyes occurs, flush with water
• Advise patient that sexual contacts should be treated simultaneously
• Inform the patient of CNS toxicity: dizziness, cramps, anxiety, nausea, vomiting, seizures

Evaluation
Positive therapeutic outcome
• Decreased crusts, nits, brownish trails on skin, itching papules in skinfolds
• Decreased itching after several wk

Treatment of ingestion: Gastric lavage, saline laxatives, **IV** diazepam (Valium) for seizures (if taken orally)

---

linezolid (Rx)
(lih-nee'zoh-lid)
Zyvox
Func. class.: Broad-spectrum antiinfective
Chem. class.: Oxazolidinone

Pregnancy category C

Action: Inhibits protein synthesis by interfering with translation; binds to bacterial 23S ribosomal RNA of the 50S subunit preventing formation of the bacterial translation process in primarily gram-positive organisms

Therapeutic outcome: Negative blood cultures, absence of signs/symptoms of infection

Uses: Vancomycin-resistant *Enterococcus faecium* infections, nosocomial pneumonia, uncomplicated or complicated skin and skin structure infections, community-acquired pneumonia

Dosage and routes
Vancomycin-resistant E. faecium infections
Adult: **IV**/PO 600 mg q12hr × 14-28 days; max 1200 mg/day

Nosocomial pneumonia/complicated skin infections/community-acquired pneumonia/concurrent bacterial infection
Adult: **IV**/PO 600 mg q12hr × 10-14 days; max 1200 mg/day
Child birth-11 yr: PO 10 mg/kg q8hr × 10-14 days

Uncomplicated skin infections
Adult: **IV**/PO 400 mg q12hr × 10-14 days; max 1200 mg/day
Adolescent: PO 600 mg q12hr × 10-14 days, max 1200 mg/day
Infant, preterm <7 days old: PO 10 mg/kg q12hr × 10-14 days

Available forms: Tabs 600 mg; oral susp 100 mg/5 ml; inj 2 mg/ml

Adverse effects
CNS: Headache, dizziness, insomnia
GI: Nausea, diarrhea, increased ALT, AST, *vomiting,* taste change, tongue color change, **pseudomembranous colitis**
HEMA: **Myelosuppression**
MISC: Vaginal moniliasis, fungal infection, oral moniliasis, **lactic acidosis**

Contraindications: Hypersensitivity

Precautions: Pregnancy **C**, breastfeeding, children, thrombocytopenia, bone marrow suppression

---

Adverse effects: *italic* = common, **bold** = life-threatening

Pharmacokinetics	
Absorption	Rapidly, excessively
Distribution	Protein binding 31%
Metabolism	Oxidation of the morpholine ring
Excretion	Unknown
Half-life	Unknown

Pharmacodynamics
Unknown

Interactions
Individual drugs
Amoxapine, cyclobenzaprine, maprotiline, mirtazapine, trazodone: increased hypertensive crisis, seizures, coma

Levodopa: increased hypertensive crisis

Drug classifications
Adrenergic blockers: increased effects of adrenergics

Antidepressants (tricyclics): increased hypertensive crisis, seizures, coma

MAOIs or those that possess MAOI-like action (flurazolidone, isoniazid, INH, procarbazine): do not use together; hypertensive crisis may occur

SSRIs: increased serotonin syndrome

Serotonergic agents: increased effect

Drug/herb
Acidophilus: do not use with antiinfectives; separate by several hours

Green tea: avoid use

Drug/food
Tyramine foods: avoid; increased pressor response

NURSING CONSIDERATIONS
Assessment
- Assess CNS symptoms: headache, dizziness
- Monitor liver function tests: AST, ALT
- Monitor allergic reactions: fever, flushing, rash, urticaria, pruritus
- Assess for pseudomembranous colitis: severe diarrhea, cramping
- Monitor CBC weekly, assess for myelosuppression (anemia, leukopenia, pancytopenia, thrombocytopenia)

Nursing diagnoses
- Infection, risk for (uses)
- Knowledge, deficient (teaching)

Implementation
PO route
- Store reconstituted oral susp at room temperature, use within 3 wk

IV route
- Give over 30-120 min; do not use **IV** inf bag in series connections, do not use with additives in sol, do not use with another product, administer separately

Y-site compatibilities: Acyclovir, alfentanil, amikacin, aminophylline, ampicillin, aztreonam, bretylium, buprenorphine, butorphanol, calcium gluconate, carboplatin, cefazolin, cefoperazone, cefotetan, cefoxitin, ceftazidime, ceftizoxime, ceftriaxone, cefuroxime, cimetidine, ciprofloxacin, cisatracurium, cisplatin, clindamycin, cyclophosphamide, cycloSPORINE, cytarabine, hydromorphone, ifosfamide, labetalol, leucovorin, levofloxacin, lidocaine, lorazepam, magnesium sulfate, mannitol, meperidine, meropenem, mesna, methotrexate, methylPREDNISolone, metoclopramide, metronidazole, midazolam, minocycline, mitoxantrone, morphine, nalbuphine, naloxone, nitroglycerin, ofloxacin, ondansetron, paclitaxel, pentobarbital, piperacillin, potassium chloride, prochlorperazine, promethazine, propranolol, ranitidine, remifentanil, theophylline, ticarcillin, tobramycin, vancomycin, vecuronium, verapamil, vinCRIStine, zidovudine

Solution compatibilities: D₅, 0.9% NaCl, LR

Patient/family education
- Advise patient if dizziness occurs, to ambulate, perform activities with assistance
- Advise patient to complete full course of product therapy
- Advise patient to contact prescriber if adverse reaction occurs
- Advise patient to avoid large amounts of tyramine-containing foods (give list)

Evaluation
Positive therapeutic outcome
- Decreased symptoms of infection, blood cultures negative

---

liothyronine (T₃) (Rx)
(lye-oh-thye'roe-neen)
Cytomel, l-Triiodothyronine, liothyronine sodium, Triostat, T₃
Func. class.: Thyroid hormone
Chem. class.: Synthetic T₃

Pregnancy category A

Action: Controls protein synthesis; increases metabolic rates, cardiac output, renal blood flow, O₂ consumption, body temp, blood volume, growth, development at cellular level; exact mechanism unknown

Therapeutic outcome: Correction of lack of thyroid hormone

Uses: Hypothyroidism, myxedema coma, thyroid hormone replacement, nontoxic goiter, T_3 suppression test, congenital hypothyroidism

Dosage and routes
Adult: PO 25 mcg/day, increase by 12.5-25 mcg q1-2wk until desired response; maintenance dose 25-75 mcg/day; max 100 mcg/day
Geriatric: PO 5 mcg/day, increase by 5 mcg/day q1-2wk, maintenance 25-75 mcg/day

Congenital hypothyroidism
Child >3 yr: PO 50-100 mcg/day
Child <3 yr: PO 5 mcg/day, increase by 5 mcg q3-4day titrated to response; maintenance 20 mcg/day

Myxedema, severe hypothyroidism
Adult: PO 25-50 mcg, then may increase by 5-10 mcg q1-2wk; maintenance dose 50-100 mcg/day

Myxedema coma/precoma
Adult: **IV** 25-50 mcg initially; 5 mcg in geriatric; 10-20 mcg in cardiac disease; give doses q4-12hr

Nontoxic goiter
Adult: PO 5 mcg/day, increase by 12.5-25 mcg q1-2wk; maintenance dose 75 mcg/day

Suppression test (T_3)
Adult: PO 75-100 mcg daily × 1 wk; ¹³¹I is given before and after 1st wk dose

Available forms: Tabs 5, 25, 50 mcg; inj 10 mcg/ml

Adverse effects
CNS: Insomnia, tremors, headache, **thyroid storm**
CV: Tachycardia, palpitations, angina, dysrhythmias, hypertension, **cardiac arrest**
GI: Nausea, diarrhea, increased or decreased appetite, cramps
MISC: Menstrual irregularities, weight loss, sweating, heat intolerance, fever, alopecia

Contraindications: Adrenal insufficiency, MI, thyrotoxicosis, untreated hypertension

Black Box Warning: Obesity treatment

Precautions: Pregnancy **A**, breastfeeding, geriatric, angina pectoris, hypertension, ischemia, cardiac disease, diabetes

Pharmacokinetics
Absorption	Well (PO); complete (**IV**)
Distribution	Widely distributed; does not cross placenta
Metabolism	Liver
Excretion	Feces via bile, breast milk
Half-life	1-2 days

Pharmacodynamics
	PO/IV
Onset	Unknown
Peak	12-24 hr
Duration	72 hr

Interactions
Individual drugs
Cholestyramine, colestipol: decreased absorption of thyroid hormone
Digoxin: decreased effects of digoxin
Insulin: increased requirement for insulin
Drug classifications
Amphetamines, anticoagulants (oral), antidepressants (tricyclics), decongestants, sympathomimetics, vasopressors: increased effect of each specific product
Calcium, iron, aluminum, magnesium products: decreased absorption of liothyronine
Estrogens: decreased effects of liothyronine
Hypoglycemics: decreased effect of each specific product
Drug/herb
Agar, bugleweed, carnitine, kelpware, soy, spirulina: decreased thyroid hormone effect
Drug/lab test
Increased: CPK, LDH, AST, PBI, blood glucose
Decreased: thyroid function tests

NURSING CONSIDERATIONS
Assessment
• Determine if the patient is taking anticoagulants, antidiabetic agents; document on patient record
• Take B/P, pulse before each dose; monitor I&O ratio and weight every day in same clothing, using same scale, at same time of day
• Monitor height, weight, psychomotor development, and growth rate if given to a child
• Monitor T_3, T_4, FTIs, which are decreased; radioimmunoassay of TSH, which is increased; radioactive iodine uptake, which is increased if medication dose is too low
• Monitor protime; may require decreased anticoagulant; check for bleeding, bruising
• Assess for increased nervousness, excitability, irritability, which may indicate too high a dose, usually after 1-3 wk of treatment
• Assess cardiac status: angina, palpitations, chest pain, change in VS; geriatric patients may have undetected cardiac problems, and baseline ECG should be completed before treatment

L

Adverse effects: *italic* = common, **bold** = life-threatening

Nursing diagnoses
• Knowledge, deficient (teaching)
• Noncompliance (teaching)

Implementation
PO route
• Give in AM if possible as a single dose to decrease sleeplessness; give at same time each day to maintain product level
• Do not take with food or absorption will be decreased
• Give only for hormone imbalances; not to be used for obesity, male infertility, menstrual conditions, lethargy; give lowest dose that relieves symptoms; give lower dose to the geriatric and those with cardiac diseases
• Store in airtight, light-resistant container
IV route
• Administer **IV** for myxedema coma and precoma; do not give IM or SUBCUT; give q4-12hr; use PO dose as soon as feasible

Patient/family education
• Teach patient that product is not a cure but controls symptoms, and treatment is long term
• Instruct patient to report excitability, irritability, anxiety, sweating, heat intolerance, chest pain, palpitations, which indicate overdose
• Advise patient not to switch brands unless approved by prescriber; bioavailability may differ
• Teach patient that product may be discontinued after giving birth; thyroid panel will be evaluated after 1-2 mo
• Teach patient that hyperthyroid child will show almost immediate behavior/personality change; that hair loss will occur in child but is temporary
• Caution patient that product is not to be taken to reduce weight
• Caution patient to avoid OTC preparations with iodine; read labels; other medications should not be used unless approved by prescriber
• Teach patient to avoid iodine-rich food: iodized salt, soybeans, tofu, turnips, high iodine seafood, some bread

Evaluation
Positive therapeutic outcome
• Absence of depression
• Weight loss
• Increased diuresis, pulse, appetite
• Absence of constipation, peripheral edema, cold intolerance, pale, cool dry skin, brittle nails, alopecia, coarse hair, menorrhagia, night blindness, paresthesias, syncope, stupor, coma, rosy cheeks
• Improved levels of T_3, T_4 by laboratory tests

• Child: age-appropriate weight, height, and psychomotor development

Treatment of overdose: Withhold dose for up to 1 wk; for acute overdose: gastric lavage or induce emesis, then activated charcoal; provide supportive treatment to control symptoms

liotrix (Rx)
(lye'oh-trix)
T_3/T_4, Thyrolar
Func. class.: Thyroid hormone
Chem. class.: Levothyroxine/liothyronine (synthetic T_4, T_3)

Pregnancy category A

Do not confuse:
Thyrolar/Thyrar

Action: Increases metabolic rates, cardiac output, O_2 consumption, body temp, blood volume, growth, development at cellular level; exact mechanism unknown

Therapeutic outcome: Correction of lack of thyroid hormone

Uses: Hypothyroidism, thyroid hormone replacement

Dosage and routes
Adult: **PO** a single dose of Thyrolar ¼ or ½ adult dose, adjust as needed at 2-wk intervals
Geriatric: **PO** ¼ tab, initially, adjust q6-8wk

Available forms: Tabs levothyroxine 12.5 mcg/liothyronine 3.1 mcg; levothyroxine 25 mcg/liothyronine 6.25 mcg (Thyrolar-½); levothyroxine 50 mcg/liothyronine 12.5 mcg (Thyrolar-1); levothyroxine 100 mcg/liothyronine 25 mcg (Thyrolar-2); levothyroxine 150 mcg/liothyronine 37.5 mcg (Thyrolar-3)

Adverse effects
CNS: Insomnia, tremors, headache, **thyroid storm,** nervousness
CV: Tachycardia, palpitations, angina, dysrhythmias, hypertension, **cardiac arrest**
GI: Nausea, diarrhea, increased or decreased appetite, cramps, vomiting
MISC: Menstrual irregularities, weight loss, sweating, heat intolerance, fever

Contraindications: Adrenal insufficiency, MI, thyrotoxicosis, obesity treatment

Precautions: Pregnancy **A**, breastfeeding, geriatric, angina pectoris, hypertension, ischemia, cardiac disease, diabetes

Pharmacokinetics

Absorption	50%-80% (T_4); 95% (T_3)
Distribution	Widely distributed; does not cross placenta
Metabolism	Liver, tissues
Excretion	Feces via bile; breast milk
Half-life	6-7 days (T_4); 2 days (T_3)

Pharmacodynamics

	PO (T_4)	PO (T_3)
Onset	Unknown	Unknown
Peak	Unknown	24-72 hr
Duration	Unknown	72 hr

Interactions
Individual drugs
Carbamazepine, phenytoin, rifampin: decreased effects of liotrix
Cholestyramine: decreased absorption of thyroid hormone
Colestipol: decreased absorption of liotrix
Digoxin: decreased effect of digoxin
Insulin: increased requirement for insulin
Theophylline: decreased effect of theophylline
Drug classifications
Amphetamines, decongestants, vasopressors: increased effect of each specific product
Anticoagulants (oral): increased effect of anticoagulants
Antidepressants (tricyclics): increased tricyclic effect
Catecholamines: increased catecholamine effect
Estrogens: decreased liotrix effect
Hypoglycemics: decreased hypoglycemic effect
Sympathomimetics: increased sympathomimetic effect
Drug/herb
Agar, bugleweed, carnitine, kelpware, soy, spirulina: decreased thyroid hormone effect
Drug/lab test
Increased: CPK, LDH, AST, PBI, blood glucose
Decreased: thyroid function tests

NURSING CONSIDERATIONS
Assessment
- Determine if the patient is taking anticoagulants, antidiabetic agents; document on chart
- Take B/P, pulse before each dose; monitor I&O ratio and weight every day in same clothing, using same scale, at same time of day
- Monitor height, weight, psychomotor development, and growth rate if given to a child
- Monitor T_3, T_4, FTIs, which are decreased; radioimmunoassay of TSH, which is increased; radioactive iodine uptake (RA international units), which is increased if medication dose is too low
- Monitor pro-time; may require decreased anticoagulant; check for bleeding, bruising
- Assess for increased nervousness, excitability, irritability, which may indicate too high a dose of medication, usually after 1-3 wk of treatment
- Assess cardiac status: angina, palpitations, chest pain, change in VS; the geriatric patient may have undetected cardiac problems, and baseline ECG should be completed before treatment

Nursing diagnoses
- Knowledge, deficient (teaching)
- Noncompliance (teaching)

Implementation
- Give in AM if possible as a single dose to decrease sleeplessness; give at same time each day to maintain product level
- Do not take with food or absorption will be decreased
- Give only for hormone imbalances; not to be used for obesity, male infertility, menstrual conditions, lethargy; give lowest dose that relieves symptoms; give lower dose to the geriatric and those with cardiac diseases
- Store in airtight, light-resistant container
- Remove medication 4 wk before RAIU test

Patient/family education
- Teach patient that product is not a cure but controls symptoms, and treatment is long term
- Instruct patient to report excitability, irritability, anxiety, sweating, heat intolerance, chest pain, palpitations, which indicate overdose
- Advise patient not to switch brands unless approved by prescriber; bioavailability may differ
- Teach patient that product may be discontinued after giving birth; thyroid panel will be evaluated after 1-2 mo
- Teach patient that hyperthyroid child will show almost immediate behavior/personality change; that hair loss will occur in child but is temporary
- Caution patient that product is not to be taken to reduce weight
- Caution patient to avoid OTC preparations with iodine; read labels; other medications should not be used unless approved by prescriber
- Teach patient to avoid iodine-rich food: iodized salt, soybeans, tofu, turnips, high iodine seafood, some bread

L

Adverse effects: *italic* = common, **bold** = life-threatening

Evaluation
Positive therapeutic outcome
- Absence of depression
- Weight loss
- Increased diuresis, pulse, appetite
- Absence of constipation, peripheral edema, cold intolerance, pale, cool dry skin, brittle nails, alopecia, coarse hair, menorrhagia, night blindness, paresthesias, syncope, stupor, coma, rosy cheeks
- Improved levels of T_3, T_4 by laboratory tests
- Child: age-appropriate weight, height, and psychomotor development

Treatment of overdose: Withhold dose for up to 1 wk; acute overdose: gastric lavage or induce emesis, then activated charcoal; provide supportive treatment to control symptoms

---

lisdexamfetamine (Rx)
(lis-dex′am-fet′a-meen)
Vyvanse
Func. class.: CNS stimulant
Chem. class.: Amphetamine

Pregnancy category C
Controlled substance schedule II

Action: Increases release of norepinephrine, dopamine in cerebral cortex to reticular activating system

Therapeutic outcome: Ability to focus, decreased hyperactivity

Uses: Attention deficit disorder with hyperactivity (ADHD)

Dosage and routes
Child 6-12 yr: PO 30 mg/day in the AM, may increase by 20 mg/day at weekly intervals; max 70 mg/day

Available forms: Caps 30, 50, 70 mg
Adverse effects
CNS: Hyperactivity, insomnia, restlessness, talkativeness, dizziness, headache, dysphoria, irritability, aggressiveness, CNS tumor, dependence, addiction, mild euphoria, somnolence, lability, psychosis, mania, hallucinations, aggression
CV: Palpitations, tachycardia, hypertension, decrease in heart rate, **dysrhythmias,** MI, **cardiomyopathy**
EENT: Blurred vision, mydriasis, diplopia
ENDO: Growth inhibition
GI: Anorexia, dry mouth, diarrhea, weight loss
GU: Impotence, change in libido

INTEG: Urticaria, **angioedema, Stevens-Johnson syndrome, toxic epidermal necrolysis**

Contraindications: Hyperthyroidism, hypertension, glaucoma, severe arteriosclerosis, CV disease, anxiety, breastfeeding, hypersensitivity to sympathomimetic amines
Black Box Warning: Substance abuse

Precautions: Pregnancy C, children <6 yr, Gilles de la Tourette's disorder, depression, anorexia nervosa

Pharmacokinetics
Absorption	Unknown
Distribution	Crosses placenta, breast milk
Metabolism	Liver
Excretion	Urine pH dependent
Half-life	<1 hr

Pharmacodynamics
Unknown

Interactions
Individual drugs
AcetaZOLAMIDE, sodium bicarbonate: increased lisdexamfetamine effect
Ascorbic acid, ammonium chloride: decreased lisdexamfetamine effect
Haloperidol, meperidine, modafinil, phenobarbital, phenytoin: increased CNS effect
Melatonin: increased CNS stimulation
Phenytoin: decreased absorption
Drug classifications
Adrenergic blockers, antidiabetics: decreased effect
Antacids: increased lisdexamfetamine effect
⬧MAOIs or within 14 days of MAOIs: hypertensive crisis
Phenothiazines, tricyclics: increased CNS effect
Drug/herb
Eucalyptus: decreased stimulant effect
Green tea, guarana, khat, melatonin: increased stimulant effect
St. John's wort: serotonin syndrome
Drug/food
Caffeine: increased amine effect

NURSING CONSIDERATIONS
Assessment
- Monitor VS, B/P; this product may reverse antihypertensives; check patients with cardiac disease often
- Monitor CBC, urinalysis; in diabetes: blood glucose; insulin changes may be required, since eating may decrease

---

- Monitor height, growth rate in children; growth rate may be decreased
- Assess mental status: mood, sensorium, affect, stimulation, insomnia, irritability
- Assess for tolerance or dependency: an increased amount may be used to get same effect; will develop after long-term use
- Assess for overdose: pain, fever, dehydration, insomnia, hyperactivity

Nursing diagnoses
- Knowledge, deficient (teaching)
- Noncompliance (teaching)

Implementation
- Provide gum, hard candy, frequent sips of water for dry mouth

Patient/family education
- Advise patient to decrease caffeine consumption (coffee, tea, cola, chocolate); may increase irritability, stimulation
- Advise patient to avoid OTC preparations unless approved by prescriber
- Teach patient to taper product over several weeks; depression, increased sleeping, lethargy
- Advise to take every day in AM
- Give without regard to meals
- Caps: may take whole or opened with contents dissolved in water and taken
- Avoid breastfeeding
- Advise to use as part of a comprehensive treatment program
- Caution patient to avoid alcohol ingestion
- Advise patient to avoid hazardous activities until stabilized on medication
- Instruct patient to get needed rest; patient will feel more tired at end of day

Evaluation
Positive therapeutic outcome
- Ability to stay on task, decreased hyperactivity

Treatment of overdose: Administer fluids, antihypertensive for increased B/P, ammonium chloride for increased excretion, chlorpromazine to antagonize CNS effect

lisinopril (Rx)
(lyse-in'oh-pril)
Prinivil, Zestril
Func. class.: Antihypertensive, angiotensin converting enzyme (ACE) inhibitor
Chem. class.: Enalaprilat lysine analog

Pregnancy category
C (1st trimester),
D (2nd/3rd trimesters)

Do not confuse:
lisinopril/Risperdal, Prinivil/Plendil/Prilosec/Proventil

Action: Selectively suppresses renin-angiotensin-aldosterone system; inhibits ACE; prevents conversion of angiotensin I to angiotensin II; results in dilatation of arterial, venous vessels

Therapeutic outcome: Decreased B/P in hypertension, decreased preload, afterload in CHF

Uses: Mild to moderate hypertension, adjunctive therapy of systolic CHF, acute MI

Dosage and routes
Hypertension
Adult: PO 10-40 mg/day; may increase to 80 mg/day if required
Geriatric: PO 2.5-5 mg/day, increase q7day

CHF
Adult: PO 5 mg initially with diuretics/digoxin, range 5-20 mg

Available forms: Tabs 2.5, 5, 10, 20, 30 40 mg

Adverse effects
CNS: **Vertigo,** depression, **stroke,** insomnia, paresthesias, *headache,* fatigue, asthenia, dizziness
CV: Chest pain, hypotension
EENT: Blurred vision, nasal congestion
GI: Nausea, vomiting, anorexia, constipation, flatulence, GI irritation, diarrhea
GU: **Proteinuria, renal insufficiency,** sexual dysfunction, impotence
INTEG: Rash, pruritus
MISC: Muscle cramps, hyperkalemia
RESP: Dry cough, dyspnea
SYST: **Angioedema**

Contraindications: Hypersensitivity, angioedema

Black Box Warning: Pregnancy **D** (2nd/3rd trimesters)

Precautions: Pregnancy **C** (1st trimester), breastfeeding, renal disease, hyperkalemia, renal artery stenosis, CHF

Adverse effects: *italic* = common, **bold** = life-threatening

Pharmacokinetics

Absorption	Variable
Distribution	Unknown
Metabolism	Not metabolized
Excretion	Kidneys, unchanged
Half-life	12 hr

Pharmacodynamics

Onset	1 hr
Peak	6-8 hr
Duration	24 hr

Interactions
Individual drugs
Alcohol (large amounts), probenecid: increased hypotension
Allopurinol: increased hypersensitivity
Aspirin: decreased lisinopril effect
CycloSPORINE: increased hyperkalemia
Digoxin: increased serum levels, toxicity
Indomethacin: decreased antihypertensive effect
Lithium: increased levels of lithium, toxicity
Drug classifications
Antihypertensives, diuretics, nitrates, phenothiazines: increased hypotension
Diuretics, potassium-sparing, potassium salt substitutes, potassium supplements: increased hyperkalemia
NSAIDs: decreased lisinopril effect
Drug/herb
Aconite: increased toxicity, death
Astragalus, cola tree: increased or decreased antihypertensive effect
Barberry, betony, black catechu, black cohosh, bloodroot, broom, burdock, cat's claw, dandelion, goldenseal, hawthorn, Irish moss, Jamaican dogwood, kelp, khella, mistletoe, parsley: increased antihypertensive effect
Coltsfoot, guarana, khat, licorice, yohimbe: decreased antihypertensive effect
Drug/food
High-potassium diet (bananas, orange juice, avocados, broccoli, nuts, spinach) should be avoided; hyperkalemia may occur
Drug/lab test
Interference: glucose/insulin tolerance tests, ANA titer

NURSING CONSIDERATIONS
Assessment
• Assess blood studies: platelets, WBC with differential, baseline, periodically q3mo; if neutrophils <1000/mm^3, discontinue treatment

• Monitor B/P, check for orthostatic hypotension, syncope; if changes occur, dosage change may be required
• Establish baselines in renal, liver function tests before therapy begins
• Monitor renal, liver function tests: protein, BUN, creatinine; watch for increased levels that may indicate nephrotic syndrome and renal failure; monitor renal symptoms: polyuria, oliguria, frequency, dysuria
• Check potassium levels throughout treatment, although hyperkalemia rarely occurs
• Check for edema in feet, legs daily
• Assess for allergic reactions: rash, fever, pruritus, urticaria; product should be discontinued if antihistamines fail to help

Nursing diagnoses
• Cardiac output, decreased (uses)
• Injury, risk for (side effects)
• Knowledge, deficient (teaching)
• Noncompliance (teaching)

Implementation
• Store in airtight container at 86° F (30° C) or less
• Severe hypotension may occur after 1st dose of this medication; may be prevented by reducing or discontinuing diuretic therapy 3 days before beginning lisinopril therapy

Patient/family education
• Caution patient not to discontinue product abruptly; advise patient to inform all health care providers about taking this product
• Teach patient not to use OTC products (cough, cold, allergy) unless directed by prescriber; serious side effects can occur
• Teach patient the importance of complying with dosage schedule, even if feeling better; to continue with medical regimen to decrease B/P: exercise, cessation of smoking, decreasing stress, diet modifications
• Teach patient to notify prescriber of mouth sores, sore throat, fever, swelling of hands or feet, irregular heartbeat, chest pain, coughing, shortness of breath
• Caution patient to report excessive perspiration, dehydration, vomiting, diarrhea; may lead to fall in B/P
• Emphasize the need to rise slowly to sitting or standing position to minimize orthostatic hypotension; not to exercise in hot weather or increased hypotension can occur
• Caution patient that product may cause dizziness, fainting, light-headedness; may occur during 1st few days of therapy; to avoid activities that may be hazardous

- Teach patient how to take B/P, and normal readings for age-group; advise patient to take B/P regularly
- Instruct patient to avoid increasing potassium in the diet

Evaluation
Positive therapeutic outcome
- Decreased B/P in hypertension
- Decreased CHF symptoms

Treatment of overdose: 0.9% NaCl **IV** inf, hemodialysis

lithium (Rx)
(li'thee-um)
Carbolith ✤, Duralith ✤, Eskalith, Eskalith-CR, lithium carbonate, Lithizine ✤, Lithobid, Lithonate, Lithotabs
Func. class.: Antimanic, antipsychotic
Chem. class.: Alkali metal ion salt

Pregnancy category D

Action: May alter sodium, potassium ion transport across cell membrane in nerve, muscle cells; may balance biogenic amines of norepinephrine, serotonin in CNS areas involved in emotional responses

Therapeutic outcome: Stable mood

Uses: Bipolar disorders (manic phase), prevention of bipolar manic-depressive psychosis

Dosage and routes
Adult: PO 300-600 mg tid; maintenance 300 mg tid or qid; SLOW REL Tab 300 mg bid; dosage should be individualized to maintain blood levels at 0.5-1.5 mEq/L
Geriatric: PO 300 mg bid, increase q7day by 300 mg to desired dose
Child: PO 15-20 mg/kg/day in 2-3 divided doses; increase as needed; do not exceed adult doses; maintain blood levels at 0.4-0.5 mEq/L

Renal dose
Adult: PO CCr 10-50 ml/min 50%-75% of dose; CCr <10 ml/min 25%-50% of dose

Available forms: Caps 150, 300, 600 mg; tabs 300 mg; ext rel tabs 300, 450 mg; syr 300 mg/5 ml (8 mEq/5 ml); slow rel caps 150, 300 mg ✤

Adverse effects
CNS: Headache, drowsiness, dizziness, tremors, twitching, ataxia, **seizures,** slurred speech, restlessness, *confusion,* stupor, memory loss, clonic movements, *fatigue*

CV: Hypotension, ECG changes, **dysrhythmias, circulatory collapse, edema**
EENT: Tinnitus, blurred vision
ENDO: Hypothyroidism, goiter, hyperglycemia, hyperthyroidism, hyponatremia
GI: Dry mouth, anorexia, nausea, vomiting, diarrhea, incontinence, abdominal pain, metallic taste
GU: **Polyuria, glycosuria, proteinuria, albuminuria,** urinary incontinence, polydipsia
HEMA: **Leukocytosis**
INTEG: Drying of hair, alopecia, rash, pruritus, hyperkeratosis, *acneiform rash, folliculitis*
MS: Muscle weakness

Contraindications: Pregnancy **D**, breast-feeding, children <12 yr, hepatic disease, brain trauma, organic brain syndrome, schizophrenia, severe cardiac/renal disease, severe dehydration

Precautions: Geriatric, thyroid disease, seizure disorders, diabetes mellitus, systemic infection, urinary retention

Black Box Warning: Lithium level >1.5 mmol/L

Pharmacokinetics
Absorption	Completely absorbed
Distribution	Reabsorbed by renal tubules (80%); crosses blood-brain barrier; crosses placenta
Metabolism	Unknown
Excretion	Urine, unchanged
Half-life	18-36 hr depending on age

Pharmacodynamics
Onset	Rapid
Peak	½-12 hr
Duration	Unknown

Interactions
Individual drugs
Acetazolamide, aminophylline, mannitol, sodium bicarbonate: increased renal clearance
Calcium iodide, iodinated glycerol, potassium iodide: increased hypothyroid effect
Carbamazepine, fluoxetine, methyldopa, probenecid: increased lithium effect/toxicity
Haloperidol: increased neurotoxicity
Indomethacin, losartan: increased toxicity
Thioridazine: brain damage
Urea: decreased lithium effect
Drug classifications
Antithyroid agents: increased hypothyroid effects

*Adverse effects: italic = common, **bold** = life-threatening*

Neuromuscular blocking agents: increased effect of neuromuscular blocking effects

NSAIDs, thiazides: increased lithium toxicity

Phenothiazines: increased effect of phenothiazines

Theophyllines, urinary alkalinizers: decreased effect of lithium

Drug/herb

Broom, buchu, dandelion, goldenrod, horsetail, juniper, nettle, parsley: increased lithium effect, increased toxicity

Coffee, cola nut, guarana, plantain, tea (black/green), yerba maté: decreased lithium effect

Drug/food

Significant changes in sodium intake will alter lithium excretion

Drug/lab test

Increased: potassium excretion, urine glucose, blood glucose, protein, BUN

Decreased: VMA, T_3, T_4, PBI, ^{131}I

NURSING CONSIDERATIONS
Assessment

• Assess for minor lithium toxicity: vomiting, diarrhea, poor coordination, fine motor tremors, weakness, lassitude; major toxicity: coarse tremors, severe thirst, tinnitus, dilute urine

• Assess weight daily; check for edema in legs, ankles, wrists; report if present; check skin turgor at least daily

• Monitor sodium intake; decreased sodium intake with decreased fluid intake may lead to lithium retention; increased sodium and fluids may decrease lithium retention

• Monitor urine for albuminuria, glycosuria, uric acid during beginning treatment, q2mo thereafter

• Assess neurologic status: LOC, gait, motor reflexes, hand tremors

• Monitor serum lithium levels weekly initially, then q2mo (therapeutic level: 0.5-1.5 mEq/L); toxic level >1.5 mcg/L; toxicity and therapeutic levels are very close; toxicity may occur rapidly; blood levels are measured before the AM dose

Nursing diagnoses

• Coping, ineffective (uses)
• Knowledge, deficient (teaching)
• Noncompliance (teaching)

Implementation

• Do not break, crush, or chew caps and slow rel caps

• Administer reduced dosage to geriatric; give with meals to avoid GI upset

• Provide adequate fluids (2-3 L/day) to prevent dehydration during initial treatment, 1-2 L/day during maintenance

• Give list of products that interact with lithium

Patient/family education

• Provide patient with written information on symptoms of minor toxicity: vomiting, diarrhea, poor coordination, fine motor tremors, weakness, lassitude; major toxicity: coarse tremors, severe thirst, tinnitus, dilute urine

• Advise patient to monitor urine specific gravity; emphasize need for follow-up care to determine lithium effects

• Advise patient that contraception is necessary, since lithium may harm fetus

• Caution patient not to operate machinery until lithium levels are stable and response determined; that beneficial effects may take 1-3 wk

• Provide to the patient a list of products that interact with lithium and discuss need for adequate, stable intake of salt and fluid

• Advise to have lithium levels monitored to ensure effectiveness

Evaluation
Positive therapeutic outcome

• Decrease in excitement, poor judgment, insomnia (manic phase)

• Decreased mood swings and lability

Treatment of overdose: Induce emesis or lavage, maintain airway, respiratory function; dialysis for severe intoxication

---

Iodoxamide ophthalmic
See Appendix B

---

lomustine (Rx)
(loe-mus'teen)
CCNU, CeeNU
Func. class.: Antineoplastic alkylating agent
Chem. class.: Nitrosourea

Pregnancy category D

Action: Changes essential cellular ions to covalent bonding with resultant alkylation; this interferes with normal biologic function of DNA; activity is not phase specific; action is due to myelosuppression

Therapeutic outcome: Prevention of rapid growth of malignant cells in chronic myelocytic leukemia

Uses: Hodgkin's disease, malignant glioma

Unlabeled uses: Brain, breast, renal, GI tract, bronchogenic carcinoma; melanomas

Dosage and routes
Adult: PO 100-130 mg/m² as a single dose q6wk or 75-100 mg/m² q6wk in combination; titrate dosage to WBC level; do not give repeat dose unless WBCs are >4000/mm³, platelet count >100,000/mm³

Available forms: Caps 10, 40, 100 mg

Adverse effects
CNS: Lethargy
GI: Nausea, vomiting, anorexia, stomatitis, **hepatotoxicity**
GU: **Azotemia, renal failure**
HEMA: **Thrombocytopenia, leukopenia, myelosuppression, anemia**
INTEG: Alopecia
RESP: **Fibrosis, pulmonary infiltrate**

Contraindications: Pregnancy **D**, breast-feeding, "blastic" phase of chronic myelocytic leukemia, hypersensitivity

Black Box Warning: Leukopenia, thrombocytopenia

Precautions: Radiation therapy, pulmonary disease

Pharmacokinetics	
Absorption	Rapidly absorbed
Distribution	Widely
Metabolism	Liver
Excretion	Kidneys, breast milk
Half-life	16-48 hr

Pharmacodynamics
Unknown

Interactions
Individual drugs
Allopurinol: increased bone marrow suppression
Aspirin: increased bleeding
Cimetidine, chloral hydrate, phenytoin: increased toxicity
Phenobarbital: increased lomustine metabolism
Succinylcholine: increased lomustine effect
Drug classifications
Anticoagulants: increased bleeding
Barbiturates: increased toxicity
Drug/lab test
False positive: cytology tests for breast, bladder, cervix, lung

NURSING CONSIDERATIONS
Assessment
◆ Monitor CBC, differential, platelet count weekly; withhold product if WBC is <4000/mm³ or platelet count is <100,000/mm³; notify prescriber of results if WBC <20,000/mm³, platelets <150,000/mm³; these may occur after 4-6 wk and with cumulative dose >600 mg
• Monitor pulmonary function tests, chest x-ray films before, during therapy; chest film should be obtained q2wk during treatment; assess for dyspnea, crackles, unproductive cough, chest pain, tachypnea
• Monitor renal function tests: BUN, serum uric acid, urine CCr before, during therapy; I&O ratio; report fall in urine output of 30 ml/hr; check for decreased hyperuricemia
• Monitor for cold, fever, sore throat (may indicate beginning of infection), usually after 4 wk; identify edema in feet, joint and stomach pain, shaking; prescriber should be notified
• Assess for bleeding: hematuria, guaiac, bruising or petechiae, mucosa or orifices q8hr, no rectal temp

Nursing diagnoses
• Body image, disturbed (adverse reactions)
• Infection, risk for (adverse reactions)
• Injury, risk for (adverse reactions)
• Knowledge, deficient (teaching)

Implementation
• Give product after evening meal, before bedtime; administer antiemetic and dexamethasone 30-60 min before giving product to prevent vomiting; no food or drinks for ≥2 hr after administration
• Store in tight container

Patient/family education
• Teach patient to avoid use of products containing aspirin or ibuprofen, razors, commercial mouthwash, since bleeding may occur; to report symptoms of bleeding (hematuria, tarry stools)
• Advise patient to report signs of anemia (fatigue, headache, irritability, faintness, shortness of breath)
• Caution patient to report any changes in breathing or coughing even several mo after treatment; to avoid crowds and persons with respiratory tract or other infections
• Caution patient not to have any vaccinations without the advice of prescriber; serious reactions can occur
• Tell patient contraception is needed during treatment and for several mo after the completion of therapy; to avoid breastfeeding

L

Evaluation
Positive therapeutic outcome
- Decreased tumor sizes
- Decreased spread of malignancy

loperamide (OTC, Rx)
(loe-per'a-mide)
Imodium, Imodium A-D, Imodium A-D
Caplet, Loperamide, loperamide solution,
Kaopectate II Caplets, Maalox
Antidiarrheal Caplets, Neo-Diaral, Pepto
Diarrhea Control
Func. class.: Antidiarrheal
Chem. class.: Piperidine derivative

Pregnancy category B

Do not confuse:
Imodium/Indocin, Loperimide/furosemide

Action: Direct action on intestinal muscles
to decrease GI peristalsis; reduces volume,
increases bulk; electrolytes are not lost

Therapeutic outcome: Absence of
diarrhea

Uses: Diarrhea (cause undetermined),
chronic diarrhea, to decrease amount of
ileostomy discharge, traveler's diarrhea, IBD

Dosage and routes
Adult: PO 4 mg, then 2 mg after each loose
stool, max 16 mg/24 hr
Child 9-11 yr: PO 2 mg, then 1 mg after
each loose stool, max 6 mg/24 hr
Child 2-5 yr: PO 1 mg, then 0.1 mg/kg
after each loose stool, max 4 mg/24 hr

Available forms: Caps 2 mg; liquid 1
mg/5 ml; tabs 2 mg

Adverse effects
CNS: Dizziness, drowsiness, fatigue
*GI: Nausea, dry mouth, vomiting, constipa-
tion,* abdominal pain, anorexia, **toxic mega-
colon,** bacterial enterocolitis, flatulence
INTEG: Rash
MISC: Hyperglycemia
SYST: **Anaphylaxis,** angioedema, **toxic
epidermal necrolysis**

Contraindications: Hypersensitivity,
pseudomembranous colitis, constipation,
dysentery, GI bleeding/obstruction/perforation,
ileus, vomiting

Precautions: Pregnancy **B**, breastfeeding,
children <2 yr, hepatic disease, gastroenteritis,
toxic megacolon, geriatric patients, dehydration, bacterial disease, AIDS, severe ulcerative
colitis

Pharmacokinetics
Absorption	Poor
Distribution	Unknown
Metabolism	Liver
Excretion	Feces, unchanged; small amount in urine
Half-life	9-14 hr

Pharmacodynamics
Onset	½-1 hr
Peak	Unknown
Duration	4-5 hr

Interaction
Individual drugs
Alcohol: increased CNS depression
Drug classifications
Antihistamines, analgesics (opioids), sedative/
  hypnotics: increased CNS depression
Drug/herb
Chamomile, hops, kava, skullcap, valerian:
  increased CNS depression
Nutmeg: increased antidiarrheal effect

NURSING CONSIDERATIONS
Assessment
- Monitor electrolytes (potassium, sodium,
chloride) if patient is on long-term therapy;
check fluid status, skin turgor
- Assess bowel pattern before, during
treatment; check for rebound constipation
after termination of medication; check bowel
sounds
- Check response after 48 hr; if no response,
product should be discontinued and other
treatment initiated
- Assess for abdominal distention, toxic
megacolon, which may occur in ulcerative
colitis
- Assess for dehydration, CNS symptoms in
children or those with hepatic disease

Nursing diagnoses
- Constipation (adverse reactions)
- Diarrhea (uses)
- Knowledge, deficient (teaching)
- Noncompliance (teaching)

Implementation
- Do not break, crush, or chew caps
- Store in airtight containers
- Do not mix oral sol with other sol

Patient/family education
- Caution patient to avoid alcohol and OTC
products unless directed by prescriber; may
cause increased CNS depression
- Advise patient not to exceed recommended
dosage; product may be habit forming; ileos-

tomy patient may take this product for extended time

• Advise patient that product may cause drowsiness and to avoid hazardous activities until response to product is determined

• Teach patient that dry mouth can be decreased by frequent sips of water, hard candy, sugarless gum

Evaluation
Positive therapeutic outcome
• Decreased diarrhea

loracarbef
See cephalosporins—2nd generation

loratadine (Rx, OTC)
(lor-a'ti-deen)
Alavert, Children's Loratadine, Children's ND Non-Drowsy Allergy, Claritin, Claritin Non-Drowsy Allergy, Clear-Atadine, Dimetapp, Tavist ND
Func. class.: Antihistamine (2nd generation)
Chem. class.: Selective histamine (H_1) receptor antagonist

Pregnancy category B

Do not confuse:
loratadine/lovastatin/lorazepam/losartan

Action: Binds to peripheral histamine receptors, which provides antihistamine action without sedation

Therapeutic outcome: Decreased nasal stuffiness, itching, swollen eyes

Uses: Seasonal rhinitis, chronic idiopathic urticaria for those ≥2 yr

Dosage and routes
Adult and child ≥6 yr: PO 10 mg/day
Child 2-5 yr: PO 5 mg/day

Renal dose
Adult: PO CCr <30 ml/min 10 mg every other day

Hepatic dose
Adult: PO 10 mg every other day

Available forms: Tabs 10 mg; rapid-disintegrating tabs 10 mg; orally disintegrating tabs 10 mg; syr 1 mg/ml; susp 5 mg/ml

Adverse effects
CNS: Sedation (more common with increased dosages), headache, fatigue, restlessness
CV: Sinus tachycardia
RESP: Wheezing

Contraindications: Hypersensitivity, acute asthma attacks, lower respiratory tract disease

Precautions: Pregnancy **B**, increased intraocular pressure, bronchial asthma, breastfeeding, hepatic/renal disease

Pharmacokinetics	
Absorption	Well absorbed
Distribution	Unknown
Metabolism	Liver, extensively, to active metabolite desloratadine
Excretion	Kidneys
Half-life	17-28 hr

Pharmacodynamics	
Onset	1-3 hr
Peak	8-12 hr
Duration	>24 hr

Interactions
Individual drugs
Alcohol: increased CNS depression
Cimetidine, ketoconazole: increased loratadine level
Drug classifications
Antidepressants, antihistamines (other), sedative/hypnotics: increased CNS depression
Macrolides (clarithromycin, erythromycin): increased loratadine level
MAOIs: increased antihistamine effects
Drug/herb
Chamomile, hops, Jamaican dogwood, kava, khat, senega, skullcap, valerian: increased CNS depression
Corkwood, henbane: increased anticholinergic effect
Drug/lab test
False negative: skin allergy tests (discontinue antihistamine 3 days before testing)

NURSING CONSIDERATIONS
Assessment
• Assess allergy: hives, rash, rhinitis
• Assess respiratory status: rate, rhythm, increase in bronchial secretions, wheezing, chest tightness; provide fluids to 2 L/day to decrease secretion thickness
• Monitor LFTs, serum creatinine/bun

Nursing diagnoses
• Airway clearance, ineffective (uses)
• Knowledge, deficient (teaching)
• Noncompliance (teaching, overuse)

Implementation
• Give on an empty stomach, 1 hr before or 2 hr after meals to facilitate absorption

L

Adverse effects: *italic* = common, **bold** = life-threatening

- Place rapidly disintegrating tabs on tongue, then swallow after disintegrated with or without water
- Use within 6 mo of opening pouch; immediately after opening blister pack
- Store in airtight, light-resistant container

Patient/family education

- Teach all aspects of product uses; to notify prescriber if confusion, sedation, hypotension occur; to avoid driving and other hazardous activity if drowsiness occurs; to avoid alcohol and other CNS depressants that may potentiate effect
- Teach patient to take 1 hr before or 2 hr after meals to facilitate absorption
- Advise patient to use sunscreen or stay out of the sun to prevent burns
- Caution patient not to exceed recommended dosage; dysrhythmias may occur
- Teach patient that hard candy, gum, frequent rinsing of mouth may be used for dryness

Evaluation

Positive therapeutic outcome

- Absence of runny or congested nose, other allergy symptoms

---

lorazepam (Rx)

(lor-az′e-pam)
Apo-Lorazepam ✢, Ativan, lorazepam, Novo-Lorazem ✢, Nu-Loraz ✢
Func. class.: Sedative/hypnotic, antianxiety agent
Chem. class.: Benzodiazepine, short acting

Pregnancy category D

Controlled substance schedule IV

Do not confuse:
lorazepam/alprazolam/clonazepam

Action: Potentiates the actions of GABA, an inhibitory neurotransmitter, especially in the limbic system and reticular formation, which depresses the CNS

Therapeutic outcome: Decreased anxiety, relaxation

Uses: Anxiety, irritability in psychiatric or organic disorders, preoperatively; insomnia; adjunct in endoscopic procedures

Unlabeled uses: Antiemetic before chemotherapy, status epilepticus, rectal use

Dosage and routes
Anxiety
Adult: PO 2-6 mg/day in divided doses, max 10 mg/day

Geriatric: PO 1-2 mg/day in divided doses, or 0.5-1 mg at bedtime
Child ≥12 yr: PO 0.05 mg/kg/dose, q4-8hr
Insomnia
Adult: PO 2-4 mg at bedtime; only minimally effective after 2 wk continuous therapy
Geriatric: PO 0.5-1 mg initially

Preoperatively
Adult: IM 50 mcg/kg 2 hr before surgery; **IV** 44 mcg/kg 15-20 min before surgery, max 2 mg 15-20 min prior to surgery
Child ≥12 yr: **IV** 0.05 mg/kg

Status epilepticus
Neonate: **IV** 0.05 mg/kg
Child: **IV** 0.1 mg/kg up to 4 mg/dose; RECT (unlabeled) 0.05-0.1 mg × 2; wait 7 min before giving 2nd dose

Available forms: Tabs 0.5, 1, 2 mg; inj 2, 4 mg/ml; conc sol 2 mg/ml

Adverse effects

CNS: Dizziness, drowsiness, confusion, headache, anxiety, tremors, stimulation, fatigue, depression, insomnia, hallucinations, weakness, unsteadiness
CV: Orthostatic hypotension, **ECG changes, tachycardia,** hypotension, **apnea, cardiac arrest (IV, rapid)**
EENT: Blurred vision, tinnitus, mydriasis
GI: Constipation, dry mouth, nausea, vomiting, anorexia, diarrhea
INTEG: Rash, dermatitis, itching
MISC: Acidosis

Contraindications: Pregnancy **D,** breastfeeding, hypersensitivity to benzodiazepines, closed-angle glaucoma, psychosis, history of drug abuse, COPD, sleep apnea

Precautions: Geriatric, debilitated patients, children <12 yr, renal/hepatic disease, addiction, suicidal ideation

Pharmacokinetics

Absorption	Well absorbed (PO); completely absorbed (IM)
Distribution	Widely distributed; crosses placenta, blood-brain barrier
Metabolism	Liver, extensively
Excretion	Kidneys, breast milk
Half-life	14 hr

Pharmacodynamics

	PO	IM	IV
Onset	½ hr	15-30 min	5-15 min
Peak	1-3 hr	1-1½ hr	Unknown
Duration	12-24 hr	6-8 hr	6-8 hr

Interactions
Individual drugs
Alcohol: increased CNS depression
Disulfiram: increased lorazepam effects
Valproic acid: decreased lorazepam effects
Drug classifications
CNS depressants, oral contraceptives: increased lorazepam effects
Drug/herb
Black cohosh: increased hypotension
Catnip, chamomile, clary, cowslip, hops, kava, lavender, mistletoe, nettle, pokeweed, poppy, Queen Anne's lace, senega, skullcap, valerian: increased CNS depression
Drug/lab test
Increased: AST, ALT, serum bilirubin
Decreased: radioactive iodine uptake
False increase: 17-OHCS

NURSING CONSIDERATIONS
Assessment
- Assess degree of anxiety; what precipitates anxiety and whether product controls symptoms; other signs of anxiety: dilated pupils, inability to sleep, restlessness, inability to focus
- Assess for alcohol withdrawal symptoms, including hallucinations (visual, auditory), delirium, irritability, agitation, fine to coarse tremors
- Monitor B/P (with patient lying/standing), pulse; check respiratory rate; if systolic B/P drops 20 mm Hg, hold product, notify prescriber; respirations q5-15min if given **IV**
- Monitor CBC during long-term therapy; blood dyscrasias have occurred (rarely)
- Monitor for seizure control; type, duration, and intensity of seizures; what precipitates seizures
- Monitor hepatic studies: AST, ALT, bilirubin, creatinine, LDH, alkaline phosphatase
- Assess mental status: mood, sensorium, affect, sleeping pattern, drowsiness, dizziness, suicidal tendencies, and ability of product to control these symptoms; check for tolerance, withdrawal symptoms: headache, nausea, vomiting, muscle pain, weakness after long-term use

Nursing diagnoses
- Coping, ineffective (uses)
- Knowledge, deficient (teaching)
- Noncompliance (teaching)
- Sleep deprivation (uses)

Implementation
PO route
- Give largest dose before bedtime if giving in divided dose
- Concentrate: use calibrated dropper; add to food/drink, consume immediately
- Give with food or milk for GI symptoms; crush tab if patient is unable to swallow medication whole; provide sugarless gum, hard candy, frequent sips of water for dry mouth
SUBCUT route
- Use by SL route for rapid response (investigational use)
IM route
- Give deep in muscle mass; if using for preoperative sedation, give 2 hr or more before surgical procedure
IV route
- Prepare immediately before use; short stability time
- Dilute with sterile water for inj, 0.9% NaCl, or D_5W just before using; give by Y-site or 3-way stopcock at 2 mg/min
- Do not use sol that is discolored or contains a precipitate

Syringe compatibilities: Cimetidine, hydromorphone

Y-site compatibilities: Acyclovir, albumin, allopurinol, amifostine, amikacin, amoxicillin, amoxicillin/clavulanate, amsacrine, atracurium, bumetanide, cefepime, cefmetazole, cefotaxime, ciprofloxacin, cisatracurium, cisplatin, cladribine, clonidine, cyclophosphamide, cytarabine, dexamethasone, diltiazem, DOBUTamine, DOPamine, DOXOrubicin, epinephrine, erythromycin, etomidate, famotidine, fentanyl, filgrastim, fluconazole, fludarabine, furosemide, gentamicin, granisetron, haloperidol, heparin, hydrocortisone, hydromorphone, ketanserin, labetalol, melphalan, methotrexate, metronidazole, midazolam, milrinone, morphine, niCARdipine, nitroglycerin, norepinephrine, paclitaxel, pancuronium, piperacillin, piperacillin/tazobactam, potassium chloride, propofol, ranitidine, tacrolimus, teniposide, thiotepa, trimethoprim/sulfamethoxazole, vancomycin, vecuronium, vinorelbine, zidovudine

Y-site incompatibilities: Idarubicin, ondansetron, sargramostim

Patient/family education
- Advise patient that product may be taken with food; that product is not to be used for everyday stress or used longer than 4 mo unless directed by a prescriber; to take no more than prescribed amount; may be habit forming
- Caution patient to avoid OTC preparations unless approved by prescriber; to avoid alcohol, other psychotropic medications

Adverse effects: *italic* = common, **bold** = life-threatening

unless prescribed by physician; not to discontinue medication abruptly after long-term use
• Inform patient to avoid driving and activities that require alertness; drowsiness may occur; to rise slowly or fainting may occur, especially in geriatric
• Inform patient that drowsiness may worsen at beginning of treatment

Evaluation
Positive therapeutic outcome
• Decreased anxiety, restlessness, insomnia

Treatment of overdose: Lavage, VS, supportive care

losartan (Rx)
(low-sar'tan)
Cozaar
Func. class.: Antihypertensive
Chem. class.: Angiotensin II receptor (type AT_1)

Pregnancy category
C (1st trimester),
D (2nd/3rd trimesters)

Do not confuse:
losartan/valsartan, Cozaar/Zocor

Action: Blocks the vasoconstrictor and aldosterone-secreting effects of angiotensin II; selectively blocks the binding of angiotensin II to the AT_1 receptor found in tissues

Therapeutic outcome: Decreased B/P

Uses: Hypertension, alone or in combination; nephropathy in type 2 diabetes, hypertension with left ventricular hypertrophy

Dosage and routes
Hypertension
Adult: PO 50 mg/day alone or 25 mg/day when used in combination with diuretic; maintenance 25-100 mg/day

Hepatic dose
Adult: PO 25 mg/day as starting dose

Hypertension with left ventricular hypertrophy
Adult: PO 50 mg/day, add hydrochlorothiazide 12.5 mg/day and/or increase losartan to 100 mg/day, then increase hydrochlorothiazide to 25 mg/day

Nephropathy in type 2 diabetes patients
Adult: PO 50 mg/day, may increase to 100 mg/day

Available forms: Tabs 25, 50, 100 mg

Adverse effects
CNS: Dizziness, insomnia, anxiety, confusion, abnormal dreams, migraine, tremor, vertigo, headache, malaise
CV: Angina pectoris, 2nd-degree AV block, **CVA,** hypotension, **MI, dysrhythmias**
EENT: Blurred vision, burning eyes, conjunctivitis
GI: Diarrhea, dyspepsia, anorexia, constipation, dry mouth, flatulence, gastritis, vomiting
GU: Impotence, nocturia, urinary frequency, urinary tract infection, **renal failure**
HEMA: Anemia, **thrombocytopenia**
INTEG: Alopecia, dermatitis, dry skin, flushing, photosensitivity, rash, pruritus, sweating **angioedema**
META: Gout
MS: Cramps, myalgia, pain, stiffness
RESP: Cough, upper respiratory infection, congestion, dyspnea, bronchitis

Contraindications: Hypersensitivity

Black Box Warning: Pregnancy **D** (2nd/3rd trimesters)

Precautions: Pregnancy **C** (1st trimester), breastfeeding, children, geriatric, hypersensitivity to ACE inhibitors, hepatic disease, angioedema, renal artery stenosis

Pharmacokinetics
Absorption	Well
Distribution	Bound to plasma proteins
Metabolism	Extensive
Excretion	Feces, urine
Half-life	Biphasic, 2 hr, 6-9 hr

Pharmacodynamics
Unknown

Interactions
Individual drugs
Fluconazole: increased antihypertensive effect
Lithium: increased toxicity
Phenobarbital, rifamycin: decreased antihypertensive effect
Drug classifications
ACE inhibitors, diuretics (potassium-sparing), potassium supplements: increased hyperkalemia
NSAIDs, salicylates: decreased antihypertensive effect
Drug/herb
Aconite: increased toxicity, death
Astragalus, cola tree: increased or decreased antihypertensive effect
Barberry, betony, black catechu, black cohosh, bloodroot, broom, burdock, cat's claw,

 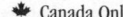

dandelion, goldenseal, hawthorn, Irish moss, Jamaican dogwood, kelp, khella, mistletoe, parsley: increased antihypertensive effect

Coltsfoot, guarana, khat, licorice, yohimbe: decreased antihypertensive effect

NURSING CONSIDERATIONS
Assessment
• Assess B/P with position changes, pulse q4hr; note rate, rhythm, quality
• Monitor electrolytes: potassium, sodium, chloride
• Obtain baselines for renal, liver function tests before therapy begins
• Monitor for edema in feet, legs daily
• Assess for skin turgor, dryness of mucous membranes for hydration status

Nursing diagnoses
• Fluid volume, deficient (side effects)
• Noncompliance (teaching)
• Knowledge, deficient (teaching)

Implementation
• Administer without regard to meals

Patient/family education
• Teach patient to avoid sunlight or wear sunscreen if in sunlight; photosensitivity may occur
• Advise patient to comply with dosage schedule, even if feeling better
• Teach patient to notify prescriber of mouth sores, fever, swelling of hands or feet, irregular heartbeat, chest pain
• Advise patient that excessive perspiration, dehydration, vomiting, diarrhea may lead to fall in blood pressure, consult prescriber if these occur
• Inform patient that product may cause dizziness, fainting; light-headedness may occur
• Caution patient to rise slowly to sitting or standing position to minimize orthostatic hypotension
• Advise patient to use contraception while taking this product

Evaluation
Positive therapeutic outcome
• Decreased B/P

loteprednol ophthalmic
See Appendix B

lovastatin ⊚ (Rx)
(loe′va-sta-tin)
Altocor, Altoprev, Mevacor
Func. class.: Antilipemic
Chem. class.: HMG-CoA reductase inhibitor
Pregnancy category X

Do not confuse:
lovastatin/Lotensin

Action: By inhibiting HMG-CoA reductase, inhibits biosynthesis of VLDL and LDL, which are responsible for cholesterol development

Therapeutic outcome: Decreased cholesterol levels and LDLs, increased HDLs

Uses: As an adjunct in primary hypercholesterolemia (types IIa, IIb), atherosclerosis, primary and secondary prevention of coronary events

Dosage and routes
(Patient should first be consuming a cholesterol-lowering diet)
Adult: PO 20 mg/day with evening meal; may increase to 20-80 mg/day in single or divided doses; max 80 mg/day; dosage adjustments should be made monthly; reduce dose in renal disease; EXT REL 20-60 mg/day at bedtime

Available forms: Tabs 10, 20, 40 mg; ext rel tab (Altocor) 10, 20, 40, 60 mg

Adverse effects
CNS: Dizziness, headache, tremor, insomnia, paresthesia, **ALS (Lou Gehrig's disease)**
EENT: Blurred vision, lens opacities
GI: Nausea, constipation, diarrhea, dyspepsia, *flatus,* abdominal pain, heartburn, **liver dysfunction,** vomiting, acid regurgitation, dry mouth, dysgeusia
***HEMA:* Thrombocytopenia, hemolytic anemia, leukopenia**
INTEG: Rash, pruritus, photosensitivity
MS: Muscle cramps, myalgia, **myositis, rhabdomyolysis,** leg, shoulder or localized pain

Contraindications: Pregnancy **X,** breastfeeding, hypersensitivity, active liver disease

Precautions: Past liver disease, alcoholism, severe acute infections, trauma, hypotension, uncontrolled seizure disorders, severe metabolic disorders, electrolyte imbalances, visual condition, children

L

Adverse effects: *italic* = common, **bold** = life-threatening

Interactions
Individual drugs

Bosentan, exonatide: decreased action of lovastatin

Clarithromycin, clofibrate, cycloSPORINE, dalfopristin, danazol, diltiazem, erythromycin, gemfibrozil, niacin, quinupristin, telithromycin, verapamil: increased myalgia, myositis

Digoxin: increased digoxin effect

Warfarin: increased bleeding

Drug classifications

Azole antifungals, protease inhibitors: increased myositis, myalgia

Bile acid sequestrants: decreased lovastatin effects

Drug/herb

Glucomannan: increased effect

Gotu kola, St. John's wort: decreased effect

Drug/food

Increased levels of lovastatin with food, must be taken with food

Grapefruit juice: increased toxicity

Oat bran: decreased absorption

Drug/lab test

Increased: CPK, liver function tests

NURSING CONSIDERATIONS
Assessment

• Assess nutrition: fat, protein, carbohydrates; nutritional analysis should be completed by dietitian before treatment

• Monitor bowel pattern daily; diarrhea may be a problem

• Monitor triglycerides, fasting cholesterol LDL, HDL at baseline, throughout treatment; watch LDL and VLDL closely; if increased, product should be discontinued

• Assess for muscle pain, tenderness, obtain CPK; if these occur, product may need to be discontinued

Nursing diagnoses

• Diarrhea (adverse reactions)
• Knowledge, deficient (teaching)
• Noncompliance (teaching)

Implementation

• Give with evening meal; if dosage is increased, take with breakfast and evening meal

• Store in cool environment in airtight, light-resistant container

Patient/family education

• Inform patient that compliance is needed for positive results to occur; not to double doses

• Inform patient that blood work and ophthalmic exam will be necessary during treatment

• Teach patient that risk factors should be decreased: high-fat diet, smoking, alcohol consumption, absence of exercise

• Advise patient to report if pregnancy is suspected

• Advise patient to notify prescriber if the GI symptoms of diarrhea, abdominal or epigastric pain, nausea, vomiting occur; or if chills, fever, sore throat, blurred vision, dizziness, headache, muscle pain, weakness occur

• Advise patient to stay out of the sun or use sunscreen to prevent burns

Evaluation

Positive therapeutic outcome

• Decreased cholesterol, serum triglyceride levels

• Improved ratio of HDLs

---

loxapine (Rx)
(lox'a-peen)
Loxapac ✤, loxapine succinate ✤, Loxitane, Loxitane IM
Func. class.: Antipsychotic/neuroleptic
Chem. class.: Dibenzoxazepine

Pregnancy category C

Do not confuse:
Loxitane/Soriatane

Action: Depresses cerebral cortex, hypothalamus, limbic system, which control activity and aggression; blocks neurotransmission produced by DOPamine at synapse; exhibits strong α-adrenergic, anticholinergic blocking action; mechanism for antipsychotic effects is unclear

Therapeutic outcome: Decreased psychotic behavior

Uses: Psychotic disorders, nonpsychotic symptoms associated with dementia

Unlabeled uses: Depression, anxiety

Dosage and routes
Adult: PO 10 mg bid-qid initially; may be rapidly increased depending on severity of condition; maintenance 60-100 mg/day; IM 12.5-50 mg q4-6hr or more until desired response, then start PO form; max 250 mg/day
Geriatric: PO 5-10 mg/day bid, increase q4-7day by 5-10 mg, max 250 mg/day

Available forms: Caps 5, 10, 25, 50 mg; conc 25 mg/ml; inj 50 mg/ml; tabs 5, 10, 25, 50 mg

Adverse effects
CNS: *EPS: pseudoparkinsonism, akathisia, dystonia, tardive dyskinesia, drowsiness, headache,* **seizures,** *confusion,* **neuroleptic malignant syndrome**
CV: *Orthostatic hypotension,* **cardiac arrest,** *ECG changes, tachycardia*
EENT: *Blurred vision, glaucoma*
GI: *Dry mouth, nausea, vomiting, anorexia, constipation,* diarrhea, jaundice, weight gain
GU: Urinary retention, urinary frequency, enuresis, impotence, amenorrhea, gynecomastia
HEMA: **Anemia, leukopenia, leukocytosis, agranulocytosis**
INTEG: *Rash,* photosensitivity, dermatitis
RESP: **Laryngospasm,** dyspnea, **respiratory depression**

Contraindications: Hypersensitivity, blood dyscrasias, coma, severe CNS depression, brain damage, bone marrow depression, alcohol and barbiturate withdrawal states, closed-angle glaucoma

Precautions: Pregnancy **C,** breastfeeding, children <16 yr, geriatric, seizure disorders, cardiac/renal/hepatic disease, prostatic hypertrophy, cardiac conditions

Black Box Warning: Dementia

Pharmacokinetics

Absorption	Well absorbed (PO)
Distribution	Unknown
Metabolism	Liver, extensively
Excretion	Kidneys
Half-life	Biphasic 5 hr, 19 hr

Pharmacodynamics

	PO	IM
Onset	½ hr	15-30 min
Peak	2-4 hr	15-20 min
Duration	12 hr	12 hr

Interactions
Individual drugs
Alcohol: increased CNS depression
epinephrine: increased toxicity
Guanadrel, guanethidine, levodopa: decreased effects
Drug classifications
Antidepressants, MAOIs: increased CNS depression
Antipsychotics: increased EPS
Drug/herb
Betel palm, kava: increased EPS
Chamomile, cola tree, hops, kava, nettle, nutmeg, skullcap, valerian: increased CNS depression

NURSING CONSIDERATIONS
Assessment
• Assess mental status: orientation, mood, behavior, presence and type of hallucinations before initial administration, monthly; this product should significantly reduce psychotic behavior
• Check for swallowing of PO medication; check for hoarding or giving of medication to other patients
• Monitor I&O ratio; palpate bladder if low urinary output occurs, especially in geriatric; urinalysis recommended before, during prolonged therapy, urinary retention may be cause
• Monitor bilirubin, CBC, liver function tests monthly
• Assess affect, orientation, LOC, reflexes, gait, coordination, sleep pattern disturbances
• Monitor B/P with patient sitting, standing, and lying; take pulse and respirations q4hr during initial treatment; establish baseline before starting treatment; report drops of 30 mm Hg
• Check for dizziness, faintness, palpitations, tachycardia on rising; severe orthostatic hypotension is common
⦿ Identify for neuroleptic malignant syndrome: hyperpyrexia, muscle rigidity, increased CPK, altered mental status; product should be discontinued
• Assess for EPS, including akathisia (inability to sit still, no pattern to movements), tardive dyskinesia (bizarre movements of the jaw, mouth, tongue, extremities), pseudoparkinsonism (ragged tremors, pill rolling, shuffling gait); an antiparkinsonian product should be prescribed
• Assess for constipation, urinary retention daily; if these occur, increase bulk, water in diet

Nursing diagnoses
- Coping, ineffective (uses)
- Knowledge, deficient (teaching)
- Noncompliance (teaching)

Implementation
PO route
- Administer product in liquid form mixed in glass of juice or cola if hoarding is suspected; do not mix in caffeine drinks, tannics, pectins
- Administer lowered dose in geriatric, since metabolism is slowed
- Administer with full glass of water or milk; or give with food to decrease GI upset
- Give antacids 2 hr before or after taking this product
- Store in airtight, light-resistant container, oral sol in amber bottle

IM route
- Inject deep in muscle mass; do not give SUBCUT; do not administer sol with a precipitate; amber-colored sol can be used
- Patient should remain lying down after IM inj for at least 30 min

Patient/family education
- Teach patient to use good oral hygiene; suggest frequent rinsing of mouth, sugarless gum for dry mouth; oral candidiasis can occur
- Caution patient to avoid hazardous activities until product response is determined; dizziness, blurred vision may occur
- Inform patient that orthostatic hypotension occurs often and to rise from sitting or lying position gradually; caution patient to avoid hot tubs, hot showers, tub baths, since hypotension may occur; tell patient that in hot weather heat stroke may occur; take extra precautions to stay cool
- Advise patient to avoid abrupt withdrawal of this product, or EPS may result; product should be withdrawn slowly
- Advise patient to avoid use with alcohol, CNS depressants; increased drowsiness may occur
- Advise patient to use a sunscreen and sunglasses to prevent burns
- Suggest patient take antacids 2 hr before or after taking this product
- Instruct patient to report sore throat, malaise, fever, bleeding, mouth sores; if these occur, CBC should be performed and product discontinued

Evaluation
Positive therapeutic outcome
- Decrease in emotional excitement, hallucinations, delusions, paranoia
- Reorganization of patterns of thought, speech

Treatment of overdose: Lavage if orally ingested; barbiturates; provide airway, **IV** fluids; do not use epinephrine, which may increase hypotension

lubiprostone (Rx)
(loo-bee-pros′-tone)
Amitiza
Func. class.: Miscellaneous gastrointestinal agent

Pregnancy category C

Action: Locally acting chloride channel activator, enhances a chloride-rich intestinal fluid secretion without altering other electrolytes; increases motility in the intestine, increasing softening and passage of stool

Therapeutic outcome: Decreased constipation

Uses: Chronic idiopathic constipation, constipation-predominant irritable bowel syndrome in women >18 yr

Dosage and routes
Chronic idiopathic constipation
Adult: PO 24 mcg bid with food

IBS with constipation (females)
Adult and adolescent ≥18 yr: PO 8 mcg bid with food and water

Available forms: Caps 8, 24 mcg

Adverse effects
CNS: *Headache,* dizziness, depression, fatigue, insomnia
CV: Hypertension, chest pain
GI: *Nausea, abdominal pain, eructation,* abdominal distention, constipation, diarrhea, dry mouth, dyspepsia, flatulence, viral gastroenteritis, gastroesophageal reflux disease, vomiting, fecal incontinence, fecal urgency
GU: UTI
MISC: Chest pain, peripheral edema, influenza, pyrexia, viral infection
MS: Back pain, arthralgia, muscle cramps, pain in extremities
RESP: Bronchitis; cough, dyspnea, nasopharyngitis, sinusitis, URI

Contraindications: Hypersensitivity, GI obstruction

Precautions: Pregnancy **C**, breastfeeding, children, diarrhea, IBD

Pharmacokinetics	
Absorption	Unknown
Distribution	Protein binding 94%
Metabolism	Rapid in stomach, jejunum
Excretion	Unknown
Half-life	0.9-1.4 hr

Pharmacodynamics	
Onset	Unknown
Peak	1.14 hr
Duration	Unknown

Interactions
Individual drugs
Anticholinergics, antidiarrheals: decreased effects of lubiprostone

NURSING CONSIDERATIONS
Assessment
- Assess GI symptoms: nausea, abdominal pain
- Assess periodically for need for continued treatment

Nursing diagnoses
- Constipation (uses)
- Knowledge, deficient (teaching)

Implementation
- Give with foods, bid
- Store at room temperature

Patient/family education
- Teach patient to notify prescriber of GI symptoms, diarrhea, hypersensitivity reactions

Evaluation
Positive therapeutic outcome
- Decreased constipation

lymphocyte immune globulin (antithymocyte) (Rx)
Atgam, Thymoglobulin
Func. class.: Immune globulin immunosuppressant

Pregnancy category C

Action: Produces immunosuppression by inhibiting the function of T-lymphocytes

Therapeutic outcome: Absence of transplant rejection; hematologic remission (aplastic anemia)

Uses: Organ transplants to prevent rejection, aplastic anemia

Unlabeled uses: Multiple sclerosis, myasthenia gravis, immunosuppressant in liver, bone marrow, heart and other organ transplants, pure red cell aplasia, scleroderma

Dosage and routes
Renal allograft
Adult: **IV** 10-30 mg/kg/day
Child: **IV** 5-25 mg/kg/day

Delay of renal allograft rejection
Adult: **IV** 15 mg/kg/day × 14 days, then every other day × 14 days for a total of 21 doses in 28 days

Aplastic anemia
Adult: **IV** 10-20 mg/kg/day × 8-14 days, then every other day for up to 21 total doses

Available forms: Inj 50 mg horse gamma globulin/ml

Adverse effects
Renal transplant
CNS: Fever, chills, headache, dizziness, weakness, faintness, **seizures**
CV: Chest pain, hypertension, tachycardia
GI: Diarrhea, nausea, vomiting, epigastric pain, **GI bleeding**
INTEG: Rash, pruritus, urticaria, wheal
SYST: **Anaphylaxis**
Aplastic anemia
CNS: Fever, chills, headache, **seizures**, light-headedness, encephalitis, postviral encephalopathy
CV: Bradycardia, myocarditis, irregularity
GI: Nausea, liver function test abnormality
HEMA: **Thrombocytopenia**

Contraindications: Hypersensitivity to this product or equine/porcine protein

Precautions: Pregnancy **C**, breastfeeding, children, severe renal/hepatic disease, leukopenia, thrombocytopenia

Black Box Warning: Infection, neoplastic disease

Pharmacokinetics	
Absorption	Unknown
Distribution	Unknown
Metabolism	Unknown
Excretion	Unknown
Half-life	5.7 days

Pharmacodynamics	
Onset	Rapid
Peak	Unknown
Duration	Unknown

L

Adverse effects: *italic* = common, **bold** = life-threatening

NURSING CONSIDERATIONS

Assessment

- Assess for infection; if infection occurs, evaluation will be needed to continue treatment
- Monitor renal function tests: BUN, creatinine at least monthly during treatment, 3 mo after treatment
- Monitor liver function tests: alkaline phosphatase, AST, ALT, bilirubin

Nursing diagnoses

- Infection, risk for (uses)
- Knowledge, deficient (teaching)
- Mobility, impaired physical (uses)

Implementation

IV route

- Do not infuse <4 hr
- Keep emergency equipment nearby for severe allergic reactions
- Skin testing must be completed before treatment; use intradermal inj of 0.1 ml of a 1:1000 dilution (5 mcg of horse IgG) in 0.9% NaCl; if a wheal or rash or both >10 mm, use caution during inf
- Dilute in saline sol before inf; invert **IV** bag, so undiluted product does not contact the air inside; concentration should not be >1 mg/ml

Patient/family education

- Advise patient to report fever, rash, chills, sore throat, fatigue, since serious infections may occur
- Caution patient to use contraceptive measures during treatment and for 12 wk after ending therapy; product is teratogenic
- Caution patient to avoid crowds and persons with known infections to reduce risk of infection

Evaluation

Positive therapeutic outcome

- Absence of graft rejection
- Hematologic recovery (aplastic anemia)

mafenide topical

See Appendix B

magaldrate (OTC)

(mag′al-drate)

Isopan, Losapan ✤, Riopan, Riopan Extra Strength ✤

Func. class.: Antacid

Chem. class.: Aluminum/magnesium hydroxide

Pregnancy category C

Action: Neutralizes gastric acidity; product is dissolved in gastric contents; this product is a combination of aluminum and magnesium

Therapeutic outcome: Decreased pain of ulcers

Uses: Antacid, hiatal hernia, indigestion/heartburn, hyperacidity

Unlabeled uses: Duodenal and gastric ulcers, peptic ulcer disease (adjunct), reflex esophagitis

Dosage and routes

Adult/child/geriatric: SUSP 5-10 ml (480-1080 mg) with water between meals, at bedtime

Available forms: Susp 540 mg/5 ml

Adverse effects

GI: Constipation, diarrhea, anorexia

META: Hypermagnesemia, hypophosphatemia

Contraindications: Hypersensitivity to this product or benzyl alcohol

Precautions: Pregnancy **C**, geriatric, fluid restriction, decreased GI motility, GI obstruction, dehydration, renal disease, sodium-restricted diets, bone disease, hypertension, appendicitis, diverticulitis, ulcerative colitis, neonates/infants, hypermagnesemia, hypophosphatemia

Pharmacokinetics

Absorption	Not absorbed
Distribution	Not distributed
Metabolism	Not metabolized
Excretion	Kidneys
Half-life	Unknown

Pharmacodynamics

Onset	Unknown
Peak	½ hr
Duration	1 hr

Interactions

Individual drugs

Chlordiazepoxide, cimetidine, isoniazid, ketoconazole, phenytoin, tetracycline:

decreased absorption of each specific product

Flecainide, quinidine: increased action when taken in large amounts

Drug classifications

Amphetamines: increased action when taken in large amounts

Anticholinergics, corticosteroids, fluoroquinolones, iron salts, phenothiazines, salicylates: decreased absorption of each specific product

Salicylates: decreased action when taken in large amounts

NURSING CONSIDERATIONS
Assessment
• Assess GI status: location of pain, intensity, characteristics, what aggravates, ameliorates pain; heartburn/indigestion; hematemesis
• Monitor serum magnesium, calcium, phosphate, potassium if using long term or with impaired renal function
• Assess for constipation: increase bulk in diet if needed or obtain order for stool softener

Nursing diagnoses
• Knowledge, deficient (teaching)
• Pain, acute (uses)

Implementation
• Take antacids 2 hr before or 2 hr after taking enteric-coated products
• Give laxatives or stool softeners if constipation occurs
• Give susp after shaking; give between meals and at bedtime
• Give when stomach is empty after meals and at bedtime

Patient/family education
• Advise patient to separate ingestion of enteric-coated products and antacid by 2 hr
• Advise patient to use 2 wk or less; product should not be used for long periods
• Teach patient to notify prescriber immediately if coffee-ground emesis, emesis with frank blood, or black tarry stools occur

Evaluation
Positive therapeutic outcome
• Absence of abdominal pain
• Decreased acidity

magnesium salts (OTC)
(mag-neez'ee-um)
magnesium chloride (Rx)
Chloromag, Slo-Mag
magnesium citrate (OTC)
Citrate of Magnesia, Citroma, CitroMag ✦
magnesium gluconate (OTC)
Almoate Magonate, Magtrate OTC
magnesium hydroxide (OTC)
Phillips Magnesia Tablets, Phillips Milk of Magnesia, MOM
magnesium oxide (OTC)
Mag-Ox 400, Maox, Uro-Mag
magnesium sulfate (OTC, Rx)
epsom salt, magnesium sulfate (**IV**)—
HIGH ALERT
Func. class.: Electrolyte; anticonvulsant, laxative, saline; antacid

Pregnancy category A, B

Action: Increases osmotic pressure, draws fluid into colon, neutralizes HCl

Therapeutic outcome: Magnesium levels WNL, absence of constipation

Uses: Constipation, bowel preparation before surgery or exam, electrolyte, anticonvulsant, in preeclampsia, eclampsia (magnesium sulfate), electrolyte

Dosage and routes
Laxative
Adult: PO 15-60 ml at bedtime (Milk of Magnesia)
Adult and child >12 yr: PO 15 g in 8 oz of H_2O (magnesium sulfate); PO 10-20 ml (Concentrated Milk of Magnesia); PO 15-30 oz at bedtime (magnesium citrate)
Child 6-11 yr: PO 15-30 ml (1.2-2.4 g) (magnesium hydroxide) as a single dose or divided
Child 2-5 yr: 5-15 ml/day (Milk of Magnesia)

Prevention of magnesium deficiency
Adult and child ≥10 yr: PO (male): 350-400 mg/day; (female): 280-300 mg/day; (breastfeeding): 335-350 mg/day; (pregnancy): 320 mg/day
Child 8-10 yr: PO 170 mg/day
Child 4-7 yr: PO 120 mg/day

M

*Magnesium sulfate
deficiency*
Adult: PO 200-400 mg in divided doses
tid-qid; IM 1 g q6hr × 4 doses; **IV** 5 g (severe)
Child 6-12 yr: 3-6 mg/kg/day in divided
doses tid-qid

*Preeclampsia/eclampsia
magnesium sulfate*
Adult: IM/**IV** INF 4-5 g; with 5 g IM in each
gluteus, then 5 g q4hr or 4 g **IV** INF, then 1-2
g/hr cont INF, max 40 g/day or 20 g/48 hr in
severe renal disease

Available forms: Chloride: sus rel tabs
535 mg (64 mg Mg); enteric tabs 833 mg
(100 mg Mg); hydroxide: liquid 400 mg/5 ml
(164 mg Mg/5 ml); conc liquid 800 mg/5 ml
(328 mg Mg/5 ml); chew tabs 300, 600 mg;
oxide: tabs 400 mg (241.3 mg Mg); caps 140
mg (84.5 mg Mg); sulfate: powder for oral;
bulk packages; (epsom salts) bulk packages;
inj 10, 12.5, 25, 50%; citrate: oral sol 240,
296, 300 ml bottles (77 mEq/100 ml)

Adverse effects
CNS: Muscle weakness, flushing, sweating,
confusion, sedation, depressed reflexes,
flaccid paralysis, hypothermia
CV: Hypotension, heart block, **circulatory
collapse,** vasodilatation
GI: Nausea, vomiting, anorexia, cramps,
diarrhea
HEMA: Prolonged bleeding time
META: Electrolyte, fluid imbalances
RESP: **Respiratory depression/paralysis**

Contraindications: Hypersensitivity,
abdominal pain, nausea/vomiting, obstruction,
acute surgical abdomen, rectal bleeding, heart
block, myocardial damage

Precautions: Pregnancy **A, B** (magnesium
sulfate), renal disease/cardiac disease

Pharmacokinetics	
Absorption	Unknown
Distribution	Unknown
Metabolism	Unknown
Excretion	Kidneys
Half-life	Unknown
	effective anticonvulsant levels
	2.5-7.5 mEq/L

Pharmacodynamics			
	PO	IM	IV
Onset	3-6 hr	1 hr	Unknown
Peak	Unknown	Unknown	Unknown
Duration	Unknown	4 hr	½ hr

Interactions
Individual products
Digoxin: decreased effect of digoxin
Nitrofurantoin: decreased absorption
Drug classifications
Antihypertensives: increased hypotension
Antiinfectives (fluoroquinolones),
    tetracyclines: decreased absorption
Neuromuscular blockers: increased effect

NURSING CONSIDERATIONS
Assessment
• Assess I&O ratio; check for decrease in
urinary output
• Assess cause of constipation; lack of fluids,
bulk, exercise
• Assess cramping, rectal bleeding, nausea,
vomiting; product should be discontinued
◆ Assess Mg toxicity: thirst, confusion, decrease in reflexes
• Assess visual changes: blurring, halos,
corneal and retinal damage
• Assess edema in feet, ankles, legs
• Assess prior product history; there are many
product interactions

Nursing diagnoses
• Constipation (uses)
• Injury, risk for, physical
• Knowledge, deficient (teaching)

Implementation
PO route
• Administer with 8 oz of H_2O
• Refrigerate magnesium citrate before
administration
• Shake susp before using
• Administer to patient crushed or whole;
chewable tablets may be chewed
• Administer with food or milk to decrease
gastric symptoms; give 30 min before or 2 hr
after antacids
IV route
• Administer only when calcium gluconate
available for magnesium toxicity
• Administer **IV** undiluted 1.5 ml of 10% sol
over 1 min; may dilute to 20% sol, inf over
3 hr
• Administer **IV** at less than 150 mg/min;
circulatory collapse may occur
Y-site compatibilities: Acyclovir,
aldesleukin, amifostine, amikacin, ampicillin,
aztreonam, cefamandole, cefazolin, cefmetazole, cefoperazone, cefotaxime, cefoxitin,
cephalothin, cephapirin, chloramphenicol,
cisatracurium, DOBUTamine, doxycycline,
DOXOrubicin liposome, enalaprilat, erythromycin, esmolol, famotidine, fludarabine,
gallium, gentamicin, granisetron, heparin,

hydromorphone, idarubicin, insulin, kanamycin, labetalol, meperidine, metronidazole, minocycline, morphine, moxalactam, nafcillin, ondansetron, oxacillin, paclitaxel, penicillin G potassium, piperacillin, piperacillin/tazobactam, potassium chloride, propofol, remifentanil, sargramostim, thiotepa, ticarcillin, tobramycin, trimethoprim/sulfamethoxazole, vancomycin, vit B complex/C

Additive compatibilities: Cephalothin, chloramphenicol, cisplatin, heparin, hydrocortisone, isoproterenol, meropenem, methyldopate, norepinephrine, penicillin G potassium, potassium phosphate, verapamil

Patient/family education

• Inform patient to report any symptoms of hepatotoxicity, renal toxicity, visual changes, ototoxicity, allergic reactions, bleeding (long-term therapy)
• Inform patient not to exceed recommended dosage; acute poisoning may result
• Inform patient to read label on other OTC products; many contain aspirin
• Inform patient that therapeutic response takes 2 wk (arthritis)
• Inform patient to avoid alcohol ingestion; GI bleeding may occur
• Inform patient that if anticoagulants are given with this product, both should be discontinued 2 wk before surgery

Evaluation
Positive therapeutic outcome
• Decreased pain, fever

Treatment of overdose: Lavage, activated charcoal, monitor electrolytes, VS

---

mannitol (Rx)
(man'i-tole)
mannitol, Osmitrol, Resectisol
Func. class.: Diuretic-osmotic
Chem. class.: Hexahydric alcohol

Pregnancy category C

Action: Increases osmolarity of glomerular filtrate, which raises osmotic pressure of fluid in renal tubules; there is a decrease in reabsorption of water, electrolytes; increases in urinary output, sodium, chloride, potassium, calcium, phosphorus, uric acid, urea, magnesium

Uses: Edema; promote systemic diuresis in cerebral edema, decrease intraocular pressure, improve renal function in acute renal failure, chemical poisoning

Dosage and routes
Oliguria, prevention
Adult: IV 50-100 g of a 5%-25% SOL, may use test dose 0.2 g/kg over 3-5 min

Oliguria, treatment
Adult: IV 300-400 mg/kg of a 20%-25% SOL up to 100 g of a 15%-20% SOL over 30-60 min
Child (unlabeled): IV 0.25-2 g/kg as a 15%-20% SOL, run over 2-6 hr (maintenance)

Intraocular pressure/ICP
Adult: IV 1.5-2 g/kg of a 15%-25% SOL over 30-60 min
Child: IV 1-2 g/kg (30-60 g/m^2) as a 15%-20% SOL run over 2-6 hr

Renal failure
Adult: IV 50-200 g/24 hr, adjusting to maintain output of 30-50 ml/hr

Diuresis in product intoxication
Adult and child >12 yr: 5%-10% SOL continuously up to 200 g **IV**, while maintaining 100-500 ml urine output/hr

Available forms: Inj 5%, 10%, 15%, 20%, 25%; GU irrigation 5%

Adverse effects
CNS: Dizziness, headache, **seizures, rebound increased ICP,** confusion
CV: Edema, hypotension, hypertension, **tachycardia, CHF,** thrombophlebitis, angina-like chest pains, fever, chills, **circulatory overload**
EENT: Loss of hearing, blurred vision, nasal congestion, decreased intraocular pressure
ELECT: Fluid, electrolyte imbalances, **acidosis,** electrolyte loss, dehydration, hyper/hypokalemia
GI: Nausea, vomiting, dry mouth, diarrhea
GU: Marked diuresis, urinary retention, thirst
RESP: Pulmonary congestion

Contraindications: Active intracranial bleeding, hypersensitivity, anuria, severe pulmonary congestion, edema, severe dehydration, progressive heart disease, renal failure

Precautions: Pregnancy **C,** breastfeeding, dehydration, severe renal disease, CHF, electrolyte imbalances

Pharmacokinetics	
Absorption	Complete
Distribution	Extracellular spaces
Metabolism	Minimal
Excretion	Renal
Half-life	100 min

Adverse effects: *italic* = common, **bold** = life-threatening

Pharmacodynamics	
Onset	½-1 hr
Peak	1 hr
Duration	6-8 hr

Interactions
Individual drugs
Lithium: increased elimination of mannitol
Drug/food
Potassium foods: increased hyperkalemia
Drug/lab test
Interference: inorganic phosphorus, ethylene glycol

NURSING CONSIDERATIONS
Assessment
* Assess neurologic status: LOC, ICP reading, pupil size and reaction when product is given for increased ICP
* Assess for visual changes or eye discomfort or pain before, during treatment (increases intraocular pressure); neurologic checks, ICP during treatment (increased ICP)
* Assess patient for tinnitus, hearing loss, ear pain; periodic testing of hearing is needed when high doses of this product are given by **IV** route
* Monitor manifestations of hypokalemia: acidic urine, reduced urine osmolality, nocturia, polyuria, polydipsia; hypotension, broad T-wave, U-wave, ectopy, tachycardia, weak pulse; muscle weakness, altered LOC, drowsiness, apathy, lethargy, confusion, depression; anorexia, nausea, cramps, constipation, distention, paralytic ileus; hypoventilation, respiratory muscle weakness
* Monitor for manifestations of hyponatremia: increased B/P, cold, clammy skin, hypovolemia or hypervolemia; anorexia, nausea, vomiting, diarrhea, abdominal cramps; lethargy, increased ICP, confusion, headache, seizures, coma, fatigue, tremors, hyperreflexia
* Assess fluid volume status: check I&O ratios and record hourly urine values, CVP, breath sounds, weight, distended red veins, crackles in lung, color, quality, and specific gravity of urine, skin turgor, adequacy of pulses, moist mucous membranes, bilateral lung sounds, peripheral pitting edema
* Assess for dehydration; symptoms of decreasing output, thirst, hypotension, dry mouth and mucous membranes should be reported
* Monitor electrolytes: potassium, sodium, calcium, magnesium; also include BUN, ABGs, CVP, PAP, CBC; regularly monitor serum and urine levels of sodium and potassium
* Assess B/P before, during therapy with patient lying, standing, and sitting as appropriate; orthostatic hypotension can occur rapidly
* Monitor for rebound ICP: headache, confusion

Nursing diagnoses
* Fluid volume, deficient (adverse reactions)
* Fluid volume, excess (uses)
* Knowledge, deficient (teaching)
* Urinary elimination, impaired (adverse reactions)

Implementation
* Administer potassium replacement if potassium level is <3 mg/ml
* Use an in-line filter for 15%, 20%, 25%; give with inf pump; check **IV** patency at inf site before, during administration; do not use sol that is yellow or has a precipitate or crystals; to redissolve, run bottle under hot water and shake vigorously; cool to body temp before giving
* Run at 30-50 ml/hr in oliguria
* Run over 30-60 min in increased ICP
* Run over 30 min for intraocular pressure; 60-90 min after surgery
Irrigation
* Use 100 ml of 25%/900 ml of sterile water for inj (2.5% sol)
Y-site compatibilities: Allopurinol, amifostine, aztreonam, cladribine, fludarabine, fluorouracil, gallium, idarubicin, melphalan, ondansetron, paclitaxel, piperacillin, propofol, sargramostim, teniposide, thiotepa, vinorelbine
Y-site incompatibilities: Amsacrine, bleomycin, DOXOrubicin, fluconazole, gentamicin, quinidine, vinBLAStine, vinCRIStine
Additive compatibilities: Amikacin, bretylium, cefamandole, cefoxitin, cimetidine, cisplatin, DOPamine, fosphenytoin, furosemide, gentamicin, metoclopramide, netilmicin, nizatidine, ofloxacin, ondansetron, sodium bicarbonate, tobramycin, verapamil
Additive incompatibilities: Blood, blood products, imipenem-cilastatin, potassium chloride, sodium chloride

Patient/family education
* Teach patient reason for and method of treatment

Evaluation
Positive therapeutic outcome
* Decreased intraocular pressure
* Prevention of hypokalemia (diuretic use)
* Decreased edema

- Decreased ICP
- Increased diuresis of >30 ml/hr
- Increased excretion of toxic substances

Treatment of overdose: Discontinue infusion; correct fluid, electrolyte imbalances; hemodialysis; monitor hydration, CV, renal function

---

maraviroc (Rx)
(mah-rav'er-rock)
Selzentry
Func. class.: Antiretroviral
Chem. class.: Fusion inhibitor

Pregnancy category B

Action: Interferes with entry into HIV-1 by inhibiting the fusion of the virus and cell membrane

Therapeutic outcome: Improvement in CD_4, viral load, T-cell count

Uses: CCR5-tropic HIV in combination with other antiretroviral agents in treating experienced patients

Dosage and routes
Those not taking any CYP3A inducers/inhibitors
Adult: PO 300 mg bid

Those taking CYP3A4 inhibitors with/without a CYP3A inducer
Adult: PO 150 mg bid

Those taking CYP3A4 inducers without a strong CYP3A inhibitor
Adult: PO 600 mg bid

Available forms: Tabs 150, 300 mg

Adverse effects
CNS: Dizziness, depression, **viral meningitis**, disturbances in consciousness, peripheral neuropathy, paresthesia, dysesthesia, fever
CV: **MI, cardiac ischemia, orthostatic hypotension**
EENT: Gingival hyperplasia
GI: Diarrhea, constipation, dyspepsia, **pseudomembranous colitis, hepatotoxicity**
INTEG: Rash, urticaria, pruritus, folliculitis
MS: Joint pain, leg pain, muscle cramps
RESP: Cough, URI, sinusitis, bronchitis, pneumonia, **bronchospasm, obstruction**
SYST: Herpes virus

Contraindications: Hypersensitivity

Precautions: Pregnancy **B,** breastfeeding, Asian patients, renal/hepatic/cardiac disease, electrolyte imbalance, dehydration, immune reconstitution syndrome, infection, MI, orthostatic hypotension, children, elderly, hepatitis

Pharmacokinetics

Absorption	Unknown
Distribution	Unknown
Metabolism	By P450 system, CYP3A metabolism
Excretion	Urine 20%, feces 76%
Half-life	Unknown

Pharmacodynamics
Unknown

Interactions
Drug classifications
CYP3A inhibitors (amiodarone, aprepitant, chloramphenicol, clarithromycin, conivaptan, cycloSPORINE, dalfopristin, danazol, diltiazem, erythromycin, estradiol, fluconazole, fluvoxamine, imatinib, isoniazid, itraconazole, ketoconazole, miconazole, nefazodone, niCARdipine, propoxyphene, RU-486, tamoxifen, telithromycin, troleandomycin, verapamil, voriconazole, zafirlukast): increased maraviroc levels
CYP3A4 inducers (aminoglutethimide, barbiturates, bexaroten, bosentan, carbamazepine, dexamethasone, efavirenz, fosphenytoin, griseofulvin, modafinil, nafcillin, oxcarbazepine, phenytoin, rifabutin, rifampin, rifapentine, topiramate, tipranavir): decreased maraviroc effect
Drug/food
High-fat meal: decreased absorption 33%

NURSING CONSIDERATIONS
Assessment
- Assess for signs of infection
- Monitor blood tests: CD_4, T-cell count, plasma HIV RNA
- Monitor renal tests: serum creatinine
- Monitor C&S before product therapy; product may be taken as soon as culture is taken; repeat C&S after treatment; determine the presence of other infections
- Assess bowel pattern before, during treatment
- Assess skin eruptions: rash, urticaria, itching
- Assess allergies before treatment and before each dose

Nursing diagnoses
- Injury, risk for (uses, adverse reactions)
- Knowledge, deficient (teaching)

Implementation
- May give without regard to meals, with 8 oz of water
- Store at room temperature

M

Adverse effects: *italic* = common, **bold** = life-threatening

Patient/family education
- Advise patient to take as prescribed; if dose is missed, take as soon as remembered up to 1 hr before next dose; do not double dose
- Teach patient that product does not cure infection, just controls symptoms, and does not prevent infecting others
◆ Teach patient to report sore throat, fever, fatigue; may indicate superinfection
- Advise patient that product must be taken in equal intervals around the clock to maintain blood levels for duration of therapy
- Teach patient to notify prescriber of side effects

Evaluation
Positive therapeutic outcome
- Improvement in CD4, viral load, T-cell count

---

mebendazole (Rx)
(me-ben′da-zole)
Func. class.: Anthelmintic
Chem. class.: Carbamate

Pregnancy category C

Action: Inhibits glucose uptake, degeneration of cytoplasmic microtubules in the cell; interferes with absorption, secretory function

Therapeutic outcome: Parasite, cyst, egg death

Uses: Infestation with pinworms, roundworms, hookworms, whipworms, threadworms, pork tapeworms, dwarf tapeworms, beef tapeworms; hydatid cyst

Dosage and routes
Adult and child >2 yr: PO 100 mg as a single dose (pinworms) or bid × 3 days (whipworms, roundworms, or hookworms); course may be repeated in 3 wk if needed, max 200 mg/day

Available forms: Chew tabs 100 mg

Adverse effects
CNS: Dizziness, fever, headache, **seizures (rare)**
GI: Transient diarrhea, abdominal pain, nausea, vomiting, constipation, **hepatitis**
INTEG: Rash

Contraindication: Hypersensitivity

Precautions: Pregnancy **C** (1st trimester), breastfeeding, children <2 yr, Crohn's disease, hepatic disease, IBD, ulcerative colitis

---

Pharmacokinetics
Absorption	Minimal
Distribution	Highly bound to plasma proteins
Metabolism	Liver
Excretion	Feces in metabolites (>95%); urine, unchanged
Half-life	2½-9 hr; increased in hepatic disease

Pharmacodynamics
Onset	Unknown
Peak	½-7 hr
Duration	Unknown

Interactions
Individual drugs
Carbamazepine: decreased effect of mebendazole
Drug classifications
Hydantoins: decreased effect of mebendazole
Drug/food
High-fat foods: increased absorption

NURSING CONSIDERATIONS
Assessment
- Assess stools during entire treatment, also 1-3 wk after treatment is completed; specimens must be sent to lab while still warm; monitor for diarrhea during expulsion of worms; avoid self-contamination with patient's feces
- Assess for allergic reaction: rash (rare)
- Identify infestation in other family members, since transmission from person to person is common
- If pinworms are suspected, place a piece of cellophane tape over the anal area at night for 1 wk after treatment at night to identify ova; negative perianal swabs taken every AM for 3 days confirm that the patient is no longer infested
- Monitor blood tests: AST, ALT, alkaline phosphatase, BUN, CBC during treatment

Nursing diagnoses
- Infection, risk for (uses)
- Knowledge, deficient (teaching)

Implementation
- Tabs may be chewed or crushed and mixed with food if patient is unable to swallow whole
- Give PO after meals to avoid GI symptoms
- Give second course after 3 wk if needed; usually recommended (pinworms)
- Store in airtight container

Patient/family education
- Teach patient proper hygiene after bowel movements, including hand-washing

---

technique; tell patient to avoid putting fingers in mouth; clean fingernails
• Advise patient that infested person should sleep alone; do not shake bed linen; wash bed linen daily in hot water; change and wash undergarments daily; that all members of the family should be treated (pinworms)
• Advise patient to clean toilet daily with disinfectant (green soap sol)
• Inform patient that compliance is needed with dosage schedule, duration of treatment
• Tell patient to wear shoes, wash all fruits and vegetables well before eating, use commercial fruit and vegetable cleaner solution
• Advise patient to report jaundice, liver pain

Evaluation
Positive therapeutic outcome
• Expulsion of worms
• Three negative stool cultures after completion of treatment

---

mecasermin (Rx)
(mec-a′sir-men)
Increlex
Func. class.: Biologic response modifier; insulin-like growth factor

Pregnancy category C

Action: Stimulates growth; IGF-1 is the principal hormonal mediator of statural growth; GH binds to its receptor in the liver and other tissues

Therapeutic outcome: Increased height

Uses: Growth failure in children with severe primary insulin-like growth factor-1 (IGF-1) deficiency (primary IGFD) or with growth hormone (GH) gene deletion who have developed neutralizing antibodies to GH

Unlabeled uses: ALS

Dosage and routes
Child: SUBCUT 0.04-0.08 mg/kg (40-80 mcg/kg) bid; if well tolerated for 1 wk, may increase by 0.04 mg/kg/dose, max 0.12 mg/kg bid

Available forms: Inj 10 mg/ml

Adverse effects
CNS: Headache, **seizures,** dizziness, cardiac valvulopathy, increased intracranial pressure
CV: Cardiac murmur
EENT: Ear pain, otitis media, abnormal tympanometry, papilledema, visual impairment, tonsillar hypertrophy
ENDO: Hypoglycemia, ketosis, **hypothyroidism**

GI: Vomiting
HEMA: Thymus hypertrophy
MISC: Bruising, lipohypertrophy, hypersensitivity reactions, inj site reaction
MS: Arthralgia, joint pain, slipped upper femoral epiphysis
RESP: Snoring, **apnea**
SYST: **Antibodies to growth hormone**

Contraindications: Hypersensitivity, benzyl alcohol, closed epiphyses, active/suspected neoplasia, **IV** use

Precautions: Pregnancy **C**, breastfeeding, children <2 yr, diabetes mellitus, hypothyroidism, lymphoid tissue hypertrophy, increased ICP, malnutrition, scoliosis, sleep apnea

Pharmacokinetics
Absorption	Near 100%
Distribution	Unknown
Metabolism	Liver/kidneys
Excretion	Unknown
Half-life	5.8 hr

Pharmacodynamics
Unknown

Interactions
Drug classifications
Antidiabetics, corticosteroids: increased hypoglycemia

NURSING CONSIDERATIONS
Assessment
• Monitor preprandial glucose at beginning of treatment and until well tolerated
• Monitor by funduscopic exam at beginning, periodically during treatment
• Assess for allergic reactions; if present, interrupt treatment and notify prescriber
• Assess growth rate of child at intervals during treatment

Nursing diagnoses
• Knowledge, deficient (teaching)

Implementation
SUBCUT route
• Give within 20 min of a meal or snack
• Rotate inj site; use sterile, disposable syringe/needles; use small-volume syringe for accurate measurement
• Store in refrigerator before opening, avoid freezing; after opening, stable for 30 days after initial vial entry, store in refrigerator, do not use if particulate matter is present, avoid direct light, do not use after expiration date

M

Adverse effects: *italic* = common, **bold** = life-threatening

Patient/family education
- Teach patient that treatment may continue for years; regular assessments are required
- Advise patient to avoid hazardous activities, driving within 2-3 hr of dosing
- Teach patient correct administration and needle disposal

Evaluation
Positive therapeutic outcome
- Growth in children

---

mechlorethamine (Rx)
(me-klor-eth'a-meen)
Mustargen, nitrogen mustard
Func. class.: Antineoplastic alkylating agent
Chem. class.: Nitrogen mustard

Pregnancy category D

Action: Responsible for cross-linking DNA strands leading to cell death, rapidly degraded; activity is not cell cycle phase specific; a vesicant

Therapeutic outcome: Prevention of rapidly growing malignant cells

Uses: Hodgkin's disease, lymphomas, leukemias, lymphosarcoma; ovarian, breast, lung carcinoma; neoplastic effusions, pericardial/peritoneal/pleural effusion; polycythemia vera

Dosage and routes
Adult: **IV** 0.2-0.4 mg/kg or 6 mg/m² as a single dose or 2-4 divided doses over 2-4 days; second course after 3 wk depending on blood cell count

Neoplastic effusions
Adult: Intracavity 0.4 mg/kg

Polycythemia vera
Adult: **IV** 0.4 mg/kg or 6 mg/m² as a single dose qmo or as needed

Available forms: Inj 10 mg/vial

Adverse effects
CNS: Headache, dizziness, drowsiness, paresthesia, peripheral neuropathy, **coma**
EENT: Tinnitus, hearing loss
GI: Nausea, vomiting, diarrhea, stomatitis, weight loss, colitis, **hepatotoxicity**
HEMA: **Thrombocytopenia, leukopenia, agranulocytosis,** anemia
INTEG: Alopecia, pruritus, herpes zoster, extravasation

Contraindications: Breastfeeding, acute herpes zoster, infection

Black Box Warning: Pregnancy **D**, myelosuppression

Precautions: Radiation therapy, chronic lymphocytic leukopenia

Black Box Warning: Accidental exposure, extravasation

Pharmacokinetics
Absorption	Complete (**IV**)
Distribution	Unknown
Metabolism	Tissues/fluids
Excretion	Kidneys
Half-life	Unknown

Pharmacodynamics
	IV
Onset	1 day
Peak	1-2 wk
Duration	1-3 wk

Interactions
Individual drugs
Amphotericin B: increased blood dyscrasia
Aspirin: increased bleeding
Radiation: increased toxicity
Drug classifications
Anticoagulants, NSAIDs: increased bleeding
Antineoplastics: increased toxicity
Live virus vaccines: decreased antibody reaction

NURSING CONSIDERATIONS
Assessment
- Monitor CBC, differential, platelet count weekly; withhold product if WBC is <1000/mm³ or platelet count is <75,000/mm³; notify prescriber of results if WBC <20,000/mm³, platelets <150,000/mm³; recovery of WBC platelets within 20 days
- Monitor pulmonary function tests, chest x-ray films before, during therapy; chest film should be obtained q2wk during treatment; assess for dyspnea, crackles, unproductive cough, chest pain, tachypnea
- Assess for increased uric acid levels, swelling, joint pain primarily in extremities; patient should be well hydrated to prevent urate deposits
- Monitor renal function tests: BUN, serum uric acid, urine CCr before, during therapy; I&O ratio; report fall in urine output of 30 ml/hr; for decreased hyperuricemia
- Monitor for cold, fever, sore throat (may indicate beginning of infection); identify edema in feet, joint and stomach pain, shaking; prescriber should be notified

- Assess for bleeding: hematuria, guaiac, bruising or petechiae, mucosa or orifices; no rectal temp

Nursing diagnoses
- Body image, disturbed (adverse reactions)
- Infection, risk for (adverse reactions)
- Injury, risk for (adverse reactions)
- Knowledge, deficient (teaching)

Implementation
- Give fluids **IV** or PO before chemotherapy to hydrate patient
- Give antacid before oral agent; give product after evening meal, before bedtime; administer antiemetic 30-60 min and dexamethasone before giving product and prn to prevent vomiting; give antibiotics for prophylaxis of infection
- Give topical or systemic analgesics for pain
- Give in AM so product can be eliminated before bedtime
- Use a liquid diet: carbonated beverages; gelatin may be added if patient is not nauseated or vomiting

Intracavity route
- Further dilute in 100 ml of 0.9% NaCl; administration is completed by prescriber
- Watch for infiltration; if infiltration occurs, infiltrate area with isotonic sodium thiosulfate; apply ice for 6-12 hr; a vesicant

IV route
- Give **IV** after diluting 10 mg/10 ml sterile water or 0.9% NaCl; leave needle in vial, shake, withdraw dose, give through Y-tube or 3-way stopcock or directly over 3-5 min into running **IV** of 0.9% NaCl

Y-site compatibilities: Amifostine, aztreonam, filgrastim, fludarabine, granisetron, melphalan, ondansetron, sargramostim, teniposide, vinorelbine

Additive incompatibilities: Methohexital

Solution incompatibilities: D₅W, 0.9% NaCl (**IV** only)

Patient/family education
- Teach patient to avoid use of products containing aspirin or ibuprofen, razors, commercial mouthwash, since bleeding may occur; to report symptoms of bleeding (hematuria, tarry stools)
- Teach patient to report signs of anemia (fatigue, headache, irritability, faintness, shortness of breath)
- Advise patient to report any changes in breathing or coughing even several months after treatment; to avoid crowds and persons with respiratory tract or other infections
- Tell patient hair loss is common; discuss the use of wigs or hairpieces
- Caution patient not to have any vaccinations without the advice of the prescriber; serious reactions can occur
- Advise patient that contraception is needed during treatment and for several months after the completion of therapy
- Have patient rinse mouth tid-qid with water, club soda; brush teeth bid-qid with soft brush or cotton-tipped applicators for stomatitis; use unwaxed dental floss

Evaluation
Positive therapeutic outcome
- Decreased size of tumor
- Decreased spread of malignancy
- Improved blood values
- Absence of sweating at night
- Increased appetite, increased weight

meclizine (OTC, Rx)
(mek′li-zeen)
Antivert, Bonamine ✤, Bonine, Dramamine Less Drowsy Formula, meclizine HCl, Medivert, Travel Sickness, Wal-Dram II
Func. class.: Antiemetic, antihistamine, anticholinergic
Chem. class.: H₁-receptor antagonist, piperazine derivative
Pregnancy category B

Action: Acts centrally by blocking chemoreceptor trigger zone, which in turn acts on vomiting center

Therapeutic outcome: Decreased nausea in motion sickness; decreased vertigo

Uses: Vertigo, motion sickness

Dosage and routes
Vertigo
Adult/adolescent: PO 25-100 mg/day in divided doses

Motion sickness
Adult/adolescent: PO 25-50 mg 1 hr before traveling; repeat dose q24hr prn

Available forms: Tabs 12.5, 25, 50 mg; chew tabs 25 mg; caps 25, 30 mg

Adverse effects
CNS: Drowsiness, fatigue, restlessness, headache, insomnia
CV: Hypotension
EENT: Dry mouth, blurred vision

GI: Nausea, anorexia, constipation, increased appetite
GU: Urinary retention

Contraindications: Hypersensitivity to cyclizines, shock

Precautions: Pregnancy **B**, breastfeeding, children, geriatric, closed-angle glaucoma, glaucoma, urinary retention, prostatic hypertrophy, CV disease, hypertension, seizure disorder

Pharmacokinetics
Absorption	Well
Distribution	Unknown
Metabolism	Unknown
Excretion	Unknown
Half-life	6 hr

Pharmacodynamics
Onset	1 hr
Peak	Unknown
Duration	8-24 hr

Interactions
Individual drugs
Alcohol: increased effects
Drug classifications
CNS depressants, opioids: increased CNS depression
Drug/herb
Corkwood, henbane leaf: increased anticholinergic effect
Hops, Jamaican dogwood, khat, senega: increased sedative effect
Drug/lab test
False negative: allergy skin testing

NURSING CONSIDERATIONS
Assessment
• Monitor VS, B/P
❹ Assess for signs of toxicity of other products or masking of symptoms of disease: brain tumor, intestinal obstruction
• Observe for drowsiness, dizziness, LOC

Nursing diagnoses
• Injury, risk for (adverse reactions)
• Knowledge, deficient (teaching)

Implementation
• Tabs may be swallowed whole, chewed, or allowed to dissolve; give with food to decrease GI upset
• Give lowest possible dose in geriatric, anticholinergic effects

Patient/family education
• Teach patient that a false-negative result may occur with skin testing for allergies; these procedures should not be scheduled for 4 days after discontinuing use
• Teach patient to avoid hazardous activities, activities requiring alertness; dizziness may occur; instruct patient to request assistance with ambulation
• Teach patient to avoid alcohol, other depressants, breastfeeding

Evaluation
Positive therapeutic outcome
• Absence of dizziness, vomiting

---

*medroxyPROGESTERone (Rx)
(me-drox-ee-proe-jess'te-rone)
Amen, Depo-Provera, medroxyPROGESTERone, Provera
Func. class.: Hormone—progestogen; contraceptive; antineoplastic
Chem. class.: Progesterone derivative

Pregnancy category X

Do not confuse:
medroxyPROGESTERone/methylPREDNISolone, Amen/Ambien, Provera/Premarin/Covera

Action: Inhibits secretion of pituitary gonadotropins, which prevents follicular maturation and ovulation; stimulates growth of mammary tissue; antineoplastic action against endometrial cancer

Therapeutic outcome: Decreased abnormal uterine bleeding, absence of amenorrhea

Uses: Uterine bleeding (abnormal), secondary amenorrhea, contraceptive, prevention of endometrial changes associated with estrogen replacement therapy (ERT)

Dosage and routes
Secondary amenorrhea
Adult: PO 5-10 mg/day × 5-10 days

Uterine bleeding
Adult: PO 5-10 mg/day × 5-10 days starting on 16th or 21st day of menstrual cycle

With ERT
Adult: PO 5-10 mg qd × 10-14 or more days/mo (sequential estrogen); 2.5-5 mg qd (continuous estrogen)

Contraceptive
Adult: IM 150 mg q12wk

Available forms: Tabs 2.5, 5, 10 mg; inj susp 50, 150, 400 mg/ml; 104 mg/0.65 ml

Adverse effects
CNS: Dizziness, headache, migraines, depression, fatigue, nervousness

 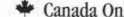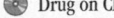

CV: Hypotension, thrombophlebitis, edema, **thromboembolism, stroke, pulmonary embolism, MI**
EENT: Diplopia
GI: Nausea, vomiting, anorexia, cramps, increased weight, **cholestatic jaundice,** abdominal pain
GU: Amenorrhea, cervical erosion, breakthrough bleeding, dysmenorrhea, vaginal candidiasis, breast changes, *gynecomastia, testicular atrophy, impotence,* endometriosis, **spontaneous abortion**
INTEG: Rash, urticaria, acne, hirsutism, alopecia, oily skin, seborrhea, purpura, melasma, photosensitivity
META: Hyperglycemia
MS: Decreased bone density
SYST: **Angioedema, anaphylaxis**

Contraindications: Pregnancy **X**, breast cancer, hypersensitivity, thrombocmbolic disorders, reproductive cancer, genital bleeding (abnormal, undiagnosed), missed abortion

Precautions: Breastfeeding, hypertension, asthma, blood dyscrasias, gallbladder disease, CHF, diabetes mellitus, bone disease, depression, migraine headache, seizure disorders, renal/hepatic disease, family history of cancer of breast or reproductive tract, bone mineral density loss, ocular disorders

Black Box Warning: Cardiac disease, dementia, osteoporosis

Pharmacokinetics
Unknown

Pharmacodynamics

	PO	IM
Onset	Unknown	Unknown
Peak	Unknown	Unknown
Duration	2-4 hr	Unknown

Interactions
Individual drugs
Aminoglutethimide: decreased contraceptive effect
Drug/lab test
Increased: alkaline phosphatase, pregnanediol, amino acids, sodium
Decreased: GTT, HDL

NURSING CONSIDERATIONS
Assessment
• Assess for symptoms indicating severe allergic reaction, angioedema; have epinephrine and resuscitative equipment available

• Monitor B/P at beginning of treatment and periodically; check weight daily; notify prescriber of weekly weight gain >5 lb; bone mineral density
• Monitor I&O ratio: be alert for decreasing urinary output, increasing edema, hypertension
• Assess liver function tests: ALT, AST, bilirubin, periodically during long-term therapy
• Assess for edema, hypertension, cardiac symptoms, jaundice
• Assess mental status: affect, mood, behavioral changes, depression

Nursing diagnoses
• Injury, risk for (adverse reactions)
• Knowledge, deficient (teaching)
• Sexual dysfunction (uses)
• Tissue perfusion, ineffective (adverse reactions)

Implementation
PO route
• Give with food or milk to decrease GI symptoms
IM route
• Store in dark area
• Give titrated dosage; usc lowest effective dosage; give oil sol deep in large muscle mass (IM); rotate sites; use after warming to dissolve crystals

Patient/family education
• Advise patients to avoid sunlight or use sunscreen; photosensitivity and melasma (brown patches on the face) can occur
• Teach patient about cushingoid symptoms: weight gain, moon face, buffalo hump, acne
• Teach women patients to report breast lumps, vaginal bleeding, edema, jaundice, dark urine, clay-colored stools, dyspnea, headache, blurred vision, abdominal pain, sudden changes in speech/coordination, numbness or stiffness in legs, chest pain; men to report impotence or gynecomastia
• Teach patient to report suspected pregnancy immediately; fertility returns in 6-12 mo after discontinuing
• Teach patient that long-term use decreases bone density; exercise, calcium supplements can help lessen this

Evaluation
Positive therapeutic outcome
• Decreased abnormal uterine bleeding
• Absence of amenorrhea
• Prevention of pregnancy
• Arrested spread of malignant cells

M

medrysone ophthalmic
See Appendix B

megestrol (Rx)
(me-jess'trole)
Megace, Megace ES, megestrol
Func. class.: Antineoplastic hormone
Chem. class.: Progestin

Pregnancy category
D (tabs),
X (susp)

Do not confuse:
Megace/Reglan

Action: Affects endometrium by antiluteinizing effect; this is thought to bring about cell death

Therapeutic outcome: Prevention of rapidly growing malignant cells; weight gain, increased appetite in AIDS

Uses: Breast, endometrial, renal cell cancer; increased weight, decreased cachexia and anorexia associated with AIDS

Unlabeled uses: Hot flashes, prostate cancer

Dosage and routes
Endometrial/ovarian carcinoma
Adult: PO 40-320 mg/day in divided doses

Breast carcinoma
Adult: PO 40 mg qid or 160 mg/day

Anorexia (AIDS)
Adult: PO 800 mg/day (oral SUSP) or 625 mg/day (ES)

Hot flashes (unlabeled)
Adult: PO 20 mg bid

Available forms: Tabs 20, 40 mg; oral susp 40, 125 mg/ml

Adverse effects
CNS: Mood swings, insomnia
CV: **Thrombophlebitis, thromboembolism,** hypertension
ENDO: Adrenal insufficiency
GI: Nausea, vomiting, diarrhea, abdominal cramps, weight gain, flatus, indigestion
GU: Gynecomastia, fluid retention, hypercalcemia, vaginal bleeding, discharge, impotence, decreased libido
INTEG: Alopecia, rash, pruritus, purpura, itching, sweating
META: Hyperglycemia

Contraindications: Pregnancy X (susp), D (tabs), hypersensitivity

Precautions: Diabetes, thrombosis, adrenal insufficiency

Pharmacokinetics
Absorption	Well absorbed; food increases oral sol
Distribution	Unknown
Metabolism	Liver, completely
Excretion	Unknown
Half-life	1 hr

Pharmacodynamics
Onset	Several wk-mo
Peak	Unknown
Duration	1-3 days

Interactions
Individual drugs
Dofetilide: do not use with megestrol
Drug/lab test
Increased: alkaline phosphatase, urinary pregnanediol, plasma amino acids, urinary sodium
Decreased: HDL, GTT
False positive: urine glucose

NURSING CONSIDERATIONS
Assessment
• Monitor effects of alopecia on body image; discuss feelings about body changes
• In AIDS patients monitor calorie counts, weight, appetite
• Assess for thrombophlebitis: pain, redness, swelling in legs; notify prescriber immediately if these occur

Nursing diagnoses
• Knowledge, deficient (teaching)

Implementation
• Administer with meals for GI symptoms
• Oral susp is usually used for AIDS patients; shake well
• Give tablets for carcinoma

Patient/family education
• Teach patient to report any complaints or side effects to prescriber
• Advise patient that contraceptive measures must be used during and several mo after treatment; product is teratogenic
• Explore with patient the need for wig or a hairpiece for hair loss
• Caution patient to report vaginal bleeding to prescriber
• Review with patient the need to comply with dosage schedule, not to miss or double doses; missed doses may be taken up to 1 hr before next dose

 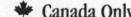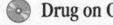

- Teach patient how to recognize signs of fluid retention, thromboembolism and report immediately
- Teach that gynecomastia and alopecia can occur; reversible after discontinuing treatment
- Advise to monitor blood glucose if diabetic

Evaluation
Positive therapeutic outcome
- Decreased spread of malignant cells
- Weight gain, increased appetite in AIDS patients
- Resolved dysfunctional uterine bleeding

---

meloxicam (Rx)
(mel-ox'i-kam)
Mobic
Func. class.: Nonsteroidal antiinflammatory/nonopioid analgesic (NSAIDs)
Chem. class.: Oxicam

Pregnancy category
C (1st trimester),
D (2nd/3rd trimesters)

Action: Inhibits prostaglandin synthesis by decreasing an enzyme needed for biosynthesis; analgesic, antiinflammatory, antipyretic effects

Therapeutic outcome: Decreased pain, swelling of joints; improved mobility

Uses: Osteoarthritis, rheumatoid arthritis, juvenile arthritis

Dosage and routes
Adult: PO 7.5 mg/day, may increase to 15 mg/day; max 15 mg/day

Available forms: Tabs 7.5, 15 mg; susp 7.5 mg/5 ml

Adverse effects
CNS: Dizziness, drowsiness, tremors, headache, nervousness, malaise, fatigue, insomnia, depression, **seizures**
CV: Hypertension, angina, **cardiac failure, MI,** hypotension, palpitations, **dysrhythmias,** tachycardia, stroke
EENT: Tinnitus, hearing loss, blurred vision
GI: Pancreatitis, nausea, colitis, GERD, vomiting, diarrhea, constipation, flatulence, cramps, dry mouth, peptic ulcer, **GI bleeding, perforation,** jaundice
GU: **Nephrotoxicity: dysuria, hematuria, oliguria, azotemia**
HEMA: **Blood dyscrasias,** anemia, prolonged bleeding
INTEG: Rash, urticaria, photosensitivity

SYST: **Angioedema, anaphylaxis, Stevens-Johnson syndrome, toxic epidermal necrolysis**

Contraindications: Pregnancy **D** (2nd/3rd trimesters), labor and delivery, breastfeeding, hypersensitivity, asthma, severe renal/hepatic disease, peptic ulcer disease, CV bleeding

Black Box Warning: Perioperative pain in CABG surgery

Precautions: Pregnancy **C** (1st trimester), children, geriatric, bleeding/GI/cardiac disorders, hypersensitivity to other antiinflammatory agents, CCr <25 ml/min

Black Box Warning: GI bleeding, MI, stroke

Pharmacokinetics
Absorption	Unknown
Distribution	Protein binding 99.4%
Metabolism	Liver <50%
Excretion	Breast milk, kidneys, feces
Half-life	15-20 hr

Pharmacodynamics
	PO	IM
Onset	Unknown	Unknown
Peak	4-5 hr	50 min
Duration	Unknown	Unknown

Interactions
Individual drugs
Cholestyramine: decreased action of meloxicam
CycloSPORINE, tacrolimus: increased nephrotoxicity
Lithium, methotrexate: increased action of each of these
Phenytoin: increased action of meloxicam
Drug classifications
Aminoglycosides, anticoagulants, diuretics, hydantoins: increased action of each specific product
β-Adrenergic blockers, ACE inhibitors, thiazides, other antihypertensives: decreased action of β-blockers
Salicylates, sulfonamides: increased action of meloxicam
Drug/herb
Arginine, gossypol: increased gastric irritation
Bearberry, bilberry: increased NSAIDs effect
Bogbean, chondroitin: increased bleeding risk

NURSING CONSIDERATIONS
Assessment
• Monitor renal, liver, blood tests: BUN, creatinine, AST, ALT, Hgb before treatment, periodically thereafter
• Assess for bleeding times; check for bruising, bleeding; test for occult blood in urine
◆ Assess for anaphylaxis and angioedema; emergency equipment should be nearby
◆ Assess for hepatic dysfunction: jaundice, yellow sclera and skin, clay-colored stools
• Assess for audiometric, ophth exam before, during, after treatment
• Assess for GI condition, hypertension, cardiac conditions

Nursing diagnoses
• Knowledge, deficient (teaching)
• Mobility, impaired physical (uses)
• Pain, chronic (uses)

Implementation
• May take without regard to meals; take with food for GI upset
• Take with full glass of water and sit upright for ½ hr
• Store at room temperature

Patient/family education
• Advise patient to report blurred vision or ringing, roaring in ears (may indicate toxicity)
• Advise patient to avoid driving, other hazardous activities if dizziness or drowsiness occurs
• Teach patient to report change in urine pattern, weight increase, edema, pain increase in joints, fever, blood in urine (indicates nephrotoxicity); to report rash, black stools, or continuing headache
• Teach patient to not use alcohol, aspirin, acetaminophen without consulting prescriber
• Advise to report use to all health care providers

Evaluation
Positive therapeutic outcome
• Decreased pain, stiffness, swelling in joints, able to move more easily

---

❗ HIGH ALERT

melphalan (Rx)
(mel'fa-lan)
Alkeran
Func. class.: Antineoplastic, alkylating agent
Chem. class.: Nitrogen mustard
Pregnancy category D

Do not confuse:
melphalan/myleran

Action: Responsible for cross-linking DNA strands leading to cell death; activity is not cell cycle phase specific

Therapeutic outcome: Prevention of rapidly growing malignant cells

Uses: Multiple myeloma, malignant melanoma, advanced ovarian cancer

Unlabeled uses: Breast, testicular, prostate carcinoma; osteogenic sarcoma, chronic myelogenous leukemia, non-Hodgkin's lymphoma

Dosage and routes
Multiple myeloma
Adult: PO 6 mg qd × 2-3 wk, adjust dose based on blood counts or 10 mg qd × 7-10 day and 2 mg qd once WBC >4000 cells/mm³, platelets >100,000 cells/mm³
Adult: IV INF 16 mg/m²; reduce in renal insufficiency; give over 15-20 min; give at 2-wk intervals × 4 doses, then at 4-wk intervals

Ovarian carcinoma
Adult: PO 200 mcg/kg/day × 5 days q4-5wk

Available forms: Tabs 2 mg; powder for inj 50 mg

Adverse effects
GI: Nausea, *vomiting,* stomatitis, diarrhea, **hepatitis**
GU: Amenorrhea, hyperuricemia, gonadal suppression
HEMA: **Thrombocytopenia, neutropenia, leukopenia,** anemia
INTEG: Rash, urticaria, alopecia, pruritus
RESP: **Fibrosis, dysplasia,** dyspnea, pneumonitis
SYST: **Anaphylaxis,** allergic reaction, **secondary malignancies,** edema

Contraindications: Pregnancy **D,** breastfeeding, or other nitrogen mustards

Black Box Warning: Hypersensitivity to this product

Precautions: Children, radiation therapy, infection, renal disease

Black Box Warning: Bone marrow depression, secondary malignancy

Pharmacokinetics
Absorption	Variable; incompletely absorbed
Distribution	Rapidly distributed, protein binding 80%-90%
Metabolism	Bloodstream
Excretion	Kidneys, unchanged (10%)
Half-life	1½ hr

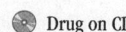

Pharmacodynamics
Unknown

Interactions
Individual drugs
Carmustine: increased pulmonary toxicity
CycloSPORINE: increased renal failure risk
Nalidixic acid: increased enterocolitis risk
Radiation: increased toxicity
Drug classifications
Anticoagulants, NSAIDs: increased bleeding risk
Antineoplastics: increased toxicity
Live virus vaccines: increased adverse reactions; decreased antibody reaction

NURSING CONSIDERATIONS
Assessment
• Monitor CBC, differential, platelet count weekly; withhold product if WBC is <3000/mm^3 or platelet count is <100,000/mm^3; notify prescriber of results if WBC <20,000/mm^3, platelets <100,000/mm^3; recovery usually occurs in 6 wk
• Monitor pulmonary function tests, chest x-ray films before, during therapy; chest film should be obtained q2wk during treatment; check for dyspnea, crackles, unproductive cough, chest pain, tachypnea
• Assess for increased uric acid levels, swelling, joint pain primarily in extremities; patient should be well hydrated to prevent urate deposits
• Monitor renal function tests: BUN, serum uric acid, before, during therapy; check I&O ratio; report fall in urine output of 30 ml/hr; check for decreased hyperuricemia; monitor AST, ALT
• Monitor for cold, fever, sore throat (may indicate beginning of infection); identify edema in feet, joint and stomach pain, shaking; prescriber should be notified
• Assess for bleeding: hematuria, guaiac, bruising or petechiae, from mucosa or orifices q8hr; no rectal temp
• Assess for symptoms indicating severe allergic reaction: rash, pruritus, urticaria, purpuric skin lesions, itching, flushing; assess allergy to chlorambucil; cross-sensitivity may occur

Nursing diagnoses
• Body image, disturbed (adverse reactions)
• Infection, risk for (adverse reactions)
• Injury, risk for (adverse reactions)
• Knowledge, deficient (teaching)

Implementation
• Give fluids **IV** or PO before chemotherapy to hydrate patient
• Give antacid before oral agent; give product after evening meal, before bedtime; provide antiemetic 30-60 min before giving product and prn to prevent vomiting; give antibiotics for prophylaxis of infection
• Give in AM so product can be eliminated before bedtime
• Use a liquid diet: carbonated beverages; gelatin may be added if patient is not nauseated or vomiting
PO route
• Give 1 hr before or 2 hr after meals to prevent nausea/vomiting
Intermittent **IV** INF route
• Use gloves during administration; if skin exposure occurs, wash immediately with soap and water
• Reconstitute with provided diluent (10 ml) to 5 mg/ml; shake until clear; further dilute with 0.9% NaCl to <0.45 mg/ml; give over 15 min, give within 1 hr
Y-site compatibilities: Acyclovir, amikacin, aminophylline, ampicillin, aztreonam, bleomycin, bumetanide, buprenorphine, butorphanol, calcium gluconate, carboplatin, carmustine, cefazolin, cefepime, cefoperazone, cefotaxime, cefotetan, ceftazidime, ceftizoxime, ceftriaxone, cefuroxime, cimetidine, cisplatin, clindamycin, cyclophosphamide, cytarabine, dacarbazine, dactinomycin, DAUNOrubicin, dexamethasone, diphenhydrAMINE, DOXOrubicin, doxycycline, droperidol, enalaprilat, etoposide, famotidine, floxuridine, fluconazole, fludarabine, fluorouracil, furosemide, gallium, ganciclovir, gentamicin, granisetron, haloperidol, heparin, hydrocortisone sodium phosphate, hydromorphone, hydrOXYzine, idarubicin, ifosfamide, imipenem-cilastatin, lorazepam, mannitol, mechlorethamine, meperidine, mesna, methylPREDNISolone, metoclopramide, methotrexate, metronidazole, miconazole, minocycline, mitomycin, mitoxantrone, morphine, nalbuphine, netilmicin, ondansetron, pentostatin, piperacillin, plicamycin, potassium chloride, prochlorperazine, promethazine, ranitidine, sodium bicarbonate, streptozocin, teniposide, thiotepa, ticarcillin, ticarcillin/clavulanate, tobramycin, trimethoprim/sulfamethoxazole, vancomycin, vinBLAStine, vinCRIStine, vinorelbine, zidovudine

Patient/family education
• Teach patient to avoid use of products containing aspirin or ibuprofen, razors,

M

Adverse effects: *italic* = common, **bold** = life-threatening

commercial mouthwash, since bleeding may occur; to report symptoms of bleeding (hematuria, tarry stools)
• Instruct patient to report signs of anemia (fatigue, headache, irritability, faintness, shortness of breath)
• Instruct patient to report any changes in breathing or coughing even several mo after treatment; to avoid crowds and persons with respiratory tract or other infections
• Tell patient hair loss is common; discuss the use of wigs or hairpieces
• Caution patient not to have any vaccinations without the advice of the prescriber, serious reactions can occur
• Advise patient that contraception is needed during treatment and for several mo after the completion of therapy
• Teach patient to rinse mouth tid-qid with water, club soda; brush teeth bid-qid with soft brush or cotton-tipped applicators for stomatitis; use unwaxed dental floss

Evaluation
Positive therapeutic outcome
• Decreased size of tumor
• Decreased spread of malignancy

---

memantine (Rx)
(me-man′teen)
Namenda
Func. class.: Anti-Alzheimer's disease agent
Chem. class.: NMDA receptor antagonist

Pregnancy category B

Action: Antagonist action of CNS NMDA receptors that may contribute to the symptoms of Alzheimer's disease

Therapeutic outcome: Improved mood, orientation, decreasing confusion

Uses: Treatment of moderate to severe dementia in Alzheimer's disease

Unlabeled uses: Vascular dementia

Dosage and routes
Adult: PO 5 mg/day, may increase dose in 5-mg increments ≥1-wk intervals; recommended target dose 20 mg/day as 10 mg bid

Available forms: Tabs 5, 10 mg; tab titration pak 5, 10 mg; oral sol 2 mg/ml, 10 mg/5 ml

Adverse effects
CNS: Dizziness, confusion, somnolence, headache, hallucinations
CV: Hypertension
GI: Vomiting, constipation

INTEG: Rash
MISC: Back pain, fatigue, pain
RESP: Coughing, dyspnea

Contraindications: Hypersensitivity, breastfeeding, children, renal failure

Precautions: Pregnancy **B**, renal disease, seizures, severe hepatic disease, GU conditions that raise urine pH

Pharmacokinetics
Absorption	Rapidly absorbed PO
Distribution	44% protein binding
Metabolism	Very little
Excretion	57%-82% excreted unchanged in urine
Half-life	Terminal elimination half-life 60-80 hr

Pharmacodynamics
Unknown

Interactions
Individual drugs
Cimetidine, hydrochlorothiazide, nicotine, quinidine, ranitidine, triamterene: may alter levels of both products
Ergot, levodopa: increased effect of each
Drug classifications
Drugs that make the urine alkaline (sodium bicarbonate, carbonic anhydrase inhibitors): decreased clearance

NURSING CONSIDERATIONS
Assessment
• Monitor B/P: hypertension; respiratory status: dyspnea
• Assess mental status: affect, mood, behavioral changes; hallucinations, confusion
• Assess GI status: vomiting, constipation, add bulk, increase fluids for constipation
• Assess GU status: urinary frequency

Nursing diagnoses
• Injury, risk for (uses)
• Knowledge, deficient (teaching)
• Noncompliance (teaching)

Implementation
• Can be taken without regard to meals
• Give twice a day if dose >5 mg
• Dosage is adjusted to response no more than q1wk
• Provide assistance with ambulation during beginning therapy; dizziness may occur

Patient/family education
• Advise to report side effects: restlessness, psychosis, visual hallucinations, stupor, loss of consciousness; indicate overdose

- Advise to use product exactly as prescribed; product is not a cure

Evaluation
Positive therapeutic outcome
- Decrease in confusion, improved mood

---

menotropins (Rx)
(men-oh-troe′pinz)
Menopur, Pergonal, Repronex
Func. class.: Gonadotropin
Chem. class.: Exogenous gonadotropin

Pregnancy category X

Action: In women, increases follicular growth, maturation; in men, when given with hCG, stimulates spermatogenesis; contains FSH and LH

Therapeutic outcome: Pregnancy, ovulation

Uses: Infertility, anovulation in women; stimulates spermatogenesis in men; usually used with hCG

Dosage and routes
Infertility
Adult (men): IM 1 ampule 3 ×/wk with hCG 2000 units 2 ×/wk × 4 mo
Adult (women): IM 75 international units of FSH, LH daily × 9-12 days, then 10,000 units of hCG 1 day after these products; repeat × 2 menstrual cycles, then increase to 150 international units of FSH, LH daily × 9-12 days, then 10,000 units of hCG 1 day after these products × 2 menstrual cycles

Anovulation
Adult (women): IM (Humegon, Pergonal) 75 international units FSH, LH daily × 7-12 days, then 10,000 units hCG 1 day after last dose of these products: repeat × 1-3 menstrual cycles; IM/subcut (Repronex only) 75 international units FSH/LH activity daily × 5 days, adjust dose by no more than 75-150 international units/day q2days

Available forms: Powder for inj lyophilized 75, 150 international units FSH, LH activity

Adverse effects
CNS: Fever, hot flashes, dizziness
CV: **Hypovolemia,** tachycardia
GI: *Nausea,* vomiting, diarrhea, anorexia
GU: **Ovarian hyperstimulation syndrome (OHSS),** multiple births, abdominal distention, pain, sudden ovarian enlargement, ascites with or without pain, ectopic pregnancy, gynecomastia in men
HEMA: **Hemoperitoneum, arterial thromboembolism**
INTEG: Rash, swelling of inj site
OTHER: **Anaphylaxis**
RESP: **ARDS, pulmonary embolism, pulmonary infarction, pleural effusion,** atelectasis, dyspnea, tachypnea

Contraindications: Pregnancy **X**, primary ovarian failure, abnormal bleeding, thyroid/adrenal dysfunction, organic intracranial lesion, ovarian cysts, primary testicular failure, high FSH

Pharmacokinetics
Absorption	Well absorbed
Distribution	Unknown
Metabolism	Unknown
Excretion	Kidneys, unchanged (8%)
Half-life	70 hr (FSH); 4 hr (LH)

Pharmacodynamics
Unknown

NURSING CONSIDERATIONS
Assessment
- Monitor weight daily; notify prescriber if weight gain increases rapidly
- Monitor estrogen excretion level; if >100 mcg/24 hr, product is withheld; serum progesterone, LH, estradiol level, pelvic exam, ovarian ultrasound; hyperstimulation syndrome may occur
- Monitor I&O ratio; be alert for decreasing urinary output
- Assess for ovarian enlargement, abdominal distention/pain; report symptoms immediately

Nursing diagnoses
- Knowledge, deficient (teaching)
- Sexual dysfunction (uses)

Implementation
- Give after reconstituting with 1-2 ml of sterile saline inj; use immediately

Patient/family education
- Advise patient that multiple births are possible; if pregnancy occurs, it is usually 4-6 wk after start of treatment
- Instruct patient to keep daily appointment for 2 wk during treatment

Evaluation
Positive therapeutic outcome
- Pregnancy

M

! HIGH ALERT

meperidine (Rx)
(me-per'i-deen)
Demerol, meperidine, Meperitab
Func. class.: Opioid analgesic
Chem. class.: Phenylpiperidine derivative

Pregnancy category B

Controlled substance schedule II

Do not confuse:
meperidine/hydromorphone/meprobamate/
morphine, Demerol/Dilaudid

Action: Depresses pain impulse transmission at the spinal cord level by interacting with opioid receptors; produces CNS depression

Therapeutic outcome: Relief of pain

Uses: Moderate to severe pain, preoperatively, postoperatively

Dosage and routes
Pain
Adult: PO/SUBCUT/IM 50-150 mg q3-4hr prn; **IV** 15-35 mg/hr as a CONT INF; PCA 10 mg, then 1-5 mg incremental dose; lockout interval 6-10 min
Elderly: PO/SUBCUT/IM start with 50 mg, increase as needed q3-4hr
Child: PO/SUBCUT/IM 1-1.8 mg/kg q3-4hr prn, max 100 mg q4hr

Preoperatively
Adult: IM/SUBCUT 50-100 mg 30-90 min before surgery; dosage should be reduced if given **IV**
Child: IM/SUBCUT 1-2 mg/kg 30-90 min before surgery

Labor analgesia
Adult: SUBCUT/IM 50-100 mg given when contractions are regulary spaced, repeat q1-3hr prn

Available forms: Inj 10, 25, 50, 75, 100 mg/ml; tabs 50, 100 mg; syr 50 mg/5 ml

Adverse effects
CNS: Drowsiness, dizziness, confusion, headache, sedation, euphoria, **increased ICP, seizures,** serotonin syndrome
CV: Palpitations, bradycardia, hypotension, change in B/P, tachycardia **(IV)**
EENT: Tinnitus, blurred vision, miosis, diplopia, depressed corneal reflex
GI: Nausea, vomiting, anorexia, constipation, cramps, biliary spasm, paralytic ileus
GU: Urinary retention, dysuria
INTEG: Rash, urticaria, bruising, flushing, diaphoresis, pruritus

RESP: **Respiratory depression**
SYST: **Anaphylaxis**

Contraindications: Hypersensitivity, addiction (opiate)

Precautions: Pregnancy **B**, breastfeeding, child <18 yr, geriatric, addictive personality, increased ICP, MI (acute), severe heart disease, respiratory depression, renal/hepatic disease, seizure disorder, abrupt discontinuation

Pharmacokinetics

Absorption	Well absorbed (IM, SUBCUT); 50% (PO)
Distribution	Widely distributed; crosses placenta; protein binding 65%-75%; toxic by-product accumulation can result from regular use or in renal disease
Metabolism	Liver, extensively to active/inactive metabolites
Excretion	Kidneys; breast milk
Half-life	3-4 hr

Pharmacodynamics

	PO	IM/ SUBCUT	IV
Onset	15 min	10 min	5 min
Peak	½-1 hr	½-1 hr	5-7 min
Duration	2-4 hr	2-4 hr	2 hr

Interactions
Individual drugs
Alcohol: increased respiratory depression, hypotension, sedation
Phenytoin: decreased meperidine effect
Procarbazine: fatal reaction, do not use together
Drug classifications
CNS depressants, opioids, sedative/hypnotics, antipsychotics, skeletal muscle relaxants: increased effects
MAOIs: do not use for 2 wk before taking meperidine; may cause fatal reaction
Protease inhibitor antiretrovirals: increased adverse reactions
Drug/herb
Chamomile, gotu kola, hops, Jamaican dogwood, kava, lavender, mistletoe, nettle, pokeweed, poppy, senega, skullcap, St. John's wort, valerian: increased CNS depression
Parsley: may promote serotonin syndrome, avoid concurrent medicinal use
Drug/lab test
Increased: amylase, lipase

 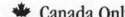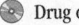

NURSING CONSIDERATIONS
Assessment
- Assess pain: location, duration, intensity before and 1 hr (IM, SUBCUT, PO), 5-10 min (**IV**) after administration
- Assess renal function before initiating therapy; poor renal function can lead to accumulation of toxic metabolite and seizures
- Monitor VS after parenteral route; note muscle rigidity, product history, liver, kidney function tests, respiratory dysfunction: respiratory depression, character, rate, rhythm; notify prescriber if respirations are <10/min
- Monitor CNS changes: dizziness, drowsiness, hallucinations, euphoria, LOC, pupil reaction; these are due to metabolite produced; CNS stimulation occurs with chronic or high doses
- Monitor allergic reactions: rash, urticaria
- Assess for constipation; increase fluids, bulk in diet; give stimulant laxatives if needed

Nursing diagnoses
- Breathing pattern, ineffective (adverse reactions)
- Injury, risk for (adverse reactions)
- Knowledge, deficient (teaching)
- Pain, acute (uses)
- Sensory perception, disturbed: visual, auditory (adverse reactions)

Implementation
- Give with antiemetic if nausea, vomiting occur
- Administer when pain is beginning to return; determine dosage interval by patient response; continuous dosing of medication is more effective given prn
- Medication should be slowly withdrawn after long-term use to prevent withdrawal symptoms
- Store in light-resistant container at room temperature

PO route
- May be given with food or milk to lessen GI upset
- Syr should be mixed with 4 oz of water

IM/SUBCUT route
- Do not give if cloudy or a precipitate has formed
- Patient should remain recumbent for 1 hr after administration

IV route
- Give by direct **IV** after diluting to 10 mg/ml with sterile water, 0.9% NaCl for inj; give slowly at 25 mg/min; rapid administration may cause respiratory depression, hypotension, circulatory collapse
- Give cont inf after diluting to 1 mg/ml with D_5W, $D_{10}W$, dextrose/saline combinations, dextrose/Ringer's, inj combinations, 0.45% NaCl, 0.9% NaCl, Ringer's, LR; give by inf pump; titrate according to response

Syringe compatibilities: Butorphanol, chlorproMAZINE, cimetidine, dimenhyDRINATE, diphenhydrAMINE, droperidol, fentanyl, glycopyrrolate, hydrOXYzine, ketamine, metoclopramide, midazolam, pentazocine, perphenazine, prochlorperazine, promazine, promethazine, ranitidine, scopolamine

Syringe incompatibilities: Heparin, morphine, pentobarbital

Y-site compatibilities: Amifostine, amikacin, ampicillin, atenolol, aztreonam, bumetanide, cefamandole, cefazolin, cefmetazole, cefotaxime, cefotetan, cefoxitin, ceftazidime, ceftizoxime, ceftriaxone, cefuroxime, cephalothin, cephapirin, chloramphenicol, cladribine, clindamycin, dexamethasone, diltiazem, diphenhydrAMINE, DOBUTamine, DOPamine, doxycycline, droperidol, erythromycin lactobionate, famotidine, filgrastim, fluconazole, fludarabine, gallium, gentamicin, granisetron, heparin, hydrocortisone, regular insulin, kanamycin, labetalol, lidocaine, magnesium sulfate, melphalan, methyldopate, methylPREDNISolone, metoclopramide, metoprolol, metronidazole, moxalactam, ondansetron, oxacillin, oxytocin, paclitaxel, penicillin G potassium, piperacillin, potassium chloride, propofol, propranolol, ranitidine, sargramostim, teniposide, thiotepa, ticarcillin, ticarcillin/clavulanate, tobramycin, trimethoprim/sulfamethoxazole, vancomycin, verapamil, vinorelbine

Y-site incompatibilities: Cefoperazone, idarubicin, imipenem/cilastatin, mezlocillin, minocycline

Additive compatibilities: Cefazolin, clonidine, DOBUTamine, metoclopramide, ondansetron, parecoxib, scopolamine, succinylcholine, triflupromazine, verapamil

Patient/family education
- Advise patients to avoid CNS depressants (alcohol, sedative/hypnotics) for at least 24 hr after taking this product
- Discuss with patient that dizziness, drowsiness, and confusion are common; to avoid getting up without assistance
- Discuss in detail with patient all aspects of the product, including its purpose and what to expect
- Caution patient to make position changes carefully to lessen orthostatic hypotension

M

Adverse effects: *italic* = common, **bold** = life-threatening

Evaluation
Positive therapeutic outcome
- Decreased pain

Treatment of overdose: Naloxone 0.2-0.8 mg **IV**, O_2, **IV** fluids, vasopressors

---

mercaptopurine (Rx)
(mer-kap-toe-pyoor'een)
6-MP, Purinethol
Func. class.: Antineoplastic, antimetabolite
Chem. class.: Purine analog

Pregnancy category D

Action: Inhibits purine metabolism at multiple sites, which inhibits DNA and RNA synthesis S phase of cell cycle

Therapeutic outcome: Prevention of rapidly growing malignant cells

Uses: Chronic myelocytic leukemia, acute lymphoblastic leukemia in children

Unlabeled uses: Polycythemia vera, psoriatic arthritis, colitis, lymphoma, acute myelogenous leukemia

Dosage and routes
Acute lymphocytic leukemia
Adult: PO 2.5-5 mg/kg/day or 80-100 mg/m²/day, maintenance 1.5-2.5 mg/kg/day
Child: PO 2.5-5 mg/kg/day, maintenance 1.5-2.5 mg/kg/day or 70-100 mg/m²/day

Available forms: Tabs 50 mg

Adverse effects
CNS: Weakness
GI: Nausea, vomiting, anorexia, diarrhea, stomatitis, **hepatotoxicity** (with high doses), jaundice, gastritis, **pancreatitis**
GU: **Renal failure,** hyperuricemia, **oliguria,** crystalluria, **hematuria**
HEMA: **Thrombocytopenia, leukopenia, myelosuppression, anemia**
INTEG: Rash, dry skin, urticaria, alopecia

Contraindications: Pregnancy **D**, breastfeeding, patients with prior product resistance, leukopenia, thrombocytopenia, anemia

Precautions: Renal/hepatic disease

Pharmacokinetics
Absorption	Variable
Distribution	Widely—body water
Metabolism	Liver—extensively
Excretion	Kidneys unchanged (small amounts)
Half-life	Terminal 1-1.5 hr

Pharmacodynamics
Onset	Unknown
Peak	1-2 hr
Duration	Unknown

Interactions
Individual products
Allopurinol, cotrimoxazole: increased bone marrow depression
Radiation: increased effects
Warfarin: increased effect of warfarin
Drug classifications
Anticoagulants, NSAIDs, platelet inhibitors, thrombolytics: increased bleeding risk
Antineoplastics, immunosuppressants: increased effects
Live virus vaccines: decreased antibodies

NURSING CONSIDERATIONS
Assessment
- Assess buccal cavity for dryness, sores or ulceration, white patches, oral pain, bleeding, dysphagia; obtain prescription for viscous lidocaine (Xylocaine)
- ⬥ Assess symptoms indicating severe allergic reaction: rash, pruritus, urticaria, purpuric skin lesions, itching, flushing
- Monitor CBC, differential, platelet count weekly; withhold product if WBC is <4000/mm³ or platelet count is <100,000/mm³; notify prescriber of results if WBC <20,000/mm³, platelets <150,000/mm³
- Assess for increased uric acid levels, swelling, joint pain primarily in extremities; patient should be well hydrated to prevent urate deposits
- Monitor renal function tests: BUN, creatinine, serum uric acid, urine CCr before, during therapy; check I&O ratio; report fall in urine output to <30 ml/hr
- Monitor temp q4hr (may indicate beginning of infection)
- Monitor liver function tests before, during therapy (bilirubin, AST, ALT, LDH) as needed or monthly; check for yellowing of skin or sclera, dark urine, clay-colored stools, itchy skin, abdominal pain, fever, diarrhea
- Assess for bleeding: hematuria, stool guaiac, bruising or petechiae, mucosa or orifices q8hr; check for inflammation of mucosa, breaks in skin

Nursing diagnoses
- Body image, disturbed (adverse reactions)
- Infection, risk for (adverse reactions)
- Injury, risk for (adverse reactions)
- Knowledge, deficient (teaching)

Implementation
- Give fluids **IV** or PO before chemotherapy to hydrate patient
- Give antiemetic 30-60 min before giving product and prn to prevent vomiting
- Give in PM on empty stomach
- Give entire dose at one time
- Provide liquid diet: carbonated beverages; gelatin may be added if patient is not nauseated or vomiting
- Tab may be crushed and added to fluids or food to facilitate swallowing

Patient/family education
- Encourage patient to rinse mouth tid-qid with water, club soda; brush teeth bid-qid with soft brush or cotton-tipped applicators for stomatitis; use unwaxed dental floss
- Advise patient that contraceptive measures are recommended during therapy; serious teratogenic effects may occur, to avoid breastfeeding
- Teach patient to avoid use of products containing aspirin or NSAIDs, razors, commercial mouthwash, since bleeding may occur; to report symptoms of bleeding (hematuria, tarry stools)
- Instruct patient to report signs of anemia (fatigue, headache, irritability, faintness, shortness of breath)
- Instruct patient to report any changes in breathing or coughing even several mo after treatment; to avoid crowds and persons with respiratory tract or other infections
- Caution patient not to have any vaccinations without the advice of the prescriber; serious reactions can occur
- Advise patient to take entire dose at one time

Evaluation
Positive therapeutic outcome
- Prevention of rapid division of malignant cells

---

meropenem (Rx)
(mer-oh-pen′em)
Merrem **IV**
Func. class.: Antiinfective—miscellaneous

Pregnancy category B

Action: Interferes with cell wall replication of susceptible organisms; osmotically unstable cell wall swells and bursts from osmotic pressure

Therapeutic outcome: Bactericidal action against the following: *Streptococcus pneumoniae*, group A β-hemolytic streptococci, *viridans* group streptococci, enterococcus; gram-negative organisms *Klebsiella*, Proteus, *Escherichia coli, Pseudomonas aeruginosa, Bacteroides fragilis, Bacteroides thetaiotamicron*, bacterial meningitis (>3 mo old)

Uses: Serious infections caused by gram-positive or gram-negative organisms (appendicitis, peritonitis)

Unlabeled uses: Febrile neutropenic, community-acquired pneumonia

Dosage and routes
Adult: **IV** 1 g q8hr, given over 15-30 min or as an **IV** BOL 5-20 ml given over 3-5 min
Child ≥ 3 mo: **IV** 20-40 mg/kg q8hr (max 2 g q8hr meningitis)
Child >50 kg: **IV** 1 g q8hr (intraabdominal infection) or 2 g q8hr (meningitis) given over 15-30 min or as an **IV** BOL 5-20 ml over 3-5 min; max 2 g q8hr

Renal dose
Adult: **IV** CCr 26-50 ml/min 1 g q12hr; CCr 10-25 ml/min 500 mg q12hr; CCr <10 ml/min 500 mg q24hr

Available forms: Powder for inj 500 mg, 1 g

Adverse effects
CNS: Fever, somnolence, *seizures*, dizziness, weakness, *headache*, myoclonia, confusion
CV: Hypotension, palpitations, tachycardia
GI: Diarrhea, nausea, vomiting, **pseudomembranous colitis, hepatitis**, glossitis
HEMA: **Eosinophilia, neutropenia,** decreased Hgb, Hct, **agranulocytosis**
INTEG: Rash, urticaria, *pruritus*, pain at inj site, phlebitis, erythema at inj site
RESP: Chest discomfort, dyspnea, hyperventilation, **pulmonary embolism**
SYST: **Anaphylaxis, Stevens-Johnson syndrome, angioedema**

Contraindications: Hypersensitivity to meropenem or imipenem

Precautions: Pregnancy **B**, breastfeeding, geriatric, renal disease, seizure disorder

Pharmacokinetics	
Absorption	Complete bioavailability
Distribution	Widely distributed
Metabolism	Liver
Excretion	Kidneys
Half-life	1 hr; increased in renal disease

M

Pharmacodynamics	
Onset	Rapid
Peak	Dose dependent
Duration	Unknown

Interactions
Individual drugs
Probenecid: increased meropenem levels
Valproic acid: decreased effect of valproic acid
Drug/herb
Do not use acidophilus with antiinfectives; separate by several hours
Drug/lab test
Increased: AST, ALT, LDH, BUN, alkaline phosphatase, bilirubin, creatinine
False positive: direct Coombs' test

NURSING CONSIDERATIONS
Assessment
• Assess patient for previous sensitivity reaction to carbapenem antiinfectives, penicillins
• Assess patient for signs and symptoms of infection, including characteristics of wounds, sputum, urine, stool, WBC >10,000/100 mm^3, fever; obtain baseline information before, during treatment
• Complete C&S tests before beginning product therapy to identify if correct treatment has been initiated
• Assess for allergic reactions, anaphylaxis: rash, urticaria, pruritus, chills, fever, joint pain; angioedema may occur a few days after therapy begins; epinephrine and resuscitation equipment should be available for anaphylactic reaction
• Identify urine output; if decreasing, notify prescriber (may indicate nephrotoxicity); also check for increased BUN, creatinine
• Monitor blood studies: AST, ALT, CBC, Hct, bilirubin, LDH, alkaline phosphatase, Coombs' test monthly if patient is on long-term therapy
• Monitor electrolytes: potassium, sodium, chloride monthly if patient is on long-term therapy
• Assess bowel pattern daily; if severe diarrhea occurs, product should be discontinued; may indicate pseudomembranous colitis
• Monitor for bleeding: ecchymosis, bleeding gums, hematuria, stool guaiac daily if on long-term therapy
• Assess for overgrowth of infection: perineal itching, fever, malaise, redness, pain, swelling, drainage, rash, diarrhea, change in cough, sputum

Nursing diagnoses
• Diarrhea (adverse reactions)
• Infection, risk for (uses)
• Injury, risk for (adverse reactions)
• Knowledge, deficient (teaching)
• Noncompliance (teaching)

Implementation
IV route
• Reconstitute with 0.9% NaCl, D$_5$W, LR, dilute in 5-20 ml of compatible sol; give by direct **IV** over 3-5 min
• Give by intermittent inf, dilute in 5-20 ml of compatible sol, give over 15-30 min
Y-site compatibilities: Aminophylline, atenolol, atropine, cimetidine, dexamethasone, digoxin, diphenhydrAMINE, enalaprilat, fluconazole, furosemide, gentamicin, heparin, insulin (regular), metoclopramide, morphine, norepinephrine, phenobarbital, vancomycin
Additive compatibilities: Aminophylline, atropine, cimetidine, dexamethasone, DOBUTamine, DOPamine, enalaprilat, fluconazole, furosemide, gentamicin, heparin, insulin (regular), magnesium sulfate, metoclopramide, morphine, norepinephrine, phenobarbital, ranitidine, vancomycin

Patient/family education
• Teach patient to report sore throat, bruising, bleeding, joint pain; may indicate blood dyscrasias (rare)
• Advise patient to contact prescriber if vaginal itching, loose foul-smelling stools, furry tongue occur; may indicate superinfection
• Advise patient to avoid breastfeeding; product is excreted in breast milk
• Advise patient to notify prescriber of diarrhea with blood or pus; may indicate pseudomembranous colitis

Evaluation
Positive therapeutic outcome
• Absence of signs/symptoms of infection (WBC <10,000/mm^3, temp WNL, absence of red draining wounds)
• Reported improvement in symptoms of infection

Treatment of anaphylaxis:
epinephrine, antihistamines, resuscitate if needed

mesalamine, 5-ASA (Rx)
(mez-al'a-meen)
Apriso, Asacol, Lialda, Pentasa, Rowasa, Salofalk ✦
Func class.: GI antiinflammatory
Chem class.: 5-Aminosalicylic acid

Pregnancy category B

Do not confuse:
Asacol/Ansaid/Os-Cal

Action: May diminish inflammation by blocking cyclooxygenase, inhibiting prostaglandin production in colon, local action only

Therapeutic outcome: Decreased cramping, pain in GI conditions

Uses: Mild to moderate active distal ulcerative colitis, proctosigmoiditis, proctitis

Unlabeled uses: Crohn's disease

Dosage and routes
Adult: RECT 60 ml (4 g) at bedtime, retained for 8 hr × 3-6 wk; PO 1000 mg qid for up to 8 wk; DEL REL tab 1.2 g/day; DEL REL tab (Lialda) 2.4 g/day; DEL REL tab (Asacol) 800 mg tid × 6 wk; CONT REL cap (Pentasa) 1 g qid up to 8 wk, EXT REL cap (Apriso) 1500 mg (4 caps) qd AM up to 6 mo

Available forms: Enema 4 g/60 ml; del rel tabs 400 mg; ext rel tab 500 mg; ext rel cap 250 mg, 500 mg; del rel tab (Lialda) 1.2 g; 0.375 g (Apriso); RECT supp 500 mg bid retained for 1-3 hr × 3-6 wk until remission, may increase to tid if needed

Adverse effects
CNS: Headache, fever, dizziness, insomnia, asthenia, weakness, fatigue
CV: Pericarditis, myocarditis, chest pain, palpitations
EENT: Sore throat, cough, pharyngitis, rhinitis
GI: Cramps, gas, nausea, diarrhea, rectal pain, constipation
INTEG: Rash, itching, acne
SYST: Flulike symptoms, malaise, back pain, peripheral edema, leg and joint pain, arthralgia, dysmenorrhea, **anaphylaxis,** acute intolerance syndrome

Contraindications: Hypersensitivity to this product or salicylates

Precautions: Pregnancy **B,** breastfeeding, children, geriatric, renal disease, sulfite sensitivity, pyloric stenosis

Pharmacokinetics
Absorption	20%-30% (PO), 10%-25% (RECT)
Distribution	Unknown
Metabolism	Unknown
Excretion	Feces
Half-life	1 hr; metabolite 5-10 hr

Pharmacodynamics
Unknown

Interactions
Individual drugs
Azathioprine: increased azathioprine action
Digoxin: decreased digoxin level
Lactulose: decreased mesalamine absorption
Omeprazole: increased mesalamine absorption
Drug/lab test
Increased: AST, ALT, alkaline phosphatase, LDH, GGTP, amylase, lipase

NURSING CONSIDERATIONS
Assessment
• Assess for GI symptoms: cramping, gas, nausea, diarrhea, rectal pain, abdominal pain; if severe, the product should be discontinued
• Assess for allergy to salicylates, sulfonamides; if allergic reactions occur, discontinue product
• Assess renal function before, during treatment: BUN, creatinine
• Monitor I&O ratios, increase fluids to 1500 ml daily to prevent crystalluria

Nursing diagnoses
• Diarrhea (uses)
• Knowledge, deficient (teaching)
• Pain, chronic (uses)

Implementation
PO route
• Do not break, crush, or chew del rel tabs
• May give orally
Rectal route (susp)
• Give at bedtime, retained until AM; empty bowel before insertion
• Store at room temperature
• Usual course of therapy is 3-6 wk
• Give after shaking bottle well

Patient/family education
• Advise patient to notify prescriber if abdominal pain, cramping, diarrhea with blood, headache, fever, rash, chest pain occur; product should be discontinued
• Teach correct administration for PO or enema

Evaluation
Positive therapeutic outcome
• Absence of pain, bleeding from GI tract

M

Adverse effects: *italic* = common, **bold** = life-threatening

metaproterenol (Rx)
(met-a-proe-ter'e-nole)
Func. class.: Selective β₂-agonist, broncho-dilator

Pregnancy category C

Action: Relaxes bronchial smooth muscle by direct action on β₂-adrenergic receptors, with increased levels of cAMP and increased bronchodilatation, diuresis, and cardiac and CNS stimulation

Therapeutic outcome: Bronchodilatation with ease of breathing

Uses: Bronchial asthma, bronchospasm

Dosage and routes
Adult and child >12 yr: INH 2-3 puffs, may repeat q3-4hr, max 12 puffs/day; IPPB or NEB 0.2-0.3 ml of 5% SOL diluted in 2.5 ml of ½ NS or NS, or 2.5 mil of 0.4, 0.6% SOL q4hr prn
Child 6-12 yr: IPPB/NEB 0.1-0.2 ml of a 5% SOL diluted in NS to a final volume of 3 ml q4hr prn
Adult: PO 20 mg q6-8hr
Geriatric: PO 10 mg tid-qid, initially
Child >9 yr or >27 kg: PO 20 mg q6-8hr or 0.4-0.9 mg/kg tid
Child 6-9 yr or <27 kg: PO 10 mg q6-8hr or 0.4-0.9 mg/kg tid
Child 2-6 yr: PO 1.3-2.6 mg/kg divided q6-8hr
Child 1-2 yr: PO 0.4 mg/kg q6-8hr

Available forms: Tabs 10, 20 mg; aerosol 0.65 mg/dose; syr 10 mg/5 ml; inh sol 0.4%, 0.6%, 5%

Adverse effects
CNS: Tremors, anxiety, insomnia, headache, dizziness, stimulation
CV: Palpitations, tachycardia, hypertension, **dysrhythmias, cardiac arrest** (high dose)
GI: Nausea, vomiting, dry mouth
MISC: Hypokalemia, pyrosis
RESP: **Paradoxical bronchospasm**

Contraindications: Hypersensitivity to sympathomimetics, closed-angle glaucoma, cardiac dysrhythmias with tachycardia

Precautions: Pregnancy C, children <6 yr, (NEB), children <12 yr (INH), geriatric, cardiac disorders, hyperthyroidism, diabetes mellitus, prostatic hypertrophy, seizure disorder

Pharmacokinetics
Absorption	Well absorbed (PO)
Distribution	Unknown
Metabolism	Liver, tissues
Excretion	Unknown
Half-life	2-4 hr

Pharmacodynamics
	PO	INH
Onset	15 min	5 min
Peak	1 hr	1 hr
Duration	4 hr	1-6 hr

Interactions
Drug classifications
β-Adrenergic blockers: block therapeutic effect
Bronchodilators, aerosol: increased action of both products
MAOIs, antidepressants (tricyclics): increased chance of hypertensive crisis
Sympathomimetics: increased effects of both products
Drug/herb
Coffee, cola nut, guarana, tea (black/green), yerba maté: increased effect
Drug/lab test
Decreased: potassium

NURSING CONSIDERATIONS
Assessment
● Monitor respiratory function: vital capacity, FEV, ABGs, lung sounds, heart rate, rhythm (baseline)
● Determine that patient has not received theophylline therapy before giving dose; identify client's ability to self-medicate
● Monitor for evidence of allergic reactions, paradoxic bronchospasm; withhold dose; notify prescriber

Nursing diagnoses
● Airway clearance, ineffective (uses)
● Gas exchange, impaired (uses)
● Knowledge, deficient (teaching)

Implementation
● Give this medication before other medications and allow 5 min between each to prevent overstimulation
PO route
● Give PO with meals to decrease gastric irritation; syr to children (no alcohol, sugar)
Aerosol route
● Give after shaking, exhale, place mouthpiece in mouth, inhale slowly, hold breath, remove, exhale slowly; allow at least 1 min between inhalations

- Store in light-resistant container, do not expose to temperature over 86° F (30° C)
- Provide spacer device for geriatric

Patient/family education

- Advise patient not to use OTC medications; excess stimulation may occur; to use this medication before other medications and allow at least 5 min between each to prevent overstimulation
- Teach patient use of inhaler; review package insert with patient; teach patient to avoid getting aerosol in eyes, since blurring may result; to wash inhaler in warm water daily and dry; to avoid smoking, smoke-filled rooms, persons with respiratory tract infections
- Advise patient that paradoxic bronchospasm may occur and to stop product immediately and notify prescriber; to limit caffeine products such as chocolate, coffee, tea, and colas
- Instruct patient on administration of dose; not to use more than prescribed; serious side effects may occur

Evaluation

Positive therapeutic outcome

- Absence of dyspnea, wheezing after 1 hr
- Improved airway exchange
- Improved ABGs

Treatment of overdose: Administer a β_1 adrenergic blocker

---

metformin (Rx)
(met-for'min)
Fortamet, Glucophage, Glucophage XR, Glumetza, Novo-Metformin ✤, Riomet
Func. class.: Antidiabetic, oral
Chem. class.: Biguanide

Pregnancy category B

Action: Inhibits hepatic glucose production and increases sensitivity of peripheral tissue to insulin

Therapeutic outcome: Blood glucose at normal levels

Uses: Type 2 diabetes mellitus

Dosage and routes
Diabetes mellitus
Adult: PO 500 mg bid initially, then increase to desired response 1-2 g; dosage adjustment q2-3wk or 850 mg/day with morning meal with dosage increased every other week, max 2550 mg/day; EXT REL (Glucophage XR) 500 mg qd with evening meal; may increase by 500 mg qwk, max 2000 mg/day; (Glumetza) 1000 mg qd with food, preferably with the PM meal,

may increase by 500 mg qwk, max 2000 mg/day; (Fortamet) 500-1000 mg qd with PM meal, may increase by 500 mg qwk, max 2550 mg/day
Geriatric: PO use lowest effective dose

Available forms: Tabs 500, 850, 1000 mg; ext rel tabs 500, 1000 mg; oral sol (Riomet) 500 mg/5 ml

Adverse effects:
CNS: Headache, weakness, dizziness, drowsiness, tinnitus, fatigue, vertigo, *agitation*
CV: **Heart failure**
ENDO: **Lactic acidosis,** hypoglycemia
GI: Nausea, vomiting, diarrhea, heartburn, anorexia, metallic taste
HEMA: **Thrombocytopenia,** decreased vit B_{12} levels
INTEG: Rash

Contraindications: Hypersensitivity; hepatic disease; creatinine >1.5 mg/ml (males), ≥1.4 (females); alcoholism; cardiopulmonary disease; acidemia; acute MI; cardiogenic shock; diabetic ketoacidosis; metabolic acidosis

Black Box Warning: History of lactic acidosis

Precautions: Pregnancy **B,** geriatric, thyroid disease, previous hypersensitivity, CHF

Pharmacokinetics	
Absorption	Unknown
Distribution	Unknown
Metabolism	Unknown
Excretion	Kidneys, unchanged (35%-50%)
Half-life	1½-5 hr, terminal 6-20 hr

Pharmacodynamics	
Onset	Unknown
Peak	1-3 hr
Duration	Unknown

Interactions
Individual drugs
Acetazolamide: increased blood glucose levels
Cimetidine, digoxin, morphine, procainamide, quinidine, ranitidine, triamterone, vancomycin: increased metformin level
Cimetidine, phenytoin: increased hypoglycemia
Radiologic contrast media: do not give together; may cause renal failure
Drug classifications
Calcium channel blockers, contraceptives (oral), corticosteroids, diuretics, estrogens,

M

phenothiazines, sympathomimetics: increased hypoglycemia

Drug/herb

Alfalfa, aloe, basil, bay, bilberry, bitter melon, black catechu, buchu, burdock, coriander, dandelion, eyebright (po), fenugreek, garlic, ginseng, glucomannan, glucosamine, goat's rue, gymnema, horehound, horse chestnut, jambul, myrrh, myrtle, rue: increased antidiabetic effect

Bee pollen, blue cohosh, broom, chromium, elecampane, eucalyptus, gotu kola: decreased antidiabetic effect

Chromium, coenzyme Q10, fenugreek: increased hypoglycemia

Glucosamine: increased hyperglycemia

Quinine: increased metformin level

NURSING CONSIDERATIONS
Assessment

• Assess for hypoglycemic reactions (sweating, weakness, dizziness, anxiety, tremors, hunger), hyperglycemic reactions soon after meals; these occur rarely with this product

• Monitor CBC (baseline, q3mo) during treatment; check liver function tests (AST, LDH) and renal tests (BUN, creatinine) periodically during treatment; glucose, A1c

◆ Monitor for lactic acidosis: malaise, myalgia, abdominal distress; risk increases with age, poor renal function; monitor electrolytes, lactate, pyruvate, blood pH, ketones, glucose

Nursing diagnoses

• Knowledge, deficient (teaching)

Implementation

• Do not break, crush, or chew ext rel tabs

• Conversion from other oral hypoglycemic agents; change may be made without gradual dosage change; monitor serum or urine glucose and ketones tid during conversion

• Give twice a day with meals to decrease GI upset and provide best absorption; may also be taken as a single dose; titrate slowly to therapeutic response, side effect tolerance

• Give in ᴀᴍ to prevent hypoglycemic reactions in ᴘᴍ

• Give immediate rel tabs crushed and mixed with meal or fluids for patients with difficulty swallowing

• Store in tight container in cool environment

Patient/family education

• Teach patient to regularly self-monitor blood glucose using blood glucose meter

• Teach patient symptoms of hypo/hyperglycemia, what to do about each (rare)

• Advise patient that product must be continued on daily basis; explain consequence of discontinuing product abruptly

• Advise patient to take product in morning to prevent hypoglycemic reactions at night

• Advise patient to avoid OTC medications, alcohol unless approved by the prescriber

• Teach patient that diabetes is a lifelong illness; that this product controls symptoms, but does not cure the condition

• Teach patient symptoms of lactic acidosis: hyperventilation, fatigue, malaise, myalgia, chills, somnolence and to notify prescriber immediately

• Teach patient to carry/wear emergency ID and glucagon emergency kit for emergencies

• Advise patient that glucophage XR tab may appear in stool

• Advise patient to take with first meal of the day

Evaluation
Positive therapeutic outcome

• Decrease in polyuria, polydipsia, polyphagia; clear sensorium; absence of dizziness; stable gait; blood glucose, A1c at normal level

---

! HIGH ALERT

methadone (Rx)
(meth′a-done)
Dolophine, methadone, Methadose
Func. class.: Opioid analgesic
Chem. class.: Synthetic diphenylheptane derivative

Pregnancy category C
Controlled substance schedule II

Do not confuse:
methadone/methylphenidate

Action: Depresses pain impulse transmission at the spinal cord level by interacting with opioid receptors; produces CNS depression

Therapeutic outcome: Relief of pain; successful opioid withdrawal

Uses: Severe pain, opiate withdrawal

Dosage and routes
Severe pain
Adult: PO/SUBCUT/IM 2.5-10 mg q8-12hr prn

Opiate withdrawal
Adult: PO 15-40 mg/day individualized initially, then 20-120 mg/day titrated to patient response

---

 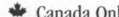

Renal dose
Adult: PO may need to be modified, no quantitative recommendations

Available forms: Inj 10 mg/ml; tabs 5, 10 mg; oral sol 5, 10 mg/5 ml, 10 mg/ml

Adverse effects
CNS: Drowsiness, dizziness, confusion, headache, sedation, euphoria, **seizures**
CV: Palpitations, bradycardia, change in B/P, **cardiac arrest, shock,** hypotension, **torsades de pointes, QT prolongation**
EENT: Tinnitus, blurred vision, miosis, diplopia
GI: Nausea, vomiting, anorexia, constipation, cramps, biliary tract spasm
GU: Increased urinary output, dysuria, urinary retention, impotence
INTEG: Rash, urticaria, bruising, flushing, diaphoresis, pruritus
RESP: **Respiratory depression, respiratory arrest**

Contraindications: Hypersensitivity to this product, or hypersensitivity to chlorobutanol (inj route), asthma, ileus

Black Box Warning: Respiratory depression

Precautions: Pregnancy **C,** breastfeeding, children <18 yr, geriatric, addictive personality, increased ICP, MI (acute), severe heart disease, respiratory depression, renal/hepatic disease, respiratory insufficiency, torsades de pointes, pulmonary disease, COPD

Black Box Warning: QT prolongation, pain

Pharmacokinetics

Absorption	Well absorbed (PO, SUBCUT, IM)
Distribution	Widely distributed; crosses placenta, half as active PO, as inj
Metabolism	Liver, extensively
Excretion	Kidneys, breast milk
Half-life	8-59 hr; extended interval with continued dosing

Pharmacodynamics

	PO	IM/SUBCUT
Onset	½-1 hr	20 min
Peak	1-1.5 hr	1½-2 hr
Duration	4-12 hr	4-6 hr

Interactions
Individual drugs
Alcohol: increased respiratory depression, hypotension, sedation
Nalbuphine, pentazine, phenytoin, rifampin: decreased analgesia

Drug classifications
Antipsychotics, opiates, sedative/hypnotics, skeletal muscle relaxants: increased respiratory depression, hypotension
Class IA antiarrhythmics (disopyramide, procainamide, quinidine), class III antiarrhythmics (amiodarone, bretylium, dofetilide, ibutilide, sotalol), astemizole, arsenic trioxide, bepridil, cisapride, chloroquine, clarithromycin, levomethadyl, pentamidine, some phenothiazines, pimozide, probucol, sparfloxacin, terfenadine: increased QT prolongation
CYP3A4 inducers (barbiturates, bosentan, carbamazepine, efavirenz, phenytoins, nevirapine, rifabutin, rifampin): decreased methadone effect
CYP3A4 inhibitors (aprepitant, antiretroviral protease inhibitors, clarithromycin, danazol, delavirdine, diltiazem, erythromycin, fluconazole, fluoxetine, fluvoxamine, imatinib, ketoconazole, mibefradil, nefazodone, telithromycin, voriconazole): increased toxicity
MAOIs: do not use for 2 wk before taking methadone: unpredictable reactions
Drug/herb
Chamomile, hops, Jamaican dogwood, kava, lavender, mistletoe, nettle, pokeweed, poppy, senega, skullcap, valerian: increased CNS depression
Corkwood: increased anticholinergic effect
St. John's wort: avoid use
Drug/lab test
Increased: amylase, lipase

NURSING CONSIDERATIONS
Assessment
• Assess for pain: type, location, intensity, grimacing before and 1½-2 hr after administration; use pain scoring
• Monitor VS after parenteral route; note muscle rigidity, product history, liver, kidney function tests, respiratory dysfunction: respiratory depression, character, rate, rhythm; notify prescriber if respirations are <10/min
• Monitor CNS changes: dizziness, drowsiness, hallucinations, euphoria, LOC, pupil reaction
• Monitor allergic reactions: rash, urticaria
• Monitor opioid detoxification: no analgesia occurs, only prevention of withdrawal symptoms
• Monitor B/P, pulse, ECG; QT prolongation, hypotension, palpitations may occur
• Monitor bowel changes; bulk, fluids, laxatives should be used for constipation

M

Adverse effects: *italic* = common, **bold** = life-threatening

Nursing diagnoses
- Breathing pattern, ineffective (adverse reactions)
- Knowledge, deficient (teaching)
- Pain, acute (uses)
- Sensory perception, disturbed: visual, auditory (adverse reactions)

Implementation
- Medication should be slowly withdrawn after long-term use to prevent withdrawal symptoms

PO route
- May be given with food or milk to lessen GI upset
- Store in light-resistant container at room temperature

IM/SUBCUT route
- Do not give if cloudy or a precipitate has formed
- Give deeply in large muscle mass; rotate inj sites

Patient/family education
- Instruct patient to report any symptoms of CNS changes, allergic reactions; to avoid CNS depressants: alcohol, sedative/hypnotics for at least 24 hr after taking this product
- Discuss with patient that dizziness, drowsiness, and confusion are common; to avoid getting up without assistance
- Discuss in detail with patient all aspects of the product
- Caution patient to make position changes slowly to prevent orthostatic hypotension

Evaluation
Positive therapeutic outcome
- Decreased pain
- Successful opioid withdrawal

Treatment of overdose: Naloxone (Narcan) 0.2-0.8 mg **IV**, O_2, **IV** fluids, vasopressors

---

methimazole (Rx)
(meth-im′a-zole)
Tapazole
Func. class.: Thyroid hormone antagonist (antithyroid)
Chem. class.: Thioamide
Pregnancy category D

Do not confuse:
methimazole/metoprolol/minoxidil

Action: Inhibits synthesis of thyroid hormones by decreasing iodine use in the manufacture of thyroglobin and iodothyronine; does not affect already formed hormones, does not affect circulatory T_4, T_3

Therapeutic outcome: Decreased T_4 levels, hyperthyroid symptoms

Uses: Hyperthyroidism, preparation for thyroidectomy, thyrotoxic crisis, thyroid storm

Dosage and routes
Hyperthyroidism
Adult: PO 15 mg/day (mild hyperthyroidism); 30-40 mg/day (moderate-severe); 60 mg/day (severe); maintenance dosage 5-15 mg/day, may be divided
Child: PO 0.4 mg/kg/day in divided doses q8hr; continue until euthyroid; maintenance dosage 0.2 mg/kg/day in divided doses q8hr, max 30 mg/24 hr

Preparation for thyroidectomy
Adult and child: PO same as above; iodine may be added for 10 days before surgery

Thyrotoxic crisis
Adult and child: PO same as hyperthyroidism with iodine and propranolol

Available forms: Tabs 5, 10, 15, 20 mg

Adverse effects
CNS: Drowsiness, headache, vertigo, fever, paresthesias, neuritis
ENDO: Enlarged thyroid
GI: Nausea, diarrhea, vomiting, jaundice, **hepatitis,** *loss of taste*
GU: **Nephritis**
HEMA: **Agranulocytosis, leukopenia, thrombocytopenia, hypothrombinemia, lymphadenopathy,** *bleeding, vasculitis*
INTEG: Rash, urticaria, pruritus, alopecia, hyperpigmentation, lupus-like syndrome
MS: Myalgia, arthralgia, nocturnal muscle cramps

Contraindications: Pregnancy **D**, breastfeeding, hypersensitivity

Precautions: Infection, bone marrow depression, hepatic disease, bleeding disorders

Pharmacokinetics
Absorption	Rapidly absorbed
Distribution	Crosses placenta
Metabolism	Liver, extensively
Excretion	Kidneys, unchanged; breast milk
Half-life	5-13 hr

Pharmacodynamics
Onset	½ hr
Peak	Unknown
Duration	2-4 hr

 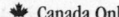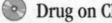

Interactions
Individual drugs
Amiodarone, potassium iodide: decreased effectiveness

Digoxin, warfarin: increased response

Radiation: increased bone marrow depression

Drug classifications
Antineoplastics: increased bone marrow depression

Phenothiazines: increased agranulocytosis

Drug/lab test
Increased: protime, AST, ALT, alkaline phosphatase

NURSING CONSIDERATIONS
Assessment
• Monitor pulse, B/P, temp; check I&O ratio; check for edema (puffy hands, feet, periorbititis); indicates hypothyroidism

• Check weight daily; same clothing, scale, time of day

• Monitor T_3, T_4, which are increased; serum TSH, which is decreased; free thyroxine index, which is increased if dosage is too low; discontinue product 3-4 wk before radioactive iodine uptake

◆ Monitor blood studies: CBC for blood dyscrasias (leukopenia, thrombocytopenia, agranulocytosis); if these occur, product should be discontinued and other treatment initiated; liver function tests

• Assess for hypersensitivity (rash, enlarged cervical lymph nodes); product may have to be discontinued

• Assess for hypoprothrombinemia (bleeding, petechiae, ecchymosis)

• Monitor clinical response: after 3 wk should include increased weight, pulse, decreased T_4

◆ Assess for bone marrow depression: sore throat, fever, fatigue

Nursing diagnoses
• Knowledge, deficient (teaching)
• Noncompliance (teaching)

Implementation
• Give with meals to decrease GI upset; give at same time each day to maintain product level

• Give lowest dosage that relieves symptoms

• Store in light-resistant container

• Increase fluids to 3-4 L/day, unless contraindicated

Patient/family education
• Advise patient to abstain from breastfeeding after delivery; product appears in breast milk

• Instruct patient to take pulse daily; to keep graph of weight, pulse, mood

• Advise patient to report redness, swelling, sore throat, mouth lesions, which indicate blood dyscrasias

• Caution patient to avoid OTC products that contain iodine; that seafood and other iodine-containing products may be restricted by prescriber

• Caution patient not to discontinue this medication abruptly; thyroid crisis may occur; stress patient compliance

• Advise patient that response may take several mo if thyroid is large

• Teach patient symptoms/signs of overdose: periorbital edema, cold intolerance, mental depression; notify prescriber at once

• Teach patient symptoms of inadequate dosage: tachycardia, diarrhea, fever, irritability; prescriber should be notified to adjust

• Teach patient to take medication exactly as prescribed, not to skip or double doses; missed doses should be taken when remembered up to 1 hr before next dose

• Instruct patient to carry ID describing medication taken and condition being treated

Evaluation
Positive therapeutic outcome
• Decreased weight gain
• Decreased pulse
• Decreased T_4
• Decreased B/P

M

methocarbamol (Rx)
(meth-oh-kar'ba-mole)
methocarbamol, Relaxin, Robaxin
Func. class.: Skeletal muscle relaxant, central acting
Chem. class.: Carbamate derivative
Pregnancy category C

Do not confuse:
Relaxin/Reglan/Relafen/Rolephin

Action: Depresses multisynaptic pathways in the spinal cord, causing skeletal muscle relaxation

Therapeutic outcome: Decreased pain, spasm, resolution of tetanic spasms

Uses: Adjunct for relief of spasm and pain in musculoskeletal conditions, tetanus

Dosage and routes
Musculoskeletal pain
Adult: PO 1.5 g qid × 2-3 days, then 1 g qid; IM 500 mg in each gluteal region; may repeat

Adverse effects: *italic* = common, **bold** = life-threatening

q8hr; **IV** BOL 1-3 g/day max at 3 ml/min; **IV** INF 1 g/250 ml D_5W or 0.9% NaCl, max 3 g/day
Geriatric: PO 500 mg qid, titrate to needed dose

Tetanus management
Adult: **IV** DIRECT 1-2 g or **IV** INF 1-3 g q6hr, max 3 g
Child: **IV** 15 mg/kg q6hr prn, max 1-8 g/m^2/day for 3 consecutive days, max 3 ml/min **IV**

Available forms: Tabs 500, 750 mg; inj 100 mg/ml

Adverse effects
CNS: Dizziness, weakness, drowsiness, syncope, flushing, headache, tremor, depression, insomnia, **seizures (IV,** IM only)
CV: Postural hypotension, *bradycardia*
EENT: Diplopia, temporary loss of vision, conjunctivitis, nasal congestion, blurred vision, nystagmus
GI: Nausea, vomiting, hiccups, anorexia, metallic taste, dyspepsia, jaundice
GU: Brown, black, green urine
HEMA: Hemolysis, increased hemoglobin, **leukopenia (IV** only)
INTEG: Rash, pruritus, fever, facial flushing, urticaria, phlebitis, extravasation
MISC: **Anaphylaxis, angioneurotic edema** (IM, **IV**)

Contraindications: Hypersensitivity to this product or PEG300 (inj), children <12 yr, intermittent porphyria, renal disease (IM/**IV**)

Precautions: Pregnancy **C,** renal/hepatic disease, addictive personalities, myasthenia gravis, epilepsy

---

Pharmacokinetics

Absorption	Rapidly absorbed (PO)
Distribution	Widely distributed; crosses placenta
Metabolism	Liver, partially
Excretion	Kidney, unchanged
Half-life	1-2 hr

Pharmacodynamics

	PO	IM	IV
Onset	½ hr	Rapid	Rapid
Peak	1-2 hr	Unknown	Inf end
Duration	>8 hr	Unknown	Unknown

Interactions
Individual drugs
Alcohol: increased CNS depression

Drug classifications
Antidepressants (tricyclic), barbiturates, opioids, sedative/hypnotics: increased CNS depression
Drug/herb
Chamomile, hops, kava, skullcap, St. John's wort, valerian: increased CNS depression
Drug/lab test
False increase: VMA, urinary 5-HIAA

NURSING CONSIDERATIONS
Assessment
• Assess for pain and spasm: location, duration, intensity, range of motion
• Assess blood studies: CBC, WBC differential; blood dyscrasias may occur
• Assess hepatic studies: AST, ALT, alk phos; hepatitis may occur; renal studies: BUN, creatinine with **IV** use
• Monitor during and after inj: CNS effects, rash, conjunctivitis, and nasal congestion may occur
• Monitor EEG in epileptic patients; poor seizure control has occurred in patients taking this product
• Assess allergic reactions: rash, fever, respiratory distress; check for severe weakness, numbness in extremities
• Assess for tolerance: increased need for medication, more frequent requests for medication, increased pain
• Assess for CNS depression: dizziness, drowsiness, psychiatric symptoms

Nursing diagnoses
• Injury, risk for (adverse reactions)
• Knowledge, deficient (teaching)
• Mobility, impaired physical (uses)

Implementation
• Methocarbamol incompatible with any product in sol or syringe
PO route
• Give with meals if GI symptoms occur
• Store in airtight container at room temperature
IM route
• Give inj deep in large muscle mass; rotate sites
• Do not give SUBCUT
IV route
• Give **IV** undiluted over 1 min or more; give 300 mg or less 1 min or longer; may be diluted in 250 ml or less D_5 or isotonic NaCl sol for slow **IV** inf
• Give by slow **IV** to prevent phlebitis; keep recumbent during and for 15 min after to prevent orthostatic hypotension; check for extravasation

---

Patient/family education
• Advise patient not to discontinue medication quickly; insomnia, nausea, headache, spasticity, tachycardia will occur; product should be tapered off over 1-2 wk
• Inform patient that urine may turn green, black, or brown
• Caution patient not to take with alcohol, other CNS depressants; increased CNS depression can occur
• Advise patient to avoid altering activities while taking this product
• Caution patient to avoid hazardous activities if drowsiness, dizziness occur; driving should be avoided until product response is known
• Advise patient to avoid using OTC medications that are CNS depressants (cough preparations, antihistamines) unless directed by prescriber; CNS depression can occur

Evaluation
Positive therapeutic outcome
• Decreased pain, spasticity

Treatment of overdose: Activated charcoal, dialysis; have epinephrine, antihistamines, and corticosteroids available, enhance elimination with osmotic diureses, **IV** fluids for hypotension

---

⚠ HIGH ALERT

methotrexate
(amethopterin, MTX)
💿 (Rx)
(meth-oh-trex'ate)
Dose Pack, Methotrexate, Rheumatrex, Trexall
Func. class.: Antineoplastic, antimetabolite
Chem. class.: Folic acid antagonist

Pregnancy category X

Do not confuse:
methotrexate/metolazone/mitoxantene

Action: Inhibits an enzyme that reduces folic acid, which is needed for nucleic acid synthesis in all cells; cell cycle specific (S phase); immunosuppressive

Therapeutic outcome: Prevention of rapidly growing malignant cells; immunosuppression

Uses: Acute lymphocytic leukemia, in combination for breast, lung, head, neck carcinoma, lymphosarcoma, gestational choriocarcinoma, hydatidiform mole, psoriasis, rheumatoid arthritis, mycosis fungoides, osteosarcoma

Unlabeled uses: Used investigationally to produce abortion

Dosage and routes
Acute lymphocytic leukemia
Adult and child: PO/IM/**IV** 3.3 mg/m^2/day × 4-6 wk until remission, then 20-30 mg/m^2 PO/IM qwk in 2 divided doses or 2.5 mg/kg **IV** × 2 wk

Burkitt's lymphoma (stages I, II, III)
Adult: PO 10-25 mg/day × 4-8 days with 7-day rest period

Lymphosarcoma (stage III)
Adult: PO/IM/**IV** 0.625-2.5 mg/kg/day

Meningeal leukemia
Adult and child: 12 mg/m^2 IT q2-5day until CSF is normal, then one additional dose, max 15 mg

Choriocarcinoma
Adult and child: PO/IM 15-30 mg/kg/day × 5 days, then off 1 wk; may repeat

Breast cancer
Adult: **IV** 40-60 mg/m^2 on day 1 of every 21-28 days with other antineoplastics

Rheumatoid arthritis
Adult: PO 7.5 mg/wk or divided doses of 2.5 mg q12hr × 3 given qwk, max 20 mg/wk

Polyarticular-course juvenile RA
Child: PO/IM 10 mg/m^2 qwk

Osteosarcoma
Adult and child: **IV** 12 g/m^2 given over 4 hr, then leucovorin rescue is given

Mycosis fungoides
Adult: PO 2.5-10 mg/day until cleared (may be many mo), IM 50 mg qwk or 25 mg 2 ×/wk

Psoriasis
Adult: PO/IM/**IV** 10-25 mg qwk or 2.5 mg PO q12hr × 3 doses qwk; may increase to 25 mg qwk

Available forms: Tabs 2.5, 5, 7.5, 10, 15 mg; inj 25 mg/ml; powder for inj 20 mg, 1 g

Adverse effects
CNS: Dizziness, **seizures,** headache, confusion, hemiparesis, malaise, fatigue, chills, fever, **leukoencephalopathy; arachnoiditis** (intrathecal)
GI: *Nausea, vomiting, anorexia, diarrhea, ulcerative stomatitis,* **hepatotoxicity,** cramps, ulcer, gastritis, **GI hemorrhage,** abdominal pain, hematemesis, **hepatic fibrosis, acute toxicity**
GU: Urinary retention, **renal failure,** menstrual irregularities, defective spermatogenesis,

M

Adverse effects: *italic* = common, **bold** = life-threatening

hematuria, azotemia, uric acid nephrop-athy
HEMA: **Leukopenia, thrombocytopenia, myelosuppression, anemia**
INTEG: *Rash, alopecia,* dry skin, urticaria, photosensitivity, folliculitis, vasculitis, pete-chiae, ecchymosis, acne, alopecia, **severe fatal skin reactions**
RESP: **Methotrexate-induced lung disease**
SYST: **Sudden death,** ***Pneumocystis jiroveci*** **pneumonia**

Contraindications: Hypersensitivity, leukopenia (<3500/mm^3), thrombocytopenia (<100,000/mm^3), anemia, psoriatic patients with severe renal disease, alcoholism, HIV infection

Black Box Warning: Pregnancy **X**, hepatic disease

Precautions: Breastfeeding, children

Black Box Warning: Renal disease, ascites, diarrhea, exfoliative dermatitis, infection, intrathecal administration, lymphoma, pleural effusion, pulmonary disease, radiation therapy, stomatitis, tumor lysis syndrome

Pharmacokinetics

Absorption	Well absorbed (GI)
Distribution	Widely distributed; crosses placenta
Metabolism	Not metabolized
Excretion	Kidneys, unchanged; breast milk (minimal)
Half-life	Terminal 10-12 hr; increased in renal disease

Pharmacodynamics

	PO	IM/IV	IT
Onset	Unknown	Unknown	Unknown
Peak	1-4 hr	½-2 hr	Unknown
Duration	Unknown	Unknown	Unknown

Interactions
Individual drugs
Alcohol, phenylbutazone, probenecid, radia-tion, theophylline: increased toxicity
Digoxin (PO), fosphenytoin, phenytoin: decreased effect of each specific product
Folic acid: decreased effect of methotrexate
Radiation: increased bone marrow suppres-sion
Drug classifications
Anticoagulants (oral): increased hypopro-thrombinemia
Antineoplastics, NSAIDs, penicillins, salicylates, sulfa products: increased toxicity
Live virus vaccines: decreased antibodies

NURSING CONSIDERATIONS
Assessment
• Assess buccal cavity q8hr for dryness, sores or ulceration, white patches, oral pain, bleed-ing, dysphagia; obtain prescription for viscous lidocaine (Xylocaine)
• Assess symptoms indicating severe allergic reaction: rash, pruritus, urticaria, purpuric skin lesions, itching, flushing
• Assess tachypnea, ECG changes, dyspnea, edema, fatigue; identify dyspnea, crackles, unproductive cough, chest pain, tachypnea
• Monitor CBC, differential, platelet count weekly; withhold product if WBC is <3500/mm^3 or platelet count is <100,000/mm^3; notify prescriber of results if WBC <20,000/mm^3, platelets <150,000/mm^3; WBC, platelet nadirs occur on day 7
• Assess for increased uric acid levels, swell-ing, joint pain primarily in extremities; patient should be well hydrated to prevent urate deposits
• Monitor renal function studies: BUN, creati-nine, serum uric acid, urine CCr before, during therapy; check I&O ratio; report fall in urine output to <30 ml/hr
• Monitor temp (may indicate beginning of infection)
• Monitor liver function tests before, during therapy (bilirubin, AST, ALT, LDH) as needed or monthly; check for jaundice of skin and sclera, dark urine, clay-colored stools, itchy skin, abdominal pain, fever, diarrhea (hepato-toxicity)
• Assess for bleeding: hematuria, stool guaiac, bruising or petechiae, mucosa or orifices; check for inflammation of mucosa, breaks in skin
• Identify effects of alopecia on body image; discuss feelings about body changes
• Identify edema in feet, joint and stomach pain, shaking; prescriber should be notified
• Monitor methotrexate levels, adjust leu-covorin dose based on the level

Nursing diagnoses
• Body image, disturbed (adverse reactions)
• Infection, risk for (adverse reactions)
• Injury, risk for (adverse reactions)
• Knowledge, deficient (teaching)

Implementation
• Avoid contact with skin, since product is very irritating; wash completely to remove
◆ Administer leucovorin calcium within 24 hr of giving this product to prevent tissue damage; check agency policy; continue until methotrex-ate level <10^{-8} m

- Give fluids **IV** or PO before chemotherapy to hydrate patient
- Give antiemetic 30-60 min before giving product and prn to prevent vomiting; administer antibiotics for infection prophylaxis
- Give in AM so product can be eliminated before bedtime
- Provide liquid diet: carbonated beverages; gelatin may be added if patient is not nauseated or vomiting

PO route

- Give 1 hr before or 2 hr after meals to prevent vomiting
- Make sure product is taken weekly in RA, JRA

IM route

- Give deeply in large muscle mass

IV route

- Give **IV** after diluting 5 mg/2 ml of sterile water for inj; give through Y-tube or 3-way stockcock
- Give **IV** inf after diluting in 0.9% NaCl, D₅W, D₅/0.9% NaCl and give as prescribed
- Give sodium bicarbonate tabs or **IV** fluids to prevent precipitation of product at high doses; urine pH should be >7; may need to reduce dose if BUN is 20-30 mg/dl or creatinine is 1.2-2 mg/dl; stop product if BUN >30 mg/dl or creatinine is >2 mg/dl

Syringe compatibilities: Bleomycin, cisplatin, cyclophosphamide, doxapram, DOXOrubicin, fluorouracil, furosemide, heparin, leucovorin, mitomycin, vinBLAStine, vinCRIStine

Syringe incompatibilities: Droperidol, ranitidine

Y-site compatibilities: Allopurinol, amifostine, asparaginase, aztreonam, bleomycin, cefepime, ceftriaxone, cimetidine, cisplatin, cyclophosphamide, cytarabine, DAUNOrubicin, dexchlorpheniramine, diphenhydrAMINE, DOXOrubicin, etoposide, famotidine, filgrastim, fludarabine, fluorouracil, furosemide, gallium, ganciclovir, granisetron, heparin, hydromorphone, imipenem-cilastatin, leucovorin, lorazepam, melphalan, mesna, methylPREDNISolone, metoclopramide, mitomycin, morphine, ondansetron, oxacillin, paclitaxel, piperacillin/tazobactam, prochlorperazine, ranitidine, sargramostim, teniposide, thiotepa, vinBLAStine, vinCRIStine, vinorelbine

Y-site incompatibilities: Droperidol, idarubicin

Additive compatibilities: Cephalothin, cyclophosphamide, cytarabine, fluorouracil, hydrOXYzine, mercaptopurine, ondansetron, sodium bicarbonate, vinCRIStine

Additive incompatibilities: Bleomycin, prednisoLONE

Solution compatibilities: Amino acids, 4.25%/D₂₅, D₅W, sodium bicarbonate 0.05 mol/L, sodium chloride 0.9%

Patient/family education

- Encourage patient to rinse mouth tid-qid with water, club soda; brush teeth bid-qid with soft brush or cotton-tipped applicators for stomatitis; use unwaxed dental floss
- Advise patient that contraceptive measures are recommended during therapy; product is teratogenic; contraception should be used for 3 mo (male) and 4-6 wk (female); to discontinue breastfeeding; toxicity to infant may occur
- Teach patient to avoid use of products containing aspirin or NSAIDs, razors, commercial mouthwash, since bleeding may occur; to report symptoms of bleeding (hematuria, tarry stools)
- Caution patient to report signs of anemia (fatigue, headache, irritability, faintness, shortness of breath)
- Advise patient to report any changes in breathing or coughing even several mo after treatment; to avoid crowds and persons with respiratory tract or other infections
- Advise patient to report stomatitis: any bleeding, white spots, ulcerations in mouth to prescriber; tell patient to examine mouth daily, report symptoms, use good oral hygiene
- Teach patient that hair may be lost during treatment; a wig or hairpiece may make patient feel better; new hair may be different in color, texture
- Caution patient not to have any vaccinations without the advice of the prescriber; serious reactions can occur
- Advise patient to use sunblock or protective clothing to prevent burns

Evaluation

Positive therapeutic outcome

- Prevention of rapid division of malignant cells
- Decreased joint inflammation in RA

M

methoxy polyethylene glycol-epoetin beta (Rx)
(meth-ox′ee pol′ee-eth′i-leen glye′kol-e-poe′e-tin bay′ta)

Mircera

Func. class.: Antianemic, biologic modifier, hormone

Chem. class.: Amino acid polypeptide

Pregnancy category C

Action: Erythropoietin is one factor controlling rate of red cell production; product is developed by recombinant DNA technology

Therapeutic outcome: Increase in reticulocyte count in 2-6 wk, Hgb/Hct; increased appetite, enhanced sense of wellbeing

Uses: Anemia caused by reduced endogenous erythropoietin production, primarily end-stage renal disease; to correct hemostatic defect in uremia on all dosages

Dosage and routes
For all dosages
Adult and geriatric: Reduce by 25% if Hgb >1 g/dl in any 2 wk period or if Hgb is close to 12 g/dl; if Hgb continues to rise after decrease, hold until Hgb starts to decrease

Treatment of anemia in chronic renal failure (dialysis dependant/independent)—not currently using ESA
Adult and geriatric: **IV**/SUBCUT 0.6 mcg q2wk

Using >80 mcg/wk darbepoetin or >16000 units/wk epoetin
Adult and geriatric: **IV**/SUBCUT 180 mcg q2wk or 360 mcg q4wk

Using 40-80 mcg/wk darbepoetin or 8000-16,000 units/wk epoetin
Adult and geriatric: **IV**/SUBCUT 100 mcg q2wk

Using <40 mcg/wk darbepoetin or <8000 units/wk epoetin
Adult and geriatric: **IV**/SUBCUT 60 mcg q2wk or 120 mcg q4wk

Adverse effects
CNS: **Seizures, encephalopathy,** headache
CV: *Hypertension,* edema, **heart failure,** hypotension, **sinus tachycardia, stroke, myocardial infarction**
GI: Diarrhea
HEMA: **Anemia, red cell aplasia, thrombocytopenia, thromboembolism, thrombosis**
INTEG: Pruritus, rash, erythema, inj site reaction
MS: Muscle spasms, back pain
SYST: Antibody formation

Contraindications: Red cell aplasia, neoplastic disease, hypersensitivity to mannitol

Black Box Warning: Hgb >12 g/dl

Precautions: Pregnancy **C**, seizure disorder, porphyria, children <1 mo, breastfeeding, multidose preserved formulation contains benzyl alcohol and should not be used in premature infants, CV disease, hemodialysis, latex allergy, surgery, hypertension, history of CABG

Black Box Warning: Neoplastic disease

Pharmacokinetics
Absorption	Unknown
Distribution	Unknown
Metabolism	Unknown
Excretion	Unknown
Half-life	Half-life 139 +/- 67 hr rise in reticulocytes on day 7, rise in Hgb in 7-14 days (SUBCUT); Half-life 134 +/- 65 hr (**IV**)

Pharmacodynamics
Unknown

Interactions
Drug classifications
Androgens: increased action of methoxy polyethylene gycol-epoetin
Other erythropoiesis stimulating agents (ESA) (epoetin, darbepoetin): adverse reactions; do not give concurrently

NURSING CONSIDERATIONS
Assessment
- Monitor renal studies: urinalysis, protein, blood, BUN, creatinine; I&O, report drop in output <50 ml/hr

 Assess CBC, blood studies: ferritin, transferrin monthly; transferrin ≥20%, ferritin ≥100 ng/ml; Hct 2 ×/wk until stabilized in target range (30%-36%) then at regular intervals; those with endogenous erythropoietin levels of <500 units/L respond to this agent; monitor Hct 2 ×/wk in chronic renal failure; patients treated with zidovudine or cancer patients should be monitored weekly, then periodically after stabilization; death may occur in Hgb >12 g/dl

- Monitor B/P; check for rising B/P as Hct rises, antihypertensives may be needed;

 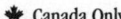

hypertension may occur rapidly leading to hypertensive encephalopathy
• Assess CNS symptoms: for seizures if Hct is increased within 2 wk by 4 pts
• Assess for hypersensitivity reactions: skin rashes, urticaria (rare), antibody development
◆ For pure cell aplasia (PRCA) in absence of other causes, evaluate by testing sera for recombinant erythropoetin antibodies; any loss of response to epoetin should be evaluated
• Assess dialysis patients: thrill, bruit of shunts, monitor for circulation impairment

Nursing diagnoses
• Injury, risk for (uses)
• Knowledge, deficient (teaching)
• Urinary elimination, impaired (uses)

Implementation
• Do not shake vial
• Give iron supplements as needed; adequate iron stores are needed for this agent to work properly
SUBCUT route
• Inject into outer aspect of upper arms, abdomen (except for 2 inches around navel) or front aspect of middle thigh; do not inject in areas that have stretch marks or are scarred or bruised
• Rotate inj sites
IV route
• Give additional heparin to lower chance of clots
• Give by direct inj or bolus into venous line at end of dialysis

Solution compatibilities: Do not dilute or administer with other solutions

Patient/family education
• Caution patient to avoid driving or hazardous activities during beginning of treatment
• Instruct patient to monitor B/P
• Instruct patient to take iron supplements, vitamin B_{12}, folic acid as directed

Evaluation
Positive therapeutic outcome
• Increase in reticulocyte count in 2-6 wk, Hgb/Hct; increased appetite, enhanced sense of wellbeing

methyldopa/ methyldopate (Rx)
(meth-ill-doe′pa)
Apo-methyldopa ✦, Dopamet ✦, methyldopa/methyldopate, Novo-medopa ✦, Nu-Medopa ✦
Func. class.: Antihypertensive
Chem. class.: Centrally acting α-adrenergic inhibitor

Pregnancy category
B (PO)
C (IV)

Do not confuse:
methyldopa/ʟ-dopa (levodopa)

Action: Stimulates central α_2-adrenergic receptors in the CNS, resulting in decreased sympathetic outflow from the brain with decreased peripheral resistance

Therapeutic outcome: Decreased B/P in hypertension

Uses: Hypertension, hypertensive crisis

Dosage and routes
Adult: PO 250-500 mg bid or tid, then adjusted q2day prn, 0.5-2 g/day in 2-4 divided doses (maintenance), max 3 g/day; **IV** 250-500 mg in 100 ml D_5W q6hr, run over 30-60 min, max 1 g q6hr, switch to PO as soon as possible
Geriatric: PO 125 mg bid tid, increase q2day as needed, max 3 g/day
Child: PO 10 mg/kg/day in 2-4 divided doses, max 65 mg/kg or 3 g/day, whichever is less; **IV** 20-40 mg/kg/day in 4 divided doses, max 65 mg/kg or 3 g, whichever is less

Available forms: Methyldopa: tabs 125, 250, 500 mg; oral susp 50 mg/ml; methyldopate: inj 50 mg/ml (250 mg/5 ml)

Adverse effects
CNS: Drowsiness, weakness, dizziness, sedation, headache, depression, psychosis, paresthesias, parkinsonism, Bell's palsy, nightmares
CV: Bradycardia, **myocarditis,** orthostatic hypotension, angina, edema, weight gain, **CHF,** paradoxical pressor response (**IV** use)
EENT: Nasal congestion
ENDO: Breast enlargement, gynecomastia, breastfeeding, amenorrhea
GI: Nausea, vomiting, diarrhea, constipation, **hepatic dysfunction,** sore or "black" tongue, **pancreatitis,** colitis, flatulence
GU: Impotence, failure to ejaculate

HEMA: **Leukopenia, thrombocytopenia, hemolytic anemia, granulocytopenia,** positive Coombs' test

INTEG: Lupus-like syndrome, rash, **toxic epidural necrolysis**

Contraindications: Active hepatic disease, hypersensitivity

Precautions: Pregnancy **B**, geriatric patients, cardiac disease, autoimmune disease, depression, dialysis, hemolytic anemia, Parkinson's disease, pheochromocytoma, sulfite hypersensitivity

Pharmacokinetics

Absorption	50% (PO)
Distribution	Crosses placenta, blood-brain barrier
Metabolism	Liver, moderately
Excretion	Kidneys, unchanged (partially)
Half-life	1½ hr

Pharmacodynamics

	PO	IV
Onset	Unknown	Unknown
Peak	2-4 hr	2 hr
Duration	12-24 hr	10-16 hr

Interactions

Individual drugs

Alcohol: CNS depression
Haloperidol: increased psychosis
Iron: decreased methyldopa absorption
Levodopa: increased CNS toxicity, hypotension
Lithium: increased lithium toxicity
TOLBUTamide: increased hypoglycemia

Drug classifications

Amphetamines, antidepressants (tricyclics), barbiturates, NSAIDs, phenothiazines: decreased antihypertensive effect
Analgesics, antidepressants, antihistamines, sedative/hypnotics: increased CNS depression
Antihypertensives, diuretics: increased hypotension
β-Adrenergic blockers: increased B/P
MAOIs: increased pressor effect
Sympathomimetic amines: increased pressor effect

Drug/herb

Aconite: increased toxicity, death
Astragalus, cola tree: increased or decreased antihypertensive effect
Barberry, betony, black catechu, black cohosh, bloodroot, broom, burdock, cat's claw, dandelion, goldenseal, hawthorn, Irish moss, Jamaican dogwood, kelp, khella, mistletoe, parsley: increased antihypertensive effect
Capsicum, Indian snakeroot: decreased effect
Coltsfoot, guarana, khat, licorice, yohimbe: decreased antihypertensive effect

Drug/lab test

Interference: urinary uric acid, serum creatinine, AST
False increase: urinary catecholamines

NURSING CONSIDERATIONS

Assessment

• Monitor blood tests: neutrophils, decreased platelets; direct Coombs' test before, after 6, 12 mo of therapy
• Monitor renal studies: protein, BUN, creatinine; watch for increased levels that may indicate nephrotic syndrome: polyuria, oliguria, frequency; report weight gain >5 lb
• Obtain baselines in renal, liver function tests before therapy begins; check potassium levels, although hyperkalemia rarely occurs
• Monitor B/P, pulse if the product is being used for hypertension; notify prescriber of changes
• Monitor edema in feet, legs daily; monitor I&O; check weight for decreasing output
• Assess for allergic reaction: rash, fever, pruritus, urticaria; product should be discontinued if antihistamines fail to help
• Monitor CNS symptoms, especially in the geriatric; depression; change in mental status

Nursing diagnoses

• Cardiac output, decreased (uses)
• Injury, risk for (side effects)
• Knowledge, deficient (teaching)
• Noncompliance (teaching)

Implementation

PO route

• Give before meals
• Shake susp before using
• Store in airtight container at room temperature

IV route

• Give by intermittent inf after diluting in 100 ml of 0.9% NaCl, D₅W, D₅/0.9% NaCl, 5% sodium bicarbonate, Ringer's; administer over 30-60 min

Y-site compatibilities: Esmolol, heparin, meperidine, morphine, theophylline

Additive compatibilities: Aminophylline, ascorbic acid, chloramphenicol, diphenhydrAMINE, heparin, magnesium sulfate, multivitamins, netilmicin, potassium chloride, promazine, sodium bicarbonate, succinylcholine, verapamil, vit B/C

Additive incompatibilities: Amphotericin B, barbiturates, methohexital, sulfonamides
Solution compatibilities: D_5W, D_5/0.9% NaCl, Ringer's, sodium bicarbonate 5%, 0.9% NaCl, amino acids 4.25%/D_{25}, Dextran$_6$/0.9% NaCl, Normosol R, Normosol M/D_5W

Patient/family education

• Instruct patient not to discontinue product abruptly, or withdrawal symptoms may occur: anxiety, increased B/P, headache, insomnia, increased pulse, tremors, nausea, sweating
• Caution patient not to use OTC (cough, cold, or allergy) products unless directed by prescriber
• Teach patient to comply with dosage schedule even if feeling better; product controls symptoms, does not cure
• Caution patient to change position slowly, to rise slowly to sitting or standing position to minimize orthostatic hypotension, especially geriatric
• Teach patient about excessive perspiration, dehydration, vomiting, diarrhea; may lead to fall in B/P; consult prescriber if these occur
• Advise patient that product may cause dizziness, fainting; light-headedness may occur during 1st few days of therapy; that product may cause dry mouth; use hard candy, saliva product, or frequent rinsing of mouth
• Caution patient that compliance is necessary; not to skip or stop product unless directed by prescriber
• Teach patient that product may cause skin rash
• Teach patient to avoid hazardous activities, since product may cause drowsiness, dizziness

Evaluation

Positive therapeutic outcome
• Decreased B/P

Treatment of overdose: Gastric evacuation, sympathomimetics, may be indicated if severe; hemodialysis

---

methylergonovine (Rx)
(meth-ill-er-goe-noe′veen)
Methergine, methylergonovine
Func. class.: Oxytocic
Chem. class.: Ergot alkaloid

Pregnancy category C

Action: Stimulates uterine and vascular smooth muscle, causing contractions, decreased bleeding, arterial vasoconstriction

Therapeutic outcome: Absence of hemorrhage

Uses: Treatment of hemorrhage postpartum or after abortion, uterine contractions

Dosage and routes
Adult: PO 200 mcg tid-qid up to 7 days; IM/IV 200 mcg q2-4hr for 1-5 doses

Available forms: Inj 200 mcg/ml; tabs 200 mcg

Adverse effects
CNS: Headache, dizziness, **seizures**
CV: **Hypotension,** chest pain, palpitations, *hypertension,* **dysrhythmias; CVA (IV)**
EENT: Tinnitus
GI: Nausea, vomiting
GU: Cramping
INTEG: Sweating, rash, allergic reactions
RESP: Dyspnea

Contraindications: Pregnancy (4th stage of labor), hypersensitivity to ergot preparations, angina, arteriosclerosis, CAD, dysfunctional uterine bleeding, eclampsia, MI, neonates, Raynaud's disease, sepsis, stroke, Buerger's disease, thrombophlebitis, hypertension, PID, respiratory disease, cardiac disease, peripheral vascular disease

Precautions: Pregnancy C, severe renal/hepatic disease, jaundice, diabetes mellitus, seizure disorders, sepsis, CAD

Pharmacokinetics	
Absorption	Well absorbed (PO, IM)
Distribution	Unknown
Metabolism	Liver, possibly
Excretion	Unknown
Half-life	½-2 hr

Pharmacodynamics			
	PO	IM	IV
Onset	5-15 min	5 min	Immediate
Peak	Unknown	Unknown	Unknown
Duration	3 hr	3 hr	Unknown

Interactions
Individual drugs
Smoking: increased vasoconstriction
Drug classifications
Vasopressors: increased vasoconstriction

NURSING CONSIDERATIONS
Assessment
• Monitor B/P, pulse; watch for change that may indicate hemorrhage; check respiratory rate, rhythm, depth; notify prescriber of abnormalities
• Assess fundal tone, nonphasic contractions; check for relaxation or severe cramping

Adverse effects: *italic* = common, **bold** = life-threatening

- Assess for ergotism or overdose: nausea, vomiting, weakness, muscular pain, insensitivity to cold, paresthesia of extremities; product should be decreased or infusion discontinued
- Before administering ergonovine, check calcium levels; if hypocalcemia is present, correction should be made to increase effectiveness of this product
- Monitor prolactin levels and for decreased breast milk production

Nursing diagnoses
- Injury, risk for (adverse reactions)
- Knowledge, deficient (teaching)
- Tissue perfusion, ineffective (uses)

Implementation
PO route
- PO is the preferred route

IM route
- Give inj deeply in large muscle mass

IV route
- Give by this route for severe, life-threatening hemorrhage
- Give directly undiluted or diluted with 5 ml of 0.9% NaCl given through Y-site or 3-way stopcock; give 0.2 mg/min; use clear, colorless sol
- Store up to 2 mo if unused

Y-site compatibilities: Heparin, hydrocortisone sodium succinate, potassium chloride, vit B/C

Patient/family education
- Advise patient to stop smoking, since increased vasoconstriction will result
- Inform patient that abdominal cramps are a side effect of this medication
- Instruct patient to notify prescriber if chest pain, nausea, vomiting, headache, muscle pain, weakness, or cold, numb extremities occur

Evaluation
Positive therapeutic outcome
- Prevention of hemorrhage

---

methylnaltrexone (Rx)
(meth-il-nal-trex'one)
Relistor
Func. class.: Opioid antagonist

Pregnancy category B

Action: Peripheral mu-opioid receptor antagonist that reduces constipation associated with opiate agonists

Therapeutic outcome: Decreased constipation

Uses: Treatment of opioid-induced constipation in patients with advanced illness who are receiving palliative care when response to laxative therapy has been insufficient

Dosage and routes
Opiate-agonist induced constipation
Adult >114 kg: SUBCUT 0.15 mg/kg every other day prn
Adult 62-114 kg: SUBCUT 12 mg every other day prn
Adult 38-62 kg: SUBCUT 8 mg every other day prn
Adult <38 kg: SUBCUT 0.15 mg/kg every other day prn

Renal dose
Adult: SUBCUT CCr <30 ml/min, reduce normal adult dose by 50%

Available forms: Solution for inj 12 mg/0.6 ml

Adverse effects
CNS: Dizziness, migraines, obsessive-compulsive disorder
GI: Nausea, vomiting, diarrhea, flatulence, abdominal pain

Contraindications: Hypersensitivity, GI obstruction, **IV** route

Precautions: Pregnancy **B**, breastfeeding, renal disease, children, diarrhea, driving, operating machinery, geriatric patients

Pharmacokinetics	
Absorption	Unknown
Distribution	Protein binding 11%-15.3%
Metabolism	Unknown
Excretion	Unknown
Half-life	Terminal 8 hr

Pharmacodynamics	
Onset	Unknown
Peak	30 min (SUBCUT)
Duration	Unknown

NURSING CONSIDERATIONS
Assessment
- Monitor serum creatinine
- Assess for stool characteristics

Nursing diagnoses
- Constipation (uses)
- Knowledge, deficient (teaching)

Implementation
- Give SUBCUT only; oral dose is investigational and not currently available

---

- Do not give **IV; IV** dosing for urinary retention is investigational
- Store at 15°-30° C (59°-86° F); do not freeze
- Store away from light

SUBCUT route
- Inspect the solution before use; it should be a clear, colorless to pale yellow aqueous solution; do not use if particulate matter or discoloration are present
- Withdraw the needed amount of solution into a sterile syringe; if immediate administration is impossible, the syringe may be kept at room temperature for up to 24 hrs; the syringe does not need to be kept away from light during the 24-hr period; immediately discard any unused portion in the vile; no preservatives are present
- Administer into the upper arm, abdomen, or thigh no more than 1 ×/24 hr; rotate inj sites; do not inject the same spot each time; do not inject into areas where skin is tender, bruised, red, or hard; avoid areas with scars or stretch marks
- If using with retractable needle, slowly push down on the plunger past the resistance point until the syringe is empty and a click is heard

Patient/family education
- Caution patient not to drive or operate machinery until effect is known

Evaluation
Positive therapeutic outcome
- Decreasing constipation

---

methylphenidate 🌐 **(Rx)**
(meth-ill-fen′i-date)
Concerta, Daytrana, Metadate CD, Methidate, Methylin, Methylin ER, PMS-Methylphenidate ✿, Riphenidate ✿, Ritalin, Ritalin LA, Ritalin SR
Func. class.: Cerebral stimulant
Chem. class.: Piperidine derivative

Pregnancy category C

Controlled substance schedule II

Do not confuse:
methylphenidate/methadone

Action: Increases release of norepinephrine and dopamine in cerebral cortex to reticular activating system; exact action not known

Therapeutic outcome: Increased alertness, decreased fatigue, ability to stay awake (narcolepsy), increased attention span, decreased hyperactivity (ADHD)

Uses: Attention deficit disorder with hyperactivity (ADHD), narcolepsy (except Concerta, Metadate CD, Ritalin LA), attention deficit disorder (ADD)

Dosage and routes
ADHD
Adult: PO 20-30 mg/day; EXT REL (Concerta) 18-36 mg/day
Child >6 yr: PO (immediate-release tab, chew tabs, oral SOL) 5 mg before breakfast and lunch, increasing by 5-10 mg/wk, max 60 mg/day; EXT REL 20 mg daily-tid

Attention deficit hyperactivity disorder, conversion from PO to transdermal
Child 6-12 yr: Week 1, 12.5 cm² (10 mg); week 2, 18.75 cm² (15 mg); week 3, 25 cm² (20 mg); week 4, 37.5 cm² (30 mg)

Narcolepsy
Adult: PO 10 mg bid-tid, 30-45 min before meals; may increase up to 60 mg/day

Available forms: Tabs 5, 10, 20 mg; ext rel tabs 10, 20 mg; ext rel tabs (Concerta) 18, 27, 36, 54 mg; chew tabs (Methylin) 2.5, 5, 10 mg; ext rel cap 10, 20, 30, 40 mg; oral sol 5 mg, 10 mg/ml; transdermal patch 12.5 cm² (10 mg), 18.75 cm² (15 mg), 25 cm² (20 mg), 37.5 cm² (30 mg)

Adverse effects
CNS: Hyperactivity, insomnia, restlessness, talkativeness, dizziness, headache, akathisia, dyskinesia, masking or worsening of Gilles de la Tourette's syndrome, **seizures,** drowsiness, toxic psychosis, hallucinations, **neuroleptic malignant syndrome**
CV: Palpitations, tachycardia, B/P changes, angina, **dysrhythmias**
ENDO: Growth retardation
GI: Nausea, anorexia, dry mouth, weight loss, abdominal pain
HEMA: **Leukopenia, anemia, thrombocytopenic purpura**
INTEG: **Exfoliative dermatitis,** urticaria, rash, erythema multiforme, **hypersensitivity reactions**
MISC: Fever, arthralgia, scalp hair loss

Contraindications: Hypersensitivity, anxiety, history of Gilles de la Tourette's syndrome, children <6 yr, glaucoma, anorexia nervosa, tartrazine dye hypersensitivity

Precautions: Pregnancy C, breastfeeding, hypertension, depression, seizures
Black Box Warning: Substance abuse

M

Pharmacokinetics

Absorption	Well absorbed (PO); delayed (ext rel)
Distribution	Widely distributed; crosses placenta
Metabolism	Liver
Excretion	Kidneys
Half-life	1-3 hr

Pharmacodynamics

	PO	PO–EXT REL
Onset	½-1 hr	2 hr
Peak	1-3 hr	4 hr
Duration	4-6 hr	6-8 hr

Interactions
Individual drugs
Guanethidine: decreased effect of guanethidine
Drug classifications
Anticonvulsants, antidepressants (tricyclics), selective serotonin reuptake inhibitors: increased effects
MAOIs (or within 14 days of MAOIs), vasopressors: hypertensive crisis
Drug/herb
Cola nut, guarana, horsetail, yerba maté, yohimbe: increased CNS stimulation
Melatonin: synergistic effect
Drug/food
Caffeine: increased stimulation

NURSING CONSIDERATIONS
Assessment
• Monitor VS, B/P, since this product may reverse antihypertensives; check patients with cardiac disease more often for increased B/P
• Perform CBC, urinalysis; for diabetic patients monitor blood glucose, urine glucose; insulin changes may be required, since eating will decrease
• Monitor height and weight q3mo since growth rate in children may be decreased; appetite is suppressed, weight loss is common during the first few mo of treatment
• Monitor mental status: mood sensorium, affect, stimulation, insomnia; aggressiveness may occur; depression with crying spells may occur after product has worn off
• Assess for tolerance; should not be used for extended time except in ADHD; dosage should be discontinued gradually to prevent withdrawal symptoms
• Assess for narcoleptic symptoms before medication and after; ability to stay awake should increase significantly
• In children or adults with ADHD, monitor for improved organizational skills, attention span, attending to tasks, impulse control, socialization, and ability to get along better with others
◆ Assess for withdrawal symptoms: headache, nausea, vomiting, muscle pain, weakness; product tolerance will develop after long-term use; dosage should not be increased if tolerance develops
• Assess appetite, sleep, speech patterns

Nursing diagnoses
• Coping, compromised family (uses)
• Coping, ineffective (uses)
• Knowledge, deficient (teaching)

Implementation
PO route
• Do not chew, crush time rel tabs; caps may be opened and beads sprinkled over spoonful of applesauce
• Give at least 6 hr before bedtime (regular release); at least 10 hr (ext rel) to avoid sleeplessness; titrate to patient's response; lowest dosage should be used to control symptoms
• Give gum, hard candy, frequent sips of water for dry mouth at beginning of treatment; these symptoms tend to lessen with time
• Avoid Metadate CD on day of surgery
Transdermal route
• Place on clean, dry area of the hip; avoid waist; removal is 9 hr after application; fold after removal and flush down toilet
• If patch falls off, apply a new patch to a different site; total wear time should be 9 hr

Patient/family education
• Teach patient to decrease caffeine consumption (coffee, tea, cola, chocolate); not to use guarana, cola nut, yerba maté, which may increase irritability and stimulation; to avoid OTC preparations unless approved by prescriber; to avoid alcohol ingestion; these may cause serious product interactions
• Advise patient to taper off product over several wk, or depression, increased sleeping, lethargy may occur
• Caution patient to avoid hazardous activities until stabilized on medication
• Instruct patient not to double doses if medication is missed; prescriber may suggest product holidays (ADHD) during the school year to assess progress and determine continued product necessity
• Instruct patient/family to notify presciber if significant side effects occur: tremors, insomnia, palpitations, restlessness; product changes may be needed
• Inform patient that if dry mouth occurs to use frequent sips of water, sugarless gum, hard

candy during beginning therapy; dry mouth lessens with continued treatment
- Encourage patient to get needed rest; patient will feel more tired at end of day; to take last dose at least 6 hr before bedtime to avoid insomnia
- Advise patient that shell of Concerta tab may appear in stools

Evaluation
Positive therapeutic outcome
- Decreased hyperactivity in ADHD
- Improved attention span in ADHD
- Absence of sleeping during day in narcolepsy

Treatment of overdose: Administer fluids, hemodialysis, peritoneal dialysis, antihypertensives for increased B/P

---

*methylPREDNISolone (Rx)
(meth-ill-pred-niss'oh-lone)
A-Methapred, depMedalone, Depoject, Depo-Medrol, Depopred, Depo-Predate, Duralone, Medralone, Medrol, Rep-Pred, Solu-Medrol
Func. class.: Corticosteroid, synthetic
Chem. class.: Glucocorticoid, immediate acting

Pregnancy category C

Do not confuse:
methylPREDNISolone/medroxyPROGESTERone, predniSONE/methylTESTOSTERone

Action: Decreases inflammation by suppression of migration of polymorphonuclear leukocytes, fibroblasts; reverses increased capillary permeability and lysosomal stabilization

Therapeutic outcome: Decreased inflammation

Uses: Severe inflammation, shock, adrenal insufficiency, collagen disorders, management of acute spinal cord injury, multiple sclerosis

Dosage and routes
Adrenal insufficiency/ inflammation
Adult: PO 2-60 mg in 4 divided doses; IM 10-80 mg (acetate); IM/IV 10-250 mg (succinate); intraarticular 4-30 mg (acetate); RECT 40 mg 3-7 ×/wk for ≥2 wk
Child: IV 0.5-1.7 mg/kg in 3-4 divided doses (succinate); RECT 0.5-1 mg/kg (15-30 mg/m^2) daily or every other day × 1 wk or more

Shock
Adult: **IV** 100-250 mg q2-6hr or 30 mg/kg, then q4-6hr prn × 2-3 days (succinate)

Multiple sclerosis
Adult: PO 160 mg/day × 1 wk, then 64 mg every other day × 30 days

Available forms: Tabs 2, 4, 6, 8, 16, 24, 32 mg; inj 20, 40, 80 mg/ml acetate; inj 40, 125, 500, 1000, 2000 mg/vial succinate; dose pack 4 mg tabs; susp for inj 20, 40, 80 mg/ml; enema 40 mg

Adverse effects
CNS: Depression, flushing, sweating, headache, mood changes
CV: Hypertension, **circulatory collapse, thrombophlebitis, embolism,** tachycardia
EENT: Fungal infections, increased intraocular pressure, blurred vision, cataracts
GI: Diarrhea, nausea, abdominal distention, **GI hemorrhage,** increased appetite, **pancreatitis**
HEMA: **Thrombocytopenia**
INTEG: Acne, poor wound healing, ecchymosis, petechiae
MS: Fractures, osteoporosis, weakness

Contraindications: Hypersensitivity, Cushing's syndrome, measles, varicella, fungal infections

Precautions: Pregnancy C, breastfeeding, diabetes mellitus, glaucoma, osteoporosis, seizure disorders, ulcerative colitis, CHF, myasthenia gravis, renal disease, esophagitis, peptic ulcer, tartrazine, benzyl alcohol, corticosteroid hypersensitivity, viral infection, TB, traumatic brain injury

Pharmacokinetics	
Absorption	Well absorbed (PO); systemic (topical)
Distribution	Crosses placenta
Metabolism	Liver, extensively
Excretion	Kidney
Half-life	3-5 hr (plasma) 18-36 hr (tissue), adrenal suppression 3-4 days

Pharmacodynamics				
	PO	IM	IV	TOPICAL
Onset	Unknown	Unknown	Rapid	Min to hr
Peak	2 hr	4-8 days	Unknown	Hr to days
Duration	1½ days	1-4 wk	Unknown	Hr to days

Interactions
Individual drugs
Amphotericin B: increased side effects

Insulin: increased need for insulin

Phenytoin, rifampin: decreased action; increased metabolism

Somatrem: decreased effect

Drug classifications
Contraceptives, oral: increased methylPRED-NISolone action

CYP3A4 inducers (barbiturates, bosentan, carbamazepine, efavirenz, phenytoins, nevirapine, rifabutin, rifampin): decreased methylPREDNISolone effect

CYP3A4 inhibitors (aprepitant, antiretroviral protease inhibitors, clarithromycin, danazol, delavirdine, diltiazem, erythromycin, fluconazole, fluoxetine, fluvoxamine, imatinib, ketoconazole, mibefradil, nefazodone, telithromycin, voriconazole): increased adrenal suppression

Diuretics: increased side effects

Hypoglycemic agents: increased need for hypoglycemic agents

Vaccines: decreased effects of vaccines

Drug/herb
Aloe, buckthorn, cascara sagrada, Chinese rhubarb, senna: increased hypokalemia

Aloe, licorice, perilla: increased corticosteroid effect

St. John's wort: avoid use

Drug/food
Grapefruit juice: increased methylPREDNISolone level; do not use concurrently

Drug/lab test
Increased: cholesterol, sodium, blood glucose, uric acid, calcium, urine glucose

Decreased: calcium, potassium, T_4, T_3, thyroid radioactive iodine uptake test, urine 17-OHCS, 17-KS

False negative: skin allergy tests

NURSING CONSIDERATIONS
Assessment
- Monitor potassium, blood glucose, urine glucose while patient is on long-term therapy; hypokalemia and hyperglycemia
- Monitor weight daily; notify prescriber of weekly gain >5 lb
- Monitor B/P q4hr, pulse; notify prescriber if chest pain occurs
- Monitor I&O ratio; be alert for decreasing urinary output and increasing edema
- Monitor plasma cortisol levels during long-term therapy (normal level 138-635 nmol/L when drawn at 8 AM)
- Monitor adrenal function periodically for hypothalamic-pituitary-adrenal axis suppression
- Assess for infection: increased temp, WBC even after withdrawal of medication; product masks infection symptoms
- Assess for potassium depletion: paresthesias, fatigue, nausea, vomiting, depression, polyuria, dysrhythmias, weakness
- Assess for edema, hypertension, cardiac symptoms
- Assess mental status: affect, mood, behavioral changes, aggression
- Check temp; if fever develops, product should be discontinued
- Assess for systemic absorption: increased temp, inflammation, irritation (topical)

Nursing diagnoses
- Infection, risk for (adverse reactions)
- Knowledge, deficient (teaching)
- Noncompliance (teaching)

Implementation
PO route
- Give with food or milk to decrease GI symptoms

IM route
- Give IM inj deep in large muscle mass; rotate sites; avoid deltoid; use 21-G needle
- Give in one dose in AM to prevent adrenal suppression; avoid SUBCUT administration; may damage tissue

Inhalation route
- Give inh with water to decrease possibility of fungal infections
- Give titrated dosage; use lowest effective dosage
- Clean aerosol topically daily with warm water; dry thoroughly
- Store in cool environment; do not puncture or incinerate container

Topical route
- Cleanse area before applying product
- Apply only to affected areas; do not get in eyes
- Apply medication, then cover with occlusive dressing (only if prescribed); seal to normal skin; change q12hr; systemic absorption may occur
- Apply only to dermatoses; do not use on weeping, denuded, or infected area
- Apply treatment for a few days after area has cleared
- Store at room temperature

IV route
- Give **IV**, use only sodium phosphate product; give >1 min; may be given by **IV** inf in compatible sol

- Give after shaking susp (parenteral)
- Give titrated dosage; use lowest effective dosage

Syringe compatibilities: Granisetron, metoclopramide

Y-site compatibilities: Acyclovir, amifostine, aztreonam, cefepime, cisplatin, cladribine, cyclophosphamide, cytarabine, DOPamine, DOXOrubicin, enalaprilat, famotidine, fludarabine, granisetron, heparin, inamrinone, melphalan, meperidine, methotrexate, metronidazole, midazolam, morphine, piperacillin/tazobactam, sodium bicarbonate, tacrolimus, teniposide, theophylline, thiotepa, vit B with C

Y-site incompatibilities: Ondansetron, paclitaxel, sargramostim, vinorelbine

Additive compatibilities: Chloramphenicol, cimetidine, clindamycin, DOPamine, granisetron, heparin, norepinephrine, penicillin G potassium, ranitidine, theophylline, verapamil

Patient/family education
- Teach patient that emergency ID as corticosteroid user should be carried/worn
- Advise patient to notify prescriber if therapeutic response decreases; dosage adjustment may be needed
- Caution patient not to discontinue abruptly; adrenal crisis can result
- Caution patient to avoid OTC products: salicylates, alcohol in cough products, cold preparations unless directed by prescriber
- Teach patient all aspects of product usage including cushingoid symptoms
- Teach patient symptoms of adrenal insufficiency: nausea, anorexia, fatigue, dizziness, dyspnea, weakness, joint pain
- Inform patient that long-term therapy may be needed to clear infection (1-2 mo depending on type of infection)

Nasal route
- Advise patient to clear nasal passages if sneezing attack occurs; repeat dose
- Advise patient to continue using product even if mild nasal bleeding occurs; is usually transient
- Teach patient method of instillation after providing written instructions from manufacturer

Topical route
- Advise patient to avoid sunlight on affected area; burns may occur

Evaluation
Positive therapeutic outcome
- Ease of respirations, decreased inflammation
- Absence of severe itching, patches on skin, flaking (top)

metipranolol ophthalmic
See Appendix B

metoclopramide (Rx)
(met-oh-kloe-pra′mide)
Apo-Metoclop ✦, Emex ✦, Maxeran ✦, metoclopramide, metozol, Octamide, Reglan
Func. class.: Cholinergic, antiemetic
Chem. class.: Central dopamine receptor antagonist
Pregnancy category B

Do not confuse:
metoclopramide/metolazone, Reglan/Megace/Renagel

Action: Enhances response to acetylcholine of tissue in upper GI tract, which causes contraction of gastric muscle, relaxes pyloric, duodenal segments, increases peristalsis without stimulating secretions, blocks dopamine in chemoreceptor trigger zone of CNS

Therapeutic outcome: Decreased symptoms of delayed gastric emptying, decreased nausea, vomiting

Uses: Prevention of nausea, vomiting induced by chemotherapy, radiation; delayed gastric emptying, gastroesophageal reflux

Unlabeled uses: Hiccups, migraines, breastfeeding induction, lung cancer

Dosage and routes
Nausea/vomiting (chemotherapy)
Adult: **IV** 1-2 mg/kg 30 min before administration of chemotherapy, then q2hr × 2 doses, then q3hr × 3 doses
Child (unlabeled): **IV** 1-2 mg/kg/dose

Facilitation of small bowel intubation in radiologic exams
Adult and child >14 yr: **IV** 10 mg over 1-2 min
Child 6-14 yr: **IV** 2.5-5 mg
Child <6 yr: **IV** 0.1 mg/kg

Diabetic gastroparesis
Adult: **PO** 10 mg 30 min before meals, at bedtime × 2-8 wk

Adverse effects: *italic* = common, **bold** = life-threatening

Geriatric: PO 5 mg ½ hr before meals, at bedtime, increase to 10 mg if needed

Gastroesophageal reflux
Adult: PO 10-15 mg qid 30 min before meals and at bedtime
Child: PO 0.4-0.8 mg/kg/day divided in 4 doses

Hiccups (unlabeled)
Adult: PO/IM/**IV** 10 mg q6hr

Lactation induction (unlabeled)
Adult: PO 10 mg bid-tid, may increase to 20-45 mg/day in divided doses

Non–small cell lung cancer (NSCLC) radiation sensitizer (unlabeled) (Sensamide IV)
Adult: **IV** 2 mg/kg given 1 hr prior to radiation therapy 3 ×/wk

Renal dose
Adult: **IV** CCr <40 ml/min 50% of dose

Available forms: Tabs 5, 10 mg; syr 5 mg/5 ml; inj 5 mg/ml, conc sol 10 mg/ml

Adverse effects

CNS: Sedation, fatigue, restlessness, head-ache, sleeplessness, dystonia, dizziness, drowsiness, **suicidal ideation, seizures,** EPS, **neuroleptic malignant syndrome; tardive dyskinesia** (>3 mo, high doses)
CV: Hypotension, **supraventricular tachy-cardia**
GI: Dry mouth, constipation, nausea, anorexia, vomiting, diarrhea
GU: Decreased libido, prolactin secretion, amenorrhea, galactorrhea
HEMA: **Neutropenia, leukopenia, agranu-locytosis**
INTEG: Urticaria, rash

Contraindications: Hypersensitivity to this product or procaine or procainamide, seizure disorder, pheochromocytoma, breast cancer (prolactin dependent), GI obstruction

Precautions: Pregnancy **B,** breastfeeding, GI hemorrhage, CHF, Parkinson's disease

Black Box Warning: Tardive dyskinesia

Pharmacokinetics

Absorption	Well absorbed (PO)
Distribution	Widely distributed; crosses blood-brain barrier, placenta
Metabolism	Liver, minimally
Excretion	Kidneys, breast milk
Half-life	4 hr

Pharmacodynamics

	PO	IM	IV
Onset	½-1 hr	10-15 min	1-3 min
Peak	Unknown	Unknown	Unknown
Duration	1-2 hr	1-2 hr	1-2 hr

Interactions
Individual drugs
Alcohol: increased sedation
Haloperidol: increased extrapyramidal reaction

Drug classifications
Anticholinergics, opiates: decreased action of metoclopramide
CNS depressants: increased sedation
MAOIs: avoid use
Phenothiazines: increased extrapyramidal reaction

Drug/lab test
Increased: prolactin, aldosterone, thyrotropin

NURSING CONSIDERATIONS
Assessment
• Assess GI complaints: nausea, vomiting, anorexia, constipation, abdominal distention before, after administration
• Assess for EPS and tardive dyskinesia; more likely to occur in geriatric patient: rigidity, grimacing, shuffling gait, tremors, rhythmic involuntary movements of tongue, mouth, jaw, feet, hands; these side effects should be reported to prescriber immediately; some effects may be irreversible
• Assess mental status: depression, anxiety, irritability during treatment

Nursing diagnoses
• Injury, risk for (adverse reactions)
• Knowledge, deficient (teaching)

Implementation
PO route
• Use gum, hard candy, frequent rinsing of mouth for dryness of oral cavity
• Give ½-1 hr before meals for better absorption
IV route
• Give **IV** undiluted if dose is ≤10 mg; give over 2 min
• Dilute more than 10 mg in 50 ml or more D₅W, NaCl, Ringer's, LR and give over 15 min or more
• Give diphenhydrAMINE **IV** for EPS
• Discard open ampules
Syringe compatibilities: Aminophyl-line, ascorbic acid, atropine, benztropine, bleomycin, butorphanol, chlorproMAZINE, cisplatin, cyclophosphamide, cytarabine, dexamethasone, dimenhyDRINATE, diphenhy-

drAMINE, DOXOrubicin, droperidol, fentanyl, fluorouracil, heparin, hydrocortisone, hydrOXYzine, regular insulin, leucovorin, lidocaine, magnesium sulfate, meperidine, methotrimeprazine, methylPREDNISolone, midazolam, mitomycin, morphine, pentazocine, perphenazine, prochlorperazine, promazine, promethazine, ranitidine, scopolamine, sufentanil, vinBLAStine, vinCRIStine, vit B/C

Syringe incompatibilities: Ampicillin, calcium gluconate, cephalothin, chloramphenicol, furosemide, penicillin G potassium, sodium bicarbonate

Y-site compatibilities: Acyclovir, aldesleukin, amifostine, aztreonam, bleomycin, ciprofloxacin, cisplatin, cladribine, cyclophosphamide, cytarabine, diltiazem, DOXOrubicin, droperidol, famotidine, filgrastim, fluconazole, fludarabine, fluorouracil, foscarnet, gallium, granisetron, heparin, Idarubicin, leucovorin, melphalan, meperidine, meropenem, methotrexate, mitomycin, morphine, ondansetron, paclitaxel, piperacillin/tazobactam, propofol, sargramostim, sufentanil, tacrolimus, teniposide, thiotepa, vinBLAStine, vinCRIStine, vinorelbine, zidovudine

Y-site incompatibilities: Furosemide
Additive compatibilities: Clindamycin, meropenem, morphine, multivitamins, potassium acetate/chloride/phosphate, verapamil
Additive incompatibilities: Cisplatin, erythromycin, tetracycline

Patient/family education
• Instruct patient to avoid driving, other hazardous activities until stabilized on this medication
• Advise patient to avoid alcohol and other CNS depressants that enhance sedating properties of this product
• Advise patient to notify prescriber if involuntary movements occur

Evaluation
Positive therapeutic outcome
• Absence of nausea, vomiting, anorexia, fullness

metolazone (Rx)
(me-tole′a-zone)
Zaroxolyn
Func. class.: Diuretic, antihypertensive
Chem. class.: Thiazide-like quinazoline derivative

Pregnancy category B

Do not confuse:
metolazone/methotrexate/metoclopramide

Action: Acts on the distal tubule and cortical thick ascending limb of the loop of Henle in the kidney, increasing excretion of sodium, water, chloride, magnesium, potassium, and bicarbonate

Therapeutic outcome: Decreased B/P, decreased edema in lung tissue and peripherally

Uses: Edema in CHF, nephrotic syndrome; may be used alone or as adjunct with antihypertensives for mild to moderate hypertension

Dosage and routes
Edema
Adult: PO 2.5-20 mg/day; max 20 mg/day

Hypertension
Adult: PO 2.5-5 mg/day

Available forms: Tabs 2.5, 5, 10 mg

Adverse effects
CNS: Anxiety, depression, headache, *dizziness, fatigue, weakness*
CV: Orthostatic hypotension, palpitations, volume depletion, chest pain, hypotension
EENT: Blurred vision
ELECT: Hypokalemia, hypercalcemia, hyponatremia
GI: Nausea, vomiting, anorexia, constipation, diarrhea, cramps, **pancreatitis,** GI irritation, dry mouth, jaundice
GU: Frequency, polyuria, **uremia,** glucosuria, nocturia, impotence
HEMA: **Aplastic anemia, hemolytic anemia, leukopenia, agranulocytosis, neutropenia**
INTEG: Rash, urticaria, purpura, photosensitivity, fever, dry skin
META: Hyperglycemia, increased creatinine, BUN

Contraindications: Hypersensitivity to thiazides or sulfonamides, anuria

Black Box Warning: Hepatic encephalopathy

Precautions: Pregnancy **B**, breastfeeding, geriatric, hypokalemia, renal/hepatic disease, gout, COPD, lupus erythematosus, diabetes

M

Adverse effects: *italic* = common, **bold** = life-threatening

mellitus, hypotension, history of pancreatitis, hypersensitivity to sulfonamides, thiazides

Pharmacokinetics

Absorption	GI tract (10%-20%)
Distribution	Crosses placenta
Metabolism	Urine, unchanged
Excretion	Breast milk
Half-life	8 hr (extended); 14 hr (prompt)

Pharmacodynamics

Onset	1 hr
Peak	2 hr
Duration	12-24 hr

Interactions
Individual drugs
Alcohol: increased hypotension (large amounts)

Amphotericin B, digoxin, mezlocillin, piperacillin: increased hypokalemia

Lithium: increased toxicity

Drug classifications
Antihypertensives: increased antihypertensive effect

Barbiturates, nitrates, opioids: increased hypotension

Diuretics (loop): increased metolazone effect

Glucocorticoids, laxatives (stimulant): increased hypokalemia

NSAIDs, salicylates: decreased action of metolazone

Drug/herb
Aconite: increased toxicity, death

Aloe, buckthorn, cascara sagrada, rhubarb, senna: increased hypokalemia

Astragalus, cola tree: increased or decreased antihypertensive effect

Barberry, betony, black catechu, black cohosh, bloodroot, broom, burdock, cat's claw, dandelion, goldenseal, Irish moss, Jamaican dogwood, kelp, khella, mistletoe, parsley: increased antihypertensive effect

Coltsfoot, guarana, khat, licorice: decreased antihypertensive effect

NURSING CONSIDERATIONS
Assessment
• Monitor blood glucose if patient is diabetic
• Check for rashes, temp elevation daily
• Monitor patients receiving cardiac glycosides for increased hypokalemia
• Monitor manifestations of hypokalemia; acidic urine, reduced urine, osmolality, nocturia; hypotension, broad T-wave, U-wave, ectopy, tachycardia, weak pulse; muscle weakness, altered LOC, drowsiness, apathy, lethargy, confusion, depression; anorexia, nausea, cramps, constipation, distention, paralytic ileus; hypoventilation, respiratory muscle weakness
• Monitor for manifestations of hypomagnesemia: agitation, muscle twitching, paresthesias, hyperactive reflexes, positive Babinski reflex, dysphagia, nystagmus seizures, tetany; nausea, vomiting, diarrhea, anorexia, abdominal distention; ectopy, tachycardia, broad, flat, or inverted T-waves, depressed ST segment, prolonged QT interval, decreased cardiac output, hypotension
• Monitor for manifestations of hyponatremia; increased B/P, cold, clammy skin, hypovolemia or hypervolemia; anorexia, nausea, vomiting, diarrhea, abdominal cramps; lethargy, increased ICP, confusion, headache, seizures, coma, fatigue, tremors, hyperreflexia
• Monitor for manifestations of hyperchloremia: weakness, lethargy, coma, deep rapid breathing
• Assess and record fluid volume status: I&O ratios; monitor weight, distended red veins, crackles in lung, color, quality and specific gravity of urine, skin turgor, adequacy of pulses, moist mucous membranes, bilateral lung sounds, peripheral pitting edema; dehydration symptoms of decreasing output, thirst, hypotension, dry mouth and mucous membranes should be reported
• Monitor electrolytes: potassium, sodium, calcium, magnesium; also include BUN, blood pH, ABGs, uric acid, CBC, blood glucose
• Assess B/P before, during therapy with patient lying, standing, and sitting as appropriate; orthostatic hypotension can occur rapidly

Nursing diagnoses
• Fluid volume, deficient (adverse reactions)
• Fluid volume, excess (uses)
• Knowledge, deficient (teaching)
• Urinary elimination, impaired (adverse reactions)

Implementation
• Give in AM to avoid interference with sleep
• Provide potassium replacement if potassium level is 3.0; product may be crushed if patient is unable to swallow
• Give with food; if nausea occurs, absorption may be increased; extended-release product is Zaroxolyn; prompt action product is Mykrox; the two formulations are not equivalent

Patient/family education
• Teach patient to take the medication early in the day to prevent nocturia
• Instruct patient to take with food or milk if GI symptoms of nausea and anorexia occur

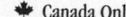 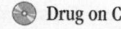

- Teach patient to maintain a weekly record of weight and notify prescriber of weight loss >5 lb
- Caution patient that this product causes a loss of potassium, so foods rich in potassium should be added to the diet; refer to a dietitian for assistance in planning
- Caution the patient to rise slowly from sitting or reclining positions, not to exercise in hot weather or stand for prolonged periods, since orthostatic hypotension will be enhanced; lie down if dizziness occurs
- Teach patient not to use alcohol or any OTC medications without prescriber's approval; serious product reactions may occur
- Emphasize the need to contact prescriber immediately if muscle cramps, weakness, nausea, dizziness, or numbness occur
- Teach patient to take own B/P and pulse and record
- Advise patient to use sunscreen to prevent burns
- Teach patient to continue taking medication even if feeling better; this product controls symptoms but does not cure the condition
- Advise patient with hypertension to continue other medical regimen (exercise, weight loss, relaxation techniques, cessation of smoking)

Evaluation
Positive therapeutic outcome
- Decreased edema
- Decreased B/P

Treatment of overdose: Lavage if taken orally, monitor electrolytes; administer dextrose in saline; monitor hydration, CV, renal status

metoprolol (Rx)
(met-oh-proe'lole)
Betaloc ✤, Betaloc Durules ✤, Lopresor ✤, Lopressor, Lopressor SR ✤, Novometoprol ✤, Nu-Metop ✤, Toprol-XL
Func. class.: Antihypertensive, antianginal
Chem. class.: β₁-Adrenergic blocker

Pregnancy category C

Do not confuse:
metoprolol/misoprostol

Action: Competitively blocks stimulation of β₁-adrenergic receptor within vascular smooth muscle; produces chronotropic, inotropic activity (decreases rate of SA node discharge, increases recovery time), slows conduction of AV node, decreases heart rate, which decreases O_2 consumption in myocardium; also decreases renin-aldosterone-angiotensin system at high doses, negative chronotropic effect

Therapeutic outcome: Decreased B/P, heart rate, AV conduction

Uses: Mild to moderate hypertension, acute MI to reduce cardiovascular mortality, angina pectoris, New York Heart Association class II, III heart failure

Dosage and routes
Hypertension
Adult: PO 50 mg bid, or 100 mg/day; may give 200-450 mg in divided doses; EXT REL 25-100 mg qd, titrate at weekly intervals
Child/adolescent 6-16 yr: PO EXT REL 1 mg/kg up to 50 mg qd
Geriatric: PO 25 mg/day initially, increase weekly as needed

MI
Adult: **IV** BOL (early treatment) 5 mg q2 min × 3 doses, then 50 mg PO 15 min after last dose and q6hr × 48 hr (late treatment); PO maintenance 100 mg bid for ≥3 mo

Heart failure (NYHA class II/III)
Adult: PO EXT REL 25 mg qd × 2 wk (class II); 12.5 mg qd (class III)

Angina
Adult: PO 100 mg/day as a single dose or in 2 divided doses, increase qwk as needed, or 100 mg EXT REL tab daily

Migraine prevention (unlabeled)
Adult: PO 50-100 mg bid-qid

Available forms: Tabs 50, 100 mg; inj 1 mg/ml; ext rel tabs (tartrate) 100 mg; ext rel tabs (succinate) (XL) 25, 50, 100, 200 mg

Adverse effects
CNS: Insomnia, dizziness, mental changes, hallucinations, depression, anxiety, headaches, nightmares, confusion, fatigue
CV: **CHF,** *palpitations,* dysrhythmias, **cardiac arrest, AV block,** hypotension, **bradycardia, pulmonary/peripheral edema, chest pain**
EENT: Sore throat, dry burning eyes
GI: Nausea, vomiting, colitis, cramps, *diarrhea,* constipation, flatulence, dry mouth, *hiccups*
GU: Impotence
HEMA: **Agranulocytosis, eosinophilia, thrombocytopenic purpura**
INTEG: Rash, purpura, alopecia, dry skin, urticaria, pruritus
RESP: **Bronchospasm,** dyspnea, wheezing

Adverse effects: *italic* = common, **bold** = life-threatening

Contraindications: Hypersensitivity to β-blockers, cardiogenic shock, heart block (2nd- and 3rd-degree), sinus bradycardia, pheochromocytoma, sick sinus syndrome

Precautions: Pregnancy **C**, breastfeeding, geriatric, major surgery, diabetes mellitus, thyroid/renal/hepatic disease, COPD, CAD, nonallergic bronchospasm, CHF, bronchial asthma, CVA, children, depression, vasospastic angina

Pharmacokinetics

Absorption	Well absorbed (PO); completely absorbed (**IV**)
Distribution	Crosses blood-brain barrier, placenta
Metabolism	Liver, extensively
Excretion	Kidneys, breast milk
Half-life	3-4 hr

Pharmacodynamics

	PO	IV
Onset	15 min	Immediate
Peak	2-4 hr	20 min
Duration	6-19 hr	5-8 hr

Interactions
Individual drugs
Cimetidine: increased metoprolol level
DOBUTamine: decreased effect of DOBUTamine
DOPamine: decreased DOPamine
epinephrine, hydrALAZINE, methyldopa prazosin, reserpine: increased hypotension, bradycardia
Insulin: increased hypoglycemia
Drug classifications
Antidiabetics (oral): increased hypoglycemia
Amphetamines, calcium channel blockers, histamine H$_2$ antagonists: increased hypotension, bradycardia
Barbiturates: decreased metoprolol level
Benzodiazepines: increased effect of benzodiazepines
MAOIs: do not use together
NSAIDs, salicylates: decreased antihypertensive effect
Xanthines: decreased effects of xanthines
Drug/herb
Aconite: increased toxicity, death
Astragalus, cola tree: increased or decreased antihypertensive effect
Barberry, betony, black catechu, black cohosh, bloodroot, broom, burdock, cat's claw, dandelion, goldenseal, Irish moss, Jamaican dogwood, kelp, khella, mistletoe, parsley: increased antihypertensive effect

Coltsfoot, guarana, khat, licorice: decreased antihypertensive effect
Drug/food
Increased: absorption with food
Drug/lab test
Increased: BUN, potassium, ANA titer, serum lipoprotein, triglycerides, uric acid, alkaline phosphatase, LDH, AST, ALT

NURSING CONSIDERATIONS
Assessment
• Monitor B/P during beginning treatment, periodically thereafter; pulse q4hr; note rate, rhythm, quality; check apical/radial pulse before administration; notify prescriber of any significant changes (pulse <50 bpm)
• Check for baselines in renal, liver function tests before therapy begins and periodically thereafter
• Assess for edema in feet, legs daily; monitor I&O, daily weight; check for jugular vein distention, crackles bilaterally, dyspnea (CHF)
• Monitor skin turgor, dryness of mucous membranes for hydration status, especially geriatric

Nursing diagnoses
• Cardiac output, decreased (uses)
• Injury, risk for (adverse reactions)
• Knowledge, deficient (teaching)
• Noncompliance (teaching)

Implementation
PO route
• Do not break, crush, or chew ext rel tabs
• Give regular release tab before meals, at bedtime; tab may be crushed or swallowed whole; give with food to prevent GI upset; reduced dosage in renal dysfunction; take at same time each day
• Store protected from light, moisture; place in cool environment
IV route
• Give by direct **IV** 5 mg/2 min or more × 3 doses at 2 min intervals, start PO 15 min after last **IV** dose
Y-site compatibilities:
Alteplase, meperidine, morphine

Patient/family education
• Teach patient not to discontinue product abruptly; taper over 2 wk; may cause precipitate angina if stopped abruptly
• Teach patient not to use OTC products containing α-adrenergic stimulants (such as nasal decongestants, cold preparations); to avoid alcohol, smoking and to limit sodium intake as prescribed
• Teach patient how to take pulse and B/P at home; advise when to notify prescriber

• Instruct patient to comply with weight control, dietary adjustments, modified exercise program
• Tell patient to carry/wear emergency ID to identify product being taken, allergies; tell patient product controls symptoms but does not cure
• Caution patient to avoid hazardous activities if dizziness, drowsiness is present, to avoid driving until product response is known
• Teach patient to report symptoms of CHF; difficult breathing, especially with exertion or when lying down, night cough, swelling of extremities or bradycardia, dizziness, confusion, depression, fever, decreased vision
• Teach patient to take product as prescribed, not to double doses or skip doses; take any missed doses as soon as remembered if at least 4 hr until next dose
• Advise to monitor blood glucose closely if diabetic
• Advise to report Raynaud's symptoms

Evaluation
Positive therapeutic outcome
• Decreased B/P in hypertension (after 1-2 wk)
• Absence of dysrhythmias
• Decreased anginal pain

Treatment of overdose. Lavage, **IV** atropine for bradycardia, **IV** theophylline for bronchospasm, digoxin, O₂, diuretic for cardiac failure, hemodialysis, **IV** glucose for hyperglycemia, **IV** diazepam (or phenytoin) for seizures

---

metronidazole (Rx)
(me-troe-ni′da-zole)
Apo-Metronidazole ✦, Flagyl, Flagyl ER, Flagyl IV, Flagyl IV RTU, Metronidazole, Novonidazole ✦
Func. class.: Trichomonacide, amebicide, antiinfective
Chem. class.: Nitroimidazole derivative

Pregnancy category B
(2nd, 3rd trimesters)

Action: Direct-acting amebicide/ trichomonacide; binds, degrades DNA structure, inhibiting bacterial nucleic acid synthesis

Therapeutic outcome: Trichomonacidal, amebicidal, bactericidal for the following susceptible organisms: *Bacteroides, Clostridium, Trichomonas vaginalis, Giardia lamblia, Entamoeba histolytica*

Uses: Intestinal amebiasis, amebic abscess, trichomoniasis, refractory trichomoniasis, bacterial anaerobic infections, giardiasis; septicemia, endocarditis, bone, joint, and lower respiratory tract infections, rosacea

Unlabeled uses: Crohn's disease

Dosage and routes
Trichomoniasis
Adult: PO 250 mg tid × 7 days or 2 g in single dose; do not repeat treatment for 4-6 wk
Child (unlabeled): PO 15 mg/kg/day divided in 3 doses × 7-10 days

Refractory trichomoniasis
Adult: PO 250 mg bid × 10 days

Amebic hepatic abscess
Adult: PO 500-750 mg tid × 5-10 days
Child: PO 35-50 mg/kg/day in 3 divided doses × 10 days

Intestinal amebiasis
Adult: PO 750 mg tid × 5-10 days
Child: PO 35-50 mg/kg/day in 3 divided doses × 10 days; then oral iodoquinol

Anaerobic bacterial infections
Adult: **IV** INF 15 mg/kg/over 1 hr, then 7.5 mg/kg **IV** or PO q6hr, max 4 g/day; first maintenance dose should be administered 6 hr after loading dose

Bacterial vaginosis
Adult: PO EXT REL 750 mg/day × 7 days

Giardiasis (unlabeled)
Adult: PO 250 mg tid × 5 days
Child: PO 5 mg/kg tid × 5 days

Antibiotic-associated pseudomembranous colitis
Adult (unlabeled): PO 250-500 mg 3-4 ×/day × 10-14 days
Child: PO 20 mg/kg/day (max 2 g) divided q6hr

Available forms: Tabs 250, 500 mg; ext rel tabs 750 mg; caps 375, 500 mg; inj 500 mg/100 ml; powder for inj 500 mg single dose

Adverse effects
CNS: Headache, dizziness, confusion, irritability, restlessness, ataxia, depression, fatigue, drowsiness, insomnia, paresthesia, peripheral neuropathy, **seizures,** incoordination, depression, encephalopathy
CV: Flat T-waves
EENT: Blurred vision, sore throat, retinal edema, dry mouth, metallic taste, furry tongue, glossitis, stomatitis, photophobia
GI: Nausea, vomiting, diarrhea, epigastric distress, *anorexia,* constipation, *abdominal cramps,* **pseudomembranous colitis**

M

Adverse effects: *italic* = common, **bold** = life-threatening

GU: Darkened urine, vaginal dryness, polyuria, **albuminuria,** dysuria, cystitis, decreased libido, **nephrotoxicity,** incontinence, dyspareunia, candidiasis
HEMA: **Leukopenia, bone marrow depression, aplasia**
INTEG: Rash, pruritus, urticaria, flushing

Contraindications: Pregnancy (1st trimester), breastfeeding, hypersensitivity to this product, renal/hepatic/GI disease, contracted visual or color fields, blood dyscrasias, CNS disorders

Precautions: Pregnancy **B** (2nd/3rd trimesters), candidal infections, heart failure, fungal infection, geriatric, dental disease, bone marrow suppression, hematologic disease

Black Box Warning: Secondary malignancy

Pharmacokinetics

Absorption	80% (PO)
Distribution	Widely distributed, crosses placenta
Metabolism	Liver
Excretion	Urine, unchanged; feces
Half-life	6-11 hr

Pharmacodynamics

	PO	IV
Onset	Rapid	Immediate
Peak	1-2 hr	Infusion's end
Duration	Unknown	Unknown

Interactions
Individual drugs
Alcohol: increased disulfiram-like reaction
Azathioprine, fluorouracil: increased leukopenia
Cimetidine: increased metronidazole level
Cimetidine, phenobarbital, phenytoin: decreased effect of metronidazole
Warfarin: increased action of warfarin
Drug/herb
Acidophilus: do not use with antiinfectives; separate by several hours
Drug/lab test
Altered: AST, ALT, LDH

NURSING CONSIDERATIONS
Assessment
• Assess patient for signs and symptoms of infection including characteristics of wounds, WBC >10,000/mm^3, vaginal secretions, fever; obtain baseline information and during treatment
• Obtain C&S before beginning product therapy to identify if correct treatment has been initiated

• Assess for allergic reactions: rash, urticaria, pruritus
• Identify urine output; if decreasing, notify prescriber (may indicate nephrotoxicity); also check for increased BUN, creatinine
• Assess bowel pattern daily; if severe diarrhea occurs, product should be discontinued
• Assess for overgrowth of infection: perineal itching, fever, malaise, redness, pain, swelling, drainage, rash, diarrhea, change in cough, sputum

Nursing diagnoses
• Diarrhea (adverse reactions)
• Infection, risk for (uses)
• Injury, risk for (adverse reactions)
• Knowledge, deficient (teaching)
• Noncompliance (teaching)

Implementation
PO route
• Give with or after a meal to avoid GI symptoms, metallic taste; crush tab if needed
• Store in light-resistant container; do not refrigerate
Topical route
• A thin coating should be applied to affected area after cleaning with soap and water and patting dry
IV route
• Give intermittent **IV** prediluted; for Flagyl **IV** dilute with 4.4 ml of sterile water or 0.9% NaCl; must be diluted further with 8 mg/ml or more 0.9% NaCl, D$_5$W, or LR; must neutralize with 5 mEq of NaCO$_3$/500 mg; CO$_2$ gas will be generated and may require venting; run over 1 hr or more; primary **IV** must be discontinued; may be given as cont inf; do not use aluminum products; **IV** may require venting
Y-site compatibilities: Acyclovir, allopurinol, amifostine, amiodarone, cefepime, cyclophosphamide, diltiazem, DOPamine, enalaprilat, esmolol, fluconazole, foscarnet, granisetron, heparin, hydromorphone, labetalol, lorazepam, magnesium sulfate, melphalan, meperidine, methylPREDNISolone, midazolam, morphine, perphenazine, piperacillin/ tazobactam, sargramostim, tacrolimus, teniposide, theophylline, thiotepa, vinorelbine
Additive compatibilities: Amikacin, aminophylline, cefazolin, cefotaxime, ceftazidime, ceftizoxime, ceftriaxone, cefuroxime, chloramphenicol, ciprofloxacin, clindamycin, disopyramide, floxacillin, fluconazole, gentamicin, heparin, moxalactam, multielectrolyte concentrate, multivitamins, netilmicin, penicillin G potassium, tobramycin

---

Patient/family education
- Teach patient to report sore throat, bruising, bleeding, joint pain; may indicate blood dyscrasias (rare)
- Advise patient to contact prescriber if vaginal itching, loose foul-smelling stools, furry tongue occur; may indicate superinfection
- Advise patient to notify physician of numbness or tingling of extremities
- Teach trichomoniasis patient that both partners need to be treated; condoms should be used during intercourse to prevent reinfection
- Advise patient of disulfiram-like reaction to alcohol ingestion; alcohol should not be used within 48 hr of this product
- Inform patient product has a metallic taste and urine may turn dark
- Advise patient to contact prescriber if pregnancy is suspected
- Advise patient to use sips of water, sugarless gum, candy for dry mouth

Evaluation
Positive therapeutic outcome
- Decreased symptoms of infection

metronidazole topical
See Appendix B

mexiletine (Rx)
(mex-il′e-teen)
Func. class.: Antidysrhythmic (class IB)
Chem. class.: Lidocaine analog

Pregnancy category C

Action: Increases electrical stimulation threshold of ventricle and His-Purkinje system, which stabilizes cardiac membrane and decreases automaticity

Therapeutic outcome: Decreased ventricular dysrhythmia

Uses: Life-threatening ventricular tachycardia; because of proarrhythmic effects, use with lesser dysrhythmias is not recommended

Unlabeled uses: Neuropathic pain

Dosage and routes
Adult: PO 200-400 mg (loading dose), then 200 mg q8hr, then 200-400 mg q8hr

Neuropathic pain (unlabeled)
Adult: PO 450-600 mg/day

Available forms: Caps 150, 200, 250 mg

Adverse effects
CNS: Headache, dizziness, confusion, **seizures**, tremors, psychosis, nervousness, paresthesias, weakness, fatigue, coordination difficulties, change in sleep habits
CV: Hypotension, bradycardia, angina, PVCs, **heart block, cardiovascular collapse, arrest**, sinus node slowing, **left ventricular failure**, syncope, **cardiogenic shock, AV conduction disturbances, CHF, atrial dysrhythmias, palpitations, ventricular dysrhythmias, ventricular tachycardia, other ventricular arrhythmias in acute phase of MI**
EENT: Blurred vision, tinnitus
GI: Nausea, vomiting, anorexia, diarrhea, abdominal pain, **hepatitis**, dry mouth, peptic ulcer, altered taste, **GI bleeding**, constipation
GU: Urinary hesitancy, decreased libido
HEMA: **Thrombocytopenia, leukopenia, agranulocytosis**
INTEG: Rash, alopecia, dry skin
MISC: Edema, arthralgia, fever, systemic lupus erythematosus syndrome
RESP: Dyspnea

Contraindications: Hypersensitivity, cardiogenic shock, severe heart block (if no pacemaker)

Precautions: Pregnancy C, breastfeeding, children, hepatic disease, CHF, seizure disorders, hypotension, renal disease, blood dyscrasias, electrolyte imbalances, Parkinson's disease

Black Box Warning: MI, cardiac arrhythmias

Pharmacokinetics
Absorption	Well absorbed
Distribution	Body tissues
Metabolism	Liver, extensively
Excretion	Kidneys, unchanged (10%)
Half-life	12 hr

Pharmacodynamics
Onset	½-2 hr
Peak	2-3 hr
Duration	8-12 hr

Interactions
Individual drugs
Atropine, aluminum/magnesium hydroxide, phenobarbital, phenytoin, rifampin: decreased mexiletine levels
Caffeine, theophylline: increased levels of each
Cimetidine: increased or decreased mexiletine effects

Adverse effects: *italic* = common, **bold** = life-threatening

Metoclopramide: increased effects of mexiletine

Drug classifications

Acidifers (urinary), opiates: decreased mexiletine levels

Alkalinizers (urinary): increased mexiletine levels

Smoking: decreased mexiletine effect

Drug/herb

Aconite: increased toxicity, death

Aloe, broom, buckthorn (chronic use), cascara sagrada (chronic use), Chinese rhubarb, figwort, fumitory, goldenseal, kudzu, licorice: increased effect

Aloe, buckthorn, cascara sagrada, rhubarb, senna: increased hypokalemia, increased antidysrhythmic action

Coltsfoot: decreased effect

Horehound: increased serotonin effect

Drug/lab test

Increased: CPK, LFTs

NURSING CONSIDERATIONS
Assessment

• Assess for oxygenation or perfusion deficit: decreased B/P, chest pain, dizziness, loss of consciousness

• Assess respiratory status: auscultate lung fields for bibasilar crackles in patients with advanced CHF

• Assess for urinary retention: check for pain, abdominal absorption, palpate bladder; check males with benign prostatic hypertrophy; anticholinergic reaction may cause retention

• Monitor I&O ratio; electrolytes; potassium, sodium, chloride; watch for decreasing urinary output, possible retention

• Monitor liver function tests: AST, ALT, bilirubin, alkaline phosphatase

• Monitor ECG periodically to determine product effectiveness; measure PR, QRS, QT intervals; check for PVCs, other dysrhythmias; assess B/P for hypo/hypertension, for rebound hypertension after 1-2 hr; for prolonged PR/QT intervals, QRS complex; if QT or QRS increase by 50% or more, withhold next dose, notify prescriber

• Monitor for dehydration and hypovolemia

• Monitor blood levels (therapeutic level 0.5-2 mcg/ml), notify prescriber of abnormal results

• Assess pulmonary toxicity: dyspnea, fatigue, cough, fever, chest pain; product should be discontinued

• Assess cardiac rate, respiration: rate, rhythm, character, chest pain, ventricular tachycardia, supraventricular tachycardia, fibrillation

Nursing diagnoses

• Cardiac output, decreased (uses)
• Gas exchange, impaired (adverse reactions)
• Knowledge, deficient (teaching)

Implementation

• Give with meals for GI upset

Patient/family education

• Teach patient to report side effects immediately to prescriber; to take exactly as prescribed; if dose is missed, take when remembered if within 3-4 hr of next dose; do not double doses

• Caution patient to avoid temperature extremes; impairment of heat-regulating mechanism can occur

• Encourage patient to complete follow-up appointment with health care provider, including pulmonary function tests, chest x-ray

• Instruct patient that dry mouth may be relieved by frequent sips of water, hard candy, sugarless gum

• Caution patient to make position changes from lying to standing slowly to prevent orthostatic hypotension

Evaluation
Positive therapeutic outcome

• Decreased B/P, dysrhythmias
• Decreased heart rate
• Normal sinus rhythm

Treatment of overdose: O$_2$, artificial ventilation, ECG monitoring, administer DOPamine for circulatory depression, administer diazepam or thiopental for seizures, isoproterenol

micafungin (Rx)
(my-ca-fun'gin)
Mycamine
Func. class.: Antifungal, systemic
Chem. class.: Echinocandin
Pregnancy category C

Action: Inhibits an essential component in fungal cell walls; causes direct damage to fungal cell wall

Therapeutic outcome: Prevention of *Candida* infection in HSTC; or decreased symptoms of candida infection, negative culture

Uses: Treatment of esophageal candidiasis; prophylaxis of *Candida* infections in patients undergoing hematopoietic stem cell transplantation (HSCT); susceptible *Candida* species: *C.*

albicans, C. glabrata, C. krusei, C. parapsilosis, C. tropicalis

Dosage and routes
Esophageal candidiasis
Adult: IV 150 mg/day, given over 1 hr
Prophylaxis of Candida infections
Adult: IV 50 mg/day, given over 1 hr

Available forms: Powder for injection 50 mg, in single-dose vials; 50, 100 mg vial

Adverse effects
CNS: Convulsions, dizziness, *headache, somnolence*
CV: Flushing, hypertension, phlebitis
GI: Abdominal pain, *nausea, anorexia, vomiting, diarrhea, increased AST, ALT, alkaline phosphatase, blood dehydrogenase, hyperbilirubinemia*
HEMA: Neutropenia, thrombocytopenia, leukopenia, coagulopathy, anemia, hemolytic anemia
INTEG: *Rash, pruritus, inj site pain*
META: Hypokalemia, hypocalcemia, hypomagnesemia
MS: *Rigors*

Contraindications: Hypersensitivity to this product or other echinocandins

Precautions: Pregnancy **C**, breastfeeding, children, geriatric, severe hepatic disease

Pharmacokinetics

Absorption	Unknown
Distribution	Protein binding 99%
Metabolism	Liver
Excretion	Feces, urine
Half-life	Terminal 14-20 hr

Pharmacodynamics

Unknown

Interactions
Individual drugs
Sirolimus, nifedipine: increased plasma concentrations; may need dosage reduction

NURSING CONSIDERATIONS
Assessment
- Assess for signs and symptoms of infection, clearing of cultures during treatment; obtain culture baseline, throughout; product may be started as soon as culture is taken (esophageal candidiasis); monitor cultures during HSCT, for prevention of *Candida* infections
- Monitor CBC (RBC, Hct, Hgb), differential, platelet count periodically; notify prescriber of results

- Monitor renal studies: BUN, urine CCr, electrolytes before, during therapy
- Monitor hepatic studies before, during treatment: bilirubin, AST, ALT, alkaline phosphatase, as needed
- Assess for bleeding: hematuria, heme-positive stools, bruising or petechiae, mucosa or orifices; blood dyscrasias can occur
- Assess for hypersensitivity: rash, pruritus, facial swelling; also for phlebitis
- Assess for hemolytic anemia
- Assess GI symptoms: frequency of stools, cramping; if severe diarrhea occurs, electrolytes may need to be given

Nursing diagnoses
- Infection, risk for (uses)
- Injury, risk for (adverse reactions)
- Knowledge, deficient (teaching)

Implementation
- Do not use if cloudy or precipitated; do not admix product
- Flush line before, after administration with 0.9% NaCl
IV route
- For *Candida* prevention, reconstitute with provided diluent 0.9% NaCl without bacteriostatic product; 50 mg vial/5 ml (10 mg/ml), swirl to dissolve, do not shake; further dilute with 100 ml 0.9% NaCl, only, run over 1 hr
- For *Candida* infection, reconstitute with provided diluent 50 mg/5 ml (10 mg/ml); further dilute 3 reconstituted vials in 100 ml of 0.9% NaCl, run over 1 hr
- Store at room temperature, away from light; do not freeze; discard unused solution

Patient/family education
- Advise patient to notify prescriber if pregnancy is suspected or planned; use nonhormonal form of contraception while taking this product
- Teach patient to avoid breastfeeding while taking this product
- Teach patient to inform prescriber of renal or hepatic disease
- Teach patient to report bleeding, facial swelling, wheezing, difficulty breathing, itching, rash, hives, increasing warmth, flushing
- Instruct patient to report signs of infection: increased temp, sore throat, flulike symptoms
- Advise patient to notify prescriber of nausea, vomiting, diarrhea, jaundice, anorexia, clay-colored stools, dark urine; hepatotoxicity may occur

M

Adverse effects: *italic* = common, **bold** = life-threatening

Evaluation
Positive therapeutic outcome
- Prevention of *Candida* infection in HSTC; or decreased symptoms of *Candida* infection, negative culture

---

miconazole (Rx, OTC)
(mi-kon'a-zole)
Femizole-M, Monistat, Monistat 3, Monistat 7, Monistat-Derm, Monistat Dual-Pak, M-Zole 7 Dual Pack, topical: Micatin, Micatin Liquid, miconazole nitrate
Func. class.: Antifungal
Chem. class.: Imidazole

Pregnancy category C

Action: Alters cell membranes, inhibits fungal enzymes, inhibits sterols so intracellular contents are lost, prevents biosynthesis of phospholipids/triglycerides

Therapeutic outcome: Fungistatic/ fungicidal against *Aspergillus, Coccidioides, Cryptococcus, Candida, Dermatophytes, Histoplasma*

Uses: Coccidioidomycosis, candidiasis, cryptococcosis, paracoccidioidomycosis, chronic mucocutaneous candidiasis, fungal meningitis; **IV** used for severe infections only; (topical) tinea pedis, tinea cruris, tinea corporis, tinea versicolor, vaginal or vulva candidal infections

Dosage and routes
Adult: **IV** INF 200-3600 mg/day; may be divided in 3 INF at 200-1200 mg/INF; may have to repeat course; IT 20 mg given simultaneously with **IV** for fungal meningitis q1-2day
Child: **IV** 20-40 mg/kg/day, max 15 mg/kg/day
Adult and child: TOP apply to affected area bid × 2-4 wk
Adult: Intravaginal 200 mg SUPP at bedtime × 3 days or 100 mg SUPP × 1 wk

Available forms: Inj 10 mg/ml; aerosol 2%; cream 2%; lotion 2%; powder 2%; spray 2%; vag cream 2%; vag supp 100, 200 mg

Adverse effects
CNS: Drowsiness, headache, lethargy
CV: Tachycardia, **dysrhythmias** (rapid **IV**)
GI: Nausea, vomiting, anorexia, diarrhea, cramps
GU: Vulvovaginal burning, itching, hyponatremia, pelvic cramps (topical forms)
HEMA: **Decreased Hct, thrombocytopenia, hyperlipidemia**
INTEG: Pruritus, rash, fever, flushing, hives
SYST: **Anaphylaxis**

Contraindications: Hypersensitivity
Precautions: Pregnancy **C**, renal/hepatic disease

Pharmacokinetics
Absorption	Poorly absorbed (PO)
Distribution	Widely distributed (**IV**); bound to serum proteins (90%)
Metabolism	Liver, extensively
Excretion	Unknown
Half-life	Triphasic: 0.4, 2.1, 24 hr

Pharmacodynamics
	IV	TOPICAL	VAG
Onset	Rapid	Unknown	Unknown
Peak	Infusion's end	Unknown	Unknown
Duration	Unknown	Unknown	Unknown

Interactions
Individual drugs
Amphotericin B: decreased effect of amphotericin B
Amphotericin B, isoniazid, rifampin: decreased effect of miconazole
Phenytoin: increased effect
Warfarin: increased anticoagulant effect
Drug classifications
Sulfonylureas: increased effect
Drug/lab test
False positive: urine glucose, urine protein

NURSING CONSIDERATIONS
Assessment
- Assess for signs and symptoms of infection: drainage, sore throat, urinary pain, hematuria, fever
- Obtain C&S before beginning treatment; therapy may be started after culture is taken; monitor signs of infection before, throughout treatment
- Monitor bowel pattern before, during treatment; diarrhea may occur
- Monitor cardiac system: B/P, pulse; watch for increasing pulse, cardiac dysrhythmias; product should be discontinued
- Monitor blood studies: WBC, RBC, Hgb, Hct, bleeding time; patients taking anticoagulants may need a decreased dosage; monitor liver and renal studies periodically for patients on long-term therapy
- Monitor I&O ratio; watch for decreasing urinary output, change in specific gravity; discontinue product to prevent renal damage;

 Alert   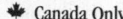 Canada Only   Drug on CD   * "Tall Man" lettering (See Preface)

patients with renal disease may require lowered dose

- Monitor **IV** site for thrombophlebitis; site should be changed q48-72hr
- Monitor for allergies before initiation of treatment and reaction to each medication; highlight allergies on chart; check for allergic reaction: burning, stinging, swelling, redness (topical); observe for skin eruptions after administration of product to 1 wk after discontinuing product

Nursing diagnoses
- Infection, risk for (uses)
- Injury, risk for (adverse reactions)
- Knowledge, deficient (teaching)
- Skin integrity, impaired (uses)

Implementation
- Have adrenalin, suction, tracheostomy set, endotracheal intubation equipment available

Topical route
- Apply after cleansing area with soap and water before each application; use enough medication to cover lesions completely; dry well
- Store at room temperature in dry place

Vaginal route
- Administer 1 applicator full every night high into the vagina
- Store at room temperature in dry place

IV route
- Give 200 mg initially to prevent severe hypersensitive reaction
- Give **IV** after diluting ≤1 g/10 ml of sterile water, D₅W, or 0.45% NaCl over 3-5 min
- Give by intermittent **IV** after diluting in 200 ml or more D₅W or 0.9% NaCl; give over 30-60 min
- Store at room temperature; reconstituted sol is stable for 24 hr refrigerated

Y-site compatibilities: Allopurinol, filgrastim, foscarnet, granisetron, melphalan, ondansetron, propofol, sargramostim, teniposide, thiotepa, vinorelbine

Y-site incompatibilities: Fludarabine

Patient/family education
- Inform patient that culture may be performed after completed course of medication
- Advise patient to notify nurse of diarrhea, symptoms of candidal vaginitis

Topical route
- Teach patient to use medical asepsis (hand washing) before, after each application; to apply with glove to prevent further infection; to avoid contact with eyes; not to use occlusive dressings
- Caution patient to avoid use of OTC creams, ointments, lotions unless directed by prescriber

- Instruct patient to notify prescriber if no improvement in condition in 4 wk or if symptoms return in 2 mo; pregnancy or a serious medical condition may be the cause
- Teach patient to use for full prescribed treatment time, or reinfection may occur

Vaginal route
- Instruct patient in asepsis (hand washing) before, after each application
- Teach patient to apply with applicator only; to avoid use of any other vaginal product unless directed by prescriber; sanitary napkin may prevent soiling of undergarments; to abstain from sexual intercourse until treatment is completed; reinfection and irritation may occur
- Instruct patient to notify prescriber if symptoms persist

Evaluation
Positive therapeutic outcome
- Decreasing oral candidiasis, fever, malaise, rash
- Negative C&S for infectious organism
- Decrease in size, number of lesions
- Decrease in itching or white discharge (vaginal)

Treatment of overdose: Withdraw product; maintain airway; administer epinephrine, aminophylline, O₂, **IV** corticosteroids for anaphylaxis

---

miconazole topical
See Appendix B

---

miconazole vaginal antifungal
See Appendix B

---

midazolam (Rx)
(mid′ay-zoe-lam)
Func. class.: Sedative/hypnotic, antianxiety
Chem. class.: Benzodiazepine, short-acting

Pregnancy category D
Controlled substance schedule **IV**

Action: Depresses subcortical levels in CNS; may act on limbic system, reticular formation; may potentiate GABA by binding to specific benzodiazepine receptors

M

Therapeutic outcome: Sedation for anesthesia induction and procedures

Uses: Preoperative sedation, general anesthesia induction, sedation for diagnostic endoscopic procedures, intubation, anxiety

Unlabeled uses: Refractory status epilepticus

Dosage and routes
Preoperative sedation
Adult and child ≥12 yr: IM 0.07-0.08 mg/kg 30-60 min before general anesthesia
Child 1-6 mo: IM 0.1-0.15 mg/kg, may give up to 0.5 mg/kg if needed, max 10 mg
Child 6 mo-5 yr: IV 0.05-0.1 mg/kg, a total dose of 0.6 mg/kg may be needed
Child 6-11 yr: IV 0.025-0.05 mg/kg, a total dose of 0.4 mg/kg may be needed

Induction of general anesthesia
Adult >55 yr: (ASA I/II) IV 150-300 mcg/kg over 30 sec; (ASA III/IV) limit dose to 250 mcg/kg (nonpremedicated) or 150 mcg/kg (premedicated)
Adult <55 yr: IV 200-350 mcg/kg over 20-30 sec; if patient has not received premedication, may repeat by giving 20% of original dose; if patient has received premedication reduce dose by 50 mcg/kg
Child: No safe and effective dose established; however, doses of 50-200 mcg/kg IV have been used

Continuous infusion for intubation (critical care)
Adult: IV 0.01-0.05 mg/kg over several min; repeat at 10-15 min intervals, until adequate sedation; then 0.02-0.10 mg/kg/hr maintenance; adjust as needed
Child: IV 0.05-0.2 mg/kg over 2-3 min, then 0.06-0.12 mg/kg/hr by CONT INF; adjust as needed
Neonates: IV 0.03-0.06 mg/kg/hr titrate using lowest dose

Available forms: Inj 1, 5 mg/ml; syr 2 mg/ml

Adverse effects
CNS: Retrograde amnesia, euphoria, confusion, headache, anxiety, insomnia, slurred speech, paresthesia, tremors, weakness, chills, agitation, paradoxical reactions
CV: Hypotension, PVCs, tachycardia, bigeminy, nodal rhythm, **cardiac arrest**
EENT: Blurred vision, nystagmus, diplopia, loss of balance
GI: *Nausea, vomiting,* increased salivation, hiccups

INTEG: Urticaria, pain at injection site, swelling at inj site, rash, pruritus at injection site
RESP: Coughing, **apnea, bronchospasm, laryngospasm,** dyspnea, **respiratory depression**

Contraindications: Pregnancy **D,** hypersensitivity to benzodiazepines, acute closed-angle glaucoma, status asthmaticus

Precautions: Breastfeeding, children, geriatric, COPD, CHF, chronic renal failure, chills, debilitated, hepatic disease, shock, coma, alcohol intoxication

Black Box Warning: Neonates (contains benzyl alcohol), **IV** administration, respiratory depression/insufficiency

Pharmacokinetics
Absorption	Well absorbed
Distribution	Crosses placenta, blood-brain barrier, protein binding 97%
Metabolism	Liver
Excretion	Kidneys, breast milk
Half-life	1.8-6.4 hr

Pharmacodynamics
	PO	IM	IV
Onset	20-30 min	15 min	3-5 min
Peak	Unknown	½-1 hr	Unknown
Duration	Unknown	2-3 hr	<2 hr

Interactions
Individual drugs
Alcohol: increased respiratory depression
Cimetidine, erythromycin, ranitidine, theophylline: decreased midazolam metabolism
Fluvoxamine, indinavir, ritonavir, verapamil: increased respiratory depression
Drug classifications
Antifungals, azole, CYP3A4 inhibitors: increased levels of midazolam
Barbiturates, opiate analgesics, other CNS depressants: increased respiratory depression
CYP3A4 inducers (azole antifungals, theophylline): increased half-life of midazolam
Drug/herb
Black cohosh: increased hypotension
Catnip, chamomile, clary, cowslip, hops, kava, lavender, mistletoe, nettle, pokeweed, poppy, Queen Anne's lace, senega, skullcap, St. John's wort, tan-shen, valerian: increased CNS depression

 Alert   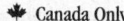 Canada Only   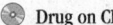 Drug on CD   * "Tall Man" lettering (See Preface)

Drug/food
Grapefruit juice: increased midazolam effect (PO)

NURSING CONSIDERATIONS
Assessment
- Monitor B/P, pulse, respiration during **IV**; O_2 and emergency equipment should be nearby
- Monitor inj site for redness, pain, swelling
- Assess degree of amnesia in geriatric; may be increased
- Assess anterograde amnesia
- Assess vital signs for recovery period in obese patient, since half-life may be extended
- Assess for apnea, respiratory depression, which may be increased in the geriatric

Nursing diagnoses
- Knowledge, deficient (teaching)

Implementation
PO route
- Remove cap of press-in bottle adaptor and push adaptor into neck of bottle; close with cap, remove cap, and insert tip of dispenser and insert into adaptor; turn upside-down and withdraw correct dose; place in mouth

IM route
- Give inj deep into large muscle mass
- Store at room temperature; protect from light

IV route
- Give **IV** undiluted or after diluting with D_5W or 0.9% NaCl to a conc of 0.25 mg/ml; give over 2 min (conscious sedation) or over 30 sec (anesthesia induction)
- Ensure immediate availability of resuscitation equipment, O_2 to support airway; do not give by rapid bol

Syringe compatibilities: Alfentanil, atracurium, atropine, benzquinamide, buprenorphine, butorphanol, chlorproMAZINE, cimetadine, cisatracurium, diphenhyDRAMINE, droperidol, fentanyl, glycopyrrolate, hydromorphine, hydrOXYzinc, ketamine, meperidine, metoclopramide, morphine, nalbuphine, promazine, promethazine, remifentanil, scopolamine, sufentanil, thiethylperazine, trimethobenzamide

Syringe incompatibilities: Dimenhydrinate, pentobarbital, perphenazine, prochlorperazine, ranitidine

Y-site compatibilities: Abciximab, alfentamil, amikacin, amiodarone, argatroban, atracurium, atropine, aztreonam, benzotropine, calcium gluconate, cefazolin, cefotaxime, cefoxitine, ceftriaxone, cimetidine, ciprofloxacin, cisplatin, clindamycin, clonidine, cyanocobalamin, cycloSPORINE, dactinomycin, digoxin, diltiazem, diphenhydramine, docetaxal, DOPamine, doxycycline, enalaprilat, epinephrine, erythromycin, esmolol, etomidate, etoposide, famotidine, fentanyl, fluconazole, folic acid, gatifloxacin, gemcitabine, gentamicin, glycopyrrolate, granisetron, heparin, hetastarch, hydromorphone, hydrOXYzine, inamrinone, isoproterenol, labetalol, lactated Ringer's, levofloxacin, lidocaine, linezolid, lorazepam, magnesium, mannitol, meperidine, methadone, methyldopa, methylPREDNISolone, metoclopramide, metomolol, metronidazole, milrinone, morphine, nalbuphine, naloxone, niCARdipine, nitroglycerin, nitroprusside, norepinephrine, ondansetron, oxacillin, oxytocin, paclitaxel, palonosetron, pancuronium, papaverin, phentolamine, phytonadione, piperacillin, potassium chloride, propanolol, protamine, pyridoxine, ranitidine, remifentanil, sodium nitroprusside, streptokinase, succinylcholine, sufentanil, teniposide, theophylline, thiotepa, ticarcillin, tobramycin, vancomycin, vasopressin, vecuronium, verapamil, voriconazole

Y-site incompatibilities: Foscarnet

Patient/family education
- Inform patient that amnesia occurs; events may not be remembered
- Caution patient to avoid CNS depressants including alcohol for 24 hr after taking this product

Evaluation
Positive therapeutic outcome
- Induction of sedation, amnesia

Treatment of overdose: O_2, flumazenil

---

midodrine (Rx)
(mye'doh-dreen)
ProAmatine
Func. class.: Proproduct

Pregnancy category C

Do not confuse:
ProAmatine/Protamine

Action: Activates α-adrenergic receptors of arteriolar, venous vasculature; increases vascular tone

Therapeutic outcome: Decreased feeling of faintness upon rising, absence of significant change in B/P

Uses: Orthostatic hypotension

Dosage and routes
Adult: PO 10 mg tid, max 40 mg/day

M

Adverse effects: *italic* = common, **bold** = life-threatening

Renal dose
Adult: PO 2.5 mg tid

Available forms: Tabs 2.5, 5, 10 mg

Adverse effects
CNS: Drowsiness, restlessness, headache, paresthesia, pain, chills, confusion
CV: **Supine hypertension,** vasodilatation, flushing face
EENT: Dry mouth, blurred vision
GI: Nausea, anorexia
GU: Dysuria
INTEG: Pruritus, piloerection, rash

Contraindications: Hypersensitivity, acute renal disease, urinary retention, pheochromocytoma, thyrotoxicosis

Black Box Warning: Severe organic heart disease, persistent/excessive supine hypertension

Precautions: Pregnancy C, breastfeeding, children, hepatic impairment, orthostatic diabetic patients, renal disease, thyroid disease, visual disturbance, dialysis, diabetes, heart failure

Pharmacokinetics

Absorption	Bioavailability 90%
Distribution	Unknown
Metabolism	Unknown
Excretion	Urine 80%, active metabolite
Half-life	3-4 hr

Pharmacodynamics

Onset	Unknown
Peak	1-2 hr
Duration	Unknown

Interactions
Individual drug
Fludrocortisone: increased supine hypertension
Metformin: increased lactic acidosis
Drug classifications
α-Adrenergic agonists: increased pressor effects
β-Adrenergic blockers, cardiac glycosides, psychotropics, tricyclics: increased bradycardia
MAOIs or products with MAOI-type activity: do not use concurrently

NURSING CONSIDERATIONS
Assessment
• Monitor VS, B/P (standing, supine); notify prescriber if B/P supine is increased
• Observe for drowsiness, dizziness, LOC

Nursing diagnoses
• Knowledge, deficient (teaching)

Implementation
• Tablets may be swallowed whole, chewed, or allowed to dissolve
• Administer upon rising, at midday, and in late afternoon (no later than 6 PM)
• Avoid administering if patient is to be supine during day

Patient/family education
• Advise patient to avoid hazardous activities; activities requiring alertness; dizziness may occur; instruct patient to request assistance with ambulation
• Advise patient to avoid alcohol, other depressants, OTC products; multiple drug-drug interactions

Evaluation
Positive therapeutic outcome
• Decreased orthostatic hypotension

---

mifepristone, RU-486 (Rx)
(mif-ee-press'tone)
Mifeprex
Func. class.: Abortifacient
Chem. class.: Antiprogestational

Pregnancy category C

Action: Stimulates uterine contractions, causing complete abortion

Therapeutic outcome: Termination of pregnancy

Uses: Abortion through 49 days gestation

Unlabeled uses: Postcoital contraception/contragestation, intrauterine fetal death, endometriosis, Cushing's syndrome, unresectable meningioma

Dosage and routes
Coadministration of mifepristone/ misoprostol
Adult: Day 1: PO single dose 600 mg mifepristone, 400 mcg misoprostol day 3 if needed

Available forms: Tabs 200 mg

Adverse effects
CNS: Dizziness, insomnia, anxiety, syncope, fainting, headache
GI: *Nausea, vomiting, diarrhea,* dyspepsia
GU: Uterine cramping, uterine hemorrhage, vaginitis, pelvic pain
MISC: Fatigue, back pain, fever, viral infections, chills, sinusitis

Contraindications: Hypersensitivity to this product, misoprostol, or prostaglandins;

severe renal/hepatic disease, PID, respiratory/
cardiac disease, IUD, ectopic pregnancy,
chronic adrenal failure, bleeding disorder,
inherited porphyrias

Precautions: Pregnancy **C,** women >35
yr/smoking ≥10 cigarettes/day, asthma, anemia, jaundice, diabetes mellitus, seizure
disorders, past uterine surgery

Black Box Warning: Infection, sepsis,
vaginal bleeding

Pharmacokinetics

Absorption	Rapidly
Distribution	98% protein binding, albumin, glycoprotein
Metabolism	Unknown
Excretion	Feces, urine
Half-life	Unknown

Pharmacodynamics

Onset	Unknown
Peak	90 min
Duration	Unknown

Interactions
Individual drugs

Erythromycin, itraconazole, ketoconazole:
decreased metabolism of each specific
product
Drug classifications

Anticoagulants, long-term corticosteroids: do
not use together
Drug/herb

St. John's wort: decreased mifepristone action
Drug/food

Grapefruit juice: decreased metabolism of
mifepristone

NURSING CONSIDERATIONS
Assessment
• Monitor B/P, pulse; watch for change that
may indicate hemorrhage
• Monitor respiratory rate, rhythm, depth;
notify prescriber of abnormalities
• Assess for length, duration of contraction;
notify prescriber of contractions lasting over 1
min or absence of contractions
• Assess for incomplete abortion; pregnancy
must be terminated by another method;
product is teratogenic

Nursing diagnoses
• Knowledge, deficient (teaching)
• Pain, acute (adverse reactions)

Implementation
• Provide emotional support before and after
abortion

Patient/family education
• Advise patient to report increased blood
loss, abdominal cramps, increased temp,
foul-smelling lochia
• Teach patient some methods of comfort
control and pain control
• Advise patient to continue with follow-up
• Advise patient that cramping and vaginal
bleeding will occur

Evaluation
Positive therapeutic outcome
• Expulsion of fetus

miglitol (Rx)
(mig′le-tol)
Glyset
Func. class.: Oral hypoglycemic
Chem. class.: α-Glucosidase inhibitor

Pregnancy category B

Action: Delays the digestion/absorption of
ingested carbohydrates, results in a smaller
rise in blood glucose after meals; does not
increase insulin production

Therapeutic outcome: Decreased
blood glucose levels in diabetes mellitus

Uses: Type 2 diabetes mellitus

Dosage and routes
Initial dose
Adult: PO 25 mg tid initially, with first bite of
meal

Maintenance dose
Adult: PO may be increased to 50 mg tid;
may increase to 100 mg tid if needed with
dosage adjustment at 4-8 wk intervals

Available forms: Tabs 25, 50, 100 mg

Adverse effects
GI: Abdominal pain, diarrhea, flatulence,
hepatotoxicity
HEMA: Low iron
INTEG: Rash

Contraindications: Hypersensitivity,
diabetic ketoacidosis, cirrhosis, IBD, colonic
ulceration, partial intestinal obstruction,
chronic intestinal disease, ileus

Precautions: Pregnancy **B,** breastfeeding,
children, renal/hepatic disease

Pharmacokinetics	
Absorption	Unknown
Distribution	Unknown
Metabolism	Not metabolized
Excretion	Kidneys, unchanged product
Half-life	2 hr

Pharmacodynamics	
Onset	Unknown
Peak	2-3 hr
Duration	Unknown

Interactions
Individual drugs
Digoxin: decreased levels of digoxin
Propranolol: decreased levels of propranolol
Ranitidine: decreased levels of ranitidine
Drug classifications
Adsorbents (intestinal), enzymes (digestive): decreased miglitol levels; do not use together
Drug/herb
Broom, buchu, dandelion, juniper: decreased hypoglycemia
Chromium, fenugreek, ginseng: increased or decreased hypoglycemic effect
Karela: improved glucose tolerance
Drug/food
Carbohydrates: increased diarrhea

NURSING CONSIDERATIONS
Assessment
• Assess for hypo/hyperglycemia; even though this product does not cause hypoglycemia, if taking a sulfonylurea or insulin, hypoglycemia may be additive (rare)
• Monitor blood glucose levels, A1C, liver function tests; if hypoglycemia occurs with monotherapy, treat with glucose

Nursing diagnoses
• Knowledge, deficient (teaching)
• Noncompliance (teaching)
• Nutrition: less than body requirements, imbalanced (adverse reactions)
• Nutrition: more than body requirements, imbalanced (uses)

Implementation
• Give tid with first bite of each meal
• Provide storage in airtight container at room temperature

Patient/family education
• Teach patient the symptoms of hypo/hyperglycemia and what to do about each
• Instruct that medication must be taken as prescribed; explain consequences of discontinuing the medication abruptly; that during periods of stress, infection, surgery, insulin may be required
• Tell patient to avoid OTC medications unless approved by prescriber
• Teach patient that diabetes is a lifelong illness; product will not cure condition
• Instruct patient to carry/wear emergency ID as diabetic
• Teach patient that diet and exercise regimen must be followed
• Teach patient GI side effects and what to do about them

Evaluation
Positive therapeutic outcome
• Decreased signs, symptoms of diabetes mellitus (polyuria, polydipsia, polyphagia, clear sensorium, absence of dizziness, stable gait)
• Improved blood glucose, A1c

❗ HIGH ALERT

milrinone (Rx)
(mill-re′none)
Func. class.: Inotropic/vasodilator agent with phosphodiesterase activity
Chem. class.: Bipyridine derivative
Pregnancy category C

Action: Positive inotropic agent with vasodilator properties; increases contractility of cardiac muscle; reduces preload and afterload by direct relaxation of vascular smooth muscle; increases myocardial contractility

Therapeutic outcome: Increased inotropic effect resulting in increased cardiac output

Uses: Short-term management of advanced CHF that has not responded to other medication; can be used with digoxin

Dosage and routes
Adult: **IV** BOL 50 mcg/kg given over 10 min; start INF of 0.375-0.75 mcg/kg/min; reduce dosage in renal impairment

Available forms: Inj 1 mg/ml; premixed inj 200 mcg/ml in D_5W

Adverse effects
CV: Dysrhythmias, hypotension, chest pain
GI: Nausea, vomiting, anorexia, abdominal pain, **hepatotoxicity**, jaundice
HEMA: **Thrombocytopenia**
MISC: Headache, hypokalemia, tremor, injection site reactions

---

 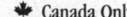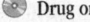

Contraindications: Hypersensitivity to this product, severe aortic disease, severe pulmonic valvular disease, acute MI

Precautions: Pregnancy **C**, breastfeeding, children, geriatric, renal/hepatic disease, atrial flutter/fibrillation

Pharmacokinetics

Absorption	Completely absorbed
Distribution	Unknown
Metabolism	Liver (50%)
Excretion	Kidney, unchanged (83%), metabolites (12%)
Half-life	2.4 hr; increased in CHF

Pharmacodynamics

Onset	2-5 min
Peak	10 min
Duration	Variable

NURSING CONSIDERATIONS
Assessment
• Monitor manifestations of hypokalemia: acidic urine, reduced urine, osmolality, nocturia; hypotension, broad T-wave, U-wave, ectopy, tachycardia, weak pulse; muscle weakness, altered LOC, drowsiness, apathy, lethargy, confusion, depression; anorexia, nausea, cramps, constipation, distention, paralytic ileus; hypoventilation, respiratory muscle weakness
• Assess fluid volume status: complete I&O ratio and record; note weight, distended red veins, crackles in lung, color, quality, and specific gravity of urine, skin turgor, adequacy of pulses, moist mucous membranes, bilateral lung sounds, peripheral pitting edema; dehydration symptoms of decreasing output, thirst, hypotension, dry mouth and mucous membranes should be reported
◆ Monitor electrolytes: potassium, sodium, calcium, magnesium; also include BUN, blood pH, ABGs
• Monitor B/P and pulse, ECG continuously during **IV**; ventricular dysrhythmia can occur; PCWP, CVP, index often during inf; if B/P drops 30 mm Hg, stop inf and call prescriber
• Monitor ALT, AST, bilirubin daily; if these are elevated, hepatoxicity is suspected
• Monitor platelets; if <150,000/mm³, product is usually discontinued and another product started
• Assess for extravasation: change site q48hr

Nursing diagnoses
• Cardiac output, decreased (uses)
• Fluid volume, excess (uses)
• Knowledge, deficient (teaching)

Implementation
IV route
• Give **IV** loading dose undiluted over 10 min
• Do not mix directly with glucose sol; chemical reaction occurs over 24 hr; precipitate forms if milrinone and furosemide come in contact
• Administer by direct **IV** into inf through Y-connector or directly into tubing; may give undiluted over 2-3 min
• Give by cont inf diluted with 0.9% NaCl to conc of 1-3 mg/ml, run at prescribed rate; give by inf pump for doses other than bol
• Administer potassium supplements if ordered for potassium levels <3.0 mg/dl
Syringe compatibilities: Atropine, calcium chloride, digoxin, epinephrine, lidocaine, morphine, propranolol, sodium bicarbonate, verapamil
Y-site compatibilities: Digoxin, diltiazem, DOBUTamine, DOPamine, epinephrine, fentanyl, heparin, hydromorphone, labetalol, lorazepam, midazolam, morphine, niCARdipine, nitroglycerin, norepinephrine, propranolol, quinidine, ranitidine, thiopental, vecuronium
Additive compatibilities: Quinidine

Patient/family education
• Teach patient reason for medication and expected results
• Instruct patient to make position changes slowly; orthostatic hypotension may occur
• Teach patient signs and symptoms of hypersensitivity reactions and hypokalemia

Evaluation
Positive therapeutic outcome
• Increased cardiac output
• Decreased PCWP, adequate CVP
• Decreased dyspnea, fatigue, edema, ECG

Treatment of overdose: Discontinue product, support circulation

M

---

minocycline (Rx)
(min-oh-sye′kleen)
Arestin, Dynacin, Minocin, Myrac, Soledyn
Func. class.: Antiinfective
Chem. class.: Tetracycline

Pregnancy category D

Action: Inhibits protein synthesis and phosphorylation in microorganisms by binding

Adverse effects: *italic* = common, **bold** = life-threatening

to 30S ribosomal subunits and reversibly binding to 50S ribosomal subunits; bacteriostatic

Therapeutic outcome: Bactericidal action against susceptible organisms, including *Neisseria meningitidis, Neisseria gonorrhoeae, Treponema pallidum, Chlamydia trachomatis, Ureaplasma urealyticum, Mycoplasma pneumoniae, Nocardia, Rickettsia*

Uses: Syphilis, chlamydial infection, gonorrhea, lymphogranuloma venereum, rickettsial infections, inflammatory acne, meningitis carriers, periodontitis, methicillin-resistant *Staphylococcus aureus* (MRSA) infections

Unlabeled uses: Rheumatoid arthritis

Dosage and routes
Adult: PO/**IV** 200 mg, then 100 mg q12hr or 50 mg q6hr, max 400 mg/24 hr **IV**; subgingival insert into periodontal pocket
Child >8 yr: PO/**IV** 4 mg/kg then 4 mg/kg/day PO in divided doses q12hr

Gonorrhea
Adult: PO 200 mg, then 100 mg q12hr × 4 days or more

C. trachomatis *infection*
Adult: PO 100 mg bid × 7 days

Syphilis
Adult: PO 200 mg, then 100 mg q12hr × 10-15 days

Uncomplicated gonococcal urethritis in men
Adult: PO 100 mg q12hr × 5 days

Rheumatoid arthritis (unlabeled)
Adult: PO 100 mg bid for ≤48 wk

Available forms: Caps 50, 75, 100 mg; oral susp 50 mg/5 ml; powder for inj 100 mg; pellet filled caps 50, 100 mg; tabs 50, 75, 100 mg; ext rel tabs 45, 90, 135 mg

Adverse effects
CNS: Dizziness, fever, light-headedness, vertigo, seizures, **increased intracranial pressure**
CV: Pericarditis
EENT: Dysphagia, glossitis, decreased calcification, permanent discoloration of teeth, oral candidiasis
GI: Nausea, abdominal pain, *vomiting, diarrhea,* anorexia, enterocolitis, **hepatotoxicity,** flatulence, abdominal cramps, epigastric burning, stomatitis
GU: Increased BUN, polyuria, polydipsia, **renal failure, nephrotoxicity**

HEMA: **Eosinophilia, neutropenia, thrombocytopenia, hemolytic anemia,** pancytopenia
INTEG: Rash, urticaria, photosensitivity, increased pigmentation, **exfoliative dermatitis,** pruritus, blue-gray color of skin and mucous membranes
MS: Myalgia, arthritis, bone discoloration, joint stiffness
SYST: **Angioedema, Stevens-Johnson syndrome**

Contraindications: Pregnancy **D,** hypersensitivity to tetracyclines, children <8 yr

Precautions: Breastfeeding, hepatic disease

Pharmacokinetics

Absorption	Well absorbed (PO)
Distribution	Widely distributed (70%-75% protein bound); some distribution in CSF, crosses placenta
Metabolism	Liver, some
Excretion	Kidneys, unchanged (20%), bile, feces
Half-life	11-17 hr

Pharmacodynamics

	PO	IV
Onset	Rapid	Rapid
Peak	2-3 hr	Infusion's end
Duration	Unknown	Unknown

Interactions
Individual drugs
Calcium: forms chelates, decreased absorption
Carbamazepine, phenytoin: decreased effect
Digoxin: increased effect
Insulin: increased effect
Kaolin/pectin, sodium bicarbonate, cimetidine, iron: decreased minocycline effect
Theophylline: increased effect
Warfarin: increased effect
Drug classifications
Alkali products, antacids: decreased minocycline effect
Anticoagulants (oral): increased effect
Barbiturates, penicillins: decreased effect
Oral contraceptives: decreased effect of oral contraception
Drug/herb
Acidophilus: do not use with antiinfectives; separate by several hours
Drug/lab test
False negative: urine glucose with Clinistix, Tes-Tape

NURSING CONSIDERATIONS
Assessment
- Assess patient for previous sensitivity reaction
- Assess patient for signs and symptoms of infection including characteristics of wounds, sputum, urine, stool, WBC >10,000/mm^3, fever; obtain baseline information before, during treatment
- Obtain C&S before beginning product therapy to identify if correct treatment has been initiated
- Assess for allergic reactions: rash, urticaria, pruritus
- Monitor blood studies: AST, ALT, CBC, Hct, bilirubin, alkaline phosphatase, amylase monthly if patient is on long-term therapy
- Assess bowel pattern daily; if severe diarrhea occurs, product should be discontinued
- Monitor for bleeding: ecchymosis, bleeding gums, hematuria, stool guaiac daily if on long-term therapy; blood dyscrasias may occur
- Assess for overgrowth of infection: perineal itching, fever, malaise, redness, pain, swelling, drainage, rash, diarrhea, change in cough, sputum; black, furry tongue

Nursing diagnoses
- Diarrhea (adverse reactions)
- Infection, risk for (uses)
- Knowledge, deficient (teaching)
- Noncompliance (teaching)

Implementation
PO route
- Give around the clock to maintain proper blood levels; give with food to increase absorption of product; do not give within 3 hr of other agents; product interactions may occur
- Give with 8 oz of water 1 hr before bedtime to prevent ulceration
- Shake liquid preparation well before giving; use calibrated device for proper dosing
- Do not give with iron, calcium, magnesium products, or antacids, which decrease absorption and form insoluble chelate
IV route
- Check for irritation, extravasation, phlebitis daily; change site q72hr
- For intermittent inf, dilute each 100 mg/10 ml of 0.9% NaCl, sterile water for inj; further dilute in 500-1000 ml of 0.9% NaCl, D$_5$W, Ringer's, LR, D$_5$/LR; give over 6 hr

Y-site compatibilities: Alfentanil, amikacin, atracurium, benztropine, bretylium, buprenorphine, butorphanol, calcium chloride, carboplatin, caspofungin, cefonicid, chlorpromazine, cimetidine, codeine, cyclophosphamide, cyclosporine, cytarabine, dactinomycin, dexmedetomidine, diltiazem, diphenhydramine, dobutamine, docetaxel, doxacurium, doxycycline, enalaprilat, ephedrine, epinephrine, eptifibatide, etoposide, fenoldopam, fentanyl, fludarabine, gatifloxacin, gemcitabine, gentamicin, glycopyrrolate, granisetron, heparin, hetastarch, idarubicin, ifosfamide, inamrinone, isoproterenol, labetalol, levofloxacin, lidocaine, linezolid, lorazepam, magnesium sulfate, mannitol, melphalan, metaraminol, methotrexate, methyldopa, metoclopramide, metoprolol, midazolam, mitoxantrone, nalbuphine, naloxone, perphenazine, potassium chloride, sargramostim, sodium succinate, vinorelbine, vit B/C

Y-site incompatibilities: Aztreonam, filgrastim, hydromorphone, meperidine, morphine, teniposide

Patient/family education
- Teach patient to use sunscreen when outdoors to decrease photosensitivity reaction
- Teach patient to report sore throat, bruising, bleeding, joint pain; may indicate blood dyscrasias (rare)
- Advise patient to contact prescriber if vaginal itching, loose foul-smelling stools, furry tongue occur; may indicate superinfection; report itching, rash, pruritus, urticaria
- Instruct patient to take all medication prescribed for the length of time ordered; product must be taken around the clock to maintain blood levels; do not give medication to others; take with a full glass of water; may take with food; not to use outdated product, Fanconi's syndrome may occur
- Advise patient to use a form of contraception other than hormonal

Evaluation
Positive therapeutic outcome
- Absence of signs/symptoms of infection (WBC <10,000/mm^3, temp WNL, absence of red, draining wounds)
- Reported improvement in symptoms of infection

M

minoxidil (Rx, OTC)
(mi-nox'i-dill)
minoxidil, Rogaine (top)
Func. class.: Antihypertensive, hair growth stimulant
Chem. class.: Vasodilator, peripheral

Pregnancy category C

Do not confuse:
minoxidil/Monopril

Action: Directly relaxes arteriolar smooth muscle, causing vasodilatation; increased cutaneous blood flow; stimulation of hair follicles

Therapeutic outcome: Decreased B/P in hypertension; hair growth

Uses: Severe hypertension unresponsive to other therapy (use with diuretic); topically to treat alopecia

Dosage and routes
Severe hypertension
Adult: PO 2.5-5 mg/day in 1-2 divided doses, max 100 mg/day; usual range 10-40 mg/day in single doses
Geriatric: PO 2.5 mg/day, may be increased gradually
Child <12 yr: PO initial 0.1-0.2 mg/kg/day; effective range, 0.25-1 mg/kg/day; max, 50 mg/day

Alopecia
Adult: TOP 1 ml bid, rub into scalp daily, max 2 ml/day

Available forms: Tabs 2.5, 10 mg; topical 2% sol

Adverse effects
Systemic
CNS: Headache, fatigue
CV: *Severe rebound hypertension (on withdrawal in children),* tachycardia, angina, increased T-wave, **CHF, pulmonary edema, pericardial effusion,** edema, sodium retention, water retention
GI: Nausea, vomiting
GU: Breast tenderness
HEMA: Hct, Hgb, erythrocyte count may decrease initially
INTEG: Pruritus, **Stevens-Johnson syndrome,** rash, hirsutism

Contraindications: Dissecting aortic aneurysm, hypersensitivity, pheochromocytoma

Black Box Warning: Acute MI

Precautions: Pregnancy C, breastfeeding, children, geriatric, renal disease, CVD

Black Box Warning: CAD, CHF, cardiac disease, cardiac tamponade, edema, hypotension, orthostatic hypotension, pericardial effusion

Pharmacokinetics
Absorption	Well absorbed (PO); minimally absorbed (topical)
Distribution	Widely distributed
Metabolism	Liver
Excretion	Kidneys, breast milk
Half-life	4.2 hr

Pharmacodynamics
	PO	TOPICAL
Onset	½ hr	4 mo
Peak	2-3 hr	Unknown
Duration	75 hr	4 mo

Interactions
Drug classifications
Antihypertensives: increased orthostatic hypotension
NSAIDs, salicylates: decreased antihypertensive effect
Drug/herb
Hawthorn: increased antihypertensive effect
Yohimbe: decreased antihypertensive effect
Drug/lab test
Increased: renal function tests
Decreased: Hgb, Hct, RBC

NURSING CONSIDERATIONS
Assessment
 Monitor closely; usually given with β-blocker to prevent tachycardia and increased myocardial workload; usually given with diuretic to prevent serious fluid accumulation; patient should be hospitalized during beginning treatment
- Monitor B/P, pulse, jugular venous distention periodically throughout treatment
- Monitor electrolytes, blood studies: potassium, sodium, chloride, carbon dioxide, CBC, serum glucose
 Monitor weight daily, I&O; assess edema in feet, legs daily; check skin turgor, dryness of mucous membranes for hydration status
- Assess for crackles, dyspnea, orthopnea, peripheral edema, fatigue, weight gain, jugular vein distention (CHF)
- Assess for signs of hyperglycemia: acetone breath, increased urinary output, severe thirst, lethargy, dizziness

 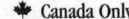

Nursing diagnoses
- Cardiac output, decreased (adverse reactions)
- Injury, risk for (side effects)
- Knowledge, deficient (teaching)

Implementation
PO route
- Give with meals to decrease GI symptoms
- Give with β-blockers and/or diuretic for hypertension
- Store protected from light and heat

Topical route
- Administer 1 ml dose no matter how much balding has occurred; increasing dose does not speed hair growth
- Treatment must continue long term or new hair will be lost again

Patient/family education
Topical route
- Teach patient that new hair will be soft and hardly visible
- Caution patient not to use on other parts of the body; product is to be used on the scalp only
- Instruct patient that hair should be clean before applying medication; do not get on clothing
- Caution patient not to get medication near mucous membranes (mouth, nose, eyes) and to contact prescriber if burning, stinging, or rash occurs

Evaluation
Positive therapeutic outcome
- Decreased B/P in hypertension
- Hair growth (Top)

---

mirtazapine (Rx)
(mer-ta′za-peen)
Remeron, Remeron Soltab
Func. class.: Antidepressant
Chem. class.: Tetracyclic

Pregnancy category C

Action: Blocks reuptake of norepinephrine, serotonin into nerve endings, increasing action of norepinephrine, serotonin in nerve cells; antagonist of central α_2-receptors, blocks histamine receptors; has anticholinergic action

Therapeutic outcome: Decreased symptoms of depression after 2-3 wk

Uses: Depression, dysthymic disorder, bipolar disorder: depression, agitated depression

Dosage and routes
Adult: PO 15 mg/day at bedtime, maintenance to continue for 6 mo, titrate up to 45 mg/day; orally disintegrating tabs open blister pack, place tab on tongue, allow to disintegrate, swallow
Geriatric: PO 7.5 mg nightly, increase by 7.5 mg q1-2wk to desired dose, max 45 mg/day

Available forms: Tabs 15, 30, 45 mg; orally disintegrating tabs (soltab) 15, 30, 45 mg

Adverse effects
CNS: Dizziness, drowsiness, confusion, headache, anxiety, tremors, stimulation, weakness, nightmares, EPS (geriatric), increased psychiatric symptoms, **seizures**
CV: Orthostatic hypotension, ECG changes, tachycardia, hypertension, palpitations
EENT: Blurred vision, tinnitus, mydriasis
GI: Diarrhea, dry mouth, nausea, vomiting, **paralytic ileus,** increased appetite, cramps, epigastric distress, **jaundice, hepatitis,** stomatitis, constipation, increased cholesterol levels
GU: Retention, **acute renal failure**
HEMA: **Agranulocytosis, thrombocytopenia, eosinophilia, leukopenia**
INTEG: Rash, urticaria, sweating, pruritus, photosensitivity
SYST: Flulike symptoms

Contraindications: Hypersensitivity to tricyclics, recovery phase of MI, agranulocytosis, jaundice

Precautions: Pregnancy C, geriatric, suicidal patients, severe depression, increased intraocular pressure, closed-angle glaucoma, urinary retention, cardiac/renal/hepatic disease, hypo/hyperthyroidism, electroshock therapy, elective surgery, seizure disorder, bone marrow suppression, thrombocytopenia

Black Box Warning: Suicidal ideation, children

Pharmacokinetics
Absorption	Slow, complete
Distribution	Widely distributed; crosses placenta
Metabolism	Liver, extensively
Excretion	Feces; breast milk
Half-life	20-40 hr

Pharmacodynamics
Onset	Unknown
Peak	2 hr
Duration	Unknown

M

Adverse effects: *italic* = common, **bold** = life-threatening

Interactions
Individual drugs
Alcohol: increased CNS depression
Clonidine: decreased effects
Drug classifications
Barbiturates, benzodiazepines, CNS depressants (other): increased effects
MAOIs: hypertensive episode, seizures, hyperpyretic crisis
Sympathomimetics, indirect acting (ephedrine): decreased effects
Drug/herb
Belladonna, henbane: increased anticholinergic effect
Chamomile, hops, kava, skullcap, valerian: increased CNS depression
Scopolia: increased antidepressant effect
St. John's wort, SAM-e: serotonin syndrome
Drug/lab test
Increased: serum bilirubin, blood glucose, alkaline phosphatase
Decreased: VMA, 5-HIAA
False increase: urinary catecholamines

NURSING CONSIDERATIONS
Assessment
• Monitor B/P (with patient lying, standing), pulse q4hr during beginning treatment; if systolic B/P drops 20 mm Hg, hold product, notify prescriber; take VS q4hr in patients with CV disease
• Monitor blood studies: CBC, leukocytes, differential, cardiac enzymes if patient is receiving long-term therapy
• Monitor liver function tests: AST, ALT, bilirubin
• Check weight weekly; product may increase appetite
• Assess ECG for flattening of T-wave, bundle branch block, AV block, dysrhythmias in cardiac patients
• Assess for EPS primarily in geriatric: rigidity, dystonia, akathisia
• Assess mental status: mood, sensorium, affect, suicidal tendencies; assess increase in psychiatric symptoms: depression, panic
• Identify alcohol consumption; if alcohol is consumed, hold dose until AM

Nursing diagnoses
• Coping, ineffective (uses)
• Injury, risk for (side effects)
• Knowledge, deficient (teaching)
• Noncompliance (teaching)

Implementation
• Give with food or milk for GI symptoms; crush if patient is unable to swallow medication whole
• Give dose at bedtime if oversedation occurs during day; may take entire dose at bedtime; geriatric may not tolerate once/day dosing
• Store at room temperature; do not freeze
• Allow orally disintegrating tablets to dissolve on tongue; no water needed; do not split

Patient/family education
• Inform patient that therapeutic effects may take 2-3 wk; take at bedtime
• Advise patient to use caution in driving and other activities requiring alertness because of drowsiness, dizziness, blurred vision; to avoid rising quickly from sitting to standing, especially geriatric
• Caution patient to avoid alcohol ingestion, other CNS depressants
• Teach patient to increase fluids, bulk in diet if constipation, urinary retention occur, especially geriatric
• Teach patient to use gum, hard sugarless candy, or frequent sips of water for dry mouth
• Teach patient to report immediately urinary retention, worsening of depression, suicidal thoughts/behavior
• Advise not to use within 14 days of MAOIs

Evaluation
Positive therapeutic outcome
• Decrease in depression
• Absence of suicidal thoughts

Treatment of overdose: ECG monitoring, lavage, activated charcoal, administer anticonvulsant

misoprostol (Rx)
(mye-soe-prost'ole)
Cytotec
Func. class.: Gastric mucosa protectant; antiulcer
Chem. class.: Prostaglandin E₁ analog
Pregnancy category X

Do not confuse:
misoprostol/metoprolol, Cytotec/Cytoxan

Action: Inhibits gastric acid secretion; may protect gastric mucosa; can increase bicarbonate, mucus production

Therapeutic outcome: Prevention of gastric ulcers

Uses: Prevention of NSAID-induced gastric ulcers

Dosage and routes
Adult: PO 200 mcg qid with food for duration of NSAID therapy with last dose at

bedtime; if 200 mcg is not tolerated, 100 mcg may be given

Available forms: Tabs 100, 200 mcg

Adverse effects

GI: Diarrhea, nausea, vomiting, flatulence, constipation, dyspepsia, abdominal pain
GU: Spotting, cramps, hypermenorrhea, menstrual disorders

Contraindications: Hypersensitivity to this product or prostaglandins

Black Box Warning: Pregnancy X, females

Precautions: Breastfeeding, children, geriatric, renal disease, CV disease

Pharmacokinetics	
Absorption	Well absorbed
Distribution	Unknown
Metabolism	Liver
Excretion	Kidneys
Half-life	½-1 hr

Pharmacodynamics	
Onset	½ hr
Peak	Unknown
Duration	3 hr

Interactions
Drug/food
Decreased absorption with food

NURSING CONSIDERATIONS
Assessment
• Assess patient for GI symptoms: hematemesis, occult or frank blood in stools, also severe abdominal pain, cramping, severe diarrhea
• Obtain a negative pregnancy test in women of childbearing age before starting medication; miscarriages are common

Nursing diagnoses
• Knowledge, deficient (teaching)
• Pain, chronic (uses)

Implementation
• Give with meals for prolonged product effect; avoid use of magnesium antacids

Patient/family education
• Advise patient to avoid black pepper, caffeine, alcohol, harsh spices, extremes in temperature of food, which may aggravate condition
• Caution patient to avoid OTC preparations: aspirin, cough, cold preparations; condition may worsen
• Teach patient that product must be continued for prescribed time to be effective and

taken exactly as prescribed; doses are not to be doubled
• Instruct patient to report to prescriber diarrhea, black tarry stools, abdominal pain, cramping, menstrual disorders
• Caution patient to prevent pregnancy while taking this product; spontaneous abortion may occur

Evaluation
Positive therapeutic outcome
• Prevention of ulcers

⚠ HIGH ALERT

mitomycin (Rx)
(mye-toe-mye'sin)
mitomycin
Func. class.: Antineoplastic, antibiotic

Pregnancy category D

Do not confuse:
mitomycin/mithramycin/mitotane/mitoxantrone

Action: Inhibits DNA synthesis, primarily; derived from *Streptomyces caespitosus;* appears to cause cross-linking of DNA; a vesicant

Therapeutic outcome: Prevention of rapidly growing malignant cells

Uses: Pancreas, stomach, colorectal, bladder cancer

Dosage and routes
Adult: **IV** 10-20 mg/m^2 q6-8wk

Available forms: Inj 5, 20, 40 mg/vial

Adverse effects
CNS: Fever, headache, confusion, drowsiness, syncope, fatigue
EENT: Blurred vision
GI: Nausea, vomiting, anorexia, stomatitis, **hepatotoxicity,** diarrhea
GU: Urinary retention, **renal failure,** edema
HEMA: **Thrombocytopenia, leukopenia, anemia**
INTEG: Rash, alopecia, **extravasation,** nail discoloration
MISC: **Hemolytic uremic syndrome, CHF**
RESP: **Fibrosis, pulmonary infiltrate,** dyspnea

Contraindications: Pregnancy **D** (1st trimester), breastfeeding, hypersensitivity, as a single agent, coagulation disorders

Black Box Warning: Thrombocytopenia

Adverse effects: *italic* = common, **bold** = life-threatening

Precautions: Accidental exposure, acute bronchospasm, anemia, children, dental disease/work, extravasation, females, hemolytic-uremic syndrome, infection, radiation therapy, surgery, vaccines, renal/respiratory disease

Black Box Warning: Bone marrow suppression, hemolytic uremic syndrome

Pharmacokinetics

Absorption	Complete bioavailability
Distribution	Widely distributed; concentrates in tumor
Metabolism	Liver, extensively
Excretion	Kidneys, unchanged
Half-life	1 hr

Pharmacodynamics
Unknown

Interactions
Individual drugs
Radiation: increased toxicity
Drug classifications
Anticoagulants, NSAIDs: increased bleeding risk
Antineoplastics: increased toxicity
Drug/herb
Black cohosh: avoid use

NURSING CONSIDERATIONS
Assessment

⬥ Assess for fatal hemolytic uremic syndrome: hypertension, thrombocytopenia, microangiopathic hemolytic anemia; occurs during long-term therapy
• Assess buccal cavity q8hr for dryness, sores or ulceration, white patches, oral pain, bleeding, dysphagia; obtain prescription for viscous lidocaine (Xylocaine)
• Assess symptoms indicating severe allergic reaction: rash, pruritus, urticaria, purpuric skin lesions, itching, flushing
• Monitor CBC, differential, platelet count weekly; withhold product if WBC is <2000/mm^3 or platelet count is <100,000/mm^3 or granulocyte count is <1000/mm^3; notify prescriber of results if WBC <20,000/mm^3, platelets <150,000/mm^3
• Monitor renal function tests: BUN, creatinine, serum uric acid, urine CCr before, during therapy; check I&O ratio; report fall in urine output to <30 ml/hr; adjust dose based on renal function
⬥ Assess for pulmonary fibrosis, bronchospasm, dyspnea, crackles, unproductive cough, chest pain, tachypnea, fatigue, increased pulse, pallor, lethargy
• Monitor temp q4hr (may indicate beginning of infection)
• Monitor liver function tests before, during therapy (bilirubin, AST, ALT, LDH) as needed or monthly; check for jaundiced skin and sclera, dark urine, clay-colored stools, itchy skin, abdominal pain, fever, diarrhea
• Assess for bleeding: hematuria, stool guaiac, bruising or petechiae, mucosa or orifices q8hr; inflammation of mucosa, breaks in skin
• Identify effects of alopecia on body image; discuss feelings about body changes
• Identify edema in feet, joint pain, stomach pain, shaking; check for inflammation of mucosa, breaks in skin

Nursing diagnoses
• Body image, disturbed (adverse reactions)
• Infection, risk for (adverse reactions)
• Injury, risk for (adverse reactions)
• Knowledge, deficient (teaching)

Implementation
IV route
• Avoid contact with skin, since medication is very irritating; wash completely to remove
• Give fluids **IV** or PO before chemotherapy to hydrate patient
• Provide antacid before oral agent; give product after evening meal, before bedtime; administer antiemetic 30-60 min before giving product and prn to prevent vomiting; use antibiotics for prophylaxis of infection
• Give topical or systemic analgesics for pain
• Give in ᴀᴍ so product can be eliminated before bedtime
• Provide a liquid diet: carbonated beverages; gelatin may be added if patient is not nauseated or vomiting
• Product should be prepared by experienced personnel using proper precautions in a biologic cabinet using gown, gloves, mask
• Give by direct **IV** after diluting 5 mg/1 ml or 10 mg/40 ml sterile water for inj; shake, allow to stand, give through Y-tube or 3-way stopcock; give slow **IV** push or inf over 15-30 min through running D₅W, 0.9% NaCl **IV**; color of reconstituted sol is gray
• Apply ice compress for extravasation
Syringe compatibilities: Bleomycin, cisplatin, cyclophosphamide, DOXOrubicin, droperidol, fluorouracil, furosemide, heparin, leucovorin, methotrexate, metoclopramide, vinBLAStine, vinCRIStine
Y-site compatibilities: Allopurinol, amifostine, bleomycin, cisplatin, cyclophosphamide, DOXOrubicin, droperidol, fluoroura-

cil, furosemide, granisetron, heparin, leucovorin, melphalan, methotrexate, metoclopramide, ondansetron, teniposide, thiotepa, vinBLAStine, vinCRIStine
Y-site incompatibilities: Sargramostim, vinorelbine
Additive compatibilities: Dexamethasone, hydrocortisone
Additive incompatibilities: Bleomycin
Solution compatibilities: LR, 0.3% NaCl, 0.5% NaCl

Patient/family education
• Advise patient to get adequate fluids 2-3 L/day unless contraindicated
• Encourage patient to rinse mouth tid-qid with water, club soda, brush teeth bid-qid with soft brush or cotton-tipped applicators for stomatitis, use unwaxed dental floss
• Teach patient to avoid use of products containing aspirin or ibuprofen, razors, commercial mouthwash, since bleeding may occur; to report symptoms of bleeding (hematuria, tarry stools)
• Caution patient to report signs of anemia (fatigue, headache, irritability, faintness, shortness of breath)
• Advise patient to report any changes in breathing or coughing even several mo after treatment; to avoid crowds and persons with respiratory tract or other infections
• Inform patient that hair may be lost during treatment; a wig or hairpiece may make patient feel better; new hair may be different in color, texture
• Advise patient not to have any vaccinations without the advice of the prescriber; serious reactions can occur
• Teach patient that contraception is needed during treatment and for several mo after completion of therapy
• Teach patient to report immediately urine retention, absence of urine, dyspnea, bleeding, jaundice

Evaluation
Positive therapeutic outcome
• Prevention of rapid division of malignant cells

⚠ **HIGH ALERT**

mitoxantrone (Rx)
(mye-toe-zan′trone)
Novantrone
Func. class.: Antineoplastic-antibiotic, immunomodulator
Chem. class.: Synthetic anthraquinone
Pregnancy category D

Action: DNA reactive agent; cytocidal effect on both proliferating and nonproliferating cells; topoisomerase II inhibitor; a vesicant

Therapeutic outcome: Prevention of rapidly growing malignant cells

Uses: Acute myelogenous leukemia (adult), relapsed leukemia, breast cancer, multiple sclerosis; used with steroids to treat bone pain (advanced prostate cancer); multiple sclerosis

Unlabeled uses: Liver malignancies, non-Hodgkin's lymphoma, breast cancer, ALL

Dosage and routes
Acute nonlymphatic leukemia/induction
Adult: **IV** INF 12 mg/m^2/day on days 1-3, and 100 mg/m^2 cytosine arabinoside × 7 days as a CONT 24-hr INF

Consolidation
Adult: **IV** INF 12 mg/m^2 given as a short 5-15 min INF

Advanced prostate cancer
Adult: **IV** 12-14 mg/m^2 as a single dose or short INF q21day

Multiple sclerosis
Adult: **IV** INF 12 mg/m^2 as a 5-15 min INF q3mo

Available forms: Inj 2, 10, 12.5, 15 mg/ml

Adverse effects
CNS: Headache, **seizures,** fatigue
CV: **CHF, cardiomyopathy, dysrhythmias**
EENT: Conjunctivitis, blue-green sclera, blurred vision
GI: Nausea, vomiting, diarrhea, anorexia, mucositis, **hepatoxicity**
GU: Amenorrhea, menstrual disorders
HEMA: **Thrombocytopenia, leukopenia, myelosuppression, anemia, secondary leukemia**
INTEG: Rash, necrosis at inj site, alopecia, dermatitis, thrombophlebitis at inj site, alopecia
MISC: Fever
RESP: Cough, dyspnea

M

Adverse effects: *italic* = common, **bold** = life-threatening

Contraindications: Pregnancy **D**, hypersensitivity

Precautions: Breastfeeding, children, myelosuppression, cardiac/renal/hepatic disease, gout

Black Box Warning: Secondary malignancy, neutropenia, intrathecal administration, extravasation, heart failure

Pharmacokinetics

Absorption	Completely absorbed
Distribution	Widely distributed, protein binding 78%
Metabolism	Liver
Excretion	Bile; kidneys, unchanged (<10%)
Half-life	23-215 hr

Pharmacodynamics
Unknown

Interactions
Individual drugs
Heparin: do not mix; precipitate will form
Radiation: increased toxicity, bone marrow suppression
Drug classifications
Do not mix with any other product
Anticoagulants, NSAIDs: increased bleeding risk
Antineoplastics: increased toxicity, bone marrow suppression
Live virus vaccines: increased adverse reactions
Drug/herb
Black cohosh, dong quai: avoid use

NURSING CONSIDERATIONS
Assessment
• Multiple sclerosis: obtain baseline multigated angiogram, left ventricular ejection fraction (LVEF) if symptoms of CHF occur, repeat LVEF or if cumulative dose is >100 mg/m^2; do not administer to patients who have received a lifetime dose of ≥140 mg/m^2 or if LVEF <50% or significant decrease in LVEF
• Do not administer in multiple sclerosis if neutrophils <1500/mm^3
• Obtain pregnancy test in all women of childbearing age
 Monitor ECG; watch for ST-T wave changes, low QRS and T, possible dysrhythmias (sinus tachycardia, heart block, PVCs); also monitor ECHO, MUGA, chest x-ray, RAI angiography to assess ejection fraction before, during treatment; product is cardiotoxic: may develop during treatment or months to years after treatment

• Assess buccal cavity q8hr for dryness, sores or ulceration, white patches, oral pain, bleeding, dysphagia; obtain prescription for viscous lidocaine (Xylocaine)
• Assess symptoms indicating severe allergic reaction: rash, pruritus, urticaria, purpuric skin lesions, itching, flushing
• Assess tachypnea, ECG changes, dyspnea, edema, fatigue
• Monitor CBC, differential, platelet count weekly; withhold product if WBC is <4000/mm^3 or platelet count is <75,000/mm^3, notify prescriber of results if WBC <20,000/mm^3, platelets <150,000/mm^3; neutrophil count or ANC
• Assess for increased uric acid levels, swelling, joint pain primarily in extremities; patient should be well hydrated to prevent urate deposits
• Monitor renal function tests: BUN, creatinine, urine CCr before, during therapy; determine I&O ratio
• Monitor temp q4hr (may indicate beginning of infection)
• Monitor liver function tests before, during therapy (bilirubin, AST, ALT, LDH) as needed or monthly; dose reduction needed in hepatic disease; check for jaundiced skin and sclera, dark urine, clay-colored stools, itchy skin, abdominal pain, fever, diarrhea
• Assess for bleeding: hematuria, stool guaiac, bruising or petechiae, mucosa or orifices q8hr; check for inflammation of mucosa, breaks in skin
• Identify effects of alopecia on body image; discuss feelings about body changes
 Assess for MS: obtain MUGA, LVEF baselines; repeat LVEF if symptoms of CHF occur or if cumulative dose is >100 mg/m^2; do not give to patients who have received a lifetime dose of ≥140 mg/m^2 or if LVEF <50% or significant LVEF
 Assess for secondary acute myelogenous leukemia (AML) that can develop after taking this product

Nursing diagnoses
• Body image, disturbed (adverse reactions)
• Infection, risk for (adverse reactions)
• Injury, risk for (adverse reactions)
• Knowledge, deficient (teaching)

Implementation
 Do not mix with any other product
• Avoid contact with skin, since medication is very irritating; wash completely to remove
• Give fluids **IV** or PO before chemotherapy to hydrate patient

---

 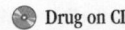

- Give antacid before oral agent; give product after evening meal, before bedtime; provide antiemetic 30-60 min before giving product and prn to prevent vomiting; administer antibiotics for prophylaxis of infection
- Give topical or systemic analgesics for pain
- Liquid diet: carbonated beverages; gelatin may be added if patient is not nauseated or vomiting
- Sol should be prepared by qualified personnel only under controlled conditions in a biologic cabinet using mask, gloves, gown
- Use Luer-Lok tubing to prevent leakage; do not let sol come in contact with skin; if contact occurs, wash well with soap and water
- Give by direct **IV** after diluting with 50 ml or more of 0.9% NaCl or D₅W; give over 3-5 min, running **IV** of D₅W or 0.9% NaCl
- Intermittent inf may be diluted further in D₅W, 0.9% NaCl and run over 15-30 min; check for extravasation

Y-site compatibilities: Allopurinol, amifostine, cladribine, filgrastim, fludarabine, granisetron, melphalan, ondansetron, sargramostim, teniposide, thiotepa, vinorelbine
Y-site incompatibilities: Paclitaxel
Additive compatibilities: Cyclophosphamide, cytarabine, fluorouracil, hydrocortisone, potassium chloride
Additive incompatibilities: Heparin
Solution compatibilities: D₅/0.9 NaCl, D₅W, 0.9% NaCl

Patient/family education
- Encourage patient to rinse mouth tid-qid with water, club soda; brush teeth bid-qid with soft brush or cotton-tipped applicators for stomatitis; use unwaxed dental floss
- Teach patient to avoid use of products containing aspirin or NSAIDs, razors, commercial mouthwash, since bleeding may occur; to report symptoms of bleeding (hematuria, tarry stools)
- Caution patient to report signs of anemia (fatigue, headache, irritability, faintness, shortness of breath)
- Inform patient that hair may be lost during treatment; a wig or hairpiece may make patient feel better; new hair may be different in color, texture
- Caution patient not to have any vaccinations without the advice of the prescriber; serious reactions can occur
- Advise patient that contraception is needed during treatment and for several mo after completion of therapy
- Advise patient that sclera, urine may turn blue or green
- Advise patient to increase fluids to 2-3 L/day unless contraindicated
- Teach patient to avoid crowds, persons with infections
- Teach patient to report immediately bleeding, dyspnea, possible infections, seizure, jaundice

Evaluation
Positive therapeutic outcome
- Prevention of rapid division of malignant cells

modafinil (Rx)
(mo-daf'i-nil)
Alertec ✦, Provigil
Func. class.: CNS stimulant
Chem. class.: Racemic compound

Pregnancy category C
Controlled substance IV

Action: Similar action as sympathomimetics; doesn't alter release of dopamine, norepinephrine

Therapeutic outcome: Ability to stay awake

Uses: Narcolepsy, shift work sleep disturbance, obstructive sleep apnea

Dosage and routes
Adult: PO 200 mg qd

Hepatic dose (severe hepatic disease)
Adult: PO 100 mg qd

Available forms: Tabs 100, 200 mg
Adverse effects
CNS: *Headache,* anxiety, cataplexy, depression, dizziness, insomnia, amnesia, confusion, ataxia, tremors, paresthesia, dyskinesia, **suicidal ideation**
CV: Dysrhythmias, hyper-hypotension, chest pain, vasodilation
EENT: Change in vision, *rhinitis,* pharyngitis, epistaxis
GI: Nausea, vomiting, changes in LFTs, anorexia, diarrhea, thirst, mouth ulcers
GU: Ejaculation disorder, urinary retention, albuminuria
HEMA: Eosinophilia
INTEG: Rash, dry skin, herpes simplex, **Stevens-Johnson syndrome**
MISC: Infection, hyperglycemia, neck pain
RESP: *Dyspnea,* lung changes

Contraindications: Hypersensitivity, ischemic heart disease, left ventricular hypertrophy, chest pain, dysrhythmias

Adverse effects: *italic* = common, **bold** = life-threatening

Precautions: Pregnancy **D,** breastfeeding, child <16 yr, geriatrics, unstable angina, history of MI, severe hepatic disease

Pharmacokinetics	
Absorption	Rapid
Distribution	60% protein binding
Metabolism	Liver (90%)
Excretion	Unknown
Half-life	15 hr

Pharmacodynamics	
Onset	Unknown
Peak	2-4 hr
Duration	Unknown

Interactions
Individual drugs
Diazepam, phenytoin, propranolol, tricyclic antidepressants, warfarin: increased effects of these drugs

Cyclosporine, hormonal contraceptives, theophylline: decreased effects of these drugs
Drug/herb
Coffee, cola nut, guarana, mate, tea: increased stimulation
Drug/lab test
Increased: eosinophils, glucose, LFTs

NURSING CONSIDERATIONS
Assessment
- For narcolepsy, shift work, history of sleep apnea
- For depression, suicidal ideation
- Monitor B/P in those with hypertension

Nursing diagnosis
- Sleep pattern disturbance (uses)

Implementation
- Give 1 hr before start of shift work, or in the AM for those with narcolepsy or sleep apnea
- Store at room temperature

Patient/family education
- Advise patient to take only as directed; may be taken with or without food
- Advise patient to use other form of contraception during and at least 30 days after discontinuing medication, if using hormonal birth control
- Advise patient to notify prescriber if pregnancy is planned or suspected, or if breastfeeding
- Advise patient to notify prescriber of allergic reaction, tremors, confusion
- Teach patient to avoid all OTC medications unless approved by prescriber
- Teach patient to avoid hazardous activities until drug effect is known

Evaluation
- Ability to stay awake

moexipril (Rx)
(moe-ex'i-pril)
Univasc
Func. class.: Antihypertensive
Chem. class.: Angiotensin-converting enzyme (ACE) inhibitor

Pregnancy category D

Action: Selectively suppresses renin-angiotensin-aldosterone system; inhibits ACE; prevents conversion of angiotensin I to angiotensin II; results in dilatation of arterial, venous vessels

Therapeutic outcome: Decreased B/P in hypertension

Uses: Hypertension, alone or in combination with thiazide diuretics

Dosage and routes
Initial treatment
Adult: PO 7.5 mg 1 hr before meals initially, may be increased or divided depending on B/P response

Maintenance
Adult: PO 7.5-30 mg/day in 1-2 divided doses 1 hr before meals

Renal dose
Adult: PO CCr <40 ml/min 3.75 mg/day titrate to desired dose, max 15 mg/day

Available forms: Tabs 7.5, 15 mg

Adverse effects
CNS: Fever, chills
CV: Hypotension, postural hypotension
GI: Loss of taste
GU: Impotence, dysuria, nocturia, proteinuria, nephrotic syndrome, acute reversible renal failure, polyuria, oliguria, frequency
HEMA: **Neutropenia**
INTEG: Rash
META: Hypokalemia
RESP: **Bronchospasm,** dyspnea, dry cough
SYST: **Angioedema, anaphylaxis**

Contraindications: Pregnancy **D,** breastfeeding, hypersensitivity, children, heart block, bilateral renal stenosis, history of angioedema

Precautions: Dialysis patients, hypovolemia, leukemia, scleroderma, lupus erythematosus, blood dyscrasias, CHF, diabetes mellitus, renal/thyroid disease, COPD, asthma, potassium-sparing diuretics

Pharmacokinetics

Absorption	Unknown
Distribution	Unknown
Metabolism	Liver to metabolites
Excretion	Via kidneys, crosses placenta, excreted in breast milk
Half-life	Unknown

Pharmacodynamics

Unknown

Interactions

Individual drugs
Azathioprine: increased myelosuppression
CycloSPORINE: increased hyperkalemia
Digoxin, lithium: increased toxicity

Drug classification
Adrenergic blockers, antihypertensives, diuretics, ganglionic blockers, phenothiazines: increased hypotension
Diuretics (potassium-sparing), potassium supplements, sympathomimetics: do not use together
NSAIDs: decreased antihypertensive effect

Drug/herb
Hawthorn: increased antihypertensive effect
Yohimbe: decreased antihypertensive effect

Drug/lab test
False positive: urine acetone

NURSING CONSIDERATIONS
Assessment
• Monitor blood studies: neutrophils, decreased platelets
• Monitor B/P
• Monitor renal function tests: protein, BUN, creatinine; watch for increased levels that may indicate nephrotic syndrome
• Monitor baselines in renal, liver function tests before therapy begins
• Monitor potassium levels, although hyperkalemia rarely occurs
• Assess edema in feet, legs daily
• Assess allergic reaction: rash, fever, pruritus, urticaria; product should be discontinued if antihistamines fail to help
• Assess for symptoms of CHF: edema, dyspnea, wet crackles, B/P
• Monitor for renal symptoms: polyuria, oliguria, frequency

Nursing diagnoses
• Knowledge, deficient (teaching)

Implementation
• Give PO 1 hr before meals
• Store in airtight container at 86° F or less

Patient/family education
• Instruct patient not to discontinue product abruptly
• Tell patient not to use OTC (cough, cold, allergy) products unless directed by prescriber
• Teach patient to comply with dosage schedule, even if feeling better
• Encourage patient to rise slowly to sitting or standing position to minimize orthostatic hypotension
• Teach patient to notify prescriber of mouth sores, sore throat, fever, swelling of hands or feet, irregular heartbeat, chest pain, signs of angioedema
• Tell patient that excessive perspiration, dehydration, vomiting, diarrhea may lead to fall in B/P; consult prescriber if this occurs
• Teach patient that dizziness, fainting, lightheadedness may occur during first few days of therapy
• Tell patient that skin rash or impaired perspiration may occur
• Teach patient how to take B/P

Evaluation
Positive therapeutic outcome
• Decreased B/P in hypertension

Treatment of overdose: 0.9% NaCl **IV** inf, hemodialysis

M

montelukast (Rx)
(mon tch-loo′kast)
Singulair
Func. class.: Bronchodilator
Chem. class.: Leukotriene antagonist, cysteinyl
Pregnancy category B

Action: Inhibits leukotriene (LTD_4) formation; leukotrienes exert their effects by increasing neutrophil, eosinophil migration; aggregation of neutrophils, monocytes; smooth muscle contraction, capillary permeability; these actions further lead to bronchoconstriction, inflammation, edema

Therapeutic outcome: Ability to breathe with ease

Uses: Chronic asthma in adults and children, seasonal allergic rhinitis

Unlabeled uses: Chronic urticaria

Dosage and routes
Asthma
Adult and child ≥15 yr: PO 10 mg/day PM

Child 6-14 yr: PO 5 mg chew tabs/day PM

Adverse effects: *italic* = common, **bold** = life-threatening

Child 2-5 yr: PO chew tabs 4 mg/day
Child 12-23 mo: PO 1 packet of granules taken PM

Exercise-induced bronchoconstriction
Adult and adolescent ≥15 yr: PO 10 mg 2 hr prior to exercise; do not take another dose within 24 hr

Available forms: Tabs 10 mg; chewable tabs 4, 5 mg; oral granules 4 mg/packet

Adverse effects
CNS: Dizziness, fatigue, headache, behavior changes, **suicidal ideation, suicide, seizures,** agitation, anxiety, depression, fever, hallucinations
GI: Abdominal pain, dyspepsia, nausea, vomiting, diarrhea
INTEG: Rash
MS: Asthenia
RESP: Influenza, cough, nasal congestion
SYST: **Anaphylaxis, angioedema**

Contraindications: Hypersensitivity

Precautions: Pregnancy **B**, breastfeeding, children <6 yr, acute attacks of asthma, alcohol consumption, aspirin sensitivity, severe hepatic disease

Pharmacokinetics

Absorption	Rapidly
Distribution	Protein binding 99%
Metabolism	Liver
Excretion	Bile
Half-life	2.7-5.5 hr

Pharmacodynamics

Onset	Unknown
Peak	3-4 hr
Duration	Unknown

Interactions
Individual drugs
Phenobarbital, rifampin: decreased montelukast levels
Drug/herb
Tea (green, black), guarana: increased stimulation
Drug/lab test
Increased: ALT, AST

NURSING CONSIDERATIONS
Assessment
🔷 Assess adult patients carefully for symptoms of Churg-Strauss syndrome (rare), including eosinophilia, vasculitic rash, worsening pulmonary symptoms, cardiac complications and/or neuropathy

• Monitor CBC, blood chemistry during treatment
• Assess respiratory rate, rhythm, depth; auscultate lung fields bilaterally; notify prescriber of abnormalities
• Assess allergic reactions: rash, urticaria; product should be discontinued

Nursing diagnoses
• Activity intolerance (uses)
• Airway clearance, ineffective (uses)
• Knowledge, deficient (teaching)

Implementation
PO route
• Give PO in PM daily for all uses except exercise-induced bronchoconstriction; then take 2 hr prior to exercise
• Do not open packet until ready to use; mix whole dose, give within 15 min
• Granules may be given directly in mouth or mixed with a spoonful of soft food (carrots, applesauce, ice cream, rice)

Patient/family education
• Advise patient to avoid hazardous activities; dizziness may occur
• Teach patient that product is not to be used for acute asthma attacks
• Advise patient to avoid NSAIDs if sensitive to aspirin
• Advise patient to continue to use inhaled β-agonists if exercise-induced asthma occurs

Evaluation
Positive therapeutic outcome
• Increased ease of breathing
• Decreased bronchospasm

morphine 🔵 (Rx)
(mor'feen)

Astramorph, Astramorph PF, Avinza, Duramorph, Epimorph ✦, Infumorph, Kadian, morphine sulfate, Morphitec ✦, M.O.S. ✦, M.O.S.-S.R. ✦, MS Contin, MSIR, OMS Concentrate, Oramorph SR, RMS, Roxanol, Roxanol Rescudose, Roxanol-T, Statex ✦

Func. class.: Opioid analgesic
Chem. class.: Alkaloid

Pregnancy category C

Controlled substance schedule II

Do not confuse:
morphine/hydromorphone, Roxanol/Roxicet

Action: Depresses pain impulse transmission at the spinal cord level by interacting with opioid receptors

Therapeutic outcome: Decreased pain

Uses: Moderate to severe pain

Dosage and routes
Adult: SUBCUT/IM 5-20 mg q4hr prn; PO 10-30 mg q4hr prn; EXT REL 15-30 mg q8-12hr; RECT 10-20 mg q4hr prn; **IV** 2.5-15 mg diluted in 4-5 ml of water for inj, over 5 min; SUS REL cap (Kadian), EXT REL cap (Avinza) give total daily dose q24hr; for those with no tolerance to opioids, 30 mg/day, may adjust by no more than 30 mg q4day
Child: SUBCUT/**IV** 0.05-0.2 mg/kg, max 15 mg; PO 0.2-0.5 mg/kg q4-6hr (regular REL), q12hr (SUS REL)

Available forms: Inj 0.5, 1, 2, 3, 4, 5, 8, 10, 15, 25, 50 mg/ml; sol tabs 10, 15, 30 mg; oral sol 10, 20 mg/5 ml, 20 mg/10 ml, 20 mg/ml; oral tabs 15, 30 mg; rect supp 5, 10, 20, 30 mg; ext rel tabs 15, 30, 60, 100, 200 mg; caps 15, 30 mg; syr 1, 5 mg/ml; cont rel cap pellets (Kadian) 20, 30, 50, 60, 100 mg; ext rel caps (Avinza) 30, 60, 90, 120 mg

Adverse effects
CNS: Drowsiness, dizziness, *confusion,* headache, *sedation,* euphoria, insomnia, **seizures**

CV: Palpitations, **bradycardia,** change in B/P, **shock, cardiac arrest,** chest pain, hyper/hypotension, edema, **tachycardia**
EENT: Tinnitus, blurred vision, miosis, diplopia
GI: Nausea, vomiting, anorexia, *constipation,* cramps, biliary tract pressure
GU: Urinary retention
HEMA: **Thrombocytopenia**
INTEG: Rash, urticaria, bruising, flushing, diaphoresis, pruritus
RESP: **Respiratory depression, respiratory arrest, apnea**

Contraindications: Hypersensitivity, addiction (opioid), hemorrhage, bronchial asthma, increased ICP

Black Box Warning: Respiratory depression

Precautions: Pregnancy C, breastfeeding, children <18 yr, geriatric, addictive personality, acute MI, severe heart disease, renal/hepatic disease, bowel impaction

Black Box Warning: Abrupt discontinuation, accidental exposure, epidural/intrathecal administration, opioid-naive patients, substance abuse

Pharmacokinetics

Absorption	Variably absorbed (PO); well absorbed (IM, SUBCUT, RECT); completely absorbed (**IV**)
Distribution	Widely distributed; crosses placenta
Metabolism	Liver, extensively
Excretion	Kidneys
Half-life	1½-2 hr

Interactions
Individual drugs
Alcohol: increased effects with other CNS depressants
Rifampin: decreased analgesic action
Drug classifications
Antipsychotics, opiates, sedative/hypnotics, skeletal muscle relaxants: increased effects with other CNS depressants
MAOIs: unpredictable reaction may occur; avoid use

Pharmacodynamics

	PO	PO–EXT REL	IM	SUBCUT	RECT	IV	IT
Onset	Variable	Unknown	10-30 min	20 min	Unknown	Rapid	Rapid
Peak	1 hr	Unknown	½-1 hr	1-1½ hr	½-1 hr	20 min	Unknown
Duration	4-5 hr	8-12 hr	3-7 hr	4-5 hr	4-5 hr	4-5 hr	Ext

Adverse effects: *italic* = common, **bold** = life-threatening

M

Drug/herb
Chamomile, hops, Jamaican dogwood, kava, lavender, mistletoe, nettle, pokeweed, poppy, senega, skullcap, St. John's wort, valerian: increased CNS depression
Corkwood: increased anticholinergic effect
Drug/food
Cranberry juice (excessive amounts), oats: decreased morphine effect
Drug/lab test
Increased: amylase

NURSING CONSIDERATIONS
Assessment
- Assess pain: location, type, character, intensity; give dose before pain becomes extreme
- Monitor I&O ratio; check for decreasing output; may indicate urinary retention; check for constipation; increase fluids, bulk in diet if needed, or stimulant laxatives may be prescribed
- Monitor CNS changes: dizziness, drowsiness, hallucinations, euphoria, LOC, pupil reactions
- Monitor allergic reactions: rash, urticaria
- Assess respiratory dysfunction: depression, character, rate, rhythm; notify prescriber if respirations are <10/min

Nursing diagnoses
- Breathing pattern, ineffective (adverse reactions)
- Knowledge, deficient (teaching)
- Pain, acute (uses)
- Sensory perception, disturbed: visual, auditory (adverse reactions)

Implementation
- Give with antiemetic if nausea, vomiting occur
- Administer when pain is beginning to return; determine dosage interval by patient response; continuous dosing of medication is more effective than giving prn
- Withdraw medication slowly after long-term use to prevent withdrawal symptoms
- Store in light-resistant container at room temperature
- Kadian is not bioequivalent to other controlled release forms

PO route
- Swallow ext rel tabs whole; do not break, crush, or chew
⬥ Kadian tabs may be opened and sprinkled on applesauce immediately before use; do not break, crush, chew, or dissolve pellets in Kadian cap, which may lead to an overdose; adjustments may need to be made when converting from another form of morphine
- May be given with food or milk to lessen GI upset; other forms may be crushed and mixed with food or fluids

IM/SUBCUT route
- Do not give if cloudy or a precipitate has formed

IV route
- Give direct **IV** by diluting with ≥5 ml of sterile water or 0.9% NaCl for inj; give 2.5-15 mg/4-5 min; rapid administration may lead to increased respiratory depression, death
- Give cont inf by adding to D_5W, $D_{10}W$, 0.9% NaCl, 0.45% NaCl, Ringer's, LR, any dextrose/ saline sol, or any dextrose/Ringer's, 0.1-1 mg/ml
- Give by inf pump to deliver correct dosage; titrate to provide adequate pain relief without serious sedation, respiratory depression, hypotension
- May be given by patient-controlled analgesia (PCA) pump in terminal illnesses; patient is able to control amount of morphine
- Administer epidurally with caution in the geriatric

Syringe compatibilities: Atropine, benzquinamide, bupivacaine, butorphanol, cimetidine, dimenhyDRINATE, diphenhydrA-MINE, droperidol, fentanyl, glycopyrrolate, hydrOXYzine, ketamine, metoclopramide, midazolam, milrinone, pentazocine, perphenazine, promazine, ranitidine, scopolamine
Syringe incompatibilities: Meperidine, thiopental
Y-site compatibilities: Allopurinol, amifostine, amikacin, aminophylline, amiodarone, ampicillin, ampicillin/sulbactam, amsacrine, atenolol, atracurium, aztreonam, bumetanide, calcium chloride, cefamandole, cefazolin, cefmetazole, cefoperazone, cefotaxime, cefotetan, cefoxitin, ceftazidime, ceftizoxime, ceftriaxone, cefuroxime, cephalothin, cephapirin, chloramphenicol, cisplatin, cladribine, clindamycin, cyclophosphamide, cytarabine, dexamethasone, digoxin, diltiazem, dobutamine, DOPamine, doxycycline, enalaprilat, epinephrine, erythromycin, esmolol, etomidate, famotidine, fentanyl, filgrastim, fluconazole, fludarabine, foscarnet, gentamicin, granisetron, heparin, hydrocortisone, hydromorphone, IL-2, insulin (regular), kanamycin, labetalol, lidocaine, lorazepam, magnesium sulfate, melphalan, meropenem, methotrexate, methyldopa, methylPREDNISolone, metoclopramide, metoprolol, metronidazole, mezlocillin, midazolam, milrinone, moxalactam, nafcillin, niCARdipine, nitroglycerin, norepinephrine, ondansetron, oxacillin, oxytocin, paclitaxel, pancuronium, penicillin G

potassium, piperacillin, piperacillin/tazobactam, potassium chloride, propofol, propranolol, ranitidine, sodium bicarbonate, sodium nitroprusside, teniposide, thiotepa, ticarcillin, ticarcillin/clavulanate, tobramycin, trimethoprim/sulfamethoxazole, vancomycin, vecuronium, vinorelbine, vit B/C, warfarin, zidovudine

Y-site incompatibilities: Furosemide, minocycline, tetracycline

Additive compatibilities: Alteplase, atracurium, baclofen, bupivacaine, DOBUTamine, fluconazole, furosemide, meropenem, metoclopramide, ondansetron, succinylcholine, verapamil

Additive incompatibilities: Aminophylline

Patient/family education
• Advise patient to report any symptoms of CNS changes, allergic reactions
• Caution patients to avoid CNS depressants (alcohol, sedative/hypnotics) for at least 24 hr after taking this product
• Discuss with patient that dizziness, drowsiness, and confusion are common; to avoid getting up without assistance
• Discuss in detail all aspects of the product and expected response

Evaluation
Positive therapeutic outcome
• Decreased pain

Treatment of overdose: Naloxone (Narcan) 0.2-0.8 **IV**, O₂, **IV** fluids, vasopressors

---

moxifloxacin (Rx)
(mox-i-floks'a-sin)
Avelox, Avelox IV
Func. class.: Antiinfective
Chem. class.: Fluoroquinolone

Pregnancy category C

Action: Interferes with conversion of intermediate DNA fragments into high molecular weight DNA in bacteria; DNA gyrase inhibitor

Therapeutic outcome: Bactericidal action against the following: *Staphylococcus aureus, Streptococcus pneumoniae, Haemophilus influenzae, Haemophilus parainfluenzae, Moraxella catarrhalis, Klebsiella pneumoniae, Mycoplasma pneumoniae, Chlamydia pneumoniae; Streptococcus pyogenes, E. coli, Bacteroides fragilis, Streptococcus arginosus, Streptococcus constellatus, Enterococcus faecalis, Proteus mirabilis, Clostridium perfringens, Bacteroides thetalomicron, Peptostreptococcus, Enterobacter cloacae*

Uses: Acute bacterial sinusitis, acute bacterial exacerbation of chronic bronchitis, community-acquired pneumonia (mild to moderate), uncomplicated skin/skin structure infections, complicated intraabdominal infections including polymicrobial infections, complicated skin/skin structure infections

Dosage and routes
Acute bacterial sinusitis
Adult: PO/**IV** 400 mg q24hr × 10 days

Acute bacterial exacerbation of chronic bronchitis
Adult: PO/**IV** 400 mg q24hr × 5 days

Community-acquired pneumonia
Adult: PO/**IV** 400 mg q24hr × 7-14 days

Uncomplicated skin/skin structure infections
Adult: PO/**IV** 400 mg q24hr × 7 days

Complicated intraabdominal infections
Adult: **IV** 400 mg/day × 5-14 days

Complicated skin, skin structure infections
Adult: PO/**IV** 400 mg/day × 7-21 days

Available forms: Tabs 400 mg; inj premix 400 mg/250 ml

Adverse effects
CNS: Headache, dizziness, fatigue, insomnia, depression, restlessness, **seizures**, confusion, **increased intracranial pressure**, peripheral neuropathy
CV: **Prolonged QT interval, dysrhythmias, torsades de pointes,** tachycardia
EENT: Blurred vision, tinnitus, taste changes
GI: Nausea, increased ALT, AST, flatulence, heartburn, vomiting, diarrhea, oral candidiasis, dysphagia, **pseudomembranous colitis**
INTEG: Rash, pruritus, urticaria, photosensitivity, flushing, fever, chills
MS: Tremor, arthralgia, tendon rupture, myalgia
SYST: **Anaphylaxis, Stevens-Johnson syndrome**

Contraindications: Hypersensitivity to quinolones

Precautions: Pregnancy **C**, breastfeeding, children, renal/hepatic/cardiac disease, epilepsy, uncorrected hypokalemia, prolonged QT interval, patients receiving class IA, III antidysrhythmics, GI disease, seizure disorder

M

Adverse effects: *italic* = common, **bold** = life-threatening

Black Box Warning: Tendon pain/rupture, tendonitis

Pharmacokinetics

Absorption	Well absorbed (75%) (PO)
Distribution	Widely distributed
Metabolism	Liver
Excretion	Kidneys
Half-life	Increased in renal disease

Pharmacodynamics

	PO
Onset	Rapid
Peak	1 hr
Duration	Unknown

Interactions
Individual drugs
Aluminum hydroxide, calcium, didanosine, iron, sucralfate, zinc sulfate: decreased absorption of moxifloxacin

CycloSPORINE: increased cycloSPORINE effect

Probenecid: increased blood levels

Warfarin: increased warfarin effect

Drug classifications
Antacids (magnesium), iron salts: decreased absorption of moxifloxacin

Antidysrhythmics IA, III, other drugs that increase QT prolongation: prolonged QT interval

NSAIDs: increased seizure risk

Drug/herb
Acidophilus: do not use with antiinfectives; separate by several hours

Cola tree: increased antiinfective effect

Drug/food
Enteral feeding: decreased absorption of moxifloxacin

NURSING CONSIDERATIONS
Assessment
• Assess patient for previous sensitivity reaction

• Assess patient for signs and symptoms of infection including characteristics of wounds, sputum, urine, stool, WBC >10,000/mm^3, fever baseline, during treatment

• Obtain C&S before beginning product therapy to identify if correct treatment has been initiated

• Assess for allergic reactions, Stevens-Johnson syndrome, toxic epidermal necrolysis, and anaphylaxis: rash, urticaria, pruritus, chills, fever, joint pain; may occur a few days after therapy begins; epinephrine and resuscitation equipment should be available for anaphylactic reaction

• Assess for CNS symptoms: headache, dizziness, fatigue, insomnia, depression, **seizures**

• Identify urine output; if decreasing, notify prescriber (may indicate nephrotoxicity); also check for increased BUN, creatinine

• Monitor blood tests: AST, ALT, CBC, Hct, bilirubin, LDH, alkaline phosphatase, Coombs' test monthly if patient is on long-term therapy

• Monitor electrolytes: potassium, sodium chloride monthly if patient is on long-term therapy

• Assess bowel pattern daily; if severe diarrhea occurs, product should be discontinued; may indicate pseudomembranous colitis

• Monitor for bleeding: ecchymosis, bleeding gums, hematuria, stool guaiac daily if on long-term therapy

• Assess for overgrowth of infection: perineal itching, fever, malaise, redness, pain, swelling, drainage, rash, diarrhea, change in cough, sputum

⬥ Assess for tendon pain, rupture, tendonitis; if tendon becomes inflamed, drug should be discontinued

⬥ Assess cardiac status; prolonged QT; or use of drugs that increase QT prolongation

Nursing diagnoses
• Diarrhea (side effects)
• Infection, risk for (uses)
• Injury, risk for (side effects)
• Knowledge, deficient (teaching)
• Noncompliance (teaching)

Implementation
• Do not use theophylline with this product; may cause toxicity

PO route
• Give once a day for 5-10 days depending on condition

IV route
• Discontinue primary **IV** while administering moxifloxacin

• Do not give SUBCUT, IM

Solution compatibilities: 0.9% NaCl, D$_5$, D$_{10}$, LR, sterile water for inj

Patient/family education
• Teach patient to report sore throat, bruising, bleeding, joint pain; may indicate blood dyscrasias (rare)

• Advise patient to contact prescriber if vaginal itching, loose foul-smelling stools, furry tongue occur; may indicate superinfection; report itching, rash, pruritus, urticaria

• Instruct patient to take all medication prescribed for the length of time ordered; do not give medication to others

• Advise patient to notify prescriber of diarrhea with blood or pus

- Advise patient to rinse mouth frequently, use sugarless candy or gum for dry mouth
- Advise patient to take as prescribed, not to double or miss doses

Evaluation
Positive therapeutic outcome
- Absence of signs/symptoms of infection (WBC <10,000/mm^3, temp WNL)
- Reported improvement in symptoms of infection

moxifloxacin ophthalmic
See Appendix B

multivitamins
(PO, OTC, **IV**, Rx)
Adavite, Dayalets, LKV Drops, Multi-75, Multi-Day, One-A-Day, Optilets, Poly-Vi-Sol, Quintabs, Rulets, Sesame Street Vitamins, Tab-A-Vite, Therabid, Theragran, Unicaps, Vita-Bob, Vita-Kid, many other brands
Func. class.: Vitamins, multiple

Pregnancy category A

Do not confuse:
Theragran/Phenergan

Action: Needed for adequate metabolism

Therapeutic outcome: Prevention and treatment of vitamin deficiencies

Uses: Prevention and treatment of vitamin deficiencies

Dosage and routes
Adult and child: PO/**IV**—depends on brand

Available forms: Many forms available

Adverse effects
Rare at recommended dosage

Precautions: Pregnancy A

Pharmacokinetics	
Absorption	Well absorbed (PO)
Distribution	Widely distributed; crosses placenta
Metabolism	Widely metabolized
Excretion	Kidney, unchanged (water soluble)
Half-life	Unknown

Pharmacodynamics
Unknown

NURSING CONSIDERATIONS
Assessment
- Assess patient for vitamin deficiency; usually more than one vitamin deficiency is present

Nursing diagnoses
- Knowledge, deficient (teaching)
- Nutrition: less than body requirements, imbalanced (uses)

Implementation
PO route
- Liquid multivitamins can be diluted or dropped into patient's mouth using dropper provided with some brands
- Chew tabs should be chewed and not swallowed whole
IV route
- Give by cont inf only after diluting 5-10 ml (multivitamins)/500-1000 ml of D$_5$W, D$_{10}$W, D$_{20}$W, LR, D$_5$/LR, D$_5$/0.9% NaCl, 0.9% NaCl, 3% NaCl
- Do not use sol with crystals, precipitate, or color other than bright yellow
Y-site compatibilities: Acyclovir, ampicillin, cefazolin, cephalothin, cephapirin, diltiazem, erythromycin, fludarabine, gentamicin, tacrolimus, tetracycline
Additive compatibilities: Cefoxitin, isoproterenol, methyldopate, metoclopramide, metronidazole, netilmicin, norepinephrine, sodium bicarbonate, verapamil
Additive incompatibilities: Penicillin G, erythromycin, tetracycline, kanamycin, streptomycin, doxycycline, lincomycin should not be admixed

Patient/family education
- Advise patient that adequate nutrition must be maintained to prevent further deficiencies; to comply with treatment regimen
- Advise patient to avoid treating flavored multivitamins as candy; child may overdose
- Caution patient to store vitamins out of children's reach

Evaluation
Positive therapeutic outcome
- Check each individual vitamin for guidelines
- Absence of vitamin deficiencies

mupirocin topical
See Appendix B

muromonab-CD3 (Rx)

(mur-oe-mone'ab)
Orthoclone OKT3
Func. class.: Immunosuppressive
Chem. class.: Murine monoclonal antibody

Pregnancy category C

Action: Reverses graft rejection by blocking T-cell function

Therapeutic outcome: Prevention of graft rejection

Uses: Acute allograft rejection in renal, cardiac, hepatic transplant patients

Dosage and routes
Adult: **IV** BOL 5 mg/day × 10-14 days
Child ≤30 kg: **IV** 2.5 mg qd × 10-14 day

Cardiac/hepatic allograft rejection, steroid resistant
Adult: **IV** BOL 5 mg/day × 10-14 days; begin when it is known that rejection has not been reversed by steroids

Available forms: Inj 5 mg/5 ml

Adverse effects
CNS: Pyrexia, chills, tremors, **aseptic meningitis,** fever, headache
CV: Chest pain
EENT: Vision impairment
GI: Vomiting, nausea, diarrhea
MISC: **Infection, cytokine release syndrome, anaphylaxis,** malaise
RESP: Dyspnea, wheezing, **pulmonary edema**

Contraindications: Hypersensitivity to murine origin, CHF, uncontrolled hypertension

Black Box Warning: Fluid overload, seizures

Precautions: Pregnancy C, children <2 yr, fever, cerebral edema, thrombus, CV/vascular disease

Black Box Warning: Angioedema, immunosuppressants

Pharmacokinetics

Absorption	Completely absorbed
Distribution	Unknown
Metabolism	Unknown
Excretion	Unknown
Half-life	Unknown

Pharmacodynamics
Unknown

Interactions
Individual drugs
Azathioprine, cycloSPORINE: increased risk of infection
Indomethacin: increased CNS symptoms
Drug classifications
Corticosteroids: increased risk of infection
Immunosuppressants: increased immunosuppression
Live virus vaccines: decreased antibody response
Drug/herb
Astragalus, echinacea, melatonin: interference with immunosuppression
Ginseng, maitake, mistletoe, schisandra, St. John's wort, turmeric: decreased effect

NURSING CONSIDERATIONS
Assessment
◆ Assess for cytosine release syndrome (CRS): nausea, vomiting, chills, fever, joint pain, weakness, dizziness, diarrhea, tremors, abdominal pain; occurs 30-60 min after first dose; methylPREDNISolone sodium succinate may be prescribed to lessen this reaction
• Assess for hypersensitivity reaction, anaphylaxis: dyspnea, bronchospasm, urticaria, tachycardia, hypotension, angioedema; discontinue product; emergency equipment must be nearby
• Assess for headache, photophobia, fever, rigidity; indicate aseptic meningitis has developed
• Assess for sore throat, fever, chills, rash, dysuria, which may indicate infection; therapy may be discontinued
• Assess for fluid overload: edema, pulmonary edema, increasing weight
• Monitor blood studies: CBC with differential, platelets, BUN, creatinine, alkaline phosphatase, bilirubin during treatment monthly
• Monitor AST, ALT, BUN, creatinine, alkaline phosphatase, bilirubin
• Obtain human-mouse antibody; if titer is >1:1000, this product should not be used
• Monitor T-cells with CD3, CD4, CD8 antigen daily; report should be CD3 positive and T-cells <25/mm³

Nursing diagnoses
• Infection, risk for (uses)
• Knowledge, deficient (teaching)

Implementation
• Give by direct **IV** undiluted; withdraw with a 0.2-0.22 low–protein binding μm filter; discard and use new needle for administration; give over 1 min

 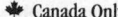

- Give for several days before transplant surgery

Patient/family education
- Instruct patient to report fever, chills, sore throat, fatigue, since serious infections may occur; rash, rapid heartbeat
- Advise patient to use contraceptive measures during treatment and for 12 wk after ending therapy; product is mutagenic
- Advise patient to avoid crowds and persons with known infections to reduce risk of infection
- Advise patient to report symptoms of cytokine release syndrome, aseptic meningitis, give list of symptoms
- Instruct patient to avoid vaccinations during treatment

Evaluation
Positive therapeutic outcome
- Absence of graft rejection

---

mycophenolate (Rx)
(mie-koe-feen'oh-late)
CellCept, Myfortic
Func. class.: Immunosuppressant

Pregnancy category C

Action: Inhibits inflammatory responses that are mediated by the immune system; prolongs survival of allogenic transplants

Therapeutic outcome: Absence of graft rejection

Uses: Organ transplants to prevent rejection (renal); prophylaxis of rejection in allogenic cardiac, hepatic, renal transplants

Unlabeled uses: Refractory uveitis, 2nd-line therapy for Churg-Strauss syndrome, diffuse proliferative lupus nephritis (in combination), rheumatoid arthritis, psoriasis

Dosage and routes
Renal transplant
Adult: PO/**IV** give initial dose 72 hr before transplantation; 1 g bid given to renal transplant patients in combination with corticosteroids and cycloSPORINE; ER tab 720 mg bid on empty stomach
Child: PO-ER 400 mg/m^2 bid, max 720 mg bid

Renal dose
Adult: PO/**IV** GFR <25 ml/min, max 2 g/day

Cardiac transplant
Adult: PO/**IV** 1.5 g bid, **IV** can be started ≤24 hr after transplant, switch to PO when able

Hepatic transplant
Adult: PO 1.5 g bid, **IV** 1 g over ≥2 hr

Available forms: Caps 250 mg; tabs 500 mg; inj (powder) 500 mg/20 ml vial; powder for oral susp 200 mg/ml; ext rel tab (Myfortic) 180, 360 mg

Adverse effects
CNS: Tremor, dizziness, insomnia, headache, fever, progressive multifocal leukoencephalopathy
CV: Hypertension, chest pain
GI: Nausea, vomiting, stomatitis, *diarrhea, constipation,* **GI bleeding**
GU: UTI, *hematuria,* **renal tubular necrosis**
HEMA: **Leukopenia, thrombocytopenia, anemia, pancytopenia,** pure red cell aplasia
INTEG: Rash
META: Peripheral edema, hypercholesterolemia, hypophosphatemia, edema, hypo/hyperkalemia, hyperglycemia, hypocalcemia, hypomagnesemia
MS: Arthralgia, muscle wasting
RESP: Dyspnea, respiratory infection, increased cough, pharyngitis, bronchitis, pneumonia
SYST: **Lymphoma, nonmelanoma skin carcinoma, sepsis**

Contraindications: Hypersensitivity to this product or mycophenolic acid

Precautions: Breastfeeding, lymphomas, neutropenia, renal disease

Black Box Warning: Pregnancy **D**, infection, neoplastic disease

M

Pharmacokinetics	
Absorption	Rapidly and completely absorbed
Distribution	Unknown
Metabolism	To active metabolite (MPA)
Excretion	Urine, feces
Half-life	Unknown

Pharmacodynamics
Unknown

Interactions
Individual drugs
Acyclovir, ganciclovir: increased concentration of both products
Azathioprine: avoid use
Cholestyramine: decreased levels of mycophenolate
Phenytoin: increased effects; decreased protein binding of phenytoin

---

Adverse effects: *italic* = common, **bold** = life-threatening

Probenecid: increased levels of mycophenolate

Theophylline: increased effects; decreased protein binding of theophylline

Drug classifications

Antacids: decreased levels of mycophenolate

Contraceptives (oral), live attenuated vaccines: decreased effects

Salicylates: increased levels of mycophenolate

Drug/herb

Astragalus, echinacea, melatonin: interferes with immunosuppression

Drug/food

Decreased absorption if taken with food

NURSING CONSIDERATIONS
Assessment
- Monitor blood tests: CBC monthly during treatment
- Monitor liver function tests: alkaline phosphatase, AST, ALT, bilirubin

Nursing diagnoses
- Infection, risk for (uses)
- Knowledge, deficient (teaching)

Implementation
- Give 72 hr before transplantation; may be given in combination with corticosteroids and cycloSPORINE

PO route
- Do not crush, chew tabs; do not open caps; avoid inhalation or direct contact with skin, mucous membranes; tetratogenic in animals
- Give alone for better absorption

IV route
- Do not give by rapid or bolus inj: reconstitute and dilute to 6 mg/ml with D$_5$, give over ≥2 hr
- Do not admix with mycophenolate **IV** in inf catheter or with other **IV** product or inf admixtures

Patient/family education
- Teach patient to report fever, rash, severe diarrhea, chills, sore throat, fatigue, since serious infections may occur
- Instruct patient to avoid crowds to reduce risk of infection
- Advise patient that repeated lab tests are necessary
- Advise patient to limit exposure to sunlight/UV light
- Instruct patient to use contraception before, during, and 6 wk after therapy

Evaluation
Positive therapeutic outcome
- Absence of graft rejection

nabilone (Rx)
(nab′-ih-lohn)
Cesamet
Func. class.: Antiemetic
Chem. class.: Miscellaneous—cannabinoid

Pregnancy category C

Action: Orally, active cannabinoid, chemically related to marijuana; may decrease nausea by action on cannabinoid receptors in the CNS

Therapeutic outcome: Decreased nausea and vomiting associated with chemotherapy

Uses: Prevention of nausea, vomiting associated with cancer chemotherapy, in those that have not responded to other treatment; not to be used on an as-needed basis

Dosage and routes
Adult: PO 1-2 mg bid; give initial dose 1-3 hrs prior to chemotherapy; start with lower dose and increase as needed; may give dose of 1-2 mg the night before chemotherapy; may give 2-3 times daily during chemotherapy cycle

Available forms: Caps 1 mg

Adverse effects
CNS: Headache, ataxia, drowsiness, dysphoria, euphoria, sleep disturbance, vertigo, asthenia, concentration difficulties, depression, syncope, hallucinations
CV: Chest discomfort, **tachycardia,** orthostatic hypotension
GI: Dry mouth, nausea, *anorexia,* increased appetite
INTEG: Allergic reactions, rash, photosensitivity, pruritus
MS: Back, joint, muscle, neck pain

Contraindications: Hypersensitivity to this product or cannabinoids

Precautions: Pregnancy C, breastfeeding, depression, mental disorders, severe heptic/renal disease, hypertension, tachycardia, CV disorders

Pharmacokinetics

Absorption	Rapid 10%-20%
Distribution	Unknown
Metabolism	Liver
Excretion	Biliary system in feces
Half-life	Terminal 2 hr

Pharmacodynamics

Onset	Unknown
Peak	Unknown
Duration	Unpredictable; psychiatric symptoms may occur for up to 72 hr after treatment concludes

Interactions
Individual drugs
Disulfiram, possibly fluoxetine: hypomanic reaction

Naltrexone: increased action or nabilone

Theophylline: decreased metabolism of theophylline

Drug classifications
Anticholinergics (antihistamines, atropine, scopolamine): increased tachycardia, drowsiness

CNS depressants (alcohol, barbiturates, benzodiazepines, buspirone, lithium, muscle relaxants, opioids): increased drowsiness, CNS depression

Opioids: increased action of both products

Sympathomimetics (amphetamines, cocaine): increased hypertension, tachycardia, and possibly cardiotoxicity

Tricyclic antidepressants: increased tachycardia, hypertension, drowsiness

NURSING CONSIDERATIONS
Assessment
• Assess for absence of nausea and vomiting during chemotherapy

• Assess for CNS symptoms: headache, depression, ataxia, drowsiness, dysphoria, euphoria, sleep disturbances, concentration difficulties

• Assess for CV symptoms, cardiac status: tachycardia, orthostatic hypotension, hypertension

Nursing diagnoses
• Injury, risk for (uses, adverse reactions)
• Knowledge, deficient (teaching)
• Nutrition: less than body requirements, imbalanced (uses)

Implementation
• Give PO, not to be used on an as needed basis

• Store capsules at room temperature, away from light and moisture

Patient/family education
• Teach patient that mood, behavioral changes may occur while taking this product

• Advise patient to notify prescriber if pregnancy is suspected

• Advise patient to avoid breastfeeding while taking this product

• Instruct patient not to use alcohol or other CNS depressants unless approved by prescriber

• Instruct patient not to operate machinery or perform other hazardous activities while taking this product

Evaluation
Positive therapeutic outcome
• Decreased nausea and vomiting associated with chemotherapy

nabumetone (Rx)
(na-byoo'me-tone)
Relafen
Func. class.: Nonsteroidal antiinflammatory
Chem. class.: Acetic acid derivative
Pregnancy category C

Action: Metabolite inhibits COX-1, COX-2 by blocking arachidonate; analgesic, antiinflammatory, antipyretic

Therapeutic outcome: Decreased pain, swelling of joints

Uses: Osteoarthritis, rheumatoid arthritis, acute or chronic treatment

Dosage and routes
Adult: PO 1 g as a single dose or divided bid; may increase to 2 g/day if needed; may give daily or bid (as a divided dose)

Available forms: Tabs 500, 750 mg

Adverse effects
CNS: Dizziness, headache, drowsiness, fatigue, tremors, confusion, insomnia, anxiety, depression, nervousness
CV: Tachycardia, peripheral edema, palpitations, **dysrhythmias, CHF, MI, stroke**
EENT: Tinnitus
GI: Nausea, anorexia, vomiting, diarrhea, jaundice, cholestatic hepatitis, constipation, flatulence, cramps, dry mouth, peptic ulcer, gastritis, **ulceration, perforation,** bleeding
GU: **Nephrotoxicity, dysuria, hematuria, oliguria, azotemia,** cystitis
HEMA: **Blood dyscrasias**
INTEG: Purpura, rash, pruritus, sweating, photosensitivity
RESP: Dyspnea, pharyngitis, **bronchospasm**
SYST: **Anaphylaxis, angioneurotic edema**

Contraindications: Pregnancy **D** (3rd trimester), hypersensitivity to this product or aspirin, iodides, NSAIDs

N

Adverse effects: *italic* = common, **bold** = life-threatening

Black Box Warning: Perioperative pain in CABG surgery

Precautions: Pregnancy **C**, breastfeeding, children, geriatric, bleeding disorders, GI/cardiac/renal disorders, hepatic dysfunction, asthma, bone marrow suppression, lupus (SLE), ulcerative colitis, blood dyscrasias

Black Box Warning: MI, stroke, GI bleeding

Pharmacokinetics

Absorption	Well absorbed
Distribution	Unknown
Metabolism	Liver, extensively, to inactive metabolite
Excretion	Unknown
Half-life	22-30 hr

Pharmacodynamics

Onset	Unknown
Peak	2½-4 hr
Duration	Unknown

Interactions
Individual drugs
Alcohol, potassium: increased GI reactions
Cefamandole, cefoperazone, cefotetan, clopidogrel, eptifibatide, plicamycin, ticlopidine, valproic acid: increased risk of bleeding
Lithium, methotrexate: increased effect of each
Radiation: increased risk of hematologic reactions
Drug classifications
Anticoagulants, thrombolytics: increased risk of bleeding
Antihypertensives: decreased effect of antihypertensives
Antineoplastics: increased risk of hematologic reactions
Corticosteroids, NSAIDs, potassium supplements, salicylates: increased GI reactions
Diuretics: decreased effectiveness of diuretics
Drug/herb
Arginine, gossypol: increased gastric irritation
Bearberry, bilberry: increased NSAID effect
Garlic, ginger, ginkgo: increased bleeding risk
Drug/lab test
Increased: bleeding time, K, BUN, AST, ALT, LDH, alkaline phosphatase, creatinine
Decreased: CCr, blood glucose, Hct, Hgb

NURSING CONSIDERATIONS
Assessment
• Assess for pain: frequency, characteristics, location, duration, intensity, relief of pain after medication; and for inflammation of joints, ROM
• Monitor blood counts during therapy; watch for decreasing platelets; if low, therapy may need to be discontinued, restarted after hematologic recovery; check for blood dyscrasias (thrombocytopenia): bruising, fatigue, bleeding, poor healing; monitor liver function tests: AST, ALT, alkaline phosphatase; LDH, blood glucose, WBC, CCr
• Assess for asthma, aspirin sensitivity, nasal polyps; increased hypersensitivity reactions

Nursing diagnoses
• Injury, risk for (adverse reactions)
• Knowledge, deficient (teaching)
• Mobility, impaired physical (uses)
• Pain, acute (uses)
• Pain, chronic

Implementation
• Administer tab to patient crushed or whole
• Give with food or milk to decrease gastric symptoms
• Patient should take with a full glass of water and sit upright

Patient/family education
• Tell patient that product must be continued for prescribed time to be effective; to avoid aspirin, alcoholic beverages, NSAIDs, and OTC medications unless approved by prescriber
• Caution patient to report bleeding, bruising, fatigue, malaise, since blood dyscrasias do occur
• Instruct patient to use caution when driving; drowsiness, dizziness may occur
• Advise patient to use sunscreen, hat, and other protective clothing to prevent burns
• Advise patient to report dark stools, a change in urine pattern, increased weight, edema, increased pain in joints, fever, blood in urine, blurred vision, ringing or roaring in ears
• Advise to report use to all health care providers

Evaluation
Positive therapeutic outcome
• Decreased pain
• Decreased inflammation
• Increased mobility

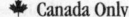

nadolol (Rx)

(nay-doe'lole)

Corgard, Syn-Nadolol ✦

Func. class.: Antihypertensive, antianginal

Chem. class.: β-Adrenergic receptor blocker

Pregnancy category C

Do not confuse:

Corgard/Cognex

Action: Long-acting, nonselective β-adrenergic receptor blocking agent, blocks β_1 in the heart and β_2 in the lungs, uterus, and circulatory system; mechanism is similar to that of propranolol

Therapeutic outcome: Decreased B/P, heart rate

Uses: Chronic stable angina pectoris, mild to moderate hypertension

Unlabeled uses: Tachydysrhythmias, aggression, anxiety, tremors, esophageal varices (rebleeding only), prophylaxis of migraine headaches, hyperthyroidism adjunctive therapy

Dosage and routes

Adult: PO 40 mg/day; increase by 40-80 mg q3-7day, maintenance 40-240 mg/day for angina, 40-320 mg/day for hypertension

Geriatric: PO 20 mg/day, may increase by 20 mg until desired dose

Renal dose

Adult: PO CCr 31-50 ml/min give q24-36hr; CCr 10-30 ml/min give q24-48hr; CCr <10 ml/min give q40-60hr

Available forms: Tabs 20, 40, 80, 120, 160 mg

Adverse effects

CNS: Depression, dizziness, fatigue, lethargy, paresthesia, headache, *weakness,* insomnia, memory loss, nightmares

CV: **Bradycardia,** *hypotension,* **CHF,** palpitations, AV block, chest pain, peripheral ischemia, flushing, edema, vasodilatation, conduction disturbances

EENT: Blurred vision, dry eyes, nasal congestion

ENDO: Hyperglycemia, hypoglycemia

GI: Nausea, vomiting, diarrhea, colitis, constipation, cramps, dry mouth, flatulence, hepatomegaly, **pancreatitis,** taste distortion

GU: Impotence, decreased libido

HEMA: **Agranulocytosis, thrombocytopenia**

INTEG: Rash, pruritus, fever, alopecia

RESP: Dyspnea, respiratory dysfunction, **bronchospasm,** cough, wheezing, pharyngitis, **laryngospasm, pulmonary edema**

Contraindications: Hypersensitivity to this product, cardiac failure, cardiogenic shock, 2nd- or 3rd-degree heart block, bronchospastic disease, sinus bradycardia, CHF, COPD

Precautions: Pregnancy **C,** breastfeeding, diabetes mellitus, renal disease, hyperthyroidism, peripheral vascular disease, myasthenia gravis, major surgery, nonallergic bronchospasm

Black Box Warning: Abrupt discontinuation

Pharmacokinetics

Absorption	Variably absorbed
Distribution	Crosses placenta; minimal concentration in CNS, protein binding 30%
Metabolism	Unknown
Excretion	Kidneys, unchanged
Half-life	10-24 hr; increased in renal disease

Pharmacodynamics

Onset	Variable
Peak	3-4 hr
Duration	20-24 hr

N

Interactions

Individual drugs

Clonidine, epinephrine: increased hypotension, bradycardia

Digoxin: increased bradycardia

Thyroid: decreased β-blocking effect

Drug classifications

Antihypertensives: increased hypotension

Ergots: peripheral ischemia

MAOIs: increased bradycardia; do not use together

NSAIDs: decreased antihypertensive effect

Phenothiazines: increased hypotensive effects

Drug/herb

Aconite: increased toxicity, death

Astragalus, cola tree: increased or decreased antihypertensive effect

Barberry, betony, black catechu, black cohosh, bloodroot, broom, burdock, cat's claw, dandelion, goldenseal, Irish moss, Jamaican dogwood, kelp, khella, mistletoe, parsley: increased antihypertensive effect

Coltsfoot, guarana, khat, licorice: decreased antihypertensive effect

Adverse effects: *italic* = common, **bold** = life-threatening

Drug/lab test
Increased: serum potassium, serum uric acid, ALT, AST, alkaline phosphatase, LDH, blood glucose, cholesterol, ANA, triglycerides

NURSING CONSIDERATIONS
Assessment
• Monitor B/P at beginning of treatment, periodically thereafter; note rate, rhythm, quality of apical/radial pulse before administration; notify prescriber of any significant changes (pulse <55 bpm), orthostatic hypotension
• Check for baselines in renal, liver function tests before therapy begins
• Assess for edema in feet, legs daily; monitor I&O, daily weight; check for jugular vein distention and crackles bilaterally, dyspnea (CHF)
• Monitor skin turgor, dryness of mucous membranes for hydration status, especially geriatric

Nursing diagnoses
• Cardiac output, decreased (uses)
• Injury, risk for (adverse reactions)
• Knowledge, deficient (teaching)
• Noncompliance (teaching)

Implementation
• Give before meals, at bedtime; tab may be crushed or swallowed whole; give with food to prevent GI upset; give reduced dosage in renal dysfunction
• Store protected from light, moisture; place in cool environment

Patient/family education
• Teach patient not to discontinue product abruptly; taper over 2 wk; may cause precipitate angina, serious dysrhythmias if stopped abruptly
• Teach patient not to use OTC products containing α-adrenergic stimulants (such as nasal decongestants, cold preparations); to avoid alcohol, smoking and to limit sodium intake as prescribed
• Teach patient how to take pulse and B/P at home; to hold dose if pulse ≤50 bpm, systolic B/P <90 mm Hg; advise when to notify prescriber
• Instruct patient to comply with weight control, dietary adjustments, modified exercise program; to report weight gain >5 lb, swelling, unusual bruising, bleeding
• Advise patient to carry/wear emergency ID to identify product being taken, allergies; teach patient product controls symptoms but does not cure condition

• Caution patient to avoid hazardous activities if dizziness, drowsiness are present; to rise slowly to prevent orthostatic hypotension
• Teach patient to report symptoms of CHF: difficult breathing, especially on exertion or when lying down, night cough, swelling of extremities or bradycardia, dizziness, confusion, depression, fever
• Teach patient to take product as prescribed, not to double doses, skip doses; take any missed doses as soon as remembered if at least 4 hr until next dose

Evaluation
Positive therapeutic outcome
• Decreased B/P in hypertension

nafarelin (Rx)
(naf-ah-rell′in)
Synarel
Func. class.: Gonadotropin
Chem. class.: Analog of gonadotropin-releasing hormone

Pregnancy category X

Action: Stimulates the release of LH and FSH, which increases ovarian steroid production; repeated dosing prevents stimulation of the pituitary gland

Therapeutic outcome: Decreased symptoms of endometriosis; resolution of central precocious puberty

Uses: Endometriosis, gonadotropin-dependent precocious puberty

Dosage and routes
Endometriosis
Adult: NASAL 400 mcg/day as one spray (200 mcg) into one nostril in morning and 1 spray into other nostril in evening; start treatment between days 2 and 4 of menstrual cycle; may increase to 800 mcg/day (1 spray into each nostril twice a day); recommended duration of treatment is 6 mo

Central precocious puberty
Child: NASAL 2 sprays in each nostril ᴀᴍ and ᴘᴍ, may increase to 3 sprays after alternating nostril tid

Available forms: Nasal spray 2 mg/ml (200 mcg/spray)

Adverse effects
CNS: Headache, flushing, depression, insomnia, emotional lability, hot flashes
GU: Decreased libido, vaginal dryness, breast tenderness, increased pubic hair, *impaired*

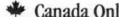

fertility, reduction in breast size, absence of menses, impotence, irregular periods
INTEG: Acne
META: Decreased bone density, increased cholesterol, triglycerides
MISC: Body odor, seborrhea, rhinitis, *nasal irritation*
SENSITIVITY: Shortness of breath, chest pain, urticaria, pruritus

Contraindications: Pregnancy **X;** breastfeeding; hypersensitivity to this product, GnRH, sorbitol; undiagnosed abnormal vaginal bleeding

Precautions: Children, females, menstruation, osteoporosis, pituitary insufficiency

Pharmacokinetics

Absorption	Well
Distribution	Unknown
Metabolism	Unknown
Excretion	20%-40% feces, 3% urine, unchanged
Half-life	3 hr

Pharmacodynamics

Onset	Up to 4 wk
Peak	3-4 wk
Duration	Several months

Interactions
Drug classifications
Nasal decongestants (nasal sprays): decreased nafarelin absorption

NURSING CONSIDERATIONS
Assessment
• Assess abdominal pain in endometriosis during treatment
• Assess endocrine studies, bone age, sex steroids, RHCG, GnRH, baseline q8wk
• Assess for precocious puberty including secondary sex characteristics
• Assess test results: pituitary/hypothalamus dysfunction (decreased LH); postmenopausal (increased LH)

Nursing diagnoses
• Knowledge, deficient (teaching)
• Pain, acute (uses)
• Sexual dysfunction (uses, adverse reactions)

Implementation
• Repeated doses may be necessary to elevate pituitary gonadotropin reserve
• Tilt head back slightly, wait 30 sec between sprays; do not use decongestant until 2 hr later
• Store at room temperature; protect from light

Patient/family education
• Teach patient to use nonhormonal contraception
• Teach patient about correct nasal use, 1 spray in right nostril AM, 1 in left nostril PM
• Teach patient that medication may cause hot flashes, decreased libido, vaginal dryness
• Advise to avoid use of nasal decongestants or separate by 12 hr
• Inform that growth of facial hair, increased body odor, and vaginal discharge may occur in females

Evaluation
Positive therapeutic outcome
• Decreased symptoms of endometriosis; adequate resolution of central precocious puberty

---

nafcillin (Rx)
(naf-sill′in)
Nafcillin sodium, Unipen
Func. class.: Antiinfective—broad-spectrum
Chem. class.: Penicillinase-resistant penicillin

Pregnancy category B

Action: Interferes with cell wall replication of susceptible organisms; osmotically unstable cell wall swells, bursts from osmotic pressure

Therapeutic outcome: Bactericidal effects for gram-positive cocci *Staphylococcus aureus, Streptococcus viridans, Streptococcus pneumoniae* and infections caused by penicillinase-producing *Staphylococcus*

Uses: Infections caused by penicillinase-producing staphylococci, streptococci; respiratory tract, skin, skin structure, urinary tract, bone, joint infections; sinusitis; endocarditis; septicemia; meningitis

Dosage and routes
Adult: **IV** 500-2000 mg q4hr
Infant and child >1 mo: **IV** 50-200 mg/kg/day in divided doses q4-6hr
Neonate >7 days (weight >2 kg): **IV** 25 mg/kg q8hr
Neonate ≤7 days (weight <2 kg): **IV** 25 mg/kg q12hr

Meningitis
Adult: **IV** 100-200 mg/kg/day divided q4-6hr, max 12 g/day
Neonate >7 days (weight >2 kg): **IV** 50 mg/kg q6hr
Neonate ≤7 days (weight <2 kg): **IV** 50 mg/kg q12hr

N

Adverse effects: *italic* = common, **bold** = life-threatening

Available forms: Powder for inj 1, 2, 10 g

Adverse effects

CNS: Lethargy, hallucinations, anxiety, depression, muscle twitching, **coma, seizures**

GI: Nausea, vomiting, diarrhea, increased AST, ALT, abdominal pain, glossitis, **pseudomembranous colitis**

GU: Oliguria, **proteinuria, hematuria,** vaginitis, moniliasis, **glomerulonephritis,** interstitial nephritis

HEMA: Anemia, increased bleeding time, **bone marrow depression, granulocytopenia**

SYST: **Anaphylaxis, serum sickness, Stevens-Johnson syndrome**

Contraindications: Hypersensitivity to penicillins

Precautions: Pregnancy **B**, breastfeeding, neonates, GI disease, asthma, hypersensitivity to cephalosporins

Pharmacokinetics

Absorption	Well absorbed (IM); erratic (PO)
Distribution	Widely distributed; crosses placenta
Metabolism	Not metabolized
Excretion	Kidneys, unchanged; breast milk
Half-life	1 hr; increased in renal disease

Pharmacodynamics

	PO	IM	IV
Onset	½ hr	½ hr	Immediate
Peak	1-2 hr	1-2 hr	Infusion end
Duration	Unknown	Unknown	Unknown

Interactions

Individual drugs

Cyclosporine: decreased effect of cyclosporine
Probenecid: increased nafcillin levels

Drug classifications

Tetracyclines: avoid use

Drug/herb

Acidophilus: do not use with antiinfectives; separate by several hours
Khat: decreased absorption

Drug/food

Food, carbonated drinks, citrus fruit juices: decreased absorption

Drug/lab test

False positive: urine glucose, urine protein

NURSING CONSIDERATIONS
Assessment

• Assess patient for previous sensitivity reaction to penicillins or other cephalosporins; cross-sensitivity between penicillins and cephalosporins is common

• Assess patient for signs and symptoms of infection including characteristics of wounds, sputum, urine, stool, WBC >10,000/mm³, earache, fever; obtain information baseline, during treatment

• Obtain C&S before beginning product therapy to identify if correct treatment has been initiated

• Assess for allergic reactions, anaphylaxis: rash, urticaria, pruritus, chills, fever, dyspnea, laryngeal edema, joint pain; angioedema may occur a few days after therapy begins; epinephrine, resuscitation equipment should be available for anaphylactic reaction

• Assess renal function tests: urinalysis, protein, blood, BUN, creatinine

◆ Identify urine output; if decreasing, notify prescriber (may indicate nephrotoxicity)

• Monitor blood studies: AST, ALT, CBC, Hct, bilirubin, LDH, alkaline phosphatase, Coombs' test monthly if patient is on long-term therapy

• Monitor electrolytes: potassium, sodium, chloride monthly if patient is on long-term therapy

• Assess bowel pattern daily; if severe diarrhea occurs, product should be discontinued; may indicate pseudomembranous colitis

• Monitor for bleeding: ecchymosis, bleeding gums, hematuria, stool guaiac daily if on long-term therapy

• Assess for overgrowth of infection: perineal itching, fever, malaise, redness, pain, swelling, drainage, rash, diarrhea, change in cough, sputum

Nursing diagnoses

• Diarrhea (adverse reactions)
• Infection, risk for (uses)
• Injury, risk for (adverse reactions)
• Knowledge, deficient (teaching)
• Noncompliance (teaching)

Implementation
PO route

• Give in even doses around the clock; if GI upset occurs, give with food; product must be given for 10-14 days to ensure organism death and prevent superinfection; store in airtight container.

• Shake susp; store in refrigerator for 2 wk, 1 wk at room temperature

IM route

• Reconstitute 500 mg/1.7-1.8 ml; 1 g/3.4 ml; 2 g/6.6-6.8 ml with sterile water or bacteriostatic water for a conc of 250 mg/ml; store unused portion in refrigerator for up to 7 days

• Give deep in large muscle mass

 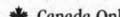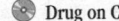

IV route

- Reconstitute 1 g/3.4 ml, 2 g/6.6-6.8 ml with sterile water or bacteriostatic water for a conc of 250 mg/ml; store unused portion in refrigerator for up to 7 days
- Give by direct **IV** by diluting reconstituted sol with 15-30 ml of sterile water or 0.9% NaCl; give over 5-10 min
- Give by intermittent inf by diluting to a conc of 2-40 mg/ml with 0.9% NaCl, D$_5$W, D$_{10}$W, D$_5$/0.9% NaCl, D$_5$/LR, LR, Ringer's; store in refrigerator for up to 96 hr or 24 hr room temperature; run over 30-60 min

Syringe compatibilities: Cimetidine, heparin

Y-site compatibilities: Acyclovir, atropine, cyclophosphamide, diazepam, enalaprilat, esmolol, famotidine, fentanyl, fluconazole, foscarnet, hydromorphone, magnesium sulfate, morphine, perphenazine, propofol, theophylline, zidovudine

Y-site incompatibilities: Droperidol, fentanyl/droperidol, labetalol, nalbuphine, pentazocine, regular insulin, verapamil

Additive compatibilities: Chloramphenicol, chlorothiazide, dexamethasone, diphenhydrAMINE, ephedrine, heparin, hydrOXYzine, lidocaine, potassium chloride, prochlorperazine, sodium bicarbonate, sodium lactate

Additive incompatibilities: Ascorbic acid, aztreonam, bleomycin, cytarabine, gentamicin, hydrocortisone sodium succinate, methylPREDNISolone sodium succinate, promazine

Patient/family education

- Teach patient to report sore throat, bruising, bleeding, joint pain; may indicate blood dyscrasias (rare)
- Advise patient to contact prescriber if vaginal itching, loose foul-smelling stools, furry tongue occur; may indicate superinfection
- Instruct patient to take all medication prescribed for the length of time ordered
- Advise patient to notify prescriber of diarrhea with blood or pus, which may indicate pseudomembranous colitis
- Advise patient to carry/wear emergency ID if allergic to penicillins

Evaluation

Positive therapeutic outcome

- Absence of signs/symptoms of infection (WBC <10,000/mm^3, temp WNL, absence of red, draining wounds, earache)
- Reported improvement in symptoms of infection

Treatment of anaphylaxis: Withdraw product, maintain airway, administer epinephrine, aminophylline, O$_2$, **IV** corticosteroids

---

⚠ HIGH ALERT

nalbuphine (Rx)
(nal′byoo-feen)
nalbuphine HCl
Func. class.: Opioid analgesic
Chem. class.: Synthetic opioid agonist/antagonist

Pregnancy category C

Action: Inhibits ascending pain pathways in limbic system, thalamus, midbrain, hypothalamus by binding to opiate receptor sites, thus altering pain perception and response

Therapeutic outcome: Relief of pain

Uses: Moderate to severe pain

Dosage and routes
Analgesic
Adult: SUBCUT/IM/**IV** 10 mg q3-6hr prn, max 160 mg/day

Balanced anesthesia supplement
Adult: **IV** 0.3-3 mg/kg given over 10-15 min; may give 0.25-0.5 mg/kg as needed (maintenance)

Available forms: Inj 10, 20 mg/ml

Adverse effects
CNS: Drowsiness, dizziness, confusion, headache, sedation, euphoria, dysphoria (high doses), hallucinations, increased dreaming, tolerance, physical and psychologic dependency
CV: Palpitations, bradycardia, change in B/P, orthostatic hypotension, **cardiac arrest**
EENT: Tinnitus, blurred vision, miosis (high doses), diplopia
GI: Nausea, vomiting, anorexia, constipation, cramps, abdominal pain, dyspepsia, xerostomia, bitter taste
GU: Increased urinary output, dysuria, urinary retention, urgency
INTEG: Rash, urticaria, bruising, flushing, *diaphoresis,* pruritus
RESP: **Respiratory depression,** pulmonary edema

Contraindications: Hypersensitivity, addiction (opioid)

Precautions: Pregnancy **C**, breastfeeding, addictive personality, increased ICP, MI (acute), severe heart disease, respiratory

N

depression, renal/hepatic disease, bowel impaction

Pharmacokinetics

Absorption	Well absorbed (SUBCUT, IM); completely absorbed (**IV**)
Distribution	Crosses placenta
Metabolism	Liver, extensively
Excretion	Feces, kidneys, unchanged (small amounts); breast milk
Half-life	3-6 hr

Pharmacodynamics

	IM	SUBCUT	IV
Onset	Up to 15 min	Up to 15 min	Rapid
Peak	1 hr	Unknown	½ hr
Duration	3-6 hr	3-6 hr	3-6 hr

Interactions
Individual drugs
Alcohol: increased respiratory depression, hypotension, sedation
Drug classifications
Antipsychotics, CNS depressants, sedative/hypnotics, skeletal muscle relaxants: increased respiratory depression, hypotension
MAOIs: avoid use, results are unpredictable
Opiates: increased effects with other CNS depressants
Drug/herb
Chamomile, gotu kola, hops, Jamaican dogwood, kava, lavender, mistletoe, nettle, pokeweed, poppy, senega, skullcap, St. John's wort, valerian: increased CNS depression
Corkwood: increased anticholinergic effect
Drug/lab test
Increased: amylase

NURSING CONSIDERATIONS
Assessment
• Assess pain characteristics (location, intensity, type) before medication administration, after treatment
• Assess bowel status; constipation is common
• Monitor VS after parenteral route; note muscle rigidity, product history, liver, kidney function tests; respiratory dysfunction: respiratory depression, character, rate, rhythm; notify prescriber if respirations are <10/min
• Monitor CNS changes: dizziness, drowsiness, hallucinations, euphoria, LOC, pupil reaction
• Monitor allergic reactions: rash, urticaria

Nursing diagnoses
• Breathing pattern, ineffective (adverse reactions)

• Knowledge, deficient (teaching)
• Pain, acute (uses)
• Sensory perception, disturbed: visual, auditory (adverse reactions)

Implementation
• Give by inj (IM, **IV**), only with resuscitative equipment available; give slowly to prevent rigidity
• Store in light-resistant area at room temperature
IM route
• Give inj deeply in large muscle mass; rotate inj sites
IV route
• Give direct **IV** undiluted 10 mg or less over 3-5 min or more
Syringe compatibilities: Atropine, cimetidine, diphenhydrAMINE, droperidol, glycopyrrolate, hydrOXYzine, lidocaine, midazolam, prochlorperazine, promethazine, ranitidine, scopolamine, trimethobenzamide
Syringe incompatibilities: Diazepam, pentobarbital
Y-site compatibilities: Amifostine, aztreonam, cefmetazole, cladribine, filgrastim, fludarabine, granisetron, melphalan, paclitaxel, propofol, teniposide, thiotepa, vinorelbine
Y-site incompatibilities: Nafcillin, sargramostim

Patient/family education
• Instruct patient to report any symptoms of CNS changes, allergic reactions
• Caution patients to avoid CNS depressants: alcohol, sedative/hypnotics for at least 24 hr after taking this product
• Discuss with patient that dizziness, drowsiness, confusion are common; to avoid getting up without assistance
• Discuss in detail all aspects of the product: reason for taking product and expected results
• Instruct patient to change position slowly to prevent orthostatic hypotension
• Teach patient to turn, cough, deep breathe after surgery to prevent atelectasis

Evaluation
Positive therapeutic outcome
• Relief of pain

Treatment of overdose: Naloxone (Narcan) 0.2-0.8 **IV**, O$_2$, **IV** fluids, vasopressors

naloxone (Rx)
(nal-oks'one)
naloxone HCl
Func. class.: Opioid antagonist, antidote
Chem. class.: Thebaine derivative

Pregnancy category C

Action: Competes with opioids at opioid receptor sites

Therapeutic outcome: Absence of opioid overdose

Uses: Respiratory depression induced by opioids, pentazocine, propoxyphene; refractory circulatory shock, asphyxia neonatorum, coma, hypotension

Unlabeled uses: IBS, opiate agonist dependence, opiate agonist-induced constipation, pruritus

Dosage and routes
Opioid-induced respiratory depression
Adult: **IV**/SUBCUT/IM 0.4-2 mg; repeat q2-3min if needed, max 10 mg
Child <5 yr or ≤20 kg: **IV**/SUBCUT/IM 0.01 mg/kg slowly followed by 0.1 mg/kg if needed or as an INF titrated to response

Postoperative opioid-induced respiratory depression
Adult: **IV** 0.1-0.2 mg q2-3min prn
Child: **IV**/IM/SUBCUT 0.005-0.01 mg/kg q2-3min prn

Opioid overdose
Adult: **IV**/SUBCUT/IM 0.4 mg (10 mcg/kg) (not opioid dependent), may repeat q2-3min; 0.1-0.2 mg q2-3min (opioid dependent)

Available forms: Inj 0.02, 0.4 mg/ml

Adverse effects
CNS: Drowsiness, nervousness, **seizures,** tremor
CV: Rapid pulse, **ventricular tachycardia, fibrillation,** increased systolic B/P (high doses), hypo/hypertension, **cardiac arrest, sinus tachycardia**
GI: Nausea, vomiting, **hepatotoxicity**
RESP: Hyperpnea, **pulmonary edema**

Contraindications: Hypersensitivity

Precautions: Pregnancy C, breastfeeding, neonates, children, CV disease, opioid dependency, seizure disorder, drug dependency

Pharmacokinetics

Absorption	Well absorbed (SUBCUT, IM); completely absorbed (**IV**)
Distribution	Rapidly distributed; crosses placenta
Metabolism	Liver
Excretion	Kidneys
Half-life	1 hr; up to 3 hr (neonates)

Pharmacodynamics

	IV	IM/SUBCUT
Onset	1 min	2-5 min
Peak	Unknown	Unknown
Duration	45 min	45-60 min

Interactions
Drug classifications
Analgesics (opioids): decreased effects of opioid analgesics
Drug/lab test
Interference: urine VMA, 5-HIAA, urine glucose

NURSING CONSIDERATIONS
Assessment
- Assess for signs of opioid withdrawal in drug-dependent individuals: cramping, hypertension, anxiety, vomiting; may occur up to 2 hr after administration
- Monitor VS q3-5min; ABGs including Po_2, Pco_2
- Assess cardiac status: tachycardia, hypertension; monitor ECG
- Assess for pain: duration, intensity, location before, after administration; may be used for respiratory depression
- Assess for respiratory dysfunction: respiratory depression, character, rate, rhythm; if respirations are <10/min, probably due to opioid overdose, administer naloxone; monitor LOC

Nursing diagnoses
- Breathing pattern, ineffective (uses)
- Coping, ineffective (uses)
- Knowledge, deficient (teaching)
- Pain, acute (adverse reactions)

Implementation
IV route
- Give by direct **IV** undiluted; give 0.4 mg or less over 15 sec or titrate inf to response
- Give cont inf **IV** further diluted with 0.9% NaCl and D$_5$ and give as an inf
- Give only with resuscitative equipment, O$_2$ nearby
- Use only sol prepared within 24 hr
- Store at room temperature in darkness
Syringe compatibilities: Benzquinamide, heparin

N

Adverse effects: *italic* = common, **bold** = life-threatening

Y-site compatibilities: Propofol
Additive compatibilities: Verapamil

Patient/family education
- Explain reason for and expected results of medication when patient alert

Evaluation
Positive therapeutic outcome
- Reversal of respiratory depression
- LOC: alert

---

nandrolone (Rx)
(nan′droe-lone)
Deca-Durabolin, Hybolin Decanoate, Kabolin
Func. class.: Androgenic anabolic steroid, antianemic
Chem. class.: Halogenated testosterone derivative

Pregnancy category X
Controlled substance schedule III

Action: May stimulate bone marrow development, stimulates erythropoietin production, increases Hgb and RBCs

Therapeutic outcome: Increased Hgb, RBCs

Uses: Anemia associated with renal disease

Dosage and routes
Adult and child ≥14 yr: IM (women) 50-100 mg q1-4wk; (men) 100-200 mg q1-4wk
Child 2-13 yr: IM 25-50 mg q3-4wk

Available forms: Inj 50, 100, 200 mg/ml

Adverse effects
CNS: Dizziness, headache, fatigue, tremors, paresthesias, flushing, sweating, anxiety, lability, insomnia, carpal tunnel syndrome, chills, depression
CV: Increased B/P, edema
EENT: Conjunctival edema, nasal congestion
ENDO: Abnormal GTT, *virilism (women, prepubescent boys)*
GI: Nausea, vomiting, constipation, weight gain, **cholestatic jaundice**, diarrhea, **hepatic necrosis/failure, peliosis, hepatitis**
GU: **Hematuria**, amenorrhea, vaginitis, decreased libido, decreased breast size, clitoral hypertrophy, testicular atrophy, priapism, voiding change, impotence
INTEG: Rash, acneiform lesions, oily hair/skin, flushing, sweating, acne vulgaris, alopecia, hirsutism

MISC: Hypercalcemia, chills, blood coagulation disorder, electrolyte imbalances
MS: Cramps, spasms

Contraindications: Pregnancy X, breast-feeding, males with cancer of breast, prostate, severe cardiac disease, hypersensitivity to this product or benzyl alcohol, abnormal genital bleeding, females

Black Box Warning: Hepatic disease, hypercholesterolemia

Precautions: Diabetes mellitus, CV disease, MI, prostatic hypertrophy, renal disease, hypercalcemia

Black Box Warning: Hepatocellular cancer

Pharmacokinetics
Absorption	Well
Distribution	Unknown
Metabolism	Unknown
Excretion	Unknown
Half-life	Unknown

Pharmacodynamics
Onset	Unknown
Peak	Up to 6 days
Duration	Unknown

Interactions
Drug classifications
Anticoagulants, NSAIDs, salicylates: increased bleeding risk
Hepatotoxics: increased hepatotoxicity
Drug/lab test
Increased: serum cholesterol, blood glucose, urine glucose, LDL
Decreased: serum calcium, serum potassium, T_4, T_3, thyroid ^{131}I uptake test, urine 17-OHCS, 17-KS, BPI, HDL

NURSING CONSIDERATIONS
Assessment
- Assess for anemia symptoms: dyspnea, fatigue, weakness, pallor
- Monitor weight daily; notify prescriber if weekly weight gain is >5 lb
- Monitor B/P q4hr
- Monitor I/O ratio; be alert for decreasing urinary output, increasing edema
- Assess growth rate in children, since growth rate may be uneven (linear/bone growth) with extended use
- Monitor electrolytes: K, Na, Cl, Ca; cholesterol
- Monitor blood studies: CBC, Hct, Hgb, lipid panel

 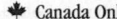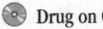

- Monitor liver function tests: ALT, AST, bilirubin
- Assess edema, hypertension, cardiac symptoms, jaundice
- Assess mental status: affect, mood, behavioral changes, aggression
- Assess signs of masculinization in female: increased libido, deepening of voice, decreased breast tissue, enlarged clitoris, menstrual irregularities; male: gynecomastia, impotence, testicular atrophy
- Assess hypercalcemia: lethargy, polyuria; polydipsia, nausea, vomiting, constipation; product may have to be decreased
- Assess for hypoglycemia in diabetics, since oral antidiabetic is increased

Nursing diagnoses
- Knowledge, deficient (teaching)

Implementation
- Give titrated dose; use lowest effective dose
- Inject deeply, use large muscle mass

Patient/family education
- Teach patient that product must be combined with complete health plan: diet, rest, exercise
- Teach patient to notify prescriber if therapeutic response decreases
- Teach patient not to discontinue abruptly
- Teach patient about changes in sex characteristics
- Teach patient that females should report menstrual irregularities
- Teach patient to increase calories, protein; decrease sodium if edema occurs

Evaluation
Positive therapeutic outcome
- Increased appetite, increased stamina

naphazoline nasal
See Appendix B

naphazoline ophthalmic
See Appendix B

naproxen (Rx, OTC)
(na-prox′en)
Apo-Naproxen ✦, EC-Naprosyn, Naprosyn, Naprosyn-E ✦, Naprosyn-SR ✦, Naxen ✦, Novo-Naprox ✦, Nu-Naprox ✦
naproxen sodium (Rx, OTC)
Aleve, Anaprox, Anaprox DS, Apo-Napro-Na ✦, Midol Extended Relief, Naprelan, Novo-Naprox Sodium ✦, Novo-Naprox Sodium DS ✦, Synflex ✦, Synflex DS ✦
Func. class.: Nonsteroidal antiinflammatory, nonopioid analgesic
Chem. class.: Propionic acid derivative

Pregnancy category
B (1st trimester),
D (2nd/3rd trimesters)

Do not confuse:
Naprosyn/Natacyn/Naprelan

Action: Completely inhibits COX-1, COX-2 by blocking arachidonate; analgesic, antiinflammatory, antipyretic

Therapeutic outcome: Decreased pain, inflammation

Uses: Mild to moderate pain, osteoarthritis, rheumatoid arthritis, gouty arthritis, juvenile arthritis, primary dysmenorrhea, tendonitis, ankylosing spondylitis, bursitis

Dosage and routes
Antiinflammatory/analgesic/antidysmenorrheal
Adult: PO 250-500 mg bid, max 1250 mg/day; DEL REL TAB 375-500 mg bid
Child ≥2 yr: PO 5-7 mg/kg/day

Antigout
Adult: PO 750 mg, then 250 mg q8hr

OTC use
Adult: PO 200 mg q8-12hr or 400 mg, then 200 mg q12hr, max 600 mg/24 hr, taken no longer than 10 days

Geriatric >65 yr: PO max 200 mg q12hr

Available forms: Naproxen: tabs: 250, 375, 500 mg; del rel tabs (EC-Naprosyn, Naprosyn-E) 250✦, 375, 500 mg; oral susp 125 mg/5 ml; ext rel tabs (SR) 375, 500, 750 mg✦; naproxen sodium; tabs 220, 275, 375, 500, 550 mg; ext rel tab 220 mg

Adverse effects
CNS: Dizziness, drowsiness, fatigue, tremors, confusion, insomnia, anxiety, depression
CV: Tachycardia, peripheral edema, palpitations, **dysrhythmias, MI, stroke**

N

Adverse effects: *italic* = common, **bold** = life-threatening

EENT: Tinnitus, hearing loss, blurred vision
GI: Nausea, anorexia, vomiting, diarrhea, jaundice, **cholestatic hepatitis,** constipation, flatulence, cramps, peptic ulcer, **GI ulceration, bleeding, perforation**
GU: **Nephrotoxicity: dysuria, hematuria, oliguria, azotemia**
HEMA: **Blood dyscrasias**
INTEG: Purpura, rash, pruritus, sweating
SYST: **Anaphylaxis**

Contraindications: Pregnancy **D** (2nd/ 3rd trimesters), hypersensitivity to NSAIDs, salicylates, asthma, severe renal/hepatic/ulcer disease

Black Box Warning: Perioperative pain in CABG surgery

Precautions: Pregnancy **B** (1st trimester), breastfeeding, children <2 yr, geriatric, bleeding disorders, GI/cardiac disorders, hypersensitivity to other antiinflammatory agents, CCr <30 ml/min

Black Box Warning: MI, GI bleeding, stroke

Pharmacokinetics

Absorption	Completely absorbed
Distribution	Crosses placenta, 99% protein binding
Metabolism	Liver, extensively
Excretion	Breast milk
Half-life	10-20 hr

Pharmacodynamics

Onset	1 hr
Peak	2-4 hr
Duration	<7 hr

Interactions
Individual drugs
Alcohol, aspirin: increased risk of GI side effects
Cefamandole, cefoperazone, cefotetan, clopidogrel, eptifibatide, plicamycin, ticlopidine, tirofiban, valproic acid: increased bleeding risk
Lithium: increased toxicity
Methotrexate: increased toxicity
Probenecid: increased toxicity
Radiation: increased risk of hematologic toxicity
Sucralfate: decreased/delayed absorption of naproxen
Drug classifications
ACE inhibitors: possible renal impairment
Antacids, antilipidemics: decreased/delayed absorption of naproxen

Anticoagulants, SSRIs, thrombolytics, tricyclics: increased risk of bleeding
Antihypertensives: decreased effect of antihypertensives
Antineoplastics: increased risk of hematologic toxicity
Corticosteroids, NSAIDs: increased risk of GI adverse reactions
Diuretics: decreased effectiveness of diuretics
Drug/herb
Anise, arnica, bogbean, chamomile, chondroitin, clove, dong quai, fenugreek, feverfew, garlic, ginger, ginkgo, ginseng *(Panax),* licorice, horse chestnut, red clover: increased bleeding risk
Arginine, gossypol: increased gastric irritation
Bearberry, bilberry: increased NSAIDs effect
Drug/lab test
Increased: BUN, alkaline phosphatase
False: increased 5-HIAA, 17KS

NURSING CONSIDERATIONS
Assessment
• Monitor liver function, renal function, other blood tests: AST, ALT, bilirubin, creatinine, BUN, CBC, Hct, Hgb, protime, LDH, blood glucose, WBC, platelets; if patient is on long-term therapy
• Check I&O ratio; decreasing output may indicate renal failure (long-term therapy)
• Assess hepatotoxicity: dark urine, clay-colored stools, yellowing of the skin and sclera, itching, abdominal pain, fever, diarrhea if patient is on long-term therapy
• Assess for allergic reactions: rash, urticaria; if these occur, product may have to be discontinued
• Assess for ototoxicity: tinnitus, ringing, roaring in ears; audiometric testing needed before, after long-term therapy
• Assess for visual changes: blurring, halos; may indicate corneal, retinal damage
• Check for edema in feet, ankles, legs
• Identify prior product history; there are many product interactions
• Monitor pain: location, frequency, duration, characteristics, type, intensity before dose and 1 hour after; assess ROM before dose and after
• Assess for asthma, aspirin hypersensitivity, or nasal polyps, increased risk of hypersensitivity

Nursing diagnoses
• Injury, risk for (adverse reactions)
• Knowledge, deficient (teaching)
• Mobility, impaired physical (uses)
• Pain, acute (uses)
• Pain, chronic

 Alert   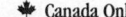 Canada Only   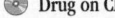 Drug on CD   * "Tall Man" lettering (See Preface)

Implementation

• Administer to patient crushed or whole (regular release); do not crush, break, or chew del rel tab

• Give OTC for 10 days or less unless approved by prescriber

• Give with food or milk to decrease gastric symptoms; give ½ hr before or 2 hr after meals for better absorption

• Patient should take with 8 oz of water and sit upright for 30 min after dose to prevent ulceration

Patient/family education

• Teach patient to report any symptoms of renal/hepatic toxicity, visual changes, ototoxicity, allergic reactions, bleeding (long-term therapy); to report use to all health care providers

• Caution patient not to exceed recommended dosage; acute poisoning may result; to take as prescribed, do not double dose

• Advise patient to use sunscreen to prevent photosensitivity reactions

• Teach patient to read label on other OTC products; many contain other antiinflammatories; caution patient to avoid alcohol ingestion; GI bleeding may occur

• Inform patient that the therapeutic response takes 2 wk (arthritis)

• Teach patient to report tinnitus, confusion, diarrhea, sweating, hyperventilation, blurred vision, fever, joint aches, black stools, flulike symptoms

Evaluation

Positive therapeutic outcome

• Decreased pain
• Decreased inflammation
• Increased mobility

---

naratriptan (Rx)

(nair'ah-trip-tan)

Amerge

Func. class.: Migraine agent

Chem. class.: 5-HT$_1$-like receptor agonist

Pregnancy category C

Action: Binds selectively to the vascular 5-HT$_1$ receptor subtype, exerts antimigraine effect; causes vasoconstriction in cranial arteries

Therapeutic outcome: Decreased intensity and incidence of migraines

Uses: Acute treatment of migraine with or without aura

Dosage and routes

Adult: PO 1 or 2.5 mg with fluids; if headache returns, repeat once after 4 hr, max 5 mg/24 hr

Renal/hepatic dose

Max 2.5 mg/24 hr

Available forms: Tabs 1, 2.5 mg

Adverse effects

CNS: Dizziness, sedation, fatigue

CV: Increased B/P, palpitations, **tachydysrhythmias, PR, QT$_C$ prolongation, ST/T wave changes, PVCs, atrial flutter, fibrillation, coronary vasospasm**

EENT: EENT infections, photophobia

GI: Nausea, vomiting

MISC: Temp change sensations, tightness, pressure sensations

MS: Weakness, neck stiffness, myalgia

Contraindications: Angina pectoris, history of MI, documented silent ischemia, ischemic heart disease, concurrent ergotamine-containing preparations, uncontrolled hypertension, hypersensitivity, severe renal disease (CCr <15 ml/min), severe hepatic disease (Child-Pugh grade C), CV syndromes, hemiplegic or basilar migraines

Precautions: Pregnancy C, breastfeeding, children, postmenopausal women, men >40 yr, risk factors for CAD, hypercholesterolemia, obesity, diabetes, impaired renal/hepatic function, peripheral vascular disease

Pharmacokinetics	
Absorption	Unknown
Distribution	28%-31% protein binding
Metabolism	Liver (metabolite)
Excretion	Urine/feces
Half-life	6 hr

Pharmacodynamics	
Onset	Unknown
Peak	2-3 hr
Duration	Unknown

Interactions

Individual drugs

Sibutramine: increased naratriptan effect

Drug classifications

5-HT agonists, ergot derivatives: increased vasospastic effect

MAOIs: increased risk of adverse reactions, do not use together

Selective serotonin release inhibitors (fluoxetine, fluvoxamine, paroxetine, sertraline): increased weakness, hyperreflexia, incoordination

---

Adverse effects: *italic* = common, **bold** = life-threatening

Drug/herb
Butterbur: increased effect
SAM-e, St. John's wort: increased serotonin syndrome

NURSING CONSIDERATIONS
Assessment
- Assess for stress level, activity, recreation, coping mechanisms
- Assess neurologic status: LOC, blurred vision, nausea, tics preceding headache

Nursing diagnoses
- Knowledge, deficient (teaching)
- Noncompliance (teaching)
- Pain, acute (uses)

Implementation
- Do not use product if another 5-HT agonist or an ergot preparation has been used in past 24 hr
- Give with fluids as soon as symptoms appear; may take another dose after 4 hr; max 5 mg in any 24-hr period
- Provide a quiet, calm environment with decreased stimulation for noise, bright light, excessive talking

Patient/family education
- Teach patient to report pain, tightness in chest, neck, throat, or jaw; notify prescriber immediately if sudden, severe abdominal pain occurs
- Teach patient to use contraception while taking product, to notify prescriber if pregnancy is planned or suspected

Evaluation
Positive therapeutic outcome
- Absence of migraine headaches

---

natalizumab (Rx)
(na-ta-liz'u-mab)
Tysabri
Func. class.: Biological response modifier, immunoglobulins, monoclonal antibody
Pregnancy category C

Action: Action not clearly understood; biologic response modifying properties mediated through specific receptors on cells, may be secondary of blockade of the interaction by inflammatory cells on vascular endothelial cells

Therapeutic outcome: Decreased symptoms of multiple sclerosis

Uses: Ambulatory patients with relapsing-remitting multiple sclerosis who have not responded to other treatment, moderate-severe Crohn's disease

Dosage and routes
Adult: **IV** INF 300 mg q4wk, give over 1 hr, observe during and for 1 hr after inf

Available forms: Single-use vial, 300 mg/100 ml 0.9% NaCl

Adverse effects
CNS: Headache, fatigue, rigors, syncope, tremors, *depression,* **PML (progressive multifocal leukoencephalopathy), suicidal ideation,** anxiety
CV: Chest discomfort, hyper/hypotension, tachycardia
GI: Abdominal discomfort, abnormal liver function tests, gastroenteritis, severe hepatic injury
GU: Amenorrhea, *UTI, irregular menses,* vaginitis, urinary frequency
INTEG: Rash, dermatitis, pruritus, **skin melanoma,** infusion-related reactions
MS: Arthralgia, myalgia
RESP: Lower respiratory tract infection, dyspnea
SYST: **Anaphylaxis, angioedema**

Contraindications: Hypersensitivity, immunocompromised individuals (HIV, AIDS, leukemia, lymphoma, transplants), PML, murine (mouse) protein allergy

Black Box Warning: Progressive multifocal leukoencephalopathy

Precautions: Pregnancy C, breastfeeding, geriatric, chronic progressive multiple sclerosis, depression, mental disorders, diabetes, TB, active infections, hepatotoxicity

Pharmacokinetics

Absorption	Unknown
Distribution	Unknown
Metabolism	Unknown
Excretion	Unknown
Half-life	Approximately 11 days

Pharmacodynamics
Unknown

Interactions
Drug classifications
Do not use with vaccines
Immunosuppressants, antineoplastics, immunomodulators: increased infection

NURSING CONSIDERATIONS
Assessment
- Monitor blood, renal, hepatic tests: CBC, differential, platelet counts, BUN, creatinine, ALT, urinalysis, for hypersensitivity reactions

---

 Alert   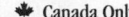 Canada Only    Drug on CD   * "Tall Man" lettering (See Preface)

- Assess CNS symptoms: headache, fatigue, depression, rigors, tremors
- Assess GI status: abdominal discomfort
- Assess mental status: depression, depersonalization, suicidal thoughts, insomnia
- Assess for multiple sclerosis symptoms; this product should only be used in patients who have not responded to other treatments
⚠ Assess for anaphylaxis: shortness of breath, hives; swelling, tightness in throat, chest pain; usually within 2 hr of inf
- Monitor PML using gadolinium-enhanced MRI scan of the brain, possibly CSF for JC viral DNA

Nursing diagnoses
- Injury, risk for (uses, adverse reactions)
- Knowledge, deficient (teaching)
- Mobility, impaired physical (uses)

Implementation
- Give acetaminophen for fever, headache
- Give only after being enrolled in the TOUCH Prescribing Program
Intermittent IV inf
- Use only clear, colorless solution, without particulates
- Withdraw 15 ml from the vial using aseptic technique: inject conc into 100 ml 0.9% NaCl; do not use other diluents; mix completely; do not shake; infuse immediately or refrigerate for up to 8 hr; warm to room temperature before using; flush with 0.9% NaCl before, after inf; do not admix or use in same line with other agents
- Withhold product at first sign of PML
- Store solution in refrigerator; do not freeze or shake; protect from light; use within 8 hr of preparation

Patient/family education
- Provide patient or family member with written, detailed information about the product
- Teach female patients they may experience irregular menses, amenorrhea
- Advise patient to use sunscreen to prevent photosensitivity
- Instruct patient to notify prescriber if pregnancy is suspected
- Instruct patient to avoid breastfeeding while taking this product
- Instruct patient to notify prescriber of possible infection: sore throat, cough, increased temp

Evaluation
Positive therapeutic outcome
- Decreased symptoms of multiple sclerosis

natamycin ophthalmic
See Appendix B

nebivolol (Rx)
(ne-biv'oh-lol)
Bystolic
Func. class.: Antihypertensive
Chem. class.: β₁-Blocker
Pregnancy category C

Action: Competitively blocks stimulation of β-adrenergic receptors within vascular smooth muscle; decreases rate of SA node discharge, increases recovery time, slows conduction of AV node resulting in decreased heart rate (negative chronotropic effect), which decreases O_2 consumption in myocardium due to β₁-receptor antagonism; also decreases renin-aldosterone-angiotensin system at high doses, inhibits β₂-receptors in bronchial system (high doses)

Therapeutic outcome: Decreased B/P after 1-2 wk

Uses: Hypertension alone or in combination

Unlabeled uses: Heart failure

Dosage and routes
Hypertension
Adult: PO 5 mg/day, may be increased to desired response q2wk; max 40 mg/day
Geriatric: PO max 40 mg/day

Renal dose
Adult: PO CCr <30 ml/min, 2.5 mg/day; may increase cautiously

Hepatic dose
Adult: PO (Child-Pugh class B) 2.5 mg qd; use dose escalation cautiously

Heart failure (unlabeled)
Adult: PO 1.25 mg titrated to max 10 mg/day

Available forms: Tabs 2.5, 5, 10, 20 mg

Adverse effects
CNS: Insomnia, fatigue, dizziness, mental changes, drowsiness, headache
CV: **Bradycardia, MI,** AV heart block, edema
GI: Nausea, diarrhea, vomiting, abdominal pain
GU: Impotence
HEMA: **Thrombocytopenia**
INTEG: Rash, pruritus, vasculitis, urticaria, psoriasis, **angioedema**
MISC: **Renal failure, pulmonary edema,** hyperuricemia, hypercholesterolemia
RESP: **Bronchospasm,** dyspnea

N

Adverse effects: *italic* = common, **bold** = life-threatening

Contraindications: Cardiogenic shock, sick sinus syndrome, AV heart block, hypersensitivity to this agent or β-blockers, heart failure, severe hepatic disease, severe bradycardia

Precautions: Pregnancy **C**, breastfeeding, children, major surgery, peripheral vascular disease, diabetes mellitus, thyrotoxicosis disease, COPD, asthma, well-compensated heart failure, renal/hepatic disease, abrupt discontinuation, acute bronchospasm

Pharmacokinetics

Absorption	Unknown
Distribution	Unknown
Metabolism	In liver by CYP2D6
Excretion	38% excreted in urine, 44% in feces
Half-life	12 hr

Pharmacodynamics

Onset	Unknown
Peak	1.5-4 hr
Duration	Unknown

Interactions
Individual drugs
Cimetidine: increased nebivolol action
Mefloquine: do not give
Sildenafil: decreased nebivolol action
Drug classifications
β-blockers, others: do not use concurrently
Calcium channel blockers (nondihydropyridine), CYP2D6 inhibitors (amiodarone, buPROPion, chloroquine, chlorpheniramine, chlorproMAZINE, cinacalcet, diphenhydrAMINE, duloxetine, fluoxetine, haloperidol, imatinib, paroxetine, promethazine, propoxyphene, quinidine, quinine, ritonavir, terbinafine, thioridazine): increased nebivolol action
CYP2D6 inducers (rifampin): decreased nebivolol action
Drug/herb
Hawthorn: may increase nebivolol effect
Drug/lab test
Increased: serum lipoprotein levels, BUN, potassium, triglyceride, uric acid, LDH, AST, ALT, blood glucose, alkaline phosphatase
Positive: ANA titer

NURSING CONSIDERATIONS
Assessment
- Monitor B/P during beginning treatment, periodically thereafter; pulse q4hr; note rate, rhythm, quality
- Assess apical/radial pulse before administration; notify prescriber of any significant changes (pulse <50 bpm); signs of CHF (dyspnea, crackles, weight gain, jugular vein distention)
- Assess baselines in renal/hepatic studies before therapy begins, periodically
- Monitor I&O, edema in feet, legs daily
- Monitor skin turgor, dryness of mucous membranes for hydration status, especially geriatric patients

Nursing diagnoses
- Cardiac output, decreased (uses)
- Knowledge, deficient (teaching)
- Noncompliance (teaching)

Implementation
PO route
- Give without regard for meals; tab may be crushed or swallowed whole; give with food to prevent GI upset
- Store protected from light, moisture; place in cool environment

Patient/family education
◆ Caution patient not to discontinue product abruptly; severe cardiac reactions may occur; taper over 2 wk; do not double dose; if a dose is missed, take as soon as remembered up to 4 hr before next dose
- Inform patient product may mask signs of hypoglycemia or alter blood glucose levels
- Advise patient not to use OTC products containing α-adrenergic stimulants (such as nasal decongestants, OTC cold preparations) unless directed by prescriber
- Instruct patient to report low pulse, dizziness, confusion, depression, fever
- Teach patient to take pulse, B/P at home; advise when to notify prescriber
- Advise patient to comply with weight control, dietary adjustments, modified exercise program
- Instruct patient to carry emergency ID to identify product, allergies
- Caution patient to avoid hazardous activities if dizziness, drowsiness are present
- Instruct patient to report symptoms of CHF: difficulty breathing, especially on exertion or when lying down, night cough, swelling of extremities
- Teach patient to continue with required lifestyle changes (exercise, diet, weight loss, stress reduction)

Evaluation
Positive therapeutic outcome
- Decreased B/P after 1-2 wk
- Decreased dysrhythmias

Treatment of overdose: Lavage, **IV** atropine for bradycardia, **IV** theophylline for bronchospasm, digoxin, O_2, diuretic for cardiac failure, **IV** glucose for hypoglycemia, **IV** diazepam (or phenytoin) for seizures, **IV** fluids, **IV** pressors

nelarabine (Rx)
(nella-ra'ben)
Arranon
Func. class.: Antineoplastic
Chem. class.: Purine analog

Pregnancy category D

Action: Leukemic blasts allow for incorporation into DNA, thus interfering with cell replication, leading to cell death

Therapeutic outcome: Decreased growth of malignant cells

Uses: T-cell lymphoblastic leukemia, T-cell lymphoblastic lymphoma post relapse or treatment failure with at least two chemotherapeutic agents

Dosage and routes
Adult: **IV** 1500 mg/m² over 2 hr on days 1, 3, 5 repeated q21day
Child: **IV** 650 mg/m² over 1 hr/day × 5 days, repeated q21day

Available forms: Sol for inj 5 mg/ml (50 ml)

Adverse effects
CNS: Dizziness, *fatigue,* insomnia, rigors, **seizures,** peripheral neuropathy, **paralysis,** confusion, headache, **Guillain-Barré syndrome,** depression, drowsiness, encephalopathy
CV: Edema
GI: Nausea, vomiting, anorexia, diarrhea, stomatitis, constipation
HEMA: **Neutropenia,** leukopenia, **thrombocytopenia,** anemia
META: Decreased potassium, calcium, magnesium, albumin, bilirubin, AST, ALT, hyperuricemia; increased glucose
MS: Myalgia, arthralgia, back pain, weakness
RESP: **Pleural effusion,** cough, dyspnea, wheezing, epistaxis
SYST: Tumor lysis syndrome (TLS)

Contraindications: Pregnancy **D**, hypersensitivity

Black Box Warning: Severe neurotoxicity

Precautions: Breastfeeding, children, geriatric, renal/hepatic disease

Black Box Warning: Seizure disorder, IM administration, neurological disease, peripheral neuropathy

Pharmacokinetics
Absorption	Unknown
Distribution	Unknown
Metabolism	Liver
Excretion	Kidneys
Half-life	30 min-3hr

Pharmacodynamics
Unknown

Interactions
Drug classifications
Anticoagulants, NSAIDs, platelet inhibitors, salicylates: increased bleeding risk
Toxoids, vaccinations (live virus): do not use

NURSING CONSIDERATIONS
Assessment
• Monitor CBC (RBC, Hct, Hgb), differential platelet count weekly; withhold products if WBC is <4000/mm³, platelet count is <75,000/mm³, or RBC, Hct, Hgb low; notify prescriber of these results
• Monitor renal function tests: BUN, serum uric acid, urine CCr, electrolytes before, during therapy
• Monitor temp; fever may indicate beginning infection; no rectal temps
• Monitor liver function tests before, during therapy: bilirubin, ALT, AST, alkaline phosphatase as needed or monthly
• Assess for bleeding: hematuria, heme-positive stools, bruising or petechiae, mucosa or orifices
• Assess for neurotoxicity: somnolence, confusion, seizures, ataxia, paresthesias, hypoesthesia, coma, status epilepticus, craniospinal demyelination; contact prescriber immediately
• Assess for dyspnea, crackles, unproductive cough, chest pain, tachypnea, fatigue, increased pulse, pallor, lethargy, personality changes
• Assess buccal cavity q8hr for dryness, sores or ulceration, white patches, oral pain, bleeding, dysphagia
• Assess for GI symptoms: frequency of stools, cramping; if severe diarrhea occurs, fluid and electrolytes may need to be given

Nursing diagnoses
• Injury, risk for (uses, adverse reactions)

N

Implementation
- Provide **IV** hydration, and allopurinol in risk of hyperuricemia
- Use procedures for proper handling/disposal of anticancer products
- Provide for rinsing of mouth tid-qid with water, club soda; brushing of teeth bid-tid with soft brush or cotton-tipped applicators for stomatitis; use unwaxed dental floss
- Store at room temperature

Patient/family education
- Advise patient to avoid foods with citric acid, hot or rough texture if stomatitis is present; OTC products
- Advise patient to use contraception while taking this product
- Advise patient to avoid using while breast-feeding
- Teach patient to report signs of infection: increased temp, sore throat, flulike symptoms
- Teach patient to report signs of anemia: fatigue, headache, faintness, shortness of breath, irritability
- Teach patient to report bleeding; to avoid use of razors, commercial mouthwash
- Advise patient that seizures may occur; do not operate machinery or drive until effects are known; to report numbness, paresthesias, weakness
- Advise patient not to receive vaccinations while taking this product

Evaluation
Positive therapeutic outcome
- Decreased spread of malignancy

---

nelfinavir (Rx)
(nell-fin'a-ver)
Viracept
Func. class.: Antiretroviral
Chem. class.: HIV protease inhibitor
Pregnancy category B

Action: Inhibits HIV-1 protease

Therapeutic outcome: Prevents maturation of the infectious virus

Uses: HIV-1 in combination with other antiretrovirals

Dosage and routes
HIV infection
Adult and child >13 yr: PO 750 mg tid or 1250 mg bid
Child 2-13 yr: PO 20-30 mg/kg tid, max 2500 mg/day

Prevention of HIV infection after exposure
Adult: PO 1250 mg bid with two other antiretroviral agents × 4 wk

Available forms: Tabs 250, 625 mg; oral powder 50 mg/g/scoop

Adverse effects
CNS: Headache, asthenia, poor concentration, **seizures, suicidal ideation**
CV: Bleeding
ENDO: Hyperglycemia, hyperlipidemia
GI: Diarrhea, nausea, anorexia, dyspepsia, *flatulence,* **hepatitis, pancreatitis**
HEMA: **Anemia, leukopenia, thrombocytopenia, Hgb abnormalities**
INTEG: Rash, dermatitis
MS: Pain, arthralgia, myalgia, myopathy
OTHER: **Hypoglycemia,** redistribution/accumulation of body fat

Contraindications: Hypersensitivity to protease inhibitors

Precautions: Pregnancy **B**, breastfeeding, hemophilia, PKU, renal/hepatic disease, pancreatitis, diabetes, infection

Pharmacokinetics
Absorption	Unknown
Distribution	98% protein binding
Metabolism	Liver (minimal)
Excretion	Feces/urine
Half-life	3½-5 hr

Pharmacodynamics
Onset	Unknown
Peak	2-4 hr
Duration	Unknown

Interactions
Individual drugs
Amiodarone, lovastatin, midazolam, pimozide, quinidine, simvastatin, triazolam: increased serious dysrhythmias
Alfentanil, alosetron, atorvastatin, azithromycin, bortezomib, buprenorphine, buspirone, calcium channel blockers, cilostazol, cycloSPORINE, disopyramide, docetaxel, dofetilide, donepezil, ethosuximide, fentanyl, galantamine, gefitinib, halofantrine, indinavir, levomethadyl, systemic lidocaine, paclitaxel, rifabutin, saquinavir, sibutramine, sildenafil, sirolimus, sufentanil, tacrolimus, ziprasidone, zonisamide: increased effect
Carbamazepine, nevirapine, phenobarbital, phenytoin, rifamycin: decreased nelfinavir levels

Delavirdine: increased protease inhibitor levels

Didanosine, methadone, phenytoin: decreased effect

Indinavir, ketoconazole, ritonavir: increased nelfinavir levels

Drug classifications
Contraceptives (oral): decreased effect
Ergots: increased serious dysrhythmias
HIV protease inhibitors: increased protease inhibitor levels

Drug/herb
St. John's wort: decreased antiretroviral effect

Drug/food
Increased: absorption with food

Drug/lab test
Increased: AST, ALT, alkaline phosphatase, total bilirubin, CPK, LDH

NURSING CONSIDERATIONS
Assessment
- Assess resistance testing at initiation and failure of treatment
- Assess signs of infection, anemia
- Monitor liver function tests: ALT, AST
- Monitor C&S before product therapy; product may be taken as soon as culture is performed; repeat C&S after treatment; determine the presence of other STDs
- Assess bowel pattern before, during treatment; if severe abdominal pain with bleeding occurs, product should be discontinued; monitor hydration
- Assess skin eruptions, rash, urticaria, itching
- Assess allergies before treatment, reaction of each medication; place allergies on chart
- Monitor blood studies: serum lipid profile, plasma HIV RNA, blood glucose, viral load, CD$_4$ cell counts baseline, throughout treatment

Nursing diagnoses
- Infection, risk for (uses)
- Knowledge, deficient (teaching)

Implementation
- Administer with food
- Oral powder can be mixed with fluids; do not mix with juice or acidic fluids; stable mixed for 6 hr

Patient/family education
- Advise patient to take with meal or snack; if dose is missed, take as soon as remembered up to 1 hr before next dose; do not double dose
- Advise patient to avoid taking with other medications, unless directed by prescriber

- Teach patient that product does not cure, but manages symptoms; does not prevent transmission of HIV to others
- Teach patient to use nonhormonal form of contraception while taking this product
- Teach to report symptoms of hyperglycemia

Evaluation
Positive therapeutic outcome
- Decreasing symptoms of HIV
- Improving viral load and CD4 cell counts

neomycin topical
See Appendix B

neostigmine (Rx)
(nee-oh-stig'meen)
neostigmine, Prostigmin
Func. class.: Cholinergic stimulant; anticholinesterase
Chem. class.: Quaternary compound

Pregnancy category C

Action: Inhibits destruction of acetylcholine, which increases concentration at sites where acetylcholine is released; this facilitates transmission of impulses across the myoneural junction

Therapeutic outcome: Increased strength in myasthenia gravis, reversal of nondepolarizing muscular blockers

Uses: Diagnosis/treatment of myasthenia gravis, nondepolarizing neuromuscular blocker antagonist, postoperative ileus, urinary retention

Dosage and routes
Myasthenia gravis diagnosis
Adult: IM 0.02 mg/kg as a single dose
Child: IM 0.04 mg/kg as a single dose

Myasthenia gravis treatment
Adult: PO 15 mg tid, may increase to 375 mg/day; IM/**IV** 0.5-2.5 mg q1-3hr up to 10 mg/day
Child: PO 2.5 mg/kg/day q3-4hr; IM/**IV**/SUBCUT 0.01-0.04 mg/kg q2-4hr

Nondepolarizing neuromuscular blocker antagonist
Adult: IV 0.5-2 mg slowly; may repeat if needed, max 5 mg (give 0.6-1.2 mg atropine several min before this product)
Infant and child: **IV** 0.025-0.08 mg/kg/dose (give atropine several min before this product)

N

Abdominal distention/ postoperative ileus

Adult: IM/SUBCUT 0.25-1 mg (1 : 4000) q4-6hr depending on condition × 2-3 days

Urinary retention treatment

Adult: IM/SUBCUT 0.25-1 mg q3hr × 5 days after bladder is emptied

Renal dose

Adult: PO/IM/**IV** CCr 10-50 ml/min 50% of dose; CCr <10 ml/min 25% of dose

Available forms: Tabs 15 mg; inj 1 : 1000, 1 : 2000, 1 : 4000

Adverse effects

CNS: Dizziness, headache, sweating, weakness, **seizures,** incoordination, **paralysis,** drowsiness, LOC

CV: Tachycardia, **dysrhythmias,** bradycardia, hypotension, AV block, ECG changes, **cardiac arrest,** syncope

EENT: Miosis, blurred vision, lacrimation, visual changes

GI: *Nausea, diarrhea, vomiting, cramps,* increased peristalsis, salivary and gastric secretions

GU: Frequency, incontinence, urgency

INTEG: Rash, urticaria, flushing

RESP: **Respiratory depression, bronchospasm, constriction, laryngospasm, respiratory arrest, dyspnea**

Contraindications: Obstruction of intestine, renal system, bromide sensitivity, peritonitis, urinary tract obstruction, ileus

Precautions: Pregnancy **C**, breastfeeding, children, bradycardia, hypotension, seizure disorders, bronchial asthma, coronary occlusion, hyperthyroidism, dysrhythmias, peptic ulcer, megacolon, poor GI motility

Pharmacokinetics

Absorption	Poorly absorbed (PO), completely absorbed (**IV**)
Distribution	Unknown
Metabolism	Liver
Excretion	Kidneys
Half-life	40-90 min

Pharmacodynamics

	PO	IM	IV
Onset	45-75 min	10-30 min	4-8 min
Peak	Unknown	30 min	30 min
Duration	2½-4 hr	2½-4 hr	2-4 hr

Interactions

Individual drugs

Atropine, disopyramide, haloperidol, quinidine: decreased neostigmine action

Decamethonium, succinylcholine: increased action of each specific product

Digoxin: increased bradycardia

Drug classifications

Aminoglycosides, anticholinergics, antidepressants, antihistamines, corticosteroids, local general anesthetics, phenothiazines: decreased neostigmine action

β-blockers, calcium channel blockers: increased bradycardia

Drug/herb

Pill bearing spurge: increased effect

NURSING CONSIDERATIONS

Assessment

- Monitor VS, respiration during rest
- Monitor for bradycardia, hypotension, bronchospasm, headache, dizziness, seizures, respiratory depression; product should be discontinued if toxicity occurs

Nursing diagnoses

- Breathing pattern, ineffective (uses)
- Knowledge, deficient (teaching)

Implementation

PO route

- Give only after all other cholinergics have been discontinued
- Increased dosage as ordered may be needed if tolerance develops
- Give larger doses as ordered after exercise or fatigue
- Administer on empty stomach for better absorption
- Store at room temperature

IV route

- Give direct **IV** undiluted, through Y-tube or 3-way stopcock; give 0.5 mg or less over 1 min
- Give only with atropine sulfate available for cholinergic crisis

Syringe compatibilities: Glycopyrrolate, heparin, pentobarbital, thiopental

Y-site compatibilities: Heparin, hydrocortisone sodium succinate, potassium chloride, vit B/C

Additive compatibilities: Netilmicin

Patient/family education

- Teach patient to carry/wear emergency ID specifying myasthenia gravis, products taken, prescriber's phone number

Evaluation

Positive therapeutic outcome

- Increased muscle strength, hand grasp
- Improved gait
- Absence of labored breathing (if severe)

Treatment of overdose: Respiratory support, **IV** atropine 1-4 mg

nepafenac ophthalmic
See Appendix B

nesiritide (Rx)
(nes-eer'ih-tide)
Natrecor
Func. class.: Vasodilator
Chem. class.: Human B-type natriuretic peptide

Pregnancy category C

Action: Uses DNA technology; human B-type natriuretic peptide binds to the receptor in vascular smooth muscle and endothelial cells, leading to smooth muscle relaxation

Therapeutic outcome: Improvement in symptoms of CHF

Uses: Acutely decompensated CHF

Dosage and routes
Adult: BOL **IV** 2 mcg/kg, then CONT **IV** INF 0.01 mcg/kg/min

Available forms: Powder for inj, 1.5 mg single-use vial

Adverse effects
CNS: Headache, insomnia, dizziness, anxiety, confusion, paresthesia, tremor
CV: Hypotension, **tachycardia,** dysrhythmias, bradycardia, ventricular tachycardia, ventricular extrasystoles, **atrial fibrillation**
GI: Vomiting, nausea
INTEG: Rash, sweating, pruritus, inj site reaction
MISC: Back pain, abdominal pain
RESP: Increased cough, hemoptysis, **apnea**

Contraindications: Hypersensitivity to this product or *E. coli* protein, cardiogenic shock or B/P <90 mm Hg as primary therapy

Precautions: Pregnancy C, breastfeeding, children, mitral stenosis; significant valvular stenosis, restriction, or obstructive cardiomyopathy, or any condition that depends on venous return; renal disease, constrictive pericarditis

Pharmacokinetics
Absorption	Vascular smooth muscle and endothelial cells
Distribution	Unknown
Metabolism	Unknown
Excretion	Bound to cell surfaces, internalized, and proteolyzed; cleaved by endopeptidases on vascular lumenal surface; renal filtration
Half-life	18 min

Pharmacodynamics
Onset	15 min
Peak	1 hr
Duration	Unknown

Interactions
Drug classifications
ACE inhibitors: increased symptomatic hypotension

NURSING CONSIDERATIONS
Assessment
• Assess PCWP, RAP, cardiac index, MPAP
• Assess B/P, pulse during treatment until stable
• Monitor I&O, daily weight, serum creatinine, BUN
• Assess for CHF: weight gain, dyspnea, crackles, edema

Nursing diagnoses
• Knowledge, deficient (teaching)
• Tissue perfusion, ineffective (uses)

Implementation
IV route
• Do not administer nesiritide through a central heparin-coated catheter; heparin should be administered through a separate catheter
• Prime **IV** fluid with inf of 25 ml before connecting to patient's vascular access port and before bolus dose or **IV** inf
• Reconstitute one 1.5 mg vial/5 ml of diluent from prefilled 250 ml plastic **IV** bag with diluent of choice (D₅, 0.9% NaCl, D₅/0.9% NaCl, D₅/0.2% NaCl); do not shake vial, roll gently; use only clear sol
• Withdraw all contents of reconstituted vial and add to the 250-ml plastic **IV** bag (6 mcg/ml); invert bag several times
• Use within 24 hr of reconstituting

Patient/family education
• Explain purpose of medication and expected results

Evaluation
Positive therapeutic outcome
• Improvement in CHF with improved PCWP, RAP, MPAP

---

nevirapine (Rx)
(ne-veer′a-peen)
Viramune
Func. class.: Antiretroviral
Chem. class.: Non-nucleoside reverse transcriptase inhibitor (NNRTI)

Pregnancy category B

Do not confuse:
nevirapine/nelfinavir, Viramune/Viracept

Action: Binds directly to reverse transcriptase and blocks RNA, DNA, causing a disruption of the enzyme's site

Therapeutic outcome: Improvement of HIV-1 infection

Uses: HIV-1 in combination with other highly active antiretroviral treatments (HAART)

Dosage and routes
Treatment of HIV infection in combination with other antiretroviral agents
Adult and adolescent: PO 200 mg/day × 2 wk, then 200 mg bid in combination
Neonate ≥15 days old/infant/child: PO 150 mg/m²/day × 14 days, then 150 mg/m² bid; max 400 mg/day

Perinatal transmission prophylaxis (unlabeled)
Females with no previous antiretroviral therapy: PO 200 mg as a single dose at onset of labor with zidovudine 2 mg/kg over 1 hr followed by zidovudine 1 mg/kg/hr until delivery
Neonate ≥34 wk gestation: PO Nevirapine 2 mg/kg as a single dose at age 48-72 hr and PO zidovudine 2 mg/kg q6hr for 6 wk

Available forms: Tabs 200 mg; oral susp 50 mg/5 ml

Adverse effects
CNS: Paresthesia, headache, fever, peripheral neuropathy
GI: Diarrhea, abdominal pain, *nausea, stomatitis,* **hepatotoxicity, hepatic failure**
HEMA: **Neutropenia, anemia, thrombocytopenia**
INTEG: Rash, **toxic epidermal necrolysis**

MISC: **Stevens-Johnson syndrome, anaphylaxis**
MS: Pain, myalgia, **rhabdomyolysis**

Contraindications:

Black Box Warning: Hypersensitivity

Precautions: Pregnancy **B**, breastfeeding, children, renal disease

Black Box Warning: Hepatic disease, females, hepatitis

Pharmacokinetics
Absorption	Rapid
Distribution	Protein binding 60%
Metabolism	Liver, by hepatic P450 enzyme system
Excretion	91% urine
Half-life	25-30 hr 50% removed by peritoneal dialysis; slower clearance rate in Hispanics, African Americans

Pharmacodynamics
Onset	Unknown
Peak	4 hr
Duration	Unknown

Interactions
Individual drugs
Cimetidine: increased nevirapine levels
Clonazepam, diazepam, warfarin: decreased nevirapine level
Itraconazole: decreased effect of itraconazole
Ketoconazole: decreased effect of ketoconazole
Methadone: decreased effect of methadone
Drug classifications
Anticonvulsants, rifamycins: decreased nevirapine levels
Antiinfectives, macrolides: increased nevirapine levels
Oral contraceptives, protease inhibitors: decreased action
Drug/herb
St. John's wort: decreased nevirapine levels, do not use together
Drug/lab test
Increased: ALT, AST, GGT, bilirubin, Hgb
Decreased: neutrophil count

NURSING CONSIDERATIONS
Assessment
• Use resistance testing prior to starting and when therapy fails
• Assess signs of infection, anemia, hepatotoxicity, immune reconstitution syndrome
• Assess liver, renal, blood tests: ALT, AST, viral load, CD4, plasma HIV RNA, glucose

---

 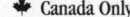

levels in diabetic patients; if liver function tests are elevated significantly, product should be withheld
• Assess C&S before product therapy; product may be taken as soon as culture is performed; repeat C&S after treatment; determine the presence of other sexually transmitted disease
• Assess bowel pattern before, during treatment; if severe abdominal pain with bleeding occurs, product should be discontinued; monitor hydration
⬥ Assess skin eruptions; rash, urticaria, itching; if rash is severe or systemic symptoms occur, discontinue immediately
• Assess allergies before treatment, reaction to each medication

Nursing diagnoses
• Diarrhea (side effects)
• Infection, risk for (uses)
• Knowledge, deficient (teaching)

Implementation
• Do not initiate treatment in females when CD4 counts >250 cells/mm^3, or in males when >400 cells/mm^3 unless benefit outweighs risks
• Give without regard to meals
• Give at equal intervals around the clock to maintain blood levels

Patient/family education
• Instruct patient to report any right quadrant pain, jaundice, rash immediately
• Inform patient that product may be taken with food, antacids, didanosine
• Advise patient to take as prescribed; if dose is missed, take as soon as remembered up to 1 hr before next dose; do not double dose
• Advise patient that product must be taken in equal intervals around the clock to maintain blood levels for duration of therapy
• Advise patient that product is not a cure, controls symptoms of HIV, does not prevent transmission
• Instruct patient to avoid OTC agents unless approved by prescriber
• Advise patient to use a nonhormonal form of contraception during treatment

Evaluation
Positive therapeutic outcome
• Improving viral load and CD4 cell counts
• Absence of AIDs defining symptoms
• Improvement in quality of life

niacin (Rx, OTC)
(nye'a-sin)
Edur-Acin, Nia-Bid, Niac, Niacels, Niacor, Niaspan, Nico-400, Nicobid, Nicolar, Nicotinex
nicotinic acid (Rx, OTC)
(nick-oh-tin'ick)
Novo-Niacin ✤, Slo-Niacin, vitamin B
niacinamide (Rx, OTC)
(nye-a-sin'a-mide)
nicotinamide (Rx, OTC)
(nick-oh-tin'ah-mide)
Func. class.: Vitamin B$_3$
Chem. class.: Water-soluble vitamin, lipid-lowering product

Pregnancy category C

Do not confuse:
Nicobid/Nitro-Bid

Action: Needed for conversion of fats, protein, carbohydrates by oxidation-reduction; acts directly on vascular smooth muscle, causing vasodilatation; reduces LDL, VLDL, total cholesterol, triglycerides, and lipoprotein A; increases HDL

Therapeutic outcome: Decreasing cholesterol and LDL levels, B$_3$ supplementation

Uses: Pellagra, hyperlipidemias (types IV, V), peripheral vascular disease that presents a risk for pancreatitis

Dosage and routes
Niacin deficiency
Adult: PO 100-500 mg/day in divided doses; IM/SUBCUT 5-100 mg 5 or more times a day; **IV** 25-100 mg bid or tid
Child: PO up to 300 mg/day in divided doses

Adjunct in hyperlipidemia
Adult: 250 mg after evening meal, may increase dose at 1-4 wk intervals to 1-2 g tid, max 6 g/day; EXT REL 500 mg at bedtime, ×4 wk, then 1000 mg at bedtime for wk 5-8, do not increase by more than 500 mg q4wk, max 2000 mg/day

Pellagra
Adult: PO 300-500 mg/day in divided doses
Child: PO 100-300 mg/day in divided doses

Peripheral vascular disease
Adult: PO 250-800 mg/day in 3-5 divided doses

Available forms: Niacin: tabs 25, 50, 100, 250, 500, 1000 mg; time rel tabs 250, 500 mg; elix 50 mg/5 ml; ext rel caps 250, 400 mg; sus

N

rel tabs 500 mg; cont rel tabs 250, 500, 750 mg; sus rel cap 125, 500 mg; nicotinamide: tabs 100, 250, 500 mg

Adverse effects

CNS: Paresthesias, headache, dizziness, anxiety
CV: Postural hypotension, vasovagal attacks, dysrhythmias, vasodilatation
EENT: Blurred vision, ptosis
GI: Nausea, vomiting, anorexia, *jaundice,* diarrhea, peptic ulcer, **hepatotoxicity,** dyspepsia, **hepatitis**
GU: Hyperuricemia, **glycosuria, hypoalbuminemia**
INTEG: Flushing, dry skin, rash, pruritus, itching, tingling

Contraindications: Breastfeeding, hypersensitivity, peptic ulcer, hepatic disease, hemorrhage, severe hypotension

Precautions: Pregnancy **C**, breastfeeding, glaucoma, CV disease, CAD, diabetes mellitus, gout, schizophrenia

Pharmacokinetics

Absorption	Well absorbed (PO)
Distribution	Widely distributed
Metabolism	Converted to niacinamide
Excretion	Urine, unchanged (30%); breast milk
Half-life	45 min

Pharmacodynamics

	PO	IV
Onset	Unknown	Unknown
Peak	30-70 min	Unknown
Duration	Unknown	Unknown

Interactions

Individual drugs
Alcohol: increased flushing, pruritus, avoid use
Drug classifications
Ganglionic blockers: increased postural hypotension
HMG-CoA reductase inhibitors: increased myopathy, rhabdomyolysis
Drug/herb
Red yeast rice: increased myopathy, rhabdomyolysis
Drug/lab test
Increased: bilirubin, alkaline phosphatase, liver enzymes, LDH, uric acid, glucose
Decreased: cholesterol
False increase: urinary catecholamines
False positive: urine glucose

NURSING CONSIDERATIONS

Assessment

- Assess for niacin deficiency (pellagra): nausea, vomiting, stomatitis, confusion, hallucinations before, throughout treatment
- Assess for symptoms of niacin deficiency: nausea, vomiting, anemia, poor memory, confusion, dermatitis
- Assess for lipid, triglyceride, cholesterol level, if using for hyperlipidemia
- Assess nutrition: fat, protein, carbohydrates, nutritional analysis should be completed by dietitian
- Monitor liver function tests: AST, ALT, bilirubin, uric acid, alkaline phosphatase; blood glucose before, during treatment; liver dysfunction: clay-colored stools, itching, dark urine, jaundice
- Monitor niacin levels during administration of this product
- Monitor cardiac status: rate, rhythm, quality; postural hypotension, dysrhythmias
- Monitor nutritional status: liver, yeast, legumes, organ meat, lean poultry; high-level niacin products should be included in the diet
- Assess for CNS symptoms: headache, paresthesias, blurred vision

Nursing diagnoses

- Knowledge, deficient (teaching)
- Noncompliance (teaching)
- Nutrition: less than body requirements, imbalanced (uses)

Implementation

PO route
- Do not break, crush, or chew ext rel products
- Give with meals or milk for GI symptoms, and 81-325 mg of aspirin or NSAIDs ½ hr before dose to decrease flushing

IV route
- Give by direct **IV** after diluting to 2 mg/ml at a rate of ≤2 mg/min
- Give by inf by adding 500 ml of 0.9% NaCl at a rate of ≤2 mg/min

Additive incompatibilities: Acids (strong), alkalis, erythromycin, kanamycin, streptomycin
Additive compatibilities: TPN sol

Patient/family education

- Advise patient that flushing and increase in feelings of warmth will occur several hr after taking product (PO); after 2 wk of therapy these side effects diminish
- Instruct patient to remain recumbent if postural hypotension occurs; to rise slowly from sitting or recumbent

---

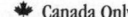 Alert   Canada Only   Drug on CD   * "Tall Man" lettering (See Preface)

- Caution patient to abstain from alcohol if product is prescribed for hyperlipidemia
- Caution patient to avoid sunlight if skin lesions are present
- Advise patient to report clay-colored stools, anorexia, jaundiced sclera, skin, dark urine; hepatotoxicity may occur

Evaluation
Positive therapeutic outcome
- Decreased lipid levels
- Warm extremities
- Absence of numbness in extremities

---

*niCARdipine (Rx)
(nye-card'i-peen)
Cardene IV, Cardene SR
Func. class.: Calcium channel blocker, antianginal, antihypertensive
Chem. class.: Dihydropyridine

Pregnancy category C

Do not confuse:
niCARdipine/NIFEdipine, Cardene/Cardizem, Cardene SR/Cardizem SR

Action: Inhibits calcium ion influx across cell membrane during cardiac depolarization, produces relaxation of coronary vascular smooth muscle and peripheral vascular smooth muscle, dilates coronary arteries, increases myocardial oxygen delivery in patients with vasospastic angina

Therapeutic outcome: Decreased angina pectoris, decreased B/P in hypertension

Uses: Chronic stable angina pectoris, hypertension

Dosage and routes
Hypertension
Adult: PO 20 mg tid initially; may increase after 3 days (range 20-40 mg tid) or SUS REL 30 mg bid; may increase to 60 mg bid **IV** 5 mg/hr; may increase by 2.5 mg/hr q15min; max 15 mg/hr

Angina
Adult: PO 20 mg tid, may be adjusted q3day, may use 20-40 mg tid

Renal dose
Adult: PO 20 mg tid or SUS REL 30 mg bid

Hepatic dose
Adult: PO 20 mg bid

Available forms: Caps 20, 30 mg; sus rel caps 30, 45, 60 mg; inj 2.5 mg/ml

Adverse effects
CNS: Headache, dizziness, anxiety, depression, confusion, paresthesia, somnolence, *flushing*
CV: Edema, bradycardia, hypotension, palpitations, **pulmonary edema,** chest pain, tachycardia, increased angina, **arrhythmias, CHF**
GI: Nausea, vomiting, gastric upset, constipation, **hepatitis,** abdominal cramps, dry mouth, sore throat
GU: Nocturia, polyuria
INTEG: Rash, infusion site discomfort, **Stevens-Johnson syndrome**
MISC: Blurred vision, flushing, sweating, SOB, impotence

Contraindications: Sick sinus syndrome, 2nd- or 3rd-degree heart block, hypersensitivity, advanced aortic stenosis

Precautions: Pregnancy C, breastfeeding, children, geriatric, CHF, hypotension, hepatic injury, renal disease

Pharmacokinetics
Absorption	Well absorbed (PO); bioavailability poor
Distribution	Unknown
Metabolism	Liver, extensively
Excretion	Kidneys 60%, feces 35%
Half-life	2-5 hr

Pharmacodynamics
	PO	PO-SUS REL
Onset	½ hr	Unknown
Peak	1-2 hr	2-6 hr
Duration	8 hr	10-12 hr

Interactions
Individual drugs
Alcohol: increased hypotension
Carbamazepine, cycloSPORINE, prazosin, propranolol, quinidine: increased risk of toxicity
Cimetidine: increased niCARdipine effects
Digoxin, quinidine, theophylline: increased effects
Rifampin: decreased antihypertensive effect
Drug classifications
Antihypertensives, neuromuscular blocking agents, nitrates: increased hypotension
NSAIDs: decreased antihypertensive effect
Drug/herb
Barberry, betel palm, burdock, goldenseal, khat, khella, lily of the valley, plantain: increased effect
Yohimbe: decreased effect

Adverse effects: *italic* = common, **bold** = life-threatening

Drug/food
Grapefruit juice: increased hypotensive effect

NURSING CONSIDERATIONS
Assessment
• Assess fluid volume status (I&O ratio) and record weight, color, quality, and specific gravity of urine, skin turgor, adequacy of pulses, moist mucous membranes, bilateral lung sounds, peripheral pitting edema; dehydration symptoms of decreasing output, thirst, hypotension, dry mouth, and mucous membranes should be reported
• Monitor for CHF: weight gain, crackles, jugular venous distention, dyspnea
• Monitor B/P and pulse
• Assess anginal pain: intensity, location, duration, alleviating factors
• Monitor potassium, renal/liver function tests, periodically

Nursing diagnoses
• Cardiac output, decreased (uses)
• Knowledge, deficient (teaching)

Implementation
PO route
• Do not break, crush, chew, or open sus rel caps
• Give with or without regard to meals
• Store in airtight container at room temperature
IV route
• Dilute each 25 mg/240 ml of compatible sol (0.1 mg/ml), give slowly, stable for 24 hr at room temperature
Solution compatibilities: D_5W, $D_5/0.45\%$ NaCl, $D_5/0.9\%$ NaCl
Y-site compatibilities: Diltiazem, DOBUTamine, DOPamine, epinephrine, fentanyl, hydromorphone, labetalol, lorazepam, midazolam, milrinone, morphine, nitroglycerin, norepinephrine, ranitidine, vecuronium

Patient/family education
• Advise patient to avoid hazardous activities until stabilized on product and dizziness is no longer a problem
• Instruct patient to limit caffeine consumption; to avoid alcohol and OTC products unless directed by a prescriber
◆ Instruct patient to comply in all areas of medical regimen: diet, exercise, stress reduction, product therapy; to notify prescriber of irregular heartbeat, shortness of breath, swelling of feet and hands, pronounced dizziness, constipation, nausea, hypotension, change in severity/pattern/incidence of angina

• Teach patient to use medication as directed even if feeling better; may be taken with other cardiovascular products (nitrates, β-blockers)
• Teach patient to take medication exactly as prescribed
• Advise patient to contact prescriber if anginal attacks continue or become worse

Evaluation
Positive therapeutic outcome
• Decreased angina attacks
• Decreased B/P

Treatment of overdose: Defibrillation, atropine for AV block, vasopressor for hypotension

---

nicotinamide
See niacin

---

nicotine (OTC)
(nik′o-teen)
nicotine chewing gum (OTC)
Nicorette
nicotine inhaler (Rx)
Nicotrol Inhaler
nicotine lozenge (OTC)
Commit
nicotine nasal spray (Rx)
Nicotrol NS
nicotine transdermal (OTC)
Clear Nicoderm CQ, Habitrol, NicoDerm CQ, Nicotrol, Nicotrol TD
Func. class.: Smoking deterrent
Chem. class.: Ganglionic cholinergic agonist

Pregnancy category
D (transdermal)
X (gum)

Action: Agonist at nicotinic receptors in the peripheral and central nervous systems; acts at sympathetic ganglia, on chemoreceptors of the aorta and carotid bodies; also affects adrenalin-releasing catecholamines

Therapeutic outcome: Decreased withdrawal effects when smoking cessation is attempted

Uses: Deter cigarette smoking

Unlabeled uses: Gilles de la Tourette's syndrome

Dosage and routes
Nicotine chewing gum
Adult: If patient smokes <25 cigarettes/day, start with 2 mg gum; if >25 cigarettes/day, start with 4 mg gum; then 1 piece of gum q1-2hr × 6 wk, then 1 piece of gum q2-4hr × 2 wk, then 1 piece of gum q4-8hr × 2 wk, then discontinue; max 24/day

Nicotine inhaler
Adult: Inhale 6 cartridges/day for first 3-6 wk, max 16/day × 12 wk

Nicotine lozenge
Adult: If cigarette is desired >30 min after awakening, start with 1-2–mg lozenge; if <30 min after awakening, start with 4-mg lozenge; then 1 q1-2hr, max 20 lozenges/day or 5 lozenges/6 hr × 6 wk, then 1 lozenge q2-4hr × 2 wk, then 1 lozenge q4-8hr × 2 wk, then discontinue

Nicotine nasal spray
Adult: 1 spray in each nostril 1-2 ×/hr, max 5 ×/hr or 40 ×/day, max 3 mo

Nicotine transdermal/inhaler system
Habitrol, NicoDerm
Adult: 21 mg/day × 4-8 wk; 14 mg/day × 2-4 wk; 7 mg/day × 2-4 wk

Nicotrol
Adult: 15 mg/day × 12 wk; 10 mg/day × 2 wk; 5 mg/day × 2 wk

Nicotrol inhaler
Adult: Delivers 30% of what a smoker receives from an actual cigarette

Gilles de la Tourette's syndrome (unlabeled)
Adult and child: Chewing gum 2 mg chewed × ½ hr bid × 1-6 mo; transdermal 7 or 10 mg patch daily × 2 days

Available forms: Gum: 2 mg/piece; nicotine transdermal system (Habitrol, Nico-Derm, Nicotine Transdermal System); 7, 14, 21 mg/day delivered; (NicoDerm) 5, 10, 15 mg/day; nicotine inhaler: 4 mg delivered; nasal spray: 0.5 mg of nicotine/actuation; lozenge: 2 mg, 4 mg

Adverse effects
CNS: Dizziness, vertigo, insomnia, headache, confusion, **seizures**, depression, euphoria, numbness, tinnitus, strange dreams
CV: **Dysrhythmias,** tachycardia, palpitations, edema, flushing, hypertension
EENT: Jaw ache, irritation in buccal cavity
GI: *Nausea, vomiting, anorexia, indigestion,* diarrhea, abdominal pain, constipation, eructation, irritation
RESP: Breathing difficulty, cough, hoarseness, sneezing, wheezing, bronchial spasm

Contraindications: Pregnancy **X** (gum), **D** (transdermal), hypersensitivity, immediate post-MI recovery period, severe angina pectoris

Precautions: Breastfeeding, vasospastic disease, dysrhythmias, diabetes mellitus, hyperthyroidism, pheochromocytoma, coronary disease, esophagitis, peptic ulcer, renal/hepatic disease; MRI (patch)

Pharmacokinetics
Absorption	Slowly absorbed, buccal cavity
Distribution	Unknown
Metabolism	Liver; some by lungs, kidneys
Excretion	Kidneys, unchanged (20%); breast milk
Half-life	1-2 hr

Pharmacodynamics
Onset	Rapid
Peak	½ hr
Duration	Unknown

Interactions
Individual drugs
Acetaminophen, caffeine, furosemide, imipramine, oxazepam, pentazocine, propranolol: increased effects of each specific product with cessation of smoking
Glutethimide: decreased absorption
Insulin (SUBCUT): increased absorption
Propoxyphene: decreased propoxyphene metabolism
Theophylline: increased blood levels with cessation of smoking
Drug/herb
Blue cohosh, lobelia: increased effect
Oats: decreased effect

NURSING CONSIDERATIONS
Assessment
• Assess for adverse reaction to gum: irritation of buccal cavity, dislike of taste, jaw ache
• Assess for withdrawal symptoms: headache, fatigue, drowsiness, restlessness, irritability, severe cravings for nicotine products before, during, and after treatment
• Obtain a nicotine assessment: brand of cigarettes, chewing tobacco, cigars, number of each used per day; what increases need or activities performed when each is used
• Gum should not be used if temporomandibular condition exists
• Assess for nicotine toxicity: GI symptoms (nausea, vomiting, diarrhea), cardiopulmo-

nary symptoms (decreased B/P, dyspnea, change in pulse), weakness, abdominal cramping, headache, blurred vision, tinnitus; product should be discontinued

Nursing diagnoses
• Coping, ineffective (uses)
• Knowledge, deficient (teaching)
• Noncompliance (teaching)

Implementation
• Give only prescribed amount, or toxicity may occur
• Protect gum from light and heat

Patient/family education
• Advise patient to begin product withdrawal after 3 mo use; max 6 mo
• Teach patient all aspects of product; give package insert to patient and explain; caution patient not to exceed prescribed dose
• Caution patient not to use during pregnancy; birth defects may occur

Gum
• Advise patient to chew gum slowly for 30 min to promote buccal absorption of the product; do not chew over 45 min
• Inform patient that gum will not stick to dentures, dental appliances
• Caution patient that gum is as toxic as cigarettes; it is to be used only to deter smoking

Transdermal patch
• Caution patient that patch is as toxic as cigarettes; to be used only to deter smoking
• Caution patient not to use during pregnancy; birth defects may occur
• Instruct patient to keep used and unused system out of reach of children and pets
• Instruct patient to apply once a day to a nonhairy, clean, dry area of skin on upper body or upper outer arm; to rotate sites to prevent skin irritation
• Instruct patient to stop smoking immediately when beginning patch treatment
• Teach patient to apply promptly after removing from protective pouch; system may lose strength

Inhaler
• Advise patient that puffing on mouthpiece delivers nicotine through the mouth lining

Evaluation
Positive therapeutic outcome
• Decrease in urge to smoke
• Decreased need for gum after 3-6 mo

---

*NIFEdipine (Rx)
(nye-fed′i-peen)
Adalat, Adalat CC, Apo-Nifed PA ✖,
Nifediac CC, Nifedical XL, NIFEdipine,
Novo-Nifedin ✖, Nu-Nifedin ✖,
Procardia, Procardia XL
Func. class.: Calcium channel blocker, antianginal, antihypertensive
Chem. class.: Dihydropyridine
Pregnancy category C

Do not confuse:
NIFEdipine/niCARdipine/nimodipine

Action: Inhibits calcium ion influx across cell membrane during cardiac depolarization, produces relaxation of coronary vascular smooth muscle and peripheral vascular smooth muscle, dilates coronary vascular arteries, increases myocardial oxygen delivery in patients with vasospastic angina

Therapeutic outcome: Decreased angina pectoris, decreased B/P in hypertension

Uses: Chronic stable angina pectoris, vasospastic angina, hypertension

Dosage and routes
Adult: PO immediate release, 10 mg tid; increase in 10 mg increments q7-14day, max 180 mg/24 hr or single dose of 30 mg; SUS REL 30-60 mg/day; may increase q7-14day; doses >120 mg not recommended

Hypertension
Adult: PO EXT REL 30-60 mg qd, titrate upward as needed; max 90 mg/day (Adalat CC); 120 mg/day (Procardia XL)
Adolescent/child (unlabeled): PO 0.25-0.5 mg/kg/day, max 3 mg/kg/day

Available forms: Caps 5 ✖, 10, 20 mg; ext rel tabs (CC, XL) 10 ✖, 20 ✖, 30, 60, 90 mg; tabs 10 mg ✖

Adverse effects
CNS: Headache, fatigue, drowsiness, *dizziness,* anxiety, depression, weakness, insomnia, *light-headedness,* paresthesia, tinnitus, blurred vision, nervousness, tremor, flushing
CV: **Dysrhythmias,** edema, hypotension, palpitations, tachycardia
GI: Nausea, vomiting, diarrhea, gastric upset, constipation, increased liver function tests, dry mouth, flatulence, gingival hyperplasia, **hepatotoxicity**
GU: Nocturia, polyuria
HEMA: Bruising, bleeding, petechiae
INTEG: Rash, pruritus, *flushing,* hair loss
MISC: Sexual difficulties, cough, fever, chills
SYST: **Stevens-Johnson syndrome**

Contraindications: Hypersensitivity to this product or dihydropyridine

Precautions: Pregnancy **C,** breastfeeding, children, CHF, hypotension, sick sinus syndrome, 2nd- or 3rd-degree heart block, hypotension less than 90 mm Hg systolic, hepatic injury, renal disease, acute MI, aortic stenosis, cardiogenic shock, GERD, heart failure

Pharmacokinetics

Absorption	Well absorbed (PO)
Distribution	Unknown
Metabolism	Liver, extensively
Excretion	Unknown
Half-life	2-5 hr

Pharmacodynamics

	PO	PO–EXT REL
Onset	½ hr	Unknown
Peak	Unknown	Unknown
Duration	6-8 hr	24 hr

Interactions
Individual drugs
Carbamazepine, cimetidine, cycloSPORINE, phenytoin, prazosin, ranitidine: increased risk of toxicity
Digoxin: increased digoxin levels
Quinidine: decreased effects
Smoking: decreased NIFEdipine level
Drug classifications
Antihypertensives, β-adrenergic blockers: increased effects
NSAIDs: decreased antihypertensive effect
Drug/herb
Barberry, betel palm, burdock, goldenseal, khat, khella, lily of the valley, plaintain: increased effect
Yohimbe: decreased effect
Drug/food
Grapefruit juice: increased NIFEdipine level
Drug/lab test
Positive: ANA titer, direct Coombs' test
Increased: CPK, LDH, AST

NURSING CONSIDERATIONS
Assessment
• Assess anginal pain: location, intensity, duration, character, alleviating, aggravating factors
• Assess for bruising, petechiae, bleeding
• Monitor potassium, renal/liver function tests periodically during treatment
• Assess fluid volume status (I&O ratio) and record weight, distended red veins, crackles in lung, color, quality, and specific gravity of urine, skin turgor, adequacy of pulses, moist mucous membranes, bilateral lung sounds, peripheral pitting edema; dehydration symptoms of decreasing output, thirst, hypotension, dry mouth, and mucous membranes should be reported
• Monitor ALT, AST, bilirubin daily; if these are elevated, hepatotoxicity is suspected
• Monitor cardiac status: B/P, pulse, respirations, ECG

Nursing diagnoses
• Cardiac output, decreased (uses)
• Knowledge, deficient (teaching)
• Pain, acute (uses)

Implementation
PO route
• Give without regard to meals
• Store in airtight container at room temperature
Sublingual route
• Using a sterile needle puncture the cap and squeeze medication in buccal area (not an FDA-approved use)

Patient/family education
• Advise patient to avoid hazardous activities until stabilized on product and dizziness is no longer a problem
• Instruct patient to limit caffeine consumption; to avoid alcohol and OTC products unless directed by prescriber
• Tell patient that ext rel tab has nonabsorbable shell, may appear in stools
• Instruct patient to comply in all areas of medical regimen: diet, exercise, stress reduction, product therapy; to notify prescriber of irregular heartbeat, SOB, swelling of feet and hands, pronounced dizziness, constipation, nausea, hypotension, severe rash, changes in pattern/frequency/severity of angina
• Teach patient to use as directed even if feeling better; may be taken with other cardiovascular products (nitrates, β-blockers)
• Advise patient to increase fluid intake to prevent constipation
• Teach patient to check for gingival hyperplasia and report promptly
• Teach patient not to discontinue abruptly; gradually taper

Evaluation
Positive therapeutic outcome
• Decreased angina attacks
• Decreased B/P

Treatment of overdose: Defibrillation, atropine for AV block, vasopressor for hypotension

N

Adverse effects: *italic* = common, **bold** = life-threatening

nilotinib (Rx)
(nye-loe'ti-nib)
Tasigna
Func. class.: Antineoplastic—miscellaneous
Chem. class.: Protein-tyrosine kinase
inhibitor

Pregnancy category D

Action: Inhibits BCR-ABL tyrosine kinase
created in chronic myeloid leukemia (CML)

Therapeutic outcome: Decrease in
progression of disease

Uses: Chronic phase/accelerated phase
Philadelphia chromosome-positive chronic
myelogenous leukemia that is resistant/
intolerant to imatinib

Dosage and routes
Adult: PO 400 mg q12h; continue until
disease progression or unacceptable toxicity

*Escalation regimen for those
taking a strong CYP3A4 inducer*
Adult: PO increase dose as required

*Adjustment following
discontinuation of a strong
CYP3A4 inducer*
Adult: PO reduce to 400 mg/bid

*For those taking a strong CYP3A4
inhibitor*
Adult: PO reduce dose to 400 mg/day

QT prolongation
QTc >480 msec: Withhold dose

Myelosuppression
*ANC 1 x 10^9/L or platelets <50 x
10^9/L:* Withhold dose

Available forms: Caps 200 mg

Adverse effects
CNS: Headache, dizziness, fatigue, fever,
flushing, paresthesia
CV: **QT prolongation,** palpitations, **torsades
de pointes**
GI: *Nausea,* **hepatotoxicity, vomiting,
dyspepsia,** *anorexia, abdominal pain,*
constipation, **pancreatitis,** diarrhea
HEMA: **Neutropenia, thrombocytopenia,
anemia, pancytopenia**
INTEG: *Rash,* alopecia, erythema
META: Hyperamylasemia, hyperbilirubinemia,
hyperglycemia, hyperkalemia, hypocalcemia,
hyponatremia, hypomagnesemia
MISC: Diaphoresis
MS: Arthralgia, myalgia, back/bone pain,
muscle cramps
RESP: Cough, dyspnea
SYST: **Bleeding**

Contraindications: Pregnancy **D**, breastfeeding, hypersensitivity

Black Box Warning: Hypokalemia, hypomagnesemia, QT prolongation

Precautions: Children, women, geriatric
patients, active infections, anemia, cardiac
disease, bone marrow suppression, cholestasis, diabetes, gelatin hypersensitivity, infertility,
galactose-free diet, lactase deficiency, neutropenia, pancreatitis, thrombocytopenia

Black Box Warning: Hepatic disease

Pharmacokinetics
Absorption	Unknown
Distribution	Protein binding 98%, plasma levels 3 hr
Metabolism	By CYP3A4
Excretion	Unknown
Half-life	Elimination 17 hr

Pharmacodynamics
Unknown

Interactions
Individual drugs
• Product interactions are numerous
Acetaminophen: increased hepatotoxicity
Carbamazepine, dexamethasone, phenobarbi-
tal, phenytoin, rifampin: decreased concen-
trations
Clarithromycin, erythromycin, itraconazole,
ketoconazole: increased concentrations
Pimozide, ziprasidone: do not use concur-
rently
Simvastatin: increased plasma concentrations
Warfarin: increased plasma concentration;
avoid use with warfarin, use low-molecular-
weight anticoagulants instead
Drug classifications
Calcium channel blockers: increased plasma
concentrations
Phenothiazines: do not use concurrently
Drug/herb
St. John's wort: decreased concentration
Drug/food
Grapefruit juice: increased plasma concentra-
tions

NURSING CONSIDERATIONS
Assessment
• Assess ANC and platelets; if ANC <1 × 10^9/L
and/or platelets <50 × 10^9/L, stop until ANC
>1.5 × 10^9/L and platelets >75 × 10^9/L
• Monitor CV status: hypertension, QT prolongation can occur; monitor left ventricular
ejection fraction (LVEF) baseline periodically

 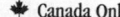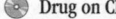

- Assess for renal toxicity: if bilirubin >3 × IULN, withhold until bilirubin levels return to <1.5 × IULN
- Assess for hepatotoxicity: monitor hepatic function tests, before treatment and qmo; if liver transaminases >5 × IULN, withhold until transaminase levels return to <2.5 × IULN
- Monitor CBC, differential, platelet count weekly; withhold product if WBC is <3500/mm^3 or platelet count <100,000/mm^3; notify prescriber of these results; product should be discontinued
- Monitor for bleeding: epistaxis, rectal, gingival, upper GI, genital, and wound bleeding; tumor-related hemorrhage may occur rapidly
- Monitor electrolytes: calcium, potassium, magnesium, sodium; lipase, phosphate; hypokalemia, hypomagnesemia should be corrected prior to use

Nursing diagnoses
- Knowledge, deficient (teaching)

Implementation
- Do not break, crush, or chew caps
- Give on an empty stomach; separate doses by 12 hr; a make-up dose should not be taken if a dose is missed
- Store at 15°-30° C (59°-86° F)

Patient/family education
- Instruct patient to report adverse reactions immediately: SOB, bleeding
- Inform patient reason for treatment, expected result
- Advise patient that many adverse reactions may occur
- Teach patient to avoid persons with known upper respiratory infections; immunosuppression is common
- Instruct in signs/symptoms of low potassium or magnesium

Evaluation
Positive therapeutic outcome
- Decrease in progression of disease

---

nilutamide (Rx)
(nil-u′ta-mide)
Anandron ✤, Nilandron
Func. class.: Antineoplastic, hormone
Chem. class.: Antiandrogen

Pregnancy category C

Action: Interferes with testosterone uptake in the nucleus or testosterone activity in target tissues; arrests tumor growth in androgen-sensitive tissue (prostate gland); prostatic carcinoma is androgen-sensitive, so tumor growth is arrested

Therapeutic outcome: Decreased tumor size

Uses: Metastatic prostatic carcinoma, stage D2 in combination with surgical castration (only to be used by men)

Dosage and routes
Adult: PO 300 mg/day × 30 days, then 150 mg/day

Available forms: Tabs 50, 100 ✤, 150 mg

Adverse effects
CNS: Hot flashes, drowsiness, insomnia, dizziness, hyperthesia, depression
CV: **Heart failure,** hypertension
EENT: Delay in adaptation to dark
GI: Diarrhea, nausea, vomiting, elevated liver function tests, constipation, dyspepsia, **hepatotoxicity**
GU: Decreased libido, impotence, testicular atrophy, UTI, hematuria, nocturia, gynecomastia
HEMA: Anemia
INTEG: Rash, sweating, alopecia, dry skin
MISC: Edema
RESP: Dyspnea, URI, pneumonia, **interstitial pneumonitis**

Contraindications: Women, hypersensitivity, severe hepatic impairment, severe respiratory disease

Precautions: Pregnancy C

Pharmacokinetics

Absorption	Rapidly, completely
Distribution	Unknown
Metabolism	Unknown
Excretion	Urine, feces
Half-life	Unknown

Pharmacodynamics
Unknown

Interactions
Individual drugs
Phenytoin, theophylline, vitamin K: increased toxicity

NURSING CONSIDERATIONS
Assessment
◆ Monitor liver function tests: AST, ALT, alkaline phosphatase, which may be elevated; if elevated 3 × normal, discontinue product
- Monitor PSA, improvement in bone pain
- Monitor for CNS symptoms: drowsiness, insomnia, dizziness

Adverse effects: *italic* = common, **bold** = life-threatening

N

- Monitor chest x-rays routinely, baseline pulmonary function tests; dyspnea, cough may indicate interstitial pneumonitis; discontinue treatment if this condition is suspected
- Monitor for hyperglycemia, increased BUN, creatinine, alkaline phosphatase leukopenia

Nursing diagnoses
- Infection, risk for (side effects)
- Knowledge, deficient (teaching)

Implementation
- Administer without regard to meals
- Start therapy on day of or after surgery
- Store at room temperature

Patient/family education
⬥ Advise patient to report side effects: decreased libido, impotence, breast enlargement, hot flashes, diarrhea, dyspnea, cough; symptoms of hepatotoxicity (dark urine, abdominal pain, clay-colored stools, jaundiced eyes, skin); notify prescriber immediately if shortness of breath occurs
- Advise patient to wear tinted lenses to alleviate delay in adapting to the dark
- Advise patient that product is started on day of or day after surgical removal of testes
- Advise patient to avoid alcohol consumption

Evaluation
Positive therapeutic outcome
- Decrease in prostatic tumor size, decrease in spread of cancer

Treatment of overdose: Induce vomiting, provide supportive care

---

nimodipine (Rx)
(ni-moe'dip-een)
Nimotop
Func. class.: Calcium channel blocker
Chem. class.: Dihydropyridine
Pregnancy category C

Action: Unknown, may have greater effect on cerebral arteries

Therapeutic outcome: Prevention of vascular spasm (subarachnoid hemorrhage)

Uses: Prevention of cerebrovascular spasm in subarachnoid hemorrhage

Dosage and routes
Adult: PO begin therapy within 96 hr, 60 mg q4hr × 21 days

Available forms: Caps 30 mg

Adverse effects
CNS: Headache, fatigue, drowsiness, dizziness, anxiety, depression, weakness, insomnia, confusion, paresthesia, somnolence
CV: Dysrhythmia, edema, CHF, bradycardia, hypotension, palpitations, **MI, pulmonary edema**
GI: Nausea, vomiting, diarrhea, gastric upset, constipation, **hepatitis,** abdominal cramps
GU: Nocturia, polyuria, **acute renal failure**
INTEG: Rash, pruritus, urticaria, photosensitivity, hair loss
MISC: Blurred vision, flushing, nasal congestion, sweating, shortness of breath, gynecomastia, hyperglycemia, sexual difficulties

Contraindications: Sick sinus syndrome, 2nd- or 3rd-degree heart block, hypotension less than 90 mm Hg systolic, hypersensitivity

Precautions: Pregnancy **C**, breastfeeding, children, geriatric, CHF, hypotension, hepatic injury, renal disease

Pharmacokinetics
Absorption	Well absorbed, bioavailability poor
Distribution	Crosses blood-brain barrier
Metabolism	Liver, extensively
Excretion	Kidneys
Half-life	1-2 hr

Pharmacodynamics
Onset	Unknown
Peak	1 hr
Duration	Unknown

Interactions
Individual drugs
Alcohol: increased hypotension
Digoxin: increased digoxin levels, bradycardia
Phenobarbital, phenytoin: decreased effectiveness
Propranolol: increased toxicity
Drug classifications
Antihypertensives: increased hypotension
β-Adrenergic blockers: increased bradycardia
Nitrates: increased nitrates
Drug/herb
Barberry, betel palm, burdock, goldenseal, khat, khella, lily of the valley, plantain: increased effect
Yohimbe: decreased effect

NURSING CONSIDERATIONS
Assessment
- Assess fluid volume status (I&O ratio) and record weight; distended red veins; crackles in lung; color, quality, and specific gravity of

urine; skin turgor; adequacy of pulses; moist mucous membranes; bilateral lung sounds; peripheral pitting edema; dehydration symptoms of decreasing output, thirst, hypotension, dry mouth and mucous membranes should be reported
• Monitor B/P and pulse; if B/P drops 30 mm Hg, call prescriber
• Monitor ALT, AST, bilirubin daily; if these are elevated, hepatotoxicity is suspected

Nursing diagnoses
• Injury, risk for (uses)
• Knowledge, deficient (teaching)

Implementation
• May puncture cap and dilute in water and give through nasogastric tube; flush tube with 0.9% NaCl
• Store in airtight container at room temperature

Evaluation
Positive therapeutic outcome
• Prevention of neurologic damage from subarachnoid hemorrhage

---

nisoldipine (Rx)
(nye′sol-dye peen)
Sular
Func. class.: Antihypertensive, calcium channel blocker
Chem. class : Dihydropyridine

Pregnancy category C

Action: Inhibits calcium ion influx across cell membrane, resulting in dilatation of peripheral arteries

Therapeutic outcome: Decreased B/P in hypertension

Uses: Essential hypertension, alone or with other antihypertensives

Dosage and routes
Adult: PO 17 mg/day initially, may increase by 8.5 mg/wk, usual dose 17-34 mg/day, max 34 mg/day
Geriatric/hepatic dose: PO 8.5 mg/day, increase based on response

Available forms: Ext rel tabs 8.5, 17, 20, 25.5, 30, 34, 40 mg

Adverse effects
CNS: Headache, fatigue, drowsiness, dizziness, anxiety, depression, nervousness, insomnia, light-headedness, paresthesia, tinnitus, psychosis, somnolence, ataxia, confusion, malaise, migraine

CV: **Dysrhythmias,** edema, **CHF,** hypotension, palpitations, **MI, pulmonary edema,** tachycardia, syncope, AV block, angina, chest pain, ECG abnormalities
GI: Nausea, vomiting, diarrhea, gastric upset, constipation, elevated liver function tests, dry mouth, dyspepsia, dysphagia, flatulence
GU: Nocturia, hematuria, dysuria
HEMA: **Anemia, leukopenia,** petechiae
INTEG: Rash, pruritus
MISC: Sexual difficulties, gingival hyperplasia, chills, fever, gout, sweating, cough, nasal congestion, shortness of breath, wheezing, epistaxis, dyspnea

Contraindications: Hypersensitivity, sick sinus syndrome, 2nd- or 3rd-degree heart block, aortic stenosis

Precautions: Pregnancy **C,** breastfeeding, children, geriatric, CHF, hypotension <90 mm Hg systolic, hepatic injury, renal disease, acute MI, unstable angina, CAD, cardiogenic shock

Pharmacokinetics
Absorption	Well absorbed
Distribution	Highly protein bound
Metabolism	Liver
Excretion	Kidneys
Half-life	Unknown

Pharmacodynamics
Onset	Unknown
Peak	6-12 hr
Duration	Unknown

Interactions
Individual drugs
Cimetidine, ranitidine: increased nisoldipine level
Digoxin: increased effects
Drug classifications
Antifungals (azole), CYP3A4 inhibitors: increased nisoldipine level
Antihypertensives: increased hypotension
β-Adrenergic blockers: increased effects
Hydantoins, CYP3A4 inducers: decreased nisoldipine effect
Drug/herb
Barberry, betel palm, burdock, goldenseal, hawthorn, khat, khella, lily of the valley, plantain: increased effect
St. John's wort, yohimbe: decreased effect
Drug/food
Grapefruit juice: increased hypotension
High-fat foods: increased nisoldipine level

N

Adverse effects: *italic* = common, **bold** = life-threatening

NURSING CONSIDERATIONS
Assessment
- Assess fluid volume status: I&O ratio and record; weight; skin turgor; adequacy of pulses; moist mucous membranes; bilateral lung sounds; peripheral pitting edema; dehydration symptoms of decreasing output, thirst, hypotension, dry mouth and mucous membranes should be reported
- Monitor ALT, AST, bilirubin daily if these are elevated and hepatotoxicity is suspected
- Monitor cardiac status: B/P, pulse, respiration, ECG

Nursing diagnoses
- Cardiac output, decreased (uses)
- Knowledge, deficient (teaching)

Implementation
- Give once a day, with food to decrease GI symptoms; avoid high-fat foods, grapefruit

Patient/family education
- Caution patient to avoid hazardous activities until stabilized on product and dizziness is no longer a problem
- Instruct patient to limit caffeine consumption; to avoid alcohol and OTC products unless directed by prescriber
- Urge patient to comply in all areas of medical regimen: diet, exercise, stress reduction, product therapy; to notify prescriber of irregular heartbeat, SOB, swelling of feet and hands, pronounced dizziness, constipation, nausea, hypotension
- Teach patient to use as directed even if feeling better; may be taken with other cardiovascular products (nitrates, β-blockers)
- Advise patient to rise slowly to prevent orthostatic hypotension
- Teach patient to report nausea, dizziness, edema, SOB, palpitations

Evaluation
Positive therapeutic outcome
- Decreased B/P

---

nitazoxanide (Rx)
(nye-taz-ox′a-nide)
Alinia
Func. class.: Antiprotozoal

Pregnancy category B

Action: Interferes with DNA/RNA synthesis in protozoa

Therapeutic outcome: C&S negative for organism

Uses: Diarrhea caused by *Cryptosporidium parvum* or *Giardia lamblia*

Dosage and routes
Adult: PO 500 mg q12hr × 3 days
Child 4-11 yr: PO 10 ml (200 mg) q12hr × 3 days
Child 12-47 mo: PO 5 ml (100 mg) q12hr × 3 days

Available forms: Powder for oral susp 100 mg/5 ml; tab 500 mg

Adverse effects
CNS: Dizziness, fever, headache
CV: Hypotension
GI: Nausea, anorexia, flatulence, increased appetite, enlarged salivary glands, abdominal pain, diarrhea, vomiting
HEMA: Anemia, **leukopenia**, neutropenia
INTEG: Pruritus, sweating
MISC: Increased creatinine, pale yellow eye discoloration, rhinitis, discolored urine, infection, malaise

Contraindications: Hypersensitivity

Precautions: Pregnancy **B**, breastfeeding, children <1 yr or >11 yr, renal/hepatic disease, diabetes mellitus (contains sucrose), HIV, immunocompromised patients

Pharmacokinetics
Absorption	Unknown
Distribution	Metabolite protein binding >99%
Metabolism	Hydrolyzed to active metabolite, undergoes conjugation
Excretion	Urine, bile, feces
Half-life	Unknown

Pharmacodynamics
Unknown

Interactions
Drug classifications
Other highly protein bound products (phenytoin, aspirin): competes for binding sites

NURSING CONSIDERATIONS
Assessment
- Assess for signs of infection
- Assess bowel pattern before, during treatment

Nursing diagnoses
- Infection, risk for (uses)
- Knowledge, deficient (teaching)

Implementation
PO route
- Give with food
- Shake oral susp before giving

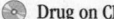

Patient/family education
- Advise to take with food; shake susp well before each dose

Evaluation
Positive therapeutic outcome
- C&S negative for organism
- Decreased diarrhea

---

nitrofurantoin (Rx)
(nye-troe-fyoor'an-toyn)
Apo-Nitrofurantoin ✿, Furadantin, Macrobid, Macrodantin, nitrofurantoin
Func. class.: Urinary tract antiinfective
Chem. class.: Synthetic nitrofuran derivative

Pregnancy category B

Action: Inhibits bacterial acetyl-CoA from interfering with carbohydrate metabolism

Therapeutic outcome: Resolution of infection

Uses: Urinary tract infections caused by *Escherichia coli, Klebsiella, Pseudomonas, Proteus vulgaris, Proteus morganii, Serratia, Citrobacter, Staphylococcus aureus, Staphylococcus epidermidis, Enterococcus, Salmonella, Shigella*

Dosage and routes
Active infections
Adult: PO 50-100 mg qid after meals or 50-100 mg at bedtime for long-term treatment
Child: PO 5-7 mg/kg/day in 4 divided doses; 1-2 mg/kg/day for long-term treatment; max 7 mg/kg/day

Chronic suppression
Adult: PO 50-100 mg qPM
Child: PO 2 mg/kg/day qPM or 0.5-1 mg/kg q12hr if dose is not well tolerated

Available forms: Caps 25, 50, 100 mg; tabs 50, 100 mg; susp 25 mg/ml; macrocrystal caps (Macrodantin) 25, 50, 100 mg; cap (Macrobid) 100 mg (25 macrocrystals, 75 monohydrate)

Adverse effects
CNS: **Dizziness, headache,** drowsiness, peripheral neuropathy, chills, confusion, vertigo
CV: **Bundle branch block,** chest pain
GI: **Nausea, vomiting, abdominal pain, diarrhea, cholestatic jaundice,** loss of appetite, **pseudomembranous colitis, hepatitis,** pancreatitis
HEMA: **Anemia, agranulocytosis, hemolytic anemia, leukopenia, thrombocytopenia**

INTEG: Pruritus, rash, urticaria, **angioedema,** alopecia, tooth staining, **exfoliative dermatitis**
MS: Arthralgia, myalgia, numbness, peripheral neuropathy
RESP: Cough, dyspnea, pneumonitis, pulmonary fibrosis/infiltrate
SYST: **Stevens-Johnson syndrome, superinfection,** SLE-like syndrome

Contraindications: Infants <1 mo, hypersensitivity, anuria, severe renal disease, CCr <60 ml/min

Precautions: Pregnancy **B,** breastfeeding, geriatric, G6PD deficiency, GI disease, diabetes, cholestatic jaundice due to nitrofurantoin therapy

Pharmacokinetics
Absorption	Readily
Distribution	Crosses placenta, excreted in breast milk
Metabolism	Liver, partially
Excretion	Kidneys, 30%-50% unchanged
Half-life	20-60 min

Pharmacodynamics
Onset	Unknown
Peak	30 min
Duration	6-12 hr

Interactions
Individual products
Magnesium trisilicate: decreased absorption
Norfloxacin: antagonist effect
Probenecid: increased nitrofurantoin levels
Drug/herb
Acidophilus: do not use with antiinfectives; separate by several hours
Drug/lab test
Increased: BUN, alkaline phosphatase, bilirubin, creatinine, blood glucose

NURSING CONSIDERATIONS
Assessment
- Monitor blood count during chronic therapy
- Monitor I/O ratio: C&S before treatment, after completion; symptoms of UTI
- Assess CNS symptoms: insomnia, vertigo, headache, drowsiness, seizures
- Assess allergy: fever, flushing, rash, urticaria, pruritus

Nursing diagnoses
- Infection, risk for (uses)
- Knowledge, deficient (teaching)

N

Adverse effects: *italic* = common, **bold** = life-threatening

Implementation
• Do not break, crush, chew, or open tabs, caps
• Give after clean-catch urine for C&S
• Give two daily doses if urine output is high or if patient has diabetes

Patient/family education
• Teach patient to take with food or milk; avoid alcohol
• Teach patient to protect susp from freezing and shake well before taking
• Teach patient that product may cause drowsiness; instruct client to seek aid in walking and other activities; advise patient not to drive or operate machinery while on medication
• Teach patient that diabetics should monitor blood glucose level
• Teach patient that product may turn urine rust-yellow to brown
◆ Teach patient to notify prescriber of symptoms of pseudomembranous colitis: fever, diarrhea with mucous, pus, or blood

Evaluation
Positive therapeutic outcome
• Decreased dysuria, fever; negative C&S

---

nitrofurazone topical
See Appendix B

---

nitroglycerin 💿 (Rx)
(nye-troe-gli'ser-in)
transmucosal tablets (Rx)
Nitrogard, Nitrogard SR ✦
extended release caps (Rx)
Nitroglyn E-R, Nitro-par, Nitro-Time
extended release buccal tabs (Rx)
Nitrogard, Nitrogard SR ✦
intravenous (Rx)
Nitro-Bid IV, Tridil
spray (Rx)
Nitrolingual Translingual Spray
sublingual (Rx)
Nitrostat, NitroQuick
topical ointment (Rx)
Nitro-Bid, Nitrol
transdermal (Rx)
Deponit, Minitran, Nitrek, Nitrocine, Nitrodisc, Nitro-Dur, Transderm-Nitro
Func. class.: Coronary vasodilator, antianginal
Chem. class.: Nitrate

Pregnancy category C

Do not confuse:
Nitro-Bid/Nicobid

Action: Decreases preload and afterload, which thus decreases left ventricular end-diastolic pressure and systemic vascular resistance; dilates coronary arteries and improves blood flow through coronary vasculature, dilates arterial, venous beds systemically

Therapeutic outcome: Prevention of anginal attack

Uses: Chronic stable angina pectoris, prophylaxis of angina pain, CHF associated with acute MI, controlled hypotension in surgical procedures

Dosage and routes
Adult: SL dissolve tab under tongue when pain begins; may repeat q5min until relief occurs; take no more than 3 tab/15 min; use 1 tab prophylactically 5-10 min before activities; SUS REL cap q6-12hr on empty stomach; TOP 1-2 in q8hr; increase to 4 in q4hr as needed; **IV** 5 mcg/min, then increase by 5 mcg/min q3-5min; if no response after 20 mcg/min, increase by 10-20 mcg/min until desired response; transdermal apply a pad daily to a site free from hair; remove patch at bedtime to

---

provide 10-12 hr nitrate-free interval to avoid tolerance; BUCCAL 1 mg q5hr

Child: **IV** initial 0.25-0.5 mcg/kg/min, titrate to patient response, usual dose 1-3 mcg/kg/min transmucosal

Available forms: Buccal tabs 1, 2, 3 mg; translingual aerosol 0.4 mg/m spray; sus rel caps 2.5, 6.5, 9, 13 mg; sus rel tabs 2.6, 6.5, 9 mg; SL tabs 0.3, 0.4, 0.6 mg; oint 2%; trans syst 0.1, 0.2, 0.3, 0.4, 0.6, 0.8 mg/hr; inj 25 mg/250 ml, 50 mg/250 ml, 100 mg/250 ml, 50 mg/500 ml, 100 mg/500 ml, 200 mg/500 ml

Adverse effects
CNS: Headache, flushing, dizziness
CV: Postural hypotension, tachycardia, **collapse,** syncope, palpitations
GI: Nausea, vomiting
INTEG: Pallor, sweating, rash

Contraindications: Hypersensitivity to this product or nitrites, severe anemia, increased ICP, cerebral hemorrhage, closed-angle glaucoma

Precautions: Pregnancy **C,** breastfeeding, children, postural hypotension, severe renal/hepatic disease

Pharmacokinetics
Absorption	Well absorbed (PO, buccal, SL)
Distribution	Unknown
Metabolism	Liver, extensively
Excretion	Kidney
Half-life	1-4 min

Interactions
Individual drugs
Alcohol: increased hypotension, CV collapse
Aspirin: increased nitrate level
Heparin: decreased effects (with IV nitroglycerin)
Sildenafil, tadalafil, vardenafil: increased hypotension
Drug classifications
Antihypertensives, β-adrenergic blockers, calcium channel blockers, diuretics: increased hypotension
Drug/lab test
Increased: urine catecholamine, urine VMA
False increase: cholesterol

NURSING CONSIDERATIONS
Assessment
● Monitor orthostatic B/P, pulse
● Assess pain: duration, time started, activity being performed, character; check for tolerance if taken over long period
● Monitor for headache, light-headedness, decreased B/P; may indicate a need for decreased dosage

Nursing diagnoses
● Cardiac output, decreased (uses)
● Knowledge, deficient (teaching)
● Noncompliance (teaching)
● Poisoning, risk for (uses)
● Tissue perfusion, ineffective (uses)

Implementation
PO route
● Swallow sus rel tabs whole; do not break, crush, or chew sus rel tabs
● Give 1 hr before or 2 hr after meals with 8 oz of water
Transmucosal route
● Tab should be placed between cheek and gum line
● Do not take anything PO when tab is in place
Topical route
● Apply ointment using dose-measuring papers supplied; apply to an area without hair; ointment should cover 2-3-In area; may apply an occlusive dressing as directed
Transdermal route
● Apply transdermal patches to area without hair; press hard to adhere; if patch becomes dislodged, apply a new one
SL route
● Keep tab in original container
● If 3 SL tab in 15 min do not relieve pain, consider diagnosis of MI
● SL tab should be held under tongue until dissolved (a few min); do not take anything by mouth when SL tab is in place
IV route
● Give **IV** diluted in amount specified D₅W, or 0.9% NaCl for inf; use glass inf bottles, non–polyvinyl chloride inf tubing; titrate to patient response; do not use filters
Y-site compatibilities: Amiodarone, amphotericin B cholesteryl, atracurium,

N

Pharmacodynamics
	SUS REL	SL	TD	IV	TRANSMU-COSAL	AEROSOL	TOPICAL OINT
Onset	20-45 min	1-3 min	½-1 hr	1-2 min	1-2 min	2 min	½-1 hr
Peak	Unknown	Unknown	Unknown	Unknown	Unknown	Unknown	Unknown
Duration	3-8 hr	½ hr	12-24 hr	3-5 min	3-5 hr	½-1 hr	2-12 hr

Adverse effects: *italic* = common, **bold** = life-threatening

cefmetazole, cisatracurium, diltiazem, DO-BUTamine, DOPamine, epinephrine, esmolol, famotidine, fentanyl, fluconazole, furosemide, haloperidol, heparin, hydromorphone, inamrinone, regular insulin, labetalol, lidocaine, lorazepam, midazolam, milrinone, morphine, niCARdipine, nitroprusside, norepinephrine, pancuronium, ranitidine, remifentanil, streptokinase, tacrolimus, theophylline, vecuronium
Y-site incompatibilities: Alteplase
Additive compatibilities: Alteplase, aminophylline, DOBUTamine, DOPamine, enalaprilat, furosemide, lidocaine, verapamil
Additive incompatibilities: Manufacturer recommends that nitroglycerin not be admixed with other medications

Patient/family education
• Instruct patient to avoid alcohol
• Advise patient that product may cause headache; tolerance usually develops; use nonopioid analgesic
• Teach patient that product may be taken before stressful activity, exercise, sexual activity
• Inform patient that SL tab may sting when product comes in contact with mucous membranes
• Caution patient to avoid hazardous activities if dizziness occurs
• Instruct patient to comply with complete medical regimen
• Advise patient to make position changes slowly to prevent fainting

Evaluation
Positive therapeutic outcome
• Decreased, prevention of anginal pain

! HIGH ALERT

nitroprusside (Rx)
(nye-troe-pruss′ide)
Nitropress, Sodium nitroprusside
Func. class.: Antihypertensive, vasodilator
Pregnancy category C

Action: Directly relaxes arteriolar, venous smooth muscle, resulting in reduction in cardiac preload, afterload

Therapeutic outcome: Decreased B/P in hypertensive crisis, decreased preload, afterload

Uses: Hypertensive crisis, to decrease bleeding by creating hypotension during surgery, acute CHF

Dosage and routes
Adult and child: **IV** INF 0.25-1.0 mcg/kg/min; max 10 mcg/kg/min

Available forms: Inj 50 mg

Adverse effects
CNS: Dizziness, headache, agitation, twitching, decreased reflexes, restlessness
CV: Bradycardia, ECG changes, tachycardia, hypotension
GI: Nausea, vomiting, abdominal pain
INTEG: Pain, irritation at inj site, sweating
MISC: **Cyanide, thiocyanate toxicity,** flushing, hypothyroidism

Contraindications: Hypersensitivity, hypertension (compensatory) due to aortic coarctation or AV shunting, acute CHF associated with reduced peripheral vascular resistance, AV shunt, Leber's disease, toxic amblyopia

Black Box Warning: Cyanide toxicity

Precautions: Pregnancy C, breastfeeding, children, geriatric, fluid, electrolyte imbalances, renal/hepatic disease, hypothyroidism

Black Box Warning: Hypotension

Pharmacokinetics	
Absorption	Complete bioavailability
Distribution	Not known
Metabolism	RBCs, tissues
Excretion	Kidneys
Half-life	3 days; circulating half-life 2 min

Pharmacodynamics	
Onset	1-2 min
Peak	Rapid
Duration	1-10 min

Interactions
Individual drugs
Enflurane, halothane; severe hypotension
Drug classifications
Circulatory depressants, ganglionic blockers, volatile liquid anesthetics: severe hypotension
Drug/herb
Aconite: increased toxicity, death
Astragalus, cola tree: increased or decreased antihypertensive effect
Barberry, betony, black catechu, black cohosh, bloodroot, broom, burdock, cat's claw, dandelion, goldenseal, Irish moss, Jamaican dogwood, kelp, khella, mistletoe, parsley: increased antihypertensive effect
Coltsfoot, guarana, khat, licorice: decreased antihypertensive effect

---

NURSING CONSIDERATIONS
Assessment
- Monitor B/P q5min × 2 hr, then qhr × 2 hr; monitor pulse q4hr; monitor jugular venous distention q4hr; ECG should be monitored continuously; monitor PCWP; rebound hypertension may occur after nitroprusside is discontinued
- Monitor electrolytes, blood studies: potassium, sodium, chloride, CO_2, CBC, serum glucose, serum methemoglobin if pulmonary oxygen levels are decreased
- Check weight, I&O, edema in feet and legs daily; assess skin turgor, dryness of mucous membranes for hydration status
- Assess for signs of CHF: dyspnea, edema, wet crackles
- ◊ Monitor for increased lactate, cyanide, thiocyanate levels if on long-term treatment; thiocyanate level should be ≤1 millimole/L
- Monitor for decrease in bicarbonate, Pco_2, and blood pH; acidosis may occur with this product

Nursing diagnoses
- Injury, risk for (adverse reactions)
- Knowledge, deficient (teaching)
- Tissue perfusion, ineffective (uses)

Implementation
- Give by cont inf after diluting 50 mg/2-3 ml of D_5W; further dilute in 250 ml of D_5W; use an inf pump only; wrap bottle with aluminum foil to protect from light; observe for color change in inf; discard if highly discolored (blue, green, red); titrate to patient response; avoid extravasation

Syringe compatibilities: Heparin
Y-site compatibilities: Atracurium, diltiazem, DOBUTamine, DOPamine, enalaprilat, famotidine, inamrinone, lidocaine, nitroglycerin, pancuronium, tacrolimus, theophylline, vecuronium
Additive incompatibilities: Do not give with any other products

Patient/family education
- Teach patient to report headache, dizziness, loss of hearing, blurred vision, dyspnea, faintness; may indicate adverse reactions

Evaluation
Positive therapeutic outcome
- Decreased B/P in hypertension
- Absence of bleeding in surgery

Treatment of overdose: Administer amyl nitrate inh until 3% sodium nitrate sol can be prepared for **IV** administration, then inject sodium thiosulfate **IV**; correct drop in B/P with vasopressor

---

nizatidine (Rx, OTC)
(ni-za'ti-deen)
Axid, Axid AR
Func. class.: H_2-receptor antagonist
Chem. class.: Substituted thiazole

Pregnancy category B

Action: Blocks H_2 receptors, thereby reducing gastric acid output

Therapeutic outcome: Healing of duodenal ulcers or gastric ulcers; prevention of duodenal ulcers; decreases symptoms of gastroesophageal reflux disease (GERD)

Uses: Benign gastric and duodenal ulceration, prevention of duodenal ulcer recurrence, symptomatic relief of gastroesophageal reflux, heartburn prevention

Dosage and routes
Prophylaxis of duodenal ulcer
Adult: PO 150 mg/day at bedtime

Gastric and duodenal ulcer disease
Adult: PO 300 mg at night or 150 mg bid for 4-8 wk; maintenance 150 mg at night

Gastroesophageal reflux
Adult and child ≥12 yr: PO 150 mg bid, up to 12 wk, max 300 mg/day

Heartburn prevention
Adult: PO 75 mg before eating bid

Renal dose
Adult: PO CCr 20-50 ml/min give 150 mg every other day; CCr <20 ml/min give 150 mg q72hr

Available forms: Caps 150, 300 mg; tabs 75 mg

Adverse effects
CNS: Headache, somnolence, confusion, abnormal dreams, dizziness
CV: **Dysrhythmias, cardiac arrest**
ENDO: Gynecomastia
GI: Elevated liver enzymes, **hepatitis**, jaundice, nausea
HEMA: **Thrombocytopenia, agranulocytosis, aplastic anemia**
INTEG: Pruritus, sweating, urticaria, **exfoliative dermatitis**
META: Hyperuricemia
MS: Myalgia
RESP: **Bronchospasm, laryngeal edema, pneumonia**
Contraindications: Hypersensitivity

N

Adverse effects: *italic* = common, **bold** = life-threatening

Precautions: Pregnancy **B**, breastfeeding, renal/hepatic impairment (reduce dose in renal impairment)

Pharmacokinetics

Absorption	70%
Distribution	Breast milk, crosses placenta
Metabolism	Liver, partially
Excretion	Kidney
Half-life	1½ hr

Pharmacodynamics

Onset	Variable
Peak	½-3 hr
Duration	Unknown

Interactions
Individual drugs
Ketoconazole, itraconazole: decreased effect of each of these drugs

NURSING CONSIDERATIONS
Assessment
• Assess patient with ulcers or suspected ulcers: epigastric or abdominal pain, hematemesis, occult blood in stools, blood or gastric aspirate before, throughout treatment, monitor gastric pH (5 should be maintained)
◆ Monitor I&O ratio, BUN, creatinine, CBC with differential monthly; agranulocytosis may occur

Nursing diagnoses
• Knowledge, deficient (teaching)
• Pain, chronic (uses)

Implementation
• May be given with or without meals
• Give antacids 1 hr before or 1 hr after this product

Patient/family education
• Caution patient that gynecomastia, impotence may occur and are reversible after treatment is discontinued
• Advise patient to avoid driving, other hazardous activities until stabilized on this medication; drowsiness or dizziness may occur
• Caution patient to avoid black pepper, caffeine, alcohol, harsh spices, extremes in temperature of food; tell patient to avoid OTC preparations: aspirin, cough, cold preparations because condition may worsen
• Caution patient not to take OTC and Rx forms concurrently
• Inform patient that smoking decreases the effectiveness of the product; that smoking cessation should be considered

• Instruct patient that product must be continued for prescribed time to be effective and taken exactly as prescribed; doses should not be doubled; a missed dose should be taken as soon as remembered up to 1 hr before next dose
• Advise patient to report bruising, fatigue, malaise; blood dyscrasias may occur
• Advise patient to report diarrhea, black tarry stools, sore throat, rash, dizziness, confusion, or delirium to prescriber immediately

Evaluation
Positive therapeutic outcome
• Decreased pain in abdomen
• Healing of ulcers
• Absence of gastroesophageal reflux

norfloxacin (Rx)
(nor-flox'a-sin)
Noroxin
Func. class.: Antiinfective—urinary
Chem. class.: Fluoroquinolone antibacterial
Pregnancy category C

Action: Interferes with conversion intermediate DNA fragments into high-molecular weight DNA in bacteria; inhibits DNA gyrase

Therapeutic outcome: Bactericidal action against gram-positive methicillin-resistant strains of *Staphylococcus aureus*, group D streptococci; gram-negative *Escherichia coli, Klebsiella pneumoniae, Enterobacter cloacae, Proteus mirabilis, Citrobacter freundii*

Uses: Adult UTIs (including complicated), uncomplicated gonorrhea, prostatitis, cystitis

Dosage and routes
Uncomplicated infections
Adult: PO 400 mg bid × 3-10 days 1 hr before or 2 hr after meals

Complicated infections
Adult: PO 400 mg bid × 10-21 days; 400 mg/day × 7-10 days in impaired renal function

Uncomplicated gonorrhea
Adult: PO 800 mg as a single dose

Prostatitis
Adult: PO 400 mg bid × 6 wk

Renal dose
Adult: PO CCr ≤30 ml/min 400 mg/day

Available forms: Tabs 400 mg

Adverse effects
CNS: Headache, dizziness, fatigue, somnolence, depression, insomnia

CV: **QT prolongation,** torsades de pointes, dysrhythmias
EENT: Visual disturbances
GI: Nausea, constipation, **hepatic necrosis,** increased ALT, AST, flatulence, heartburn, vomiting, diarrhea, dry mouth, **pseudomembranous colitis**
HEMA: **Agranulocytosis**
INTEG: Rash, photosensitivity
SYST: **Stevens-Johnson syndrome, angioedema**

Contraindications: Hypersensitivity to quinolones

Black Box Warning: Tendon pain/rupture, tendonitis

Precautions: Pregnancy **C,** breastfeeding, children, renal disease, seizure disorders, acute MI, atrial fibrillation, dehydration, females, QT prolongation, pseudomembranous colitis, torsades de pointes

Pharmacokinetics
Absorption	30% (PO)
Distribution	Concentration in urinary system
Metabolism	Liver (minimal)
Excretion	Kidneys, unchanged (30%)
Half-life	3-4 hr; increased in renal disease

Pharmacodynamics
	PO
Onset	Unknown
Peak	1 hr
Duration	Unknown

Interactions
Individual drugs
Bepridil, chloroquine, clarithromycin, droperidol, erythromycin, grepafloxacin, halofantrine, haloperidol, methadone, pentamidine, probucol, sparfloxacin: increased QT prolongation
Caffeine, theophylline: possible increased levels, toxicity; do not use together
CycloSPORINE: increased serum concentrations
Nitrofurantoin: decreased effects of norfloxacin; monitor closely
Probenecid: increased norfloxacin level
Sucralfate: decreased absorption of norfloxacin, give 2 hr apart
Warfarin: increased anticoagulation
Drug classifications
Antacids, iron salts: decreased absorption of norfloxacin; give 2 hr apart
Anticoagulants (oral): increased effect of anticoagulants

β-agonists, class IA/III antidysrhythmics, local anesthetics, phenothiazines (some), tricyclics: increased QT prolongation
Drug/herb
Acidophilus: do not use with antiinfectives; separate by several hours
Drug/lab test
Increased: AST, ALT, BUN, creatinine, alkaline phosphatase

NURSING CONSIDERATIONS
Assessment
• Assess patient for previous sensitivity reaction
• Assess patient for signs and symptoms of infection including characteristics of urine, WBC >10,000/mm^3, temp; obtain baseline information before, during treatment
• Obtain C&S before beginning product therapy to identify if correct treatment has been initiated
• Assess for allergic reactions: rash, urticaria, pruritus
• Monitor blood studies: AST, ALT, BUN, creatinine, alkaline phosphatase monthly if patient is on long-term therapy
• Assess bowel pattern daily; if severe diarrhea occurs, product should be discontinued
• Assess for overgrowth of infection: perineal itching, fever, malaise, redness, pain, swelling, drainage, rash, diarrhea, change in cough, sputum

Nursing diagnoses
• Diarrhea (adverse reactions)
• Infection, risk for (uses)
• Injury, risk for (adverse reactions)
• Knowledge, deficient (teaching)
• Noncompliance (teaching)

Implementation
• Give in equal intervals q12hr around the clock to maintain proper blood levels; give with food to increase absorption of product; do not give within 3 hr of other agents; product interactions may occur; give with 8 oz of water
• Do not give with iron, zinc products, or antacids, which decrease absorption

Patient/family education
• Instruct patient to take all medication prescribed for the length of time ordered; product must be taken at same time of day to maintain blood levels; do not give medication to others; do not double doses; take any missed dose when remembered
• Advise patient to increase fluids to 2 L/day to prevent crystalluria

Adverse effects: *italic* = common, **bold** = life-threatening

- Caution patient to avoid driving and other hazardous activities until response is known; dizziness may occur
- Instruct patient to use sunglasses to prevent photophobia
- Have patient use hard candy, frequent sips of water for dry mouth
- Teach patient correct instillation procedure (ophth)

Evaluation
Positive therapeutic outcome
- Reported improvement in symptoms of infection
- Absence of red or itching eyes (ophth)

norfloxacin ophthalmic
See Appendix B

nortriptyline (Rx)
(nor-trip′ti-leen)
Pamelor
Func. class.: Antidepressant, tricyclic
Chem. class.: Dibenzocycloheptene, secondary amine
Pregnancy category D

Do not confuse:
nortriptyline/amitriptyline

Action: Blocks reuptake of norepinephrine, serotonin into nerve endings, increasing action of norepinephrine, serotonin in nerve cells; has anticholinergic effects

Therapeutic outcome: Decreased symptoms of depression after 2-3 wk

Uses: Major depression

Unlabeled uses: Chronic pain management

Dosage and routes
Adult: PO 25 mg tid or qid; may increase to 150 mg/day; may give daily dose at bedtime
Adolescent: PO 1-3 mg/kg/day in 3-4 divided doses or qd at bedtime; max 150 mg/day
Geriatric: PO 10-25 mg nightly, increase by 10-25 mg at weekly intervals to desired dose; usual maintenance 75 mg/day

Available forms: Caps 10, 25, 50, 75 mg; sol 10 mg/5 ml

Adverse effects
CNS: Dizziness, drowsiness, confusion, headache, anxiety, tremors, stimulation, weakness, insomnia, nightmares, EPS (geriatric), increased psychiatric symptoms, **seizures**
CV: Orthostatic hypotension, ECG changes, tachycardia, **hypertension,** palpitations, **dysrhythmias**
EENT: Blurred vision, tinnitus, mydriasis
GI: Constipation, dry mouth, nausea, vomiting, **paralytic ileus,** increased appetite, cramps, epigastric distress, jaundice, **hepatitis,** stomatitis
GU: Retention, **acute renal failure**
HEMA: **Agranulocytosis, thrombocytopenia, eosinophilia, leukopenia**
INTEG: Rash, urticaria, sweating, pruritus, photosensitivity

Contraindications: Pregnancy **D,** hypersensitivity to tricyclics, recovery phase of MI, seizure disorders, prostatic hypertrophy

Precautions: Breastfeeding, suicidal patients, severe depression, increased intraocular pressure, closed-angle glaucoma, urinary retention, cardiac/hepatic disease, hyperthyroidism, electroshock therapy, elective surgery

Black Box Warning: Children, suicidal ideation

Pharmacokinetics
Absorption	Well absorbed
Distribution	Widely distributed; crosses placenta
Metabolism	Liver, extensively
Excretion	Kidneys, breast milk
Half-life	18-28 hr; steady state 4-19 days

Pharmacodynamics
Unknown

Interactions
Individual drugs
Alcohol: increased CNS depression
Clonidine, guanethidine: decreased effects
Smoking (heavy): decreased product effect
Drug classifications
Barbiturates, benzodiazepines, CNS depressants: increased effects
MAOIs: hypertensive episode, hyperpyretic crisis, seizures
Sympathomimetics (direct-acting), products increasing QT interval: increased effects
Sympathomimetics (indirect-acting): decreased effects
Drug/herb
Belladonna, corkwood, henbane, jimsonweed: increased anticholinergic effect
Hops, lavender: increased CNS effect
SAM-e, St. John's wort: serotonin syndrome
Scopolia: increased antidepressant action

Drug/lab test
Increased: serum bilirubin, blood glucose, alkaline phosphatase
Decreased: VMA, 5-HIAA
False increase: urinary catecholamines

NURSING CONSIDERATIONS
Assessment
• Monitor B/P (with patient lying, standing), pulse q4hr; if systolic B/P drops 20 mm Hg, hold product, notify prescriber; take VS q4hr of patients with CV disease
• Monitor blood studies: CBC, leukocytes, differential, cardiac enzymes if patient is receiving long-term therapy
• Monitor liver function tests: AST, ALT, bilirubin
• Check weight weekly; appetite may increase with product
• Assess ECG for flattening of T-wave, bundle branch block, AV block, dysrhythmias in cardiac patients
• Assess for EPS primarily in geriatric: rigidity, dystonia, akathisia
• Assess mental status: mood, sensorium, affect, suicidal tendencies; increase in psychiatric symptoms: depression, panic
• Monitor urinary retention, constipation; constipation is more likely to occur in children or geriatric
◆ Assess for withdrawal symptoms: headache, nausea, vomiting, muscle pain, weakness; do not usually occur unless product was discontinued abruptly
• Identify alcohol consumption; if alcohol is consumed, hold dose until AM

Nursing diagnoses
• Coping, ineffective (uses)
• Injury, risk for (adverse reactions)
• Knowledge, deficient (teaching)
• Noncompliance (teaching)

Implementation
• Give with food or milk to decrease GI symptoms; mix conc with water, milk, fruit juice to disguise taste
• Give dose at bedtime if oversedation occurs during day; may take entire dose at bedtime; geriatric may not tolerate once/day dosing
• Store at room temperature; do not freeze

Patient/family education
• Teach patient that therapeutic effects may take 2-3 wk
• Teach patient to use caution in driving and other activities requiring alertness because of drowsiness, dizziness, blurred vision; to avoid rising quickly from sitting to standing, especially geriatric
• Teach patient to avoid alcohol ingestion, MAOIs within 14 days, other CNS depressants; teach patient not to discontinue medication quickly after long-term use; may cause nausea, headache, malaise
• Teach patient to wear sunscreen or large hat to avoid burns, because photosensitivity occurs
• Teach patient to increase fluids, bulk in diet if constipation, urinary retention occur, especially geriatric, worsening depression, suicidal thoughts/behavior
• Teach patient to take gum, hard sugarless candy, or frequent sips of water for dry mouth

Evaluation
Positive therapeutic outcome
• Decrease in depression
• Absence of suicidal thoughts

Treatment of overdose: ECG monitoring, lavage, activated charcoal, administer anticonvulsant

nystatin (Rx, OTC)
(nis′ta-tin)
Bio-Statin, Mycostatin, Nadostine ✦, Nilstat, nystatin, Nystex, Pastilles, PMS-Nystatin ✦; topical: Mycostatin, Nadostine ✦, Nyaderm ✦, Nystex vaginal
Func. class.: Antiinfective
Chem. class.: Antifungal
Pregnancy category B

Action: Interferes with fungal DNA replication; binds sterols in fungal cell membrane, which increases permeability, resulting in leaking of cell nutrients

Therapeutic outcome: Fungistatic/fungicidal against *Candida* organisms

Uses: *Candida* species causing oral, vaginal, intestinal infections; vaginal: cutaneous vulvovaginal candidiasis; topical: mucocutaneous fungal infections, infant eczema, pruritus ani and vulvae

Dosage and routes
Oral infection
Adult: Susp 400,000-600,000 units qid, use ½ dose in each side of mouth, swish and swallow
Infant: 200,000 units qid (100,000 units in each side of mouth)
Newborn and premature infant: SUSP 100,000 units qid
Adult and child: Troches 200,000-400,000 units qid × up to 2 wk

GI infection
Adult: PO 500,000-1,000,000 units tid

Available forms: Tabs 500,000 units; powder 50, 150, 500 million, 1, 2, 5 billion units; troches 200,000 units; susp 100,000 units/ml; oral caps 500,000, 1,000,000 units

Adverse effects
GI: Nausea, vomiting, anorexia, diarrhea, cramps
INTEG: Rash, urticaria (rare)

Contraindication: Hypersensitivity

Precautions: Pregnancy **B**

Pharmacokinetics
Absorption	Poorly absorbed
Distribution	Unknown
Metabolism	Not metabolized
Excretion	Feces, unchanged
Half-life	Unknown

Pharmacodynamics
Onset	Rapid
Peak	Unknown
Duration	6-12 hr

NURSING CONSIDERATIONS
Assessment
• Assess for allergic reaction: rash, urticaria; product may have to be discontinued
• Assess for predisposing factors for candidal infection: antibiotic therapy, pregnancy, diabetes mellitus, sexual partner infection (vag infections), AIDS

Nursing diagnoses
• Infection, risk for (uses)
• Knowledge, deficient (teaching)
• Skin integrity, impaired (uses)

Implementation
PO route
• Give oral susp dose by placing ½ in each cheek, swish for several min, then swallow; shake susp before use
• Store oral susp in refrigerator, tab in airtight, light-resistant containers at room temperature
Topical route
• Administer by moistening lesions with a swab coated with cream or ointment; use enough medication to cover lesions completely; give after cleansing with soap, water before each application; dry well
Vaginal route
• Insert vag tab high into vagina with applicator provided; administer in gravid client 3-6 wk before term to decrease candidiasis in the newborn
• Store at room temperature in dry place; protect from light, air, heat

Patient/family education
• Instruct patient that long-term therapy may be needed to clear infection; to complete entire course of medication
• Teach patient proper hygiene: use no commercial mouthwashes for mouth infection
• Advise patient to avoid getting preparation on hands
• Instruct patient to wear light-day pad for vag preparations to avoid soiling clothing; to avoid sexual contact during treatment to minimize reinfection
• Instruct patient to notify prescriber if irritation occurs; product may have to be discontinued
• Inform patient that relief from itching may occur after 24-72 hr
Topical route
• Advise patient to discontinue use and notify prescriber if irritation occurs
• Teach patient to apply with glove to prevent further infection; product may stain
• Caution patient not to use occlusive dressings; to avoid use of OTC creams, ointments, lotions unless directed by prescriber

Evaluation
Positive therapeutic outcome
• Culture negative for *Candida*
• Decrease in size, number of lesions
• Decreased itching, white patches on vulva (vaginal)

---

nystatin topical
See Appendix B

---

nystatin vaginal antifungal
See Appendix B

---

octreotide (Rx)
(ok-tree'-o-tide)
Sandostatin, Sandostatin LAR Depot
Func. class.: Hormone, antidiarrheal
Chem. class.: Octapeptide

Pregnancy category B

Action: Action similar to somatostatin

Therapeutic outcome: Decreased diarrhea; decreased symptoms of acromegaly,

---

carcinoid tumors, vasoactive intestinal peptide tumors (VIPomas)

Uses: Sandostatin: acromegaly, carcinoid tumors, VIPomas; LAR Depot: long-term maintenance of acromegaly, carcinoid tumors, VIPomas

Unlabeled uses: GI fistula, variceal bleeding, diarrheal conditions, pancreatic fistula, IBS, dumping syndrome

Dosage and routes
Acromegaly
Adult: SUBCUT/**IV** 50-100 mcg bid-tid, adjust q2wk based on growth hormone levels (Sandostatin) or IM 20 mg q4wk × 3 mo, adjust by growth hormone levels (Sandostatin LAR)

VIPomas
Adult: SUBCUT/**IV** 200-300 mcg/day in 2-4 doses for 2 wk, max 450 mcg/day; (Sandostatin) or IM 20 mg q2wk × 2 mo, adjust dose (Sandostatin LAR)

Carcinoid tumors
Adult: SUBCUT/**IV** 100-600 mcg/day in 2-4 doses for 2 wk, titrated to patient response (Sandostatin) or IM 20 mg q4wk × 2 mo, adjust dose (Sandostatin LAR)

GI fistula
Adult: SUBCUT 50-200 mcg q8hr

Antidiarrheal in AIDS patients (unlabeled)
Adult: SUBCUT 50 mcg q8h PRN, increase to 500 mcg q8h

Irritable bowel syndrome (unlabeled)
Adult: SUBCUT 100 mcg single dose to 125 mcg bid

Dumping syndrome (unlabeled)
Adult: SUBCUT 50-150 mcg/day

Variceal bleeding (unlabeled)
Adult: **IV** 25-50 mcg/hr CONT **IV** INF for 18 hr-5 days

Available forms: Sandostatin: inj 0.05, 0.1, 0.2, 0.5, 1 mg/ml; LAR Depot: inj 10 mg, 20, 30 mg/5 ml

Adverse effects
CNS: Headache, dizziness, fatigue, weakness, depression, anxiety, tremors, **seizures,** paranoia
CV: Sinus bradycardia, conduction abnormalities, **dysrhythmias,** chest pain, shortness of breath, thrombophlebitis, ischemia, **CHF,** hypertension, palpitations, **QT prolongation, ST-T wave changes**
ENDO: Hypo/hyperglycemia, ketosis, hypothyroidism, galactorrhea, diabetes insipidus

GI: Diarrhea, nausea, abdominal pain, vomiting, flatulence, distension, constipation, **hepatitis,** elevated liver function tests, **GI bleeding, pancreatitis,** cholelithiasis, ileus
GU: UTI
HEMA: Hematoma of inj site, bruise
INTEG: Rash, urticaria, pain, inflammation at inj site
MS: Joint and muscle pain

Contraindications: Hypersensitivity

Precautions: Pregnancy **B,** breastfeeding, children, geriatric, diabetes mellitus, hypothyroidism, renal disease

Pharmacokinetics
Absorption	Rapidly, completely
Distribution	Unknown
Metabolism	Little
Excretion	Urine, unchanged
Half-life	1.7 hr

Pharmacodynamics
Onset	Unknown
Peak	½ hr
Duration	12 hr

Interactions
Individual drugs
Other products that prolong QT: increased QT prolongation
CycloSPORINE: decreased effect of cycloSPORINE
Drug/food
Decreased: absorption of dietary fat, vit B_{12} levels
Drug/lab test
Decreased: T_4

NURSING CONSIDERATIONS
Assessment
• Identify growth hormone antibodies, IGF-1, 1-4 hr intervals for 8-12 hr after dose in acromegaly; 5-HIAA; blood glucose, serotonin levels (carcinoid tumors), plasma substance P, plasma vasoactive intestinal peptide (VIP) (VIPomas)
• Monitor for fecal fat, serum carotene
• Monitor thyroid function tests: T_3, T_4, T_7, TSH to identify hypothyroidism
• Assess for allergic reaction: rash, itching, fever, nausea, wheezing
• Assess for cardiac status: bradycardia, conduction abnormalities, dysrhythmias; monitor ECG for QT prolongation, low voltage, axis shifts, early repolarization, R/S transition, early wave progression

Adverse effects: *italic* = common, **bold** = life-threatening

Nursing diagnoses
• Body image, disturbed (uses)
• Knowledge, deficient (teaching)

Implementation
• Store unopened amps, vials in refrigerator; or room temperature for 2 wk, protect from light; do not use discolored or cloudy sol

SUBCUT route
• Rotate inj sites, use hip, thigh, abdomen
• Avoid using medication that is cold; allow to reach room temperature

IM route
• Reconstitute with diluent provided; inj into gluteal muscle

IV route
• May use **IV** bolus if required; give over 3 min
• To use by intermittent inf, dilute in 50-200 ml D₅W, 0.9% NaCl, give over 15-30 min
• In an emergency carcinoid crisis, give rapid bolus

Patient/family education
• Explain reason for medication and expected results
• Advise patient that routine follow-up is needed
• Instruct parents on procedure for medication preparation and inj use; request demonstration, return demonstration; provide written instructions
• Advise patient to change position slowly to prevent orthostatic hypotension

Evaluation
Positive therapeutic outcome
• Decreased symptoms of acromegaly, carcinoid, VIPoma
• Decreased diarrhea in AIDS

---

ofloxacin (Rx)
(o-flox'a-sin)
Func. class.: Antiinfective
Chem. class.: Fluoroquinolone

Pregnancy category C

Action: Interferes with conversion of intermediate DNA fragments into high molecular weight DNA in bacteria, inhibits DNA gyrase

Therapeutic outcome: Bactericidal action against gram-positive pathogens *Staphylococcus epidermidis,* methicillin-resistant strains of *Staphylococcus aureus, Streptococcus pyogenes, Streptococcus pneumoniae;* gram-negative pathogens *Escherichia coli, Klebsiella* species, *Enterobacter, Salmonella,*

Shigella, Proteus vulgaris, Proteus rettgeri, Providencia stuartii, Morganella morganii, Pseudomonas aeruginosa, Serratia, Haemophilus species, *Acinetobacter, Neisseria gonorrhoeae, Neisseria meningitidis, Yersinia, Vibrio, Brucella, Campylobacter,* and *Aeromonas* species; anaerobic pathogens *Bacteroides fragilis intermedius, Clostridium perfringens, Gardnerella vaginalis, Peptococcus niger, Peptostreptococcus* species; *Chlamydia pneumoniae, Chlamydia trachomatis, Legionella pneumoniae, Mycobacterium tuberculosis, Mycoplasma pneumoniae*

Uses: Treatment of lower respiratory tract infections (pneumonia, bronchitis), genitourinary infections (prostatitis, UTIs), skin and skin structure infections, conjunctivitis (ophth)

Dosage and routes
Lower respiratory tract infection/ skin and skin structure infections
Adult: PO/**IV** 400 mg q12hr × 10 days

Cervicitis, urethritis
Adult: PO/**IV** 300 mg q12hr × 7 days

Prostatitis
Adult: PO 300 mg q12hr × 6 wk

Urinary tract infection
Adult: PO/**IV** 200 mg q12hr × 3-10 days

Pelvic inflammatory disease
Adult: PO 400 mg q12hr × 10-14 days

Renal dose
Adult: PO CCr 20-50 ml/min give q24hr; CCr <20 ml/min give ½ of dose q24hr

Available forms: Tabs 200, 300, 400 mg; inj 20, 40 mg/ml, 200 mg/50 ml, 400 mg/100 ml

Adverse effects
CNS: Dizziness, headache, fatigue, somnolence, depression, insomnia, lethargy, malaise, **seizures,** vertigo
CV: **QT prolongation, dysrhythmias,** chest pain
EENT: Visual disturbances
GI: Diarrhea, nausea, vomiting, anorexia, flatulence, heartburn, dry mouth, increased AST, ALT, abdominal pain, constipation, **pseudomembranous colitis,** abnormal taste
HEMA: **Blood dyscrasias**
INTEG: Rash, pruritus, photosensitivity
SYST: **Anaphylaxis, Stevens-Johnson syndrome, toxic epidermal necrosis**

Contraindication: Hypersensitivity to quinolones, QT prolongation

---

 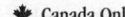

Precautions: Pregnancy C, breastfeeding, children, geriatric, renal disease, seizure disorders, excessive sunlight, hypokalemia
Black Box Warning: Tendon pain/rupture, tendonitis

Pharmacokinetics

Absorption	Well absorbed (PO)
Distribution	Widely distributed
Metabolism	Unknown
Excretion	Kidneys, unchanged; breast milk
Half-life	5-9 hr; increased in renal disease

Pharmacodynamics

	PO	IV	OPHTH
Onset	Rapid	Rapid	Unknown
Peak	1-2 hr	Inf end	Unknown
Duration	Unknown	Unknown	Unknown

Interactions
Individual drugs
Bepridil, chloroquine, clarithromycin, droperidol, erythromycin, grepafloxacin, halofantrine, haloperidol, methadone, pentamidine, probucol, sparfloxacin: increased QT prolongation
Sucralfate, zinc sulfate: decreased absorption of ofloxacin, separate by 2 hr
Theophylline: increased toxicity, do not use together
Warfarin: increased anticoagulation
Drug classifications
Antacids with aluminum, iron salts, magnesium: decreased absorption of ofloxacin, separate by 2 hr
Antidiabetics: altered blood glucose levels
β-agonists, class IA/III antidysrhythmics, local anesthetics, some phenothiazines, tricyclics: increased QT prolongation
NSAIDs: increased CNS stimulation, seizures
Drug/herb
Acidophilus: do not use with antiinfectives; separate by several hours
Cola nut: increased effect

NURSING CONSIDERATIONS
Assessment
- Assess patient for previous sensitivity reaction
- Assess patient for signs and symptoms of infection including characteristics of wounds, sputum, urine, stool, WBC >10,000/mm³, fever; obtain baselines and monitor during treatment
- Obtain C&S before beginning product therapy to identify if correct treatment has been initiated
- Assess for allergic reactions: rash, urticaria, pruritus
- Monitor blood studies: AST, ALT, CBC, serum glucose monthly if patient is on long-term therapy
- Assess bowel pattern daily; if severe diarrhea occurs, product should be discontinued
- Assess for overgrowth of infection: perineal itching, fever, malaise, redness, pain, swelling, drainage, rash, diarrhea, change in cough, sputum
- Assess for CNS symptoms: seizures, vertigo, drowsiness, agitation, confusion, tremors

Nursing diagnoses
- Diarrhea (adverse reactions)
- Infection, risk for (uses)
- Injury, risk for (adverse reactions)
- Knowledge, deficient (teaching)
- Noncompliance (teaching)

Implementation
PO route
- Give in equal intervals q12hr around the clock to maintain proper blood levels; do not give within 2 hr of other agents, since product interactions are possible; give with 8 oz of water
- Do not give with iron, aluminum, zinc products or antacids, which decrease absorption and form insoluble chelate
IV route
- For intermittent inf, dilute to 4 mg/ml with D₅W, D₅/0.9% NaCl, 0.9% NaCl, D₅/LR, sodium bicarbonate, sodium lactate, D₅/Plasmalyte 56; give over 1 hr or more
- Store for 2 wk refrigerated or 6 mo frozen, after reconstitution
Syringe compatibilities: Cefotaxime
Y-site compatibilities: Ampicillin, cisatracurium, docetaxel, etoposide, gemcitabine, granisetron, linezolid, propofol, remifentanil, thiotepa
Additive compatibilities: Amoxicillin, ceftazidime, clindamycin, gentamicin, piperacillin, tobramycin, vancomycin

Patient/family education
- Instruct patient to take all medication prescribed for the length of time ordered; product must be taken around the clock to maintain blood levels; do not give medication to others
- Teach patient to use sunscreen when outdoors to decrease phototoxicity
- Advise patient to increase fluids to 2 L/day to prevent crystalluria
- Caution patient to avoid driving and other hazardous activities until response is known; dizziness, confusion, drowsiness may occur

O

Adverse effects: *italic* = common, **bold** = life-threatening

Evaluation
Positive therapeutic outcome
- Absence of signs/symptoms of infection
- Reported improvement in symptoms of infection
- Absence of red or itching eyes (ophth)

ofloxacin ophthalmic
See Appendix B

olanzapine (Rx)
(oh-lanz'a-peen)
Zydis, Zyprexa, Zyprexa Intramuscular
Func. class.: Antipsychotic/neuroleptic
Chem. class.: Thienobenzodiazepine

Pregnancy category C

Do not confuse:
olanzapine/osalazine, zyprexa/Celexa/zyrtec

Action: Unknown; may mediate antipsychotic activity by both dopamine and serotonin type 2 (5-HT$_2$) antagonism; also, may antagonize muscarinic receptors, histaminic (H$_1$)- and α-adrenergic receptors

Therapeutic outcome: Decreased psychotic symptoms

Uses: Schizophrenia, acute manic episodes in bipolar disorder

Unlabeled uses: Dementia related to Alzheimer's disease, OCD

Dosage and routes
Schizophrenia
Adult: PO 5-10 mg/day initially, may increase dosage by 5 mg at 1 wk or more intervals; orally disintegrating tabs open blister pack, place tab on tongue, let disintegrate, swallow; max 20 mg/day
Geriatric: PO 5 mg, may increase cautiously at 1 wk intervals, max 20 mg/day

Bipolar mania
Adult: PO 10-15 mg/day, may increase dose after 24 hr by 5 mg

Agitation associated with schizophrenia, bipolar I mania
Adult: IM 10 mg

Available forms: Tabs 2.5, 5, 7.5, 10, 15, 20 mg; orally disintegrating tabs 5, 10, 15, 20 mg; powder for injection 10 mg

Adverse effects
CNS: EPS (pseudoparkinsonism, akathisia, dystonia, tardive dyskinesia), **seizures,** headache, **neuroleptic malignant syn-**
drome (**rare**), agitation, nervousness, hostility, dizziness, hypertonia, tremor, euphoria, confusion, *drowsiness,* fatigue, *abnormal gait, insomnia, fever*
CV: Hypotension, tachycardia, chest pain, **heart failure, sudden death (geriatric, IM),** orthostatic hypotension
ENDO: Increased prolactin levels, hypoglycemia
GI: Dry mouth, nausea, vomiting, anorexia, constipation, abdominal pain, weight gain, appetite, dyspepsia, jaundice, **hepatitis**
GU: Urinary retention, urinary frequency, enuresis, impotence, amenorrhea, gynecomastia, breast engorgement, premenstrual syndrome
HEMA: **Neutropenia**
INTEG: Rash
MISC: Peripheral edema, accidental injury, hypertonia, hyperlipidemia
MS: Joint pain, twitching
RESP: Cough, pharyngitis, **fatal pneumonia (geriatric, IM)**

Contraindications: Hypersensitivity

Precautions: Pregnancy **C,** breastfeeding, geriatric, hypertension, cardiac/renal/hepatic disease, diabetes, agranulocytosis, abrupt discontinuation, Asian patients, closed-angle glaucoma, coma, leukopenia, QT prolongation, tardive dyskinesia, torsades de pointes

Black Box Warning: Dementia

Pharmacokinetics	
Absorption	Well
Distribution	93% plasma protein binding
Metabolism	Liver
Excretion	Kidneys
Half-life	Unknown

Pharmacodynamics	
Onset	Unknown
Peak	6 hr
Duration	Unknown

Interactions
Individual drugs
Alcohol: increased sedation, hypotension
Bromocriptine, levodopa: decreased antiparkinson activity
Carbamazepine, omeprazole, rifampin: decreased levels of olanzapine
Diazepam: increased hypotension
Fluvoxamine: increased olanzapine levels
Drug classifications
Anesthetics (barbiturates), antidepressants, antihistamines, CNS depressants, sedative/hypnotics: increased sedation

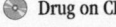

Anticholinergics: increased anticholinergic effects

Antihypertensives: increased hypotension

Dopamine agonists: decreased antiparkinson activity

Drug/herb

Betel palm, kava: increased EPS

Cola tree, hops, nettle, nutmeg: increased action

Drug/lab test

Increased: liver function tests, prolactin, CPK

NURSING CONSIDERATIONS
Assessment
- Assess mental status, orientation, mood, behavior, presence of hallucinations and type before initial administration and monthly
- Monitor swallowing of PO medication: check for hoarding or giving of medication to other patients
- Monitor I&O ratio; palpate bladder if low urinary output occurs, especially in geriatric
- Monitor bilirubin, CBC
- Monitor urinalysis; recommended before, during prolonged therapy
- Assess affect, orientation, LOC, reflexes, gait, coordination, sleep pattern disturbances
- Monitor B/P sitting, standing, lying; take pulse and respirations q4hr during initial treatment; establish baseline before starting treatment; report drops of 30 mm Hg; obtain baseline ECG
- Assess dizziness, faintness, palpitations, tachycardia on rising
- Assess for neuroleptic malignant syndrome: hyperpyrexia, muscle rigidity, increased CPK, altered mental status, for acute dystonia (check chewing, swallowing, eyes, pin rolling)
- EPS including akathisia (inability to sit still, no pattern to movements), tardive dyskinesia (bizarre movements of the jaw, mouth, tongue, extremities), pseudoparkinsonism (rigidity, tremors, pill rolling, shuffling gait)
- Monitor skin turgor daily
- Monitor constipation, urinary retention daily; increase bulk, H_2O in diet

Nursing diagnoses
- Knowledge, deficient (teaching)
- Noncompliance (teaching)

Implementation
- Give antiparkinsonian agent for EPS
- Give decreased dose in geriatric
- Give PO with full glass of water, milk; or with food to decrease GI upset
- Provide decreased stimuli by dimming light, avoiding loud noises

- Provide supervised ambulation until stabilized on medication; do not involve in strenuous exercise program because fainting is possible; patients should not stand still for long periods
- Give increased fluids to prevent constipation
- Give sips of water, candy, gum for dry mouth
- Store in airtight, light-resistant container
- Give orally disintegrating tabs: open blister pack, place tab on tongue until dissolved, swallow; no water needed

Patient/family education
- Teach patient to use good oral hygiene; frequent rinsing of mouth, candy, ice chips, sugarless gum for dry mouth
- Advise patient to avoid hazardous activities until product response is determined
- Advise patient that orthostatic hypotension occurs often and to rise from sitting or lying position gradually
- Advise patient to avoid hot tubs, hot showers, tub baths, since hypotension may occur
- Advise patient to avoid abrupt withdrawal of this product, or EPS may result; product should be withdrawn slowly
- Advise patient to avoid OTC preparations (cough, hay fever, cold) unless approved by prescriber, since serious product interactions may occur; avoid use with alcohol, CNS depressants, increased drowsiness may occur
- Advise patient that in hot weather, heat stroke may occur; take extra precautions to stay cool

Evaluation
Positive therapeutic outcome
- Decrease in emotional excitement, hallucinations, delusions, paranoia, reorganization of patterns of thought, speech

Treatment of overdose: Lavage if orally ingested; provide airway; do not induce vomiting or use epinephrine

---

olmesartan (Rx)
(ol-meh-sar′tan)

Benicar

Func. class.: Antihypertensive

Pregnancy category
C (1st trimester),
D (2nd/3rd trimesters)

Action: Blocks the vasoconstrictor and aldosterone-secreting effects of angiotensin II; selectively blocks the binding of angiotensin II to the AT_1 receptor found in tissues

Therapeutic outcome: Decreased B/P

Adverse effects: *italic* = common, **bold** = life-threatening

Uses: Hypertension, alone or in combination with other antihypertensives

Dosage and routes
Adult: PO sngle agent 20 mg/day initially in patients who are not volume depleted; may be increased to 40 mg/day if needed after 2 wk

Available forms: Tabs 5, 20, 40 mg

Adverse effects
CNS: *Dizziness,* fatigue, headache, insomnia
CV: Chest pain, peripheral edema, tachycardia
EENT: Sinusitis, rhinitis, pharyngitis
GI: *Diarrhea,* abdominal pain
MS: Arthralgia, pain
RESP: *Upper respiratory infection,* bronchitis
SYST: **Angioedema**

Contraindications: Hypersensitivity

Black Box Warning: Pregnancy **D** (2nd/ 3rd trimesters)

Precautions: Pregnancy **C** (1st trimester), breastfeeding, children, geriatric, hepatic disease, CHF

Pharmacokinetics
Absorption	Unknown
Distribution	Unknown
Metabolism	Unknown
Excretion	Urine, feces
Half-life	Unknown

Pharmacodynamics
Unknown

Interactions
Individual drugs
Lithium: increased effect
Drug classifications
Antihypertensives (other), diuretics: increased antihypertensive effects
NSAIDs, salicylates: decreased antihypertensive effect
Potassium supplements, potassium-sparing diuretics: increased hyperkalemia
Drug/herb
Aconite: increased toxicity, death
Astragalus, cola tree: increased or decreased antihypertensive effect
Barberry, betony, black catechu, black cohosh, bloodroot, broom, burdock, cat's claw, dandelion, goldenseal, hawthorn, Irish moss, Jamaican dogwood, kelp, khella, mistletoe, parsley: increased antihypertensive effect
Coltsfoot, guarana, khat, licorice, yohimbe: decreased antihypertensive effect

NURSING CONSIDERATIONS
Assessment
- Assess for pregnancy; this product can cause fetal death when given in pregnancy
- Assess response and adverse reactions, especially in renal disease
- Monitor B/P, pulse q4hr; note rate, rhythm, quality; electrolytes: K, Na, Cl; baselines in renal, liver function tests before therapy begins
- Assess skin turgor, dryness of mucous membranes for hydration status; for angioedema: facial swelling, dyspnea

Nursing diagnoses
- Cardiac output, decreased (uses)
- Knowledge, deficient (teaching)
- Noncompliance (teaching)
- Tissue perfusion, ineffective (uses)

Implementation
- Give without regard to meals

Patient/family education
- Advise to comply with dosage schedule, even if feeling better
- Advise patient to notify prescriber of mouth sores, fever, swelling of hands or feet, irregular heartbeat, chest pain
- Teach that excessive perspiration, dehydration, vomiting, diarrhea may lead to fall in B/P; to consult prescriber if these occur
- Teach that product may cause dizziness, fainting; light-headedness may occur
- Advise to rise slowly to sitting or standing position to minimize orthostatic hypotension
- Teach to notify prescriber immediately if pregnant; not to use during breastfeeding
- Advise to avoid all OTC medications, unless approved by prescriber
- Advise to inform all health care providers of medication use
- Advise to use proper technique for obtaining B/P and acceptable parameters

Evaluation
Positive therapeutic outcome
- Decreased B/P

olopatadine ophthalmic
See Appendix B

olsalazine (Rx)
(ohl-sal'ah-zeen)
Dipentum ✦
Func. class.: Antiinflammatory
Chem. class.: Salicylate derivative
Pregnancy category C

Action: Bioconverted to 5-aminosalicylic acid, which decreases inflammation

Therapeutic outcome: Lessening of loose, diarrhea stools and cramping

Uses: Maintenance of remission of ulcerative colitis in patients intolerant to sulfasalazine

Dosage and routes
Adult: PO 500 mg bid

Available forms: Caps 250 mg

Adverse effects
CNS: Headache, hallucinations, depression, vertigo, fatigue, dizziness
GI: Nausea, vomiting, abdominal pain, **hepatitis,** diarrhea, bloating, **pancreatitis**
HEMA: Leukopenia, neutropenia, **thrombocytopenia, agranulocytosis, anemia**
INTEG: Rash, dermatitis, urticaria

Contraindications: Hypersensitivity to salicylates

Precautions: Pregnancy **C,** breastfeeding, children <14 yr, impaired renal/hepatic function, severe allergy, bronchial asthma

Pharmacokinetics	
Absorption	Colon 99% converted to mesalamine
Distribution	Colon
Metabolism	Liver
Excretion	Feces
Half-life	0.9 hr

Pharmacodynamics	
Onset	Unknown
Peak	1 hr
Duration	12 hr

Interactions
Drug/lab test
Increased: AST, ALT

NURSING CONSIDERATIONS
Assessment
⬥ Assess for blood dyscrasias: skin rash, fever, sore throat, bruising, bleeding, fatigue, joint pain (rare)
• Assess for allergic reaction: rash, dermatitis, urticaria, pruritus, dyspnea, bronchospasm

Nursing diagnoses
• Diarrhea (uses)
• Knowledge, deficient (teaching)
• Pain, acute (uses)

Implementation
• Give total daily dose evenly spaced to minimize GI intolerance, with food
• Store in tight, light-resistant container at room temperature

Patient/family education
• Advise patient to take as prescribed, take missed dose as soon as remembered
• Inform patient not to operate machinery or drive until effects are known, may cause dizziness
• Advise patient to notify prescriber if symptoms do not improve or if allergic reaction or sore throat occurs

Evaluation
Positive therapeutic outcome
• Absence of fever, mucus in stools

omalizumab (Rx)
(oh-mah-lye-zoo'mab)
Xolair
Func. class.: Monoclonal antibody
Pregnancy category B

Action: Recombinant DNA-derived humanized IgG murine monoclonal antibody that selectively binds to IgE to limit the release of mediators in the allergic response

Therapeutic outcome: Ability to breathe more easily

Uses: Moderate to severe persistent asthma

Unlabeled uses: Seasonal allergic rhinitis, food allergy

Dosage and routes
Adult/adolescent/child ≥12 yr:
SUBCUT 150-375 mg × 2-4 wk, divide inj into 2 sites, if dose is >150 mg; dose is adjusted based on IgE levels and significant changes in body weight

Available forms: Powder for inj, lyophilized 202.5 mg (150 mg/1.2 ml after reconstitution)

Adverse effects
CV: **Heart failure,** cardiomyopathy, hypotension
HEMA: Serious systemic eosinophilia
INTEG: Pruritus, dermatitis, inj site reactions, rash

Adverse effects: *italic* = common, **bold** = life-threatening

MISC: Earache, dizziness, fatigue, pain, **malignancies,** viral infections, **anaphylaxis, thrombocytopenia,** headache
MS: Arthralgia, fracture, leg, arm pain
RESP: Sinusitis, upper respiratory tract infections, pharyngitis, pulmonary hypertension, **bronchospasm**

Contraindications: Hamster protein

Black Box Warning: Hypersensitivity to this product

Precautions: Pregnancy **B,** breastfeeding, children <12 yr, acute attacks of asthma, lymphoma, nephrotic disease, bronchospasm, neoplastic disease, status asthmaticus

Pharmacokinetics

Absorption	Slow
Distribution	Unknown
Metabolism	Degradation by liver
Excretion	In bile
Half-life	26 days

Pharmacodynamics

Onset	Unknown
Peak	7-8 days
Duration	Unknown

Interactions
Drug classifications
Vaccines (live virus): use cautiously

NURSING CONSIDERATIONS
Assessment
• Monitor respiratory rate, rhythm, depth; auscultate lung fields bilaterally; notify prescriber of abnormalities; monitor pulmonary function tests; serum IgE
• Assess for anaphylaxis, allergic reactions: rash, urticaria, inability to breathe, edema of throat; observe for 2 hr, reaction can occur up to 24 hr; have emergency equipment available; product should be discontinued

Nursing diagnoses
• Gas exchange, impaired (uses)
• Knowledge, deficient (teaching)

Implementation
SUBCUT route
• Given q2-4wk; product is viscous; if >150 mg is given, divide into two sites; the inj may take 5-10 sec to administer
• Do not give more than 150 mg/inj site

Patient/family education
• Advise that improvement will not be immediate

• Teach not to stop taking or decrease current asthma medications unless instructed by prescriber
• To report signs of allergic reaction

Evaluation
Positive therapeutic outcome
• Ability to breathe more easily

---

omeprazole (Rx, OTC)
(oh-mep′ra-zole)
Losec ✤, Prilosec, Prilosec OTC
Func. class.: Antiulcer, proton pump inhibitor
Chem. class.: Benzimidazole

Pregnancy category C

Do not confuse:
Prilosec/Prinivil/predniSONE/Prozac

Action: Suppresses gastric secretion by inhibiting hydrogen/potassium ATPase enzyme system in the gastric parietal cell; characterized as a gastric acid pump inhibitor, since it blocks the final step of acid production

Therapeutic outcome: Absence of duodenal ulcers; decreased gastroesophageal reflux

Uses: Gastroesophageal reflux disease (GERD), severe erosive esophagitis, poorly responsive systemic GERD, pathologic hypersecretory conditions (Zollinger-Ellison syndrome, systemic mastocytosis, multiple endocrine adenomas); possibly effective for treatment of duodenal ulcers with or without antiinfectives for *Helicobacter pylori*

Unlabeled uses: GERD-related laryngitis, enhancing pancreatin

Dosage and routes
Active duodenal ulcers
Adult: PO 20 mg/day × 4-8 wk; associated with *H. pylori* 40 mg q$_{AM}$ and clarithromycin 500 mg tid on days 1-14, then 20 mg/day days 15-28

Severe erosive esophagitis/poorly responsive GERD
Adult: PO (DEL REL cap/SUSP) 20 mg/day × 4-8 wk

Pathologic hypersecretory conditions
Adult: PO 60 mg/day; may increase to 120 mg tid; daily doses >80 mg should be divided

Gastric ulcer
Adult: PO 40 mg/day × 4-8 wk
Geriatric: PO max 20 mg/day

Heartburn (OTC)
Adult: PO 1 DEL REL tab (20 mg) daily before AM meal with glass of water

Laryngitis (unlabeled)
Adult: PO 20-40 mg nightly × 6-24 wk or 20 mg bid × 4-12 wk

Available forms: Del rel caps 10, 20, 40 mg, del rel tabs (Prilosec OTC) 20 mg; granules for oral susp 2.5, 10 mg (del rel)

Adverse effects
CNS: Headache, dizziness, asthenia
CV: Chest pain, angina, tachycardia, bradycardia, palpitations, peripheral edema, **heart failure**
EENT: Tinnitus, taste perversion
GI: Diarrhea, abdominal pain, vomiting, nausea, constipation, flatulence, acid regurgitation, abdominal swelling, anorexia, irritable colon, esophageal candidiasis, dry mouth, **hepatic failure**
GU: UTI, frequency, increased creatinine, **proteinuria, hematuria,** testicular pain, glycosuria
HEMA: **Pancytopenia, thrombocytopenia, neutropenia, leukocytosis,** anemia
INTEG: Rash, dry skin, urticaria, pruritus, alopecia
META: Hypoglycemia, increased hepatic enzymes, weight gain
MISC: Back pain, fever, fatigue, malaise
RESP: Upper respiratory tract infections, cough, epistaxis, **pneumonia**
SYST: **Angioedema, exfoliative dermatitis, Stevens-Johnson syndrome, toxic epidermal necrosis**

Contraindications: Hypersensitivity

Precautions: Pregnancy **C,** breastfeeding, children

Pharmacokinetics
Absorption	Rapidly absorbed
Distribution	Protein binding (95%); gastric parietal cells
Metabolism	Liver, extensively; by CYP450 enzyme system
Excretion	Kidneys, feces
Half-life	½-1 hr; increased in the geriatric, hepatic disease

Pharmacodynamics
Onset	1 hr
Peak	½-3½ hr
Duration	3-4 days

Interactions
Individual drugs
Ampicillin: decreased effect of ampicillin
Calcium carbonate: decreased absorption of calcium carbonate
Cyanocobalamin: decreased absorption of cyanocobalamin
CycloSPORINE: increased cycloSPORINE levels
Diazepam: increased serum levels of diazepam
Digoxin: increased serum levels, delayed absorption of digoxin
Disulfiram: increased disulfiram levels
Flurazepam: increased flurazepam level
Gefitinib: decreased effect of gefitinib
Indinavir: decreased effect of indinavir
Iron salts: decreased absorption
Ketoconazole: decreased absorption of ketoconazole
Phenytoin: increased serum levels of phenytoin
Triazolam: increased triazolam level
Warfarin: increased bleeding tendencies
Drug classifications
Iron products: decreased absorption of iron
Drug/lab test
Increased: alkaline phosphatase, AST, ALT, bilirubin, gastrin

NURSING CONSIDERATIONS
Assessment
- Assess GI system: bowel sounds q8hr, abdomen for pain and swelling, anorexia
- Monitor hepatic enzymes: AST, ALT, increased alkaline phosphatase during treatment

Nursing diagnoses
- Knowledge, deficient (teaching)
- Pain, chronic (uses)

Implementation
- Swallow sus rel caps whole; do not break, crush, chew, or open
- Give before patient eats; may give with antacids

Patient/family education
- Advise patient to report severe diarrhea; product may have to be discontinued
- Caution patient to avoid driving and other hazardous activities until response to product is known
- Caution patient to avoid alcohol, salicylates, ibuprofen; may cause GI irritation

Evaluation
Positive therapeutic outcome
- Absence of epigastric pain, swelling, fullness

O

ondansetron (Rx)
(on-dan'sa-tron)
Zofran, Zofran ODT
Func. class.: Antiemetic
Chem. class.: 5-HT receptor antagonist

Pregnancy category B

Do not confuse:
Zofran/Zantac

Action: Prevents nausea, vomiting by blocking serotonin (5-HT) peripherally, centrally, and in the small intestine

Therapeutic outcome: Control of nausea, vomiting

Uses: Prevention of nausea, vomiting associated with cancer chemotherapy, radiotherapy, and prevention of postoperative nausea, vomiting

Unlabeled uses: Bulimia, pruritus (rectal use), alcoholism, hyperemesis gravidarum

Dosage and routes
Prevention of nausea/vomiting associated with cancer chemotherapy
Adult and child 4-18 yr: **IV** 0.15 mg/kg infused over 15 min, 30 min before start of cancer chemotherapy; 0.15 mg/kg is given 4 hr and 8 hr after first dose or 32 mg as a single dose; dilute in 50 ml of D_5 or 0.9% NaCl before giving; RECT (unlabeled) 16 mg daily 2 hr before chemotherapy; PO 8 mg ½ hr prior to chemotherapy, repeat 8 hr later
Child ≥4 yr: PO 4 mg ½ hr prior to chemotherapy

Prevention of nausea/vomiting from radiotherapy
Adult: PO 8 mg tid, may repeat 4, 8 hr after 1st dose

Prevention of postoperative nausea/vomiting
Adult: **IV**/IM 4 mg undiluted over >30 sec prior to induction of anesthesia
Child 2-12 yr: **IV** 0.1 mg/kg (≤40 kg); 4 mg (≥40 kg), give ≥30 sec

Hepatic dose
Adult: PO/IM/**IV** max dose 8 mg daily

Hyperemesis gravidarum (unlabeled)
Adult: PO/**IV** 4-8 mg bid-tid

Pruritus (unlabeled)
Adult: PO 4 mg bid

Alcoholism (unlabeled)
Adult: PO 4 mcg/kg bid

Available forms: Inj 2 mg/ml, 32 mg/50 ml (premixed); tabs 4, 8 mg; oral sol 4 mg/5 ml; oral disintegrating tabs 4, 8 mg

Adverse effects
CNS: *Headache*, dizziness, drowsiness, fatigue, EPS
GI: *Diarrhea, constipation, abdominal pain,* dry mouth
MISC: Rash, **bronchospasm** (rare), *musculoskeletal pain, wound problems, shivering, fever, hypoxia, urinary retention*

Contraindications: Hypersensitivity; phenylketonuric hypersensitivity (oral disintegrating tab), torsades de pointes

Precautions: Pregnancy **B**, breastfeeding, children, geriatric, granisetron hypersensitivity

Pharmacokinetics	
Absorption	Completely absorbed (**IV**)
Distribution	Unknown
Metabolism	Liver, extensively
Excretion	Kidneys
Half-life	3.5-4.7 hr

Pharmacodynamics
Unknown

Interactions
Individual drugs
Carbamazepine, phenytoin, rifampin: decreased ondansetron effect

NURSING CONSIDERATIONS
Assessment
• Assess for absence of nausea, vomiting during chemotherapy
• Assess for hypersensitivity reaction: rash, bronchospasm
• Assess for EPS shuffling gait, tremors, grimacing, rigidity

Nursing diagnoses
• Knowledge, deficient (teaching)
• Noncompliance (teaching)

Implementation
IV route
• Give **IV** after diluting a single dose in 50 ml of 0.9% NaCl or D_5W, 0.45% NaCl; give over 15 min
• Store at room temperature for 48 hr after dilution
Y-site compatibilities: Aldesleukin, amifostine, amikacin, aztreonam, bleomycin, carboplatin, carmustine, cefazolin, ceforanide, cefotazime, cefoxitin, ceftazidime, ceftizoxime,

 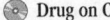

cefuroxime, chlorproMAZINE, cimetidine, cisatracurium, cisplatin, cladribine, clindamycin, cyclophosphamide, cytarabine, dacarbazine, dactinomycin, DAUNOrubicin, dexamethasone, diphenhydrAMINE, DOXOrubicin, DOXOrubicin liposome, doxycycline, droperidol, etoposide, famotidine, filgrastim, floxuridine, fluconazole, fludarabine, gentamicin, haloperidol, heparin, hydrocortisone, hydromorphone, hydrOXYzine, ifosfamide, imipenem/cilastatin, magnesium sulfate, mannitol, mechlorethamine, melphalan, meperidine, mesna, methotrexate, metoclopramide, miconazole, mitomycin, mitoxantrone, morphine, paclitaxel, pentostatin, potassium chloride, prochlorperazine, ranitidine, remifentanil, streptozocin, teniposide, thiotepa, ticarcillin, ticarcillin/clavulanate, vancomycin, vinBLAStine, vinCRIStine, vinorelbine, zidovudine

Y-site incompatibilities: Acyclovir, aminophylline, amphotericin B, ampicillin, ampicillin/sulbactam, cefoperazone, furosemide, ganciclovir, lorazepam, methylPREDNISolone, mezlocillin, piperacillin, sargramostim, sodium bicarbonate

Additive compatibilities: Cisplatin, cyclophosphamide, cytarabine, dacarbazine, dexamethasone, DOXOrubicin, etoposide, meperidine, methotrexate

Solution compatibilities: May also be diluted with D_5W, LR, D_5/0.9% NaCl, D_5/0.45% NaCl

Patient/family education
• Instruct patient to report diarrhea, constipation, rash, changes in respirations, or discomfort at insertion site
• Teach patient reason for medication and expected results

Evaluation
Positive therapeutic outcome
• Absence of nausea, vomiting during cancer chemotherapy

---

orlistat (Rx, OTC)
(or-li′-stat)
Alli, Xenical
Chem. class.: Weight control agent, lipase inhibitor
Pregnancy category B

Action: Inhibits the absorption of dietary fat
Therapeutic outcome: Decrease in weight

Uses: Obesity management

Dosage and routes
Adult: PO 60 mg (Alli)-120 mg (Xenical) tid with each main meal containing fat, max 360 mg/day

Available forms: Caps 60 mg (Alli), 120 mg (Xenical)

Adverse effects
CNS: Insomnia, dizziness, headache, depression, anxiety, fatigue
GI: Oily spotting, flatus with discharge, fecal urgency, fatty/oily stool, oily evacuation, fecal incontinence, frequent defecation, nausea, vomiting, abdominal pain, infectious diarrhea, rectal pain, tooth disorder, hypovitaminosis, **hepatic failure, hepatitis, pancreatitis**
GU: UTI, vaginitis, menstrual irregularity
INTEG: Dry skin, rash
MS: Back pain, arthritis, myalgia, tendinitis
RESP: Influenza, upper, lower respiratory tract infection, EENT symptoms

Contraindications: Breastfeeding, hypersensitivity, chronic malabsorption syndrome, cholestasis

Precautions: Pregnancy **B,** children, hypothyroidism, other organic causes of obesity, anorexia nervosa, bulimia, nephrolithiasis, GI disease, diabetes, fat-soluble vitamin deficiency

Pharmacokinetics	
Absorption	Minimal
Distribution	99% protein binding
Metabolism	Unknown
Excretion	Feces
Half-life	1-2 hr

Pharmacodynamics	
Onset	Unknown
Peak	8 hr
Duration	Unknown

Interactions
Individual drugs
Cyclosporine: decreased absorption
Pravastatin: increased lipid-lowering effect
Warfarin: increased effects of warfarin
Drug classifications
Fat-soluble vitamins: decreased absorption

NURSING CONSIDERATIONS
Assessment
• Monitor weight weekly, diabetic patients may need reduction in oral hypoglycemics

Adverse effects: *italic* = common, **bold** = life-threatening

- Assess for misuse in certain populations (anorexia nervosa, bulimia)
- Assess for liver injury: jaundice, weakness, abdominal pain

Nursing diagnoses
- Knowledge, deficient (teaching)
- Noncompliance (teaching)

Implementation
- Patient should be on a diet with 30% of calories from fat; omit dose of orlistat if a meal contains no fat

Patient/family education
- Advise patient that 60 mg cap can be obtained OTC; 60 mg tid is the highest OTC dose
- Warn patient that safety and effectiveness beyond 2 yr have not been determined
- Instruct patient to read patient's information sheet, discuss unpleasant GI side effects
- Advise patient to avoid hazardous activities until stabilized on medication
- Instruct patient to take a multivitamin containing fat-soluble vitamins, take 2 hr before or after orlistat; psyllium taken with each dose or at bedtime may decrease GI symptoms
- Instruct patient/family to notify prescriber if significant side effects occur
- Advise prescriber if pregnancy is planned or suspected

Evaluation
Positive therapeutic outcome
- Decreased weight

---

oseltamivir (Rx)
(oh-sell-tam'ih-ver)
Tamiflu
Func. class.: Antiviral
Chem. class.: Neuramidase inhibitor

Pregnancy category C

Action: Inhibits influenza virus neuraminidase with possible alteration of virus particle aggregation and release

Therapeutic outcome: Decreased symptoms of influenza type A

Uses: Prevention/treatment of influenza type A or B

Unlabeled uses: Avian influenzae (H5N1), swine flu (H1N1), encephalitis

Dosage and routes
Treatment
Adult and child >40 kg: PO 75 bid mg × 5 days, begin treatment within 2 days of onset of symptoms

Child 23-40 kg and ≥1 yr: PO 60 mg bid
Child 15-23 kg and ≥1 yr: PO 45 mg bid
Child ≤15 kg and ≥1 yr: PO 30 mg bid
Prevention
Adult and child ≥13 yr: PO 75 mg/day × ≥7 days; begin treatment within 2 days of contact, max use 6 wk
Renal dose
Adult: PO CCr 10-30 ml/min 75 mg/day × 5 days (treatment); 75 mg every other day or 30 mg/day (prophylaxis)

H1N1 influenzae A virus (unlabeled)
Adult/adolescent/child >40 kg: PO 75 mg bid × 5 days
Child/adolescent 24-40 kg: PO 60 mg bid × 5 days
Child >1 yr and 15-23 kg: PO 45 mg bid × 5 days
Child >1 yr and <15 kg: PO 30 mg bid × 5 days

Available forms: Caps 30, 45, 75 mg; powder for oral susp 12 mg/ml after reconstitution

Adverse effects
CNS: Headache, fatigue, insomnia, dizziness, delirium, **self-injury (children)**
GI: Nausea, vomiting, diarrhea, abdominal pain
INTEG: Toxic epidermal necrolysis, Stevens-Johnson syndrome, erythema multiforme
RESP: Cough

Contraindications: Hypersensitivity

Precautions: Pregnancy **C**, geriatric, renal/hepatic/pulmonary/cardiac disease, infants, children, neonates, psychosis, viral infection, breastfeeding

Pharmacokinetics	
Absorption	Rapidly absorbed
Distribution	Protein binding 3%
Metabolism	Converted to oseltamivir carboxylate
Excretion	Eliminated by conversion, urine 99%
Half-life	1-3 hr

Pharmacodynamics	
Unknown	

 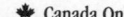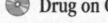

NURSING CONSIDERATIONS
Assessment
- Assess for symptoms of influenza A: increased temperature, malaise, aches and pains

Nursing diagnoses
- Infection, risk for (uses)
- Knowledge, deficient (teaching)

Implementation
- Give within 2 days of symptoms of influenza; continue for 5 days
- Give at least 4 hr before bedtime to prevent insomnia
- Administer after meals for better absorption, to decrease GI symptoms: caps may be opened and mixed with food for easy swallowing
- Store in airtight, dry container

Patient/family education
- Teach patient about aspects of product therapy: the need to report dyspnea, weight gain, dizziness, poor concentration, dysuria, behavioral changes
- Teach patient to avoid hazardous activities if dizziness occurs
- Advise patient to take missed dose as soon as remembered if within 2 hr of next dose

Evaluation
Positive therapeutic outcome
- Absence of fever, malaise, cough, dyspnea in influenza A

oxacillin (Rx)
(ox-a-sill'in)
oxacillin sodium
Func. class.: Broad-spectrum antiinfective
Chem. class.: Penicillinase-resistant penicillin

Pregnancy category B

Action: Interferes with cell wall replication of susceptible organisms; osmotically unstable cell wall swells, bursts from osmotic pressure

Therapeutic outcome: Bactericidal effects for gram-positive cocci: *Staphylococcus aureus, Streptococcus pneumoniae,* infections caused by penicillinase-producing staphylococci

Uses: Infections caused by penicillinase-producing staphylococci, streptococci; respiratory tract, skin, skin structure, urinary tract, bone, joint infections; sinusitis; endocarditis; septicemia; meningitis

Dosage and routes
Adult: IM/**IV** 2-12 g/day in divided doses q4-6hr
Child: IM/**IV** 50-100 mg/kg/day in divided doses q4-6hr, max 4 g/day

Available forms: Powder for inj 250, 500 mg, 1, 2, 4, 10 g

Adverse effects
CNS: Lethargy, hallucinations, anxiety, depression, twitching, **coma, seizures**
GI: Nausea, vomiting, diarrhea, increased AST, ALT, abdominal pain, glossitis, colitis, **pseudomembranous colitis,** hepatotoxicity
GU: **Oliguria, proteinuria, hematuria,** vaginitis, moniliasis, **glomerulonephritis,** acute interstitial nephritis
HEMA: Anemia, increased bleeding time, **bone marrow depression, granulocytopenia,** eosinophilia
INTEG: **Exfoliative dermatitis, Stevens-Johnson syndrome**
SYST: **Anaphylaxis, serum sickness**

Contraindications: Hypersensitivity to penicillins or corn

Precautions: Pregnancy **B,** breastfeeding, neonates, hypersensitivity to cephalosporins, renal/hepatic/GI disease, hypersensitivity to cephalosporins/carbapenem

Pharmacokinetics
Absorption	Rapid, incomplete (PO); well absorbed (IM); completely (**IV**)
Distribution	Widely distributed; crosses placenta
Metabolism	Liver
Excretion	Kidneys, unchanged (51%); breast milk
Half-life	20-50 min; increased in severe hepatic disease

Pharmacodynamics
	PO	IM	IV
Onset	Rapid	Rapid	Rapid
Peak	½-1 hr	½ hr	Inf end
Duration	Unknown	Unknown	Unknown

Interactions
Individual drugs
Chloramphenicol, cholestyramine, colestipol: decreased effectiveness of oxacillin
Probenecid: increased oxacillin levels
Rifampin: decreased oxacillin effect
Drug classifications
Aminoglycosides: do not mix or give together
Erythromycins, sulfonamides, tetracyclines: decreased antimicrobial effectiveness

Adverse effects: *italic* = common, **bold** = life-threatening

Drug/herb
Acidophilus: do not use with antiinfectives; separate by several hours
Khat: decreased absorption, separate by ≥2 hr
Drug/lab test
False positive: urine glucose, urine protein

NURSING CONSIDERATIONS
Assessment

• Assess patient for previous sensitivity reaction to penicillins or other cephalosporins; cross-sensitivity between penicillins and cephalosporins is common
• Assess patient for signs and symptoms of infection including characteristics of wounds, sputum, urine, stool, WBC >10,000/mm^3, fever; obtain information baseline during treatment
• Obtain C&S before beginning product therapy to identify if correct treatment has been initiated
• Assess for allergic reactions: rash, urticaria, pruritus, chills, fever, joint pain; angioedema may occur a few days after therapy begins; epinephrine, resuscitation equipment should be available for anaphylactic reaction
◆ Assess urine output; if decreasing, notify prescriber (may indicate nephrotoxicity); also check for increased BUN, creatinine
• Monitor blood studies: AST, ALT, CBC, Hct, bilirubin, LDH, alkaline phosphatase, Coombs' test monthly if patient is on long-term therapy
• Monitor electrolytes: potassium, sodium, chloride monthly if patient is on long-term therapy
• Assess bowel pattern daily; if severe diarrhea occurs, product should be discontinued; may indicate pseudomembranous colitis
• Monitor for bleeding: ecchymosis, bleeding gums, hematuria, stool guaiac daily if on long-term therapy
• Assess for overgrowth of infection: perineal itching, fever, malaise, redness, pain, swelling, drainage, rash, diarrhea, change in cough, sputum

Nursing diagnoses
• Diarrhea (adverse reactions)
• Infection, risk for (uses)
• Injury, risk for (adverse reactions)
• Knowledge, deficient (teaching)
• Noncompliance (teaching)

Implementation
PO route
• Give in even doses around the clock; if GI upset occurs, give with food; product must be given for 10-14 days to ensure organism death

and prevent superinfection; store in airtight container
• Shake susp; store in refrigerator for 2 wk, 1 wk at room temperature
IM route
• Reconstitute 250 mg/1.4 ml, 500 mg/2.7-2.8 ml, 1 g/5.7 ml, 2 g/11.4-11.5 ml, 4 g/21.8-23 ml of sterile water for a conc of 250 mg/1.5 ml; store unused portion in refrigerator for 1 wk or 3 days at room temperature
• Inject deeply in large muscle mass
IV route
• Reconstitute 250 mg/1.4 ml, 500 mg/2.7-2.8 ml, 1 g/5.7 ml, 2 g/11.4-11.5 ml, 4 g/21.8-23 ml of sterile water for a conc of 250 mg/1.5 ml; store unused portion in refrigerator for 1 week or 3 days at room temperature
• Give direct **IV** by diluting reconstituted sol with 250-500 mg/5 ml, 1 g/10 ml, 2 g/20 ml, 4 g/40 ml of sterile water or 0.9% NaCl, give over 10 min
• Give intermittent inf by diluting to a conc of 0.5-40 mg/ml with D$_5$W, 0.9% NaCl, D$_5$/0.9% NaCl, LR; give over 6 hr or less
Y-site compatibilities: Acyclovir, cyclophosphamide, diltiazem, famotidine, fluconazole, foscarnet, heparin, hydrocortisone, hydromorphone, labetalol, magnesium sulfate, meperidine, methotrexate, morphine, perphenazine, potassium chloride, tacrolimus, vit B with C, zidovudine
Y-site incompatibilities: Verapamil
Additive compatibilities: Cephapirin, chloramphenicol, DOPamine, potassium chloride, sodium bicarbonate
Additive incompatibilities: Cytarabine, tetracycline

Patient/family education
• Teach patient to report sore throat, bruising, bleeding, joint pain; may indicate blood dyscrasias (rare)
• Advise patient to contact prescriber if vaginal itching, loose foul-smelling stools, furry tongue occur; may indicate superinfection
• Instruct patient to take all medication prescribed for the length of time ordered
• Advise patient to notify prescriber of diarrhea with blood or pus, which may indicate pseudomembranous colitis

Evaluation
Positive therapeutic outcome
• Absence of signs/symptoms of infection (WBC <10,000/mm^3, temp WNL, absence of red, draining wounds)
• Reported improvement in symptoms of infection

Treatment of anaphylaxis: Withdraw product, maintain airway, administer epinephrine, aminophylline, O$_2$, **IV** corticosteroids

oxaliplatin (Rx)
(ox-al-i'plat-in)
Eloxitin
Func. class.: Antineoplastic
Chem. class.: 3rd generation platinum analog
Pregnancy category D

Action: Forms cross links, inhibiting DNA replication and transcription, cell-cycle nonspecific

Therapeutic outcome: Decreased size of tumor, spread of malignancy

Uses: Metastatic carcinoma of the colon or rectum in combination with 5-FU/leucovorin

Unlabeled uses: Relapsed or refractory non-Hodgkin's lymphoma, advanced ovarian cancer

Dosage and routes
Colorectal cancer
Dosage protocols may vary
Adult: **IV** INF *Day 1:* oxaliplatin 85 mg/m^2 in 250-500 ml D$_5$W and leucovorin 200 mg/m^2 in D$_5$W, give both over 2 hr at the same time in separate bags using a Y-line, followed by 5-FU 400 mg/m^2 **IV** BOL over 2-4 min, then 5-FU 600 mg/m^2 **IV** INF in 500 ml D$_5$W as a 22-hr CONT INF; *Day 2:* leucovorin 200 mg/m^2 **IV** INF over 2 hr, then 5-FU 400 mg/m^2 **IV** BOL over 2-4 min, then 5-FU 600 mg/m^2 **IV** INF in 500 ml D$_5$W as a 22-hr CONT INF; repeat cycle q2wk

Available forms: Powder for inj 50, 100 mg single-use vials

Adverse effects
CNS: Peripheral neuropathy, fatigue, headache, dizziness, insomnia
CV: Cardiac abnormalities, **thromboembolism**
EENT: Decreased visual acuity, tinnitus, hearing loss
GI: Severe nausea, vomiting, diarrhea, weight loss, stomatitis, anorexia, gastroesophageal reflux, constipation, dyspepsia, mucositis, flatulence
GU: Hematuria, dysuria, creatinine
HEMA: **Thrombocytopenia, leukopenia, pancytopenia, neutropenia, anemia, hemolytic uremic syndrome**

INTEG: Alopecia, rash, flushing, extravasation, redness, swelling, pain at inj site
META: Hypokalemia
RESP: **Fibrosis,** dyspnea, cough, rhinitis, URI, pharyngitis
SYST: **Anaphylaxis, angioedema**

Contraindications: Pregnancy **D**, breastfeeding, radiation therapy or chemotherapy within 1 mo, thrombocytopenia, smallpox vaccination

Black Box Warning: Hypersensitivity to this product or other platinum products

Precautions: Children, geriatric, pneumococcus vaccination, renal disease

Pharmacokinetics
Absorption	Unknown
Distribution	15% of platinum in systemic circulation; 85% is either in tissues or being eliminated in urine
Metabolism	Liver
Excretion	Urine
Half-life	40 days

Pharmacodynamics
Unknown

Interactions
Individual drugs
Alcohol, aspirin: increased risk of bleeding
Radiation: increased myelosuppression
Drug classifications
Aminoglycosides, diuretics (loop): increased nephrotoxicity
Anticoagulants, NSAIDs: increased risk of bleeding
Live virus vaccines: decreased antibody response
Myelosuppressives: increased myelosuppression
Tannins: increased oxaliplatin toxicity
Drug/lab test
Increased: ALT, AST, bilirubin, creatinine
Decreased: potassium, neutrophils, WBC, platelets

NURSING CONSIDERATIONS
Assessment
For bone marrow depression
• Monitor CBC, differential, platelet count weekly; withhold product if WBC is <4000 or platelet count is <100,000; notify prescriber of results
• Monitor renal function tests: BUN, creatinine, serum uric acid, urine CCr before, electrolytes during therapy; dose should not be given if BUN >19 mg/dl; creatinine <1.5

mg/dl; I&O ratio; report fall in urine output of <30 ml/hr

🔶 Assess for anaphylaxis: wheezing, tachycardia, facial swelling, fainting; discontinue product and report to prescriber; resuscitation equipment should be nearby
• Monitor temp (may indicate beginning infection)
• Monitor liver function tests before, during therapy (bilirubin, AST, ALT, LDH) as needed or monthly
• Assess for bleeding: hematuria, guaiac, bruising or petechiae, mucosa or orifices q8hr; obtain prescription for viscous lidocaine (Xylocaine)
• Assess effects of alopecia on body image; discuss feelings about body changes
• Assess for jaundice of skin, sclera; dark urine; clay-colored stools; itchy skin; abdominal pain; fever; diarrhea
• Assess for edema in feet, joint pain, stomach pain, shaking

Nursing diagnoses
• Infection, risk for (adverse reactions)
• Knowledge, deficient (teaching)
• Nutrition: less than body requirements, imbalanced (adverse reactions)

Implementation
• Provide comprehensive oral hygiene
• Provide all medications PO, if possible; avoid IM inj when platelets <100,000/mm^3
• Increase fluid intake to 2-3 L/day to prevent urate deposits, calculi formation, elimination of product

IV route
• Do not reconstitute or dilute with sodium chloride or any chloride-containing solutions
• Do not use aluminum equipment during any preparation or administration, will degrade platinum; do not refrigerate unopened powder or solution
• Prepare in biologic cabinet using gown, gloves, mask; do not allow product to come in contact with skin, use soap and water if contact occurs
• Hydrate patient with 0.9% NaCl over 8-12 hr before treatment
• Have epinephrine, antihistamines, corticosteroids for hypersensitivity reaction
• Give antiemetic 30-60 min before giving product and prn
• Give diuretic (furosemide 40 mg **IV**) or mannitol after inf
• Provide blankets, hat, gloves for cold prevention

Patient/family education
• Advise to report signs of infection: increased temp, sore throat, flulike symptoms
• Advise to report signs of anemia: fatigue, headache, faintness, shortness of breath, irritability
• Advise to report bleeding; avoid use of razors, commercial mouthwash
• Advise to avoid aspirin, ibuprofen, NSAIDs, alcohol; may cause GI bleeding
• Advise to report any complaints or side effects to nurse or prescriber
• Advise to report any changes in breathing, coughing
• Advise that hair may be lost during treatment; a wig or hairpiece may make patient feel better; new hair may be different in color, texture
• Advise to report numbness, tingling in face or extremities, poor hearing or joint pain, swelling
• Advise not to receive vaccines during treatment
• Advise to use contraception during treatment and 4 mo after; this product may cause infertility
• Teach patient to avoid contact with cold (air, ice, liquid); causes acute dysesthesias

Evaluation
Positive therapeutic outcome
• Decreased tumor size, spread of malignancy

---

oxaprozin (Rx)
(ox-a-proe′zin)
Daypro
Func. class.: Nonsteroidal antiinflammatory, antirheumatic
Chem. class.: Propionic acid derivative

Pregnancy category C

Do not confuse:
Daypro/Diupres

Action: Completely inhibits COX-1, COX-2 by blocking arachidonate, analgesic, antiinflammatory, antipyretic

Therapeutic outcome: Decreased pain, inflammation

Uses: Acute and long-term management of osteoarthritis, rheumatoid arthritis, juvenile rheumatoid arthritis

Dosage and routes
Adult: PO 600-1200 mg/day; max 1800 mg/day or 26 mg/kg, whichever is lower
Adult <50 kg: PO 600 mg/day

Juvenile rheumatoid arthritis
Child 6-16 yr: PO 22-31 kg, 600 mg/dose; 32-54 kg, 900 mg/dose; ≥55 kg, 1200 mg/dose

Available forms: Tabs 600 mg; tabs oxaprozin potassium 678 mg (equal to 600 mg oxaprozin); caps 600 mg

Adverse effects
CNS: Dizziness, headache, drowsiness, fatigue, tremors, confusion, insomnia, anxiety, depression
CV: Tachycardia, peripheral edema, palpitations, dysrhythmias, **MI, stroke**
EENT: Tinnitus, hearing loss, blurred vision
GI: Nausea, *anorexia,* vomiting, *diarrhea,* jaundice, **cholestatic hepatitis,** constipation, flatulence, *cramps,* dry mouth, peptic ulcer, **GI bleeding,** perforation, ulceration, dyspepsia
GU: **Nephrotoxicity: dysuria, hematuria, oliguria, azotemia**
HEMA: Increased bleeding time, **pancytopenia**
INTEG: Purpura, rash, pruritus, sweating, photosensitivity
SYST: **Anaphylaxis, angioneurotic edema, toxic epidermal necrolysis, Stevens-Johnson syndrome**

Contraindications: Pregnancy D (3rd trimester), hypersensitivity, asthma, patients in whom aspirin and iodides have induced symptoms of allergic reactions or asthma

Black Box Warning: Perioperative pain in CABG surgery

Precautions: Pregnancy C, breastfeeding, children, geriatric, bleeding/GI/cardiac disorders, CHF, hypersensitivity to other antiinflammatory agents, severe renal/hepatic disease

Black Box Warning: GI bleeding, MI, stroke

Pharmacokinetics
Absorption	Well absorbed
Distribution	99% protein binding
Metabolism	Liver, extensively
Excretion	Breast milk/urine/feces
Half-life	40-50 hr

Pharmacodynamics
Onset	Unknown
Peak	2 hr
Duration	Unknown

Interactions
Individual drugs
Alcohol: increased GI side effects
Aspirin: increased GI adverse reactions, toxicity
Cefamandole, cefoperazone, cefotetan, clopidogrel, eptifibatide, plicamycin, ticlopidine, tirofiban: increased bleeding risk
Cyclosporine, methotrexate, probenecid: increased toxicity
Lithium: increased lithium levels, avoid concomitant use
Phenytoin: increased phenytoin level, avoid concomitant use
Drug classifications
Anticoagulants, thrombolytics: increased risk of bleeding
Antihypertensives: decreased effect of antihypertensives
Corticosteroids, NSAIDs: increased GI side effects
Diuretics: decreased effectiveness of diuretics
Potassium supplements: increased GI side effects
Drug/herb
Anise, arnica, bogbean, chamomile, chondroitin, clove, dong quai, fenugreek, feverfew, garlic, ginger, ginkgo, ginseng *(Panax),* licorice: increased bleeding risk
Arginine, gossypol: increased gastric irritation
Bearberry, bilberry: increased NSAIDs effect
Drug/lab test
Increased: BUN, alkaline phosphatase
False positive: Increased 5-HIAA
False increase: 17-KS

NURSING CONSIDERATIONS
Assessment
- Assess for pain and ROM: intensity, location, duration
- Monitor blood studies: alkaline phosphatase, LDH, AST, ALT, and bleeding time (may be increased)
- Assess for asthma, aspirin hypersensitivity, nasal polyps; increased hypersensitivity reactions

Nursing diagnoses
- Injury, risk for (adverse reactions)
- Knowledge, deficient (teaching)
- Mobility, impaired physical (uses)
- Pain, chronic (uses)

Implementation
- Do not break, crush, or chew tabs
- Give with full glass of water to enhance absorption
- Give with food, antacids, milk to decrease gastric symptoms

Adverse effects: *italic* = common, **bold** = life-threatening

• Sit upright for 30 min to prevent stomach irritation and ulceration

Patient/family education

• Teach patient that product must be continued for prescribed time to be effective; to avoid aspirin, alcoholic beverages
• Instruct patient to use caution when driving; drowsiness, dizziness may occur
• Teach patient to take with a full glass of water to enhance absorption; patient should sit upright for 30 min to prevent stomach irritation and ulceration
• Instruct patient to use sunscreen and protective clothing to prevent burns
• Advise patient to report to prescriber severe abdominal pain, rash, itching, yellowing of skin or eyes, depression
• Advise to avoid prolonged sun exposure, use sunscreens, protective clothing
• Teach to avoid ASA, alcohol, other OTC products without prescriber approval
• Advise to inform all health care providers that product is being used

Evaluation

Positive therapeutic outcome

• Decreased pain
• Decreased inflammation
• Increased mobility

oxazepam (Rx)

(ox-az'e-pam)

Apo-Oxazepam ✤, Novoxapam ✤, oxazepam

Func. class.: Sedative/hypnotic; antianxiety
Chem. class.: Benzodiazepine, short-acting

Pregnancy category D

Controlled substance schedule IV

Action: Depresses subcortical levels of CNS, including limbic system, reticular formation; potentiates GABA

Therapeutic outcome: Decreased anxiety, successful alcohol withdrawal, relaxation

Uses: Anxiety, alcohol withdrawal, insomnia

Dosage and routes

Anxiety

Adult: PO 10-30 mg tid-qid, max 120 mg/day

Geriatric: PO 5 mg daily-bid initially, may increase, max 15 mg qid

Alcohol withdrawal

Adult: PO 15-30 mg tid-qid

Available forms: Caps 10, 15, 30 mg; tab 15 mg

Adverse effects

CNS: *Dizziness, drowsiness,* confusion, headache, anxiety, tremors, fatigue, depression, insomnia, hallucinations, paradoxic excitement, transient amnesia
CV: *Orthostatic hypotension,* **ECG changes, tachycardia,** hypotension
EENT: *Blurred vision,* tinnitus, mydriasis
GI: Nausea, vomiting, anorexia
HEMA: Leukopenia
INTEG: Rash, dermatitis, itching
SYST: Dependence

Contraindications: Pregnancy **D,** breastfeeding, children <12 yr, hypersensitivity to benzodiazepines, closed-angle glaucoma, psychosis

Precautions: Geriatric, debilitated, renal/hepatic disease, depression, suicidal ideation, dementia, sleep apnea, seizure disorder

Pharmacokinetics	
Absorption	Well absorbed
Distribution	Widely distributed; crosses placenta, blood-brain barrier
Metabolism	Liver
Excretion	Kidneys, breast milk
Half-life	5-15 hr

Pharmacodynamics	
Onset	½-1½ hr
Peak	Unknown
Duration	6-12 hr

Interactions

Individual drugs

Alcohol: increased CNS depression
Disulfiram: increased oxazepam effects
Levodopa: decreased effects of levodopa
Phenytoin, theophylline, valproic acid: decreased oxazepam effects

Drug classifications

CNS depressants: increased oxazepam effects
Oral contraceptives: increased or decreased oxazepam effect

Drug/herb

Black cohosh: increased hypotension
Catnip, chamomile, clary, cowslip, hops, kava, lavender, mistletoe, nettle, pokeweed, poppy, Queen Anne's lace, senega, skullcap, valerian: increased CNS depression

Drug/lab test

Increased: AST, ALT, serum bilirubin
Decreased: radioactive iodine uptake
False increase: 17-OHCS

NURSING CONSIDERATIONS
Assessment
- Assess mental status: mood, sensorium, anxiety, affect, sleeping pattern, drowsiness, dizziness, especially geriatric; physical dependency, withdrawal symptoms: anxiety, panic attacks, agitation, seizures, headache, nausea, vomiting, muscle pain, weakness; suicidal tendencies; indications of increasing tolerance and abuse
- Monitor B/P with patient lying, standing; pulse; if systolic B/P drops 20 mm Hg, hold product, notify prescriber
- Monitor blood tests: CBC during long-term therapy; blood dyscrasias have occurred rarely; decreased hematocrit, neutropenia may occur
- Monitor hepatic tests: AST, ALT, bilirubin, creatinine LDH, alkaline phosphatase if taking long term
- Monitor I&O; indicate renal dysfunction

Nursing diagnoses
- Anxiety (uses)
- Injury, risk for (adverse reactions)
- Knowledge, deficient (teaching)

Implementation
- Give with food or milk for GI symptoms; tab may be crushed if patient is unable to swallow medication whole

Patient/family education
- Teach patient that product may be taken with food or fluids; tab may be crushed or swallowed whole
- Caution patient not to use for everyday stress or longer than 3 mo unless directed by prescriber; not to take more than prescribed amount; not to double doses or skip doses
- Advise patient to avoid OTC preparations unless approved by prescriber; alcohol and CNS depressants will increase CNS depression
- Caution patient to avoid driving and activities that require alertness, since drowsiness may occur; to avoid alcohol and other psychotropic medications; to rise slowly or fainting may occur, especially geriatric; that drowsiness may worsen at beginning of treatment
- Caution patient not to discontinue medication abruptly after long-term use; withdrawal symptoms include vomiting, cramping, tremors, seizures
- Advise patient to use sugarless gum, hard candy, frequent sips of water for dry mouth

Evaluation
Positive therapeutic outcome
- Decreased anxiety, restlessness, sleeplessness (short-term treatment only)

Treatment of overdose: Lavage, VS, supportive care

---

oxcarbazepine (Rx)
(ox'kar-baz'uh-peen)
Trileptal
Func. class.: Anticonvulsant
Pregnancy category C

Action: May inhibit nerve impulses by limiting influx of sodium ions across cell membrane in motor cortex

Therapeutic outcome: Absence of seizures

Uses: Partial seizures

Unlabeled uses: Trigeminal neuralgia, atypical panic disorder, bipolar disorder

Dosage and routes
Seizures adjunctive therapy
Adult: PO 300 mg bid, may be increased by 600 mg/day in divided doses bid at weekly intervals; maintenance 1200 mg/day
Child 4-16 yr: PO 8-10 mg/kg/day divided bid, max 600 mg/day; dose is determined by weight

Conversion to monotherapy in partial seizures
Adult: PO 300 mg bid with reduction in other anticonvulsants, increase oxcarbazepine by 600 mg/day qwk over 2-4 wk; withdraw other anticonvulsants over 3-6 wk, max 2400 mg/day

Initiation of monotherapy in partial seizures
Adult: PO 300 mg bid, increase by 300 mg/day q3day to 1200 mg divided bid

Renal dose
Adult: PO CCr <30 ml/min 150 mg bid and increase slowly

Available forms: Film-coated tabs 150, 300, 600 mg; oral susp 300 mg/5 ml

Adverse effects
CNS: Headache, dizziness, confusion, fatigue, feeling abnormal, ataxia, abnormal gait, tremors, anxiety, agitation, **worsening of seizures, suicidal ideation/behavior**
CV: Hypotension, chest pain, edema
EENT: Blurred vision, diplopia, nystagmus, rhinitis, sinusitis
GI: Nausea, constipation, diarrhea, anorexia, vomiting, abdominal pain, gastritis, dry mouth, thirst, **rectal hemorrhage**
GU: Frequency, UTI, vaginitis

Adverse effects: *italic* = common, **bold** = life-threatening

INTEG: Purpura, rash, acne
RESP: Rhinitis, URI
SYST: **Angioedema, anaphylaxis, Stevens-Johnson syndrome, toxic epidermal necrolysis**

Contraindications: Hypersensitivity

Precautions: Pregnancy **C**, breastfeeding, children <4 yr, hypersensitivity to carbamazepine, renal disease, fluid restriction, hyponatremia

Pharmacokinetics

Absorption	Unknown
Distribution	Unknown
Metabolism	Liver
Excretion	Unknown
Half-life	Unknown

Pharmacodynamics

Onset	Unknown
Peak	4-6 hr
Duration	Unknown

Interactions
Individual products
Alcohol: increased CNS depression
Carbamazepine: decreased carbamazepine level, decreased oxcarbazepine levels
Felodipine: decreased effects of felodipine
Nisoldipine, ranolazine: do not use concurrently
Phenobarbital, valproic acid, verapamil: decreased oxcarbazepine level
Phenytoin: decreased oxcarbazepine level
Drug classifications
Contraceptives (oral): decreased oral contraceptive level
MAOIs: do not use concurrently
Drug/herb
Ginkgo: increased anticonvulsant effect
Ginseng, santonica: decreased anticonvulsant effect

NURSING CONSIDERATIONS
Assessment
• Assess seizure activity, including frequency, duration, and aura; provide seizure precautions
• Assess mental status including mood, sensorium, affect, behavioral changes; if mental status changes, notify prescriber
• Assess eye problems: ophthalmic examinations (slit lamp, funduscopy, tonometry) are needed before, during, after treatment
• Assess patient for hypersensitivity to carbamazepine
• Assess for serious reactions: angioedema, anaphylaxis, Stevens-Johnson syndrome

Nursing diagnoses
• Injury, risk for (side effects)
• Knowledge, deficient (teaching)

Implementation
• Store product at room temperature
• Provide assistance with ambulation during early part of treatment; dizziness may occur
• Give product with food, milk to decrease GI symptoms

Patient/family education
• Caution patient to avoid driving, other activities that require alertness
• Advise patient not to discontinue medication quickly after long-term use
• Instruct patient to avoid use of alcohol while taking this medication
• Instruct patient to use alternate contraception if using hormonal method
• Advise patient to use hard candy or gum for dry mouth, rinse mouth frequently
• Advise patient to carry/wear emergency ID stating name, products taken, condition, prescriber's name and phone number

Evaluation
Positive therapeutic outcome
• Decreased seizure activity

Treatment of overdose: Activated charcoal, give 0.9% NaCl (hypotensive state), atropine (bradycardia); use benzodiazepines, barbiturates for seizures

---

oxybutynin (Rx)
(ox-i-byoo´ti-nin)
Ditropan, Ditropan XL, Gelnique, oxybutynin, Oxytrol Transdermal
Func. class.: Anticholinergic
Chem. class.: Synthetic tertiary amine
Pregnancy category B

Do not confuse:
Ditropan/diazepam

Action: Relaxes smooth muscles in urinary tract by inhibiting acetylcholine at postganglionic sites

Therapeutic outcome: Decreased symptoms of urgency, nocturia, incontinence

Uses: Antispasmodic for neurogenic bladder, overactive bladder

Dosage and routes
Adult: PO 5 mg bid-tid, max 5 mg qid; EXT REL tabs 5-10 mg/day, may increase by 5 mg, max 30 mg/day; transdermal apply one patch to abdomen, hip, buttock 2 ×/wk (q3-4day);

GEL apply contents of 1 packet to abdomen, upper arms, shoulders, thighs

Geriatric: PO 2.5-5 mg tid, increase by 2.5 mg q several days

Child >6 yr: PO 5 mg bid, not to exceed 5 mg tid; EXT REL 5 mg/day, max 20 mg/day

Child 1-5 yr: PO 0.2 mg/kg/dose 2-4 ×/day

Available forms: Syr 5 mg/5 ml; tabs 5 mg; ext rel tabs 5, 10, 15 mg; transdermal 3.9 mg/day; top gel 10% (Gelnique)

Adverse effects

CNS: Anxiety, restlessness, dizziness, somnolence, insomnia, nervousness, **seizures,** headache, drowsiness, confusion

CV: Palpitations, sinus tachycardia, hypertension, peripheral edema

EENT: Blurred vision, increased intraocular tension; dry mouth, throat, dry eyes

GI: Nausea, vomiting, anorexia, abdominal pain, constipation, *dyspepsia,* diarrhea, taste perversion, GERD

GU: Dysuria, impotence, retention, hesitancy

Contraindications: Hypersensitivity, GI obstruction, GU obstruction, glaucoma, severe colitis, myasthenia gravis, unstable CV, infants

Precautions: Pregnancy **B**, breastfeeding, children <12 yr, geriatric, suspected glaucoma, cardiac disease, dementia

Pharmacokinetics	
Absorption	Rapidly absorbed
Distribution	Unknown
Metabolism	Liver
Excretion	Unknown
Half-life	Unknown

Pharmacodynamics	
Onset	½-1 hr
Peak	3-4 hr
Duration	6-10 hr

Interactions

Individual drugs

Acetaminophen: decreased levels of acetaminophen

Amantadine: increased anticholinergic effects

Atenolol: increased levels of atenolol

Digoxin: increased levels of digoxin

Haloperidol: decreased levels of haloperidol

Levodopa: decreased levels of levodopa

Nitrofurantoin: increased levels of nitrofurantoin

Drug classifications

Antihistamines, other anticholinergics: increased anticholinergic effects

CYP3A4 inducers: decreased effects of oxybutynin

CYP3A4 inhibitors: altered pharmacokinetic parameters

Phenothiazines: increased or decreased levels of phenothiazines

Drug/herb

Black catechu: increased constipation

Butterbur, jimsonweed, scopolia: increased anticholinergic action

Jamborandi tree, pill-bearing spurge: decreased anticholinergic effect

NURSING CONSIDERATIONS

Assessment

- Assess for allergic reactions: rash, urticaria; if these occur, product should be discontinued
- Assess urinary patterns: distention, nocturia, frequency, urgency, incontinence; catheterization may be required to remove residual urine

Nursing diagnoses

- Knowledge, deficient (teaching)
- Pain, acute (uses)
- Urinary elimination, impaired (uses)

Implementation

PO route

- Do not break, crush, or chew ext rel tabs
- May be given with meals or fluids or on an empty stomach

Topical route

- Rotate sites
- Delivers 100 mg

Transdermal route

- Delivers 3.9 mg/day

Patient/family education

- Advise patient to avoid hazardous activities until response to product is known; dizziness, blurred vision may occur
- Caution patient to avoid OTC medication with alcohol or other CNS depressants
- Advise patient to prevent photophobia by wearing sunglasses
- Teach patient to use frequent rinsing of mouth, sips of water for dry mouth
- Teach patient to stay cool; avoid hot weather, strenuous activity since overheating may occur; product decreases perspiration
- Advise patient to report CNS effects: confusion, anxiety, anticholinergic effect in the geriatric

Evaluation

Positive therapeutic outcome

- Absence of dysuria, frequency, nocturia, incontinence

Adverse effects: *italic* = common, **bold** = life-threatening

! HIGH ALERT

oxycodone (Rx)
(ox-i-koe'done)
Endocodone, M-oxy, OxyContin, OxyFast, Oxyl R, Roxicodone, Roxicodone SR, Supeudol ✦

oxycodone/acetaminophen (Rx)
Endocet ✦, Oxycocet ✦, Percocet, Roxicet, Roxilox, Tylox

oxycodone/aspirin (Rx)
Endodan ✦, Oxycodan ✦, Percodan, Percodan-Demi, Roxiprin

oxycodone/ibuprofen (Rx)
Combunox
Func. class.: Opiate analgesic
Chem. class.: Semisynthetic derivative

Pregnancy category B
Controlled substance schedule II

Do not confuse:
Percodan/Decadron, Roxicet/Roxanol, Tylox/Trimox/Wymox/Xanax

Action: Inhibits ascending pain pathways in CNS, increases pain threshold, alters pain perception

Therapeutic outcome: Decreased pain

Uses: Moderate to severe pain

Unlabeled uses: Postherpetic neuralgia (cont rel)

Dosage and routes
Adult: PO 10-30 mg q4hr (5 mg q6hr for Oxyl R, OxyFast); **OxyFast CONC SOL is extremely concentrated, do not use interchangeably;** CONT REL 10 mg q12hr in opiate-naïve patients

Available forms: Oxycodone: cont rel tabs (OxyContin) 10, 20, 40, 80, 160 mg; immediate rel tabs 15, 30 mg; tabs 5 mg; immediate rel caps 5 mg; oral sol 5 mg/5 ml, 20 mg/ml; oxycodone with acetaminophen: tabs 5 mg/325 mg; caps 5 mg/500 mg; oral sol 5 mg/325 mg/5 ml; oxycodone with aspirin: 2.44, 4.88 mg/325 mg

Adverse effects
CNS: Drowsiness, dizziness, confusion, headache, sedation, euphoria, fatigue, abnormal dreams, thoughts, hallucinations
CV: Palpitations, bradycardia, change in B/P
EENT: Tinnitus, blurred vision, miosis, diplopia
GI: Nausea, vomiting, anorexia, constipation, cramps, gastritis, dyspepsia, biliary spasms

GU: Increased urinary output, dysuria, urinary retention
INTEG: Rash, urticaria, bruising, flushing, diaphoresis, pruritus
RESP: **Respiratory depression**

Contraindications: Hypersensitivity, addiction (opiate), asthma, ileus

Black Box Warning: Respiratory depression

Precautions: Pregnancy **B**, breastfeeding, children <18 yr, addictive personality, increased ICP, MI (acute), severe heart disease, renal/hepatic disease, bowel impaction

Black Box Warning: Opioid-naïve patients, substance abuse

Pharmacokinetics
Absorption	Well absorbed
Distribution	Widely distributed; crosses placenta, protein binding 45%
Metabolism	Liver, extensively
Excretion	Kidneys, breast milk
Half-life	3-5 hr

Pharmacodynamics
	PO	RECT
Onset	15-30 min	Unknown
Peak	½-1 hr	Unknown
Duration	3-4 hr	4-6 hr

Interactions
Individual drugs
Alcohol: increased respiratory depression, hypotension, sedation
Cimetidine: increased toxicity
Drug classifications
Antipsychotics, CNS depressants, opioids, sedative/hypnotics, skeletal muscle relaxants: increased respiratory depression, hypotension
MAOIs: increased toxicity
Drug/herb
Corkwood: increased anticholinergic effect
Gotu kola, Jamaican dogwood, kava, lavender, mistletoe, nettle, pokeweed, poppy, senega, St. John's wort, valerian: increased sedative effect
Drug/lab test
Increased: amylase, lipase

NURSING CONSIDERATIONS
Assessment
• Monitor VS after parenteral route; note muscle rigidity, product history, renal, liver function tests, respiratory dysfunction: respira-

tory depression, character, rate, rhythm; notify prescriber if respirations are <10/min
• Monitor CNS changes: dizziness, drowsiness, hallucinations, euphoria, LOC, pupil reaction
• Monitor allergic reactions: rash, urticaria
• Assess bowel status: constipation; stimulant laxative may be needed

Nursing diagnoses
• Breathing pattern, ineffective (adverse reactions)
• Injury, risk for (adverse reactions)
• Knowledge, deficient (teaching)
• Pain, acute (uses)
• Pain, chronic
• Sensory perception, disturbed: visual, auditory (adverse reactions)

Implementation
• Give with antiemetic if nausea, vomiting occur
• Give when pain is beginning to return; determine dosage interval by patient response; continuous dosing of medication is more effective than when given prn
• Medication should be slowly withdrawn after long-term use to prevent withdrawal symptoms
• Store in light-resistant container at room temperature

PO route
• Do not break, crush, or chew cont rel tabs; give q12hr, no more frequently
• May be given with food or milk to lessen GI upset
• Use 80, 160 mg cont rel tabs only in opioid-tolerant patients

Rectal route
• Store supp in the refrigerator; run under warm water before insertion

Patient/family education
• Advise patients to avoid CNS depressants: alcohol, sedative/hypnotics
• Discuss with patient that dizziness, drowsiness, and confusion are common; to avoid getting up without assistance
• Discuss in detail all aspects of the product, including purpose and what to expect
• Advise patient to make position changes slowly to lessen orthostatic hypotension
• Advise patient to avoid CNS depressants, alcohol
• Advise patient to avoid operating machinery, driving if drowsiness occurs

Evaluation
Positive therapeutic outcome
• Decreased pain

Treatment of overdose: Naloxone 0.2-0.8 **IV**, O_2, **IV** fluids, vasopressors

oxymetazoline nasal agent
See Appendix B

oxymetazoline ophthalmic
See Appendix B

⚠ HIGH ALERT

oxymorphone (Rx)
(ox-i-mor'fone)
Numorphan, Opana, Opana ER
Func. class.: Opiate analgesic
Chem. class.: Semisynthetic phenanthrene derivative

Pregnancy category B
Controlled substance schedule II

Action: Depresses pain impulse transmission at the spinal cord level by interacting with opioid receptors

Therapeutic outcome: Decreased pain

Uses: Moderate to severe pain

Dosage and routes
Adult: IM/SUBCUT 1-1.5 mg q4-6hr prn; **IV** 0.5 mg q4-6hr prn; RECT 5 mg q4-6hr prn; PO (immediate release only) 5-20 mg q4-6hr prn; PO-ER 5 mg q12hr in those requiring around the clock dosing

Labor analgesia
Adult: IM 0.5-1 mg

Available forms: Inj 1, 1.5 mg/ml; supp 5 mg; ER tab 5, 10, 20, 40 mg; tabs 5, 10 mg

Adverse effects
CNS: Drowsiness, dizziness, confusion, headache, sedation, euphoria (geriatric), **seizures,** hallucinations, **increased ICP**
CV: Palpitations, **bradycardia,** change in B/P, hypotension
EENT: Tinnitus, blurred vision, miosis, diplopia
GI: Nausea, vomiting, anorexia, constipation, cramps
GU: Dysuria, urinary retention
INTEG: Rash, urticaria, bruising, flushing, diaphoresis, pruritus
RESP: **Respiratory depression**

O

Adverse effects: *italic* = common, **bold** = life-threatening

Contraindications: Hypersensitivity, addiction (opioid), asthma, hepatic disease, ileus, intrathecal use, surgery

Black Box Warning: Respiratory depression, alcoholism, opioid-naïve patients, substance abuse

Precautions: Pregnancy **B** (short-term), breastfeeding, children <18 yr, addictive personality, increased ICP, MI (acute), severe heart disease, respiratory depression, renal/hepatic disease, bowel impaction

Pharmacokinetics

Absorption	Well absorbed (RECT, IM, SUBCUT); completely absorbed **(IV)**
Distribution	Widely distributed; crosses placenta
Metabolism	Liver, extensively
Excretion	Kidneys
Half-life	2½-4 hr

Pharmacodynamics

	IM/SUBCUT	IV	RECT
Onset	15 min	10 min	30 min
Peak	1-1½ hr	15-30 min	Unknown
Duration	3-6 hr	3-4 hr	3-6 hr

Interactions
Individual drugs
Alcohol: increased respiratory depression, hypotension, sedation
Drug classifications
CNS depressants, opiates, antipsychotics, skeletal muscle relaxants, sedative/hypnotics: increased respiratory depression, hypotension
MAOIs: do not use 2 wk before oxymorphone; unpredictable effects
Drug/herb
Corkwood: increased anticholinergic effect
Gotu kola, Jamaican dogwood, kava, lavender, mistletoe, nettle, pokeweed, poppy, senega, St. John's wort, valerian: increased sedative effect
Drug/lab test
Increased: amylase

NURSING CONSIDERATIONS
Assessment
• Assess for pain: location, intensity, type, other characteristics, before and 1 hr after (IM); 30 min **(IV)**; need for pain medication, physical dependence
• Assess bowel/bladder status: constipation, may need stimulant laxative; I&O ratio for decreasing output, may indicate urinary retention

• Monitor VS after parenteral route; note muscle rigidity, product history, liver, kidney function tests, respiratory dysfunction: respiratory depression, character, rate, rhythm; notify prescriber if respirations are <10/min
• Monitor CNS changes: dizziness, drowsiness, hallucinations, euphoria, LOC, pupil reaction
• Monitor allergic reactions: rash, urticaria

Nursing diagnoses
• Breathing pattern, ineffective (adverse reactions)
• Injury, risk for (adverse reactions)
• Knowledge, deficient (teaching)
• Pain, acute (uses)
• Sensory perception, disturbed: visual, auditory (adverse reactions)

Implementation
• Give 1 hr before or 2 hr after food (PO)
• Give with antiemetic if nausea, vomiting occur
• Do not break, crush, chew ER product
• Give when pain is beginning to return; determine dosage interval by patient response; continuous dosing of medication is more effective than when given prn
• Medication should be slowly withdrawn after long-term use to prevent withdrawal symptoms
• Store in light-resistant container at room temperature
Rectal route
• Store in refrigerator
IV route
• Give by direct **IV** undiluted over 2-3 min
Y-site compatibilities: Glycopyrrolate, hydrOXYzine, ranitidine

Patient/family education
• Advise patients to avoid CNS depressants: alcohol, sedative/hypnotics
• Discuss with patient that dizziness, drowsiness, and confusion are common; to avoid getting up without assistance
• Discuss in detail all aspects of the product, including purpose and what to expect
• Advise patient to make position changes slowly to lessen orthostatic hypotension
• Advise patient not to drive, operate machinery if drowsiness occurs
• Advise patient to avoid CNS depressants, alcohol

Evaluation
Positive therapeutic outcome
• Decreased pain

Treatment of overdose: Naloxone (Narcan) 0.2-0.8 mg **IV**, O_2, **IV** fluids, vasopressors

! HIGH ALERT

oxytocin 😊 (Rx)
(ox-i-toe'sin)
Pitocin
Func. class.: Oxytocic hormone

Pregnancy category N/A

Action: Acts directly on myofibrils, producing uterine contraction; stimulates breast milk letdown, vasoactive antidiuretic effect

Therapeutic outcome: Stimulation of labor, control of bleeding; stimulation of milk letdown

Uses: Stimulation, induction of labor; missed or incomplete abortion; postpartum bleeding

Dosage and routes
Labor induction
Adult: **IV** 0.5-2 milliunit/min, increase by 1-2 milliunit q15-60min until regular contractions occur, then decrease dosage

Postpartum hemorrhage
Adult: **IV** 10-40 units in 1000 ml nonhydrating diluent infused at 20-40 milliunit/min
Adult: IM 3-10 units after placenta delivery

Incomplete abortion
Adult: **IV** INF 10 units/500 ml D₅W or 0.9% NaCl run at 10-20 milliunit/min, max 30 units/12 hr

Fetal stress test
Adult: **IV** 0.5 milliunit/min; increase q20min until 3 contractions occur at 10 min

Available forms: Inj 10 units/ml

Adverse effects
CNS: **Seizures, tetanic contractions**
CV: Hypo/hypertension, dysrhythmias, increased pulse, bradycardia, tachycardia, premature ventricular contractions
FETUS: Dysrhythmias, jaundice, hypoxia, **intracranial hemorrhage**
GI: Anorexia, nausea, vomiting, constipation
GU: **Abruptio placentae, decreased uterine blood flow**
HEMA: Increased hyperbilirubinemia
INTEG: Rash
RESP: **Asphyxia**
SYST: Water intoxication of mother

Contraindications: Hypersensitivity, serum toxemia, cephalopelvic disproportion, fetal distress, hypertonic uterus, prolapsed umbilical cord, active genital herpes

Precautions: Cervical/uterine surgery, uterine sepsis, primipara >35 yr, 1st/2nd stage of labor

Black Box Warning: Elective induction of labor

Pharmacokinetics
Absorption	Well absorbed (nasal); completely absorbed (**IV**)
Distribution	Widely distributed (extracellular fluid)
Metabolism	Liver, rapidly
Excretion	Kidneys
Half-life	3-12 min

Pharmacodynamics
	NASAL	IV	IM
Onset	5 min	Rapid	3-7 min
Peak	Unknown	Unknown	Unknown
Duration	20 min	1 hr	1 hr

Interactions
Drug classifications
Vasopressors: increased hypertension
Drug/herb
Ephedra: hypertension

NURSING CONSIDERATIONS
Assessment
• Assess labor contractions: fetal heart tones, frequency, duration, intensity of contractions; if fetal heart tones increase or decrease significantly or if contractions are longer than 1 min, notify prescriber; turn patient on left side to increase oxygen to fetus
🔷 Assess for water intoxication: confusion, anuria, drowsiness, headache; notify prescriber
• Watch for fetal distress, acceleration, deceleration, fetal presentation, pelvic dimensions
• Monitor B/P, pulse, respiratory rate, rhythm, depth
• Monitor I&O ratio
• Provide an environment conducive to letdown reflex

Nursing diagnoses
• Breastfeeding, ineffective (uses)
• Injury, risk for (uses)
• Knowledge, deficient (teaching)

Implementation
IV route
• Use an inf pump; rotate sol for mixing; have magnesium sulfate available
• For labor induction administer after diluting 10 units/L of D₅W, 0.9% NaCl, 0.45% NaCl, LR, Ringer's for a conc of 10 units/ml; start at 1-2 milliunits/min (0.1-0.2 ml); may increase by 1-2 milliunits/min q15-30min until labor begins

Adverse effects: *italic* = common, **bold** = life-threatening

- For threatened abortion administer after diluting 10 units/500 ml of D_5W, $D_{10}W$, 0.9% NaCl, 0.45% NaCl, LR, Ringer's for a conc of 20 units/ml; give at 10-40 milliunits/min
- For postpartum bleeding administer after diluting 10-40 milliunits/L of D_5W, $D_{10}W$, 0.9% NaCl, 0.45% NaCl, LR, Ringer's for a conc of 10-40 units/ml; may titrate to response

Y-site compatibilities: Heparin, regular insulin, hydrocortisone, meperidine, morphine, potassium chloride, vit B/C, warfarin
Additive compatibilities: Chloramphenicol, metaraminol, netilmicin, sodium bicarbonate, thiopental, verapamil
Additive incompatibilities: Fibrinolysin, warfarin

Patient/family education

- Teach patient to report increased blood loss, abdominal cramps, increased temp or foul-smelling lochia
- Advise patient that contractions will be similar to menstrual cramps, gradually increasing in intensity

Evaluation
Positive therapeutic outcome

- Stimulation of milk letdown (nasal)
- Induction of labor
- Decreased postpartum bleeding

---

paclitaxel (Rx)
(pa-kli-tax′el)
Onxol, Taxol
paclitaxel protein-bound particles (Rx)
Abraxane
Func. class.: Antineoplastic—miscellaneous
Chem. class.: Natural diterpene, antimicrotubule

Pregnancy category D

Do not confuse:
paclitaxel/paroxetine/Paxil, Taxol/Paxil/Taxotere

Action: Inhibits the reorganization of the microtubule network needed for interphase and mitotic cellular functions; also causes abnormal bundles of microtubules during cell cycle and multiple esters of microtubules during mitosis

Therapeutic outcome: Prevention of rapidly growing malignant cells

Uses: Taxol: metastatic carcinoma of the ovary unresponsive to other treatment, breast carcinoma, AIDS-related Kaposi's sarcoma

(second line), non–small cell lung cancer (first line), adjuvant treatment for node-positive breast cancer; Onxol: failure of other treatment in breast cancer, advanced ovarian cancer, bladder cancer

Unlabeled uses: Advanced head, neck, small cell lung cancer; non-Hodgkin's lymphoma, adenocarcinoma of the upper GI tract, hormone-refractory prostate cancer

Dosage and routes
Paclitaxel
Ovarian carcinoma
Adult: **IV** INF 135 mg/m² given over 24 hr q3wk, then cisplatin 75 mg/m² or 175 mg/m² over 3 hr q3wk or 175 mg/m² over 3 hr

Advanced ovarian carcinoma
Adult: **IV** INF 175 mg/m² with cisplatin 75 mg/m² over 3 hr q3wk

Breast carcinoma
Adult: **IV** INF 175 mg/m² over 3 hr q3wk × 4 courses

AIDS-related Kaposi's sarcoma
Adult: **IV** INF 135 mg/m² over 3 hr q3wk or 100 mg/m² over 3 hr q2wk

1st line non–small cell lung cancer
Adult: **IV** INF 135 mg/m²/24 hr with cisplatin 75 mg/m² × 3 wk

Paclitaxel protein-bound particles
Adult: **IV** 260 mg/m² q3wk

Available forms: Inj 30 mg/5-ml vial, 100 mg/16.7-ml vial, 150 mg/24-ml vial, 300 mg/5-ml vials; powder for inj, lyophilized 100 mg in single-use vials (Abraxane)

Adverse effects
CNS: Peripheral neuropathy
CV: Bradycardia, hypotension, abnormal ECG, supraventricular tachycardia (SVT)
GI: Nausea, vomiting, diarrhea, mucositis; increased bilirubin, alkaline phosphatase, AST
HEMA: **Neutropenia, leukopenia, thrombocytopenia, anemia,** bleeding, infections
INTEG: Alopecia, tissue necrosis, generalized urticaria
MS: Arthralgia, myalgia
RESP: **Pulmonary embolism,** dyspnea
SYST: Hypersensitivity reactions, **anaphylaxis, Stevens-Johnson syndrome, toxic epidermal necrolysis, angioedema**

Contraindications: Pregnancy **D,** hypersensitivity to paclitaxel or other products with polyoxyethylated castor oil, albumin

Black Box Warning: Neutropenia (neutrophils <1500/mm³)

Precautions: Breastfeeding, children, CV/hepatic disease, CNS disorder, renal disease, bone marrow suppression, dental disease/work, extravasation, females, geriatric patients, herpes, infection, infertility, jaundice, ocular exposure, radiation therapy, thrombocytopenia, vaccination

Black Box Warning: Taxane hypersensitivity

Pharmacokinetics

Absorption	Completely absorbed
Distribution	89%-98% protein binding
Metabolism	Liver, extensively
Excretion	Unknown
Half-life	5-17 hr

Pharmacodynamics

Onset	Unknown
Peak	1-2 wk
Duration	3 wk

Interactions
Individual drugs
CycloSPORINE, dexamethasone, diazepam, etoposide, quinidine, teniposide, testosterone, verapamil, vinCRIStine: decreased metabolism of paclitaxel
DOXOrubicin: increased levels of DOXOrubicin
Ketoconazole: increased toxicity, decreased metabolism; avoid concurrent use
Radiation: increased myelosuppression
Drug classifications
Anticoagulants, NSAIDs: increased bleeding risk
Antineoplastics: increased myelosuppression
CYP2C8, CYP2C9 inducers: decreased paclitaxel level
Vaccines (live virus): decreased immune response

NURSING CONSIDERATIONS
Assessment
• Assess CNS changes: confusion, paresthesias, psychosis, tremors, seizures, neuropathies; product should be discontinued
• Check buccal cavity q8hr for dryness, sores or ulceration, white patches, oral pain, bleeding, dysphagia; obtain prescription for viscous lidocaine (Xylocaine) to use in mouth
• Assess symptoms indicating severe allergic reaction, anaphylaxis: rash, pruritus, urticaria, purpuric skin lesions, itching, flushing
• Monitor CBC, differential, platelet count weekly; withhold product if WBC is <1500/mm^3 or platelet count is <100,000/mm^3, notify prescriber of results

• Monitor renal function tests: BUN, creatinine, serum uric acid, urine CCr before, during therapy; check I&O ratio; report fall in urine output to <30 ml/hr
• Monitor temp q4hr (may indicate beginning of infection)
• Monitor liver function tests before, during therapy (bilirubin, AST, ALT, LDH) as needed or monthly; check for jaundice of skin and sclera, dark urine, clay-colored stools, itchy skin, abdominal pain, fever, diarrhea
• Assess for bleeding: hematuria, stool guaiac, bruising or petechiae, mucosa or orifices q8hr; check for inflammation of mucosa, breaks in skin
• Assess effects of alopecia on body image; discuss feelings about body changes

Nursing diagnoses
• Body image, disturbed (adverse reactions)
• Infection, risk for (adverse reactions)
• Injury, risk for (adverse reactions)
• Knowledge, deficient (teaching)

Implementation
• Give fluids PO before chemotherapy to hydrate patient
• Confirm that dexamethasone was given 12 hr and 6 hr before inf begins; provide antiemetic 30-60 min before giving product and prn to prevent vomiting; administer antibiotics for prophylaxis of infection
• Give topical or systemic analgesics for pain to lessen effects of stomatitis
• Give liquid diet: carbonated beverages; gelatin may be added if patient is not nauseated or vomiting
IV route
• Check for extravasation, if given by regular **IV**, not port
• Give after diluting in 0.9% NaCl, D$_5$, D$_5$ and 0.9% NaCl, D$_5$LR to a concentration of 0.3-1.2 mg/ml
• Use an in-line filter ≤0.22 mcg
• Give after premedicating with dexamethasone 20 mg PO 12 and 6 hr before paclitaxel, diphenhydrAMINE 50 mg **IV** ½-1 hr before paclitaxel and cimetidine 300 mg or ranitidine 50 mg **IV** ½-1 hr before paclitaxel
• Use only glass bottles, polypropylene, polyolefin bags and administration sets; do not use PVC inf bags or sets
• Use gloves and cytotoxic handling precautions
Abraxane
• Reconstitute vial by injecting 20 ml of 0.9% NaCl
• Slowly inject the 20 ml of 0.9% NaCl over at least 1 min to direct the sol flow on wall of vial

P

- Do not inject 0.9% NaCl directly onto lyophilized cake (foaming will occur)
- Allow vial to sit for at least 5 min to ensure proper wetting of lyophilized cake
- Gently swirl or invert vial slowly for at least 2 min until completely dissolved
- Calculate dosing by: Dosing volume (ml) = total dose (mg) ÷ 5 (mg/ml)

Y-site compatiblilities: Acyclovir, amikacin, aminophylline, bleomycin, butorphanol, calcium chloride, carboplatin, cefepime, cefotetan, ceftazidime, ceftriaxone, cimetidine, cisplatin, cyclophosphamide, cytarabine, dacarbazine, dexamethasone, diphenhydrAMINE, DOXOrubicin, droperidol, etoposide, famotidine, floxuridine, fluconazole, fluorouracil, furosemide, ganciclovir, gentamicin, haloperidol, heparin, mannitol, meperidine, mesna, methotrexate, metoclopramide, morphine, nalbuphine, ondansetron, pentostatin, potassium chloride, prochlorperazine, propofol, ranitidine, sodium bicarbonate, vancomycin, vinBLAStine, vinCRIStine, zidovudine

Patient/family education

- Inform patient that nonhormonal contraceptive measures are recommended during therapy and >4 mo after; teratogenic effects are possible
- Teach patient to avoid use of products containing aspirin or ibuprofen, razors, commercial mouthwash, since bleeding may occur; to report symptoms of bleeding (hematuria, tarry stools)
- Instruct patient to report signs of anemia (fatigue, headache, irritability, faintness, shortness of breath) and CNS reactions (confusion, psychosis, nightmares, seizures, severe headaches)
- Teach patient to rinse mouth tid-qid with water, club soda; brush teeth bid-qid with soft brush or cotton-tipped applicators for stomatitis; use unwaxed dental floss
- Inform patient that hair may be lost during treatment; a wig or hairpiece may make patient feel better; new hair may be different in color, texture
- Inform patient that receiving vaccinations during therapy may cause serious reactions

Evaluation
Positive therapeutic outcome
- Prevention of rapid division of malignant cells

paliperidone (Rx)
(pal-ee-per′i-done)
Invega, Invega Sustenna
Func. class.: Antipsychotic
Chem. class.: Benzisoxazole derivative

Pregnancy category C

Do not confuse:
Invega/Iveegan, paliperidone/risperidone

Action: Mediated through both dopamine type 2 (D_2) and serotonin type 2 (5-HT_2) antagonism

Therapeutic outcome: Decrease in emotional excitement, hallucinations, delusions, paranoia; reorganization of patterns of thought, speech

Uses: Schizophrenia

Dosage and routes
Adult: PO 6 mg/day; IM 234 mg on day 1, then 156 mg 1 wk later, after 2nd dose, give 117 mg qmo, range 39-234 mg, max 12 mg/day

Renal dose
Adult: PO CCr 50-79 ml/min, max 6 mg/day; CCr 10-49 ml/min, max 3 mg/day

Available forms: Ext rel tabs 3, 6, 9 mg; ext rel susp for inj 39 mg/0.25 ml, 78 mg/0.5 ml, 117 mg/0.75 ml, 156 mg/1 ml, 234 mg/1.5 ml

Adverse effects
CNS: EPS, pseudoparkinsonism, akathisia, dystonia, tardive dyskinesia; drowsiness, insomnia, agitation, anxiety, headache, **seizures, neuroleptic malignant syndrome,** dizziness
CV: Orthostatic hypotension, **tachycardia, heart failure, QT prolongation,** heart block, dysrhythmias
EENT: Blurred vision
ENDO: Insulin increase
GI: Nausea, vomiting, *anorexia, constipation,* weight gain, xerostomia

Contraindications: Breastfeeding, seizure disorders, AV block, geriatric, QT prolongation, torsades de pointes, hypersensitivity to this product or risperidone

Precautions: Pregnancy C, children, renal/hepatic disease, obesity, Parkinson's disease

Black Box Warning: Dementia

Pharmacokinetics

Absorption	Unknown
Distribution	Unknown
Metabolism	Unknown
Excretion	80% urine, 11% feces
Half-life	Elimination 23 hr

Pharmacodynamics

Onset	Unknown
Peak	24 hr
Duration	Unknown

Interactions
Individual drugs
Abarelix, alfuzosin, amoxapine, apomorphine, chloroquine, dasatinib, dolasetron, droperidol, flecainide, pimozide, probucol: increased QT prolongation
Alcohol: increased sedation
Levodopa: decreased levodopa effect
Paliperidone: increased excretion
Drug classifications
Azole antifungals; β-blockers; class IA, III antidysrhythmics; halogenated anesthetics; some antipsychotics; some phenothiazines; tricyclics (high doses): increased QT prolongation
Other antipsychotics: increased EPS
Other CNS depressants, sedatives/hypnotics, opiates: increased sedation
Drug/herb
Betel palm, kava: increased EPS
Cola tree, hops, nettle, nutmeg: increased action
Kava: increased CNS depression
Drug/lab test
Increased: prolactin levels

NURSING CONSIDERATIONS
Assessment
- Assess mental status before initial administration
- Monitor for swallowing of PO medication; check for hoarding or giving of medication to other patients
- Monitor I&O ratio; palpate bladder if urinary output is low
- Assess affect, orientation, LOC, reflexes, gait, coordination, sleep pattern disturbances
- Monitor B/P standing and lying; also pulse, respirations; take these q4hr during initial treatment; establish baseline before starting treatment; report drops of 30 mm Hg; watch for ECG changes
- Assess for dizziness, faintness, palpitations, tachycardia on rising
- Assess for EPS, including akathisia, tardive dyskinesia (bizarre movements of the jaw, mouth, tongue, extremities), pseudoparkinsonism (rigidity, tremors, pill rolling, shuffling gait)
- ◆ Assess for serious reactions in the geriatric patient
- ◆ Assess for neuroleptic malignant syndrome: hyperthermia, increased CPK, altered mental status, muscle rigidity
- Assess skin turgor daily
- Assess for constipation, urinary retention daily; if these occur, increase bulk and water in diet

Nursing diagnoses
- Knowledge, deficient (teaching)
- Noncompliance (teaching)

Implementation
- Do not break, crush, or chew ext rel tabs
- Give without regard for food
- Give a reduced dose to the geriatric patient
- Give antiparkinsonian agent on order from prescriber; to be used for EPS
- Avoid use with CNS depressants
- Supervise ambulation until patient is stabilized on medication; do not involve in strenuous exercise program, because fainting is possible; patient should not stand still for a long time
- Increase fluids to prevent constipation
- Decrease stimulus by dimming lights, avoiding loud noise
- Provide sips of water, candy, gum for dry mouth
- Store in airtight, light-resistant container

Patient/family education
- Advise patient that orthostatic hypotension may occur and to rise from sitting or lying position gradually
- Advise patient to avoid hot tubs, hot showers, tub baths; hypotension may occur
- Caution patient to avoid abrupt withdrawal of this product; EPS may result; product should be withdrawn slowly
- Teach patient to avoid OTC preparations (cough, hay fever, cold) unless approved by prescriber; serious product interactions may occur; avoid use of alcohol; increased drowsiness may occur
- Advise patient to avoid hazardous activities if drowsy or dizzy
- Teach patient compliance with product regimen; non-absorbable tab shell is expelled in stool
- Teach patient to report impaired vision, tremors, muscle twitching

P

- Caution patient that heat stroke may occur in hot weather; take extra precautions to stay cool
- Teach patient to use contraception, inform prescriber if pregnancy is planned or suspected

Evaluation
Positive therapeutic outcome
- Decrease in emotional excitement, hallucinations, delusions, paranoia; reorganization of patterns of thought, speech

Treatment of overdose: Lavage if orally ingested; provide airway; *do not induce vomiting*

---

palivizumab (Rx)
(pal-ih-viz′uh-mab)
Synagis
Func. class.: Monoclonal antibody

Pregnancy category C

Action: A humanized monoclonal antibody that exhibits neutralizing and fusion-inhibitory activity against respiratory syncytial virus (RSV)

Therapeutic outcome: Absence of RSV

Uses: Prevention of serious lower respiratory tract disease caused by RSV in pediatric patients

Dosage and routes
Child: IM 15 mg/kg monthly; those patients who develop RSV should continue to receive monthly doses during RSV season (November-April)

Available forms: Powder for reconstitution 50, 100 mg; sol 50 mg/0.5 ml, 100 mg/1 mg

Adverse effects
CNS: Fever
EENT: Otitis media, rhinitis, pharyngitis
GI: Nausea, vomiting, diarrhea, increased AST
INTEG: Rash, inj site reaction
RESP: Upper respiratory tract infection, **apnea,** cough
SYST: **Anaphylaxis, angioedema**

Contraindications: Hypersensitivity, adults, cyanotic congenital heart disease

Precautions: Pregnancy C, thrombocytopenia, coagulation disorders, established RSV, congenital heart disease, chronic lung disease, systemic allergic reactions

---

Absorption	Unknown
Distribution	Unknown
Metabolism	Unknown
Excretion	Unknown
Half-life	20 days

Unknown

NURSING CONSIDERATIONS
Assessment
- Assess for presence of RSV infection; product is given to prevent infection
- Assess for side effects and report if allergic reaction is evident
◆ Assess for anaphylaxis: difficulty breathing; product should be discontinued; have emergency equipment nearby

Nursing diagnoses
- Infection, risk for (uses)
- Knowledge, deficient (teaching)

Implementation
- Give IM only
- Do not dilute prior to IM use
- Dosage >1 ml should be divided and injected in different sites
- Do not shake

Patient/family education
- Teach patient to report upper respiratory infections, earaches, rash, sore throat

Evaluation
Positive therapeutic outcome
- Absence of RSV

---

palonosetron (Rx)
(pa-lone-o′se-tron)
Aloxi
Func. class.: Antiemetic
Chem. class.: 5-HT$_3$ receptor antagonist

Pregnancy category B

Action: Prevents nausea, vomiting by blocking serotonin peripherally, centrally, and in the small intestine at the 5-HT$_3$ receptor

Therapeutic outcome: Decreased nausea, vomiting during chemotherapy

Uses: Prevention of nausea, vomiting associated with cancer chemotherapy; postoperative nausea/vomiting

Dosage and routes
Adult: PO 0.5 mg as a single dose 1 hr prior to chemotherapy; **IV** 0.25 mg as a single dose

over 30 sec, 30 min prior to chemotherapy, max 0.25 mg **IV** as a single dose

Postoperative nausea/vomiting prophylaxis for up to 24 hr after surgery
Adult: **IV** 0.075 mg given over 10 sec immediately before induction

Available forms: Inj 0.25 mg/5 ml

Adverse effects
CNS: Headache, dizziness, drowsiness, fatigue, insomnia
GI: Diarrhea, constipation, abdominal pain
MISC: Weakness, hyperkalemia, anxiety, rash, **bronchospasm** (rare), arthralgia, *fever, urinary retention*

Contraindications: Hypersensitivity

Precautions: Pregnancy **B**, breastfeeding, children, geriatric, with hypokalemia, hypomagnesemia

Pharmacokinetics

Absorption	Unknown
Distribution	62% protein bound
Metabolism	Liver
Excretion	Unchanged product and metabolites excreted by kidney
Half-life	40 hr

Pharmacodynamics
Unknown

Interactions
Individual drugs
Bepridil, chloroquine, clarithromycin, droperidol, erythromycin, grepafloxacin, halofantrine, haloperidol, methadone, pentamidine: possible QT prolongation
Drug classifications
Class 1A antidysrhythmics (disopyramide, procainamide, quinidine), class III antidysrhythmics (amiodarone, bretylium, dofetilide, ibutilide, sotalol), diuretics (except potassium sparing), some phenothiazines: possible QT prolongation

NURSING CONSIDERATIONS
Assessment
• Monitor for absence of nausea, vomiting during chemotherapy
• Assess hypersensitivity reaction: rash, bronchospasm

Nursing diagnoses
• Knowledge, deficient (teaching)

Implementation
IV route
• Give as a single dose over 30 sec
• Do not mix with other products; flush **IV** line before, after administration
• Store at room temperature

Patient/family education
• Teach to report diarrhea, constipation, rash, or changes in respirations or discomfort at insertion site

Evaluation
Positive therapeutic outcome
• Absence of nausea, vomiting during cancer chemotherapy

---

pamidronate (Rx)
(pam-i-drone'ate)
Aredia
Func. class.: Bone resorption inhibitor, electrolyte modifier
Chem. class.: Bisphosphonate
Pregnancy category D

Do not confuse:
Aredia/Adriamycin

Action: Inhibits bone resorption, apparently without inhibiting bone formation and mineralization; absorbs calcium phosphate crystals in bone and may directly block dissolution of hydroxyapatite crystals of bone

Therapeutic outcome: Serum calcium at normal level

Uses: Moderate to severe Paget's disease, hypercalcemia, osteolytic bone metastases in breast cancer patients, multiple myeloma

Unlabeled uses: Postmenopausal osteoporosis, hyperparathyroidism

Dosage and routes
Hypercalcemia of malignancy
Adult: **IV** INF 60-90 mg as a single dose in moderate hypercalcemia, 90 mg in severe hypercalcemia given over 2-24 hr; dose should be diluted in 1000 ml 0.45% NaCl, 0.9% NaCl, or D_5W; wait 7 days before 2nd course

Osteolytic lesions
Adult: **IV** 90 mg/500 ml of D_5W, 0.45% NaCl, or 0.9% NaCl given over 4 hr on a monthly basis (multiple myeloma) or over 2 hr q3-4wk (breast carcinoma)

Paget's disease
Adult: **IV** INF 30 mg/day given over 4 hr × 3 days

P

Available forms: Powder for inj 30, 90 mg/vial; inj 3, 6, 9 mg/ml

Adverse effects

CNS: Fatigue, fever

CV: Hypertension, **atrial fibrillation**

EENT: Ocular pain, inflammation, vision impairment

GI: Abdominal pain, anorexia, constipation, nausea, vomiting, dyspepsia

GU: **Renal failure**

INTEG: Redness, swelling, induration, pain on palpation at site of catheter insertion

META: Anemia, hypokalemia, hypomagnesemia, hypophosphatemia, hypocalcemia, hypothyroidism

MS: Severe bone pain, myalgia, **osteonecrosis of the jaw**

RESP: Coughing, dyspnea, URI

SYST: **Angioedema, anaphylaxis**

Contraindications: Pregnancy **D**, hypersensitivity to bisphosphonates

Precautions: Children, nursing mothers, renal dysfunction, poor dentition

Pharmacokinetics

Absorption	Rapidly cleared from circulation
Distribution	Mainly to bones, primarily in areas of high bone turnover
Metabolism	Unknown
Excretion	Kidneys, unchanged (50%)
Half-life	Biphasic 27 hr; from bone to 300 days

Pharmacodynamics

Onset	1 day
Peak	1 wk
Duration	Unknown

Interactions

Individual drugs

Calcium, vitamin D: decreased pamidronate effect

CycloSPORINE, tacrolimus, vancomycin: increased nephrotoxicity

Entecavir: increased effect of entecavir

Drug classifications

Aminoglycosides, NSAIDs, radiopaque contrast agents: increased nephrotoxicity

Loop diuretics: increased hypokalemia

NURSING CONSIDERATIONS

Assessment

• Assess for hypocalcemia: Chvostek's, Trousseau's sign, paresthesia, twitching, laryngospasm

• Assess dental health; cover with antiinfectives for dental extractions

• Assess for atrial fibrillation

• Monitor manifestations of hypocalcemia: personality changes, anxiety, disturbances, depression, psychosis; nausea, vomiting, constipation, abdominal pain from muscle spasm; decreased contractility, decreased cardiac output, hypotension, lengthened ST segment, prolonged QT interval; scaling eczema, alopecia, hyperpigmentation; tetany, muscle twitching, cramping, grimacing, seizure, altered deep tendon reflexes, spasm

• Monitor manifestations of hypomagnesemia: agitation; muscle twitching, paresthesia, hyperactive reflexes, positive Babinski reflex, dysphagia, nystagmus, seizures, tetany; nausea, vomiting, diarrhea, anorexia, abdominal distention; ectopy, tachycardia, broad, flat, or inverted T-waves, depressed ST segment, prolonged QT interval, decreased cardiac output, hypotension

• Monitor manifestations of hypokalemia: acidic urine, reduced urine osmolality, nocturia, polyuria, polydipsia; hypotension, broad T-wave, U-wave, ectopy, tachycardia, weak pulse; muscle weakness, altered LOC, drowsiness, apathy, lethargy, confusion, depression; anorexia, nausea, cramps, constipation, distention, paralytic ileus; hypoventilation, respiratory muscle weakness

• Assess fluid volume status: check I&O ratio and record, assess for distended red veins, crackles in lung, color, quality, and specific gravity of urine, skin turgor, adequacy of pulses, moist mucous membranes, bilateral lung sounds, peripheral pitting edema

• Monitor electrolytes: phosphorus, potassium, sodium, calcium, magnesium; also include BUN, creatinine, CBC, platelets, hemoglobin

• Assess B/P before, during therapy

• Assess for pain: in joints or on exertion, duration and characteristics; analgesics may be ordered

• Assess for phlebitis at **IV** site: swelling, redness, pain, warmth

Nursing diagnoses

• Fluid volume, excess (side effects)

• Injury, risk for (uses, adverse reactions)

• Knowledge, deficient (teaching)

Implementation

• Give by **IV** inf after reconstituting by adding 10 ml of sterile water for inj to each vial, then adding to 1000 ml of sterile 0.45%, 0.9% NaCl, D₅W, run over 4 hr for hypercalcemia or 60 mg ≥4 hr, 90 mg/24 hr; dilute reconstituted sol in 500 ml of 0.9% NaCl, 0.45% NaCl, or

 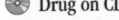

D_5W, give over 4 hr (multiple myeloma, Paget's disease)

• Do not mix with calcium-containing inf sol such as Ringer's sol
• Store inf sol for up to 24 hr at room temperature
• Reconstituted sol with sterile water may be stored under refrigeration for up to 24 hr
Additive incompatibilities:
Calcium products, sol

Patient/family education
• Advise patient to report hypercalcemic relapse: nausea, vomiting, bone pain, thirst; unusual muscle twitching, muscle spasms, severe diarrhea, constipation, ocular symptoms
• Advise patient to continue with dietary recommendations, including calcium and vit D
• To obtain an analgesic from provider for bone pain
• Advise patient that, small, frequent meals may help nausea/vomiting

Evaluation
Positive therapeutic outcome
• Decreased calcium levels to normal

---

pancrelipase (Rx)
(pan-kre-li'pase)
Cotazym, Cotazym-65B ✤, Cotazym E.C.S. 8, Cotazym E.C.S. 20, Cotazym Capsules, Cotazym-S, Creon, Ilozyme, Ku-Zyme HP, Lipram-CR20, Lipram-PN10, Lipram-PN16, Lipram-UL12, Pancrease Capsules, Pancrease MT 4, Pancrease MT 10, Pancrease MT 16, Protilase, Ultrase MT 12, Ultrase MT 20, Viokase, Zenpep, Zymase
Func. class.: Digestant
Chem. class.: Pancreatic enzyme (bovine/porcine)

Pregnancy category B

Action: Pancreatic enzyme needed for breakdown of substances released from the pancreas

Therapeutic outcome: Increases protein, fat, carbohydrate digestion

Uses: Exocrine pancreatic secretion insufficiency, cystic fibrosis (digestive aid), steatorrhea, pancreatic enzyme deficiency

Dosage and routes
Many products listed above are not interchangeable
Adult and child: PO 1-3 cap/tab before or with meals, or 1 cap/tab with snack or 1-2 powder packets before meals

Available forms: Powder 16,800 units lipase/70,000 units protease and amylase; caps 8000 units lipase/30,000 units protease and amylase; del rel caps, 4000 units lipase/12,000 units protease and amylase, 4000 units lipase/25,000 units protease/20,000 units amylase, 5000 units lipase/20,000 units protease and amylase, 10,000 units lipase/30,000 units protease and amylase, 12,000 units lipase/24,000 units protease and amylase, 12,000 units lipase/39,000 units protease and amylase, 16,000 units lipase/48,000 units protease and amylase 20,000 units lipase/65,000 units protease and amylase, 24,000 units lipase/78,000 units protease and amylase; del rel cap 5000, 15,000 units

Adverse effects
GI: Anorexia, nausea, vomiting, diarrhea, cramping, bloating
GU: Hyperuricuria, hyperuricemia

Contraindications: Allergy to pork

Precautions: Pregnancy **B**, ileus, pancreatitis, Crohn's disease

Pharmacokinetics
Unknown

Pharmacodynamics
Unknown

Interactions
Individual drugs
Acarbose, miglitol: decreased effects of each specific drug
Cimetidine, iron (oral): decreased absorption of pancrelipase
Drug classifications
Antacids: decreased absorption of pancrelipase

NURSING CONSIDERATIONS
Assessment
• Monitor I&O ratio; watch for increasing urinary output
• Monitor fecal fat, nitrogen, pro-time during treatment
• Monitor for polyuria, polydipsia, polyphagia (may indicate diabetes mellitus)
• Assess for allergy to pork; patient may also be sensitive to this product
• Assess for appropriate weight, height, development; there may be a developmental lag
• Check stools for steatorrhea, which signifies undigested fat content

P

Nursing diagnoses
• Knowledge, deficient (teaching)
• Nutrition: less than body requirements, imbalanced (uses)

Implementation
• Avoid inhaling powder
• Give tab with 8 oz of water and sitting up only; do not let tab sit in mouth; give with meals
• Give after antacid or cimetidine; decreased pH inactivates product
• Give powder mixed in prepared fruit for infants, children
• Administer low-fat diet to decrease GI symptoms
• Provide adequate hydration
• Store in airtight container at room temperature

Patient/family education
• Teach patient to take tab with 8 oz or more water, not to let tab sit in mouth; have patient take tab sitting up only
• Advise patient to notify prescriber of allergic reactions, abdominal pain, cramping, or hematuria
• Teach patient not to inhale powder, very irritating to mucous membranes, some powder may irritate skin

Evaluation
Positive therapeutic outcome
• Absence of steatorrhea
• Improved digestion of carbohydrates, proteins, fat

⚠ HIGH ALERT

pancuronium (Rx)
(pan-cure-oh'nee-yum)
pancuronium bromide
Func. class.: Neuromuscular blocker (nondepolarizing)
Chem. class.: Synthetic curariform

Pregnancy category C

Action: Inhibits transmission of nerve impulses by binding with cholinergic receptor sites, antagonizing action of acetylcholine; no analgesic response

Therapeutic outcome: Paralysis of all skeletal muscles

Uses: Facilitation of endotracheal intubation, skeletal muscle relaxation during mechanical ventilation, surgery, or general anesthesia

Dosage and routes
Adult/child/infant >1 mo: IV 0.06-0.1 mg/kg initially or 0.05 mg/kg after initial dose of succinylcholine; maintenance 0.01 mg/kg 60-100 min after initial dose, then 0.01 mg/kg q25-60min as needed; in obese patients, use ideal body weight

Neonate <1 mo: IV test dose 0.02 mg/kg, then 0.03 mg/kg/dose initially, repeat 2 × as needed at 5-10 min intervals; maintenance 0.03-0.09 mg/kg/dose q30min-4hr as needed

Available forms: Inj 1, 2 mg/ml

Adverse effects
CV: Bradycardia, tachycardia, increased, decreased B/P, ventricular extrasystoles, edema, hypotension
EENT: Increased secretions
INTEG: Rash, flushing, pruritus, urticaria, sweating, salivation
MS: Weakness to prolonged skeletal muscle relaxation
RESP: Prolonged apnea, bronchospasm, cyanosis, respiratory depression, dyspnea
SYST: **Anaphylaxis**

Contraindications: Hypersensitivity to bromide ion

Precautions: Pregnancy C, breastfeeding, children <2 yr, renal/hepatic/cardiac/neuromuscular disease, electrolyte imbalances, dehydration, previous anaphylactic reactions (other neuromuscular blockers)

Black Box Warning: Respiratory insufficiency

Pharmacokinetics
Absorption	Complete bioavailability
Distribution	Extracellular space; crosses placenta
Metabolism	Plasma
Excretion	Kidneys, unchanged
Half-life	2 hr

Pharmacodynamics
Onset	3-5 min, dose dependent
Peak	3-5 min
Duration	35-40 min

Interactions
Individual products
Clindamycin, enflurane, isoflurane, lincomycin, lithium, quinidine: increased neuromuscular blockade
Theophylline: dysrhythmias
Drug classifications
Aminoglycosides, anesthetics (local), analgesics (opioid), polymyxin antiinfectives, thiazides: increased neuromuscular blockade

---

 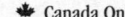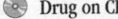

Drug/lab test
Decreased: cholinesterase

NURSING CONSIDERATIONS
Assessment
• Monitor vital signs (B/P, pulse, respirations, airway) until fully recovered; note rate, depth, pattern of respirations, strength of hand grip; patient should be intubated before use
• Monitor for electrolyte imbalances (potassium, magnesium) before product is used; electrolyte imbalances may lead to increased action of this product
• Monitor for recovery: decreased paralysis of face, diaphragm, leg, arm, rest of body; residual weakness and respiratory problems may occur during recovery period
❶ Assess for hypersensitive reactions, anaphylaxis: rash, fever, respiratory distress, pruritus; product should be discontinued

Nursing diagnoses
• Breathing pattern, ineffective (uses)
• Communication, impaired verbal (adverse reactions)
• Fear (adverse reactions)
• Knowledge, deficient (teaching)

Implementation
• Use peripheral nerve stimulator (anesthesiologist) to determine neuromuscular blockade; deep tendon reflexes should be monitored during extended periods
• Give direct **IV** undiluted over 1-2 min, or diluted in D₅W or 0.9% NaCl and give as an inf at prescribed rate; titrate to patient response; should be administered only by qualified person, usually an anesthesiologist; do not administer IM
• Store in light-resistant area
• Give anticholinesterase to reverse neuromuscular blockade
Syringe compatibilities: Heparin
Y-site compatibilities: Aminophylline, cefazolin, cefuroxime, cimetidine, DOBUTamine, DOPamine, epinephrine, esmolol, fentanyl, fluconazole, gentamicin, heparin, hydrocortisone, isoproterenol, lorazepam, midazolam, morphine, nitroglycerin, nitroprusside, ranitidine, sulfamethoxazole/trimethoprim, vancomycin
Y-site incompatibilities: Diazepam
Additive compatibilities: Verapamil
Additive incompatibilities: Barbiturates

Patient/family education
• Provide reassurance if communication is difficult during recovery from neuromuscular blockade

• Provide explanation to patients regarding all procedures or treatments; patient will remain conscious if anesthesia is not given also

Evaluation
Positive therapeutic outcome
• Paralysis of jaw, eyelid, head, neck, rest of body as evaluated by peripheral nerve stimulator

Treatment of overdose: Edrophonium or neostigmine, atropine; monitor VS; may require mechanical ventilation

---

panitumumab (Rx)
(pan-i-tue′moo-mab)
Vectibix
Func. class.: Antineoplastic—miscellaneous
Chem. class.: Multikinase inhibitor, signal transduction inhibitor
Pregnancy category C

Action: Decreases growth and survival of cancer cells by competitive inhibition of EGF receptor

Therapeutic outcome: Decrease in colon carcinoma progression

Uses: EGFR expressing metastatic colorectal cancer, not beneficial in KRAS mutations in Codon 12 or 13

Dosage and routes
Adult: **IV** INF 6 mg/kg over 60 min q2wk

Available forms: Sol for inj 20 mg/ml

Adverse effects
CNS: Fatigue
CV: Peripheral edema
EENT: Ocular irritation, ocular hyperemia
GI: Nausea, diarrhea, vomiting, anorexia, mouth ulceration, abdominal pain, constipation
HEMA: Thrombophlebitis
INTEG: Rash, pruritus, **exfoliative dermatitis,** skin fissure, **angioedema, severe/fatal infusion reactions**
META: Hypocalcemia, hypomagnesemia, antibody formation
RESP: **Bronchospasm, cough,** dyspnea, **hypoxia, pulmonary fibrosis/embolism,** pneumonitis, wheezing

Contraindications: Hypersensitivity

Precautions: Pregnancy C, breastfeeding, children, hepatic disease, acute bronchospasm, diarrhea, hamster protein allergy, hypomagnesemia, hypotension, pulmonary fibrosis, sepsis, KRAS mutations

P

Adverse effects: *italic* = common, **bold** = life-threatening

Black Box Warning: Exfoliative dermatitis, infusion-related reactions

Pharmacokinetics

Absorption	38%-49%, high-fat meal decreases absorption
Distribution	Protein binding 99.5%
Metabolism	Liver, oxidative metabolism by CYP3A4, glucuronidation by UGT1A9
Excretion	Feces 77%
Half-life	Elimination 7.5 day

Pharmacodynamics

Onset	Unknown
Peak	3 hr
Duration	Unknown

Interactions
Drug classifications
Antineoplastics, other: do not use with other products

NURSING CONSIDERATIONS
Assessment
• Monitor serum electrolytes periodically (calcium, magnesium)
• Assess for signs of infection: increased temperature
• Assess for signs of infusion reactions: bronchospasm, fever, chills, hypotension
• Assess for signs of ocular toxicity: ocular irritation, hyperemia

Nursing diagnoses
• Infection, risk for (uses)
• Knowledge, deficient (teaching)
• Nutrition: less than body requirements, imbalanced (adverse reactions)

Implementation
• Give in hospital or clinic setting with full resuscitation equipment
• Give only as IV inf using controlled IV inf pump; do not give **IV** push or bolus; use low-protein binding 0.2 or 0.22 micron in-line filter; flush line with 0.9% NaCl before, after administration
• Give over 60 min through a peripheral line or in-dwelling catheter; inf doses of >1000 mg over 90 min
• Dilute in 100 ml of 0.9% NaCl; dilute doses >1000 mg in 150 ml of 0.9% NaCl; mix by inverting; max 10 mg/ml; use within 6 hr if stored at room temperature; can be stored between 2°-8° C for up to 24 hr
• Store unopened vials in refrigerator; do not shake; protect from direct sunlight; do not freeze

Patient/family education
◆ Instruct patient to report adverse reactions immediately: difficulty breathing, mouth sores, skin rash, ocular toxicity
• Teach patient reason for treatment, expected results, adverse reactions
• Teach males/females to use contraception while taking this product and for 6 mo after treatment; do not breastfeed for at least 2 mo after treatment
• Advise to use sunscreen while taking, 2 mo after

Evaluation
Positive therapeutic outcome
• Decrease in colon carcinoma progression

pantoprazole (Rx)
(pan-toe-pray´zole)
Protonix, Protonix IV
Func. class.: Proton pump inhibitor
Chem. class.: Benzimidazole

Pregnancy category C

Action: Suppresses gastric secretion by inhibiting hydrogen/potassium ATPase enzyme system in gastric parietal cell; characterized as gastric acid pump inhibitor, since it blocks final step of acid production

Therapeutic outcome: Absence of epigastric fullness, pain, swelling

Uses: Gastroesophageal reflux disease (GERD), severe erosive esophagitis, maintenance, long-term pathological hypersecretory conditions including Zollinger-Ellison syndrome

Dosage and routes
GERD
Adult: PO 40 mg/day × 8 wk, may repeat course

Erosive esophagitis
Adult: IV 40 mg/day × 7-10 days; PO 40 mg/day × 8 wk; may repeat PO course

Pathologic hypersecretory conditions
Adult: PO 40 mg bid; IV 80 mg q12hr; max 240 mg/day

Available forms: Del rel tabs 20, 40 mg; powder for inj, freeze dried 40 mg/vial

Adverse effects
CNS: Headache, insomnia
GI: Diarrhea, abdominal pain, flatulence
INTEG: Rash
META: Hyperglycemia
RESP: **Pneumonia**

 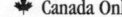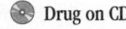

Contraindications: Hypersensitivity

Precautions: Pregnancy **C**, breastfeeding, children, proton pump hypersensitivity

Pharmacokinetics

Absorption	Unknown
Distribution	Protein binding 97%
Metabolism	Unknown
Excretion	Urine-metabolites, feces, decreased rate in geriatric
Half-life	1½ hr

Pharmacodynamics

Onset	Unknown
Peak	2.4 hr
Duration	>24 hr

Interactions
Individual drugs
Calcium carbonate, sucralfate, vit B$_{12}$: decreased absorption of pantoprazole
Clarithromycin, diazepam, flurazepam, phenytoin, triazolam: increased levels of pantoprazole
Warfarin: increased risk of bleeding

NURSING CONSIDERATIONS
Assessment
• Assess GI system: bowel sounds q8hr, abdomen for pain, swelling, anorexia
• Monitor hepatic enzymes: AST, ALT, alkaline phosphatase during treatment

Nursing diagnoses
• Knowledge, deficient (teaching)

Implementation
• Swallow del rel tabs whole; do not break, crush, or chew
• May take with or without food
IV route
• Reconstitute with 10 ml 0.9% NaCl, further dilute with 80 ml LR, D$_5$, 0.9% NaCl (0.8 mg/ml), give over 15 min (≤6 mg/min) or as **IV** push over 2 min

Patient/family education
• Advise patient to report severe diarrhea; product may have to be discontinued
• Advise patient with diabetes that hyperglycemia may occur
• Advise patient to avoid hazardous activities; dizziness may occur
• Advise patient to avoid alcohol, salicylates, ibuprofen; may cause GI irritation

Evaluation
Positive therapeutic outcome
• Absence of epigastric pain, swelling, fullness

---

paricalcitol (Rx)
(par-ih-cal'sih-tol)
Zemplar
Func. class.: Vitamin D analog
Chem. class.: Fat-soluble vitamin

Pregnancy category C

Action: Reduces parathyroid hormone (PTH) levels; suppresses PTH levels in patients with chronic renal failure with absence of hypercalcemia/hyperphosphatemia; serum PO$_4$, Ca, calcium-phosphate product (CaxP) may increase

Therapeutic outcome: Decreased symptoms of hyperparathyroidism

Uses: Hyperparathyroidism in chronic renal failure

Dosage and routes
Adult: **IV** BOL 0.04-0.1 mcg/kg (2.8-7 mcg) no more than every other day during dialysis; may increase by 2-4 mcg q2-4wk until target serum intact PTH (1.5-3 × nonuremic upper limit of normal) is achieved; PO 1 mcg/day or 2 mcg 3 ×/wk

Available forms: Inj 5 mcg/ml; caps 1, 2, 4 mcg

Adverse effects
CNS: Light-headedness
CV: Palpitations
GI: Nausea, vomiting, anorexia, dry mouth
MISC: Pneumonia, edema, chills, fever, flu, **sepsis**

Contraindications: Hypersensitivity, hypercalcemia

Precautions: Pregnancy **C**, breastfeeding, children, geriatric, CV disease, renal calculi

Pharmacokinetics

Excretion	Crosses placenta, enters breast milk

Pharmacodynamics
Unknown

Interactions
Individual products
Digitalis: increased toxicity

NURSING CONSIDERATIONS
Assessment
• Monitor Ca, PO$_4$, 2 ×/wk qwk during initial therapy; after dose is established measure calcium and phosphorus qmo

Nursing diagnoses
• Knowledge, deficient (teaching)

P

Implementation
- Give by **IV** bol only

Patient/family education
- Advise patient to report weakness, lethargy, headache, anorexia, loss of weight
- Teach patient to report nausea, vomiting, palpitations

Evaluation
Positive therapeutic outcome
- Decreased hypoparathyroidism in chronic renal disease

---

paroxetine (Rx)
(par-ox'e-teen)
Paxeva, Paxil, Paxil CR
Func. class.: Antidepressant, selective serotonin reuptake inhibitor (SSRI)
Chem. class.: Phenylpiperidine derivative
Pregnancy category D

Do not confuse:
paroxetine/paclitaxel, Paxil/paclitaxel/Taxol

Action: Inhibits CNS neuron reuptake of serotonin but not of norepinephrine or DOPamine

Therapeutic outcome: Relief of depression

Uses: Major depressive disorder, obsessive-compulsive disorder, panic disorder, generalized anxiety disorder, posttraumatic stress disorder, premenstrual disorders, social anxiety disorder

Unlabeled uses: Premature ejaculation

Dosage and routes
Depression
Adult: PO 20 mg/day in AM; after 4 wk if no clinical improvement is noted, dosage may be increased by 10 mg/day weekly to desired response; max 50 mg/day; or CONT REL 25 mg/day, may increase by 12.5 mg/day weekly up to 62.5 mg/day
Geriatric: PO 10 mg/day, increase by 10 mg to desired dose, max 40 mg/day

Obsessive-compulsive disorder
Adult: PO 40 mg/day in AM; start with 20 mg/day, increase 10 mg/day increments, max 60 mg/day

Panic disorder
Adult: Start with 10 mg/day and increase in 10 mg/day increments to 40 mg/day, max 60 mg/day; or CONT REL 12.5 mg/day max 75 mg/day

Generalized anxiety disorder
Adult: PO 20 mg/day in AM, range 20-50 mg/day

Posttraumatic stress disorder
Adult: PO 20 mg/day, range 20-60 mg/day

Premenstrual disorders
Adult: CONT REL 12.5 mg/day in AM

Renal dose
Adult: PO CCr <30 ml/min 10 mg/day in AM, may increase by 10 mg/day qwk, max 50 mg/day; or CONT REL 12.5 mg/day max 40 mg/day

Available forms: Tabs 10, 20, 30, 40 mg; oral susp 10 mg/5 ml; cont rel 12.5, 25, 37.5 mg

Adverse effects
CNS: Headache, nervousness, insomnia, drowsiness, anxiety, tremor, dizziness, fatigue, sedation, abnormal dreams, agitation, apathy, euphoria, hallucinations, delusions, psychosis, **seizures, malignant neuroleptic syndrome–like reactions**
CV: Vasodilatation, postural hypotension, palpitations
EENT: Visual changes
GI: Nausea, diarrhea, constipation, dry mouth, anorexia, dyspepsia, vomiting, taste changes, flatulence, decreased appetite, cramps
GU: Dysmenorrhea, decreased libido, urinary frequency, UTI, amenorrhea, cystitis, impotence, *abnormal ejaculation* (male)
INTEG: Sweating, rash
MS: Pain, arthritis, myalgia, myopathy, myasthenia
RESP: Infection, pharyngitis, nasal congestion, sinus headache, sinusitis, cough, dyspnea, yawning
SYST: Asthenia, fever, abrupt withdrawal syndrome

Contraindications: Pregnancy **D**, hypersensitivity, MAOI use, alcohol use

Precautions: Breastfeeding, geriatric, seizure history, patients with history of mania, renal/hepatic disease

Black Box Warning: Children, suicidal ideation

Pharmacokinetics

Absorption	Well absorbed
Distribution	Widely distributed; crosses blood-brain barrier, protein-binding 95%
Metabolism	Liver, mostly by CYP2D6 enzyme system
Excretion	Kidneys, unchanged (2%); breast milk
Half-life	21 hr (reg rel); 15-20 hr (cont rel)

Pharmacodynamics	
Onset	Unknown
Peak	5.2 hr
Duration	Unknown

Interactions
Individual drugs
Cimetidine: increased paroxetine levels
Digoxin: decreased effect of digoxin
L-tryptophan: increased agitation
Phenobarbital: decreased paroxetine levels
Phenytoin: decreased effect of paroxetine
◆Pimozide: potentially fatal reactions
Theophylline: increased theophylline levels
◆Thioridazine: do not use with paroxetine; hypertensive crisis, seizures, potentially fatal reactions can occur
Warfarin: increased bleeding

Drug classifications
CYP2D6 inhibitors (aprepitant, delavirdine, imatinib, nefazodone): increased toxicity
Highly protein-bound products: increased side effects
◆MAOIs: hypertensive crisis, seizures; do not use together; potentially fatal reactions can occur

Drug/herb
Corkwood, jimsonweed: increased anticholinergic effect
Ephedra: hypertensive crisis
Hops, lavender: increased sedation
Kava, St. John's wort: avoid use
SAM-e, St. John's wort: possible serotonin syndrome
Yohimbe: increased CNS stimulation

Drug/lab test
Increased: serum bilirubin, blood glucose, alkaline phosphatase
Decreased: VMA, 5-HIAA
False increase: urinary catecholamines

NURSING CONSIDERATIONS
Assessment
- Assess mental status: mood, sensorium, affect, suicidal tendencies; increase in psychiatric symptoms: depression, panic
- Assess for withdrawal symptoms: headache, nausea, vomiting, muscle pain, weakness; do not usually occur unless product was discontinued abruptly
- Monitor B/P (with patient lying, standing), pulse q4hr; if systolic B/P drops 20 mm Hg, hold product, notify prescriber; take VS q4hr in patients with CV disease
- Monitor blood studies: CBC, leukocytes, differential, cardiac enzymes if patient is receiving long-term therapy
- Monitor hepatic studies: AST, ALT, bilirubin
- Check weight weekly; appetite may increase with product
- Assess ECG for flattening of T-wave, bundle branch block, AV block, dysrhythmias in cardiac patients
- Assess for EPS primarily in geriatric: rigidity, dystonia, akathisia
- Monitor urinary retention, constipation; constipation is more likely to occur in children or geriatric
- Identify alcohol consumption; if alcohol is consumed, hold dose until AM

Nursing diagnoses
- Coping, ineffective (uses)
- Injury, risk for (adverse reactions)
- Knowledge, deficient (teaching)
- Noncompliance (teaching)

Implementation
- Give with food or milk for GI symptoms; store at room temperature; do not freeze
- Give crushed if patient is unable to swallow whole, regular release only

Patient/family education
- Advise patient that therapeutic effects may take 1-4 wk
- Teach patient to use caution in driving and other activities requiring alertness because of drowsiness, dizziness, blurred vision; to avoid rising quickly from sitting to standing, especially geriatric
- Caution patient to avoid alcohol ingestion, other CNS depressants, and OTC medication unless prescribed
- Caution patient not to discontinue medication quickly after long-term use; may cause nausea, anxiety, headache, malaise; do not double doses if one is missed
- Advise patient to use gum, hard sugarless candy, or frequent sips of water for dry mouth; if dry mouth continues an artificial saliva product may be used
- Advise patient that depression may worsen, suicidal thoughts/behavior occur

Evaluation
Positive therapeutic outcome
- Decrease in depression
- Absence of suicidal thoughts

Treatment of overdose: Activated charcoal, gastric lavage, maintain airway; for seizures give diazepam, symptomatic treatment

P

Adverse effects: *italic* = common, **bold** = life-threatening

pegaptanib (Rx)
(peg-ap′ta-nib)
Macugen
Func. class: Ophthalmic agent—
miscellaneous
Pregnancy category B

Action: Binds to vascular endothelial growth factor (VEGF), thereby inhibiting angiogenesis

Therapeutic outcome: Stabilization of vision in macular degeneration

Uses: Treatment of neovascular (wet) age-related macular degeneration; may be used alone or with photodynamic therapy (PDT)

Dosage and routes
Adult: Intravitreal inj 0.3 mg inj q6wk

Available forms: Inj 0.3 mg, single glass syringes

Adverse effects
EENT: *Anterior chamber inflammation, blurred vision, conjunctival hemorrhage, corneal edema, cataract, eye discharge, eye pain, increased intraocular pressure, punctate keratitis, reduced visual acuity, vitreous floaters, vitreous opacities, blepharitis, conjunctivitis, photophobia,* retinal detachment, iatrogenic traumatic cataract

Contraindications: Hypersensitivity, ocular or periocular infections

Precautions: Pregnancy **B**, inflammatory eye disease, ocular hypertension

Pharmacokinetics	
Absorption	Unknown
Distribution	Unknown
Metabolism	Unknown
Excretion	Unknown
Half-life	87-100 hr in vitreous humor of the monkey

Pharmacodynamics	
Onset	Unknown
Peak	Unknown
Duration	May remain fully active in the eye for 7-28 days

NURSING CONSIDERATIONS
Assessment
• Test visual acuity periodically
• Assess treated eye for increased intraocular pressure, infection, endophthalmitis
• Monitor perfusion of the optic nerve head immediately after injection, tonometry ½ hr after inj, biomicroscopy 2-7 days after inj

Nursing diagnoses
• Knowledge, deficient (teaching)
• Sensory perception, disturbed: visual (uses)

Implementation
• Administer anesthesia and a broad-spectrum antiinfective prior to injection
• The inj should be done under aseptic conditions
• Remove all air bubbles prior to use
• Store at 36°-46° F, do not freeze or shake vigorously

Patient/family education
• Instruct patient to report any inflammation, bleeding, eye discharge, opacities to prescriber
• Instruct patient to continue with follow-up care during treatment

Evaluation
Positive therapeutic outcome
• Macular degeneration stabilized

⚠ HIGH ALERT

pegaspargase (Rx)
(peg-as′per-gase)
Oncaspar, PEG-L-asparaginase
Func. class.: Antineoplastic
Chem. class.: *Escherichia coli* enzyme
Pregnancy category C

Action: Indirectly inhibits protein synthesis in tumor cells; without amino acid, DNA, RNA synthesis is halted; asparagine, protein synthesis is halted; G_1 phase of cell cycle specific; a nonvesicant; a modified version of L-asparaginase

Therapeutic outcome: Prevention of rapidly growing malignant cells

Uses: Acute lymphocytic leukemia unresponsive to other agents in combination with other antineoplastics

Dosage and routes
In combination
Adult and child: **IV**/IM 2500 international units/m² q14day, run **IV** over 1-2 hr in 100 ml of NaCl or D_5 through a running **IV**; IM should be no more than 2 ml in one inj site used in combination with other chemotherapeutics

Available forms: Inj 750 international units/ml in a phosphate-buffered saline sol

Adverse effects
CNS: Neuritis, dizziness, headache, **coma, depression,** fatigue, confusion, hallucinations, **seizures, intracranial bleeding**
CV: Chest pain, **hypotension**
ENDO: Hyperglycemia
GI: Nausea, vomiting, anorexia, cramps, stomatitis, **hepatotoxicity, pancreatitis,** *diarrhea*
GU: Urinary retention, **renal failure,** glycosuria, polyuria, azotemia, uric acid neuropathy
HEMA: **Thrombocytopenia, leukopenia, myelosuppression, anemia, decreased clotting factors, pancytopenia, DIC**
INTEG: Rash, urticaria, chills, fever
RESP: **Fibrosis, pulmonary infiltrate, severe bronchospasm**
SYST: **Anaphylaxis, hypersensitivity, angioedema**

Contraindications: Breastfeeding, infants, hypersensitivity, pancreatitis, acute bronchospasm, bleeding, coagulopathy, coronary thrombosis, DIC, hypotension

Precautions: Pregnancy C, renal/hepatic/CNS disease, *E. coli* protein hypersensitivity, hemophilia, tumor lysis syndrome, infection

Pharmacokinetics
Absorption	Complete bioavailability
Distribution	Intravascular spaces
Metabolism	Unknown
Excretion	Reticuloendothelial system
Half-life	5½ days

Pharmacodynamics
Onset	Rapid
Peak	Unknown
Duration	2 wk

Interactions
Individual drugs
Aspirin, heparin, warfarin: coagulation factor imbalances
Methotrexate: decreased action of methotrexate
Radiation: do not use together
Drug classifications
NSAIDs: coagulation factor imbalances

NURSING CONSIDERATIONS
Assessment
🔴 Assess for signs and symptoms of pancreatitis (nausea, vomiting, severe abdominal pain), anaphylaxis (bronchospasm, dyspnea), cyanosis; monitor amylase, glucose
🔴 Assess symptoms indicating severe allergic reaction: rash, pruritus, urticaria, purpuric skin lesions, itching, flushing; monitor for joint pain, bronchospasm, hypotension; epinephrine and crash carts should be nearby
• Monitor for frequency of stools, characteristics: cramping, acidosis; signs of dehydration: rapid respirations, poor skin turgor, decreased urine output, dry skin, restlessness, weakness
• Monitor CBC, differential, platelet count weekly; withhold product if WBC is <4000/mm³ or platelet count is <100,000/mm³; notify physician of results; also assess protime, PTT, and thrombin time, which may be increased
• Monitor renal function tests: BUN, creatinine, serum uric acid, urine CCr before, during therapy; check I&O ratio; report fall in urine output to <30 ml/hr; patient should be well hydrated with 2-3 L/day to prevent urate deposits
• Monitor temp q4hr (may indicate beginning of infection)
• Monitor liver function tests before, during therapy (bilirubin, AST, ALT, LDH) as needed or monthly; check for jaundice of skin and sclera, dark urine, clay-colored stools, itchy skin, abdominal pain, fever, diarrhea; also monitor cholesterol, alkaline phosphatase
• Assess for bleeding: hematuria, stool guaiac, bruising or petechiae, mucosa or orifices q8hr; check for inflammation of mucosa, breaks in skin
• Identify edema in feet, joint pain, stomach pain, shaking

Nursing diagnoses
• Infection, risk for (adverse reactions)
• Injury, risk for (adverse reactions)
• Knowledge, deficient (teaching)

Implementation
• Preparation by trained personnel is required in controlled environment
• Give fluids **IV** or PO before chemotherapy to hydrate patient
• Provide antiemetic 30-60 min before giving product and prn to prevent vomiting; administer antibiotics for prophylaxis of infection
• Provide a liquid diet: carbonated beverages; gelatin may be added if patient is not nauseated or vomiting
IM route
• Dilute 10,000 international units/2 ml of 0.9% NaCl with preservatives; give 2 ml or less per site
Intradermal route
• After intradermal skin testing and desensitization, give 0.1 ml (2 international units) intradermally after reconstituting with 5 ml of

P

sterile water or 0.9% NaCl for inj; then add 0.1 ml of reconstituted product to 9.9 ml of diluent (20 international units/ml); observe for 1 hr, check for wheal; desensitization may be required

IV route
• For direct **IV** dilute 10,000 international units/5 ml of sterile water for inj or 0.9% NaCl without preservatives; give through 5-μm filter if fibers are present; do not use if sol cloudy or discolored, give over 30 min through Y-site of full-flowing **IV** of 0.9% NaCl or D₅W; run **IV** sol for at least 2 hr after direct administration
• Give **IV** inf using 21, 23, 25-G needle; administer by slow **IV** inf via Y-tube or 3-way stopcock of flowing D₅W or 0.9% NaCl inf over 30 min after diluting 10,000 international units/5 ml of sterile water or 0.9% NaCl (no preservatives) to 2000 international units/ml; filter may be necessary if fibers are present
• Provide allopurinol or sodium bicarbonate to reduce uric acid levels, alkalinization of urine

Patient/family education
• Advise patient that contraceptive measures are recommended during therapy; product is teratogenic
• Teach patient to avoid use of products containing aspirin or NSAIDs, razors, commercial mouthwash, since bleeding may occur; to report symptoms of bleeding (hematuria, tarry stools)
• Teach patient to report signs of anemia (fatigue, headache, irritability, faintness, shortness of breath)
• Tell patient to avoid crowds and persons with respiratory tract infections to prevent patient infection
• Advise patient to avoid vaccinations, since serious reactions can occur
• Teach patient to report nausea, vomiting, bruising, bleeding, stomatitis, severe diarrhea, jaundice, chest pain, abdominal pain, trouble breathing, rash

Evaluation
Positive therapeutic outcome
• Prevention of rapid division of malignant cells

---

pegfilgrastim (Rx)
(peg-fill-grass′stim)
Neulasta
Func. class.: Hematopoietic agent

Pregnancy category C

Action: Stimulates proliferation and differentiation of neutrophils

Therapeutic outcome: Absence of infection

Uses: To decrease infection in patients receiving antineoplastics that are myelosuppressive; to increase WBC in patients with product-induced neutropenia

Dosage and routes
Adult: SUBCUT 6 mg give once per chemotherapy cycle

Available forms: Sol for inj 10 mg/0.6 ml

Adverse effects
CNS: Fever, fatigue, headache, dizziness, insomnia, peripheral edema
GI: Nausea, vomiting, diarrhea, mucositis, anorexia, constipation, dyspepsia, abdominal pain, stomatitis, **splenic rupture**
HEMA: **Leukocytosis, granulocytopenia, sickle cell crisis, hemoglobin S disease with crisis**
INTEG: Alopecia
MISC: Chest pain, hyperuricemia, **anaphylaxis, influenza-like syndrome**
MS: Skeletal pain
RESP: **Respiratory distress syndrome**

Contraindications: Hypersensitivity to proteins of *E. coli,* filgrastim

Precautions: Pregnancy **C,** breastfeeding, child <45 kg, adolescents, myeloid malignancies, sickle cell disease, leukocytosis, splenic rupture, allergic-type reactions, ARDS, peripheral blood stem cell mobilization (PBSC)

Pharmacokinetics
Absorption	Unknown
Distribution	Unknown
Metabolism	Unknown
Excretion	Unknown
Half-life	15-80 hr; 20-38 hr (child)

Pharmacodynamics
Unknown

Interactions
Individual drug
Lithium: increased release of neutrophils
Drug classifications
Cytotoxic chemotherapy agents: do not use this product concomitantly or 2 wk before or 24 hr after administration of cytotoxics
Drug/lab test
Increased: uric acid, LDH, alkaline phosphatase

 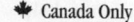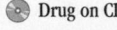

NURSING CONSIDERATIONS
Assessment
• Assess for allergic reactions, anaphylaxis: rash, urticaria; discontinue this product, have emergency equipment nearby
• Monitor blood studies: CBC, platelet count before treatment and twice weekly; neutrophil counts may be increased for 2 days after therapy
• Monitor B/P, respirations, pulse before, during therapy
• Assess for bone pain, give mild analgesics

Nursing diagnoses
• Infection, risk for (uses)
• Knowledge, deficient (teaching)

Implementation
• Give using single-use vials; after dose is withdrawn, do not reenter vial
• Do not use 6-mg fixed dose in infants, children, or others <45 kg
• Inspect sol for discoloration, particulates; if present, do not use
• Do not administer in the period 14 days before and 24 hr after cytotoxic chemotherapy
• Store in refrigerator; do not freeze; may store at room temperature up to 6 hr, avoid shaking, protect from light

Patient/family education
• Teach the technique for self-administration: dose, side effects, disposal of containers and needles; provide instruction sheet

Evaluation
Positive therapeutic outcome
• Absence of infection

---

peginterferon alfa-2a (Rx)
(peg-in-ter-feer'on)
Pegasys
peginterferon alfa-2b (Rx)
PegIntron
Func. class.: Immunomodulator

Pregnancy category C

Action: Stimulates genes to modulate many biologic effects, including inhibition of viral replication; inhibits ion cell proliferation, immunomodulation, stimulates effector proteins, decreases leukocyte, platelet counts

Therapeutic outcome: Undetectable viral load; decreasing signs, symptoms of chronic hepatitis C

Uses: Chronic hepatitis C infections in adults with compensated liver disease, chronic hepatitis B in adults with HBe AG–positive, HBe AG–negative; HCV patients coinfected with HIV, nonresponders, or relapsers with chronic hepatitis C

Dosage and routes
Pegasys
Adult: SUBCUT 180 mcg qwk × 48 wk; if poorly tolerated, reduce dose to 135 mcg qwk; in some cases reduction to 90 mcg may be needed

PegIntron
Each dose × 1 yr
Adult 137-160 kg: SUBCUT 1 mcg/kg/wk (0.5 ml of 150 mcg vial or Redipen)
Adult 107-136 kg: SUBCUT 1 mcg/kg/wk (0.5 ml of 120 mcg vial or Redipen)
Adult: 89-106 kg: SUBCUT 1 mcg/kg/wk (0.4 ml of 120 vial or Redipen)
Adult 73-88 kg: SUBCUT 1 mcg/kg/wk (0.5 ml of 80 mcg vial or Redipen)

Available forms: Inj 180 mcg/0.5 ml, 180 mcg/ml (2a); powder for inj 50, 80, 120, 150 mcg (2b)

Adverse effects
CNS: Headache, insomnia, dizziness, anxiety, hostility, lability, nervousness, depression, fatigue, poor concentration, pyrexia, **suicidal ideation, homicidal ideation,** relapse of drug addiction
CV: **Ischemic CV events**
ENDO: Hypothyroidism, diabetes
GI: Abdominal pain, nausea, diarrhea, anorexia, vomiting, dry mouth, **fatal colitis, fatal pancreatitis**
HEMA: **Thrombocytopenia,** neutropenia, anemia, lymphopenia
INTEG: Alopecia, pruritus, rash, dermatitis
MISC: Blurred vision, inj site reaction, rigors
MS: Back pain, myalgia, arthralgia
RESP: Cough, dyspnea

Contraindications: Hypersensitivity to interferons, neonates, infants, autoimmune hepatitis, decompensated hepatic disease before use of this product

Precautions: Pregnancy C, breastfeeding, children <18 yr, geriatric, thyroid disorders, myelosuppression, renal/hepatic disease, suicidal/homicidal ideation, preexisting ophthalmologic disorders, pancreatitis, hemodialysis

Black Box Warning: Cardiac/autoimmune disease, depression, infection, use with ribavirin

P

Pharmacokinetics

Absorption	Large variability
Distribution	Large variability
Metabolism	Large variability
Excretion	Large variability
Half-life	15-80 hr

Pharmacodynamics

Unknown

Interactions
Individual drugs
Theophylline: use caution if giving together
Drug classifications
Myelosuppressives: use caution if giving together
Drug/lab test
Increased: triglycerides, ALT, neutrophils, platelets
Abnormal: thyroid function test

NURSING CONSIDERATIONS
Assessment
• Monitor ALT, HCV viral load; patients who show no reduction in ALT, HCV are unlikely to show benefit of treatment after 6 mo
• Monitor platelet counts, heme concentration, ANC, serum creatinine concentration, albumin, bilirubin, TSH, T_4, AFP
• Assess for myelosuppression, hold dose if neutrophil count is $<500 \times 10^6$/L or if platelets are $<50 \times 10^9$/L
• Assess for hypersensitivity: discontinue immediately if hypersensitivity occurs

Nursing diagnoses
• Infection, risk for (uses)
• Knowledge, deficient (teaching)

Implementation
• Give in PM to reduce discomfort, sleep through side effects
• Continue pediatric dose in those who turn 18 yr

Patient/family education
• Provide patient or family member with written, detailed information about product
• Give instructions for home use if appropriate
• Advise to take in evening to reduce discomfort, sleep through some side effects

Evaluation
Positive therapeutic outcome
• Decreased chronic hepatitis C signs/symptoms, undetectable viral load

---

! HIGH ALERT

pemetrexed (Rx)
(pem-ah-trex'ed)
Alimta
Func. class.: Antineoplastic-antimetabolite
Chem. class.: Folic acid antagonist

Pregnancy category D

Action: Inhibits multiple enzymes that reduce folic acid, which is needed for cell replication

Therapeutic outcome: Decreased spread of mesothelioma, decreased tumor size

Uses: Malignant pleural mesothelioma in combination with cisplatin; non–small cell lung cancer as a single agent; non-squamous non–small cell lung cancer (first-line treatment)

Dosage and routes
Adult: **IV** INF 500-600 mg/m² given over 10 min on day 1 of a 21-day cycle with cisplatin 75 mg/m² INF over 2 hr beginning ½ hr after end of pemetrexed INF ANC < 500/mm³ and platelets $= 50,000$/mm³ 75% of previous dose

Available forms: Inj, single-use vials, 500 mg

Adverse effects
CNS: Fatigue, fever, mood alteration, neuropathy
CV: **Thrombosis/embolism,** *chest pain*
GI: Nausea, vomiting, anorexia, diarrhea, ulcerative stomatitis, constipation, dysphagia, dehydration
GU: **Renal failure,** *creatinine elevation*
HEMA: **Neutropenia, leukopenia, thrombocytopenia, myelosuppression, anemia**
INTEG: Rash, desquamation
RESP: Dyspnea
SYST: **Infection with/without neutropenia,** radiation recall reaction

Contraindications: Pregnancy **D**, hypersensitivity, ANC <1500 cells/mm³, CCr < 45 ml/min, thrombocytopenia ($<100,000$/mm³), anemia

Precautions: Breastfeeding, children, renal/hepatic disease

Pharmacokinetics

Absorption	Unknown
Distribution	81% protein binding
Metabolism	Not metabolized
Excretion	Excreted in urine (unchanged 70%-90%) Not known if it is excreted in breast milk
Half-life	3.5 hr

Pharmacodynamics
Unknown

Interactions
Individual drugs
Mannitol: do not use concurrently
Drug classifications
Anticoagulants, NSAIDs: increased bleeding risk

Nephrotoxic products (NSAIDs): decreased pemetrexed clearance

NURSING CONSIDERATIONS
Assessment
◆ Monitor CBC, differential, platelet count; monitor for nadir and recovery; a new cycle should not begin if ANC < 1500 cells/mm³, platelets are < 100,000 cells/mm³, creatinine clearance < 45 ml/min
• Monitor renal tests: BUN, serum uric acid, urine CCr, electrolytes before, during therapy
• Monitor I&O ratio; report fall in urine output to <30 ml/hr
• Monitor temp q4hr; fever may indicate beginning infection; no rectal temps
• Assess bleeding time, coagulation time during treatment; bleeding: hematuria, guaiac, bruising or petechiae, mucosa or orifices q8hr
• Assess buccal cavity q8hr for dryness, sores, ulceration, white patches, oral pain, bleeding, dysphagia
◆ Assess for symptoms indicating severe allergic reaction: rash, urticaria, itching, flushing

Nursing diagnoses
• Body image, disturbed (adverse reactions)
• Infection, risk for (adverse reactions)
• Injury, risk for (adverse reactions)
• Knowledge, deficient (teaching)

Implementation
• Administer vit B_{12} and low-dose folic acid as a prophylactic measure to treat related hematologic, GI toxicity; at least 5 daily doses of folic acid must be taken in the 7 days preceding first dose
• Premedicate with a corticosteroid (dexamethasone) given PO bid the day before, day of, and day after administration of pemetrexed
IV route
• Use aseptic technique during reconstitution, dilution
• Reconstitute 500 mg vial/20 ml 0.9% NaCl injection (preservative free) = 25 mg/ml, swirl until dissolved, further dilute with 100 ml 0.9% NaCl injection (preservative free), give as **IV** inf over 10 mg
• Use only 0.9% NaCl inj (preservative free) for reconstitution, dilution

• Follow strict medical asepsis and protective isolation if WBC levels are low
• Use a liquid diet: carbonated beverage, Jell-O; dry toast, crackers may be added when patient is not nauseated or vomiting
• Assist patient with rinsing of mouth tid-qid with water, club soda; brushing of teeth bid-tid with soft brush or cotton-tipped applicators for stomatitis; use unwaxed dental floss
• Store at 77° F, excursions permitted 59°-86° F, not light sensitive, discard unused portions

Patient/family education
• Instruct patient to report any complaints, side effects to nurse or prescriber: black tarry stools, chills, fever, sore throat, bleeding, bruising, cough, shortness of breath, dark or bloody urine
• Instruct patient to avoid foods with citric acid, hot or rough texture if stomatitis is present
• Instruct patient to report stomatitis: any bleeding, white spots, ulcerations in mouth to prescriber; tell patient to examine mouth daily, report symptoms to nurse, use good oral hygiene
• Advise patient that contraceptive measures are recommended during therapy and for at least 8 wk following cessation of therapy, to discontinue breastfeeding; toxicity to infant may occur
• Advise patient to avoid alcohol, salicylates, live vaccines
• Advise patient to avoid use of razors, commercial mouthwash
• Teach to eat foods high in folic acid and take supplements as prescribed

Evaluation
Positive therapeutic outcome
• Decreased spread of malignancy

penciclovir topical
See Appendix B

PENICILLINS

penicillin G benzathine (Rx)
(pen-i-sill'in)
Bicillin L-A, Megacillin ✤, Permapen
penicillin G (Rx)
Pfizerpen
penicillin G procaine (Rx)
Ayercillin ✤, Wycillin
penicillin V (Rx)
Apo-Pen-VK ✤, Beepen-VK, Nadopen-V ✤, Novopen-VK ✤, Pen-Vee K ✤, PVFK ✤, Veetids
Func. class.: Broad-spectrum antiinfective
Chem. class.: Natural penicillin

Pregnancy category B

Action: Interferes with cell wall replication of susceptible organisms; osmotically unstable cell wall swells and bursts from osmotic pressure, resulting in cell death

Therapeutic outcome: Bactericidal effects on the gram-positive cocci *Staphylococcus, Streptococcus pyogenes, Streptococcus viridans, Streptococcus faecalis, Streptococcus bovis, Streptococcus pneumoniae;* gram-negative cocci *Neisseria gonorrhoeae;* gram-positive bacilli *Actinomyces, Bacillus anthracis, Clostridium perfringens, Clostridium tetani, Corynebacterium diphtheriae, Listeria monocytogenes;* gram-negative bacilli *Escherichia coli, Proteus mirabilis, Salmonella, Shigella, Enterobacter, Streptobacillus moniliformis;* spirochete *Treponema pallidum*

Uses: Respiratory tract infections, scarlet fever, erysipelas, otitis media, pneumonia, skin and soft tissue infections, gonorrhea; prevention of rheumatic fever, glomerulonephritis, syphilis

Dosage and routes
Penicillin G benzathine
Early syphilis
Adult: IM 2.4 million units in single dose

Congenital syphilis
Child <2 yr: IM 50,000 units/kg in single dose

Prophylaxis of rheumatic fever, glomerulonephritis
Adult and child: IM 1.2 million units in single dose q3-4wk or 600,000 units q2wk

Upper respiratory tract infections (group A streptococcal)
Adult: IM 1.2 million units in single dose

Child >27 kg: IM 900,000 units in single dose
Child <27 kg: IM 300,000-600,000 units in single dose
Available forms: Inj 300,000 units/ml; 600,000 units/ml

Penicillin G
Pneumococcal/streptococcal infections (serious)
Adult: IM/**IV** 5-24 million units in divided doses q4-6hr
Child <12 yr: **IV** 150,000-300,000 units/kg/day in 4-6 divided doses; max 24 million units/day

Renal dose
CCr <10 ml/min, give full loading dose, then ½ of loading dose q8-10hr

Available forms: Inj 1, 2, 3 million units/50 ml; powder for inj 1, 5, 20 million units/vial

Penicillin G procaine
Moderate to severe pneumococcal infections
Adult and child: IM 600,000-1.2 million units in 1 or 2 doses/day for 10 days to 2 wk
Newborn: Avoid use in newborns

Pneumococcal pneumonia
Adult and child >12 yr: IM 600,000-1.2 million units/day × 7-10 days

Available forms: Inj 600,000, 1,200,000 units/dose

Penicillin V
Pneumococcal/staphylococcal infections
Adult: PO 250-500 mg q6hr
Child <12 yr: PO 25-50 mg/kg/day in divided doses q6-8hr, max 3 g/day

Streptococcal infections
Adult: PO 125 mg q6-8hr × 10 days

Prevention of recurrence of rheumatic fever/chorea
Adult: PO 125-250 mg bid continuously

Vincent's gingivitis/pharyngitis
Adult: PO 250 mg q6-8hr

Renal dose
CCr <50 ml/min dosage reduction indicated based on clinical response, degree of impairment

Available forms: Tabs 250, 500 mg; powder for oral sol 125, 250 mg/5 ml

Adverse effects
CNS: Lethargy, hallucinations, anxiety, depression, twitching, **coma, seizures,** hyperreflexia

GI: *Nausea, vomiting, diarrhea,* increased AST, ALT, abdominal pain, glossitis, colitis, **pseudomembranous colitis**
GU: **Oliguria, proteinuria, hematuria,** *vaginitis, moniliasis,* **glomerulonephritis,** renal tubular damage
HEMA: Anemia, increased bleeding time, **bone marrow depression, granulocytopenia,** hemolytic anemia
META: Hyperkalemia, hypokalemia, alkalosis, hypernatremia
MISC: Local pain, tenderness and fever with IM inj, **anaphylaxis serum sickness, Stevens-Johnson syndrome**

Contraindications: Hypersensitivity to penicillins, corn; neonates

Precautions: Pregnancy **B,** breastfeeding, hypersensitivity to cephalosporins/carbapenem/sulfite, severe renal disease, GI disease, asthma

Penicillin G benzathine

Pharmacokinetics

Absorption	Delayed; prolonged drug levels
Distribution	Widely distributed; crosses placenta
Metabolism	Liver, minimally
Excretion	Kidneys, unchanged; breast milk
Half-life	½-1 hr

Pharmacodynamics

Onset	Slow
Peak	12-24 hr
Duration	1-4 wk

Penicillin G

Pharmacokinetics

Absorption	Variably absorbed (PO); well absorbed (IM)
Distribution	Widely distributed; crosses placenta
Metabolism	Liver, minimally
Excretion	Kidneys, unchanged; breast milk
Half-life	½-1 hr

Pharmacodynamics

	PO	IM	IV
Onset	Rapid	Rapid	Rapid
Peak	1 hr	¼-½ hr	Immediate
Duration	Unknown	Unknown	Unknown

Penicillin G procaine

Pharmacokinetics

Absorption	Delayed; prolonged drug levels
Distribution	Widely distributed; crosses placenta
Metabolism	Liver, minimally
Excretion	Kidneys, unchanged; breast milk
Half-life	½-1 hr

Pharmacodynamics

Onset	Slow
Peak	1-4 hr
Duration	15 hr

Penicillin V

Pharmacokinetics

Absorption	Widely absorbed
Distribution	Widely distributed; crosses placenta
Metabolism	Liver, minimally
Excretion	Kidneys, unchanged; breast milk
Half-life	½-1 hr

Pharmacodynamics

Onset	Rapid
Peak	½ hr
Duration	Unknown

Interactions
Individual drugs
Aspirin, probenecid: increased penicillin levels
Heparin: increased effect of heparin
Methotrexate: increased effect of methotrexate
Typhoid vaccine: decreased effect of toxoid vaccine
Drug classifications
Contraceptives (oral): decreased contraceptive effectiveness
Tetracyclines: decreased antimicrobial effectiveness of penicillin
Drug/herb
Acidophilus: do not use with antiinfectives; separate by several hours
Khat: decreased absorption of penicillin; separate doses by 2 hr or more
Drug/lab test
False positive: urine glucose, urine protein

NURSING CONSIDERATIONS
Assessment
• Assess patient for previous sensitivity reaction to penicillins or cephalosporins; cross-sensitivity between penicillins and cephalosporins is common
• Assess patient for signs and symptoms of infection including characteristics of wounds, sputum, urine, stool, WBC >10,000/mm^3, earache, fever; obtain information baseline, during treatment
• Obtain C&S before beginning drug therapy to identify if correct treatment has been initiated
• Assess for allergic reactions: rash, urticaria, pruritus, chills, fever, joint pain; angioedema may occur a few days after therapy begins; epinephrine, resuscitation equipment should be available for anaphylactic reaction

Adverse effects: *italic* = common, **bold** = life-threatening

● Identify urine output; if decreasing, notify prescriber (may indicate nephrotoxicity); also check for increased BUN, creatinine

● Monitor blood studies: AST, ALT, CBC, Hct, bilirubin, LDH, alkaline phosphatase, Coombs' test monthly if patient is on long-term therapy

● Monitor electrolytes: potassium, sodium, chloride monthly if patient is on long-term therapy

● Assess bowel pattern daily; if severe diarrhea occurs, product should be discontinued; may indicate pseudomembranous colitis

● Monitor for bleeding: ecchymosis, bleeding gums, hematuria, stool guaiac daily if on long-term therapy

● Assess for overgrowth of infection: perineal itching, fever, malaise, redness, pain, swelling, drainage, rash, diarrhea, change in cough, sputum

Nursing diagnoses
● Diarrhea (adverse reactions)
● Infection, risk for (uses)
● Injury, risk for (adverse reactions)
● Knowledge, deficient (teaching)
● Noncompliance (teaching)

Implementation
Penicillin G benzathine
PO route
● Give in even doses around the clock; if GI upset occurs, give with food, avoid acidic juices; carbonated beverages may decrease PO absorption; product must be given for 10-14 days to ensure organism death and prevent superinfection
● Shake susp
IM route
● Do not give **IV**
● Give inj deep in large muscle mass
● Reconstitute with 0.9% NaCl, sterile water for inj, D₅W; refrigerate unused portion

Penicillin G
IM route
● Reconstitute with D₅W, 0.9% NaCl, sterile water for inj; shake well
● Give deep in large muscle mass; massage
● Do not give SUBCUT; may cause severe pain
● If injected near a nerve, loss of function and severe pain may occur

IV route
● Change **IV** sites q48hr to prevent pain and phlebitis
● Give by intermittent inf by diluting 3 million units or less/50 ml or more; dilute 3 million units or more/100 ml of D₅W, D₁₀W, 0.45% NaCl, 0.9% NaCl, LR, Ringer's, or any combination run over 1-2 hr (adult), 15-30 min (child)

● Give by cont inf by diluting and infusing over 24 hr

Syringe compatibilities: Heparin
Syringe incompatibilities: Metoclopramide
Y-site compatibilities: Acyclovir, amiodarone, cyclophosphamide, diltiazem, enalaprilat, esmolol, fluconazole, foscarnet, heparin, hydromorphone, labetalol, magnesium sulfate, meperidine, morphine, perphenazine, potassium chloride, tacrolimus, theophylline, verapamil, vit B/C
Additive compatibilities: Ascorbic acid, calcium chloride, calcium gluconate, cephapirin, chloramphenicol, cimetidine, clindamycin, colistimethate, corticotropin, dimenhyDRINATE, diphenhydrAMINE, ephedrine, erythromycin, furosemide, hydrocortisone, kanamycin, lidocaine, magnesium sulfate, methicillin, methylPREDNISolone, metronidazole, polymyxin B, prednisoLONE, potassium chloride, procaine, prochlorperazine, verapamil
Additive incompatibilities: Aminoglycosides, aminophylline, amphotericin B, chlorproMAZINE, DOPamine, floxacillin, hydrOXYzine, metaraminol, oxytetracycline, pentobarbital, prochlorperazine mesylate, promazine, tetracycline, thiopental

Penicillin G procaine
● Do not give **IV**
● Give deeply in large muscle mass
● Reconstitute with 0.9% NaCl, sterile water for inj, D₅W; refrigerate unused portion
● Shake medication before administering
● IM route may include procaine reactions: fear of death, depression, seizures, anxiety, confusion, hallucinations

Penicillin V
● Give in even doses around the clock; if GI upset occurs, give with food; product must be given for 10-14 days to ensure organism death and prevent superinfection; store in tight container
● Shake susp; store in refrigerator for 2 wk or for 1 wk at room temperature

Patient/family education
● Teach patient to report sore throat, bruising, bleeding, joint pain; may indicate blood dyscrasias (rare)
● Advise patient to contact prescriber if vaginal itching, loose foul-smelling stools, furry tongue occur; may indicate superinfection
● Instruct patient to take all medication prescribed for the length of time ordered

- Advise patient to notify prescriber of diarrhea with blood or pus, which may indicate pseudomembranous colitis

Evaluation
Positive therapeutic outcome
- Absence of signs/symptoms of infection (WBC <10,000/mm^3, temp WNL, absence of red, draining wounds, earache)
- Reported improvement in symptoms of infection

Treatment of anaphylaxis: Withdraw product, maintain airway, administer epinephrine, aminophylline, O_2, **IV** corticosteroids

---

pentamidine (Rx)
(pen-tam'i-deen)
Nebupent, Pentacarinat ✦, Pentam 300, Pneumopent ✦
Func. class.: Antiprotozoal
Chem. class.: Aromatic diamide derivative

Pregnancy category C

Action: Interferes with DNA/RNA synthesis in protozoa; has direct effect on islet cells in the pancreas

Therapeutic outcome: Protozoa death

Uses: Treatment/prevention of *Pneumocystis jiroveci* infections

Unlabeled uses: Leishmaniasis, African trypanosomiasis

Dosage and routes
Adult and child ≥4 mo: **IV**/IM 4 mg/kg/day × 2-3 wk; NEB 300 mg via specific nebulizer given q4wk for prevention

Available forms: Inj; aerosol 300 mg/vial; sol for aerosol 60 mg/vial ✦

Adverse effects
CNS: Disorientation, hallucinations, dizziness, confusion, drowsiness
CV: Hypotension, ventricular tachycardia, **QT prolongation, dysrhythmias**
GI: *Nausea, vomiting, anorexia,* increased AST, ALT, **acute pancreatitis,** metallic taste
GU: **Acute renal failure, increased serum creatinine, renal toxicity,** decreased urination
HEMA: Anemia, **leukopenia, thrombocytopenia**
INTEG: Sterile abscess, pain at inj site, pruritus, urticaria, rash
META: Hyperkalemia, hypocalcemia, *hypoglycemia,* hypomagnesemia

MISC: Fatigue, fever, chills, night sweats, **anaphylaxis, Stevens-Johnson syndrome**
RESP: Cough, shortness of breath, **bronchospasm** (with aerosol), sore throat

Contraindications: Hypersensitivity

Precautions: Pregnancy C, breastfeeding, children, blood dyscrasias, cardiac/renal/hepatic disease, diabetes mellitus, hypocalcemia, hyper/hypotension, anemia

Pharmacokinetics
Absorption	Well absorbed (IM); minimally absorbed (inh); completely absorbed (**IV**)
Distribution	Widely distributed; does not appear in CSF
Metabolism	Not known
Excretion	Kidneys, unchanged (up to 30%)
Half-life	6½-9½ hr; increased in renal disease

Pharmacodynamics
	IM	IV	INH
Onset	Unknown	Unknown	Unknown
Peak	½-1 hr	Inf end	Unknown
Duration	Unknown	Unknown	Unknown

Interactions
Individual drugs
Amphotericin B, cisplatin, vancomycin: increased nephrotoxicity
⬥ Erythromycin **IV:** fatal dysrhythmias
Radiation: bone marrow suppression
Drug classifications
Aminoglycosides NSAIDs: increased nephrotoxicity
Antineoplastics: increased bone marrow depression
Class IA, class III antidysrhythmics, phenothiazines, any agent that increases QT interval: increased QT prolongation

NURSING CONSIDERATIONS
Assessment
⬥ Assess any patient with compromised renal system: product is excreted slowly in poor renal system function; toxicity may occur rapidly
- Assess patient for infection, including increased temp, thick sputum, WBC >10,000/mm^3; monitor these signs of infection throughout treatment; obtain C&S before beginning therapy; treatment may begin after culture is obtained
- Assess respiratory system including rate, rhythm, bilateral lung sounds, SOB, wheezing, dyspnea

P

- Monitor ECG for cardiac dysrhythmias; ECG and pulse should be checked frequently during treatment, since cardiotoxicity can occur
- Assess for hypoglycemia including nausea, tremors, anxiety, chills, diaphoresis, headache, hunger, cold, pale skin; this side effect can last for several mo after treatment is completed
- Monitor for hyperglycemia including flushed, dry skin, acetone breath, thirst, anorexia, drowsiness, polyuria; this side effect can last for several mo after treatment is completed
- Monitor renal function tests including BUN, urinalysis, creatinine; obtain at baseline and frequently during treatment; nephrotoxicity may occur; check I&O, report hematuria, oliguria
- Monitor blood studies including blood glucose, CBC, platelets; blood glucose fluctuations are common; anemia, leukopenia, thrombocytopenia can occur
- Monitor liver function studies including AST, ALT, alkaline phosphatase, bilirubin before beginning treatment and every 3 days during therapy
- Monitor calcium and magnesium before beginning treatment and every 3 days during therapy; hypocalcemia may occur

Nursing diagnoses
- Infection, risk for (uses)
- Knowledge, deficient (teaching)

Implementation
IM route
- Reconstitute 300 mg/3 ml of sterile water for inj; give deep in large muscle mass by Z-track; IM is a painful route
- Do not mix in normal saline

Inhalation route
- Dilute 300 mg/600 ml sterile water for inj; put reconstituted sol into nebulizer (use Respirgard II jet nebulizer); do not use with other products or sol precipitate may occur; sol stable for 48 hr at room temperature; protect from light; administer over 30-45 min

IV route
- For intermittent inf reconstitute 300 mg/3-5 ml of sterile water for inj, D_5W; withdraw dose and further dilute in 50-250 ml of D_5W; diluted sol is stable for 48 hr; discard unused sol; give over 1 hr or more

Y-site compatibilities: Alfentanil, atracurium, atropine, benztropine, buprenorphine, calcium gluconate, carboplatin, caspofungin, chlorpromazine, cimetidine, cisplatin, cyclophosphamide, cyclosporine, cytarabine, dactinomycin, diltiazem, gatifloxacin, zidovudine

Y-site incompatibilities: Foscarnet, fluconazole

Patient/family education
- Teach patient to report sore throat, fever, fatigue; could indicate superinfection
- Advise patient not to drink alcohol or take aspirin, since gastric bleeding may occur
- Teach patient to make position changes slowly to prevent orthostatic hypotension
- Advise patient to maintain adequate fluid intake

Evaluation
Positive therapeutic outcome
- Decreased signs and symptoms of protozoan infections
- Decreased signs and symptoms of *P. jiroveci* pneumonia in HIV infections

---

⚠ HIGH ALERT

pentazocine (Rx)
(pen-taz′oh-seen)
Talwin, Talwin NX
Func. class.: Opiate analgesic
Chem. class.: Synthetic benzomorphan (agonist/antagonist)

Pregnancy category C

Controlled substance schedule IV

Action: Inhibits ascending pain pathways in limbic system, thalamus, midbrain, hypothalamus by binding to opiate receptor sites, altering pain perception and response

Therapeutic outcome: Relief of pain

Uses: Moderate to severe pain

Dosage and routes
Adult: PO 50-100 mg q3-4hr prn, max 600 mg/day; IV/IM/SUBCUT 30 mg q3-4hr prn, max 360 mg/day

Labor
Adult: IM 30-60 mg; **IV** 30 mg q2-3hr when contractions are regular

Renal dose
Adult: CCr 10-50 ml/min reduce dose by 25%; CCr <10 ml/min reduce dose by 50%

Available forms: SUBCUT, IM, **IV** 30 mg/ml; tabs 50 mg

Adverse effects
CNS: Drowsiness, dizziness, confusion, headache, sedation, euphoria, hallucinations, dreaming, insomnia, light-headedness
CV: Palpitations, bradycardia, change in B/P, tachycardia, increased B/P (high doses), hypotension, syncope, flushing

EENT: Tinnitus, blurred vision, miosis, diplopia
GI: *Nausea,* vomiting, anorexia, constipation, cramps, dry mouth
GU: Urinary retention, increased urinary output, dysuria
HEMA: Eosinophilia, decreased WBC
INTEG: *Rash,* urticaria, bruising, flushing, diaphoresis, pruritus, severe irritation at inj sites, **Stevens-Johnson syndrome**
RESP: Respiratory depression

Contraindications: Hypersensitivity to this product or sulfites, addiction (opioid)

Precautions: Pregnancy **C,** breastfeeding, child <18 yr, addictive personality, increased ICP, MI (acute), severe heart disease, respiratory depression, renal/hepatic disease, seizure disorder, head trauma, bowel impaction, geriatric patients

Pharmacokinetics

Absorption	Well absorbed (PO, SUBCUT, IM); completely absorbed (**IV**)
Distribution	Widely distributed; crosses placenta
Metabolism	Liver, extensively
Excretion	Kidneys, small amounts (unchanged)
Half-life	2-3 hr

Pharmacodynamics

	PO	SUBCUT/IM	IV
Onset	15-30 min	15-30 min	Rapid
Peak	1-3 hr	1-2 hr	15 min
Duration	3 hr	2-4 hr	1 hr

Interactions
Individual drugs
Alcohol: increased effects
Drug classifications
Antipsychotics, CNS depressants, sedative/hypnotics, skeletal muscle relaxants: increased effects
MAOIs: use cautiously; results are unpredictable
Opiates: decreased effects
Drug/lab test
Increased: amylase

NURSING CONSIDERATIONS
Assessment
• Assess pain: location, intensity, type of pain before, after treatment
• Assess bowel status: constipation; may need stimulant laxative/stool softener
• Monitor VS after parenteral route; note muscle rigidity, product history, liver, kidney function tests, respiratory dysfunction: respiratory depression, character, rate, rhythm; notify prescriber if respirations are <10/min

• Monitor CNS changes: dizziness, drowsiness, hallucinations, euphoria, LOC, pupil reaction
• Monitor allergic reactions: rash, urticaria
• Assess for withdrawal symptoms in opiate-dependent patients

Nursing diagnoses
• Breathing pattern, ineffective (adverse reactions)
• Knowledge, deficient (teaching)
• Pain, acute (uses)
• Sensory perception, disturbed: visual, auditory (adverse reactions)

Implementation
• Give by inj (IM, **IV**), only when resuscitative equipment available; give slowly to prevent rigidity
• Store in light-resistant area at room temperature
PO route
• Tabs made in the United States contain naloxone 0.5 mg to prevent abuse if the PO preparation is used **IV**
IM/SUBCUT route
• Give IM inj deeply in large muscle mass; rotate inj sites; repeated SUBCUT inj may cause necrosis
IV route
• Give by direct **IV** after diluting 5 mg/ml of sterile water for inj; give 5 mg or less over 1 min
Syringe compatibilities: Atropine, benzquinamide, butorphanol, chlorproMAZINE, cimetidine, dimenhyDRINATE, diphenhydrAMINE, droperidol, fentanyl, hydromorphone, hydrOXYzine, meperidine, metoclopramide, morphine, perphenazine, prochlorperazine, promazine, promethazine, propiomazine, ranitidine, scopolamine
Syringe incompatibilities: Glycopyrrolate, heparin, pentobarbital, other barbiturates
Y-site compatibilities: Heparin, hydrocortisone, potassium chloride, vit B/C
Y-site incompatibilities: Nafcillin
Additive incompatibilities: Aminophylline, amobarbital, pentobarbital, phenobarbital, secobarbital, sodium bicarbonate

Patient/family education
• Teach patient to report any symptoms of CNS changes, allergic reactions
• Advise patients to avoid CNS depressants: alcohol, sedative/hypnotics for at least 24 hr after taking this product
• Discuss with patient that dizziness, drowsiness, and confusion are common; to avoid getting up without assistance
• Discuss in detail all aspects of the product

Adverse effects: *italic* = common, **bold** = life-threatening

- Instruct patient to change position slowly to prevent orthostatic hypotension
- Teach patient to turn, cough, deep breathe after surgery to prevent atelectasis
- Advise patient to avoid CNS depressants, alcohol
- Teach patient to avoid operating machinery if drowsiness occurs

Evaluation
Positive therapeutic outcome
- Relief of pain

Treatment of overdose: Naloxone (Narcan) 0.2-0.8 mg **IV**, O₂, **IV** fluids, vasopressors

---

! HIGH ALERT

pentobarbital (Rx)
(pen-toe-bar′bi-tal)
Nembutal, Nova-Rectal ✤,
Novopentobarb ✤, pentobarbital sodium
Func. class.: Sedative/hypnotic barbiturate; anticonvulsant, anesthetic adjunct
Chem. class.: Barbitone, short acting

Pregnancy category D

Controlled substance schedule II (USA), schedule G (Canada)

Do not confuse:
pentobarbital/phenobarbital

Action: Depresses activity in brain cells, primarily in reticular activating system in brain stem; also selectively depresses neurons in posterior hypothalamus, limbic structures; may decrease cerebral blood flow, ICP (**IV**), and cerebral edema; may potentiate GABA, an inhibitory neurotransmitter

Therapeutic outcome: Sedation, sleep

Uses: Insomnia, sedation, preoperative medication, increased ICP, dental anesthetic, status epilepticus

Dosage and routes
Insomnia
Adult: PO 100-200 mg at bedtime; IM 150-200 mg at bedtime; **IV** 100 mg initially, then up to 500 mg; RECT 120-200 mg at bedtime
Child: IM 2-6 mg/kg, max 100 mg; PO 2-6 mg/kg/day in divided doses; PO preoperatively 2-6 mg/kg, max 100 mg/dose; **IV** 100 mg (hypnotic/anticonvulsant)

Status epilepticus
Adult, child, infant: IM/**IV** 15-18 mg/kg, then 10 mg/kg, then 5 mg/kg q30-60 min after 1st dose

Available forms: Caps 50, 100 mg; elix 20 mg/5 ml; rectal supp 30, 60, 120, 200 mg; inj 50 mg/ml

Adverse effects
CNS: Lethargy, drowsiness, hangover, dizziness, paradoxic stimulation in geriatric and children, light-headedness, dependence, **CNS depression,** mental depression, slurred speech, agitation
CV: Hypotension, bradycardia
GI: Nausea, vomiting, diarrhea, constipation, hepatic injury
HEMA: **Agranulocytosis, thrombocytopenia, megaloblastic anemia** (long-term treatment)
INTEG: Rash, urticaria, pain, abscesses at inj site, **angioedema, thrombophlebitis**
RESP: **Respiratory depression, apnea, laryngospasm, bronchospasm**
SYST: **Stevens-Johnson syndrome**

Contraindications: Pregnancy **D**, hypersensitivity to barbiturates, respiratory depression, addiction to barbiturates, severe renal/hepatic impairment, porphyria, uncontrolled pain

Precautions: Breastfeeding, geriatric, anemia, renal/hepatic disease, hypertension, acute/chronic pain, suicidal ideation, depression, angioedema

Pharmacokinetics
Absorption	Well absorbed
Distribution	Widely distributed; crosses placenta, enters breast milk
Metabolism	Liver
Excretion	Kidneys, unchanged (minimally)
Half-life	15-48 hr

Pharmacodynamics
	PO	IM	IV	RECT
Onset	15-30 min	10-25 min	Immediate	Slow
Peak	3-4 hr	Unknown	1 min	Unknown
Duration	4-6 hr	1-4 hr	15 min	4-6 hr

Interactions
Individual drugs
Alcohol: increased CNS depression
CycloSPORINE, voriconazole: avoid concurrent use
Doxycycline: increased half-life
Griseofulvin, quinidine: decreased effectiveness

Drug classifications
Anticoagulants: decreased effectiveness
Antihistamines, CNS depressants, MAOIs, opiates, sedative/hypnotics: increased CNS depression
Corticosteroids: decreased effectiveness

Drug/herb
Eucalyptus, Jamaican dogwood, kava, lemon balm, nettle, pill-bearing spurge, poppy, quinine, senega, valerian: increased pentobarbital level

Drug/lab test
False increase: sulfobromophthalein

NURSING CONSIDERATIONS
Assessment
• Assess mental status: mood, sensorium, affect, memory (long, short), especially geriatric; if using as a hypnotic, assess sleep patterns during therapy, product suppresses REM sleep with dreaming; withdrawal insomnia may occur after short-term use; do not start using product again; insomnia will improve in 1-3 nights; may experience increased dreaming
• Monitor for respiratory dysfunction: respiratory depression, character, rate, rhythm (when using **IV**); hold product if respirations are < 10/min or if pupils are dilated; also check VS q30min after parenteral route for 2 hr
• Assess for blood dyscrasias: fever, sore throat, bruising, rash, jaundice, epistaxis (long-term treatment only)
• Assess seizure activity including type, location, duration, and character; provide seizure precaution
• Assess for pain in postoperative patients; pain threshold is lowered when patients are taking this medication

Nursing diagnoses
• Injury, risk for (side effects)
• Knowledge, deficient (teaching)

Implementation
• Administer only after removal of cigarettes, to prevent fires
• Reserve use until after trying conservative measures for insomnia

PO route
• Give 30 min before bedtime for expected sleeplessness
• May dilute elixir in juice, milk, or water if needed
• Give on empty stomach for best absorption

IM route
• Give deeply in muscle mass (gluteal) to minimize irritation to tissues; split inj >5 ml

into 2 inj since irritation to tissues may occur; do not administer SUBCUT

IV route
• Use large vein to prevent extravasation; if extravasation occurs, use moist heat to the area and 5% procaine sol injected into area; give at 50 mg/1 min or more
• Give **IV** only with resuscitative equipment available (and only by qualified personnel)

Syringe compatibilities: Aminophylline, ephedrine, hydromorphone, neostigmine, scopolamine, sodium bicarbonate, thiopental

Syringe incompatibilities: Benzquinamide, butorphanol, chlorproMAZINE, cimetidine, dimenhyDRINATE, diphenhydrAMINE, droperidol, fentanyl, glycopyrrolate, hydrOXYzine, meperidine, midazolam, nalbuphine, pentazocine, perphenazine, prochlorperazine, promazine, promethazine, ranitidine

Y-site compatibilities: Acyclovir, propofol, regular insulin

Additive compatibilities: Amikacin, aminophylline, calcium chloride, cephapirin, chloramphenicol, dimenhyDRINATE, erythromycin, lidocaine, thiopental, verapamil

Additive incompatibilities: Chlorpheniramine, codeine, ephedrine, erythromycin gluceptate, hydrocortisone, hydrOXYzine, levorphanol, methadone, norepinephrine, pentazocine, penicillin G potassium, phenytoin, promazine, promethazine, regular insulin, sodium succinate, streptomycin, triflupromazine, vancomycin

Patient/family education
• Teach patient to carry/wear emergency ID stating name, products taken, condition, prescriber's name, phone number
• Caution patient to avoid driving and other activities that require alertness
• Caution patient to avoid alcohol ingestion and CNS depressants; increased sedation may occur
• Teach patient not to discontinue medication quickly after long-term use; taper off over several wk

Evaluation
Positive therapeutic outcome
• Improved sleeping patterns
• Decreased seizure activity
• Improved energy

Treatment of overdose: Lavage, activated charcoal, warming blanket, vital signs, hemodialysis

Adverse effects: *italic* = common, **bold** = life-threatening

! HIGH ALERT

pentostatin (Rx)
(pen'toe-sta-tin)
Nipent
Func. class.: Antineoplastic, enzyme inhibitor
Chem. class.: Streptomyces antibioticus derivative

Pregnancy category D

Action: Inhibits the enzyme adenosine deaminase (ADA), which is able to block DNA synthesis and some RNA synthesis

Therapeutic outcome: Prevention of rapidly growing malignant cells

Uses: α-Interferon–refractory hairy cell leukemia

Unlabeled uses: Chronic lymphocytic leukemia, non-Hodgkin's lymphoma

Dosage and routes
Adult: **IV** 4 mg/m² every other wk; may be given **IV** BOL or diluted in a larger volume and given over 20-30 min

Available forms: Powder for inj 10 mg/vial

Adverse effects
CNS: Headache, anxiety, confusion, depression, dizziness, insomnia, nervousness, paresthesia
GI: Nausea, vomiting, anorexia, diarrhea, constipation, flatulence, stomatitis, elevated liver function tests
GU: **Hematuria,** dysuria, increased BUN/creatinine, **acute renal failure**
HEMA: **Leukopenia, anemia, thrombocytopenia, ecchymosis, lymphadenopathy,** petechiae
INTEG: Rash, eczema, dry skin, pruritus, sweating, herpes simplex/zoster
RESP: Cough, upper respiratory tract infection, bronchitis, dyspnea, epistaxis, pneumonia, pharyngitis, rhinitis, sinusitis, **pulmonary edema**
SYST: Fever, infection, fatigue, pain, allergic reaction, chills, **death, sepsis,** chest pain, flulike symptoms

Contraindications: Pregnancy **D,** hypersensitivity to this product or mannitol

Precautions: Breastfeeding, children, renal disease, bone marrow depression

Black Box Warning: Hepatic disease, pulmonary edema, renal failure, seizures

Pharmacokinetics

Absorption	Completely absorbed
Distribution	Unknown; low protein binding
Metabolism	Unknown
Excretion	Kidneys
Half-life	5-7 hr; increased in renal disease

Pharmacodynamics

Onset	4-5 mo
Peak	Unknown
Duration	1½-34 mo

Interactions
Individual drugs
Black Box Warning: Fludarabine: fatal pulmonary reaction

Vidarabine: increased adverse reactions

Drug classifications
Anticoagulants, NSAIDs: increased bleeding risk
Drug/lab test
Increased: uric acid

NURSING CONSIDERATIONS
Assessment
• Assess CNS changes: confusion, paresthesias, psychosis, tremors, seizures, neuropathies; product should be discontinued
• Assess for toxicity: facial flushing, epistaxis, increased pro-time, thrombocytopenia; product should be discontinued
• Assess acidosis, signs of dehydration: rapid respirations, poor skin turgor, decreased urine output, dry skin, restlessness, weakness
• Check buccal cavity q8hr for dryness, sores or ulceration, white patches, oral pain, bleeding, dysphagia; obtain prescription for viscous lidocaine (Xylocaine) to use in mouth
• Assess symptoms indicating severe allergic reaction: rash, pruritus, urticaria, purpuric skin lesions, itching, flushing
• Assess tachypnea, ECG changes, dyspnea, edema, fatigue; respiratory and CV reaction can be severe
• Monitor CBC, differential, platelet count weekly; withhold product if WBC is <2000/mm³ or platelet count is <100,000/mm³, notify prescriber of results
• Monitor renal function tests: BUN, creatinine, serum uric acid, urine CCr before, during therapy; I&O ratio; report fall in urine output to <30 ml/hr
• Monitor temp q4hr (may indicate beginning of infection)
• Monitor liver function tests before, during therapy (bilirubin, AST, ALT, LDH) as needed

or monthly; check for jaundice of skin and sclera, dark urine, clay-colored stools, itchy skin, abdominal pain, fever, diarrhea
• Assess for bleeding: hematuria, stool guaiac, bruising or petechiae, mucosa or orifices q8hr; check for inflammation of mucosa, breaks in skin
• Assess effects of alopecia on body image; discuss feelings about body changes

Nursing diagnoses
• Body image, disturbed (adverse reactions)
• Infection, risk for (adverse reactions)
• Injury, risk for (adverse reactions)
• Knowledge, deficient (teaching)

Implementation
• Give fluids **IV** or PO before chemotherapy to hydrate patient
• Antiemetic 30-60 min before giving product and prn to prevent vomiting; allopurinol to prevent uric acid increases
• Give TOP or systemic analgesics for pain to lessen effects from stomatitis
• Avoid use of higher doses than recommended; toxicity can occur
• Give liquid diet: carbonated beverages; gelatin may be added if patient is not nauseated or vomiting
• Preparation should be done by personnel knowledgeable in preparing antineoplastics wearing gloves, gown, mask in biologic cabinet
• Give by direct **IV** by reconstituting 10 mg/5 ml of sterile water for inj (2 mg/ml); shake well
• Give over 5 min
• Give by intermittent inf after diluting 10 mg/25-50 ml of 0.9% NaCl, D₅W; give over 30 min
• Diluted sol should be used within 8 hr at room temperature
Y-site compatibilities: Fludarabine, melphalan, ondansetron, paclitaxel, sargramostim
Solution compatibilities: D₅W, 0.9% NaCl, LR

Patient/family education
• Teach patient to avoid use of products containing aspirin or NSAIDs, razors, commercial mouthwash, since bleeding may occur; to report symptoms of bleeding (hematuria, tarry stools)
• Encourage patient to rinse mouth tid-qid with water, club soda; brush teeth bid-qid with soft brush or cotton-tipped applicators for stomatitis; use unwaxed dental floss
• Advise patient to report signs of anemia (fatigue, headache, irritability, faintness, shortness of breath); CNS reactions including

confusion, psychosis, nightmares, seizures, severe headaches
• Inform patient that hair may be lost during treatment; a wig or hairpiece may make patient feel better; new hair may be different in color, texture
• Advise patient to use sunscreen and protective clothing to prevent photosensitive reactions

Evaluation
Positive therapeutic outcome
• Prevention of rapid division of malignant cells
• Decreased bone marrow hairy cells

---

pentoxifylline (Rx)
(pen-tox-if'i-lin)
Pentoxil, Trental
Func. class.: Hemorheologic agent
Chem. class.: Dimethylxanthine derivative

Pregnancy category C

Action: Decreases blood viscosity, stimulates prostacyclin formation, increases blood flow by increasing flexibility of RBCs; decreases RBC hyperaggregation; reduces platelet aggregation, decreases fibrinogen concentration

Therapeutic outcome: Decreased claudication and improved blood flow

Uses: Intermittent claudication related to chronic occlusive vascular disease

Unlabeled uses: Diabetic neuropathies, sickle cell anemia

Dosage and routes
Adult: PO 400 mg tid with meals, may decrease to bid if side effects occur, must be taken for ≥8 wk for maximal effect

Available forms: Cont rel tabs 400 mg; ext rel tabs 400 mg

Adverse effects
CNS: Headache, anxiety, *tremors,* confusion, *dizziness*
CV: Angina, dysrhythmias, palpitations, hypotension, chest pain, dyspnea, edema
EENT: Blurred vision, earache, increased salivation, sore throat, conjunctivitis
GI: Dyspepsia, nausea, vomiting, anorexia, bloating, belching, constipation, cholecystitis, dry mouth, thirst, bad taste, flatulence
INTEG: Rash, pruritus, urticaria, brittle fingernails
MISC: Epistaxis, flulike symptoms, laryngitis, nasal congestion, **leukopenia,** malaise, weight changes

P

Adverse effects: *italic* = common, **bold** = life-threatening

Contraindications: Hypersensitivity to this product or xanthines, retinal/cerebral hemorrhage, severe hepatic disease

Precautions: Pregnancy **C**, breastfeeding, children, angina pectoris, impaired renal function, recent surgery, peptic ulcer, cardiac/hepatic disease, bleeding disorders

Pharmacokinetics

Absorption	Well absorbed
Distribution	Unknown
Metabolism	Liver, degradation
Excretion	Kidneys
Half-life	½-1 hr

Pharmacodynamics

Onset	Unknown
Peak	2-4 hr
Duration	Unknown

Interactions
Individual drugs

Abciximab, clopidogrel, eptifibatide, ticlopidine, tirofiban, warfarin: increased bleeding risk

Cimetidine, ciprofloxacin: increased pentoxifylline level

Theophylline: increased theophylline level
Drug classifications

Antihypertensives, nitrates: increased hypotension

NSAIDs, salicylates, heparins, thrombin inhibitor, thrombolytics: increased bleeding risk
Drug/herb

Anise, arnica, chamomile, clove, dong quai, fenugreek, feverfew, garlic, ginger, ginkgo, ginseng *(Panax),* licorice: increased bleeding risk

NURSING CONSIDERATIONS
Assessment
* Monitor B/P, respirations in patient taking antihypertensives
* Assess for intermittent claudication baseline, during treatment
* Monitor blood tests: PT, Hgb, Hct in patients at risk for hemorrhage

Nursing diagnoses
* Activity intolerance (uses)
* Knowledge, deficient (teaching)
* Noncompliance (teaching)
* Pain, chronic (uses)

Implementation
* Do not break, crush, or chew cont rel or ext rel tab
* Give with meals to prevent GI upset

Patient/family education
* Teach patient that therapeutic response may take 2-4 wk
* Instruct patient to observe feet for arterial insufficiency
* Instruct patient to use cotton socks, well-fitted shoes; not to go barefoot
* Advise patient to watch for bleeding, bruises, petechiae, epistaxis
* Advise that there are many drug, herb interactions

Evaluation
Positive therapeutic outcome
* Decreased pain, cramping
* Increased ambulation

---

perindopril (Rx)
(per-in-doe-pril)
Aceon
Func. class.: Antihypertensive
Chem. class.: Angiotensin-converting enzyme (ACE) inhibitor
Pregnancy category D

Action: Selectively suppresses renin-angiotensin-aldosterone system; inhibits ACE; prevents conversion of angiotensin I to angiotensin II, resulting in dilatation of arterial and venous vessels

Therapeutic outcome: Decreased B/P in hypertension

Uses: Hypertension alone or in combination, stable artery disease

Dosage and routes
Hypertension
Adult: PO 4 mg/day, may increase or decrease to desired response; range 4-8 mg/day may give in 2 divided doses or as a single dose; max 16 mg/day

Patients taking diuretics
Discontinue diuretic 2-3 days before perindopril, then resume diuretic if needed

Stable CAD
Adult: PO 4 mg/day × 2 wk, then increase as tolerated to 8 mg/day

Renal dose
Adult: PO CCr 16-29 ml/min, 2 mg every other day; CCr 30-59 ml/min 2 mg/day

Available forms: Tabs, scored 2, 4, 8 mg

Adverse effects
CNS: Insomnia, dizziness, paresthesias, headache, fatigue, anxiety, depression

---

 Alert   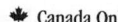 Canada Only   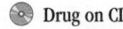 Drug on CD   * "Tall Man" lettering (See Preface)

CV: Hypotension, chest pain, tachycardia, dysrhythmias, syncope
EENT: Tinnitus, visual changes, sore throat, double vision, dry burning eyes
GI: Nausea, vomiting, colitis, cramps, diarrhea, constipation, flatulence, dry mouth, loss of taste
GU: **Proteinuria, renal failure,** increased frequency of polyuria or oliguria
HEMA: **Agranulocytosis, neutropenia**
INTEG: Rash, purpura, alopecia, hyperhidrosis
META: Hyperkalemia
RESP: Dyspnea, dry cough, crackles
SYST: **Angioedema**

Contraindications: Hypersensitivity, history of angioedema

Black Box Warning: Pregnancy **D**

Precautions: Breastfeeding, renal disease, hyperkalemia, hepatic failure, dehydration, bilateral renal artery stenosis, cough, angioedema, severe CHF

Pharmacokinetics	
Absorption	Well absorbed
Distribution	Unknown
Metabolism	Liver
Excretion	Kidneys
Half-life	Unknown

Pharmacodynamics
Unknown

Interactions
Individual drugs
Allopurinol: increased hypersensitivity
Lithium: increased serum levels
Drug classifications
Antihypertensives, diuretics: increased hypotension
Antihypertensives, neuromuscular blocking agents: increased effects
Diuretics (potassium-sparing), potassium supplements, salt substitutes: hyperkalemia
NSAIDs: decreased effects
NSAIDs, salicylates: decreased antihypertensive effect
Drug/herb
Aconite: increased toxicity, death
Astragalus, cola tree: increased or decreased antihypertensive effect
Barberry, betony, black catechu, black cohosh, bloodroot, broom, burdock, cat's claw, dandelion, goldenseal, hawthorn, Irish moss, Jamaican dogwood, kelp, khella,

mistletoe, parsley: increased antihypertensive effect
Coltsfoot, guarana, khat, licorice, yohimbe: decreased antihypertensive effect
Drug/lab test
Interference: glucose/insulin tolerance tests

NURSING CONSIDERATIONS
Assessment
• Monitor blood studies: neutrophils, decreased platelets
• Monitor B/P, orthostatic hypotension, syncope; if changes occur dosage change may be required
• Monitor renal studies: protein, BUN, creatinine; increased levels may indicate nephrotic syndrome and renal failure
• Monitor renal symptoms: polyuria, oliguria, frequency, dysuria
• Establish baselines in renal, liver function tests before therapy begins
• Check potassium levels throughout treatment, although hyperkalemia rarely occurs
• Check for edema in feet, legs daily
• Assess for allergic reactions: rash, fever, pruritus, urticaria; product should be discontinued if antihistamines fail to help

Nursing diagnoses
• Cardiac output, decreased (uses)
• Injury, risk for (adverse reactions)
• Knowledge, deficient (teaching)
• Noncompliance (teaching)

Implementation
• Store in airtight container at 86° F (30° C) or less
• Severe hypotension may occur after 1st dose of this medication; decreased hypotension may be prevented by reducing or discontinuing diuretic therapy 3 days before beginning perindopril therapy
• Give by **IV** inf of 0.9% NaCl (as ordered) to expand fluid volume if severe hypotension occurs

Patient/family education
• Advise patient not to discontinue product abruptly; advise patient to tell all persons associated with health care
• Teach patient not to use OTC products (cough, cold, allergy medications) unless directed by physician; serious side effects can occur; xanthines, such as coffee, tea, chocolate, cola can prevent action of product
• Instruct patient on the importance of complying with dosage schedule, even if feeling better; to continue with medical regimen to decrease B/P: exercise, cessation of smoking, decreasing stress, diet modifications

Adverse effects: *italic* = common, **bold** = life-threatening

- Emphasize the need to rise slowly to sitting or standing position to minimize orthostatic hypotension; not to exercise in hot weather, which can cause increased hypotension
- Advise patient to notify prescriber of mouth sores, sore throat, fever, swelling of hands or feet, irregular heartbeat, chest pain, coughing, shortness of breath
- Caution patient to report excessive perspiration, dehydration, vomiting, diarrhea; may lead to fall in B/P
- Caution patient that product may cause dizziness, fainting, light-headedness; may occur during 1st few days of therapy; to avoid activities that may be hazardous
- Teach patient how to take B/P, and normal readings for age-group

Evaluation
Positive therapeutic outcome
- Decreased B/P in hypertension

Treatment of overdose: Lavage, **IV** atropine for bradycardia, **IV** theophylline for bronchospasm, digoxin, O₂; diuretic for cardiac failure, hemodialysis

---

perphenazine (Rx)
(per-fen'a-zeen)
Apo-Perphenazine ✤, perphenazine, PMS Perphenazine ✤
Func. class.: Antipsychotic/neuroleptic
Chem. class.: Phenothiazine piperidine

Pregnancy category C

Action: Depresses cerebral cortex, hypothalamus, limbic system, which control activity, aggression; blocks neurotransmission produced by dopamine at synapse; exhibits strong α-adrenergic, anticholinergic blocking action; as antiemetic inhibits medullary chemoreceptor trigger zone; receptor affinity DOPamine D_2, histamine H_1, α-adrenergic

Therapeutic outcome: Decreased signs and symptoms of psychosis; decreased nausea and vomiting

Uses: Psychotic disorders, schizophrenia, nausea, vomiting

Dosage and routes
Nausea/vomiting
Adult and child >12 yr: PO 8-16 mg/day in divided doses, up to 24 mg

Psychiatric use in hospitalized patients
Adult: PO 4-16 mg bid-qid, gradually increased to desired dose, max 64 mg/day

Geriatric: PO 2-4 mg daily-bid, increase by 2-4 mg/wk to desired dose
Child >12 yr: PO 6-12 mg in divided doses

Nonhospitalized patients
Adult: PO 4-8 mg tid

Available forms: Tabs 2, 4, 8, 16 mg

Adverse effects
CNS: EPS (pseudoparkinsonism, akathisia, dystonia, tardive dyskinesia), **neuroleptic malignant syndrome, seizures,** *headache,* dizziness
CV: Orthostatic hypotension (geriatric), **cardiac arrest,** ECG changes, **tachycardia**
EENT: Blurred vision, glaucoma
GI: Dry mouth, nausea, vomiting, anorexia, constipation, diarrhea, jaundice, weight gain
GU: Urinary retention, urinary frequency, enuresis, impotence, amenorrhea, gynecomastia, ejaculatory dysfunction
HEMA: Anemia, **leukopenia, leukocytosis, agranulocytosis**
INTEG: Rash, photosensitivity, dermatitis
RESP: **Laryngospasm,** dyspnea, **respiratory depression**

Contraindications: Child <12 yr, hypersensitivity, blood dyscrasias, coma, brain damage, bone marrow depression, CNS depression

Precautions: Pregnancy **C,** breastfeeding, geriatric, seizure disorders, hypertension, renal/hepatic/cardiac disease, closed-angle glaucoma

Black Box Warning: Dementia

Pharmacokinetics
Absorption	Variably absorbed (PO); well absorbed (IM)
Distribution	Widely distributed; high concentrations in CNS; crosses placenta; 91%-99% protein binding
Metabolism	Liver, extensively; GI mucosa
Excretion	Kidneys
Half-life	Unknown

Pharmacodynamics
	PO
Onset	Erratic
Peak	4-8 hr
Duration	6-12 hr

Interactions
Individual drugs
Alcohol: increased effects of both products, oversedation

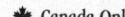 Alert   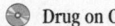 Canada Only   🔵 Drug on CD   * "Tall Man" lettering (See Preface)

Aluminum hydroxide, magnesium hydroxide: decreased absorption
Epinephrine: increased toxicity
Levodopa: decreased antiparkinson activity
Lithium: increased risk of EPS
Ritonavir: increased perphenazine effect
Meperidine: increased hypotension

Drug classifications

Anesthetics, CNS depressants, barbiturate anesthetics: increased sedation
Anticholinergics: increased anticholinergic effects
Anticoagulants (oral): decreased anticoagulant effect
β-Adrenergic blockers: increased effects of both products
Diuretics (thiazide): increased hypotension

Drug/herb

Betel palm, kava: increased EPS
Cola tree, hops, nettle, nutmeg: increased action
Henbane: increased anticholinergic effect

Drug/lab test

Increased: liver function tests, cardiac enzymes, cholesterol, blood glucose, prolactin, bilirubin, PBI, cholinesterase, iodine
Decreased: hormones (blood and urine)
False positive: pregnancy tests, PKU
False negative: urinary steroids, 17-OHCS

NURSING CONSIDERATIONS
Assessment

• Assess mental status: orientation, mood, behavior, presence and type of hallucinations before initial administration and monthly; this product should significantly reduce psychotic behavior
• Check for swallowing of PO medication; check for hoarding or giving medication to other patients
• Monitor I&O ratio; palpate bladder if low urinary output occurs, especially in geriatric; urinalysis recommended before, during prolonged therapy
• Monitor bilirubin, CBC, liver function tests monthly
• Assess affect, orientation, LOC, reflexes, gait, coordination, sleep pattern disturbances
• Monitor B/P with patient sitting, standing, and lying; take pulse and respirations q4hr during initial treatment; establish baseline before starting treatment; report drops of 30 mm Hg; obtain baseline ECG, with Q- and T-wave changes
• Check for dizziness, faintness, palpitations, tachycardia on rising; severe orthostatic hypotension is common

◆ Identify for neuroleptic malignant syndrome: hyperpyrexia, muscle rigidity, increased CPK, altered mental status; product should be discontinued
• Assess for EPS including akathisia (inability to sit still, no pattern to movements), tardive dyskinesia (bizarre movements of the jaw, mouth, tongue, extremities), pseudoparkinsonism (ragged tremors, pill rolling, shuffling gait); an antiparkinsonian product should be prescribed
• Assess for constipation, urinary retention daily; if these occur, increase bulk, water in diet

Nursing diagnoses
• Coping, ineffective (uses)
• Knowledge, deficient (teaching)
• Noncompliance (teaching)

Implementation
PO route
• Administer decreased dose in geriatric, in whom metabolism is slowed

Patient/family education
• Teach patient to use good oral hygiene; frequent rinsing of mouth, sugarless gum for dry mouth
• Advise patient to avoid hazardous activities until product response is determined, dizziness, blurred vision may occur
• Inform patient that orthostatic hypotension occurs often and to rise from sitting or lying position gradually; to remain lying down after IM inj for at least 30 min; tell patient to avoid hot tubs, hot showers, tub baths, since hypotension may occur; teach patient that in hot weather heat stroke may occur; take extra precautions to stay cool
• Teach patient to avoid abrupt withdrawal of this product, or EPS may result; product should be withdrawn slowly
• Teach patient to avoid OTC preparations (cough, hay fever, cold) unless approved by prescriber, since serious product interactions may occur; avoid use with alcohol, CNS depressants; increased drowsiness may result
• Caution patient to use a sunscreen and sunglasses to prevent burns
• Teach patient about EPS and necessity of meticulous oral hygiene, since oral candidiasis may occur
• Instruct patient to take antacids 2 hr before or after taking this product
• Teach patient to report sore throat, malaise, fever, bleeding, mouth sores; if these occur, CBC should be performed and product discontinued

Adverse effects: *italic* = common, **bold** = life-threatening

• Teach patient that urine may turn reddish brown

Evaluation
Positive therapeutic outcome
• Decrease in emotional excitement, hallucinations, delusions, paranoia
• Reorganization of patterns of thought, speech

Treatment of overdose: Lavage if orally ingested; provide airway; *do not induce vomiting or use epinephrine*

---

phenazopyridine (Rx, OTC)
(fen-az-o-peer′i-deen)
AZO-100, AZO-Gesic, AZO-Standard, Baridium, Eridium, Geridium, Phenazo ✤, Phenazodine, phenazopyridine, Prodium, Pyridiate, Pyridium, Urinary Analgesic, Urodine, Urogesic, Walgreen's Urinary Pain Relief
Func. class.: Nonopioid analgesic, urinary
Chem. class.: Azodye

Pregnancy category B

Action: Exerts analgesic, anesthetic action on the urinary tract mucosa

Therapeutic outcome: Decreased pain, burning when urinating

Uses: Urinary tract irritation, infection (for symptoms only of pain, burning, itching) used with urinary antiinfectives

Dosage and routes
Adult: PO 200 mg tid × 2 days or less when used with antibacterial for UTI
Child 6-12 yr: PO 4 mg/kg tid × 2 days

Renal dose
Adult: PO CCr 50-80 ml/min give dose 8-16 hr; CCr <50 ml/min do not use

Available forms: Tabs 95, 97.2, 100, 200 mg

Adverse effects
CNS: Headache, **aseptic meningitis**
GI: Nausea, vomiting, diarrhea, heartburn, anorexia, **hepatic toxicity**
GU: **Renal toxicity,** *orange-red urine*
HEMA: **Thrombocytopenia, agranulocytosis, leukopenia, neutropenia, hemolytic anemia, methemoglobinemia**
INTEG: Rash, pruritus, skin pigmentation
SYST: **Anaphylaxis,** body fluid staining

Contraindications: Hypersensitivity, renal insufficiency, hepatic disease, uremia

Precautions: Pregnancy **B,** breastfeeding, children <12 yr, geriatric patient, contact lens use

Pharmacokinetics
Absorption	Well absorbed
Distribution	Unknown; crosses placenta
Metabolism	Unknown
Excretion	Kidneys, unchanged
Half-life	Unknown

Pharmacodynamics
Onset	Unknown
Peak	5-6 hr
Duration	8 hr

Interactions
Drug/lab test
Interference: urinalysis

NURSING CONSIDERATIONS
Assessment
• Assess urinary status: burning, pain, itching, urgency, frequency, hematuria before, during, after completion of product therapy
• Monitor liver function tests: AST, ALT, bilirubin if patient is on long-term therapy
◆ Assess for hepatotoxicity: dark urine, clay-colored stools, yellowing of skin and sclera, itching, abdominal pain, fever, diarrhea if patient is on long-term therapy
• Assess for allergic reactions: rash, urticaria; if these occur, product may have to be discontinued

Nursing diagnoses
• Knowledge, deficient (teaching)
• Pain, acute (uses)
• Urinary elimination, impaired (uses)

Implementation
• Give to patient crushed or whole; chew tab should be chewed
• Give with food or milk to decrease gastric symptoms

Patient/family education
• Advise patient to report any symptoms of hepatotoxicity
• Caution patient not to exceed recommended dosage and to take with meals; to read label on other OTC products
• Teach patient not to discontinue after pain is relieved but continue to take concurrent prescribed antiinfective until finished
• Inform patient urine may turn red-orange; body fluids may stain clothing or contact lenses

---

Evaluation
Positive therapeutic outcome
• Decrease in pain, burning, itching when urinating

Treatment of overdose: Methylene blue 1-2 mg/kg **IV** or vit C 100-200 mg PO

❗ HIGH ALERT

phenobarbital 😊 **(Rx)**
(fee-noe-bar′bit-tal)
Ancalixir ✦, Luminal, phenobarbital sodium
Func. class.: Anticonvulsant, sedative/hypnotic
Chem. class.: Barbiturate

Pregnancy category D
Controlled substance schedule IV

Do not confuse:
phenobarbital/pentobarbital

Action: Depresses activity in brain cells primarily in reticular activating system in brain stem; also selectively depresses neurons in posterior hypothalamus, limbic structures; able to decrease seizure activity by inhibition of impulses in CNS; decreases motor activity

Therapeutic outcome: Sedation, anticonvulsant, improved energy

Uses: All forms of epilepsy, status epilepticus, febrile seizures in children, sedation, insomnia

Unlabeled uses: Hyperbilirubinemia, chronic cholestasis

Dosage and routes
Seizures
Adult: PO 1-3 mg/kg/day in divided doses tid or total dose at bedtime
Child 5-12 yr: PO 3-6 mg/kg/day in 1-2 divided doses
Child 1-5 yr: PO 6-8 mg/kg/day in 1-2 divided doses
Infant: PO 5-6 mg/kg/day in 1-2 divided doses
Neonate: PO 3-4 mg/kg/day as a single dose

Status epilepticus
Adult: **IV** INF 10 mg/kg; run no faster than 50 mg/min; may give up to 30 mg/kg
Child: **IV** INF 5-10 mg/kg; may repeat q10-15min up to 20 mg/kg; run no faster than 50 mg/min

Insomnia
Adult: PO/IM/SUBCUT 100-200 mg
Child (unlabeled): PO/IM/SUBCUT 3-5 mg/kg

Sedation
Adult: PO 30-120 mg/day in 2-3 divided doses
Child: PO 3-5 mg/kg/day in 3 divided doses

Preoperative sedation
Adult: IM 100-200 mg 1-1½ hr before surgery
Child: PO/IM/**IV** 1-3 mg/kg 1-1½ hr before surgery

Available forms: Caps 15 mg; elix 20 mg/5 ml; tabs 15, 30, 32, 60, 65, 100 mg; inj 30, 60, 65, 130 mg/ml

Adverse effects
CNS: Paradoxic excitement (geriatric), drowsiness, lethargy, *hangover headache,* flushing, hallucinations, **coma**
GI: Nausea, vomiting, diarrhea, constipation
HEMA: **Agranulocytosis, megaloblastic anemia, thrombocytopenia, thrombophlebitis**
INTEG: Rash, urticaria, **Stevens-Johnson syndrome, angioedema,** local pain, swelling, necrosis, scaling eczema

Contraindications: Pregnancy **D,** breastfeeding, geriatric, hypersensitivity to barbiturates, porphyria, hepatic/respiratory disease, nephritis, hyperthyroidism, diabetes mellitus

Precautions: Anemia, renal disease

Pharmacokinetics	
Absorption	Slow (70%-90%) (PO/IM/**IV**)
Distribution	Not known; crosses placenta
Metabolism	Liver (75%)
Excretion	Kidneys (25% unchanged)
Half-life	2-6 days

Pharmacodynamics			
	PO	IM	IV
Onset	30-60 min	10-30 min	5 min
Peak	Unknown	Unknown	30 min
Duration	6-8 hr	4-6 hr	4-6 hr

Interactions
Individual drugs
Alcohol: increased CNS depression
Chloramphenicol, disulfiram: increased effects
Doxycycline, metronidazole, quinidine, theophylline: decreased effectiveness
Furosemide: increased orthostatic hypotension
Valproic acid: increased sedation
Drug classifications
Anticoagulants, glucocorticoids, estrogens, hormonal contraceptives: decreased effectiveness
CNS depressants: increased effects

Adverse effects: *italic* = common, **bold** = life-threatening

MAOIs, skeletal muscle relaxants (nondepolarizing), sulfonamides: increased effects

Drug/herb

Chamomile, eucalyptus, hops, Jamaican dogwood, kava, lemon balm, nettle, pill-bearing spurge, poppy, senega, skullcap, valerian: increased CNS depression

Quinine: increased phenobarbital levels

St. John's wort: decreased barbiturate effect

NURSING CONSIDERATIONS
Assessment
• Assess mental status: mood, sensorium, affect, memory (long, short), especially geriatric; if using as a hypnotic, assess sleep patterns during therapy; product suppresses REM sleep with dreaming
• Withdrawal insomnia may occur after short-term use; do not start using product again; insomnia improves in 1-3 nights; may experience increased dreaming
• Assess respiratory dysfunction: respiratory depression, character, rate, rhythm when using **IV**; hold product if respirations are <10/min or if pupils are dilated; also check VS q30min after parenteral route for 2 hr
• Assess for barbiturate toxicity: hypotension, pulmonary constriction, cold, clammy skin, cyanosis of lips, CNS depression, nausea, vomiting, hallucinations, delirium, weakness, coma, pupillary constriction; mild symptoms occur in 8-12 hr without product
• Assess for pain in postoperative patients; pain threshold is lowered when patients are taking this medication
• Assess for blood dyscrasias: fever, sore throat, bruising, rash, jaundice, epistaxis (long-term treatment only)
• Assess seizure activity including type, location, duration, and character; provide seizure precaution

Nursing diagnoses
• Injury, risk for (adverse reactions)
• Knowledge, deficient (teaching)
• Sleep deprivation (uses)

Implementation
• Give medication after removal of cigarettes to prevent fires
• Give medication after trying conservative measures for insomnia

PO route
• Tab may be crushed and mixed with food if swallowing is difficult; also may be mixed with other fluids 30-60 min before bedtime for expected sleeplessness; on empty stomach for best absorption

IM route
• Give inj in deep muscle mass (gluteal) to minimize irritation to tissues
• Split inj of >5 ml into two, since irritation to tissues may occur

IV, direct route
• Use large vein to prevent extravasation; if extravasation occurs, use moist heat to the area and 5% procaine sol injected into area; give at 65 mg or less/min; titrate to patient response

Syringe compatibilities: Heparin

Syringe incompatibilities: Benzquinamide, ranitidine

Y-site compatibilities: Enalaprilat, meropenem, propofol, sufentanil

Y-site incompatibilities: Hydromorphone

Additive compatibilities: Amikacin, aminophylline, calcium chloride, calcium gluceptate, cephapirin, colistimethate, dimenhyDRINATE, meropenem, polymyxin B, sodium bicarbonate, thiopental, verapamil

Additive incompatibilities: Cephalothin, chlorproMAZINE, codeine, ephedrine, hydrALAZINE, hydrocortisone sodium succinate, hydrOXYzine, insulin, levorphanol, meperidine, methadone, morphine, norepinephrine, pentazocine, procaine, prochlorperazine mesylate, promazine, promethazine, streptomycin, vancomycin

Solution compatibilities: D_5W, $D_{10}W$, 0.45% NaCl, 0.9% NaCl, Ringer's, dextrose/saline combinations, dextrose/Ringer's, dextrose/LR combinations, sodium lactate

Patient/family education
• Teach patient that hangover is common
• Instruct patient that product is indicated only for short-term treatment of insomnia and is probably ineffective after 2 wk
• Inform patient that physical dependency may result when used for extended time (45-90 days depending on dosage)
• Teach patient to avoid driving and other activities requiring alertness
• Caution patient to avoid alcohol ingestion and CNS depressants; serious CNS depression may result
• Instruct patient not to discontinue medication quickly after long-term use; may cause seizures; product should be tapered over 1 wk; take exactly as prescribed
• Emphasize the need to tell all prescribers that a barbiturate is being taken
• Teach the patient to make position changes slowly; orthostatic hypotension may occur

- Teach patient that response may take 4 days to 2 wk
- Instruct patient to notify prescriber immediately if bruising, bleeding occur, which may indicate blood dyscrasias

Evaluation
Positive therapeutic outcome
- Improved sleeping patterns
- Decreased seizure activity
- Sedative preoperatively

Treatment of overdose: Lavage, activated charcoal, warming blanket, VS, hemodialysis, alkalinize urine, give **IV** volume expanders, **IV** fluids

---

phentolamine (Rx)
(fen-tole'a-meen)
Func. class.: Antihypertensive
Chem. class.: α-Adrenergic blocker
Pregnancy category C

Do not confuse:
phentolamine/phentermine

Action: α-Adrenergic blocker; binds to α-adrenergic receptors, dilating peripheral blood vessels, lowering peripheral resistance, lowering blood pressure

Therapeutic outcome: Decreased B/P, reversal of vasoconstriction (dermal necrosis)

Uses: Hypertension; pheochromocytoma; prevention, treatment of dermal necrosis after extravasation of norepinephrine, DOPamine, epinephrine

Unlabeled uses: Impotence, hypertensive crisis due to MAOIs

Dosage and routes
Treatment of hypertensive episodes in pheochromocytoma
Adult: **IV**/IM 5 mg; repeat if necessary
Child: **IV** 0.05-0.1 mg/kg; repeat if necessary, max 5 mg

Diagnosis of pheochromocytoma
Adult: **IV** 2.5 mg; if negative, repeat with 5 mg **IV**
Child: **IV** 0.05 mg/kg; if negative, repeat with 0.1 mg/kg **IV**

Treatment of necrosis
Adult: 5-10 mg/10 ml NS injected into area of extravasation within 12 hr
Child: 0.1-0.2 mg/kg; max 5 mg

Prevention of dermal necrosis
Adult: **IV** 10 mg/L of norepinephrine-containing sol
Child: **IV** 0.1-0.2 mg/kg, max 5 mg

Available forms: Inj 5 mg/ml

Adverse effects
CNS: Dizziness, flushing, weakness, **cerebrovascular spasm**
CV: Hypotension, **tachycardia,** *angina,* **dysrhythmias, MI**
EENT: Nasal congestion
GI: Dry mouth, nausea, vomiting, diarrhea, abdominal pain

Contraindications: Hypersensitivity, MI, coronary insufficiency, angina

Precautions: Pregnancy **C**, breastfeeding, dysrhythmia

Pharmacokinetics

Absorption	Well absorbed (IM); completely absorbed (**IV**)
Distribution	Unknown
Metabolism	Unknown
Excretion	Kidneys, unchanged (10%)
Half-life	Unknown

Pharmacodynamics

	IM	IV
Onset	Unknown	Rapid
Peak	20 min	2 min
Duration	½-1 hr	½ hr

Interactions
Individual drugs
EpINEPHrine: increased effects of epinephrine
Drug classifications
Antihypertensives: increased effects of antihypertensives
Drug/herb
Aconite: increased toxicity, death
Astragalus, cola tree: increased or decreased antihypertensive effect
Barberry, betony, black catechu, black cohosh, bloodroot, broom, burdock, cat's claw, dandelion, goldenseal, hawthorn, Irish moss, Jamaican dogwood, kelp, khella, mistletoe, parsley: increased antihypertensive effect
Coltsfoot, guarana, khat, licorice, yohimbe: decreased antihypertensive effect

NURSING CONSIDERATIONS
Assessment
- Monitor B/P, orthostatic hypotension, syncope, pulse and ECG until stable

P

Nursing diagnoses
- Cardiac output, decreased (uses)
- Injury, risk for (adverse reactions)
- Knowledge, deficient (teaching)
- Noncompliance (teaching)

Implementation
- Give with vasopressor nearby

IV route
- Give by direct **IV** after diluting 5 mg/1 ml of sterile water for inj or 0.9% NaCl; give 5 mg or less/min
- Give by cont inf by further diluting 5-10 mg/500 ml of D_5W, titrate to patient response
- Add 10 mg/L to norepinephrine in **IV** sol for prevention of dermal necrosis

Syringe compatibilities: Papaverine
Y-site compatibilities: Amiodarone
Additive compatibilities: DOBUTamine, verapamil

Patient/family education
- Caution patient not to discontinue product abruptly
- Teach patient not to use OTC products (cough, cold, allergy) unless directed by prescriber
- Teach patient the importance of complying with dosage schedule, even if feeling better
- Emphasize the need to rise slowly to sitting or standing position to minimize orthostatic hypotension
- Teach patient to notify prescriber of mouth sores, sore throat, fever, swelling of hands or feet, irregular heartbeat, chest pain
- Caution patient to report excessive perspiration, dehydration, vomiting, diarrhea; may lead to fall in B/P
- Caution patient that product may cause dizziness, fainting, light-headedness; may occur during 1st few days of therapy
- Teach patient how to take B/P, and normal readings for age-group

Evaluation
Positive therapeutic outcome
- Decreased B/P in hypertension
- Resolution of impotence
- Prevention of dermal necrosis

Treatment of overdose: Administer norepinephrine; discontinue product

---

phenylephrine (Rx)
(fen-ill-ef'rin)
Neo-Synephrine
Func. class.: Adrenergic, direct acting
Chem. class.: Direct sympathomimetic amine (α-agonist)

Pregnancy category C

Action: Powerful and selective receptor agonist causing contraction of blood vessels, vasoconstriction of eye arterioles; decreases eye engorgement by stimulation of α-adrenergic receptors

Therapeutic outcome: Increased B/P, decreased nasal congestion, decreased eye irritation

Uses: Hypotension, paroxysmal supraventricular tachycardia, shock, B/P maintenance during spinal anesthesia, topical ocular vasoconstrictor in uveitis, open-angle glaucoma, preoperatively, diagnostic procedures, refraction without cycloplegia, nasal congestion

Dosage and routes
Hypotension
Adult: SUBCUT/IM 2-5 mg; may repeat q10-15min if needed, do not exceed initial dose; **IV** 0.1-0.5 mg; may repeat q10-15min if needed, do not exceed initial dose
Child: IM/SUBCUT 0.1 mg/kg/dose q1-2hr prn

Supraventricular tachycardia
Adult: **IV** max 0.5 mg given rapidly, max single dose 1 mg

Shock
Adult: **IV** INF 10 mg/500 ml of D_5W given 100-180 mcg/min (if 20 gtt/ml device is used), then maintenance of 40-60 mcg/min (if 20 gtt/ml device is used); use inf pump
Child: **IV** BOL 5-20 mcg/kg/dose q10-15min; **IV** INF 0.1-0.5 mg/kg/min

Available forms: Inj 1% (10 mg/ml)

Adverse effects
CNS: Headache, dizziness, anxiety, tremor, insomnia
CV: Reflex bradycardia, **dysrhythmias, hypertension, tachycardia,** palpitations, ectopic beats, angina
GI: Nausea, vomiting
INTEG: Necrosis, tissue sloughing with extravasation, **gangrene**
MISC: **Anaphylaxis**

Contraindications: Hypersensitivity, closed-angle glaucoma, ventricular fibrillation, tachydysrhythmias, pheochromocytoma, severe hypertension

Precautions: Pregnancy **C**, breastfeeding, geriatric, hyperthyroidism, severe arteriosclerosis, arterial embolism, peripheral vascular disease, bradycardia, myocardial disease, partial heart block

Black Box Warning: Cardiac disease, extravasation

Pharmacokinetics

Absorption	Well absorbed (IM); completely absorbed (**IV**); minimally absorbed (nasal, ophth)
Distribution	Unknown
Metabolism	Liver
Excretion	Unknown
Half-life	Unknown

Pharmacodynamics

	SUBCUT/IM	IV
Onset	15 min	Rapid
Peak	Unknown	Unknown
Duration	45-60 min	20-30 min

Interactions
Individual drugs
Bretylium, digoxin: increased dysrhythmias
Drug classifications
α-Blockers: decreased phenylephrine action
Antidepressants (tricyclics), β-adrenergic blockers, H₁ antihistamines: increased pressor effect
General anesthetics: increased dysrhythmias
MAOIs: do not use within 2 wk, hypertensive crisis may result
Oxytocics: increased B/P

NURSING CONSIDERATIONS
Assessment
• Monitor I&O ratio; notify prescriber if output <30 ml/hr
• Monitor ECG during administration continuously; if B/P increases, product is decreased
• Monitor B/P and pulse q5min after parenteral route; CVP or PWP during inf if possible
• Assess for paresthesias and coldness of extremities; peripheral blood flow may decrease

Nursing diagnoses
• Cardiac output, decreased (uses)
• Knowledge, deficient (teaching)
• Tissue perfusion, ineffective (uses)

Implementation
IV route
• Give plasma expanders for hypovolemia
• Give **IV** after diluting 1 mg/9 ml of sterile water for inj; give dose over 30-60 sec; may be diluted 10 mg/500 ml of D₅W or 0.9% NaCl; titrate to patient response; low normal B/P; check for extravasation; check site for infiltration; use inf pump
• Store reconstituted sol in refrigerator for no longer than 24 hr
• Do not use discolored sol
Y-site compatibilities: Famotidine, haloperidol, inamrinone, zidovudine
Additive compatibilities: Chloramphenicol, DOBUTamine, lidocaine, potassium chloride, sodium bicarbonate

Patient/family education
• Inform patient of reason for product administration and expected result
• Advise patient to report pain at inf site immediately
• Instruct patient to report change in vision, blurring, loss of sight; breathing trouble, sweating, flushing

Evaluation
Positive therapeutic outcome
• Increased B/P with stabilization

phenylephrine nasal agent
See Appendix B

phenylephrine ophthalmic
See Appendix B

phenytoin (Rx)
(fen'i-toyn)
Dilantin, Dilantin Infatab, Phenytek
Func. class.: Anticonvulsant/antidysrhythmic (class IB)
Chem. class.: Hydantoin
Pregnancy category D

Action: Inhibits spread of seizure activity in motor cortex by altering ion transport; increases AV conduction to decrease dysrhythmias

Therapeutic outcome: Decreased seizures, absence of dysrhythmias

Uses: Generalized tonic-clonic seizures, status epilepticus, nonepileptic seizures associated with Reye's syndrome or after head trauma, Bell's palsy, complex/partial seizures

Adverse effects: *italic* = common, **bold** = life-threatening

Dosage and routes
Seizures
Adult: PO 1 g or 20 mg/kg (EXT REL) in 3-4 divided doses given q2hr or 400 mg, then 300 mg q2hr × 2 doses, maintenance 300-400 mg/day; max 600 mg/day; **IV** 15-20 mg/kg, max 25-50 mg/min then 100 mg q6-8hr
Child: PO 5 mg/kg/day in 2-3 divided doses, maintenance 4-8 mg/kg/day in 2-3 divided doses, max 300 mg/day; **IV** 15-20 mg/kg at 1-3 mg/kg/min

Status epilepticus
Adult: IV 15-20 mg/kg, max 25-50 mg/min; may give 100 mg q6-8hr thereafter
Child: IV 15-20 mg/kg, max in divided doses 1-3 mg/kg/min

Ventricular dysrhythmias
Adult: PO loading dose 1 g divided over 24 hr, then 500 mg/day × 2 days; **IV** 250 mg given over 5 min until dysrhythmias subside or 1 g is given, or 100 mg q15min until dysrhythmias subside or 1 g is given
Child: PO 3-8 mg/kg or 250 mg/m²/day as single dose or divided in 2 doses; **IV** 3-8 mg/kg given over several min, or 250 mg/m²/day as single dose or divided in 2 doses

Renal dose
Adult: Do not use loading dose CCr <10 ml/min or hepatic failure

Available forms: Susp 25 mg/5 ml; chew tabs 50 mg; inj 50 mg/ml; ext rel caps 100, 200, 300 mg; prompt rel caps 100 mg

Adverse effects
CNS: Drowsiness, dizziness, insomnia, paresthesias, depression, **suicidal tendencies,** aggression, headache, confusion, slurred speech, peripheral neuropathy
CV: Hypotension, **ventricular fibrillation**
EENT: Nystagmus, diplopia, blurred vision
ENDO: Diabetes insipidus
GI: Nausea, vomiting, constipation, anorexia, weight loss, **hepatitis,** jaundice, gingival hyperplasia
GU: Nephritis, urine discoloration
HEMA: Agranulocytosis, leukopenia, aplastic anemia, thrombocytopenia, megaloblastic anemia
INTEG: Rash, **lupus erythematosus, Stevens-Johnson syndrome,** hirsutism, **toxic epidermal necrolysis**
SYST: Hypocalcemia, **purple glove syndrome (IV)**

Contraindications: Pregnancy **D,** hypersensitivity, psychiatric condition, bradycardia, SA and AV block, Stokes-Adams syndrome, hepatic failure, acute intermittent porphyria

Precautions: Geriatric, allergies, renal/hepatic disease, petit mal seizures, hypotension, myocardial insufficiency, Asian patients positive for HLA-B 1502

Pharmacokinetics
Absorption	Slowly absorbed from GI tract; erratic (IM)
Distribution	Crosses placenta, 90%-95% protein binding
Metabolism	Liver, extensively
Excretion	Kidneys, minimally; enters breast milk
Half-life	7-42 hr, dose dependent

Pharmacodynamics
	PO	PO-EXT REL	IM	IV
Onset	2-24 hr	2-24 hr	Erratic	1-2 hr
Peak	1½-3 hr	4-12 hr	Erratic	Unknown
Duration	6-12 hr	12-36 hr	12-24 hr	12-24 hr

Interactions
Individual drugs
Alcohol (chronic use), carbamazepine, diazoxide, folic acid, rifampin: decreased effects of phenytoin
Chloramphenicol, cimetidine, cycloSERINE, diazepam, valproate: increased phenytoin effect
Drug classifications
Antacids, barbiturates: decreased effect of phenytoin
Antidepressants (tricyclics), benzodiazepines, salicylates: increased phenytoin level
Drug/herb
Aloe, buckthorn, cascara sagrada, senna: increased hypokalemia, antidysrhythmic action
Ginkgo: increased effect
Ginseng, santonica, valerian: decreased anticonvulsant effect
Drug/lab test
Increased: glucose, alkaline phosphatase, BSP
Decreased: dexamethasone, metyrapone test serum, urinary steroids

NURSING CONSIDERATIONS
Assessment
* Assess product level: toxic level 30-50 mcg/ml; therapeutic level 7.5-20 mcg/ml, wait ≥1 wk to determine level
🔷 Assess mental status: mood, sensorium, affect, memory (long, short), especially geriatric; suicidal thoughts/behaviors
* Assess for beginning rash that may lead to Stevens-Johnson syndrome or toxic epidermal necrolysis; phenytoin should not be used again

- Assess for blood dyscrasias: fever, sore throat, bruising, rash, jaundice, epistaxis (long-term treatment only)
- Assess seizure activity including type, location, duration, and character; provide seizure precaution
- Assess renal studies: urinalysis, BUN, urine creatinine
- Monitor blood studies: RBC, Hct, Hgb, reticulocyte counts weekly for 4 wk then monthly; also check thyroid function tests, serum calcium
- Monitor liver function tests for renal failure: ALT, AST, bilirubin, creatinine
- Assess for signs of physical withdrawal if medication suddenly discontinued
- Assess eye problems: need for ophth exam before, during, after treatment (slit lamp, funduscopy, tonometry)
- Assess allergic reaction: red raised rash, increased temp, lymphadenopathy; if this occurs, product should be discontinued, usually occurs 3-12 wk after start of treatment; may also cause hepatotoxicity, rhabdomyolysis
- Monitor for toxicity: bone marrow depression, nausea, vomiting, ataxia, diplopia, CV collapse, slurred speech, confusion

Nursing diagnoses
- Injury, risk for (uses, adverse reactions)
- Knowledge, deficient (teaching)
- Noncompliance (teaching)

Implementation
PO route
- Give with meals to decrease GI upset
- Chew tab can be crushed or chewed; cap can be opened and mixed with foods or fluids; cap and tab are not interchangeable, only ext rel cap are to be used for once a day dosing
- Do not take antacids or antidiarrheals within 2-3 hr of taking phenytoin
- Give by gastric/NG tube: dilute susp before administration, flush tube with 20 ml of H₂O after dose
- Shake oral susp well; use measuring device for correct dose
- Allow 7-10 days between dosage changes
IV route
- Administer by direct **IV** after diluting with special diluent provided (1 ml/50 mg, 2.2 ml/100 mg, 5.2 ml/250 mg); shake; give through Y-tube or 3-way stopcock; inject slowly <50 mg/min
- Give intermittent **IV** after diluting to a conc of 1-10 mg/ml
- Clear **IV** tubing first with 0.9% NaCl sol; use in-line filter; discard sol 4 hr after preparation;

inject into large veins to prevent purple glove syndrome
Additive compatibilities: Bleomycin, verapamil
Y-site compatibilities: Esmolol, famotidine, fluconazole, foscarnet, tacrolimus
Y-site incompatibilities: Enalaprilat, potassium chloride, vit B/C

Patient/family education
- Teach patient to carry/wear emergency ID stating name, products taken, condition, prescriber's name and phone number
- Advise patient to avoid driving and other activities that require alertness until product response is known; dizziness, drowsiness can occur
- Advise patient to avoid alcohol ingestion and CNS depressants unless approved by prescriber; increased sedation may occur
- Teach patient not to discontinue medication quickly after long-term use; taper off over several wk
- Advise patient that urine may turn pink, red, or brown
- Caution patient to avoid antacids or antidiarrheals within 2-3 hr of taking phenytoin
- Instruct patient in proper oral hygiene to prevent gingival hyperplasia; to visit dentist routinely

Evaluation
Positive therapeutic outcome
- Decreased seizure activity
- Decreased dysrhythmias
- Relief of pain

P

physostigmine ophthalmic
See Appendix B

phytonadione (vit K₁) (Rx)
(fye-toe-na-dye'one)
Mephyton
Func. class.: Vitamin K₁, fat-soluble vitamin
Pregnancy category C

Action: Needed for adequate blood clotting (factors II, VII, IX, X)

Therapeutic outcome: Prevention of bleeding

Uses: Vitamin K malabsorption, hypoprothrombinemia, prevention of hypoprothrombinemia caused by oral anticoagulants, prevention of hemorrhagic disease of the newborn

---

Adverse effects: *italic* = common, **bold** = life-threatening

Dosage and routes
Hypoprothrombinemia caused by vitamin K malabsorption
Adult: PO/IM 2.5-25 mg; may repeat or increase to 50 mg
Child: PO 2.5-5 mg
Infant: PO/IM 2 mg

Prevention of hemorrhagic disease of the newborn
Neonate: IM 0.5-1 mg within 1 hr after birth; repeat in 2-3 wk if required

Hypoprothrombinemia caused by oral anticoagulants
Adult and child: PO/SUBCUT/IM 1-10 mg, may repeat 12-48 hr after PO dose or 6-8 hr after SUBCUT/IM dose, based on INR

Available forms: Tabs 5 mg; inj 2 mg/10 ml; aqueous colloidal (IM, **IV**); inj aqueous dispersion 10 mg/ml (IM), 1 mg/0.5 ml

Adverse effects
CNS: Headache, **brain damage** (large doses)
GI: Nausea, decreased liver function tests
HEMA: **Hemolytic anemia, hemoglobin-uria, hyperbilirubinemia**
INTEG: Rash, urticaria
RESP: **Bronchospasm,** dyspnea, chest constriction, **respiratory arrest**

Contraindications: Hypersensitivity, severe hepatic disease, last few wk of pregnancy

Precautions: Pregnancy **C,** neonates, hepatic disease

Black Box Warning: IV use

Pharmacokinetics
Absorption	Well absorbed (PO, IM, SUBCUT)
Distribution	Crosses placenta
Metabolism	Liver, rapidly
Excretion	Breast milk
Half-life	Unknown

Pharmacodynamics
	PO	SUBCUT/IM
Onset	6-12 hr	1-2 hr
Peak	Unknown	6 hr
Duration	Unknown	14 hr

Interactions
Individual drugs
Cholestyramine, mineral oil: decreased action of phytonadione
Drug classifications
Oral anticoagulants: decreased anticoagulant effect
Drug/food
Olestra: decreased vit K levels

NURSING CONSIDERATIONS
Assessment
• Monitor protime during treatment (2-sec deviation from control time, bleeding time, and clotting time)
• Monitor for bleeding, INR pulse, and B/P
• Assess nutritional status: liver (beef), spinach, tomatoes, coffee, asparagus, broccoli, cabbage, lettuce, greens
• Assess for bleeding or bruising: hematuria, black tarry stools, hematemesis

Nursing diagnoses
• Knowledge, deficient (teaching)
• Nutrition: less than body requirements, imbalanced (uses)
• Tissue perfusion, ineffective (uses)

Implementation
IV route
• Give **IV** after diluting with D₅ NS 10 ml or more; give 1 mg/min or more
• Give **IV** only when other routes not possible (deaths have occurred)
• Store in airtight, light-resistant container
Syringe compatibilities: Doxapram
Y-site compatibilities: Alfentanil, amikacin, aminophylline, ampicillin, epineph-rine, famotidine, heparin, hydrocortisone, potassium chloride, tolazoline, vit B/C
Additive compatibilities: Amikacin, calcium gluconate, chloramphenicol, cimeti-dine, netilmicin, sodium bicarbonate

Patient/family education
• Teach patient not to take other supplements, unless directed by prescriber; to take this medication as directed
• Teach patient necessary foods high in vit K to be included in diet
• Advise patient to avoid IM inj, hard tooth-brush, flossing; use electric razor until treat-ment is terminated
• Instruct patient to report symptoms of bleeding: bruising, nosebleeds, blood in urine, heavy menstruation, black tarry stools
• Caution patient not to use OTC medications unless approved by prescriber
• Stress the need for periodic lab tests to monitor coagulation levels
• Stress the need for patient to carry/wear emergency ID with condition, treatment, and medications taken

Evaluation
Positive therapeutic outcome
• Decreased bleeding tendencies
• Decreased protime
• Decreased clotting time

pilocarpine ophthalmic
See Appendix B

pimecrolimus topical
See Appendix B

pindolol (Rx)
(pin'doe-lole)
Novo-Pindol ✦, Syn-Pindol ✦, Visken
Func. class.: Antihypertensive
Chem. class.: Nonselective β-blocker

Pregnancy category B

Do not confuse:
pindolol/Parlodel/Plendil

Action: Competitively blocks stimulation of β-adrenergic receptor within vascular smooth muscle; produces chronotropic, inotropic activity (decreases rate of SA node discharge, increases recovery time), slows conduction of AV node, decreases heart rate, which decreases O_2 consumption in myocardium; also decreases renin-aldosterone-angiotensin system and at high doses inhibits $β_2$ receptors in bronchial system

Therapeutic outcome: Decreased B/P in hypertension, heart rate

Uses: Mild to moderate hypertension

Dosage and routes
Adult: PO 5 mg bid; usual dose 15 mg/day (5 mg tid); may increase by 10 mg/day q3-4wk to a max of 60 mg/day
Geriatric: PO 5 mg/day increase by 5 mg q3-4wk

Available forms: Tabs 5, 10 mg

Adverse effects
CNS: Insomnia, dizziness, hallucinations, anxiety, fatigue, headache, depression
CV: Hypotension, bradycardia, **CHF,** edema, chest pain, palpitations, claudication, tachycardia, **AV block, pulmonary edema, bradycardia, dysrhythmias**
EENT: Visual changes, sore throat, *double vision,* dry burning eyes, nasal stuffiness
GI: Nausea, vomiting, **ischemic colitis,** diarrhea, *abdominal pain,* **mesenteric arterial thrombosis,** flatulence, constipation
GU: Impotence, urinary frequency
HEMA: **Agranulocytosis, thrombocytopenia, purpura**
INTEG: Rash, alopecia, pruritus, fever
MISC: Joint pain, muscle pain

RESP: **Bronchospasm,** *dyspnea,* cough, crackles

Contraindications: Hypersensitivity to β-blockers, cardiogenic shock, 2nd- or 3rd-degree heart block, sinus bradycardia, sick sinus syndrome, acute bronchospasm

Precautions: Pregnancy **B,** breastfeeding, major surgery, diabetes mellitus, renal/hepatic disease, thyroid disease, COPD, well-compensated heart failure, CAD, nonallergic bronchospasm, peripheral vascular disease

Black Box Warning: Abrupt discontinuation

Pharmacokinetics
Absorption	Well absorbed
Distribution	Crosses placenta; some penetration in CNS, protein binding 40%
Metabolism	Liver, moderately (60%-65%)
Excretion	Kidneys, unchanged (30%-45%)
Half-life	3-4 hr

Pharmacodynamics
Onset	Unknown
Peak	2-4 hr
Duration	8-24 hr

Interactions
Individual drugs
Hydralazine, methyldopa, prazosin, reserpine: increased hypotension, bradycardia
Insulin: may alter hypoglycemic effect
Thyroid: decreased effect of β-blockers
Drug classifications
Anticholinergics: increased hypotension, bradycardia
$β_2$-Adrenergic agonists: increased effect of β-blockers
Calcium channel blockers: increased effects of calcium channel blockers
NSAIDs, salicylates, sympathomimetics: decreased antihypertensive effect
Oral hypoglycemics: may alter hypoglycemic effect
Theophyllines, $β_2$-agonists: decreased bronchodilatation
Drug/herb
Aconite: increased toxicity, death
Astragalus, cola tree: increased or decreased antihypertensive effect
Barberry, betony, black catechu, black cohosh, bloodroot, broom, burdock, cat's claw, dandelion, goldenseal, hawthorn, Irish moss, Jamaican dogwood, kelp, khella, mistletoe, parsley: increased antihypertensive effect

P

Adverse effects: *italic* = common, **bold** = life-threatening

Coltsfoot, guarana, khat, licorice, St. John's wort, yohimbe: decreased antihypertensive effect

Drug/lab test
Increased: renal/liver function tests
Interference: glucose, insulin tolerance test

NURSING CONSIDERATIONS
Assessment
• Monitor B/P during beginning treatment, periodically thereafter; pulse q4hr; note rate, rhythm, quality: apical/radial pulse before administration; notify prescriber of any significant changes (pulse <50 bpm)
• Obtain baselines in renal, liver function tests before therapy begins
• Assess for edema in feet, legs daily; monitor I&O, daily weight; check for jugular vein distention, crackles bilaterally, dyspnea (CHF)
• Monitor skin turgor, dryness of mucous membranes for hydration status, especially geriatric

Nursing diagnoses
• Cardiac output, decreased (uses)
• Injury, risk for (adverse reactions)
• Knowledge, deficient (teaching)
• Noncompliance (teaching)

Implementation
• Give before meals, at bedtime; tab may be crushed or swallowed whole; give with food to prevent GI upset
• Store protected from light, moisture; place in cool environment

Patient/family education
◆ Teach patient not to discontinue product abruptly; taper over 2 wk; may cause precipitate angina if stopped abruptly
• Teach patient not to use OTC products containing α-adrenergic stimulants (such as nasal decongestants, cold preparations); to avoid alcohol, smoking, and to limit sodium intake as prescribed
• Teach patient how to take pulse and B/P at home; advise when to notify prescriber
• Instruct patient to comply with weight control, dietary adjustments, modified exercise program
• Tell patient to carry/wear emergency ID to identify product being taken, allergies; tell patient product controls symptoms but does not cure
• Caution patient to avoid hazardous activities if dizziness, drowsiness present
• Teach patient to report symptoms of CHF: difficult breathing, especially on exertion or when lying down, night cough, swelling of extremities or bradycardia, dizziness, confusion, depression, fever

• Teach patient to take product as prescribed, not to double doses, skip doses; take any missed doses as soon as remembered if at least 4 hr until next dose; to take with or immediately after meals if GI symptoms occur

Evaluation
Positive therapeutic outcome
• Decreased B/P in hypertension (after 1-2 wk)

Treatment of overdose: Lavage, **IV** atropine for bradycardia, **IV** theophylline for bronchospasm, digoxin, O_2, diuretic for cardiac failure, hemodialysis, **IV** glucose for hyperglycemia, **IV** diazepam (or phenytoin) for seizures

---

pioglitazone (Rx)
(pie-oh-glye′ta-zone)
Actos
Func. class.: Antidiabetic, oral
Chem. class.: Thiazolidinedione
Pregnancy category C

Action: Specifically targets insulin resistance, an insulin sensitizer; regulates the transcription of a number of insulin responsive genes

Therapeutic outcome: Decreased symptoms of diabetes mellitus

Uses: Type 2 diabetes mellitus

Dosage and routes
Monotherapy
Adult: PO 15-30 mg/day, may increase to 45 mg/day

Combination therapy
Adult: PO 15-30 mg/day with a sulfonylurea, metformin, or insulin; decrease sulfonylurea dose if hypoglycemia occurs; decrease insulin dose by 10%-25% if hypoglycemia occurs or if plasma glucose is <100 mg/dl; max 45 mg/day

Hepatic dose
Do not use in active liver disease or if ALT >2.5 × ULN

Available forms: Tabs 15, 30, 45 mg

Adverse effects
CNS: Headache
CV: **MI, heart failure, death** (geriatric patients)
ENDO: Hyper/hypoglycemia
MISC: Myalgia, sinusitis, upper respiratory tract infection, pharyngitis, **hepatotoxicity,** edema, weight gain, anemia, macular edema
MS: Fractures (females), myalgia

 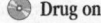

Contraindications: Breastfeeding, children, hypersensitivity to thiazolidinediones, diabetic ketoacidosis

Black Box Warning: CHF

Precautions: Pregnancy C, thyroid/renal/hepatic disease, edema, geriatric patients with CV disease

Pharmacokinetics

Absorption	Unknown
Distribution	Unknown
Metabolism	Unknown
Excretion	Kidneys
Half-life	3-7 hr, terminal 16-24 hr

Pharmacodynamics

Onset	Unknown
Peak	6-12 wk
Duration	Unknown

Interactions
Individual drugs

Fluconazole, itraconazole, ketoconazole, miconazole, voriconazole: decreased pioglitazone effect

Gatifloxacin: poor glucose control; avoid concurrent use

Drug classifications

CYP2C8 inducers: decreased pioglitazone effect

Oral contraceptives: decreased effect, use an alternative contraceptive method

Drug/herb

Alfalfa, aloe, basil, bay, bilberry, bitter melon, black catechu, buchu, burdock, coriander, dandelion, eyebright (po), fenugreek, garlic, ginseng, glucomannan, glucosamine, goat's rue, gymnema, horehound, horse chestnut, jambul, myrrh, myrtle: increased antidiabetic effect

Bee pollen, blue cohosh, broom, chromium, elecampane, eucalyptus, gotu kola: decreased antidiabetic effect

Chromium, coenzyme Q10, fenugreek: increased hypoglycemia

Glucosamine: decreased blood glucose control

NURSING CONSIDERATIONS
Assessment

- Assess for hypoglycemic reactions (sweating, weakness, dizziness, anxiety, tremors, hunger), hyperglycemic reactions soon after meals (rare)
- Check liver function tests periodically; AST, LDH, FBS, glycosylated Hgb, plasma lipids, lipoproteins, B/P, body weight during treatment

Nursing diagnoses

- Knowledge, deficient (teaching)
- Nutrition: more than body requirements, imbalanced (uses)

Implementation

- Convert from other oral hypoglycemic agents; change may be made with gradual dosage change; monitor serum glucose during conversion
- Give once a day; give with meals to decrease GI upset
- Give tabs crushed and mixed with meal or fluids for patients with difficulty swallowing
- Store in airtight container in cool environment

Patient/family education

- Teach patient to self-monitor using a blood glucose meter
- Teach patient symptoms of hypo/hyperglycemia, what to do about each (rare)
- Advise patient that product must be continued on daily basis; explain consequence of discontinuing product abruptly
- Advise patient to avoid OTC medications or herbal preparations unless approved by prescriber; to report weight gain, edema
- Advise patient that diabetes is life-long illness; that this product is not a cure, only controls symptoms
- Instruct patient to notify prescriber if oral contraceptives are used
- Teach patient not to use if breastfeeding

Evaluation
Positive therapeutic outcome

- Decrease in polyuria, polydipsia, polyphagia; clear sensorium; absence of dizziness; stable gait; blood glucose, A1c improvement

---

piperacillin (Rx)
(pi-per′a-sill-in)
Func. class.: Broad-spectrum antiinfective
Chem. class.: Extended-spectrum penicillin

Pregnancy category B

Action: Interferes with cell wall replication of susceptible organisms; osmotically unstable cell wall swells and bursts from osmotic pressure

Therapeutic outcome: Bactericidal effects for gram-positive cocci *Staphylococcus aureus, Streptococcus pyogenes, Streptococcus viridans, Streptococcus faecalis, Streptococcus bovis, Streptococcus pneumoniae;*

gram-negative cocci *Neisseria gonorrhoeae, Neisseria meningitidis;* gram-positive bacilli *Acinetobacter, Clostridium perfringens, Clostridium tetani;* gram-negative bacilli *Bacteroides, Fusobacterium nucleatum, Escherichia coli, Klebsiella, Proteus mirabilis, Proteus vulgaris, Proteus rettgeri, Morganella morganii, Enterobacter, Citrobacter, Pseudomonas aeruginosa, Serratia, Peptococcus, Peptostreptococcus, Eubacterium*

Uses: Respiratory tract, skin, skin structure, urinary tract, bone, and joint infections; gonorrhea, pneumonia, endocarditis, septicemia, meningitis, sinusitis; infections caused by penicillinase-producing staphylococci, streptococci; may be combined with an aminoglycoside for *Pseudomonas* infection

Dosage and routes
Urinary tract infections
Adult: IM/**IV** 6-8 g/day (100-125 mg/kg/day) in divided doses q6-12hr, max 24 g/day

Serious systemic infections
Adult and child >12 yr: IM/**IV** 2-4 g q4-6hr (2 g/site IM)
Child <12 yr: IM/**IV** 200-300 mg/kg/day in divided doses q4-6hr

Prophylaxis of surgical infections
Adult: **IV** 2 g 30-60 min before procedure; may be repeated during or after surgery

Renal dose
Adult: **IV** CCr 20-40 ml/min give q8hr, CCr <20 ml/min give q12hr

Available forms: Powder for inj 2, 3, 4, 40 g

Adverse effects
CNS: Lethargy, hallucinations, anxiety, depression, twitching, **coma, seizures**
GI: Nausea, vomiting, diarrhea, increased AST, ALT, abdominal pain, glossitis, colitis, **pseudomembranous colitis, hepatitis**
GU: **Oliguria, proteinuria, hematuria,** vaginitis, moniliasis, **glomerulonephritis,** acute renal failure
HEMA: Anemia, increased bleeding time, **bone marrow depression, thrombocytopenia,** hemolytic anemia
META: Hypokalemia, hypernatremia
SYST: **Serum sickness, anaphylaxis, Stevens-Johnson syndrome, exfoliative dermatitis, toxic epidermal necrolysis**

Contraindications: Neonates, hypersensitivity to penicillins

Precautions: Pregnancy **B**, breastfeeding, hypersensitivity to cephalosporins/carbapenems, CHF, renal/GI disease, seizures

Pharmacokinetics

Absorption	Well absorbed (80%)
Distribution	Widely distributed; crosses placenta
Metabolism	Not metabolized
Excretion	Kidneys, unchanged (90%); bile (10%); breast milk
Half-life	0.7-1.3 hr

Pharmacodynamics

	IM	IV
Onset	Rapid	Rapid
Peak	30-50 min	Inf end
Duration	Unknown	Unknown

Interactions
Individual drugs
Aspirin, probenecid: increased piperacillin levels
Methotrexate: increased levels of methotrexate
Drug classifications
Aminoglycosides: decreased antimicrobial effect of piperacillin
Contraceptives (oral): decreased contraceptive effectiveness
Neuromuscular blockers: increased levels of neuromuscular blockers
Tetracyclines: decreased antimicrobial effectiveness (with high concentrations of piperacillin)
Drug/herb
Acidophilus: do not use with antiinfectives; separate by several hours
Khat: decreased absorption
Drug/lab test
False positive: urine glucose, urine protein, Coombs' test

NURSING CONSIDERATIONS
Assessment
• Assess patient for previous sensitivity reaction to penicillins or other cephalosporins; cross-sensitivity between penicillins and cephalosporins is common
• Assess patient for signs and symptoms of infection, including characteristics of wounds, sputum, urine, stool, WBC >10,000/mm^3, fever; obtain information baseline, during treatment
• Obtain C&S before beginning product therapy to identify if correct treatment has been initiated
• Assess for allergic reactions: rash, urticaria, pruritus, chills, fever, joint pain; angioedema may occur a few days after therapy begins;

epinephrine, resuscitation equipment should be available for anaphylactic reaction

⬥ Identify urine output; if decreasing, notify prescriber (may indicate nephrotoxicity); also check for increased BUN, creatinine

• Monitor blood studies: AST, ALT, CBC, Hct, bilirubin, LDH, alkaline phosphatase, Coombs' test monthly if patient is on long-term therapy

• Monitor electrolytes: potassium, sodium, chloride monthly if patient is on long-term therapy

• Assess bowel pattern daily; if severe diarrhea occurs, product should be discontinued; may indicate pseudomembranous colitis

• Monitor for bleeding: ecchymosis, bleeding gums, hematuria, stool guaiac daily if on long-term therapy

• Assess for overgrowth of infection: perineal itching, fever, malaise, redness, pain, swelling, drainage, rash, diarrhea, change in cough, sputum

Nursing diagnoses
• Diarrhea (adverse reactions)
• Infection, risk for (uses)
• Injury, risk for (adverse reactions)
• Knowledge, deficient (teaching)
• Noncompliance (teaching)

Implementation
IM route
• Reconstitute 2 g/4 ml, 3 g/6 ml, 4 g/7.8 ml with sterile water, 0.9% NaCl, bacteriostatic water, 0.5% or 1% lidocaine without epinephrine
• Inject deep in large muscle mass, massage; split inj >2 g into 2 inj
IV route
• Reconstitute with 5 ml or more 0.9% NaCl, bacteriostatic water; shake sol to dissolve
• Change **IV** sites q48hr to prevent phlebitis and pain
• Give direct **IV** over 3-5 min
• Give by intermittent inf by diluting in 50 ml or more D₅W, 0.9% NaCl, D₅/0.9% NaCl, LR, give over 20-30 min by Y-site; discontinue primary inf during intermittent inf
Syringe compatibilities: Heparin
Y-site compatibilities: Acyclovir, aldesleukin, allopurinol, amifostine, aztreonam, ciprofloxacin, cyclophosphamide, diltiazem, enalaprilat, esmolol, famotidine, fludarabine, foscarnet, heparin, hydromorphone, IL-2, labetalol, lorazepam, magnesium sulfate, melphalan, meperidine, midazolam, morphine, perphenazine, propofol, ranitidine, tacrolimus, teniposide, theophylline, thiotepa, verapamil, zidovudine

Y-site incompatibilities: Ondansetron, fluconazole, sargramostim, vinorelbine
Additive compatibilities: Ciprofloxacin, clindamycin, fluconazole, hydrocortisone sodium succinate, ofloxacin, potassium chloride, verapamil
Additive incompatibilities: Aminoglycosides

Patient/family education
• Teach patient to report sore throat, bruising, bleeding, joint pain; may indicate blood dyscrasias (rare)
• Advise patient to contact prescriber if vaginal itching, loose foul-smelling stools, furry tongue occur; may indicate superinfection
• Advise patient to notify prescriber of diarrhea with blood or pus, which may indicate pseudomembranous colitis

Evaluation
Positive therapeutic outcome
• Absence of signs/symptoms of infection (WBC <10,000/mm³, temp WNL, absence of red, draining wounds)
• Reported improvement in symptoms of infection

Treatment of anaphylaxis: Withdraw product, maintain airway, administer epinephrine, aminophylline, O₂, **IV** corticosteroids

---

piperacillin/tazobactam (Rx)
Zosyn
Func. class.: Broad-spectrum antiinfective
Chem. class.: Extended-spectrum penicillin
Pregnancy category B

Action: Interferes with cell wall replication of susceptible organisms; osmotically unstable cell wall swells and bursts from osmotic pressure; tazobactam is a β-lactamase inhibitor, protects piperacillin from enzymatic degradation

Therapeutic outcome: Bactericidal effects for piperacillin-resistant β-lactamase, *Escherichia coli, Staphylococcus aureus, Bacteroides fragilis, Bacteroides ovatus, Bacteroides thetaiotaomicron, Bacteroides vulgatus, Haemophilus influenzae*

Uses: Moderate to severe infections: piperacillin-resistant, β-lactamase strains causing infections in respiratory tract, skin, skin structure, urinary tract, bone, and joint; gonorrhea, pneumonia, infections from penicillinase-producing staphylococci, streptococci

P

Adverse effects: *italic* = common, **bold** = life-threatening

Dosage and routes
Nosocomial pneumonia
Adult: IV 3.375 g q24h with an aminoglycoside × 1-2 wk; continue aminoglycoside only if *Pseudomonas aeruginosa* is isolated

Other infections
Adult: IV INF 6-12 g/day, given 2.25 g q8hr to 3.375 g q6hr over 30 min × 7-10 days

Renal dose
Adult: IV CCr 20-40 ml/min 2.25 g q6hr; CCr <20 ml/min 2.25 g q8hr

Available forms: Powder for inj 2 g piperacillin/0.25 g tazobactam; 3 g piperacillin/0.375 g tazobactam, 4 g piperacillin/0.5 g tazobactam, 36 g piperacillin/4.5 g tazobactam

Adverse effects
CNS: Headache, insomnia, dizziness, fever, lethargy, hallucinations, anxiety, depression, twitching, **seizures,** vertigo
CV: **Cardiac toxicity**
GI: *Nausea, vomiting, diarrhea,* increased AST, ALT, abdominal pain, glossitis, constipation, **pseudomembranous colitis**
GU: **Oliguria, proteinuria, hematuria,** *vaginitis, moniliasis,* **glomerulonephritis, renal failure**
HEMA: Anemia, increased bleeding time, **bone marrow depression, agranulocytosis,** hemolytic anemia
INTEG: Rash, pruritus, **exfoliative dermatitis**
META: Hypokalemia, hypernatremia
SYST: **Serum sickness, anaphylaxis, Stevens-Johnson syndrome**

Contraindications: Hypersensitivity to penicillins; neonates, carbapenem allergy

Precautions: Pregnancy **B,** breastfeeding, CHF, seizures, hypersensitivity to cephalosporins, renal insufficiency in children, GI disease, electrolyte imbalances

Pharmacokinetics
Absorption	Well absorbed (80%)
Distribution	Widely distributed; crosses placenta
Metabolism	Not metabolized
Excretion	Kidneys, unchanged (90%); bile (10%); breast milk
Half-life	0.7-1.3 hr

Pharmacodynamics
Onset	Rapid
Peak	Inf end
Duration	Unknown

Interactions
Individual drugs
Aspirin, probenecid: increased piperacillin levels
Methotrexate: increased effect of methotrexate
Drug classifications
Aminoglycosides (**IV**): decreased piperacillin effect
Contraceptives (oral): decreased contraceptive effectiveness
Neuromuscular blockers: increased effects
Tetracyclines: decreased antimicrobial effectiveness of piperacillin
Drug/herb
Acidophilus: do not use with antiinfectives; separate by several hours
Khat: decreased absorption
Drug/lab test
Increased: platelet count, eosinophilia, neutropenia, leucopenia, serum creatinine, PTT, AST, ALT, alkaline phosphatase, bilirubin, BUN, electrolytes
Decreased: Hct, Hgb, electrolytes
False positive: urine glucose, urine protein, Coombs' test

NURSING CONSIDERATIONS
Assessment
• Assess patient for previous sensitivity reaction to penicillins or other cephalosporins; cross-sensitivity between penicillins and cephalosporins is common
• Assess patient for signs and symptoms of infection, including characteristics of wounds, sputum, urine, stool, WBC >10,000/mm^3, fever; obtain information baseline, during treatment
• Obtain C&S before beginning product therapy to identify if correct treatment has been initiated
• Assess for allergic reactions: rash, urticaria, pruritus, chills, fever, joint pain; angioedema may occur a few days after therapy begins; epinephrine, resuscitation equipment should be available for anaphylactic reaction
◆ Identify urine output; if decreasing, notify prescriber (may indicate nephrotoxicity); also check for increased BUN, creatinine
• Monitor blood studies: AST, ALT, CBC, Hct, bilirubin, LDH, alkaline phosphatase, Coombs' test monthly if patient is on long-term therapy
• Monitor electrolytes: potassium, sodium, chloride monthly if patient is on long-term therapy
• Assess bowel pattern daily; if severe diarrhea occurs, product should be discontinued; may indicate pseudomembranous colitis
• Monitor for bleeding: ecchymosis, bleeding gums, hematuria, stool guaiac daily if on long-term therapy

- Assess for overgrowth of infection: perineal itching, fever, malaise, redness, pain, swelling, drainage, rash, diarrhea, change in cough, sputum

Nursing diagnoses
- Diarrhea (adverse reactions)
- Infection, risk for (uses)
- Injury, risk for (adverse reactions)
- Knowledge, deficient (teaching)
- Noncompliance (teaching)

Implementation
- Reconstitute with 5 ml or more 0.9% NaCl, bacteriostatic water; shake sol to dissolve
- Give by intermittent inf by diluting in 50 ml or more D$_5$W, 0.9% NaCl, D$_5$/0.9% NaCl, LR; give over 20-30 min by Y-site; discontinue primary inf during intermittent inf
- Change **IV** sites q48hr to prevent phlebitis and pain
- Give direct **IV** over 3-5 min

Y-site compatibilities: Aminophylline, aztreonam, bleomycin, bumetanide, buprenorphine, butorphanol, calcium gluconate, carboplatin, carmustine, cefepime, cimetidine, clindamycin, cyclophosphamide, cytarabine, dexamethasone, diphenhydrAMINE, DOPamine, enalaprilat, etoposide, floxuridine, fluconazole, fludarabine, fluorouracil, furosemide, gallium, granisetron, heparin, hydrocortisone, hydromorphone, ifosfamide, leucovorin, lorazepam, magnesium sulfate, mannitol, meperidine, mesna, methotrexate, methylPREDNISolone, metoclopramide, metronidazole, morphine, ondansetron, plicomycin, potassium chloride, ranitidine, sargramostim, sodium bicarbonate, thiotepa, trimethoprim/sulfamethoxazole, vinBLAStine, vinCRIStine, zidovudine

Y-site incompatibilities: Fluconazole, ondansetron, sargramostim, vinorelbine

Patient/family education
- Teach patient to report sore throat, bruising, bleeding, joint pain; may indicate blood dyscrasias (rare)
- Advise patient to contact prescriber if vaginal itching, loose foul-smelling stools, furry tongue occur; may indicate superinfection
- Advise patient to notify prescriber of diarrhea with blood or pus, which may indicate pseudomembranous colitis

Evaluation
Positive therapeutic outcome
- Absence of signs/symptoms of infection (WBC <10,000/mm^3, temp WNL, absence of red, draining wounds)

- Reported improvement in symptoms of infection

Treatment of anaphylaxis: Withdraw product, maintain airway, administer epinephrine, aminophylline, O$_2$, **IV** corticosteroids

---

pirbuterol (Rx)
(peer-byoo'ter-ole)
Maxair
Func. class.: Bronchodilator
Chem. class.: β-Adrenergic agonist
Pregnancy category C

Action: Relaxes bronchial smooth muscle by direct action on β$_2$-adrenergic receptors, with increased levels of cAMP and increased bronchodilatation, diuresis, and cardiac and CNS stimulation

Therapeutic outcome: Bronchodilatation with ease of breathing

Uses: Reversible bronchospasm (prevention, treatment), including asthma; may be given with theophylline or steroids

Dosage and routes
Adult and child >12 yr: INH 1-2 (0.4 mg) q4-6hr; max 12 inh/day

Available forms: Aerosol delivers 0.2 mg pirbuterol/actuation

Adverse effects
CNS: Tremors, anxiety, insomnia, headache, dizziness, stimulation, restlessness, hallucinations, drowsiness, irritability
CV: Palpitations, tachycardia, hypo/hypertension, angina, **dysrhythmias**
EENT: Dry nose and mouth, irritation of nose, throat
GI: Gastritis, nausea, vomiting, anorexia
MS: Muscle cramps
RESP: **Paradoxical bronchospasm**, dyspnea, coughing

Contraindications: Hypersensitivity to sympathomimetics, tachycardia

Precautions: Pregnancy **C**, breastfeeding, cardiac disorders, hyperthyroidism, hypertension, diabetes mellitus, prostatic hypertrophy

Pharmacokinetics	
Absorption	Minimally absorbed
Distribution	Unknown
Metabolism	Liver
Excretion	Unknown
Half-life	2 hr

P

Adverse effects: *italic* = common, **bold** = life-threatening

Pharmacodynamics	
Onset	5-15 min
Peak	1-1½ hr
Duration	5 hr

Interactions
Individual drugs
Levothyroxine: increased pirbuterol action
Drug classifications
Antidepressants (tricyclics), antihistamines: increased pirbuterol action

β-Adrenergic blockers: block therapeutic effect

Bronchodilators (aerosol): increased action of bronchodilator

MAOIs: increased chance of hypertensive crisis
Drug/herb
Cola nut, guarana, yerba maté: increased action of both

Green tea (large amounts), guarana: increased effect

NURSING CONSIDERATIONS
Assessment
• Monitor respiratory function: vital capacity, FEV, ABGs, lung sounds, heart rate, rhythm (baseline)
• Monitor for evidence of allergic reactions, paradoxic bronchospasm (can occur rapidly); withhold dose and notify prescriber

Nursing diagnoses
• Airway clearance, ineffective (uses)
• Gas exchange, impaired (uses)
• Knowledge, deficient (teaching)

Implementation
• Give after shaking; have patient exhale, place mouthpiece in mouth, inhale slowly, hold breath, remove, exhale slowly; allow at least 1 min between inhalations
• Give this medication before other medications and allow at least 1 min between each to prevent overstimulation
• Store in light-resistant container; do not expose to temperature over 86° F (30° C)

Patient/family education
• Advise patient not to use OTC medications; extra stimulation may occur; to use this medication before other medications and allow at least 1 min between each to prevent overstimulation
• Teach patient use of inhaler; to avoid getting aerosol in eyes: blurring may result; to wash inhaler in warm water and dry daily; to avoid smoking, smoke-filled rooms, persons with respiratory tract infections; review package insert with patient

• Teach patient that paradoxic bronchospasm may occur and to stop product immediately and notify prescriber; to limit caffeine products such as chocolate, coffee, tea, and colas
• Instruct patient on administration of dose; not to use more than prescribed; serious side effects may occur

Evaluation
Positive therapeutic outcome
• Absence of dyspnea, wheezing after 1 hr
• Improved airway exchange
• Improved ABGs

Treatment of overdose: Administer a β₂-adrenergic blocker

---

piroxicam (Rx)
(peer-ox'i-kam)
Apo-Piroxicam ✲, Feldene, Gen-Piroxicam ✲, Novopirocam ✲, PMS-Piroxicam ✲
Func. class.: Nonsteroidal antiinflammatory
Chem. class.: Oxicam derivative

Pregnancy category C

Action: Inhibits prostaglandin synthesis by decreasing an enzyme needed for biosynthesis; analgesic, antiinflammatory; antipyretic properties

Therapeutic outcome: Decreased pain, inflammation

Uses: Mild to moderate pain, osteoarthritis, rheumatoid arthritis

Dosage and routes
Adult: PO 20 mg/day or 10 mg bid

Available forms: Caps 10, 20 mg

Adverse effects
CNS: Dizziness, *drowsiness,* fatigue, tremors, confusion, insomnia, anxiety, depression, *headache*
CV: Tachycardia, peripheral edema, palpitations, **dysrhythmias,** hypertension, **MI, stroke,** CHF
EENT: Tinnitus, hearing loss, blurred vision
GI: Nausea, anorexia, vomiting, diarrhea, jaundice, **cholestatic hepatitis,** constipation, flatulence, cramps, dry mouth, peptic ulcer, **bleeding, ulceration, perforation,** dyspepsia
GU: **Nephrotoxicity: dysuria, hematuria, oliguria, azotemia**
HEMA: **Blood dyscrasias**
INTEG: Purpura, rash, pruritus, sweating, photosensitivity

MISC: Hyperkalemia, hypoglycemia
SYST: **Anaphylaxis**

Contraindications: Pregnancy **D** (3rd trimester); hypersensitivity to this product, NSAIDs, salicylates; asthma

Black Box Warning: Perioperative pain in CABG surgery

Precautions: Pregnancy **C**, breastfeeding, children, bleeding disorders, GI/cardiac disorders, hypersensitivity to other antiinflammatory agents, CHF

Black Box Warning: GI bleeding, MI, stroke

Pharmacokinetics

Absorption	Well absorbed
Distribution	Unknown
Metabolism	Liver, extensively
Excretion	Kidneys, minimal; breast milk
Half-life	50 hr

Pharmacodynamics

Onset	1 hr
Peak	3-5 hr
Duration	48-72 hr

Interactions
Individual drugs
Alcohol, aspirin, cycloSPORINE, lithium, methotrexate: increased toxicity
Drug classifications
Anticoagulants (oral), corticosteroids: increased toxicity
Anticoagulants, antiplatelets, NSAIDs, SSRIs, thrombin inhibitors: increased bleeding risk
Antidiabetics (oral): hypoglycemia
Antihypertensives: decreased effect of antihypertensives
Diuretics: decreased effectiveness of diuretics
Drug/herb
Arginine, gossypol: increased gastric irritation
Bearberry, bilberry: increased NSAIDs effect
Bogbean, chondroitin: increased bleeding risk

NURSING CONSIDERATIONS
Assessment
• Monitor blood counts during therapy; watch for decreasing platelets; if low, therapy may need to be discontinued, restarted after hematologic recovery; check for blood dyscrasia (thrombocytopenia): bruising, fatigue, bleeding, poor healing
• Assess for pain: location, duration, ROM, before, 1-2 hr after administration
• Assess for aspirin sensitivity, asthma, nasal polyps; these may develop into allergic reactions

Nursing diagnoses
• Injury, risk for (adverse reactions)
• Knowledge, deficient (teaching)
• Mobility, impaired physical (uses)
• Pain, chronic (uses)

Implementation
• Swallow caps whole; do not break, crush, or chew
• Give with food or milk to decrease gastric symptoms, water to enhance absorption
• Store at room temp, in light-resistant container

Patient/family education
• Teach patient that product must be continued for prescribed time to be effective; to avoid aspirin, alcoholic beverages, and other OTC medications unless approved by prescriber
• Caution patient to report bleeding, bruising, fatigue, malaise, since blood dyscrasias do occur
• Instruct patient to use caution when driving; drowsiness, dizziness may occur
• Teach patient to take with a full glass of water to enhance absorption
• Instruct to inform all health care providers about product use

Evaluation
Positive therapeutic outcome
• Decreased pain
• Decreased inflammation
• Increased mobility

pitavastatin
Livalo
See Appendix A, Selected New Drugs

plasma protein fraction (Rx)
Plasmanate
Func. class.: Hematological agent
Chem. class.: Plasma volume expander
Pregnancy category C

Action: Exerts similar oncotic pressure as human plasma, expands blood volume, shifts water from extravascular space to intravascular space

Therapeutic outcome: Shift of fluid from extravascular into intravascular space

Uses: Hypovolemic shock, hypoproteinemia, ARDS, preoperative cardiopulmonary bypass,

Adverse effects: *italic* = common, **bold** = life-threatening

acute liver failure, nephrotic syndrome, cardiogenic shock

Dosage and routes
Hypovolemia
Adult: IV INF 250-500 ml (12.5-25 g of protein), max 10 ml/min
Child: IV INF 10-30 ml/kg max 5-10 ml/min

Hypoproteinemia
Adult: IV INF 1000-1500 ml/day, max 8 ml/min

Available forms: Inj 5%

Adverse effects
CNS: Fever, chills, headache, paresthesias, flushing
CV: **Fluid overload,** hypotension, erratic pulse
GI: Nausea, vomiting, increased salivation
INTEG: Rash, urticaria, cyanosis
RESP: Altered respirations, dyspnea, **pulmonary edema**

Contraindications: Hypersensitivity to
this product or albumin, CHF, severe anemia, renal insufficiency, hyponatremia, cardiopulmonary bypass

Precautions: Pregnancy C, decreased salt
intake, decreased cardiac reserve, lack of albumin deficiency, hepatic disease

Pharmacokinetics	
Absorption	Completely absorbed
Distribution	Intravascular space
Metabolism	Unknown
Excretion	Unknown
Half-life	Unknown

Pharmacodynamics	
Onset	15-30 min
Peak	Unknown
Duration	Unknown

Interactions
Drug/lab test
False increase: alkaline phosphatase

NURSING CONSIDERATIONS
Assessment
• Monitor blood studies: Hct, Hgb; electrolytes, serum protein; if serum protein declines, dyspnea, hypoxemia can result
• Monitor B/P (decreased), pulse (erratic), respiration during inf; CVP, jugular vein distention, PWP (increases if overload occurs); shortness of breath, anxiety, insomnia, expiratory crackles, frothy blood-tinged cough, cyanosis indicate pulmonary overload

• Monitor I&O ratio; urinary output may decrease
• Assess for allergy: fever, rash, itching, chills, flushing, urticaria, nausea, vomiting, or hypotension require discontinuation of inf; use new lot if therapy reinstituted, premedicate with diphenhydrAMINE

Nursing diagnoses
• Cardiac output, decreased (uses)
• Fluid volume, deficient (uses)
• Fluid volume, excess (adverse reactions)

Implementation
• Give by **IV;** no dilution required; use inf pump, large-gauge needle (≥20-G); discard unused portion; inf slowly to prevent hypotension; give within 4 hr of opening
• Provide adequate hydration before administration
• Do not use sol that has been frozen
• Adjust rate to changes in B/P
• Store at room temp, max 86° F
Additive compatibilities:
Carbohydrate and electrolyte sol, whole blood, packed RBCs, chloramphenicol, tetracycline
Additive incompatibilities:
Protein hydrolysate sol, amino acid sol, alcohol, norepinephrine

Patient/family education
• Explain reason for and expected result of medication

Evaluation
Positive therapeutic outcome
• Increased B/P
• Decreased edema
• Increased serum albumin

plerixafor (Rx)
(pler-ix′a-fore)
Mozobil
Func. class.: Biologic modifier
Chem. class.: Colony-stimulating factor
Pregnancy category D

Action: Competitively inhibits the binding of stromal-derived factors, allowing hematopoietic stem cells to mobilize into peripheral blood

Therapeutic outcome: Successful collection of stem cells

Uses: For peripheral blood stem cell (PBSC) mobilization for collection and autologous transplant in non-Hodgkin's lymphoma, multiple myeloma; used with a granulocyte colony stimulating factor (G-CSF)

Dosage and routes
Adult: SUBCUT 0.24 mg/kg qd about 11 hr prior to initiation of apheresis; give up to 4 consecutive days; give filgrastim 10 mcg/kg SUBCUT qd each AM beginning 4 days prior to the 1st evening dose of plerixafor and on each day of apheresis; give filgrastim before procedure

Available forms: Inj 300 mcg/ml, 480 mcg/1.6 ml, 480 mcg/0.8 ml, 3000 mcg/ 0.5 ml

Adverse effects
CNS: Syncope, dizziness, fatigue, headache, insomnia, malaise, paresthesias
GI: Nausea, vomiting, diarrhea, abdominal pain, constipation
HEMA: **Thrombocytopenia,** leukocytosis
INTEG: Rash, skin irritation, pruritus, inj site reaction, erythema, urticaria
MS: Musculoskeletal pain
RESP: Dyspnea, hypoxia

Contraindications: Hypersensitivity, breastfeeding

Precautions: Pregnancy **D,** children, renal disease, thrombocytopenia

Pharmacokinetics
Absorption	Unknown
Distribution	Protein binding 58%
Metabolism	Unknown
Excretion	70% kidney as parent drug
Half-life	Terminal 3-5 hr

Pharmacodynamics
Onset	30-60 min
Peak	6-9 hr mobilization
Duration	Unknown

Interactions
Individual drugs
Lithium: increased adverse reactions, increased leukocytosis

NURSING CONSIDERATIONS
Assessment
- Monitor blood studies: CBC/differential
- Monitor B/P, respirations, pulse before, during therapy
- Assess for bone pain; give mild analgesics

Nursing diagnoses
- Knowledge, deficient (teaching)

Implementation
- Each single use vial contains 24 mg of plerixafor (1.2 ml of 20 mg/ml sol); the volume is calculated by multiplying 0.012 by the actual body wt (kg)
- Give 11 hr before apheresis
- Max 40 mg/day, or 27 mg/day in renal disease
- Store at room temperature

Patient/family education
- Explain reason for use and expected results

Evaluation
Positive therapeutic outcome
- Collection of stem cells

---

porfimer (Rx)
(pour'fih-mur)
Photofrin
Func. class.: Antineoplastic—miscellaneous
Chem. class.: Photosensitizing agent, hematoporphyrin derivative

Pregnancy category C

Action: Used in photodynamic treatment (PDT) of tumors; antitumor and cytotoxic actions are light and O_2 dependent; used with 630-nm laser light

Therapeutic outcome: Prevention of growth of tumor

Uses: Esophageal cancer (completely obstructing), endobronchial non–small-cell lung cancer, Barrett's esophagus

Dosage and routes
Refer to Optiguide for complete instructions
Adult: **IV** 2 mg/kg over 3-5 min, then illumination with laser light 40-50 hr after inj; a second laser light application may be given 96-120 hr after inj; may repeat q30day × 3

Endobronchial cancer
Adult: 200 joules/cm of tumor length

Available forms: Cake/powder for inj 75 mg; 15-, 75-mg vials

Adverse effects
CNS: Anxiety, confusion, insomnia
CV: Hypo/hypertension, **atrial fibrillation, cardiac failure,** *tachycardia,* chest pain
GI: Abdominal pain, constipation, diarrhea, dyspepsia, dysphagia, eructation, esophageal edema/bleeding, hematemesis, melena, nausea, vomiting, anorexia
MISC: Dehydration, weight decrease, anemia, photosensitivity reaction, UTI, moniliasis
RESP: **Pleural effusion,** pneumonia, dyspnea, respiratory insufficiency, **tracheoesophageal fistula,** stricture/ulceration

Contraindications: Porphyria, porphyrin allergy (porfirmer); tracheoesophageal,

P

bronchoesophageal fistula; major blood vessels with eroding tumors (PDT)

Precautions: Pregnancy **C,** breastfeeding, children, geriatric

Pharmacokinetics
Absorption	Unknown
Distribution	In tissues
Metabolism	Unknown
Excretion	Cleared by biliary excretion
Half-life	250 hr

Pharmacodynamics
Onset	Unknown
Peak	5-10 hr
Duration	Unknown

Interactions
Drug classifications

Anticoagulants, corticosteroids, calcium channel blockers, NSAIDs, platelet inhibitors, thrombolytics: decreased porfimer effect

Phenothiazines, sulfonamides, sulfonylureas, tetracyclines, thiazides: increased photosensitivity

NURSING CONSIDERATIONS
Assessment
- Assess for ocular sensitivity; sensitivity to sun, bright lights, car headlights; patients should wear dark sunglasses with an average white light transmittance of <4%
- Assess for chest pain: may be so severe as to necessitate opiate analgesics
- Assess for extravasation at inj site: take care to protect from light

Nursing diagnoses
- Infection, risk for (adverse reactions)
- Knowledge, deficient (teaching)

Implementation
- Give as a single slow **IV** inj over 3-5 min at 2 mg/kg; reconstitute each vial with 31.8 ml of D₅ or 0.9% NaCl (2.5 mg/ml), shake well, do not mix with other products or sol, protect from light, and use immediately
- Laser light is initiated; 630-nm wavelength laser light, 40-50 hr after inj; 2nd laser if indicated at 96-120 hr
- Wipe spills with damp cloth, avoid skin/eye contact, use rubber gloves, eye protection; dispose of material in polyethylene bag according to policy

Patient/family education
- Advise patient to report chest pain, eye sensitivity, signs/symptoms of infection, respiratory distress, bleeding
- Advise patient to wear sunglasses; avoid exposure to sunlight or bright light for 30 days, report severe sunburn, blistering

Evaluation
Positive therapeutic outcome
- Reducing number and spread of malignant cells

---

posaconazole (Rx)
(poe′sa-kon′a-zole)
Noxafil
Func. class.: Antifungal, systemic
Chem. class.: Triazole derivative
Pregnancy category C

Action: Inhibits a portion of cell wall synthesis; alters cell membranes and inhibits several fungal enzymes

Therapeutic outcome: Decreased fever, malaise, rash; negative C&S for infecting organism

Uses: Prevention of aspergillus, candida infection, oropharyngeal candidiasis in the immunocompromised

Dosage and routes
Adult: PO 800 mg/day in 2-4 divided doses
Child: PO 100 mg tid

Available forms: Oral susp 200 mg/5 ml

Adverse effects
CNS: Headache, dizziness, insomnia, fever, rigors, weakness, anxiety
CV: Hypo/hypertension, tachycardia, anemia
GI: Nausea, vomiting, anorexia, diarrhea, cramps, abdominal pain, flatulence, **GI bleeding, hepatotoxicity**
GU: Gynecomastia, impotence, decreased libido
INTEG: Pruritus, fever, *rash,* **toxic epidermal necrolysis**
MISC: Edema, fatigue, malaise, hypokalemia, tinnitus, **rhabdomyolysis**

Contraindications: Hypersensitivity to this product or other systemic antifungal or azoles, fungal meningitis, onchomycosis or dermatomycosis in cardiac dysfunction

Precautions: Pregnancy **C,** breastfeeding, children, hepatic/cardiac disease

---

Pharmacokinetics

Absorption	Well, enhanced by food
Distribution	Protein binding 98%-99%
Metabolism	Liver
Excretion	Feces, 77% unchanged
Half-life	19-35 hr

Pharmacodynamics

Onset	Unknown
Peak	4-11 hr
Duration	Unknown

Interactions
Individual drugs
⬥BusPIRone, busulfan, clarithromycin, cycloSPORINE, diazepam, digoxin, felodipine, indinavir, isradipine, niCARdipine, niFEDipine, nimodipine, phenytoin, quinidine, ritonavir, saquinavir, tacrolimus, warfarin: increased levels, toxicity

Didanosine, rifamycin: decreased posaconazole action

⬥Dofetilide, pimozide, quinidine: life threatening reactions

Midazolam (oral), triazolam: increased sedation

Quinidine: increased tinnitus, hearing loss
Drug classifications
Antacids, H₂-receptor antagonists, rifamycins: decreased posaconazole action

Calcium channel blockers: increased edema

⬥Ergots: life-threatening reactions

Other hepatotoxic products: increased hepatotoxicity

Oral contraceptives: decreased effect, use other contraceptives

Oral hypoglycemics: increased severe hypoglycemia
Drug/herb
Gossypol: nephrotoxicity
Drug/food
Food: increased absorption

NURSING CONSIDERATIONS
Assessment
• Assess for type of infection; may begin treatment prior to obtaining results
• Assess for infection: temp, WBC, sputum, baseline, periodically
• Monitor I&O ratio, potassium levels
• Monitor liver function tests (ALT, AST, bilirubin) if on long-term therapy
• Assess for allergic reaction: rash, photosensitivity, uricaria, dermatitis
⬥ Assess for hepatotoxicity: nausea, vomiting, jaundice, clay-colored stools, fatigue

Nursing diagnoses
• Infection, risk for (uses)
• Knowledge, deficient (teaching)

Implementation
• Give after shaking well; use calibrated measuring device; take only with a full meal or liquid nutritional supplements such as Ensure; rinse measuring device after each use
• Store in a tight container in refrigerator; do not freeze

Patient/family education
• Teach patient that long-term therapy may be needed to clear infection (1 wk-6 mo depending on infection)
• Advise patient to avoid hazardous activities if dizziness occurs
• Advise patient to take 2 hr before administration of other products that increase gastric pH (antacids, H₂-blockers, omeprazole, sucralfate, anticholinergics); to notify health care provider of all medications taken
• Teach the patient the importance of compliance with product regimen; to use alternative method of contraception
• Teach patient to notify prescriber of GI symptoms, signs of hepatic dysfunction (fatigue, nausea, anorexia, vomiting, dark urine, pale stools)

Evaluation
Positive therapeutic outcome
• Decreased fever, malaise, rash, negative C&S for infecting organism

P

Adverse effects: *italic* = common, **bold** = life-threatening

**potassium acetate/
potassium bicarbonate
(Rx, OTC)**

K+ Care ET, K-Electrolyte, K-Ide, Klor-Con EF, K-Lyte, K-Vescent

**potassium bicarbonate/
potassium chloride
(Rx, OTC)**

Klorvess, Klorvess Effervescent Granules, K-Lyte/Cl, Neo-K ✤

**potassium bicarbonate/
potassium citrate** (Rx, OTC)

Effer-K, K-Lyte DS

**potassium chloride
(Rx, OTC)**

Apo-K ✤, Cena-K, Gen-K, K+ Care, K+10, Kalium Duriles ✤, Kaochlor, Kaochlor S-F, Kaon-Cl, Kay Ciel, KCl, K-Dur, K-Lease, K-Long ✤, K-Lor, Klor-Con, Klorvess, Klotrix, K-Lyte/Cl powder, K-med, K-Norm, K-Sol, K-Tab, Micro-K, Micro-LS, Potasalan, Roychlor, Rum-K, Slow-K, Ten-K

**potassium chloride/
potassium bicarbonate/
potassium citrate** (Rx, OTC)

Kaochlor Eff

**potassium gluconate
(Rx, OTC)**

Kaon, Kaylixir, K-G Elixir, Potassium-Rougier ✤

**potassium gluconate/
potassium chloride
(Rx, OTC)**

Kolyum

**potassium gluconate/
potassium citrate** (Rx, OTC)

Twin-K

Func. class.: Electrolyte, mineral replacement

Chem. class.: Potassium

Pregnancy category C

Action: Needed for adequate transmission of nerve impulses and cardiac contraction, renal function, intracellular ion maintenance

Therapeutic outcome: Potassium level 3.0-5.0 mg/dl

Uses: Prevention and treatment of hypokalemia

Dosage and routes
Potassium bicarbonate
Adult: PO dissolve 25-50 mEq in water daily-qid

Hypokalemia (prevention)
Adult and child: PO 20 mEq/day in 2-4 divided doses

Potassium acetate—hypokalemia
Adult and child: PO 40-100 mEq/day in divided doses × 2-4 days

Potassium chloride
Adult: PO 40-100 mEq in divided doses tid-qid; **IV** 20 mEq/hr when diluted as 40 mEq/1000 ml, max 150 mEq/day
Child: PO 1-2 mEq/kg/day

Potassium gluconate
Adult: PO 40-100 mEq in divided doses tid-qid

Potassium phosphate
Adult: **IV** 1 mEq/hr in SOL of 60 mEq/L, max 150 mEq/day; PO 40-100 mEq/day in divided doses
Child: **IV** max rate of INF 1 mEq/kg/min

Available forms: Tabs for sol 6.5, 25 mEq; ext rel caps 8, 10 mEq; powder for sol 3.3, 5, 6.7, 10, 13.3 mEq/5 ml; tabs 2, 4, 5, 13.4 mEq; ext rel tabs 6.7, 8, 10 mEq; elix 6.7 mEq/5 ml; oral sol 2.375 mEq/5 ml; inj for prep of **IV** 1.5, 2, 2.4, 3, 3.2, 4.4, 4.7 mEq

Adverse effects
CNS: Confusion
CV: Bradycardia, *cardiac depression,* **dysrhythmias, arrest, peaking T waves, lowered R and depressed RST, prolonged P–R interval, widened QRS complex**
GI: Nausea, vomiting, cramps, pain, *diarrhea,* ulceration of small bowel
GU: Oliguria
INTEG: Cold extremities, rash

Contraindications: Renal disease (severe), severe hemolytic disease, Addison's disease, hyperkalemia, acute dehydration, extensive tissue breakdown

Precautions: Pregnancy C, cardiac disease, potassium-sparing diuretic therapy, systemic acidosis

Pharmacokinetics	
Absorption	Unknown
Distribution	Unknown
Metabolism	Unknown
Excretion	Kidneys, feces
Half-life	Unknown

Pharmacodynamics		
	PO	IV
Onset	30 min	Immediate
Peak	Unknown	Unknown
Duration	Unknown	Unknown

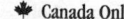

Interactions
Drug classifications
Angiotensin-converting enzyme inhibitors, calcium, diuretics (potassium-sparing), magnesium, potassium phosphate, **IV**, other potassium products: increased hyperkalemia

NURSING CONSIDERATIONS
Assessment
• Assess ECG for peaking T-waves, lowered R, depressed RST, prolonged PR interval, widening QRS complex, hyperkalemia; product should be reduced or discontinued
• Monitor potassium level during treatment (3.5-5.0 mg/dl is normal level)
• Monitor I&O ratio; watch for decreased urinary output; notify prescriber immediately; check urinary pH in patients receiving the product as a urinary acidifier
• Assess cardiac status: rate, rhythm, CVP, PWP, PAWP if being monitored directly

Nursing diagnoses
• Knowledge, deficient (teaching)
• Nutrition: less than body requirements, imbalanced (uses)

Implementation
PO route
• Do not break, crush, or chew ext rel tabs/caps or enteric-coated products
• Give with meal or after meal; take cap with full glass of liquid; dissolve effervescent tab, powder in 8 oz of cold water or juice; do not give IM, SUBCUT
• Store at room temperature

IV route
• Give through large-bore needle to decrease vein inflammation; check for extravasation; administer in large vein, avoiding scalp vein in child
• After diluting in large volume of **IV** sol give as an **IV** inf slowly to prevent toxicity; never give **IV** bol or IM

Potassium acetate
Additive compatibilities: Metoclopramide

Potassium chloride
Y-site compatibilities: Acyclovir, aldesleukin, allopurinol, amifostine, aminophylline, amiodarone, ampicillin, atropine, aztreonam, betamethasone, calcium gluconate, cefmetazole, cephalothin, cephapirin, chlordiazepoxide, chlorproMAZINE, ciprofloxacin, cladribine, cyanocobalamin, dexamethasone, digoxin, diltiazem, diphenhydrAMINE, DOBUTamine, DOPamine, droperidol, edrophonium, enalaprilat, epinephrine, esmolol, estrogens, ethacrynate, famotidine, fentanyl, filgrastim, fludarabine, fluorouracil, furosemide, gallium, granisetron, heparin, hydrALAZINE, idarubicin, indomethacin, inamrinone, regular insulin, isoproterenol, kanamycin, labetalol, lidocaine, lorazepam, magnesium sulfate, melphalan, meperidine, methicillin, methoxamine, methylergonovine, midazolam, minocycline, morphine, neostigmine, norepinephrine, ondansetron, oxacillin, oxytocin, paclitaxel, penicillin G potassium, pentazocine, phytonadione, piperacillin/tazobactam, prednisoLONE, procainamide, prochlorperazine, propofol, propranolol, pyridostigmine, sargramostim, scopolamine, sodium bicarbonate, succinylcholine, tacrolimus, teniposide, theophylline, thiotepa, trimethaphan, trimethobenzamide, vinorelbine, zidovudine

Additive compatibilities: Aminophylline, amiodarone, atracurium, bretylium, calcium chloride, cefepime, cephalothin, cephapirin, chloramphenicol, cimetidine, ciprofloxacin, clindamycin, cloxacillin, corticotropin, cytarabine, dimenhyDRINATE, DOPamine, enalaprilat, erythromycin, floxacillin, fluconazole, furosemide, heparin, hydrocortisone, isoproterenol, lidocaine, metaraminol, methicillin, methyldopate, metoclopramide, mitoxantrone, nafcillin, netilmicin, norepinephrine, oxacillin, penicillin G potassium or sodium, phenylephrine, piperacillin, ranitidine, sodium bicarbonate, thiopental, vancomycin, verapamil, vit B/C

Potassium chloride
Y-site compatibilities: Aldesleukin, amifostine, granisetron, lorazepam, midazolam, thiotepa

Patient/family education
• Teach patient to eat foods rich in potassium after medication is discontinued
• Advise patient to avoid OTC products: antacids, salt substitutes, analgesics, vit preparations, unless specifically directed by prescriber; avoid licorice in large amounts, may cause hypokalemia, sodium retention
• Advise patient to report hyperkalemia symptoms or continued hypokalemia symptoms
• Tell patient to take cap with full glass of liquid; to dissolve powder or tab completely in at least 120 ml of water or juice; not to crush, chew caps or tabs
• Emphasize importance of regular follow-up and periodic potassium levels

P

Evaluation
Positive therapeutic outcome
- Absence of fatigue, muscle weakness, and decreased thirst and urinary output, cardiac changes
- Potassium level normal

! High Alert

pralatrexate (Rx)
(pra-luh-treks'ate)
Folotyn
Func. class.: Antineoplastic/antimetabolite
Chem. class.: Folate analog

Pregnancy category D

Action: Inhibits an enzyme that reduces folic acid, which is needed for nucleic acid synthesis in all cells; S phase of cell cycle specific; immunosuppressive

Therapeutic outcome: Decreased tumor size, spread of malignancy

Uses: Non-Hodgkin's lymphoma (NHL)

Dosage and routes
Adult: **IV** direct 30 mg/m² as a slow push over 3-5 min, via the side port of free-flowing 0.9% NaCL qwk × 6 wk in a 7-wk cycle

Available forms: Inj 20 mg/ml, 40 mg/2 ml

Adverse effects
CNS: Fatigue, fever; asthenia
CV: Sinus tachycardia
GI: Nausea, vomiting, anorexia, diarrhea, stomatitis, constipation, abdominal pain, mucositis
HEMA: **Leukopenia, thrombocytopenia, myelosuppression, anemia, epistaxis, neutropenia**
INTEG: Rash, pruritus
META: Hypokalemia
MS: Back pain
RESP: Cough, dyspnea
SYST: **Edema, infection, night sweats**

Contraindications: Pregnancy **D**, hypersensitivity, leukopenia (<3500/mm³), thrombocytopenia (<100,000/mm³), anemia, bone marrow suppression

Precautions: Breastfeeding, children, renal/hepatic disease

Pharmacokinetics	
Absorption	Unknown
Distribution	Crosses placenta, blood-brain barrier, protein binding 67%
Metabolism	Unknown
Excretion	Urine 34%
Half-life	Terminal 12-18 hr

Pharmacodynamics
Unknown

Interactions
Individual drugs
Radiation, trimethoprim, SMX-TMP: increased toxicity
Drug classifications
Folic acid supplements: decreased effect of pralatrexate
NSAIDs, salicylates, sulfa products, other antineoplastics: increased toxicity
Oral vaccines, toxoids: decreased effect of these agents

NURSING CONSIDERATIONS
Assessment
◆ Monitor CBC, differential, platelet count weekly; withhold product if WBC is <3500/mm³ or platelet count is <100,000/mm³; notify prescriber; WBC, platelet nadirs occur on day 7
- Monitor renal studies: BUN, serum uric acid, urine CCr, electrolytes before, during therapy
- Monitor temp; fever may indicate beginning infection; no rectal temps
- Monitor hepatic studies before, during therapy: bilirubin, ALK phos, AST, ALT; liver biopsy should be done before start of therapy (psoriasis patients)
- Assess buccal cavity for dryness, sores, ulceration, white patches, oral pain, bleeding, dysphagia
◆ Assess for symptoms indicating severe allergic reaction: rash, urticaria, itching, flushing

Nursing diagnoses
- Infection, risk for (adverse reaction)
- Knowledge, deficient (teaching)

Implementation
- Use strict medical asepsis and protective isolation if WBC levels are low
- Provide liquid diet: carbonated beverage, Jell-O; dry toast, crackers may be added when patient is not nauseated or vomiting
- Provide for rinsing of mouth tid-qid with water, club soda; brushing of teeth bid-tid with soft brush or cotton-tipped applicators for stomatitis; use unwaxed dental floss

- Give nutritious diet with iron, vitamin supplements, no folic acid
- Give antiemetic 30-60 min before giving product
- Use cytotoxic handling precautions
- Supplement patients with vit B_{12} IM 1 mg q8-10wk, and folic acid PO 1-1.25 mg qd

IV route
- Do not dilute
- Inspect for particulate/discoloration; it should be clear yellow
- Withdraw calculated dose; discard remaining drug
- Protect from light, refrigerate until use

Patient/family education
- Teach to report any complaints, side effects to nurse or prescriber: chills, fever, sore throat, bleeding, bruising, cough, dark or bloody urine
- Advise to avoid foods with citric acid, hot flavor or rough texture if stomatitis is present
- Advise to report stomatitis: any bleeding, white spots, ulcerations in mouth to prescriber; tell patient to examine mouth daily, report symptoms to nurse, use good oral hygiene
- Inform that contraceptive measures are recommended during therapy and for at least 8 wk following cessation of therapy, to discontinue breastfeeding; toxicity to infant may occur
- Teach to drink 10-12 glasses of fluid/day
- Teach to avoid alcohol, salicylates, live vaccines
- Teach to avoid use of razors, commercial mouthwash
- Advise to use sunblock to prevent burns

Evaluation
Positive therapeutic outcome
- Decreased tumor size, spread of malignancy

pramipexole (Rx)
(pra-mi-pex'ol)
Mirapex, Mirapex ER
Func. class.: Antiparkinsonian agent
Chem. class.: Dopamine receptor agonist, nonergot

Pregnancy category C

Action: Selective agonist for D_2 receptors (presynaptic/postsynaptic sites); binding at D_3 receptor contributes to antiparkinson effects

Therapeutic outcome: Decreased symptoms of Parkinson's disease (involuntary movements)

Uses: Parkinsonism, restless leg syndrome

Dosage and routes
Initial treatment
Adult: PO from a starting dose of 0.375 mg/day given in 3 divided doses, increase gradually by 0.125 mg/dose at 5-7–day intervals until total daily dose of 4.5 mg is reached; ER 0.375 mg qd, may increase up to 0.75 mg/day, then increments of 0.75 mg/day ≤5-7 days, max 4.5 mg/day

Maintenance treatment
Adult: PO 1.5-4.5 mg/day in 3 divided doses

Restless leg syndrome
Adult: PO 0.125 mg 2-3 hr before bedtime, increase gradually

Renal dose
Adult: PO CCr 35-59 ml/min 0.125 mg bid, may increase q5-7day to 1.5 mg bid; CCr 15-34 ml/min 0.125 mg/day, may increase q5-7day to 1.5 mg/day

Available forms: Tabs 0.125, 0.25, 0.5, 1, 1.5 mg; cap ER 0.375 mg

Adverse effects
CNS: Agitation, insomnia, psychosis, hallucinations, depression, dizziness, headache, confusion, amnesia, dream disorder, asthenia, dyskinesia, hypersomnolence, sudden sleep onset
CV: Orthostatic hypotension, edema, syncope, tachycardia
EENT: Blurred vision
GI: Nausea, anorexia, constipation, dysphagia, dry mouth
GU: Impotence, urinary frequency
HEMA: **Hemolytic anemia, leukopenia, agranulocytosis**

Contraindications: Hypersensitivity

Precautions: Pregnancy **C**, renal/cardiac disease, MI with dysrhythmias, affective disorders, psychosis, preexisting dyskinesias, history of falling asleep during daily activities

Pharmacokinetics
Absorption	Well absorbed
Distribution	Widely distributed
Metabolism	Liver, minimally
Excretion	Kidneys, unchanged
Half-life	8 hr; 12 hr in geriatric

Pharmacodynamics
Onset	Unknown
Peak	2 hr
Duration	Unknown

Adverse effects: *italic* = common, **bold** = life-threatening

Interactions
Individual drugs
Cimetidine, diltiazem, levodopa, quinidine, ranitidine, triamterine, verapamil: increased pramipexole levels
Metoclopramide: decreased pramipexole levels
Drug classifications
Butyrophenones, DOPamine agonists, phenothiazines: decreased pramipexole effect
Drug/herb
Chaste tree fruit, kava: decreased pramipexole effect

NURSING CONSIDERATIONS
Assessment
• Monitor B/P, ECG, respiration during initial treatment; hypo/hypertension should be reported
• Assess mental status: affect, mood, behavioral changes, depression; complete suicide assessment
• Monitor renal function tests
• Assess for involuntary movements in parkinsonism: akinesia, tremors, staggering gait, muscle rigidity, drooling; these symptoms should improve with therapy
◆ Assess for sleep attacks: may fall asleep during activities, without warning; may need to discontinue medication

Nursing diagnoses
• Injury, risk for (uses)
• Knowledge, deficient (teaching)
• Mobility, impaired physical (uses)
• Noncompliance (teaching)

Implementation
• Adjust dosage to patient response
• Give with meals to decrease GI upset

Patient/family education
• Advise patient that therapeutic effects may take several wk to a few mo
• Caution patient to change positions slowly to prevent orthostatic hypotension
• Instruct patient to use product exactly as prescribed; if product is discontinued abruptly, parkinsonian crisis may occur; if treatment is to be discontinued, taper over 1 wk; avoid alcohol, OTC sleeping products
• Advise patient to notify prescriber if pregnancy is planned or suspected

Evaluation
Positive therapeutic outcome
• Decreased akathisia, other involuntary movements
• Improved mood

---

pramlintide (Rx)
(pram'lin-tide)
Symlin
Func. class.: Antidiabetic
Chem. class.: Synthetic human amylin analog

Pregnancy category C

Action: Modulates and slows stomach emptying, prevents postprandial rise in plasma glucagon, decreases appetite, leads to decreased caloric intake and weight loss

Therapeutic outcome: Decreased polyuria, polydipsia, polyphagia; improved A1c

Uses: As an adjunct to insulin therapy with uncontrolled type 1 or type 2 diabetes

Dosage and routes
Type 1 diabetes
Adult: SUBCUT prior to each meal (≥30 g CHO), titrate up from 15 mcg to target dose of 60 mcg/dose, each dose titration should occur after no nausea for 3 days

Type 2 diabetes
Adult: SUBCUT 60 mcg prior to each meal (≥30 g CHO), titrate up to 120 mcg SUBCUT with each meal after no nausea for 3-7 days

Available forms: Inj 5 ml vials (0.6 mg/ml)

Adverse effects
CNS: Headache, fatigue, dizziness
GI: Nausea, vomiting, anorexia, abdominal pain
INTEG: Inj site reactions
META: Hypoglycemia
MS: Arthralgia
RESP: Cough, pharyngitis
SYST: Systemic allergy

Contraindications: Hypersensitivity to this product or cresol, gastroparesis

Black Box Warning: Hypoglycemia

Precautions: Pregnancy **C**, breastfeeding

Pharmacokinetics
Absorption	30%-40%
Distribution	Extensively bound to blood cells or albumin
Metabolism	Kidneys
Excretion	Unknown
Half-life	48 min

Pharmacodynamics
Unknown

 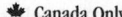

Interactions
Individual drugs
Acetaminophen: may increase effect of acetaminophen

Alcohol, disopyramide, insulin: increased hypoglycemia

Dextrothyroxine, niacin, triamterene: decreased hypoglycemia

Diphenoxylate, loperamide, octreotide: increased pramlintide action

Erythromycin, metoclopramide: do not use

Drug classifications
ACE inhibitors, anabolic steroids, androgens, corticosteroids, fibric acid derivatives: increased hypoglycemia

α-Glucosidase inhibitors, antimuscarinics, opiate agonist, tricyclics: increased pramlintide action

Estrogens, MAOIs, oral contraceptives, progestins, thiazide diuretics: decreased hypoglycemia

Phenothiazines: increased hyperglycemia

NURSING CONSIDERATIONS
Assessment
• Monitor fasting blood glucose, 2 hr PP (80-150 mg/dl, normal fasting level; 70-130 mg/dl, normal 2 hr level); A1c may also be drawn to identify treatment effectiveness; also monitor weight, appetite

• Assess for hypoglycemic reaction (sweating, weakness, dizziness, chills, confusion, headache, nausea, rapid weak pulse, fatigue, tachycardia, memory lapses, slurred speech, staggering gait, anxiety, tremors, hunger)

• Assess for hyperglycemia: acetone breath, polyuria, fatigue, polydipsia, flushed, dry skin, lethargy

Nursing diagnoses
• Injury, risk for (uses)
• Knowledge, deficient (teaching)
• Noncompliance (teaching)

Implementation
• Pre-meal insulin should be decreased by 50% when starting and adjusted to therapeutic dose to prevent hypoglycemia

SUBCUT route
• Give immediately before mealtime or if 30 g of carbohydrates will be consumed
• Do not use if a meal is skipped
• Do not use if discolored; do not give in arm; absorption is variable
• Store at room temperature for up to 30 days; keep away from heat and sunlight; refrigerate all other supply

Syringe compatibilities: Do not mix with insulin, give separately

Patient/family education
• Advise patient that product does not cure diabetes but controls symptoms
• Advise patient to carry emergency ID as diabetic
• Teach patient to recognize hypoglycemia reaction: headache, fatigue, weakness
• Teach patient the dosage, route, mixing instructions, if any diet restrictions, disease process
• Advise patient to carry a glucose source (candy or lump sugar) to treat hypoglycemia
• Teach patient symptoms of ketoacidosis: nausea, thirst, polyuria, dry mouth, decreased B/P, dry, flushed skin, acetone breath, drowsiness, Kussmaul respirations
• Advise patient that a plan is necessary for diet, exercise; all food on diet should be eaten; exercise routine should not vary
• Teach patient about blood glucose testing; make sure patient is able to determine glucose level
• Advise patient to avoid OTC products unless directed by prescriber, avoid alcohol
• Advise patient not to operate machinery or drive until effect is known

Evaluation
Positive therapeutic outcome
• Decrease in polyuria, polydipsia, polyphagia, clear sensorium; improved A1c, blood glucose; absence of dizziness; stable gait

Treatment of overdose: Glucose 25 g **IV,** via dextrose 50% sol, 50 ml or glucagon 1 mg SUBCUT

P

pramoxine topical
See Appendix B

prasugrel (Rx)
(pra′soo-grel)
Effient
Func. class.: Platelet aggregation inhibitor
Chem. class.: ADP receptor antagonist

Pregnancy category B

Action: Inhibits ADP-induced platelet aggregation

Therapeutic outcome: Absence of MI, stroke

Uses: Reducing the risk of stroke, MI, vascular death, peripheral arterial disease in high-risk patients

Adverse effects: *italic* = common, **bold** = life-threatening

Dosage and routes
Adult/geriatric <75 yr and ≥60 kg:
PO 60 mg loading dose, then 10 mg qd with aspirin (75-325 mg/day)
Adult/geriatric <75 yr and <60 kg:
PO 60 mg loading dose, then 5 mg qd
Geriatric >75 yr: Not recommended

Available forms: Tabs 5, 10 mg

Adverse effects
CNS: Headache, dizziness
CV: Edema, atrial fibrillation, bradycardia, chest pain, hyper/hypotension
GI: Nausea, vomiting, diarrhea
HEMA: Epistaxis, **leukopenia, thrombocytopenia, neutropenia, anaphylaxis, angioedema, anemia**
INTEG: Rash, hypercholesterolemia
MISC: Fatigue, **intracranial hemorrhage, secondary malignancy**
MS: Back pain

Contraindications: Hypersensitivity, stroke, TIA

Black Box Warning: Active bleeding

Precautions: Pregnancy **B**, breastfeeding, children, hepatic disease, increased bleeding risk, neutropenia, agranulocytosis, renal disease, surgery, trauma, thrombotic thrombocytopenia purpura, Asian patients, weight <60 kg, CABG, geriatric

Black Box Warning: Abrupt discontinuation

Pharmacokinetics	
Absorption	Rapidly absorbed
Distribution	Unknown
Metabolism	Liver CYP3A4, CYP2B6
Excretion	Urine feces
Half-life	7-8 hr

Pharmacodynamics	
Onset	Unknown
Peak	30 min
Duration	Unknown

Interactions
Individual drugs
Abciximab, aspirin, eptifibatide, rifampin, tirofiban, ticlopidine, treprostinil: increased bleeding risk
Drug classifications
Anticoagulants, NSAIDs, SSRIs: increased bleeding risk

Drug/herb
Bogbean, dong quai, feverfew, garlic, ginger, ginkgo biloba, green tea, horse chestnut: increased prasugrel effect

NURSING CONSIDERATIONS
Assessment:
◆ Assess for thrombotic/thrombocytic purpura: fever, thrombocytopenia, neurolytic anemia
• Assess for symptoms of stroke, MI during treatment
• Monitor hepatic studies: AST, ALT, bilirubin, creatinine (long-term therapy)
• Monitor blood studies: CBC, differential, Hct, Hgb, PT, cholesterol (long-term therapy)

Nursing diagnoses
• Injury, risk for (uses)
• Knowledge, deficient (teaching)

Implementation
• Give with food to decrease gastric symptoms
• Do not break tablets
• Do not discontinue therapy abruptly

Patient/family education
• Advise that blood work will be necessary during treatment
• Teach to report any unusual bruising, bleeding to prescriber; that it may take longer to stop bleeding
• Advise to take with food or just after eating to minimize GI discomfort
• Advise to report diarrhea, skin rashes, subcutaneous bleeding, chills, fever, sore throat
• Teach to tell all health care providers that prasugrel is used; may be held before surgery

Evaluation
Positive therapeutic outcome
• Absence of stroke, MI

pravastatin (Rx)
(pra'va-sta-tin)
Pravachol
Func. class.: Antilipidemic
Pregnancy category X

Do not confuse:
Pravachol/Prevacid

Action: Inhibits biosynthesis of VLDL, LDL, which are responsible for cholesterol development, by inhibiting the enzyme HMG-CoA reductase

Therapeutic outcome: Decreasing cholesterol levels and LDL, increased HDL

Uses: As an adjunct in primary hypercholesterolemia types IIa, IIb, III, IV, artherosclerosis; to reduce the risk of recurrent MI, primary/secondary CV events; reduce stroke, TIAs

Dosage and routes
Adult: PO 40-80 mg/day at bedtime (range 20-80 mg/day), start at 10 mg/day if also on immunosuppressants
Adolescent 14-18 yr: PO 40 mg/day
Child 8-13 yr: PO 20 mg/day
Geriatric/renal/hepatic dose: PO 10 mg/day, initially

Available forms: Tabs 10, 20, 40, 80 mg

Adverse effects
CNS: Headache, dizziness, fatigue, **ALS (Lou Gehrig's disease)**
CV: Chest pain
EENT: Lens opacities
GI: Nausea, constipation, diarrhea, flatus, abdominal pain, heartburn, **liver dysfunction, pancreatitis, hepatitis**
INTEG: Rash, pruritus, photosensitivity
MS: Muscle cramps, myalgia, **myositis, rhabdomyolysis**
RESP: Common cold, rhinitis, cough

Contraindications: Pregnancy **X**, breastfeeding, hypersensitivity, active liver disease

Precautions: Past liver disease, alcoholism, severe acute infections, trauma, severe metabolic disorders, electrolyte imbalances

Pharmacokinetics
Absorption	Poorly absorbed, erratic
Distribution	Protein binding 80%
Metabolism	Liver, extensively
Excretion	Feces (70%-75%); kidneys, unchanged (20%); breast milk (minimal)
Half-life	2 hr

Pharmacodynamics
Onset	Unknown
Peak	1-1½ hr
Duration	Unknown

Interactions
Individual drugs
Clarithromycin, clofibrate, cycloSPORINE, erythromycin, gemfibrozil, itraconazole, niacin: increased risk for myopathy
Digoxin: increased effects of digoxin
Warfarin: increased bleeding
Drug classifications
Bile acid sequestrants: decreased pravastatin bioavailability
Protease inhibitors: increased risk of myopathy

Drug/herb
Glucomannan: increased effect
Gotu kola, oat bran, St. John's wort: decreased effect
Drug/lab test
Increased: CPK, liver function tests
Altered: thyroid function tests

NURSING CONSIDERATIONS
Assessment
• Assess nutrition: fat, protein, carbohydrates; nutritional analysis should be completed by dietitian before treatment
• Monitor triglycerides, esterol, cholesterol at baseline, throughout treatment; LDL and HDL should be watched closely; if increased, product should be discontinued
⬥ Assess for muscle tenderness, pain; obtain CPK; rhabdomyolysis may occur; therapy should be discontinued
• Monitor ophth status yearly

Nursing diagnoses
• Knowledge, deficient (teaching)
• Noncompliance (teaching)

Implementation
• Give at bedtime only; give 1 hr before or 2 hr after bile acid sequestrants
• Store in cool environment in airtight, light-resistant container

Patient/family education
• Inform patient that compliance is needed for positive results to occur; not to double doses or skip doses
• Teach patient that risk factors should be decreased: high-fat diet, smoking, alcohol consumption, absence of exercise
• Advise patient to notify prescriber of weakness, tenderness, or limited mobility
• Explain to patient that contraception is necessary, since product produces teratogenic effects
• Advise patient to use sunscreen, protective clothing to prevent burns

Evaluation
Positive therapeutic outcome
• Decreased cholesterol, serum triglyceride levels and improved ratio with HDL

P

Adverse effects: *italic* = common, **bold** = life-threatening

prazosin (Rx)
(pra´zoe-sin)
Minipress, prazosin
Func. class.: Antihypertensive
Chem. class.: α₁-Adrenergic blocker

Pregnancy category C

Action: Blocks α-mediated vasoconstriction of adrenergic receptors, inducing peripheral vasodilatation

Therapeutic outcome: Decreased B/P in hypertension; decreased cardiac preload, afterload

Uses: Hypertension, refractory CHF, Raynaud's vasospasm

Unlabeled uses: Benign prostatic hypertrophy to decrease urine outflow obstruction

Dosage and routes
Hypertension
Adult: PO 1 mg bid or tid, increasing to 20 mg/day in divided doses if required, usual range 6-15 mg/day; max 1 mg initially, or 15 mg/day
Child: PO 5 mcg/kg q6hr; max 400 mcg/kg/day

Benign prostatic hyperplasia (unlabeled)
Adult: PO 2 mg bid

Available forms: Caps 1, 2, 5 mg

Adverse effects
CNS: Dizziness, headache, drowsiness, anxiety, depression, vertigo, weakness, fatigue
CV: Palpitations, orthostatic hypotension, tachycardia, edema, rebound hypertension
EENT: Blurred vision, epistaxis, tinnitus, dry mouth, red sclera
GI: Nausea, vomiting, diarrhea, constipation, abdominal pain
GU: Urinary frequency, incontinence, impotence, priapism, water and sodium retention

Contraindications: Hypersensitivity

Precautions: Pregnancy **C**, breastfeeding, children, geriatric patients, renal/hepatic disease, prostate cancer, ocular surgery, orthostatic hypotension

Pharmacokinetics
Absorption	60%
Distribution	Widely distributed
Metabolism	Liver, extensively; protein binding 97%
Excretion	Kidneys, unchanged (10%); bile (90%)
Half-life	2-3 hr

Pharmacodynamics
Onset	2 hr
Peak	1-3 hr
Duration	6-12 hr

Interactions
Individual drugs
Alcohol, nitroglycerin, verapamil: increased hypotension
Clonidine: decreased antihypertensive effect
Drug classifications
Antihypertensives, β-adrenergic blockers: increased hypotension
NSAIDs, salicylates: decreased antihypertensive effect
Drug/herb
Aconite: increased toxicity, death
Astragalus, cola tree: increased or decreased antihypertensive effect
Barberry, betony, black catechu, black cohosh, bloodroot, broom, burdock, cat's claw, dandelion, goldenseal, hawthorn, Irish moss, Jamaican dogwood, kelp, khella, mistletoe, parsley: increased antihypertensive effect
Coltsfoot, guarana, khat, licorice, yohimbe: decreased antihypertensive effect
Drug/lab test
Increased: urinary norepinephrine, VMA

NURSING CONSIDERATIONS
Assessment
• Monitor B/P, orthostatic hypotension, syncope; check for edema in feet, legs daily; monitor I&O, weight daily; notify prescriber of changes
• Assess for allergic reactions: rash, fever, pruritus, urticaria; product should be discontinued if antihistamines fail to help
• Assess for orthostatic hypotension; tell patient to rise slowly from sitting or lying position

Nursing diagnoses
• Cardiac output, decreased (uses)
• Injury, risk for (adverse reactions)
• Knowledge, deficient (teaching)
• Noncompliance (teaching)

Implementation
• Severe hypotension may occur after first dose of this medication; hypotension may be prevented by reducing or discontinuing diuretic therapy 3 days before beginning prazosin therapy
• Give same time each day
• Store in airtight container at 86° F (30° C) or less

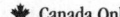 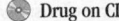

Patient/family education

• Instruct patient not to discontinue product abruptly; stress the importance of complying with dosage schedule, even if feeling better; if dose is missed, take as soon as remembered; take at same time each day

• Advise patient not to use OTC products (cough, cold, allergy) unless directed by prescriber; also to avoid large amounts of caffeine

• Emphasize the need to rise slowly to sitting or standing position to minimize orthostatic hypotension

• Teach patient to notify prescriber of mouth sores, sore throat, fever, swelling of hands or feet, irregular heartbeat, chest pain

• Caution patient to report excessive perspiration, dehydration, vomiting, diarrhea; may lead to fall in B/P

• Caution patient that product may cause dizziness, fainting, light-headedness; may occur during 1st few days of therapy; to avoid hazardous activities

• Teach patient how to take B/P and normal readings for age-group; instruct to take B/P q7day

Evaluation

Positive therapeutic outcome

• Decreased B/P in hypertension

Treatment of overdose: Administer volume expanders or vasopressors, discontinue product, place patient in supine position

---

*prednisoLONE (Rx)

(pred-niss'oh-lone)

Articulose-50, Delta-Cortef, Hydeltrasol, Hydeltra-T.B.A., Key-Pred 25, Key-Pred 50, Key-Pred SP, Orapred, Pediapred, Predaject-50, Predalone 50, Predalone-T.B.A., Predcor-25, Predcor-50, Prednisol TBA, prednisoLONE, PrednisoLONE Acetate, Prelone

Func. class.: Corticosteroid, synthetic
Chem. class.: Intermediate-acting glucocorticoid

Pregnancy category   C

Do not confuse:
prednisoLONE/predniSONE

Action: Decreases inflammation by suppressing migration of polymorphonuclear leukocytes, fibroblasts; reversal to increase capillary permeability and lysosomal stabilization, minimal mineralocorticoid

Therapeutic outcome: Decreased inflammation, decreased adrenal insufficiency

Uses: Severe inflammation, immunosuppression, neoplasms

Dosage and routes
Rheumatic disorders
Adult: PO 5-60 mg/day or in divided doses

Asthma/antiinflammatory
Adult: PO 40-80 mg/day in 1-2 divided doses
Child: PO 1 mg/kg/day in 2 divided doses

Available forms: Tabs 5 mg; syr 5 mg/5 ml, 15 mg/15 ml; oral liquid 5 mg/ml; tabs 1, 2.5, 5, 10, 20, 50 mg; oral sol 5 mg/ml, 5 mg/5 ml; syr 5 mg/5 ml; oral dissolving tab 10, 15, 30 mg

Adverse effects
CNS: Depression, flushing, sweating, headache, mood changes
CV: Hypertension, **circulatory collapse, thrombophlebitis, embolism,** tachycardia
EENT: Fungal infections, increased intraocular pressure, blurred vision
GI: Diarrhea, nausea, abdominal distention, **GI hemorrhage,** increased appetite, **pancreatitis**
HEMA: **Thrombocytopenia**
INTEG: Acne, poor wound healing, ecchymosis, petechiae
MS: Fractures, osteoporosis, weakness, arthralgia, myopathy, tendon rupture

Contraindications: Child <2 yr, psychosis, hypersensitivity, idiopathic thrombocytopenia, acute glomerulonephritis, amebiasis, fungal infections, nonasthmatic bronchial disease, measles, varicella, Cushing's syndrome

Precautions: Pregnancy **C**, breastfeeding, children, diabetes mellitus, glaucoma, osteoporosis, seizure disorders, ulcerative colitis, CHF, myasthenia gravis

Pharmacokinetics

Absorption	Well absorbed (PO, IM), completely absorbed (**IV**)
Distribution	Widely distributed, crosses placenta
Metabolism	Liver, extensively
Excretion	Kidney, breast milk
Half-life	2-4 hr

Pharmacodynamics

	PO	IM (phosphate)	IV	IA/IL
Onset	1 hr	Rapid	Rapid	Slow
Peak	2 hr	1 hr	Unknown	Unknown
Duration	1½ days	Unknown	Unknown	Up to 1 mo

P

Adverse effects: *italic* = common, **bold** = life-threatening

Interactions
Individual drugs
Alcohol, amphotericin B, cycloSPORINE, digitalis, indomethacin: increased side effects

Ambenonium, isoniazid, neostigmine, somatrem: decreased effects of each specific product

Cholestyramine, colestipol, ephedrine, phenytoin, rifampin, theophylline: decreased action of prednisoLONE

Indomethacin, ketoconazole: increased action of prednisoLONE

Drug classifications
Antibiotics (macrolide), contraceptives (oral), estrogens, salicylates: increased action of prednisoLONE

Anticholinesterases, anticoagulants, anticonvulsants, antidiabetics, salicylates, toxoids, vaccines: decreased effects of each specific product

Barbiturates: decreased action of prednisoLONE

Diuretics, salicylates: increased side effects
Drug/herb
Aloe, buckthorn, cascara sagrada, Chinese rhubarb, senna: increased hypokalemia

Aloe, licorice, perilla: increased effect
Drug/lab test
Increased: cholesterol, sodium, blood glucose, uric acid, calcium, urine glucose

Decreased: calcium, potassium, T_4, T_3, thyroid ^{131}I uptake test, urine 17-OHCS, 17-KS

False negative: skin allergy tests

NURSING CONSIDERATIONS
Assessment
• Monitor potassium, blood glucose, urine glucose while patient is on long-term therapy; hypokalemia and hyperglycemia may occur

• Monitor weight daily; notify prescriber of weekly gain >5 lb; monitor I&O ratio; be alert for decreasing urinary output and increasing edema

• Monitor B/P q4hr, pulse; notify prescriber if chest pain occurs

• Monitor plasma cortisol levels during long-term therapy (normal level 138-635 nmol/L [SI units] when measured at 8 AM)

• Assess adrenal function periodically for hypothalamic-pituitary-adrenal axis suppression

• Assess infection: increased temp, WBC even after withdrawal of medication; product masks infection symptoms

• Assess for potassium depletion: paresthesias, fatigue, nausea, vomiting, depression, polyuria, dysrhythmias, weakness, edema, hypertension, cardiac symptoms

• Assess mental status: affect, mood, behavioral changes, aggression

• Monitor temp; if fever develops, product should be discontinued

• Assess for systemic absorption: increased temp, inflammation, irritation (topical)

Nursing diagnoses
• Infection, risk for (adverse reactions)
• Knowledge, deficient (teaching)
• Noncompliance (teaching)

Implementation
• Oral sol: use calibrated measuring devices
• Orally disintegrating tabs: place on tongue, allow to dissolve, swallow; or swallow whole; do not cut, split

Patient/family education
• Advise patient to carry/wear emergency ID as steroid user

• Advise patient to notify prescriber if therapeutic response decreases; dosage adjustment may be needed

• Caution patient not to discontinue abruptly; adrenal crisis can result; take exactly as prescribed

• Caution patient to avoid OTC products: salicylates, cough products with alcohol, cold preparations unless directed by prescriber

• Teach patient all aspects of product usage including cushingoid symptoms

• Teach patient symptoms of adrenal insufficiency: nausea, anorexia, fatigue, dizziness, dyspnea, weakness, joint pain

• Advise patient that long-term therapy may be needed to clear infection (1-2 mo depending on type of infection)

Evaluation
Positive therapeutic outcome
• Decreased inflammation

---

*prednisoLONE ophthalmic
See Appendix B

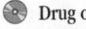

*predniSONE 😊 (Rx)
(pred'ni-sone)
Func. class.: Corticosteroid
Chem. class.: Intermediate-acting glucocorticoid

Pregnancy category C

Do not confuse:
predniSONE/methylPREDNISolone/
prednisoLONE/Prilosec

Action: Decreases inflammation by suppressing migration of polymorphonuclear leukocytes, fibroblasts; reversal to increase capillary permeability and lysosomal stabilization, minimal mineralocorticoid activity

Therapeutic outcome: Decreased inflammation, decreased adrenal insufficiency

Uses: Severe inflammation, immunosuppression, neoplasms, multiple sclerosis, collagen disorders, dermatologic disorders

Dosage and routes
Adult: PO 5-60 mg/day or divided bid-qid
Child: PO 0.05-2 mg/kg/day divided 1-4 ×/day

Nephrosis
Child: PO 2 mg/kg/day in divided doses, max 28 days, then 1-1.5 mg/kg/day every other day × 4 wk

Multiple sclerosis
Adult: PO 200 mg/day × 1 wk, then 80 mg every other day × 1 mo

Available forms: Tabs 1, 2.5, 5, 10, 20, 50 mg; oral sol 5 mg/5 ml; syr 5 mg/5 ml

Adverse effects
CNS: Depression, flushing, sweating, headache, mood changes
CV: Hypertension, **circulatory collapse, thrombophlebitis, embolism,** tachycardia
EENT: Fungal infections, increased intraocular pressure, blurred vision
GI: Diarrhea, nausea, abdominal distention, **GI hemorrhage,** increased appetite, **pancreatitis**
HEMA: **Thrombocytopenia**
INTEG: Acne, poor wound healing, ecchymosis, petechiae
META: Hyperglycemia
MS: Fractures, osteoporosis, weakness

Contraindications: Psychosis, hypersensitivity, idiopathic thrombocytopenia, acute glomerulonephritis, amebiasis, fungal infections, nonasthmatic bronchial disease, child <2 yr, AIDS, TB, measles

Precautions: Pregnancy **C,** diabetes mellitus, glaucoma, osteoporosis, seizure disorders, ulcerative colitis, CHF, myasthenia gravis, renal disease, esophagitis, peptic ulcer, cataracts, coagulopathy

Pharmacokinetics
Absorption	Well absorbed
Distribution	Widely distributed, crosses placenta
Metabolism	Liver, extensively
Excretion	Kidney, breast milk
Half-life	3-4 hr

Pharmacodynamics
Onset	Unknown
Peak	1-2 hr
Duration	1½ days

Interactions
Individual drugs
Alcohol, amphotericin B, cycloSPORINE, digoxin: increased side effects
Ambenonium, isoniazid, neostigmine, sometrem: decreased effects of each specific product
Cholestyramine, colestipol, ephedrine, phenytoin, rifampin, theophylline: decreased action of predniSONE
Indomethacin: increased side effects, increased action of predniSONE
Ketoconazole: increased action of predniSONE
Drug classifications
Anticholinesterases, anticoagulants, anticonvulsants, antidiabetics, toxoids, vaccines: decreased effects of each specific product
Antiinfectives (macrolide), contraceptives (oral), estrogens: increased action of predniSONE
Barbiturates: decreased action of predniSONE
Diuretics: increased side effects
Salicylates: increased side effects, increased action of predniSONE, decreased effects of salicylates
Drug/herb
Aloe, buckthorn, Chinese rhubarb, senna: increased hypokalemia
Aloe, licorice, perilla: increased effect
Ephedra (Ma huang): decreased predniSONE effect
Drug/lab test
Increased: cholesterol, sodium, blood glucose, uric acid, calcium, urine glucose
Decreased: calcium, potassium, T_4, T_3, thyroid ^{131}I uptake test, urine 17-OHCS, 17-KS, PBI
False negative: skin allergy tests

P

Adverse effects: *italic* = common, **bold** = life-threatening

NURSING CONSIDERATIONS
Assessment
- Monitor potassium, blood glucose, urine glucose while on long-term therapy; hypokalemia and hyperglycemia may occur
- Monitor weight daily; notify prescriber of weekly gain >5 lb; monitor I&O ratio; be alert for decreasing urinary output and increasing edema
- Monitor B/P q4hr, pulse; notify prescriber if chest pain occurs
- Monitor plasma cortisol levels during long-term therapy (normal level 138-635 nmol/L when measured at 8 AM)
- Assess adrenal function periodically for hypothalamic-pituitary-adrenal axis suppression
- Assess infection: increased temp, WBC even after withdrawal of medication; product masks infection symptoms
- Assess for potassium depletion: paresthesias, fatigue, nausea, vomiting, depression, polyuria, dysrhythmias, weakness, edema, hypertension, cardiac symptoms
- Assess mental status: affect, mood, behavioral changes, aggression
- Monitor temp; if fever develops, product should be discontinued
- Assess for systemic absorption: increased temp, inflammation, irritation (topical)

Nursing diagnoses
- Infection, risk for (adverse reactions)
- Knowledge, deficient (teaching)
- Noncompliance (teaching)

Implementation
- Give with food or milk to decrease GI symptoms; use measuring device for liquid route
- For long-term use, alternative product therapy is recommended, to decrease adverse reactions

Patient/family education
- Advise patient that emergency ID as corticosteroid user should be carried or worn
- Advise patient to notify prescriber if therapeutic response decreases; dosage adjustment may be needed
- ⚠ Caution patient not to discontinue abruptly; adrenal crisis can result
- Caution patient to avoid OTC products: salicylates, cough products with alcohol, cold preparations unless directed by prescriber
- Teach patient all aspects of product usage including cushingoid symptoms
- Teach patient symptoms of adrenal insufficiency: nausea, anorexia, fatigue, dizziness, dyspnea, weakness, joint pain
- Advise patient that long-term therapy may be needed to clear infection (1-2 mo depending on type of infection)

Evaluation
Positive therapeutic outcome
- Decreased inflammation

pregabalin (Rx)
(pre-gab′a-lin)
Lyrica
Func. class.: Anticonvulsant

Pregnancy category C

Controlled substance schedule V

Action: Binds to high-voltage–gated calcium channels in CNS tissues; this may lead to anticonvulsant action, similar to the inhibitory neurotransmitter GABA, anxiolytic, analgesics, and antiepileptic properties

Therapeutic outcome: Decreased seizure activity, decreased neuropathic pain

Uses: Neuropathic pain associated with diabetic peripheral neuropathy, partial onset seizures, postherpetic neuralgia, fibromyalgia

Unlabeled uses: Generalized anxiety disorder (GAD), moderate pain, social anxiety disorder

Dosage and routes
Diabetic peripheral neuropathic pain
Adult: PO 50 mg tid, may increase to 300 mg/day (max) within 1 wk, adjust in renal disease

Partial onset seizures
Adult: PO 75 mg bid or 50 mg tid; may increase to 600 mg/day (max)

Postherpetic neuralgia
Adult: 150 mg/day in 2-3 doses, may increase to 300 mg/day in 2-3 divided doses, if higher dose is needed in 2-4 wk, may increase to 600 mg/day in 2-3 divided doses

Fibromyalgia
Adult: PO 75 mg bid, may increase to 150 mg bid within 1 wk and 225 mg bid after 1 wk

Renal dose
PO CCr 30-60 ml/min 75-300 mg/day in 2-3 divided doses; CCr 15-30 ml/min 25-150 mg/day in 1-2 divided doses, CCr <15 ml/min 25-75 mg/day in a single dose

Available forms: Caps 25, 50, 75, 100, 150, 200, 225, 300 mg

 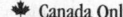

Adverse effects

CNS: Dizziness, fatigue, confusion, euphoria, incoordination, nervousness, neuropathy, tremor, vertigo, somnolence, ataxia, amnesia, abnormal thinking
EENT: Dry mouth, blurred vision, nystagmus, amblyopia, sinusitis
GI: Constipation, flatulence, abdominal pain, weight gain
HEMA: Ecchymosis, **thrombocytopenia**
MS: Back pain, **rhabdomyolysis**, myopathy
MISC: Pruritus, impotence, peripheral edema, **angioedema, suicidal ideation**
RESP: Dyspnea

Contraindications: Hypersensitivity, abrupt discontinuation

Precautions: Pregnancy **C,** breastfeeding, children <12 yr, geriatric, renal disease, PR interval prolongation, creatine kinase elevations, CHF (class III, IV), decreased platelets, drug abuse, dependence, glaucoma, myopathy, angioedema history, suicidal behavior

Pharmacokinetics

Absorption	Well, decreased by food
Distribution	Not bound to plasma proteins
Metabolism	Negligible
Excretion	90% unchanged, urine
Half-life	6 hr

Pharmacodynamics

Onset	Unknown
Peak	1.5 hr
Duration	Unknown

Interactions
Individual drugs
Alcohol: increased CNS depression
Drug classifications
Anxiolytics, barbiturates, general anesthetics, hypnotics, opiate agonists, phenothiazines, sedating H₁ blockers, sedatives, thiazolidinediones, tricyclics: increased CNS depression
Thiazolidinediones: increased weight gain/fluid retention; avoid use if possible
Drug/herb
Gotu kola, kava, St. John's wort, valerian: increased CNS depression
Drug/lab test
Increased: creatine kinase
Decreased: platelets

NURSING CONSIDERATIONS
Assessment
• Assess for seizures: aura, location, duration, activity at onset
• Assess for pain: location, duration, characteristics if using for diabetic neuropathy
• Monitor renal function tests: urinalysis, BUN, urine creatinine q3mo, creatine kinase; if markedly increased, discontinue
• Assess mental status: mood, sensorium, affect, behavioral changes; if mental status changes, notify prescriber

Nursing diagnoses
• Knowledge, deficient (teaching)
• Pain, chronic (uses)

Implementation
• Do not crush or chew caps; caps may be opened and contents put in applesauce or dissolved in juice
• Give without regard to meals
• Gradually withdraw over 7 days; abrupt withdrawal may precipitate seizures
• Store at room temperature away from heat and light
• Give hard candy, frequent rinsing of mouth, gum for dry mouth
• Provide assistance with ambulation during early part of treatment; dizziness occurs
• Provide seizure precautions: padded side rails; move objects that may harm patient
• Provide increased fluids, bulk in diet for constipation

Patient/family education
• Advise patient to carry emergency ID stating patient's name, products taken, condition, prescriber's name and phone number
• Advise patient to avoid driving, other activities that require alertness: dizziness, drowsiness may occur
• Teach patient not to discontinue medication quickly after long-term use, taper over ≥1 wk; withdrawal-precipitated seizures may occur, not to double doses if dose is missed, take if 2 hr or more before next dose
• Teach patient to notify prescriber if pregnancy planned or suspected; avoid breastfeeding
• Teach patient to report muscle pain, tenderness, weakness, when accompanied by fever, malaise
• Advise patient to avoid alcohol

Evaluation
Positive therapeutic outcome
• Decreased seizure activity; decrease in neuropathic pain

Treatment of overdose: Lavage, VS, hemodialysis

P

primidone (Rx)
(pri'mi-done)

Apo-Primidone ✤, Mysoline, PMS-Primidone ✤, primidone, Sertan ✤
Func. class.: Anticonvulsant
Chem. class.: Barbiturate derivative

Pregnancy category D

Action: Raises seizure threshold by conversion of product to phenobarbital; decreases neuron firing

Therapeutic outcome: Reduction in seizure activity

Uses: Generalized tonic-clonic (grand mal), complex

Dosage and routes
Adult and child >8 yr: PO 125-250 mg at bedtime, increase by 125-250 mg/day q3-7day, usual dose 750-1500 mg/day in 3-4 divided doses, max 2 g/day in divided doses
Child <8 yr: PO 50-125 mg at bedtime, increase by 50-125 mg/day q3-7day, usual dose 10-25 mg/kg/day in 3-4 divided doses
Neonate: PO 12-20 mg/kg/day in 2-4 divided doses, start at lower dose and titrate

Renal dose
Adult: CCr 10-15 ml/min increase interval between doses to 8-12 hr, CCr <10 ml/min increase interval to 12-24 hr

Available forms: Tabs 50, 250 mg; susp 250 mg/5 ml ✤; chew tabs 125 mg ✤

Adverse effects
CNS: Stimulation, drowsiness, irritability, fatigue, emotional disturbances, mood changes, paranoia, psychosis, ataxia, *vertigo,* **suicidal ideation**
EENT: Diplopia, nystagmus, edema of eyelids
GI: Nausea, vomiting, anorexia, **hepatitis**
GU: Impotence
HEMA: **Thrombocytopenia, leukopenia, neutropenia, eosinophilia, megaloblastic anemia,** decreased serum folate level, lymphadenopathy
INTEG: Rash, edema, alopecia, lupus-like syndrome

Contraindications: Pregnancy **D**, hypersensitivity, porphyria, hepatic encephalopathy, breastfeeding

Precautions: COPD, renal/hepatic disease, hyperactive children, suicidal ideation/behavior

Pharmacokinetics
Absorption	60%-80%
Distribution	Widely distributed, crosses placenta
Metabolism	Liver, converted to phenobarbital + PEMA
Excretion	Kidneys, breast milk
Half-life	3-12 hr

Pharmacodynamics
Onset	Unknown
Peak	4 hr
Duration	Unknown

Interactions
Individual drugs
Acebutolol, lamotrigine, metoprolol, propranolol: decreased effectiveness
Acetazolamide, carbamazepine: decreased primidone levels
Alcohol, heparin, isoniazid, nicotinamide, phenobarbital, phenytoin: increased primidone levels
Drug classifications
Antidepressants (tricyclic), oral contraceptives, phenothiazines: decreased effectiveness
CNS depressants: increased primidone levels
CYP3A4 inducers (barbiturates, carbamazepine, efavirenz, nevirapine), phenytoins: decreased primidone effect
CYP3A4 inhibitors (aprepitant, antiretroviral protease inhibitors, delavirdine, fluconazole, imatinib, voriconazole): increased toxicity
Succinimides: decreased primidone levels
Drug/herb
Ginkgo: increased effect
Ginseng, santonica: decreased effect
Kava, St. John's wort, valerian: avoid use

NURSING CONSIDERATIONS
Assessment
• Assess mental status: mood, sensorium, affect, memory (long, short), especially geriatric; suicidal thoughts/behaviors
• Assess for blood dyscrasias: fever, sore throat, bruising, rash, jaundice, epistaxis (long-term treatment only)
• Assess seizure activity including type, location, duration, and character; provide seizure precaution
• Assess renal function tests: urinalysis, BUN, urine creatinine
• Monitor blood studies: RBC, Hct, Hgb, reticulocyte counts weekly for 4 wk then monthly
• Monitor liver function tests: ALT, AST, bilirubin, creatinine

- Monitor product levels during initial treatment: therapeutic level 5-15 mcg/ml; CBC, LFTs should be done q6mo
- Assess for signs of physical withdrawal if medication is suddenly discontinued
- Assess eye problems: need for ophth exam before, during, after treatment (slit lamp, funduscopy, tonometry)
- Assess allergic reaction: red raised rash; if this occurs, product should be discontinued
- Monitor for toxicity: bone marrow depression, nausea, vomiting, ataxia, diplopia, CV collapse

Nursing diagnoses
- Injury, risk for (side effects)
- Knowledge, deficient (teaching)

Implementation
- May give with food to decrease gastric irritation
- May crush tab and mix with food or fluid

Patient/family education
- Teach patient to carry/wear emergency ID stating name, products taken, condition, prescriber's name, phone number
- Advise patient to avoid driving and other activities that require alertness
- Caution patient to avoid alcohol and CNS depressants, increased sedation may occur
- Teach patient not to discontinue medication quickly after long-term use; taper off over several wk

Evaluation
Positive therapeutic outcome
- Decreased seizure activity

---

probenecid (Rx)
(proe-ben′e-sid)
Benuryl ✦, probenecid
Func. class.: Uricosuric; antigout
Chem. class.: Sulfonamide derivative

Pregnancy category B

Action: Inhibits tubular reabsorption of urates, with increased excretion of uric acids

Therapeutic outcome: Decreased uric acid levels

Uses: Hyperuricemia in gout, gouty arthritis; adjunct to cephalosporin, cidofovir, or penicillin treatment (gonorrhea)

Dosage and routes
Gonorrhea
Adult: PO 1 g with 3.5 g of ampicillin or 1 g 30 min before 4.8 million units of aqueous penicillin G procaine injected into 2 sites IM

Gout/gouty arthritis
Adult: PO 250 mg bid for 1 wk, then 500 mg bid; max 2 g/day; maintenance 500 mg/day × 6 mo

Adjunct in penicillin/cephalosporin treatment
Adult and child >50 kg: PO 500 mg qid
Child <50 kg: PO 25 mg/kg, then 40 mg/kg in divided doses qid

Minimize toxicity in cidofovir therapy
Adult: PO 2 g 3 hr prior to cidofovir dose, followed by 1 g at 2 and 8 hr after end of cidofovir inf

Renal dose
Adult: PO CCr <50 ml/min avoid use

Available forms: Tabs 0.5 g

Adverse effects
CNS: Drowsiness, headache
CV: Bradycardia
GI: Gastric irritation, nausea, vomiting, anorexia, **hepatic necrosis**
GU: Glycosuria, thirst, frequency, **nephrotic syndrome**
INTEG: Rash, dermatitis, pruritus, fever
META: Acidosis, hypokalemia, hyperchloremia, hyperglycemia
RESP: **Apnea,** irregular respirations

Contraindications: Hypersensitivity, severe renal/hepatic disease, CCr <50 mg/min, history of uric acid calculus

Precautions: Pregnancy **B,** children <2 yr, sulfonamide hypersensitivity

P

Pharmacokinetics	
Absorption	Well absorbed
Distribution	Crosses placenta
Metabolism	Liver
Excretion	Kidneys
Half-life	5-8 hr

Pharmacodynamics	
Onset	½ hr
Peak	2-4 hr
Duration	8 hr

Interactions
Individual drugs
Acyclovir, allopurinol, dyphylline, zidovudine: increased effect
Clofibrate, dapsone, indomethacin, methotrexate, naproxen, rifampin: increased toxicity

Adverse effects: *italic* = common, **bold** = life-threatening

Drug classifications
Barbiturates, benzodiazepines: increased effect
Salicylates: decreased action of probenecid
Sulfa products: increased toxicity

Drug/lab test
Increased: BSP/urinary PSP, theophylline levels
False positive: urine glucose with copper sulfate test (Clinitest)

NURSING CONSIDERATIONS
Assessment
• Monitor I&O ratio; observe for decrease in urinary output; increase fluids to 2-3 L/day; urine may be alkalized with sodium bicarbonate acetaZOLAMIDE
• Assess mobility, joint pain, and swelling in the joints
• Monitor CBC, urine pH, uric acid and BUN, creatinine before, periodically during treatment

Nursing diagnoses
• Knowledge, deficient (teaching)
• Mobility, impaired physical (uses)
• Pain, chronic (uses)

Implementation
• Give with food or antacid to decrease GI upset
• Reduce dosage gradually if uric acid levels are normal after 6 mo

Patient/family education
• Advise patient to increase fluids to 2-3 L/day, avoid caffeine, alcohol
• Caution patient to avoid salicylates; probenecid levels will be decreased
• Advise patient to report any pain, redness, or hard area, usually in legs
• Instruct patient on importance of complying with medical regimen including weight loss program, diet restrictions, and alcohol intake

Evaluation
Positive therapeutic outcome
• Decreased pain in joints
• Normal serum uric acid levels
• Increased duration of antiinfectives

---

procainamide 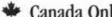 **(Rx)**
(proe'kane-ah-mide)
Func. class.: Antidysrhythmic (class IA)
Chem. class.: Procaine HCl amide analog
Pregnancy category C

Action: Depresses excitability of cardiac muscle to electrical stimulation and slows conduction in atrium, bundle of His, and ventricle; increases refractory period

Therapeutic outcome: Prevention of dysrhythmias

Uses: Life-threatening ventricular dysrhythmias

Dosage and routes
Atrial fibrillation/PAT
Adult: PO 1-1.25 g; may give another 750 mg if needed; if no response, 500 mg-1g q2hr until desired response; maintenance 50 mg/kg in divided doses q6hr

Ventricular tachycardia
Adult: PO 1 g; maintenance 50 mg/kg/day given in 3-hr intervals

Other dysrhythmias
Adult: **IV** BOL 100 mg q5min, given 25-50 mg/min, max 500 mg; or 17 mg/kg total, then **IV** INF 2-6 mg/min

Renal dose
Adult: **IV** CCr 35-59 ml/min give 70% of maintenance dose; CCr 15-34 ml/min give 40%-60% maintenance dose; CCr <15 ml/min individualized

Available forms: Caps 250, 375, 500 mg; tabs 250, 500 mg; inj **IV** 100, 500 mg/ml

Adverse effects
CNS: *Headache, dizziness,* confusion, psychosis, restlessness, irritability, weakness, depression
CV: *Hypotension,* **heart block, cardiovascular collapse, arrest**
GI: Nausea, vomiting, anorexia, diarrhea, hepatomegaly, pain, bitter taste
HEMA: Systemic lupus erythematosus syndrome, **agranulocytosis, thrombocytopenia, neutropenia, hemolytic anemia**
INTEG: Rash, urticaria, edema, swelling (rare), pruritus, flushing, **angioedema**
SYST: SLE

Contraindications: Hypersensitivity, severe heart block, torsades de pointes

Black Box Warning: Lupus erythromatosis

Precautions: Pregnancy C, breastfeeding, children, renal/hepatic disease, CHF, respiratory depression, cytopenia, dysrhythmia associated with digoxin toxicity, myasthenia gravis, digoxin toxicity

Black Box Warning: Bone marrow failure, cardiac arrhythmias

Pharmacokinetics

Absorption	Well absorbed
Distribution	Rapidly distributed
Metabolism	Liver
Excretion	Kidneys, unchanged (50%-70%)
Half-life	2½-4½ hr; increased in renal disease

 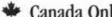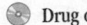

Pharmacodynamics

	PO	PO-EXT REL	IV
Onset	½ hr	Unknown	Rapid
Peak	1-1½ hr	Unknown	½-1 hr
Duration	3 hr	Up to 8 hr	3-4 hr

Interactions
Individual drugs
Cimetidine, quinidine, ranitidine, trimethoprim: increased procainamide effect
Thioridazine: increased toxicity
Drug classifications
Antidysrhythmics, quinolones: increased toxicity
β-Adrenergic blockers: increased procainamide effects
Neuromuscular blockers: increased neuromuscular blocking effect
Drug/herb
Aconite: increased toxicity, death
Aloe, broom, buckthorn (chronic use), cascara sagrada (chronic use), Chinese rhubarb, figwort, fumitory, goldenseal, kudzu, licorice: increased effect
Coltsfoot: decreased effect
Henbane: increased anticholinergic effect
Horehound: increased serotonin effect
Drug/lab test
Increased: ALT, AST, alkaline phosphatase, LDH, bilirubin

NURSING CONSIDERATIONS
Assessment
• Assess for oxygenation or perfusion deficit: decreased B/P, chest pain, dizziness, loss of consciousness
• Assess respiratory status: auscultate lung fields for bibasilar crackles in patients with advanced CHF
• Monitor I&O ratio; electrolytes: potassium, sodium, chloride; watch for decreasing urinary output, possible retention
• Monitor liver function tests: AST, ALT, bilirubin, alkaline phosphatase
◆ Monitor ECG continuously to determine product effectiveness; measure PR, QRS, QT intervals; check for PVCs, other dysrhythmias; check B/P continuously for hypo/hypertension; for rebound hypertension after 1-2 hr; prolonged PR/QT intervals, QRS complex; if QT or QRS increases by 50% or more, withhold next dose, notify prescriber
• Monitor ANA titer; during long-term treatment, watch for lupuslike symptoms
• Monitor for dehydration or hypovolemia
◆ Monitor for CNS symptoms: confusion, seizures, psychosis, numbness, depression, involuntary movements; if these occur, product should be discontinued
• Monitor blood levels (therapeutic level 3-10 mcg/ml), ANA titer or *N*-acetylprocainamide levels 10-20 mcg/ml; notify prescriber of abnormal results; assess for toxicity: confusion, drowsiness, nausea, vomiting, tachydysrhythmias, oliguria
• Assess cardiac rate, respiration: rate, rhythm, character, chest pain, ventricular tachycardia, supraventricular tachycardia or fibrillation

Nursing diagnoses
• Cardiac output, decreased (uses)
• Gas exchange, impaired (adverse reactions)
• Knowledge, deficient (teaching)

Implementation
PO route
• Do not break, crush, or chew sus rel tab
• Give on an empty stomach with a full glass of water
• May be given with meals if GI irritation occurs; absorption will be decreased
• Tab may be crushed and mixed with fluid or foods for patients with swallowing difficulties
IV route
• Give by direct **IV** after diluting 100 mg/10 ml of D₅W or sterile water for inj; give 50 mg/min or less
• Give by intermittent inf after diluting to a conc of 2-4 mg/ml, 200 mg up to 1 g/50-500 ml of D₅W; give over 30 min (2-6 mg/min maintenance); use inf pump for correct dosage
• Do not use if sol is dark or if precipitate is present
Y-site compatibilities: Amiodarone, famotidine, heparin, hydrocortisone, potassium chloride, ranitidine, vit B/C
Y-site incompatibilities: Milrinone
Additive compatibilities: Amiodarone, DOBUTamine, flumazenil, lidocaine, netilmicin, verapamil
Additive incompatibilities: Esmolol, ethacrynate, milrinone
Solution compatibilities: D₅W, D₅/0.9% NaCl, 0.45% NaCl, 0.9% NaCl, water for inj

Patient/family education
• Advise patient to report side effects immediately to prescriber; to take exactly as prescribed; if dose is missed take when remembered if within 3-4 hr of next dose, do not double doses
• Caution patient that dark glasses may be needed for photophobia; to use sunscreen or stay out of sun to prevent burns; avoid temper-

ature extremes; impairment of heat-regulating mechanism can occur
- Advise patient to complete follow-up appointment with prescriber, including pulmonary function tests, chest x-ray
- Instruct patient that dry mouth may be relieved by frequent sips of water, hard candy, sugarless gum
- Caution patient to make position changes from lying to standing slowly to prevent orthostatic hypotension
◆ Advise prescriber immediately if lupuslike symptoms (joint pain, butterfly rash, fever, chills, dyspnea), leukopenia symptoms (sore mouth, gums, throat), or thrombocytopenia symptoms (bleeding, bruising) occur
- Teach patient how to take pulse and when to report to prescriber

Evaluation
Positive therapeutic outcome
- Decreased PVCs, ventricular tachycardia

Treatment of overdose: O_2, artificial ventilation, ECG, administer DOPamine for circulatory depression, diazepam or thiopental for seizures, isoproterenol

---

procarbazine (Rx)
(proe-kar′ba-zeen)
Matulane, Natulan ✤
Func. class.: Antineoplastic, alkylating agent
Chem. class.: Hydrazine derivative
Pregnancy category D

Action: Inhibits DNA, RNA, protein synthesis, cell cycle S phase specific; has multiple sites of action; a nonvesicant

Therapeutic outcome: Prevention of rapidly growing malignant cells

Uses: Lymphoma, Hodgkin's disease, cancers resistant to other therapy

Unlabeled uses: Brain, lung malignancies, other lymphomas, multiple myeloma, malignant melanoma, polycythemia vera

Dosage and routes
Adult: PO 2-4 mg/kg/day for first wk; maintain dosage of 4-6 mg/kg/day until platelets and WBC fall; after recovery, 1-2 mg/kg/day
Child: PO 50 mg/m^2/day for 7 days, then 100 mg/m^2 until desired response, leukopenia, or thrombocytopenia occurs; 50 mg/m^2/day is maintenance after bone marrow recovery

Available forms: Caps 50 mg

Adverse effects
CNS: Headache, dizziness, **seizures,** insomnia, hallucinations, confusion, **coma,** pain, chills, fever, sweating, paresthesias, peripheral neuropathy
EENT: Retinal hemorrhage, nystagmus, photophobia, diplopia, dry eyes
GI: Nausea, vomiting, anorexia, diarrhea, constipation, dry mouth, stomatitis, elevated hepatic enzymes
GU: Azoospermia, cessation of menses
HEMA: **Thrombocytopenia, anemia, leukopenia, myelosuppression, bleeding tendencies,** purpura, petechiae, epistaxis, **hemolysis**
INTEG: Rash, pruritus, dermatitis, alopecia, herpes, hyperpigmentation
MS: Arthralgias, myalgias
RESP: Cough, pneumonitis
SYST: **Secondary malignancy**

Contraindications: Pregnancy **D**, breastfeeding, hypersensitivity, thrombocytopenia, bone marrow depression

Precautions: Cardiac/renal/hepatic disease, radiation therapy, seizure disorder, anemia

Pharmacokinetics
Absorption	Well absorbed
Distribution	Widely distributed, crosses blood-brain barrier
Metabolism	Liver
Excretion	Kidneys
Half-life	1 hr

Pharmacodynamics
Unknown

Interactions
Individual drugs
Alcohol: increased CNS depression, disulfiram-like reaction
Caffeine, guanethidine, levodopa, methyldopa, reserpine: increased hypertension
Meperidine: hypotension; do not use together
Drug classifications
Anticoagulants, NSAIDs, platelet inhibitors, thrombolytics: increased bleeding risk
Antidepressants (tricyclics), MAOIs: disulfiram-like reaction
Antihistamines, barbiturates, hypotensive agents, opiates, phenothiazines: increased CNS depression
Selective serotonin reuptake inhibitors: confusion, seizures, hypertension
Sympathomimetics: disulfiram-like reaction, life-threatening hypertensive crisis

---

Drug/food
Tyramine-containing foods: increased disulfiram-like reaction, hypertensive crisis

NURSING CONSIDERATIONS
Assessment
- Monitor CBC, differential, platelet count weekly; withhold product if WBC is <4000/mm^3 or platelet count is <75,000/mm^3; notify prescriber of results if WBC <20,000/mm^3, platelets <150,000/mm^3
- Monitor pulmonary function tests, chest x-ray films before, during therapy; chest film should be obtained q2wk during treatment; check for dyspnea, crackles, unproductive cough, chest pain, tachypnea
- Monitor renal function tests: BUN, serum uric acid, urine CCr before, during therapy; I&O ratio; report fall in urine output of 30 ml/hr; check for decreased hyperuricemia
- Monitor hepatic studies before, during therapy: bilirubin, AST, ALT, ALK phos, LDH, PRN or qmo
- Monitor for cold, fever, sore throat (may indicate beginning of infection); identify edema in feet, joint and stomach pain, shaking; prescriber should be notified
- Assess for bleeding: hematuria, guaiac, bruising or petechiae, mucosa or orifices; no rectal temp
- Assess for tyramine-containing foods in the diet; hypertensive crisis can occur

Nursing diagnoses
- Body image, disturbed (adverse reactions)
- Infection, risk for (adverse reactions)
- Injury, risk for (adverse reactions)
- Knowledge, deficient (teaching)

Implementation
- Give with foods, fluids for GI upset; open cap and give with food/fluids for swallowing difficulty; administer as directed

Patient/family education
- Teach patient to avoid use of products containing aspirin or NSAIDs, razors, commercial mouthwash, since bleeding may occur; to report symptoms of bleeding (hematuria, tarry stools)
- Caution patient to report signs of anemia (fatigue, headache, irritability, faintness, shortness of breath); CNS changes, diarrhea
- Advise patient to report any changes in breathing or coughing even several mo after treatment; to avoid crowds and persons with respiratory tract or other infections
- Inform patient hair loss is common; discuss the use of wigs or hairpieces
- Caution patient not to have any vaccinations without the advice of the prescriber; serious reactions can occur
- Advise patient that contraception is needed during treatment and for several mo after the completion of therapy; may cause infertility; avoid breastfeeding
- Teach patient to avoid sunlight, UV exposure; wear sunscreen or protective clothing

Evaluation
Positive therapeutic outcome
- Absence of swelling at night
- Increased appetite, increased weight
- Decreasing malignancy

prochlorperazine (Rx)
(proe-klor-pair′a-zeen)
Compro
Func. class.: Antiemetic/antipsychotic
Chem. class.: Phenothiazine, piperazine derivative

Pregnancy category C

Do not confuse:
prochlorperazine/chlorproMAZINE, Compazine/Coumadin

Action: Depresses cerebral cortex, hypothalamus, limbic system, which control activity aggression; blocks neurotransmission produced by DOPamine at synapse; exhibits a strong α-adrenergic, anticholinergic blocking action; mechanism for antipsychotic effects is unclear; acts centrally by blocking chemoreceptor trigger zone, which in turn acts on vomiting center

Therapeutic outcome: Decreased nausea, vomiting, decreased signs and symptoms of psychosis

Uses: Nausea, vomiting, psychosis

Dosage and routes
Postoperative nausea/vomiting
Adult: IM 5-10 mg 1-2 hr before anesthesia; may repeat in 30 min; **IV** 5-10 mg 15-30 min before anesthesia; **IV** INF 20 mg/L D$_5$W or 0.9% NaCl 15-30 min before anesthesia, max 40 mg/day

Severe nausea/vomiting
Adult: PO 5-10 mg tid-qid; SUS REL 15 mg/day in AM or 10 mg q12hr; RECT 25 mg/bid; IM 5-10 mg; may repeat q3-4hr prn, max 40 mg/day

P

Adverse effects: *italic* = common, **bold** = life-threatening

Child 18-39 kg: PO 2.5 mg tid or 5 mg bid; IM 0.132 mg/kg, q3-4hr prn, max 15 mg/day

Child 14-17 kg: PO/RECT 2.5 mg bid-tid; IM 0.132 mg/kg, q3-4hr prn, max 10 mg/day

Child 9-13 kg: PO/RECT 2.5 mg daily-bid; IM 0.132 mg/kg, q3-4hr prn, max 7.5 mg/day

Antipsychotic

Adult and child ≥12 yr: PO 5-10 mg tid-qid; may increase q2-3day, max 150 mg/day; IM 10-20 mg q2-4hr up to 4 doses, then 10-20 mg q4-6hr, max 200 mg/day; RECT 10 mg tid-qid may increase by 5-10 mg q2-3day as needed

Child 2-12 yr: PO 2.5 mg bid-tid; IM 0.132 mg/kg

Antianxiety

Adult and child ≥12 yr: PO 5 mg tid-qid, max 20 mg/day or >12 wk; IM 5-10 mg q3-4hr, max 40 mg/day; **IV** 2.5-10 mg; max 40 mg/day

Child 2-12 yr: IM 132 mcg/kg

Available forms: Syr 5 mg/ml; inj 5 mg/ml; tabs 5, 10, 25 mg; sus rel caps 10, 15 mg; supp 2.5, 5, 25 mg

Adverse effects

CNS: Tardive dyskinesia, *euphoria,* **depression, EPS,** restlessness, tremor, dizziness, **neuroleptic malignant syndrome,** drowsiness, headache

CV: **Circulatory failure, tachycardia,** hypotension, ECG changes

EENT: Blurred vision

GI: Nausea, vomiting, anorexia, dry mouth, diarrhea, constipation, weight loss, metallic taste, cramps

HEMA: **Agranulocytosis**

MISC: Impotence

RESP: **Respiratory depression**

Contraindications: Hypersensitivity to phenothiazines, coma, infants/neonates/child <2 yr, surgery

Precautions: Pregnancy **C**, breastfeeding, geriatric, seizure, encephalopathy, hepatic disease, Parkinson's disease, BPH

Black Box Warning: Dementia

Pharmacokinetics

Absorption	Variably absorbed (PO); well absorbed (IM)
Distribution	Widely distributed, high concentration in CNS, crosses placenta
Metabolism	Liver, extensively; GI mucosa
Excretion	Kidneys, breast milk
Half-life	Unknown

Pharmacodynamics

	PO	PO-SUS REL	RECT	IM	IV
Onset	½ hr	½ hr	1 hr	10-20 min	4-5 min
Peak	Unkn	Unkn	Unkn	Unkn	Unkn
Duration	3-4 hr	10-12 hr	3-4 hr	3-4 hr	3-4 hr

Interactions

Drug classifications

Antacids, barbiturates: decreased prochlorperazine effect

Anticholinergics, antidepressants, antiparkinson products: increased anticholinergic effects

CNS depressants: increased CNS depression

Drug/herb

Betel palm, kava: increased EPS

Chamomile, cola nut, hops, kava, nettle, nutmeg, St. John's wort, skullcap, valerian: increased CNS depression

Dong quai: avoid use

Henbane, jimsonweed, scopolia: increased anticholinergic effect

Drug/lab test

Increased: liver function tests, cardiac enzymes, cholesterol, blood glucose, prolactin, bilirubin, PBI, ^{131}I, alkaline phosphatase, leukocytes, granulocytes, platelets

Decreased: hormones (blood and urine)

False positive: pregnancy tests, urine bilirubin

False negative: urinary steroids, 17-OHCS, pregnancy tests

NURSING CONSIDERATIONS

Assessment

• Assess mental status: orientation, mood, behavior, presence and type of hallucinations before initial administration and monthly; this product should significantly reduce psychotic behavior

• Check for swallowing of PO medication; check for hoarding or giving of medication to other patients

• Monitor I&O ratio; palpate bladder if low urinary output occurs, especially in geriatric; urinalysis recommended before, during prolonged therapy

◆ Monitor bilirubin, CBC, liver function tests monthly; blood dyscrasias, hepatotoxicity may occur

• Assess affect, orientation, LOC, reflexes, gait, coordination, sleep pattern disturbances

• Monitor B/P with patient sitting, standing, and lying; take pulse and respirations q4hr during initial treatment; establish baseline before starting treatment; report drops of 30

---

mm Hg; obtain baseline ECG, Q-wave and T-wave changes
- Check for dizziness, faintness, palpitations, tachycardia on rising; severe orthostatic hypotension is common

◆ Identify neuroleptic malignant syndrome: hyperpyrexia, muscle rigidity, increased CPK, altered mental status, seizures, fever, tachycardia, dyspnea, fatigue, loss of bladder control; notify prescriber immediately; product should be discontinued

- Assess for EPS including akathisia (inability to sit still, no pattern to movements), tardive dyskinesia (bizarre movements of the jaw, mouth, tongue, extremities), pseudoparkinsonism (ragged tremors, pill rolling, shuffling gait); an antiparkinsonism product should be prescribed
- Assess for constipation, urinary retention daily; if these occur, increase bulk, water in diet

Nursing diagnoses
- Coping, ineffective (uses)
- Knowledge, deficient (teaching)
- Noncompliance (teaching)

Implementation
PO route
- Do not break, crush, or chew sus rel caps
- Give product in liquid form mixed in glass of juice if hoarding is suspected; do not mix in caffeine drinks, tannics, pectins
- Give decreased dosage in geriatric since metabolism is slowed
- Give PO with full glass of water, milk; or give with food to decrease GI upset
- Give antacids 2 hr before or after taking this product
- Store in airtight, light-resistant container; oral sol in amber bottle

IM route
- Inject slowly in deep muscle mass; do not give SUBCUT; aspirate to avoid **IV** administration; do not administer sol with a precipitate; have patient lie down afterward for at least 30 min

IV route
- Give by direct **IV** after diluting **IV** using 0.9% NaCl to 1 mg/1 ml; administer at 1 mg/min or less
- Administer by intermittent inf after diluting 20 mg/L or less LR, Ringer's, dextrose, saline, or any combination

Syringe compatibilities: Atropine, butorphanol, chlorproMAZINE, cimetidine, diamorphine, diphenhydrAMINE, droperidol, fentanyl, glycopyrrolate, hydrOXYzine, meperidine, metoclopramide, nalbuphine, pentazocine, perphenazine, promazine, promethazine, ranitidine, scopolamine, sufentanil

Syringe incompatibilities: DimenhyDRINATE, midazolam, pentobarbital, thiopental

Y-site compatibilities: Amsacrine, calcium gluconate, cisplatin, cladribine, cyclophosphamide, cytarabine, DOXOrubicin, fluconazole, granisetron, heparin, hydrocortisone, melphalan, methotrexate, ondansetron, paclitaxel, potassium chloride, propofol, sargramostim, sufentanil, teniposide, thiotepa, vinorelbine, vit B/C

Y-site incompatibilities: Foscarnet

Additive compatibilities: Amikacin, ascorbic acid, dexamethasone, dimenhyDRINATE, erythromycin, ethacrynate, lidocaine, nafcillin, netilmicin, sodium bicarbonate, vit B/C

Additive incompatibilities: Aminophylline, amphotericin B, ampicillin, calcium gluceptate, cefoperazone, cephalothin, chloramphenicol, chlorothiazide, floxacillin, furosemide, hydrocortisone sodium succinate, methohexital sodium, penicillin G sodium, phenobarbital, thiopental

Patient/family education
- Teach patient to use good oral hygiene; frequent rinsing of mouth, sugarless gum for dry mouth since oral candidiasis may occur
- Caution patient to avoid hazardous activities until product response is determined; dizziness, blurred vision may occur
- Inform patient that orthostatic hypotension occurs often and to rise from sitting or lying position gradually; to remain lying down after IM inj for at least 30 min; tell patient to avoid hot tubs, hot showers, tub baths, since hypotension may occur; tell patient that in hot weather heat stroke may occur; take extra precautions to stay cool
- Advise patient to avoid abrupt withdrawal of this product, or EPS may result; product should be withdrawn slowly
- Teach patient to avoid OTC preparations (cough, hay fever, cold) unless approved by prescriber, since serious product interactions may occur; avoid use with alcohol, CNS depressants; increased drowsiness may occur; avoid activities requiring mental alertness
- Instruct patient to avoid sun or use sunscreen, sunglasses, and protective clothing to prevent burns
- Advise patient to take antacids 2 hr before or after taking this product

P

- Advise patient to report sore throat, malaise, fever, bleeding, mouth sores; if these occur, CBC should be done and product discontinued
- Teach patient not to double or skip doses
- Teach patient urine may turn pink to reddish brown
- Instruct patient to report dark urine, clay-colored stools, bleeding, bruising, rash, blurred vision
- Advise patient that suppositories may contain coconut/palm oil

Evaluation
Positive therapeutic outcome
- Relief of nausea and vomiting
- Decrease in emotional excitement, hallucinations, delusions, paranoia
- Reorganization of patterns of thought, speech

Treatment of overdose: Lavage if orally ingested; provide airway; *do not induce vomiting or use epinephrine*

---

progesterone (Rx)
(proe-jess'ter-one)
Crinone, Endometrin, Prochieve, progesterone, Prometrium
Func. class.: Progestogen
Chem. class.: Progesterone derivative

Pregnancy category D

Action: Inhibits secretion of pituitary gonadotropins, which prevents follicular maturation, ovulation; stimulates growth of mammary tissue; antineoplastic action against endometrial cancer

Therapeutic outcome: Decreased abnormal uterine bleeding, absence of amenorrhea

Uses: Contraception, amenorrhea, premenstrual syndrome, abnormal uterine bleeding, endometrial hyperplasia prevention, assisted reproductive technology (ART) gel

Unlabeled uses: Corpus luteum insufficiency

Dosage and routes
Infertility
Adult: Vag 90 mg/day (micronized gel); 100 mg 2-3 times/day, starting day after oocyte retrieval and up to 10 wk total

Amenorrhea/uterine bleeding
Adult: IM 5-10 mg/day × 6-8 doses

Endometrial hyperplasia prevention
Adult: PO 200 mg/day × 12 days

Assisted reproductive technology
Adult: GEL 90 mg (8%) vaginally daily, for supplementation; 90 mg (8%) vaginally bid for replacement; if pregnancy occurs, continue × 10-12 wk

Corpus luteum insufficiency (unlabeled)
Adult: VAG insert 100 mg bid-tid starting at oocyte retrieval and continuing up to 10-12 wk gestation

Available forms: Caps 100, 200 mg; inj 50 mg/ml; powder micronized; vag gel 4%, 8%; vag insert 100 mg; supp 25, 100, 200, 500 mg

Adverse effects
CNS: Dizziness, headache, migraines, depression, fatigue, mood swings, dementia
CV: Hypotension, **thrombophlebitis**, edema, **thromboembolism, stroke, pulmonary embolism, MI**
EENT: Diplopia, retinal thrombosis
GI: Nausea, vomiting, anorexia, cramps, increased weight, **cholestatic jaundice,** constipation
GU: Amenorrhea, cervical erosion, breakthrough bleeding, dysmenorrhea, vaginal candidiasis, breast changes, *gynecomastia, testicular atrophy, impotence,* endometriosis, **spontaneous abortion,** breast pain, ectopic pregnancy
INTEG: Rash, urticaria, acne, hirsutism, alopecia, oily skin, seborrhea, purpura, melasma
META: Hyperglycemia
SYST: **Angioedema, anaphylaxis**

Contraindications: Pregnancy **D,** thromboembolic disorders, reproductive cancer, genital bleeding (abnormal, undiagnosed), cerebral hemorrhage, ectopic pregnancy, PID, STDs, hypersensitivity to this product or peanut oil

Black Box Warning: Breast cancer

Precautions: Breastfeeding, hypertension, asthma, blood dyscrasias, gallbladder disease, CHF, diabetes mellitus, bone disease, depression, migraine headache, seizure disorders, renal/hepatic disease, family history of breast or reproductive tract cancer

Black Box Warning: Cardiac disease, dementia

 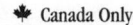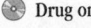

Pharmacokinetics

Absorption	Unknown
Distribution	Unknown
Metabolism	Unknown
Excretion	Breast milk
Half-life	Unknown

Pharmacodynamics

	IM	RECT	VAG
Onset	Unknown	Unknown	Unknown
Peak	Unknown	Unknown	Unknown
Duration	24 hr	24 hr	24 hr

Interactions
Drug classifications
Barbiturates, phenytoins: decreased progesterone effect

CYP3A4 inhibitors (cimetidine, clarithromycin, danazol, diltiazem, erythromycin, fluconazole, itraconazole, ketoconazole, troleandomycin, verapamil, voriconazole): increased progesterone effect
Drug/herb
Alfalfa: increased hormonal effect
Drug/lab test
Increased: alkaline phosphatase, nitrogen (urine), pregnanediol, amino acids, factors VII, VIII, IX, X

Decreased: GTT, HDL

NURSING CONSIDERATIONS
Assessment
• Monitor B/P at beginning of treatment and periodically; check weight daily; notify prescriber of weekly weight gain >5 lb
• Monitor I&O ratio: be alert for decreasing urinary output, increasing edema, hypertension
• Assess liver function tests: ALT, AST, bilirubin periodically during long-term therapy
• Assess edema, hypertension, cardiac symptoms, jaundice
• Assess mental status: affect, mood, behavioral changes, depression
• Assess for hypercalcemia
• Assess cervical cytology

Nursing diagnoses
• Injury, risk for (adverse reactions)
• Knowledge, deficient (teaching)
• Sexual dysfunction (uses)
• Tissue perfusion, ineffective (adverse reactions)

Implementation
• Wait at least 6 hr after any vaginal treatment before using vaginal gel
• Start progesterone 14 days after estrogen dose, if given concomitantly

IM route
• Store in dark area
• Give titrated dose; use lowest effective dosage; give oil sol deep in large muscle mass; rotate sites; use after warming to dissolve crystals

Patient/family education
• Teach patient to report breast lumps, vaginal bleeding, edema, jaundice, dark urine, clay-colored stools, dyspnea, headache, blurred vision, abdominal pain, numbness or stiffness in legs, chest pain
• Teach patient to report suspected pregnancy

Evaluation
Positive therapeutic outcome
• Decreased abnormal uterine bleeding
• Absence of amenorrhea
• Prevented pregnancy

promethazine (Rx)
(proe-meth'a-zeen)
Histanil ✦, Phenadoz, Phenergan, promethazine HCl
Func. class.: Antihistamine, H₁-receptor antagonist; antiemetic; sedative/hypnotic
Chem. class.: Phenothiazine derivative

Pregnancy category C

Do not confuse:
Phenergan/Theragran

Action: Acts on blood vessels, GI, respiratory system by competing with histamine for H₁-receptor site; decreases allergic response by blocking histamine; also acts on chemoreceptor trigger zone to decrease vomiting; increases CNS stimulation, has anticholinergic response

Therapeutic outcome: Absence of allergy symptoms and rhinitis, absence of nausea/vomiting, sedation

Uses: Motion sickness, rhinitis, allergy symptoms, sedation, nausea, preoperative and postoperative sedation

Dosage and routes
Nausea
Adult: PO/IM/**IV**/RECT 12.5-25 mg; q4-6hr prn
Child >2 yr: PO/IM/**IV**/RECT 0.25-0.5 mg/kg q4-6hr prn

Motion sickness
Adult: PO 25 mg bid; give 30-60 min before departure and q8-12hr prn
Child >2 yr: PO/IM/RECT 12.5-25 mg bid; give 30-60 min before departure and q8-12hr prn

P

Adverse effects: *italic* = common, **bold** = life-threatening

Allergy/rhinitis (unlabeled)
Adult: PO 12.5 mg qid, or 25 mg at bedtime
Child ≥2 yr: PO 6.25-12.5 mg tid or 25 mg at bedtime

Sedation
Adult: PO/IM 25-50 mg at bedtime
Child ≥2 yr: PO/IM/RECT 12.5-25 mg at bedtime

Sedation (preoperative/ postoperative)
Adult: PO/IM/**IV** 25-50 mg
Child ≥2 yr: PO/IM/**IV** 0.5-1.1 mg/kg

Available forms: Tabs 12.5, 25, 50 mg; supp 12.5, 25, 50 mg; inj 25, 50 mg/ml; syr 6.25 mg/5 ml

Adverse effects
CNS: *Dizziness, drowsiness,* poor coordination, fatigue, anxiety, euphoria, confusion, paresthesia, neuritis, EPS, **neuroleptic malignant syndrome**
CV: Hyper/hypotension, palpitations, tachycardia
EENT: Blurred vision, dilated pupils, tinnitus, nasal stuffiness, dry nose, throat, mouth, photosensitivity
GI: *Constipation,* dry mouth, nausea, vomiting, anorexia, diarrhea
GU: *Retention,* dysuria, frequency
HEMA: **Thrombocytopenia, agranulocytosis, hemolytic anemia**
INTEG: Rash, urticaria, photosensitivity
RESP: Increased thick secretions, wheezing, chest tightness, **apnea in pediatric patients**

Contraindications: Hypersensitivity to H₁-receptor antagonist, agranulocytosis, bone marrow suppression, breastfeeding, coma, jaundice, Reye's syndrome

Black Box Warning: Infants, intraarterial use, neonates, subcut use, children

Precautions: Pregnancy **C**, renal/cardiac/ hepatic disease, asthma, seizure disorder, prostatic hypertrophy, bladder obstruction, glaucoma, COPD, GI obstruction, ileus, CNS depression, diabetes, sleep apnea, urinary retention

Black Box Warning: IV use

Pharmacokinetics	
Absorption	Well absorbed (PO, IM); erratically absorbed (RECT)
Distribution	Widely distributed; crosses the blood-brain barrier, placenta
Metabolism	Liver
Excretion	Kidneys, breast milk
Half-life	Unknown

Pharmacodynamics		
	PO/IM/RECT	IV
Onset	20 min	3-5 min
Peak	Unknown	Unknown
Duration	4-12 hr	4-6 hr

Interactions
Individual drugs
Alcohol: increased CNS depression
Heparin: decreased oral anticoagulants effect
Drug classifications
Antidepressants (tricyclics), barbiturates, CNS depressants, opiates, sedative/hypnotics: increased CNS depression
MAOIs: increased promethazine effect
Drug/herb
Henbane, jimsonweed, scopolia: increased anticholinergic effect
Drug/lab test
False negative: skin allergy tests (discontinue antihistamines 3 days before testing)
False positive: urine pregnancy test
Interference: blood grouping (ABO), GTT

NURSING CONSIDERATIONS
Assessment
• Assess respiratory status: rate, rhythm, increase in bronchial secretions, wheezing, chest tightness; provide fluids to 2 L/day to decrease secretion thickness
• Monitor I&O ratio: be alert for urinary retention, frequency, dysuria, especially geriatric; product should be discontinued if these occur
• Monitor CBC during long-term therapy; blood dyscrasias may occur but are rare
• Monitor cardiac status: VS, palpitations, increased pulse, hypo/hypertension

Nursing diagnoses
• Airway clearance, ineffective (uses)
• Injury, risk for (adverse reactions)
• Knowledge, deficient (teaching)
• Noncompliance (teaching, overuse)

Implementation
PO route
• Give 1 hr before or 2 hr after meals to facilitate absorption
• Give with meals to decrease GI upset
• Store in airtight, light-resistant container
IM route
• Give IM inj in large muscle mass; aspirate to avoid **IV** administration; do not give SUBCUT; necrosis may occur
IV route
• Do not use if precipitate is present
• Rapid administration may cause transient decrease in B/P

 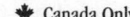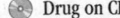

- Give **IV** directly; give 25 mg or less over 1 min; rapid drop in B/P may occur with rapid administration

Syringe compatibilities: Atropine, butorphanol, chlorproMAZINE, cimetidine, diphenhydrAMINE, droperidol, fentanyl, glycopyrrolate, hydromorphone, hydrOXYzine, meperidine, metoclopramide, midazolam, pentazocine, perphenazine, prochlorperazine, promazine, ranitidine, scopolamine

Syringe incompatibilities: Dimenhy-DRINATE, heparin, pentobarbital, thiopental

Y-site compatibilities: Amifostine, amsacrine, aztreonam, ciprofloxacin, cisplatin, cladribine, cyclophosphamide, cytarabine, DOXOrubicin, filgrastim, fluconazole, fludara-bine, granisetron, melphalan, ondansetron, sargramostim, teniposide, thiotepa, vinorel-bine

Y-site incompatibilities: Cefoperazone, foscarnet, heparin

Additive compatibilities: Amikacin, ascorbic acid, chloroquine, hydromorphone, netilmicin, vit B/C

Additive incompatibilities: Aminoph-ylline, carbenicillin, chloramphenicol, chloro-thiazide, floxacillin, furosemide, heparin, hydrocortisone sodium succinate, methicillin, methohexital, penicillin G, pentobarbital, phenobarbital, thiopental

Patient/family education

- Inform patient that a false-negative result may occur with skin testing; these procedures should not be scheduled until 3 days after discontinuing use
- Advise patient to take 30 min before depar-ture to prevent motion sickness
- Caution patient to avoid hazardous activities, activities requiring alertness, since dizziness may occur; instruct patient to request assis-tance with ambulation
- Advise patient to avoid alcohol, other depressants; serious CNS depression may occur
- Teach patient all aspects of product use; to notify prescriber if confusion, sedation, hypotension, jaundice, fever occur; to avoid driving and other hazardous activity if drowsi-ness occurs
- Advise patient to take 1 hr before or 2 hr after meals to facilitate absorption
- Caution patient not to exceed recommended dosage; dysrhythmias may occur
- Inform patient hard candy, gum, frequent rinsing of mouth may be used for dryness
- Advise that product may reduce sweating (heat stroke)

Evaluation

Positive therapeutic outcome

- Absence of motion sickness
- Absence of nausea, vomiting

---

propafenone (Rx)

(pro-faff'e-nown)
Rythmol, Rythmol SR
Func. class.: Antidysrhythmic (Class IC)

Pregnancy category C

Action: Slows conduction velocity; reduces membrane responsiveness; inhibits automaticity; increases ratio of effective refractory period to action potential duration; β-blocking activity

Therapeutic outcome: Absence of arrhythmias

Uses: Atrial fibrillation, life-threatening dysrhythmias, sustained ventricular tachycar-dia

Dosage and routes

Adult: PO 150 mg q8hr; allow a 3-4 day interval before increasing dose, max 900 mg/day

Atrial fibrillation

Adult: PO 450 or 600 mg as a single dose; SR 225 mg q12hr, may increase to 325 mg q12hr, max 425 mg q12hr

Available forms: Tabs 150, 225, 300 mg

Adverse effects

CNS: Headache, dizziness, abnormal dreams, syncope, confusion, **seizures,** insomnia, tremor, anxiety, fatigue

CV: **Supraventricular dysrhythmia, ven-tricular dysrhythmia, bradycardia,** pro-dysrhythmia, palpitations, AV block, intraven-tricular conduction delay, AV dissociation, hypotension, chest pain

EENT: Blurred vision, altered taste, tinnitus

GI: *Nausea, vomiting,* constipation, dyspep-sia, cholestasis, abnormal hepatic studies, dry mouth

HEMA: **Leukopenia, agranulocytosis, granulocytopenia, thrombocytopenia,** anemia, bruising

INTEG: Rash

RESP: Dyspnea

Contraindications: 2nd-, 3rd-degree AV block, right bundle branch block, cardiogenic shock, hypersensitivity, bradycardia, uncon-trolled CHF, sick sinus syndrome, marked hypotension, bronchospastic disorders

P

Adverse effects: *italic* = common, **bold** = life-threatening

Precautions: Pregnancy C, breastfeeding, children, geriatric, CHF, hypo/hyperkalemia, nonallergic bronchospasm, renal/hepatic disease, hematologic disorders

Black Box Warning: Recent MI, cardiac arrhythmias, QT prolongation, torsades de pointes

Pharmacokinetics

Absorption	Well
Distribution	Widely, crosses placenta
Metabolism	Rapid, liver, CYP1A2, CYP2D6, CYP3A4
Excretion	Kidneys
Half-life	2-32 hr

Pharmacodynamics (antiarrhythmic)

Onset	Hours-several days
Peak	4-5 days
Duration	Several hr

Interactions
Individual products
Cimetidine, quinidine, rifampin: decreased propafenone effect
CycloSPORINE, digoxin: increased serum levels
Metropolol, propranolol: increased β-blocker effect
Warfarin: increased anticoagulation
Drug classifications
Local anesthetics: increased CNS effects
Drug/herb
Aconite: increased toxicity, death
Aloe, broom, buckthorn (chronic use), cascara sagrada (chronic use), Chinese rhubarb, figwort, fumitory, goldenseal, kudzu, licorice: increased effect
Aloe, buckthorn, cascara sagrada, senna pod/leaf: hypokalemia, increased antidysrhythmic action, hypokalemia
Coltsfoot: decreased effect
Horehound: increased serotonin effect
Drug/lab test
Increased: CPK

NURSING CONSIDERATIONS
Assessment
• Monitor GI status: bowel pattern, number of stools
🔷 Assess cardiac status: rate, rhythm, quality; ECG or Holter monitor prior to, during therapy; watch for PR, QT prolongation
• Monitor chest x-ray film, pulmonary function test during treatment
• Monitor I&O ratio; check for decreasing output; daily weight
• Monitor B/P for fluctuations
• Assess lung fields; bilateral crackles, dyspnea, peripheral edema, weight gain, jugular venous distention may occur in CHF patient
🔷 Assess toxicity: fine tremors, dizziness, hypotension, drowsiness, abnormal heart rate

Nursing diagnoses
• Cardiac output, decreased (uses)
• Knowledge, deficient (teaching)

Implementation
• Begin treatment in hospital
• Remove other antiarrhythmics before starting propafenone
• Adjust dosage q3-4day, no sooner

Patient/family education
• Advise patient to avoid hazardous activities until response is known
• Advise patient to report fever, chills, sore throat, bleeding, shortness of breath, chest pain, palpitations, blurred vision
• Advise patient to take medication with food
• Advise patient to carry emergency ID identifying medication and prescriber

Evaluation
Positive therapeutic outcome
• Absence of dysrhythmias

Treatment of overdose: O₂, artificial ventilation, defibrillation ECG; administer DOPamine for circulatory depression, diazepam or thiopental for seizures, isoproterenol

---

propantheline (Rx)
(proe-pan'the-leen)
Propanthel ✦
Func. class.: GI anticholinergic; antiulcer agent
Chem. class.: Synthetic quaternary ammonium compound

Pregnancy category C

Action: Inhibits muscarinic actions of acetylcholine at postganglionic parasympathetic neuroeffector sites

Therapeutic outcome: Absence of peptic ulcer disease symptoms

Uses: Treatment of peptic ulcer disease, irritable bowel syndrome, duodenography, urinary incontinence

Dosage and routes
Adult: PO 15 mg tid before meals, 30 mg at bedtime
Geriatric/small patients: PO 7.5 mg tid before meals
Child: 1-2 mg/kg/day in 3-4 doses

Available forms: Tabs 7.5, 15 mg

Adverse effects

CNS: Confusion, stimulation in geriatric, headache, insomnia, dizziness, drowsiness, anxiety, weakness, hallucinations

CV: Palpitations, tachycardia, orthostatic hypotension (geriatric)

EENT: Blurred vision, photophobia, mydriasis, cycloplegia, increased ocular tension

GI: Dry mouth, constipation, **paralytic ileus,** heartburn, nausea, vomiting, dysphagia, absence of taste

GU: Hesitancy, retention, impotence

INTEG: Urticaria, rash, pruritus, anhidrosis, fever, allergic reactions

Contraindications: Hypersensitivity to anticholinergics, closed-angle glaucoma, GI obstruction, myasthenia gravis, paralytic ileus, GI atony, toxic megacolon, urinary tract obstruction

Precautions: Pregnancy **C,** geriatric, hyperthyroidism, CAD, dysrhythmias, CHF, ulcerative colitis, hypertension, hiatal hernia, renal/hepatic disease, urinary retention, prostatic hypertrophy

Pharmacokinetics	
Absorption	Moderately absorbed
Distribution	Unknown
Metabolism	Unknown
Excretion	Unknown
Half-life	Unknown

Pharmacodynamics	
Onset	½ hr
Peak	2-6 hr
Duration	4-6 hr

Interactions

Individual products

Disopyramide, procainamide, quinidine: increased anticholinergic effect

Drug classifications

Antidepressants (tricyclics), H_1-antihistamines, belladonna alkaloids, MAOIs, opioids, phenothiazenes: increased anticholinergic effect

Drug/herb

Henbane, jimsonweed, scopolia: increased anticholinergic effect

NURSING CONSIDERATIONS

Assessment

• Assess for the pain of peptic ulcer disease before, during, after treatment

Nursing diagnoses

• Constipation (adverse reactions)
• Knowledge, deficient (teaching)
• Pain, chronic (uses)

Implementation

• Give 30 min before meals and at bedtime; do not give with antacids; separate by at least 1 hr

Patient/family education

• Teach patient to report blurred vision, chest pain, allergic reactions

• Advise patient not to perform strenuous activity in high temperatures; heat stroke may result due to decreased perspiration

• Instruct patient to take as prescribed; not to skip doses

• Instruct patient to report change in vision; blurring or loss of sight; product should be discontinued

• Advise patient not to operate machinery or drive if dizziness occurs

• Caution patient not to take OTC products without approval of prescriber

Evaluation

Positive therapeutic outcome

• Decreased pain in peptic ulcer disease

proparacaine ophthalmic
See Appendix B

⚠ HIGH ALERT

propofol (Rx)

(pro'poh-fole)

Diprivan, Fresenius, Propoven

Func. class.: General anesthetic

Pregnancy category B

Action: Produces dose-dependent CNS depression by activation of GABA receptor

Therapeutic outcome: Induction of anesthesia

Uses: Induction or maintenance of anesthesia as part of balanced anesthetic technique; sedation in mechanically ventilated patients

Dosage and routes

Induction

Adult: **IV** 2-2.5 mg/kg, approximately 40 mg q10sec until induction onset

Child 3-16 yr: **IV** 2.5-3.5 mg/kg over 20-30 sec

P

Adverse effects: *italic* = common, **bold** = life-threatening

Geriatric: **IV** 1-1.5 mg/kg, approximately 20 mg q10sec until induction onset

Maintenance
Adult: **IV** 0.1-0.2 mg/kg/min (6-12 mg/kg/hr)
Child ≥3 yr: **IV** 0.125-0.3 mg/kg/min (7.5-18 mg/kg/hr)
Geriatric: **IV** 0.05-0.1 mg/kg/min (3-6 mg/kg/hr)

ICU sedation
Adult: **IV** 5 mcg/kg/min over 5 min; may increase by 5-10 mcg/kg/min over 5-10 min until desired response

Available forms: Inj 10 mg/ml in 20 ml ampule, 50 ml, 100 ml vials

Adverse effects
CNS: Involuntary movement, headache, jerking, fever, dizziness, shivering, tremor, confusion, somnolence, paresthesia, agitation, abnormal dreams, euphoria, fatigue, **increased ICP, impaired cerebral flow, seizures**
CV: Bradycardia, hypotension, hypertension, PVC, PAC, tachycardia, abnormal ECG, ST segment depression, **asystole, bradydysrhythmias**
EENT: Blurred vision, tinnitus, eye pain, strange taste, diplopia
GI: Nausea, vomiting, abdominal cramping, dry mouth, swallowing, hypersalivation, **pancreatitis**
GU: Urine retention, green urine, cloudy urine, oliguria
INTEG: Flushing, phlebitis, hives, burning/stinging at inj site, rash, pain of extremities
MS: Myalgia
RESP: **Apnea**, *cough, hiccups,* dyspnea, hypoventilation, sneezing, wheezing, tachypnea, hypoxia, respiratory acidosis

Contraindications: Hypersensitivity to product or soybean oil, egg, benzyl alcohol (some products)

Precautions: Pregnancy **B**, breastfeeding, children, geriatric, respiratory depression, severe respiratory disorders, cardiac dysrhythmias, labor and delivery, renal disease, hyperlipidemia

Pharmacokinetics

Absorption	Completely
Distribution	Rapid
Metabolism	Liver, conjugation to active metabolites; 95%-99% protein binding
Excretion	Urine
Half-life	3-12 hr

Pharmacodynamics

Onset	15-30 sec
Peak	Unknown
Duration	Unknown

Interactions
Individual drugs
Alcohol: increased CNS depression

Drug classifications
Antipsychotics, CNS depressants (sedative/hypnotics, opioid analgesics), inhalational anesthetics, skeletal muscle relaxants: increased CNS depression
MAOIs: do not use within 10 days

Drug/herb
St. John's wort: increased propofol effect

NURSING CONSIDERATIONS
Assessment
• Assess inj site: phlebitis, burning, stinging
• Monitor ECG for changes: PVC, PAC, ST segment changes; monitor VS
• Assess CNS changes: movement, jerking, tremors, dizziness, LOC, pupil reaction
• Assess allergic reactions: hives
◆ Assess respiratory dysfunction: respiratory depression, character, rate, rhythm; notify prescriber if respirations are <10/min

Nursing diagnoses
• Breathing pattern, ineffective (adverse reactions)
• Injury, risk for (adverse reactions)
• Knowledge, deficient (teaching)

Implementation
• Shake well before use; if diluted, use only D$_5$W to not less than 2 mg/ml; give over 3-5 min, titrate to needed level of sedation; use only glass containers when mixing, not stable in plastic
• May be given by cont inf; give by inf pump
• Give only with resuscitative equipment available
• Give only by qualified persons trained in anesthesia
• Store in light-resistant area at room temperature; use within 6 hr of opening
• If transferred from original container to another container, complete inf within 12 hr (Dipravan), 6 hr (generic propofol)
Y-site compatibilities: Acyclovir, alfentanil, aminophylline, ampicillin, aztreonam, bumetanide, buprenorphine, butorphanol, calcium gluconate, carboplatin, cefazolin, cefoperazone, cefotaxime, cefotetan, cefoxitin, ceftizoxime, ceftriaxone, cefuroxime, chlorproMAZINE, cimetidine, cisplatin, clindamycin,

cyclophosphamide, cycloSPORINE, cytarabine, dexamethasone, diphenhydrAMINE, DOBUTamine, DOPamine, doxycycline, droperidol, enalaprilat, ephedrine, epinephrine, esmolol, famotidine, fentanyl, fluconazole, fluorouracil, furosemide, ganciclovir, glycopyrrolate, granisetron, haloperidol, heparin, hydrocortisone, hydromorphone, hydrOXYzine, ifosfamide, imipenem/cilastatin, inamrinone, insulin (regular), isoproterenol, ketamine, labetalol, levorphanol, lidocaine, lorazepam, magnesium sulfate, mannitol, meperidine, mezlocillin, miconazole, morphine, nafcillin, nalbuphine, naloxone, nitroglycerin, norepinephrine, ofloxacin, paclitaxel, pentobarbital, phenobarbital, piperacillin, potassium chloride, prochlorperazine, propranolol, ranitidine, scopolamine, sodium bicarbonate, sodium nitroprusside, succinylcholine, sufentanil, thiopental, ticarcillin, ticarcillin/clavulanate, vecuronium, verapamil

Solution compatibilities: (is given together via Y-site) D₅W, D₅LR, LR, D₅/0.45% NaCl, D₅/0.2% NaCl

Patient/family education
• Teach patient that this medication will cause dizziness, drowsiness, sedation

Evaluation
Positive therapeutic outcome
• Induction of anesthesia

Treatment of overdose: Discontinue product; administer vasopressor agents or anticholinergics, artificial ventilation

---

！HIGH ALERT

propoxyphene (Rx)
(proe-pox'i-feen)
Darvon, Darvon-N, Dolene, Novapropoxyn ✦
Func. class.: Opiate analgesics
Chem. class.: Synthetic opiate

Pregnancy category C

Controlled substance schedule IV

Action: Depresses pain impulse transmission at the spinal cord level by interacting with opioid receptors

Therapeutic outcome: Decreased pain

Uses: Mild to moderate pain

Dosage and routes
Adult: PO (HCl) 65 mg q4hr prn, max 390 mg/day
Adult: PO (napsylate) 100 mg q4hr prn, max 600 mg/day

Available forms: Propoxyphene HCl: caps 32, 65 mg; propoxyphene napsylate: tabs 100 mg; oral susp 50 mg/5 ml

Adverse effects
CNS: Drowsiness, dizziness, confusion, **increased ICP,** *headache, sedation,* euphoria, **seizures, hyperthermia (geriatric)**
CV: Palpitations, bradycardia, change in B/P, **dysrhythmias**
EENT: Tinnitus, blurred vision, miosis, diplopia
GI: Nausea, vomiting, anorexia, constipation, cramps, abdominal pain, jaundice
GU: Urinary retention, dysuria
INTEG: Rash, urticaria, bruising, flushing, diaphoresis, pruritus
RESP: **Respiratory depression, pulmonary edema**

Contraindications: Hypersensitivity to acetylsalicylic acid products (some preparations)

Black Box Warning: Alcoholism, substance abuse, suicidal ideation

Precautions: Pregnancy C, breastfeeding, children <18 yr, geriatric, addictive personality, increased ICP, MI (acute), severe heart disease, respiratory depression, renal/hepatic disease

Black Box Warning: Potential for overdose/poisoning

Pharmacokinetics
Absorption	Well absorbed
Distribution	Widely distributed, crosses placenta
Metabolism	Liver, extensively
Excretion	Kidneys, breast milk
Half-life	6-12 hr

Pharmacodynamics
Onset	½-1 hr
Peak	2-3 hr
Duration	4-6 hr

Interactions
Individual drugs
Alcohol: possible fatal reactions
Drug classifications
Antipsychotics, CNS depressants, opioids, sedative/hypnotics, skeletal muscle relaxants: increased effects
MAOIs: possible fatal reactions
Drug/herb
Chamomile, hops, kava, Jamaican dogwood, lavender, mistletoe, nettle, pokeweed, poppy,

P

Adverse effects: *italic* = common, **bold** = life-threatening

senega, skullcap, valerian: increased CNS depression

Corkwood: increased anticholinergic effects

Drug/lab test

Increased: amylase

False positive: methadone test

NURSING CONSIDERATIONS
Assessment

- Assess pain: location, duration, intensity before and 1 hr after administration
- Monitor bowel/bladder status: constipation may need stimulant laxative; I&O ratio, check for decreasing output, may indicate retention
- Monitor CNS changes: dizziness, drowsiness, euphoria, LOC, pupil reaction
- Monitor allergic reactions: rash, urticaria

Nursing diagnoses

- Breathing pattern, ineffective (adverse reactions)
- Injury, risk for (adverse reactions)
- Knowledge, deficient (teaching)
- Pain, acute (uses)
- Sensory perception, disturbed: visual, auditory (adverse reactions)

Implementation

- Give with antiemetic if nausea, vomiting occur
- Give when pain is beginning to return; determine dosage interval by patient response; continuous dosing of medication is more effective than when given prn
- Withdraw medication slowly after long-term use to prevent withdrawal symptoms
- Store in light-resistant container at room temperature
- May be given with food or milk to lessen GI upset

Patient/family education

- Teach patient to avoid CNS depressants: alcohol, sedative/hypnotics for at least 24 hr after taking this product
- Advise that physical dependency may result when used for extended periods of time; significant potential for overdose exists
- Discuss with patient that dizziness, drowsiness, and confusion are common; to avoid getting up without assistance
- Discuss in detail all aspects of the product, including purpose and what to expect after anesthesia
- Advise patient to make position changes slowly to lessen orthostatic hypotension

Evaluation
Positive therapeutic outcome

- Decreased pain

Treatment of overdose: Naloxone 0.2-0.8 mg **IV**, O_2, **IV** fluids, vasopressors

---

propranolol 😳 (Rx)
(proe-pran'oh-lole)

Apo-Propranolol ✦, Betaclinron E-R ✦, Detensol ✦, Inderal, Inderal LA, InnoPran XL, NovoPranol ✦, PMS-Propranolol ✦, propranolol HCl

Func. class.: Antihypertensive, antianginal, antidysrhythmic (class III)

Chem. class.: β-Adrenergic blocker

Pregnancy category C

Do not confuse:
Inderal/Toradol/Inderide/Adderall/Imuran, Propranolol/Pravachol

Action: Competitively blocks stimulation of β-adrenergic receptor within vascular smooth muscle; produces chronotropic, inotropic activity (decreases rate of SA node discharge, increases recovery time), slows conduction of AV node, decreased heart rate, which decreases O_2 consumption in myocardium; also suppresses renin-aldosterone-angiotensin system at high doses, inhibits $β_2$-receptors in bronchial system (high doses)

Therapeutic outcome: Decreased B/P, heart rate

Uses: Chronic stable angina pectoris, hypertension, supraventricular dysrhythmias, migraine prophylaxis, pheochromocytoma, cyanotic spells related to hypertrophic subaortic stenosis

Unlabeled uses: Parkinson's tremor, prevention of variceal bleeding caused by portal hypertension, akathisia induced by antipsychotics

Dosage and routes
Dysrhythmias

Adult: PO 10-30 mg tid-qid; **IV** BOL 0.5-3 mg given 1 mg/min; may repeat in 2 min; may repeat q4hr thereafter

Child: PO 1 mg/kg/day divided in 2 doses, **IV** 0.01-0.1 mg/kg over 5 min

Hypertension

Adult: PO 40 mg bid or 80 mg/day (SUS REL) initially; usual dosage 120-240 mg/day bid-tid or 120-160 mg/day (SUS REL)

Child: PO 0.5-1 mg/kg/day divided q6-12hr

Angina

Adult: PO 80-320 mg in divided doses bid-qid or 80 mg/day (SUS REL); usual dosage 160 mg/day (SUS REL)

MI prophylaxis
Adult: PO 180-240 mg/day tid-qid starting 5 days to 2 wk after MI

Pheochromocytoma
Adult: PO 60 mg/day × 3 days preoperatively in divided doses or 30 mg/day in divided doses (inoperable tumor)

Migraine
Adult: PO 80 mg/day (EXT REL) or in divided doses; may increase to 160-240 mg/day in divided doses
Child: PO 0.6-1.5 mg/kg/day divided q8hr

Essential tremor
Adult: PO 40 mg bid; usual dosage 120 mg/day

Available forms: Ext rel caps 60, 80, 120, 160 mg; tabs 10, 20, 40, 60, 80, 90 mg; inj 1 mg/ml; oral sol 4 mg, 8 mg/ml; conc oral sol 80 mg/ml

Adverse effects
CNS: Depression, hallucinations, dizziness, *fatigue,* lethargy, paresthesia, bizarre dreams, disorientation
CV: **Bradycardia,** *hypotension,* **CHF,** palpitations, AV block, peripheral vascular insufficiency, vasodilatation, **pulmonary edema, dysrhythmias,** cold extremities
EENT: Sore throat, **laryngospasm,** blurred vision, dry eyes
GI: Nausea, vomiting, diarrhea, colitis, constipation, cramps, dry mouth, hepatomegaly, gastric pain, acute pancreatitis
GU: Impotence, decreased libido, UTIs
HEMA: **Agranulocytosis, thrombocytopenia**
INTEG: Rash, pruritus, fever
META: Hyperglycemia, hypoglycemia
MISC: Facial swelling, weight change, Raynaud's phenomenon
MS: Joint pain, arthralgia, muscle cramps, pain
RESP: Dyspnea, respiratory dysfunction, **bronchospasm,** cough

Contraindications: Hypersensitivity to this product, cardiogenic shock, AV heart block, bronchospastic disease, sinus bradycardia, bronchospasm, asthma

Precautions: Pregnancy **C,** breastfeeding, children, diabetes mellitus, renal/hepatic disease, hyperthyroidism, COPD, myasthenia gravis, peripheral vascular disease, hypotension, cardiac failure, Raynaud's disease, sick sinus syndrome, vasospastic angina, smoking, Wolff-Parkinson-White syndrome

Black Box Warning: Abrupt discontinuation

Pharmacokinetics

Absorption	Well absorbed (PO); slowly absorbed (ext rel); completely absorbed (**IV**)
Distribution	Widely distributed, crosses blood-brain barrier, protein binding 90%
Metabolism	Liver, extensively
Excretion	Kidneys
Half-life	3-5 hr; ext rel 8-11 hr

Pharmacodynamics

	PO	PO-EXT REL	IV
Onset	½ hr	Unknown	Rapid
Peak	1-1½ hr	6 hr	1 min
Duration	6-12 hr	24 hr	4-6 hr

Interactions
Individual drugs
Cimetidine: increased β-blocking effect
Disopyramide: increased negative inotropic effects
Haloperidol, prazosin, quinidine: increased hypotension
Phenothiazines: increased toxicity
Propafenone: increased propranolol levels
Smoking: decreased propranolol levels
Drug classifications
Barbiturates: decreased β-blocking effect
Calcium channel blockers, neuromuscular blockers: increased effects
Phenothiazines: increased toxicity
Drug/herb
Aconite: increased toxicity, death
Astragalus, cola tree: increased or decreased antihypertensive effect
Barberry, betony, black catechu, black cohosh, bloodroot, broom, burdock, cat's claw, dandelion, goldenseal, Irish moss, Jamaican dogwood, kelp, khella, mistletoe, parsley: increased antihypertensive effect
Betel palm, coltsfoot, guarana, khat, licorice, ma huang: decreased antihypertensive effect
Drug/lab test
Increased: serum potassium, serum uric acid, AST, ALT, alkaline phosphatase, LDH
Decreased: blood glucose
Interference: glaucoma testing

NURSING CONSIDERATIONS
Assessment
• Monitor B/P during beginning treatment, periodically thereafter; pulse q4hr; note rate, rhythm, quality; check apical/radial pulse before administration; notify prescriber of any

P

significant changes (pulse <50 bpm or systolic B/P <90 mm Hg)
• Check for baselines in renal, liver function tests before therapy begins and periodically thereafter
• Assess for edema in feet, legs daily; monitor I&O, weight daily; check for jugular vein distention, crackles bilaterally; dyspnea (CHF)
• Monitor skin turgor, dryness of mucous membranes for hydration status, especially geriatric
• Assess for headache, light-headedness, decreased B/P; may indicate need for decreased dose; may aggravate symptoms of arterial insufficiency

Nursing diagnoses
• Cardiac output, decreased (uses)
• Injury, risk for (adverse reactions)
• Knowledge, deficient (teaching)
• Noncompliance (teaching)

Implementation
PO route
• Do not break, crush, or chew sus rel cap
• Given before meals, at bedtime, tab may be crushed or swallowed whole; give with food to prevent GI upset; reduce dosage in renal dysfunction
• May mix oral sol with liquid or semisolid food, rinse container to get entire dose
• Store protected from light, moisture; placed in cool environment
IV route
• Give by direct **IV** undiluted or diluted 1 mg/10 ml of D_5W for inj; administer over 1 min or more
• Give by intermittent inf after diluting in 50 ml of D_5W, 0.9% NaCl, D_5/0.45% NaCl, D_5/0.9% NaCl, LR; administer over 15 min
Y-site compatibilities:
Heparin, hydrocortisone, inamrinone, meperidine, milrinone, morphine, potassium chloride, tacrolimus, vit B/C
Y-site incompatibilities: Diazoxide
Additive compatibilities: DO-BUTamine, verapamil
Solution compatibilities: 0.9% NaCl, 0.45% NaCl, Ringer's, D_5W, D_5/0.9% NaCl, D_5/0.45% NaCl

Patient/family education
🔴 Teach patient not to discontinue product abruptly (life-threatening dysrhythmias, exacerbation of angina, MI); to take at same time of day either with or without food consistently; taper over 2 wk
• Teach patient not to use OTC products containing α-adrenergic stimulants (such as nasal decongestants, cold preparations); to

avoid alcohol, smoking and to limit sodium intake as prescribed
• Teach patient how to take pulse and B/P at home; advise when to notify prescriber
• Instruct patient to comply with weight control, dietary adjustments, modified exercise program
• Instruct patient to carry/wear emergency ID to identify product being taken, allergies; tell patient product controls symptoms but does not cure
• Caution patient to avoid hazardous activities if dizziness, drowsiness are present
• Teach patient to report symptoms of CHF: difficult breathing, especially on exertion or when lying down, night cough, swelling of extremities or bradycardia, dizziness, confusion, depression, fever
• Advise patient that sensitivity to cold may occur
• Teach patient to monitor blood glucose; may mask symptoms of hypoglycemia
• Teach patient how to take pulse, B/P; withhold if <50 bpm or systolic B/P <90 mm Hg

Evaluation
Positive therapeutic outcome
• Decreased B/P in hypertension (after 1-2 wk)
• Decreased tremors
• Absence of dysrhythmias
• Decreased migraine headaches

Treatment of overdose: Lavage, **IV** atropine for bradycardia, **IV** theophylline for bronchospasm, digoxin, O_2, diuretic for cardiac failure, hemodialysis, **IV** glucose for hyperglycemia, **IV** diazepam (or phenytoin) for seizures

propylhexadrine nasal
See Appendix B

propylthiouracil (Rx)
(proe-pill-thye-oh-yoor′a-sill)
PIV, propylthiouracil, Propyl-Thyracil ✣, PTU
Func. class.: Thyroid hormone antagonist (antithyroid)
Chem. class.: Thioamide
Pregnancy category D

Action: Blocks synthesis peripherally of T_3, T_4, inhibits organification of iodine

Therapeutic outcome: Decreased T$_3$, T$_4$ levels, hyperthyroid symptoms

Uses: Preparation for thyroidectomy, thyrotoxic crisis, hyperthyroidism, thyroid storm

Dosage and routes
Thyrotoxic crisis
Adult and child: PO same as hyperthyroidism with iodine and propranolol

Preparation for thyroidectomy
Adult: PO 600-1200 mg/day
Child: PO 10 mg/kg/day in divided doses

Hyperthyroidism
Adult: PO 100 mg tid increasing to 300 mg q8hr if condition is severe; continue to euthyroid state, then 100 mg daily-tid
Child >10 yr: PO 100 mg tid; continue to euthyroid state, then 25 mg tid to 100 mg bid
Child 6-10 yr: PO 50-150 mg in divided doses q8hr
Neonate: PO 10 mg/kg/day in divided doses

Available forms: Tabs 50 mg

Adverse effects
CNS: Drowsiness, headache, vertigo, fever, paresthesias, neuritis
GI: Nausea, diarrhea, vomiting, jaundice, **hepatitis,** loss of taste, **liver failure, death**
GU: **Nephritis**
HEMA: **Agranulocytosis, leukopenia, thrombocytopenia, hypothrombinemia, lymphadenopathy,** bleeding, vasculitis, periarteritis
INTEG: Rash, urticaria, pruritus, alopecia, hyperpigmentation, lupus-like syndrome
MS: Myalgia, arthralgia, nocturnal muscle cramps, osteoporosis

Contraindications: Pregnancy **D,** breastfeeding, hypersensitivity, agranulocytosis, hepatitis, jaundice

Precautions: Infection, bone marrow depression, hepatic disease, fever

Pharmacokinetics
Absorption	Rapidly absorbed
Distribution	Crosses placenta, concentration in thyroid gland
Metabolism	Liver
Excretion	Urine, bile, breast milk
Half-life	1-2 hr

Pharmacodynamics
Onset	30-40 min
Peak	Unknown
Duration	2-4 hr

Interactions
Individual drugs
Heparin: decreased anticoagulant effect
Lithium: increased antithyroid effect
Potassium/sodium iodide: increased effects
Radiation: increased bone marrow depression
Drug classifications
Anticoagulants (oral): decreased anticoagulant effect
Antineoplastics: increased bone marrow depression
Phenothiazines: increased agranulocytosis
Drug/lab test
Increased: pro-time, AST, ALT, alkaline phosphatase

NURSING CONSIDERATIONS
Assessment
• Monitor pulse, B/P, temp; I&O ratio; check for edema (puffy hands, feet, periorbits); indicates hypothyroidism
• Check weight daily with same clothing, scale, time of day
• Monitor T$_3$, T$_4$, which are increased; check serum TSH, which is decreased; assess free thyroxine index, which is increased if dosage is too low; discontinue product 3-4 wk before radioactive iodine uptake test
• Monitor blood tests: CBC for blood dyscrasias (leukopenia, thrombocytopenia, agranulocytosis); liver function tests
◆ Assess overdose (peripheral edema, heat intolerance, diaphoresis, palpitations, dysrhythmias, severe tachycardia, increased temp, delirium, CNS irritability); product should be discontinued
• Assess for hypersensitivity (rash, enlarged cervical lymph nodes); product may have to be discontinued
• Assess for hypoprothrombinemia (bleeding, petechiae, ecchymosis)
• Monitor clinical response: after 3 wk should include increased weight, decreased pulse, decreased T$_4$
• Assess for bone marrow depression: sore throat, fever, fatigue

Nursing diagnoses
• Knowledge, deficient (teaching)
• Noncompliance (teaching)

Implementation
• Give with meals to decrease GI upset
• Give at same time each day to maintain product level
• Give lowest dosage that relieves symptoms
• Store in light-resistant container
• Increase fluids to 3-4 L/day, unless contraindicated

P

Adverse effects: *italic* = common, **bold** = life-threatening

Patient/family education

• Advise patient to abstain from breastfeeding after delivery; product appears in breast milk
• Teach patient to take pulse daily and to keep graph of weight, pulse, mood
• Advise patient to report redness, swelling, sore throat, mouth lesions, which indicate blood dyscrasias
• Caution patient to avoid OTC products that contain iodine; that seafood, other iodine-containing foods may be restricted by prescriber
• Caution patient not to discontinue this medication abruptly; thyroid crisis may occur; stress patient compliance
• Teach patient that response may take several mo if thyroid is large
• Teach patient symptoms/signs of overdose: periorbital edema, cold intolerance, mental depression; notify prescriber at once
• Teach patient symptoms of inadequate dose: tachycardia, diarrhea, fever, irritability; prescriber should be notified to adjust dosage
• Teach patient to take medication exactly as prescribed, not to skip or double doses; missed doses should be taken when remembered up to 1 hr before next dose
• Instruct patient to carry/wear emergency identification indicating medication taken and condition being treated

Evaluation

Positive therapeutic outcome
• Weight gain
• Decreased pulse
• Decreased T_4
• Decreased B/P

protamine (Rx)
(proe'ta-meen)
Func. class.: Heparin antagonist
Chem. class.: Low-molecular-weight protein

Pregnancy category C

Action: Binds heparin, making it ineffective

Therapeutic outcome: Prevention of heparin overdose

Uses: Heparin overdose; neutralizes heparin in procedures, hemorrhage

Dosage and routes
Adult and child: **IV** 1 mg of protamine/100 units of heparin given or 100 anti-XA units of LMWH; administer slowly over 1-3 min; max 50 mg/10 min

Available forms: Inj 10 mg/ml

Adverse effects
CNS: Lassitude, flushing
CV: Hypotension, bradycardia, **circulatory collapse,** capillary leak
GI: Nausea, vomiting, anorexia
HEMA: Bleeding
INTEG: Rash, dermatitis, urticaria
RESP: Dyspnea, **pulmonary edema, severe respiratory distress, bronchospasm**
SYST: **Anaphylaxis, angioedema**

Contraindication: Hypersensitivity

Precautions: Pregnancy **C**, breastfeeding, fish allergy, diabetes, previous exposure to protamine, insulins, heparin rebound or bleeding

Pharmacokinetics
Absorption	Completely absorbed
Distribution	Unknown
Metabolism	Unknown
Excretion	Unknown
Half-life	Unknown

Pharmacodynamics
Onset	5 min
Peak	Unknown
Duration	2 hr

NURSING CONSIDERATIONS
Assessment
• Monitor blood studies (Hct, platelets, occult blood stools) q3mo
• Monitor coagulation tests (APTT, ACT) 15 min after dose, then in several hr
• Monitor VS, B/P, pulse q30min, plus 3 hr after dose
◆ Assess for hypersensitivity: skin rash, urticaria, dermatitis, cough, wheezing, have emergency equipment nearby; men who have had a vasectomy may be more prone to hypersensitivity
◆ Assess for allergy to salmon; use with caution in these patients

Nursing diagnoses
• Injury, risk for (uses)
• Knowledge, deficient (teaching)
• Tissue perfusion, ineffective (uses)

Implementation
• Give by direct **IV** after diluting 50 mg/5 ml of sterile bacteriostatic water for inj; shake; give 20 mg or less over 1-3 min
• Give by intermittent inf after further diluting with equal volume of NaCl or D_5W and run over 2-3 hr; titrate to APTT, ACT; use inf pump

- Too rapid inf leads to hypotension, anaphylactoid reactions
- Store at 36°-46° F (2°-8° C)

Additive compatibilities: Cimetidine, ranitidine, verapamil

Additive incompatibilities: Penicillins, cephalosporins

Patient/family education
- Explain reason for medication and expected results; not to take if allergic to fish
- Caution patient to avoid contact activities that may result in bleeding

Evaluation
Positive therapeutic outcome
- Reversal of heparin overdose

---

pseudoephedrine (OTC)
(soo-doe-e-fed'rin)
Afrin, Allermed, Cenafed, Children's Congestion Relief, Children's Silfedrine, Congestion Relief, Decofed Syrup, DeFed-60, Dorcol Children's Decongestant, Drixoral Non-Drowsy Formula, Dynafed, Efidac/24, Eltor ♦, Genaphed, Halofed, Mini Thin Pseudo, pseudoephedrine HCl, Pseudo, Pseudogest, Scudotabs, Sinustop Pro, Sudafed, Sudafed 12 hour, Sudex, Triaminic AM Decongestant Formula
Func. class.: Adrenergic
Chem. class.: Substituted phenylethylamine

Pregnancy category C

Action: Primary activity through α-adrenergic effects on respiratory mucosal membranes reducing congestion, hyperemia, edema; minimal bronchodilatation secondary to β-adrenergic effects

Therapeutic outcome: Decreased nasal congestion, swelling

Uses: Nasal decongestant, otitis media adjustment, adjunct with antihistamines

Dosage and routes
Adult and child >12 yr: PO 60 mg q6hr; EXT REL 120 mg q12hr or 240 mg q24hr
Geriatric: PO 30-60 mg q6hr prn
Child 6-12 yr: PO 30 mg q6hr, max 120 mg/day
Child 2-6 yr: PO 15 mg q6hr, max 60 mg/day

Available forms: Ext rel caps 120, 240 mg; oral sol 15 mg, 30 mg/5 ml; drops 7.5 mg/0.8 ml; tabs 30, 60 mg; caps 60 mg; ext rel tabs 120, 240 mg

Adverse effects
CNS: Tremors, anxiety, stimulation, insomnia, headache, dizziness, hallucinations, **seizures** (geriatric)
CV: Palpitations, tachycardia, hypertension, chest pain, **dysrhythmias, CV collapse**
EENT: Dry nose, irritation of nose and throat
GI: Anorexia, nausea, vomiting, dry mouth
GU: Dysuria

Contraindications: Hypersensitivity to sympathomimetics, closed-angle glaucoma

Precautions: Pregnancy **C,** breastfeeding, cardiac disorders, hyperthyroidism, diabetes mellitus, prostatic hypertrophy, hypertension

Pharmacokinetics	
Absorption	Well absorbed
Distribution	Enters CSF, crosses placenta
Metabolism	Liver, partially
Excretion	Kidneys, unchanged (75%); breast milk
Half-life	7 hr

Pharmacodynamics		
	PO	PO-EXT REL
Onset	15-30 min	1 hr
Peak	Unknown	Unknown
Duration	4-6 hr	12 hr

Interactions
Individual products
Methyldopa: decreased effect of pseudoephedrine
Drug classifications
Antidepressants (tricyclics), MAOIs: hypertensive crisis, do not use together
Rauwolfia alkaloids, urinary acidifiers: decreased effect of pseudoephedrine
Urinary alkalizers: increased effect of pseudoephedrine

NURSING CONSIDERATIONS
Assessment
- Assess for CNS side effects in the geriatric: excitation, seizures, hallucinations
- Monitor for nasal congestion; auscultate lung sounds; check for tenacious bronchial secretions; children with otitis media should be assessed for eustachian tube congestion
- Monitor B/P and pulse throughout treatment

Nursing diagnoses
- Airway clearance, ineffective (uses)
- Knowledge, deficient (teaching)

Implementation
- Swallow tab and ext rel cap whole; do not break, crush, or chew

P

Adverse effects: *italic* = common, **bold** = life-threatening

- Give several hr before bedtime if insomnia occurs
- Store at room temperature

Patient/family education
- Teach patient reason for product administration and expected results
- Instruct patient not to use continuously, or more than recommended dose; rebound congestion may occur
- Advise patient to check with prescriber before using other products, as product interactions may occur
- Advise patient to avoid taking near bedtime; stimulation can occur
- Caution patient not to use if stimulation, restlessness, tremors occur
- Notify parents of possible excessive agitation in children
🔶 Advise patient to notify prescriber of anxiety, slow or fast heart rate, dyspnea, seizures

Evaluation
Positive therapeutic outcome
- Decreased nasal congestion

---

pseudoephedrine nasal agent
See Appendix B

---

psyllium (OTC)
(sill'i-um)
Fiberall, Fiberall Natural Flavor and Orange Flavor, Genfiber, Hydrocil Instant, Karacil ✤, Konsyl, Konsyl Orange, Maalox Daily Fiber Therapy, Metamucil, Metamucil Lemon Lime, Metamucil Orange Flavor, Metamucil Sugar Free, Metamucil Sugar Free Orange Flavor, Modane Bulk, Mylanta Natural Fiber Supplement, Natural Fiber Laxative, Natural Fiber Laxative Sugar Free, Natural Vegetable Reguloid, Prodiem Plain ✤, Reguloid Natural, Reguloid Orange, Reguloid Sugar Free Orange, Reguloid Sugar Free Regular, Restore, Restore Sugar Free, Serutan, Syllact
Func. class.: Laxative, bulk-forming
Chem. class.: Psyllium colloid

Pregnancy category C

Action: Promotes peristalsis by combining with water in the intestine to form a gel-like substance that is easily evacuated

Therapeutic outcome: Decreased constipation, decreased diarrhea in colitis

Uses: Chronic constipation, ulcerative colitis, irritable bowel syndrome

Dosage and routes
Adult: PO 1-2 tsp in 8 oz of water bid or tid, then 8 oz of water or 1 premeasured packet in 8 oz of water bid or tid, then 8 oz of water
Child >6 yr: 1 tsp in 4 oz of water at bedtime

Available forms: Chew pieces 1.7, 3.4 g/piece; powder effervescent 3.4, 3.7 g/packet; powder 3.3, 3.4, 3.5, 4.94 g/tsp; wafers 3.4 g/wafer

Adverse effects
GI: *Nausea, vomiting, anorexia, diarrhea,* cramps, intestinal/esophageal blockage

Contraindications: Hypersensitivity, intestinal obstruction, abdominal pain, nausea/vomiting, fecal impaction

Precautions: Pregnancy **C**

Pharmacokinetics
Absorption	None
Distribution	None
Metabolism	Unknown
Excretion	Feces
Half-life	Unknown

Pharmacodynamics
Onset	12-24 hr
Peak	2-4 days
Duration	Unknown

Interactions
Drug classifications
Cardiac glycosides, oral anticoagulants, salicylates: decreased absorption of each specific product
Drug/herb
Flax, senna: increased laxative

NURSING CONSIDERATIONS
Assessment
- Monitor blood, urine electrolytes if used often by patient; check I&O ratio to identify fluid loss
- Assess for cramping, rectal bleeding, nausea, vomiting; if these symptoms occur, product should be discontinued; identify cause of constipation; identify whether fluids, bulk, or exercise is missing from lifestyle
- Assess stool for color, consistency, amount, presence of flatulence

Nursing diagnoses
- Constipation (uses)
- Knowledge, deficient (teaching)
- Noncompliance (teaching)

Implementation
- Give alone for better absorption; give after mixing with water immediately before use; administer with 8 oz of water or juice followed by another 8 oz of fluid
- Administer in AM or PM (oral dose)
- Shake susp well

Patient/family education
- Discuss with patient that adequate fluid consumption is necessary
- Teach patient that normal bowel movements do not always occur daily
- Caution patient not to use in presence of abdominal pain, nausea, vomiting; tell patient to notify prescriber if constipation is unrelieved or if symptoms of electrolyte imbalance occur (muscle cramps, pain, weakness, dizziness, excessive thirst)
- Teach patient not to use laxatives for long-term therapy; bowel tone will be lost and will decrease
- Teach patient not to take at bedtime as a laxative; may interfere with sleep; also problems with lipid pneumonia
- Teach patient not to use with food or vitamin preparations; delays digestion and absorption of fat-soluble vitamins

Evaluation
Positive therapeutic outcome
- Decreased constipation in 12-24 hr

---

pyrazinamide (Rx)
(peer-a-zin′a-mide)
PMS Pyrazinamide ✤, pyrazinamide, Tebrazid ✤
Func. class.: Antitubercular agent
Chem. class.: Pyrazinoic acid amine/nicoturimide analog

Pregnancy category C

Action: Bactericidal interference with lipid; nucleic acid biosynthesis is possible

Therapeutic outcome: Bactericidal for *Mycobacterium* species

Uses: Tuberculosis, as an adjunct when other products are not feasible

Dosage and routes
HIV negative
Adult: PO 15-30 mg/kg/day, max 2 g/day
Child: PO 7.5-15 mg/kg bid or 15-30 mg/kg/day, max 2 g

HIV positive
Adult: PO 15-30 mg/kg/day, max 2 g × 2 mo used with a rifamycin

Child: PO 20-40 mg/kg/day, max 2 g/day × 2 mo given with a rifamycin

Renal dose
Adult: PO CCr 10-50 ml/min, give dose q48-72hr; CCr <10 ml/min give dose q72hr

Available forms: Tabs 500 mg

Adverse effects
CNS: Headache
GI: **Hepatotoxicity,** abnormal liver function tests, peptic ulcer, nausea, vomiting, anorexia, cramps, diarrhea
GU: Urinary difficulty, increased uric acid
HEMA: **Hemolytic anemia**
INTEG: Photosensitivity, urticaria

Contraindications: Hypersensitivity, severe hepatic damage, acute gout

Precautions: Pregnancy C, child <13 yr, renal failure, diabetes, porphyria, chronic gout

Pharmacokinetics
Absorption	Well absorbed
Distribution	Widely distributed
Metabolism	Liver, extensively
Excretion	Kidneys, breast milk
Half-life	9-10 hr

Pharmacodynamics
Onset	Unknown
Peak	2 hr
Duration	9½ hr; metabolites 12 hr

Interactions
Drug/lab test
Increased: PBI
Decreased: 17-KS

NURSING CONSIDERATIONS
Assessment
- C&S studies should be done before treatment begins, periodically during treatment
- Monitor serum uric acid, which may be elevated and cause gout symptoms
- Monitor liver function tests weekly: ALT, AST, bilirubin; hepatic status: decreased appetite, jaundice, dark urine, fatigue
- Monitor renal status before treatment, monthly thereafter: BUN, creatinine, output, specific gravity, urinalysis, uric acid
- Monitor mental status often: affect, mood, behavioral changes; psychosis may occur

Nursing diagnoses
- Diarrhea (adverse reactions)
- Infection, risk for (uses)
- Injury, risk for (adverse reactions)
- Knowledge, deficient (teaching)
- Noncompliance (teaching)

P

Adverse effects: *italic* = common, **bold** = life-threatening

Implementation

- Give with meals to decrease GI symptoms
- Give antiemetic if vomiting occurs
- May be given with other antitubercular products

Patient/family education

- Instruct patient that compliance with dosage schedule, duration is necessary; that scheduled appointments must be kept or relapse may occur
- Advise diabetic patient to use blood glucose monitor to obtain correct result
- Advise patient to report weakness, fatigue, loss of appetite, nausea, vomiting, yellowing of skin or eyes, tingling/numbness of hands/feet

Evaluation

Positive therapeutic outcome

- Decreased symptoms of TB
- Sputum culture negative × 3

---

pyridostigmine (Rx)

(peer-id-oh-stig′meen)

Mestinon, Mestinon SR, Mestinon Timespan, Regonol

Func. class.: Cholinergic, anticholinesterase
Chem. class.: Tertiary amine carbamate

Pregnancy category C

Action: Inhibits destruction of acetylcholine, which increases concentration at sites where acetylcholine is released; this facilitates transmission of impulses across myoneural junction

Therapeutic outcome: Decreased action of nondepolarizing muscle relaxant; increased muscle strength in myasthenia gravis

Uses: Nondepolarizing muscle relaxant antagonist, myasthenia gravis

Dosage and routes

Myasthenia gravis

Adult: PO 600 mg/day in 5-6 divided doses, max 1.5 g/day; IM/**IV** 2 mg or 1/30 of PO dose; SUS REL 180-540 mg/day or bid at intervals of at least 6 hr

Child: PO 7 mg/kg/day in 5-6 divided doses; IM/**IV** 0.05-0.15 mg/kg/dose

Nondepolarizing neuromuscular blocker antagonist

Adult: 0.6-1.2 mg **IV** atropine, then 0.1-0.25 mg/kg/dose

Child: IV 0.1-0.25 mg/kg/dose

Available forms: Tabs 60 mg; ext rel tabs 180 mg; syr 60 mg/5 ml; inj 5 mg/ml

Adverse effects

CNS: Dizziness, headache, sweating, weakness, **seizures,** uncoordination, paralysis, drowsiness, LOC

CV: Tachycardia, dysrhythmias, bradycardia, AV block, hypotension, ECG changes, **cardiac arrest,** syncope

EENT: Miosis, blurred vision, lacrimation, visual changes

GI: Nausea, diarrhea, vomiting, cramps, increased salivary and gastric secretions, peristalsis

GU: Frequency, incontinence, urgency

INTEG: Rash, urticaria, flushing

RESP: **Respiratory depression, bronchospasm, constriction, laryngospasm, respiratory arrest**

Contraindications: Bradycardia, hypotension, obstruction of intestine, renal system, bromide, benzyl alcohol sensitivity, cholinesterase inhibitor toxicity

Precautions: Pregnancy C, seizure disorders, bronchial asthma, coronary occlusion, hyperthyroidism, dysrhythmias, peptic ulcer, megacolon, poor GI motility

Pharmacokinetics

Absorption	Poorly absorbed (PO)
Distribution	Widely distributed, crosses placenta
Metabolism	Liver, plasma cholinesterase
Excretion	Kidneys
Half-life	2 hr (**IV**); 4 hr (PO)

Pharmacodynamics

	PO	PO-EXT REL	IM/IV
Onset	20-30 min	½-1 hr	2-15 min
Peak	Unknown	Unknown	Unknown
Duration	3-6 hr	3-6 hr	2-4 hr

Interactions

Individual drugs

Atropine, gallamine, metocurine, pancuronium, tubocurarine: decreased action

Decamethonium, succinylcholine: increased action of pyridostigmine

Magnesium, mecamylamine, polymyxin, procainamide, quinidine: decreased action of pyridostigmine

Drug classifications

Aminoglycosides, anesthetics, antidysrhythmics, corticosteroids, quinolones: decreased action of pyridostigmine

Drug/herb

Jaborandi tree, pill-bearing spurge: increased effect

NURSING CONSIDERATIONS
Assessment
- Monitor VS, respiration; increased B/P during test and at baseline
- Monitor diabetic patient carefully, since this product lowers blood glucose

Nursing diagnoses
- Breathing pattern, ineffective (uses)
- Knowledge, deficient (teaching)

Implementation
PO route
- Give only after all other cholinergics have been discontinued
- Give increased doses as ordered if tolerance occurs
- Give larger doses as ordered after exercise or fatigue
- Give on empty stomach for better absorption
- Store at room temperature

IV route
- Give **IV** undiluted, give through Y-tube or 3-way stopcock; give 0.5 mg or less/min
- Give only when atropine sulfate available for cholinergic crisis

Syringe compatibilities: Glycopyrrolate
Y-site compatibilities: Heparin, hydrocortisone, potassium chloride, vit B/C

Patient/family education
- Advise patient to carry/wear emergency ID specifying myasthenia gravis, products taken

Evaluation
Positive therapeutic outcome
- Increased muscle strength, hand grasp
- Improved gait
- Absence of labored breathing (if severe)

Treatment of overdose: Discontinue product, atropine 1-4 mg **IV**

---

pyridoxine (vitamin B₆)
(OTC, Rx)
(peer-i-dox'een)
Beesix, Doxine, Nestrex, Pyri, pyridoxine HCl, Rodex, Vitabee 6, Vitamin B₆
Func. class.: Vitamin B₆, water soluble

Pregnancy category A

Action: Needed for fat, protein, carbohydrate metabolism; enhances glycogen release from liver and muscle tissue; needed as coenzyme for metabolic transformations of a variety of amino acids

Therapeutic outcome: Absence of vit B₆ deficiency

Uses: Vitamin B₆ deficiency associated with the following: inborn errors of metabolism, seizures, cycloSERINE, hydrALAZINE penicillamine, isoniazid therapy, oral contraceptives, alcoholism, polyneuritis

Unlabeled uses: Palmar-plantar erythrodysesthesia syndrome

Dosage and routes
RDA
Adult: PO (male) 1.7-2 mg; (female) 1.4-1.6 mg
Child 9-13 yr: PO 1 mg/day
Child 4-8 yr: PO 0.6 mg/day
Child 1-3 yr: PO 0.5 mg/day
Infant 7-12 mo: PO 0.3 mg/day

Vitamin B₆ deficiency
Adult: PO/IM/**IV** 2.5-25 mg/day × 3 wk
Child: PO/IM/**IV** 10 mg until desired response

Deficiency caused by isoniazid, cycloSERINE, hydrALAZINE, penicillamine
Adult: PO 100-300 mg/day
Child: PO 10-50 mg/day

Prevention of deficiency caused by isoniazid, cycloSERINE, hydrALAZINE, penicillamine
Adult: PO 25-100 mg/day
Child: PO 1.2 mg/kg/day

Palmar-plantar erythrodysesthesia syndrome (unlabeled)
Adult: PO 50-150 mg/day

Available forms: Tabs 10, 25, 50, 100 mg; ext rel tabs 100 mg; inj 100 mg/ml; ext rel caps 150 mg

Adverse effects
CNS: Paresthesia, flushing, warmth, lethargy (rare with normal renal function)
INTEG: Pain at inj site

Contraindication: Hypersensitivity

Precautions: Pregnancy A, breastfeeding, children, Parkinson's disease, patients taking levodopa should avoid supplemental vitamins with >5 mg pyridoxine

P

Pharmacokinetics

Absorption	Well absorbed (PO)
Distribution	Stored in liver, muscle, brain; crosses placenta
Metabolism	Unknown
Excretion	Kidneys, unchanged (not used)
Half-life	Unknown

Pharmacodynamics

Unknown

Interactions
Individual drugs
Chloramphenicol, cycloSERINE, hydrALAZINE, isoniazid, penicillamine: decreased effects of pyridoxine
Levodopa: decreased effects of levodopa
Drug classifications
Contraceptives (oral), immunosuppressants: decreased effects of pyridoxine

NURSING CONSIDERATIONS
Assessment
• Monitor pyridoxine levels throughout treatment
• Assess nutritional status: yeast, liver, legumes, bananas, green vegetables, whole grains
• Assess for pyridoxine (B_6) deficiency: nausea, vomiting, dermatitis, cheilosis, seizures, irritability, dermatitis before, during treatment
• Assess neurologic status: paresthesia, lethargy
• Monitor blood tests: Hct, Hgb

Nursing diagnoses
• Knowledge, deficient (teaching)
• Noncompliance (teaching, overuse)
• Nutrition: less than body requirements, imbalanced (uses)

Implementation
PO route
• Swallow ext rel cap and ext rel tabs whole; do not break, crush, or chew
IM route
• Rotate sites to avoid pain; burning or stinging at site may occur; give by Z-track to minimize pain
• Store in airtight, light-resistant container
IV route
• Give **IV** undiluted or added to most **IV** sol; give 50 mg or less/1 min if undiluted
Syringe compatibilities:
Doxapram
Additive incompatibilities:
Erythromycin, iron salts, kanamycin, riboflavin, streptomycin

Patient/family education
• Teach patient to avoid other vitamin supplements unless directed by prescriber
• Advise patient to increase meat, bananas, potatoes, lima beans, whole grain cereals in diet which are high in vit B_6
• Caution patient not to increase dosage, since serious reactions may occur

Evaluation
Positive therapeutic outcome
• Absence of nausea, vomiting, anorexia, skin lesions, glossitis, stomatitis, edema, seizures, restlessness, paresthesia

---

pyrimethamine (Rx)
(peer-i-meth′a-meen)
Daraprim, Fansidar (with sulfadoxine)
Func. class.: Antimalarial, antiprotozoal
Chem. class.: Folic acid antagonist
Pregnancy category C

Action: Inhibits folic acid metabolism in parasite; prevents transmission by stopping growth of fertilized gametes

Therapeutic outcome: Prevention of malaria

Uses: Malaria prophylaxis, antiprotozoal action against *Plasmodium vivax, Pneumocystis jiroveci*

Dosage and routes
Prophylaxis of malaria
• Begin 2 wk before entering endemic area and continue for 6-10 wk after return
Adult and child >10 yr: PO 25 mg qwk
Child 4-10 yr: PO 12.5 mg qwk
Child <4 yr: PO 6.25 mg qwk

Toxoplasmosis
Adult: PO 50-75 mg, then reduce by about 50% for 4-5 wk, with 4 g sulfADIAZINE q6hr
Child: PO 1 mg/kg/day in 2 divided doses or 2 mg/kg/day × 3 days, then 1 mg/kg/day or divided twice daily × 4 wk, max 25 mg/day

Toxoplasmosis in AIDS patients
Adult: PO 100-200 mg/day × 1-2 days, then 50-100 mg/day × 3-6 wk, then 25-50 mg/day for life (given with clindamycin or sulfADIAZINE)

Available forms: Tabs 25 mg; combo tabs 500 mg sulfadoxine/25 mg pyrimethamine

Adverse effects
CNS: Stimulation, irritability, **seizures,** tremors, ataxia, fatigue, fever
CV: **Dysrhythmias**

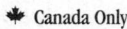 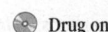

GI: *Nausea, vomiting, cramps, anorexia,* diarrhea, atrophic glossitis, gastritis
HEMA: Thrombocytopenia, leukopenia, pancytopenia, megaloblastic anemia, decreased folic acid, **agranulocytosis**
INTEG: Skin eruptions, photosensitivity, **Stevens-Johnson syndrome**
RESP: Respiratory failure

Contraindications: Hypersensitivity, chloroquine-resistant malaria, megaloblastic anemia caused by folate deficiency

Precautions: Pregnancy C, breastfeeding, geriatric patients, blood dyscrasias, seizure disorder, glucose-6-phosphate dehydrogenase disease, renal/hepatic disease

Pharmacokinetics

Absorption	Well absorbed
Distribution	Widely; crosses placenta
Metabolism	Liver, extensively
Excretion	Kidneys, unchanged (30%); breast milk
Half-life	4 days

Pharmacodynamics

Onset	Unknown
Peak	2 hr
Duration	Unknown

Interactions
Individual drugs
Folic acid: increased synergistic action
Radiation: increased bone marrow suppression
Zidovudine: increased risk of megaloblastic anemia, agranulocytosis, thrombocytopenia
Drug classifications
Bone marrow depressants, folate antagonists: increased bone marrow suppression

NURSING CONSIDERATIONS
Assessment
• C&S studies should be done before treatment begins and periodically during treatment
• Monitor serum uric acid, which may be elevated and cause gout symptoms
• Monitor liver function tests weekly: ALT, AST, bilirubin; hepatic status: decreased appetite, jaundice, dark urine, fatigue
• Monitor renal status before therapy, monthly thereafter: BUN, creatinine, output, specific gravity, urinalysis
• Monitor mental status often: affect, mood, behavioral changes; psychosis may occur

Nursing diagnoses
• Diarrhea (adverse reactions)
• Infection, risk for (uses)

• Injury, risk for (adverse reactions)
• Knowledge, deficient (teaching)
• Noncompliance (teaching)

Implementation
• Give with meals to decrease GI symptoms
• Give antiemetic if vomiting occurs

Patient/family education
• Instruct patient that compliance with dosage schedule, duration is necessary; that scheduled appointments must be kept or relapse may occur
• Advise diabetic patient to use blood glucose monitor to obtain correct result
• Advise patient to report weakness, fatigue, loss of appetite, nausea, vomiting, yellowing of skin or eyes, sore throat, glossitis

Evaluation
Positive therapeutic outcome
• Decreased symptoms of toxoplasmosis
• Decreased symptoms of *Pneumocystis jiroveci* pneumonia

---

quetiapine (Rx)
(kwe-tie'a-peen)
Seroquel, Seroquel XR
Func. class.: Antipsychotic
Chem. class.: Dibenzodiazepine
Pregnancy category C

Action: Functions as an antagonist at multiple neurotransmitter receptors in the brain including 5-HT$_{1A}$, 5-HT$_2$, dopamine D$_1$, D$_2$, H$_1$, adrenergic α_1, α_2 receptors

Therapeutic outcome: Decreased hallucinations and disorganized thought

Uses: Bipolar disorder, bipolar I disorder, depression, mania, schizophrenia

Dosage and routes
Bipolar I disorder
Adult: PO (monotherapy or as adjunct to lithium or divalproex) 50 mg bid on day 1, 100 mg on day 2 in 2 divided doses as tolerated to 400 mg on day 4; range 400-800 mg/day

Psychotic disorders
Adult: PO 25 mg bid, titrate upward; XR: 300 mg/day in PM

Available forms: Tabs 25, 50, 100, 200, 300, 400 mg; ext rel tab 200, 300, 400 mg

Adverse effects
CNS: EPS, pseudoparkinsonism, akathisia, dystonia, tardive dyskinesia, drowsiness, insomnia, agitation, anxiety, *headache*, sei-

Adverse effects: *italic* = common, **bold** = life-threatening

zures, **neuroleptic malignant syndrome,** dizziness, dystonia, restless legs syndrome
CV: Orthostatic hypotension, **tachycardia,** QT prolongation, CV disease, Parkinson's disease, cardiomyopathy, myocarditis
ENDO: SIADH, hyperglycemia
GI: Nausea, anorexia, constipation, abdominal pain, dry mouth
HEMA: **Leukopenia, agranulocytosis**
INTEG: Rash
META: Hyponatremia
MISC: Asthenia, back pain, fever, ear pain
MS: **Rhabdomyolysis**
RESP: Rhinitis
SYST: **Stevens-Johnson syndrome, anaphylaxis**

Contraindications: Hypersensitivity

Precautions: Pregnancy **C**, breastfeeding, geriatric, long-term use, seizures, hepatic disease, breast cancer, QT prolongation, CV disease, Parkinson's, brain tumor, hematological disease, torsades de pointes, cataracts, dehydration

Black Box Warning: Children, suicidal ideation, dementia

Pharmacokinetics

Absorption	Rapidly
Distribution	Widely
Metabolism	Liver, extensively; inhibits P450 CYP3A4 enzyme system; 83% protein binding
Excretion	Urine, feces
Half-life	≥6 hr

Pharmacodynamics

Onset	Unknown
Peak	1.5 hr
Duration	Up to 12 hr

Interactions
Individual drugs
Alcohol: increased CNS depression
Bepridil, chloroquine, clarithromycin, droperidol, erythromycin, grepafloxacin, halofantrine, haloperidol, methadone, pentamidine, probucol, sparfloxacin: increased QT prolongation
Carbamazepine, phenytoin, rifampin, thioridazine: increased quetiapine clearance
Cimetidine: decreased quetiapine clearance
Erythromycin: increased effects of erythromycin
Fluconazole, itraconazole, ketoconazole: increased action of quetiapine
Levodopa: decreased effect of levodopa
Lorazepam: decreased effect of lorazepam

Drug classifications
Analgesics (opioid), antihistamines, sedatives/hypnotics: increased CNS depression
Barbiturates, glucocorticoids: increased clearance of quetiapine
β-agonists, class IA/III antidysrhythmics, local anesthetics, phenothiazines (some), tricyclics: increased QT prolongation
DOPamine agonists: decreased effects of DOPamine agonists
Drug/herb
Cola tree, hops, nettle, nutmeg: increased action
Betel palm, kava: increased EPS

NURSING CONSIDERATIONS
Assessment
• Assess CV status: QT prolongation, tachycardia, orthostatic B/P
• Assess mental status: orientation, mood, AIMS assessment, presence and type of hallucinations before initial administration, monthly; this product should significantly reduce psychotic behavior
• Check that patient swallows all PO medication; check for hoarding or giving of medication to other patients
• Obtain baselines in blood glucose, liver function tests, neurologic status, ophthalmologic exam, cholesterol profile, weight
• Assess affect, orientation, LOC, reflexes, gait, coordination, sleep pattern disturbances
• Monitor B/P with patient in sitting, standing, and lying positions; take pulse and respirations q4hr during initial treatment; establish baseline before starting treatment; report drops of 30 mm Hg; obtain baseline ECG and monitor Q- and T-wave changes
• Check for dizziness, faintness, palpitations, tachycardia on rising; severe orthostatic hypotension is common
◆ Identify for neuroleptic malignant syndrome: hyperpyrexia, muscle rigidity, increased CPK, altered mental status, seizures, tachycardia, diaphoresis, hyper/hypotension, fatigue; product should be discontinued and prescriber notified immediately
• Assess for EPS including akathisia (inability to sit still, no pattern to movements), tardive dyskinesia (bizarre movements of the jaw, mouth, tongue, extremities), pseudoparkinsonism (rigidity, tremors, pill rolling, shuffling gait); an antiparkinson product should be prescribed

Nursing diagnoses
• Coping, ineffective (uses)
• Knowledge, deficient (teaching)
• Noncompliance (teaching)

 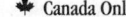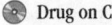

quinapril   863

Implementation
- PO with full glass of water, milk; or give with food to decrease GI upset
- Store in airtight, light-resistant container

Patient/family education
- Teach patient to use good oral hygiene; frequent rinsing of mouth, sugarless gum for dry mouth
- Caution patient to avoid hazardous activities until product response is determined; dizziness, blurred vision may occur
- Inform patient that orthostatic hypotension occurs often; patient should rise from sitting or lying position gradually; avoid hot tubs, hot showers, and tub baths because hypotension may occur
- Inform patient that heat stroke may occur in hot weather, and to take extra precautions to stay cool
- Advise patient to avoid abrupt withdrawal of this product or EPS may result; product should be withdrawn slowly
- Teach patient to avoid OTC preparations (cough, hayfever, cold) unless approved by prescriber; serious product interactions may occur; avoid use with alcohol, CNS depressants because increased drowsiness may occur

Evaluation
Positive therapeutic outcome
- Decrease in emotional excitement, hallucinations, delusions, paranoia
- Reorganization of patterns of thought, speech

Treatment of overdose: Lavage, provide airway

---

quinapril (Rx)
(kwin′a-pril)
Accupril
Func. class.: Antihypertensive
Chem. class.: Angiotensin-converting enzyme (ACE) inhibitor
Pregnancy category D

Action: Selectively suppresses renin-angiotensin-aldosterone system; inhibits ACE, prevents conversion of angiotensin I to angiotensin II; results in dilatation of arterial, venous vessels

Therapeutic outcome: Decreased B/P in hypertension

Uses: Hypertension, alone or in combination with thiazide diuretics, systolic CHF

Dosage and routes
Hypertension (monotherapy)
Adult: PO 10-20 mg/day initially, then 20-80 mg/day divided bid or daily
Geriatric: PO 10 mg/day, titrate to desired response

Congestive heart failure
Adult: PO 5 mg bid, may increase qwk until 20-40 mg/day in 2 divided doses

Renal dose
Adult: PO CCr 30-60 ml/min 5 mg/day initially; CCr <30 ml/min 2.5 mg/day initially

Available forms: Tabs 5, 10, 20, 40 mg

Adverse effects
CNS: Headache, dizziness, fatigue, somnolence, depression, malaise, nervousness, vertigo
CV: Hypotension, postural hypotension, syncope, palpitations, angina pectoris, **MI, tachycardia,** vasodilatation, chest pain
GI: Nausea, diarrhea, constipation, vomiting, gastritis, **GI hemorrhage,** dry mouth
GU: Increased BUN, creatinine, decreased libido, impotence
HEMA: **Thrombocytopenia, agranulocytosis**
INTEG: **Angioedema,** rash, sweating, photosensitivity, pruritus
META: Hyperkalemia
MISC: Back pain, amblyopia
MS: Myalgia
RESP: Cough, pharyngitis, dyspnea

Contraindications: Children, hypersensitivity to ACE inhibitors, angioedema
Black Box Warning: Pregnancy **D**

Precautions: Breastfeeding, geriatric, impaired renal/liver function, dialysis patients, hypovolemia, blood dyscrasias, COPD, asthma, bilateral renal stenosis, cough

Pharmacokinetics
Absorption	Well absorbed
Distribution	Unknown, crosses placenta
Metabolism	Unknown
Excretion	Urine (60%), feces (37%)
Half-life	2 hr

Pharmacodynamics
Onset	½-1 hr
Peak	2-6 hr
Duration	12-24 hr

Adverse effects: *italic* = common, **bold** = life-threatening

Interactions
Individual drugs
Alcohol: increased hypotension (large amounts)

Digoxin, lithium: increased toxicity

Hydralazine, prazosin: use caution

Indomethacin: decreased antihypertensive effect of quinapril

Tetracycline: decreased absorption of tetracycline

Drug classifications
Adrenergic blockers, antihypertensives, diuretics, ganglionic blockers, nitrates, phenothiazines: increased hypotension

Diuretics (potassium sparing), potassium supplements, sympathomimetics, vasodilators: use caution

Drug/herb
Aconite: increased toxicity, death

Astragalus, cola tree: increased or decreased antihypertensive effect

Barberry, betony, black catechu, black cohosh, bloodroot, broom, burdock, cat's claw, dandelion, goldenseal, hawthorn, Irish moss, Jamaican dogwood, kelp, khella, mistletoe, parsley: increased antihypertensive effect

Coltsfoot, guarana, khat, licorice, yohimbe: decreased antihypertensive effect

Drug/lab test
False positive: urine acetone, ANA titer

NURSING CONSIDERATIONS
Assessment
• Monitor blood studies: neutrophils, decreased platelets; WBC with differential baseline, periodically q3mo; if neutrophils <1000/mm³ discontinue treatment

• Monitor B/P, check for orthostatic hypotension, syncope; if changes occur, dosage change may be required

• Monitor renal function tests (protein, BUN, creatinine) and periodically liver function tests, uric acid; glucose may be elevated; watch for increased levels that may indicate nephrotic syndrome and renal failure; monitor renal symptoms: polyuria, oliguria, frequency, dysuria

• Check potassium levels throughout treatment, although hyperkalemia rarely occurs

• Check for edema in feet, legs daily, weight daily in CHF

• Assess for allergic reactions: rash, fever, pruritus, urticaria; product should be discontinued if antihistamines fail to help

Nursing diagnoses
• Cardiac output, decreased (uses)
• Injury, risk for (adverse reactions)

• Knowledge, deficient (teaching)
• Noncompliance (teaching)

Implementation
• Tabs may be crushed if necessary
• Store in airtight container at 86° F (30° C) or less
• Severe hypotension may occur after 1st dose of this medication; may be prevented by reducing or discontinuing diuretic therapy 3 days before beginning quinapril therapy

Patient/family education
• Advise patient not to discontinue product abruptly; advise patient to tell all persons associated with care

• Teach patient not to use OTC products (cough, cold, allergy) unless directed by physician; serious side effects can occur

• Inform patient that xanthines such as coffee, tea, chocolate, cola can prevent action of product

• Caution patient on the importance of complying with dosage schedule, even if feeling better; to continue with medical regimen to decrease B/P: exercise, cessation of smoking, decreasing stress, diet modifications

• Emphasize the need to rise slowly to sitting or standing position to minimize orthostatic hypotension; not to exercise in hot weather or increased hypotension can occur

• Teach patient to notify prescriber of mouth sores, sore throat, fever, swelling of hands or feet, irregular heartbeat, chest pain, coughing, shortness of breath

• Caution patient to report excessive perspiration, dehydration, vomiting, diarrhea; may lead to fall in B/P

• Caution patient that product may cause dizziness, fainting, light-headedness; may occur during 1st few days of therapy; to avoid activities that may be hazardous

• Teach patient how to take B/P, and normal readings for age group

Evaluation
Positive therapeutic outcome
• Decreased B/P in hypertension

Treatment of overdose: 0.9% NaCl **IV** inf, hemodialysis

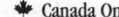

quinidine (Rx)
(kwin'i-deen)
quinidine gluconate (Rx)
Quinaglute Dura-Tabs, Quinalan,
Quinate ✤
**quinidine
polygalacturonate** (Rx)
Cardioquin
quinidine sulfate (Rx)
Apo-Quinidine ✤, Cin-Quin,
Novoquinidine ✤, Quinidex Extentabs,
Quinora
Func. class.: Antidysrhythmic (class IA)
Chem. class.: Quinine dextro isomer

Pregnancy category C

Action: Prolongs action potential duration and effective refractory period, thus decreasing myocardial excitability; anticholinergic properties

Therapeutic outcome: Treatment of dysrhythmias

Uses: Premature ventricular contractions (PVCs), atrial fibrillation, flutter; paroxysmal atrial tachycardia, ventricular tachycardia, malaria (**IV** quinidine gluconate)

Dosage and routes
Quinidine sulfate
Atrial fibrillation/flutter
Adult: PO 200 mg q2-3hr × 5-8 doses; may increase daily until sinus rhythm is restored; max 4 g/day given only after digitalization; local anesthetics, maintenance 200-300 mg tid-qid or 300-600 mg q8-12hr (SUS REL)

Paroxysmal supraventricular tachycardia
Adult: PO 400-600 mg q2-3hr, then 200-300 mg q6-8hr or 300-600 mg q8-12hr (SUS REL)

Premature atrial/ventricular contraction
Adult: PO 200-300 mg q6-8hr or 300-600 mg (SUS REL) q8-12hr, max 4 g/day
Child: PO 30 mg/kg/day or 900 mg/m²/day in 5 divided doses

Quinidine gluconate
Adult: PO 324-648 mg q8-12hr (SUS REL);

IM 600 mg, then 400 mg q2hr; **IV** give 16 mg/min

Available forms: Gluconate: sus rel tabs 324, 330 mg; inj gluconate 80 mg/ml; sulfate: tabs 200, 300 mg; sus rel tabs 300 mg; polygalacturonase: tabs 275 mg

Adverse effects
CNS: Headache, dizziness, involuntary movement, confusion, psychosis, restlessness, irritability, syncope, excitement, depression, ataxia
CV: **Hypotension,** *bradycardia, PVCs,* **heart block, cardiovascular collapse, arrest, torsades de pointes,** widening QRS complex, **ventricular tachycardia**
EENT: Cinchonism: tinnitus, blurred vision, hearing loss, mydriasis, disturbed color vision
GI: Nausea, vomiting, anorexia, *diarrhea,* **hepatotoxicity,** abdominal pain
HEMA: **Thrombocytopenia, hemolytic anemia, agranulocytosis,** hypoprothrombinemia
INTEG: Rash, urticaria, **angioedema,** swelling, photosensitivity, flushing with severe pruritus
RESP: Dyspnea, **respiratory depression**

Contraindications: Hypersensitivity or idiosyncratic response, digoxin toxicity, blood dyscrasias, myasthenia gravis

Black Box Warning: History of long QT syndrome, product-induced torsades de pointes, severe heart block

Precautions: Pregnancy C, breastfeeding, children, geriatric, renal/hepatic disease, potassium imbalance, CHF, respiratory depression, bradycardia, hypotension, syncope

Black Box Warning: Cardiac arrhythmias, MI

Pharmacokinetics	
Absorption	Well absorbed (PO, IM), slowly absorbed (sus rel)
Distribution	Widely distributed, crosses placenta, protein binding 80%-90%
Metabolism	Liver
Excretion	Kidney unchanged, 10%-50% breast milk
Half-life	6-8 hr

Pharmacodynamics					
	PO (SULFATE)	PO-SUS REL	PO (GLUCONATE)	IM	IV
Onset	½ hr	Unknown	Unknown	½ hr	5 min
Peak	1-1½ hr	4 hr	4 hr	½-1½ hr	Unknown
Duration	6-8 hr	8-12 hr	6-8 hr	6-8 hr	6-8 hr

Adverse effects: *italic* = common, **bold** = life-threatening

Q

Interactions
Individual drugs
Amiodarone, cimetidine, NIFEdipine: increased quinidine level

Digoxin: increased digoxin level

NIFEdipine, sodium bicarbonate, verapamil: increased quinidine effect

Phenytoin, rifampin, sucralfate: decreased effects of quinidine

Propranolol: increased effect of propranolol

Reserpine: increased cardiac depression

Warfarin: increased levels of warfarin

Drug classifications
Antacids, carbonic anhydrase inhibitors, hydroxide suspensions: increased effects of quinidine

Anticholinergic blockers: increased vagolytic effects

Anticoagulants (oral): increased levels of anticoagulant

Antidepressants (tricyclics): increased effect of antidepressant

Antidysrhythmics: increased cardiac depression

Barbiturates, cholinergics: decreased effects of quinidine

Neuromuscular blockers: increased neuromuscular blocking

Phenothiazines: increased cardiac depression

Drug/herb
Aconite: increased toxicity, death

Aloe, broom, buckthorn (chronic use), cascara sagrada (chronic use), Chinese rhubarb, figwort, fumitory, goldenseal, kudzu, licorice: increased effect

Aloe, buckthorn, cascara sagrada, senna: increased hypokalemia, increased antidysrhythmic action

Coltsfoot: decreased effect

Horehound: increased serotonin effect

Drug/food
Grapefruit juice: decreased absorption, decreased metabolism

Drug/lab test
Increased: CPK

Interference: triamterene therapy interferes with quinidine test levels

NURSING CONSIDERATIONS
Assessment
• Monitor ECG continuously to determine product effectiveness, measure PR, QRS, QT intervals, check for PVCs, other dysrhythmias; monitor B/P continuously for hypo/hypertension; for rebound hypertension after 1-2 hr; check for dehydration or hypovolemia

• Monitor blood levels (therapeutic level 2-7 mcg/ml)

• Monitor I&O ratio, electrolytes (potassium, sodium, chloride); check weight daily; check for signs of CHF or pulmonary toxicity: dyspnea, fatigue, cough, fever, chest pain; if these occur, product should be discontinued

• Monitor liver function tests: AST, ALT, bilirubin, alkaline phosphatase

• Assess for CNS symptoms: confusion, psychosis, numbness, depression, involuntary movements; if these occur, product should be discontinued

• Monitor cardiac rate, respiration: rate, rhythm, character, chest pain; watch for ventricular tachycardia, supraventricular tachycardia, or fibrillation that indicates toxicity

Nursing diagnoses
• Cardiac output, decreased (uses)
• Gas exchange, impaired (adverse reactions)
• Knowledge, deficient (teaching)

Implementation
PO route
• Do not break, crush, or chew sus rel tab
• Give on an empty stomach with a full glass of water
• May be given with meals if GI irritation occurs, absorption will be decreased
• Sus rel forms not interchangeable
• Tab may be crushed and mixed with fluid or foods for patients with swallowing difficulties

IV route
• Give by intermittent inf after diluting 800 mg/50 ml of D_5W; gluconate: (16 mg/ml) give at 1 ml/min or less using an inf pump for correct dose
• Do not use colored sol or sol with precipitate
• Diluted quinidine is stable for 24 hr at room temperature

Y-site compatibilities: Diazepam, milrinone

Y-site incompatibilities: Furosemide

Additive compatibilities: Bretylium, cimetidine, milrinone, ranitidine, verapamil

Additive incompatibilities: Amiodarone

Patient/family education
• Instruct patient to report adverse effects immediately to prescriber

• Caution patient that sunglasses may be needed for photophobia; to use sunscreen, protective clothing, or stay out of sun to prevent burns

• Instruct patient to complete follow-up appointments with health care provider including pulmonary function tests, chest x-ray, ophth and otoscopic exams

Evaluation
Positive therapeutic outcome
- Resolution of dysrhythmias

quinine (OTC, Rx)
(kwye'nine)
Novoquine ✤, Qualaquin
Func. class.: Antimalarial
Chem. class.: Cinchona tree alkaloid

Pregnancy category C

Action: Inhibits parasite replications, transcription of DNA to RNA by forming complexes with DNA of parasite

Therapeutic outcome: Reduction/death of *Plasmodium falciparum*; decreased leg cramps

Uses: *P. falciparum*, malaria

Dosage and routes
Malaria
Adult: PO 648 mg q8hr × 3 days or 7 days in SE Asia, given with tetracycline 250 mg q5hr × 7 days or clindamycin 900 mg q8hr × 7 days or doxycycline 100 mg q12hr × 7 days
Child: PO 25 mg/kg/day divided q8hr for 3-7 days in conjunction with another agent

Available forms: Tabs 325 mg

Adverse effects
CNS: Headache, stimulation, fatigue, irritability, **seizures,** bad dreams, dizziness, fever, confusion, anxiety
CV: Angina, dysrhythmias, tachycardia, hypotension, **acute circulatory failure**
EENT: Blurred vision, corneal changes, retinal changes, difficulty focusing, tinnitus, vertigo, deafness, photophobia, diplopia, night blindness
ENDO: Hypoglycemia
GI: Nausea, vomiting, anorexia, diarrhea, epigastric pain
GU: Renal tubular damage, **anuria**
HEMA: **Thrombocytopenia, purpura, hypothrombinemia, hemolysis**
INTEG: Pruritus, pigmentary changes, skin eruptions, lichen planus–like eruptions, flushing, facial edema, sweating
MISC: **Hemolytic uremic syndrome**
RESP: Dyspnea

Contraindications: Breastfeeding, hypersensitivity, G6PD deficiency, retinal field changes, myasthenia gravis

Precautions: Pregnancy **C,** blood dyscrasias, severe GI/hepatic disease, neurologic disease, psoriasis, cardiac dysrhythmias, tinnitus, hypoglycemia, nocturnal leg cramps

Pharmacokinetics
Absorption	Rapidly, 80%
Distribution	Crosses placenta, excreted breast milk, protein binding >90% in malaria
Metabolism	Liver, extensively 80%
Excretion	Urine, 20% unchanged
Half-life	11 hr, increases in malaria

Pharmacodynamics
Onset	Unknown
Peak	3½-6 hr
Duration	8 hr

Interactions
Individual products
Acetazolamide, NaHCO$_3$: increased toxicity
Digoxin: increased levels
Rifampin: increased treatment failure
Warfarin: increased bleeding risk
Drug classifications
Antacids: decreased absorption of quinine
Anticoagulants: increased levels of anticoagulants
Neuromuscular blockers: increased effect of neuromuscular blockers
Drug/lab test
Increased: 17-KS

NURSING CONSIDERATIONS
Assessment
- Monitor B/P, pulse; watch for hypotension, tachycardia
- Assess liver studies qwk: ALT, AST, bilirubin
- Assess blood tests, CBC, since blood dyscrasias occur
- Assess for cinchonism: nausea, blurred vision, tinnitus, headache, difficulty focusing; quinidine levels >10 mcg/ml
- Assess for symptoms of malaria and improvement
- Assess frequency/duration of nocturnal leg cramps

Nursing diagnoses
- Infection, risk for (uses)
- Knowledge, deficient (teaching)
- Noncompliance (teaching)

Implementation
- Give before or after meals at same time each day to maintain level
- Store in airtight, light-resistant container

Patient/family education
- Advise patient to avoid OTC preparations: cold preparations, tonic water
- Advise patient to take only as prescribed

Q

Adverse effects: italic = common, **bold** *= life-threatening*

- Teach patient visual changes may occur, to avoid driving or hazardous activities until response is known
- Teach patient to stop product and call prescriber if difficulty breathing, ringing in the ears, or allergic reaction occurs
- Teach patient to use insect repellant, protective clothing if in area with mosquitoes

Evaluation
Positive therapeutic outcome
- Decreased symptoms of malaria

rabeprazole (Rx)
(rab-ee-pray'zole)
Aciphex
Func. class.: Proton pump inhibitor
Chem. class.: Benzimidazole

Pregnancy category C

Action: Suppresses gastric secretion by inhibiting hydrogen/potassium ATPase enzyme system in the gastric parietal cell; characterized as a gastric acid pump inhibitor, since it blocks the final step of acid production

Therapeutic outcome: Absence of duodenal ulcers; decreased gastroesophageal reflux

Uses: Gastroesophageal reflux disease (GERD), severe erosive esophagitis, poorly responsive systemic GERD, pathologic hypersecretory conditions (Zollinger-Ellison syndrome, systemic mastocytosis, multiple endocrine adenomas); treatment of duodenal ulcers with or without antiinfectives for *Helicobacter pylori;* daytime, nighttime heartburn

Dosage and routes
Healing of duodenal ulcers
Adult: PO 20 mg/day × ≤4 wk, to be taken after breakfast

Erosive esophagitis/GERD
Adult: PO 20 mg/day × 4-8 wk
Adolescent: PO 20 mg/day up to 8 wk

Pathologic hypersecretory conditions
Adult: PO 60 mg/day; may increase to 120 mg in 2 divided doses

Available forms: Del rel tabs 20 mg
Adverse effects
CNS: Headache, dizziness, asthenia
CV: Chest pain, angina, tachycardia, bradycardia, palpitations, peripheral edema
EENT: Tinnitus, taste perversion
GI: Diarrhea, abdominal pain, vomiting, nausea, constipation, flatulence, acid regurgitation, abdominal swelling, anorexia, irritable colon, esophageal candidiasis, dry mouth
GU: UTI, frequency, increased creatinine, **proteinuria, hematuria,** testicular pain, glycosuria
HEMA: **Pancytopenia, thrombocytopenia, neutropenia, leukocytosis,** anemia
INTEG: Rash, dry skin, urticaria, pruritus, alopecia
META: Hypoglycemia, increased hepatic enzymes, weight gain
MISC: Back pain, fever, fatigue, malaise
RESP: Upper respiratory tract infections, cough, epistaxis, **pneumonia**

Contraindications: Hypersensitivity

Precautions: Pregnancy **C,** breastfeeding, children

Pharmacokinetics
Absorption	Unknown
Distribution	Unknown
Metabolism	Liver, extensively
Excretion	Kidneys, feces
Half-life	Unknown

Pharmacodynamics
Unknown

Interactions
Individual drugs
Calcium carbonate, sucralfate, vitamin B_{12}: decreased rabeprazole levels
Clarithromycin, phenytoin: increased levels of rabeprazole
Warfarin: increased bleeding risk
Drug classifications
Benzodiazepines: increased levels of rabeprazole

NURSING CONSIDERATIONS
Assessment
- Assess GI system: bowel sounds q8hr, abdomen for pain and swelling, anorexia
- Monitor hepatic enzymes: AST, ALT, increased alkaline phosphatase during treatment

Nursing diagnoses
- Knowledge, deficient (teaching)
- Pain, chronic (uses)

Implementation
- Do not break, crush, or chew del rel tab
- Give after breakfast daily

Patient/family education
- Advise patient to report severe diarrhea; product may have to be discontinued

- Caution patient to avoid driving and other hazardous activities until response to product is known
- Caution patient to avoid alcohol, salicylates, NSAIDs; may cause GI irritation
- Advise patient to wear sunscreen, protective clothing to prevent burns

Evaluation
Positive therapeutic outcome
- Absence of epigastric pain, swelling, fullness

---

raloxifene (Rx)
(ral-ox'ih-feen)
Evista
Func. class.: Hormone modifier, selective estrogen receptor modulator (SERM)
Chem. class.: Benzothiophene
Pregnancy category X

Action: Tissue-selective estrogen agonist/antagonist; agonist activity in bone and lipid metabolism, antagonistic activity on breast and uterus, reduces resorption of bone and decreases bone turnover; mediated through estrogen receptor binding

Therapeutic outcome: Absence or decrease of osteoporosis in postmenopausal women

Uses: Prevention, treatment of osteoporosis in postmenopausal women, breast cancer prophylaxis

Dosage and routes
Hormone replacement
Adult: PO 60 mg/day, max 60 mg/day

Available forms: Tabs 60 mg

Adverse effects
CNS: Insomnia, **CVA**
CV: Hot flashes, peripheral edema, **thromboembolism**
GI: *Nausea,* vomiting, diarrhea, dyspepsia
GU: Vaginitis, leukorrhea, *hot flashes,* cystitis, vaginal bleeding
INTEG: Rash, sweating
META: Weight gain, peripheral edema
MS: Arthralgia, myalgia, *leg cramps,* arthritis
RESP: Sinusitis, pharyngitis, increased cough, pneumonia, laryngitis, rhinitis, bronchitis, **pulmonary embolism,** flulike symptoms

Contraindications: Pregnancy **X,** breastfeeding, hypersensitivity

Black Box Warning: Women with active or history of venous thromboembolic events

Precautions: Hepatic/CV disease, cervical/uterine cancer, elevated triglycerides, pulmonary embolism

Black Box Warning: Stroke

Pharmacokinetics
Absorption	Unknown
Distribution	Highly protein bound
Metabolism	Unknown
Excretion	Feces, breast milk
Half-life	28-32 hr (elimination)

Pharmacodynamics
Unknown

Interactions
Individual drugs
Ampicillin, cholestyramine: decreased action of raloxifene
Drug classifications
Anticoagulants, thyroid replacement hormones: decreased action of anticoagulants
Highly protein-bound products: administer cautiously
Drug/food
Soy: decreased effect of raloxifene
Drug/lab test
Increased: apolipoprotein, corticosteroid-binding globulin, thyroxine binding globulin (TBG)
Decreased: lipoprotein, fibrinogen, LDL cholesterol, total cholesterol, calcium, total protein, albumin, platelets

NURSING CONSIDERATIONS
Assessment
- Obtain bone density test baseline, periodically throughout treatment; bone-specific alkaline phosphatase; osteocalcin, collagen breakdown
- Monitor weight daily; notify prescriber of weekly weight gain >5 lb
- Monitor B/P q4hr, watch for increase caused by H_2O and sodium retention
- Monitor liver function tests: AST, ALT, bilirubin, alkaline phosphatase
- Monitor I&O ratio; decreasing urinary output, increasing edema

Nursing diagnoses
- Knowledge, deficient (teaching)
- Mobility, impaired physical (uses)

Implementation
- Administer without regard to meals
- Add calcium supplement, vit D if lacking

R

Adverse effects: *italic* = common, **bold** = life-threatening

Patient/family education
• Teach patient to weigh weekly, report gain >5 lb
• Teach patients to discontinue product 72 hr before prolonged bedrest
• Advise patient to avoid maintaining one position for long periods
• Advise patient to take calcium supplements, vit D if intake is inadequate
• Advise patient to increase exercise using weights
• Advise patient to stop smoking and to decrease alcohol consumption
• Inform patient that this product does not help control hot flashes
• Teach patient to report fever, acute migraine, insomnia, emotional distress; UTI or vaginal burning/itching; swelling, warmth, or pain in calves

Evaluation
Positive therapeutic outcome
• Prevention, treatment of osteoporosis

---

raltegravir (Rx)
(ral-teg′ra-vir)
Isentress
Func. class.: Antiretroviral
Chem. class.: HIV integrase strand transfer inhibitor (ISTIs)

Pregnancy category C

Action: Inhibits catalytic activity of HIV integrase, which is an HIV-encoded enzyme needed for replication

Therapeutic outcome: Improvement in CD4, T-cell counts

Uses: HIV in combination with other antiretrovirals

Dosage and routes
Adult and adolescent ≥16 yr: PO 400 mg bid, max 800 mg/day with or without food

Available forms: Tabs 400 mg

Adverse effects
CNS: Fatigue, fever, *dizziness, headache,* asthenia, **suicidal ideation**
CV: **MI**
GI: Nausea, vomiting, diarrhea, abdominal pain, gastritis, **hepatitis**
GU: **Oliguria, proteinuria, hematuria, glomerulonephritis, acute renal failure, renal tubular necrosis**
HEMA: **Anemia, neutropenia**
INTEG: Rash, urticaria, pruritus, pain or phlebitis at IV site, unusual sweating, alopecia

META: Hyperamylasia, hyperglycemia
MS: Myopathy, **rhabdomyolysis**

Contraindications: Hypersensitivity, breastfeeding

Precautions: Pregnancy **C**, children, geriatric, hepatic disease, immune reconstitution syndrome, hepatitis, antimicrobial resistance, lactase deficiency

Pharmacokinetics

Absorption	Max 3 hr if taken on empty stomach
Distribution	Unknown
Metabolism	Liver
Excretion	51% feces, 32% urine
Half-life	Terminal 9 hr

Pharmacodynamics
Unknown

Interactions
Individual drugs
Rifampin: decreased raltegravir levels
Drug classifications
Fibric acid derivatives, HMG-CoA reductase inhibitors: increased rhabdomyolysis, myopathy, elevated CPK
H_2 blockers, protein pump inhibitors: increased raltegravir effect

NURSING CONSIDERATIONS
Assessment
• Assess for signs of infection, anemia
• Resistance testing prior to therapy and at treatment failure
• Monitor blood tests: viral load, CD4, T-cell count, plasma HIV RNA
• Assess skin eruptions: rash, urticaria, itching
• Assess for allergies before treatment, reaction of each medication; place allergies on chart in bright red letters

Nursing diagnoses
• Infection, risk for (uses)
• Knowledge, deficient (teaching)
• Noncompliance (teaching)

Implementation
• Do not break, crush, or chew tabs
• May give without regard to meals, with 8 oz of water
• Store at room temperature

Patient/family education
• Teach patient to take as prescribed; if dose is missed, take as soon as remembered up to 1 hr before next dose; do not double dose
• Teach patient that sexual partners need to be told that patient has HIV

- Advise patient that product does not cure infection, just controls symptoms, and does not prevent infecting others
◆ Teach patient to report sore throat, fever, fatigue (may indicate superinfection)
- Advise patient that product must be taken in equal intervals around the clock to maintain blood levels for duration of therapy

Evaluation
Positive therapeutic outcome
- Improvement in CD4, T-cell counts

ramelteon (Rx)
(rah-mel′tee-on)
Rozerem
Func. class.: Sedative/hypnotic, antianxiety
Chem. class.: Melatonin receptor agonist

Pregnancy category C

Action: Binds selectively to melatonin receptors (MT$_1$, MT$_2$); thought to be involved in circadian rhythm and the normal sleep/wake cycle

Therapeutic outcome: Ability to fall asleep easily and decrease early-morning awakenings

Uses: Insomnia

Dosage and routes
Adult: PO 8 mg at bedtime

Hepatic dose
Do not use in severe hepatic disease; use with caution in mild to moderate hepatic disease

Available forms: Tabs 8 mg

Adverse effects
CNS: Dizziness, somnolence, fatigue, headache, insomnia, depression, complex sleep-related reactions: sleep driving, sleep eating
GI: Nausea, diarrhea, dysgeusia, vomiting
MISC: Myalgia, arthralgia, decreased blood cortisol, influenza, upper respiratory tract infection
SYST: **Severe allergic reactions, angioedema**

Contraindications: Breastfeeding, infants, children, hypersensitivity, alcohol intoxication, hepatic encephalopathy

Precautions: Pregnancy C, hepatic disease, alcoholism, COPD, seizure disorder, sleep apnea, suicidal ideation, angioedema, depression, sleep-related behavior (sleepwalking), schizophrenia, bipolar disorder

Pharmacokinetics
Absorption	Rapidly
Distribution	Protein binding 82%
Metabolism	Rapid first pass metabolism, liver
Excretion	84% urine, 4% feces
Half-life	2-5 hr

Pharmacodynamics
Onset	Unknown
Peak	0.75 hr
Duration	Unknown

Interactions
Individual drugs
Alcohol, ciprofloxacin, fluconazole, fluvoxamine, ketoconazole: increased ramelteon effect
Rifampin: decreased effect of ramelteon
Drug classifications
Antiretroviral protease inhibitors: possible toxicity
Anxiolytics, azole antifungals, barbiturates, CYP1A2 inhibitors, hypnotics, sedatives: increased ramelteon effect
Drug/herb
Do not use with melatonin
Catnip, chamomile, clary, cowslip, hops, kava, lavender, mistletoe, nettle, pokeweed, poppy, Queen Anne's lace, senega, skullcap, valerian: increased CNS depression
Drug/food
High-fat/heavy meal: prolonged absorption, sleep onset reduced

NURSING CONSIDERATIONS
Assessment
- Assess mental status: mood, sensorium, affect, memory (long, short)
- Assess type of sleep problem: falling asleep, staying asleep

Nursing diagnoses
- Injury, risk for (adverse reactions)
- Knowledge, deficient (teaching)
- Sleep deprivation (uses)

Implementation
- Give after removal of cigarettes to prevent fires
- Give after trying conservative measures for insomnia
- Give within 30 min of bedtime for sleeplessness
- Give on empty stomach for fast onset
- Provide assistance with ambulation after receiving dose
- Provide safety measure: nightlight, call bell within easy reach

Adverse effects: *italic* = common, **bold** = life-threatening

- Check to see if PO medication has been swallowed
- Store in tight container in cool environment

Patient/family education

- Advise patient to avoid driving or other activities requiring alertness until product is stabilized
- Advise patient to avoid alcohol ingestion or CNS depressants
- Teach patient alternative measures to improve sleep: reading, exercise several hr before bedtime, warm bath, warm milk, TV, self-hypnosis, deep breathing
- Advise patient to take immediately before going to bed
- Advise patient not to ingest a high-fat/heavy meal before taking
- Teach patient to report cessation of menses, galactorrhea (women), decreased libido, infertility, worsening of insomnia, or behavioral changes

Evaluation
Positive therapeutic outcome

- Ability to sleep at night, decreased amount of early-morning awakening

---

ramipril (Rx)
(ra-mi'pril)
Altace
Func. class.: Antihypertensive
Chem. class.: Angiotensin-converting enzyme (ACE) inhibitor

Pregnancy category D

Do not confuse:
ramipril/enalapril, Altace/alteplase/Artane

Action: Selectively suppresses renin-angiotensin-aldosterone system; inhibits ACE; prevents conversion of angiotensin I to angiotensin II; results in dilatation of arterial, venous vessels

Therapeutic outcome: Decreased B/P in hypertension

Uses: Hypertension, alone or in combination with thiazide diuretics; CHF (after MI), reduction in risk of MI, stroke, death from CV disorders

Dosage and routes
Hypertension
Adult: PO 2.5 mg/day initially, then 2.5-20 mg/day divided bid or daily

CHF/Post MI
Adult: PO 1.25-2.5 mg bid, may increase to 5 mg bid

Reduction in risk of MI, stroke, death
Adult: PO 2.5 mg/day × 7 days, then 5 mg/day × 21 days, then may increase to 10 mg/day

Renal impairment
Adult: PO CCr <40 ml/min; reduce by 50%, titrate upwards to max 5 mg/day

Available forms: Caps 1.25, 2.5, 5, 10 mg

Adverse effects
CNS: Headache, dizziness, anxiety, insomnia, paresthesia, fatigue, depression, malaise, vertigo, **seizures**
CV: Hypotension, chest pain, palpitations, angina, syncope, **dysrhythmia**
EENT: Hearing loss
GI: Nausea, constipation, vomiting, dyspepsia, dysphagia, anorexia, diarrhea, abdominal pain
GU: **Proteinuria,** increased BUN, creatinine, impotence
HEMA: Decreased Hct, Hgb, **eosinophilia, leukopenia**
INTEG: Rash, sweating, photosensitivity, pruritus
META: Hyperkalemia
MISC: **Angioedema**
MS: Arthralgia, arthritis, myalgia
RESP: Cough, dyspnea

Contraindications: Breastfeeding, children, hypersensitivity to ACE inhibitors, history of angioedema

Black Box Warning: Pregnancy **D**

Precautions: Impaired renal/liver function, dialysis patients, hypovolemia, blood dyscrasias, COPD, CHF, asthma, geriatric, renal artery stenosis, cough

Pharmacokinetics	
Absorption	Well absorbed
Distribution	Not known, crosses placenta
Metabolism	Liver, extensively; protein binding 73%
Excretion	Urine
Half-life	Ramipril (5 hr), ramiprilat (24 hr)

Pharmacodynamics	
Onset	½-1 hr
Peak	6-8 hr
Duration	24-72 hr

Interactions
Individual drugs
Alcohol: increased hypotension (large amounts)
Digoxin, lithium: increased serum levels

Hydralazine, prazocin: increased toxicity

Indomethacin: decreased antihypertensive effect

Drug classifications

Adrenergic blockers, antihypertensives, diuretics, ganglionic blockers, nitrates: increased hypotension

Antacids: decreased absorption

Diuretics (potassium sparing), potassium supplements, sympathomimetics, vasodilators: increased toxicity

NSAIDs, salicylates: decreased antihypertensive effect

Drug/herb

Aconite: increased toxicity, death

Astragalus, cola tree: increased or decreased antihypertensive effect

Barberry, betony, black catechu, black cohosh, bloodroot, broom, burdock, cat's claw, dandelion, goldenseal, hawthorn, Irish moss, Jamaican dogwood, kelp, khella, mistletoe, parsley: increased antihypertensive effect

Coltsfoot, guarana, khat, licorice, yohimbe: decreased antihypertensive effect

Drug/lab test

False positive: urine acetone, ANA titer

NURSING CONSIDERATIONS

Assessment

• Monitor blood tests: neutrophils, decreased platelets; WBC with differential baseline, periodically q3mo; if neutrophils <1000/mm^3, discontinue treatment

• Monitor B/P, check for orthostatic hypotension, syncope; if changes occur, dosage may need to be changed

• Monitor renal function tests: protein, BUN, creatinine; watch for increased levels that may indicate nephrotic syndrome and renal failure; monitor renal symptoms: polyuria, oliguria, frequency, dysuria

• Establish baselines in renal, liver function tests before therapy begins and monitor periodically; liver function tests, uric acid, and glucose may be increased

• Check potassium levels throughout treatment, although hyperkalemia rarely occurs

• Check for edema in feet, legs daily, weight daily in CHF

• Assess for allergic reactions: rash, fever, pruritus, urticaria; product should be discontinued if antihistamines fail to help

Nursing diagnoses

• Cardiac output, decreased (uses)

• Injury, risk for (side effects)

• Knowledge, deficient (teaching)

• Noncompliance (teaching)

Implementation

• Caps can be opened and added to food

• Store in airtight container at 86° F (30° C) or less

• Severe hypotension may occur after 1st dose of this medication; decreased hypotension may be prevented by reducing or discontinuing diuretic therapy 3 days before beginning benazepril therapy

• Give **IV** inf of 0.9% NaCl (as ordered) to expand fluid volume if severe hypotension occurs

Patient/family education

• Caution patient not to discontinue product abruptly; advise patient to tell all persons associated with care

• Teach patient not to use OTC products (cough, cold, allergy) unless directed by physician; serious side effects can occur; xanthines such as coffee, tea, chocolate, cola can prevent action of product

• Instruct patient on the importance of complying with dosage schedule, even if feeling better; to continue with medical regimen to decrease B/P: exercise, cessation of smoking, decreasing stress, diet modifications

• Emphasize the need to rise slowly to sitting or standing position to minimize orthostatic hypotension; not to exercise in hot weather because increased hypotension can occur

• Teach patient to notify prescriber of mouth sores, sore throat, fever, swelling of hands or feet, irregular heartbeat, chest pain, coughing, shortness of breath

• Caution patient to report excessive perspiration, dehydration, vomiting, diarrhea; may lead to fall in B/P

• Caution patient that product may cause dizziness, fainting, light-headedness; may occur during 1st few days of therapy; to avoid activities that may be hazardous

• Teach patient how to take B/P, and normal readings for age group

Evaluation

Positive therapeutic outcome

• Decreased B/P in hypertension

Treatment of overdose: 0.9% NaCl **IV** inf, hemodialysis

R

ranibizumab (Rx)
(ran-ih-biz'oo-mab)
Lucentis
Func. class.: Ophthalmic
Chem. class.: Selective vascular endothelial growth factor antagonist

Pregnancy category C

Action: Binds to receptor-binding site of active forms of vascular endothelial growth factor A (VEGF-A) that causes angiogenesis and cell proliferation

Therapeutic outcome: Prevention of increasing neovascular macular degeneration

Uses: Macular degeneration (neovascular) (wet)

Dosage and routes
Adult: Intravitreal 0.5 mg (0.05 ml) qmo

Available forms: Sol for inj 0.5 mg/ 0.05 ml

Adverse effects
CNS: Dizziness, headache
EENT: Blepharitis, cataract, conjunctival hemorrhage/hyperemia, detachment of the retinal pigment epithelium, dryness/irritation/ pain in the eye, visual impairment, vitreous floaters, ocular infection
GI: Constipation, nausea
MISC: Hypertension, UTI, **thromboembolism, non-ocular bleeding**
RESP: Bronchitis, cough, sinusitis, URI

Contraindications: Hypersensitivity, ocular infections

Precautions: Pregnancy **C**, breastfeeding, children, retinal detachment, increased intraocular pressure

Pharmacokinetics	
Absorption	Minimal
Distribution	None
Metabolism	None
Excretion	None
Half-life	Elimination 9 days

Pharmacodynamics
Unknown

Interactions
Individual drugs
Verteporfin photodynamic therapy (PDT): increased severe inflammation

NURSING CONSIDERATIONS
Assessment
• Assess for eye changes: redness, sensitivity to light, vision change, intraocular pressure change; report to ophthalmologist immediately

Nursing diagnoses
• Knowledge, deficient (teaching)

Implementation
• Given by ophthalmologist via intravitreal injection using adequate anesthesia; use 19-gauge filter
• Store in refrigerator; do not freeze
• Protect from light

Patient/family education
• Teach patient that if eye becomes red, sensitive to light, or painful or if there is a change in vision, seek immediate care from ophthalmologist
• Teach patient reason for treatment, expected results

Evaluation
Positive therapeutic outcome
• Prevention of increasing neovascular macular degeneration

ranitidine (Rx)
(ra-nit'i-deen)
Apo-Ranitidine ✤, Equaline, Gen-Ranitidine ✤, Leader Ranitidine, Novo-Ranidine ✤, Nu-Ranit ✤, PMS-Ranitidine ✤, Wal-Zan, Zantac, Zantac-C ✤, Zantac EFFER-dose, Zantac GELdose
ranitidine bismuth citrate
Tritec
Func. class.: H$_2$ histamine receptor antagonist

Pregnancy category B

Do not confuse:
ranitidine/amantadine, Zantac/Xanax/Zofran

Action: Inhibits histamine at H$_2$ receptor site in the gastric parietal cells, which inhibits gastric acid secretion

Therapeutic outcome: Healing of duodenal ulcers or gastric ulcers; prevention of duodenal ulcers; decreased symptoms of gastroesophageal reflux disease (GERD), Zollinger-Ellison syndrome, or heartburn

Uses: Short-term treatment of duodenal and gastric ulcers and maintenance; management of GERD, Zollinger-Ellison syndrome, active duodenal ulcers with *Helicobacter pylori* in

 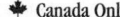

combination with clarithromycin, hypersecretory conditions, stress ulcers, erosive esophagitis (maintenance), systemic mastocytosis, multiple endocrine adenoma syndrome, heartburn

Unlabeled uses: Prevention of aspiration pneumonitis, stress ulcers, upper GI bleeding

Dosage and routes
Ranitidine
Erosive esophagitis
Adult: PO 150 mg qid for up to 12 wk
Child ≥1 mo: PO 5-10 mg/kg/day in 2-3 divided doses

Duodenal ulcer
Adult: PO 150 mg bid or 300 mg/day after PM meal or at bedtime, maintenance 150 mg at bedtime
Infant and child: PO 2-4 mg/kg bid, max 300 mg/day

Zollinger-Ellison syndrome
Adult: PO 150 mg bid, may increase if needed

Gastric ulcer
Adult: PO 150 mg bid × 6 wk, then 150 mg at bedtime

GERD
Adult: PO 150 mg bid

Renal dose
Adult: CCr <50 ml/min give 50% of dose or extend dosing interval

Ranitidine bismuth citrate
Adult: PO 400 mg bid × 4 wk with clarithromycin 500 mg tid × first 2 wk

Available forms: Ranitidine: tabs 75, 150, 300 mg; caps 150, 300 mg; syr 15 mg/ml; sol for inj 25 mg/ml; effervescent tabs 25 mg; ranitidine bismuth citrate: tabs 400 mg

Adverse effects
CNS: Headache, sleeplessness, dizziness, confusion, agitation, depression; hallucinations (geriatric)
CV: Tachycardia, bradycardia, premature ventricular contractions
EENT: Blurred vision, increased ocular pressure
GI: Constipation, abdominal pain, diarrhea, nausea, vomiting, **hepatotoxicity**
GU: Impotence, gynecomastia, **acute interstitial nephritis (rare)**
INTEG: Urticaria, rash, fever
RESP: **Pneumonia**
SYST: **Anaphylaxis (rare)**

Contraindications: Hypersensitivity

Precautions: Pregnancy **B**, breastfeeding, child <12 yr, renal/hepatic disease

Pharmacokinetics

Absorption	Well absorbed (PO, IM), completely absorbed (**IV**)
Distribution	Widely distributed, crosses placenta
Metabolism	Liver (30%)
Excretion	Kidneys unchanged (70%)
Half-life	2-3 hr, increased renal disease

Pharmacodynamics

	PO	IM/IV
Onset	Unknown	Unknown
Peak	2-3 hr	15 min
Duration	8-12 hr	8-12 hr

Interactions
Individual drugs
Diazepam, metoclopramide: decreased absorption of ranitidine
Ketoconazole: decreased effect of ketoconazole
Procainamide: increased absorption, toxicity
Drug classifications
Anticholinergics, antacids: decreased ranitidine absorption
Anticoagulants, sulfonylureas: increased absorption, toxicity
Benzodiazepines: increased effects of benzodiazepines
Calcium channel blockers: increased effect of calcium channel blockers
Cephalosporins: decreased effects of cephalosporins
Iron salts: decreased effects of iron salts
Drug/lab test
Increased: alkaline phosphatase, AST, creatinine, LDH, ALT, bilirubin
False positive: urine protein

NURSING CONSIDERATIONS
Assessment
• Assess patient with ulcers or suspected ulcers: epigastric or abdominal pain, hematemesis, occult blood in stools, blood in gastric aspirate before, throughout treatment; monitor gastric pH (5 should be maintained)
• Monitor I&O ratio, BUN, creatinine, CBC with differential monthly

Nursing diagnoses
• Knowledge, deficient (teaching)
• Pain, chronic (uses)

Implementation
PO route
• May be given with or without meals
• Give antacids 1 hr before or 1 hr after this product

R

IV, direct route
- Give by direct **IV** after diluting 50 mg/20 ml of 0.9% D₅W, NaCl over 5 min or more

Intermittent IV inf route
- Give by intermittent inf over 15 min after diluting 50 mg/100 ml of D₅W, 0.9% NaCl

Continuous inf route
- Give by continuous inf for a concentration 150 mg/250 ml, give 6.25 mg/hr
- Give Zollinger-Ellison patients up to a conc of 2.5 mg/ml at 1 mg/kg/hr initially

Syringe compatibilities: Atropine, cyclizine, dexamethasone, dimenhyDRINATE, diphenhydrAMINE, DOBUTamine, DOPamine, fentanyl, glycopyrrolate, hydromorphone, meperidine, metoclopramide, morphine, nalbuphine, oxymorphone, pentazocine, perphenazine, prochlorperazine, promethazine, scopolamine

Syringe incompatibilities: Hydroxyzine, methotrimeprazine, midazolam, pentobarbital, phenobarbital

Y-site compatibilities: Acyclovir, aldesleukin, allopurinol, amifostine, aminophylline, atracurium, aztreonam, bretylium, DOBUTamine, DOPamine, DOXOrubicin, enalaprilat, epinephrine, esmolol, fentanyl, filgrastim, fluconazole, fludarabine, foscarnet, furosemide, gallium, granisetron, heparin, hydromorphone, idarubicin, labetalol, lorazepam, melphalan, meperidine, methotrexate, midazolam, milrinone, morphine, niCARdipine, nitroglycerin, norepinephrine, ondansetron, paclitaxel, pancuronium, piperacillin, piperacillin/tazobactam, procainamide, propofol, sargramostim, vecuronium, zidovudine

Additive compatibilities: Acetazolamide, amikacin, aminophylline, chloramphenicol, chlorothiazide, ciprofloxacin, colistimethate, dexamethasone, digoxin, DOBUTamine, DOPamine, doxycycline, furosemide, gentamicin, heparin, lidocaine, penicillin G sodium, potassium chloride, ticarcillin, tobramycin, vancomycin

Additive incompatibilities: Amphotericin B, clindamycin

Patient/family education
- Caution patient that gynecomastia, impotence may occur and are reversible after treatment is discontinued
- Advise patient to avoid driving, other hazardous activities until stabilized on this medication; drowsiness or dizziness may occur
- Inform patient that smoking decreases the effectiveness of the product; that smoking cessation should be considered
- Instruct patient that product must be continued for prescribed time to be effective and taken exactly as prescribed; doses should not be doubled; a missed dose should be taken when remembered up to 1 hr before next dose
- Advise patient to report bruising, fatigue, malaise; blood dyscrasias may occur
- Inform patient to report diarrhea, black tarry stools, sore throat, rash, dizziness, confusion, rash, or delirium to prescriber immediately

Evaluation
Positive therapeutic outcome
- Decreased pain in abdomen, heartburn
- Healing of ulcers
- Absence of gastroesophageal reflux

---

ranolazine (Rx)
(ruh-no′luh-zeen)
Ranexa
Func. class: Antianginal
Pregnancy category C

Action: Antianginal, antiischemic; unknown, may work by inhibiting portal fatty-acid oxidation

Therapeutic outcome: Decreased anginal pain and number of episodes

Uses: Chronic stable angina pectoris; use in those that have not responded to other treatment options; should be used in combination with other antianginals such as amlodipine, beta blockers, or nitrates

Dosage and routes
Adult: PO 500 mg bid and increased to 1000 mg bid based on response; max 1000 mg bid

Available forms: Ext rel tabs 500 mg

Adverse effects
CNS: Headache, dizziness
CV: Palpitations, **QT prolongation**
GI: Nausea, vomiting, constipation, dry mouth
MISC: Peripheral edema
RESP: Dyspnea

Contraindications: Preexisting QT prolongation, hepatic disease (Child-Pugh class A, B, C), hypersensitivity, hypokalemia, renal failure, torsades de pointes, ventricular dysrhythmia, ventricular tachycardia

Precautions: Pregnancy C, breastfeeding, children, geriatric, renal disease, hypotension

---

Pharmacokinetics

Absorption	Varied
Distribution	Protein binding 62%
Metabolism	By CYP3A, CYP2D6 (lesser)
Excretion	Urine 75%, feces 25%
Half-life	7 hr

Pharmacodynamics

Onset	Unknown
Peak	2-5 hr
Duration	Unknown

Interactions
Individual drugs
Arsenic trioxide, chloroquine, chlorpromazine, droperidol, grepafloxacin, halofantrine, haloperidol, levomethadyl, mesoridazine, methadone, pentamidine, pimozide, probucol, thioridazine: increased QT prolongation and torsades de pointes

Digoxin, simvastatin: increased action of digoxin, simvastatin

Diltiazem, dofetilide, ketoconazole, paroxetine, quinidine, sotalol, thioridazine, verapamil, ziprasidone: increased ranolazine action

Drug classifications
Anti-retroviral protease inhibitors: increased ranolazine absorption, toxicity

Class IA/III antidysrhythmics: increased QT prolongation and torsades de pointes

CYP3A4 inhibitors (ketoconazole, fluconazole, itraconazole, IV miconazole, voriconazole, diltiazem, verapamil): increased ranolazine action and QT prolongation; do not use concurrently

Macrolide antibiotics, protease inhibitors: increased ranolazine action

Macrolides (clarithromycin, erythromycin, troleandomycin): increased QTc interval

Drug/food
Do not use with grapefruit or grapefruit juice

NURSING CONSIDERATIONS
Assessment
- Assess cardiac status: B/P, pulse, respiration, ECG; watch for prolongation of QT

Nursing diagnoses
- Knowledge, deficient (teaching)
- Pain, acute (uses)
- Tissue perfusion, ineffective (uses)

Implementation
- Do not break, crush, or chew tabs; give products as prescribed; do not double or skip dose
- Give bid, without regard to meals

Patient/family education
- Teach patient to avoid hazardous activities until stabilized on product, dizziness is no longer a problem
- Advise patient to avoid OTC drugs, grapefruit juice, drugs prolonging QTc (quinidine, dofetilide, sotalol, erythromycin, thioridazine, ziprasidone or protease inhibitors, diltiazem, ketoconazole, macrolide antibiotics, verapamil) unless directed by prescriber
- Advise patient to comply in all areas of medical regimen
- Teach patient to notify prescriber of palpitations, fainting
- Teach patient to notify all health care providers of this product use

Evaluation
Positive therapeutic outcome
- Decreased anginal pain and number of episodes

---

rasagiline (Rx)
(ra-sa′-ji-leen)
Azilect
Func. class.: Antiparkinson agent
Chem. class.: MAOI

Pregnancy category C

Action: Inhibits MAOI type B; may increase dopamine levels

Therapeutic outcome: Improved symptoms in those with Parkinson's disease

Uses: Idiopathic Parkinson's disease monotherapy or with levodopa

Dosage and routes
Monotherapy
Adult: PO 1 mg/day

Adjunctive therapy
Adult: PO 0.5 mg/day, may be increased to 1 mg/day; change of levodopa dose in adjunct therapy; reduced levodopa dose may be needed

Hepatic dose
Adult: PO 0.5 mg in mild hepatic disease

Concomitant ciprofloxacin, other CYP1A2 inhibitors
Adult: PO 0.5 mg; plasma concentrations of rasagiline may double

Available forms: Tabs 0.5, 1 mg

Adverse effects
CNS: Drowsiness, hallucinations, depression, headache, malaise, paresthesia, vertigo, syncope

R

Adverse effects: italic = common, bold = life-threatening

CV: Angina, **hypertensive crisis** (ingestion of tyramine products), orthostatic hypotension
GI: *Nausea,* diarrhea, dry mouth, dyspepsia
GU: Impotence, decreased libido
MISC: Conjunctivitis, fever, flu syndrome, neck pain, allergic reaction, alopecia
MS: Arthralgia, arthritis, dyskinesia, falls
RESP: Rhinitis

Contraindications: Breastfeeding, hypersensitivity to this product or MAOIs, pheochromocytoma

Precautions: Pregnancy **C,** children, psychiatric disorders, severe hepatic disorders

Pharmacokinetics

Absorption	Well
Distribution	Protein binding >88%-94%
Metabolism	Liver, CYP1A2
Excretion	Kidneys
Half-life	Unknown

Pharmacodynamics
Unknown

Interactions
Individual drugs
Ciprofloxacin: increased levels of rasagiline up to twofold
◆ Meperidine: do not give; serious reaction including coma and death may occur
Drug classifications
◆ Analgesics, sympathomimetics: do not give; serious reaction including coma and death may occur
◆ Antidepressants (tricyclics, selective serotonin reuptake inhibitors, SNRIs, mirtazapine, cyclobenzaprine): increased severe CNS toxicity
CYP1A2 inhibitors (atazanavir, mexiletine, taurine): increased levels of rasagiline up to twofold
◆ MAOIs: increased hypertensive crisis
Drug/herb
◆ St. John's wort: do not give

NURSING CONSIDERATIONS
Assessment
• Assess for Parkinson's symptoms: tremor, ataxia, muscle weakness and rigidity; baseline, periodically
• Assess mental status: hallucinations, confusion, notify prescriber
• Assess for hypertensive crisis: severe headache, blurred vision, seizures, chest pain, difficulty thinking, nausea/vomiting, signs of stroke; any unexplained severe headache should be considered to be hypertensive crisis

• Assess for increased dyskinesia and postural hypotension if used in combination with levodopa
• Assess for melanomas frequently, perform periodic skin exams by a dermatologist
• Monitor cardiac status: B/P, ECG; periodically during beginning treatment

Nursing diagnoses
• Injury, risk for (uses, adverse reactions)
• Knowledge, deficient (teaching)
• Mobility, impaired physical (uses)

Implementation
• Give with meals to prevent nausea; continuing therapy usually reduces or eliminates nausea
• Give reduced dose of carbidopa/levodopa, cautiously

Patient/family education
• Advise patient to change positions slowly to prevent orthostatic hypotension
• Instruct patient to avoid hazardous activities until stabilized; dizziness can occur
• Advise patient to rinse mouth frequently, use sugarless gum to alleviate dry mouth
• Teach patient to take as prescribed, not to miss dose or double doses; take missed dose as soon as remembered, if several hours before next dose
• Teach patient to prevent hypertensive crisis by avoiding tyramine foods
• Teach patient to report signs of hypertensive crisis

Evaluation
Positive therapeutic outcome
• Improved symptoms in those with Parkinson's disease (decreasing tremors, ataxia, muscle weakness/rigidity)

rasburicase (Rx)
(rass-burr'i-case)
Elitek
Func. class.: Enzyme
Chem. class.: Recombinant urate-oxidase enzyme

Pregnancy category C

Action: Catalyzes enzymatic oxidation of uric acid into an inactive and a soluble metabolite (allantoin)

Therapeutic outcome: Decreased uric acid levels

Uses: To reduce uric acid levels in children with leukemia, lymphoma, solid tumor malignancies who are receiving chemotherapy

 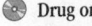

Dosage and routes
Adult/adolescent/child/infant: **IV**
INF 0.2 mg/kg as a single daily dose given as **IV** INF over ½ hr × 5 days

Available forms: Powder for inj 1.5 mg/vial

Adverse effects
CNS: Headache, fever
CV: Chest pain, hypotension
GI: Nausea, vomiting, anorexia, diarrhea, abdominal pain, constipation, dyspepsia, mucositis
HEMA: Neutropenia with fever, hemolysis, methemoglobinemia
INTEG: Rash
MISC: Edema
RESP: **Bronchospasm,** wheezing, dyspnea
SYST: **Anaphylaxis, hemolysis, methemoglobinemia, sepsis**

Contraindications: Hypersensitivity

Black Box Warning: G6PD deficiency, hemolytic reactions, or methemoglobinemia reactions to this product

Precautions: Pregnancy **C,** breastfeeding, children <2 yr, anemia

Black Box Warning: Acute bronchospasm, angina, angioedema, patients of African or Mediterranean ancestry, hypotension, urticaria

Pharmacokinetics

Absorption	Unknown
Distribution	Unknown
Metabolism	Unknown
Excretion	Unknown
Half-life	Elimination 16-21 hr

Pharmacodynamics
Unknown

Interactions
Individual drugs
Allopurinol: increased toxicity

NURSING CONSIDERATIONS
Assessment
• Monitor blood studies: BUN, serum uric acid, urine CCr, electrolytes, CBC with differential before, during therapy
• Monitor temp q4hr; fever may indicate beginning infection; no rectal temp
• Assess for anaphylaxis, have emergency equipment nearby
• Assess for G6PD deficiency, hemolytic reactions, methemoglobinemia; these patients should not be given this agent

• Assess for toxicity: severe diarrhea, nausea, vomiting
• Assess GI symptoms: frequency of stools, cramping; if severe diarrhea occurs, fluid and electrolytes may need to be given

Nursing diagnoses
• Injury, risk for (adverse reactions, uses)
• Knowledge, deficient (teaching)

Implementation
• Give antiemetic 30-60 min before giving product and prn
• Reconstitute with diluent provided; add 1 ml of diluent/vial, swirl; may dilute further
• Infuse over 30 min; do not filter, do not give as bolus

Patient/family education
• Advise of reason for therapy, expected results
• Advise to report trouble breathing, jaundice, chest pain

Evaluation
Positive therapeutic outcome
• Decreased uric acid levels

⚠ HIGH ALERT

remifentanil (Rx)
(re-me-fin′ta-nill)
Ultiva
Func. class.: Opiate agonist analgesic
Chem. class.: µ-Opioid agonist

Pregnancy category C
Controlled substance schedule II

Action: Inhibits ascending pain pathways in limbic system, thalamus, midbrain, hypothalamus

Therapeutic outcome: Maintenance of anesthesia

Uses: In combination with other products in general anesthesia to provide analgesia

Dosage and routes
Adult: Induction **IV** 0.5-1 mcg/kg/min with a hypnotic or volatile agent; maintenance with isoflurane (0.4-1.5 MAC) or propofol (100-200 mcg/kg/min); CONT INF 0.25-0.4 mcg/kg/min
Child 1-12 yr: CONT **IV** INF 0.25 mcg/kg/min with isoflurane
Full-term neonate and infant up to 2 mo: CONT **IV** INF 0.4 mcg/kg/min with nitrous oxide

Available forms: Powder for inj, lyophilized 1 mg/ml after reconstitution

R

Adverse effects: *italic* = common, **bold** = life-threatening

Adverse effects

CNS: Drowsiness, *dizziness,* confusion, *headache,* sedation, euphoria, delirium, agitation, anxiety

CV: Palpitations, **bradycardia,** change in B/P; facial flushing, syncope, **asystole**

EENT: Tinnitus, blurred vision, miosis, diplopia

GI: *Nausea, vomiting,* anorexia, constipation, cramps, dry mouth

GU: Urinary retention, dysuria

INTEG: Rash, urticaria, bruising, flushing, diaphoresis, pruritus

MS: Rigidity

RESP: **Respiratory depression, apnea**

Contraindications: Hypersensitivity

Precautions: Pregnancy **C**, breastfeeding, geriatric, increased ICP, acute MI, severe heart disease, GI/renal/hepatic disease, asthma, respiratory conditions, seizure disorders, bradyarrhythmias, child <12 yr

Pharmacokinetics	
Absorption	Complete
Distribution	70% protein binding
Metabolism	Unknown
Excretion	Unknown
Half-life	Terminal 3-10 min

Pharmacodynamics	
Onset	Immediate
Peak	Unknown
Duration	Unknown

Interactions
Individual drugs
Alcohol: increased respiratory depression, hypotension, profound sedation
Drug classifications
Antihistamines, CNS depressants, phenothiazines, sedative/hypnotics: increased respiratory depression, hypotension, profound sedation
Drug/herb
Kava: increased CNS depression

NURSING CONSIDERATIONS
Assessment
• Monitor I&O ratio, check for decreasing output; may indicate urinary retention, especially in geriatric
• Assess CNS changes: dizziness, drowsiness, hallucinations, euphoria, LOC pupil reaction
• Assess allergic reactions: rash, urticaria
• Assess respiratory dysfunction: respiratory depression, character, rate, rhythm; notify prescriber if respirations are <12/min; CV status, bradycardia, syncope
• Monitor GI status: nausea, vomiting, anorexia, constipation
• Use pain scoring to determine pain perception

Nursing diagnoses
• Knowledge, deficient (teaching)

Implementation
• Add 1 ml diluent/remifentanil
• Interruption of inf results in rapid reversal (no residual opioid effect within 5-10 min)
• Store in light-resistant area at room temperature

Y-site compatibilities: Acyclovir, alfentanil, amikacin, aminophylline, ampicillin, ampicillin/sulbactam, aztreonam, bretylium, bumetanide, buprenorphine, butorphanol, calcium gluconate, cefazolin, cefepime, cefotaxime, cefotetan, cefoxitin, ceftazidime, ceftizoxime, ceftriaxone, cefuroxime, cimetidine, ciprofloxacin, cisatracurium, cisplatin, clindamycin, dactinomycin, dexamethasone, digoxin, diltiazem, diphenhydrAMINE, DOBUTamine, docetaxel, DOPamine, doxacurium, doxycycline, droperidol, enalaprilat, epinephrine, esmolol, etoposide, famotidine, fentanyl, fluconazole, furosemide, ganciclovir, gatifloxacin, gemcitabine, gentamicin, granisetron, haloperidol, heparin, hetastarch, hydrocortisone sodium succinate, hydromorphone, hydrOXYzine, imipenem/cilastatin, inamrinone, isoproterenol, ketorolac, levofloxacin, lidocaine, lorazepam, magnesium sulfate, mannitol, meperidine, methylprednisoLONE sodium succinate, metoclopramide, metronidazole, mezlocillin, midazolam, minocycline, morphine, nalbuphine, netilmicin, nitroglycerin, norepinephrine, ofloxacin, ondansetron, paclitaxel, palonsetron, phenylephrine, piperacillin, potassium chloride, procainamide, prochlorperazine, promethazine, ranitidine, sulfamethoxazole/trimethoprim, sulfentanil, teniposide, theophylline, thiopental, thiotepa, ticarcillin, ticarcillin/clavulate, tobramycin, vancomycin, voriconazole, zidovudine

Solution compatibilities: D₅, 0.45% NaCl, LR, D₅LR, 0.9% NaCl

Patient/family education
• Advise patient to call for assistance when ambulating or smoking; drowsiness, dizziness may occur
• Advise patient to make position changes slowly to prevent orthostatic hypotension

 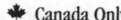

Evaluation
Positive therapeutic outcome
• Maintenance of anesthesia

---

repaglinide (Rx)
(re-pag'lih-nide)
Gluco Norm ✤, Prandin
Func. class.: Antidiabetic
Chem. class.: Meglitinides

Pregnancy category C

Action: Causes functioning β-cells in pancreas to release insulin, leading to drop in blood glucose levels; closes ATP-dependent potassium channels in the β-cell membrane; this leads to opening of calcium channels; increased calcium influx induces insulin secretion

Therapeutic outcome: Blood glucose controlled

Uses: Type 2 diabetes mellitus

Dosage and routes
Adult: PO 1-2 mg with each meal, max 16 mg/day, adjust at weekly intervals; oral hypoglycemic-naïve patients or those with A1c <8% should start with 0.5 mg with each meal

Renal/hepatic dose
Adult: PO CCr 20-39 ml/min: 0.5 mg/day; titrate upward cautiously

Available forms: Tabs 0.5, 1, 2 mg

Adverse effects
CNS: Headache, weakness, paresthesia
ENDO: **Hypoglycemia**
GI: Nausea, vomiting, diarrhea, constipation, dyspepsia
INTEG: Rash, allergic reactions
MISC: Chest pain, UTI, allergy
MS: Back pains, arthralgia
RESP: URI, sinusitis, rhinitis, bronchitis

Contraindications: Hypersensitivity to meglitinides, diabetic ketoacidosis, type 1 diabetes

Precautions: Pregnancy **C**, breastfeeding, children, geriatric, cardiac disease, severe renal/hepatic disease, thyroid disease, severe hypoglycemic reactions

Pharmacokinetics
Absorption	Complete
Distribution	98% protein binding, crosses placenta
Metabolism	Liver
Excretion	Urine/feces
Half-life	1 hr

Pharmacodynamics
Onset	30 min
Peak	1-1½ hr
Duration	<4 hr

Interactions
Individual drugs
Carbamazepine, rifampin: increased repaglinide metabolism
Chloramphenicol, fenofibrate, gemfibrozil, probenecid, simvastatin: increased effect of repaglinide
Erythromycin, ketoconazole, miconazole: decreased repaglinide metabolism
Isoniazid, phenobarbital, phenytoin, rifampin: decreased action of repaglinide
Levonorgestrel/ethinyl estradol: increase in both
Drug classifications
Antifungals, CYP450 inhibitors, macrolides: decreased repaglinide metabolism
Barbiturates, CYP450 inducers: increased repaglinide metabolism
β-Adrenergic blockers, coumarins, MAOIs, NSAIDs, salicylates, sulfonamides: increased repaglinide effect
Calcium channel blockers, contraceptives (oral), corticosteroids, diuretics (thiazide), estrogens, phenothiazines, sympathomimetics, thyroid preparations: decreased repaglinide effect
Drug/herb
Alfalfa, aloe, basil, bay, bilberry, bitter melon, black catechu, buchu, burdock, coriander, dandelion, eyebright (po), fenugreek, garlic, ginseng, glucomannan, glucosamine, goat's rue, gymnema, horehound, horse chestnut, jambul, myrrh, myrtle: increased antidiabetic effect
Bee pollen, blue cohosh, broom, chromium, elecampane, eucalyptus, gotu kola: decreased antidiabetic effect
Broom, buchu, dandelion, juniper: decreased hypoglycemia
Chromium, fenugreek, ginseng: increased or decreased hypoglycemia
Karela: decreased glucose tolerance
Drug/food
Decreased: repaglinide level; give before meals

NURSING CONSIDERATIONS
Assessment
⬥ Assess for hypoglycemic or hyperglycemic reaction, which can occur soon after meals; dizziness, weakness, headache, tremor, anxiety, tachycardia, hunger, sweating, abdominal pain

R

Adverse effects: *italic* = common, **bold** = life-threatening

- Monitor A1c, fasting, postprandial glucose during treatment

Nursing diagnoses
- Knowledge, deficient (teaching)
- Noncompliance (teaching)
- Nutrition: more than body requirements, imbalanced (uses)

Implementation
- 15 min before meals: 2, 3, or 4 ×/day preprandially
- Skip dose if meal is skipped; add dose if meal is added
- Store in airtight container at room temperature

Patient/family education
- Teach patient technique of blood glucose monitoring using blood glucose meter
- Teach patient the symptoms of hypoglycemia and hyperglycemia, what to do about each
- Teach patient that product must be continued on daily basis; explain consequence of discontinuing product abruptly
- Advise patient to avoid OTC medications unless ordered by prescriber
- Advise patient that diabetes is a lifelong illness; product will not cure disease
- Advise patient to eat all food included in diet plan to prevent hypoglycemia; to have glucagon emergency kit available
- Instruct patient to carry/wear emergency ID for emergency purposes

Evaluation
Positive therapeutic outcome
- Decrease in polyuria, polydipsia, polyphagia; clear sensorium; absence of dizziness; stable gait; blood glucose, A1c improvement

---

retapamulin topical
See Appendix B

---

retinoic acid
See tretinoin

Rh$_o$ (D) immune globulin, standard dose IM
BayRho (HyperRHO SD), Rho Gam Ultra Filtered Plus Solution for Injection

Rh$_o$ (D) immune globulin microdose IM
MICRhoGAM Ultra Filtered Plus Solution for Injection

Rh$_o$ (D) immune globulin IV
Rhophylac Pre-Filled Syringes, WinRho SDF
Func. class.: Immune globulins

Pregnancy category C

Action: Suppresses immune nonsensitized Rh$_o$ (D or D^u)-negative patients who are exposed to Rh$_o$ (D or D^u)-positive blood

Therapeutic outcome: Absence of Rh factor and transfusion error

Uses: Prevention of isoimmunization in Rh-negative women exposed to Rh-positive blood given after abortions, miscarriages, amniocentesis, chronic idiopathic thrombocytopenic purpura (Rhophylac)

Dosage and routes
To reduce risk of Rh isoimmunization antepartum/suppression of Rh isoimmunization postpartum following delivery of full-term infant
Adult and adolescent ≥16 yr: IM (BayRho-D [HyperRHO SD] [full dose only]) 300 mcg (1500 international units) at 28 wk gestation, repeat within 72 hr of delivery of confirmed Rho(D)-positive infant; a dose is not needed after delivery, if delivery is within 3 wk of last dose and no fetal maternal hemorrhage of >15 ml of RBC; IM (RhoGam only) 300 mcg (1500 international units) at 26-28 wk gestation, repeat within 72 hr even if status of Rho is unknown or if 72 hr have passed; IM/**IV** (WinRho SDF only) 300 mcg (1500 international units) at 28 wk gestation; if given earlier in pregnancy, give at 12-wk intervals during pregnancy, a 120-mcg (600 international units) dose; IM/**IV** should be given as soon as possible and preferably within 72 hr of delivery of a confirmed Rho(D)-positive infant, and even if status is unknown give up to 28 days after delivery

Known or suspected massive fetomaternal hemorrhage (>15 ml of fetal RBC or >30 ml of fetal whole blood)
Adult and adolescent ≥16 yr: IM (BayRho-D [HyperRHO SD] [full dose only]) 300 mcg (1500 international units) per every

---

15 ml of fetal blood cells or 30 ml of whole blood, multiple syringes may be injected IM at the same time in different sites, give within 72 hr of exposure, repeat dose within 72 hr of delivery; IM (RhoGAM only) 300 mcg (1500 international units) for every 15 ml of fetal blood cells or 30 ml of whole blood, give total dose within 72 hr of exposure; IM/**IV** (Win-Rho SDF only) if large fetomaternal hemorrhage is suspected, give **IV** 9 mcg (45 international units) or IM 12 mcg (60 international units) for every ml of fetal whole blood, give **IV** 600 mcg (3000 international units) q8hr or IM 1200 mcg (6000 international units) q12hr until total dose is given, total dose should be given within 72 hr of exposure

Threatened abortion at any stage of pregnancy
Adult and adolescent ≥16 yr: IM (BayRho-D [HyperRHO SD] [full dose only]) 300 mcg (1500 international units) as soon as possible; if given 13-18 wk gestation, give another 300 mcg (1500 international units) at 26-28 wk gestation; repeat dose within 72 hr of delivery; IM (RhoGam only) 300 mcg (1500 international units) as soon as possible and within 72 hr; IM/**IV** (Rhophylac only) 300 mcg (1500 international units) as soon as possible and within 72 hr; IM/**IV** (WinRho SDF only) 300 mcg (1500 international units) as soon as possible and within 72 hr, repeat dose at 12-wk intervals during pregnancy and 120 mcg (600 international units) as soon as possible after delivery and within 72 hr

Following spontaneous abortion, induced termination of pregnancy, or ectopic pregnancy that occurs ≤12 wk gestation
Adult and adolescent ≥16 yr: IM (BayRho-D Minidose, HYperRHO Minidose, MICRORhoGAM only) 50 mcg (250 international units) as soon as possible, give within 3 hr of spontaneous or surgical removal, if possible within 72 hr

Following spontaneous abortion, induced termination of pregnancy, or ruptured tubal pregnancy that occurs ≥13 wk
Adult and adolescent ≥16 yr: IM (BayRho-D full dose [HyperRHO SD full dose] RhoGAM only) 300 mcg (1500 international units) as soon as possible and within 72 hr of event

Following spontaneous abortion, induced termination of pregnancy, aminocentesis, chorionic villus sampling, abdominal trauma, ruptured tubal pregnancy, or percutaneous umbilical cord sampling up to 34 wk gestation
Adult and adolescent ≥16 wk: IM/**IV** (WinRho SDF only) 300 mcg (1500 international units) within 72 hr, repeat at 12-wk intervals during pregnancy, give 120 mcg (600 international units) as soon as possible and preferably within 72 hr of delivery

Available forms: BayRho-D sol for inj 300 mcg/ml (HyperRHO SD solution for injection); MICRhoGAM Ultra Filtered Plus Solution for inj 50 mcg/ml; RhoGam Ultra Filtered Plus Solution for inj 50 mcg; Rhophylac Pre-Filled Syringes Solution for inj 300 mcg/2 ml; WinRho SDF Liquid for inj; WinRho powder for inj

Adverse effects
CNS: Lethargy
INTEG: Irritation at inj site, fever
MS: Myalgia

Contraindications: Previous immunization with this product, Rh₀ (O) positive/D^u^-positive patient

Precautions: Pregnancy C

Pharmacokinetics	
Absorption	Well absorbed
Distribution	Unknown
Metabolism	Unknown
Excretion	Unknown
Half-life	Unknown

Pharmacodynamics	
Onset	Rapid
Peak	Unknown
Duration	Unknown

Interactions
Drug classifications
Live virus vaccines (measles, mumps, rubella): decreased antibody response to vaccine

NURSING CONSIDERATIONS
Assessment
🔴 Assess for allergies, reactions to immunizations; previous immunization with this product
• Obtain type and cross-match of mother's blood and of neonate's cord blood; neonate must be Rh₀(D)-positive, mother must be

Rh$_o$(D)-negative and (D^u)-negative, medication should be given if there is a doubt

◆ Assess for intravascular hemolysis: back pain, chills, hemoglobinuria, renal insufficiency, idiopathic thrombocytopenic purpura

Nursing diagnoses
• Knowledge, deficient (teaching)

Implementation
• BayRho-D is being changed to HyperRHO SD
• BayRho-D (HyperRHO SD), MICRhoGAM, RhoGAM are given by IM only; do not give **IV**
• WinRho SDF and Rhophylac can be given IM or **IV**
• Inspect for particulate matter; do not use if particulate matter is present
• Reconstitution/dilution: no reconstitution or dilution is needed for BayRho-D (HyperRHO SD), Rhophylac, MICRoGAM, RhoGAM, or the liquid formulation of WinRho SDF
• WinRho SDF powder for **IV** use: if giving **IV**, reconstitute 600 international units or 1500 international units immediately before use with 2.5 ml of sterile diluent; reconstitute 5000 international units with 8.5 ml sterile diluent; add diluent to vial slowly down the wall of the vial; gently swirl until powder is dissolved; do not shake
• WinRho SDF powder for IM use: **IV** giving IM, reconstitute 600 international units or 1500 international units immediately before use with 1.25 ml of sterile diluent; 5000 international units with 8.5 ml of sterile diluent; add diluent to the vial slowly down the wall of the vial; gently swirl until powder is dissolved; do not shake

IM route
• Use aseptic technique, observe for 20 min after administration
• Bring Rhophylac to room temperature before using
• Inject into the deltoid muscle of upper arm or anterolateral portion of the upper thigh; do not inject into gluteal muscle
• If dose calculated will need multiple vials or syringes, use different site at the same time

IV route
• Use aseptic technique
• WinRhoSDF: remove entire contents of vial to obtain calculated dose; if partial vial contents are required for dosage calculation, withdraw the entire vial contents to ensure correct calculation; inf correct calculated dose over 3-5 min; do not inf with other fluids or products
• Rhophylac: bring to room temperature; inf by slow **IV**; observe for 20 min

Patient/family education
• Teach patient how product works; that product must be given after subsequent deliveries if subsequent babies are Rh-positive

Evaluation
Positive therapeutic outcome
• Prevention of Rh$_o$(D) sensitization in transfusion error
• Prevention of erythroblastosis fetalis in subsequent Rh$_o$(D)-positive neonates

---

ribavarin (Rx)
(rye-ba-vye′rin)
Virazole
Func. class.: Synthetic antiviral
Chem. class.: Tricyclic amine

Pregnancy category X

Action: Prevents replication of DNA and RNA synthesis

Therapeutic outcome: Resolution of severe lower respiratory tract infections

Uses: Severe lower respiratory tract infections in infants and children

Unlabeled uses: Influenza A or B (early)

Dosage and routes
Infant and young child: INH 20 mg/ml × 12-18 hr/day × 3-7 days

Available forms: Powder for reconstitution for aerosol 6 g/vial

Adverse effects
CNS: Dizziness, faintness
CV: Hypotension, cardiac arrest
EENT: Eye irritation, conjunctivitis, blurred vision, photosensitivity
INTEG: Rash

Contraindications: Pregnancy **X**, breastfeeding, children <1 yr, hypersensitivity

Precautions: Epilepsy, renal/hepatic disease

Pharmacokinetics	
Absorption	Inh (systemic)
Distribution	To respiratory tract
Metabolism	Liver
Excretion	Respiratory tract
Half-life	9½ hr

Pharmacodynamics	
Onset	Unknown
Peak	Inh end
Duration	Unknown

 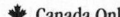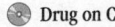

Interactions
Individual products
Zidovudine: decreased antiviral action, increased toxicity
Drug classification
Cardiac glycosides: increased toxicity

NURSING CONSIDERATIONS
Assessment
• Assess allergies before initiation of treatment, reaction of each medication; list allergies on chart in bright red letters
• Monitor respiratory status: rate, character, wheezing, tightness in chest
• Obtain C&S test results before starting treatment

Nursing diagnoses
• Gas exchange, impaired (uses)
• Infection, risk for (uses)
• Knowledge, deficient (teaching)

Implementation
• Give by the Viratek small particle aerosol generator (SPAG-2), do not use other inhalation equipment
• May be given by an oxygen hood for infants, or a face mask may be attached to the SPAG-2
• Reconstitute 6 g of sterile water for inj or inh, place sol in the Erlenmeyer flask and dilute further to 20 mg/ml

Patient/family education
• Teach patient and parents aspects of product therapy

Evaluation
Positive therapeutic outcome
• Absence of respiratory syncytial virus

riboflavin
(vitamin B₂) (OTC)
(rye'boo-flay-vin)
Func. class.: Vitamin B₂, water soluble
Pregnancy category A

Action: Needed for respiratory reactions (catalyzes proteins) and for normal vision

Therapeutic outcome: Prevention or treatment of riboflavin deficiency

Uses: Vitamin B₂ deficiency or polyneuritis; cheilosis adjunct with thiamine

Dosage and routes
Deficiency
Adult: PO 5-30 mg/day
Child ≥3 yr: PO 2-10 mg/day, then 0.6 mg/1000 cal ingested

RDA
Adult: PO (Males) 1.3 mg; (females) 1.1 mg

Available forms: Tabs 5, 10, 25, 50, 100, 250 mg

Adverse effects
GU: Yellow discoloration of urine (large doses)

Precautions: Pregnancy A

Pharmacokinetics
Absorption	Well absorbed (by active transport)
Distribution	60% protein bound, widely distributed, crosses placenta
Metabolism	Unknown
Excretion	Kidneys (unchanged), excess amounts
Half-life	1-1½ hr

Pharmacodynamics
Unknown

Interactions
Individual drugs
Alcohol, probenecid: increased riboflavin need
Tetracycline: decreased action of tetracycline
Drug classifications
Antidepressants (tricyclics), phenothiazines: increased riboflavin need
Drug/lab test
False increase: urinary catecholamines

NURSING CONSIDERATIONS
Assessment
• Assess patient's nutritional status: liver, eggs, dairy products, yeast, whole grain, green vegetables
• Assess for vit B₂ deficiency: photophobia, cheilosis, stomatitis, ocular swelling

Nursing diagnoses
• Knowledge, deficient (teaching)
• Nutrition: less than body requirements, imbalanced (uses)

Implementation
• Give with food for better absorption
• Store in airtight, light-resistant container

Patient/family education
• Inform patient that urine may turn bright yellow
• Instruct patient about needed addition of foods that are rich in riboflavin

Evaluation
Positive therapeutic outcome
• Absence of headache, GI problems, cheilosis, skin lesions, depression, burning, itchy eyes, anemia

Adverse effects: *italic* = common, **bold** = life-threatening

rifabutin (Rx)
(riff'a-byoo-tin)
Mycobutin
Func. class.: Antimycobacterial
Chem. class.: Rifamycin S derivative

Pregnancy category B

Do not confuse:
rifabutin/rifampin

Action: Inhibits DNA-dependent RNA polymerase in susceptible strains

Therapeutic outcome: Antimycobacterial death of *Escherichia coli, Bacillus subtilis,* and *Mycobacterium avium*

Uses: Prevention of *M. avium* complex (MAC) in patients with advanced HIV infection

Unlabeled uses: *Helicobacter pylori* that has not responded to other treatment

Dosage and routes
Adult: PO 300 mg/day (may take as 150 mg bid); max 600 mg/day

Renal dose
Adult: PO CCr <30 ml/min reduce dose by 50%

Available forms: Caps 150 mg

Adverse effects
CNS: Headache, fatigue, anxiety, confusion, insomnia
GI: Nausea, vomiting, anorexia, diarrhea, heartburn, **hepatitis,** discolored saliva
GU: Hematuria, discolored urine
HEMA: **Hemolytic anemia, eosinophilia, thrombocytopenia, leukopenia**
INTEG: Rash
MISC: Flulike syndrome, shortness of breath, chest pressure
MS: Asthenia, arthralgia, myalgia

Contraindications: Hypersensitivity, active TB, WBC <1000/mm^3, platelets <50,000/mm^3

Precautions: Pregnancy **B**, breastfeeding, children, hepatic disease, blood dyscrasias

Pharmacokinetics

Absorption	Well absorbed
Distribution	Widely distributed
Metabolism	Liver
Excretion	Kidney
Half-life	45 hr

Pharmacodynamics

Onset	Unknown
Peak	2-3 hr
Duration	Unknown

Interactions
Individual drugs
Amprenavir, busPIRone, clofibrate, cycloSPORINE, dapsone, delavirdine, digoxin, disopyramide, doxycycline, efavirenz, fluconazole, indinavir, ketoconazole, losartan, nelfinavir, nevirapine, phenytoin, quinidine, saquinavir, theophylline, tocainide, verapamil, zidovudine, zolpidem: decreased action of each specific product
Ritonavir: increased rifabutin level

Drug classifications
Analgesics (opioid), anticoagulants, antidepressants (tricyclics), barbiturates, β-blockers, contraceptives (oral), corticosteroids, estrogens, sulfonylureas: decreased action of each specific product

Drug/food
High-fat foods: decreased absorption

Drug/lab test
Interference: folate level, vit B$_{12}$, BSP, gallbladder tests

NURSING CONSIDERATIONS
Assessment
• Assess for active TB: chest x-ray, sputum culture, blood culture, biopsy of lymph nodes, obtain PPD test; product should be given only for MAC and never for TB
• Monitor CBC for neutropenia, thrombocytopenia, eosinophilia

Nursing diagnoses
• Diarrhea (adverse reaction)
• Infection, risk for (uses)
• Injury, risk for (adverse reaction)
• Knowledge, deficient (teaching)
• Noncompliance (teaching)

Implementation
• Give with meals to decrease GI symptoms; better to take on empty stomach 1 hr before or 2 hr after meals; high-fat food slows absorption
• Give antiemetic if vomiting occurs

Patient/family education
• Caution patient that compliance with dosage schedule and duration is necessary
• Instruct patient that scheduled appointments must be kept or relapse may occur
• Instruct patient to notify prescriber if hepatitis, neutropenia, or thrombocytopenia occurs: sore throat, fever, bleeding, bruising, yellow sclera, anorexia, nausea, vomiting, fatigue, weakness; myositis: muscle or bone pain
• Advise patient that urine, feces, saliva, sputum, sweat, tears may be colored red-orange; soft contact lenses may become permanently stained

 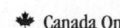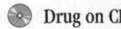

- Caution patients using oral contraceptives to use a nonhormonal method of birth control because rifabutin may decrease efficiency of oral contraceptives

Evaluation
Positive therapeutic outcome
- Decreased symptoms of *M. avium* in patients with HIV

rifampin (Rx)
(rif'am-pin)
Rifadin, Rofact ✦
Func. class.: Antitubercular
Chem. class.: Rifamycin B derivative

Pregnancy category C

Do not confuse:
rifampin/rifabutin

Action: Inhibits DNA-dependent polymerase, decreases tubercle bacilli replication

Therapeutic outcome: Bactericidal against the following organisms: mycobacteria, *Staphylococcus aureus*, *Haemophilus influenzae*, *Neisseria meningitidis*, *Legionella pneumophila*

Uses: Pulmonary TB, meningococcal carriers (prevention)

Dosage and routes
Tuberculosis
Adult: PO/IV max 600 mg/day as single dose 1 hr before or 2 hr after meals, or 10 mg/kg/day 2-3 ×/wk
Child >5 yr: PO/IV 10-20 mg/kg/day as single dose 1 hr before or 2 hr after meals, max 600 mg/day, with other antitubercular products

6-mo regimen: 2-mo treatment of isoniazid, rifampin, pyrazinamide, and possibly streptomycin or ethambutol; then rifampin and isoniazid × 4 mo

9-mo regimen: Rifampin and isoniazid supplemented with pyrazinamide, or streptomycin or ethambutol

Meningococcal carriers
Adult: PO/IV 600 mg bid × 2 days, max 600 mg/dose
Child >5 yr: PO/IV 10-20 mg/kg bid × 2 days, max 600 mg/dose
Infant 3 mo-1 yr: PO 5 mg/kg bid for 2 days

Available forms: Caps 150, 300 mg; powder for inj 600 mg/vial

Adverse effects
CNS: Headache, fatigue, anxiety, drowsiness, confusion
EENT: Visual disturbances
GI: Nausea, vomiting, anorexia, diarrhea, **pseudomembranous colitis,** *heartburn,* sore mouth and tongue, **pancreatitis,** elevated liver function tests
GU: **Hematuria, acute renal failure, hemoglobinuria**
HEMA: **Hemolytic anemia, eosinophilia, thrombocytopenia, leukopenia**
INTEG: Rash, pruritus, urticaria
MISC: Flulike syndrome, menstrual disturbances, edema, shortness of breath
MS: Ataxia, weakness

Contraindications: Hypersensitivity to this product or rifamycins, active *Neisseria meningitidis* infection

Precautions: Pregnancy **C,** breastfeeding, children <5 yr, hepatic disease, blood dyscrasias

Pharmacokinetics
Absorption	Well absorbed (PO), completely absorbed (**IV**)
Distribution	Widely distributed, crosses placenta
Metabolism	Liver—extensively
Excretion	Feces
Half life	3 hr

Pharmacodynamics
	PO	IV
Onset	Rapid	Rapid
Peak	2-3 hr	Inf end
Duration	Unknown	Unknown

R

Interactions
Individual drugs
Acetaminophen, alcohol, chloramphenicol, clofibrate, cycloSPORINE, dapsone, digoxin, diltiazem, doxycycline, haloperidol, NIFEdipine, phenytoin, theophylline, verapamil, zidovudine: decreased effect of specific product
Imidazole: decreased antifungal action
Isoniazid: increased hepatotoxicity
Lithium: increased lithium toxicity
Sodium lactate: products are incompatible
Drug classifications
Anticoagulants: decreased action of anticoagulants

Adverse effects: *italic* = common, **bold** = life-threatening

Antidiabetics: decreased action of antidiabetics

Barbiturates: decreased action of barbiturates

Benzodiazepines: decreased action of benzodiazepines

β-blockers: decreased action of β-blockers

Contraceptives (oral), glucocorticoids: decreased effect

Fluroquinolones: decreased action of fluoroquinolones

Hormones: decreased action of hormones

Imidazole antifungals: decreased antifungal action

Sulfonamides: decreased action of sulfonamides

Protease inhibitors: decreased action of protease inhibitors

Drug/lab test

Interference: folate level, vit B_{12} gallbladder studies, dexamethasone suppression test

False positive: direct Coombs' test

NURSING CONSIDERATIONS
Assessment

• Monitor liver function tests qmo: ALT, AST, bilirubin

• Monitor renal status: before, qmo: BUN, creatinine, output, specific gravity, urinalysis

• Monitor mental status often: affect, mood, behavioral changes; psychosis may occur

• Monitor hepatic status: decreased appetite, jaundice, dark urine, fatigue

• Assess for infection: sputum culture, lung sounds

• C&S should be performed before beginning treatment, during, and after therapy is completed

Nursing diagnoses

• Diarrhea (adverse reactions)

• Infection, risk for (uses)

• Injury, risk for (adverse reactions)

• Knowledge, deficient (teaching)

• Noncompliance (teaching)

Implementation

• Administer with meals to decrease GI symptoms; better to take on empty stomach 1 hr before or 2 hr after meals, with full glass of water

Intermittent IV route

• Give by intermittent inf after reconstituting 600 mg/10 ml of sterile water for inj, agitate gently; dilute further in 100 or 500 ml of 0.9% NaCl or D_5W; give 100 ml/30 min or 500 ml/3 hr

• Do not mix with other products or sols

Patient/family education

• Instruct patient that compliance with dosage schedule, duration is necessary

• Instruct patient that scheduled appointments must be kept or relapse may occur

• Instruct patient to notify prescriber if hepatitis, neutropenia, or thrombocytopenia occurs: sore throat, fever, bleeding, bruising, yellow sclera, anorexia, nausea, vomiting, fatigue, weakness

• Advise patient that urine, feces, saliva, sputum, sweat, tears may be colored redorange; soft contact lenses may be permanently stained

• Caution patients using oral contraceptives to use a nonhormonal method of birth control because rifabutin may decrease the efficiency of oral contraceptives

• Advise patient to avoid alcohol; hepatotoxicity may occur

Evaluation
Positive therapeutic outcome

• Decreased symptoms of TB

---

rifapentine (Rx)
(riff'ah-pen-teen)
Priftin
Func. class.: Antitubercular
Chem. class.: Rifamycin derivative

Pregnancy category C

Action: Inhibits DNA-dependent polymerase, decreases tubercule bacilli replication

Therapeutic outcome: Resolution of pulmonary TB

Uses: Pulmonary TB; must be used with at least one other antitubercular product

Dosage and routes
Intensive phase

Adult: PO 600 mg (4 150-mg tabs) 2 ×/wk, with an interval of 72 hr between doses × 2 mo; must be given with at least one other antitubercular product

Continuation phase

Adult: 600 mg qwk × 4 mo in combination with isoniazid or other appropriate antitubercular product

Available forms: Tabs 150 mg

Adverse effects

CNS: Headache, fatigue, anxiety, dizziness

EENT: Visual disturbances

GI: Nausea, vomiting, anorexia, diarrhea, bilirubinemia, hepatitis, increased ALT, AST, *heartburn,* **pancreatitis**

GU: **Hematuria,** pyuria, proteinuria, urinary casts, urine discoloration
HEMA: **Thrombocytopenia, leukopenia, neutropenia, lymphopenia,** anemia, **leukocytosis,** purpura, hematoma
INTEG: Rash, pruritus, urticaria, acne
MISC: Edema, aggressive reaction, increased B/P
MS: Gout, arthrosis

Contraindications: Hypersensitivity to rifamycins, porphyria

Precautions: Pregnancy **C,** breastfeeding, children <12 yr, geriatric, hepatic disease, blood dyscrasias, HIV

Pharmacokinetics
Unknown

Pharmacodynamics
Unknown

Interactions
Individual drugs
Amitriptyline, chloramphenicol, clarithromycin, clofibrate, cycloSPORINE, dapsone, delaviridine, diazepam, digoxin, diltiazem, disopyramide, doxycycline, fentanyl, fluconazole, haloperidol, indinavir, itraconazole, ketoconazole, methadone, mexiletine, nelfinavir, NIFEdipine, nortriptyline, phenytoin, quinidine, quinine, ritonavir, saquinavir, sildenafil, tacrolimus, theophylline, tocainide, verapamil, warfarin, zidovudine: decreased action of each specific product
Drug classifications
Anticoagulants, antidiabetics, barbiturates, β-adrenergic blockers, corticosteroids, fluoroquinolones, oral contraceptives, phenothiazines, progestins, thyroid preparations: decreased action of each product class
Protease inhibitors: use extreme caution
Drug/food
Food: increased absorption with food
Drug/lab test
Interference: folate level, vit B$_{12}$

NURSING CONSIDERATIONS
Assessment
- Obtain baselines in CBC, AST, ALT, bilirubin, platelets
- Assess for infection: sputum culture, lung sounds
- Assess signs of anemia: Hct, Hgb, fatigue
- Monitor liver function tests qmo: ALT, AST, bilirubin

- Monitor renal status qmo: BUN, creatinine, output, specific gravity, urinalysis
- Assess hepatic status: decreased appetite, jaundice, dark urine, fatigue

Nursing diagnoses
- Diarrhea (side effects)
- Infection, risk for (uses)
- Knowledge, deficient (teaching)
- Noncompliance (teaching)

Implementation
- May be given with food for GI upset
- Give antiemetic if vomiting occurs
- Administer after C&S is completed; qmo to detect resistance

Patient/family education
- Advise patient that compliance with dosage schedule, duration is necessary
- Instruct patient that scheduled appointments must be kept; relapse may occur
- Teach patient that urine, feces, saliva, sputum, sweat, tears may be colored red-orange; soft contact lenses, dentures may be permanently stained
- Teach patient to use alternative method of contraception; oral contraceptive action may be decreased
- Teach patient to report flulike symptoms: excessive fatigue, anorexia, vomiting, sore throat; unusual bleeding, jaundice of skin, eyes

Evaluation
Positive therapeutic outcome
- Decreased symptoms of TB
- Negative culture

rifaximin (Rx)
(rif-ax'i-min)
Xifaxan
Func. class.: Misc. antiinfective
Chem. class.: Analog of rifampin
Pregnancy category C

R

Action: Binds to bacterial DNA dependent RNA polymerase, thereby inhibiting bacterial RNA synthesis

Therapeutic outcome: Bacterial action against *E. coli*

Uses: Traveler's diarrhea in those ≥12 yr old, caused by *E. coli*

Dosage and routes
Adult and child ≥12 yr: PO 200 mg tid × 3 days without regard to meals

Available forms: Tabs 200 mg

Adverse effects
CNS: Abnormal dreams, dizziness, insomnia
GI: Abdominal pain, constipation, defecation urgency, flatulence, nausea, rectal tenesmus, vomiting
MISC: Headache, pyrexia, motion sickness, tinnitus, rash, photosensitivity, **exfoliative dermatitis**

Contraindications: Hypersensitivity, diarrhea with fever, blood in stool

Precautions: Pregnancy **C**, breastfeeding, children

Pharmacokinetics	
Absorption	Unknown
Distribution	Unknown
Metabolism	Induces P450 3A4 (CYP3A4)
Excretion	Feces
Half-life	6 hr

Pharmacodynamics
Unknown

Interactions
Drug/herb
Acidophilus: do not use with antiinfectives; separate by several hours

NURSING CONSIDERATIONS
Assessment
• Assess for GI symptoms: amount and character of diarrhea, abdominal pain, nausea, vomiting
⬥ Assess for overgrowth of infection and pseudomembranous colitis

Nursing diagnoses
• Infection, risk for (uses)
• Knowledge, deficient (teaching)
• Noncompliance (teaching)

Implementation
• May be administered without regard to food

Patient/family education
• Instruct patient to discontinue rifaximin and notify prescriber if diarrhea persists for more than 24-48 hr, if diarrhea worsens, or if blood is in stools and fever is present

Evaluation
Positive therapeutic outcome
• Absence of infection

---

rilonacept (Rx)
(ril-on′a-sept)
Func. class.: Biologic response modifier
Chem. class.: Interleukin-1 inhibitor

Pregnancy category C

Action: Inhibits interleukin-1 by binding IL-1 and preventing its interaction with receptors, thus reducing inflammation

Therapeutic outcome: Reduction in joint pain, fever, chills, fatigue, rash, eye redness

Uses: Cryopyrin-associated periodic syndromes (CAPS) including familial cold autoinflammatory syndrome (FCAS) and Muckle-Wells syndrome (MWS) in adults and children ≥12 yr

Dosage and routes
Adult: SUBCUT 320 mg given as two 2-ml inj of 160 mg on the same day at two different sites, continue qwk with 160 mg as a single 2 ml inj starting on day 8, max 320 mg qwk
Child 12-17 yr: SUBCUT 4.4 mg/kg (max 320 mg) given as one or two inj with no more volume than 2 ml, then 2.2 mg/kg (max 160 mg) 1×wk starting on day 8

Available forms: Inj, lyophilized powder, vial 220 mg

Adverse effects
EENT: Sinusitis
GI: Nausea, vomiting, abdominal pain, stomach discomfort
HEMA: **Neutropenia, bleeding**
INTEG: Inj site reactions, rash, pruritus, ecchymosis
META: Hypercholesterolemia, hypertriglyceridemia
RESP: Upper respiratory infection, cough
SYST: **Malignancies,** meningitis

Contraindications: Hypersensitivity, IM/**IV** administration

Precautions: Pregnancy **C**, breastfeeding, children <12 yr, geriatric patients, hepatic/renal disease, HIV/AIDS, asthma, bone-marrow suppression, diabetes mellitus, hamster protein hypersensitivity, hepatitis, hypercholesterolemia, hypertriglyceridemia, immunosuppression, infection, TB, live vaccines

Pharmacokinetics	
Absorption	Unknown
Distribution	Steady state 8 days
Metabolism	Unknown
Excretion	Unknown
Half-life	Unknown

Pharmacodynamics
Unknown

Interactions
Individual drugs
Adalimumab, anakinra, tumor necrosis factor modifiers: avoid concurrent use
Warfarin: change in effect
Drug classifications
Toxoids, vaccines: avoid concurrent use
Immunosuppressives: increased infections

NURSING CONSIDERATIONS
Assessment
• Monitor serum cholesterol/serum triglycerides baseline and periodically during treatment
• Assess for symptoms of CAPS: fever, chills, rash, fatigue, joint pain, eye redness

Nursing diagnoses
• Pain, chronic (uses)
• Knowledge, deficient (teaching)

Implementation
• Give as subcut inj only
• Reconstitute each vial with 2.3 ml of supplied sterile water for inj (80 mg/ml); shake for 1 min and let stand for 1 min; do not use if particulate is present or if color is anything other than clear to pale yellow; use a new syringe/needle to withdraw needed amount; discard unused amount
• Maximum single inj is 2 ml (160 mg); if giving 4 ml (320 mg), give in two divided inj
• Rotate inj sites; do not use areas that are hard, bruised, red, or tender
• Store reconstituted solution for up to 3 hr at room temperature

Patient/family education
• Teach reason for use and expected result

Evaluation
• Therapeutic response: absence of joint pain, fever, chills, fatigue, rash, eye redness

---

riluzole (Rx)
(ri-loo′zole)
Rilutek
Func. class.: Amyotropic lateral sclerosis (ALS) agent
Chem. class.: Benzathiazole

Pregnancy category C

Action: Unknown; may act by inhibiting glutamate, interfering with binding of amino acid receptors, inactivation of voltage-dependent sodium channels

Therapeutic outcome: Decreased symptoms of ALS

Uses: ALS

Dosage and routes
Adult: PO 50 mg q12hr; take 1 hr before or 2 hr after meals

Available forms: Tabs 50 mg

Adverse effects
CNS: Hypertonia, depression, dizziness, insomnia, somnolence, vertigo, paresthesia
CV: Hypertension, tachycardia, phlebitis, palpitation, postural hypertension
GI: Nausea, vomiting, dyspepsia, anorexia, diarrhea, flatulence, stomatitis, dry mouth, increased liver function tests, jaundice, abdominal pain
GU: UTI, dysuria
HEMA: **Neutropenia**
INTEG: Pruritus, eczema, alopecia, **exfoliative dermatitis**
MS: Arthralgia
RESP: Decreased lung function; rhinitis, increased cough, pneumonia

Contraindications: Hypersensitivity

Precautions: Pregnancy C, breastfeeding, children, geriatric, neutropenia, renal/hepatic disease, cigarette smoking, febrile illness, pneumonia

Pharmacokinetics	
Absorption	Well
Distribution	Unknown
Metabolism	Extensively—live
Excretion	Urine, feces
Half-life	Unknown

Pharmacodynamics
Unknown

R

Interactions
Individual drugs
Allopurinol, leflunomide, methotrexate, methyldopa, sulfasalazine, tacrine: increased hepatic injury
Amitriptyline, caffeine, theophylline: decreased elimination of riluzole
Carbamazepine: increased liver function tests
Cigarette smoke, omeprazole, rifampin: increased elimination of riluzole
Drug classifications
Barbiturates: increased liver function tests
Quinolones: decreased elimination of riluzole

Adverse effects: *italic* = common, **bold** = life-threatening

Drug/food
Charcoal-broiled foods: increased elimination of riluzole
High-fat meal: decreased absorption

NURSING CONSIDERATIONS
Assessment
- Assess for clinical improvement in neurologic function
- Monitor liver function tests: AST, ALT, bilirubin, GGT, baseline and qmo × 3 mo, then q3mo
- Assess for neutropenia (neutrophils <500/mm³)

Nursing diagnoses
- Knowledge, deficient (teaching)
- Mobility, impaired physical (uses)

Implementation
- Give 1 hr before or 2 hr after meals; a high-fat meal decreases absorption

Patient/family education
- Advise to report febrile illness, may indicate neutropenia; cardiac/respiratory changes
- Teach reason for product and expected results

Evaluation
Positive therapeutic outcome
- Decreasing symptoms of ALS

rimantadine (Rx)
(ri-man'ti-deen)
Flumadine
Func. class.: Synthetic antiviral
Chem. class.: Tricyclic amine

Pregnancy category C

Do not confuse:
rimantadine/amantadine/ranitidine

Action: Prevents uncoating of nucleic acid in viral cell, preventing penetration of virus to host; causes release of dopamine from neurons

Therapeutic outcome: Prevention of influenza type A

Uses: Prophylaxis or treatment of influenza type A

Dosage and routes
Influenza type A prophylaxis
Adult and child >10 yr: PO 100 mg bid
Child 1-10 yr: PO 5 mg/kg/day, max 150 mg

Treatment
Adult: PO 100 mg bid; start treatment at onset of symptoms, continue for at least 1 wk
Geriatric: PO 100 mg/day

Renal/hepatic dose
Adult: PO ≤10 ml/min 100 mg qd

Available forms: Tabs 100 mg; syr 50 mg/5 ml

Adverse effects
CNS: *Headache, dizziness,* fatigue, depression, hallucinations, tremors, **seizures,** insomnia, poor concentration, asthenia, gait abnormalities, anxiety, confusion
CV: Pallor, palpitations, edema
EENT: Tinnitus, taste abnormality, eye pain
GI: *Nausea, vomiting,* constipation, *dry mouth, anorexia, abdominal pain, diarrhea,* dyspepsia
INTEG: Rash

Contraindications: Hypersensitivity to products of adamantine class (this product, amantadine)

Precautions: Pregnancy C, breastfeeding, children <1 yr, epilepsy, renal/hepatic disease

Pharmacokinetics
Absorption	Minimally absorbed (PO)
Distribution	Widely distributed, crosses placenta, CSF concentration 50% plasma
Metabolism	Liver
Excretion	95% unchanged—kidneys
Half-life	13-65 hr, increased in renal disease

Pharmacodynamics
	PO
Onset	Unknown
Peak	1½-2½
Duration	Unknown

Interactions
Individual drugs
Acetaminophen, aspirin, intranasal influenza vaccine: decreased peak concentration of rimantadine
Cimetidine: increased rimantidine concentration

NURSING CONSIDERATIONS
Assessment
- Assess for seizures; if seizures occur, product should be discontinued
- Assess allergies before initiation of treatment, patient's reaction to each medication; list allergies on chart

 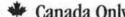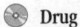

- Monitor respiratory status: rate, character, wheezing, tightness in chest

Nursing diagnoses
- Infection, risk for (uses)
- Knowledge, deficient (teaching)

Implementation
- Give before exposure to influenza; continue for 10 days after contact
- Give at least 4 hr before bedtime to prevent insomnia
- Administer after meals for better absorption, to decrease GI symptoms; cap may be opened and mixed with food for easy swallowing
- Give in divided doses to prevent CNS disturbances: headache, dizziness, fatigue, drowsiness
- Store in airtight, dry container

Patient/family education
- Instruct patient about aspects of product therapy: need to report dyspnea, dizziness, poor concentration, behavioral changes
- Advise patient to avoid hazardous activities if dizziness occurs
- Caution patient to consult prescriber before taking OTC medications, alcohol; serious product interactions may result

Evaluation
Positive therapeutic outcome
- Absence of fever, malaise, cough, dyspnea

---

risedronate (Rx)
(rih-sed'roh-nate)
Actonel
Func. class.: Bone resorption inhibitor
Chem. class.: Bisphosphonate
Pregnancy category C

Action: Inhibits bone resorption; absorbs calcium phosphate crystal in bone and may directly block dissolution of hydroxyapatite crystals of bone

Therapeutic outcome: Increased bone mass, activity without fractures

Uses: Paget's disease; prevention, treatment of osteoporosis in postmenopausal women; glucocorticoid-induced osteoporosis; osteoporosis in men

Dosage and routes
Paget's disease
Adult: PO 30 mg/day × 2 mo; give calcium and vit D if dietary intake is lacking; if relapse occurs, retreatment is advised

Treatment/prevention of postmenopausal osteoporosis
Adult: PO 5 mg/day or 35 mg qwk or 75 mg/day × 2 consecutive days 2 × mo or 150 mg qmo

Glucocorticoid osteoporosis
Adult: PO 5 mg/day

Osteoporosis in men
Adult: PO 35 mg qwk

Renal dose
Adult: PO CCr <30 mg/min, avoid use

Available forms: Tabs 5, 30, 35, 75, 150 mg

Adverse effects
CNS: Dizziness, headache, depression
CV: Chest pain, hypertension, **atrial fibrillation**
GI: Abdominal pain, diarrhea, *nausea,* constipation, esophagitis
MS: Severe muscle/joint/bone pain, arthralgia, osteonecrosis of the jaw
MISC: Rash, UTI, pharyngitis, hypocalcemia, hypophosphatemia, increased PTH
SYST: **Angioedema**

Contraindications: Hypersensitivity to bisphosphonates, inability to stand or sit upright for ≥30 min

Precautions: Pregnancy **C**, breastfeeding, children, renal disease, active upper GI disorders, dental disease

Pharmacokinetics
Absorption	Unknown
Distribution	To bones (50%)
Metabolism	Unknown
Excretion	Kidneys
Half-life	Terminal 220 hr

Pharmacodynamics
Unknown

Interactions
Drug classifications
Aluminum, antacids, calcium, iron, magnesium salts: decreased absorption of risedronate
NSAIDs, salicylates: increased GI irritation
Drug/food
Food: decreased bioavailability; take ½ hr before food or drinks other than water
Drug/lab test
Increased: bone imaging agents

R

NURSING CONSIDERATIONS
Assessment
- Assess for symptoms of Paget's disease: headache, bone pain, increased head circumference
- Monitor phosphate, alkaline phosphatase, calcium; creatinine, BUN (renal disease)
- Assess for hypercalcemia: paresthesia, twitching, laryngospasm, Chvostek's/Trousseau's signs
- Assess for serious skin reactions; angioedema
- Assess dental health, cover with antiinfectives prior to dental extraction
- Assess for atrial fibrillation

Nursing diagnoses
- Knowledge, deficient (teaching)
- Mobility, impaired physical (uses)
- Nutrition: less than body requirements, imbalanced (uses)

Implementation
- Give PO for 2 mo to be effective in Paget's disease
- Give with a full glass of water; patient should be in upright position
- Administer supplemental calcium and vit D in Paget's disease
- Give daily ≥30 min before meals
- Store in cool environment, out of direct sunlight

Patient/family education
- Advise patient to sit upright for ½ hr after dose to prevent irritation
- Instruct patient to comply with dietary restrictions, maintain good oral hygiene
- Advise patient to notify prescriber if pregnancy is planned or suspected

Evaluation
Positive therapeutic outcome
- Increased bone mass, absence of fractures

---

risperidone (Rx)
(res-pare′a-done)
Risperdal, Risperdal Consta, Risperdal M-TAB
Func. class.: Antipsychotic
Chem. class.: Benzisoxazole derivative

Pregnancy category C

Do not confuse:
Risperdal/reserpine

Action: Unknown; may be mediated through both dopamine type 2 (D_2) and serotonin type 2 (5-HT_2) antagonism

Therapeutic outcome: Decreased hallucinations and disorganized thought

Uses: Irritability associated with autism, bipolar disorder, mania, schizophrenia

Dosage and routes
Adult: PO 1 mg bid, with incremental increases of 1 mg bid on days 2 and 3 to a dose of 3 mg bid by day 3, then do not increase dose for at least 1 wk; IM 25 mg q2wk, may increase to max 50 mg q2wk
Geriatric: PO 0.5 mg daily-bid, increase by 1 mg qwk

Hepatic dose/renal dose
Adult: PO 0.5 mg, increase by 0.5 mg bid, then increase to 1.5 mg bid

Available forms: Tabs 0.25, 0.5, 1, 2, 3, 4 mg; oral sol 1 mg/ml; orally disintegrating tabs 0.5, 1, 2, 3, 4 mg; oral sol 1 mg/ml (30 ml); long-acting inj kit (Risperdal Consta) 12.5, 25, 37.5, 50 mg

Adverse effects
CNS: EPS (pseudoparkinsonism, akathisia, dystonia, tardive dyskinesia), drowsiness, *insomnia, agitation, anxiety, headache,* **neuroleptic malignant syndrome,** dizziness, **seizures**
CV: Orthostatic hypotension, **tachycardia, heart failure, sudden death (geriatric)**
EENT: Blurred vision
GI: Nausea, vomiting, *anorexia, constipation,* jaundice, weight gain
GU: Hyperprolactinemia, gynecomastia
MISC: **Renal artery disease;** weight gain, hyperprolactinemia (child)
RESP: Rhinitis, sinusitis, upper respiratory infection, cough

Contraindications: Breastfeeding, hypersensitivity, seizure disorders

Precautions: Pregnancy C, children, geriatric, cardiac/renal/hepatic disease, breast cancer, Parkinson's disease, CNS depression, brain tumor, dehydration, diabetes, hematologic disease

Black Box Warning: Dementia with Lewy bodies

Pharmacokinetics
Absorption	Unknown
Distribution	Unknown
Metabolism	Liver, extensively
Excretion	Urine 90%
Half-life	3-24 hr

 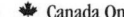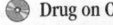

Pharmacodynamics	
Onset	Unknown
Peak	1-2 hr
Duration	Up to 12 hr

Interactions
Individual drugs
Alcohol: increased sedation

◆Bepridil, chloroquine, clarithromycin, droperidol, erythromycin, grepafloxacin, halofantrine, haloperidol, methadone, pentamidine, probucol, sparfloxacin: increased QT prolongation

Carbamazepine: increased risperidone excretion

◆Furosemide: possible death in dementia-related psychosis

Levodopa: decreased levodopa effect

Drug classifications
Antipsychotics: increased EPS

◆β-agonists, class IA/III antidysrhythmics, local anesthetics, some phenothiazines, tricyclics: increased QT prolongation

CNS depressants: increased sedation

CYP2D6 inducers (carbamazepine, barbiturates, phenytoin, rifampin): decreased risperidone action

CYP2D6 inhibitors (selective serotonin reuptake inhibitors): increased EPS

Drug/herb
Betel palm, kava: increased EPS

Cola tree, hops, nettle, nutmeg: increased action

Kava: increased CNS depression

Drug/lab test
Increased: prolactin levels

NURSING CONSIDERATIONS
Assessment
- Assess mental status: orientation, mood, behavior, presence and type of hallucinations before initial administration, monthly; this product should significantly reduce psychotic behavior
- Check that patient swallows all PO medication; check for hoarding or giving of medication to other patients
- Monitor I&O ratio; palpate bladder if low urinary output occurs, especially in geriatric; urinalysis recommended before, during prolonged therapy
- Monitor bilirubin, CBC, liver function tests monthly
- Assess affect, orientation, LOC, reflexes, gait, coordination, sleep pattern disturbances
- Monitor B/P with patient in sitting, standing, and lying positions; take pulse and respirations q4hr during initial treatment; establish baseline before starting treatment; report drops of 30 mm Hg; obtain baseline ECG and monitor Q- and T-wave changes
- Check for dizziness, faintness, palpitations, tachycardia on rising; severe orthostatic hypotension is common

◆ Identify for neuroleptic malignant syndrome: hyperpyrexia, muscle rigidity, increased CPK, altered mental status; product should be discontinued

- Assess for EPS including akathisia (inability to sit still, no pattern to movements), tardive dyskinesia (bizarre movements of the jaw, mouth, tongue, extremities), pseudoparkinsonism (rigidity, tremors, pill rolling, shuffling gait); an antiparkinsonian product should be prescribed
- Assess for constipation, urinary retention daily; if these occur, increase bulk, water in diet

Nursing diagnoses
- Coping, ineffective (uses)
- Knowledge, deficient (teaching)
- Noncompliance (teaching)

Implementation
PO route
- Give with full glass of water, milk; or give with food to decrease GI upset
- Do not open blister pack or orally disintegrating tabs until ready to use; tear one of the four units apart at perforation; bend corner where indicated; peel back foil; do not push tab through foil; remove from pack and place on tongue; tab disintegrates in seconds and can be swallowed with or without liquids
- Store in airtight, light-resistant container

IM route
- Only use provided diluent and needle; do not substitute
- Do not give **IV**
- Inject deeply in large muscle mass
- Store unopened vials in refrigerator; protect from light; do not freeze
- Patient should lie down 30 min after IM inj

Patient/family education
- Teach patient to use good oral hygiene; frequent rinsing of mouth, sugarless gum for dry mouth
- Caution patient to avoid hazardous activities until product response is determined; dizziness, blurred vision may occur
- Inform patient that orthostatic hypotension occurs often; patient should rise from sitting or lying position gradually and remain lying down for at least 30 min after IM inj

R

- Instruct patient to avoid hot tubs, hot showers, tub baths; hypotension may occur
- Inform patient that heat stroke may occur in hot weather, and to take extra precautions to stay cool
- Advise patient to avoid abrupt withdrawal of this product, or EPS may result; product should be withdrawn slowly
- Teach patient to avoid OTC preparations (cough, hay fever, cold) unless approved by prescriber; serious product interactions may occur; avoid use with alcohol, CNS depressants because increased drowsiness may occur
- Advise patient to use contraception, to inform prescriber if pregnancy is planned or suspected

Evaluation
Positive therapeutic outcome
- Decrease in emotional excitement, hallucinations, delusions, paranoia
- Reorganization of patterns of thought, speech

Treatment of overdose: Lavage, provide airway

---

ritonavir (Rx)
(ri-toe′na-veer)
Norvir
Func. class.: Antiretroviral
Chem. class.: Protease inhibitor
Pregnancy category B

Do not confuse:
ritonavir/retrovir

Action: Inhibits HIV-1 protease and prevents maturation of the infectious virus

Therapeutic outcome: Improvement of HIV-1 infection

Uses: HIV-1 in combination with other antiretrovirals

Dosage and routes
Adult/adolescent >16 yr: PO 600 mg bid; if nausea occurs, begin dose at ½ and gradually increase
Adolescent ≤16 yr/child/infant: PO 400 mg/m² bid up to 1200 mg/day; may start lower and escalate

Available forms: Caps 100 mg; oral sol 80 mg/ml

Adverse effects
CNS: Paresthesia, headache, **seizures,** dizziness, insomnia, fever
CV: **QT, PR interval prolongation**

GI: Diarrhea, buccal mucosa ulceration, *abdominal pain, nausea, taste perversion,* dry mouth, *vomiting, anorexia*
INTEG: Rash
MISC: Asthenia, **angioedema, anaphylaxis, Stevens-Johnson syndrome,** increased lipids, lipodystrophy
MS: Pain

Contraindications: Hypersensitivity

Black Box Warning: Coadministration with other drugs

Precautions: Pregnancy B, breastfeeding, children, liver disease, pancreatitis, diabetes, hemophilia, AV block, hypercholesterolemia, immune reconstitution syndrome, neonates, cardiomyopathy

Pharmacokinetics
Absorption	Well
Distribution	Unknown
Metabolism	98% protein binding, liver
Excretion	Unknown
Half-life	3-5 hr

Pharmacodynamics
Onset	Unknown
Peak	2-4 hr
Duration	Unknown

Interactions
Individual drugs
Amiodarone, astemizole, bepridil, buPROPion, cisapride, clozapine, desipramine, dihydro-ergotamine, encainide, ergotamine, flecainide, meperedine, midazolam, pimozide, piroxicam, propafenone, propoxyphene, quinidine, ranolazine, saquinavir, terfenadine, triazolam, zolpidem: toxicity, do not use together
Atovaquone, ethinyl estradiol, lamotrigine, phenytoin, sulfamethoxazole, theophylline, voriconazole, zidovudine: decreased levels of each drug
Bosentan: increased levels of bosentan
Clarithromycin: increased level of both products
ddI: increased levels of both products
Fluconazole: increased ritonavir level
Divalproex: decreased levels of divalproex
Nevirapine, phenytoin: decreased ritonavir levels
Drug classifications
Anticoagulants: decreased levels of anticoagulants
Azole antifungals, benzodiazepines, HMG-CoA reductase inhibitors, interleukins: toxicity, do not use together

---

Barbiturates, rifamycins: decreased ritonavir level

Drug/herb
Red yeast rice: avoid use
St. John's wort: decreased ritonavir levels, avoid concurrent use

Drug/lab test
Increased: ALT, GGT, AST, CPK, cholesterol, triglycerides, uric acid
Decreased: Hct, RBC, Hgb, neutrophils, WBC

NURSING CONSIDERATIONS
Assessment
- Assess for QT, PR prolongation, ECG
- Assess signs of infection, anemia
- Monitor viral load and CD4, blood glucose, plasma HIV RNA, serum cholesterol, lipid profile baseline, throughout therapy
- Resistance testing prior to starting therapy and after treatment failure
- Assess liver function tests: ALT, AST
- Monitor C&S before product therapy; product may be taken as soon as culture is done; repeat C&S after treatment; determine the presence of other STDs
- Assess bowel pattern before, during treatment; if severe abdominal pain with bleeding occurs, product should be discontinued; monitor hydration
- Assess skin eruptions, rash
- Assess allergies before treatment, reaction to each medication; place allergies on chart

Nursing diagnoses
- Infection, risk for (uses)
- Knowledge, deficient (teaching)

Implementation
- Administer with food at equal intervals around the clock
- Shake oral sol well
- Mix oral powder with high-calorie drink
- Store caps in refrigerator

Patient/family education
- Teach patient to take as prescribed; if dose is missed, take as soon as remembered up to 1 hr before next dose; do not double dose
- Teach patient that product must be taken in equal intervals around the clock to maintain blood levels for duration of therapy
- Teach patient that product is not a cure for HIV; opportunistic infections may continue to be acquired, and others may continue to contract HIV from the patient
- Advise patient not to use St. John's wort, that it decreases this product's effect
- Inform that redistribution of body fat or accumulation of body fat may occur

Evaluation
Positive therapeutic outcome
- Decreasing symptoms of HIV
- Improving viral load and CD4 cell counts

rituximab (Rx)
(rih-tuks'ih-mab)
Rituxan
Func. class.: Antineoplastic—miscellaneous; DMARDs
Chem. class.: Murine/human monoclonal antibody

Pregnancy category C

Action: Directed against the CD20 antigen that is found on malignant B lymphocytes; CD20 regulates a portion of cell cycle initiation/differentiation

Therapeutic outcome: Decreased tumor size, prevention of spread of cancer

Uses: Non-Hodgkin's lymphoma (CD20 positive, B-cell), bulky disease (tumors >10 cm), rheumatoid arthritis

Dosage and routes
Non-Hodgkin's Lymphoma (NHL), Chronic Lymphocytic Leukemia (CLL)
Adult: **IV** INF 375 mg/m^3 qwk × 4 doses; give at 50 mg/hr for 1st INF; if hypersensitivity does not occur, increase rate by 50 mg/hr q½hr, max 400 mg/hr; slow/interrupt INF if hypersensitivity occurs; other INF can be given at 100 mg/hr and increased by 100 mg/hr, max 400 mg/hr

Rheumatoid Arthritis
Adult: **IV** 100 mg on days 1, 15

Available forms: Inj 10 mg/ml

Adverse effects
CNS: **Life-threatening brain infection**
CV: **Cardiac dysrhythmias, heart failure, MI, superventricular tachycardia, hyper-tension,** angina
GI: *Nausea, vomiting, anorexia,* **GI obstruction/perforation**
GU: **Renal failure**
HEMA: **Leukopenia, neutropenia, throm-bocytopenia,** anemia
INTEG: *Irritation at inj site, rash,* **fatal mucocutaneous infections (rare)**
MISC: *Fever,* chills, asthenia, *headache,* **angioedema,** hypotension, myalgia, broncho-spasm, ARDs
SYST: **Stevens-Johnson syndrome, exfoli-ative dermatitis, toxic epidermal necroly-sis, tumor lysis syndrome**

R

Adverse effects: *italic* = common, **bold** = life-threatening

Contraindications: Hypersensitivity, murine proteins

Precautions: Pregnancy **C,** breastfeeding, children, geriatric, cardiac/renal/pulmonary conditions

Black Box Warning: Exfoliative dermatitis, infusion-related reactions, progressive multifocal leukoencephalopathy

Pharmacokinetics
Absorption	Unknown
Distribution	Unknown
Metabolism	Unknown
Excretion	Unknown
Half-life	31-152 hr

Pharmacodynamics
Unknown

Interactions
Drug classifications
Anticoagulants, NSAIDs: increased bleeding risk

NURSING CONSIDERATIONS
Assessment
⬥ Assess for signs of fatal inf reaction: hypoxia, pulmonary infiltrates, ARDS, MI, ventricular fibrillation, cardiogenic shock; most fatal inf reactions occur with first inf, discontinue product
⬥ Assess for signs of severe mucocutaneous reactions: Stevens-Johnson syndrome, lichenoid dermatitis, toxic epidermal lysis; signs occur 1-13 wk after product was given
⬥ Assess for tumor lysis syndrome: acute renal failure requiring hemodialysis, hyperkalemia, hypocalcemia, hyperuricemia, hyperphosphatasemia
• Monitor CBC, differential, platelet count weekly; withhold product if WBC is <3500/mm^3 or platelet count <100,000/mm^3; notify prescriber of these results; product should be discontinued
• Monitor ECG, serum creatinine/BUN, electrolytes, uric acid
• Assess GI symptoms: frequency of stools
• Assess signs of dehydration: rapid respirations, poor skin turgor, decreased urine output, dry skin, restlessness, weakness

Nursing diagnoses
• Injury, risk for (side effects)
• Knowledge, deficient (teaching)

Implementation
IV route
• Hold antihypertensive 2 hr prior to administration

• Administer after diluting to a final conc of 1-4 mg/ml; use 0.9% NaCl, D$_5$W, gently invert bag to mix; do not mix with other products
• Increase fluid intake to 2-3 L/day to prevent dehydration, unless contraindicated
• Provide nutritious diet with iron, vitamin supplement, low fiber, few dairy products
• Store vials at 36°-40° F, protect vials from direct sunlight, inf sol is stable at 36°-46° F × 24 hr and room temperature for another 12 hr

Patient/family education
• Teach patient to report adverse reactions
• Advise to avoid OTC products
• Teach to use contraception during and up to 12 mo after therapy
• Avoid use with vaccines, toxoids

Evaluation
Positive therapeutic outcome
• Prevention of increasing cancer progression

---

rivastigmine (Rx)
(riv-as-tig′mine)
Exelon, Exelon Patch
Func. class.: Anti-Alzheimer's agent
Chem. class.: Cholinesterase inhibitor
Pregnancy category B

Action: Potent, selective inhibitor of brain acetylcholinesterase (AChE) and butycholinerase (BChE)

Therapeutic outcome: Decreased signs and symptoms of Alzheimer's dementia

Uses: Mild-moderate Alzheimer's dementia, dementia associated with Parkinson's disease

Dosage and routes
Adult: PO 1.5 mg bid for 4 wk or more, may increase to 3 mg bid after 4 wk or more; may increase to 4.5 mg bid and thereafter 6 mg bid, max 12 mg/day; transdermal apply 4.6 mg/24 hr after 4 wk or more, may increase to 9.5 mg/24 hr

Available forms: Caps 1.5, 3, 4.5, 6 mg; sol 2 mg/ml; transdermal patch 4.6, 9.5 mg/24 hr

Adverse effects
CNS: Tremors, confusion, insomnia, psychosis, hallucination, depression, dizziness, headache, anxiety, somnolence, fatigue, syncope, EPS, exacerbation of Parkinson's disease
GI: Nausea, vomiting, anorexia, abdominal distress, flatulence, diarrhea, constipation, dyspepsia
MISC: UTI, asthenia, increased sweating,

---

hypertension, influenza-like symptoms, weight change

Contraindications: Hypersensitivity to this product, other carbamates; GI bleeding, jaundice

Precautions: Pregnancy **B**, breastfeeding, children, renal/hepatic/respiratory disease, seizure disorder, asthma, urinary obstruction, peptic ulcer, increased intracranial pressure, surgery

Pharmacokinetics

Absorption	Rapidly, completely
Distribution	40% protein binding
Metabolism	To decarbamylated metabolite
Excretion	Kidney—metabolites, clearance lowered in geriatric, hepatic disease, increased nicotine use
Half-life	1½ hr

Pharmacodynamics
Unknown

Interactions
Individual drugs
Nicotine: increased metabolism, decreased blood level of rivastigmine

Drug classifications
Anticholinergics, phenothiazines, sedating H_1 blockers, tricyclics: decreased rivastigmine effect
Cholinergic agonists, other cholinesterase inhibitors: increased synergistic effect
NSAIDs: increased GI effects

NURSING CONSIDERATIONS
Assessment
• Monitor liver function tests: AST, ALT, alkaline phosphatase, LDH, bilirubin, CBC
• Assess for severe GI effects: nausea, vomiting, anorexia, weight loss
• Monitor B/P, respiration during initial treatment; hypo/hypertension should be reported
• Assess mental status: affect, mood, behavioral changes, depression; complete suicide assessment

Nursing diagnoses
• Knowledge, deficient (teaching)

Implementation
• Give with meals; take with AM and PM meal even though absorption may be decreased
• Provide assistance with ambulation during beginning therapy

• Discontinue treatment for several doses and restart at same or next lower dosage level if adverse reactions cause intolerance
• If treatment is interrupted for longer than several days treatment should be initiated with the lowest daily dose and titrated as indicated above
Transdermal route
• Apply to clean, hairless, dry skin; not in an area that clothing will rub; rotate sites daily; remove liner; apply firmly; may be used during water activities; avoid saunas

Patient/family education
• Teach patient procedure for giving oral sol; use instruction sheet provided
• Teach patient to notify prescriber of severe GI effects
• Teach patient that product may cause dizziness, anorexia, weight loss

Evaluation
Positive therapeutic outcome
• Increased coherence, decreased symptoms of Alzheimer's disease, improved mood

---

rizatriptan (Rx)
(rye-zah-trip′tan)
Maxalt, Maxalt-MLT
Func. class.: Migraine agent
Chem. class.: 5-HT₁-like receptor agonist

Pregnancy category C

Action: Binds selectively to the vascular serotonin type 1 (5-HT₁) receptor, exerts antimigraine effect; causes vasoconstriction in cranial arteries

Therapeutic outcome: After treatment, relief of migraine

Uses: Acute treatment of migraine

Dosage and routes
Adult: **PO** 5-10 mg single dose, redosing separate by 2 hr or more; max 30 mg/24 hr, use 5 mg in patient on propanolol; max 15 mg/24 hr

Available forms: Tabs (Maxalt) 5, 10 mg; orally disintegrating tabs (Maxalt-MLT) 5, 10 mg

Adverse effects
CNS: Dizziness, drowsiness, *headache, fatigue,* warm/cold sensation, flushing
CV: **MI, ventricular fibrillation, ventricular tachycardia, coronary artery vasospasm**
ENDO: Hot flashes, mild increase in growth hormone

R

Adverse effects: *italic* = common, **bold** = life-threatening

GI: *Nausea,* dry mouth, diarrhea, abdominal pain
RESP: Chest tightness, pressure, dyspnea

Contraindications: Angina pectoris, history of MI, documented silent ischemia, Prinzmetal's angina, ischemic heart disease, concurrent ergotamine-containing preparations, uncontrolled hypertension, hypersensitivity, basilar or hemiplegic migraine

Precautions: Pregnancy **C**, breastfeeding, children, postmenopausal women, men >40 yr, geriatric, risk factors for CAD, hypercholesterolemia, obesity, diabetes, impaired renal/hepatic function

Pharmacokinetics
Absorption	Unknown
Distribution	Unknown
Metabolism	Liver (metabolite)
Excretion	Urine/feces
Half-life	2-3 hr

Pharmacodynamics
Onset	10 min-2 hr
Peak	Unknown
Duration	Unknown

Interactions
Individual drugs
Cimetidine, isocarboxazide, pargyline, phenelzine, propranolol, trancyclomine: increased rizatriptan action
Ergot: increased vasospastic effects
Sibutramine: increased levels of sibutramine
Drug classifications
Contraceptives (oral), MAOIs, MAOIs (nonselective types A and B): increased rizatriptan action
Ergot derivatives, 5-HT$_1$ receptor agonists: increased vasospastic effects
Selective serotonin reuptake inhibitors: increased weakness, hyperreflexia, incoordination
Drug/herb
Butterbur, feverfew: increased effect
SAM-e, St. John's wort: serotonin syndrome

NURSING CONSIDERATIONS
Assessment
• Assess for stress level, activity, recreation, coping mechanisms
• Assess neurologic status: LOC, blurring vision, nausea, vomiting, tingling in extremities preceding headache
• Monitor for ingestion of tyramine-containing foods (pickled products, beer, wine, aged cheese), food additives, preservatives, colorings, artificial sweeteners, chocolate, caffeine, which may precipitate these types of headaches

Nursing diagnoses
• Knowledge, deficient (teaching)
• Pain, acute (uses)

Implementation
• Provide quiet, calm environment with decreased stimulation for noise, bright light, excessive talking
• Do not open blister pack until ready to use
• Put orally disintegrating tab on tongue to dissolve; swallow with saliva

Patient/family education
• Teach patient use of orally disintegrating tab: instruct patient not to open blister until use, to peel blister open with dry hands, to place tab on tongue, where it will dissolve, and to swallow with saliva (contains phenylalanine)
• Advise patient to report any side effects to prescriber
• Advise patient to use alternate contraception while taking product if oral contraceptives are being used

Evaluation
Positive therapeutic outcome
• Decrease in frequency, severity of headache

romiplostim (Rx)
(roe-mi-ploe'stim)
Nplate
Func. class.: Thrombopoietin receptor agonist

Pregnancy category C

Action: A thrombopoietin-like fusion protein produced by DNA recombinant technology

Therapeutic outcome: Increase in platelet counts, absence of bleeding

Uses: Chronic idiopathic thrombocytopenic purpura in patients who have had an insufficient response to corticosteroids, immunoglobulins, or splenectomy

Dosage and routes
Adult: SUBCUT 1 mcg/kg qwk, increase qwk by 1 mcg/kg until platelets ≥50,000/mm^3, max 10 mcg/kg/wk

Available forms: Inj vials 250, 500 mcg

Adverse effects
CNS: *Dizziness, insomnia, headache,* fatigue
GI: Abdominal pain, dyspepsia, diarrhea
HEMA: Thromboembolism, thrombosis, bleeding, myelofibrosis
MS: Myalgia

SYST: **Secondary malignancy,** antibody formation

Contraindications: Hypersensitivity to this product or mannitol

Precautions: Pregnancy **C**, breastfeeding, malignancies, bleeding, bone marrow suppression, children

Pharmacokinetics

Absorption	Unknown
Distribution	Unknown
Metabolism	Unknown
Excretion	Unknown
Half-life	Terminal 1-34 days

Pharmacodynamics

Onset	Unknown
Peak	7-50 hr
Duration	Unknown

Interactions
Drug classifications
Anticoagulants, NSAIDs, platelet inhibitors, thrombolytics, salicylates: possible risk of bleeding

NURSING CONSIDERATIONS
Assessment
• Assess blood studies: CBC during treatment weekly and for 2 wks after discontinuing

Nursing diagnoses
• Injury, risk for (uses)
• Knowledge, deficient (teaching)

Implementation
• Romiplostim is only available through Nplate NEXUS Program; call 1-877-675-2831 to enroll
• Store vials in refrigerator, do not freeze; protect from light; diluted sol is stable refrigerated or at room temperature for 24 hrs
SUBCUT route
• Use 0.01 ml graduations syringe
• Discard any unused portion in vial; do not pool unused portions from vials
• Dilute 250 mcg/0.72 preservative-free sterile water for inj; 500 mcg/1.2 preservative-free sterile water for inj; final concentration 500 mcg/ml
• Gently swirl until dissolved; do not shake
• Do not use if discolored or if particulate matter is present
• Inj into outer aspect of upper arm or abdomen except for 2 inches around navel or front aspect of middle thigh; do not use areas that are bruised, scratched, or scarred
• Rotate inj sites

Patient/family education
• Instruct patient to report bleeding
• Inform the patient the reason for product and expected results
• Advise patient to report a missed dose to prescriber due to increased risk of bleeding

Evaluation
Positive therapeutic outcome
• Increase in platelet counts, absence of bleeding

---

ropinirole (Rx)
(roe-pin'e-role)
Requip, Requip XL
Func. class.: Antiparkinsonian agent
Chem. class.: Dopamine-receptor agonist, nonergot
Pregnancy category C

Action: Selective agonist for dopamine D_2 receptors (presynaptic/postsynaptic sites); binding at D_3 receptor contributes to antiparkinson effects

Therapeutic outcome: Decreased symptoms of Parkinson's disease (involuntary movements)

Uses: Parkinsonism, restless leg syndrome

Dosage and routes
Adult: PO 0.25 mg tid, titrate weekly to max of 24 mg/day; (XL) 2 mg/day × 1-2wk, may increase by 2 mg/day qwk

Restless leg syndrome
Adult: PO 0.25 mg 1-3 hr before bedtime, may increase until symptoms resolve

Available forms: Tabs 0.25, 0.5, 1, 2, 3, 4, 5 mg; ext rel tab 2, 4, 8, 12 mg

Adverse effects
CNS: Dystonia, *agitation, insomnia,* dizziness, psychosis, hallucinations, depression, somnolence, **sleep attacks**
CV: Orthostatic hypotension, hypotension, syncope, palpitations, **tachycardia,** hypertension
EENT: Blurred vision
GI: Nausea, vomiting, anorexia, dry mouth, constipation, dyspepsia, flatulence
GU: Impotence, urinary frequency
HEMA: **Hemolytic anemia, leukopenia, agranulocytosis**
INTEG: Rash, sweating
RESP: Pharyngitis, rhinitis, sinusitis, bronchitis, dyspnea

Contraindications: Hypersensitivity

R

Precautions: Pregnancy C, cardiac/renal/hepatic disease, dysrhythmias, affective disorders, psychosis

Pharmacokinetics

Absorption	Well absorbed
Distribution	Widely distributed
Metabolism	Liver, extensively by the liver by CYP450 CYP1A2 enzyme system
Excretion	Kidneys
Half-life	6 hr

Pharmacodynamics

Unknown

Interactions
Individual drugs
Cimetidine, ciprofloxacin, digoxin, diltiazem, enoxacin, erythromycin, fluvoxamine, levodopa, mexiletine, norfloxacin, tacrine, theophylline: increased effect of ropinirole

Metoclopramide: decreased ropinirole effect
Drug classifications
Butyrophenones, phenothiazines, thioxanthenes: decreased ropinirole effect
Drug/herb
Chaste tree fruit, kava: decreased ropinirole action

NURSING CONSIDERATIONS
Assessment
• Monitor B/P, respiration during initial treatment; hypotension or hypertension should be reported

• Assess mental status: affect, mood, behavioral changes, depression; complete suicide assessment

• Assess for involuntary movements in parkinsonism: akinesia, tremors, staggering gait, muscle rigidity, drooling; these symptoms should improve with therapy

◆ Assess for sleep attacks, drowsiness, falling asleep without warning even during hazardous activities

Nursing diagnoses
• Injury, risk for (uses)
• Knowledge, deficient (teaching)
• Mobility, impaired physical (uses)
• Noncompliance (teaching)

Implementation
• Give product until NPO before surgery
• Adjust dosage to patient response
• Give with meals to decrease GI upset

Patient/family education
• Advise patient that therapeutic effects may take several wk to a few mo

• Caution patient to change positions slowly to prevent orthostatic hypotension

• Instruct patient to use product exactly as prescribed; if product is discontinued abruptly, parkinsonian crisis may occur

Evaluation
Positive therapeutic outcome
• Decreased akathisia, other involuntary movements
• Increased mood

ropivacaine (Rx)
(roe-pi′va-kane)
Naropin
Func. class.: Local anesthetic
Chem. class.: Amide

Pregnancy category B

Action: Competes with calcium for sites in nerve membrane that control sodium transport across cell membrane; decreases rise of depolarization phase of action potential

Therapeutic outcome: Maintenance of local anesthesia

Uses: Peripheral nerve block, caudal anesthesia, central neural block, vaginal, epidural, spinal block

Dosage and routes
Lumbar epidural block for C-section
Adult: 20-30 ml of 0.5% SOL, or 15-20 ml of 0.75% SOL

Thoracic epidural
Adult: 5-15 ml of 0.5%-0.75% SOL

Major nerve block
Adult: 35-50 ml of 0.5% SOL or 10-40 ml of 0.75% SOL

Labor pain epidural
Adult: 10-20 ml of 0.2% SOL, then 6-14 ml/hr

Postoperative (lumbar/thoracic epidural)
Adult: 6-14 ml/hr of 0.2% SOL

Infiltration/minor nerve block
Adult: 1-100 ml of 0.2% SOL or 1-40 ml of 0.5% SOL

Available forms: Inj 2, 5, 7.5 mg/ml

Adverse effects
CNS: Anxiety, restlessness, **seizures, loss of consciousness,** drowsiness, disorientation, tremors, shivering, paresthesia

CV: **Myocardial depression, cardiac arrest, dysrhythmias,** bradycardia, *hypo/*hypertension, **fetal bradycardia**
EENT: Blurred vision, tinnitus, pupil constriction
ENDO: Hypokalemia
GI: Nausea, vomiting
GU: Urinary retention
INTEG: Rash, urticaria, allergic reactions, edema, burning, skin discoloration at injection site, tissue necrosis
RESP: **Status asthmaticus, respiratory arrest, anaphylaxis**

Contraindications: Children <12 yr, geriatric, hypersensitivity to amide local anesthetics, severe liver disease, severe hypotension, complete heart block

Precautions: Pregnancy **B**, severe product allergies, hyperthyroidism, CV, hepatic/neurologic disease

Pharmacokinetics

Absorption	Complete
Distribution	Unknown
Metabolism	Liver
Excretion	Kidneys
Half-life	Unknown

Pharmacodynamics

Onset	2-8 min
Peak	Unknown
Duration	3 hr, varies with inj site

Interactions
Individual drugs
Amiodarone, cimetidine, ciprofloxacin, fluvoxamine, imipramine, theophylline: increased effect
Chloroprocaine: decreased action of ropivacaine
Enflurane, epinephrine, halothane: increased dysrhythmias
Drug classifications
Antidepressants (tricyclics), MAOIs, phenothiazines: increased hypertension
Azole antifungals: increased effect

NURSING CONSIDERATIONS
Assessment
• Assess B/P, pulse, respiration during treatment
• Assess fetal heart tones during labor
• Assess allergic reactions: rash, urticaria, itching
• Assess cardiac status: ECG for dysrhythmias, pulse, B/P during anesthesia

Nursing diagnoses
• Knowledge, deficient (teaching)
Implementation
• Give only with resuscitative equipment nearby
• Give only products without preservatives for epidural or caudal anesthesia
• Use new sol; discard unused portions

Evaluation
Positive therapeutic outcome
• Anesthesia necessary for procedure

Treatment of overdose: Airway, O_2, vasopressor, **IV** fluids, anticonvulsants for seizures

---

rosiglitazone (Rx)
(roes-i-glye′ta-zone)
Avandia
Func. class.: Antidiabetic, oral
Chem. class.: Thiazolidinedione
Pregnancy category C

Action: Improves insulin resistance by hepatic glucose metabolism, insulin receptor kinase activity, insulin receptor phosphorylation

Therapeutic outcome: Decreased symptoms of diabetes mellitus

Uses: Stable type 2 diabetes mellitus alone or in combination with sulfonylureas, metformin, or insulin

Unlabeled uses: Increased ovulation frequency in those with polycystic ovary syndrome; reduced in-stent restenosis in those with diabetes

Dosage and routes
Adult: PO 4 mg/day or in 2 divided doses, may increase to 8 mg/day or in 2 divided doses after 12 wk; may be added to metformin, sulfonylureas at the adult dose

Available forms: Tabs 2, 4, 8 mg

Adverse effects
CNS: Fatigue, *headache*
CV: **CHF, MI, death (geriatric patients)**
ENDO: Hyper/hypoglycemia
GI: Weight gain, **hepatotoxicity**
MISC: Accidental injury, upper respiratory tract infection, sinusitis, anemia, back pain, diarrhea, edema, bone fractures (female)
SYST: **Anaphylaxis, Stevens-Johnson syndrome**

Contraindications: Breastfeeding, children, hypersensitivity to thiazolidinediones,

R

diabetic ketoacidosis, jaundice, CAD, T1DM
type 1 diabetes

Precautions: Pregnancy **C**, geriatric,
thyroid/renal/hepatic disease, heart failure, MI

Pharmacokinetics

Absorption	Unknown
Distribution	Protein binding 99.8%
Metabolism	Unknown
Excretion	Urine, feces, breast milk
Half-life	Elimination 3-4 hr

Pharmacodynamics

Onset	Unknown
Peak	6-12 wk
Duration	Unknown

Interactions
Individual drugs
Insulin: avoid concurrent use
Drug classifications
CYP2CS inducers/inhibitors: may increase/
decrease effect

Nitrates: avoid concurrent use
Drug/herb
Alfalfa, aloe, basil, bay, bilberry, bitter melon,
black catechu, buchu, burdock, coriander,
dandelion, eyebright (po), fenugreek, garlic,
ginseng, glucomannan, glucosamine, goat's
rue, gymnema, horehound, horse chestnut,
jambul, myrrh, myrtle: increased antidiabetic effect

Bee pollen, blue cohosh, broom, chromium,
elecampane, eucalyptus, gotu kola: decreased antidiabetic effect

Chromium, coenzyme Q10, fenugreek: hypoglycemia

Glucosamine: decreased glucose control

NURSING CONSIDERATIONS
Assessment
⬥ Assess for CV status; those with CV disease
should be monitored carefully
• Assess for hypoglycemic reactions (sweat-
ing, weakness, dizziness, anxiety, tremors,
hunger), hyperglycemic reactions soon after
meals
• Assess for systemic reactions: anaphylaxis,
Stevens-Johnson syndrome
• Check liver function tests periodically; AST,
FBS, ALT (if ALT >2.5 × ULN, do not use),
HbA$_{2c}$, plasma lipids, lipoproteins, B/P, body
weight during treatment
Nursing diagnoses
• Knowledge, deficient (teaching)
• Nutrition: more than body requirements,
imbalanced (uses)

Implementation
• Convert from other oral hypoglycemic
agents if needed; change may be made without
gradual dosage change; monitor blood glucose
during conversion
• Give tabs crushed and mixed with meal or
fluids for patients with difficulty swallowing
• Store in airtight container in cool environment
Patient/family education
• Teach patient to monitor capillary blood
glucose test, that periodic liver function tests
are mandatory; to report edema, weight gain
• Teach patient symptoms of hypo/
hyperglycemia, what to do about each
• Advise patient that product must be continued on daily basis; explain consequence of
discontinuing product abruptly
• Advise patient to avoid OTC medications or
herbal preparations unless approved by
prescriber
• Advise patient that diabetes is lifelong
illness; that this product is not a cure, only
controls symptoms
• Advise patient that all food included in diet
plan must be eaten to prevent hypoglycemia
• Advise patient to carry/wear emergency ID
and glucagon emergency kit for emergencies
• Instruct patient to notify prescriber if oral
contraceptives are used
• Teach patient not to use if breastfeeding;
may be secreted in breast milk
Evaluation
Positive therapeutic outcome
• Decrease in polyuria, polydipsia,
polyphagia; clear sensorium; absence of
dizziness; stable gait; blood glucose, A1c
improvement

---

rosuvastatin (Rx)
(roe-soo'va-sta-tin)
Crestor
Func. class.: Antilipemic
Chem. class.: HMG-CoA reductase inhibitor

Pregnancy category X

Action: Inhibits HMG-CoA reductase enzyme, which reduces cholesterol synthesis

Therapeutic outcome: Decreasing
cholesterol levels

Uses: As an adjunct in primary hypercholesterolemia (types IIa, IIb), mixed dyslipidemia
elevated serum triglycerides, homozygous
familial hypercholesterolemia (FH), slowing of
atherosclerosis

Dosage and routes
Patient should first be placed on a cholesterol-lowering diet

Hypercholesterolemia
Adult: PO 5-40 mg/day; initial dose 10 mg/day, reanalyze lipid levels at 2-4 wk and adjust dosage accordingly

Homozygous FH
Adult: PO 20 mg/day, max 40 mg

Dose in patients taking cycloSPORINE
Adult: 5 mg/day

Dose when taken with gemfibrozil
Adult: Max 10 mg/day

Asian patients/predisposition for myopathy
Adult: PO 5 mg/day

Atherosclerosis slowing
Adult: PO 10 mg/day (for those not taking cycloSPORINE or gemfibrozil)

Renal dose
Adult: PO CCr <30 ml/min 5 mg daily; max 10 mg daily

Available forms: Tabs 5, 10, 20, 40 mg

Adverse effects
CNS: Headache, dizziness, insomnia, paresthesia, **ALS (Lou Gehrig's disease)**
GI: Nausea, constipation, abdominal pain, flatus, diarrhea, dyspepsia, heartburn, **kidney failure, liver dysfunction,** vomiting
HEMA: **Thrombocytopenia, hemolytic anemia, leukopenia**
INTEG: Rash, pruritus, photosensitivity
MS: Asthenia, muscle cramps, arthritis, arthralgia, myalgia, **myositis, rhabdomyolysis,** leg, shoulder or localized pain
RESP: Rhinitis, sinusitis, *pharyngitis,* bronchitis, increased cough

Contraindications: Pregnancy **X,** breastfeeding, hypersensitivity, active liver disease

Precautions: Children, geriatric, past liver disease, alcoholism, severe acute infections, trauma, hypotension, uncontrolled seizure disorders, severe metabolic disorders, electrolyte imbalances, severe renal impairment, hypothyroidism

Pharmacokinetics
Absorption	Unknown
Distribution	88% protein bound, crosses placenta
Metabolism	Minimal liver metabolism (about 10%)
Excretion	Primarily in feces (90%)
Half-life	19 hr

Pharmacodynamics
Onset	Unknown
Peak	3-5 hr
Duration	Unknown

Interactions
Individual drugs
Clofibrate, cycloSPORINE, gemfibrozil, niacin: increased myalgia, myositis
Warfarin: increased bleeding
Drug classifications
Antifungals (azole): increased myalgia, myositis
Bile acid sequestrants: increased effects
Drug/herb
St. John's wort: decreased rosuvastatin effect
Drug/food
Grapefruit juice: possible toxicity
Drug/lab test
Increased: CPK, liver function tests

NURSING CONSIDERATIONS
Assessment
• Assess diet: obtain diet history including fat, cholesterol in diet
• Monitor fasting cholesterol, LDL, HDL, triglycerides periodically during treatment
• Monitor liver function tests q1-2mo during the first 1½ yr of treatment; AST, ALT, liver function tests may increase
• Monitor renal function in patients with compromised renal system: BUN, creatinine, I&O ratio
• Obtain ophthalmic exam before, 1 mo after treatment begins, annually; lens opacities may occur
◆ Assess for muscle pain, tenderness, obtain CPK; if these occur, product may need to be discontinued

Nursing diagnoses
• Knowledge, deficient (teaching)
• Noncompliance (teaching)

Implementation
• May be taken at any time of day, with or without food
• Store in cool environment in airtight, light-resistant container

Patient/family education
• Advise to report suspected pregnancy
• Advise that blood work and ophthalmic exam will be necessary during treatment
• Teach to report blurred vision, severe GI symptoms, dizziness, headache, muscle pain, weakness
• Teach to use sunscreen or stay out of the sun to prevent photosensitivity

R

Adverse effects: *italic* = common, **bold** = life-threatening

- Teach that previously prescribed regimen will continue: low-cholesterol diet, exercise program, smoking cessation

Evaluation
Positive therapeutic outcome
- Cholesterol at desired level after 8 wk

rufinamide (Rx)
(roo-fin′a-mide)
Banzel
Func. class.: Anticonvulsant
Chem. class.: Triazole derivative

Pregnancy category C

Action: May act through action at sodium channels; exact action is unknown

Therapeutic outcome: Decrease in severity of seizures

Uses: Lennox-Gastaut syndrome

Dosage and routes
Adult: PO 400-800 mg/day divided bid, increase by 400-800 mg/day q2day to 3200 mg/day
Child ≥4 yr: PO 10 mg/kg/day divided equally bid; increase by 10 mg/kg/day every other day to 45 mg/kg/day or 3200 mg/day, whichever is less

Available forms: Tabs 200, 400 mg

Adverse effects
CNS: Dizziness, ataxia, drowsiness, fever, seizures, tremor, fatigue, headache, gait disturbance
EENT: Diplopia, blurred vision, nystagmus
GI: Nausea, hepatitis, vomiting
HEMA: **Anemia, leukopenia, neutropenia, thrombocytopenia,** lymphadenopathy
INTEG: Rash, urticaria
MISC: Edema, hematuria, influenzae, nephrolithiasis

Contraindications: Hypersensitivity

Precautions: Pregnancy C, breastfeeding, renal/hepatic disease, geriatric patients, child <16 yr, depression, dialysis, hazardous activities, suicidal ideation

Pharmacokinetics
Absorption	Unknown
Distribution	Unknown
Metabolism	Liver
Excretion	Kidneys
Half-life	Terminal 6-10 hr

Pharmacodynamics
Onset	Unknown
Peak	4-6 hr
Duration	Unknown

Interactions
Individual drugs
Carbamazepine, phenobarbital, phenytoin, primidone: decreased effect of rufinamide
Valproate: increased rufinamide effect
Drug classifications
Hormonal contraceptives: decreased effect
Drug/lab test
Increased: LFTs

NURSING CONSIDERATIONS
Assessment
- Assess for seizures: duration, type, intensity precipitating factors
- Assess mental status: mood, sensorium, affect, memory (long, short), increased suicidal thoughts/actions

Nursing diagnoses
- Injury, risk for (uses)
- Knowledge, deficient (teaching)

Patient/family education
- Caution patient not to discontinue product abruptly; seizures may occur
- Advise patient to avoid hazardous activities until stabilized on product
- Instruct patient to carry emergency ID stating product use
- Instruct patient to notify prescriber if pregnancy is planned or suspected
- Teach patient to use alternate form of contraception; hormonal contraceptives may be decreased
- Inform patient to take adequate fluids

Evaluation
Positive therapeutic outcome
- Decrease in severity of seizures

salicylic acid topical
See Appendix B

salmeterol (Rx)
(sal-met′er-ole)
Serevent, Serevent Diskus
Func. class.: Adrenergic β₂ agonist, bronchodilator

Pregnancy category C

Action: Causes bronchodilatation by action on β₂ (pulmonary) receptors by increasing levels of cAMP, which relaxes smooth muscle; with very little effect on heart rate, maintains improvement in FEV from 3 to 12 hr; prevents nocturnal asthma symptoms

Therapeutic outcome: Ease of breathing

Uses: Prevention of exercise-induced asthma, bronchospasm, COPD

Dosage and routes
Adult: INH 50 mcg (one inhalation as dry powder); exercise-induced bronchospasm: 50 mcg (2 INH) ½-1 hr prior to exercise
Child 4-12 yr: INH 50 mcg as dry powder bid; exercise-induced bronchospasm 50 mcg as dry powder ½-1 hr prior to exercise

Available forms: Inhalation powder 50 mcg/blister

Adverse effects
CNS: Tremors, anxiety, insomnia, headache, dizziness, stimulation, restlessness, hallucinations, flushing, irritability
CV: Palpitations, **tachycardia**, angina, hypo/hypertension, **dysrhythmias**
EENT: Dry nose, irritation of nose and throat
GI: Heartburn, nausea, vomiting
MS: Muscle cramps
RESP: **Bronchospasm**

Contraindications: Hypersensitivity to sympathomimetics, tachydysrhythmias, severe cardiac disease

Precautions: Pregnancy **C**, breastfeeding, cardiac disorders, hyperthyroidism, diabetes mellitus, hypertension, prostatic hypertrophy, closed-angle glaucoma, seizures, acute asthma, as a substitute for corticosteroids

Black Box Warning: Respiratory insufficiency

Pharmacokinetics
Unknown

Pharmacodynamics

Onset	5-15 min
Peak	4 hr
Duration	12 hr

Interactions
Drug classifications
Antidepressants (tricyclics): increased salmeterol action
β-Adrenergic blockers: block therapeutic effect
Bronchodilators, aerosol: increased action of bronchodilator
MAOIs: increased action of salmeterol

Drug/herb
Betel palm, butterbur, coffee, cola nut, figwort, fumitory, guarana, hawthorn, lily of the valley, motherwort, plantain, tea (black, green), yerba maté: increased stimulation

NURSING CONSIDERATIONS
Assessment
• Monitor respiratory function tests: vital capacity, FEV, ABGs, lung sounds, heart rate, rhythm (baseline)
Nursing diagnoses
• Airway clearance, ineffective (uses)
• Gas exchange, impaired (uses)
• Knowledge, deficient (teaching)
Implementation
• Shake aerosol container, ask patient to exhale, then place mouthpiece in mouth, inhale slowly, hold breath, remove, exhale slowly; allow at least 1 min between inhalations
• Use this medication before other medications and allow at least 1 min between each
• Use spacing device for pediatric/geriatric patients
• Store in light-resistant container, do not expose to temperatures over 86° F (30° C)
Patient/family education
• Caution patient not to use OTC medications because extra stimulation may occur
• Instruct patient to use this medication before other medications and to allow at least 1 min between each, to prevent overstimulation
• Teach patient how to use inhaler; to avoid getting aerosol in eyes; blurring may result; to wash inhaler in warm water daily and dry; to avoid smoking, smoke-filled rooms, and persons with respiratory infections; review package insert with patient
• Instruct patient on administration of dose, not to use more than prescribed; serious side effects may occur
Evaluation
Positive therapeutic outcome
• Absence of dyspnea, wheezing
• Improved airway exchange
• Improved ABGs

Treatment of overdose: Administer a β₂-adrenergic blocker

salsalate (Rx)

(sal-sa'late)

Amigesic, Anaflex, Disalcid, Marthritic, Mono-Gesic, Salflex, Salgesic, Salsalate, Salsitab

Func. class.: Nonopioid analgesic; nonsteroidal antiinflammatory agent

Chem. class.: Salicylate

Pregnancy category C

Action: Blocks formation of peripheral prostaglandins, which cause pain and inflammation; antipyretic action results from inhibition of hypothalamic heat-regulating center; does not inhibit platelet aggregation

Therapeutic outcome: Decreased pain, inflammation

Uses: Mild to moderate pain or fever, including arthritis (osteoarthritis, rheumatoid arthritis)

Dosage and routes
Adult: PO 3 g/day in divided doses

Available forms: Caps 500 mg; tabs 500, 750 mg

Adverse effects
CNS: Stimulation, drowsiness, dizziness, confusion, **seizures,** headache, flushing, hallucinations, coma

CV: Rapid pulse, **pulmonary edema**

EENT: Tinnitus, hearing loss

ENDO: Hypoglycemia, hyponatremia, hypokalemia, alteration in acid-base balance

GI: Nausea, vomiting, GI bleeding, diarrhea, heartburn, anorexia, **hepatotoxicity**

HEMA: **Thrombocytopenia, agranulocytosis, leukopenia, neutropenia, hemolytic anemia,** increased protime

INTEG: Rash, urticaria, bruising

RESP: Wheezing, hyperpnea

Contraindications: Children <3 yr, hypersensitivity to salicylates, NSAIDs, GI bleeding, bleeding disorders, vit K deficiency

Precautions: Pregnancy **C** (1st trimester), breastfeeding, geriatric, anemia, renal/hepatic disease, Hodgkin's disease

Pharmacokinetics

Absorption	Absorbed in small intestine, full benefit 3-4 days
Distribution	Rapidly and widely distributed, crosses placenta
Metabolism	Not metabolized
Excretion	Unchanged—kidneys
Half-life	2-3 hr (low doses), 15-30 hr (high doses)

Pharmacodynamics

Onset	30 min
Peak	1-3 hr
Duration	3-6 hr

Interactions
Individual drugs

Alcohol, heparin, warfarin: increased bleeding

Insulin, methotrexate, phenytoin, probenecid: increased effects

p-Aminobenzoic acid: increased toxic effects

Spironolactone, sulfinpyrazone: decreased effects

Drug classifications

Antacids, steroids, urinary alkalizers: decreased effects of salsalate

Anticoagulants, penicillins: increased effects

Salicylates: decreased blood glucose levels

Diuretics (loop), sulfonylamides: decreased effects

NSAIDs, platelet inhibitors, thrombolytics: increased bleeding risk

Drug/herb

Feverfew: decreased effect of this herb

Drug/food

Foods causing acidic urine may increase level

Drug/lab test

Increased: coagulation studies, liver function tests, serum uric acid, amylase, CO_2, urinary protein

Decreased: serum potassium, cholesterol, blood glucose

Interference: urine catecholamines, pH, pregnancy test

NURSING CONSIDERATIONS
Assessment

• Monitor liver function tests: AST, ALT, bilirubin, creatinine if patient is on long-term therapy

• Monitor renal function tests: BUN, urine creatinine if patient is on long-term therapy

• Monitor blood tests: CBC, Hct, Hgb, Protime, stool guaiac, serum salicylate if patient is on long-term therapy

• Check I&O ratio; decreasing output may indicate renal failure if patient is on long-term therapy

• Assess hepatotoxicity: dark urine, clay-colored stools, yellowing of the skin and sclera, itching, abdominal pain, fever, diarrhea if patient is on long-term therapy

• Assess for allergic reactions: rash, urticaria; if these occur, product may have to be discontinued; assess for asthma, aspirin sensitivity, nasal polyps; may develop hypersensitivity

 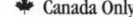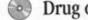

- Assess for ototoxicity: tinnitus, ringing, roaring in ears; audiometric testing needed before, after long-term therapy
- Assess for visual changes
- Check edema in feet, ankles, legs
- Identify prior product history; many product interactions are possible
- Monitor pain: location, duration, type, intensity, prior to dose and 1 hr after
- Monitor musculoskeletal status: ROM before dose
- Identify fever, length of time, and related symptoms

Nursing diagnoses
- Injury, risk for (side effects)
- Knowledge, deficient (teaching)
- Mobility, impaired physical (uses)
- Pain, chronic (uses)

Implementation
- Give with 8 oz of water and sit upright ½ hr after dose; with food or milk to decrease gastric symptoms
- Give antacids 1-2 hr after enteric products

Patient/family education
- Advise patient to report any symptoms of renal/hepatic toxicity, visual changes, ototoxicity, allergic reactions, bleeding (long-term therapy)
- Instruct patient to take with 8 oz of water and sit upright for ½ hr after dose
- Caution patient not to exceed recommended dosage; acute poisoning may result
- Advise patient to read label on other OTC products; many contain aspirin
- Inform patient that the therapeutic response takes 2 wk (arthritis)
- Teach patient to report tinnitus, confusion, diarrhea, sweating, hyperventilation
- Caution patient to avoid alcohol ingestion; GI bleeding may occur
- Inform patient that patients who have allergies may develop allergic reactions

Evaluation
Positive therapeutic outcome
- Decreased pain
- Decreased inflammation

Treatment of overdose: Lavage, activated charcoal, monitor electrolytes, VS

saquinavir (Rx)
(sa-quen'a-ver)
Invirase
Func. class.: Antiretroviral
Chem. class.: Protease inhibitor
Pregnancy category B

Action: Inhibits HIV-1 protease

Therapeutic outcome: Prevents maturation of the infectious virus

Uses: HIV-1 in combination with other antiretrovirals

Dosage and routes
Adult: PO 1000 mg bid with 100 mg ritonavir

Available forms: Caps 200, 500 mg

Adverse effects
CNS: Paresthesia, headache, **seizures**
GI: Diarrhea, buccal mucosa ulceration, *abdominal pain, nausea,* vomiting
INTEG: Rash, **Stevens-Johnson syndrome**
MISC: Asthenia, *hyperglycemia*
MS: Pain

Contraindications: Hypersensitivity

Precautions: Pregnancy **B,** breastfeeding, children, hepatic, diabetes, pancreatitis, immune reconstitution syndrome, hemophilia, hyperlipidemia

Pharmacokinetics

Absorption	Increased with food
Distribution	Protein-binding 98%
Metabolism	Extensively
Excretion	Unknown
Half-life	Terminal 12 hr

Pharmacodynamics
Unknown

Interactions
Individual drugs
Clarithromycin, delavirdine, indinavir, ketoconazole, nelfinavir, ritonavir: increased saquinavir level
Carbamazepine, dexamethasone, nevirapine, phenobarbital, phenytoin, rifamycins: decreased saquinavir levels
Clindamycin, dapsone, quinidine: increased toxicity
Midazolam, triazolam: increased toxicity, increased CNS depression; do not use concurrently

S

Drug classifications
Calcium channel blockers: increased toxicity
Ergots: toxicity, increased vasoconstriction; do not use together
HMG-CoA reductase inhibitors: avoid use with saquinavir
Drug/herb
Garlic, St. John's wort: decreased saquinavir level, avoid concurrent use
Drug/food
Increased: bioavailability after high-fat meal
Grapefruit juice: increased saquinivir level
Drug/lab test
Interference: CPK, glucose (low)

NURSING CONSIDERATIONS
Assessment
• Assess signs of infection, anemia
• Monitor blood glucose, viral load, CD4+ T cell count, plasma HIV RNA, serum cholesterol/lipid profile
• Obtain resistance testing at start of and at treatment failure
• Monitor liver function tests: ALT, AST
• Monitor C&S before product therapy; product may be taken as soon as culture is done; repeat C&S after treatment; determine the presence of other STDs
• Assess bowel pattern before, during treatment; if severe abdominal pain with bleeding occurs, product should be discontinued; monitor hydration
• Assess skin eruptions, rash, urticaria, itching
• Assess allergies before treatment, reaction of each medication; place allergies on chart

Nursing diagnoses
• Infection, risk for (uses)
• Knowledge, deficient (teaching)

Implementation
• Give in equal intervals around the clock for duration of therapy

Patient/family education
• Advise patient to take as prescribed within 2 hr of a full meal; if dose is missed, take as soon as remembered up to 1 hr before next dose; do not double dose
• Advise patient that product must be taken in equal intervals around the clock to maintain blood levels for duration of therapy; that product is not a cure
• Advise to take precautions to prevent transmission
• Teach that there are significant drug interactions

Evaluation
Positive therapeutic outcome
• Decreasing symptoms of HIV
• Improving viral load and CD4 cell counts

---

sargramostim (Rx)
(sar-gram'oh-stim)
Leukine, rhu GM-CSF
Func. class.: Biologic modifier: cytokine
Chem. class.: Granulocyte/macrophage colony stimulating factor (GM-CSF)

Pregnancy category C

Do not confuse:
Leukine/leucovorin/Leukeran

Action: Stimulates proliferation and differentiation of hematopoietic progenitor cells (granulocyte, macrophage)

Therapeutic outcome: WBC and differential recovery

Uses: Acceleration of myeloid recovery in patients with non-Hodgkin's lymphoma, acute lymphoblastic leukemia, acute myelogenous leukemia, autologous bone marrow transplantation in Hodgkin's disease; bone marrow transplantation failure or engraftment delay; mobilization and transplant of peripheral blood progenitor cells (PBPCs)

Unlabeled uses: Aplastic anemia, Crohn's disease, ganciclovir- or zidovudine-induced neutropenia

Dosage and routes
Myeloid reconstitution after autologous bone marrow transplantation
Adult: **IV** 250 mcg/m²/day × 3 wk; give over 2 hr, begin 2-4 hr after bone marrow INF, and not less than 24 hr after last dose of antineoplastics and 12 hr after last dose of radiotherapy, bone marrow transplantation failure, or engraftment delay

Acceleration of myeloid recovery
Adult: **IV** 250 mcg/m²/day × 14 days; give over 2 hr; may repeat in 7 days, may repeat 500 mcg/m²/day × 14 days after another 7 days if no improvement

Mobilization of PBPCs
Adult: **IV**/SUBCUT 250 mcg/m²/day during collection of PBPCs

After PBPC transplantation
Adult: **IV**/SUBCUT 250 mcg/m²/day until ANC >1500/mm³ × 3 days

---

Available forms: Powder for inj lyophilized 250 mcg

Adverse effects

CNS: Fever, malaise, CNS disorder, weakness, chills, dizziness, syncope, headache

CV: **Transient supraventricular tachycardia,** peripheral edema, **pericardial effusion,** hypotension, tachycardia

GI: Nausea, vomiting, diarrhea, anorexia, **GI hemorrhage,** stomatitis, **liver damage,** hyperbilirubinemia

GU: Urinary tract disorder, abnormal kidney function

HEMA: **Blood dyscrasias, hemorrhage**

INTEG: Alopecia, rash, peripheral edema

MS: Bone pain, myalgia

RESP: Dyspnea

Contraindications: Hypersensitivity to GM-CSF, benzyl alcohol, yeast products; excessive leukemic myeloid blast in the bone marrow or peripheral blood, neonates

Precautions: Pregnancy **C**, breastfeeding, children, renal/hepatic/lung/cardiac disease, pleural/pericardial effusions, peripheral edema, leukocytosis, mannitol hypersensitivity, hepatic/renal disease

Pharmacokinetics

Absorption	Completely absorbed
Distribution	Unknown
Metabolism	Unknown
Excretion	Unknown
Half-life	Elimination IV 60 min; SUBCUT 2-3 hr

Pharmacodynamics

Onset	Rapid
Peak	2 hr
Duration	Unknown

Interactions

Individual drugs

Lithium: increased myeloproliferation

Drug classifications

Antineoplastics: do not use together

Corticosteroids: increased myeloproliferation

NURSING CONSIDERATIONS

Assessment

• Monitor blood studies: CBC, differential count before treatment and twice weekly; leukocytosis may occur (WBC >50,000 cells/mm^3, ANC >20,000 cells/mm^3), platelets; if ANC >20,000/mm^3 or 10,000/mm^3 after nadir

has occurred or platelets >500,000/mm^3, reduce dose by ½ or discontinue; if blast cells occur, discontinue

• Monitor renal, liver function tests before treatment: BUN, creatinine, urinalysis; AST, ALT, alkaline phosphatase; monitoring is needed twice a week in renal/hepatic disease

• Assess for hypersensitivity reactions/rashes and local inj site reactions; usually transient

• Assess for increased fluid retention in cardiac disease, body weight, hydration status, pulmonary function

• Assess for myalgia, arthralgia in legs, feet; use analgesics

Nursing diagnoses

• Infection, risk for (uses)

• Knowledge, deficient (teaching)

Implementation

• Reconstitute with 1 ml of sterile water for inj without preservative; do not reenter vial; discard unused portion; direct reconstitution sol at side of vial; rotate contents; do not shake

SUBCUT route

• Use reconstituted sol

IV route

• Give by intermittent inf after diluting in 0.9% NaCl inj to prepare **IV** inf; if final conc is <10 mcg/ml, add human albumin to make a final conc of 0.1% to the NaCl before adding sargramostim to prevent absorption; for a final conc of 0.1% albumin, add 1 mg of human albumin/1 ml of 0.9% NaCl inj; run over 2 hr (bone marrow transplant or failure of graft); over 4 hr (chemotherapy for acute myeloid leukemia); over 24 hr as cont inf (PBPCs); give within 6 hr after reconstitution

• Store in refrigerator; do not freeze

Y-site compatibilities: Amikacin, aminophylline, aztreonam, bleomycin, butorphanol, calcium gluconate, carboplatin, carmustine, cefazolin, cefepime, cefotaxime, cefotetan, ceftizoxime, ceftriaxone, cefuroxime, cimetidine, cisplatin, clindamycin, cyclophosphamide, cycloSPORINE, cytarabine, dacarbazine, dactinomycin, dexamethasone, diphenhydrAMINE, DOPamine, DOXOrubicin, doxycycline, droperidol, etoposide, famotidine, fentanyl, floxuridine, fluconazole, fluorouracil, furosemide, gentamicin, granisetron, heparin, idarubicin, ifosfamide, immune globulin, magnesium sulfate, mannitol, mechlorethamine, meperidine, mesna, methotrexate, metoclopramide, metronidazole, minocycline, mitoxantrone, netilmicin, pentostatin, piperacillin/tazobactam, potassium

S

chloride, prochlorperazine, promethazine, ranitidine, teniposide, ticarcillin, ticarcillin/clavulanate, trimethoprim/sulfamethoxazole, vinBLAStine, vinCRIStine, zidovudine

Y-site incompatibilities: Acyclovir, ampicillin, ampicillin/sulbactam, cefonicid, cefoperazine, ceftazidime, chlorproMAZINE, ganciclovir, haloperidol, hydrocortisone, hydromorphone, hydrOXYzine, idarubicin, imipenem/cilastatin, lorazepam, methylPREDNISolone sodium succinate, mitomycin, morphine, nalbuphine, ondansetron, piperacillin, sodium bicarbonate, tobramycin

Patient/family education

• Teach patient reason for medication and expected results
• Advise patient to notify nurse or prescriber of side effects

Evaluation

Positive therapeutic outcome
• WBC and differential recovery
• Absence of infection

---

saxagliptin
See Appendix A, Selected New Drugs

---

scopolamine (Rx)
(skoe-pol'a-meen)
Scopolamine Hydrobromide, Injection Transderm-Scop, Transderm-V
Func. class.: Antiemetic, anticholinergic, mydriatic
Chem. class.: Belladonna alkaloid

Pregnancy category C

Action: Inhibits acetylcholine at receptor sites in autonomic nervous system, which controls secretions, free acids in stomach; blocks central muscarinic receptors, which decreases involuntary movements

Therapeutic outcome: Absence of vomiting, secretions (preoperatively), involuntary movements

Uses: Reduction of secretions before surgery, production of amnesia, prevention of motion sickness, Parkinson's symptoms

Unlabeled uses: Drooling (TD)

Dosage and routes
Prevention of motion sickness
Adult: Transdermal 1 patch placed behind ear 4-5 hr before travel, reapply q3day; alternate ears; not recommended for children

Parkinson's symptoms
Adult: IM/SUBCUT/**IV** 0.3-0.6 mg tid-qid diluted using dilution provided

Preoperatively
Adult: SUBCUT 0.3-0.5 mg; may repeat q4-6hr

Nausea and vomiting
Child: SUBCUT 0.006 mg/kg or 0.2 mg/m²; max 0.3 mg/dose

Drooling (unlabeled)
Adult: Transdermal 1.5 mg patch q3day

Available forms: Patch 1 mg, 1.5 mg delivered in 72 hr; inj 0.3, 0.4, 0.86, 1 mg/ml

Adverse effects
CNS: Confusion, drowsiness, disorientation, anxiety, restlessness, irritability, delusions, headache, fatigue, hallucinations, sedation, depression, incoherence, dizziness, excitement, delirium, flushing, weakness; transdermal: memory disturbances
CV: Palpitations, **tachycardia,** postural hypotension, paradoxical bradycardia
EENT: Transdermal: blurred vision, photophobia, dilated pupils, difficulty swallowing, mydriasis, cycloplegia, altered depth perception, *dry mouth,* dry, itchy red eyes, acute closed-angle glaucoma
GI: *Dryness of mouth, constipation,* nausea, vomiting, abdominal distress, **paralytic ileus**
GU: Hesitancy, retention, difficult urination (patch)
INTEG: Rash, erythema (patch), urticaria, dry skin
MISC: Suppression of breastfeeding, nasal congestion, decreased sweating

Contraindications: Hypersensitivity, closed-angle glaucoma, myasthenia gravis, GI/GU obstruction, hypersensitivity to belladonna, barbiturates

Precautions: Pregnancy **C,** breastfeeding, children, geriatric, prostatic hypertrophy, CHF, hypertension, dysrhythmias, gastric ulcer, renal/hepatic disease, hiatal hernia, GERD, ulcerative colitis, hyperthyroidism; transdermal: pyloric urinary; bladder neck, intestinal obstruction; renal/hepatic disease

Pharmacokinetics

Absorption	Well absorbed (IM, SUBCUT, Transdermal)
Distribution	Crosses placenta, blood-brain barrier
Metabolism	Liver
Excretion	Unknown
Half-life	8 hr

Pharmacodynamics

	SUBCUT/IM	IV	TRANS-DERMAL
Onset	30-45 min	10-15 min	4-5 hr
Peak	1 hr	1 hr	Unknown
Duration	6 hr	4 hr	72 hr

Interactions
Individual drugs
Alcohol: increased anticholinergic effect
Drug classifications
Antidepressants (tricyclics), antihistamines, opioids, phenothiazines: increased anticholinergic effect
Drug/herb
Henbane, jimsonweed, scopolia: increased anticholinergic effects

NURSING CONSIDERATIONS
Assessment
• Monitor I&O ratio; retention commonly causes decreased urinary output
• Assess for parkinsonism, EPS: shuffling gait, muscle rigidity, involuntary movements
• Assess for urinary hesitancy, retention; palpate bladder if retention occurs
• Assess for constipation; increase fluids, bulk, exercise if this occurs
• Assess for tolerance over long-term therapy; dose may have to be increased or changed
• Assess mental status: affect, mood, CNS depression, worsening of mental symptoms during early therapy

Nursing diagnoses
• Fluid volume, deficient (uses)
• Knowledge, deficient (teaching)

Implementation
IM/SUBCUT/IV route
• Administer parenteral dose with patient recumbent to prevent postural hypotension
Transdermal route
• Instruct patient to wash, dry hands before and after applying to surface behind ear; to change patch q72hr; to apply at least 4 hr before traveling
IV route
• Give by direct **IV** after diluting with sterile water; give slowly
Syringe compatibilities: Atropine, benzquinamide, butorphanol, chlorproMAZINE, cimetidine, dimenhyDRINATE, diphenhydrAMINE, droperidol, fentanyl, glycopyrrolate, hydromorphone, hydrOXYzine, meperidine, metoclopramide, midazolam, morphine, nalbuphine, pentazocine, pentobarbital, perphenazine, prochlorperazine, promazine, promethazine, ranitidine, sufentanil, thiopental
Y-site compatibilities: Heparin, hydrocortisone, potassium chloride, propofol, sufentanil, vit B/C
Additive compatibilities: Floxacillin, furosemide, meperidine, succinylcholine

Patient/family education
• Tell patient to avoid hazardous activities, activities requiring alertness; dizziness may occur
• Advise patient to discontinue use if blurred vision, severe dizziness, drowsiness occurs; another type of antiemetic may be used or the patch rotated to the other ear
• Instruct patient to read labels of all OTC medications; if any scopolamine is found in product, avoid use
• Advise patient to keep medication out of children's reach
• Caution patient to report change in vision, blurring or loss of sight, trouble breathing, inhibition of sweating, flushing
• Inform patient that blurred vision will decrease with repeated use of ophthalmic product
• Caution patient not to discontinue this product abruptly; to taper off over 1 wk

Evaluation
Positive therapeutic outcome
• Decreased secretions
• Absence of motion sickness

scopolamine ophthalmic
See Appendix B

S

selegiline (Rx)
(se-le′ji-leen)
Carbex, Eldepryl, Emsam, Novo-Selegiline ✦, Zelapar
Func. class.: Antiparkinson agent
Chem. class.: MAOI, type B

Pregnancy category C

Do not confuse:
Eldepryl/enalapril

Action: Increased dopaminergic activity by inhibition of MAO type B activity; not fully understood

Therapeutic outcome: Decreased symptoms of Parkinson's disease

Uses: Adjunct management of Parkinson's disease in patients being treated with levodopa/carbidopa who have responded poorly to therapy

Unlabeled use: Alzheimer's disease, depression

Dosage and routes
Adult: PO 10 mg/day in divided doses, 5 mg at breakfast and lunch with levodopa/carbidopa; after 2-3 days begin to reduce the dose of levodopa/carbidopa 10%-30%; oral disintegrating tab 2.5 mg (2 tabs) initially, then 1.25 (1 tab) dissolved on tongue daily before breakfast × 6 wk or more; max 2.5 mg/day; transdermal 6 mg/24 hr initially, increase by 3 mg/24 hr at ≥2 wk, up to 12 mg/24 hr if needed

Alzheimer's disease (unlabeled)
Adult: PO 5 mg bid AM, PM

Available forms: Tabs 5 mg, caps 5 mg; oral disintegrating tabs 1.25 mg; transdermal 6 mg/24 hr (20 mg/20 cm²), 9 mg/24 hr (30 mg/30 cm²), 12 mg/24 hr (40 mg/40 cm²)

Adverse effects
CNS: Increased tremors, chorea, restlessness, blepharospasm, increased bradykinesia, grimacing, tardive dyskinesia, dystonic symptoms, involuntary movements, increased apraxia, hallucinations, dizziness, mood changes, nightmares, delusions, lethargy, apathy, overstimulation, sleep disturbances, headache, migraine, numbness, muscle cramps, confusion, anxiety, tiredness, vertigo, personality change, back/leg pain, **suicide in children/adolescents, suicidal ideation in adults**

CV: Orthostatic hypotension, hypertension, **dysrhythmia,** palpitations; angina pectoris, hypotension, tachycardia, edema, sinus bradycardia, syncope, **hypertensive crisis (children)**
EENT: Diplopia, dry mouth, blurred vision, tinnitus
GI: Nausea, vomiting, constipation, weight loss, anorexia, diarrhea, heartburn, rectal bleeding, poor appetite, dysphagia, xerostomia
GU: Slow urination, nocturia, prostatic hypertrophy, hesitation, retention, frequency, sexual dysfunction
INTEG: Increased sweating, alopecia, hematoma, rash, photosensitivity, facial hair
RESP: Asthma, shortness of breath

Contraindications: Children/adolescents (suicide/hypertensive crisis), hypersensitivity, breastfeeding

Precautions: Pregnancy C

Pharmacokinetics	
Absorption	Well absorbed
Distribution	Widely distributed
Metabolism	Rapidly, liver
Excretion	Metabolites-*N*-desmethyldeprenyl, amphetamine, methamphetamine
Half-life	9 min

Pharmacodynamics	
Onset	Unknown
Peak	½-2 hr
Duration	Unknown

Interactions
Individual drugs
Dextromethorphan: increased unusual behavior, psychosis
Fluoxetine, fluvoxamine, paroxetine, sertraline: increased serotonin syndrome (confusion, seizures, fever, hypertension, agitation) discontinue 5 wk before selegiline
Levodopa/carbidopa: increased side effects
◆Meperidine: do not use, fatal reaction
Drug classifications
◆Antidepressants (tricyclics), opioids: do not use, fatal reaction
Antihypertensives: increased hypotension
Drug/herb
Chaste tree fruit, kava: decreased selegiline action

Drug/lab test

Decreased: VMA

False positive: urine ketones, urine glucose

False negative: urine glucose (glucose oxidase)

False increase: uric acid, urine protein

NURSING CONSIDERATIONS
Assessment

- Monitor cardiac status: tachycardia, bradycardia; B/P, respiration throughout treatment
- Assess mental status: affect, mood, behavioral changes, depression; perform suicide assessment
- Assess for decreased Parkinson's symptoms: rigidity, unsteady gait, weakness, tremors; these should decrease in severity
- Assess opioids; if patient has received, do not give selegiline; fatal reactions have occurred

Nursing diagnoses

- Knowledge, deficient (teaching)
- Mobility, impaired physical (uses)

Implementation

- Adjust dosage to patient response
- Give with meals; limit protein taken with product
- Give at doses <10 mg/day because of risks associated with nonselective inhibition of MAO

Patient/family education

- Caution patient to change positions slowly to prevent orthostatic hypotension
- Advise patient to report side effects: twitching, eye spasms; may indicate overdose
- Caution patient to use product exactly as prescribed; if product is discontinued abruptly, parkinsonian crisis may occur
- Instruct patient to avoid foods high in tyramine: cheese, pickled products, wine, beer, large amounts of caffeine
- Instruct patient not to exceed recommended dose of 10 mg; might precipitate a hypertensive crisis; report severe headache or other unusual symptoms

Evaluation

Positive therapeutic outcome

- Decreased symptoms of Parkinson's disease

Treatment of overdose: IV fluids for hypertension, **IV** dilute pressure agent for B/P titration

---

selenium topical

See Appendix B

---

senna, sennosides (OTC)

(sin'na)

Black Draught, Dr. Caldwell Dosalax, Ex-Lax Gentle, Fletcher's Castoria, Gentlax, Senexon, Senna-Gen, Senokot, Senokotxtra, Senolax

Func. class.: Laxative-stimulant

Chem. class.: Anthraquinone

Pregnancy category C

Action: Stimulates peristalsis by action on Auerbach's plexus; softens feces by increasing water and electrolytes in large intestine

Therapeutic outcome: Decreased constipation

Uses: Acute constipation; bowel preparation for surgery or exam, prevention of constipation in those taking opiates long term

Dosage and routes

Adult: PO (Senokot) 1-8 tabs/day or ½ to 4 tsp of granules added to water or juice; RECT SUPP 1-2 at bedtime; SYR 1-4 tsp at bedtime (1 tsp = 4 ml), 7.5-15 ml; (Black Draught) ¾ oz dissolved in 2.5 oz of liquid given between 2-4 PM the day before procedure (X-Prep)

Child >27 kg: PO ½ adult dose; do not use Black Draught for children

Child 1 mo-1 yr: SYR 1.25-2.5 ml (Senokot) at bedtime

Available forms: Tabs 6, 8.6, 15, 25 mg; granules 15, 20 mg/5 ml; syr 8.8 mg/5 ml; liquid 33.3 mg/ml

Adverse effects

GI: Nausea, vomiting, anorexia, abdominal cramps, diarrhea, flatulence

GU: Pink-red or brown-black discoloration of urine

META: Hypocalcemia, enteropathy, alkalosis, hypokalemia, **tetany**

Contraindications: Breastfeeding, hypersensitivity, GI bleeding, intestinal obstruction, CHF, abdominal pain, nausea/vomiting, appendicitis, acute surgical abdomen

Precautions: Pregnancy C

S

Adverse effects: *italic* = common, **bold** = life-threatening

Pharmacokinetics

Absorption	Minimally absorbed (PO)
Distribution	Unknown
Metabolism	Not metabolized
Excretion	Kidneys, feces
Half-life	Unknown

Pharmacodynamics

	PO	RECT
Onset	6-24 hr	Unknown
Peak	Unknown	Unknown
Duration	3-4 days	Unknown

Interactions
Individual drugs
Disulfiram: do not use together
Drug/herb
Flax, senna: increased laxative effect

NURSING CONSIDERATIONS
Assessment
- Monitor blood, urine electrolytes if used often by patient; check I&O ratio to identify fluid loss
- Assess cramping, rectal bleeding, nausea, vomiting; if these symptoms occur, product should be discontinued; identify cause of constipation; identify whether fluids, bulk, or exercise is missing from lifestyle
- Assess for magnesium toxicity: thirst, confusion, decrease in reflexes
- Monitor blood ammonia level (30-70 mg/100 ml); monitor for clearing of confusion, lethargy, restlessness, irritability (hepatic encephalopathy)

Nursing diagnoses
- Constipation (uses)
- Diarrhea (side effects)
- Knowledge, deficient (teaching)
- Noncompliance (teaching)

Implementation
PO route
- Administer on empty stomach for more rapid results
- Give with a full glass of water in AM or PM (oral dose); evacuation occurs 6-12 hr later
- Dissolve granules in water or juice before administration
- Shake oral sol before giving

Patient/family education
- Discuss with patient that adequate fluid consumption is necessary
- Inform patient that normal bowel movements do not always occur daily
- Teach patient not to use in presence of abdominal pain, nausea, vomiting; tell patient to notify prescriber if constipation is unrelieved or if symptoms of electrolyte imbalance occur: muscle cramps, pain, weakness, dizziness, excessive thirst

Evaluation
Positive therapeutic outcome
- Decreased constipation in 8-10 hr

sertraline (Rx)
(ser'tra-leen)
Zoloft
Func. class.: Antidepressant
Chem. class.: Selective serotonin reuptake inhibitor (SSRI)

Pregnancy category C

Do not confuse:
Zoloft/Zocor

Action: Inhibits serotonin reuptake in CNS, thus increasing action of serotonin; does not affect dopamine, norepinephrine

Therapeutic outcome: Relief of depression, obsessive-compulsive disorder (OCD), posttraumatic stress disorder (PTSD), panic disorder

Uses: Major depression, OCD, PTSD, social anxiety disorder, panic disorder, premenstrual dysphoric disorder (PMDD)

Dosage and routes
Adult/adolescent: PO 25-50 mg/day; may increase to a maximum of 200 mg/day, do not change dose at intervals of <1 wk; administer daily in AM or PM
Geriatric: PO 25 mg/day, increase by 25 mg q3day to desired dose
Child 6-12 yr: PO 25 mg/day, max 200 mg/day

Premenstrual disorders
Adult: PO 50-150 mg nightly

Available forms: Tabs 25, 50, 100 mg; oral conc 20 mg/ml

Adverse effects
CNS: Insomnia, agitation, somnolence, dizziness, headache, tremor, fatigue, paresthesia, twitching, confusion, ataxia, gait abnormality (geriatric), **seizures, neuroleptic malignant syndrome–like reactions**
CV: Palpitations, chest pain
EENT: Vision abnormalities, yawning
ENDO: Syndrome of inappropriate antidiuretic hormone (geriatric)
GI: Diarrhea, nausea, constipation, anorexia, dry mouth, dyspepsia, *vomiting, flatulence*

GU: *Male sexual dysfunction,* micturition disorder
INTEG: Increased sweating, rash, hot flashes
MISC: Hyponatremia

Contraindications: Hypersensitivity to this product or selective serotonin reuptake inhibitors

Precautions: Pregnancy **C,** breastfeeding, geriatric, renal/hepatic disease, epilepsy, recent MI, latex sensitivity (dropper of oral conc)

Black Box Warning: Suicidal ideation, children

Pharmacokinetics

Absorption	Well absorbed
Distribution	Unknown, steady state 1 wk
Metabolism	Liver, extensively
Excretion	Feces (14%)
Half-life	26 hr

Pharmacodynamics

Onset	Unknown
Peak	4.5-8.4 hr
Duration	Unknown

Interactions
Individual drugs
Cimetidine, warfarin: increased sertraline effect
Diazepam: increased diazepam effect
Disulfiram: disulfiram reaction with oral conc due to alcohol content
Lithium: altered lithium levels
Pimozide: sertraline is contraindicated with pimozide
Sumatriptan: increased sumatriptan effects
TOLBUTamide: increased effect of TOLBUTamide
Warfarin: increased warfarin effect
Drug classifications
Antidepressants (tricyclics), benzodiazepines: increased effect
Highly protein-bound products: increased sertraline levels
◆ MAOIs: fatal reactions
Drug/herb
Corkwood, jimsonweed: increased anticholinergic effect
Ephedra: hypertensive crisis
Hops, lavender: increased CNS effect
SAM-e, St. John's wort: increased effect of selective serotonin reuptake inhibitors, serotonin syndrome; do not use together
Drug/lab test
Increased: AST, ALT

NURSING CONSIDERATIONS
Assessment
• Assess mental status: mood, sensorium, affect, suicidal tendencies; increase in psychiatric symptoms: depression, panic
• Identify alcohol consumption; if alcohol is consumed, hold dose until AM

Nursing diagnoses
• Coping, ineffective (uses)
• Injury, risk for (adverse reactions)
• Knowledge, deficient (teaching)
• Noncompliance (teaching)

Implementation
• Administer dosage at bedtime if oversedation occurs during day; may take entire dose at bedtime; may crush
• Store at room temperature; do not freeze

Patient/family education
• Teach patient that therapeutic effects may take 1 wk or longer
• Instruct patient to use caution in driving or other activities requiring alertness because of drowsiness, dizziness, blurred vision; to avoid rising quickly from sitting to standing, especially geriatric
• Advise patient to avoid alcohol ingestion, other CNS depressants
◆ Teach patient not to discontinue medication quickly after long-term use; may cause nausea, headache, malaise
• Caution patient to wear sunscreen or large hat because photosensitivity can occur
• Teach patient to increase fluids, bulk in diet if constipation, urinary retention occur, especially geriatric
• Instruct patient to take gum, hard sugarless candy, or frequent sips of water for dry mouth
• Teach patient that suicidal thoughts/behavior may occur (children/adolescents)

Evaluation
Positive therapeutic outcome
• Decrease in depression, OCD
• Absence of suicidal thoughts

Treatment of overdose: ECG monitoring, induce emesis, lavage, activated charcoal, administer anticonvulsant

S

sildenafil (Rx)

(sil-den'a-fill)

Revatio, Viagra

Func. class.: Erectile agent

Chem. class.: Selective inhibitor of cGMP-PDE5

Pregnancy category B

Action: Enhances the effect of nitric oxide (NO) by inhibiting phosphodiesterase type 5 (PDE5), which is necessary for degrading cGMP in the corpus cavernosum

Therapeutic outcome: Ability to achieve and maintain erection

Uses: Treatment of erectile dysfunction, pulmonary hypertension; improvement in exercise ability

Unlabeled uses: Sexual dysfunction (women)

Dosage and routes
Erectile dysfunction (Viagra only)
Adult: PO 50 mg 1 hr before sexual activity or may be taken ½-4 hr before sexual activity; may be increased to 100 mg or decreased to 25 mg; max once/day

Renal/hepatic dose
Adult: PO (Child Pugh A, B) 25 mg, take 1 hr before sexual activity, do not use more than 1 ×/day; CCr <30 ml/min 25 mg starting dose

Pulmonary hypertension (Revatio only)
Adult: PO 20 mg tid, take 4-6 hr apart

Available forms: Tabs 20, 25, 50, 100 mg

Adverse effects
CNS: Headache, flushing, dizziness, transient global amnesia
CV: **MI, sudden death, CV collapse**
MISC: Dyspepsia, nasal congestion, UTI, abnormal vision, diarrhea, rash, **NAION (nonarteritic ischemic optic neuropathy),** hearing loss, priapism

Contraindications: Hypersensitivity to this product or nitrates

Precautions: Pregnancy **B,** anatomical penile deformities, sickle cell anemia, leukemia, multiple myeloma, retinitis pigmentosa, bleeding disorders, active peptic ulceration, CV/renal/hepatic disease, multidrug antihypertensive regimens

Pharmacokinetics
Absorption	Rapidly, bioavailability (40%)
Distribution	Unknown
Metabolism	Liver (active metabolites)
Excretion	Feces, urine
Half-life	4 hr

Pharmacodynamics
Onset	Unknown
Peak	½-1½ hr
Duration	Unknown

Interactions
Individual drugs
Alcohol, amlodipine: decreased B/P
Bosentan, rifampin: decreased sildenafil levels
Cimetidine, erythromycin, itraconazole, ketoconazole: increased sildenafil levels
Drug classifications
Antacids, barbiturates: decreased sildenafil levels
Antiretroviral protease inhibitors: increased sildenafil levels
α-Blockers, angiotensin II receptor blockers: decreased B/P
◆ Nitrates: fatal reaction; do not use together

NURSING CONSIDERATIONS
Assessment
◆ Identify organic nitrates that should not be used with this product
◆ Assess for any severe loss of vision while taking this or any similar products; these products should not be used if vision loss has occurred

Nursing diagnoses
• Knowledge, deficient (teaching)
• Noncompliance (teaching)

Implementation
• Give approximately 1 hr before sexual activity, do not use more than once a day
• Tab may be split

Patient/family education
• Teach patient that product does not protect against STDs, including HIV
• Teach patient that product absorption is reduced with a high-fat meal
• Teach patient that product should not be used with nitrates in any form
• Teach patient that tab may be split
• Teach patient to notify prescriber immediately and stop taking product if vision loss occurs

Evaluation
Positive therapeutic outcome
• Ability to achieve and maintain an erection

 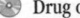

silodosin (Rx)
(si-lo'do-seen)
Rapaflo
Func. class.: Selective α_1-adrenergic blocker
Chem. class.: Sulfamoylphenethylamine derivative

Pregnancy category B

Action: Binds preferentially to α_{1A}-adrenoceptor subtype located mainly in the prostate

Therapeutic outcome: Decreased symptoms of benign prostatic hyperplasia

Uses: Symptoms of benign prostatic hyperplasia (BPH)

Dosage and routes
Adult: PO 8 mg/day with a meal; max 8 mg/day

Available forms: Tabs 8 mg

Adverse effects
CNS: Dizziness, headache, asthenia, insomnia, syncope
CV: Orthostatic hypotension
EENT: Nasal congestion, rhinorrhea, sinusitis
GI: Diarrhea, abdominal pain, jaundice
GU: Abnormal ejaculation, priapism, urinary incontinence
HEMA: Purpura

Contraindications: Hypersensitivity, renal failure

Precautions: Pregnancy **B,** breastfeeding, children, renal/hepatic disease, females, hypotension, ocular surgery, orthostatic hypotension, prostate cancer, syncope, geriatric patients

Pharmacokinetics	
Absorption	Decreased with high fat/high calorie meal
Distribution	Extensive protein binding 97%
Metabolism	Liver
Excretion	Urine
Half-life	24 hr (metabolite)

Pharmacodynamics
Unknown

Interactions
Drug classifications
CYP3A4 inhibitors (clarithromycin, itraconazole, ritonavir, anti-retroviral protease inhibitors, aprepitant, chloramphenicol, conivaptan, dalfopristin, danazol, delavirdine, efavirenz, fosaprepitant, fluconazole, fluvoxamine, imatinib, isoniazid, mifepristone, nefazodone, tamoxifen, telithromycin, troleandomycin, voriconazole, zileuton, zafirlukast): increased silodosin effect
Drug/food
Grapefruit juice: increased silodosin effect
Drug/lab test
Increased: LFTs

NURSING CONSIDERATIONS
Assessment
• Assess prostatic hyperplasia: change in urinary patterns, baseline and throughout treatment
• Monitor CBC with diff and LFTs; B/P and heart rate
• Monitor BUN, uric acid, urodynamic studies (urinary flow rates, residual volume)
• Assess I&O ratios, weight daily, edema, report weight gain or edema

Nursing diagnoses
• Urinary elimination, impaired (uses)
• Knowledge, deficient (teaching)

Implementation
• Give with meal at same time of day
• Store at room temperature; protect from light and moisture

Patient/family education
• Caution patient not to drive or operate machinery until effect is known
• Advise patient not to use with grapefruit juice

Evaluation
Positive therapeutic outcome
• Decreased symptoms of benign prostatic hyperplasia

silver nitrate 1% ophthalmic
See Appendix B

silver nitrate sulfacetamide sodium ophthalmic
See Appendix B

silver sulfADIAZINE topical
See Appendix B

S

Adverse effects: *italic* = common, **bold** = life-threatening

simethicone (Rx, OTC)
(si-meth'i-kone)

Extra Strength Gas-X, Extra Strength Maalox Anti-Gas, Extra Strength Maalox GRF Gas Relief Formula ♣, Flatulex, Gas Relief, Gas-X, Genasyme, Maalox Anti-Gas, Maalox GRF Gas Relief Formula ♣, Maximum Strength Gas Relief, Maximum Strength Mylanta Gas Relief, Maximum Strength Phazyme, Mylanta Gas, Mylicon, Ovol ♣, Phazyme, Phazyme-95, Phazyme-125

Func. class.: Antiflatulent

Pregnancy category C

Do not confuse:
Mylicon/Mylanta Gas

Action: Disperses, prevents gas pockets in GI system; lowers surface tension of gas bubbles

Therapeutic outcome: Belching or flatus

Uses: Flatulence

Unlabeled uses: Dyspepsia

Dosage and routes
Adult and child >12 yr: PO 40-125 mg after meals and at bedtime prn, max 500 mg/day
Child 2-12 yr: PO 40 mg after meals and at bedtime prn, max 240 mg/day
Child <2 yr: PO 20 mg qid prn

Available forms: Chew tabs 40, 150, 166 mg; tabs 60, 80, 95, 125 mg; drops 20 mg/0.3 ml, 95 mg/1.425 ml; caps 95, 180 mg; caps, soft gel 125, 180 mg; oral dissolving film 62.5 mg

Adverse effects
GI: Belching, rectal flatus, diarrhea

Contraindications: Hypersensitivity, GI obstruction/perforation

Precautions: Pregnancy **C**, abdominal pain, fistula, hiatal hernia

Pharmacokinetics	
Absorption	None
Distribution	None
Metabolism	None
Excretion	None
Half-life	Unknown

Pharmacodynamics	
Onset	Rapid
Peak	Unknown
Duration	3 hr

NURSING CONSIDERATIONS
Assessment
- Identify the reason for excess gas production: decreased bowel sounds, recent surgery, other GI conditions

Nursing diagnoses
- Knowledge, deficient (teaching)
- Pain, acute (uses)

Implementation
- Give after meals and at bedtime
- Shake susp well before administration
- Chew tab should be chewed and not swallowed whole

Patient/family education
- Caution patient that tab must be chewed; to shake susp well before pouring

Evaluation
Positive therapeutic outcome
- Absence of flatulence

simvastatin (Rx)
(sim-va-stat'in)
Zocor
Func. class.: Antilipidemic
Chem. class.: HMG-CoA reductase inhibitor

Pregnancy category X

Do not confuse:
Zocor/Cozaar/Zoloft

Action: Inhibits HMG-CoA reductase enzyme, which reduces cholesterol synthesis; this enzyme is needed for cholesterol production

Therapeutic outcome: Decreasing cholesterol levels and LDLs, increased HDLs

Uses: As an adjunct in primary hypercholesterolemia (types IIa, IIb), isolated hypertriglyceridemia (Frederickson type IV) and type III hyperlipoproteinemia

Dosage and routes
Adult: PO 20 mg/day in PM initially, usual range 5-40 mg/day daily in PM, max 80 mg/day; dosage adjustments may be made at 4-wk intervals or more; those taking verapamil, max 20 mg/day

Renal dose/those taking gemfibrozil, danazol
Adult: PO 5 mg day, initially; CCr <20 ml/min 5 mg qd in the evening

Cardiac/renal transplantation
Adult: PO 5 mg/day, max 10 mg/day

With amiodarone or verapamil
Adult: PO max 20 mg/day

With fibrates or niacin
Adult: PO max 10 mg/day

Available forms: Tabs 5, 10, 20, 40, 80 mg

Adverse effects
CNS: Headache, **ALS (Lou Gehrig's disease)**
EENT: Lens opacities
GI: Nausea, constipation, diarrhea, dyspepsia, flatus, abdominal pain, **liver dysfunction, pancreatitis**
INTEG: Rash, pruritus, photosensitivity
MS: Muscle cramps, myalgia, **myositis, rhabdomyolysis**
RESP: Upper respiratory tract infection

Contraindications: Pregnancy **X**, breast-feeding, hypersensitivity, active liver disease

Precautions: Past liver disease, alcoholism, severe acute infections, trauma, severe metabolic disorders, electrolyte imbalances

Pharmacokinetics

Absorption	85%
Distribution	Unknown
Metabolism	Liver—extensively
Excretion	70% feces, 20% kidneys
Half-life	3 hr

Pharmacodynamics
Unknown

Interactions
Individual drugs
Clarithromycin, clofibrate, cycloSPORINE, erythromycin, gemfibrozil, itraconazole, ketoconazole, niacin: increased myalgia, myositis
Digoxin: increased digoxin levels
Warfarin: increased risk of bleeding
Drug classifications
Protease inhibitors: increased myalgia, myositis
Drug/herb
Glucomannan: increased effect
Gotu kola, St. John's wort: decreased effect
Drug/lab test
Increased: CPK, liver function tests

NURSING CONSIDERATIONS
Assessment
• Assess nutrition: fat, protein, carbohydrates; nutritional analysis should be completed by dietitian before treatment is initiated
⬥ Assess for rhabdomyolysis: muscle tenderness, increased CPK levels; therapy should be discontinued
• Monitor bowel pattern daily; diarrhea may be a problem

• Monitor triglycerides, cholesterol baseline, throughout treatment; LDL, HDL, triglycerides and cholesterol should be watched closely at 6-8 wk and q6mo; if increased, product should be discontinued

Nursing diagnoses
• Diarrhea (adverse reactions)
• Knowledge, deficient (teaching)
• Noncompliance (teaching)

Implementation
• Give 30 min before AM and PM meals

Patient/family education
• Inform patient that compliance is needed for positive results to occur, not to double doses
• Advise patient to lower risk factors: high-fat diet, smoking, alcohol consumption, absence of exercise
• Advise patient to notify health care prescriber if the GI symptoms of diarrhea, abdominal or epigastric pain, nausea, vomiting occur; or if chills, fever, sore throat occur

Evaluation
Positive therapeutic outcome
• Decreased cholesterol levels, serum triglycerides and improved ratio with HDLs

---

sirolimus (Rx)
(seer-roe'-li-mus)
Rapamune
Func. class.: Immunosuppressant
Chem. class.: Macrolide
Pregnancy category C

Action: Produces immunosuppression by inhibiting T-lymphocyte activation and proliferation

Therapeutic outcome: Prevention of rejection in organ transplant

Uses: Organ transplants: to prevent rejection, recommended use is with cycloSPORINE and corticosteroids

Dosage and routes
Adult: PO 2 mg daily with 6 mg loading dose
Child >13 yr <40 kg (88 lb): PO 1 mg/m²/day, 3 mg/m²/loading dose

Hepatic dose
Adult and child ≥13 yr <40 kg: PO reduce by 33% in maintenance dose (mild-moderate hepatic impairment); reduce by 50% in maintenance dose (severe hepatic impairment)

S

Available forms: Oral sol 1 mg/ml; tabs 1 mg, 2 mg

Adverse effects

CNS: Tremors, headache, insomnia, paresthesia, chills, fever

CV: Hypo/hypertension, **atrial fibrillation, CHF,** palpitations, **tachycardia,** peripheral edema

EENT: Blurred vision, photophobia

GI: Nausea, vomiting, diarrhea, constipation, **hepatotoxicity**

GU: UTI, **albuminuria, hematuria, proteinuria, renal failure,** nephrotic syndrome

HEMA: Anemia, **thrombocytopenia purpura, leukopenia**

INTEG: Rash, acne, photosensitivity

META: Increased creatinine, edema, hypercholesterolemia, *hyperlipemia,* hypophosphatemia, weight gain, hyperglycemia, hypo/hyperkalemia, hyperuricemia, hypomagnesemia

RESP: **Pleural effusion, atelectasis,** *dyspnea*

SYST: **Lymphoma,** exfoliative dermatitis

Contraindications: Breastfeeding, hypersensitivity to this product or to components of the product

Precautions: Pregnancy **C,** children <13 yr, severe cardiac/renal/hepatic disease, diabetes mellitus, hyperkalemia, hyperuricemia, hypertension, interstitial lung disease, hyperlipidemia

Black Box Warning: Lymphomas, infection, other malignancies

Pharmacokinetics	
Absorption	Rapidly absorbed
Distribution	92% protein binding
Metabolism	Liver; extensively by CYP3A4 enzyme system
Excretion	Unknown
Half-life	Unknown

Pharmacodynamics	
Onset	Unknown
Peak	1 hr single dose, 2 hr multiple dosing
Duration	Unknown

Interactions

Individual drugs

Bromocriptine, cimetidine, cycloSPORINE, danazol, erythromycin, metoclopramide: increased blood level

Carbamazepine, phenobarbital, phenytoin, rifamycin, rifapentine: decreased blood levels

Drug classifications

ACE inhibitors, angiotensin II receptor antagonists, cephalosporins, iodine-containing radiopaque contrast media, neuromuscular blockers, NSAIDs, penicillins, salicylates, thrombolytics: increased angioedema

Antifungal agents, calcium channel blockers, HIV protease inhibitors: increased blood levels

Live virus vaccines: decreased effect of vaccines

Drug/herb

Astragalus, echinacea, melatonin: decreased immunosuppression

Ginseng, maitake, mistletoe: increased effect

St. John's wort: decreased sirolimus effect

Drug/food

Food: alters bioavailability, use consistently with or without food

Grapefruit juice: do not use with grapefruit juice

NURSING CONSIDERATIONS

Assessment

• Monitor blood studies: Hgb, WBC, platelets monthly during treatment; if leukocytes are <3000/mm^3 or platelets <100,000/mm^3, product should be discontinued or reduced; decreased Hgb level may indicate bone marrow suppression

• Monitor blood levels in those who may have altered metabolism, trough levels ≥15 ng/ml are associated with increased adverse reactions

• Monitor lipid profile: cholesterol, triglycerides; a lipid-lowering agent may be needed

• Assess for infection and development of lymphoma

• Monitor liver function tests: alkaline phosphatase, AST, ALT, amylase, bilirubin, and for hepatotoxicity: dark urine, jaundice, itching, light-colored stools; product should be discontinued

Nursing diagnoses

• Infection, risk for (uses)

• Knowledge, deficient (teaching)

Implementation

• Administer prophylaxis for *Pneumocystis jiroveci* pneumonia for 1 yr after transplantation; prophylaxis for cytomegalovirus (CMV) is recommended for 90 days after transplantation in those at increased risk for CMV

• Use amber oral dose syringe and withdraw amount of oral sol needed from the bottle, empty correct dose into plastic/glass container

 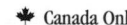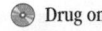

holding 60 ml of water/orange juice, stir vigorously and have patient drink at once, refill container with additional 120 ml of water/orange juice, stir vigorously, and have patient drink at once; if using a pouch squeeze entire contents into container and follow preceding directions

• Give all medications PO if possible; avoid IM inj because bleeding may occur

• Give for 3 days before transplant surgery; patients should be placed in protective isolation

• Store protected from light; refrigerate; stable for 24 months

Patient/family education

• Instruct patient to report fever, rash, severe diarrhea, chills, sore throat, fatigue because serious infections may occur; clay-colored stools, cramping may indicate hepatotoxicity

• Caution patient to avoid crowds or persons with known infections to reduce risk of infection

• Teach patient to use contraception before, during, and 12 wk after product has been discontinued, avoid breastfeeding

• Teach patient to use sunscreen, protective clothing to prevent burns

Evaluation

Positive therapeutic outcome

• Absence of graft rejection

---

sitagliptin (Rx)

(sit-a-glip'tin)

Januvia

Func. class.: Antidiabetic, oral

Chem. class.: Dipeptidyl-peptidase-4 inhibitor (DPP-4 inhibitor)

Pregnancy category C

Action: Slows the inactivation of incretin hormones; improves glucose homeostasis, improves glucose-dependent insulin secretion, lowers glucagon secretions and slows gastric emptying time

Therapeutic outcome: Decrease in polyuria, polydipsia, polyphagia; clear sensorium; absence of dizziness; stable gait; blood glucose at normal level

Uses: Type 2 diabetes mellitus as monotherapy or in combination with other antidiabetic agents

Dosage and routes

Adult: PO 100 mg/day; may use with other antidiabetic agents (metformin, pioglitazone, rosiglitazone) other than insulin

Renal dose

Adult: PO CCr 30-50 ml/min 50 mg qd; CCr <30 ml/min 25 mg qd

Available forms: Tabs 25, 50, 100 mg

Adverse effects

CNS: Headache

ENDO: Hypoglycemia

GI: Nausea, vomiting, abdominal pain, diarrhea

SYST: **Anaphylaxis, Stevens-Johnson syndrome, angioedema**

Contraindications: Hypersensitivity, diabetic ketoacidosis (DKA)

Precautions: Pregnancy **C**, geriatric, hypersensitivity, GI obstruction, thyroid disease, surgery, renal/hepatic disease, trauma

Pharmacokinetics

Absorption	Rapidly
Distribution	Unknown
Metabolism	Unknown
Excretion	Kidneys, 79% unchanged
Half-life	Terminal 12.4 hr

Pharmacodynamics

Onset	Unknown
Peak	1-4 hr
Duration	Unknown

Interactions

Individual drugs

Aripiprazole, clozapine, fosphenytoin, olanzapine, phenytoin, quetiapine, risperidone, ziprasidone: decreased antidiabetic effect

Cimetidine, disopyramide: increased sitagliptan level

Cimetidine, fluoxetine: increased hypoglycemia

Digoxin: increased levels of digoxin

Drug classifications

ACE inhibitors, estrogens, oral contraceptives, phenothiazines, protease inhibitors, sympathomimetics, thiazide diuretics: decreased antidiabetic effect

Androgens, β-blockers, corticosteroids, fibric acid derivatives, insulins, MAOIs, salicylates: increased hypoglycemia

Drug/herb

Alfalfa, aloe, basil, bay, bilberry, bitter melon, black catechu, buchu, burdock, coriander, dandelion, eyebright (po), fenugreek, garlic, ginseng, glucomannan, glucosamine, goat's rue, gymnema, horehound, horse chestnut, jambul, myrrh, myrtle: increased antidiabetic effect

S

Bee pollen, blue cohosh, broom, chromium, elecampane, eucalyptus, gotu kola: decreased antidiabetic effect

Chromium, coenzyme Q-10, fenugreek: increased hypoglycemia

Glucosamine: increased hyperglycemia

NURSING CONSIDERATIONS
Assessment
• Assess for hypoglycemic reactions (sweating, weakness, dizziness, anxiety, tremors, hunger), hyperglycemic reactions soon after meals
• Monitor CBC (baseline, q3mo) during treatment; check liver function tests periodically, AST, LDH, renal studies: BUN, creatinine during treatment; glycosylated hemoglobin A1c
• Monitor blood glucose (BG) as needed

Nursing diagnoses
• Knowledge, deficient (teaching)
• Noncompliance (teaching)
• Nutrition: more than body requirements, imbalanced (uses)

Implementation
• May be taken with or without food
• Conversion from other antidiabetic agents; change may be made with gradual dosage change
• Store in tight container at room temperature

Patient/family education
• Teach patient to use regular self-monitoring of blood glucose using blood glucose meter
• Teach patient the symptoms of hypo/hyperglycemia, what to do about each
• Teach patient that product must be continued on daily basis; explain consequence of discontinuing product abruptly
• Advise patient to avoid OTC medications, alcohol, digoxin, exenatide, insulins, nateglinide, repaglinide and other products that lower blood sugar, unless approved by prescriber
• Teach patient that diabetes is a lifelong illness; that this product is not a cure, only controls symptoms
• Teach patient that all food included in diet plan must be eaten to prevent hypo/hyperglycemia
• Teach patient to carry emergency ID

Evaluation
Positive therapeutic outcome
• Decrease in polyuria, polydipsia, polyphagia; clear sensorium; absence of dizziness; stable gait, blood glucose, A1C improvement

---

sodium bicarbonate (Rx, OTC)
baking soda, Bellans, Brosch-Neut, Citrocarbonate, Neut, Sellymin ✤, Soda Mint

Func. class.: Alkalinizer; antacid

Pregnancy category C

Action: Orally neutralizes gastric acid, which forms water, NaCl, CO_2; increases plasma bicarbonate, which buffers H^+ ion concentration; reverses acidosis **IV**

Therapeutic outcome: Correction of acidosis, gastric acid neutralization

Uses: Acidosis (metabolic), cardiac arrest, alkalinization (systemic/urinary); antacid (PO); salicylate poisoning

Dosage and routes
Acidosis, metabolic
Adult and child: IV INF 2-5 mEq/kg over 4-8 hr depending on CO_2, pH

Cardiac arrest
Adult and child: IV BOL 1 mEq/kg of 7.5% or 8.4% SOL, then 0.5 mEq/kg q5-10min, then doses based on ABGs
Infant: IV INF max 8 mEq/kg/day based on ABGs (4.2% SOL)

Alkalinization of urine
Adult: PO 325 mg-2 g qid or 48 mEq/kg (4 g), then 12-24 mEq q4hr
Child: PO 84-840 mg/kg/day (1-10 mEq/kg), in divided doses q4-6hr

Antacid
Adult: PO 300 mg-2 g chewed, taken with water daily-qid

Available forms: Tabs 300, 325, 600, 650 mg; inj 4.2%, 5%, 7.5%, 8.4%

Adverse effects
CNS: Irritability, headache, confusion, stimulation, tremors, *twitching, hyperreflexia,* **tetany,** weakness, **seizures** caused by alkalosis
CV: Irregular pulse, **cardiac arrest,** water retention, edema, weight gain
GI: Flatulence, *belching, distention,* **paralytic ileus,** acid rebound, nausea
GU: Calculi
META: Alkalosis
MS: Muscular twitching, tetany, irritability
RESP: Shallow, slow respirations, cyanosis, **apnea**

Contraindications: Respiratory/metabolic alkalosis, hypochloremia, hypocalcemia

---

Precautions: Pregnancy **C**, CHF, cirrhosis, toxemia, renal disease, hypertension, hypokalemia, breastfeeding, hypernatremia

Pharmacokinetics

Absorption	Unknown
Distribution	Widely distributed—extracellular fluids
Metabolism	Unknown
Excretion	Kidneys
Half-life	Unknown

Pharmacodynamics

	PO	IV
Onset	2 min	Rapid
Peak	½ hr	Rapid
Duration	1-3 hr	Unknown

Interactions
Individual drugs
Chlorpropamide, lithium: decreased effect of each specific product
Flecainide, mecamylamine, pseudoephedrine, quinidine, quinine: increased effects of each specific product
Drug classifications
Amphetamines, anorexiants, sympathomimetics: increased effects of each specific product
Barbiturates: decreased effects of barbiturates
Benzodiazepines: decreased effects of each specific product
Corticosteroids: increased sodium; decreased potassium
Ketoconazoles: decreased effects of ketoconazoles
Salicylates: decreased effect of salicylates
Drug/herb
Oak bark: decreased action of sodium bicarbonate
Drug/lab test
Increased: urinary urobilinogen, sodium, lactate
False positive: urinary protein, blood lactate
Decreased: potassium

NURSING CONSIDERATIONS
Assessment
• Assess respiratory and pulse rate, rhythm, depth, lung sounds; notify prescriber of abnormalities
• Assess for CO_2 in GI tract; may lead to perforation if ulcer is severe
• Monitor fluid balance (I&O ratio, weight daily, edema); notify prescriber of fluid overload
• Monitor electrolytes, blood pH, PO_2, HCO_3 during beginning treatment; ABGs frequently during emergencies

• Monitor urine pH, urinary output during beginning treatment
• Monitor extravasation with **IV** administration (tissue sloughing, ulceration, and necrosis)
• Assess for alkalosis: irritability, confusion, twitching, hyperreflexia, stimulation, slow respirations, cyanosis, irregular pulse
• Monitor manifestations of hypokalemia: *RENAL:* acidic urine, reduced urine osmolality, nocturia, polyuria, polydipsia; *CV:* hypotension, broad T-wave, U-wave, ectopy, tachycardia, weak pulse; *NEURO:* muscle weakness, altered LOC, drowsiness, apathy, lethargy, confusion, depression; *GI:* anorexia, nausea, cramps, constipation, distention, paralytic ileus; *RESP:* hypoventilation, respiratory muscle weakness
• Monitor for manifestations of hyponatremia: *CV:* increased B/P, cold, clammy skin, hypo/hypervolemia; *GI:* anorexia, nausea, vomiting, diarrhea, abdominal cramps; *NEURO:* lethargy, increased ICP, confusion, headache, seizures, coma, fatigue, tremors, hyperreflexia
• Assess for milk-alkali syndrome: confusion, headache, nausea, vomiting, anorexia, urinary stones, hypercalcemia

Nursing diagnoses
• Fluid volume, excess (adverse reactions)
• Gas exchange, impaired (uses)
• Knowledge, deficient (teaching)

Implementation
PO route
• Antacid tab must be chewed and taken with 8 oz of water
• Dissolve effervescent tab in water
• May be used to neutralize gastric acid in peptic ulcer disease, given 1 and 3 hr after meals and at bedtime
IV route
• Give **IV** bol in cardiac arrest, may be repeated q10min
• Give by intermittent or cont inf in prepared sol or diluted in an equal amount of any dextrose/saline combination; administer 2-5 mEq/kg over 4-8 hr, max 50 mEq/hr; slower rate in children
Syringe compatibilities: Milrinone, pentobarbital
Syringe incompatibilities: Glycopyrrolate, metoclopramide, thiopental
Y-site compatibilities: Acyclovir, amifostine, asparaginase, aztreonam, cefepime, cefmetazole, ceftriaxone, cladribine, cyclophosphamide, cytarabine, DAUNOrubicin, dexamethasone, dexchlorpheniramine, DOXOrubicin, etoposide, famotidine, filgrastim,

Adverse effects: *italic* = common, **bold** = life-threatening

fludarabine, gallium, granisetron, heparin, ifosfamide, indomethacin, insulin, melphalan, mesna, methylPREDNISolone, morphine, paclitaxel, piperacillin/tazobactam, potassium chloride, propofol, tacrolimus, teniposide, thiotepa, tolazoline, vancomycin, vit B/C

Y-site incompatibilities: Calcium chloride, idarubicin, imanrinone, sargramostim, verapamil, vinorelbine

Additive compatibilities: Amikacin, aminophylline, amobarbital, amphotericin B, atropine, bretylium, calcium gluceptate, cefoxitin, ceftazidime, cephalothin, cephapirin, chloramphenicol, chlorothiazide, cimetidine, clindamycin, cytarabine, droperidol/fentanyl, ergonovine, erythromycin, esmolol, floxacillin, furosemide, heparin, hyaluronidase, hydrocortisone, kanamycin, lidocaine, mannitol, metaraminol, methotrexate, methyldopate, multivitamins, nafcillin, nalmefene, netilmicin, nizatidine, ofloxacin, oxacillin, oxytocin, phenobarbital, phenylephrine, phenytoin, phytonadione, potassium chloride, prochlorperazine, thiopental, verapamil

Additive incompatibilities: Amoxicillin, ascorbic acid, carboplatin, carmustine, cefotaxime, cisplatin, codeine, DOBUTamine, epinephrine, hydromorphone, imipenem/cilastatin, insulin, isoproterenol, labetalol, levorphanol, magnesium sulfate, methadone, morphine, norepinephrine, pentazocine, pentobarbital, procaine, secobarbital, streptomycin, succinylcholine, tetracycline, vit B/C

Patient/family education

• Instruct patient to chew antacid tab and drink 8 oz of water; not to take antacid with milk because milk-alkali syndrome may result; not to use antacid for more than 2 wk
• Advise patient to notify prescriber if indigestion is accompanied by chest pain; trouble breathing; diarrhea; dark, tarry stools; coffee grounds–looking vomit; swelling of feet/ankles
• Teach patient about sodium-restricted diet; to avoid use of baking soda for indigestion

Evaluation

Positive therapeutic outcome

• ABGs, electrolytes, blood pH, HCO_3 normal levels
• Decreased gastric pain

---

sodium biphosphate/ sodium phosphate (OTC)

Fleet Enema, Phospho-soda
Func. class.: Laxative, saline

Pregnancy category C

Action: Increases water absorption in the small intestine by osmotic action; laxative effect occurs by increased peristalsis and water retention

Therapeutic outcome: Absence of constipation

Uses: Constipation, bowel or rectal preparation for surgery, examination

Dosage and routes
Adult: PO 20-30 ml (Phospho-soda)
Child: PO 5-15 ml (Phospho-soda)
Adult and child >12 yr: RECT enema (118 ml)
Child 2-12 yr: RECT ½ enema (59 ml)

Available forms: Enema 7 g/phosphate and 19 g/biphosphate/118 ml; oral sol 18 g phosphate/48 g biphosphate/100 ml

Adverse effects

CV: **Dysrhythmias, cardiac arrest,** hypotension, widening QRS complex
GI: Nausea, cramps, diarrhea
META: Electrolyte, fluid imbalances

Contraindications: Hypersensitivity, rectal fissures, abdominal pain, nausea/vomiting, appendicitis, acute surgical abdomen, ulcerated hemorrhoids, Na-restricted diets, renal failure, hyperphosphatemia, hypocalcemia, hypokalemia, hypernatremia, Addison's disease, CHF, ascites, bowel perforation, megacolon, imperforate anus

Black Box Warning: GI obstruction, renal failure

Precautions: Pregnancy C

Black Box Warning: Colitis, elderly, hypovolemia, renal disease

Pharmacokinetics

Absorption	Up to 20% (rec)
Distribution	Unknown
Metabolism	Unknown
Excretion	Kidneys
Half-life	Unknown

Pharmacodynamics

	PO	RECT
Onset	½-3 hr	5 min
Peak	Unknown	Unknown
Duration	Unknown	Unknown

NURSING CONSIDERATIONS
Assessment
- Assess stools: color, amount, consistency
- Assess for bowel pattern, bowel sounds (frequency, intensity), flatulence, distention, increased temp, dietary patterns (fluid, bulk), exercise
- Assess for cramping, rectal bleeding, nausea, vomiting; if these symptoms occur, product should be discontinued

Nursing diagnoses
- Constipation (uses)
- Knowledge, deficient (teaching)

Implementation
PO route
- Give on empty stomach
- Mix oral sol in cold water
- Take alone for better absorption; do not take within 1 hr of other products

Patient/family education
- Advise patient not to use laxatives or enema for long-term therapy; bowel tone will be lost
- Teach patient that normal bowel movements do not always occur daily
- Caution patient not to use in presence of abdominal pain, nausea, vomiting
- Caution patient to notify prescriber if constipation is unrelieved or if symptoms of electrolyte imbalance occur: muscle cramps, pain, weakness, dizziness, excessive thirst
- Instruct patient to maintain adequate fluid consumption to help prevent constipation

Evaluation
Positive therapeutic outcome
- Decrease in constipation

---

sodium polystyrene sulfonate (Rx)
(po-lee-stye′reen)
Kayexalate, K-Exit ✦, Kionex, PMS Sodium Polystyrene Sulfonate ✦, SPS
Func. class.: Potassium-removing resin
Chem. class.: Cation exchange resin

Pregnancy category C

Action: Removes potassium by exchanging sodium for potassium in body; occurs primarily in large intestine

Therapeutic outcome: Potassium levels within accepted range

Uses: Hyperkalemia in conjunction with other measures

Dosage and routes
Adult: PO 15 g daily-qid; RECT enema 30-50 q1-2hr initially prn, then q6hr prn
Child (unlabeled): PO 1 g/kg q6hr prn; RECT 1 g/kg q2-6hr prn

Available forms: Powder for susp 453.6 g, 454 g; oral susp 15 g/60 ml; rectal enema susp 15 g/60 ml

Adverse effects
GI: Constipation, anorexia, nausea, vomiting, diarrhea (sorbitol), *fecal impaction,* gastric irritation
META: Hypocalcemia, hypokalemia, hypomagnesemia, sodium retention

Contraindications: Hypersensitivity to saccharin or parabens that may be in some products; ileus

Precautions: Pregnancy C, geriatric, renal failure, CHF, severe edema, severe hypertension, sodium restriction, constipation

Pharmacokinetics
Absorption	None
Distribution	None
Metabolism	None
Excretion	Feces
Half-life	Unknown

Pharmacodynamics
	PO	RECT
Onset	2-12 hr	2-12 hr
Peak	Unknown	Unknown
Duration	6-24 hr	4-6 hr

Interactions
Drug classifications
Antacids (calcium or magnesium), laxatives: decreased effect of sodium polystyrene
Diuretics (loop): increased hypokalemia

NURSING CONSIDERATIONS
Assessment
- Assess bowel function daily: amount of stool, color, characteristics
- Assess for hypotension: confusion, irritability, muscular pain, weakness
- Monitor for manifestations of hypokalemia: *RENAL:* acidic urine, reduced urine osmolality, nocturia, polyuria, polydipsia; *CV:* hypotension, broad T-wave, U-wave, ectopy, tachycardia, weak pulse; *NEURO:* muscle weakness, altered LOC, drowsiness, apathy, lethargy, confusion, depression; *GI:* anorexia, nausea, cramps, constipation, distention, paralytic ileus; *RESP:* hypoventilation, respiratory muscle weakness

S

Adverse effects: *italic* = common, **bold** = life-threatening

- Monitor for manifestations of hyperkalemia: confusion, dyspnea, weakness, dysrhythmias
- Monitor for manifestations of hypocalcemia: *CNS:* personality changes, anxiety, disturbances, depression, psychosis, nausea, vomiting, *GI:* constipation, abdominal pain from muscle spasm; *CV:* decreased contractility, decreased cardiac output, hypotension, lengthened ST segment, prolonged QT interval; *INTEG:* scaling eczema, alopecia, hyperpigmentation; *NEURO:* tetany, muscle twitching, cramping grimacing, seizure, altered deep tendon reflexes, spasm
- Monitor for manifestations of hypomagnesemia; *CNS:* agitation; *NEURO:* muscle twitching, paresthesias, hyperactive reflexes, positive Babinski reflex, dysphagia, nystagmus, seizures, tetany; *GI:* nausea, vomiting, diarrhea, anorexia, abdominal distention; *CV:* ectopy; tachycardia, broad, flat, or inverted T-waves; depressed ST segment; prolonged QT interval; decreased cardiac output; hypotension
- Monitor electrolytes: potassium, sodium, calcium, magnesium; I&O ratio, weight daily
- Monitor ECG for spiked T-waves, depressed ST segments, prolonged QT interval and widening QRS complex

Nursing diagnoses
- Constipation (adverse reactions)
- Diarrhea (adverse reactions)
- Knowledge, deficient (teaching)

Implementation
PO route
- Give oral dose as susp mixed with H_2O or syr (20-100 ml)
- Give mild laxative as ordered to prevent constipation and fecal impaction; sorbitol as ordered to prevent constipation

Rectal route
- Give by retention enema after mixing with warm water; introduce by gravity, continue stirring, flush with 100 ml of fluid, clamp, and leave in place for at least ½-1 hr
- Complete irrigation of colon after enema with 1-2 qt of nonsodium sol, drain
- Store freshly prepared sol for 24 hr at room temperature

Patient/family education
- Explain reason for medication and expected results

Evaluation
Positive therapeutic outcome
- Potassium level 3.5-5 mg/dl

---

solifenacin (Rx)
(sol-i-fen'a-sin)
VESIcare
Func. class.: Overactive bladder product, anticholinergic
Chem. class.: Muscarinic receptor antagonist

Pregnancy category C

Action: Relaxes smooth muscles in urinary tract by inhibiting acetylcholine at postganglionic sites

Therapeutic outcome: Decreased dysuria, frequency, nocturia, incontinence

Uses: Overactive bladder (urinary frequency, urgency, incontinence)

Dosage and routes
Adult: PO 5 mg/day, max 10 mg/day

Renal/hepatic dose
Adult: PO CCr <30 ml/min 5 mg/day

Available forms: Tabs 5, 10 mg

Adverse effects
CNS: Anxiety, paresthesia, fatigue, *dizziness,* headache
CV: Chest pain, hypertension, **QTc prolongation, peripheral edema**
EENT: Vision abnormalities, xerophthalmia, nasal dryness
GI: Nausea, vomiting, anorexia, abdominal pain, *constipation,* dry mouth, dyspepsia
GU: Dysuria, urinary retention, frequency, UTI
INTEG: Rash, pruritus
RESP: Bronchitis, cough, pharyngitis, URI

Contraindications: Hypersensitivity, uncontrolled closed-angle glaucoma, urinary retention, gastric retention

Precautions: Pregnancy **C,** breastfeeding, children, geriatric patients, renal/hepatic disease, controlled closed-angle glaucoma, bladder outflow obstruction, GI obstruction, decreased GI motility, history of QT prolongation

Pharmacokinetics
Absorption	Rapid
Distribution	98% highly protein bound
Metabolism	Extensively metabolized by CYP3A4
Excretion	Excreted in urine/feces
Half-life	Terminal half-life 45-68 hr

Pharmacodynamics
Unknown

 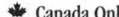

Interactions
Drug classifications
Benzodiazepines, hypnotics, opioids, sedatives: increased CNS depression

CYP3A4 inducers (carbamazepine, nevirapine, phenobarbitol, phenytoin): decreased effects of solifenacin

CYP3A4 inhibitors (clarithromycin, diclofenac, doxycycline, erythromycin, isoniazid, ketoconazole, nefazodone, propofol, protease inhibitors, verapamil): increased action of solifenacin, with max dose 5 mg
Drug/herb
Henbane, jimsonweed, scopolia: increased effects

St. John's wort: decreased effects
Drug/food
Grapefruit juice: increased effect

NURSING CONSIDERATIONS
Assessment
• Assess urinary patterns: distention, nocturia, frequency, urgency, incontinence
• Assess for allergic reactions: rash; if this occurs, product should be discontinued

Nursing diagnoses
• Knowledge, deficient (teaching)
• Urinary elimination, impaired (uses)

Patient/family education
• Caution patient to avoid hazardous activities; dizziness may occur
• Advise patient that constipation, blurred vision may occur
• Instruct patient to call prescriber if severe abdominal pain or constipation lasts for 3 or more days
• Advise patient that heat prostration may occur if used in a hot environment

Evaluation
Positive therapeutic outcome
• Urinary status: dysuria, frequency, nocturia, incontinence

---

somatropin (Rx)
(soe-ma-troe′pin)
Accretropin, Genotropin, Genotropin-MiniQuick, Humatrope, Norditropin, Nutropin, Nutropin AQ, Nutropin Depot, Omnitrope, Saizen, Serostim, Tev-Tropin, Zorbtive
Func. class.: Pituitary hormone
Chem. class.: Growth hormone
Pregnancy category C

Do not confuse: Somatropin/sumatriptan

Action: Stimulates growth; similar to natural growth hormone—both preparations are developed by recombinant DNA technique

Therapeutic outcome: Increase in height as a result of skeletal growth in pituitary growth hormone deficiency

Uses: Pituitary growth hormone deficiency (hypopituitary dwarfism), children with human growth hormone deficiency, AIDS wasting syndrome, cachexia, adults with somatropin deficiency syndrome (SDS), short stature in Noonan syndrome, SHOX deficiencies; Turner's syndrome, Prader-Willi syndrome

Dosage and routes
Genotropin
Child: SUBCUT 0.16-0.24 mg/kg/wk, divided into 6 or 7 daily inj, give in abdomen, thigh, buttocks
Adult: SUBCUT 0.4-0.8 mg/kg/wk divided in 6-7 daily doses

Humatrope
Child: SUBCUT/IM 0.18 mg/kg divided into equal doses either on 3 alternate days or 6 ×/wk, max 0.3 mg/kg/wk
Adult: IM 0.018 units/kg/day, max 0.0125 units/kg/day

Growth hormone deficiency
Nutropin/Nutropin AQ
Child: SUBCUT 0.3 mg/kg/wk

Serostim
Adult: SUBCUT at bedtime >55 kg 6 mg, 45-55 kg 5 mg, 35-45 kg 4 mg

Norditropin
Child: SUBCUT 0.024-0.034 mg/kg 6-7 ×/wk

Accretropin
Child: SUBCUT 0.18-0.3 mg/kg/wk divided into 6 or 7 equal daily inj

S

Adverse effects: *italic* = common, **bold** = life-threatening

Replacement of GH in GH deficiency

Adult: SUBCUT (Saizen) 0.005 mg/kg/day; may increase after 4 wk to max 0.01 mg/kg/day

Available forms: Powder for inj (lyophilized) 1.5 mg (4 international units/ml), 4 mg (12 international units/vial), 5 mg (13 international units/vial), 5 mg (15 international units/vial), rDNA origin, 5.8 mg (15 international units/ml), 6 mg (18 international units/ml), 8 mg (24 international units/vial), 10 mg (26 international units/vial), inj 10 mg (30 international units/vial); 5, 10, 15 mg/1.5 ml

Adverse effects

CNS: Headache, **growth of intracranial tumor,** fever, aggressive behavior
ENDO: Hyperglycemia, ketosis, hypothyroidism
GI: Nausea, vomiting
GU: Hypercalciuria
INTEG: Rash, urticaria, pain, inflammation at inj site; hematoma
MS: Tissue swelling, joint and muscle pain
SYST: Antibodies to growth hormone

Contraindications: Hypersensitivity to benzyl alcohol, closed epiphyses, intracranial lesions, acute respiratory failure, Prader-Willi syndrome with obesity, trauma

Precautions: Pregnancy **C**, breastfeeding, newborns, geriatric, diabetes mellitus, hypothyroidism, intracranial lesions, prolonged treatment in adults, scoliosis, sleep apnea, chemotherapy, diabetes, respiratory disease

Pharmacokinetics

Absorption	Well absorbed (SUBCUT/IM)
Distribution	Unknown
Metabolism	Unknown
Excretion	Unknown
Half-life	15-60 min

Pharmacodynamics

	IM/SUBCUT (GROWTH)
Onset	Unknown
Peak	Unknown
Duration	7 days

Interactions
Drug classifications
Androgens, thyroid hormones: increased epiphyseal closure
Glucocorticosteroids: decreased growth

NURSING CONSIDERATIONS
Assessment
- Assess for signs/symptoms of diabetes
- Identify growth hormone antibodies if patient fails to respond to therapy
- Monitor thyroid function tests: T_3, T_4, T_7, TSH to identify hypothyroidism
- Assess for allergic reaction: rash, itching, fever, nausea, wheezing
- Assess for hypercalciuria: urinary stones; groin, flank pain; nausea, vomiting, frequency, hematuria, chills
- Monitor growth rate, bone age of child at intervals during treatment

Nursing diagnoses
- Body image, disturbed (uses)
- Knowledge, deficient (teaching)

Implementation
- Store in refrigerator for <1 mo; if reconstituted, <1 wk; do not use discolored or cloudy sol
IM route
- Accretropin: Does not require reconstitution
- Norditropin: After reconstituting 4-8 mg/2 ml diluent
- Humatrope: 5 mg/1.5-5 ml dilute, do not shake
- Nutropin/Nutropin AQ: Reconstitute 5 mg/1-5 ml or 10 mg/1-10 ml of bacteriostatic water for inj (benzyl alcohol preserved)
- Zorbtive: Reconstitute 4, 5, 6 mg with 0.5-1 ml of sterile water for inj; reconstitute each 8.8 mg with 1-2 bacteriostatic water for inj

Patient/family education
- Explain reason for medication and expected results; that treatment may continue for yr
- Advise patient that routine follow-up is needed to monitor growth rate
- Instruct parents on procedure for medication preparation and inj use; request demonstration, return demonstration; provide written instructions
- Teach patient to maintain growth record, report knee, hip pain or limping
- Advise patient treatment is very expensive

Evaluation
Positive therapeutic outcome
- Growth in children until epiphyseal plates close

---

sorafenib (Rx)
(sore-ah-fen'ib)
Nexavar
Func. class.: Antineoplastic—miscellaneous
Chem. class.: Multikinase inhibitor, signal
transduction inhibitor

Pregnancy category D

Action: Multikinase inhibitor that decreases
tumor cell proliferation

Therapeutic outcome: Prevention of
spread of malignancy

Uses: Advanced/metastatic murine renal cell
carcinoma, unresectable hematocellular
cancer

Dosage and routes
Adult: PO 400 mg bid without food, continue until no longer benefiting or until unacceptable toxicity occurs

Available forms: Tabs 200 mg

Adverse effects
CNS: Fatigue, weight loss, headache
CV: **Hypertension, cardiac ischemia,
infarction, hypertensive crisis, cardiotoxicity, MI**
GI: Nausea, diarrhea, vomiting, anorexia,
pancreatitis, mouth ulceration, *abdominal
pain,* constipation, **GI perforation**
HEMA: **Hemorrhage, leukopenia, lymphopenia, anemia, neutropenia, thrombocytopenia, pancytopenia**
INTEG: Rash, pruritus, *dry skin,* erythema,
hand-foot syndrome, **exfoliative dermatitis,** acne, flushing, *alopecia*
META: Hypophosphatemia
MS: Arthralgia, myalgia
RESP: Hoarseness

Contraindications: Pregnancy **D,** hypersensitivity

Precautions: Breastfeeding, children,
geriatric, cardiac/renal/hepatic disease, GI
bleeding, infection, surgery, dental disease/
work

Pharmacokinetics
Absorption	38%-49%, high fat meal decreases bioavailability
Distribution	Protein binding 99.5%
Metabolism	Liver, oxidative metabolism by CYP3A4, glucuronidation by UGT1A9
Excretion	77% feces
Half-life	Elimination 1-2 day

Pharmacodynamics
Onset	Unknown
Peak	3 hr
Duration	Unknown

Interactions
Individual drugs
Carbamazepine, cimetidine, dexamethasone,
phenobarbital, phenytoin, ranitidine, rifampin, sodium bicarbonate: decreased sorafenib levels
Drug classifications
Anticoagulants, NSAIDs, platelet inhibitors,
thrombolytics: increased bleeding risk
CYP3A4 inducers (barbiturates, bosentan,
carbamazepine, efavirenz, nevirapine,
phenytoins, rifabutin, rifampin): may decrease sorafenib effect
UGT1A1 drugs (irinotecan, DOXOrubicin,
morphine, naltrexone, estradiol,
buprenorphine): increased effect of UGT1A1
substrates
Drug/lab test
Decreased: RBC, WBC, platelets
Increased: lipase, amylase, TSH, bilirubin,
WBC, platelets

NURSING CONSIDERATIONS
Assessment
• Monitor CBC with differential LFTs
• Assess for skin toxicities: grade 1, continue
therapy, topical treatment for relief; grade 2
(1st episode), continue therapy, if no improvement after 7 days, delay treatment until resolved to grade ≤1, resume dose by one dose
level; grade 2 (2nd or 3rd episode), delay
treatment until resolved to grade ≤1, resume
dose by one dose level; grade 2 (4th episode),
discontinue therapy; grade 3 (1st or 2nd
episode), delay treatment until resolved to
grade ≤1, resume dose by one dose level;
grade 3 (3rd episode), discontinue therapy
• Monitor B/P weekly × 6 wk (hypertension);
cardiac ischemia, bleeding, bruising
• Assess for hand-foot reactions during first 6
wk of therapy
• Monitor PT, INR (bleeding)

Nursing diagnoses
• Injury, risk for (uses, adverse reactions)

Implementation
• Swallow tab whole; do not break, crush, or
chew
• Give on empty stomach 1 hr before or 2 hr
after meal
• Store at room temp, in dry place

Adverse effects: italic = common, **bold** = life-threatening

Patient/family education

⬥ Teach patient to report adverse reactions immediately
• Teach patient the reason for treatment, expected results
• Advise patient to use contraception during treatment, birth defects may occur; avoid breastfeeding
• Advise patient not to double dose if missed
• Advise patient to avoid OTC products without approval of prescriber

Evaluation
Positive therapeutic outcome
• Decrease in renal cell carcinoma stabilization

---

sotalol (Rx)
(soe-ta'lole)
Betapace, Betapace AF, Sotacar ✦
Func. class.: Antidysrhythmic, group III
Chem. class.: Nonselective β-blocker

Pregnancy category B

Action: Competitively blocks stimulation of β-adrenergic receptor within vascular smooth muscle; produces chronotropic, inotropic activity (decreases rate of SA node discharge, increases recovery time), slows conduction of AV node, decreases heart rate, which decreases O_2 consumption in myocardium; also decreases renin-aldosterone-angiotensin system at high doses, inhibits β_2 receptors in bronchial system (high doses)

Therapeutic outcome: Decreased B/P, heart rate, AV conduction

Uses: Life-threatening ventricular dysrhythmias; Betapace AF: to maintain sinus rhythm in symptomatic atrial fibrillation/flutter

Dosage and routes
Adult: PO initial 80 mg bid, may increase to total of 240-320 mg/day

Renal dose
Adult: PO CCr 30-60 ml/min q24hr; CCr 10-29 ml/min q36-48hr; CCr <10 ml/min individualize dose

Betapace AF
Adult: PO initial 80 mg bid, titrate upward to 120 mg bid during initial hospitalization

Renal dose (Betapace AF)
CCr >60 ml/min q12hr; CCr 40-60 ml/min q24hr; CCr <40 ml/min do not use

Available forms: Tabs 80, 120, 160, 240 mg; (Betapace AF) 80, 120, 160 mg; inj 150 mg/10 ml (15 mg/ml)

Adverse effects
CNS: Dizziness, mental changes, drowsiness, fatigue, headache, catatonia, depression, anxiety, nightmares, paresthesia, lethargy, insomnia, decreased concentration
CV: Orthostatic hypotension, bradycardia, **CHF,** chest pain, **ventricular dysrhythmias, prolonged QT,** AV block, peripheral vascular insufficiency, palpitations, **prodysrhythmia, torsades de pointes; Betapace AF: life-threatening ventricular dysrhythmias**
EENT: Tinnitus, visual changes, sore throat, double vision, dry, burning eyes
GI: Nausea, vomiting, diarrhea, dry mouth, flatulence, constipation, anorexia, indigestion
GU: Impotence, dysuria, ejaculatory failure, urinary retention
HEMA: **Agranulocytosis, thrombocytopenic purpura (rare), thrombocytopenia, leukopenia**
INTEG: Rash, alopecia, urticaria, pruritus, fever, diaphoresis
MISC: Facial swelling, decreased exercise tolerance, weight change, Raynaud's disease
MS: Joint pain, arthralgia, muscle cramps, pain
RESP: **Bronchospasm,** dyspnea, wheezing, nasal stuffiness, pharyngitis

Contraindications: Hypersensitivity to β-blockers, cardiogenic shock, heart block (2nd or 3rd degree), sinus bradycardia, CHF, bronchial asthma, CCr <40 ml/min

Black Box Warning: Congenital or acquired long QT syndrome, hypokalemia

Precautions: Pregnancy **B,** breastfeeding, major surgery, diabetes mellitus, renal/thyroid disease, COPD, well-compensated heart failure, CAD, nonallergic bronchospasm, electrolyte disturbances, bradycardia, peripheral vascular disease

Black Box Warning: Cardiac dysrhythmias, torsades de pointes, ventricular dysrhythmias, ventricular fibrillation

---

Pharmacokinetics

Absorption	Variable (30%)
Distribution	Crosses placenta, minimal penetration in CNS
Metabolism	Liver, protein binding 0%
Excretion	70% unchanged—kidneys
Half-life	10-24 hr, increased in renal disease

  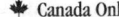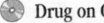

Pharmacodynamics	
Onset	Several hr
Peak	Unknown
Duration	Unknown

Interactions
Individual drugs
Insulin: increased hypoglycemia
Lidocaine: increased effects of lidocaine
Nitroglycerin: increased hypotension
Theophylline: decreased bronchodilating effects of theophylline

Drug classifications
Antihypertensives, diuretics: increased hypotension
β_2-Agonists: decreased bronchodilating effects
Sulfonylureas: decreased hypoglycemic effects
Sympathomimetics: decreased β-blocker effects

Drug/herb
Aconite: increased toxicity, death
Aloe, broom (chronic use), buckthorn, cascara sagrada (chronic use), Chinese rhubarb, figwort, fumitory, goldenseal, kudzu, licorice: increased effect
Coltsfoot: decreased effect
Horehound: increased serotonin effect

Drug/lab test
False: increased urinary catecholamines
Interference: glucose, insulin tolerance tests

NURSING CONSIDERATIONS
Assessment
• Monitor B/P during beginning treatment, periodically thereafter; pulse q4hr; note rate, rhythm, quality; apical/radial pulse before administration; notify prescriber of any significant changes (pulse <50 bpm); monitor ECG continuously (Betapace AF); use QT interval to determine patient eligibility; baseline QT must be ≤450 msec
• Check for baselines in renal function tests, before therapy begins
• Assess for edema in feet, legs daily, monitor I&O ratio, daily weight; check for jugular vein distention, crackles, bilaterally, dyspnea (CHF)
• Monitor skin turgor, dryness of mucous membranes for hydration status, especially in geriatric

Nursing diagnoses
• Cardiac output, decreased (uses)
• Injury, risk for (adverse reactions)
• Knowledge, deficient (teaching)
• Noncompliance (teaching)

Implementation
PO route
• Given before meals, at bedtime, tab may be crushed or swallowed whole; give with food to prevent GI upset; reduce dosage in renal dysfunction
• Betapace and Betapace AF are not interchangeable
• Store protected from light, moisture; place in cool environment
IV route
• Dilute to a volume of either 120 ml or 300 ml with D_5W, LR
• 75-mg dose: withdraw 6 ml sotalol inj (90 mg), add 114 ml dilute to make 120 ml (0.75% mg/ml); or withdraw 6 ml sotalol inj (90 mg), add 294 ml, dilute to make 300 ml (0.3 mg/ml)
• 112.5-mg dose: withdraw 9 ml sotalol inj, (135 ml), add 111 ml, dilute to 120 ml (1.125 mg/ml); or withdraw 9 ml sotalol (135 mg) and add 291 ml dilute to 300 ml (0.45 mg/ml)
• 150-mg dose: withdraw 12 ml sotalol (180 mg), add 108 ml to 120 ml (1.5 mg/ml); or withdraw 12 ml of sotalol (180 mg), add 288 ml to 300 ml (0.6 mg/ml)
• Use inf pump

Patient/family education
• Teach patient not to discontinue product abruptly, taper over 2 wk; may cause precipitate angina if stopped abruptly
• Teach patient not to use OTC products containing α-adrenergic stimulants (such as nasal decongestants, cold preparations); to avoid alcohol and smoking and to limit sodium intake as prescribed
• Teach patient how to take pulse and B/P at home, advise when to notify prescriber
• Instruct patient to comply with weight control, dietary adjustments, modified exercise program
• Caution patient to carry/wear emergency ID to identify product being taken, allergies
• Inform patient that product controls symptoms but does not cure
• Caution patient to avoid hazardous activities if dizziness, drowsiness are present
• Teach patient to report symptoms of CHF: difficulty breathing, especially on exertion or when lying down; night cough; swelling of extremities; bradycardia; dizziness; confusion; depression; fever
• Teach patient to take product as prescribed, not to double or skip doses; take any missed doses as soon as remembered if at least 4 hr until next dose

S

Adverse effects: *italic* = common, **bold** = life-threatening

Evaluation
Positive therapeutic outcome
- Absence of dysrhythmias

Treatment of overdose: Lavage; **IV** atropine for bradycardia; **IV** theophylline for bronchospasm; digoxin, O_2, diuretic for cardiac failure; hemodialysis; **IV** glucose for hyperglycemia; **IV** diazepam (or phenytoin) for seizures

---

spironolactone (Rx)
(speer'on-oh-lak'tone)
Aldactone, Novo-Spiroton ✦
Func. class.: Potassium-sparing diuretic
Chem. class.: Aldosterone antagonist

Pregnancy category D

Action: Competes with aldosterone at receptor sites in the distal tubule in the renal system, resulting in excretion of sodium chloride, water, potassium, and phosphate are retained

Therapeutic outcome: Diuretic and antihypertensive effect while retaining potassium; lowered aldosterone levels

Uses: Edema of CHF, hypertension, diuretic-induced hypokalemia, primary hyperaldosteronism (diagnosis, short-term treatment, long-term treatment), edema of nephrotic syndrome, cirrhosis of the liver with ascites

Unlabeled uses: CHF, hirsutism in women

Dosage and routes
Edema/hypertension
Adult: PO 25-200 mg/day in 1-2 divided doses

CHF
Adult: PO 12.5-25 mg/day, max 50 mg/day

Edema
Child: PO 1.5-3.3 mg/kg/day in single or divided doses

Hypertension
Child (unlabeled): PO 1.5-3.3 mg/kg in divided doses

Hypokalemia
Adult: PO 25-100 mg/day; if PO, potassium supplements must not be used

Primary hyperaldosteronism diagnosis
Adult: PO 400 mg/day × 4 days or 4 wk depending on the test, then 100-400 mg/day maintenance

Edema (nephrotic syndrome, CHF, hepatic disease)
Adult: PO 100 mg/day given as a single dose or in divided doses, titrate to response
Child: PO 1.5-3.3 mg/kg/day or 60 mg/m^2/day given daily or in 2-4 divided doses

Renal dose
Adult: PO CCr 10-50 ml/min; give dose q12-24hr; CCr <10 ml/min, avoid use

Polycystic ovary syndrome/hirsutism in women (unlabeled)
Adult: PO 50-200 mg in 1-2 divided doses

Available forms: Tabs 25, 50, 100 mg

Adverse effects
CNS: Headache, confusion, drowsiness, lethargy, ataxia
ELECT: Hyperchloremic metabolic acidosis, **hyperkalemia,** hyponatremia
ENDO: Impotence, gynecomastia, irregular menses, amenorrhea, postmenopausal bleeding, hirsutism, deepening voice, breast pain
GI: Diarrhea, cramps, **bleeding,** gastritis, vomiting, anorexia, nausea, **hepatocellular toxicity**
HEMA: **Agranulocytosis**
INTEG: *Rash, pruritus,* urticaria

Contraindications: Pregnancy **D,** hypersensitivity, anuria, severe renal disease, hyperkalemia

Precautions: Breastfeeding, dehydration, renal/hepatic disease, electrolyte imbalances, metabolic acidosis, gynecomastia

Black Box Warning: Secondary malignancy

Pharmacokinetics	
Absorption	GI tract; well absorbed
Distribution	Crosses placenta
Metabolism	Liver to canrenone (active metabolite)
Excretion	Renal; breast milk
Half-life	12-24 hr (canrenone)

Pharmacodynamics	
Onset	24-48 hr
Peak	48-72 hr
Duration	Unknown

Interactions
Individual drugs
Aspirin: decreased action of spironolactone
Cholestyramine: increased hyperchloremic acidosis in cirrhosis

Digoxin: increased digoxin action

Lithium: increased action, toxicity

Drug classifications

ACE inhibitors, diuretics (potassium-sparing), potassium products, salt substitute: increased hyperkalemia

Anticoagulants: decreased effects of anticoagulants

Antihypertensives: increased action

NSAIDs: decreased effect of spironolactone

Drug/herb

Arginine: fatal hypokalemia

Bearberry, gossypol: hypokalemia

Cucumber, dandelion, horsetail, licorice nettle, pumpkin, Queen Anne's lace: increased effect

Khella: increased hypotension

St. John's wort: severe photosensitivity

Drug/lab test

Interference: 17-OHCS, 17-KS, radioimmunoassay, digoxin assay

NURSING CONSIDERATIONS
Assessment

• Monitor for manifestations of hyperkalemia: *MS:* fatigue, muscle weakness; *CV:* arrhythmias, hypotension, *NEURO:* paresthesias, confusion, *RESP:* dyspnea

• Monitor for manifestations of hyponatremia: *CV:* increased B/P, cold, clammy skin, hypo- or hypervolemia; *GI:* anorexia, nausea, vomiting, diarrhea, abdominal cramps; *NEURO:* lethargy, increased ICP, confusion, headache, seizures, coma, fatigue, tremors, hyperreflexia

• Monitor for manifestations of hyperchloremia: *NEURO:* weakness, lethargy, coma; *RESP:* deep rapid breathing

• Assess fluid volume status: I&O ratios and record, count or weigh diapers as appropriate, weight, distended red veins, crackles in lung, color, quality, and specific gravity of urine, skin turgor, adequacy of pulses, moist mucous membranes, bilateral lung sounds, peripheral pitting edema; dehydration symptoms of decreasing output, thirst, hypotension, dry mouth and mucous membranes should be reported

• Monitor electrolytes: potassium, sodium, calcium, magnesium; also include BUN, ABGs, uric acid, CBC, blood glucose

Nursing diagnoses

• Fluid volume, deficient (adverse reactions)
• Fluid volume, excess (uses)
• Knowledge, deficient (teaching)
• Urinary elimination, impaired (adverse reactions)

Implementation

• Give in AM to avoid interference with sleep
• Give with food if nausea occurs; absorption may be increased; take at same time each day

Patient/family education

• Teach patient to take medication early in day to prevent nocturia

• Instruct patient to take with food or milk if GI symptoms of nausea and anorexia occur

• Teach patient to maintain a record of weight on a weekly basis and notify prescriber of weight loss of >5 lb

• Caution patient that this product causes an increase in potassium levels, that foods high in potassium should be avoided; refer to dietitian for assistance planning

• Teach patient not to use alcohol, or any OTC medications without prescriber's approval; serious product reactions may occur

• Emphasize the need to contact prescriber immediately if muscle cramps, weakness, nausea, dizziness, or numbness occur

• Teach patient to take own B/P and pulse and record

• Advise patient that dizziness and confusion may occur; avoid driving or other hazardous activities if alertness is decreased

• Teach patient to continue taking medication even if feeling better; this product controls symptoms but does not cure the condition

• Advise patient with hypertension to continue other treatment (exercise, weight loss, relaxation techniques, cessation of smoking)

Evaluation
Positive therapeutic outcome

• Prevention of hypokalemia (diuretic use)
• Decreased edema
• Decreased B/P
• Decreased aldosterone levels
• Increased diuresis

Treatment of overdose:

• Lavage if taken orally, monitor electrolytes
• Administer sodium bicarbonate
• Monitor hydration, CV, renal status

S

stavudine (Rx)
(sta'vu-deen)
d4T, Zerit
Func. class.: Antiretroviral
Chem. class.: Nucleoside reverse transcriptase inhibitor
Pregnancy category C

Action: Prevents replication of HIV-1 by the inhibition of the enzyme reverse transcriptase; causes DNA chain termination

Therapeutic outcome: Decreasing diarrhea, fatigue, night sweats; increased body weight

Uses: Treatment of HIV-1; used in combination with other antiretrovirals

Dosage and routes
Adult >60 kg: PO 40 mg q12hr
Adult <60 kg: PO 30 mg q12hr
Child <30 kg: PO 1 mg/kg q12hr
Child ≥30 kg ≤60 kg: PO 30 mg q12hr
Child >60 kg: PO 40 mg q12hr

Renal dose
Adult >60 kg: CCr 26-50 ml/min 20 mg q12hr; CCr 10-25 ml/min 20 mg q24hr
Adult <60 kg: CCr 26-50 ml/min 15 mg q12hr; CCr 10-25 ml/min 15 mg q24hr

Available forms: Caps 15, 20, 30, 40 mg; oral powder for sol 1 mg/ml

Adverse effects
CNS: Peripheral neuropathy, insomnia, anxiety, depression, dizziness, confusion, *headache,* chills/fever, malaise
CV: Chest pain, vasodilatation, hypertension
EENT: Conjunctivitis, abnormal vision
GI: **Hepatotoxicity,** *diarrhea, nausea, vomiting,* anorexia, dyspepsia, constipation, stomatitis, **pancreatitis**
HEMA: **Bone marrow suppression**
INTEG: Rash, sweating, pruritus, benign neoplasms
MISC: **Lactic acidosis,** asthenia, lipodystrophy
MS: Myalgia, arthralgia
RESP: Dyspnea, pneumonia, asthma

Contraindications: Hypersensitivity to this product or zidovudine, didanosine, zalcitabine; severe peripheral neuropathy

Black Box Warning: Lactic acidosis

Precautions: Breastfeeding, advanced HIV infections, bone marrow suppression, renal, peripheral neuropathy, osteoporosis, obesity

Black Box Warning: Pregnancy C, hepatic disease, pancreatitis

Pharmacokinetics
Absorption	Rapidly absorbed, 82% bioavailability
Distribution	Cerebrospinal fluid
Metabolism	Unknown
Excretion	Kidneys, breast milk
Half-life	Elimination: 1-1.6 hr, intracellular: 3-3.5 hr

Pharmacodynamics
Onset	Unknown
Peak	1 hr
Duration	Unknown

Interactions
Individual drugs
Chloramphenicol, cisplatin, dapsone, didanosine, ethambutol, hydrALAZINE, lithium, phenytoin, vinCRIStine, zalcitabine: increased peripheral neuropathy
Methadose: decreased stavudine effect
Probenecid: increased stavudine levels
Drug classifications
Myelosuppressants: increased myelosuppression

NURSING CONSIDERATIONS
Assessment
 Assess for lactic acidosis and severe hepatomegaly with steatosis; death may result
• Monitor viral load and CD4 counts, plasma HIV RNA baseline, throughout treatment
• Monitor for peripheral neuropathy: tingling, pain in extremities; if these occur, discontinue product
• Monitor for pancreatitis: severe upper abdominal pain, nausea, vomiting throughout treatment; if these occur, discontinue product
• Monitor blood tests: WBC, differential, RBC, Hct, Hgb, platelets, serum amylase, lipase
• Monitor renal function tests: urinalysis, protein, blood, serum creatinine
• Obtain C&S before product therapy; product may be taken as soon as culture is performed; repeat C&S after therapy
• Monitor bowel pattern before, during treatment
• Monitor fluid overload; product requires large volume to stay in sol
• Assess for weakness, tremors, confusion, dizziness, psychosis; if these occur, product may have to be decreased or discontinued

Nursing diagnoses
• Infection, risk for (uses)
• Knowledge, deficient (teaching)

 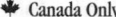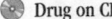

Implementation
- Give with or without meals; absorption does not appear to be lowered when taken with food
- Give product q4hr around the clock, even during night
- Shake susp well before using

Patient/family education
- Teach patient signs of peripheral neuropathy: burning, weakness, pain, pricking feeling in the extremities
- Caution patient that this product should not be given with antineoplastics
- Inform patient that GI complaints and insomnia resolve after 3-4 wk of treatment
- Inform patient that product is not a cure for AIDS, but will control symptoms
- Advise patient to call prescriber if sore throat, swollen lymph nodes, malaise, fever occur; may indicate presence of other infections
- Caution patient that even with product administration, virus is still infective and may be passed on to others
- Caution patient that follow-up visits must be continued because serious toxicity may occur; blood counts must be done q2wk
- Teach patient that product must be taken q4hr around the clock even during night
- Caution patient that serious product interactions with other medications may occur, check with prescriber first if taking chloramphenicol, dapsone, cisplatin, didanosine, ethambutol, lithium, antifungals
- Inform patient that other products may be necessary to prevent other infections
- Inform patient that product may cause fainting or dizziness

Evaluation
Positive therapeutic outcome
- Decreased symptoms of HIV infection

❗ HIGH ALERT

streptokinase 😊 (Rx)
(strep-toe-kye′nase)
Streptase
Func. class.: Thrombolytic enzyme
Chem. class.: β-Hemolytic *Streptococcus* filtrate (purified)

Pregnancy category C

Action: Activates conversion of plasminogen to plasmin (fibrinolysin): plasmin breaks down clots (fibrin), fibrinogen, factors V, VII; occlusion of venous access lines

Therapeutic outcome: Lysis of emboli, or thrombosis in various parts of the body

Uses: Deep vein thrombosis (DVT), pulmonary embolism, arterial thrombosis, arterial embolism, lysis of coronary artery thrombi after MI, acute evolving transmural MI

Unlabeled uses: Arteriovenous cannula occlusion

Dosage and routes
Lysis of coronary artery thrombi
Adult: IC 20,000 international units, then 2000 international units/min over 1 hr as **IV** INF

Thrombosis/embolism/DVT/ pulmonary embolism
Adult: **IV** INF 250,000 international units over ½ hr, then 100,000 international units/hr for 72 hr for DVT; 100,000 international units/hr over 24-72 hr for pulmonary embolism; 100,000 international units/hr × 24-72 hr for arterial thrombosis or embolism

Acute evolving transmural MI
Adult: **IV** INF 1,500,000 international units diluted to a volume of 45 ml; give within 1 hr via INF pump; intracoronary INF 20,000 international units by bol, then 2000 international units/min × 1 hr, total dose 140,000 international units

Arteriovenous cannula occlusion (unlabeled)
Adult: **IV** INF 10,000 international units/3 ml SOL into occluded limb of cannula; clamp for 1 hr distally; aspirate contents; flush with NaCl SOL and reconnect (serious reactions have been reported)

Available forms: Powder for inj, lyophilized 250,000, 750,000, 1,500,000 international units/vial

Adverse effects
CNS: Headache, fever, Guillain-Barré syndrome
CV: **Dysrhythmias,** hypotension, noncardiogenic pulmonary edema, **pulmonary embolism**
EENT: Periorbital edema
GI: Nausea
HEMA: Decreased Hct, **bleeding,** anemia
INTEG: Rash, urticaria, phlebitis at infusion site, itching, flushing
MS: Low back pain, arthralgia, myalgia
RESP: Altered respirations, shortness of breath, **bronchospasm,** pulmonary bleeding
SYST: GI, GU, **intracranial retroperitoneal bleeding, surface bleeding, anaphylaxis**

S

Adverse effects: *italic* = common, **bold** = life-threatening

Contraindications: Breastfeeding, children, hypersensitivity, active internal bleeding, intraspinal surgery, CNS neoplasms, uncontrolled severe hypertension, recent CVA, intracranial, intrapleural surgery

Precautions: Pregnancy **C**, arterial emboli from left side of heart, ulcerative colitis, enteritis, severe renal disease, hepatic disease, hypocoagulation, COPD, subacute bacterial endocarditis, rheumatic valvular disease, cerebral embolism/thrombosis/hemorrhage, intraarterial diagnostic procedure or surgery (10 days), recent major surgery

Pharmacokinetics

Absorption	Completely absorbed
Distribution	Unknown
Metabolism	>80%—liver, rapidly cleared by reticuloendothelial system
Excretion	Kidneys
Half-life	35 min

Pharmacodynamics

Onset	Immediate
Peak	Rapid
Duration	<12 hr

Interactions
Individual drugs
Abciximab, aspirin, clopidogrel, dipyridamole, eptifibatide, indomethacin, phenylbutazone, plicamycin, ticlopidine, tirofiban, valproic acid: increased bleeding risk
Drug classifications
Anticoagulants (oral), cephalosporins (some), glycoprotein IIb/IIIa inhibitors, NSAIDs: increased bleeding risk
Drug/lab test
Increased: pro-time, APTT, TT
Decreased: plasminogen, fibrinogen

NURSING CONSIDERATIONS
Assessment
• Monitor VS, B/P, pulse, respirations (including peripheral), neurologic signs, temp at least q4hr; temp >104° F (40° C) indicates internal bleeding; monitor rhythm closely; ventricular dysrhythmias may occur with hyperfusion; monitor heart, breath sounds, neurologic status, peripheral pulses

◆ Assess for bleeding during first hr of treatment: hematuria, hematemesis, bleeding from mucous membranes, epistaxis, ecchymosis; guaiac, all body fluids, stools; may require transfusion (rare); blood studies (Hct, platelets, PTT, pro-time, TT, APTT) before

starting therapy; pro-time or APTT must be less than 2 × control before starting therapy; TT or protime q3-4hr during treatment
• Assess allergy: fever, rash, itching, chills; mild reaction may be treated with antihistamines; report to prescriber
• Monitor ECG on monitor, watch for segment changes, changes in rhythm; sinus bradycardia, ventricular tachycardia, accelerated idioventricular rhythm may occur as a result of reperfusion (coronary thrombosis); cardiac enzymes, radionuclide myocardial scanning/coronary angiography
• Monitor ABGs, respiratory rate (depth, characteristics), pulse, B/P, hemodynamics (pulmonary embolism)
• Monitor peripheral pulses, assess Homans' sign, check for redness, swelling qhr; notify prescriber of changes; B/P should not be taken in extremities (deep vein thrombosis)
• Check catheter for ability to aspirate blood from port; patient must exhale and hold breath when inserting and removing syringe to prevent air embolism (catheter/cannula occlusion)
• Assess for Guillain-Barré syndrome that may occur after treatment with this product
• Assess for respiratory depression

Nursing diagnoses
• Gas exchange, impaired (uses)
• Injury, risk for (adverse reactions)
• Knowledge, deficient (teaching)
• Tissue perfusion, ineffective (uses)

Implementation
• Give after reconstituting with provided diluent; add appropriate amount of sterile water for inj (no preservatives) 20-mg vial/20 ml or 50-mg vial/50 ml to make 1 mg/ml, mix by slow inversion or dilute with NaCl, D₅W to a concentration of 0.5 mg/ml; use 18-G needle; flush line with NaCl after administration; reconstituted **IV** sol within 8 hr; within 6 hr of coronary occlusion for best results
• Give **IV** loading dose over 30 min to avoid hypotension
• Give **IV** over 1 hr after dilution with 4-5 g/250 ml of 0.9% NaCl, D₅W, LR; may give by cont inf after loading dose(s) of 1 g/hr diluted in 50-100 ml of compatible sol; use inf pump; do not give by direct **IV**
• Give heparin therapy after thrombolytic therapy is discontinued, TT, ACT, or APTT less than 2 × control (about 3-4 hr); **IV** heparin with loading dose is recommended after discontinuing streptokinase to prevent redevelopment of thrombi

---

- Avoid invasive procedures, injection, taking temp via rectal route
- Apply pressure for 30 sec to minor bleeding sites; 30 min to sites of atrial puncture, followed by pressure dressing; inform prescriber if this does not attain hemostasis; apply pressure dressing
- Store powder at room temperature or refrigerate; protect from excessive light

Y-site compatibilities: Dobutamine, DOPamine, heparin, lidocaine, nitroglycerin

Additive incompatibilities: Do not mix with other medications

Patient/family education

- Teach patient reason for medication, signs and symptoms of bleeding, allergic reactions, when to notify prescriber
- Explain that patient is to continue bed rest to avoid injury

Evaluation

Positive therapeutic outcome

- Lysis of thrombi or emboli

---

streptomycin (Rx)

(strep-toe-mye′sin)
Func. class.: Antiinfective, antituberculosis
Chem. class.: Aminoglycoside

Pregnancy category D

Action: Interferes with protein synthesis in bacterial cell by binding to ribosomal subunit, causing inaccurate peptide sequence to form in protein chain, resulting in bacterial death

Therapeutic outcome: Bactericidal effects for the following organisms: sensitive strains of *Mycobacterium tuberculosis,* nontuberculous infections caused by sensitive strains of *Yersinia pestis, Brucella, Haemophilus influenzae, Klebsiella pneumoniae, Escherichia coli, Enterobacter aerogenes, Streptococcus viridans, Francisella tularensis, Proteus*

Uses: Active TB; used in combination for streptococcal and enterococcal infections; endocarditis, tularemia, plague

Dosage and routes

Tuberculosis (HIV negative)
Adult: IM 15 mg/kg (max 1 g) daily × 2-3 mo, then 1 g 2-3 ×/wk given with other antitubercular products for up to 1 yr
Child: IM 20-40 mg/kg/day; max 1 g/day

Streptococcal endocarditis
Adult: IM 15 mg/kg/day divided q12h

Enterococcal endocarditis
Adult: IM 1 g q12hr × 2 wk, then 500 mg q12hr × 4 wk with penicillin, max 15 mg/kg/day

Available forms: Inj 500 mg ✿, 1 g/ml

Adverse effects

CNS: Confusion, dizziness, depression, numbness, tremors, **seizures,** muscle twitching, **neurotoxicity,** dizziness, headache
CV: Hypotension, myocarditis, palpitations
EENT: Ototoxicity, tinnitus, deafness, visual disturbances
GI: Nausea, vomiting, anorexia, increased ALT, AST, bilirubin, hepatomegaly, **hepatic necrosis,** splenomegaly
GU: **Oliguria, hematuria, renal damage, azotemia, renal failure, nephrotoxicity**
HEMA: **Agranulocytosis, thrombocytopenia, leukopenia,** eosinophilia, anemia
INTEG: Rash, burning, urticaria, dermatitis, alopecia
MS: Arthralgia, weakness

Contraindications: Hypersensitivity

Black Box Warning: Pregnancy **D,** severe renal disease

Precautions: Breastfeeding, geriatric, neonates, mild renal disease, myasthenia gravis, Parkinson's disease, hepatic disease

Black Box Warning: Hearing deficits, neuromuscular disease

Pharmacokinetics

Absorption	Well absorbed
Distribution	Widely distributed in extracellular fluids, poorly distributed in CSF; crosses placenta
Metabolism	Minimal—liver
Excretion	Mostly unchanged (>90%) kidneys
Half-life	2-2½ hr, increase in renal disease

Pharmacodynamics

Onset	Rapid
Peak	1-2 hr
Duration	Unknown

Interactions

Individual drugs
Amphotericin B, cidofovir, cisplatin, ethacrynic acid, furosemide, mannitol, methoxyflurane, polymyxin, vancomycin: increased ototoxicity, neurotoxicity, nephrotoxicity

S

Adverse effects: *italic* = common, **bold** = life-threatening

Succinylcholine, warfarin: increased effects of streptomycin

Drug classifications

Aminoglycosides, cephalosporins: increased ototoxicity, neurotoxicity, nephrotoxicity
Nondepolarizing neuromuscular blockers, NSAIDs: increased effects of streptomycin

Drug/herb

Acidophilus: do not use with antiinfectives; separate by several hours
Lysine (large amounts): increased toxicity

NURSING CONSIDERATIONS
Assessment
- Assess patient for previous sensitivity reaction
- Assess patient for signs and symptoms of infection including characteristics of sputum, urine, stool WBC >10,000/mm^3, temp
- Obtain baseline information before, during treatment
- Complete C&S testing before, after product therapy to identify if correct treatment has been initiated
- Assess for allergic reactions: rash, urticaria, pruritus, chills, fever, joint pain; angioedema may occur a few days after therapy begins; epinephrine, resuscitation equipment should be available for anaphylactic reaction
- Identify urine output; if decreasing, notify prescriber (may indicate nephrotoxicity); also increased BUN, creatinine, urine CCr <80 ml/min
- Monitor blood tests: AST, ALT, CBC, Hct, bilirubin, LDH, alkaline phosphatase, Coombs' test monthly if patient is on long-term therapy
- Monitor electrolytes: potassium, sodium, chloride, magnesium monthly if patient is on long-term therapy
- Monitor for bleeding: ecchymosis, bleeding gums, hematuria, stool guaiac daily if on long-term therapy
- Assess for overgrowth of infection: perineal itching, fever, malaise, redness, pain, swelling, drainage, rash, diarrhea, change in cough, sputum
- Obtain weight before treatment; calculation of dosage is usually based on ideal body weight, but may be calculated on actual body weight
- Monitor I&O ratio; urinalysis daily for proteinuria, cells, casts; report sudden change in urine output
- Obtain serum peak 60 min after IM inj; trough level obtained just before next dose; blood level should be 2-4 × bacteriostatic level
- Monitor for deafness by audiometric testing, ringing, roaring in ears, vertigo; assess hearing before, during, after treatment

- Monitor for dehydration: high specific gravity, decrease in skin turgor, dry mucous membranes, dark urine

Nursing diagnoses
- Diarrhea (adverse reactions)
- Infection, risk for (uses)
- Injury, risk for (adverse reactions)
- Knowledge, deficient (teaching)
- Noncompliance (teaching)

Implementation
- Give deeply in large muscle mass
- Reconstitute with 4.2-4.5 ml of sterile water for inj or 0.9% NaCl/1 g (200 mg/ml), 3.2-3.5 ml/1 g (250 mg/ml), 17 ml/5 g (250 mg/ml); give at 500 mg/ml or less

Syringe compatibilities: Penicillin G sodium
Syringe incompatibilities: Heparin
Y-site compatibilities: Esmolol
Additive compatibilities: Bleomycin

Patient/family education
- Teach patient to report sore throat, bruising, bleeding, joint pain, may indicate blood dyscrasias (rare); ringing, roaring in the ears
- Advise patient to contact prescriber if vaginal itching, loose foul-smelling stools, furry tongue occur; may indicate superinfection

Evaluation
Positive therapeutic outcome
- Absence of signs/symptoms of infection
- Reported improvement in symptoms of infection

Treatment of overdose: Withdraw product, hemodialysis, monitor serum levels of product, may give ticarcillin or carbenicillin

---

succimer (Rx)
(sux′i-mer)
Chemet
Func. class.: Heavy metal antagonist
Chem. class.: Chelating agent

Pregnancy category C

Action: Binds with ions of lead to form a water-soluble complex that is excreted by kidneys

Therapeutic outcome: Removal of lead from the body

Uses: Lead poisoning in children with lead levels above 45 mcg/dl; may be beneficial in mercury, arsenic poisoning

Dosage and routes
Adult: PO 10-30 mg/kg/day × 5 days
Child with lead level >45 mcg/dl:
PO 10 mg/kg or 350 mg/m^2 q8hr × 5 days,
then 10 mg/kg or 350 mg/m^2 q12hr × 2 wk;
another course may be required depending on
lead levels; allow 2 wk between courses

Available forms: Caps 100 mg

Adverse effects
CNS: Drowsiness, dizziness, paresthesia,
sensorimotor neuropathy
EENT: Otitis media, watery eyes, film in eyes,
plugged ears
*GI: Nausea, vomiting, diarrhea, metallic
taste, anorexia*
GU: **Proteinuria,** decreased urination,
voiding difficulties
HEMA: **Increased platelets, intermittent
eosinophilia**
INTEG: Rash, urticaria, pruritus
META: Increased AST, ALT, alkaline phosphatase, cholesterol
RESP: Sore throat, rhinorrhea, nasal congestion, cough
SYST: Back, stomach, head, rib, flank pain;
abdominal cramps; chills; fever; flulike symptoms, head cold; headache

Contraindications: Hypersensitivity

Precautions: Pregnancy C, breastfeeding,
children <1 yr, renal/hepatic disease

Pharmacokinetics	
Absorption	Rapidly absorbed
Distribution	Unknown
Metabolism	Liver—extensively
Excretion	Kidneys—unchanged
Half-life	2 days

Pharmacodynamics	
Onset	Up to 2 hr
Peak	2-4 hr
Duration	8-12 hr

Interactions
Drug classifications
Heavy metal antagonist, others: do not use
together

NURSING CONSIDERATIONS
Assessment
• Assess VS, B/P, pulse, respirations, weigh
daily
• Monitor I&O ratio, renal function tests,
BUN, creatinine, CCr; watch for decreasing
urine output
• Assess neurologic status: watch for pares-
thesias, beginning of seizures
• Monitor urine: pH, albumin, casts, blood,
coproporphyrins, calcium
• Assess for febrile reactions that may occur
4-8 hr after product therapy
• Monitor for cardiac abnormalities: dysrhyth-
mias, hypotension, tachycardia
• Assess for allergic reactions (rash, urticaria);
if these occur, product should be discontinued

Nursing diagnoses
• Injury, risk for (uses, adverse reactions)
• Knowledge, deficient (teaching)
• Poisoning, risk for (uses)

Implementation
• Give whole or cap contents mixed with food
or fluid

Patient/family education
• Explain reason for medication and expected
results
• Provide a referral to health department to
assess lead levels in home or workplace
• Teach patient to increase fluid intake

Evaluation
Positive therapeutic outcome
• Decreased symptoms of lead intoxication
• Decreased lead level <50 mcg/dl

⚠ HIGH ALERT

succinylcholine (Rx)
(suk-sin-ill-koe'leen)
Anectine, Anectine Flo-Pack, Quelicin,
succinylcholine chloride, Sucostrin,
Suxamethonium
Func. class.: Neuromuscular blocker
(depolarizing—ultra short)
Pregnancy category C

Action: Inhibits transmission of nerve
impulses by binding with cholinergic receptor
sites, antagonizing action of acetylcholine;
causes release of histamine

Therapeutic outcome: Paralysis of
skeletal muscles

Uses: Facilitation of endotracheal intubation,
skeletal muscle relaxation during orthopedic
manipulations

Dosage and routes
Adult: **IV** 0.3-1.1 mg/kg, max 150 mg,
maintenance 0.04-0.07 mg/kg q5-10min as
needed; CONT **IV** INF dilute to concentration
of 1-2 mg/ml in D$_5$W or NS 10-100 mcg/kg/
min

S

Adverse effects: *italic* = common, **bold** = life-threatening

Child: **IV** initially 1-2 mg/kg; CONT **IV** INF not recommended

Available forms: Inj 20, 50, 100 mg/ml; powder for inj 100, 500 mg/vial, 1 g/vial

Adverse effects
CV: Bradycardia, tachycardia; increased, decreased B/P, **sinus arrest, dysrhythmias,** edema
EENT: Increased secretions, increased intraocular pressure
HEMA: **Myoglobulinemia**
INTEG: Rash, flushing, pruritus, urticaria
MS: Weakness, muscle pain, fasciculation, prolonged relaxation, myalgia, **rhabdomyolysis**
RESP: **Prolonged apnea, bronchospasm, cyanosis, respiratory depression,** wheezing, dyspnea
SYST: **Anaphylaxis, angioedema**

Contraindications: Hypersensitivity, malignant hyperthermia, trauma

Precautions: Pregnancy **C,** breastfeeding, children <2 yr, geriatric or debilitated patients, severe burns, fractures (fasciculation may increase damage), electrolyte imbalances, dehydration, neuromuscular disease, respiratory disease, collagen diseases, glaucoma, eye surgery, renal/hepatic/cardiac disease

Black Box Warning: Hyperkalemia, myopathy, rhabdomyolysis

Pharmacokinetics

Absorption	Well absorbed (IM)
Distribution	Widely distributed, crosses placenta
Metabolism	Plasma (90%)
Excretion	Hydrolyzed in blood, excreted in urine (active/inactive metabolites)
Half-life	Unknown

Pharmacodynamics

	IM	IV
Onset	2-3 min	1 min
Peak	Unknown	2-3 min
Duration	10-30 min	6-10 min

Interactions
Individual products
Clindamycin, enflurane, isoflurane, lincomycin, lithium, oxytocin, procainamide, quinidine: increased neuromuscular blockade
Theophylline: dysrhythmias
Drug classifications
Aminoglycosides, anesthetics (local), antibiotics (polymyxin), β-adrenergic blockers, cardiac glycosides, magnesium salts, opi-

oids, thiazides: increased neuromuscular blockade
Drug/herb
Melatonin: blocks succinylcholine

NURSING CONSIDERATIONS
Assessment
• Assess for electrolyte imbalances (potassium, magnesium); may lead to increased action of this product
• Monitor VS (B/P, pulse, respirations, airway) until fully recovered; rate, depth, pattern of respirations, strength of hand grip
• Monitor I&O ratio; check for urinary retention, frequency, hesitancy
• Assess for recovery: decreased paralysis of face, diaphragm, leg, arm, rest of body
• Assess for allergic reactions: rash, fever, respiratory distress, pruritus; product should be discontinued if these occur

Nursing diagnoses
• Breathing pattern, ineffective (uses)
• Communication, impaired verbal (adverse reactions)

Implementation
IM route
• Give inj deep IM, preferably high in deltoid muscle
• Store in refrigerator; store powder at room temperature; close container tightly
IV route
• Use nerve stimulator by anesthesiologist to determine neuromuscular blockade
• Give anticholinesterase to reverse neuromuscular blockade
• Give by **IV** inf; dilute 1-2 mg/ml in D$_5$, isotonic saline sol, give 0.5-10 mg/min, titrate to patient response; may be given directly over 1 min
Syringe compatibilities: Heparin
Y-site compatibilities: Etomidate, heparin, potassium chloride, propofol, vit B/C
Additive compatibilities: Amikacin, cephapirin, isoproterenol, meperidine, methyldopate, morphine, norepinephrine, scopolamine
Additive incompatibilities: Barbiturates, nafcillin, sodium bicarbonate

Patient/family education
• Explain reason for medication and expected results
• Provide reassurance if communication is difficult during recovery from neuromuscular blockade; postoperative stiffness is normal, soon subsides

 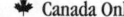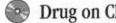

Evaluation
Positive therapeutic outcome
- Paralysis of jaw, eyelid, head, neck, rest of body

Treatment of overdose: Edrophonium or neostigmine, atropine, monitor VS; may require mechanical ventilation

---

sucralfate (Rx)
(soo-kral'fate)
Carafate, Sulcrate ✤
Func. class.: Protectant; antiulcer
Chem. class.: Aluminum hydroxide/sulfated sucrose

Pregnancy category B

Do not confuse:
Carafate/Cafergot

Action: Forms a complex that adheres to ulcer site, adsorbs pepsin

Therapeutic outcome: Healing of ulcers

Uses: Duodenal ulcer, oral mucositis, stomatitis after radiation of head and neck

Unlabeled uses: Gastric ulcers, gastroesophageal reflux

Dosage and routes
Duodenal ulcers
Adult: PO 1 g qid 1 hr before meals and at bedtime
Child: PO 40-80 mg/kg/day divided

Available forms: Tabs 1 g; oral susp 1 g/10 ml

Adverse effects
CNS: Drowsiness, dizziness
GI: *Dry mouth, constipation,* nausea, gastric pain, vomiting
INTEG: Urticaria, rash, pruritus

Contraindications: Hypersensitivity

Precautions: Pregnancy **B**, breastfeeding, children, renal failure

Pharmacokinetics
Absorption	Minimally absorbed
Distribution	Unknown
Metabolism	Not metabolized
Excretion	Feces (90%)
Half-life	6-20 hr

Pharmacodynamics
Onset	½ hr
Peak	Unknown
Duration	6 hr

Interactions
Individual drugs
Cimetidine, digoxin, ketoconazole, phenytoin, ranitidine, tetracycline, theophylline: decreased action of each specific product
Drug classifications
Antacids: decreased absorption of sucralfate
Fat-soluble vitamins: decreased action of fat-soluble vitamins
Fluoroquinolones: decreased absorption

NURSING CONSIDERATIONS
Assessment
- Monitor gastric pH (>5 should be maintained); blood in stools

Nursing diagnoses
- Constipation (adverse reactions)
- Knowledge, deficient (teaching)
- Pain, acute (uses)
- Pain, chronic (uses)

Implementation
- Do not break, crush, or chew tabs
- Give on empty stomach 1 hr before meals and at bedtime
- Avoid antacids ½ hr before or 1 hr after taking this product
- Store at room temperature

Patient/family education
- Instruct patient to take medication on empty stomach
- Caution patient to take full course of therapy, not to use >8 wk, to avoid smoking
- Caution patient to avoid antacids within ½ hr of product or 1 hr after this product

Evaluation
Positive therapeutic outcome
- Absence of pain or GI complaints

---

sulfamethoxazole (Rx)
(sul-fa-meth-ox'a-zole)
Apo-Sulfamethoxazole ✤, Gantanol, Urobak
Func. class.: Antiinfective
Chem. class.: Sulfonamide, intermediate-acting

Pregnancy category C

S

Action: Inhibits folic acid synthesis

Therapeutic outcome: Bactericidal action against susceptible organisms: streptococci and staphylococci, *Clostridium perfringens, Clostridium tetani, Nocardia asteroides;* gram-negative pathogens, including *Enterobacter, Escherichia coli, Klebsiella,*

Adverse effects: *italic* = common, **bold** = life-threatening

Proteus mirabilis, Proteus vulgaris, Salmonella, Shigella

Uses: UTIs, chancroid, inclusion conjunctivitis, malaria, meningococcal meningitis, nocardiosis, acute otitis media, toxoplasmosis, trachoma

Dosage and routes
Adult: PO 2 g, then 1 g bid or tid for 7-10 days
Child >2 mo: PO 50-60 mg/kg × 1 dose, then 25-30 mg/kg bid, max 75 mg/kg/day

Renal dose
Adult: PO CCr <10-30 ml/min 50% of dose; CCr <10 ml/min give 25% of dose or extend interval

Available forms: Tabs 500 mg; oral susp 500 mg/5 ml

Adverse effects
CNS: Headache, insomnia, hallucinations, depression, vertigo, fatigue, anxiety, seizures, product fever, chills, drowsiness
CV: **Allergic myocarditis**
EENT: Tinnitus
GI: *Nausea, vomiting, abdominal pain,* stomatitis, **hepatitis**, glossitis, **pancreatitis**, diarrhea, **enterocolitis**, anorexia
GU: **Renal failure, toxic nephrosis,** increased BUN, creatinine, crystalluria, hematuria, proteinuria
HEMA: **Leukopenia, thrombocytopenia, agranulocytosis, hemolytic anemia, aplastic anemia**
INTEG: Rash, dermatitis, urticaria, erythema, photosensitivity, alopecia
SYST: **Anaphylaxis**

Contraindications: Pregnancy at term, breastfeeding, infants <2 mo (except congenital toxoplasmosis), hypersensitivity to sulfonamides, sulfonylureas, thiazide and loop diuretics, salicylates, sunscreen with PABA, porphyria, G6PD deficiency

Precautions: Pregnancy **C**, geriatric, impaired renal/hepatic function, severe allergy, bronchial asthma, UV exposure

Pharmacokinetics
Absorption	Well absorbed
Distribution	Widely distributed, crosses placenta
Metabolism	Liver, large amounts
Excretion	Unchanged kidneys (20%), enters breast milk
Half-life	7-12 hr

Pharmacodynamics
Onset	1 hr
Peak	3-4 hr
Duration	Unknown

Interactions
Individual drugs
Bosentan, ramelteon, voriconazole: increased effects of each specific product
CycloSPORINE: increased nephrotoxicity
Indomethacin, probenecid: increased product-free concentrations
Methenamine: increased crystalluria
Methotrexate: decreased renal excretion of methotrexate
Phenytoin: decreased hepatic clearance of phenytoin
Warfarin: increased anticoagulant effect
Drug classifications
Barbiturates, uricosuric agents: increased effects
Diuretics (thiazide): increased thrombocytopenia
Salicylates: increased product-free concentrations
Sulfonylurea agents: increased hypoglycemic response
Drug/herb
Acidophilus: do not use with antiinfectives; separate by several hours
Drug/lab test
False positive: urinary glucose test (Benedict's method)

NURSING CONSIDERATIONS
Assessment
• Assess patient for previous sensitivity reaction
• Assess patient for signs and symptoms of infection including characteristics of wounds, sputum, urine, stool, WBC >10,000/mm³, elevated temp; obtain baseline information before, during treatment
• Complete C&S studies before beginning product therapy to identify if correct treatment has been initiated
• Assess for allergic reactions: rash, urticaria, pruritus, chills, fever, joint pain; angioedema may occur a few days after therapy begins; epinephrine, resuscitation equipment should be on unit for anaphylactic reaction; AIDS patients are more susceptible
• Monitor blood studies: CBC, Hct, bilirubin, alkaline phosphatase monthly if patient is on long-term therapy
• Monitor for bleeding: ecchymosis, bleeding gums, hematuria, stool guaiac daily if patient is on long-term therapy

- Assess for overgrowth of infection: perineal itching, fever, malaise, redness, pain, swelling, drainage, rash, diarrhea, change in cough, sputum

Nursing diagnoses
- Diarrhea (adverse reactions)
- Infection, risk for (uses)
- Injury, risk for (adverse reactions)
- Knowledge, deficient (teaching)
- Noncompliance (teaching)

Implementation
- Give around the clock to maintain proper blood levels; give on empty stomach to increase absorption of product; do not give within 3 hr of other agents, product actions may occur

Patient/family education
- Teach patient to report sore throat, bruising, bleeding, joint pain; may indicate blood dyscrasias (rare)
- Instruct patient to take with 8 oz of water to prevent crystalluria
- Advise patient to contact prescriber if vaginal itching, loose foul-smelling stools, furry tongue occur; may indicate superinfection; report itching, rash, pruritus, urticaria
- Instruct patient to take all medication prescribed for the length of time ordered; product must be taken around the clock to maintain blood levels; do not give medication to others

Evaluation
Positive therapeutic outcome
- Absence of signs/symptoms of infection (WBC <10,000/mm³, temp WNL, absence of urinary pain, hematuria)
- Reported improvement in symptoms of infection
- Negative C&S

---

sulfasalazine (Rx)
(sul-fa-sal'a-zeen)
Azulfidine, Azulfidine EN-tabs, PMS-Sulfasalazine ✦, S.A.S. ✦, Salazopyrin ✦, sulfasalazine
Func. class.: GI Antiinflammatory, antirheumatic (DMARD)
Chem. class.: GI Sulfonamide
Pregnancy category B

Do not confuse:
sulfasalazine/sulfiSOXAZOLE

Action: Proproduct to deliver sulfapyridine and 5-aminosalicylic acid to colon; antinflammatory in connective tissue

Therapeutic outcome: Treatment of ulcerative colitis, rheumatoid arthritis

Uses: Ulcerative colitis, rheumatoid arthritis (del rel tab) in patients who inadequately respond to or are intolerant of analgesics/NSAIDs, juvenile rheumatoid arthritis (Azulfidine EN-tabs)

Unlabeled uses: Crohn's disease

Dosage and routes
Bowel disease
Adult: PO 3-4 g/day in divided doses; maintenance 2 g/day in divided doses q6hr
Child ≥6 yr: PO 40-60 mg/kg/day in 4-6 divided doses, then 30 mg/kg/day in 4 doses, max 2 g/day

Rheumatoid arthritis
Adult: PO 0.5-1 g/day, then increase daily dose by 500 mg qwk to 2 g/day in 2-3 divided doses

Juvenile rheumatoid arthritis
Child ≥6 yr: PO 30-50 mg/kg/24 hr, divided into 2 doses

Renal dose
Adult: PO CCr 10-30 ml/min bid; CCr <10 ml/min daily

Available forms: Tabs 500 mg; oral susp 250 mg/5 ml; del rel tabs 500 mg

Adverse effects
CNS: Headache, confusion, insomnia, hallucinations, depression, vertigo, fatigue, anxiety, **seizures**, product fever, chills
CV: **Allergic myocarditis**
GI: Nausea, vomiting, abdominal pain, stomatitis, **hepatitis**, glossitis, **pancreatitis**, diarrhea
GU: **Renal failure, toxic nephrosis,** increased BUN, creatinine, crystalluria
HEMA: **Leukopenia, neutropenia, thrombocytopenia, agranulocytosis, hemolytic anemia**
INTEG: Rash, dermatitis, urticaria, **Stevens-Johnson syndrome,** erythema, photosensitivity
SYST: **Anaphylaxis**

Contraindications: Pregnancy at term, children <2 yr, hypersensitivity to sulfonamides or salicylates, intestinal, urinary obstruction, porphyria

Precautions: Pregnancy **B**, breastfeeding, impaired renal/hepatic function, severe allergy, bronchial asthma, megaloblastic anemia

S

Adverse effects: *italic* = common, **bold** = life-threatening

Pharmacokinetics	
Absorption	Partially absorbed
Distribution	Crosses placenta
Metabolism	Liver
Excretion	Kidneys, breast milk
Half-life	6 hr

Pharmacodynamics	
Onset	1 hr
Peak	1½-6 hr
Duration	6-12 hr

Interactions
Individual drugs
Azathioprine, mercaptopurine: increased leucopenia risk
CycloSPORINE: decreased effect of cyclo-SPORINE
Digoxin: decreased digoxin effect
Folic acid: decreased folic acid effect
Methotrexate: decreased renal excretion
Drug classifications
Anticoagulants (oral): increased anticoagulant effect
Hypoglycemics (oral): increased hypoglycemic response
Drug/food
Iron, folic acid will be poorly absorbed
Drug/lab test
False positive: urinary glucose test

NURSING CONSIDERATIONS
Assessment
• Monitor I&O ratio; note color, amount, character, pH of urine if product administered for UTIs; output should be 800 ml less than intake; if urine is highly acidic, alkalization may be needed
• Monitor kidney function tests: BUN, creatinine, urinalysis if on long-term therapy
• Monitor blood dyscrasias: skin rash, fever, sore throat, bruising, bleeding, fatigue, joint pain; monitor CBC before, during therapy (q3mo)
• Assess for allergic reaction: rash, dermatitis, urticaria, pruritus, dyspnea, bronchospasm
Nursing diagnoses
• Injury, risk for (uses)
• Knowledge, deficient (teaching)
Implementation
• Give with full glass of water to maintain adequate hydration; increase fluids to 2 L/day to decrease crystallization in kidneys; contact lenses, urine, skin may be yellow-orange
• Give total daily dose in evenly spaced doses and after meals to help minimize GI intolerance

• Give at bedtime
• Store in airtight, light-resistant container at room temperature
Patient/family education
• Advise patient to take each oral dose with full glass of water to prevent crystalluria
• Teach patient to avoid sunlight or to use sunscreen to prevent burns
• Teach patient to avoid OTC medication (aspirin, vit C) unless directed by prescriber
• Advise patient to notify prescriber if skin rash, sore throat, fever, mouth sores, unusual bruising, bleeding occur
• Advise patient to use rectal susp at bedtime and retain all night
Evaluation
Positive therapeutic outcome
• Absence of fever, mucus in stools or pain in joints

sulfinpyrazone (Rx)
(sul-fin-peer'a-zone)
Anturan ♣, Anturane, sulfinpyrazone
Func. class.: Uricosuric
Chem. class.: Pyrazolone
Pregnancy category C

Action: Inhibits tubular reabsorption of urates, with increased excretion of uric acid; inhibits prostaglandin synthesis, which decreases platelet aggregation

Therapeutic outcome: Decreased uric acid levels, absence of platelet aggregation

Uses: Gout, gouty arthritis

Dosage and routes
Gout/gouty arthritis
Adult: PO 100-200 mg bid × 1 wk, then 200-400 mg bid, max 800 mg/day
Child: PO 10 mg/kg/day in 3-4 divided doses

Renal dose
CCr <50 ml/min, avoid use

Available forms: Tabs 100 mg; caps 200 mg

Adverse effects
CNS: Dizziness, **seizures, coma**
EENT: Tinnitus
GI: Gastric irritation, nausea, vomiting, anorexia, **hepatic necrosis, GI bleeding**
GU: Renal calculi, hypoglycemia
HEMA: **Agranulocytosis** (rare)
INTEG: Rash, dermatitis, pruritus, fever, photosensitivity
RESP: **Apnea,** irregular respirations

Contraindications: Hypersensitivity to pyrazolone derivatives, salicylates, blood dyscrasias, CCr <50 ml/min, active peptic ulcer, GI inflammation, nephrolithiasis

Precautions: Pregnancy **C**, renal disease, NSAIDs hypersensitivity

Pharmacokinetics

Absorption	Well absorbed
Distribution	Unknown
Metabolism	Liver
Excretion	Feces (metabolites/active products)
Half-life	4 hr

Pharmacodynamics

Onset	Unknown
Peak	1-2 hr
Duration	4-6 hr

Interactions
Individual drugs
Acetaminophen: increased toxicity
Niacin: decreased effects of sulfinpyrazone
Theophylline, verapamil: decreased effect of each specific product
TOLBUTamide, warfarin: increased effect of each specific product
Drug classifications
NSAIDs: increased bleeding risk
Salicylates: decreased effect of sulfinpyrazone
Drug/lab test
Increased: PSP, aminohippuric acid
False positive: Clinitest

NURSING CONSIDERATIONS
Assessment
• Monitor I&O ratio; observe for decrease in urinary output; increase fluids to 2-3 L/day
• Monitor CBC, platelets, reticulocytes before, during therapy (q3mo)
• Assess mobility, joint pain, and swelling in the joints

Nursing diagnoses
• Knowledge, deficient (teaching)
• Mobility, impaired physical (uses)
• Pain, chronic (uses)

Implementation
• Give with food or antacid to decrease GI upset
• Reduce dose gradually if uric acid levels are normal after 6 mo

Patient/family education
• Advise patient to increase fluids to 3-4 L/day
• Caution patient to avoid alcohol, OTC preparations that contain alcohol; skin rashes may occur

• Advise patient to report any pain, redness, or hard area, usually in legs
• Instruct patient on importance of complying with medical regimen; bone marrow depression may occur

Evaluation
Positive therapeutic outcome
• Decreased pain in joints
• Normal serum uric acid levels
• Increased duration of antiinfectives

---

*sulfiSOXAZOLE (Rx)
(sul-fi-sox′a-zole)
Gantrisin, Gantrisin Pediatric, Novo-Soxazole ✦, sulfiSOXAZOLE
Func. class.: Antiinfective
Chem. class.: Sulfonamide, short-acting

Pregnancy category C

Do not confuse:
sulfiSOXAZOLE/sulfasalazine/sulfADIAZINE

Action: Inhibits folic acid synthesis

Therapeutic outcome: Bactericidal action against susceptible organisms: gram-positive pathogens, including streptococci and staphylococci, *Clostridium perfringens*, *Clostridium tetani*, *Nocardia asteroides*; gram-negative pathogens, including *Enterobacter*, *Escherichia coli*, *Klebsiella*, *Proteus mirabilis*, *Proteus vulgaris*, *Salmonella*, *Shigella*

Uses: UTIs; systemic infections, chancroid, trachoma, toxoplasmosis, acute otitis media, malaria, *Haemophilus influenzae* meningitis, meningococcal meningitis, nocardiosis, eye infections

Dosage and routes
UTIs, other systemic infections
Adult: PO 2-4 g loading dose, then 1-2 g qid × 7-10 days, max 12 g/day
Child >2 mo: PO 75 mg/kg or 2 g/m² loading dose, then 120-150 mg/kg/day or 4 g/m²/day in divided doses q6hr; max 6 g/day

Chlamydia trachomatis
Adult: PO 500 mg-1 g qid × 3 wk

Renal dose
Adult: PO CCr 10-50 ml/min q8-12hr, CCr <10 ml/min q12-24hr

Available forms: Tabs 500 mg; sulfiSOXAZOLE acetyl: liquid 500 mg/5 ml

S

Adverse effects

CNS: Headache, insomnia, hallucinations, depression, vertigo, fatigue, anxiety, **seizures**, product fever, chills, drowsiness

CV: **Allergic myocarditis, tachycardia,** vasculitis

GI: *Nausea, vomiting, abdominal pain,* stomatitis, **hepatitis**, glossitis, pancreatitis, diarrhea, **enterocolitis,** anorexia, **pseudomembranous colitis**

GU: **Renal failure, toxic nephrosis,** increased BUN, creatinine, crystalluria, hematuria, proteinuria, urinary retention

HEMA: **Leukopenia, thrombocytopenia, agranulocytosis, hemolytic anemia, aplastic anemia**

INTEG: Rash, dermatitis, urticaria, erythema, photosensitivity, alopecia

SYST: **Anaphylaxis, Stevens-Johnson syndrome, serum sickness–like symptoms, thyroid dysfunction**

Contraindications: Pregnancy at term, breastfeeding, infants <2 mo (except congenital toxoplasmosis), hypersensitivity to sulfonamides and sulfonylureas, thiazide and loop diuretics, salicylates; sunscreen with PABA, porphyria, G6PD deficiency

Precautions: Pregnancy **C**, breastfeeding, geriatric, impaired renal/hepatic function, severe allergy, bronchial asthma, UV exposure

Pharmacokinetics

Absorption	Well absorbed
Distribution	Widely distributed, crosses placenta
Metabolism	Liver, mostly
Excretion	Breast milk
Half-life	4-7 hr

Pharmacodynamics

Onset	Unknown
Peak	2-4 hr
Duration	Unknown

Interactions
Individual products

CycloSPORINE: increased nephrotoxicity

Indomethacin, probenecid: increased free drug concentrations

Methenamine: increased crystalluria risk

Methotrexate: decreased renal excretion of methotrexate

PABA: avoid use

Phenytoin: decreased hepatic clearance of phenytoin

Warfarin: increased anticoagulant effect

Drug classifications

Antidiabetics, barbiturates, uricosuric agents: increased effects of each specific product

Diuretics (thiazide): increased thrombocytopenia

Salicylates: increased free product concentrations

Sulfonylurea agents: increased hypoglycemic response

Drug/herb

Acidophilus: do not use with antiinfectives; separate by several hours

Drug/lab test

False positive: urinary glucose test

NURSING CONSIDERATIONS
Assessment

• Assess patient for previous sensitivity reaction

• Assess patient for signs and symptoms of infection including characteristics of wounds, sputum, urine, stool, WBC >10,000/mm^3, temp; obtain baseline information before, during treatment

• Complete C&S testing before beginning product therapy to identify if correct treatment has been initiated

• Assess for allergic reactions: rash, urticaria, pruritus, chills, fever, joint pain; angioedema may occur a few days after therapy begins; epinephrine, resuscitation equipment should be available for anaphylactic reaction

• Monitor blood tests: CBC, Hct, bilirubin, alkaline phosphatase monthly if patient is on long-term therapy

• Monitor for bleeding: ecchymosis, bleeding gums, hematuria, stool guaiac daily if on long-term therapy

• Assess for overgrowth of infection: perineal itching, fever, malaise, redness, pain, swelling, drainage, rash, diarrhea, change in cough, sputum

Nursing diagnoses

• Diarrhea (adverse reactions)
• Infection, risk for (uses)
• Injury, risk for (adverse reactions)
• Knowledge, deficient (teaching)
• Noncompliance (teaching)

Implementation

• Give around the clock to maintain proper blood levels; give on an empty stomach to increase absorption of product; do not give within 3 hr of other agents; product interactions may occur

• Give with 8 oz of water

Patient/family education
• Teach patient to report sore throat, bruising, bleeding, joint pain; may indicate blood dyscrasias (rare)
• Advise patient to contact prescriber if vaginal itching, loose foul-smelling stools, or furry tongue occur; may indicate superinfection; report itching, rash, pruritus, urticaria
• Instruct patient to take all medication prescribed for the length of time ordered; product must be taken around the clock to maintain blood levels; medication should not be shared with others

Evaluation
Positive therapeutic outcome
• Absence of signs/symptoms of infection (WBC <10,000/mm^3, temp WNL, absence of urinary pain, hematuria)
• Reported improvement in symptoms of infection
• Negative C&S

sulindac (Rx)
(sul-in'dak)
Apo-Sulin ✦, Clinoril, Novosundac ✦, sulindac
Func. class.: Nonsteroidal antiinflammatory, antirheumatic
Chem. class.: Indeneacetic acid derivative

Pregnancy category C

Do not confuse:
Clinoril/Clozaril/Oruvail

Action: Metabolite inhibits COX-1, COX-2 by blocking arachidonate; analgesic, antiinflammatory, antipyretic

Therapeutic outcome: Decreased pain, inflammation

Uses: Mild to moderate pain, osteoarthritis, rheumatoid, gouty arthritis, ankylosing spondylitis, bursitis, tendonitis

Dosage and routes
Arthritis
Adult: PO 150 mg bid, may increase to 200 mg bid, max 400 mg/day
Child (unlabeled): PO 2-4 mg/kg/day in divided doses, max 6 mg/kg/day or 200 mg bid, whichever is less (safe/effective dose not established)

Bursitis/acute arthritis
Adult: PO 200 mg bid × 1-2 wk, then reduce dose

Available forms: Tabs 150, 200 mg

Adverse effects
CNS: Dizziness, drowsiness, fatigue, tremors, confusion, insomnia, anxiety, depression, *headache*
CV: Tachycardia, peripheral edema, palpitations, dysrhythmias, **MI, stroke, CHF**
EENT: Tinnitus, hearing loss, blurred vision
GI: Nausea, anorexia, vomiting, diarrhea, jaundice, **cholestatic hepatitis**, constipation, flatulence, cramps, dry mouth, peptic ulcer, **bleeding, ulceration, perforation;** dyspepsia
GU: **Nephrotoxicity: dysuria, hematuria, oliguria, azotemia**
HEMA: **Blood dyscrasias with prolonged use**
INTEG: Purpura, *rash, pruritus,* sweating, photosensitivity
SYST: **Anaphylaxis, Stevens-Johnson syndrome, toxic epidermal necrolysis**

Contraindications: Hypersensitivity, asthma, severe renal/hepatic disease, active ulcers

Black Box Warning: Perioperative pain, in CABG

Precautions: Pregnancy C (1st trimester), breastfeeding, children, bleeding disorders, GI/cardiac/renal disorders, hypersensitivity to other antiinflammatory agents, renal disease

Black Box Warning: GI bleeding, MI stroke

Pharmacokinetics
Absorption	Well absorbed
Distribution	Not known
Metabolism	Converted to active product—liver
Excretion	Minimal unchanged kidneys, breast milk
Half-life	7.8 hr; 16.4 hr active metabolite

Pharmacodynamics
Onset	Unknown
Peak	2 hr
Duration	Unknown

Interactions
Individual drugs
Aspirin: increased GI reactions
Clopidogrel, eptifibatide, plicamycin, ticlopidine, tirofiban, valproic acid: increased bleeding risk
CycloSPORINE: increased nephrotoxicity
Diflunisal: decreased sulindac effect
Methotrexate, probenecid: increased toxicity
Drug classifications
Aminoglycosides, antacids: decreased sulindac effect

Adverse effects: *italic* = common, **bold** = life-threatening

Anticoagulants, cephalosporins (some), SNRIs, SSRIs, thrombolytics: increased bleeding risk

Antihypertensives: decreased antihypertensive effect

Glucocorticoids, NSAIDs: increased GI reactions

Quinolones (norfloxacin, floxacin, levofloxacin): increased CNS stimulation, seizures

Sulfonamides, sulfonylurea: increased toxicity

Drug/herb

Arginine, gossypol: increased gastric irritation

Bearberry, bilberry: increased NSAIDs effect

Bogbean, chondroitin, garlic, ginger, horse chestnut, red clover: increased bleeding risk

NURSING CONSIDERATIONS
Assessment
• Monitor blood counts during therapy; watch for decreasing platelets; if low, therapy may need to be discontinued, restarted after hematologic recovery; for blood dyscrasia (thrombocytopenia): bruising, fatigue, bleeding, poor healing
• Assess pain: frequency, intensity, characteristics, relief 1-2 hr after medication
• Assess for asthma, aspirin hypersensitivity, nasal polyps; hypersensitivity may develop, watch for rash

Nursing diagnoses
• Injury, risk for (adverse reactions)
• Knowledge, deficient (teaching)
• Mobility, impaired physical (uses)
• Pain, chronic (uses)

Implementation
• Do not break, crush, or chew tabs
• Give with full glass of water to enhance absorption
• Administer with food or milk to decrease gastric symptoms; food slows absorption slightly, does not decrease absorption

Patient/family education
• Advise patient that product must be continued for prescribed time to be effective; to avoid aspirin, NSAIDs, alcoholic beverages
• Caution patient to report bleeding, bruising, fatigue, malaise because blood dyscrasias do occur
• Instruct patient to use caution when driving; drowsiness, dizziness may occur
• Teach patient to take with a full glass of water to enhance absorption
• Advise to inform all health care providers that product is used

Evaluation
Positive therapeutic outcome
• Decreased pain
• Decreased inflammation
• Increased mobility

sumatriptan (Rx)
(soo-ma-trip′tan)
Imitrex, Sumavel Dose Pro
Func. class.: Antimigraine agent
Chem. class.: 5-HT₁ receptor agonist

Pregnancy category C

Do not confuse: Sumatriptan/somatropin

Action: Binds selectively to the vascular 5-HT₁ receptor subtype and exerts antimigraine effect; causes vasoconstriction in cranial arteries

Therapeutic outcome: Absence of migraines

Uses: Acute treatment of migraine with or without aura and cluster headache

Dosage and routes
Adult: SUBCUT 6 mg or less, may repeat in 1 hr, max 12 mg/24 hr; PO 25 mg with fluids if no relief in 2 hr, give another dose, max 200 mg/day; NASAL 1 dose of 5, 10, or 20 mg in one nostril, may repeat in 2 hr, max 40 mg/24 hr

Hepatic dose
Adult: PO 25 mg, if no response after 2 hr, give up to 50 mg

Available forms: Inj 6 mg (12 mg/ml); tabs 25, 50, 100 mg; nasal spray 5 mg/100 mcl-units dose spray device 20 mg/100 mcl-units

Adverse effects
CNS: Tingling, hot sensation, burning, feeling of pressure, tightness, numbness, dizziness, sedation, headache, anxiety, fatigue, cold sensation
CV: Flushing, **MI**
EENT: Throat, mouth, nasal discomfort, vision changes
GI: Abdominal discomfort
INTEG: Inj site reaction, sweating
MS: Weakness, neck stiffness, myalgia
RESP: Chest tightness, pressure

Contraindications: Angina pectoris, history of MI, documented silent ischemia, Prinzmetal's angina, ischemic heart disease, **IV** use, concurrent ergotamine-containing preparations, uncontrolled hypertension, hypersensitivity, basilar or hemiplegic migraine

Precautions: Pregnancy **C**, breastfeeding, children <18 yr, postmenopausal women, men >40 yr, geriatric, risk factors for CAD, hypercholesterolemia, obesity, diabetes, impaired renal/hepatic function

Pharmacokinetics

Absorption	Well absorbed (SUBCUT)
Distribution	10%-20% plasma protein binding
Metabolism	Liver (metabolite)
Excretion	Urine, feces
Half-life	2 hr

Pharmacodynamics

	SUBCUT
Onset	10-20 min
Peak	10 min-2 hr
Duration	Up to 24 hr (pain relief)

Interactions
Individual drugs
Ergotamine: increased risk of vasospastic reaction
Drug classifications
Ergot derivatives: extended vasospastic effects
MAOIs, selective serotonin reuptake inhibitors: increased sumatriptan levels
Drug/herb
Butterbur, feverfew: increased effect
SAM-e, St. John's wort: serotonin syndrome

NURSING CONSIDERATIONS
Assessment
• Assess for tingling, hot sensation, burning, feeling of pressure, numbness, flushing, inj site reaction
• Assess B/P; signs/symptoms of coronary vasospasm
• Monitor stress level, activity, reaction, coping mechanisms of patient
• Assess neurologic status: LOC, blurring vision, nausea, vomiting, tingling in extremities preceding headache
• Assess for ingestion of tyramine-containing foods (pickled products, beer, wine, aged cheese), food additives, preservatives, colorings, artificial sweeteners, chocolate, caffeine, which may precipitate these types of headaches

Nursing diagnoses
• Knowledge, deficient (teaching)
• Pain, chronic (uses)

Implementation
PO route
• Swallow tab whole; do not break, crush, or chew

• Take with fluids as soon as symptoms appear; may take a second dose >4 hr, max 200 mg/24 hr
SUBCUT route
• Give by SUBCUT route only, avoid IM or **IV** administration, use only for actual migraine attack
Nasal route
• Spray once in 1 nostril, may repeat if headache returns, do not repeat if pain continues after 1st dose

Patient/family education
• Caution patient not to take more than 2 doses/day or 12 mg/day; allow at least 1 hr between doses
• Caution patient to avoid driving or hazardous activities if dizziness or drowsiness occurs
• Teach patient to report chest tightness, heat, flushing, drowsiness, dizziness, fatigue, sudden severe abdominal pain or any allergic reactions that occur to prescriber immediately
• Inform patient to report any side effects to prescriber
• Caution patient to use contraception when taking product, to notify prescriber if pregnancy is suspected or planned

Evaluation
Positive therapeutic outcome
• Decrease in frequency, severity of headache

sunitinib (Rx)
(soo-nit'-in-ib)
Sutent
Func. class.: Antineoplastic—miscellaneous
Chem. class.: Protein-tyrosine kinase inhibitor

Pregnancy category D

Action: Inhibits multiple receptor tyrosine kinases (RTKs), some are responsible for tumor growth

Therapeutic outcome: Decrease in size of tumor

Uses: Gastrointestinal stromal tumors (GIST) after disease progression or intolerance to imatinib; advanced renal carcinoma

Dosage and routes
Adult: PO 50 mg/day × 4 wk, then 2 wk off; may increase or decrease dose by 12.5 mg; if administered with CYP3A4 inducers, give 87.5 mg/day; if given with CYP3A4 inhibitors give 37.5 mg/day

Available forms: Caps 12.5, 25, 50 mg

Adverse effects: *italic* = common, **bold** = life-threatening

Adverse effects

CNS: **CNS hemorrhage,** headache, dizziness, insomnia, **seizures,** fatigue

CV: Hypertension, **left ventricular dysfunction; QT prolongation, cardiotoxicity, thrombotic microangiopathy, torsades de pointes**

ENDO: Hyper/hypothyroidism

GI: Nausea, **hepatotoxicity, vomiting, dyspepsia,** *anorexia, abdominal pain,* altered taste, *constipation,* stomatitis, mucositis, **pancreatitis,** diarrhea, **GI bleeding/ perforation**

HEMA: **Neutropenia, thrombocytopenia,** hemolytic anemia, leukopenia

INTEG: **Rash,** skin discoloration, depigmentation of hair or skin, alopecia

MS: Pain, arthralgia, myalgia, myopathy, **rhabdomyolysis**

RESP: Cough, dyspnea, pulmonary embolism

SYST: **Bleeding,** electrolyte abnormalities, hand-foot syndrome, **serious infection**

Contraindications: Pregnancy **D,** breastfeeding, hypersensitivity

Precautions: Children, geriatric, active infections, QT prolongation, torsades de pointes, stroke, heart failure

Pharmacokinetics

Absorption	Unknown
Distribution	Protein binding 95%
Metabolism	By CYP3A4
Excretion	Feces, small amount in urine
Half-life	Terminal 40-60 hr (sunitinib); active metabolite 80-110 hr

Pharmacodynamics

Onset	Unknown
Peak	6-12 hr
Duration	Unknown

Interactions
Individual drugs

Acetaminophen: increased hepatotoxicity

Bevacizumab: microangiopathic hemolytic anemia; avoid concurrent use

Clarithromycin, erythromycin, itraconazole, ketoconazole: increased sunitinib concentrations

Dexamethasone, carbamazepine, phenobarbital, phenytoin, rifampin: decreased sunitinib concentrations

Simvastatin: increased plasma concentrations

Warfarin: increased plasma concentration; avoid use with warfarin, use low-molecular-weight anticoagulants instead

Drug classifications

Calcium channel blockers: increased plasma concentrations

Drug/herb

St. John's wort: decreased sunitinib concentration

Drug/food

Grapefruit juice: increased plasma concentrations

NURSING CONSIDERATIONS
Assessment

• Monitor ANC and platelets; if ANC <1 × 10^9/L and/or platelets <50 × 10^9/L, stop until ANC >1.5 × 10^9/L and platelets >75 × 10^9/L ; if ANC <0.5 × 10^9/L and/or platelets <10 × 10^9/L, reduce dose by 200 mg; if cytopenia continues, reduce dose by another 100 mg; if cytopenia continues for 4 wk, stop product until ANC ≥1 × 10^9/L

• Assess CV status: hypertension, QT prolongation can occur; monitor left ventricular ejection fraction (LVEF) (MUGA) baseline periodically

• Assess for renal toxicity: if bilirubin >3 × IULN, withhold sunitinib until bilirubin levels return to <1.5 × IULN; electrolytes

• Monitor for hepatic toxicity: liver function tests, before treatment and qmo; if liver transaminases >5 × IULN, withhold sunitinib until transaminase levels return to <2.5 × IULN

• Assess for CHF: adrenal insufficiency in those experiencing trauma

• Assess for bleeding: epistaxis rectal, gingival, upper GI, genital, wound bleeding; tumor-related hemorrhage may occur rapidly

Nursing diagnoses

• Injury, risk for (uses, adverse reactions)
• Knowledge, deficient (teaching)

Implementation

• Give with meal and large glass of water, to decrease GI symptoms

• Give nutritious diet with iron, vitamin supplement, low fiber, few dairy products

• Store at 25°C (77°F)

Patient/family education

• Advise patient to report adverse reactions immediately: shortness of breath, bleeding

• Teach patient reason for treatment, expected result

• Teach patient that many adverse reactions may occur: high B/P, bleeding, mouth swelling, taste change, skin discoloration, depigmentation of hair/skin

---

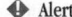 Alert   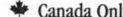 Canada Only   Drug on CD   * "Tall Man" lettering (See Preface)

- Teach patient to avoid persons with known upper respiratory infections; immunosuppression is common
- Teach to avoid grapefruit juice

Evaluation
Positive therapeutic outcome
- Decrease in size of tumor

suprofen ophthalmic
See Appendix B

tacrolimus (Rx)
(tak-roe′li-mus)
Prograf
tacrolimus topical (Rx)
Protopic
Func. class.: Immunosuppressant
Chem. class.: Macrolide

Pregnancy category C

Action: Produces immunosuppression by inhibiting lymphocytes (T)

Therapeutic outcome: Prevention of rejection in organ transplant

Uses: Organ transplants, to prevent rejection; topical: atopic dermatitis

Unlabeled uses: Severe recalcitrant psoriasis

Dosage and routes
Kidney transplant rejection prophylaxis
Adult: IV 0.03-0.05 mg/kg/day as cont INF, give no sooner than 6 hr after transplantation

Liver transplant rejection prophylaxis
Adult: PO 0.10-0.15 mg/kg/day in 2 divided doses q12h, give no sooner than 6 hr after transplantation; **IV** 0.03-0.05 mg/kg/day as a cont INF, give no sooner than 6 hr after transplantation

Heart transplant rejection prophylaxis
Adult: PO 0.075 mg/kg/day in 2 divided doses q12h, give no sooner than 6 hr after transplantation; **IV** 0.01 mg/kg/day as a cont INF, give no sooner than 6 hr after transplantation

Atopic dermatitis
Adult: TOP use 0.03% or 0.1% ointment, apply bid × 7 day
Child 2-5 yr: TOP 0.03% ointment, apply bid × 7 day

Available forms: Inj **IV** 5 mg/ml; caps 0.5, 1, 5 mg; ointment 0.03%, 0.1%

Adverse effects
CNS: Tremors, headache, insomnia, paresthesia, chills, fever, **seizures**
CV: Hypertension, myocardial hypertrophy, **prolonged QT**
EENT: Blurred vision, photophobia
GI: Nausea, vomiting, diarrhea, constipation, GI bleeding
GU: Urinary tract infections, **albuminuria, hematuria, proteinuria, renal failure**
HEMA: Anemia, **leukocytosis, thrombocytopenia, purpura**
INTEG: Rash, flushing, itching, alopecia
META: Hirsutism, hyperglycemia, hyperuricemia, hypo/hyperkalemia, hypomagnesemia
MS: Back pain, muscle spasms
RESP: **Pleural effusion, atelectasis,** dyspnea
SYST: **Anaphylaxis**

Contraindications: Hypersensitivity to this product or to some kinds of castor oil, long-term use (topical), child <2 yr (topical)

Precautions: Pregnancy C, breastfeeding, children <12 yr, severe renal/hepatic disease, diabetes mellitus, hyperkalemia, hyperuricemia, lymphomas, hypertension

Pharmacokinetics
Absorption	Erratically absorbed (PO), completely absorbed (**IV**)
Distribution	Crosses placenta, 75% protein binding
Metabolism	Liver to metabolite
Excretion	Kidney—minimal, breast milk, bile
Half-life	10 hr

Pharmacodynamics
	PO	IV
Onset	Unknown	Unknown
Peak	1-4 hr	Unknown
Duration	12 hr	12 hr

Interactions
Individual drugs
Carbamazepine, phenobarbital, phenytoin, rifamycin: decreased blood levels
Cimetidine, danazol, erythromycin, mycophenolate, mofetil: increased blood levels
Cisplatin, cycloSPORINE: increased toxicity
Ibuprofen: increased oliguria

T

Adverse effects: *italic* = common, **bold** = life-threatening

Drug classifications
Aminoglycosides: increased toxicity
Antifungals, calcium channel blockers: increased blood levels
Vaccines: decreased effect
Drug/herb
Astragalus, echinacea, melatonin: decreased immunosuppression
Ginseng, maitake, mistletoe: decreased effect

NURSING CONSIDERATIONS
Assessment
• Monitor blood studies: Hgb, WBC, platelets during treatment monthly; if WBC is <3000/mm^3 or platelet count <100,000/mm^3, product should be discontinued or reduced; decreased Hgb level may indicate bone marrow suppression
• Monitor liver function tests: alkaline phosphatase, AST, ALT, amylase, bilirubin, and for hepatotoxicity: dark urine, jaundice, itching, light-colored stools; product should be discontinued
◆ Assess for anaphylaxis: rash, pruritus, wheezing, laryngeal edema; stop inf, initiate emergency procedures

Nursing diagnoses
• Infection, risk for (uses)
• Knowledge, deficient (teaching)

Implementation
PO route
• Give all medications PO if possible; avoid IM inj because bleeding may occur
• Give with meals to reduce GI upset; nausea is common
• Give for several days before transplant surgery; patients should be placed in protective isolation
IV route
• Give after diluting in 0.9% NaCl or D$_5$W to a concentration of 0.004-0.02 mg/ml as a cont inf
Y-site compatibilities: Acyclovir, aminophylline, amphotericin B, ampicillin, ampicillin/sulbactam, benztropine, calcium gluconate, cefazolin, cefotetan, ceftazidime, ceftriaxone, cefuroxime, chloramphenicol, cimetidine, ciprofloxacin, clindamycin, dexamethasone, digoxin, diphenhydrAMINE, DOBUTamine, DOPamine, doxycycline, erythromycin, esmolol, fluconazole, furosemide, ganciclovir, gentamicin, haloperidol, heparin, hydrocortisone, imipenem/cilastatin, insulin (regular), isoproterenol, leucovorin, lorazepam, methylPREDNISolone, metoclopramide, metronidazole, mezlocillin, multivitamins, nitroglycerin, nitroprusside, oxacillin, penicillin G potassium, perphenazine, phenytoin, piperacillin, potassium chloride, propranolol,

ranitidine, sodium bicarbonate, trimethoprim/sulfamethoxazole, vancomycin

Patient/family education
• Instruct patient to report fever, rash, severe diarrhea, chills, sore throat, fatigue because serious infections may occur; clay-colored stools, cramping may indicate hepatotoxicity
• Caution patient to avoid crowds or persons with known infections to reduce risk of infection

Evaluation
Positive therapeutic outcome
• Absence of graft rejection
• Immunosuppression in autoimmune disorders

---

tadalafil (Rx)
(tah-dal′a-fil)
Adcirca, Cialis
Func. class.: Impotence agent
Chem. class.: Phosphodiesterase type 5 inhibitor
Pregnancy category B

Action: Inhibits phosphodiesterase type 5 (PDE5); enhances erectile function by increasing the amount of cGMP, which causes smooth muscle relaxation and increased blood flow into the corpus cavernosum; improves erectile function for up to 36 hr

Therapeutic outcome: Erection

Uses: Treatment of erectile dysfunction; pulmonary arterial hypertension (PAH) (Adcirca only)

Dosage and routes
Adult: PO 10 mg, taken prior to sexual activity, dose may be reduced to 5 mg or increased to a max of 20 mg; usual max dosing frequency is once per day; once daily dosing 2.5 mg/day at same time each day

Renal dose
Adult: PO CCr 31-50 ml/min 5 mg/day, max 10 mg q48hr; CCr <30 ml/min, max 5 mg q72hr

Hepatic dose
Adult: PO Child-Pugh class A, B, max 10 mg/day; Child-Pugh class C, not recommended

Concomitant medications
Ketoconazole, ritonavir, max 10 mg q72hr

Pulmonary hypertension
Adult: PO (Adcirca only) 40 mg qd; **Adult taking ritonavir:** PO 20 mg qd initially, then increase to 40 mg qd as tolerated

---

Available forms: Tabs 2.5, 5, 10, 20 mg; tab 20 mg (Adcirca)

Adverse effects

CNS: Headache, flushing, dizziness, **seizures,** transient global amnesia

CV: **MI, sudden death, CV collapse,** hypo/hypertension, tachycardia

MISC: Back pain/myalgia, *dyspepsia, nasal congestion, UTI,* blurred vision, changes in color vision, *diarrhea,* pruritus, priapism, **nonarteritic ischemic optic neuropathy (NAION),** hearing loss

Contraindications: Newborns, women, children, hypersensitivity, patients taking organic nitrates regularly or intermittently, patients taking any α-adrenergic antagonist other than 0.4 mg once-daily tamsulosin

Precautions: Pregnancy **B,** although not indicated for females, anatomic penile deformities, sickle cell anemia, leukemia, multiple myeloma, CV/renal/hepatic disease, bleeding disorders, active peptic ulcer, prolonged erection

Pharmacokinetics

Absorption	Rapid; rate and extent of absorption of tadalafil are not influenced by food
Distribution	94% protein bound
Metabolism	Liver
Excretion	Excreted primarily as metabolites, feces, urine; plasma concentration 61% in feces, 36% in urine
Half-life	17.5 hr

Pharmacodynamics

Onset	Rapid
Peak	6 hr
Duration	Unknown

Interactions

Individual drugs

Alcohol, amlodipine, enalapril: decreased B/P

Bosentan: decreased effects of tadalafil

Itraconazole, ketoconazole, ritonavir: increased levels (although not studied, may also include other HIV protease inhibitors)

Drug classifications

⬥Do not use with nitrates because of unsafe drop in B/P that could result in heart attack or stroke

α-blockers, angiotensin II receptor blockers: decreased B/P

Antacids: decreased effects of tadalafil

NURSING CONSIDERATIONS

Assessment

• Assess for organic nitrates that should not be used with this product

• Assess for severe loss of vision

Nursing diagnoses

• Knowledge, deficient (teaching)

• Sexual dysfunction (uses)

Implementation

• Sexual dysfunction: give before sexual activity; do not use more than once a day

• Pulmonary hypertension: give Adcirca without regard to meals

Patient/family education

• Advise that product does not protect against STDs, including HIV

• Instruct to tell physician if patient has a bleeding problem

• Advise that product should not be used with nitrates in any form

• Advise that product has no effect in the absence of sexual stimulation

• Instruct to seek medical help if an erection lasts more than 4 hr

• Advise to tell physician of all medicines, vitamins, and herbs patient is taking, especially α-blockers, erythromycin, indinavir, itraconazole, ketoconazole, nitrates, ritonavir

• Advise that tadalafil is contraindicated for use with α-blockers except 0.4 mg/daily tamsulosin

Evaluation

Positive therapeutic outcome

• Sustainable erection

• Improvement in exercise ability (pulmonary hypertension)

---

tamoxifen (Rx)

(ta-mox'i-fen)

Alpha-Tamoxifen ✤, Med Tamoxifen ✤, Nolvadex, Nolvadex-D ✤, Novo-Tamoxifen ✤, Soltamox, Tamofen ✤, Tamone ✤, Tamoplex ✤

Func. class.: Antineoplastic

Chem. class.: Antiestrogen hormone

Pregnancy category D

Action: Inhibits cell division by binding to cytoplasmic estrogen receptors; resembles normal cell complex but inhibits DNA synthesis and estrogen response of target tissue

Therapeutic outcome: Prevention of rapidly growing malignant cells

T

Uses: Advanced breast carcinoma that has not responded to other therapy in estrogen receptor-positive patients (usually postmenopausal), prevention of breast cancer, after breast surgery/radiation in ductal carcinoma in situ

Unlabeled uses: Mastalgia, pain/size of gynecomastia, ovulation stimulation, malignant carcinoid tumor, carcinoid syndrome, metaplastic melanoma, desmoid tumors, McCune-Albright syndrome (female pediatric patients)

Dosage and routes
Breast cancer
Adult: PO 20-40 mg/day × 5 yr, doses >20 mg/day divide AM/PM

High risk for breast cancer
Adult: PO 20 mg/day × 5 yr

Ductal carcinoma in situ
Adult: PO 20 mg/day × 5 yr

McCune-Albright syndrome (unlabeled)
Child 2-10 yr (girls): PO 20 mg/day for up to 1 yr

Available forms: Tabs 10, 20 mg

Adverse effects
CNS: *Hot flashes, headache, lightheadedness,* depression, mood changes
CV: Chest pain, stroke, fluid retention, flushing
EENT: Ocular lesions, cataracts, retinopathy, corneal opacity, blurred vision (high doses)
GI: *Nausea, vomiting,* altered taste (anorexia)
GU: Vaginal bleeding, pruritus vulvae, uterine malignancies, *altered menses, amenorrhea*
HEMA: **Thrombocytopenia, leukopenia,** deep vein thrombosis
INTEG: *Rash,* alopecia
META: Hypercalcemia
RESP: Pulmonary embolism

Contraindications: Pregnancy **D**, breast-feeding, hypersensitivity

Black Box Warning: Thromboembolic disease

Precautions: Leukopenia, thrombocytopenia, cataracts, women of childbearing age

Black Box Warning: Endometrial cancer, stroke

Pharmacokinetics
Absorption	Adequately absorbed
Distribution	Unknown
Metabolism	Liver—extensively
Excretion	Feces—slowly, small amounts (kidneys)
Half-life	1 wk

Pharmacodynamics
Onset	Unknown
Peak	4-7 hr
Duration	Unknown

Interactions
Individual drugs
Aminoglutethimide, medroxyprogesterone, rifamycin: decreased tamoxifen levels
Bromocriptine: increased tamoxifen level
Letrozole: decreased levels of letrozole
Radiation: increased myelosuppression

Drug classifications
Anticoagulants: increased risk of bleeding
Cytotoxics: increased thromboembolic action
CYP2D6 inhibitors (antidepressants): decreased tamoxifen effect
CYP3A4 inducers (barbiturates, bosentan, carbamazepine, efavirenz, phenytoin, nevirapine, rifabutin, rifampin): decreased tamoxifen effect
CYP3A4 inhibitors (aprepitant, antiretroviral protease inhibitors, clarithromycin, danazol, delavirdine, diltiazem, erythromycin, fluconazole, fluoxetine, fluvoxamine, imatinib, ketoconazole, mibefradil, nefazodone, telithromycin, voriconazole): increased toxicity

Drug/herb
Black cohosh, dong quai, St. John's wort: avoid use

Drug/lab test
Increased: serum calcium, T_4, AST, ALT, cholesterol, triglycerides

NURSING CONSIDERATIONS
Assessment
• Monitor CBC, differential, platelet count weekly; withhold product if WBC is <4000/mm^3 or platelet count is <75,000/mm^3; notify prescriber of results; monitor calcium levels (hypercalcemia is common); breast exam, mammogram, pregnancy test, bone mineral density, LFTs, serum calcium, serum lipid profile
⬥ Assess for tumor flare: increase in bone, tumor pain during beginning treatment; give analgesics as ordered to decrease pain
• Assess for bleeding: hematuria, guaiac, bruising or petechiae, mucosa or orifices q8hr, no rectal temp
⬥ Assess for uterine malignancies: symptoms of stroke, PE that may occur in women with ductal carcinoma in situ (DCIS) and women at high risk for breast cancer

Nursing diagnoses
• Injury, risk for (adverse reactions)
• Knowledge, deficient (teaching)

Implementation
- Do not break, crush, or chew tabs
- Give with food or fluids for GI upset; repeat dose may be needed if vomiting occurs
- Store in light-resistant container at room temperature

Patient/family education
- Instruct patient to report any complaints, side effects to prescriber; if dose is missed, do not double next dose; that use may be 5 yr
- Advise patient that vaginal bleeding, pruritus, hot flashes can occur and are reversible after discontinuing treatment
- Instruct patient to report immediately decreased visual acuity, which may be irreversible; stress need for routine eye exams
- Inform patient about who should be told about tamoxifen therapy
- Advise patient to report vaginal bleeding immediately; that tumor flare (increase in size or tumor, increased bone pain) may occur and will subside rapidly; may take analgesics for pain; that premenopausal women must use mechanical birth control method because ovulation may be induced (teratogenic product)
- Caution patient to use sunscreen and protective clothing to prevent burns because photosensitivity is common
- Teach patient that hair loss may occur during treatment; a wig or hairpiece may make patient feel better; new hair may be different in color, texture
- Inform patient rash or lesions are temporary and may become large during beginning therapy
- Advise patient to increase fluids to 2 L/day unless contraindicated

Evaluation
Positive therapeutic outcome
- Decreased spread of malignant cells in breast cancer

---

tamsulosin (Rx)
(tam-sue-lo′sen)
Flomax
Func. class.: Selective α-adrenergic blocker
Chem. class.: Sulfamoyl phenethylamine derivative

Pregnancy category B

Do not confuse:
Flomax/Fosamax/Volmax

Action: Binds preferentially to α IA-adrenoceptor subtype located mainly in the prostate

Therapeutic outcome: Decreased symptoms of benign prostatic hyperplasia (BPH)

Uses: Symptoms of BPH

Dosage and routes
Adult: PO 0.4 mg/day, increasing to 0.8 mg/day if required

Available forms: Caps 0.4 mg

Adverse effects
CNS: Dizziness, headache, asthenia, insomnia
CV: Chest pain
EENT: Amblyopia, floppy iris syndrome
GI: Nausea, diarrhea, dysgeusia
GU: Decreased libido, abnormal ejaculation, priapism
MS: Back pain
RESP: Rhinitis, pharyngitis, cough
SYST: **Angioedema**

Contraindications: Hypersensitivity

Precautions: Pregnancy **B,** breastfeeding, children, hepatic disease, CAD, severe renal disease

Pharmacokinetics
Absorption	Well absorbed
Distribution	Not known; 98% plasma protein bound
Metabolism	Liver, extensively
Excretion	Kidneys
Half-life	9-15 hr

Pharmacodynamics
Unknown

Interactions
Individual drugs
Cimetidine: increased toxicity
Doxazosin, prazosin, terazosin, vardenafil: do not use together
Drug classifications
β-Adrenergic blockers: do not use together
Drug/food
Decreased: absorption with food

NURSING CONSIDERATIONS
Assessment
- Monitor CBC with differential and liver function tests; B/P and heart rate
- Monitor urodynamic studies/urinary flow rates, residual volume
- Assess for BPH: change in urinary patterns, baseline, throughout treatment
- Monitor I&O ratios, weight daily, edema, report weight gain or edema

T

Adverse effects: *italic* = common, **bold** = life-threatening

Nursing diagnoses
- Cardiac output, decreased (uses)
- Injury, risk for (side effects)
- Knowledge, deficient (teaching)
- Noncompliance (teaching)

Implementation
- Swallow caps whole; do not break, crush, or chew
- Store in airtight container at 86° F (30° C) or less
- May be given with food to prevent GI symptoms; ½ hr after same meal each day

Patient/family education
- Teach patient not to discontinue product abruptly; emphasize the importance of complying with dosage schedule, even if feeling better; if dose is missed take as soon as remembered; take at same time each day
- Teach patient not to use OTC products (cough, cold, allergy) unless directed by prescriber; also to avoid large amounts of caffeine
- Caution patient that product may cause dizziness, may occur during 1st few days of therapy; to avoid hazardous activities

Evaluation
Positive therapeutic outcome
- Decreased symptoms of BPH

---

tapentadol (Rx)
(ta-pen′ta-dol)
Nucynta
Func. class.: Analgesic, miscellaneous
Chem. class.: μ-opioid receptor agonist

Controlled substance schedule II

Pregnancy category C

Action: Centrally-acting synthetic analgesic; μ-opioid agonist activity is thought to result in analgesia; inhibits norepinephrine uptake

Therapeutic outcome: Relief of pain

Uses: Moderate to severe pain

Dosage and routes
Adult: PO 50-100 mg q4-6hr; may give second dose 1 hr or more after 1st dose; max 700 mg on day 1, 600 mg/day thereafter

Available forms: Tab 50, 75, 100 mg

Adverse effects
CNS: Drowsiness, dizziness, confusion, headache, euphoria, hallucinations, restlessness, syncope, anxiety, flushing, psychological dependence, insomnia, lethargy, tremor, **seizures**

CV: Palpitations, bradycardia, hypo/hypertension, orthostatic hypotension, sinus tachycardia
GI: Nausea, vomiting, anorexia, constipation, cramps, gastritis, dyspepsia, biliary spasms
GU: Urinary retention/frequency
INTEG: Rash, urticaria, diaphoresis, pruritus
RESP: **Respiratory depression,** cough
SYST: **Anaphylaxis,** infection, serotonin syndrome

Contraindications: Hypersensitivity, asthma, ileus, respiratory depression

Precautions: Pregnancy **C**, breastfeeding, children <18 yr, increased intracranial pressure, MI (acute), severe heart disease, respiratory depression, renal/hepatic disease, GI obstruction, ulcerative colitis, sleep apnea, seizure disorder

Pharmacokinetics
Absorption	32%
Distribution	Protein binding 20%
Metabolism	Liver extensively
Excretion	Urine 99%
Half-life	Terminal 4 hr

Pharmacodynamics
Onset	Unknown
Peak	Unknown
Duration	Unknown

INTERACTIONS
Individual drugs
Alcohol: increased effects with other CNS depressants
Drug classifications
Antipsychotics, opioids, sedatives/hypnotics, skeletal muscle relaxants: increased effects with other CNS depressants
MAOIs: increased toxicity
Serotonin-receptor agonists, SSRIs, SNRIs, tricyclics: increased serotonin syndrome
Drug/herb
Gotu kola, Jamaican dogwood, kava, lavender, mistletoe, nettle, pokeweed, poppy, senega, St. John's wort, valerian: increased sedative effect

NURSING CONSIDERATIONS
Assessment
- Monitor I&O ratio; check for decreasing output; may indicate urinary retention
- Assess CNS changes: dizziness, drowsiness, hallucinations, euphoria, LOC, pupil reaction
- Assess for allergic reactions: rash, urticaria, anaphylaxis

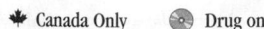

- Assess for respiratory dysfunction: respiratory depression, character, rate, rhythm; notify prescriber if respirations are <10/min; also B/P, pulse
- Assess for pain: intensity, location, type, characteristics; need for pain medication by pain/sedation scoring; physical dependence

Nursing diagnosis
- Pain, acute (uses)
- Knowledge, deficient (teaching)
- Administration

Implementation
- Give with antiemetic if nausea, vomiting occur
- Give when pain is beginning to return; determine dosage interval by response
- Store in light-resistant area at room temperature
- Provide assistance with ambulation
- Provide safety measures: night-light, call bell within easy reach

Patient/family education
- Teach patient to report any symptoms of CNS changes, allergic reactions
- Advise that physical dependency may result from extended use
- Inform that withdrawal symptoms may occur: nausea, vomiting, cramps, fever, faintness, anorexia
- Teach to avoid CNS depressants, alcohol
- Advise to avoid driving, operating machinery if drowsiness occurs

Evaluation
Positive therapeutic outcome
- Decrease in pain

---

tazobactam
See piperacillin/tazobactam

---

tegaserod (Rx)
(teg-as'er-odd)
Zelnorm
Func. class.: 5-HT$_4$ receptor partial agonist, GI agent—miscellaneous
Pregnancy category B

Action: A 5-HT$_4$ receptor partial agonist that binds 5-HT$_4$ receptors, stimulating peristalsis and intestinal secretion

Therapeutic outcome: Decreased constipation in irritable bowel syndrome (IBS)

Uses: IBS where primary bowel symptom is constipation, chronic constipation not associated with IBS

Dosage and routes
This product is only available to women ≤55 yr old who meet specific guidelines; it is off the market for the general public
Adult (females): **PO** 6 mg bid before meals × 4-6 wk

Available forms: Tabs 2, 6 mg

Adverse effects
CNS: Headache, dizziness, depression, vertigo, fatigue, suicide attempt, poor concentration
CV: Hypotension, angina, **dysrhythmias, bundle branch block, supraventricular tachycardia**
GI: Nausea, abdominal pain, increased appetite, eructation, increased AST, increased ALT, diarrhea, irritable colon, tenesmus, flatulence
GU: Polyuria, renal pain, ovarian cyst, miscarriage, albuminuria
MISC: Pain, facial edema, increased CPK, asthma, breast carcinoma
MS: Back pain, arthralgia
SYST: **Anaphylaxis**

Contraindications: Hypersensitivity, severe renal disease, moderate to severe hepatic disease, history of bowel obstruction, gallbladder disease, abdominal adhesions, sphincter of Oddi dysfunction, hypotension

Precautions: Pregnancy **B,** breastfeeding, children, diarrhea

Pharmacokinetics	
Absorption	Unknown
Distribution	98% protein binding
Metabolism	Unknown
Excretion	⅔ unchanged in feces, remainder in urine as metabolites
Half-life	11 hr

Pharmacodynamics	
Onset	Unknown
Peak	1 hr
Duration	Unknown

Interactions
Individual drug
Digoxin: decreased effect of digoxin
Drug classification
Antimuscarinics: decreased tegaserod effect
Drug/food
Food: decreased absorption, but is minimized when taken ½ hr before a meal

---

Adverse effects: *italic* = common, **bold** = life-threatening

NURSING CONSIDERATIONS
Assessment
- This product is only available to women ≤55 yrs old who meet specific guidelines; it is off the market to the general public
- Assess GI symptoms: nausea, abdominal pain
- Assess CV status: B/P, pulse, chest pain

Nursing diagnoses
- Constipation (uses)
- Knowledge, deficient (teaching)

Implementation
- Give before meals, bid
- Store at room temperature

Patient/family education
- Advise to notify prescriber of GI symptoms, hypersensitivity reactions

Evaluation
Positive therapeutic outcome
- Decreased constipation in IBS

---

telavancin (Rx)
(tel-a-van'sin)
Vibativ
Func. class.: Antiinfective—miscellaneous
Chem. class.: Lipoglycopeptide, a semi-synthetic derivative of vacomycin
Pregnancy category C

Action: Inhibits bacterial cell wall synthesis, blocks glycopeptides

Therapeutic outcome: Negative culture

Uses: Skin/skin structure infections caused by *Enterococcus faecalis, E. faecium, Staphylococcus aureus* (MSRA), *S. aureus* (MSSA), *S. epidermidis, S. haemolyticus, Streptococcus agalactiae* (group B), *S. dysgalactiae, S. pyogenes* (group A beta tremolytic), *S. anginosus, S. intermedius, S. constellates*

Unlabeled uses: Nosocomial pneumonia caused by susceptible gram-positive bacteria

Dosage and routes
Adult: **IV** INF 10 mg/kg over 60 min q24hr × 7-14 days

Nosocomial pneumonia (unlabeled)
Adult: **IV** INF 10 mg/kg q24hr × 7-21 days

Available forms: Powder for inj 250, 750 mg

Adverse effects
CNS: Anxiety, chills, flushing, headache, insomnia
CV: **QT prolongation,** irregular heartbeat

EENT: Hearing loss
GI: **Nausea,** vomiting, **pseudomembranous colitis,** abdominal pain, constipation, diarrhea, metallic taste
GU: **Nephrotoxicity,** *increased BUN, creatinine,* **renal failure,** foamy urine
HEMA: Leukopenia, **eosinophilia, anemia, thrombocytopenia**
INTEG: Chills, fever, rash, thrombophlebitis at inj site, urticaria, pruritus, necrosis (red man syndrome)
SYST: **Anaphylaxis, superinfection**

Contraindications: Hypersensitivity

Precautions: Breastfeeding, geriatric patients, renal disease, antimicrobial resistance, children, diabetes mellitus, diarrhea, GI disease, heart failure, hypertension, pseudomembranous colitis, QT prolongation, vancomycin hypersensitivity

Black Box Warning: Pregnancy C, females

Pharmacokinetics
Absorption	Unknown
Distribution	Unknown
Metabolism	Unknown
Excretion	Urine 76%
Half-life	8-9 hr

Pharmacodynamics
Onset	Rapid
Peak	Unknown
Duration	Unknown

Interactions
Individual drugs
Amphotericin B, bacitracin, cidofovir, cisplatin, colistin, polymyxin: increased toxicity, nephrotoxicity
Bepridil, chloroquine, clarithromycin, dronedarone, droperidol, erythromycin, grepafloxacin, halofantrine, haloperidol, levomethadyl, methadone, pimozide, probucol, sparfloxacin, ziprasidone: increased QT prolongation
Drug classifications
Aminoglycosides, cephalosporins, cidofovir, nondepolarizing muscle relaxants: increased toxicity, nephrotoxicity
Class IA, III antidysrhythmics, some phenothiazines: increased QT prolongation
Drug/herb
- Do not use acidophilus with antiinfectives; separate by several hours

---

 Alert   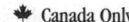 Canada Only   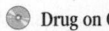 Drug on CD   * "Tall Man" lettering (See Preface)

NURSING CONSIDERATIONS
Assessment
• Assess for infection: WBC, urine, stools, sputum, characteristics of wound, throughout treatment
• Monitor I&O ratio; report hematuria, oliguria; nephrotoxicity may occur
⬥ Assess any patient with compromised renal system; product is excreted slowly in poor renal system function; toxicity may occur rapidly; BUN, creatinine
• Monitor C&S throughout treatment
• Assess auditory function during, after treatment, hearing loss, ringing, roaring in ears; product should be discontinued
• Monitor B/P during administration; sudden drop may indicate red man syndrome
• Assess for skin eruptions
• Assess respiratory status: rate, character, wheezing, tightness in chest
• Assess allergies before treatment, reaction of each medication

Nursing diagnoses
• Infection, risk for (uses)
• Knowledge, deficient (teaching)

Implementation
• Use only for susceptible organisms to prevent drug-resistant bacteria
• Give antihistamine if red man syndrome occurs: decreased B/P, flushing of neck, face
• Store in refrigerator
• Have epinephrine, suction, tracheostomy set, endotracheal intubation equipment on unit; anaphylaxis may occur
• Give adequate intake of fluids (2 L/day) to prevent nephrotoxicity
Intermittent IV route
• Administer after reconstitution with 15 ml D5W sterile water for inj; 0.9% NaCl (15 mg/ml) 250 mg vial; add 45 ml to 750 mg vial (15 mg/ml) for dose of 150-800 mg; further dilute with 100-250 ml of compatible sol; for dose <150 mg or 800 mg, further dilute to a conc of 0.6-8 mg/ml with compatible sol; give over 60 min

Solution compatibilities: D5W, LR, NS

Patient/family education
• Teach all aspects of product therapy; culture may be taken after completed course of medication
• Advise to report sore throat, fever, fatigue; could indicate superinfection

Evaluation
Positive therapeutic outcome
• Negative culture

---

telbivudine (Rx)
(tel-bi'vyoo-deen)
Tyzeka
Func. class.: Antiretroviral
Chem. class.: Nucleoside reverse transcriptase inhibitor (NRTI)

Pregnancy category B

Action: Inhibits replication of HBV DNA polymerase, which inhibits HBV replication

Therapeutic outcome: Decreased hepatitis B serology

Uses: Hepatitis B

Dosage and routes
Adult and adolescent >16 yr: PO 600 mg/day; max 600 mg/day

Available forms: Tabs 600 mg

Adverse effects
CNS: Fever, headache, malaise, weakness, *dizziness, insomnia*
EENT: Taste change, hearing loss, photophobia
GI: Nausea, vomiting, diarrhea, anorexia, abdominal pain, hepatomegaly
INTEG: Rash
MISC: Lactic acidosis
MS: Myalgia, arthralgia, muscle cramps
RESP: Cough

Contraindications: Hypersensitivity, breastfeeding

Precautions: Pregnancy B, children, severe renal disease, anemia, organ transplant, dialysis, HIV, obesity, alcoholism

Black Box Warning: Impaired hepatic function, lactic acidosis

Pharmacokinetics
Absorption	Unknown
Distribution	Steady state 5-7 days, protein binding 3.3%
Metabolism	Unknown
Excretion	Kidneys, unchanged
Half-life	Terminal 40-49 hr

Pharmacodynamics
Unknown

Interactions
Individual drugs
CycloSPORINE, erythromycin, hydrochloroquine, niacin, penicillamine, zidovudine, ZDV: increased myopathy risk
Drug classifications
Any agent altering renal function: altered telbivudine levels

---

Adverse effects: *italic* = common, **bold** = life-threatening

Azole antifungals, corticosteroids, fibric acid derivatives, HMG-CoA reductase inhibitors: increased myopathy risk

NURSING CONSIDERATIONS
Assessment
• Monitor liver function tests, hepatitis B serology, creatine kinase, periodically

Nursing diagnoses
• Infection, risk for (uses)
• Knowledge, deficient (teaching)

Implementation
• Give with or without food with a full glass of water
• Store at room temperature

Patient/family education
• Advise patient that GI complaints and insomnia may resolve after 3-4 wk of treatment
• Teach patient that product does not cure hepatitis B and does not stop the spread to others
• Teach patient that follow-up visits must be continued
• Teach patient that serious product interactions may occur if OTC products are ingested; check with prescriber before taking
• Advise patient that product may cause dizziness; avoid hazardous activities until response is known
• Teach patient to report symptoms of cough, difficulty sleeping or excessive headache

Evaluation
Positive therapeutic outcome
• Decreased hepatitis B serology

---

telithromycin (Rx)
(teh-lih-throw-my'sin)
Ketek
Func. class.: Antiinfective
Chem. class.: Ketolides
Pregnancy category C

Action: Binds to 50S ribosomal subunits of susceptible bacteria and suppresses protein synthesis

Therapeutic outcome: Bacterial action against *Streptococcus pneumoniae, Haemophilus influenzae, Moraxella catarrhalis, Staphylococcus aureus*

Uses: Acute bacterial exacerbation of chronic bronchitis caused by *Streptococcus pneumoniae, Haemophilus influenzae, Moraxella catarrhalis*; acute bacterial sinusitis caused by *S. pneumoniae, H. influenzae, M. catarrha-*

lis, Staphylococcus aureus, community-acquired pneumonia (mild to moderate)

Unlabeled uses: Acute tonsillitis/pharyngitis

Dosage and routes
Acute bacterial exacerbation of bronchitis
Adult: PO 800 mg/day × 5 days

Acute bacterial sinusitis
Adult: PO 800 mg/day × 5 days

Community-acquired pneumonia
Adult: PO 800 mg/day × 7-10 days

Available forms: Tabs 300, 400 mg

Adverse effects
CNS: Dizziness, headache, insomnia, increased sweating
CV: **QT prolongation, torsades de pointes, atrial dysrhythmias**
EENT: Blurred vision, diplopia, difficulty focusing
GI: Nausea, vomiting, diarrhea, hepatitis, abdominal pain/distension, stomatitis, anorexia, **pseudomembranous colitis, pancreatitis**
GU: Vaginitis, moniliasis
INTEG: Rash, urticaria
MS: Muscle cramps
SYST: **Anaphylaxis,** superinfection

Contraindications: Hypersensitivity to this product or macrolide antibiotics, history of hepatitis

Black Box Warning: Myasthenia gravis

Precautions: Pregnancy **C**, breastfeeding, children, geriatric, ongoing prodysrhythmias, hepatic/GI disease, QT prolongation

Pharmacokinetics
Absorption	Unknown
Distribution	Protein binding 60%-70%
Metabolism	Liver
Excretion	Bile, feces
Half-life	Unknown

Pharmacodynamics
Onset	Unknown
Peak	1 hr
Duration	Unknown

Interactions
Individual drugs
Atorvastatin, carbamazepine, cycloSPORINE, digoxin, ergots, lovastatin, metoprolol, midazolam, phenobarbital, phenytoin,

 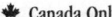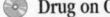

simvastatin, sirolimus, tacrolimus, theophylline: increased action

Bepridil, chloroquine, droperidol, erythromycin, grepafloxacin, halofantrine, haloperidol, methadone, pentamidine, probucol, sparfloxacin: increased QT prolongation

Carbamazepine, phenobarbital, phenytoin, rifampin: decreased action of telithromycin

Itraconazole, ketoconazole: increased telithromycin

Pimozide: serious dysrhythmias; do not use together

Sotalol: decreased action

Verapamil: increased cardiotoxicity

Drug classifications
Antidysrhythmics (amiodarone, bretylium, disopyramide, dofetilide, procainamide, quinidine, sotalol): serious dysrhythmias; do not use together

Antidysrhythmics (class IA, III), β-agonists, local anesthetics, phenothiazines (some), tricyclics: increased QT interval; do not use together

Drug/herb
Acidophilus: do not use with antiinfectives; separate by several hours

Drug/lab test
Increased: AST/ALT

NURSING CONSIDERATIONS
Assessment
• Assess for infection: temp, sputum, WBCs, baseline, periodically
• Assess for oliguria in renal disease
• Monitor liver function tests: AST, ALT if patient is on long-term therapy
• Monitor C&S before product therapy; product may be given as soon as culture is taken; C&S may be repeated after treatment
• Monitor bowel pattern before, during treatment
• Assess for skin eruptions, itching

Nursing diagnoses
• Infection, risk for (uses)

Implementation
• May take without regard to food
• Store at room temperature
• Provide adequate intake of fluids (2 L) during diarrhea episodes

Patient/family education
• Teach patient to report sore throat, fever, fatigue (could indicate superinfection)
• Teach patient to notify nurse of diarrhea, dark urine, pale stools, jaundice of eyes or skin, severe abdominal pain
• Teach patient to report blurred vision, if interfering with daily activities

• Advise patient to avoid driving, hazardous activities if blurred vision occurs
• Instruct patient to take as prescribed, do not double or skip doses
• Instruct patient not to use this product if using Class 1A or III antidysrhythmics
• Advise patient to avoid simvastatin, lovastatin, and atorvastatin
• Inform patient that medication may be taken without regard to meals

Evaluation
Positive therapeutic outcome
• Decreased symptoms of infection

Treatment of hypersensitivity:
Withdraw product; maintain airway; administer epinephrine, aminophylline, O_2, **IV** corticosteroids

---

telmisartan (Rx)
(tel-mih-sar'tan)
Micardis
Func. class.: Antihypertensive
Chem. class.: Angiotensin II receptor (type AT_1)

Pregnancy category
C (1st trimester),
D (2nd/3rd trimesters)

Action: Blocks the vasoconstrictor and aldosterone-secreting effects of angiotensin II; selectively blocks the binding of angiotensin II to the AT_1 receptor found in tissues

Therapeutic outcome: Decreased B/P

Uses: Hypertension, alone or in combination

Unlabeled uses: Heart failure

Dosage and routes
Adult: PO 40 mg/day; range 20-80 mg/day

Available forms: Tabs 20, 40, 80 mg

Adverse effects
CNS: Dizziness, insomnia, *anxiety,* headache, fatigue
GI: Diarrhea, dyspepsia, *anorexia, vomiting*
MS: Myalgia, pain
RESP: Cough, *upper respiratory tract infection,* sinusitis, pharyngitis

Contraindications: Hypersensitivity

Black Box Warning: Pregnancy **D** (2nd/3rd trimesters)

Precautions: Pregnancy C (1st trimester), breastfeeding, children, geriatric, hypersensitivity to angiotensin-converting enzyme (ACE) inhibitors, renal/hepatic disease, renal artery stenosis, dialysis, CHF

T

Adverse effects: *italic* = common, **bold** = life-threatening

Pharmacokinetics

Absorption	Unknown
Distribution	Highly protein bound
Metabolism	Liver (extensively)
Excretion	Urine/feces
Half-life	Terminal 24 hr

Pharmacodynamics
Unknown

Interactions
Digoxin: increased digoxin peak, trough concentrations
Drug classifications
Antihypertensives, diuretics: increased antihypertensive action
NSAIDs, salicylates: decreased antihypertensive effect
Potassium-sparing diuretics, potassium salt substitutes: increased hyperkalemia
Drug/herb
Aconite: increased toxicity, death
Astragalus, cola tree: increased or decreased antihypertensive effect
Barberry, betony, black catechu, black cohosh, bloodroot, broom, burdock, cat's claw, dandelion, goldenseal, hawthorn, Irish moss, Jamaican dogwood, kelp, khella, mistletoe, parsley: increased antihypertensive effect
Coltsfoot, guarana, khat, licorice, yohimbe: decreased antihypertensive effect

NURSING CONSIDERATIONS
Assessment
• Monitor B/P, pulse q4hr; note rate, rhythm, quality
• Monitor electrolytes: potassium, sodium, chloride
• Monitor baselines in renal, liver function tests before therapy begins
• Assess edema in feet, legs daily
• Assess skin turgor, dryness of mucous membranes for hydration status

Nursing diagnoses
• Knowledge, deficient (teaching)
• Noncompliance (teaching)
• Tissue perfusion, ineffective (uses)

Implementation
• Give without regard to meals
• Give increased dose to African-American patients, B/P response may be reduced

Patient/family education
• Instruct patient to comply with dosage schedule, even if feeling better

• Advise patient to notify prescriber of mouth sores, fever, swelling of hands or feet, irregular heartbeat, chest pain
• Teach patient that excessive perspiration, dehydration, vomiting, diarrhea may lead to fall in blood pressure; consult prescriber if these occur
• Teach patient that product may cause dizziness, fainting; light-headedness may occur
• Advise patient to use contraception while taking this product
• Teach patient to notify prescriber of all prescriptions, OTC preparations, and supplements taken

Evaluation
Positive therapeutic outcome
• Decreased B/P

---

temazepam (Rx)
(tem-az'a-pam)
Restoril, Temazepam
Func. class.: Sedative/hypnotic
Chem. class.: Benzodiazepine, short-intermediate acting

Pregnancy category X

Controlled substance schedule IV (USA), schedule F (Canada)

Action: Produces CNS depression at limbic, thalamic, hypothalamic levels of the CNS; may be mediated by neurotransmitter γ-aminobutyric acid (GABA); results are sedation, hypnosis, skeletal muscle relaxation, anticonvulsant activity, anxiolytic action

Therapeutic outcome: Decreased insomnia

Uses: Insomnia

Dosage and routes
Adult: PO 7.5-30 mg at bedtime
Geriatric: PO 7.5 mg at bedtime

Available forms: Caps 7.5, 15, 22.5, 30 mg

Adverse effects
CNS: Lethargy, drowsiness, daytime sedation, dizziness, confusion, light-headedness, headache, anxiety, irritability, complex sleep-related reactions (sleep driving, sleep eating), fatigue
CV: Chest pain, pulse changes, hypotension
EENT: Blurred vision
GI: Nausea, vomiting, diarrhea, heartburn, abdominal pain, constipation, anorexia

---

HEMA: Leukopenia, granulocytopenia (rare)
SYST: Severe allergic reactions

Contraindications: Pregnancy **X**, breast-feeding, hypersensitivity to benzodiazepines, intermittent porphyria

Precautions: Children <15 yr, geriatric, anemia, pulmonary/renal/hepatic disease, suicidal individuals, product abuse, psychosis, acute closed-angle glaucoma, seizure disorders, angioedema, sleep-related behaviors (sleep walking), pulmonary disease

Pharmacokinetics

Absorption	Well absorbed
Distribution	Widely distributed, crosses placenta, crosses blood-brain barrier
Metabolism	Liver
Excretion	Kidneys, breast milk
Half-life	10-20 hr

Pharmacodynamics

Onset	½ hr
Peak	2-3 hr
Duration	6-8 hr

Interactions
Individual drugs
Alcohol: increased actions of both products
Cimetidine, disulfiram: increased effect of each specific product
Rifampin: decreased action of rifampin
Theophylline: decreased effects of theophylline
Drug classifications
Antacids: decreased effect of antacids
Contraceptives (oral): increased effect
CNS depressants: increased action of both products
Drug/herb
Black cohosh: increased hypotension
Catnip, chamomile, clary, cowslip, hops, kava, lavender, mistletoe, nettle, pokeweed, poppy, Queen Anne's lace, senega, skullcap, valerian: increased CNS depression
Drug/lab test
Increased: AST/ALT, serum bilirubin
Decreased: radioactive iodine uptake
False increase: 17-OHCS

NURSING CONSIDERATIONS
Assessment
• Assess mental status: mood, sensorium, anxiety, affect, sleeping pattern, drowsiness, dizziness, especially geriatric; physical dependency, withdrawal symptoms: anxiety, panic attacks, agitation, seizures, headache, nausea, vomiting, muscle pain, weakness; suicidal tendencies; for indications of increasing tolerance and abuse
• Monitor B/P (lying, standing), pulse; if systolic B/P drops 20 mm Hg, hold product, notify prescriber
• Monitor blood studies: CBC during long-term therapy; blood dyscrasias have occurred rarely; decreased hematocrit, neutropenia may occur
• Monitor hepatic studies: AST, ALT, bilirubin, creatinine LDH, alkaline phosphatase
• Monitor I&O ratio; indicate renal dysfunction

Nursing diagnoses
• Anxiety (uses)
• Injury, risk for (adverse reactions)
• Knowledge, deficient (teaching)

Implementation
• Give with food or milk to decrease GI symptoms; if patient is unable to swallow medication whole, tab may be crushed and mixed with foods or fluids
• Give sugarless gum, hard candy, frequent sips of water for dry mouth

Patient/family education
• Inform patient that product may be taken with food, and that tab may be crushed or swallowed whole
• Advise patient not to use for everyday stress or longer than 3 mo unless directed by prescriber; not to take more than prescribed amount; may be habit forming; not to double or skip doses
• Caution patient to avoid OTC preparations unless approved by prescriber; alcohol and CNS depressants will increase CNS depression
• Advise patient to avoid driving, activities that require alertness, because drowsiness may occur; to avoid alcohol ingestion or other psychotropic medications; to rise slowly or fainting may occur, especially in geriatric; that drowsiness may worsen at beginning of treatment
• Caution patient not to discontinue medication abruptly after long-term use; withdrawal symptoms include vomiting, cramping, tremors, seizures
• Advise patient to use contraception while taking this product
• Advise patient that complex sleep-related behaviors may occur (sleep driving/eating)
• Teach patient to limit to 7-10 days continuous use

Evaluation
Positive therapeutic outcome
• Decreased anxiety, restlessness, sleeplessness (short-term treatment only)

Treatment of overdose: Lavage, VS, supportive care

---

temozolomide (Rx)
(tem-oo-zole'oo-mide)

Temodar
Func. class.: Antineoplastic alkylating agents
Chem. class.: Imidazotetrazine derivative

Pregnancy category D

Action: A proproduct that undergoes conversion to 5-(3-methyl-1-triazeno) imidazole-4-carboxamide (MTIC); MTIC action prevents DNA transcription

Therapeutic outcome: Prevention of rapidly growing malignant cells

Uses: Anaplastic astrocytoma with relapse, glioblastoma multiforme, malignant glioma

Unlabeled uses: Metastatic melanoma

Dosage and routes
Anaplastic astrocytoma
Adult: PO adjust dose based on nadir neutrophil and platelet counts 150 mg/m^2/day × 5 days during 28-day cycle

Glioblastoma multiforme
Adult: PO/**IV** 75 mg/m^2/day × 42 days with focal radiotherapy, then maintenance of 6 cycles

Malignant glioma
Adult: 150 mg/m^2/day over 90 min day 1-5, q28day; may increase to 200 mg/m^2/day on day 1-5, q28day if hematologic parameters permit

Available forms: Caps 5, 20, 100, 140, 180, 250 mg; powder for inj 100 mg

Adverse effects
CNS: **Seizures,** *hemiparesis, dizziness, poor coordination, amnesia, insomnia, paresthesia, somnolence, paresis, ataxia, anxiety, dysphagia, depression, confusion*
GI: *Nausea, anorexia, vomiting,* abdominal pain, constipation
GU: *Urinary incontinence, UTI, frequency*
HEMA: **Thrombocytopenia, leukopenia,** anemia, **myelosuppression, neutropenia**
INTEG: *Rash, pruritus*
MISC: *Headache, fatigue, asthenia, fever, edema, back pain, weight increase, diplopia*
RESP: *Upper respiratory tract infection, pharyngitis, sinusitis, coughing*
SYST: **Anaphylaxis, secondary malignancy**

Contraindications: Pregnancy **D,** breastfeeding, hypersensitivity to this product, carbazine, or gelatin

Precautions: Radiation therapy, renal/hepatic disease, bone marrow suppression, infection, geriatric, myelosuppression

Pharmacokinetics

Absorption	Rapid, complete
Distribution	Crosses blood-brain barrier
Metabolism	To MTIC and metabolite
Excretion	Urine, feces
Half-life	1.8 hr

Pharmacodynamics

Onset	Unknown
Peak	1 hr
Duration	Unknown

Interactions
Individual drugs
Digoxin: decreased action of digoxin
Filgrastim, G-CSF, pegfilgrastim, sargramostim: do not use within 24 hr of these products
Radiation: increased toxicity, bone marrow suppression
Drug classifications
Anticoagulants, NSAIDs, platelet inhibitors, thrombolytics: increased bleeding risk
Antineoplastics, bone marrow–suppressing products: increased bone marrow suppression
Live virus vaccines, toxoids: increased adverse reactions, decreased antibody reaction

NURSING CONSIDERATIONS
Assessment
• Assess symptoms indicating severe allergic reaction: rash, pruritus, urticaria, purpuric skin lesions, itching, flushing; product should be discontinued
• Assess tumor response during treatment
• Obtain CBC on day 22 (21 days after 1st dose), CBC weekly until recovery if ANC is <1.5 × 10^9/L and platelets <100 × 10^9/L, do not administer to patients that do not tolerate 100 mg/m^2; myelosuppression usually occurs late in the treatment cycle
• Assess for seizures, mental status throughout treatment
• Monitor renal function studies: BUN, creatinine, urine CCr before, during therapy; I&O ratio; report fall in urine output to <30 ml/hr
• Monitor temp q4hr (may indicate beginning of infection)

- Monitor liver function tests before, during therapy (bilirubin, AST, ALT, LDH) as needed or monthly; note jaundice of skin or sclera, dark urine, clay-colored stools, itchy skin, abdominal pain, fever, diarrhea; hepatotoxicity can be serious and fatal
- Assess for bleeding: hematuria, stool guaiac, bruising or petechiae, mucosa or orifices; check for inflammation of mucosa, breaks in skin

Nursing diagnoses
- Body image, disturbed (adverse reactions)
- Infection, risk for (adverse reactions)
- Injury, risk for (adverse reactions)
- Knowledge, deficient (teaching)

Implementation
PO route
- Give fluids **IV** or PO before chemotherapy to hydrate patient
- Give antiemetic 30-60 min before giving product to prevent vomiting, and prn; antibiotics for prophylaxis of infection
- Provide liquid diet: carbonated beverages; gelatin may be added if patient is not nauseated or vomiting
- Capsules should not be opened; if accidentally damaged, do not allow contact with skin, or inhale; take caps one at a time with 8 oz of water at the same time of day; use cytotic handling procedure
- Give on empty stomach at bedtime to prevent nausea/vomiting
IV route
- Bring vial to room temperature
- Inject sterile water for inj into vial (2.5 mg/ml)
- Gently swirl, do not shake
Intermittent IV infusion
- Withdraw up to 40 ml from each vial to make total dose and transfer to empty 250 ml PVC inf bag, flush before and after inf
- Run over 90 min
- Use reconstituted sol within 14 hr including inf time

Patient/family education
- Teach patient to avoid use of products containing aspirin or NSAIDs, razors, commercial mouthwash, since bleeding may occur; to report symptoms of bleeding (hematuria, tarry stools)
- Instruct patient to report signs of anemia (fatigue, headache, irritability, faintness, shortness of breath)
- Caution patient not to have any vaccinations without the advice of prescriber; serious reactions can occur

- Advise patient contraception is needed during treatment and for several months after completion of therapy; product has teratogenic properties

Evaluation
Positive therapeutic outcome
- Prevention of rapid division of malignant cells

temsirolimus (Rx)
(tem-sir-oh'li-mus)
Torisel
Func. class.: Biologic response modifier
Chem. class.: Kinase inhibitor, mTOR antagonist
Pregnancy category D

Action: Inhibits mammalian target of rapamycin (mTOR), a protein kinase

Therapeutic outcome: Decreased time of progression of renal cell carcinoma

Uses: Renal cell carcinoma

Dosage and routes
Adult: IV 25 mg over 30-60 min qwk; treat until disease progression or severe toxicity occurs

Available forms: 25 mg/ml sol for inj kit

Adverse effects
CNS: Headache, **seizures**
CV: Hypertension, **thrombophlebitis**
ENDO: Hypertriglyceridemia, hyperlipidemia, hyperglycemia
GI: Nausea, vomiting, diarrhea, constipation, **bowel perforation**
GU: UTIs, **albuminuria, hematuria, proteinuria, renal failure,** mucositis
HEMA: **Anemia, leukopenia, thrombocytopenia**
INTEG: Rash, pruritus
META: Metabolic acidosis, hyperglycemia, hyperlipidemia
RESP: **Interstitial lung disease**
SYST: **Lymphoma**

Contraindications: Pregnancy **D,** breastfeeding, hypersensitivity to this product or to sirolimus, polysorbate 80

Precautions: Children <13 yr, females, severe pulmonary/renal/hepatic disease, diabetes mellitus, hyperkalemia, hyperuricemia, hypertension, bone marrow suppression, hypertriglyceridemia/hyperlipidemia, surgery, brain tumors

T

Adverse effects: *italic* = common, **bold** = life-threatening

Pharmacokinetics

Absorption	Rapidly
Distribution	Unknown
Metabolism	Extensively via liver by P450 3A4
Excretion	Eliminated via feces
Half-life	Unknown

Pharmacodynamics

Onset	Unknown
Peak	0.5-2 hr
Duration	Unknown

Interactions
Individual drugs
Bromocriptine, cimetidine, clarithromycin, cycloSPORINE, danazol, erythromycin, metoclopramide: increased blood levels

Carbamazepine, dexamethasone, phenobarbital, phenytoin, rifamycin, rifapentine: decreased blood levels

Sunitinib: increased toxicity

Drug classifications
Antifungals, benzodiazepines, calcium channel blockers, CYP3A4 inhibitors, HIV-protease inhibitors, HMG-CoA reductase inhibitors: increased blood levels

CYP3A4 inducers: decreased blood levels

Vaccines: decreased effect of vaccines

Drug/herb
Astragalus, echinacea, melatonin: decreased immunosuppression

Ginseng, maitake, mistletoe: increased effect

St. John's wort: may decrease the effect of sirolimus

Drug/food
Alters bioavailability; use consistently with or without food; do not use with grapefruit juice

NURSING CONSIDERATIONS
Assessment
• Assess cardiac status: B/P, heart rate
• Assess for interstitial lung disease
• Assess for hypersensitive reactions: anaphylaxis
• Monitor lipid profile: cholesterol, triglycerides, a lipid-lowering agent may be needed; blood glucose
◆ Assess for infection and development of lymphoma
◆ Monitor blood tests: Hgb, WBC, platelets during treatment qmo
• Monitor renal function tests: BUN, creatinine, phosphate potassium; proteinuria, hematuria, albuminemia may indicate renal failure

Nursing diagnoses
• Injury, risk for (uses, adverse reactions)
• Knowledge, deficient (teaching)

Implementation
• Premedicate with 25-50 mg diphenhydramine **IV** 30 min before dose; if reaction occurs, stop for ½-1 hr; may resume at slower rate
• Use in-line filter ≤5 microns and inf pump; inf over 30-60 min; complete inf within 6 hr
• Dilute product with 1.8 ml of provided diluent; the result is 3 ml (10 mg/ml); invert to mix well; withdraw the required amount and inject rapidly into 250 ml of NS; do not use PVC infusion bags/sets
• Protect from light during preparation; use only glass

Patient/family education
• Advise patient to report fever, rash, severe diarrhea, chills, sore throat, fatigue; serious infections may occur; clay-colored stools, cramping (hepatotoxicity)
• Advise patient to avoid crowds, persons with known infections to reduce risk of infection
• Teach patient to use contraception before, during, and 12 wk after product has been discontinued; avoid breastfeeding; men should also use reliable contraception during and 12 wk after cessation of product
• Advise to report excessive thirst, urinary frequency, new or worsening breathing problems, blood in stool, abdominal pain

Evaluation
Positive therapeutic outcome
• Decreased time of progression of renal cell carcinoma

! HIGH ALERT

tenecteplase (Rx)
(ten-ek'ta-place)
TNKase
Func. class.: Thrombolytic enzyme
Chem. class.: Tissue plasminogen activator

Pregnancy category C

Action: Activates conversion of plasminogen to plasmin (fibrinolysin): plasmin breaks down clots (fibrin), fibrinogen, factors V, VII; occlusion of venous access lines

Therapeutic outcome: Resolution of MI

Uses: Acute MI

Dosage and routes
Adult <60 kg: **IV** BOL 30 mg, give over 5 sec

Adult 60-70 kg: **IV** BOL 35 mg, give over 5 sec
Adult 70-80 kg: **IV** BOL 40 mg, give over 5 sec
Adult 80-90 kg: **IV** BOL 45 mg, give over 5 sec
Adult ≥90 kg: **IV** BOL 50 mg, give over 5 sec

Available forms: Powder for inj, lyophilized 50 mg

Adverse effects
CV: Dysrhythmias, hypotension, pulmonary edema, **PE, cardiogenic shock, cardiac arrest, heart failure, myocardial reinfarction, myocardial rupture, tamponade, pericarditis, pericardial effusion, thrombosis,** CVA
HEMA: Decreased Hct, **bleeding**
INTEG: Rash, urticaria, phlebitis at **IV** inf site, itching, flushing
SYST: **GI, GU, intracranial, retroperitoneal bleeding, surface bleeding, anaphylaxis**

Contraindications: Hypersensitivity, arteriovenous malformation, aneurysm, active bleeding, intracranial, intraspinal surgery, CNS neoplasms, severe hypertension, severe renal disease, hepatic disease, history of CVA, increased ICP, stroke

Precautions: Pregnancy **C,** breastfeeding, children, geriatric, arterial emboli from left side of heart, hypocoagulation, COPD, subacute bacterial endocarditis, rheumatic valvular disease, cerebral embolism/thrombosis/hemorrhage, intraarterial diagnostic procedure or surgery (10 days), recent major surgery, dysrhythmias, hypertension

Pharmacokinetics

Absorption	Unknown
Distribution	Unknown
Metabolism	Liver
Excretion	Unknown
Half-life	20-24 min

Pharmacodynamics

Onset	Immediate
Peak	Unknown
Duration	Unknown

Interactions
Individual drugs
Aspirin, cefamandole, cefoperazone, cefotetan, clopidogrel, dipyridamole, indomethacin, phenylbutazone, ticlopidine: increased bleeding potential

Drug classifications
Anticoagulants, antithrombolytics, glycoprotein IIb, IIIa inhibitors, NSAIDs: increased bleeding potential
Drug/herb
Agrimony, alfalfa, angelica, anise, basil, bay, bilberry, black haw, bogbean, bromelain, buchu, chondroitin, cinchona bark, dong quai, fenugreek, feverfew, garlic, ginger, ginkgo, ginseng, horse chestnut, Irish moss, kelp, kelpware, khella, lovage, lungwort, meadowsweet, motherwort, mugwort, nettle, papaya, parsley (large amounts), pau d'arco, pineapple, poplar, prickly ash, safflower, saw palmetto, tonka bean, turmeric, wintergreen, yarrow: increased risk of bleeding
Chamomile, coenzyme Q10, flax, glucomannan, goldenseal, guar gum: decreased anticoagulant effect
Drug/lab test
Increased: pro-time, APTT, TT
Decreased: plasminogen, fibrinogen

NURSING CONSIDERATIONS
Assessment
• Assess for allergy: fever, rash, itching, chills; mild reaction may be treated with antihistamines
⬥Assess for bleeding during 1st hr of treatment; hematuria, hematemesis, bleeding from mucous membranes, epistaxis, ecchymosis; may require transfusion (rare), continue to assess for bleeding for 24 hr
• Monitor blood tests (Hct, platelets, PTT, pro-time, TT, APTT) before starting therapy; protime or APTT must be less than 2 × control before starting therapy; PTT or pro-time q3-4hr during treatment
• Assess for hypersensitive reactions: fever, rash, dyspnea; product should be discontinued
• Monitor VS, B/P, pulse, respirations, neurologic signs, temp at least q4hr; temp >104° F (40° C) indicates internal bleeding; systolic pressure increase >25 mm Hg should be reported to prescriber
⬥Assess for neurologic changes that may indicate intracranial bleeding
⬥Assess for retroperitoneal bleeding: back pain, leg weakness, diminished pulses

Nursing diagnoses
• Cardiac output, decreased (uses)
• Knowledge, deficient (teaching)

Implementation
IV route
• Give as soon as thrombi identified; not useful for thrombi >1 wk old

Adverse effects: *italic* = common, **bold** = life-threatening

- Administer cryoprecipitate or fresh frozen plasma if bleeding occurs
- Give heparin after fibrinogen level >100 mg/dl; heparin inf to increase PTT to 1.5-2 × baseline for 3-7 days; **IV** heparin with loading dose is recommended
- Aseptically withdraw 10 ml of sterile H₂O for inj from diluent vial, use red cannula syringe-filling device, inject all contents of syringe into product vial, direct into powder, swirl, with-draw correct dose, discard any unused solution; stand the shield with dose vertically on flat surface and passively recap the red cannula; remove entire shield assembly by twisting counterclockwise; give by **IV** bol
- **IV** therapy: use upper extremity vessel that is accessible to manual compression
- Provide bed rest during entire course of treatment
- Avoid venous or arterial puncture, inj, rectal temp, any invasive treatment
- Treat fever with acetaminophen or aspirin
- Apply pressure for 30 sec to minor bleeding sites; inform prescriber if this does not attain hemostasis; apply pressure dressing

Evaluation
Positive therapeutic outcome
- Resolution of myocardial infarction

---

tenofovir (Rx)
(ten-oh-foh′veer)
Viread
Func. class.: Antiretroviral
Chem. class.: Nucleoside analog reverse transcriptase inhibitor

Pregnancy category B

Action: Inhibits replication of HIV-1 virus by competing with the natural substrate and then incorporating into cellular DNA by viral reverse transcriptase, thereby terminating cellular DNA chain

Therapeutic outcome: Improved symptoms of HIV-1 infection

Uses: HIV-1 infection with other antiretrovirals, hepatitis B

Dosage and routes
Adult: PO 300 mg with meal; if used with didanosine, give tenofovir 2 hr before or 1 hr after didanosine

Renal dose
CCr 30-49 ml/min 300 mg q48hr
CCr 10-29 ml/min 300 mg 2 ×/wk
CCr <10 ml/min not recommended

Available forms: Tabs 300 mg (300 mg of fumarate salt equivalent to 245 mg tenofovir disoproxil)

Adverse effects
CNS: Headache, asthenia
GI: Nausea, vomiting, diarrhea, anorexia, *flatulence, abdominal pain,* **pancreatitis**
GU: **Renal failure, renal tubular acidosis/ necrosis, Fanconi syndrome**
HEMA: **Neutropenia, osteopenia**
INTEG: Rash, **angioedema**
META: **Lactic acidosis,** hypokalemia, hypo-phosphatemia
MS: Myopathy, **rhabdomyolysis**
SYST: Lipodystrophy

Contraindications: Hypersensitivity

Black Box Warning: Lactic acidosis

Precautions: Pregnancy **B**, breastfeeding, children, geriatric, renal disease, hepatic insufficiency, CCr <60 ml/min, osteoporosis, immune reconstitution syndrome

Black Box Warning: Hepatic disease, hepatitis

Pharmacokinetics
Absorption	Rapidly absorbed
Distribution	Extravascular space; bound to serum plasma <0.7%, to serum proteins <7.2%
Metabolism	Unknown
Excretion	Urine, unchanged (70%-80%)
Half-life	Terminal 17 hr

Pharmacodynamics
Onset	Unknown
Peak	0.6-1.4 hr
Duration	Unknown

Interactions
Individual drugs
Acyclovir, cidofovir, ganciclovir, valacyclovir, valganciclovir: increased level of tenofovir
Didanosine: increased level of didanosine when coadministered with tenofovir
Drug classifications
Increased: levels of tenofovir with any product that decreased renal function

NURSING CONSIDERATIONS
Assessment
- Monitor viral load, CD4+ T cell count, plasma HIV RNA, serum creatinine/BUN/ phosphate
- Resistance testing at start of therapy and at treatment failure

 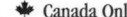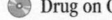

- Assess liver function tests: AST, ALT, bilirubin; amylase, lipase, triglycerides periodically during treatment
- Assess for bone, renal toxicity: if bone abnormalities are suspected, obtain tests: serum phosphorus, creatinine
- Assess for lactic acidosis, severe hepatomegaly with steatosis

Nursing diagnoses
- Infection, risk for (uses)
- Injury, risk for (adverse reactions)
- Knowledge, deficient (teaching)

Implementation
- Administer PO daily with meal
- Store at 25° C (77° F)
- Give product 2 hr before or 1 hr after taking didanosine (if used)

Patient/family education
- Instruct patient to take this product 2 hr before or 1 hr after taking didanosine (if used)
- Instruct patient to take product with meal
- Advise patients that GI complaints resolve after 3-4 wk of treatment
- Caution patient not to breastfeed while taking this product
- Inform patient that product must be taken daily even if patient feels better
- Advise patient to continue follow-up visits since serious toxicity may occur; blood counts must be done q2wk
- Inform patient that product will control symptoms but is not a cure for HIV; patient is still infectious, may pass HIV virus on to others
- Advise patient that other products may be necessary to prevent other infections
- Advise patient that changes in body fat distribution may occur

Evaluation
Positive therapeutic outcome
- Decrease in signs/symptoms of HIV

---

terazosin (Rx)
(ter-ay'zoe-sin)
Hytrin
Func. class.: Antihypertensive
Chem. class.: α-Adrenergic blocker
(peripherally acting)

Pregnancy category C

Action: Peripheral blood vessels are dilated, peripheral resistance lowered; reduction in blood pressure results from α-adrenergic receptors being blocked

Therapeutic outcome: Decreased B/P in hypertension, decreased symptoms of benign prostatic hyperplasia (BPH)

Uses: Hypertension, as a single agent or in combination with diuretics or β-blockers, BPH

Dosage and routes
Hypertension
Adult: PO 1 mg at bedtime, may increase doses slowly to desired response; max 20 mg/day

Benign prostatic hyperplasia
Adult: PO 1 mg at bedtime, gradually increase up to 5-10 mg, max 20 mg

Available forms: Caps 1, 2, 5, 10 mg

Adverse effects
CNS: Dizziness, headache, drowsiness, anxiety, depression, vertigo, weakness, fatigue
CV: Palpitations, orthostatic hypotension, tachycardia, edema, rebound hypertension
EENT: Blurred vision, epistaxis, tinnitus, dry mouth, red sclera, nasal congestion, sinusitis
GI: Nausea, vomiting, diarrhea, constipation, abdominal pain
GU: Urinary frequency, incontinence, impotence, priapism
RESP: Dyspnea, cough, pharyngitis

Contraindications: Hypersensitivity

Precautions: Pregnancy C, breastfeeding, children, prostate cancer

Pharmacokinetics	
Absorption	Well absorbed
Distribution	Not known
Metabolism	Liver (50%)
Excretion	Kidneys unchanged (10%), feces unchanged (20%)
Half-life	9-12 hr

Pharmacodynamics	
Onset	15 min
Peak	1 hr
Duration	24 hr

Interactions
Individual drugs
Alcohol, nitroglycerin, verapamil: increased hypotensive effects
Drug classifications
Antihypertensives (other): increased hypotension
β-Blockers: increased hypotensive effects
Estrogens, NSAIDs, salicylates, sympathomimetics: decreased antihypertensive effect

Adverse effects: *italic* = common, **bold** = life-threatening

NURSING CONSIDERATIONS
Assessment
- Monitor B/P, orthostatic hypotension, syncope; check for edema in feet, legs daily; I&O ratio; weight daily; notify prescriber of changes
- Assess for allergic reactions: rash, fever, pruritus, urticaria; product should be discontinued if antihistamines fail to help

Nursing diagnoses
- Cardiac output, decreased (uses)
- Injury, risk for (adverse reactions)
- Knowledge, deficient (teaching)
- Noncompliance (teaching)

Implementation
- May be used in combination with other antihypertensives
- Give at same time each day
- May be given with food to prevent GI symptoms
- Store in airtight container at 86° F (30° C) or less

Patient/family education
- Caution patient not to discontinue product abruptly; the importance of complying with dosage schedule, even if feeling better; if dose is missed take as soon as remembered; take medication at same time each day
- Teach patient not to use OTC products (cough, cold, allergy) unless directed by prescriber; also to avoid large amounts of caffeine
- Emphasize the need to rise slowly to sitting or standing position to minimize orthostatic hypotension
- Teach patient to notify prescriber of mouth sores, sore throat, fever, swelling of hands or feet, irregular heartbeat, chest pain
- Caution patient to report excessive perspiration, dehydration, vomiting, diarrhea; may lead to fall in B/P
- Caution patient that product may cause dizziness, fainting, light-headedness; may occur during 1st few days of therapy; to avoid hazardous activities
- Teach patient how to take B/P, and normal readings for age group; to take B/P q7day

Evaluation
Positive therapeutic outcome
- Decreased B/P in hypertension
- Decreased symptoms of BPH

Treatment of overdose: Administer volume expanders or vasopressors; discontinue product; place patient in supine position

terbinafine (Rx)
(ter-bin'a-feen)
Lamisil
Func. class.: Antifungal, systemic
Chem. class.: Synthetic allylamine derivative

Pregnancy category B

Do not confuse:
Lamisil/lamotrigine

Action: Interferes with cell membrane permeability in fungi such as *Trichophyton rubrum, Trichophyton mentagrophytes, Trichophyton tonsurans, Epidermophyton floccosum, Microsporum canis, Microsporum audouinii, Microsporum gypseum, Candida,* broad-spectrum antifungal

Therapeutic outcome: Resolution of fungal infection

Uses: Onychomycosis of the toenail or fingernail due to dermatophytes

Unlabeled uses: Cutaneous candidiasis, tinea versicolor

Dosage and routes
Fingernail: PO 250 mg/day × 6 wk
Toenail: PO 250 mg/day × 12 wk

Available forms: Tabs 250 mg

Adverse effects
GI: Diarrhea, dyspepsia, abdominal pain, nausea, hepatitis
HEMA: **Neutropenia**
INTEG: Rash, pruritus, urticaria, **Stevens-Johnson syndrome**
MISC: Headache, hepatic enzyme changes, taste, visual disturbance

Contraindications: Hypersensitivity, chronic/active renal/hepatic disease GFR ≤50 mg/min

Precautions: Pregnancy **B,** breastfeeding, children, renal disease

Pharmacokinetics
Absorption	80%
Distribution	Extensive, most to hair, scalp, nails; excreted in breast milk; protein binding 99%
Metabolism	Liver, extensively
Excretion	Unknown
Half-life	22 days or longer

Pharmacodynamics
Onset	Up to 1 wk
Peak	Several days-weeks
Duration	Several weeks

Interactions
Individual drugs
Cimetidine: increased effect
CycloSPORINE: increased cycloSPORINE clearance
Dextromethorphan: increased levels
Rifampin: increased terbinafine clearance
Drug/herb
Cola nut, guarana, yerba maté, tea (black, green), coffee: side effects

NURSING CONSIDERATIONS
Assessment
- Assess hepatic studies (ALT, AST) prior to beginning treatment; do not use in presence of hepatic disease
- Monitor CBC in treatment >6 wk
- Assess for continuing infection

Nursing diagnoses
- Infection, risk for (uses)
- Knowledge, deficient (teaching)
- Noncompliance (teaching)

Patient/family education
- Teach patient to notify prescriber of nausea, vomiting, fatigue, jaundice, dark urine, clay-colored stool, RUQ pain, that may indicate hepatic dysfunction
- Teach patient to avoid using OTC medication unless approved by prescriber

Evaluation
Positive therapeutic outcome
- Decrease in size, number of lesions

---

terbinafine topical
See Appendix B

---

terbutaline (Rx)
(ter-byoo'te-leen)
Brethine, Bricanye ✦
Func. class.: Selective β$_2$-agonist; broncho-dilator
Chem. class.: Catecholamine

Pregnancy category B

Action: Relaxes bronchial smooth muscle by direct action on β$_2$-adrenergic receptors through accumulation of cAMP at β-adrenergic receptor sites; results are bronchodilatation, diuresis, and CNS and cardiac stimulation; relaxes uterine smooth muscle

Therapeutic outcome: Bronchodilatation with ease of breathing

Uses: Bronchospasm, hyperkalemia

Unlabeled uses: Premature labor

Dosage and routes
Bronchospasm
Adult and child >12 yr: PO 2.5-5 mg q8hr; SUBCUT 0.25 mg q15-30min, max 0.5 mg in 4 hr

Bronchodilatation
Adult and child >15 yr: PO 2.5-5 mg q6hr during day, max 15 mg/24 hr
Child 12-15 yr: PO 2.5 mg tid q6hr

Renal dose
Adult: PO CCr 10-50 ml/min 50% of dose; CCr <10 ml/min avoid use

Severe renal failure
Adult: PO avoid if GFR <10 ml/min

Tocolytic (preterm labor) (unlabeled)
Adult: PO 2.5 mg q4-6hr until delivery

Available forms: Tabs 2.5, 5 mg; inj 1 mg/ml

Adverse effects
CNS: Tremors, anxiety, insomnia, headache, dizziness, stimulation
CV: Palpitations, tachycardia, hypertension, dysrhythmias, **cardiac arrest**
GI: Nausea, vomiting

Contraindications: Hypersensitivity to sympathomimetics; closed-angle glaucoma, tachydysrhythmias

Precautions: Pregnancy **B**, breastfeeding, geriatric, cardiac disorders, hyperthyroidism, diabetes mellitus, prostatic hypertension, hypertension, seizure disorder

Pharmacokinetics

Absorption	Well absorbed (SUBCUT), partially absorbed (PO)
Distribution	Unknown
Metabolism	Liver, partially
Excretion	Unknown
Half-life	Unknown

Pharmacodynamics

	PO	INH	SUBCUT	IV
Onset	½ hr	5-15 min	10-15 min	Rapid
Peak	1-2 hr	1-2 hr	½-1 hr	Unknown
Duration	4-8 hr	4-6 hr	1½-4 hr	Unknown

Interactions
Individual drugs
Bleomycin: products are incompatible
Drug classifications
β-Adrenergic blockers: block therapeutic effect
MAOIs: increased chance of hypertensive crisis

Adverse effects: *italic* = common, **bold** = life-threatening

Sympathomimetics: increased effects of both products

Drug/herb

Green tea (large amounts), guarana: increased effect

NURSING CONSIDERATIONS
Assessment

• Monitor respiratory function: vital capacity, FEV, ABGs, lung sounds, heart rate, rhythm (baseline)
• Determine that patient has not received theophylline therapy before giving dose; assess client's ability to self-medicate
• Monitor for evidence of allergic reactions; withhold dose and notify prescriber
• Assess for paradoxical bronchospasm: dyspnea, wheezing; keep emergency resuscitative equipment nearby
• Assess for labor: maternal heart rate, B/P, contractions, fetal heart rate

Nursing diagnoses

• Airway clearance, ineffective (uses)
• Gas exchange, impaired (uses)
• Knowledge, deficient (teaching)
• Noncompliance (teaching)

Implementation

• Use this medication before other medications and allow 5 min between each to prevent overstimulation

PO route

• Give PO with meals to decrease gastric irritation; tab may be crushed and mixed with foods and fluids

SUBCUT route

• May give by SUBCUT route; do not give by IM route

Aerosol route

• Give after shaking; ask patient to exhale, place mouthpiece in mouth, then inhale slowly; hold breath, remove, exhale slowly; allow at least 1 min between inhalations
• Store in light-resistant container, do not expose to temperatures over 86° F (30° C)

IV route

• Give at 5 mcg q10min until contractions are stopped; use inf pump for correct dose; after ½-1 hr with no contraction decrease dose by 5 mcg; switch to PO dose when possible

Syringe compatibilities: Doxapram
Y-site compatibilities: Regular insulin
Additive compatibilities: Aminophylline
Additive incompatibilities: Bleomycin

Patient/family education

• Advise patient not to use OTC medications; extra stimulation may occur; to use this medication before other medications and allow at least 5 min between each to prevent overstimulation
• Teach patient how to use inhaler; to avoid getting aerosol in eyes because blurring may result; to wash inhaler in warm water daily and dry; to avoid smoking, smoke-filled rooms, persons with respiratory infections; review package insert with patient
• Teach patient that paradoxical bronchospasm may occur; to stop product immediately and notify prescriber; to limit caffeine products such as chocolate, coffee, tea, and colas
• Instruct patient on administration of dose, not to use more than prescribed; serious side effects may occur; if taking PO regularly and dose is missed, take when remembered; space other doses on new time schedule

Evaluation
Positive therapeutic outcome

• Absence of dyspnea, wheezing after 1 hr
• Improved airway exchange
• Improved ABGs

Treatment of overdose: Administer a β_2-adrenergic blocker

---

terconazole vaginal antifungal
See Appendix B

---

teriparatide (Rx)
(tah-ree-par'ah-tide)
Forteo
Func. class.: Parathyroid hormone (rDNA)

Pregnancy category C

Action: Contains human recombinant parathyroid hormone, which stimulates new bone growth

Therapeutic outcome: Calcium levels at 9-10 mg/dl, decreased symptoms of hypocalcemia, hypoparathyroidism

Uses: Postmenopausal women with osteoporosis, men with primary or hypogonadal osteoporosis who are at high risk for fracture, glucocorticoid-induced osteoporosis

Dosage and routes
Adult: SUBCUT 20 mcg/day up to 2 yr

Available forms: Prefilled pen delivery device (delivers 20 mcg/day)

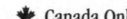

Adverse effects
CNS: Dizziness, headache, insomnia, depression, vertigo
CV: Hypertension, angina, syncope
GI: Nausea, diarrhea, dyspepsia, vomiting, constipation
INTEG: Rash, sweating
MISC: Pain, asthenia, hyperuricemia
MS: Arthralgia, leg cramps, back/leg pain, weakness, **osteosarcoma (rare)**
RESP: Rhinitis, cough, pharyngitis, pneumonia, dyspnea

Contraindications: Hypersensitivity, increased baseline risk of osteosarcoma (Paget's disease, open epiphyses, previous bone radiation), bone metastases, history of skeletal malignancies, other metabolic bone diseases, preexisting hypercalcemia

Precautions: Pregnancy **C,** breastfeeding, children, urolithiasis, hypotension, use >2 yr

Black Box Warning: Secondary malignancy

Pharmacokinetics
Absorption	Extensively, rapidly
Distribution	Unknown
Metabolism	Liver
Excretion	Kidneys
Half life	Unknown

Pharmacodynamics
Unknown

Interactions
Individual drug
Digoxin: increased digoxin toxicity
Drug/lab test
Calcium: increased levels

NURSING CONSIDERATIONS
Assessment
• Monitor uric acid, chloride, magnesium, electrolytes, urine pH, vit D, phosphate for normal serum levels; serum calcium may be transiently increased after dosing (max at 4-6 hr post-dose)
• Assess for bone pain, headache, fatigue, changes in LOC, leg cramps
• Monitor for signs of persistent hypercalcemia: nausea, vomiting, constipation, lethargy, muscle weakness
• Assess nutritional status: diet for sources of vit D (milk, some seafood), calcium (dairy products, dark green vegetables), phosphates (dairy products)

Nursing diagnoses
• Injury, risk for (uses)
• Knowledge, deficient (teaching)
• Mobility, impaired physical (uses)

Implementation
• Store refrigerated; do not freeze
SUBCUT route
• Give by SUBCUT only, rotate inj sites

Patient/family education
• Advise patient of the symptoms of hypercalcemia
• Teach about foods rich in calcium
• Teach how to use delivery device, dispose of needles, not to share pen with others
• Advise to sit or lie down if dizziness or fast heartbeat occurs after the first few doses

Evaluation
Positive therapeutic outcome
• Increased bone mineral density

testosterone ⊙ (Rx)
(tess-toss'te-rone)
testosterone, long acting (Rx)
testosterone enanthate (Rx)
Andro LA, Andropository, Andryl, Delatest, Delatestryl, Everone, Malog-x ✤, Testone LA, Testrin-PA
testosterone cypionate (Rx)
Andro-Cyp, Andronate, depAndro, Depotest, Depo-Testosterone, Dura-test, T-Cypionate, Testa-C, Testred, Testoject-LA, Virilon IM
testosterone pellets (Rx)
Testopel
testosterone transdermal (Rx)
Androderm, Androplex ✤, Testoderm, Testoderm TTS, Testoderm with Adhesive
testosterone gel (Rx)
AndroGel 1%, Testim
testosterone buccal (Rx)
Striant
Func. class.: Androgenic anabolic steroid
Chem. class.: Halogenated testosterone derivative

Pregnancy category X
Controlled substance schedule III

Action: Increases weight by building body tissue; increases potassium, phosphorus, chloride, nitrogen levels; increases bone development; responsible for maintenance of secondary sex characteristics (male)

Adverse effects: *italic* = common, **bold** = life-threatening

Therapeutic outcome: Increased hormone levels in eunuchoidism, decreased tumor growth in female breast cancer, onset of male puberty

Uses: Female breast cancer, hypogonadism, eunuchoidism, male climacteric, oligospermia, impotence, osteoporosis, weight loss in AIDS patients, vulvar dystrophies, low testosterone levels, delayed male puberty (inj)

Dosage and routes
Replacement
Adult: IM 25-50 mg 2-3 ×/wk (base or propionate) or 50-400 mg q2-4wk (enanthate or cypionate); transdermal (Testoderm) 4-6 mg applied q24hr; (Androderm, AndroGel) 5 mg applied q24hr; once daily (gel); BUCCAL 1 buccal system (30 mg) to the gum region q12hr before meals/PM

Adult (male) and child: SUBCUT (pellets) 150-450 mg (2-6 pellets) inserted q3-6mo

Breast cancer
Adult: IM 50-100 mg 3 ×/wk (propionate) or 200-400 mg q2-4wk (cypionate or enanthate)

Delayed male puberty
Child >12 yr: IM up to 100 mg/mo for up to 6 mo

Available forms: Enanthate: inj 200 mg/ml; cypionate: inj 100, 200 mg/ml; pellets 75 mg; transdermal 2.5, 4, 5, 6 mg/24 hr; gel 1% buccal system 30 mg

Adverse effects
CNS: Dizziness, headache, fatigue, tremors, paresthesias, flushing, sweating, anxiety, lability, insomnia, carpal tunnel syndrome
CV: Increased B/P
EENT: Conjunctival edema, nasal congestion
ENDO: Abnormal GTT
GI: Nausea, vomiting, constipation, weight gain, **cholestatic jaundice**
GU: Hematuria, amenorrhea, vaginitis, decreased libido, decreased breast size, clitoral hypertrophy, testicular atrophy, gynecomastia
HEMA: Polycythemia
INTEG: Rash, acneiform lesions, oily hair and skin, flushing, sweating, acne vulgaris, alopecia, hirsutism
MS: Cramps, spasms

Contraindications: Pregnancy **X**, breast-feeding, severe renal/cardiac/hepatic disease, hypersensitivity, genital bleeding (rare), male breast/prostate cancer

Precautions: Diabetes mellitus, CV disease, MI, urinary tract disorders, prostate cancer

Black Box Warning: Children, accidental exposure

Pharmacokinetics
Absorption	Well but slowly absorbed
Distribution	Crosses placenta
Metabolism	Liver
Excretion	Kidneys, breast milk
Half-life	8 days (cypionate)
	10-100 min (base)

Pharmacodynamics
	IM (base)	IM (cypionate)	IM (enanthate)	IM (propionate)
Onset	Unknown	Unknown	Unknown	Unknown
Peak	Unknown	Unknown	Unknown	Unknown
Duration	1-3 days	2-4 wk	2-4 wk	1-3 days

Interactions
Individual drugs
ACTH, buPROPion: increased edema
Insulin: decreased glucose levels may alter need for insulin
Oxyphenbutazone: increased effects of oxyphenbutazone
Drug classifications
Adrenal steroids: increased edema
Anticoagulants: increased pro-time
Antidiabetics, oral: decreased need for oral antidiabetics
Drug/lab test
Increased: serum cholesterol, blood glucose, urine glucose
Decreased: serum Ca, serum K, T_4, T_3, thyroid ^{131}I uptake test, urine 17-OHCS, 17-KS, PBI

NURSING CONSIDERATIONS
Assessment
• Monitor patient's weight daily; notify prescriber if weekly weight gain is >5 lb; assess I&O ratio; be alert for decreasing urinary output, increasing edema
• Monitor B/P q4hr, Hgb/Hct
• Assess growth rate, bone age in adolescent because growth rate may be uneven (linear/bone growth) if used for extended periods
• Monitor electrolytes: potassium, sodium, chloride, calcium; cholesterol
• Monitor liver function tests: ALT, AST, bilirubin
• Assess edema, hypertension, cardiac symptoms, jaundice
• Assess mental status: affect, mood, behavioral changes, aggression
• Assess signs of masculinization in female: increased libido, deepening of voice, de-

creased breast tissue, enlarged clitoris, menstrual irregularities; male: gynecomastia, impotence, testicular atrophy
• Assess hypercalcemia: lethargy, polyuria, polydipsia, nausea, vomiting, constipation; product may have to be decreased
• Assess hypoglycemia in diabetics because oral antidiabetic action is increased

Nursing diagnoses
• Infection, risk for (adverse reactions)
• Injury, risk for (adverse reactions)
• Knowledge, deficient (teaching)

Implementation
• Administer diet with increased calories, protein; decreased sodium if edema occurs
• Administer supportive product if anemia occurs
• Give titrated dose; use lowest effective dose
• Give IM inj deep into upper outer quadrant of gluteal muscle; route can be painful

Transdermal route
• Apply Testoderm to skin of scrotum, Androderm to skin of back, upper arms, thighs, abdomen; area must be clean and dry, free of hair

Gel route
• Apply daily to clean dry area on shoulders, upper arms, or abdomen; women, children should not touch gel or treated skin

Patient/family education
• Inform patient that product needs to be combined with complete health plan: diet, rest, exercise
• Caution patient to notify prescriber if therapeutic response decreases; not to discontinue this medication abruptly
• Inform women patients to report menstrual irregularities; about changes in sex characteristics
• Discuss that 1-3 mo course is necessary for response in breast cancer
• Inform patient about application of transdermal patches: Testoderm to skin of scrotum, Androderm to skin of back, upper arms, thighs, abdomen; area must be dry and free of hair; may be reapplied after bathing, swimming
• Teach about changes in sex characteristics: priapism, gynecomastia, increased libido

Evaluation
Positive therapeutic outcome
• Decrease size of tumor in breast cancer
• Increased androgen levels

tetracaine ophthalmic
See Appendix B

tetracaine topical
See Appendix B

tetracycline (Rx)
(tet-ra-sye′kleen)
Apo-Tetra ✤, Emtet, Nu-Tetra ✤, tetracycline HCl
Func. class.: Antiinfective—broad-spectrum
Chem. class.: Tetracycline
Pregnancy category D

Action: Inhibits protein synthesis and phosphorylation in microorganisms; bacteriostatic

Therapeutic outcome: Bactericidal action against susceptible organisms: gram-positive pathogens *Bacillus anthracis, Clostridium perfringens, Clostridium tetani, Listeria monocytogenes, Nocardia, Propionibacterium acnes, Actinomyces israelii;* gram-negative pathogens *Haemophilus influenzae, Legionella pneumophila, Yersinia entercolitica, Yersinia pestis, Neisseria gonorrhoeae, Neisseria meningitidis*

Uses: Syphilis, *Chlamydia trachomatis,* gonorrhea, lymphogranuloma venereum, uncommon gram-positive, gram-negative organisms, rickettsial infections

Dosage and routes
Susceptible gram-positive/gram-negative infections
Adult: PO 250-500 mg q6hr
Child >8 yr: PO 25-50 mg/kg/day in divided doses q6hr

Chlamydia trachomatis
Adult: PO 500 mg qid × 7 days

Syphilis
Adult and adolescent: PO 500 mg qid × 2 wk; if syphilis duration >1 yr, must treat 30 days

Brucellosis
Adult: PO 500 mg qid × 3 wk with 1 g of streptomycin IM 2 ×/day × 1 wk, and 1 ×/day the 2nd wk

T

Urethral, endocervical, rectal infections (C. trachomatis)
Adult: PO 500 mg qid × 7 days

Acne
Adult and adolescent: PO 250 mg q6hr, then 125-500 mg/day or every other day

Renal dose
Adult: PO CCr 51-90 ml/min give dose q8-12hr, CCr 10-50 ml/min give dose q12-24hr, CCr <10 ml/min give dose q24hr

Available forms: Oral susp 125 mg/5 ml, caps 250, 500 mg

Adverse effects
CNS: Fever, headache, paresthesia
CV: **Pericarditis**
EENT: Dysphagia, glossitis, decreased calcification (permanent discoloration) of deciduous teeth, oral candidiasis, oral ulcers
GI: *Nausea,* abdominal pain, *vomiting, diarrhea,* anorexia, enterocolitis, **hepatotoxicity,** flatulence, abdominal cramps, epigastric burning, stomatitis, hepatitis, **pseudomembranous colitis**
GU: *Increased BUN,* **azotemia, acute renal failure**
HEMA: **Eosinophilia, neutropenia, thrombocytopenia, leukocytosis, hemolytic anemia**
INTEG: *Rash, urticaria, photosensitivity, increased pigmentation,* **exfoliative dermatitis,** pruritus, **angioedema, Stevens-Johnson syndrome**

Contraindications: Pregnancy **D,** breastfeeding, children <8 yr, hypersensitivity to tetracyclines

Precautions: Renal/hepatic disease, UV exposure

Pharmacokinetics	
Absorption	60%-80% (PO), lower (IM)
Distribution	Widely distributed, some in CSF; crosses placenta
Metabolism	Not metabolized
Excretion	Unchanged—kidneys
Half-life	6-10 hr

Pharmacodynamics	
Onset	1-2 hr
Peak	2-3 hr
Duration	Unknown

Interactions
Individual drugs
Cimetidine, NaHCO$_3$: decreased tetracycline effect
Digoxin: increased digoxin effect
Iron: forms chelates, decreased absorption
Methoxyflurane: nephrotoxicity
Warfarin: increased warfarin effect
Drug classifications
Alkali products, antacids: decreased tetracycline effect
Contraceptives (oral): decreased oral contraceptive effect
Penicillins: decreased penicillin effect
Drug/herb
Acidophilus: do not use with antiinfectives; separate by several hours
Dong quai: increased photosensitivity
Drug/food
Decreased: absorption with dairy products; forms insoluble chelate
Drug/lab test
False increase: urinary catecholamines

NURSING CONSIDERATIONS
Assessment
• Assess patient for previous sensitivity reaction
• Assess patient for signs and symptoms of infection including characteristics of wounds, sputum, urine, stool, WBC >10,000/mm^3, temp; obtain baseline information before, during treatment
• Complete C&S testing before beginning product therapy to identify if correct treatment has been initiated
• Assess for allergic reactions: rash, urticaria, pruritus, chills, fever, joint pain; angioedema may occur a few days after therapy begins; epinephrine, resuscitation equipment should be available for anaphylactic reaction
• Identify urine output; if decreasing, notify prescriber (may indicate nephrotoxicity); increased BUN, creatinine
• Monitor blood studies: AST, ALT, CBC, Hct, bilirubin, LDH, alkaline phosphatase monthly if patient is on long-term therapy
• Assess bowel pattern daily; if severe diarrhea occurs, product should be discontinued
• Monitor for bleeding: ecchymosis, bleeding gums, hematuria, stool guaiac daily if on long-term therapy; blood dyscrasias may occur
• Assess for overgrowth of infection: perineal itching, fever, malaise, redness, pain, swelling, drainage, rash, diarrhea, change in cough, sputum

Nursing diagnoses
- Diarrhea (adverse reactions)
- Infection, risk for (uses)
- Injury, risk for (adverse reactions)
- Knowledge, deficient (teaching)
- Noncompliance (teaching)

Implementation
PO route
- Give around the clock to maintain proper blood levels; give with food to increase absorption of product; do not give within 3 hr of other agents; product interactions may occur; take on an empty stomach
- Give with 8 oz of water
- Shake liquid preparation well before giving; use calibrated device for proper dosing

Patient/family education
- Teach patient to report sore throat, bruising, bleeding, joint pain; may indicate blood dyscrasias (rare)
- Advise patient to use sunscreen when outdoors to decrease photosensitivity reaction
- Advise patient to contact prescriber if vaginal itching, loose foul-smelling stools, furry tongue occur; may indicate superinfection; report itching, rash, pruritus, urticaria
- Instruct patient to take all medication prescribed for the length of time ordered, product must be taken around the clock to maintain blood levels; do not give medication to others

Evaluation
Positive therapeutic outcome
- Absence of signs/symptoms of infection (WBC <10,000/mm³, temp WNL, absence of red, draining wounds)
- Reported improvement in symptoms of infection

---

tetrahydrozoline nasal agent
See Appendix B

---

tetrahydrozoline ophthalmic
See Appendix B

---

theophylline 🚭 (Rx)
(thee-off'i-lin)
Accurbron, Aquaphyllin, Asmalix, Bronkodyl, Elixomin, Elixophyllin, Lanophyllin, Quibron-T Dividose, Quibron-T/SR Dividose, Respbid, Slo-bid Gyrocaps, Slo-Phyllin, Sustaire, Theo-24, Theobid Duracaps, Theochron, Theoclear-80, Theoclear L.A., Theo-Dur, Theolair-SR, Theo-Sav, Theospan-SR, Theostat 80, Theovent, Theo-X, T-Phyl, Uni-Dur, Uniphyl
Func. class.: Spasmolytic, bronchodilator
Chem. class.: Xanthine, ethylenediamine

Pregnancy category C

Action: Relaxes smooth muscle of respiratory system by blocking phosphodiesterase, which increases cAMP, which increases bronchodilatation, diuresis, circulation, CNS stimulation

Therapeutic outcome: Ability to breathe without difficulty

Uses: Bronchial asthma, bronchospasm of COPD, chronic bronchitis, emphysema

Dosage and routes
Acute exacerbations of reversible airway obstructions
Adult: PO 5 mg/kg loading dose

COPD, chronic bronchitis
Adult: IV 0.4 mg/kg/hr in nonsmokers or 0.7 mg/kg/hr in smokers
Adult, child >45 kg: Maintenance PO 10 mg/kg/day, max 300 mg/day
Child 10-12 yrs: IV 0.7 mg/kg/hr, adjust based on theophylline level

Apnea of prematurity
Neonate: IV 4 mg/kg over 20-30 min, then maintenance IV/PO neonate ≥24 days 1.5 mg/kg q12h

Available forms: Caps 50, 100, 200, 250 mg; tabs 100, 125, 200, 225, 250, 300 mg; time rel tabs 100, 200, 250, 300, 400, 500 mg; time rel caps 50, 65, 100, 125, 130, 200, 250, 260, 300, 400, 500 mg; elix 80, 11.25 mg/15 mg; sol 80 mg/15 ml; liquid 80, 150, 160 mg/15 ml; susp 300 mg/15 ml

Adverse effects
CNS: Anxiety, restlessness, insomnia, dizziness, seizures, headache, light-headedness, muscle twitching, tremors

T

Adverse effects: *italic* = common, **bold** = life-threatening

CV: *Palpitations, sinus tachycardia,* hypotension, **dysrhythmias,** fluid retention with tachycardia
ENDO: Hyperglycemia
GI: *Nausea, vomiting, anorexia,* diarrhea, bitter taste, dyspepsia, gastric distress
INTEG: Flushing, urticaria
MISC: SIADH, urinary frequency
RESP: Increased rate, tachypnea

Contraindications: Hypersensitivity to xanthines, tachydysrhythmias

Precautions: Pregnancy **C,** children, geriatric, CHF, cor pulmonale, hepatic disease, active peptic ulcer disease, diabetes mellitus, hyperthyroidism, hypertension, seizure disorder

Pharmacokinetics

Absorption	Well absorbed (PO), slowly absorbed (ext rel)
Distribution	Crosses placenta, widely distributed
Metabolism	Liver
Excretion	Kidneys, breast milk
Half-life	6.5-10.5 hr; increased in liver disease, CHF, geriatric

Pharmacodynamics

	PO	PO–TIME REL	IV
Onset	Rapid	Slow	Immediate
Peak	1 hr	4-8 hr	Inf end
Duration	6 hr	12-24 hr	6-8 hr

Interactions
Individual drugs
Carbamazepine: decreased theophylline level
Cimetidine, disulfiram, erythromycin, fluvoxamine, influenza vaccine, mexiletine, propranolol: increased theophylline action
Lithium: decreased effect of lithium
Phenobarbital, phenytoin, rifampin: decreased theophylline
Drug classifications
Anticoagulants: increased anticoagulant level
β-Adrenergic blockers: cardiotoxicity
Contraceptives (oral), corticosteroids, fluoroquinolones, interferons: increased theophylline action
Smoking: decreased theophylline level
Drug/herb
Coffee, cola nut, guarana, Ma huang (ephedra), tea (black, green), yerba maté: increased toxicity
St. John's wort: decreased theophylline level

NURSING CONSIDERATIONS
Assessment
- Monitor theophylline blood levels (therapeutic level is 5-15 mcg/ml); toxicity may occur with small increase above 15 mcg/ml
- Monitor I&O; diuresis occurs; dehydration may result in children or geriatric
- Assess for signs of toxicity: irritability, insomnia, restlessness, tremors, nausea, vomiting
- Monitor respiratory rate, rhythm, depth; auscultate lung fields bilaterally; notify prescriber of abnormalities
- Assess for allergic reactions: rash, urticaria; if these occur, product should be discontinued

Nursing diagnoses
- Airway clearance, ineffective (uses)
- Knowledge, deficient (teaching)

Implementation
PO route
- Do not crush or chew time release products
- Contents of bead-filled cap may be sprinkled over food for children's use
- Give PO with 8 oz water; to decrease GI symptoms; avoid food, absorption may be affected
IV route
- Give loading dose over 20-30 min; max 20-25 mg/min; do not give by rapid **IV;** use only by cont inf
Y-site compatibilities: Acyclovir, ampicillin, aztreonam, cefazolin, cefotetan, ceftazidime, ceftriaxone, cimetidine, clindamycin, dexamethasone, diltiazem, DOBUTamine, DOPamine, doxycycline, erythromycin, famotidine, fluconazole, gentamicin, haloperidol, heparin, hydrocortisone, lidocaine, methyldopate, methylPREDNISolone, metronidazole, midazolam, nafcillin, nitroglycerin, nitroprusside, penicillin G potassium, piperacillin, potassium chloride, ranitidine, ticarcillin, ticarcillin/clavulanate, tobramycin, vancomycin
Additive compatibilities: Cefepime, chlorproMAZINE, fluconazole, methylPREDNISolone, verapamil

Patient/family education
- Advise patient to check OTC medications, current prescription medications for ephedrine, which will increase stimulation, and to avoid alcohol, caffeine
- Caution patient to avoid hazardous activities; dizziness may occur
- Inform patient that if GI upset occurs, to take product with 8 oz of water; avoid food; absorption may be decreased
- Advise patient to notify prescriber of toxicity: nausea, vomiting, anxiety, insomnia, seizures

- Advise patient to notify prescriber of change in smoking habit; dosage may have to be changed

Evaluation
Positive therapeutic outcome
- Ability to breathe more easily

---

thiamine (vitamin B₁) (PO, OTC; **IV**, IM, Rx)
Betaxin ✤, Betalin S, Biamine, Revitonus, Thiamilate, thiamine HCl
Func. class.: Vitamin B₁
Chem. class.: Water soluble

Pregnancy category A

Do not confuse:
thiamine/Tenormin

Action: Needed for pyruvate metabolism, carbohydrate metabolism

Therapeutic outcome: Prevention and treatment of thiamine deficiency

Uses: Vit B₁ deficiency or polyneuritis, cheilosis adjunct with thiamine beriberi, Wernicke-Korsakoff syndrome, pellagra, metabolic disorders, alcoholism

Dosage and routes
RDA
Adult: PO (Male) 1.2-1.5 mg; (females) 1.1 mg; (pregnancy) 1.4 mg; (breastfeeding) 1.4 mg
Child 9-13 yr: PO 0.9 mg
Child 4-8 yr: PO 0.6 mg
Child 1-3 yr: PO 0.5 mg
Infant 6 mo-1 yr: PO 0.3 mg
Neonate and infant to 6 mo: PO 0.3 mg

Beriberi
Adult: PO 5-30 mg qd or given in 3 divided doses × 1 month; IM/**IV** 5-30 mg qd or in 3 doses, then convert to PO
Child/infant: PO 10-50 mg qd × 2 wk, then 5-10 mg qd × 1 mo; **IV**/IM 10-25 mg/day × 2 wk, then 5-10 mg qd × 1 mo

Available forms: Tabs 50, 100, 250, 500 mg; inj 100 mg/ml; enteric-coated tabs 20 mg

Adverse effects
CNS: Weakness, restlessness
CV: **Collapse, pulmonary edema,** hypotension
EENT: Tightness of throat
GI: Hemorrhage, *nausea, diarrhea*
INTEG: **Angioneurotic edema,** cyanosis, sweating, warmth
SYST: **Anaphylaxis**

Contraindications: Hypersensitivity
Precautions: Pregnancy **A**

Pharmacokinetics
Absorption	Well absorbed (PO, IM), completely absorbed (**IV**)
Distribution	Widely distributed
Metabolism	Liver
Excretion	Kidneys (unchanged—excess amounts)
Half-life	Unknown

Pharmacodynamics
Unknown

NURSING CONSIDERATIONS
Assessment
- Assess nutritional status: yeast, beef, liver, whole or enriched grains, legumes

Nursing diagnoses
- Knowledge, deficient (teaching)
- Nutrition: less than body requirements, imbalanced (uses)

Implementation
IM route
- Give by IM inj; rotate sites if pain and inflammation occur; do not mix with alkaline sol; Z-track to minimize pain
- Application of cold compress may decrease pain
- Store in airtight, light-resistant container

IV route
- **IV** undiluted given over 5 min or diluted with **IV** sol and given as an inf at a rate of 100 mg or less/5 min or more

Syringe compatibilities: Doxapram
Y-site compatibilities: Famotidine
Additive incompatibilities:
Barbiturates; sol with neutral or alkaline pH, such as carbonates, bicarbonates, citrates and acetates; erythromycin, kanamycin, streptomycin

Patient/family education
- Teach patient necessary foods to be included in diet: yeast, beef, liver, legumes, whole grains

Evaluation
Positive therapeutic outcome
- Absence of nausea, vomiting, anorexia, insomnia, tachycardia, paresthesias, depression, muscle weakness

T

Adverse effects: *italic* = common, **bold** = life-threatening

thiethylperazine (Rx)
(thye-eth-il-per'a-zeen)
Norzine, Torecan
Func. class.: Antiemetic
Chem. class.: Phenothiazine, piperazine derivative

Pregnancy category X

Do not confuse:
Torecan/Toradol

Action: Acts centrally by blocking chemoreceptor trigger zone, which in turn acts on vomiting center; dopamine blocker

Therapeutic outcome: Control of nausea, vomiting

Uses: Nausea, vomiting

Dosage and routes
Adult: PO/IM 10 mg/day-tid

Available forms: Tabs 10 mg; inj 5 mg/ml

Adverse effects
CNS: *Euphoria, depression,* restlessness, tremor, EPS, **seizures,** drowsiness, confusion, **neuroleptic malignant syndrome**
CV: **Circulatory failure, tachycardia,** postural hypotension, ECG changes
GI: Nausea, vomiting, anorexia, dry mouth, diarrhea, constipation, weight loss, metallic taste, cramps
GU: Urinary retention, dark urine
HEMA: **Agranulocytosis, leukopenia**
RESP: **Respiratory depression**

Contraindications: Pregnancy **X**, hypersensitivity to phenothiazines, sulfites (inj), tartrazine (tabs), coma, seizure, encephalopathy, bone marrow depression

Precautions: Breastfeeding, children <2 yr, geriatric, Parkinson's disease

Pharmacokinetics
Absorption	Readily absorbed
Distribution	Crosses placenta
Metabolism	Liver
Excretion	Kidneys, breast milk
Half-life	Unknown

Pharmacodynamics
	PO	IM
Onset	45-60 min	Unknown
Peak	Unknown	Unknown
Duration	4 hr	Unknown

Interactions
Individual drugs
Ethanol: increased sedation
Drug classifications
Anesthetics (general), anxiolytics, sedatives/hypnotics, benzodiazepines, opiate agonists: increased sedation
Antacids: decreased effect of thiethylperazine
Anticholinergics, antiparkinson products, antidepressants (tricyclics): increased anticholinergic action
Barbiturates: decreased effect of thiethylperazine, increased sedation
Phenothiazines: avoid use, seizures may occur

NURSING CONSIDERATIONS
Assessment
• Monitor I&O ratio, palpate bladder if low urinary output occurs, especially in geriatric; urinalysis recommended before, during prolonged therapy
• Monitor bilirubin, CBC, liver function tests monthly
• Assess affect, orientation, LOC, reflexes, gait, coordination, sleep pattern disturbances
• Monitor B/P with patient in sitting, standing, and lying positions; take pulse and respirations q4hr during initial treatment; establish baseline before starting treatment; report drops of 30 mm Hg
• Check for dizziness, faintness, palpitations, tachycardia on rising; severe orthostatic hypotension is common
◆ Identify for neuroleptic malignant syndrome: hyperpyrexia, muscle rigidity, increased CPK, altered mental status, seizures, fatigue, loss of urinary control, tachycardia; product should be discontinued; have emergency equipment nearby
• Assess for EPS including akathisia (inability to sit still, no pattern to movements), tardive dyskinesia (bizarre movements of the jaw, mouth, tongue, extremities), pseudoparkinsonism (tremors, pill rolling, shuffling gait); antiparkinsonian product should be prescribed
• Assess for constipation, urinary retention daily; if these occur, increase bulk, water in diet

Nursing diagnoses
• Coping, ineffective (uses)
• Knowledge, deficient (teaching)
• Noncompliance (teaching)

Implementation
IM route
• Give IM inj in large muscle mass; aspirate to avoid **IV** administration; give slowly; have

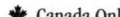

patient remain supine for at least 30 min after administration
Syringe compatibilities: Butorphanol, hydromorphone, midazolam, ranitidine
Y-site compatibilities: Aldesleukin

Patient/family education

• Teach patient to use good oral hygiene; frequent rinsing of mouth, sugarless gum for dry mouth
• Caution patient to avoid hazardous activities until product response is determined; dizziness, blurred vision may occur
• Inform patient that orthostatic hypotension often occurs and to rise gradually from sitting or lying position; avoid hot tubs, hot showers, and tub baths since hypotension may occur
• Instruct patient to remain lying down after IM inj for at least 30 min
• Inform patient that heat stroke may occur in hot weather, and to take extra precautions to stay cool
• Teach patient to avoid OTC preparations (cough, hay fever, cold) unless approved by prescriber because serious product interactions may occur; avoid use with alcohol, CNS depressants because increased drowsiness may occur
• Inform patient to use sunglasses and sunscreen to prevent burns
• Teach patient about EPS
• Instruct patient to report sore throat, malaise, fever, bleeding, mouth sores; if these occur, CBC should be performed and product discontinued

Evaluation
Positive therapeutic outcome
• Absence of nausea, vomiting

---

thioridazine (Rx)
(thye-or-rid'a-zeen)
Apo-Thioridazine ✤, Novo-Ridazine ✤, PMS-Thioridazine ✤, thioridazine HCl
Func. class.: Antipsychotic/neuroleptic
Chem. class.: Phenothiazine, piperidine
Pregnancy category C

Do not confuse:
Thioridazine/Thiothixene

Action: Depresses cerebral cortex, hypothalamus, limbic system, which control activity, aggression; blocks neurotransmission produced by dopamine at synapse; exhibits strong α-adrenergic, anticholinergic blocking action; mechanism for antipsychotic effects is unclear

Therapeutic outcome: Decreased signs and symptoms of psychosis

Uses: Psychotic disorders, schizophrenia, behavioral problems in children, anxiety, major depressive disorders, organic brain syndrome

Dosage and routes
Psychosis
Adult: PO 25-100 mg tid, max dose 800 mg/day; dose is gradually increased to desired response, then reduced to minimum maintenance

Depression/behavioral problems/ organic brain syndrome
Adult: PO 25 tid, range from 10 mg bid-qid to 50 mg tid-qid; max 800 mg/day for short period
Geriatric: PO 10-25 mg daily-bid, increase 4-7 days by 10-25 mg to desired dose, max 300 mg/day for short period
Child 2-12 yr: PO 0.5-3 mg/kg/day in divided doses, max 3 mg/kg/day

Available forms: Tabs 10, 15, 25, 50, 100, 150, 200 mg

Adverse effects
CNS: EPS (pseudoparkinsonism, akathisia, dystonia, tardive dyskinesia), **seizures,** *headache,* confusion, **neuroleptic malignant syndrome, dizziness,** drowsiness
CV: Orthostatic hypotension, **cardiac arrest,** ECG changes, **tachycardia, QT prolongation, torsades de pointes**
EENT: Blurred vision, glaucoma, dry eyes
GI: Dry mouth, nausea, vomiting, anorexia, constipation, diarrhea, jaundice, weight gain
GU: Urinary retention, urinary frequency, enuresis, impotence, amenorrhea, gynecomastia, ejaculation dysfunction, priapism
HEMA: Anemia, **leukopenia, leukocytosis, agranulocytosis**
INTEG: Rash, photosensitivity, dermatitis
RESP: **Laryngospasm,** dyspnea, **respiratory depression**

Contraindications: Children <2 yr, hypersensitivity, coma, CNS depression

Black Box Warning: QT prolongation, cardiac dysrhythmias

Precautions: Pregnancy **C,** breastfeeding, seizure disorders, hypertension, hepatic/pulmonary disease, renal failure, BPH, glaucoma, phenothiazine hypersensitivity, suicidal ideation, smoking, Reye's syndrome, Parkinson's disease

T

Black Box Warning: Cardiac disease, dementia, AV block, bundle-branch block, torsade de pointes

Pharmacokinetics

Absorption	Variably absorbed (tab)
Distribution	Widely distributed, high concentrations in CNS, crosses placenta, protein binding 91%-99%
Metabolism	Liver, extensively; GI mucosa
Excretion	Kidneys, breast milk
Half-life	26-36 hr

Pharmacodynamics

Onset	Erratic
Peak	2-4 hr
Duration	8-12 hr

Interactions
Individual drugs
Alcohol: oversedation

Aluminum hydroxide, magnesium hydroxide: decreased absorption

Lithium: decreased thioridazine levels
Drug classifications
Anesthetics (barbiturate), CNS depressants: oversedation

Antacids: decreased absorption

Anticholinergics: increased anticholinergic effects

Antiparkinson agents: decreased effect of these agents

Barbiturates: decreased thioridazine effect

Centrally acting antihypertensives: decreased antihypertensive effect

CYP2D6 inducers: decreased thioridazine levels

CYP2D6 inhibitors: increased thioridazine levels
Drug/herb
Betel palm, kava: increased EPS

Cola tree, hops, nettle, nutmeg: increased effect

Kava, St. John's wort, valerian: increased CNS depression
Drug/lab test
Increased: liver function tests, cardiac enzymes, cholesterol, blood glucose, prolactin, bilirubin, cholinesterase, ^{131}I

Decreased: hormones (blood and urine)

False positive: pregnancy tests, PKU

False negative: urinary steroids, pregnancy test

NURSING CONSIDERATIONS
Assessment
• Assess mental status: orientation, mood, behavior, presence of hallucinations, and type before initial administration and monthly; this product should significantly reduce psychotic behavior

• Check for swallowing of PO medication; check for hoarding or giving of medication to other patients

• Monitor I&O ratio; palpate bladder if low urinary output occurs, especially in geriatric; urinalysis recommended before, during prolonged therapy

• Monitor bilirubin, CBC, liver function tests monthly

• Assess affect, orientation, LOC, reflexes, gait, coordination, sleep pattern disturbances

• Monitor B/P sitting, standing, and lying, take pulse and respirations q4hr during initial treatment; establish baseline before starting treatment; report drops of 30 mm Hg; obtain baseline ECG, monitor Q- and T-wave changes

• Check for dizziness, faintness, palpitations, tachycardia on rising; severe orthostatic hypotension is common

Identify for neuroleptic malignant syndrome: hyperpyrexia, muscle rigidity, increased CPK, altered mental status, dyspnea, fatigue; product should be discontinued

• Assess for EPS including akathisia (inability to sit still, no pattern to movements), tardive dyskinesia (bizarre movements of the jaw, mouth, tongue, extremities), pseudoparkinsonism (ragged tremors, pill rolling, shuffling gate); an antiparkinsonian product should be prescribed

• Assess for constipation, urinary retention daily; if these occur, increase bulk, water in diet

Nursing diagnoses
• Coping, ineffective (uses)
• Knowledge, deficient (teaching)
• Noncompliance (teaching)

Implementation
• Decrease dose in geriatric because metabolism is slowed

• Administer PO with full glass of water, milk; or give with food to decrease GI upset

• Give antacids 2 hr before or after this product

• Store in airtight, light-resistant container, oral sol in amber bottle

Patient/family education
• Teach patient to use good oral hygiene; frequent rinsing of mouth, sugarless gum for dry mouth

• Advise patient to avoid hazardous activities until product response is determined; dizziness, blurred vision are common

 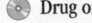

- Inform patient that orthostatic hypotension occurs often and to rise from sitting or lying position gradually; to avoid hot tubs, hot showers, tub baths because hypotension may occur
- Instruct patient that in hot weather, heat stroke may occur; take extra precautions to stay cool
- Caution patient to avoid abrupt withdrawal of this product, or EPS may result; product should be withdrawn slowly
- Teach patient to avoid OTC preparations (cough, hay fever, cold) unless approved by prescriber; serious product interactions may occur; avoid use with alcohol, CNS depressants; increased drowsiness may occur
- Advise patient to use sunglasses and sunscreen to prevent burns
- Teach patient about EPS and necessity for meticulous oral hygiene because oral candidiasis may occur
- Advise patient to take antacids 2 hr before or after this product
- Instruct patient to report sore throat, malaise, fever, bleeding, mouth sores; if these occur, CBC should be performed and product discontinued; may cause vision impairment, report to prescriber
- Advise patient that urine may be discolored

Evaluation
Positive therapeutic outcome
- Decrease in emotional excitement, hallucinations, delusions, paranoia
- Reorganization of patterns of thought, speech

Treatment of overdose: Lavage if orally ingested; provide airway; *do not induce vomiting or use epinephrine*, CV monitoring, continuous ECG

---

thyroid USP (desiccated) (Rx)
(thye′roid)
Armour Thyroid, Thyrar, Thyroid Strong, Westhroid
Func. class.: Thyroid hormone
Chem. class.: Active thyroid hormone in natural state and ratio

Pregnancy category A

Do not confuse:
Thyrar/Thyrolar

Action: Increases metabolic rates; controls protein synthesis; increases cardiac output, renal blood flow, O_2 consumption, body temp, blood volume, growth, development at cellular level

Therapeutic outcome: Correction of lack of thyroid hormone

Uses: Hypothyroidism, cretinism (juvenile hypothyroidism), myxedema

Dosage and routes
Hypothyroidism
Adult: PO 60-65 mg/day, increased by 30 mg qmo until desired response; maintenance dose 65-120 mg/day
Geriatric: PO 7.5-15 mg/day, increase dose q6-8wk until desired response

Cretinism/juvenile hypothyroidism
Child: PO 15 mg/day, then 30 mg/day after 2 wk, then 60 mg/day after another 2 wk; maintenance dose 60-180 mg/day

Myxedema
Adult: PO 15 mg/day, double dose q2wk, maintenance 60-180 mg/day

Available forms: Tabs 16, 32, 60, 65, 98, 130, 195, 260, 325 mg; enteric-coated tabs 32, 65, 130 mg; sugar-coated tabs 32, 65, 130, 195 mg; caps 65, 130, 195, 325 mg

Adverse effects
CNS: Insomnia, tremors, headache, **thyroid storm**
CV: Tachycardia, palpitations, angina, **dysrhythmias,** hypertension, **cardiac arrest**
GI: Nausea, diarrhea, increased or decreased appetite, cramps
MISC: Menstrual irregularities, weight loss, sweating, heat intolerance, fever

Contraindications: Adrenal insufficiency, MI, thyrotoxicosis, porcine protein hypersensitivity

Black Box Warning: Obesity treatment

Precautions: Pregnancy A, breastfeeding, geriatric, angina pectoris, hypertension, ischemia, cardiac disease

T

Pharmacokinetics	
Absorption	Well absorbed
Distribution	Widely distributed, does not cross placenta
Metabolism	Liver, tissues
Excretion	Feces via bile, breast milk
Half-life	T_3, 2 days; T_4, 1 wk

Pharmacodynamics	
Onset	1 hr
Peak	12-48 hr
Duration	Unknown

Adverse effects: *italic* = common, **bold** = life-threatening

Interactions
Individual drugs
Aluminum, calcium, magnesium: decreased thyroid absorption

Digoxin: decreased effect of digoxin

Insulin: increased requirement for insulin

Drug classifications
Anticoagulants, oral: increased effects of anticoagulants

Antidepressants (tricyclic): increased antidepressant (tricylics) effect

Bile acid sequestrants: decreased thyroid absorption

Catecholamines: increased effects of catecholamines

Estrogens: decreased thyroid hormone effect

Hypoglycemics: decreased effect of hypoglycemics

Sympathomimetics: increased effects of sympathomimetics

Drug/herb
Agar, bugleweed, carnitine, kelpware, soy, spirulina: decreased thyroid effect

Drug/lab test
Increased: CPK, LDH, AST, PBI, blood glucose

Decreased: thyroid function tests

NURSING CONSIDERATIONS
Assessment
• Identify if the patient is taking anticoagulants, antidiabetic agents; document on chart

• Take B/P, pulse before each dose; monitor I&O ratio and weight every day in same clothing, using same scale, at same time of day

• Monitor height, weight, psychomotor development, and growth rate if given to a child

• Monitor T_3, T_4, FTIs, which are decreased; radioimmunoassay of TSH, which is increased; radioactive iodine uptake (RAIU), which is increased if patient's dose of medication is too low

• Monitor pro-time; patient may require decreased dosage of anticoagulant; check for bleeding, bruising

• Assess for increased nervousness, excitability, irritability, which may indicate that dose of medication is too high, usually after 1-3 wk of treatment

• Assess cardiac status: angina, palpitation, chest pain, change in VS; the geriatric patient may have undetected cardiac problems; baseline ECG should be completed before treatment

Nursing diagnoses
• Knowledge, deficient (teaching)
• Noncompliance (teaching)

Implementation
• Give in AM if possible as a single dose to decrease sleeplessness; at same time each day to maintain product level

• Do not give with food as absorption will be decreased

• Give only for hormone imbalances; not to be used for obesity, male infertility, menstrual conditions, lethargy; give lowest dose that relieves symptoms; lower dose to the geriatric and in cardiac diseases

• Store in airtight, light-resistant container

• Wean patient off medication 4 wk before RAIU test

Patient/family education
• Teach patient that product is not a cure but controls symptoms and that treatment is long-term, that strong odor is normal

• Instruct patient to report excitability, irritability, anxiety, sweating, heat intolerance, chest pain, palpitations, which indicate overdose

• Advise patient not to switch brands unless approved by prescriber; bioavailability may differ; do not take with food; absorption will be decreased

• Teach patient that product may be discontinued after giving birth; thyroid panel will be evaluated after 1-2 mo

• Teach patient that hyperthyroid child will show almost immediate behavior/personality change; that hair loss will occur in child and is temporary

• Caution patient that product is not to be taken to reduce weight

• Caution patient to avoid OTC preparations containing iodine; read labels; other medications should not be used unless approved by prescriber

• Teach patient to avoid iodine-containing food: iodized salt, soybeans, tofu, turnips, certain kinds of seafood and bread

Evaluation
Positive therapeutic outcome
• Absence of depression

• Weight loss, increased diuresis, pulse, appetite

• Absence of constipation, peripheral edema, cold intolerance, pale, cool dry skin, brittle nails, alopecia, coarse hair, menorrhagia, night blindness, paresthesias, syncope, stupor, coma, rosy cheeks

• Improved levels of T_3, T_4 by laboratory tests

• Child: Age-appropriate weight, height, and psychomotor development

Treatment of overdose: Withhold dose for up to 1 wk; acute overdose—gastric lavage

or induce emesis, then activated charcoal; provide supportive treatment to control symptoms

tiagabine (Rx)
(tie-ah-ga'been)
Gabitril
Func. class.: Anticonvulsant

Pregnancy category C

Action: Inhibits reuptake and metabolism of GABA; may increase seizure threshold, structurally similar to GABA; tiagabine binding sites in neocortex, hippocampus

Uses: Adjunct treatment of partial seizures in adults and children ≥12 yr

Dosage and routes
When not given with a CYP3A4 enzyme, effect of tiagabine is doubled; lower doses are indicated
Adult: PO 4 mg/day in divided doses, may increase by 4-8 mg qwk until desired response, max 56 mg/day
Child 12-18 yr: PO 4 mg/day, may increase by 4 mg at beginning of wk 2, may increase by 4-8 mg qwk until desired response, max 32 mg/day

Available forms: Tabs 2, 4, 12, 16 mg

Adverse effects
CNS: Dizziness, anxiety, somnolence, ataxia, confusion, *asthenia,* unsteady gait, depression, **suicidal ideation**
CV: Vasodilatation
GI: Nausea, diarrhea, vomiting, increased appetite
INTEG: Pruritus, rash, **Stevens-Johnson syndrome**
RESP: Pharyngitis, coughing

Contraindications: Hypersensitivity

Precautions: Pregnancy C, breastfeeding, child <12 yr, geriatric, renal/hepatic disease, suicidal ideation/behavior, status epilepticus, mania, bipolar disorder, abrupt discontinuation, depression

Pharmacokinetics
Absorption	>95%
Distribution	Protein binding 96%
Metabolism	Liver
Excretion	Kidneys
Half-life	7-9 hr

Pharmacodynamics
Onset	Unknown
Peak	45 min
Duration	Unknown

Interactions
Individual drugs
Carbamazepine, phenobarbital, phenytoin, primidone: decreased effect of these products
Sevelamer: decreased tiagabine effect
Valproate: lower dose of tiagabine may be required
Drug classifications
CNS depressants: increased CNS depression
Drug/food
High-fat meal: decreased rate of absorption

NURSING CONSIDERATIONS
Assessment
• Monitor renal function tests: urinalysis, BUN, urine creatinine q3mo
• Monitor liver function tests: ALT, AST, bilirubin
• Assess description of seizures: location, duration, presence of aura
⊕ Assess mental status: mood, sensorium, affect, behavioral changes, suicidal thoughts; if mental status changes, notify prescriber

Nursing diagnoses
• Injury, risk for (uses, adverse reactions)
• Knowledge, deficient (teaching)
• Noncompliance (teaching)

Implementation
• Store at room temperature away from heat and light
• Provide assistance with ambulation during early part of treatment; dizziness occurs
• Provide seizure precautions: padded side rails; move objects that may harm patient

Patient/family education
• Advise patient to carry/wear emergency ID stating patient's name, products taken, condition, prescriber's name and phone number
• Advise patient to avoid driving, other activities that require alertness
• Teach patient not to discontinue medication quickly after long-term use

Evaluation
Positive therapeutic outcome
• Decreased seizure activity; document on patient's chart

Treatment of overdose: Lavage, VS

Adverse effects: *italic* = common, **bold** = life-threatening

ticarcillin (Rx)

(tye-kar-sill'in)

Ticar

Func. class.: Broad-spectrum antiinfective

Chem. class.: Extended-spectrum penicillin

Pregnancy category B

Action: Interferes with cell wall replication of susceptible organisms; osmotically unstable cell wall swells, bursts from osmotic pressure

Therapeutic outcome: Decreased symptoms of infection

Uses: Respiratory, soft tissue, urinary tract infections, bacterial septicemia; effective for gram-positive cocci *(Staphylococcus aureus, Streptococcus faecalis, Streptococcus pneumoniae)*, gram-negative cocci *(Neisseria gonorrhoeae)*, gram-positive bacilli *(Clostridium perfringens, Clostridium tetani)*, gram-negative bacilli *(Bacteroides, Fusobacterium nucleatum, Escherichia coli, Proteus mirabilis, Salmonella, Morganella morganii, Proteus rettgeri, Enterobacter, Pseudomonas aeruginosa, Serratia, Peptococcus, Peptostreptococcus, Eubacterium)*

Dosage and routes

Bacterial septicemia, respiratory, skin, soft tissue, intraabdominal, reproductive infections

Adult: **IV** INF 200-300 mg/kg/day in divided doses q4-6hr

Child <40 kg: **IV** INF 33.3-50 mg/kg/q4hr or 50-75 mg/kg q6hr

Urinary tract complicated infections

Adult and child: **IV** INF 150-200 mg/kg/day in divided doses q4-6hr

Uncomplicated urinary infections

Adult: **IM/DIRECT IV** 1 g q6hr

Child <40 kg: **IM/DIRECT IV** 50-100 mg/kg/day q6-8hr

Severe infections (Pseudomonas, Proteus, E. coli)

Neonate <2 kg: **IM/IV** 75 mg/kg q8-12hr

Neonate >2 kg: **IM/IV** 75-100 mg/kg q8hr

Renal/hepatic dose

Adult: CCr >60 ml/min 3 g q4hr; CCr 30-60 ml/min 2 g q4hr; CCr 10-30 ml/min 2 g q8hr; CCr <10 ml/min 2 g q12hr or 1 g q6hr; CCr <10 ml/min and hepatic dysfunction 2 g q24hr or 1 g q12hr

Available forms: Inj 1, 3, 6, 20, 30 g

Adverse effects

CNS: Lethargy, hallucinations, anxiety, depression, twitching, **coma, seizures,** confusion

GI: Nausea, vomiting, diarrhea; increased AST, ALT, abdominal pain, glossitis, colitis, **pseudomembranous colitis,** hepatotoxicity

GU: Oliguria, proteinuria, hematuria, *vaginitis, moniliasis,* **glomerulonephritis**

HEMA: Anemia, increased bleeding time, **bone marrow depression, granulocytopenia**

INTEG: Rash, **Stevens-Johnson syndrome**

META: Hypokalemia

SYST: **Anaphylaxis**

Contraindications: Hypersensitivity to penicillins

Precautions: Pregnancy **B,** breastfeeding, hypersensitivity to cephalosporins, renal/GI disease, diabetes, electrolyte imbalances

Pharmacokinetics

Absorption	Unknown
Distribution	Widely, breast milk
Metabolism	Liver, small amount
Excretion	Kidneys
Half-life	70 min

Pharmacodynamics

	IM	IV
Onset	Unknown	Unknown
Peak	1 hr	30-45 min
Duration	4-6 hr	4 hr

Interactions

Individual drugs

Aspirin, probenecid: increased ticarcillin concentration

Erythromycin: decreased effect of erthromycin

Heparin: increased effect of heparin

Methotrexate: increased effect of methotrexate

Drug classifications

Aminoglycosides (**IV**), tetracyclines: decreased effect of ticarcillin

Anticoagulants: increased effect of anticoagulants

Contraceptives (oral): decreased effect of oral contraceptives

Neuromuscular blockers: increased effect of neuromuscular blockers

Drug/herb

Acidophilus: do not use with antiinfectives; separate by several hours

Drug/lab test

False positive: urine glucose, urine protein

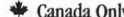

NURSING CONSIDERATIONS
Assessment
- Monitor I&O ratio; report hematuria, oliguria, since penicillin in high doses is nephrotoxic
- 🔷 Monitor any patient with compromised renal system, since product is excreted slowly in poor renal system function; toxicity may occur rapidly
- Monitor liver function tests: AST, ALT
- Monitor blood tests: WBC, RBC, Hgb, Hct, bleeding time
- Monitor renal function tests: urinalysis, protein, blood, BUN, creatinine
- Monitor C&S before product therapy; product may be given as soon as culture is performed
- Assess bowel pattern before, during treatment
- Check for skin eruptions after administration of penicillin to 1 wk after discontinuing product
- 🔷 Assess for anaphylaxis: wheezing, rash, pruritus, laryngeal edema; keep emergency equipment nearby
- Assess allergies before initiation of treatment, reaction of each medication

Nursing diagnoses
- Infection, risk for (uses)
- Knowledge, deficient (teaching)

Implementation
- Give product after C&S has been completed
- Have adrenalin, suction, tracheostomy set, endotracheal intubation equipment
- Provide adequate fluid intake (2 L) during diarrhea episodes
- Provide scratch test to assess allergy on order from prescriber; usually done when penicillin is only product of choice
- Store at room temperature, reconstituted sol 72 hr at room temperature

IM route
- Inject into well-developed muscle
- Reconstitute ticarcillin 1 g/2 ml sterile water for inj, NaCl inj, 1% lidocaine HCl without epinephrine (385 mg/ml)

IV route
- Give **IV** after diluting 1 g or less/4 ml of sterile H_2O for inj; dilute further with 10-20 ml or more D_5W, 0.9% NaCl, or sterile H_2O for inj sol; give 1 g or less/5 min or more or by intermittent inf over ½-2 hr or by continuous inf at prescribed rate

Y-site compatibilities: Acyclovir, allopurinol, amifostine, aztreonam, cyclophosphamide, diltiazem, famotidine, filgrastim, fludarabine, granisetron, hydromorphone,

heparin, IL-2, insulin (regular), magnesium sulfate, melphalan, meperidine, morphine, ondansetron, perphenazine, propofol, sargramostim, teniposide, theophylline, thiotepa, verapamil, vinorelbine

Additive compatibilities: Ranitidine, verapamil

Patient/family education
- Advise patient that culture may be done after completed course of medication
- Teach patient to report sore throat, fever, fatigue (may indicate superinfection)
- Teach patient to carry/wear emergency ID if allergic to penicillins
- Advise patient to notify nurse of diarrhea

Evaluation
Positive therapeutic outcome
- Absence of fever, purulent drainage, redness, inflammation

Treatment of overdose: Withdraw
product, maintain airway, administer epinephrine, aminophylline, O_2, **IV** corticosteroids for anaphylaxis

---

ticarcillin/clavulanate (Rx)
(tye-kar-sill'in)
Timentin
Func. class.: Extended-spectrum penicillin
Chem. class.: Antiinfective—broad-spectrum

Pregnancy category B

Action: Interferes with cell wall replication of susceptible organisms; osmotically unstable cell wall swells, bursts from osmotic pressure; clavulanate inhibits β-lactamase and protects against enzymatic degradation of ticarcillin

Therapeutic outcome: Resolution of infection

Uses: Respiratory, soft tissue, urinary tract infections; bacterial septicemia; effective for gram-positive cocci *(Staphylococcus aureus, Streptococcus faecalis, Streptococcus pneumoniae),* gram-negative cocci *(Neisseria gonorrhoeae),* gram-positive bacilli *(Clostridium perfringens, Clostridium tetani),* gram-negative bacilli *(Bacteroides, Fusobacterium nucleatum, Escherichia coli, Proteus mirabilis, Salmonella, Morganella morganii, Proteus rettgeri, Enterobacter, Pseudomonas aeruginosa, Serratia, Peptococcus, Peptostreptococcus, Eubacterium)*

T

Dosage and routes
Systemic/urinary tract infections, serious infections
Adult ≥60 kg: **IV** INF 3.1 g q4-6hr
Adult <60 kg: **IV** INF 200-300 mg/kg/day q4-6hr
Child >60 kg: **IV** INF 3.1 g q4hr
Child <60 kg: **IV** INF 300 mg/kg/day q4hr

Mild/moderate infections
Child ≥60 kg: **IV** INF 3.1 g q6hr
Child <60 kg: **IV** INF 200 mg/kg/day q6hr

Renal dose
Adult: **IV** INF loading dose 3.1 g; CCr 60 ml/min 3.1 g q4hr; CCr 30-60 ml/min 2 g q4hr; CCr 10-30 ml/min 2g q8hr; CCr <10 ml/min 2 g q12hr; CCr <10 ml/min with hepatic dysfunction 2 g q24hr

Available forms: Inj IM, **IV** 3 g ticarcillin and 0.1 g clavulanate; **IV** inf 3 g ticarcillin and 0.1 g clavulanate; powder for inj 3 g ticarcillin, 0.1 g clavulanate

Adverse effects
CNS: Lethargy, hallucinations, anxiety, depression, twitching, **coma, seizures,** confusion, drowsiness
GI: *Nausea, vomiting, diarrhea,* increased AST, ALT, abdominal pain, glossitis, colitis, **pseudomembranous colitis,** hepatotoxicity
GU: Oliguria, proteinuria, hematuria, *vaginitis, moniliasis,* **glomerulonephritis**
HEMA: Anemia, increased bleeding time, **bone marrow depression, granulocytopenia**
INTEG: Rash, urticaria, **toxic epidermal necrolysis**
META: Hypokalemia, hyperkalemia, alkalosis, hypernatremia
SYST: **Anaphylaxis, Stevens-Johnson syndrome**

Contraindications: Hypersensitivity to penicillins; neonates

Precautions: Pregnancy **B,** hypersensitivity to cephalosporins, renal disease

Pharmacokinetics	
Absorption	Completely absorbed (**IV**)
Distribution	Widely distributed, crosses blood-brain barrier
Metabolism	Liver
Excretion	Kidneys
Half-life	64-68 min

Pharmacodynamics	
	IV
Onset	Unknown
Peak	30-45 min
Duration	4 hr

Interactions
Individual drugs
Chloramphenicol: decreased antimicrobial effect of ticarcillin
Heparin: increased effect of heparin
Methotrexate: increased methotrexate level
Probenecid, sulfinpyrazone: increased ticarcillin concentration
Drug classifications
Aminoglycosides (**IV**): decreased antimicrobial effect of ticarcillin
Anticoagulants: increased bleeding
Contraceptives (oral): decreased effect of oral contraceptives
Erythromycins: decreased absorption
Macrolides, sulfonamides, tetracyclines: decreased ticarcillin effect
Drug/herb
Acidophilus: do not use with antiinfectives; separate by several hours
Drug/lab test
False positive: urine glucose, urine protein, Coombs' test

NURSING CONSIDERATIONS
Assessment
• Monitor I&O ratio; report hematuria, oliguria because penicillin in high doses is nephrotoxic
• Monitor any patient with compromised renal system because product is excreted slowly in poor renal system function; toxicity may occur rapidly
• Monitor liver function tests: AST, ALT
• Monitor blood tests: WBC, RBC, Hgb, Hct, bleeding time
• Monitor renal function tests: urinalysis, protein, blood
• Obtain C&S test results before initiating product therapy; product may be given as soon as culture is performed
• Assess bowel pattern before, during treatment
• Assess skin eruptions after administration of penicillin to 1 wk after discontinuing product
🔷 Assess for anaphylaxis: wheezing, rash, laryngeal edema; have emergency equipment nearby
• Assess allergies before initiation of treatment, reaction of each medication

Nursing diagnoses
- Infection, risk for (uses)
- Knowledge, deficient (teaching)

Implementation
- Give product after C&S has been completed
- Have adrenalin, suction, tracheostomy set, endotracheal intubation equipment available
- Give adequate fluid intake (2 L) during diarrhea episodes
- Obtain scratch test results to assess allergy after securing order from prescriber; usually done when penicillin is only product of choice
- Store at room temperature, reconstituted sol for 12-24 hr or 3-7 days refrigerated

IV route
- Give **IV** after diluting 3.1 g or less/13 ml of sterile H_2O or NaCl (200 mg/ml), shake; may further dilute in 50-100 ml or more 0.9% NaCl, D_5W, or LR sol and run over ½ hr

Y-site compatibilities: Allopurinol, aztreonam, cefepime, cyclophosphamide, diltiazem, famotidine, filgrastim, fluconazole, fludarabine, foscarnet, heparin, insulin (regular), melphalan, meperidine, morphine, ondansetron, perphenazine, sargramostim, teniposide, theophylline, vinorelbine

Patient/family education
- Advise patient that C&S may be performed after completed course of medication
- Instruct patient to report sore throat, fever, fatigue (may indicate superinfection)
- Advise patient to carry/wear emergency ID if allergic to penicillins
- Advise patient to use alternative birth control methods

Evaluation
Positive therapeutic outcome
- Absence of fever, purulent drainage, redness, inflammation

Treatment of overdose: Withdraw
product, maintain airway, administer epinephrine, aminophylline, O_2, **IV** corticosteroids for anaphylaxis

---

ticlopidine (Rx)
(tye-cloe'pi-deen)
Func. class.: Platelet aggregation inhibitor
Chem. class.: Thienopyridine compound

Pregnancy category B

Action: Irreversible inhibition of platelet aggregation through antagonism of ADP

Therapeutic outcome: Decreased stroke by decreasing platelet aggregation

Uses: Reducing the risk of stroke in high-risk patients

Unlabeled uses: Intermittent claudication, chronic arterial occlusion, subarachnoid hemorrhage, uremic patients with AV shunts/fistulas, open heart surgery, coronary artery bypass grafts, primary glomerulonephritis, diabetic neuropathy

Dosage and routes
Adult: PO 250 mg bid with food

Available forms: Tabs 250 mg

Adverse effects
CNS: Dizziness
GI: Nausea, vomiting, diarrhea, GI discomfort, **cholestatic jaundice, hepatitis,** increased cholesterol LDL, VLDL, TG, triglycerides
HEMA: **Bleeding (epistaxis, hematuria, conjunctival hemorrhage, GI bleeding), agranulocytosis, neutropenia, thrombocytopenia, thrombotic thrombocytopenic purpura**
INTEG: Rash, pruritus

Contraindications: Hypersensitivity, severe liver disease, active bleeding, coagulopathy

Black Box Warning: Agranulocytosis, neutropenia, thrombocytopenia, thrombotic thrombocytopenic purpura (TTP)

Precautions: Pregnancy **B,** breastfeeding, children, geriatric, past liver disease, renal disease, increased bleeding risk, peptic ulcer disease, surgery

Black Box Warning: Anemia, hematological disease

Pharmacokinetics
Absorption	Well absorbed
Distribution	Unknown
Metabolism	Liver, extensively; 98% protein binding
Excretion	Kidneys, unchanged product
Half-life	Increased with repeat dosing; 4-5 days (multiple doses)

Pharmacodynamics
Onset	Unknown
Peak	1-3 hr
Duration	Unknown

Interactions
Individual drugs
Abciximab, aspirin, eptifibatide, tirofiban: increased bleeding tendencies

---

Adverse effects: *italic* = common, **bold** = life-threatening

T

Ambrisenten, fosphenytoin, phenytoin, theophylline: increased levels of each specific drug

Cimetidine: increased effects of ticlopidine

CycloSPORINE: decreased plasma levels of cycloSPORINE

Digoxin: decreased plasma levels of digoxin

Drug classifications

Antacids: decreased plasma levels of ticlopidine

Anticoagulants, NSAIDs, salicylates, SSRIs, thrombin inhibitors, thrombolytics: increased bleeding risk

Drug/herb

Ginger, gingko, garlic, feverfew, horse chestnut, green tea: increased bleeding risk

NURSING CONSIDERATIONS
Assessment

• Monitor liver function tests: AST, ALT, bilirubin, creatinine if patient is on long-term therapy (4 mo or more)

• Monitor blood tests: CBC, Hct, Hgb, protime if patient is on long-term therapy; CBC q2wk × 3 mo therapy; thrombocytopenia, neutropenia may occur

• Monitor bleeding time baseline and throughout therapy, levels may be 2-5 × normal limit

Nursing diagnoses

• Injury, risk for (uses)
• Knowledge, deficient (teaching)

Implementation

• Give with food or after eating to decrease GI effects

Patient/family education

• Advise patient that blood studies will be necessary during treatment

• Advise patient to report any unusual bleeding to prescriber

• Instruct patient to take with food or just after eating to minimize GI discomfort, not to double missed dose

• Caution patient to report side effects such as diarrhea, skin rashes, subcutaneous bleeding, signs of cholestasis (yellow skin and sclera, dark urine, light-colored stools)

• Advise patient that product should be discontinued 10-14 days prior to surgery

• Advise there are many drug and herb interactions

Evaluation
Positive therapeutic outcome

• Absence of stroke

tigecycline (Rx)
(tye-ge-sye′kleen)
Tygacil
Func. class.: Broad-spectrum antiinfective
Chem. class.: Glycylcyclines

Pregnancy category D

Action: Inhibits protein synthesis and phosphorylation in microorganisms; bacteriostatic, structurally similar to the tetracyclines

Therapeutic outcome: Resolution of infection

Uses: Complicated skin/skin structure infections: *Escherichia coli, Enterococcus faecalis* (vancomycin-susceptible only) *Staphylococcus aureus, Streptococcus agalactiae, S. anginosus* group, *S. pyogenes, Bacteroides fragilis;* complicated intraabdominal infections *(Citrobacter freundii), Enterobacter cloacae, E. coli, Klebsiella oxytoca, K. pneumoniae, E. faecalis* (vancomycin-susceptible only), *S. aureus* (methicillin-susceptible only), *S. anginosus* group, *B. fragilis, Bacteroides thetaiotaomicron, B. uniformis, B. vulgatus, Clostridium perfringens, Peptostreptococcus micros,* community-acquired pneumonia

Dosage and routes
Adult: **IV** 100 mg, then 50 mg q12hr, **IV** INF is given over 30 min to 60 min q12hr; given for 5-14 days depending on infection

Hepatic dose (Child-Pugh C)
Adult: **IV** 100 mg, then 25 mg q12hr

Available forms: Powder for inj, lyophilized 50 mg

Adverse effects
CNS: Headache, dizziness, insomnia
CV: Hypo/hypertension, phlebitis
GI: Nausea, vomiting, diarrhea, anorexia, constipation, dyspepsia, **hepatotoxicity, hepatic failure**
HEMA: **Anemia, leukocytosis, thrombocytopenia**
INTEG: Rash, pruritus, sweating, photosensitivity
META: Increased ALT, AST, BUN, lactic acid, alkaline phosphatase, amylase, hyperglycemia, hypokalemia, hypoproteinemia, bilirubinemia
MISC: Back pain, fever, abnormal healing, abdominal pain, abscess, asthenia, infection, pain, peripheral edema, local reactions
RESP: Cough, dyspnea
SYST: Anaphylaxis

Contraindications: Pregnancy **D**, breast-feeding, children <18 yr, hypersensitivity to tigecycline

Precautions: Renal/hepatic disease, hypersensitivity to tetracyclines, ventricular-associated hospital-acquired pneumonias

Pharmacokinetics

Absorption	Unknown
Distribution	Protein binding 71%-89%
Metabolism	Not extensively
Excretion	22% unchanged, urine; primarily biliarily excreted
Half-life	Terminal 42 hr

Pharmacodynamics
Unknown

Interactions
Individual drugs
Warfarin: increased effect of tigecycline
Drug classifications
Oral contraceptives: decreased effect of tigecycline

NURSING CONSIDERATIONS
Assessment
◆ Assess for pseudomembranous colitis
• Assess for signs of anemia: Hct, Hgb, fatigue
• Monitor blood tests: PT, CBC, AST, ALT, BUN creatinine
• Assess for allergic reactions: rash, itching, pruritus, angioedema
• Assess for nausea, vomiting, diarrhea; administer antiemetic, antacids as ordered
• Assess for overgrowth of infection: fever, malaise, redness, pain, swelling, drainage, perineal itching, diarrhea, changes in cough or sputum

Nursing diagnoses
• Infection, risk for (use)
• Knowledge, deficient (teaching)

Implementation
• Give after C&S obtained
IV route
• Reconstitute each vial with 5.3 ml of 0.9% NaCl, or D_5 (10 mg/ml); swirl to dissolve; immediately withdraw 5 ml of the reconstituted sol and add to a 100-ml **IV** bag for inf (1 mg/ml); may be yellow or orange, if not, sol should be discarded; do not give if particulate matter is present
• Store in tight, light-resistant container at room temperature

Patient/family education
• Teach patient to avoid sun exposure; sunscreen does not seem to decrease photosensitivity
• Teach patient to avoid pregnancy while taking this product; fetal harm may occur

Evaluation
Positive therapeutic outcome
• Decreased temp, absence of lesions, negative C&S

tiludronate (Rx)
(till-oo'droe-nate)
Skelid
Func. class.: Bone resorption inhibitor
Chem. class.: Bisphosphonate

Pregnancy category C

Action: Decreases bone reabsorption and new bone development, inhibits osteoclasts

Therapeutic outcome: Decreased bone reabsorption and reduced calcium levels WNL

Uses: Paget's disease in those with alkaline phosphatase at 2 × upper limit, patients at risk of future complications of Paget's disease and those who are symptomatic

Dosage and routes
Adult: PO 400 mg/day with 8 oz of water × 3 mo

Renal dose
Adult: PO CCr <30 ml/min do not use

Available forms: Tabs 240 mg (equivalent to 200 mg tiludronic acid)

Adverse effects
CNS: Headache, dizziness, paresthesia, somnolence
CV: Chest pain, edema, peripheral edema, **atrial fibrillation**
EENT: Cataracts, ocular hypertension/pain/inflammation, conjunctivitis, visual impairment, sinusitis
ENDO: Hyperparathyroidism
GI: *Nausea, diarrhea,* dry mouth, gastritis, vomiting, flatulence, gastric ulcers, dyspepsia
GU: **Nephrotoxicity**
INTEG: Rash, epidermal necrosis, pruritus, sweating
MS: *Bone pain,* osteonecrosis of the jaw
RESP: Rhinitis, sinusitis, upper respiratory tract infection
SYST: **Stevens-Johnson syndrome**

Contraindications: Hypersensitivity to bisphosphonates, breastfeeding, severe renal disease with creatinine CCr <30 ml/min

T

Adverse effects: *italic* = common, **bold** = life-threatening

Precautions: Pregnancy **C**, GI/renal disease, restricted vit D/Ca, asthma, anemia coagulopathy, dental disease, GERD, hiatal hernia, hypocalcemia, infection

Pharmacokinetics

Absorption	Rapid
Distribution	Unknown, steady state 10 days
Metabolism	Protein binding 90%
Excretion	Feces (unabsorbed), kidney (unchanged)
Half-life	150 hr

Pharmacodynamics

Onset	Up to 4 wk
Peak	Unknown
Duration	Unknown

Interactions
Individual drugs
Aspirin: decreased tiludronate absorption
Indomethacin: increased effect of tiludronate
Drug classifications
Antacids, mineral supplements with magnesium, calcium, iron, or aluminum salicylates: decreased absorption of tiludronate, separate by ≥2 hr

NURSING CONSIDERATIONS
Assessment
• Assess for GI symptoms, polyuria, flushing, head swelling, tingling, headache; may indicate hypercalcemia; nervousness, irritability, twitching, seizures, spasm, paresthesia indicates hypocalcemia at start of treatment
• Identify nutritional status; evaluate diet for sources of vit D (milk, some seafood), calcium (dairy products, dark green vegetables), phosphates; dental health
• Monitor BUN, creatinine, uric acid, chloride, electrolytes, urine pH, urinary calcium, magnesium, phosphate, urinalysis (calcium should be kept at 9-10 mg/dl), albumin, alkaline phosphatase baseline and q3-6mo; check urine sediment for casts throughout treatment
• Assess for increased product level; toxic reactions occur rapidly; have calcium chloride or gluconate on hand if calcium level drops too low; check for tetany

Nursing diagnoses
• Injury, risk for (adverse reactions)
• Knowledge, deficient (teaching)
• Pain, chronic (uses)

Implementation
• Administer on empty stomach to improve absorption (2 hr before meals), with 6-8 oz of water; do not use with mineral water, juice, or coffee; take calcium or mineral supplements 2 hr before or 2 hr after tiludronate; take aluminum or magnesium antacids ≥2 hr after tiludronate; do not take indomethacin within 2 hr
• Remove tabs from foil strip immediately before use

Patient/family education
• Caution patient to notify prescriber of hypercalcemic relapse: renal calculi, nausea, vomiting, thirst, lethargy, deep bone or flank pain
• Teach patient to follow a low-calcium diet as prescribed (Paget's disease, hypercalcemia)
• Advise patient to notify prescriber of diarrhea, nausea; dose may be divided to lessen these symptoms
• Teach to maintain good oral hygiene

Evaluation
Positive therapeutic outcome
• Calcium levels 9-10 mg/dl
• Decreasing symptoms of Paget's disease including pain

timolol (Rx)
(tye′moe-lole)
Apo-Timol ✤, Novo-Timol ✤, timolol maleate
Func. class.: Antihypertensive; antiglaucoma
Chem. class.: Nonselective β-blocker
Pregnancy category C

Action: Competitively blocks stimulation of β-adrenergic receptor within vascular smooth muscle (decreases rate of SA node discharge, increases recovery time), slows conduction of AV node, decreases heart rate, which decreases O_2 consumption in myocardium; also decreases renin-aldosterone-angiotensin system; at high doses inhibits β_2 receptors in bronchial system

Therapeutic outcome: Decreased B/P, decreased arrhythmias, absence of death from MI, decreased aqueous humor in the eye, absence of migraine headaches

Uses: Mild to moderate hypertension, migraine prophylaxis

Unlabeled uses: Tremors, angina pectoris

Dosage and routes
Hypertension
Adult: PO 10 mg bid, or 20 mg/day, may increase by 10 mg q7day, max 60 mg/day

Myocardial infarction
Adult: 10 mg bid beginning 1-4 wk after MI

Glaucoma
Adult: Ophth 1 gtt daily or bid
Child: Ophth 1 gtt daily or bid (0.25% SOL only)

Migraine headache prevention
Adult: PO 10 mg bid, or 20 mg/day; may increase to 30 mg/day, 20 mg in AM, 10 mg in PM; discontinue if not effective after 8 wk

Available forms: Tabs 5, 10, 20 mg

Adverse effects
CNS: Insomnia, dizziness, hallucinations, anxiety, fatigue, depression, headache
CV: Hypotension, bradycardia, CHF, edema, chest pain, claudication, angina, AV block, ventricular dysrhythmias
EENT: Visual changes, sore throat, *double vision,* dry burning eyes
GI: Nausea, vomiting, **ischemic colitis,** diarrhea, *abdominal pain,* **mesenteric arterial thrombosis,** flatulence, constipation
GU: Impotence, urinary frequency
HEMA: **Agranulocytosis, thrombocytopenia, purpura**
INTEG: Rash, alopecia, pruritus, fever
META: Hypoglycemia
MUSC: Joint pain, muscle pain
RESP: **Bronchospasm,** dyspnea, cough, crackles, nasal stuffiness

Contraindications: Hypersensitivity to β-blockers, cardiogenic shock, heart block (2nd or 3rd degree), sinus bradycardia, CHF, cardiac failure, severe COPD, asthma

Precautions: Pregnancy **C,** breastfeeding, major surgery, diabetes mellitus, thyroid/renal/hepatic disease, COPD, well-compensated heart failure, CAD, nonallergic bronchospasm, peripheral vascular disease

Black Box Warning: Abrupt discontinuation

Pharmacokinetics
Absorption	Well absorbed (PO), minimal (ophth)
Distribution	Protein binding <10%
Metabolism	Liver, extensively
Excretion	Breast milk
Half-life	3 hr

Pharmacodynamics
	PO
Onset	Unknown
Peak	2-4 hr
Duration	12-24 hr

Interactions
Individual drugs
Alcohol: increased hypotension, bradycardia (large amounts)
HydrALAZINE, methyldopa, prazosin, reserpine: increased hypotension, bradycardia
Insulin: decreased hypoglycemia
Thyroid hormones: decreased antihypertensive effect

Drug classifications
Anticholinergics, nitrates: increased hypotension, increased bradycardia
β2-Adrenergic agonists: increased β-blocking effect
Calcium channel blockers: increased effects of calcium channel blockers
NSAIDs, salicylates, sympathomimetics: decreased antihypertensive effect
Sulfonylureas: decreased hypoglycemic effect
Theophyllines: decreased bronchodilatation

Drug/herb
Aconite: increased toxicity, death
Astragalus, cola tree: increased or decreased antihypertensive effect
Barberry, betony, black catechu, black cohosh, bloodroot, broom, burdock, cat's claw, dandelion, goldenseal, hawthorn, Irish moss, Jamaican dogwood, kelp, khella, mistletoe, parsley: increased antihypertensive effect
Coltsfoot, guarana, khat, licorice, yohimbe: decreased antihypertensive effect

Drug/lab test
Increased: renal, liver function tests, potassium, uric acid
Decreased: Hct, Hgb, HDL
Interference: glucose, insulin tolerance test

NURSING CONSIDERATIONS
Assessment
• Assess for headaches: location, severity, duration, frequency baseline, throughout treatment
• Monitor B/P during beginning treatment, periodically thereafter; pulse q4hr; note rate, rhythm, quality: apical/radial pulse before administration; notify prescriber of any significant changes (pulse <50 bpm)
• Check for baselines in renal, liver function tests before therapy begins

T

Adverse effects: *italic* = common, **bold** = life-threatening

- Assess for edema in feet, legs daily, monitor I&O ratio, daily weight; check for jugular vein distention, crackles bilaterally, dyspnea (CHF)
- Monitor skin turgor, dryness of mucous membranes for hydration status, especially geriatric

Nursing diagnoses
- Cardiac output, decreased (uses)
- Injury, risk for (side effects)
- Knowledge, deficient (teaching)
- Noncompliance (teaching)

Implementation
- Given before meals, at bedtime; tab may be crushed or swallowed whole; give with food to prevent GI upset; reduce dosage in renal dysfunction
- Store protected from light, moisture; place in cool environment

Patient/family education
- Teach patient not to discontinue product abruptly; taper over 2 wk; may cause precipitate angina if stopped abruptly
- Advise patient not to use OTC products containing α-adrenergic stimulants (such as nasal decongestants, cold preparations); to avoid alcohol, smoking and to limit sodium intake as prescribed
- Teach patient how to take pulse and B/P at home; advise patient when to notify prescriber
- Instruct patient to comply with weight control, dietary adjustments, modified exercise program
- Advise patient to carry/wear emergency ID to identify product being taken, any allergies; tell patient product controls symptoms but does not cure
- Caution patient to avoid hazardous activities if dizziness, drowsiness are present
- Teach patient to report symptoms of CHF; difficult breathing, especially on exertion or when lying down; night cough; swelling of extremities or bradycardia; dizziness; confusion; depression; fever
- Teach patient to take product as prescribed, not to double dose, skip doses; take any missed doses as soon as remembered if at least 4 hr until next dose

Evaluation
Positive therapeutic outcome
- Decreased B/P in hypertension (after 1-2 wk)
- Absence of dysrhythmias

Treatment of overdose: Lavage, **IV** atropine for bradycardia, **IV** theophylline for bronchospasm, digoxin, O₂, diuretic for cardiac failure, hemodialysis, **IV** glucose for hyperglycemia, **IV** diazepam (or phenytoin) for seizures

---

timolol ophthalmic
See Appendix B

---

tinidazole (Rx)
(tye-ni′da-zole)
Tindamax
Func. class.: Antiprotozoal
Chem. class.: Nitroimidazole derivative
Pregnancy category C

Action: Interferes with DNA/RNA synthesis in protozoa

Therapeutic outcome: Decrease in infection

Uses: Amebiasis, giardiasis, trichomoniasis

Dosage and routes
Amebic involvement (liver)
Adult: PO 2 g/day × 3-5 days
Child ≥3 yr: PO 50 mg/kg/day × 3-5 days, max 2 g

Giardiasis
Adult: PO 2 g as a single dose
Child ≥3 yr: PO 50 mg/kg as a single dose, max 2 g

Trichomoniasis
Adult: PO 2 g as a single dose

Bacterial vaginosis
Adult (nonpregnant woman): PO 2 g/day × 2 days with food or 1 g/day × 5 days with food

Available forms: Tabs 250, 500 mg

Adverse effects
CNS: Dizziness, headache, **seizures,** *peripheral neuropathy,* malaise, fatigue
GI: Nausea, vomiting, anorexia, increased AST and ALT, constipation, abdominal pain, indigestion, altered taste
HEMA: **Leukopenia,** neutropenia
INTEG: Pruritus, urticaria, *rash,* oral candidiasis
SYST: **Angioedema,** cramping

Contraindications: Breastfeeding, hypersensitivity to this product or nitroimidazole derivative, pregnancy

Precautions: Pregnancy **C,** children, geriatric, hepatic disease, CNS depression, blood dyscrasias, candidiasis, seizures, viral infection, alcoholism

---

Black Box Warning: Secondary malignancy

tinzaparin (Rx)
(tin-zay-par'in)
Innohep
Func. class.: Anticoagulant
Chem. class.: Unfractionated porcine heparin

Pregnancy category C

Pharmacokinetics

Absorption	Unknown
Distribution	Crosses blood/brain barrier
Metabolism	Extensively in the liver
Excretion	Unchanged (20%-25%) in urine, (12%) feces
Half-life	12-14 hr

Pharmacodynamics
Unknown

Interactions
Individual drugs
Do not use within 2 wk of taking disulfiram
Cholestyramine, oxytetracycline: decreased action of tinidazole
CycloSPORINE, fluorouracil, lithium, tacrolimus: increased action
Drug classifications
Anticoagulants, hydantoins: increased action
CYP3A4 inducers (phenobarbital, phenytoin, rifampin): decreased action of tinidazole
CYP3A4 inhibitors (cimetidine, ketoconazole): increased action of tinidazole

NURSING CONSIDERATIONS
Assessment
• Assess for amebic liver absess: CBC, ESR, amebic gel diffusion test, ultrasound, total and differential leukocyte count
• Assess for signs of infection, anemia
• Assess bowel pattern before, during treatment

Nursing diagnoses
• Infection, risk for (uses)
• Knowledge, deficient (teaching)

Implementation
• Administer to those over 3 yr old
• Give with food; tabs can be crushed and mixed with artificial cherry syrup

Patient/family education
• Instruct patient to take with food to increase plasma concentrations, minimize epigastric distress and other GI effects; not to use alcoholic beverages during or for 3 days afterward
• Advise patient that in cases of trichomoniasis, both partners should be treated at the same time

Evaluation
Positive therapeutic outcome
• Decrease in infection as evidenced by negative culture

Action: Prevents conversion of fibrinogen to fibrin and prothrombin to thrombin by enhancing inhibitory effects of antithrombin III; produces higher ratio of antifactor Xa to antifactor IIa

Therapeutic outcome: Resolution of DVT

Uses: Treatment of DVT, pulmonary emboli after abdominal, knee, hip surgery or knee, hip replacement

Unlabeled uses: DVT prophylaxis

Dosage and routes
Treatment of deep vein thrombosis
Adult: SUBCUT 175 anti-Xa international units/kg daily ≥6 days and until adequate anticoagulation with warfarin (INR ≥2 for 2 consecutive days)

Prophylaxis of DVT/ thromboembolism/PE (unlabeled)
Adult: 3500 anti-Xa units (50 anti-Xa units/ kg) daily beginning 1-2 hr prior to surgery and continued for 5-10 days

Prophylaxis of deep vein thrombosis in orthopedic procedures (unlabeled)
Adult: 75 anti-Xa units/kg/day started 12-24 hr after surgery

Available forms: Inj 20,000 international units/ml

Adverse effects
CNS: Fever, confusion, dizziness, insomnia
CV: Angina, dysrhythmias, peripheral edema, tachycardia, hypo/hypertension
GI: Nausea, constipation, flatulence, dyspepsia, **hepatitis**
GU: UTI, hematuria, urinary retention, dysuria
HEMA: Hemorrhage, **anemia, thrombocytopenia,** bleeding
INTEG: Ecchymosis, inj site reaction
MISC: Headache, chest pain, hypersensitivity
SYST: **Stevens-Johnson syndrome**

Contraindications: Hypersensitivity to this product, heparin, pork or benzyl alcohol, sulfites; hemophilia, leukemia with bleeding,

T

Adverse effects: *italic* = common, **bold** = life-threatening

peptic ulcer disease, thrombocytopenic purpura, heparin-induced thrombocytopenia

Precautions: Pregnancy **C**, breastfeeding, children, geriatric, alcoholism, severe renal/hepatic disease, blood dyscrasias, severe uncontrolled hypertension, subacute bacterial endocarditis, acute nephritis, elderly >70 yr (renal disease with DVT/PE)

Black Box Warning: Spinal/epidural anesthesia, lumbar puncture

Pharmacokinetics

Absorption	Unknown
Distribution	Unknown
Metabolism	Unknown
Excretion	Unknown
Half-life	4.5 hr

Pharmacodynamics

Onset	Unknown
Peak	3-5 hr (max antithrombin activity)
Duration	Unknown

Interactions
Individual drug
Ticlopidine: increased tinzaparin action
Drug classifications
Anticoagulants (oral), NSAIDs, platelet inhibitors, salicylates, thrombolytics: increased tinzaparin action
Drug/herb
Agrimony, alfalfa, angelica, anise, basil, bay, bilberry, black haw, bogbean, bromelain, buchu, chondroitin, cinchona bark, dong quai, fenugreek, feverfew, garlic, ginger, ginkgo, ginseng, horse chestnut, Irish moss, kelp, kelpware, khella, lovage, lungwort, meadowsweet, motherwort, mugwort, nettle, papaya, parsley (large amounts), pau d'arco, pineapple, poplar, prickly ash, safflower, saw palmetto, tonka bean, turmeric, wintergreen, yarrow: increased risk of bleeding
Chamomile, coenzyme Q10, flax, glucomannan, goldenseal, guar gum: decreased anticoagulant effect

NURSING CONSIDERATIONS
Assessment
• Monitor blood tests (Hct, platelets, occult blood in stools), anti-Xa; thrombocytopenia may occur
• Assess for bleeding gums, petechiae, ecchymosis, black tarry stools, hematuria

Nursing diagnoses
• Cardiac output, decreased (uses)
• Knowledge, deficient (teaching)

Implementation
• Give only after screening patient for bleeding disorders
• Give SUBCUT only; do not give IM
• Give SUBCUT to recumbent patient; rotate inj sites (left/right anterolateral, left/right posterolateral abdominal wall)
• Insert whole length of needle into skin fold held with thumb and forefinger
◆ Use only this product when ordered; not interchangeable with heparin or LMWHs
• Give at same time each day to maintain steady blood levels
• Do not massage area or aspirate when giving SUBCUT inj
• Avoid all IM inj that may cause bleeding
• Do not mix with other products or inf fluids
• Store at 77° F (25° C); do not freeze

Patient/family education
• Advise patient to use soft-bristle toothbrush to avoid bleeding gums, to use electric razor
• Instruct patient to report any signs of bleeding: gums, under skin, urine, stools

Evaluation
Positive therapeutic outcome
• Resolution of deep vein thrombosis

Treatment of overdose: Protamine 1 mg/100 anti-Xa international units of tinzaparin

---

tioconazole vaginal antifungal
See Appendix B

---

tiotropium (Rx)
(ty-oh'tro-pee-um)
Spiriva, HandiHaler
Func. class.: Anticholinergic, bronchodilator
Chem. class.: Synthetic quaternary ammonium compound

Pregnancy category C

Action: Inhibits interaction of acetylcholine at receptor sites on the bronchial smooth muscle, resulting in decreased cGMP and bronchodilatation

Therapeutic outcome: Improved breathing

Uses: COPD, for long-term treatment, once daily maintenance of bronchospasm, associated with COPD including chronic bronchitis and emphysema

---

Dosage and routes
Adult: INH content of 1 cap/day using HandiHaler inhalation device

Available forms: Powder for inhalation 18 mcg in blister packs containing 6 caps with inhaler; 30 caps with inhaler

Adverse effects
CNS: Depression, paresthesia
CV: Chest pain, increased heart rate
EENT: Dry mouth, blurred vision, glaucoma
GI: Vomiting, abdominal pain, constipation, dyspepsia
INTEG: Rash, **angioedema**
MISC: Urinary difficulty, urinary retention
RESP: Cough, worsening of symptoms, sinusitis, URI, epistaxis, pharyngitis

Contraindications: Hypersensitivity to this product, atropine, or its derivatives

Precautions: Pregnancy **C**, breastfeeding, children, geriatric, closed-angle glaucoma, prostatic hypertrophy, bladder neck obstruction, renal disease

Pharmacokinetics

Absorption	Unknown
Distribution	Does not cross blood-brain barrier
Metabolism	Very little metabolized in the liver
Excretion	Excreted in urine
Half-life	5-6 days in animals

Pharmacodynamics
Unknown

Interactions
Drug classifications
Anticholinergics: avoid use with other anticholinergics
Drug/herb
Black catechu: increased constipation
Butterbur, jimsonweed: increased anticholinergic effect
Green tea (large amts), guarana: increased bronchodilator effect
Jaborandi tree, pill-bearing spurge: decreased anticholinergic effect

NURSING CONSIDERATIONS
Assessment
• For tolerance over long-term therapy; dose may have to be increased or changed

Nursing diagnoses
• Breathing pattern, ineffective (uses)
• Knowledge, deficient (teaching)

Implementation
• Caps are for INH only; do not swallow
• Immediately prior to administration, peel back foil until cap is visible (until "stop" line); open dust cap of HandiHaler by pulling upward, then open mouthpiece
• Place cap in center chamber; firmly close mouthpiece until it clicks, leaving dust cap open
• Hold HandiHaler with mouthpiece upward; press button in once, completely, and release; this allows for medication to be released
• Breathe out completely; do not breathe into mouthpiece at any time
• Raise device to mouth and close lips tightly around mouthpiece
• With head upright, breathe in slowly/deeply, but allowing the cap to vibrate; breathe until lungs fill; hold breath and remove mouthpiece; resume normal breathing
• Repeat
• Remove used capsule and dispose; close the mouthpiece and dust cap; store

Patient/family education
• Teach patient how to use HandiHaler
• Teach patient signs of closed-angle glaucoma
• Advise patient that product is used for long-term maintenance, not for immediate relief of breathing problems
• Caution patient to avoid getting the powder in the eyes; may cause blurred vision and pupil dilatation

Evaluation
Positive therapeutic outcome
• Ability to breathe easier

---

tipranavir (Rx)
(ti-pran′a-veer)
Aptivus
Func. class.: Antiretroviral
Chem. class.: Protease inhibitor

Pregnancy category C

Action: Inhibits human immunodeficiency virus (HIV) protease; this prevents the maturation of virus

Therapeutic outcome: Prevention of worsening of HIV

Uses: HIV in combination with other antiretrovirals

Dosage and routes
Reduce dose in mild or moderate hepatic impairment and ketoconazole coadministration

Adult: PO 500 mg coadministered with ritonavir 200 mg bid with food

Adolescent and child ≥2 yr: PO 14 mg/kg given with ritonavir 6 mg/kg bid or 375 mg/m² given with ritonavir 150 mg/m² bid; max 500 mg with ritonavir 200 mg bid

Available forms: Caps 250 mg; oral sol 100 mg/ml

Adverse effects

CNS: Headache, insomnia, dizziness, somnolence, fatigue, *fever,* **intracranial bleeding**
GI: Diarrhea, abdominal pain, nausea, vomiting, anorexia, dry mouth, **hepatitis B or C, fatalities when given with ritonavir, pancreatitis**
GU: Nephrolithiasis
INTEG: Rash, urticaria, lipodystrophy
MS: Pain
OTHER: Asthenia, **insulin-resistant hyperglycemia,** *hyperlipidemia,* **ketoacidosis**

Contraindications: Hypersensitivity, hepatic disease (Child-Pugh B to C)

Precautions: Pregnancy **C,** breastfeeding, children, renal disease, history of renal stones, sulfa allergy, hemophilia, diabetes mellitus, pancreatitis, alcoholism, immune reconstitution syndrome, surgery, trauma, infection

Black Box Warning: Intracranial bleeding, hepatitis

Pharmacokinetics

Absorption	Unknown
Distribution	Protein binding, 99.9%, steady state 7-10 days
Metabolism	CYP3A4
Excretion	80% feces
Half-life	Terminal 6 hr

Pharmacodynamics
Unknown

Interactions
Individual drugs
◆Amiodarone, astemizole, cisapride, flecainide, midazolam, pimozide, propafenone, quinidine, rifabutin, rifampin, terfenadine, triazolam: life-threatening dysrhythmias
Clarithromycin, zidovudine: increased levels of both products
Delavirdine, itraconazole, ketoconazole: increased tipranavir levels
Efavirenz, fluconazole, nevirapine: decreased tipranavir levels
Lovastatin, simvastatin: increased myopathy, rhabdomyolysis

Drug classifications
◆ Ergots: life-threatening dysrhythmias
Oral contraceptives: increased levels of tipranavir
Rifamycins: decreased tipranavir levels
Drug/herb
St. John's wort: decreased tipranavir levels; avoid concurrent use
Drug/food
Grapefruit juice, high-fat, high-protein foods: decreased tipranavir absorption
Drug/lab test
Increased: AST, ALT

NURSING CONSIDERATIONS
Assessment
• Monitor for complaints of lower back, flank pain; indicates kidney stones
• Assess for signs of infection, anemia, the presence of other STDs
• Assess for hepatic studies: ALT, AST; total bilirubin, amylase, all may be elevated
• Monitor viral load, CD4, plasma HIV RNA, serum cholesterol/triglycerides during treatment
• Monitor bowel pattern before, during treatment; if severe abdominal pain with bleeding occurs, product should be discontinued; monitor hydration
• Monitor skin eruptions; rash, urticaria, itching
• Assess for allergies before treatment, reaction of each medication; place allergies on chart

Nursing Diagnoses
• Infection, risk for (use, adverse reactions)
• Knowledge, deficient (teaching)

Implementation
• Swallow cap whole; do not break, crush, or chew
• Give after meals
• Give in equal intervals around the clock to maintain blood levels

Patient/family education
• Teach patient to take as prescribed; if dose is missed, take as soon as remembered up to 1 hr before next dose; do not double dose
• Teach patient that product must be taken in equal intervals around the clock to maintain blood levels for duration of therapy
◆ Advise that hyperglycemia may occur; watch for increased thirst, weight loss, hunger, dry, itchy skin; notify prescriber
• Teach patient to increase fluids to prevent kidney stones; if stone formation occurs, treatment may need to be interrupted

- Advise patient that product does not cure AIDS, only controls symptoms; not to donate blood

Evaluation
Positive therapeutic outcome
- Prevention of viral replication

! HIGH ALERT

tirofiban (Rx)
(tie-roh-fee'ban)
Aggrastat
Func. class.: Antiplatelet
Chem. class.: Glycoprotein IIb/IIIa inhibitor

Pregnancy category B

Action: Antagonist of platelet glycoprotein (GP) IIb/IIIa receptor that leads to binding of fibrinogen and von Willebrand's factor, which inhibits platelet aggregation

Therapeutic outcome: Decreased platelet count

Uses: Acute coronary syndrome in combination with heparin

Dosage and routes
Adult: **IV** 0.4 mcg/kg/min × 30 min, then 0.1 mcg/kg/min for 12-24 hr after angioplasty or atherectomy

Renal dose
Adult: **IV** CCr <30 ml/min 0.2 mcg/kg/min × 30 min, then 0.05 mcg/kg/min, during angiography and for up to 24 hr after angioplasty

Available forms: Inj for sol 250 mcg/ml, inj 50 mcg/ml

Adverse effects
CNS: Dizziness, headache
CV: Bradycardia, hypotension
GI: Nausea, vomiting
HEMA: Bleeding, **thrombocytopenia**
INTEG: Rash
MISC: Dissection, coronary artery edema, pain in legs/pelvis, sweating
SYST: **Anaphylaxis**

Contraindications: Hypersensitivity, active internal bleeding, stroke, major surgery, severe trauma within 30 days, intracranial neoplasm, aneurysm, hemorrhage, acute pericarditis, platelets <100,000/mm³, history of thrombocytopenia, coagulopathy, systolic B/P >180 mm Hg or diastolic B/P >110 mm Hg

Precautions: Pregnancy **B**, breastfeeding, children, geriatric, renal disease, bleeding tendencies, hypertension, platelets <150,000/mm³

Pharmacokinetics
Absorption	Unknown
Distribution	Plasma clearance 20%-25%
Metabolism	Liver
Excretion	Urine/feces
Half-life	2 hr

Pharmacodynamics
Unknown

Interactions
Individual drugs
Abciximab, aspirin, cefamandole, cefoperazone, cefotetan, clopidogrel, dipyridamole, eptifibatide, heparin, ticlopidine, valproic acid: increased bleeding risk
Drug classifications
Heparins, NSAIDs, SNRIs, SSRIs, thrombin inhibitors: increased bleeding risk
Drug/herb
Agrimony, alfalfa, angelica, anise, basil, bay, bilberry, black haw, bogbean, bromelain, buchu, chondroitin, cinchona bark, dong quai, fenugreek, feverfew, garlic, ginger, ginkgo, ginseng, green tea, horse chestnut, Irish moss, kelp, kelpware, khella, lovage, lungwort, meadowsweet, motherwort, mugwort, nettle, papaya, parsley (large amounts), pau d'arco, pineapple, poplar, prickly ash, safflower, saw palmetto, tonka bean, turmeric, wintergreen, yarrow: increased risk of bleeding
Chamomile, coenzyme Q10, flax, glucomannan, goldenseal, guar gum: decreased anticoagulant effect

NURSING CONSIDERATIONS
Assessment
- Monitor platelet counts, Hct, Hgb before treatment, within 6 hr of loading dose and at least daily thereafter; watch for bleeding from puncture sites, catheters or in stools, urine

Nursing diagnoses
- Tissue perfusion, ineffective (uses)

Implementation
- Dilute inj: withdraw and discard 100 ml from a 500-ml bag of sterile 0.9% NaCl or D₅ and replace this vol with 100 ml of tirofiban inj from two vials
- Tirofiban inj for sol is premixed in containers of 500 ml 0.9% NaCl (50 mg/ml), give over 30 min
- Minimize other arterial/venous punctures, IM inj, catheter use, intubation to reduce bleeding risks

T

Adverse effects: *italic* = common, **bold** = life-threatening

Y-site compatibility: Heparin

Patient/family education
- Advise patient that it is necessary to quit smoking to prevent excessive vasoconstriction
- Teach signs/symptoms of bleeding, low platelets
- Advise that there are many drug and herb interactions

Evaluation
Positive therapeutic outcome
- Treatment of acute coronary syndrome

---

tizanidine (Rx)

(tye-za′na-deen)

Zanaflex

Func. class.: Skeletal muscle relaxant, central acting

Chem. class.: Imidazole

Pregnancy category C

Do not confuse:
tizanidine/tiagabine

Action: Increases presynaptic inhibition of motor neurons and reduces spasticity by α_2-adrenergic agonism

Uses: Acute/intermittent management of increased muscle tone associated with spasticity, symptoms of MS

Dosage and routes
Adult: PO 8 mg q6-8hr; max 36 mg/24 hr

Renal dose
Adult: PO CCr <25 ml/min, start with lower dose

Available forms: Tabs 2, 4 mg; caps 2, 4, 6 mg

Adverse effects
CNS: Dizziness, somnolence, speech disorder, dyskinesia, nervousness, hallucination, psychosis
CV: Hypotension, bradycardia
GI: Constipation, vomiting, dry mouth, increased ALT, abnormal liver function tests
GU: Urinary frequency
OTHER: Blurred vision, pharyngitis, rhinitis, tremor, rash, muscle weakness

Contraindications: Hypersensitivity

Precautions: Pregnancy C, breastfeeding, children, geriatric, renal/hepatic disease, hypotension

---

Pharmacokinetics

Absorption	Complete
Distribution	Widely
Metabolism	Liver, extensively
Excretion	Kidneys, feces
Half-life	2½ hr

Pharmacodynamics

Onset	Unknown
Peak	1-2 hr
Duration	3-6 hr

Interactions
Individual drugs
Alcohol: CNS depression
Amiodarone, ciprofloxacin, famotidine, fluvoxamine: increased tizanidine levels; do not use together
Drug classifications
CNS depressants: increased CNS depression
Contraceptives (oral): decreased clearance of tizanidine
Drug/herb
Black cohosh, California poppy, goldenseed, hawthorn: increased hypotension
Gotu kola, kava, St. John's wort: increased CNS depression
Drug/lab test
Increased: AST, alkaline phosphatase, ALT, serum glucose

NURSING CONSIDERATIONS
Assessment
- Assess for muscle spasticity baseline and throughout treatment
- Monitor B/P, heart rate
- Perform neurologic exam in spasticity: deep tendon reflexes, muscle tone, clonus, sensory function
- Monitor renal/liver function tests, electrolytes, CBC with differential during long-term treatment
- Assess for allergic reactions: rash, fever, respiratory distress; severe weakness, numbness in extremities
- Assess CNS depression: dizziness, drowsiness, psychiatric symptoms
- Check dosage, as individual titration is required

Nursing diagnoses
- Injury, risk for (adverse reactions)
- Knowledge, deficient (teaching)
- Mobility, impaired physical (uses)

Implementation
- Give with meals for GI symptoms
- Store in airtight container at room temperature

• Give consistently either with or without food; food may affect absorption
• Titrate dose carefully

Patient/family education

• Advise patient not to discontinue medication quickly; spasticity will occur; product should be tapered off over 1-2 wk
• Advise patient not to take with alcohol, other CNS depressants; take as directed; if dose is missed, take as soon as remembered, unless it is almost time for next dose
• Caution patient to avoid altering activities while taking this product; to avoid hazardous activities if drowsiness or dizziness occurs; to rise from sitting or lying slowly to prevent fainting
• Teach patient to use gum, frequent sips of water for dry mouth
• Advise patient to avoid using OTC medications (cough preparations, antihistamines) unless directed by prescriber
• Notify prescriber if fainting, hallucinations, dark urine, stomach pain, yellowing of skin/eyes occurs

Evaluation
Positive therapeutic outcome
• Decreased pain, spasticity

---

tobramycin (Rx)
(toe-bra-mye'sin)
tobramycin sulfate, TOBI
Func. class.: Antiinfective
Chem. class.: Aminoglycoside

Pregnancy category D

Action: Interferes with protein synthesis in bacterial cell by binding to ribosomal subunit, causing inaccurate peptide sequence to form in protein chain, causing bacterial death

Therapeutic outcome: Bactericidal effects for the following organisms: *Pseudomonas aeruginosa, Enterobacter, Escherichia coli, Providencia, Citrobacter, Staphylococcus, Proteus, Klebsiella, Serratia*

Uses: Severe systemic infections of CNS, respiratory, GI, urinary tract, bone, skin, soft tissues, eye, cystic fibrosis (nebulizer) for *P. aeruginosa*

Dosage and routes
Adult: IM/IV 3 mg/kg/day in divided doses q8hr; may give up to 6 mg/kg/day in divided doses q8-12hr; once-daily dosing (pulse dosing) (unlabeled) IV 5-7 mg/kg; dosing intervals are determined using a nomogram

and are based on random levels drawn 8-12 hr after first dose
Child: IM/IV 6-7.5 mg/kg/day in 3-4 equal divided doses
Child ≥6 yr: NEB 300 mg bid in repeating cycles of 28 days on/28 days off; give inh over 10-15 min using a hand-held PARI LC PLUS reusable nebulizer with a DeVilbiss Pulmo-Aid compressor
Neonate <1 wk: IM up to 4 mg/kg/day in divided doses q12hr; IV up to 4 mg/kg/day in divided doses q12hr diluted in 50-100 mg NS or D₅W; give over 30-60 min

Renal dose
Adult: IM/IV 1 mg/kg, then dose determined by blood levels

Available forms: Inj 10, 40 mg/ml; powder for inj 1.2 g; neb sol 300 mg/5 ml

Adverse effects
CNS: Confusion, depression, numbness, tremors, **seizures,** muscle twitching, **neurotoxicity,** dizziness, vertigo
CV: Hypo/hypertension, palpitations
EENT: Ototoxicity, deafness, visual disturbances, tinnitus
GI: Nausea, vomiting, anorexia, increased ALT, AST, bilirubin, hepatomegaly, **hepatic necrosis,** splenomegaly
GU: Oliguria, hematuria, renal damage, azotemia, renal failure, nephrotoxicity
HEMA: Agranulocytosis, thrombocytopenia, leukopenia, eosinophilia, anemia
INTEG: Rash, burning, urticaria, dermatitis, alopecia

Contraindications: Hypersensitivity to aminoglycosides

Black Box Warning: Pregnancy D, severe renal disease

Precautions: Breastfeeding, geriatric, neonates, mild renal disease, myasthenia gravis, Parkinson's disease

Black Box Warning: Hearing deficits, neuromuscular disease

Pharmacokinetics	
Absorption	Well absorbed (IM), completely absorbed (**IV**)
Distribution	Widely distributed in extracellular fluids
Metabolism	Minimal liver
Excretion	Mostly unchanged (>90%) kidneys
Half-life	2-3 hr, increased in renal disease, neonates

Adverse effects: *italic* = common, **bold** = life-threatening

Pharmacodynamics			
	IM	IV	OPHTH
Onset	Rapid	Rapid	Rapid
Peak	1 hr	Inf end	Unknown
Duration	Unknown	Unknown	Unknown

Interactions
Individual drugs
Acyclovir, amphotericin B, bacitracin, cidofovir, cisplatin, ethacrynic acid, furosemide, mannitol, methoxyflurane, polymyxin, vancomycin: increased ototoxicity, neurotoxicity, nephrotoxicity

Drug classifications
Aminoglycosides, cephalosporins, penicillins: increased ototoxicity, neurotoxicity, nephrotoxicity

Drug/herb
Acidophilus: do not use with antiinfectives; separate by several hours

Lysine (large amounts): increased toxicity

NURSING CONSIDERATIONS
Assessment
• Assess patient for previous sensitivity reaction
Systemic route
• Assess patient for signs and symptoms of infection including characteristics of wounds, sputum, urine, stool, WBC >10,000/mm^3, temp baseline, during treatment
• Complete C&S testing before beginning product therapy to identify if correct treatment has been initiated
• Assess for allergic reactions: rash, urticaria, pruritus, chills, fever, joint pain
• Identify urine output; if decreasing, notify prescriber (may indicate nephrotoxicity); also, obtain BUN, creatinine, urine CCr (<80 ml/min) values; urinalysis daily for proteinuria, cells, casts; report sudden change in urine output
• Monitor blood studies: AST, ALT, CBC, Hct, bilirubin, LDH, alkaline phosphatase, Coombs' test monthly if patient is on long-term therapy
• Monitor electrolytes: potassium, sodium, chloride, magnesium monthly if patient is on long-term therapy
• Monitor for bleeding: ecchymosis, bleeding gums, hematuria, stool guaiac daily if patient is on long-term therapy
• Assess for overgrowth of infection: perineal itching, fever, malaise, redness, pain, swelling, drainage, rash, diarrhea, change in cough, sputum
• Obtain weight before treatment; calculation of dosage is usually based on ideal body weight, but may be calculated on actual body weight
• Monitor VS during inf, watch for hypotension, change in pulse
• Assess **IV** site for thrombophlebitis including pain, redness, swelling q30min; change site if needed; apply warm compresses to discontinued site
• Obtain serum peak, drawn at 30-60 min after **IV** inf or 60 min after IM inj, trough level drawn just before next dose; peak 4-12 mcg/ml, trough 1-2 mcg/ml
• Monitor for deafness by audiometric testing, ringing, roaring in ears, vertigo; assess hearing before, during, after treatment
• Monitor for dehydration: high specific gravity, decrease in skin turgor, dry mucous membranes, dark urine
• Monitor for overgrowth of infection including increased temp, malaise, redness, pain, swelling, perineal itching, diarrhea, stomatitis, change in cough, sputum

Nursing diagnoses
• Diarrhea (adverse reactions)
• Infection, risk for (uses)
• Injury, risk for (adverse reactions)
• Knowledge, deficient (teaching)
• Noncompliance (teaching)

Implementation
IM route
• Give inj deeply in large muscle mass
Nebulizer route
• Give as close to q12hr apart as possible; do not use <6 hr apart
• Do not mix with dornase alfa in the nebulizer
• Inhale sitting or standing; breathe normally through the mouthpiece; may use nose clips
IV route
• Give **IV** diluted in 50-100 ml of 0.9% NaCl, D$_{10}$W, D$_5$/0.9% NaCl, 0.9% NaCl, Ringer's, LR, D$_5$W (adult), in over 20-60 min
• Flush after inf with D$_5$W, 0.9% NaCl
• Separate aminoglycosides and penicillins by ≥1 hr

Syringe compatibilities: Doxapram
Syringe incompatibilities: Cefamandole, clindamycin, heparin, sargramostim
Y-site compatibilities: Acyclovir, amifostine, amiodarone, amsacrine, aztreonam, ciprofloxacin, cyclophosphamide, diltiazem, enalaprilat, esmolol, filgrastim, fluconazole, fludarabine, foscarnet, furosemide, granisetron, hydromorphone, IL-2, insulin (regular), labetalol, magnesium sulfate, melphalan, meperidine, midazolam, morphine, perphenazine, tacrolimus, tenipo-

side, theophylline, thiotepa, tolazoline, vinorelbine, zidovudine

Additive compatibilities: Aztreonam, bleomycin, calcium gluconate, cefoxitin, ciprofloxacin, clindamycin, furosemide, metronidazole, ofloxacin, ranitidine, verapamil

Additive incompatibilities: Cefamandole, floxacillin

Patient/family education
• Advise patient to use multiple therapies first, then tobramycin
• Teach patient to report sore throat, bruising, bleeding, joint pain; may indicate blood dyscrasias (rare)
• Advise patient to contact prescriber if vaginal itching, loose foul-smelling stools, furry tongue occur; may indicate superinfection
• Advise patient to notify prescriber of diarrhea with blood or pus; may indicate pseudomembranous colitis

Evaluation
Positive therapeutic outcome
• Absence of signs/symptoms of infection (WBC <10,000/mm³, temp WNL, absence of red, draining wounds)
• Reported improvement in symptoms of infection

Treatment of overdose: Withdraw product, hemodialysis, exchange transfusion in the newborn, monitor serum levels of product, may give ticarcillin or carbenicillin

---

tobramycin ophthalmic
See Appendix B

---

tocainide (Rx)
(toe-kay′nide)
Tonocard
Func. class.: Antidysrhythmic (class IB)
Chem. class.: Lidocaine analog

Pregnancy category C

Action: Produces dose-dependent decreases in sodium and potassium conduction, thereby decreasing the excitability of myocardial cells; does not affect heart rate or B/P

Therapeutic outcome: Decreased ventricular dysrhythmia

Uses: Life-threatening ventricular dysrhythmias (multifocal/unifocal premature ventricular contractions [PVCs]), ventricular tachycardia

Dosage and routes
Adult: PO 400 mg q8hr, may increase to 1.2-1.8 g/day in divided doses q8-12hr

Available forms: Tabs 400, 600 mg

Adverse effects
CNS: *Headache, dizziness,* involuntary movement, confusion, psychosis, restlessness, irritability, paresthesias, tremors, **seizures**
CV: *Hypotension, bradycardia,* angina, PVCs, **heart block, CV collapse, sinus arrest, CHF,** chest pain, tachycardia, prodysrhythmias
EENT: Tinnitus, blurred vision, hearing loss
GI: Nausea, vomiting, anorexia, diarrhea, hepatitis, loss of taste
HEMA: **Blood dyscrasias: leukopenia, agranulocytosis, hypoplastic anemia, thrombocytopenia,** bone marrow depression
INTEG: Rash, urticaria, lupus, alopecia, sweating, **Stevens-Johnson syndrome**
RESP: Dyspnea, **respiratory depression, pulmonary fibrosis,** pulmonary edema, interstitial pneumonitis pneumonia

Contraindications: Hypersensitivity to amides, severe heart block

Precautions: Pregnancy C, breastfeeding, children, geriatric, pulmonary/renal/hepatic disease, CHF, myasthenia gravis, hypokalemia, atrial flutter/fibrillation

Black Box Warning: Bone marrow suppression, cardiac arrhythmias, pulmonary fibrosis

Pharmacokinetics	
Absorption	Well absorbed
Distribution	Widely distributed, crosses blood-brain barrier
Metabolism	Liver
Excretion	Kidney (up to 40% unchanged)
Half-life	10-17 hr

Pharmacodynamics	
Onset	1 hr
Peak	½-2 hr
Duration	8-12 hr

Interactions
Individual drugs
Cimetidine, rifampin: decreased effects of tocainide
Metropolol: increased tocainide effects
Drug/herb
Aconite: increased toxicity, death
Aloe, broom, buckthorn (chronic use), cascara sagrada (chronic use), Chinese

Adverse effects: *italic* = common, **bold** = life-threatening

rhubarb, figwort, fumitory, goldenseal, kudzu, licorice: increased effect

Coltsfoot: decreased effect

Horehound: increased serotonin effect

Drug/lab test

Increased: CPK

False positive: ANA titer

NURSING CONSIDERATIONS
Assessment
• Assess for oxygenation or perfusion deficit: decreased B/P, chest pain, dizziness, loss of consciousness

• Assess respiratory status: auscultate lung fields for bibasilar crackles in patients with advanced CHF

• Assess for urinary retention: check for pain, abdominal absorption, palpate bladder; check males with benign prostatic hypertrophy; anticholinergic reaction may cause retention

• Monitor I&O ratio; electrolytes (potassium, sodium, chloride); watch for decreasing urinary output, possible retention

• Monitor liver function tests: AST, ALT, bilirubin, alkaline phosphatase

• Monitor ECG to determine product effectiveness; measure PR, QRS, QT intervals; check for PVCs, other dysrhythmias; monitor B/P for hypotension, hypertension; for re-bound hypertension after 1-2 hr

• Monitor patient for CNS symptoms: confusion, psychosis, numbness, depression, involuntary movements; if these occur, product should be discontinued

• Assess pulmonary toxicity: dyspnea, fatigue, cough, fever, chest pain; product should be discontinued if these occur

• Assess cardiac rate, respiration (rate, rhythm, character), chest pain, ventricular tachycardia, supraventricular tachycardia or fibrillation

Nursing diagnoses
• Cardiac output, decreased (uses)
• Gas exchange, impaired (adverse reactions)
• Knowledge, deficient (teaching)

Implementation
• Give with meals to decrease GI upset

Patient/family education
• Inform patient or family of reason for medication and expected results

• Teach patient method for taking pulse at home and what to report to prescriber

• Advise patient to avoid hazardous activities until product response is known; dizziness, confusion, sedation may occur

• Advise patient to carry/wear emergency ID indicating medications taken, condition, and prescriber's name and phone number

• Instruct patient to report bleeding, bruising, respiratory symptoms, chills, fever, sore throat to prescriber

Evaluation
Positive therapeutic outcome
• Decreased dysrhythmias

Treatment of overdose: Defibrillation, vasopressor for hypotension

tolcapone (Rx)
(toll'cah-pone)

Tasmar

Func. class.: Antiparkinson agent

Chem. class.: Catecholamine inhibitor (COMT)

Pregnancy category C

Action: Selective, reversible inhibitor of catecholamine; used as adjunct to levodopa/carbidopa therapy

Therapeutic outcome: Increased ability to move and speak

Uses: Parkinsonism

Dosage and routes
Adult: PO 100-200 mg tid, with levodopa/carbidopa therapy; max 600 mg/day; discontinue if no benefit in 3 wk

Renal dose
Adult: PO 100 mg tid or less

Available forms: Tabs 100, 200 mg

Adverse effects
CNS: Dystonia, dyskinesia, dreaming, *fatigue, headache, confusion,* psychosis, hallucination, dizziness, sleep disorders

CV: Orthostatic *hypotension,* chest pain, hypotension

EENT: Cataract, eye inflammation

GI: Nausea, vomiting, abdominal distress, diarrhea, constipation, **fatal liver failure,** elevated liver function tests

GU: UTI, urine discoloration, uterine tumor, micturition disorder, hematuria

HEMA: **Hemolytic anemia, leukopenia, agranulocytosis**

INTEG: Sweating, alopecia

MS: **Rhabdomyolysis**

Contraindications: Hypersensitivity

Precautions: Pregnancy **C,** breastfeeding, cardiac/renal disease, hypertension, asthma, history of rhabdomyolysis

Black Box Warning: Hepatic disease

Pharmacokinetics

Absorption	Rapidly
Distribution	Protein binding 99%
Metabolism	Liver, extensively
Excretion	Urine (60%), feces (40%)
Half-life	2-3 hr

Pharmacodynamics

Onset	Unknown
Peak	2 hr
Duration	Unknown

Interactions
Individual drugs
Apomorphine, DOBUTamine, isoproterenol, α-methyldopa: may influence pharmacokinetics
Drug classifications
MAOIs: decreased normal catecholamine metabolism; MAO-B inhibitor may be used
Drug/herb
Kava: decreased effect

NURSING CONSIDERATIONS
Assessment
• Monitor liver function tests: AST, ALT, alkaline phosphatase, LDH, bilirubin, CBC
• Assess involuntary movements in parkinsonism: akinesia, tremors, staggering gait, muscle rigidity, drooling
• Monitor B/P, respiration during initial treatment; hypo/hypertension should be reported
• Monitor mental status: affect, mood, behavioral changes

Nursing diagnoses
• Injury, risk for (uses)
• Knowledge, deficient (teaching)
• Mobility, impaired physical (uses)

Implementation
• Administer tid with levodopa/carbidopa therapy
• Food taken within 1 hr before or 2 hr after meals increases action of product by 20%
• Provide assistance with ambulation during beginning therapy

Patient/family education
• Advise patient to change positions slowly to prevent orthostatic hypotension
• Advise patient that urine, sweat may change color
• Teach patient to report nausea, vomiting, anorexia

Evaluation
Positive therapeutic outcome
• Decrease in akathisia, increased mood

---

tolnaftate topical
See Appendix B

---

tolterodine (Rx)
(tol-tehr'oh-deen)
Detrol, Detrol LA
Func. class.: Overactive bladder product
Chem. class.: Muscarinic receptor antagonist

Pregnancy category C

Action: Relaxes smooth muscles in urinary tract by inhibiting acetylcholine at postganglionic sites

Therapeutic outcome: Decreased symptoms of overactive bladder

Uses: Overactive bladder (frequency, urgency), urinary incontinence

Dosage and routes
Adult and geriatric: PO 2 mg bid, EXT REL 4 mg/day, may decrease to 2 mg if needed, max 4 mg/day
Hepatic disease
Adult: PO 1 mg bid (50% dose) or EXT REL 2 mg/day
Renal dose
Adult: PO CCr ≤30 ml/min reduce by 50%

Available forms: Tabs 1, 2 mg; ext rel caps 2, 4 mg

Adverse effects
CNS: Anxiety, paresthesia, fatigue, *dizziness,* headache, increasing dementia, memory impairment
CV: Chest pain, hypertension, **QT prolongation**
EENT: Vision abnormalities, xerophthalmia
GI: Nausea, vomiting, anorexia, abdominal pain, constipation, dry mouth, dyspepsia
GU: Dysuria, retention, frequency, UTI
INTEG: Rash, pruritus
RESP: Bronchitis, cough, pharyngitis, upper respiratory tract infection
SYST: **Angioedema**

Black Box Warning: Stevens-Johnson syndrome

Contraindications: Hypersensitivity, uncontrolled closed-angle glaucoma, urinary retention, gastric retention

T

Adverse effects: *italic* = common, **bold** = life-threatening

Precautions: Pregnancy **C**, breastfeeding, children, renal/hepatic disease, controlled closed-angle glaucoma, bladder obstruction, QT prolongation, decreased GI motility

Pharmacokinetics

Absorption	Rapidly
Distribution	Highly protein bound
Metabolism	Liver, extensively
Excretion	Urine/feces
Half-life	Unknown

Pharmacodynamics

Unknown

Interactions
Individual drugs
Bepridil, chloroquine, clarithromycin, droperidol, erythromycin, grepafloxacin, halofantrine, haloperidol, methadone, pentamidine, probucol, sparfloxacin: increased QT prolongation
Drug classifications
Antibiotics (macrolide), antifungal agents, antiretroviral protease inhibitors: increased action of tolterodine
Antimuscarinics: increased anticholinergic effect
β-agonists, class IA/III antidysrhythmics, local anesthetics, tricyclics: increased QT prolongation
Diuretics: increased urinary frequency
Drug/food
Increased: bioavailability of tolterodine

NURSING CONSIDERATIONS
Assessment
• Assess urinary patterns: distension, nocturia, frequency, urgency, incontinence
• Assess allergic reactions: rash; if this occurs, product should be discontinued

Nursing diagnoses
• Activity intolerance (uses)
• Incontinence, functional urinary (uses)
• Knowledge, deficient (teaching)
• Urinary elimination, impaired (uses)

Implementation
• Swallow whole; give with liquids

Patient/family education
• Advise patient to avoid hazardous activities; dizziness may occur
• Advise patient not to drink liquids before bedtime
• Teach patient importance of bladder maintenance

• Teach patient to take with liquids; swallow whole

Evaluation
Positive therapeutic outcome
• Decreased urinary frequency, urgency

---

tolvaptan (Rx)
(tole-vap'tan)
Samsca
Func. class.: Vasopressin receptor antagonist, V2

Pregnancy category C

Action: Arginine vasopressin (AVP) antagonist with affinity for V2 receptors; level of circulating AVP in circulating blood is critical for regulation of water, electrolyte balance and is usually elevated in euvolemic/hypervolemic hyponatremia

Therapeutic outcome: Serum sodium level return to normal

Uses: Hypervolemic/euvolemic hyponatremia in heart failure, cirrhosis, SIADH

Dosage and routes
Adult: PO 15 mg qd; after 24 hr, may increase to 30 mg qd; max 60 mg/day

Available forms: Tab 15, 30 mg

Adverse effects
CNS: Fever
CV: **Ventricular fibrillation, DIC, stroke, thrombosis**
GI: Nausea, vomiting, constipation, colitis
GU: Polyuria
HEMA: **Bleeding**
META: Dehydration, hyperglycemia, hyperkalemia, hypernatremia
MS: **Rhabdomyolysis**
RESP: **Respiratory depression, pulmonary embolism**

Contraindications: Hypersensitivity, hypovolemia, anuria

Precautions: Pregnancy **C**, breastfeeding, children, dehydration, geriatric patients, hepatic disease, hyperkalemia

Black Box Warning: Alcoholism, malnutrition

Pharmacokinetics

Absorption	Unknown
Distribution	Protein binding 99%
Metabolism	CYP3A4
Excretion	Unknown
Half-life	Terminal 12 hr

Pharmacodynamics

Onset	Unknown
Peak	2-4 hr
Duration	Unknown

Interactions
Drug classifications
CYP3A4 inducers (carbamazepine, dexamethasone, etravirine, flutamide, griseofulvin, metyrapsone, modafinil, nafcillin, nevirapine, oxcarbazepine, phenytoin, rifampin, rifabutin, rifapendine, topiramate): decreased plasma concentrations of tolvaptan
CYP3A4 inhibitors (efavirenz, fosamprenavir, quinine), P-gp inhibitors (azithromycin, bepridil, cyclosporine, mefloquine, palperidone, propafenone, quinidine, testosterone): increased plasma concentrations of tolvaptan
Drug/herb
St. John's wort: decreased tolvaptan effect

NURSING CONSIDERATIONS
Assessment
• Assess renal, hepatic function
• Monitor frequent sodium volume status; overly rapid correction of sodium concentration (>12 mEq/L per 24 hr) may result in osmotic demyelination syndrome
• Assess CV status: ventricular fibrillation, hypertension, monitor B/P, pulse
• Monitor electrolytes (sodium, potassium)

Nursing diagnoses
• Injury, risk for (uses)
• Knowledge, deficient (teaching)

Implementation
• Give PO with or without food
• Avoid fluid restriction the first 24 hr
• Initiate in hospital setting

Patient/family education
• Teach patient to avoid pregnancy, breastfeeding while taking this product
• Advise of administration procedure and expected result

Evaluation
Positive therapeutic outcome
• Correction of serum sodium levels

---

topiramate (Rx)
(to-pi-ra′mate)
Topamax, Topamax Sprinkle, Topiragen
Func. class.: Anticonvulsant—miscellaneous
Chem. class.: Monosaccharide derivative

Pregnancy category C

Action: Increased GABA activity; may prevent seizure spread as opposed to an elevation of seizure threshold

Therapeutic outcome: Absence of seizures

Uses: Partial seizures in adults and children 2-16 yr old; tonic-clonic seizures; seizures in Lennox-Gastaut syndrome, migraine prophylaxis

Unlabeled uses: Infantile spasms

Dosage and routes
Adjunctive therapy
Adult/adolescent/child ≥ 10 yr: PO 25-50 mg/day initially, titrate by 25-50 mg/wk, up to 200-400 mg/day in 2 divided doses

Migraine prophylaxis
Adult: PO 25 mg/day initially, increase by 25 mg/day qwk up to 100 mg/day in 2 divided doses

Renal dose
Adult: PO CCr <70 ml/min ½ dose

Available forms: Tabs 25, 50, 100, 200 mg; sprinkle caps 15, 25 mg

Adverse effects
CNS: Dizziness, fatigue, cognitive disorder, *insomnia,* anxiety, depression, paresthesia, motor retardation, **suicidal ideation,** memory loss, tremor
EENT: Diplopia, vision abnormality
GI: Diarrhea, anorexia, nausea, dyspepsia, abdominal pain, constipation, dry mouth, **pancreatitis**
GU: Breast pain, dysmenorrhea, menstrual disorder
INTEG: Rash
MISC: Weight loss, **leukopenia,** metabolic acidosis, increased body temperature
RESP: Upper respiratory tract infection, pharyngitis

Contraindications: Hypersensitivity, metabolic acidosis

Precautions: Pregnancy C, breastfeeding, children, renal/hepatic disease, acute myopia, secondary closed-angle glaucoma, behavioral disorders

T

Adverse effects: *italic* = common, **bold** = life-threatening

Pharmacokinetics

Absorption	Well absorbed
Distribution	Crosses placenta, plasma protein binding (9%-17%), steady state 4 days
Metabolism	Unknown
Excretion	Kidneys unchanged 55%-97%
Half-life	19-25 hr

Pharmacodynamics

Onset	Unknown
Peak	2-4 hr
Duration	Unknown

Interactions
Individual drugs
Alcohol: increased CNS depression
Carbamazepine, phenytoin, probenecid: decreased levels of topiramate
Digoxin: decreased levels of digoxin
Hydrochlorothiazide, lamotrigine, metformin: increased topiramate levels
Lithium: decreased levels of lithium
Valproic acid: decreased levels of both products
Drug classifications
Carbonic anhydrase inhibitors: increased kidney stone formation
CNS depressants: increased CNS depression
Oral contraceptives: decreased level of oral contraceptives
Drug/herb
Ginkgo: increased effect
Ginseng, santonica: decreased effect

NURSING CONSIDERATIONS
Assessment
🔱 Assess mental status: mood, sensorium, affect, memory (long, short), especially in geriatric; suicidal thoughts/behaviors
• Assess for blood dyscrasias: fever, sore throat, bruising, rash, jaundice, epistaxis (long-term treatment only)
• Assess seizure activity including type, location, duration, and character; provide seizure precaution
• Monitor CBC during long-term therapy; serum bicarbonate
• Assess body weight and evidence of cognitive disorder

Nursing diagnoses
• Injury, risk for (side effects)
• Knowledge, deficient (teaching)

Implementation
• Do not break, crush, or chew tabs; very bitter
• May take without regard to meals

• Sprinkle cap can be given whole or opened and sprinkled on soft food; do not chew

Patient/family education
• Teach patient to carry/wear emergency ID stating name, products taken, condition, prescriber's name and phone number
• Advise patient to avoid driving, other activities that require alertness
• Teach patient not to discontinue medication abruptly after long-term use

Evaluation
Positive therapeutic outcome
• Decreased seizure activity

Treatment of overdose: Lavage, VS

⚠ HIGH ALERT

topotecan (Rx)
(to-poe'ti-kan)
Hycamtin
Func. class: Antineoplastic natural; topoisomerase inhibitor
Chem. class.: Camptothecin analog

Pregnancy category D

Action: Antitumor product with topoisomerase I–inhibitory activity; topoisomerase I relieves torsional strain in DNA by causing single-strand breaks; causes double-strand DNA damage

Therapeutic outcome: Decreased tumor size

Uses: Metastatic ovarian cancer after failure of traditional chemotherapy, relapsed small cell lung cancer, cervical cancer

Dosage and routes
Adult: IV INF 1.5 mg/m^2 over 30 min/day × 5 days starting on day 1 of a 21-day course × 4 courses; may be reduced to 0.25 mg/m^2 for subsequent courses if severe neutropenia occurs; PO 2.3 mg/m^2/day on days 1-5 of a 21-day course (relapsed small cell lung cancer in those with prior response)

Renal dose
Adult: IV CCr 20-39 ml/min 0.75 mg/m^2/day × 5 days on day 1 of a 21-day course

Available forms: Lyophilized powder for inj 4 mg; cap 0.25, 1 mg

Adverse effects
CNS: Arthralgia, *asthenia, headache,* myalgia, *pain,* weakness
GI: Abdominal pain, constipation, diarrhea, obstruction, *nausea,* stomatitis, *vomiting,* increased ALT, AST, anorexia

---

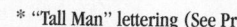

HEMA: **Neutropenia, leukopenia, thrombocytopenia, anemia, sepsis**
INTEG: *Total alopecia*
RESP: Dyspnea, cough, **interstitial lung disease**

Contraindications: Pregnancy **D**, breastfeeding, hypersensitivity, severe bone marrow depression

Black Box Warning: Neutropenia

Precautions: Children, renal disease

Pharmacokinetics

Absorption	Rapidly/completely
Distribution	7%-35% protein binding
Metabolism	Liver
Excretion	Urine, feces to metabolites
Half-life	2.8 hr

Pharmacodynamics

Unknown

Interactions
Individual drugs
Cisplatin: increased myelosuppression
Itraconazole, mefloquine, niCARdipine, quinidine, RU-486, tamoxifen, testosterone, verapamil: avoid giving together

Drug classifications
Anticoagulants, NSAIDs, platelet inhibitors, thrombolytics: increased bleeding risk
P-glycoprotein, breast cancer resistance protein inhibitors (amiodarone, clarithromycin, diltiazem, erythromycin, indinavir: avoid using together

Drug/food
Grapefruit juice: avoid use

NURSING CONSIDERATIONS
Assessment
• Monitor liver function tests: AST, ALT, alkaline phosphatase, which may be elevated; creatinine, BUN
• Monitor CBC, differential, platelet count weekly; withhold product if WBC is <3500/mm³ or platelet count is <100,000/mm³; notify prescriber of these results; product should be discontinued
• Assess buccal cavity for dryness, sores or ulceration, white patches, oral pain, bleeding, dysphagia
• Assess GI symptoms: frequency of stools, cramping
• Assess signs of dehydration: rapid respiration, poor skin turgor, decreased urine output, dry skin, restlessness, weakness

Nursing diagnoses
• Infection, risk for (adverse reactions)
• Knowledge, deficient (teaching)

Implementation
• Provide increased fluid intake to 2-3 L/day to prevent dehydration, unless contraindicated
• Change **IV** site q48hr

Patient/family education
• Advise patient to avoid foods with citric acid or hot flavor or rough texture if stomatitis is present; to drink adequate fluids
• Provide patient with nutritious diet of iron, vit K supplements, low fiber, few dairy products
• Advise patient that total alopecia may occur; hair grows back but may be different in color and texture
• Advise patient to report stomatitis; any bleeding, white spots, ulcerations in mouth; tell patient to examine mouth daily; report symptoms
• Assess patient to report signs of anemia; fatigue, headache, faintness, shortness of breath, irritability
• Teach patient to rinse mouth tid-qid with water, club soda, brush teeth bid-tid with soft brush or cotton-tipped applicator for stomatitis; use unwaxed dental floss
• Teach patient to use effective contraception during treatment and up to 6 mo after, avoid breastfeeding
• Advise patient to avoid OTC products without approval of prescriber
• Advise to avoid driving or other activities requiring alertness
• Advise to avoid vaccines, toxoids

Evaluation
Positive therapeutic outcome
• Decreased tumor size, spread of malignancy

---

toremifene (Rx)
(tore'me feen)
Fareston
Func. class.: Antineoplastic
Chem. class.: Antiestrogen hormone
Pregnancy category D

T

Action: Inhibits cell division by binding to cytoplasmic estrogen receptors; resembles normal cell complex but inhibits DNA synthesis and estrogen response of target tissue

Therapeutic outcome: Prevention of rapidly growing malignant cells

---

Adverse effects: *italic* = common, **bold** = life-threatening

Uses: Advanced breast carcinoma that has not responded to other therapy in estrogen-receptor-positive patients (usually postmenopausal)

Dosage and routes
Adult: PO 60 mg/day

Available forms: Tabs 60 mg

Adverse effects
CNS: Hot flashes, headache, light-headedness, depression
CV: Chest pain, **CHF, MI, PE,** chest pain, angina
EENT: Ocular lesions, retinopathy, corneal opacity, blurred vision (high doses)
GI: Nausea, vomiting, altered taste (anorexia)
GU: Vaginal bleeding, pruritus vulvae
HEMA: **Thrombocytopenia, leukopenia, thrombosis**
INTEG: Rash, alopecia, sweating
META: Hypercalcemia
RESP: **Pulmonary embolism**

Contraindications: Pregnancy **D,** hypersensitivity, history of thromboembolism

Precautions: Breastfeeding, children, cataracts, hypercalcemia, hepatic disease, endometrial hyperplasia

Pharmacokinetics
Absorption	Adequately absorbed
Distribution	99% protein binding
Metabolism	Liver, extensively
Excretion	Feces, slowly, small amounts (kidneys)
Half-life	Terminal 5-6 days

Pharmacodynamics
Onset	Unknown
Peak	3 hr
Duration	Unknown

Interactions
Individual drugs
Warfarin: increased warfarin effect
Drug classifications
CYP3A4 inducers (barbiturates, bosentan, carbamazepine, efavirenz, phenytoins, nevirapine, rifabutin, rifampin): decreased toremifene effect
CYP3A4 inhibitors (aprepitant, antiretroviral protease inhibitors, clarithromycin, danazol, delivirdine, diltiazem, erythromycin, fluconazole, fluoxetine, fluvoxamine, imatinib, ketoconazole, mibefradil, nefazodone, telithromycin, voriconazole): increased toxicity
Drug/herb
St. John's wort: avoid use
Drug/lab test
Increased: serum Ca

NURSING CONSIDERATIONS
Assessment
• Monitor CBC, differential, platelet count weekly; withhold product if WBC is <4000/mm^3 or platelet count is <75,000/mm^3; notify prescriber of results; monitor calcium levels (hypercalcemia is common), LFTs, serum calcium
• Assess for tumor flare: increase in bone, tumor pain during beginning treatment; give analgesics as ordered to decrease pain
• Assess for bleeding: hematuria, guaiac, bruising or petechiae, mucosa or orifices q8hr, no rectal temp

Nursing diagnoses
• Injury, risk for (adverse reactions)
• Knowledge, deficient (teaching)

Implementation
• Do not break, crush, or chew tabs
• Give with food or fluids to decrease GI upset; repeat dose may be needed if vomiting occurs
• Store in light-resistant container at room temperature

Patient/family education
• Instruct patient to report any complaints, side effects to prescriber; if dose is missed, do not double next dose
• Advise patient that vaginal bleeding, pruritus, hot flashes can occur and are reversible after discontinuing treatment
• Instruct patient to report immediately decreased visual acuity, which may be irreversible; stress need for routine eye exams
• Inform patient about who should be told about toremifene therapy
• Advise patient to report vaginal bleeding immediately; that tumor flare (increase in size of tumor, increased bone pain) may occur and will subside rapidly; may take analgesics for pain; that premenopausal women must use mechanical birth control method because ovulation may be induced (teratogenic product)
• Caution patient to use sunscreen and protective clothing to prevent burns because photosensitivity is common
• Teach patient that hair loss may occur during treatment; a wig or hairpiece may make patient feel better; new hair may be different in color, texture

- Inform patient rash or lesions are temporary and may become large during beginning therapy

Evaluation
Positive therapeutic outcome
- Decreased spread of malignant cells in breast cancer

trace elements (chromium, copper, iodide, manganese, selenium, zinc) (Rx)

Concentrated Multiple Trace Elements, ConTE-PAK-4, M.T.E.-4, M.T.E.-4 Concentrated, M.T.E.-5, M.T.E.-5 Concentrated, M.T.E.-6, M.T.E.-6 Concentrated, M.T.E.-7, MulTE-PAK-4, MulTE-PAK-5, Multiple Trace Element, Multiple Trace Element Neonatal, Multiple Trace Element Pediatric, Neotrace 4, Ped TE-PAK-4, Pedtrice-4, P.T.E.-4, P.T.E.-5
Func. class.: Mineral supplement

Pregnancy category C

Action: Needed for adequate absorption and synthesis of amino acids

Therapeutic outcome: Replacement for mineral deficiencies

Uses: Prevention of trace element deficiency, a component of TPN

Dosage and routes
Usual dosage may be given in TPN SOL

Chromium
Adult: **IV** 10-15 mcg/day
Child: **IV** 0.14-0.20 mcg/ kg/day

Copper
Adult: **IV** 0.5-1.5 mg/day
Child: **IV** 0.05-0.2 mg/kg/day

Iodide
Adult: **IV** 1 mcg/kg/day

Manganese
Adult: **IV** 0.15-0.8 mg/day

Selenium
Adult: **IV** 20-40 mcg/day
Child: **IV** 3 mcg/kg/day

Zinc
Adult: **IV** 2-4 mg/day
Child: **IV** 0.05 mg/kg/day

Available forms: Many forms available; see particular elements

Adverse effects
CHROMIUM: **Seizures, coma,** nausea, vomiting, ulcers, **renal/hepatic toxicity**

COPPER: Personality changes, diarrhea, weakness, photophobia, muscle weakness
IODINE: Headache, edema of eyelids, acne, metallic taste, sore mouth, runny nose
MANGANESE: Incoordination, headache, irritability, lability, slurred speech, impotence
SELENIUM: Alopecia, depression, vomiting, GI cramping, nervousness, garlic smell
ZINC: Vomiting, oliguria, **hypothermia,** vision changes, **tachycardia,** jaundice, **coma**

Precautions: Pregnancy C, breastfeeding, liver, biliary disease, vomiting or diarrhea

Pharmacokinetics

Absorption	Completely absorbed
Distribution	Widely distributed
Metabolism	Unknown
Excretion	Depends on element
Half-life	Unknown

Pharmacodynamics
Unknown

NURSING CONSIDERATIONS
Assessment
- Assess trace element levels; notify prescriber if low; copper 0.07-0.15 mg/ml, zinc 0.05-0.15 mg/100 ml, manganese 4 20 mcg/100 ml, selenium 0.1-0.19 mcg/ml
- Assess trace element deficiency if patient is receiving TPN for extended period
- Obtain calorie count to identify nutritional deficiencies
- Assess for toxicity to individual element (see Adverse Effects)

Nursing diagnoses
- Knowledge, deficient (teaching)
- Nutrition: less than body requirements, imbalanced (uses)

Implementation
- Give by **IV** inf, often mixed with TPN sol
- Discard unused portions
- Give by continuous inf diluted in 1 L or more **IV** sol; give at prescribed rate

Patient/family education
- Explain to patient reason for and expected results of medication

Evaluation
Positive therapeutic outcome
- Absence of element deficiency

T

Adverse effects: *italic* = common, **bold** = life-threatening

tramadol (Rx)
(trah′mah-dol)
Ryzolt, Ultram, Ultram ER
Func. class.: Analgesic, miscellaneous
Pregnancy category C

Do not confuse:
tramadol/Toradol

Action: Not completely understood, binds to opioid receptors and inhibits reuptake of norepinephrine, serotonin; does not cause histamine release or affect heart rate

Therapeutic outcome: Relief of pain

Uses: Management of moderate to severe pain, chronic pain

Dosage and routes
Mild to moderate pain
Adult: PO 50-100 mg prn q4-6hr, max 400 mg/day
Geriatric >75 yr: PO <300 mg/day in divided dose

Hepatic dose
Adult: PO 50 mg q12hr

Renal dose
Adult (Child-Pugh C): PO CCr <30 ml/min q12hr, max 200 mg/day; do not use ER tabs

Moderate to severe chronic pain
Adult: PO-ER (Ultram ER) 100 mg, titrate upward q5day by 100 mg, max 300 mg/day; (Ryzolt) 100 mg, titrate upward q2-3day in 100-mg increments; max 300 mg/day; products are not interchangeable

Available forms: Tabs 50 mg; ext rel tab 100, 200, 300 mg; orally disintegrating tab 50 mg

Adverse effects
CNS: Dizziness, CNS stimulation, somnolence, headache, anxiety, confusion, euphoria, **seizures,** hallucinations, flushing, sedation, **neuroleptic malignant syndrome–like reactions**
CV: Vasodilatation, orthostatic hypotension, tachycardia, hypertension, abnormal ECG
EENT: Visual disturbances
GI: Nausea, constipation, vomiting, dry mouth, diarrhea, abdominal pain, anorexia, flatulence, GI bleeding
GU: Urinary retention/frequency, menopausal symptoms, dysuria, menstrual disorder
INTEG: Pruritus, rash, urticaria, vesicles

SYST: **Anaphylaxis, Stevens-Johnson syndrome, toxic epidermal necrolysis, serotonin syndrome**

Contraindications: Hypersensitivity, acute intoxication with any CNS depressant

Precautions: Pregnancy **C,** breastfeeding, children, geriatric, seizure disorder, renal/hepatic disease, respiratory depression, head trauma, increased ICP, acute abdominal condition, product abuse

Pharmacokinetics

Absorption	Rapidly, almost completely absorbed
Distribution	Steady state 2 days
Metabolism	Extensively in liver, may cross blood-brain barrier
Excretion	Unchanged product 30% in urine
Half-life	Unknown

Pharmacodynamics
Unknown

Interactions
Individual drugs
Alcohol: increased CNS depression
Carbamazepine: decreased tramadol level
Drug classifications
CYP3A4 inducers (barbiturates, bosentan, carbamazepine, efavirenz, nevirapine, phenytoin, rifabutin, rifampin): decreased tramadol effect
CYP3A4 inhibitors (aprepitant, antiretroviral protease inhibitors, clarithromycin, danazol, delavirdine, diltiazem, erythromycin, fluconazole, fluoxetine, fluvoxamine, imatinib, ketoconazole, mibefradil, nefazodone, telithromycin, voriconazole): increased tramadol levels
MAOIs: inhibition of norepinephrine and serotonin reuptake; use together with caution
Opiates, sedative/hypnotics: increased CNS depression
Selective serotonin reuptake inhibitors: increased serotonin syndrome
Drug/herb
Chamomile, hops, kava, skullcap, valerian: increased CNS depression
St. John's wort: avoid use
Drug/lab test
Increased: creatinine, liver enzymes
Decreased: Hgb

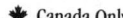

NURSING CONSIDERATIONS
Assessment
- Assess pain: location, type, character; give before pain becomes extreme
- Assess for increased side effects in renal/hepatic disease
- Monitor I&O ratio: check for decreasing output; may indicate urinary retention
- Assess need for product
- Assess for constipation and bowel pattern; increase fluids, bulk in diet
- Monitor CNS changes: dizziness, drowsiness, hallucinations, euphoria, LOC, pupil reaction
- Determine allergic reactions: rash, urticaria

Nursing diagnoses
- Injury, risk for (adverse reactions)
- Knowledge, deficient (teaching)
- Pain, acute (uses)
- Pain, chronic (uses)
- Sensory perception, disturbed: visual, auditory (adverse reactions)

Implementation
- Do not break, crush, or chew ER product
- Give with antiemetic for nausea, vomiting
- Administer when pain is beginning to return; determine dosage interval by patient response
- Ext rel products (Ryzolt/Ultram ER) are not interchangeable
- Store in cool environment, protect from sunlight

Patient/family education
- Teach patient to report any symptoms of CNS changes, allergic reactions
- Teach patient that drowsiness, dizziness, and confusion may occur; to call for assistance
- Instruct patient to make position changes slowly; orthostatic hypotension may occur
- Tell patient to avoid OTC medication and alcohol unless approved by prescriber

Evaluation
Positive therapeutic outcome
- Decreased pain

---

trandolapril (Rx)
(tran-doe'la-prill)
Mavik
Func. class.: Antihypertensive
Chem. class.: Angiotensin-converting enzyme (ACE) inhibitor

Pregnancy category D

Action: Selectively suppresses renin-angiotensin-aldosterone system; inhibits ACE; prevents conversion of angiotensin I to angiotensin II, resulting in dilatation of arterial and venous vessels and lowered B/P

Therapeutic outcome: Decreased B/P in hypertension

Uses: Hypertension alone or in combination, heart failure, after MI/left ventricular dysfunction after MI

Dosage and routes
Hypertension
Adult: PO 1 mg/day, 2 mg/day in African Americans, make dosage adjustment ≥wk; up to 8 mg/day

Heart failure (after MI/left ventricular dysfunction)
Adult: PO 1 mg/day, titrate upward to 4 mg/day if tolerated

Renal dose/hepatic dose
Adult: PO CCr <30 ml/min or hepatic disease 0.5 mg/day, may increase gradually up to 4 mg/day

Available forms: Tabs 1, 2, 4 mg

Adverse effects
CNS: Dizziness, paresthesias, headache, *syncope,* fatigue, drowsiness, depression, sleep disturbances, anxiety
CV: Hypotension, **MI,** palpitations, angina, TIAs, **stroke,** bradycardia, dysrhythmias
GI: Nausea, vomiting, cramps, diarrhea, constipation, **pancreatitis,** *dyspepsia*
GU: Proteinuria, **renal failure**
HEMA: Agranulocytosis, neutropenia, leukopenia, anemia
INTEG: Rash, purpura, pruritus
MISC: Hyperkalemia, hyponatremia, impotence, *myalgia,* **angioedema,** muscle cramps, asthenia, hypocalcemia, gout
RESP: Dyspnea, cough

Contraindications: Breastfeeding, hypersensitivity, history of angioedema

Black Box Warning: Pregnancy **D**

Precautions: Geriatric, hyperkalemia, hepatic disease, bilateral renal stenosis, post kidney transplant, aortal/mitral valve stenosis, cirrhosis, severe renal disease, untreated CHF, autoimmune diseases, cough

Pharmacokinetics
Absorption	40%-60%
Distribution	Unknown
Metabolism	Liver
Excretion	Kidneys, feces
Half-life	0.6-1.1 hr, 16-24 hr

Adverse effects: *italic* = common, **bold** = life-threatening

Pharmacodynamics	
Onset	½ hr
Peak	4-10 hr
Duration	>8 days

Interactions
Individual drugs
Levodopa, lithium, reserpine: increased effect of each specific product

Drug classifications
Antacids, NSAIDs, salicylates: decreased effect of trandolapril

Antihypertensives, diuretics: increased severe hypotension

Barbiturates, ergots, hypoglycemics, neuromuscular blocking agents: increased effects of each specific product

Diuretics (potassium-sparing): increased potassium levels

Phenothiazines: increased antihypertensive effects

Potassium supplements: increased potassium levels

Salt substitutes: increased potassium levels

Drug/herb
Aconite: increased toxicity, death

Astragalus, cola tree: increased or decreased antihypertensive effect

Barberry, betony, black catechu, black cohosh, bloodroot, broom, burdock, cat's claw, dandelion, goldenseal, hawthorn, Irish moss, Jamaican dogwood, kelp, khella, mistletoe, parsley: increased antihypertensive effect

Coltsfoot, guarana, khat, licorice, yohimbe: decreased antihypertensive effect

NURSING CONSIDERATIONS
Assessment
• Monitor blood tests: neutrophils, decreased platelets

• Monitor B/P, orthostatic hypotension, syncope; if changes occur dosage change may be required

• Monitor renal studies: protein, BUN, creatinine; increased levels may indicate nephrotic syndrome and renal failure

• Monitor renal symptoms: polyuria, oliguria, frequency, dysuria

• Establish baselines in renal, liver function tests before therapy begins

• Check potassium levels throughout treatment, although hyperkalemia rarely occurs

• Check for edema in feet, legs daily

• Assess for allergic reactions: rash, fever, pruritus, urticaria; product should be discontinued if antihistamines fail to help

Nursing diagnoses
• Cardiac output, decreased (uses)
• Injury, risk for (adverse reactions)
• Knowledge, deficient (teaching)
• Noncompliance (teaching)

Implementation
• Store in airtight container at ≤77° F (≤25° C) or less

Patient/family education
• Advise patient not to discontinue product abruptly; advise patient to tell all persons associated with health care

• Teach patient not to use OTC products (cough, cold, allergy medications) unless directed by physician; serious side effects can occur; xanthines, such as coffee, tea, chocolate, cola, can prevent action of product

• Instruct patient on the importance of complying with dosage schedule, even if feeling better; to continue with medical regimen to decrease B/P: exercise, cessation of smoking, decreasing stress, diet modifications

• Emphasize the need to rise slowly to sitting or standing position to minimize orthostatic hypotension; not to exercise in hot weather, which can cause increased hypotension

• Advise patient to notify prescriber of mouth sores, sore throat, fever, swelling of hands or feet, irregular heartbeat, chest pain, coughing, shortness of breath

• Caution patient to report excessive perspiration, dehydration, vomiting, diarrhea; may lead to fall in B/P

• Caution patient that product may cause dizziness, fainting, light-headedness; may occur during 1st few days of therapy; to avoid activities that may be hazardous

• Teach patient how to take B/P, and normal readings for age group

Evaluation
Positive therapeutic outcome
• Decreased B/P in hypertension

Treatment of overdose: Lavage, **IV** atropine for bradycardia, **IV** theophylline for bronchospasm, digoxin, O_2, diuretic for cardiac failure, hemodialysis

⚠ HIGH ALERT

trastuzumab (Rx)
(tras-tuz′uh-mab)
Herceptin
Func. class.: Antineoplastic—miscellaneous
Chem. class.: Humanized monoclonal
antibody

Pregnancy category D

Action: DNA-derived monoclonal antibody
selectively binds to extracellular portion of
human epidermal growth factor receptor 2
(HER2); it inhibits proliferation of cancer cells

Therapeutic outcome: Decreasing
symptoms of breast cancer

Uses: Breast cancer; metastatic with overexpression of HER2, early breast cancer (adjuvant, neoadjuvant)

Dosage and routes
Several regimens may be used
Adult: **IV** 4 mg/kg given over 90 min, then
maintenance 2 mg/kg given over 30 min; do
not give as **IV** PUSH or BOL; may be given in
combination with other antineoplastics

Available forms: Lyophilized powder
440 mg

Adverse effects
CNS: Dizziness, numbness, paresthesias,
depression, *insomnia,* neuropathy, peripheral
neuritis
CV: **Tachycardia, CHF**
GI: Nausea, vomiting, *anorexia, diarrhea,*
abdominal pain, **hepatotoxicity**
HEMA: Anemia, **leukopenia**
INTEG: Rash, acne, herpes simplex
META: Edema, peripheral edema
MISC: Flulike symptoms; fever, headache,
chills
MS: Arthralgia, *bone pain*
RESP: Cough, dyspnea, pharyngitis, rhinitis,
sinusitis, **pneumonia**
SYST: **Anaphylaxis, angioedema**

Contraindications: Pregnancy **D,** hypersensitivity to this product, Chinese hamster
ovary cell protein

Precautions: Breastfeeding, children,
geriatric, pulmonary disease, anemia, leukopenia

Black Box Warning: Cardiac disease,
respiratory distress syndrome, infusion-related
reactions

Pharmacokinetics
Absorption	Unknown
Distribution	Unknown
Metabolism	Unknown
Excretion	Unknown
Half-life	1-32 days

Pharmacodynamics
Unknown

Interactions
Individual drugs
Cyclophosphamide: increased cardiomyopathy
risk; avoid use
Drug classifications
Anthracyclines: increased cardiomyopathy risk
Vaccines/toxoids: decreased immune response

NURSING CONSIDERATIONS
Assessment
• Monitor CBC, HER2 overexpression
• Assess for symptoms of infection; may be
masked by product
• Assess CNS reaction: LOC, mental status,
dizziness, confusion
• Assess for CHF and other cardiac symptoms:
dyspnea, coughing, gallop; obtain a full cardiac workup including ECG, echocardiogram,
multigated angiogram
• Assess for hypersensitivity reactions, anaphylaxis
• Monitor for potentially fatal infusion reactions: fever, chills, nausea, vomiting, pain, headache, dizziness, hypotension; discontinue
product

Nursing diagnoses
• Infection, risk for (side effects)
• Knowledge, deficient (teaching)
• Nutrition: less than body requirements,
imbalanced (side effects)

Implementation
• Give acetaminophen as ordered to alleviate
fever and headache
• Increase fluid intake to 2-3 L/day
IV route
• Administer after reconstituting vial with 20
ml of bacteriostatic water for inj, 1.1% benzyl
alcohol preserved (supplied) to yield 21
mg/ml, mark date on vial 28 days from reconstitution date; if patient is allergic to benzyl
alcohol, reconstitute with sterile water for inj;
use immediately; inf over 90 min; q3wk give 8
mg/kg loading dose over 90 min; subsequent
doses 6 mg/kg may be given over 30-60 min
• Do not mix or dilute with other products or
dextrose sol

T

Adverse effects: *italic* = common, **bold** = life-threatening

Patient/family education

- Advise patient to take acetaminophen for fever
- Teach patient to avoid hazardous tasks, since confusion, dizziness may occur
- Teach patient to report signs of infection: sore throat, fever, diarrhea, vomiting
- Inform patient that emotional lability is common; instruct patient to notify prescriber if severe or incapacitating

Evaluation

Positive therapeutic outcome
- Decrease in size of tumors

---

travoprost ophthalmic
See Appendix B

---

trazodone (Rx)
(tray'zoe-done)
trazodone HCl
Func. class.: Antidepressant—miscellaneous
Chem. class.: Triazolopyridine

Pregnancy category C

Action: Selectively inhibits serotonin, norepinephrine uptake by brain, potentiates behavioral changes

Therapeutic outcome: Decreased symptoms of depression after 2-3 wk

Uses: Depression

Dosage and routes:
Adult: PO 150 mg/day in divided doses; may increase by 50 mg/day q3-4day, max 400 mg/day (outpatient), 600 mg/day (inpatient)
Geriatric: PO 25-50 at bedtime, increase by 25-50 mg q3-7day to desired dose, usual 75-150 mg/day
Child 6-18 yr: PO 1.5-2 mg/kg/day in divided doses, may increase q3-4day up to 6 mg/kg/day or 400 mg/day in divided doses, whichever is less

Available forms: Tabs 50, 100, 150, 300 mg

Adverse effects
CNS: Dizziness, drowsiness, confusion, headache, anxiety, tremors, stimulation, weakness, insomnia, nightmares, EPS (geriatric), increase in psychiatric symptoms, **suicide in children/adolescents**
CV: Orthostatic hypotension, ECG changes, tachycardia, **hypertension,** palpitations
EENT: Blurred vision, tinnitus, mydriasis

GI: Diarrhea, dry mouth, nausea, vomiting, **paralytic ileus,** increased appetite, cramps, epigastric distress, jaundice, **hepatitis,** stomatitis, constipation
GU: Retention, **acute renal failure, priapism**
HEMA: **Agranulocytosis, thrombocytopenia, eosinophilia, leukopenia**
INTEG: Rash, urticaria, sweating, pruritus, photosensitivity

Contraindications: Hypersensitivity to tricyclics, recovery phase of MI, seizure disorders, prostatic hypertrophy

Precautions: Pregnancy **C,** suicidal patients, severe depression, increased intraocular pressure, closed-angle glaucoma, urinary retention, cardiac/hepatic disease, hyperthyroidism, electroshock therapy, elective surgery, suicidal ideation in children/adolescents

Pharmacokinetics

Absorption	Well absorbed
Distribution	Widely distributed
Metabolism	Liver, extensively
Excretion	Kidneys, unchanged minimally
Half-life	4½-7½ hr

Pharmacodynamics

Onset	Unknown
Peak	1 hr without food, 2 hr with food
Duration	Unknown

Interactions
Individual drugs

Alcohol, carbamazepine, digoxin, phenytoin: increased effect of each product
Fluoxetine, nefazodone: increased levels, increased toxicity, serotonin syndrome
Warfarin: increased or decreased effects of warfarin

Drug classifications

Barbiturates, benzodiazepines, CNS depressants: increased effects
CYP3A4, 2D6 inhibitors (phenothiazenes, protease inhibitors, azole antifungals): increased effects of trazodone
MAOIs: increased hyperpyretic crisis, seizures, hypertensive episode, do not use within 14 days
Selective serotonin reuptake inhibitors: increased toxicity, serotonin syndrome
Sympathomimetics (direct-acting): increased sympathomimetic effects
Sympathomimetics (indirect-acting): decreased effects

Drug/herb
Chamomile, hops, kava, lavender, skullcap, valerian: increased CNS depression
Corkwood, jimsonweed: increased anticholinergic effect
SAM-e, St. John's wort: increased serotonin syndrome

Drug/lab test
Increased: serum bilirubin, blood glucose, alkaline phosphatase
Decreased: VMA, 5-HIAA
False increase: urinary catecholamines

NURSING CONSIDERATIONS
Assessment
- Assess for pain: location, duration, intensity before, 1-2 hr after medication
- Monitor B/P (lying, standing), pulse q4hr; if systolic B/P drops 20 mm Hg hold product, notify prescriber; take vital signs q4hr in patients with CV disease
- Monitor blood tests: CBC, leukocytes, differential, cardiac enzymes if patient is receiving long-term therapy
- Monitor liver function tests: AST, ALT, bilirubin
- Check weight qwk; appetite may increase with product
- Assess ECG for flattening of T wave, bundle branch block, AV block, dysrhythmias in cardiac patients
- Assess for EPS primarily in geriatric: rigidity, dystonia, akathisia
- Assess mental status: mood, sensorium, affect, suicidal tendencies; increase in psychiatric symptoms: depression, panic
- Monitor urinary retention, constipation; constipation is more likely to occur in children or geriatric
- Assess for withdrawal symptoms: headache, nausea, vomiting, muscle pain, weakness; do not usually occur unless product was discontinued abruptly
- Identify alcohol consumption; if alcohol is consumed, hold dose until AM

Nursing diagnoses
- Coping, ineffective (uses)
- Injury, risk for (adverse reactions)
- Knowledge, deficient (teaching)
- Noncompliance (teaching)

Implementation
- Give with food or milk for GI symptoms; crush if patient is unable to swallow medication whole
- Give dosage at bedtime if oversedation occurs during day; may take entire dose at bedtime; geriatric may not tolerate once/day dosing
- Store at room temperature; do not freeze

Patient/family education
- Teach patient that therapeutic effects may take 2-3 wk
- Teach patient to use caution in driving or other activities requiring alertness because of drowsiness, dizziness, blurred vision; to avoid rising quickly from sitting to standing, especially geriatric
- Caution patient to avoid alcohol ingestion, other CNS depressants
- Teach patient not to discontinue medication quickly after long-term use: may cause nausea, headache, malaise
- Advise patient to wear sunscreen or large hat because photosensitivity occurs
- Teach patient to increase fluids, bulk in diet if constipation, urinary retention occur, especially geriatric
- Advise patient to take gum, hard sugarless candy, or frequent sips of water for dry mouth
- Teach family to watch for suicidal ideation or tendencies, usually in children/adolescents

Evaluation
Positive therapeutic outcome
- Decrease in depression
- Absence of suicidal thoughts

Treatment of overdose: ECG monitoring, induce emesis, lavage, activated charcoal, administer anticonvulsant

---

treprostinil (Rx)
(treh-prah'stin-ill)
Remodulin, Tyvaso
Func. class.: Antiplatelet agent
Chem. class.: Tricyclic benzidine prostacyclin analog

Pregnancy category B

Action: Direct vasodilatation of pulmonary, systemic arterial vascular beds, inhibition of platelet aggregation

Therapeutic outcome: Decreased pulmonary arterial hypertension (PAH)

Uses: Pulmonary arterial hypertension (PAH) NYHA class II through IV

Dosage and routes
Adult: SUBCUT INF 1.25 ng/kg/min by cont INF, may reduce to 0.625 ng if not tolerated; may increase by 1.25 ng/kg/min qwk for first 4 wk, then 2.5 ng/kg/min qwk for remainder of INF; oral INH 3 breaths via Tyvaso INH system qid

T

Hepatic dose
Adult: SUBCUT INF 0.625 ng/kg ideal body weight/min and increase cautiously

Available forms: Inj 1, 2.5, 5, 10 mg/ml; neb sol 1.74 mg/2.9 ml

Adverse effects
CNS: Dizziness, headache
CV: Vasodilatation, hypotension, edema
GI: Nausea, *diarrhea*
INTEG: Rash, pruritus
OTHER: Jaw pain
SYST: Infusion site reactions, inf site pain, increased risk of infection

Contraindications: Hypersensitivity to this product or other prostacyclin analogs

Precautions: Pregnancy **B**, breastfeeding, children, geriatric, past hepatic disease, renal/thromboembolic disease, abrupt discontinuation, **IV** administration

Pharmacokinetics

Absorption	Unknown
Distribution	Unknown
Metabolism	Liver, 90% protein binding
Excretion	Urine, feces
Half-life	2-4 hr, terminal

Pharmacodynamics
Unknown

Interactions
Individual drug
Aspirin: increased risk of bleeding
Drug classifications
Anticoagulants, NSAIDs, SSRIs, thrombin inhibitors: increased risk of bleeding
Antihypertensives, β-blockers, calcium channel blockers, diuretics, MAOIs, vasodilators: increased hypotension

NURSING CONSIDERATIONS
Assessment
• Monitor liver function tests: AST, ALT, bilirubin, creatinine (long-term therapy)
◆ Monitor blood tests: CBC; CBC q2wk × 3 mo, Hct, Hgb, pro-time (long-term therapy)
◆ Monitor bleed time baseline and throughout; levels may be 2-5 × normal limit

Nursing diagnoses
• Knowledge, deficient (teaching)
• Tissue perfusion, ineffective (uses)

Implementation
• Give by continuous SUBCUT inf or surgically placed indwelling central venous catheter via inf pump

• Sudden decreased doses or abrupt withdrawal may worsen pulmonary atrial hypertension symptoms

Patient/family education
• Teach patient that blood work will be necessary during treatment
• Teach patient to report side effects such as diarrhea, skin rashes
• Teach patient that therapy will be needed for prolonged periods of time, sometimes years
• Advise patient that aseptic technique must be used in preparing and administration to prevent infection
• Teach that there are many drug and herb interactions
• Teach signs/symptoms of bleeding: blood in urine, stools

Evaluation
Positive therapeutic outcome
• Decreased pulmonary arterial hypertension

tretinoin (vitamin A acid, retinoic acid) (Rx)
(tret′i-noyn)
Avita, Renova, Retin-A, Retin-A Micro, Stieva-A ✿
Func. class.: Vitamin A acid/acne product, antineoplastic—miscellaneous
Chem. class.: Tretinoin derivative

Pregnancy category
C (TOPICAL),
D (PO)

Action: (Topical) Decreases cohesiveness of follicular epithelium, decreases microcomedone formation; (PO) induces maturation of acute promyelocytic leukemia, exact action is unknown

Therapeutic outcome: Decreased signs/symptoms of leukemia

Uses: (Topical) Acne vulgaris (grades 1-3); (PO) acute promyelocytic leukemia, facial wrinkles, photoaging

Unlabeled uses: Acne rosacea, actinic keratosis, ichthyosis, Kaposi's sarcoma, keloids, keratosis follicularis, melasma

Dosage and routes
Adult and child: TOP cleanse area, apply 0.025%-0.1% cream or 0.05% liquid at bedtime; cover lightly

Promyelocytic leukemia
Adult: PO 45 mg/m²/day given as 2 evenly divided doses until remission; discontinue

treatment 30 days after remission or after 90 days of treatment, whichever is first

Available forms: Topical cream 0.01%, 0.02%, 0.025%, 0.05%, 0.01%; topical gel 0.025%, 0.01%, 0.04%, 0.1%; topical liquid 0.05%; caps 10 mg

Adverse effects
PO route

CNS: Headache, fever, sweating, fatigue
CV: Cardiac dysrhythmias, pericardial effusion
GI: Nausea, vomiting, **hemorrhage**, abdominal pain, diarrhea, constipation, dyspepsia, distention, **hepatitis**
META: Hypercholesterolemia, hypertriglyceridemia
RESP: Pneumonia, upper respiratory tract disease
Topical route
INTEG: Rash, stinging, warmth, redness, erythema, blistering, crusting, peeling, contact dermatitis, hypo/hyperpigmentation, dry skin, pruritus, scaly skin

Contraindications: Hypersensitivity to retinoids or sensitivity to parabens

Black Box Warning: Pregnancy **D** (PO)

Precautions: Pregnancy **C** (topical), breastfeeding, eczema, sunburn, sun exposure

Black Box Warning: Rapid-evolving leukocytosis, respiratory compromise, acute promyelocytic leukemia differentiation syndrome

Pharmacokinetics

Absorption	Small amounts
Distribution	Unknown
Metabolism	Unknown
Excretion	Kidneys
Half-life	Unknown

Pharmacodynamics
Unknown

Interactions
Individual drugs

Aminocaproic acid, aprotinin, tranexamic acid: increased thrombotic complications
Benzoyl peroxide, resorcinol, salicylic acid (topical), sulfur: increased peeling
Ketoconazole: increased plasma concentrations of tretinoin (oral)
Drug classifications
Alcohol, astringents, cleansers with drying effect, medicated, abrasive soaps: use with caution (topical)

Diuretics (thiazide), phenothiazines, quinolones, retinoids, sulfonamides, sulfonylureas: increased photosensitivity
Tetracyclines: increased ICP, risk of pseudotumor cerebri; do not use together
Drug/lab test
Increased: AST, ALT

NURSING CONSIDERATIONS
Assessment
Topical route
• Assess part of body involved, including time involved, what helps or aggravates condition, cysts, dryness, itching; lesions may become worse at beginning of treatment

Nursing diagnoses
• Body image, disturbed (uses)
• Knowledge, deficient (teaching)
• Skin integrity, impaired (uses)

Implementation
Topical route
• Apply using gloves or cotton, once daily before bedtime; cover area lightly using gauze
• Store at room temperature
• Wash hands after application
• Apply only to affected areas

Patient/family education
Topical route
• Instruct patient to avoid application on normal skin, and to avoid getting cream in eyes, nose, other mucous membranes
• Advise patient to avoid sunlight, sunlamps or to use protective clothing or sunscreen to prevent burns
• Advise patient that treatment may cause warmth, stinging; dryness, peeling will occur
• Inform patient that cosmetics may be used over product; not to use shaving lotions
• Inform patient that rash may occur during first 1-3 wk of therapy
• Caution patient that product does not cure condition, only relieves symptoms; that therapeutic results may be seen in 2-3 wk but may not be optimal until after 6 wk

Evaluation
Positive therapeutic outcome
• Decrease in size and number of lesions

tretinoin topical
See Appendix B

T

Adverse effects: *italic* = common, **bold** = life-threatening

triamcinolone (Rx)

(trye-am-sin'oh-lone)

Amcort, Aristocort, Aristocort Forte, Aristocort Intralesional, Aristospan Intra-Articular, Aristospan Intralesional, Articulose L.A., Atolone, Azmacort, Cenocort A-40, Cenocort Forte, Kenacort, Kenaject-40, Kenalog, Kenalog-10, Kenalog-40, Tac-3, Tac-40, Triam-A, triamcinolone, triamcinolone acetonide, Triam Forte, Triamolone 40, Triamonide 40, Tri-Kort, Trilog, Trilone, Trisoject

Func. class.: Corticosteroid, synthetic; antiinflammatory

Chem. class.: Glucocorticoid, intermediate-acting

Pregnancy category C

Action: Decreases inflammation by suppression of migration of polymorphonuclear leukocytes, fibroblasts, reversal of increased capillary permeability and lysosomal stabilization

Therapeutic outcome: Decreased inflammation, normal immune response

Uses: Severe inflammation, immunosuppression, neoplasms, asthma (steroid dependent), collagen, respiratory, dermatologic disorders, rheumatic disorders

Dosage and routes

Adult: PO 4-12 mg/day in divided doses daily-qid; IM 40 mg qwk (acetonide, diacetate), 5-48 mg into neoplasms (diacetate, acetonide), 2-40 mg into joint or soft tissue (diacetate, acetonide), 0.5 mg/sq in of affected intralesional skin (hexacetonide), 2-20 mg into joint or soft tissue (hexacetonide)

Child: PO 117 mcg/kg/day in divided doses

Asthma

Adult: INH 2 tid-qid, max 16 INH/day

Child 6-12 yr: INH 1-2 tid-qid, max 12 INH/day

Severe/incapacitating allergic conditions such as asthma

Adult: IM (Trivaris) 60 mg, titrate; usual range 40-80 mg

Child: IM (Trivaris) 0.11-1.6 mg/kg/day (3.2-48 mg/m²/day) given in 3-4 divided doses

Available forms: Tabs 1, 2, 4, 8 mg; syr 2, 4.85 mg/5 ml; inj 25, 40 mg/ml diacetate; inj 3, 10, 40 mg/ml acetonide; inj 5, 20 mg/ml hexacetonide; inh 100 mcg/spray

Adverse effects

CNS: Depression, flushing, sweating, headache, mood changes

CV: Hypertension, **circulatory collapse, thrombophlebitis, embolism,** tachycardia, edema

EENT: Fungal infections, increased intraocular pressure, blurred vision

GI: Diarrhea, nausea, abdominal distention, **GI hemorrhage,** *increased appetite,* **pancreatitis**

HEMA: **Thrombocytopenia**

INTEG: Acne, poor wound healing, ecchymosis, petechiae

MS: Fractures, osteoporosis, weakness

Contraindications: Children <2 yr, psychosis, hypersensitivity, idiopathic thrombocytopenia, acute glomerulonephritis, amebiasis, fungal infections, nonasthmatic bronchial disease, AIDS, TB, adrenal insufficiency, acute bronchospasm, neonatal prematurity

Precautions: Pregnancy C, breastfeeding, diabetes mellitus, glaucoma, osteoporosis, seizure disorders, ulcerative colitis, CHF, myasthenia gravis, renal disease, esophagitis, peptic ulcer, acne, cataracts, coagulopathy, head trauma

Interactions

Individual drugs

Alcohol, amphotericin B, cycloSPORINE, digoxin, indomethacin: increased side effects

Ambenonium, isoniazid, neostigmine, somatrem: decreased effects of each specific product

Cholestyramine, colestipol, ephedrine, phenytoin, rifampin, theophylline: decreased action of triamcinolone

Indomethacin, ketoconazole: increased action of triamcinolone

Drug classifications

Anticholinesterases, anticoagulants, anticonvulsants, antidiabetics, salicylates: decreased effects of each specific product

Antidiabetic agents: increased need for antidiabetic agents

Antiinfectives (macrolide), contraceptives (oral), estrogens, salicylates: increased action of triamcinolone

Barbiturates: decreased action of triamcinolone

Diuretics, salicylates: increased side effects

Toxoids, vaccines: decreased effects of toxoids, vaccines

Drug/herb

Aloe, buckthorn, cascara sagrada, Chinese rhubarb, senna: increased hypokalemia

Drug/lab test

Increased: cholesterol, sodium, blood glucose, uric acid, calcium, urine glucose

 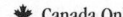

Decreased: calcium, potassium, T_4, T_3, thyroid ^{131}I uptake test, urine 17-OHCS, 17-KS

False negative: skin allergy tests

Pharmacokinetics

Absorption	Well absorbed (PO, IM)
Distribution	Crosses placenta, widely distributed
Metabolism	Liver, extensively
Excretion	Kidney, breast milk
Half-life	2-5 hr, adrenal suppression 3-4 days

NURSING CONSIDERATIONS
Assessment
• Monitor potassium, blood glucose, urine glucose while on long-term therapy; hypokalemia and hyperglycemia
• Monitor weight daily; notify prescriber of weekly gain >5 lb; I&O ratio; be alert for decreasing urinary output and increasing edema
• Monitor B/P q4hr, pulse; notify prescriber if chest pain occurs
• Monitor plasma cortisol levels during long-term therapy (normal level 138-635 nmol/L [SI units] when measured at 8 AM); adrenal function periodically for hypothalamic-pituitary-adrenal axis suppression
• Assess for infection: increased temp, WBC even after withdrawal of medication; product masks infection symptoms
• Assess for potassium depletion: paresthesias, fatigue, nausea, vomiting, depression, polyuria, dysrhythmias, weakness
• Assess mental status: affect, mood, behavioral changes, aggression
• Assess nasal passages during long-term treatment for changes in mucus (nasal)
• Monitor temp, if fever develops, product should be discontinued
• Assess for systemic absorption: increased temp, inflammation, irritation (topical)

Nursing diagnoses
• Infection, risk for (adverse reactions)
• Knowledge, deficient (teaching)
• Noncompliance (teaching)

Implementation
PO route
• Give with food or milk to decrease GI symptoms; tablet may be crushed
IM route
• Give IM inj deeply in large muscle mass; rotate sites; avoid deltoid; use 21-G needle
• Give in one dose in AM to prevent adrenal suppression; avoid SUBCUT administration; may damage tissue
Inhalation route
• Use spacer device for geriatric
• Give inh with water to decrease possibility of fungal infections; titrated dose, use lowest effective dose
• Give after cleaning aerosol top daily with warm water, dry thoroughly
• Store in cool environment; do not puncture or incinerate container
Topical route
• Apply only to affected areas; do not get in eyes
• Apply medication, then cover with occlusive dressing (only if prescribed), seal to normal skin, change q12hr; systemic absorption may occur
• Apply only to dermatoses; do not use on weeping, denuded, or infected areas
• Cleanse skin before applying product
• Continue treatment for a few days after area has cleared
• Store at room temperature
Nasal route
• Have patient clear nasal passages before administration; use decongestant if needed; shake inhaler, invert, tilt head backward, insert nozzle into nostril, away from septum; hold other nostril closed and depress activator, inhale through nose, exhale through mouth

Patient/family education
• Advise patient that emergency ID as corticosteroid user should be carried/worn
• Instruct patient to notify prescriber if therapeutic response decreases; dosage adjustment may be needed; not to discontinue abruptly; adrenal crisis can result
• Caution patient to avoid OTC products: salicylates, alcohol in cough products, cold preparations unless directed by prescriber

Pharmacodynamics

	PO	IM	TOPICAL	INH	INTRANASAL
Onset	Unknown	Unknown	Min to hr	1-2 wk	Unknown
Peak	1-2 hr	1-2 hr	Hr to days	Unknown	2-3 wk
Duration	3 days	Unknown	Hr to days	Unknown	Unknown

Adverse effects: *italic* = common, **bold** = life-threatening

- Advise patient on all aspects of product usage including cushingoid symptoms
- Teach patient symptoms of adrenal insufficiency: nausea, anorexia, fatigue, dizziness, dyspnea, weakness, joint pain
- Teach patient that long-term therapy may be needed to clear infection (1-2 mo depending on type of infection)

Inhalation route
- Teach patient proper administration technique; to wash inhaler with warm water and dry after each use
- Teach patient all aspects of product usage including cushingoid symptoms

Topical route
- Instruct patient to avoid sunlight on affected area; burns may occur

Nasal route
- Instruct patient to clear nasal passages if sneezing attack occurs, repeat dose
- Advise patient to continue using product even if mild nasal bleeding occurs; is usually transient
- Teach patient method of instillation after providing written instruction from manufacturer

Evaluation
Positive therapeutic outcome
- Decrease in runny nose (nasal)
- Decreased dyspnea, wheezing, dry crackles on auscultation (inh)
- Ease of respirations, decreased inflammation
- Absence of severe itching, patches on skin, flaking (topical)

---

triamcinolone nasal agent
See Appendix B

---

triamcinolone ophthalmic
See Appendix B

---

triamcinolone topical
See Appendix B

---

triamterene (Rx)
(try-am'ter-een)
Dyrenium
Func. class.: Potassium-sparing diuretic
Chem. class.: Pteridine derivative

Pregnancy category B

Action: Acts primarily on distal tubule to inhibit reabsorption of sodium, chloride; increases potassium retention and conserves hydrogen ions

Therapeutic outcome: Diuretic and antihypertensive effect while retaining potassium

Uses: Edema, hypertension, diuretic-induced hypokalemia

Dosage and routes
Adult: PO 50-100 mg bid after meals, max 300 mg/day
Geriatric: PO 50 mg/day, max 100 mg/day

Renal dose
CCr <10 ml/min, do not use

Available forms: Caps 50, 100 mg

Adverse effects
CNS: Weakness, headache, dizziness, fatigue
CV: Hypotension, edema, CHF, bradycardia
ELECT: Hyperkalemia, hyponatremia, hypochloremia
GI: Nausea, diarrhea, vomiting, dry mouth, jaundice, constipation
GU: **Azotemia, interstitial nephritis,** increased BUN, creatinine, renal stones, bluish discoloration of urine, **nephrotoxicity**
HEMA: **Thrombocytopenia, megaloblastic anemia, agranulocytosis**
INTEG: Photosensitivity, rash
RESP: Dyspnea

Contraindications: Breastfeeding, hypersensitivity, anuria, severe renal/hepatic disease

Black Box Warning: Hyperkalemia

Precautions: Pregnancy **B,** dehydration, renal/hepatic disease, cirrhosis, renal stenosis, hyperuricemia, electrolyte abnormalities

Pharmacokinetics

Absorption	GI tract; well absorbed
Distribution	Crosses placenta
Metabolism	Liver
Excretion	Renal; breast milk
Half-life	3 hr

Pharmacodynamics	
Onset	2 hr
Peak	6-8 hr
Duration	12-16 hr

Interactions
Drug classifications
Angiotensin-converting enzyme inhibitors, diuretics (potassium-sparing), potassium products, salt substitutes: increased hyperkalemia

Antihypertensives: increased action
Drug/herb
Arginine: fatal hypokalemia

Bearberry, gossypol: increased hypokalemia

Cucumber, dandelion, horsetail, licorice, nettle, pumpkin, Queen Anne's lace: increased diuretic effect

St. John's wort: severe photosensitivity
Drug/lab test
Interference: quinidine serum levels, LDH

NURSING CONSIDERATIONS
Assessment
• Monitor for manifestations of hyperkalemia: *RENAL:* acidic urine, reduced urine osmolality, nocturia, polyuria, polydipsia; *CV:* hypotension, broad T-wave, U-wave, ectopy, tachycardia, weak pulse, *NEURO:* muscle weakness, altered LOC, drowsiness, apathy, lethargy, confusion, depression, anorexia, nausea, cramps, constipation, distention, paralytic ileus, hypoventilation, respiratory muscle weakness

• Monitor for manifestations of hyponatremia: *CV:* increased B/P, cold, clammy skin, hypo/hypervolemia; *GI:* anorexia, nausea, vomiting, diarrhea, abdominal cramps; *NEURO:* lethargy, increased ICP, confusion, headache, seizures, coma, fatigue, tremors, hyperreflexia

• Monitor for manifestations of hyperchloremia: *NEURO:* weakness, lethargy, coma; *RESP:* deep rapid breathing

• Assess fluid volume status: I&O ratios and record, weight, distended red veins, crackles in lung, color, quality, and specific gravity of urine, skin turgor, adequacy of pulses, moist mucous membranes, bilateral lung sounds, peripheral pitting edema; dehydration symptoms of decreasing output, thirst, hypotension, dry mouth and mucous membranes should be reported

• Monitor electrolytes: potassium, sodium, calcium, magnesium; also include BUN, ABGs, uric acid, CBC, blood glucose

Nursing diagnoses
• Fluid volume, deficient (adverse reactions)
• Fluid volume, excess (uses)
• Knowledge, deficient (teaching)
• Urinary elimination, impaired (adverse reactions)

Implementation
• Give in AM to avoid interference with sleep
• Give after meals if nausea occurs

Patient/family education
• Teach patient to take medication early in the day to prevent nocturia
• Instruct the patient to take with meals if GI symptoms of nausea and anorexia occur
• Teach patient to maintain a record of weight on a weekly basis and notify prescriber of weight loss of 5 lb
• Caution the patient that this product causes an increase in potassium levels, that foods high in potassium should be avoided; refer to dietitian for assistance planning
• Caution the patient not to exercise in hot weather, stand for prolonged periods of time because orthostatic hypotension will be enhanced
• Advise patient to wear protective clothing and sunscreen in the sun to prevent photosensitivity
• Teach patient not to use alcohol or any OTC medications without prescriber's approval because serious product reactions may occur
• Emphasize the need to contact prescriber immediately if muscle cramps, weakness, nausea, dizziness, or numbness occur
• Teach patient to take own B/P and pulse and record
• Advise patient that dizziness and confusion may occur; avoid driving or other hazardous activities if alertness is decreased
• Teach patient to continue taking medication even if feeling better; this product controls symptoms but does not cure the condition
• Advise the patient with hypertension to continue other medical treatment (exercise, weight loss, relaxation techniques, cessation of smoking)

Evaluation
Positive therapeutic outcome
• Prevention of hypokalemia (diuretic use)
• Decreased edema
• Decreased B/P
• Increased diuresis

Treatment of overdose: Lavage if taken orally; monitor electrolytes; administer sodium bicarbonate for potassium 6.5 mEq/L; monitor hydration, CV, renal status

triazolam (Rx)

(trye-az'oh-lam)

Apo-Triazo ✤, Gen-Triazolam ✤, Halcion, Novotriolam ✤, Nu-Triazol ✤

Func. class.: Sedative-hypnotic, antianxiety

Chem. class.: Benzodiazepine

Pregnancy category X

Controlled substance schedule IV (USA), targeted (CDSA IV) (Canada)

Action: Produces CNS depression at limbic, thalamic, hypothalamic levels of CNS; may be mediated by neurotransmitter; γ-aminobutyric acid (GABA); results are sedation, hypnosis, skeletal muscle relaxation, anticonvulsant activity, anxiolytic action

Therapeutic outcome: Decreased anxiety, insomnia

Uses: Insomnia (short-term), sedative/hypnotic

Dosage and routes
Adult: PO 0.125-0.5 mg at bedtime, max 0.5 mg
Geriatric: PO 0.0625-0.125 mg at bedtime

Available forms: Tabs 0.125, 0.25 mg

Adverse effects
CNS: Headache, lethargy, drowsiness, daytime sedation, dizziness, confusion, lightheadedness, anxiety, irritability, amnesia, poor coordination, complex sleep-related reactions (sleep driving, sleep eating)
CV: Chest pain, pulse changes
GI: Nausea, vomiting, diarrhea, heartburn, abdominal pain, constipation, **hepatic injury**
HEMA: Leukopenia, granulocytopenia (rare)
SYST: Severe allergic reactions

Contraindications: Pregnancy **X**, breastfeeding, hypersensitivity to benzodiazepines, intermittent porphyria

Precautions: Children <15 yr, geriatric, anemia, renal/hepatic disease, suicidal individuals, product abuse, psychosis, acute closed-angle glaucoma, seizure disorders, angioedema, respiratory disease, depression, sleep-related behaviors (sleep walking)

Pharmacokinetics

Absorption	Well absorbed
Distribution	Widely distributed, crosses placenta, crosses blood-brain barrier
Metabolism	Liver
Excretion	Kidneys, breast milk
Half-life	2-3 hr

Pharmacodynamics

Onset	½ hr
Peak	Unknown
Duration	6-8 hr

Interactions
Individual drugs
Alcohol: increased action of both products
Cimetidine, disulfiram, isoniazid: increased action, do not use concurrently
Erythromycin, probenecid: increased effects, do not use concurrently
Rifampin: decreased action of rifampin
Theophylline: decreased effects of theophylline
Drug classifications
Antacids: decreased effects of antacids
Antiinfectives (clarithromycin): increased effects
CNS depressants: increased effects of both products
Contraceptives (oral): increased effects; do not use concurrently
CYP3A4 inhibitors: increased triazolam levels
Smoking: decreased hypnotic effects
Drug/herb
Black cohosh: increased hypotension
Catnip, clary, chamomile, cowslip, hops, kava, lavender, mistletoe, nettle, pokeweed, poppy, Queen Anne's lace, senega, skullcap, valerian: increased CNS depression
Drug/lab test
Increased: AST, ALT, serum bilirubin
Decreased: radioactive iodine uptake
False increase: 17-OHCS

NURSING CONSIDERATIONS
Assessment
• Assess patient's mental status: mood, sensorium, anxiety, affect, sleeping pattern, drowsiness, dizziness, especially geriatric; physical dependency, withdrawal symptoms: anxiety, panic attacks, agitation, seizures, headache, nausea, vomiting, muscle pain, weakness; suicidal tendencies; for indications of increasing tolerance and abuse
• Monitor patient's B/P (lying, standing), pulse; if systolic B/P drops 20 mm Hg, hold product, notify prescriber
• Monitor blood tests: CBC during long-term therapy; blood dyscrasias have occurred rarely; decreased hematocrit, neutropenia may occur
• Monitor liver function tests: AST, ALT, bilirubin, creatinine LDH, alkaline phosphatase
• Monitor I&O ratio; indicate renal dysfunction

Nursing diagnoses
- Anxiety (uses)
- Injury, risk for (adverse reactions)
- Knowledge, deficient (teaching)

Implementation
- Give with food or milk to decrease GI symptoms; if patient is unable to swallow medication whole, tab may be crushed and mixed with foods or fluids
- Give sugarless gum, hard candy, frequent sips of water for dry mouth

Patient/family education
- Advise patient that product may be taken with food or fluids, and tab may be crushed or swallowed whole
- Caution patient not to use for everyday stress or longer than 3 mo unless directed by prescriber; not to take more than prescribed amount; may be habit forming; not to double doses or skip doses
- Instruct patient to avoid OTC preparations unless approved by prescriber; alcohol and CNS depressants will increase CNS depression
- Caution patient to avoid driving, activities that require alertness because drowsiness may occur; to avoid alcohol ingestion or other psychotropic medications; to rise slowly or fainting may occur, especially geriatric; that drowsiness may worsen at beginning of treatment
- Teach patient to use reliable contraception
- Teach patient that complex sleep-related behaviors (sleep eating/driving) may occur
- Advise patient not to discontinue medication abruptly after long-term use; withdrawal symptoms include vomiting, cramping, tremors, seizures; decrease dose by 50% q2nights until 0.125 mg for 2 nights, then stop

Evaluation
Positive therapeutic outcome
- Decreased anxiety, restlessness, sleeplessness (short-term treatment only)

Treatment of overdose: Lavage, VS, supportive care

---

trifluoperazine (Rx)
(trye-floo-oh-per'a-zeen)
Apo-Trifluoperazine ✤, Novoflurazine ✤, Solazine ✤, Terfluzine, trifluoperazine HCl
Func. class.: Antipsychotic/neuroleptic
Chem. class.: Phenothiazine, piperazine

Pregnancy category C

Do not confuse:
trifluoperazine/trihexyphenidyl

Action: Depresses cerebral cortex, hypothalamus, limbic system, which control activity, aggression; blocks neurotransmission produced by DOPamine at synapse; exhibits strong α-adrenergic, anticholinergic blocking action; mechanism for antipsychotic effects is unclear

Therapeutic outcome: Decreased signs and symptoms of psychosis

Uses: Psychotic disorders, nonpsychotic anxiety, schizophrenia

Dosage and routes
Psychotic disorders
Adult: PO 1-5 mg bid, usual range 15-20 mg/day, may require 40 mg/day or more
Geriatric: PO 0.5-1 mg daily-bid, increase q4-7day by 0.5-1 mg/day to desired dose, max 40 mg/day
Child >6 yr: PO 1 mg/day or bid

Nonpsychotic anxiety
Adult: PO 1-2 mg bid, max 6 mg/day; do not give longer than 12 wk

Available forms: Tabs 1, 2, 5, 10 mg

Adverse effects
CNS: EPS (pseudoparkinsonism, akathisia, dystonia, tardive dyskinesia), **seizures,** **headache,** **neuroleptic malignant syndrome,** dizziness
CV: Orthostatic hypotension, hypertension, **cardiac arrest,** ECG changes, **tachycardia**
EENT: Blurred vision, glaucoma, dry eyes, pigmentary retinopathy, cornea/lens change
GI: Dry mouth, nausea, vomiting, anorexia, constipation, diarrhea, jaundice, weight gain
GU: Urinary retention, urinary frequency, enuresis, impotence, amenorrhea, gynecomastia, ejaculatory dysfunction, priapism
HEMA: Anemia, **leukopenia, leukocytosis, agranulocytosis**
INTEG: Rash, photosensitivity, dermatitis
RESP: Laryngospasm, dyspnea, **respiratory depression**

T

Adverse effects: *italic* = common, **bold** = life-threatening

Contraindications: Children <6 yr, hypersensitivity, CV disease, coma, blood dyscrasias

Precautions: Pregnancy **C**, breastfeeding, geriatric, breast cancer, seizure disorders, diabetes mellitus, respiratory conditions, prostatic hypertrophy, Parkinson's disease, renal failure, severe hepatic disease, closed-angle glaucoma, severe CNS depression

Black Box Warning: Dementia

Pharmacokinetics

Absorption	Variably absorbed (PO), well absorbed (IM)
Distribution	Widely distributed, high concentrations in CNS, crosses placenta, 91%-99% protein binding
Metabolism	Liver, extensively
Excretion	Kidneys, breast milk
Half-life	Unknown

Pharmacodynamics

	PO	IM
Onset	Rapid	Immediate
Peak	2-3 hr	1 hr
Duration	12 hr	12 hr

Interactions
Individual drugs
Alcohol: increased effects of both products, oversedation

Aluminum hydroxide, magnesium hydroxide: decreased absorption

Levodopa: decreased antiparkinson activity

Lithium: decreased effects of lithium

Drug classifications
Anesthetics, CNS depressants, opiate agonists, sedatives/hypnotics: oversedation

Anesthetics (general), opiates, sedative/hypnotic: increased CNS depression

Antacids: decreased absorption

Anticholinergics: increased anticholinergic effects

Anticonvulsants: decreased effects of anticonvulsants

β-Adrenergic blockers: increased effects of both products

CYP2D6 inducers: decreased level of trifluoperazine

CYP2D6 inhibitors: increased level of trifluoperazine

Drug/herb
Chamomile, hops, kava, skullcap, valerian: increased CNS depression

Betel palm, kava: increased EPS

Cola tree, hops, nettle, nutmeg: increased action

Drug/lab test
Increased: LFTs, cardiac enzymes, cholesterol, blood glucose, prolactin, bilirubin, cholinesterase, ^{131}I

Decreased: hormones (blood and urine)

False positive: pregnancy tests, PKU

False negative: urinary steroids, 17-OHCS, pregnancy tests

NURSING CONSIDERATIONS
Assessment
• Assess mental status: orientation, mood, behavior, presence of hallucinations and type before initial administration and monthly; product should significantly reduce psychotic behavior

• Check for swallowing of PO medication; check for hoarding or giving of medication to other patients

• Monitor I&O ratio, palpate bladder if low urinary output occurs, especially in geriatric; urinalysis recommended before, during prolonged therapy

• Monitor bilirubin, CBC, liver function tests monthly

• Assess affect, orientation, LOC, reflexes, gait, coordination, sleep pattern disturbances

• Monitor B/P sitting, standing, and lying; take pulse and respirations q4hr during initial treatment; establish baseline before starting treatment; report drops of 30 mm Hg; obtain baseline ECG, monitor Q- and T-wave changes

• Check for dizziness, faintness, palpitations, tachycardia on rising; severe orthostatic hypotension is common

◆ Identify for neuroleptic malignant syndrome: hyperpyrexia, muscle rigidity, increased CPK, altered mental status; product should be discontinued

• Assess for EPS including akathisia (inability to sit still, no pattern to movements), tardive dyskinesia (bizarre movements of the jaw, mouth, tongue, extremities), pseudoparkinsonism (ragged tremors, pill rolling, shuffling gait); an antiparkinson product should be prescribed

• Assess for constipation, urinary retention daily; if these occur, increase bulk, water in diet

• Assess for hypo/hyperglycemia; appetite patterns

Nursing diagnoses
• Coping, ineffective (uses)
• Knowledge, deficient (teaching)
• Noncompliance (teaching)

Implementation
PO route
• Give decreased dose in geriatric; metabolism is slowed in the geriatric
• Give PO with full glass of water, milk; or give with food to decrease GI upset
• Give antacids 2 hr before or after this product
• Store in airtight, light-resistant container
IV route
• Give **IV** after diluting 10 mg/9 ml of 0.9% NaCl; give 1 mg or less/2 min
Syringe compatibilities: Glycopyrrolate
Additive compatibilities: Meperidine, netilmicin

Patient/family education
• Teach patient to use good oral hygiene; frequent rinsing of mouth, sugarless gum for dry mouth; oral candidasis may occur
• Caution patient to avoid hazardous activities until product response is determined; dizziness, blurred vision is common
• Inform patient that orthostatic hypotension occurs often; to rise from sitting or lying position gradually; avoid tubs, hot showers, and tub baths because hypotension may occur
• Instruct patient that heat stroke may occur in hot weather, so take extra precautions to stay cool
• Advise patient to avoid abrups withdrawal of this product, or EPS may result; product should be withdrawn slowly
• Teach patient to avoid OTC preparations (cough, hay fever, cold) unless approved by prescriber because serious product interactions may occur; avoid use with alcohol, CNS depressants because increased drowsiness may occur
• Advise patient to use sunglasses and sunscreen to prevent burns
• Instruct patient to report sore throat, malaise, fever, bleeding, mouth sores; if these occur, CBC should be performed and product discontinued

Evaluation
Positive therapeutic outcome
• Decrease in emotional excitement, hallucinations, delusions, paranoia
• Reorganization of patterns of thought, speech

Treatment of overdose: Lavage if orally ingested; provide airway; *do not induce vomiting or use epinephrine*

---

trifluridine ophthalmic
See Appendix B

---

trihexyphenidyl (Rx)
(trye-hex-ee-fen′i-dill)
Apo-Trihex ✦, Novohexidyl ✦, PMS-Trihexyphenidyl ✦, Trihexy-2, Trihexy-5, trihexyphenidyl HCl, Trihexane
Func. class.: Cholinergic blocker; antiparkinson
Chem. class.: Synthetic tertiary amine
Pregnancy category C

Do not confuse:
trihexyphenidyl/trifluoperazine

Action: Blocks central muscarinic receptors, which decreases involuntary movements, sweating, salivation

Therapeutic outcome: Decreased involuntary movements

Uses: Parkinsonian symptoms, product-induced EPS

Unlabeled uses: Hypersalivation

Dosage and routes
Parkinsonian symptoms
Adult: PO 1 mg, increased by 2 mg q3-5day to a total of 5-15 mg/day, given in 3-4 divided doses

Drug-induced EPS
Adult: PO 1 mg/day, usual dose 5-15 mg/day, given in 3-4 divided doses

Available forms: Tabs 2, 5 mg; elix 2 mg/5 ml

Adverse effects
CNS: Confusion, anxiety, restlessness, irritability, delusions, hallucinations, headache, sedation, depression, incoherence, dizziness, flushing, weakness
CV: Palpitations, tachycardia, postural hypotension
EENT: Blurred vision, photophobia, dilated pupils, difficulty swallowing, dry eyes, increased intraocular tension, closed-angle glaucoma
GI: Dryness of mouth, constipation, nausea, vomiting, abdominal distress, **paralytic ileus**
GU: Urinary hesitancy, urinary retention, dysuria
INTEG: Urticaria, rash, dry skin, photosensitivity

T

Adverse effects: *italic* = common, **bold** = life-threatening

MISC: Suppression of lactation, nasal congestion, decreased sweating, hyperthermia, heat stroke, numbness of fingers
MS: Weakness, cramping

Contraindications: Hypersensitivity, tardive dyskinesia, closed-angle glaucoma, myasthenia gravis, GI/ GU obstruction

Precautions: Pregnancy **C**, breastfeeding, children, geriatric patients, tachycardia, abdominal obstruction, infection, gastric ulcer, myocardial ischemia, unstable CV disease, prostatic hypertrophy

Pharmacokinetics

Absorption	Well absorbed
Distribution	Unknown
Metabolism	Unknown
Excretion	Unknown
Half-life	5-10 hr

Pharmacodynamics

	PO
Onset	1 hr
Peak	2-3 hr
Duration	6-12 hr

Interactions
Individual drugs
Alcohol: increased CNS depression
Amantadine: increased cholinergic effects
Digoxin: increased levels of digoxin
Donepezil, galantamine, rivastigmine: decreased anticholinergic effect
Haloperidol: decreased action of haloperidol
Levodopa: decreased action of levodopa
Drug classifications
Analgesics, antihistamines, opioids, sedative/ hypnotics: increased CNS depression
Antidepressants (tricyclics), antihistamines, phenothiazines: increased anticholinergic effects
Drug/herb
Henbane, jimsonweed, scopolia: increased trihexyphenidyl

NURSING CONSIDERATIONS
Assessment
• Monitor I&O ratio; retention commonly causes decreased urinary output, distention, frequency, incontinence
• Assess for parkinsonism, EPS: shuffling gait, muscle rigidity, involuntary movements, pill rolling, muscle spasms, drooling before and during treatment
• Monitor for urinary hesitancy, retention; palpate bladder if retention occurs

• Monitor for constipation, cramping, pain in abdomen, abdominal distention; increase fluids, bulk, exercise if this occurs
• Assess for tolerance over long-term therapy; dose may have to be increased or changed
• Assess for mental status: affect, mood, CNS depression, worsening of mental symptoms during early therapy

Nursing diagnoses
• Knowledge, deficient (teaching)
• Mobility, impaired physical (uses)

Implementation
• Give with or after meals to prevent GI upset; may give with fluids other than water
• Give at bedtime to avoid daytime drowsiness in patient with parkinsonism
• Store at room temperature

Patient/family education
• Teach patient to use caution in hot weather; product may increase susceptibility to stroke because perspiration is decreased; patient should remain indoors
• Teach patient not to discontinue this product abruptly; to taper off over 1 wk to prevent withdrawal symptoms (insomnia, involuntary movements, anxiety, tachycardias)
• Caution patient to avoid driving or other hazardous activities; drowsiness, dizziness may occur
• Advise patient to avoid OTC medications (cough, cold preparations with alcohol, antihistamines) unless directed by prescriber; increased CNS depression may occur
• Instruct patient to rise from sitting or recumbent position slowly to minimize orthostatic hypotension
• Advise patient to use gum, hard candy, frequent sips of water to decrease dry mouth; if dry mouth continues, saliva substitutes may be prescribed
• Instruct patient that doses should not be doubled, but missed dose may be taken up to 2 hr before next dose

Evaluation
Positive therapeutic outcome
• Absence of involuntary movements (pill rolling, tremors, muscle spasms)

trimethobenzamide (Rx)

(trye-meth-oh-ben'za-mide)

Tigan, trimethobenzamide

Func. class.: Antiemetic, anticholinergic

Chem. class.: Ethanolamine derivative

Pregnancy category C

Action: Acts centrally by blocking chemoreceptor trigger zone, which in turn acts on vomiting center

Therapeutic outcome: Absence of nausea and vomiting

Uses: Nausea, vomiting, prevention of postoperative vomiting

Dosage and routes
Postoperative vomiting
Adult: IM 200 mg followed by a second dose 1 hr later

Nausea/vomiting
Adult: PO 300 mg tid-qid; IM 200 mg tid-qid

Renal dose
Adult: IM CCr 15-30 ml/min give 50% of dose

Available forms: Caps 300 mg; inj 100 mg/ml

Adverse effects
CNS: Drowsiness, headache, dizziness, confusion, *vertigo,* EPS, disorientation, **coma, seizures,** depression
CV: Hyper/hypotension, palpitations, **cardiac dysrhythmias**
EENT: Dry mouth, blurred vision, photosensitivity
GI: Nausea, diarrhea, vomiting, difficulty swallowing
INTEG: Rash, urticaria, fever, chills, flushing, hyperpyrexia

Contraindications: Children (parenterally), hypersensitivity to opioids, shock

Precautions: Pregnancy **C**, children, geriatric, cardiac dysrhythmias, acute febrile illness, encephalitis, gastroenteritis, dehydration, electrolyte imbalances, Reye's syndrome

Pharmacokinetics
Absorption	Unknown
Distribution	Unknown
Metabolism	Liver, extensively
Excretion	Kidneys
Half-life	Unknown

Pharmacodynamics
	PO	IM	RECT
Onset	20-40 min	15 min	10-40 min
Peak	Unknown	Unknown	Unknown
Duration	3-4 hr	2-3 hr	3-4 hr

Interactions
Individual drugs
Alcohol: increased effect
Drug classifications
CNS depressants: increased effect

NURSING CONSIDERATIONS
Assessment
● Monitor VS, B/P; check patients with cardiac disease more often
● Assess for signs of toxicity of other products or masking of symptoms of disease: brain tumor, intestinal obstructions
● Observe for drowsiness, dizziness
● Assess for nausea, vomiting before and after treatment

Nursing diagnoses
● Knowledge, deficient (teaching)

Implementation
PO route
● Cap may be swallowed whole or opened and mixed with food or fluids
IM route
● Administer IM inj in large muscle mass; aspirate to avoid **IV** administration
● Patient should remain lying down for 30 min after IM inj
Syringe compatibilities: Glycopyrrolate, hydromorphone, midazolam, nalbuphine
Y-site compatibilities: Heparin, hydrocortisone, potassium chloride, vit B/C

Patient/family education
● Teach patient to use good oral hygiene; frequent rinsing of mouth, sugarless gum for dry mouth
● Caution patient to avoid hazardous activities until product response is determined; drowsiness may occur
● Inform patient that orthostatic hypotension occurs often and to rise from sitting or lying position gradually; avoid hot tubs, hot showers, and tub baths because hypotension may occur
● Advise patient to remain lying down after IM inj for at least 30 min
● Inform patient that in hot weather, heat stroke may occur; take extra precautions to stay cool

T

- Teach patient to avoid OTC preparations (cough, hay fever, cold) unless approved by prescriber because serious product interactions may occur; avoid use with alcohol, CNS depressants because increased drowsiness may occur
- Teach patient about EPS
- Instruct patient to report sore throat, malaise, fever, bleeding, mouth sores; if these occur, CBC should be performed and product discontinued

Evaluation
Positive therapeutic outcome
- Decreased nausea, vomiting

---

trimethoprim/ sulfamethoxazole (cotrimoxazole) (Rx)
(trye-meth′oh-prim/sul-fa-meth-ox′a-zole [ko-trye-mox′a-zole])
Apo-Sulfatrim*, Apo-Sulfatrim DS ✿, Bactrim, Bactrim IV, Bethaprim, Cotrim, Novo-Trimel ✿, Novo-Trimel DS ✿, Nu-Cotrimox ✿, Nu-Cotrimox DS ✿, Roubac ✿, Septra, Septra DS, SMZ/TMP, Sulfatrim
Func. class.: Antiinfective
Chem. class.: Sulfonamide—miscellaneous

Pregnancy category C

Action: Sulfamethoxazole (SMZ) interferes with bacterial biosynthesis of proteins by competitive antagonism of PABA when adequate levels are maintained; trimethoprim (TMP) blocks synthesis of tetrahydrofolic acid; combination blocks two consecutive steps in bacterial synthesis of essential nucleic acids, protein

Therapeutic outcome: Absence of infection, based on C&S

Uses: UTI, otitis media, acute and chronic prostatitis, shigellosis, *Pneumocystis jiroveci* pneumonitis, chronic bronchitis, chancroid, traveler's diarrhea

Dosage and routes
Based on TMP content

UTI
Adult: PO 160 mg TMP q12hr × 10-14 days
Child: PO 8 mg/kg TMP daily in 2 divided doses q12hr

Otitis media
Child: PO 8 mg/kg TMP daily in 2 divided doses q12hr × 10 days

Chronic bronchitis
Adult: PO 160 mg TMP q12hr × 14 days

Pneumocystis jiroveci pneumonitis
Adult and child: PO 15-20 mg/kg TMP daily in 4 divided doses q6hr × 14 days; **IV** 15-20 mg/kg/day (based on TMP) in 3-4 divided doses for up to 14 days

Renal dose
Dosage reduction necessary in moderate to severe renal impairment (CCr <30 ml/min)

Available forms: Tabs 80 mg trimethoprim (TMP)/400 mg sulfamethoxazole (SMZ), 160 mg TMP/800 mg SMZ; susp 40 mg/200 mg/5 ml; **IV** 16 mg/80 mg/ml

Adverse effects
CNS: Headache, insomnia, hallucinations, depression, vertigo, fatigue, anxiety, seizures, product fever, chills, **aseptic meningitis**
CV: **Allergic myocarditis**
EENT: Tinnitus
GI: Nausea, vomiting, abdominal pain, stomatitis, **hepatitis**, glossitis, pancreatitis, diarrhea, **enterocolitis**, anorexia, **pseudomembranous colitis**
GU: **Renal failure, toxic nephrosis;** increased BUN, creatinine; crystalluria
HEMA: **Leukopenia, neutropenia, thrombocytopenia, agranulocytosis, hemolytic anemia, hypoprothrombinemia, Henoch-Schönlein purpura, methemoglobinemia, eosinophilia I**
INTEG: Rash, dermatitis, urticaria, erythema, photosensitivity, pain, inflammation at injection site, **toxic epidermal necrolysis, erythema multiforme**
RESP: Cough, shortness of breath
SYST: **Anaphylaxis, systemic lupus erythematosus, Stevens-Johnson syndrome**

Contraindications: Pregnancy at term, breastfeeding, infants <2 mo, hypersensitivity to trimethoprim or sulfonamides, megaloblastic anemia, CCr <15 ml/min, porphyria, hyperkalemia

Precautions: Pregnancy C, infants, geriatric, renal disease, glucose-6-phosphate dehydrogenase deficiency, impaired renal/hepatic function, possible folate deficiency, severe allergy, bronchial asthma, UV exposure

---

Absorption	Rapid
Distribution	Breast milk, crosses placenta, 68% protein bound
Metabolism	Liver
Excretion	Kidneys
Half-life	8-13 hr

Pharmacodynamics

Onset	Unknown
Peak	1-4 hr
Duration	Unknown

Interactions
Individual drugs
CycloSPORINE: decreased response
Dofetilide: increased levels of dofetilide
Methenamine: increased crystalluria
Methotrexate: increased bone marrow depression
Phenytoin: decreased hepatic clearance of phenytoin
Drug classifications
Anticoagulants (oral): increased anticoagulant effect
CYP2C9, CYP3A4 inducers: decreased hepatic clearance
Diuretics (potassium sparing), potassium supplements: increased potassium levels
Diuretics (thiazide): increased thrombocytopenia
Sulfonylureas: increased hypoglycemic response
Drug/herb
Acidophilus: do not use with antiinfectives; separate by several hours
Drug/lab test
Increased: alkaline phosphatase, creatinine, bilirubin, AST, ALT

NURSING CONSIDERATIONS
Assessment
• Assess allergic reactions: rash, fever (AIDS patients more susceptible)
• Monitor I&O ratio; note color, character, pH of urine if product administered for UTI; output should be 800 ml less than intake; if urine is highly acidic, alkalization may be needed
• Monitor renal function tests: BUN, creatinine, urinalysis (long-term therapy)
• Assess type of infection; obtain C&S before starting therapy
• Assess blood dyscrasias, skin rash, fever, sore throat, bruising, bleeding, fatigue, joint pain

• Assess allergic reaction: rash, dermatitis, urticaria, pruritus, dyspnea, bronchospasm

Nursing diagnoses
• Infection, risk for (uses)
• Knowledge, deficient (teaching)
• Noncompliance (teaching)

Implementation
• Give with full glass of water to maintain adequate hydration; increase fluids to 2 L/day to decrease crystallization in kidneys
• Give medication after C&S; repeat C&S after full course of medication
• Store in airtight, light-resistant container at room temp
IV route
• Dilute 5 ml ampule/100-125 ml of D$_5$W, stable for 6 hr, give over 1½ hr, do not refrigerate
Syringe compatibilities: Heparin
Y-site compatibilities: Acyclovir, aldesleukin, allopurinol, amifostine, atracurium, aztreonam, cefepime, cyclophosphamide, diltiazem, enalaprilat, esmolol, filgrastim, fludarabine, gallium, granisetron, hydromorphone, labetalol, lorazepam, magnesium sulfate, melphalan, meperidine, morphine, pancuronium, perphenazine, piperacillin/tazobactam, sargramostim, tacrolimus, teniposide, thiotepa, vecuronium, zidovudine

Patient family education
• Teach patient to take each oral dose with full glass of water to prevent crystalluria; drink 8-10 glasses of water/day
• Teach patient to complete full course of treatment to prevent superinfection
• Teach patient to avoid sunlight or use sunscreen to prevent burns
• Teach patient to avoid OTC medications (aspirin, vit C) unless directed by prescriber
• If diabetic, teach patient to use Clinistix or Tes-Tape
• Teach patient to use alternative contraceptive measures; decreased effectiveness of oral contraceptives may result
• Teach patient to notify prescriber if skin rash, sore throat, fever, mouth sores, unusual bruising, bleeding occur

Evaluation
Positive therapeutic outcome
• Absence of pain, fever, C&S negative

T

triptorelin (Rx)
(trip-toe'rel-in)
Trelstar Depot, Trelstar LA
Func. class.: Gonadotropin-releasing hormone antagonist
Chem. class.: Synthetic decapeptide analog of LHRH

Pregnancy category X

Action: Inhibitor of pituitary gonadotropin secretion; initially increases LH and FSH, with increases in testosterone, reduction in sex steroid levels

Therapeutic outcome: Decreased signs/symptoms of advanced prostate cancer

Uses: Advanced prostate cancer

Dosage and routes
Adult: IM 3.75 mg qmo; 11.25 mg q84day; ER 60 mg qam

Available forms: Microgranules, depot inj 3.75 mg, 11.25 mg; caps ER 60 mg

Adverse effects
CNS: Headache, insomnia, dizziness, lability, fatigue
CV: *Hypertension,* peripheral edema
ENDO: Gynecomastia, breast tenderness, hot flashes
GI: Nausea, vomiting, diarrhea
GU: Impotence, urinary retention, UTI
INTEG: Rash, pain on injection, pruritus, hypersensitivity
MISC: **Anaphylaxis, angioedema**
MS: Osteoneuralgia

Contraindications: Pregnancy **X**, breast-feeding, hypersensitivity to this product or other LHRH agonists or LHRH

Precautions: Metastatic vertebral lesions, urinary tract obstruction, spinal cord compression, renal disease

Pharmacokinetics	
Absorption	Unknown
Distribution	Unknown
Metabolism	CYP/450
Excretion	Liver, kidneys
Half-life	3 hr

Pharmacodynamics	
Unknown	

Interactions
Drug/lab test
Increased: alkaline phosphatase, estradiol, FSH, LH, testosterone levels
Decreased: testosterone levels, progesterone

NURSING CONSIDERATIONS
Assessment
• Assess for severe hypersensitivity: discontinue product and give antihistamines, have emergency equipment nearby
• Monitor I&O ratios; palpate bladder for distention in urinary obstruction
• Monitor for relief of bone pain (back pain)
• Assess levels of testosterone and PSA

Nursing diagnoses
• Diarrhea (adverse reactions)
• Knowledge, deficient (teaching)

Implementation
• Give IM using implant, inserted by qualified person
• Use syringe with 20-G needle, withdraw 2 ml of sterile water for inj, inject into vial, shake well, withdraw vial contents, inject immediately

Patient/family education
• Teach patient that gynecomastia may occur but will decrease after treatment is discontinued
• Advise patient to report allergic reaction immediately
• Teach patient that disease flare may occur at beginning of therapy

Evaluation
Positive therapeutic outcome
• More normal levels of PSA, acid phosphatase, alkaline phosphatase, testosterone level of <25 ng/dl, tumor response

tropicamide ophthalmic
See Appendix B

trospium (Rx)
(trose'pee-um)
Sanctura, Sanctura XR
Func. class.: Anticholinergic, overactive bladder product
Chem. class.: Muscarinic receptor antagonist

Pregnancy category C

Action: Relaxes smooth muscles in bladder by inhibiting acetylcholine effect on muscarinic receptors

Therapeutic outcome: Absence of urinary distention, nocturia, frequency, urgency, incontinence

Uses: Overactive bladder (urinary frequency, urgency)

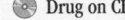

Dosage and routes
Adult: PO 20 mg bid, give 5 ml ≥1 hr prior to meals or on empty stomach

Renal dose
Adult: PO CCr < 30 ml/min 20 mg/day at bedtime
Geriatric ≥75 yr: PO titrate down to 20 mg/day based on response and tolerance

Available forms: Tabs 20 mg

Adverse effects
CNS: Fatigue, dizziness, headache
CV: Tachycardia
EENT: Dry eyes, vision abnormalities
GI: Flatulence, abdominal pain, *constipation, dry mouth,* dyspepsia
GU: Urinary retention
INTEG: Dry skin

Contraindications: Hypersensitivity, uncontrolled closed-angle glaucoma, urinary retention, gastric retention, myasthenia gravis

Precautions: Pregnancy **C**, breastfeeding, children, renal/hepatic disease, controlled closed-angle glaucoma, ulcerative colitis, intestinal atony, bladder outflow obstruction

Pharmacokinetics
Absorption	Rapidly absorbed (10%)
Distribution	Protein bound (50%-85%)
Metabolism	Not fully understood in humans; extensively metabolized
Excretion	Urine (6%), feces (85%); excreted in urine by active tubular secretion
Half-life	Unknown

Pharmacodynamics
Unknown

Interactions
Individual drugs
Alcohol: increased drowsiness
Metformin, procainamide, quinidine, ranitidine, tenofovir, triamterene, vancomycin: increased or decreased action of trospium
Drug classifications
CNS depressants: increased drowsiness
Products excreted by active renal secretion (amiloride, digoxin, morphine): increased or decreased action of trospium
Drug/herb
Herbane, jimsonweed, scopolia: increased action of these herbs
Drug/food
High-fat meal: decreased absorption

NURSING CONSIDERATIONS
Assessment
- Assess urinary patterns: distention, nocturia, frequency, urgency, incontinence

Nursing diagnoses
- Knowledge, deficient (teaching)
- Urinary elimination, impaired (uses)

Implementation
- Take 1 hr prior to meals or on empty stomach

Patient/family education
- Advise patient to avoid hazardous activities; dizziness may occur
- Caution patient that alcohol may increase drowsiness
- Inform patient about anticholinergic effects that may occur

Evaluation
Positive therapeutic outcome
- Correction of urinary status: absence of dysuria, frequency, nocturia, incontinence

---

undecylenic acid topical
See Appendix B

---

unoprostone ophthalmic
See Appendix B

⚠ HIGH ALERT

urokinase (Rx)
(yoor-oh-kin′ase)
Kinlytic
Func. class.: Thrombolytic enzyme
Chem. class.: β-Hemolytic *Streptococcus* filtrate (purified)

Pregnancy category B

Action: Promotes thrombolysis by directly converting plasminogen to plasmin

Therapeutic outcome: Lysis of emboli, or thrombosis in various parts of the body

Uses: Pulmonary embolism

Dosage and routes
Lysis of pulmonary emboli
Adult and child: **IV** 4400 international units/kg/hr over 10 min (90 ml/hr); CONT **IV** INF 4400 international units/kg/hr × 12 hr (15 ml/hr); flush line at end of INF

U

---

*Coronary artery thrombosis
(unlabeled)*
Adult: Instill 6000 international units/min
into occluded artery for 1-2 hr after giving **IV**
BOL of heparin 2500-10,000 units; may also
give as **IV** INF of 2-3 million units over 45-90
min

*Venous catheter occlusion
(unlabeled)*
Adult and child: Instill 5000 international
units into line, wait 5 min, then aspirate;
repeat aspiration attempts q5min × ½ hr; if
occlusion has not been removed, then cap line
and wait ½-1 hr, then aspirate; may need 2nd
dose if still occluded

Available forms: Powder for inj,
lyophilized: 250,000 international units/vial;
powder for catheter clearance

Adverse effects
CNS: Headache, fever
CV: Hypotension, dysrhythmias
GI: Nausea, vomiting
HEMA: Decreased Hct, **bleeding**
INTEG: Rash, urticaria, phlebitis at **IV** inf
site, itching, flushing
MS: Low back pain
RESP: Altered respirations, cyanosis, short-
ness of breath, **bronchospasm**
SYST: GI, GU, **intracranial, retroperito-
neal bleeding;** surface bleeding; **anaphy-
laxis** (rare)

Contraindications: Hypersensitivity to
this product or other thrombolytic enzymes,
internal active bleeding, intraspinal surgery,
neoplasms of CNS, ulcerative colitis/enteritis,
severe uncontrolled hypertension, renal/ hepatic
disease, hypocoagulation, COPD, subacute
bacterial endocarditis, rheumatic valvular
disease, cerebral embolism/thrombosis/
hemorrhage, intraarterial diagnostic procedure
or surgery (10 days), recent major surgery/
trauma, aneurysm, AV malformation

Precautions: Pregnancy **B,** arterial emboli
from left side of heart, hepatic disease

Pharmacokinetics	
Absorption	Completely
Distribution	Unknown
Metabolism	Liver
Excretion	Kidneys
Half-life	10-20 min

Pharmacodynamics	
Onset	Rapid
Peak	Rapid
Duration	12 hr

Interactions
Individual drugs
Abciximab, aspirin, clopidogrel, dipyridamole,
eptifibatide, heparin, indomethacin, phenyl-
butazone, plicamycin, ticlopidine, tirofiban,
valproic acid: increased bleeding potential
Drug classifications
Anticoagulants (oral), cephalosporins (some),
NSAIDs: increased bleeding potential
Glycoprotein IIb, IIIa inhibitors: increased
bleeding risk
Drug/lab test
Increased: pro-time, APTT, TT

NURSING CONSIDERATIONS
Assessment
• Monitor VS, B/P, pulse, respirations (including peripheral), neurologic signs, temp at least
q4hr; temp >104° F (40° C) indicates internal
bleeding; monitor rhythm closely; ventricular
dysrhythmias may occur with hyperfusion;
monitor heart, breath sounds, neurologic
status, peripheral pulses
• Assess for bleeding during 1st hr of
treatment: hematuria, hematemesis, bleeding
from mucous membranes, epistaxis,
ecchymosis; guaiac, all body fluids, stools;
blood studies (Hct, platelets, PTT, pro-time,
TT, APTT) before starting therapy (pro-time or
APTT must be less than 2 × control); TT or
pro-time q3-4hr during treatment
• Assess hypersensitivity: fever, rash, itching,
chills, facial swelling, dyspnea; mild reaction
may be treated with antihistamines; notify
prescriber of severe reactions, stop product,
keep resuscitative equipment nearby
• Monitor ECG on monitor, watch for segment
changes, changes in rhythm; sinus bradycardia, ventricular tachycardia, accelerated
idioventricular rhythm may occur because of
reperfusion

Nursing diagnoses
• Gas exchange, impaired (uses)
• Injury, risk for (adverse reactions)
• Tissue perfusion, ineffective (uses)

Implementation
Intermittent IV route
• Give **IV** loading dose over 30 min to avoid
hypotension
• **IV** after dilution with 4-5 g/250 ml of 0.9%
NaCl, D₅W, LR, give over 1 hr; may give by
continuous inf after loading dose(s) of 1 g/hr
diluted in 50-100 ml of compatible sol; use inf
pump; do not give by direct **IV**
• Give heparin therapy after thrombolytic
therapy is discontinued, TT, ACT, or APTT less
than 2 × control (about 3-4 hr)

- Avoid invasive procedures, inj, rectal temp
- Apply pressure for 30 sec to minor bleeding sites, 30 min to sites of atrial puncture, followed by pressure dressing; inform prescriber if this does not attain hemostasis
- Store powder at room temperature or refrigerate; protect from excessive light

Additive incompatibilities: Do not mix with other medications

Patient/family education
- Teach patient reason for medication, signs and symptoms of bleeding, allergic reactions, when to notify health care prescriber

Evaluation
Positive therapeutic outcome
- Lysis of thrombi or emboli

---

ustekinumab (Rx)
(us-te-kin′ue-mab)
Stelara
Func. class.: Antipsoriatic agent
Pregnancy category B

Action: Interleukin (IL)-12, IL-23 Antagonist

Therapeutic outcome: Decreased plaque psoriasis

Uses: Plaque psoriasis

Dosage and routes
Adult ≥100 kg: SUBCUT 90 mg, repeat in 4 wk, then 90 mg q12wk starting wk 16
Adult ≤100 kg: SUBCUT 45 mg, repeat in 4 wk, then 45 mg q12wk starting wk 16

Available forms: Sol for inj 45 mg/0.5 ml

Adverse effects
CNS: Headache, leukoencephalopathy
HEMA: **Bleeding**
INTEG: Inj site reaction, pruritus, skin irritation, erythema
SYST: **Serious infections, malignancies**

Contraindications: Hypersensitivity, sepsis, active infections

Precautions: Pregnancy **B,** breastfeeding, children ≤18 yr, surgery, TB, diabetes mellitus, geriatric patients, immunosuppression

Pharmacokinetics

Absorption	Unknown
Distribution	Unknown
Metabolism	Unknown
Excretion	Unknown
Half-life	14.9-45.6 days

Pharmacodynamics

Onset	Unknown
Peak	Unknown
Duration	Unknown

Interactions
- Vaccines: avoid concurrent use; immunizations should be brought up to date before treatment
- Immunosuppressives: avoid concurrent use

NURSING CONSIDERATIONS
Assessment
- Monitor for inj site pain, swelling

Nursing diagnoses
- Skin integrity, impaired

Implementation
- Visually inspect for particulate matter or discoloration; solution should be slightly yellow and may contain a few, small translucent or white particles; do not use if discolored or cloudy, or if foreign particulate matter is present; do not shake
- Use a 27-G, 0.5 inch needle
- May be administered subcut into upper arm, abdomen, or thigh; rotate inj sites

Patient/family education
- Inform patient that product must be continued for prescribed time to be effective
- Tell patient not to receive live vaccinations during treatment
- Tell patient to notify prescriber of possible infection (upper respiratory or other)

Evaluation
- Therapeutic response: decreased plaque psoriasis

---

valacyclovir (Rx)
(val-a-syc′kloh-vir)
Valtrex
Func. class.: Antiviral
Chem. class.: Acyclic purine nucleoside analog
Pregnancy category B

Do not confuse:
valacyclovir/valganciclovir, Valtrex/Valcyte

Action: Interferes with DNA synthesis by conversion to acyclovir, causing decreased viral replication, time of lesional healing

V

Therapeutic outcome: Absence of itching, painful lesions; crusting and healing of lesions

Uses: Treatment or suppression of herpes zoster (shingles), recurrent genital herpes, herpes labialis (cold sores), varicella, varicella-zoster

Unlabeled uses: Prevention of CMV infection in advanced HIV, posttransplant patients, Bell's palsy, herpes simplex virus prophylaxis

Dosage and routes
Genital herpes (suppressive initial)
Adult: PO 1 g bid × 10 days initially

Genital herpes (recurrent episodes)
Adult: PO 500 mg bid × 3 days

Genital herpes (suppressive therapy)
Adult: PO 1 g/day with normal immune function; 500 mg/day for those with ≤9 recurrences/yr; 500 mg bid in HIV-infected patients with CD4 ≥100

Reduction of transmission
Adult: PO 500 mg/day for source partner

Herpes zoster
Adult: PO 1 g tid × 1 wk

Herpes labialis
Adult: PO 2 g bid × 1 day

Varicella (chickenpox) in immunocompetent patients
Adolescent and child ≥2 yr: PO 20 mg/kg/dose tid × 5 days, max 3 g/day; start at first sign, preferably within 24 hr of rash

Renal dose
Adult: PO CCr 30-49 ml/min 1g q12hr (herpes zoster); 1 g q12hr × 1 day (herpes labalis); CCr 10-29 ml/min 1 g q24hr (genital herpes/herpes zoster); 500 mg q24hr (recurrent genital herpes); CCr <10 ml/min 500 mg q24hr (genital herpes/herpes zoster), 500 mg q24hr (recurrent genital herpes)

Available forms: Tabs 500, 1000 mg

Adverse effects
CNS: Tremors, lethargy, *dizziness, headache, weakness,* depression
ENDO: Dysmenorrhea
GI: Nausea, vomiting, diarrhea, abdominal pain, constipation, increased AST
HEMA: Thrombocytopenic purpura, hemolytic uremic syndrome
INTEG: Rash

Contraindications: Hypersensitivity to this product, acyclovir, valganciclovir

Precautions: Pregnancy **B**, breastfeeding, geriatric, renal/hepatic disease, electrolyte imbalance, dehydration, hypersensitivity to penciclovir, famciclovir, ganciclovir, varicella

Pharmacokinetics
Absorption	Unknown
Distribution	Crosses placenta, enters breast milk, protein binding 13.5%-17.9%
Metabolism	Converts to acyclovir
Excretion	Urine, as acyclovir
Half-life	2½-3½ hr

Pharmacodynamics
Unknown

Interactions
Individual drugs
Cimetidine, probenecid: increased blood levels of valacyclovir (only if renal disease is significant)

NURSING CONSIDERATIONS
Assessment
• Assess for signs of infection; characteristics of lesions; therapy should be started at first sign of herpes and is most effective within 72 hr of outbreak
• Assess C&S before product therapy; product may be given as soon as culture is performed; repeat C&S after treatment; determine the presence of other STDs
• Assess bowel pattern before, during treatment
• Assess for skin eruptions: rash
• Assess allergies before treatment, reaction of each medication
 Assess for thrombocytopenic purpura, hemolytic uremic syndrome, may be fatal

Nursing diagnoses
• Infection, risk for (uses)

Implementation
• Give within 72 hr of outbreak (herpes zoster); as soon as possible (herpes labialis, genital herpes)
• Give orally before infection occurs

Patient/family education
• Advise patient to take as prescribed; if dose is missed, take as soon as remembered up to 2 hr before next dose; do not double dose
• Instruct patient to take product orally before infection occurs; product should be taken when itching or pain occurs, usually before eruptions

 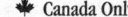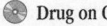

- Inform patient that partners need to be told that patient has herpes; they can become infected; condoms must be worn to prevent reinfections
- Tell patient that product does not cure infection, just controls symptoms and does not prevent infection to others

Evaluation

Positive therapeutic outcome

- Absence of itching, painful lesions; crusting and healed lesions

---

valganciclovir (Rx)

(val-gan-sy′kloh-veer)

Valcyte

Func. class.: Antiviral

Chem. class.: Synthetic nucleoside analog

Pregnancy category C

Do not confuse:

valganciclovir/valacyclovir, Valcyte/Valtrex

Action: Valganciclovir is metabolized to ganciclovir; inhibits replication of human CMV in vivo and in vitro by selectively inhibiting viral DNA synthesis

Therapeutic outcome: Decreased proliferation of virus responsible for CMV retinitis

Uses: Cytomegalovirus (CMV) retinitis in immunocompromised persons, including those with AIDS, after indirect ophthalmoscopy confirms diagnosis; prevention of CMV in transplantation; prevention of CMV in patients at risk going through transplant (kidney, heart, pancreas)

Dosage and routes

Treatment of CMV

Adult: PO induction 900 mg bid × 21 days with food; maintenance 900 mg/day with food

Transplant (CMV prophylaxis)

Adult/adolescent >16 yr: PO 900 mg/day with food starting within 10 days prior to transplantation until 100 days post transplantation

Infant ≥4 mo/child/adolescent ≤16 yr: PO give within 10 days of heart/kidney transplant; calculate dose as 7 × BSA × CCr and give a single daily dose

Renal dose

CCr ≥60 ml/min same dosage as above; CCr 40-59 ml/min 450 mg bid × 21 days, then 450 mg/day; CCr 25-39 ml/min 450 mg/day × 21 days, then 450 mg q2day; CCr 10-24 ml/min 450 mg q2day, then 450 mg 2 ×/week

Available forms: Tabs 450 mg; powder for oral sol 50 mg/ml

Adverse effects

CNS: Fever, chills, **coma,** *confusion,* abnormal thoughts, dizziness, bizarre dreams, *headache,* psychosis, tremors, somnolence, *paresthesia, weakness,* **seizures,** insomnia

EENT: Retinal detachment in CMV retinitis

GI: Abnormal liver function tests, nausea, vomiting, anorexia, diarrhea, abdominal pain, **hemorrhage**

GU: Hematuria, increased creatinine, BUN

HEMA: **Granulocytopenia, thrombocytopenia, irreversible neutropenia, anemia, eosinophilia**

INTEG: Rash, alopecia, *pruritus,* urticaria, pain at inj site, phlebitis, **Stevens-Johnson syndrome**

MISC: Local and systemic infections and **sepsis**

Contraindications: Breastfeeding, hypersensitivity to ganciclovir or valacyclovir, absolute neutrophil count <500/mm³, platelet count <25,000/mm³, hemodialysis, liver transplant

Precautions: Pregnancy **C,** children, geriatric, renal function impairment, hypersensitivity to acyclovir, penciclovir, famciclovir

Black Box Warning: Preexisting cytopenias, secondary malignancy, infertility, anemia

---

Pharmacokinetics

Absorption	Well absorbed from GI tract
Distribution	Plasma protein binding unknown; crosses blood-brain barrier, CSF
Metabolism	Rapidly metabolized in intestinal wall and liver to ganciclovir
Excretion	Kidneys (ganciclovir)
Half-life	3-4½ hr

Pharmacodynamics

Onset	Unknown
Peak	1-3 hr
Duration	Unknown

Interactions

Individual drugs

Adriamycin, amphotericin B, cycloSPORINE, dapsone, DOXOrubicin, flucytosine, pentamidine, trimethoprim/sulfamethoxazole, vinBLAStine, vinCRIStine: increased toxicity

Didanosine: increased effect

Imipenem/cilastatin: increased seizures

Probenecid: decreased renal clearance of valganciclovir

V

Adverse effects: *italic* = common, **bold** = life-threatening

Radiation, zidovudine: severe granulocyto-
penia; do not coadminister
Drug classifications
Antineoplastics: severe granulocytopenia; do
not coadminister
Nucleoside analogs, other: increased toxicity
Drug/food
Absorption: increased with high-fat meal

NURSING CONSIDERATIONS
Assessment
• Assess for leukopenia/neutropenia/
thrombocytopenia: WBCs, platelets q2day
during 2 ×/day dosing and then qwk
• Assess for leukopenia daily with WBC count
in patients with prior leukopenia using other
nucleoside analogs or for whom leukopenia
counts are <1000 cells/mm^3 at start of treatment
• Assess serum creatinine or CCr ≥q2wk
• Assess for CMV retinitis by ophthalmoscopy
before beginning treatment and q2wk
• Obtain culture for CMV
• Assess for infection: sore throat, cough,
fever, chills, back pain; notify prescriber

Nursing diagnoses
• Infection, risk for (uses)
• Injury, risk for (uses, adverse reactions)
• Knowledge, deficient (teaching)

Implementation
PO tab
• Give with food for better absorption

Oral SOL
• Measure 9 ml of purified water in graduated
cylinder, shake bottle to loosen powder, add ½
liquid, shake well, add remaining water, shake,
remove child resistant cap and push bottle
adapter into neck of bottle, close with cap, give
using the dispenser provided

Patient/family education
• Inform patient that product does not cure
condition, that regular ophthalmologic and
blood tests are necessary
• Caution patient that major toxicities may
necessitate discontinuing product
• Caution patient to use contraception during
treatment and that infertility may occur; men
should use barrier contraception for 90 days
after treatment
• Instruct patient to take with food
⊕ Instruct patient to report infection: fever,
chills, sore throat; blood dyscrasias: bruising,
bleeding, petechiae
• Advise patient to avoid crowds, persons with
respiratory infections
• Caution patient to use sunscreen to prevent
burns

Evaluation
Positive therapeutic outcome
• Decreased symptoms of CMV

Treatment of overdose: Maintain
adequate hydration; dialysis may help reduce
serum concentrations; consider use of hematopoietic growth factors

---

valproate (Rx)
(val-proh'ate)
Depacon
valproic acid (Rx)
Depakene
divalproex sodium (Rx)
Depakote, Depakote ER, Epival
Func. class.: Anticonvulsant, vascular
headache suppressant
Chem. class.: Carboxylic acid derivative

Pregnancy category D

Action: Increases levels of γ-aminobutyric
acid (GABA) in brain, which decreases seizure
activity

Therapeutic outcome: Decreased
symptoms of epilepsy, bipolar disorder

Uses: Simple (petit mal), complex (petit
mal), absence, mixed seizures, manic episode
associated with bipolar disorder, prophylaxis
of migraine, adjunct in schizophrenia, tardive
dyskinesia, aggression in children with ADHD,
organic brain syndrome, tonic-clonic (grand
mal)/myoclonic seizures

Unlabeled uses: Rectal for seizures
(valproic acid)

Dosage and routes
Epilepsy
Adult and child: PO 10-15 mg/kg/day
divided in 2-3 doses, may increase by 5-10
mg/kg/day qwk, max 60 mg/kg/day in 2-3
divided doses; **IV** ≤20 mg/min over 1 hr

Mania (divalproex sodium)
Adult: PO 750 mg/day in divided doses, max
60 mg/kg/day or 3000 mg/day

Mania (valproic acid: Stavzor)
Adult: DEL REL Cap 750 mg/day in divided
doses

Migraine (divalproex sodium)
Adult: PO 250 mg bid, may increase to 1000
mg/day; or 500 mg (Depakote ER) daily × 7
days, then 1000 mg/day

Available forms: Valproic acid: caps 250
mg; syr 250 mg/5 ml del rel cap (Stavzor) 125

---

mg; divalproex: del rel tabs 125, 250, 500 mg; ext rel tabs 250, 500 mg; sprinkle caps 125 mg; valproate: inj 100 mg/ml

Adverse effects
CNS: *Sedation, drowsiness,* dizziness, headache, incoordination, depression, hallucinations, behavioral changes, tremors, aggression, weakness, **coma, suicidal ideation**
EENT: Visual disturbances, taste perversion
GI: *Nausea, vomiting, constipation, diarrhea, dyspepsia,* anorexia, cramps, **hepatic failure, pancreatitis, toxic hepatitis,** stomatitis, weight gain
GU: Enuresis, irregular menses
HEMA: **Thrombocytopenia, leukopenia, lymphocytosis,** increased pro-time, bruising, epistaxis
INTEG: *Rash,* alopecia, photosensitivity, dry skin

Contraindications: Hypersensitivity, urea cycle disorders

Black Box Warning: Pregnancy **D**, hepatic disease, pancreatitis

Precautions: Breastfeeding, geriatric
Black Box Warning: Children <2 yr

Pharmacokinetics	
Absorption	Unknown
Distribution	Breast milk, crosses placenta, widely distributed, protein binding 90%
Metabolism	Liver
Excretion	Kidneys
Half-life	6-16 hr

Pharmacodynamics	
Onset	15-30 min
Peak	1-4 hr
Duration	4-6 hr

Interactions
Individual drugs
Abciximab, cefoperazone, cefotetan, eptifibatide, heparin, tirofiban: increased bleeding risk
Alcohol: increased CNS depression
Carbamazepine, ethosuximide, lamotrigine, lorazepam, rufinamide, zidovudine: increased action and toxicity of these products
Carbamazepine, lamotrigine, rifampin: decreased valproic acid level
Cimetidine: decreased metabolism of valproic acid
Chlorpromazine, erythromycin, felbamate: increased valproic acid level
Phenytoin: increased action of phenytoin

Drug classifications
Antidepressants (tricyclics), barbiturates: increased action
Antihistamines, barbiturates, MAOIs, opioids, sedative/hypnotics: increased CNS depression
Antiplatelets, NSAIDs, thrombolytics: increased bleeding risk
Salicylates: increased toxicity of valproic acid
Drug/lab test
False positive: ketones, urine
Interference: thyroid function tests

NURSING CONSIDERATIONS
Assessment
• Monitor blood tests: Hct, Hgb, RBC, serum folate, ammonia, platelets, pro-time, PTT, vit D if on long-term therapy
• Monitor liver function tests: AST, ALT, bilirubin, creatinine, failure
• Monitor blood levels: therapeutic level 50-100 mcg/ml
• Assess seizure disorder: location, aura, activity, duration; seizure precautions should be in place
⚠ Assess bipolar disorder: mood, activity, sleeping, eating, behavior; suicidal thoughts/behaviors
• Assess migraines: frequency, intensity
• Assess respiratory dysfunction: respiratory depression, character, rate, rhythm; hold product if respirations are <12/min or if pupils are dilated

Nursing diagnoses
• Injury, risk for (uses, adverse reactions)
• Knowledge, deficient

Implementation
• Swallow tabs and caps whole; do not break, crush, or chew; use sprinkle cap contents on food
• Give elixir alone; do not dilute with carbonated beverage; do not give syrup to patients on sodium restriction
• Give with food or milk to decrease GI symptoms

Patient/family education
• Teach patient that physical dependency may result from extended use
• Instruct patient to avoid driving, other activities that require alertness
• Advise patient not to discontinue medication quickly after long-term use; seizures may result
• Advise patient to report visual disturbances, rash, diarrhea, light-colored stools, jaundice, protracted vomiting to prescriber

V

Adverse effects: *italic* = common, **bold** = life-threatening

Evaluation
Positive therapeutic outcome
• Decreased seizures

---

valsartan (Rx)
(val-zar'tan)
Diovan
Func. class.: Antihypertensive
Chem. class.: Angiotensin II receptor
antagonist (type AT_1)

Pregnancy category D

Action: Blocks the vasoconstrictor and
aldosterone-secreting effects of angiotensin II;
selectively blocks the binding of angiotensin II
to the AT_1 receptor found in tissues

Therapeutic outcome: Decreased B/P

Uses: Hypertension, alone or in combination,
in patients >6 yr; CHF

Dosage and routes
Adult: PO 80-160 mg/day alone or in
combination with other antihypertensives, may
increase to 320 mg CHF

CHF
Adult: PO 40 mg bid, up to 60 mg bid

Available forms: Tabs 80, 160, 320 mg

Adverse effects
CNS: Dizziness, insomnia, drowsiness,
vertigo, headache, fatigue
CV: Angina pectoris, 2nd-degree AV block,
cerebrovascular accident, hypotension, **MI,
dysrhythmias**
EENT: Conjunctivitis
GI: Diarrhea, abdominal pain, nausea, **hepa-
totoxicity**
GU: Impotence, **nephrotoxicity**
HEMA: Anemia, neutropenia
META: Hyperkalemia
MISC: Vasculitis
MS: Cramps, myalgia, pain, stiffness
RESP: Cough

Contraindications: Hypersensitivity,
severe hepatic disease, bilateral renal artery
stenosis

Black Box Warning: Pregnancy **D**

Precautions: Breastfeeding, children,
geriatric, CHF, hypertrophic cardiomyopathy,
aortic/mitral valve stenosis, CAD, angioedema,
renal/hepatic disease, hypersensitivity to ACE
inhibitors

Pharmacokinetics

Absorption	Well absorbed
Distribution	Bound to plasma proteins
Metabolism	Extensive
Excretion	Feces, urine, breast milk
Half-life	9 hr

Pharmacodynamics

Onset	Up to 2 hr
Peak	4-6 hr
Duration	24 hr

Interactions
Individual drugs
Lithium: increased effects of lithium
Drug classifications
Diuretics (potassium-sparing, potassium
supplements, ACE inhibitors): increased
hyperkalemia
NSAIDs, salicylates: decreased antihypertensive
effects
Drug/herb
Aconite: increased toxicity, death
Astragalus, cola tree: increased or decreased
antihypertensive effect
Barberry, betony, black catechu, black cohosh,
bloodroot, broom, burdock, cat's claw,
dandelion, goldenseal, hawthorn, Irish
moss, Jamaican dogwood, kelp, khella,
mistletoe, parsley: increased
antihypertensive effect
Coltsfoot, guarana, khat, licorice, yohimbe:
decreased antihypertensive effect

NURSING CONSIDERATIONS
Assessment
• Assess B/P (lying, sitting, standing), pulse
q4hr; note rate, rhythm, quality periodically
• Monitor electrolytes: potassium, sodium,
chloride; total CO_2
• Assess for angioedema: facial swelling,
shortness of breath
• Obtain baselines in renal, liver function tests
before therapy begins
• Assess blood tests: BUN, creatinine, before
treatment
• Monitor for edema in feet, legs daily
• Assess for skin turgor, dryness of mucous
membranes for hydration status; correct
volume depletion before initiating therapy

Nursing diagnoses
• Fluid volume, deficient (side effects)
• Knowledge, deficient (teaching)
• Noncompliance (teaching)

Implementation
• Administer without regard to meals

Patient/family education
- Teach patient not to take this product if breastfeeding or pregnant, or have had an allergic reaction to this product
- If a dose is missed, instruct patient to take as soon as possible, unless it is within an hour before next dose
- Advise patient to comply with dosage schedule, even if feeling better
- Teach patient to notify prescriber of fever, swelling of hands or feet, irregular heartbeat, chest pain
- Advise patient excessive perspiration, dehydration, diarrhea may lead to fall in blood pressure; consult prescriber if these occur
- Inform patient that product may cause dizziness, fainting; light-headedness may occur
- Caution patient to rise slowly to sitting or standing position to minimize orthostatic hypotension; how to take B/P

Evaluation
Positive therapeutic outcome
- Decreased B/P

---

vancomycin
(van-koe-mye′sin)
Vancocin, vancomycin HCl
Func. class.: Antiinfective—miscellaneous
Chem. class.: Tricyclic glycopeptide

Pregnancy category B

Action: Inhibits bacterial cell wall synthesis, blocks glycopeptides

Therapeutic outcome: Bactericidal for the following organisms: staphylococci, streptococci, *Corynebacterium, Clostridium*

Uses: Resistant staphylococcal infections, pseudomembranous colitis, staphylococcal enterocolitis, group A β-hemolytic streptococci, endocarditis prophylaxis for dental procedures, diphtheroid endocarditis

Dosage and routes
Serious staphylococcal infections
Adult: **IV** 500 mg (7.5 mg/kg) q6-8hr or 1 g (15 mg/kg) q12hr
Child: **IV** 40-60 mg/kg/day divided q6-8hr
Neonate: **IV** 15 mg/kg initially followed by 10 mg/kg q8-24hr

Pseudomembranous/ staphylococcal enterocolitis
Adult: PO 125-500 mg q6h for 7-10 days
Child: PO 40 mg/kg/day divided q6hr × 7-14 days, max 2 g/day

Endocarditis prophylaxis for dental procedure
Adult: **IV** 1 g over 1 hr; 1 hr before dental procedure
Child: **IV** 20 mg/kg over 1 hr; 1 hr before procedure

Renal dose
Adult: **IV** CCr >70 ml/min no dosage adjustment; CCr 50-70 ml/min loading dose of 15 mg/kg, reduce dose to 750 mg-1 g q18-24hr; CCr <49 ml/min initial loading dose of 15 mg/kg, with subsequent dosing based on concentration, may be q24-72hr or longer

Available forms: Pulvules 125, 250 mg; powder for oral sol 250 mg/5 ml, 500 mg/6 ml; powder for inj **IV** 500 mg; vials 1, 5, 10 g

Adverse effects
CV: **Cardiac arrest, vascular collapse (rare),** hypotension
EENT: Ototoxicity, permanent deafness, tinnitus, nystagmus
GI: **Nausea, pseudomembranous colitis**
GU: **Nephrotoxicity: increased BUN, creatinine, albumin, fatal uremia**
HEMA: **Leukopenia, eosinophilia, neutropenia**
INTEG: Chills, fever, rash, thrombophlebitis at inj site, urticaria, pruritus, necrosis (Red Man product syndrome), skin/subcutaneous tissue disorders
RESP: Wheezing, dyspnea
SYST: **Anaphylaxis,** superinfection

Contraindications: Hypersensitivity, previous hearing loss

Precautions: Pregnancy **B,** breastfeeding, neonates, geriatric, renal disease

Pharmacokinetics

Absorption	Poorly absorbed (PO), completely absorbed (**IV**)
Distribution	Widely distributed, crosses placenta
Metabolism	Liver
Excretion	PO, feces; **IV**, kidneys
Half-life	4-8 hr

Pharmacodynamics

	IV
Onset	Immediate
Peak	Inf end
Duration	Unknown

Interactions
Individual drugs
Amphotericin B, bacitracin, cidofovir, cisplatin, colistin, polymyxin B: increased ototoxicity or nephrotoxicity

---

Adverse effects: *italic* = common, **bold** = life-threatening

Drug classifications
Aminoglycosides, cephalosporins, nondepolarizing muscle relaxants: increased ototoxicity or nephrotoxicity
Drug/herb
Acidophilus: do not use with antiinfectives; separate by several hours

NURSING CONSIDERATIONS
Assessment
• Assess for infection: WBC, urine, stools, sputum, wound characteristics, throughout treatment
• Monitor I&O ratio; report hematuria, oliguria because nephrotoxicity may occur
• Monitor any patient with compromised renal system (BUN, creatinine); product is excreted slowly in poor renal system function; toxicity may occur rapidly
• Monitor blood tests: WBC; serum levels; peak 1 hr after 1-hr inf 25-40 mg/ml; trough before next dose 5-10 mg/ml
• Obtain C&S before product therapy; product may be given as soon as culture is performed
• Assess auditory function during, after treatment; hearing loss, ringing, roaring in ears; product should be discontinued
• Monitor B/P during administration; sudden drop may indicate Red Man syndrome
• Assess for signs of infection
• Assess respiratory status: rate, character, wheezing, tightness in chest
• Identify allergies before treatment, reaction of each medication

Nursing diagnoses
• Infection, risk for (uses)
• Knowledge, deficient (teaching)

Implementation
• Give antihistamine if Red Man syndrome occurs: decreased B/P, flushing of neck, face
• Give dose based on serum concentration
• Give in equal intervals around the clock to maintain blood levels
• Store at room temperature for up to 2 wk after reconstitution
• Have adrenaline, suction, tracheostomy set, endotracheal intubation equipment on unit; anaphylaxis may occur
• Provide adequate intake of fluids (2 L) to prevent nephrotoxicity
IT route
• Use preservative-free 0.9% NaCl (2-5 mg/ml final conc)
Intermittent IV route
• Give after reconstitution with 10 ml of sterile water for inj (500 mg/10 ml); further dilution is needed for **IV**, 500 mg/100 ml of 0.9%

NaCl, D_5W given as intermittent inf over 1 hr; decrease rate of inf if Red Man syndrome occurs
Continuous IV INF route
• Reconstitute, then may inf 1-2 g in volume to give over 24 hr if intermittent **IV** route cannot be used
Y-site compatibilities: Acyclovir, allopurinol, amiodarone, amsacrine, atracurium, cyclophosphamide, diltiazem, enalaprilat, esmolol, filgrastim, fluconazole, fludarabine, gallium, granisetron, hydromorphone, insulin (regular), labetalol, lorazepam, magnesium sulfate, melphalan, meperidine, meropenem, midazolam, morphine, ondansetron, paclitaxel, pancuronium, perphenazine, propofol, sodium bicarbonate, tacrolimus, teniposide, theophylline, thiotepa, tolazoline, vecuronium, vinorelbine, warfarin, zidovudine
Additive compatibilities: Amikacin, atracurium, calcium gluconate, cefepime, cimetidine, corticotropin, dimenhyDRINATE, hydrocortisone, meropenem, ofloxacin, potassium chloride, ranitidine, verapamil, vit B/C

Patient/family education
• Teach patient aspects of product therapy: need to complete entire course of medication to ensure organism death (7-10 days); culture may be performed after completed course of medication
• Advise patient to report sore throat, fever, fatigue; could indicate superinfection
• Instruct patient that product must be taken in equal intervals around clock to maintain blood levels

Evaluation
Positive therapeutic outcome
• Absence of fever, sore throat
• Negative culture after treatment

---

vardenafil (Rx)
(var-den'a-fil)
Levitra
Func. class.: Impotence agent
Chem. class.: Phosphodiesterase type 5 inhibitor
Pregnancy category B

Action: Inhibits phosphodiesterase type 5 (PDE5); enhances erectile function by increasing the amount of cGMP, which causes smooth muscle relaxation and increased blood flow into the corpus cavernosum

Therapeutic outcome: Erection

Uses: Treatment of erectile dysfunction

Dosage and routes
Adult: PO 10 mg, taken 1 hr before sexual activity, dose may be reduced to 5 mg or increased to a max of 20 mg; max dosing frequency is once/day
Geriatric >65 yr: PO 5 mg initially, titrate as needed/tolerated

Hepatic dose (Child-Pugh B)
Adult: PO 5 mg, max 10 mg

Concomitant medications
Ritonavir, max 2.5 mg q72hr; for indinavir, ketoconazole 400 mg/day and itraconazole 400 mg/day, max 2.5 mg/day; for ketoconazole 200 mg/day, itraconazole 200 mg/day and erythromycin, max 5 mg/day

Available forms: Tabs 2.5, 5, 10, 20 mg

Adverse effects
CNS: Headache, flushing, dizziness, insomnia, **seizures,** transient global amnesia
CV: Hypertension, **MI, CV collapse,** chest pain
EENT: Conjunctivitis, tinnitus, photophobia, diminished vision, glaucoma, hearing loss
GU: Abnormal ejaculation, priapism
MISC: Rash, GERD, GGTP increased, **NAION (nonarteritic ischemic optic neuropathy),** dyspepsia
MS: Myalgia, arthralgia, neck pain
RESP: Rhinitis, sinusitis, dyspnea, pharyngitis, epistaxis

Contraindications: Hypersensitivity, coadministration of α-blockers or nitrates, renal failure, congenital or acquired QT prolongation

Precautions: Pregnancy **B**; not indicated for women, children, or newborns; hepatic impairment; retinitis pigmentosa; cardiovascular disease; anatomic penile deformities; sickle cell anemia; leukemia; multiple myeloma; bleeding disorders, active peptic ulceration; CV/renal disease

Pharmacokinetics

Absorption	Rapid; reduced absorption with high-fat meal
Distribution	Bioavailability 15%; protein binding 95%
Metabolism	Liver
Excretion	Primarily in feces (91%-95%)
Half-life	4-5 hr

Pharmacodynamics

Onset	20 min
Peak	½-1½ hr
Duration	<5 hr

Interactions
Individual drugs
Alcohol, amlodipine, metoprolol, NIFEdipine: increased hypotension, do not use concurrently
Cimetidine, erythromycin, itraconazole, ketoconazole: increased levels
Clarithromycin, droperidol, procainamide, quinidine: serious dysrhythmias; do not use concurrently
Drug classifications
⬧Do not use with nitrates because of unsafe decrease in B/P that could result in heart attack or stroke
α-Blockers, protease inhibitors: increased hypotension; do not use concurrently
Angiotensin II receptor blockers: increased hypotension; do not use concurrently
Antidysrhythmics class Ia, III, quinolones: serious dysrhythmias; do not use together
Antiretroviral protease inhibitors: increased vardenafil levels

NURSING CONSIDERATIONS
Assessment
• Assess for use of organic nitrates that should not be used with this product
• Assess for severe loss of vision while taking this or any similar products; these products should not be used if vision loss has occurred

Nursing diagnoses
• Knowledge, deficient (teaching)
• Sexual dysfunction (uses)

Implementation
• Give approximately 1 hr before sexual activity; do not use more than once a day

Patient/family education
• Advise that product does not protect against STDs, including HIV
• Teach that product absorption is reduced with a high-fat meal
• Instruct that product should not be used with nitrates in any form
• Inform that product has no effect in the absence of sexual stimulation
• Teach that patient should seek immediate medical attention if erection lasts for more than 4 hr
• Advise to inform physician of all medications being taken

V

Adverse effects: *italic* = common, **bold** = life-threatening

- Teach patient to notify prescriber immediately and stop taking product if vision loss occurs

Evaluation
Positive therapeutic outcome
- Sustainable erection

---

varenicline (Rx)
(var-e-ni'kleen)
Chantix
Func. class.: Smoking cessation agent

Pregnancy category C

Action: Partial agonist for nicotine receptors; partially activates receptors to help curb cravings; occupies receptors to prevent nicotine binding

Therapeutic outcome: Smoking cessation

Uses: Smoking deterrent

Dosage and routes
Adult: PO therapy should begin 1 week prior to smoking stop date (i.e., take product plus tobacco for 7 days); titrate for 1 wk, days 1 through 3, 0.5 mg/day; days 4 through 7, 0.5 mg bid; day 8 through end of treatment 1 mg bid; treatment is 12 wk and may repeat for another 12 wk

Available forms: Tabs 0.5, 1 mg

Adverse effects
CNS: Headache, agitation, dizziness, insomnia, abnormal dreams, fatigue, malaise, behavior changes, depression, suicidal ideation, **suicide,** amnesia, hallucinations, hostility, mania, psychosis, tremor
CV: **Dysrhythmias,** hypertension, palpitations, **tachycardia,** angina, hypotension, **MI**
EENT: *Blurred vision,* tinnitus
GI: *Nausea, vomiting,* anorexia, *dry mouth,* increased/decreased appetite, *constipation,* flatulence, GERD
GU: Erectile dysfunction, urinary frequency, menstrual irregularities
INTEG: Rash, pruritus, **angioedema, Stevens-Johnson syndrome**
MISC: Weight loss or gain
RESP: Dyspnea, rhinorrhea

Contraindications: Hypersensitivity, eating disorders

Precautions: Pregnancy **C,** breastfeeding, children <18 yr, geriatric, renal disease, recent MI

Black Box Warning: Bipolar disorder, depression, schizophrenia, suicidal ideation

Pharmacokinetics
Absorption	Unknown
Distribution	Steady state 4 days
Metabolism	Minimal
Excretion	Urine 92%, unchanged
Half-life	Elimination 24 hr

Pharmacodynamics
Unknown

NURSING CONSIDERATIONS
Assessment
- Assess for renal function in geriatric
- Assess for smoking cessation after 12 wk; if progress has not been made, product may be used for an additional 12 wk
- Assess mental status: mood, sensorium, affect

Nursing diagnoses
- Coping, ineffective (uses)
- Knowledge, deficient (teaching)

Implementation
- Do not break, crush, or chew tabs
- Give increased fluids, bulk in diet if constipation occurs
- Give after eating with a full glass of water
- Give sugarless gum, hard candy, or frequent sips of water for dry mouth

Patient/family education
- Teach patient that treatment for smoking cessation lasts 12 wk and another 12 wk may be required
- Teach patient to use caution in driving, other activities requiring alertness; blurred vision may occur
- Advise patient to set a date to quit smoking and initiate treatment 1 wk prior to that date
- Teach patient how to titrate product
- Advise patient not to use with nicotine patches unless directed by prescriber; may increase B/P
- Advise patient to notify prescriber if pregnancy is suspected or planned
- Teach patient common side effects to be expected

Evaluation
Positive therapeutic outcome
- Smoking cessation

---

vasopressin ⊕ (Rx)
(vay-soe-press'in)
Pitressin, Pressyn ✦
Func. class.: Pituitary hormone
Chem. class.: Lysine vasopressin
Pregnancy category C

Action: Promotes reabsorption of water by action on renal tubular epithelium; causes vasoconstriction on muscles in the GI system

Therapeutic outcome: Increased osmolality, decreased urine output in diabetes insipidus

Uses: Diabetes insipidus (nonnephrogenic/nonpsychogenic), abdominal distention postoperatively, bleeding esophageal varices

Dosage and routes
Diabetes insipidus
Adult: IM/SUBCUT 5-10 units bid-qid prn; CONT **IV** INF 0.0005 units/kg/hr, (0.05 milliunit/kg/hr), double dose q30min as needed
Child: IM/SUBCUT 2.5-10 units bid-qid prn; IM/SUBCUT 1.25-2.5 units q2-3day (Pitressin Tannate) for chronic therapy

Abdominal distention
Adult: IM 5 units, then q3-4hr, increasing to 10 units if needed (aqueous)

Available forms: Inj 20, 5 units/ml (tannate)

Adverse effects
CNS: Drowsiness, headache, lethargy, flushing, vertigo
CV: Increased B/P, dysrhythmias, chest pain
Black Box Warning: Cardiac arrest, shock, MI
EENT: Nasal irritation, congestion, rhinitis
GI: Nausea, heartburn, cramps, vomiting, flatus
GU: Vulval pain, uterine cramping
MISC: Tremor, sweating, vertigo, urticaria, bronchial constriction

Contraindications: Hypersensitivity, chronic nephritis

Precautions: Pregnancy C, breastfeeding, CAD, asthma, renal/vascular disease, migraines, seizures

Pharmacokinetics
Absorption	Erratically absorbed (IM)
Distribution	Widely distributed extracellular fluid
Metabolism	Liver, rapidly
Excretion	Kidneys, unchanged
Half-life	10-20 min

Pharmacodynamics
	IM	IV
Onset	1 hr	Unknown
Peak	Unknown	Unknown
Duration	3-8 hr	3-8 hr

Interactions
Individual drugs
Carbamazepine, chloropromide, clofibrate, fludrocortisone, urea: decreased antidiuretic effect
Demeclocycline, lithium: increased antidiuretic effect
Drug classifications
Tricyclics: increased antidiuretic effect

NURSING CONSIDERATIONS
Assessment
• Assess intranasal use: nausea, congestion, cramps, headache; usually decreased with decreased dose
• Monitor pulse, B/P when giving product **IV** or SUBCUT
• Monitor I&O ratio, weight daily, fluid/electrolyte balance; check for edema in extremities; if water retention is severe, diuretic may be prescribed; check for water intoxication: lethargy, behavioral changes, disorientation, neuromuscular excitability
• Small doses may precipitate coronary adverse effects; keep emergency equipment nearby

Nursing diagnoses
• Fluid volume, deficient (uses)
• Fluid volume, excess (side effects)
• Knowledge, deficient (teaching)

Implementation
IM/SUBCUT route
• May be given IM/SUBCUT for diagnosis of diabetes insipidus
• Give patient 16 oz water at administration to prevent nausea, vomiting, cramping

Patient/family education
• Teach patient technique for nasal instillation: to insert tube into nasal cavity to instill product
• Caution patient to avoid OTC products for cough, hay fever because these preparations may contain epinephrine, decrease product response; do not use with alcohol

V

Adverse effects: *italic* = common, **bold** = life-threatening

- Advise patient to carry/wear emergency ID specifying therapy, disease process (diabetes insipidus)
- Teach patient to measure/record I&O
- Teach patient to avoid alcohol, all OTC medications unless approved by prescription

Evaluation
Positive therapeutic outcome
- Absence of severe thirst
- Decreased urine output, osmolality

! HIGH ALERT

vecuronium (Rx)
(ve-kure-oh′nee-yum)
Func. class.: Neuromuscular blocker—nondepolarizing
Chem. class.: Synthetic curariform

Pregnancy category C

Action: Inhibits transmission of nerve impulses by binding with cholinergic receptor sites, antagonizing action of acetylcholine; no analgesic response

Therapeutic outcome: Skeletal muscle paralysis during anesthesia

Uses: Facilitation of endotracheal intubation; skeletal muscle relaxation during mechanical ventilation, surgery, or general anesthesia

Dosage and routes
Adult and child >1 yr: **IV** initially 0.08-0.1 mg/kg or 0.04-0.06 mg/kg if given with succinylcholine, maintenance 0.01-0.015 mg/kg 25-40 min after initial dose, then 0.01-0.015 mg/kg q12-15min
Infant 1 yr->7 wk: **IV** 0.08-0.1 mg/kg, maintenance 0.05-0.1 mg/kg q60min as needed
Neonate: **IV** 0.1 mg/kg/dose, maintenance 0.03-0.15 mg/kg/dose q1-2hr as needed

Available forms: 10 mg/5 ml vial

Adverse effects
CNS: Skeletal muscle weakness or paralysis (rarely), flushing
INTEG: Urticaria
MISC: Myopathy, hypotension
RESP: **Prolonged apnea, possible respiratory paralysis,** bronchospasm, tachycardia, flushing, wheezing, dyspnea
SYST: **Anaphylaxis**

Contraindications: Hypersensitivity

Precautions: Pregnancy **C**, breastfeeding, children <2 yr, electrolyte imbalances, dehydration, neuromuscular/cardiac/hepatic disease

Black Box Warning: Respiratory disease

Pharmacokinetics
Absorption	Completely absorbed
Distribution	Rapid, to extracellular fluids
Metabolism	Liver (20%)
Excretion	Kidneys, unchanged (35%)
Half-life	1½ hr, increased in hepatic disease

Pharmacodynamics
Onset	1 min
Peak	3-5 min
Duration	15-25 min (recovery index)

Interactions
Individual products
Amphotericin B, clindamycin, enflurane, isoflurane, lincomycin, lithium, phenytoin, piperacillin, polymyxin B, quinidine, succinylcholine, theophylline, verapamil: increased neuromuscular blockade
Drug classifications
Aminoglycosides, analgesics (opioid), local anesthetics, polymixin antibiotics, thiazides: increased neuromuscular blockade

NURSING CONSIDERATIONS
Assessment
- Monitor for electrolyte imbalances (potassium, magnesium) before product is used; electrolyte imbalances may lead to increased action of this product
- Monitor patient's vital signs (B/P, pulse, respirations, airway) until fully recovered; rate, depth, pattern of respirations, strength of hand grip; patient should be intubated before use
- Monitor patient's recovery: decreased paralysis of face, diaphragm, leg, arm, rest of body; residual weakness and respiratory problems may occur during recovery period
- Monitor allergic reactions: rash, fever, respiratory distress, pruritus; product should be discontinued

Nursing diagnoses
- Breathing pattern, ineffective (uses)
- Communication, impaired verbal (adverse reactions)
- Fear (adverse reactions)
- Knowledge, deficient (teaching)

Implementation
• Use peripheral nerve stimulator by anesthesiologist to determine neuromuscular blockade; deep tendon reflexes should be monitored during extended periods
• Give by direct **IV** after reconstituting with bacteriostatic water, over 5 min, D₅W, 0.9% NaCl or LR
• Give by direct **IV** after reconstituting dose in 5-10 ml of provided diluent; give by titrating to patient response
• Give by continuous inf after diluting to 10-20 mg/100 ml and by titrating to patient response (only by qualified person, usually an anesthesiologist); do not administer IM
• Store in light-resistant area
Syringe incompatibilities: Barbiturates
Y-site compatibilities: Aminophylline, cefazolin, cefuroxime, cimetidine, diltiazem, DOBUTamine, DOPamine, epinephrine, esmolol, fentanyl, fluconazole, gentamicin, heparin, hydrocortisone, hydromorphone, isoproterenol, labetalol, lorazepam, midazolam, milrinone, morphine, niCARdipine, nitroglycerin, nitroprusside, norepinephrine, propofol, ranitidine, trimethoprim/sulfamethoxazole, vancomycin
Y-site incompatibilities: Barbiturates

Patient/family education
• Provide patient reassurance if communication is difficult during recovery from neuromuscular blockade
• Provide explanation to patients regarding all procedures or treatments; patient will remain conscious if anesthesia is not given also

Evaluation
Positive therapeutic outcome
• Paralysis of jaw, eyelid, head, neck, rest of body as evaluated by peripheral nerve stimulator

Treatment of overdose: Edrophonium or neostigmine, atropine, monitor VS; may require mechanical ventilation

---

venlafaxine (Rx)
(ven-la-fax′een)
Effexor, Effexor XR
Func. class.: Second-generation antidepressant—miscellaneous
Pregnancy category C

Action: Potent inhibitor of neuronal serotonin and norepinephrine uptake, weak inhibitor of dopamine; no muscarinic, histaminergic, or α-adrenergic receptors in vitro

Therapeutic outcome: Relief of depression

Uses: Prevention/treatment of major depression, to treat depression at end of life; long-term treatment of generalized anxiety disorder, panic disorder, social anxiety disorder (Effexor XR only)

Dosage and routes
Depression
Adult: PO 75 mg/day in 2 or 3 divided doses; taken with food, may be increased to 150 mg/day; if needed may be further increased to 225 mg/day; increments of 75 mg/day should be made at intervals of no less than 4 days; some hospitalized patients may require up to 375 mg/day in 3 divided doses; EXT REL 37.5-75 mg PO daily, max 225 mg/day; give Effexor XR daily

Anxiety disorders
Adult: PO 75 mg/day or 37.5 mg/day × 4-7 days initially, max 225 mg/day

Hepatic dose
Adult: PO moderate impairment 50% of dose

Renal dose
Adult: PO CCr 10-70 ml/min reduce dose by 25%-50%; CCr <10 ml/min reduce by 50%

Hot flashes (unlabeled)
Adult (male, prostate cancer): PO 12.5 mg bid × 4 wk or EXT REL cap 37.5 mg × 4 wk

Available forms: Tabs scored (Effexor) 25, 37.5, 50, 75, 100 mg; ext rel caps (Effexor XR) 37.5, 75, 150, 225 mg

Adverse effects
CNS: Emotional lability, vertigo, apathy, ataxia, CNS stimulation, euphoria, hallucinations, hostility, increased libido, hypertonia, hypotonia, psychosis, insomnia, anxiety, **suicidal ideation in children/adolescents, seizures,** neuroleptic malignant syndrome–like reaction
CV: Migraine, angina pectoris, extrasystoles, postural hypotension, syncope, thrombophlebitis, hypertension, sustained hypertension, change in QTc interval, increased pulse, increased cholesterol
EENT: Abnormal vision, taste, *ear pain,* cataract, conjunctivitis, corneal lesions, dry eyes, otitis media, photophobia
GI: Dysphagia, eructation, colitis, gastritis, gingivitis, **rectal hemorrhage,** stomatitis, stomach and mouth ulceration, nausea, anorexia, dry mouth
GU: Anorgasmia, abnormal ejaculation, *dysuria, hematuria, metrorrhagia, vaginitis,*

V

Adverse effects: *italic* = common, **bold** = life-threatening

impaired urination, albuminuria, amenorrhea, kidney calculus, cystitis, nocturia, breast and bladder pain, polyuria, **uterine hemorrhage, vaginal hemorrhage,** moniliasis
HEMA: **Agranulocytosis, aplastic anemia, neutropenia, pancytopenia, abnormal bleeding**
INTEG: Ecchymosis, acne, alopecia, brittle nails, dry skin, photosensitivity, sweating
META: *Peripheral edema, weight loss or gain,* diabetes mellitus, edema, glycosuria, hyperlipemia, hypokalemia
MS: Arthritis, bone pain, bursitis, myasthenia, tenosynovitis, arthralgia
RESP: *Bronchitis, dyspnea,* asthma, chest congestion, epistaxis, hyperventilation, laryngitis
SYST: *Malaise, neck pain,* enlarged abdomen, cyst, facial edema, hangover effect, hernia

Contraindications: Hypersensitivity, bipolar disorder, interstitial lung disease

Precautions: Pregnancy **C,** breastfeeding, geriatric, mania, recent MI, cardiac/renal/hepatic disease, seizure disorder, hypertension, eosinophilic pneumonia

Black Box Warning: Children, suicidal ideation

Pharmacokinetics

Absorption	Well absorbed
Distribution	Widely distributed, 27% protein binding
Metabolism	Liver, extensively
Excretion	Kidneys, 87%
Half-life	5 hr, 11 hr (active metabolite)

Pharmacodynamics

Unknown

Interactions
Individual drugs
Alcohol: increased CNS depression
Cimetidine: increased venlafaxine effect
Clozapine, desipramine, haloperidol, warfarin: increased levels of these products
Cyproheptadine: decreased venlafaxine effect
Indinavir: decreased effect of indinavir
Sibutramine, sumatriptan, trazodone: increased serotonin syndrome
Drug classifications
Antihistamines, opioids, sedative/hypnotics: increased CNS depression
MAOIs: hyperthermia, rigidity, rapid fluctuations of vital signs, mental status changes, neuroleptic malignant syndrome

Drug/herb
Chamomile, hops, kava, lavender, skullcap, valerian: increased CNS depression
Corkwood, jimsonweed: increased anticholinergic effect
SAM-e, St. John's wort: serotonin syndrome
Yohimbe: increased hypertension
Drug/lab test
Increased: alkaline phosphatase, bilirubin, AST, ALT, BUN, creatinine, serum cholesterol, CPK, LDH

NURSING CONSIDERATIONS
Assessment
• Monitor B/P (lying, standing), pulse q4hr; if systolic B/P drops 20 mm Hg hold product, notify prescriber; take vital signs q4hr in patients with CV disease
• Monitor blood tests: CBC, leukocytes, differential, cardiac enzymes if patient is receiving long-term therapy
• Monitor liver function tests: AST, ALT, bilirubin
• Check weight qwk; weight loss or gain; appetite may increase, peripheral edema may occur
• Assess mental status: mood, sensorium, affect; increase in psychiatric symptoms: depression, panic; for suicidal ideation in children/adolescents
• Monitor urinary retention, constipation; constipation is more likely to occur in children or geriatric
• Assess for withdrawal symptoms: headache, nausea, vomiting, muscle pain, weakness; do not usually occur unless product was discontinued abruptly
• Identify alcohol consumption; if alcohol is consumed, hold dose
🔴 Assess for neuroleptic malignant syndrome–like reactions

Nursing diagnoses
• Coping, ineffective (uses)
• Injury, risk for (side effects)
• Knowledge, deficient (teaching)
• Noncompliance (teaching)

Implementation
• Give with food or milk for GI symptoms
• Crush if patient is unable to swallow medication whole
• Store at room temperature; do not freeze

Patient/family education
• Advise patient to notify prescriber of rash, hives, or allergic reactions
• Teach patient that therapeutic effects may take 2-3 wk

 Alert   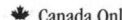 Canada Only   Drug on CD   * "Tall Man" lettering (See Preface)

- Teach patient to use caution in driving or other activities requiring alertness because of drowsiness, dizziness, blurred vision; to avoid rising quickly from sitting to standing, especially geriatric
- Teach patient to avoid alcohol ingestion, other CNS depressants
- Advise patient to avoid pregnancy, breast-feeding while taking this product
- Teach patient that worsening of symptoms, suicidal thoughts/behavior may occur in children, young adults

Evaluation
Positive therapeutic outcome
- Decreased depression, anxiety; sense of well-being
- Absence of suicidal thoughts

Treatment of overdose: ECG monitoring, induce emesis, lavage, activated charcoal, administer anticonvulsant

---

verapamil ☺ (Rx)
(ver-ap'a-mil)
Apo-Verap, Calan, Calan SR, Covera-HS, Isoptin, Isoptin SR, Novo-Verapamil ✤, Nu-Verap ✤, verapamil HCl, verapamil HCl SR, Verelan PM
Func. class.: Calcium-channel blocker; antihypertensive; antianginal, antidysrhythmic (Class IV)
Chem. class.: Diphenylalkylamine

Pregnancy category C

Action: Inhibits calcium ion influx across cell membrane during cardiac depolarization; produces relaxation of coronary vascular smooth muscle, peripheral vascular smooth muscle; dilates coronary vascular arteries; increases myocardial oxygen delivery in patients with vasospastic angina

Therapeutic outcome: Decreased angina pectoris, dysrhythmias, B/P

Uses: Chronic stable vasospastic, unstable angina; dysrhythmias, hypertension, supraventricular tachycardia, atrial flutter or fibrillation

Unlabeled uses: Prevention of migraine headaches, claudication, mania

Dosage and routes
Angina
Adult: PO 80-120 mg tid, increase qwk

Dysrhythmias
Adult: PO 240-320 mg/day in 3-4 divided doses in digitalized patients

Adult: IV BOL 5-10 mg (0.075-0.15 mg/kg) over 2 min, may repeat 10 mg (0.15 mg/kg) ½ hr after first dose
Child 1-15 yr: IV BOL 0.1-0.3 mg/kg over >2 min, repeat in 30 min, max 5 mg in a single dose
Child 0-1 yr: IV BOL 0.1-0.2 mg/kg over ≥2 min, may repeat after 30 min

Hypertension
Adult: PO 80 mg tid, may titrate upward; EXT REL 120-240 mg/day as a single dose, may increase to 240-480 mg/day

Hepatic dose/geriatric/ compromised ventricular function
Adult: PO 40 mg tid initially, increased as tolerated

Available forms: Tabs 40, 80, 120 mg; ext rel tabs 120, 180, 240 mg; inj 2.5 mg/ml in ampules, syringes, vials; ext rel caps 100, 200, 240, 300 mg

Adverse effects
CNS: Headache, drowsiness, dizziness, anxiety, depression, weakness, asthenia, fatigue, insomnia, confusion, light-headedness
CV: Edema, **CHF,** bradycardia, hypotension, palpitations, AV block, **dysrhythmias**
GI: Nausea, diarrhea, gastric upset, *constipation,* elevated liver function tests
GU: Impotence, nocturia, polyuria, gynecomastia
HEMA: Bruising, petechiae, bleeding
INTEG: Rash, bruising
MISC.: Gingival hyperplasia
SYST: **Stevens-Johnson syndrome**

Contraindications: Sick sinus syndrome, 2nd- or 3rd-degree heart block, hypotension <90 mm Hg systolic, cardiogenic shock, severe CHF

Precautions: Pregnancy **C,** breastfeeding, children, geriatric, CHF, hypotension, hepatic injury, renal disease, concomitant β-blocker therapy

Pharmacokinetics
Absorption	Well absorbed (PO)
Distribution	Not known
Metabolism	Liver, extensively
Excretion	Kidneys (70%)
Half-life	Biphasic 4 min, 3-7 hr

Pharmacodynamics
	PO	PO-EXT REL	IV
Onset	1-2 hr	Unknown	1-5 min
Peak	½-1½ hr	5-7 hr	3-5 min
Duration	3-7 hr	24 hr	2 hr

V

Adverse effects: *italic* = common, **bold** = life-threatening

Interactions
Individual drugs
Carbamazepine, cycloSPORINE, digoxin, theophylline: increased levels of each specific product

Cimetidine, telithromycin: increased effect of verapamil

Fentanyl, prazosin, quinidine: increased hypotension

Lithium: decreased lithium levels

Drug classifications
Antihypertensive, β-adrenergic blockers, nitrates: increased effects of verapamil

Nondepolarizing muscle relaxants: increased effect

NSAIDs: decreased antihypertensive effect

Drug/herb
Barberry, betel palm, burdock, goldenseal, khat, lily of the valley, plantain: increased effect

Yohimbe: decreased effect

Drug/food
Grapefruit juice: increased hypotension

Drug/lab test
Increased: alkaline phosphatase, AST, ALT, BUN, creatinine, serum cholesterol

NURSING CONSIDERATIONS
Assessment
• Assess fluid volume status: I&O ratio and record; weight; distended red veins; crackles in lung; color; quality, specific gravity of urine; skin turgor; adequacy of pulses; moist mucous membranes; bilateral lung sounds; peripheral pitting edema; dehydration symptoms of decreasing output, thirst, hypotension, dry mouth, and mucous membranes should be reported

• Monitor B/P and pulse, pulmonary capillary wedge pressure (PCWP), central venous pressure, index, often during inf; notify prescriber if <50 bpm, systolic B/P <90 mm Hg

• Monitor ALT, AST, bilirubin daily; if these are elevated, hepatotoxicity is suspected

• Monitor platelets; if <150,000/mm^3, product is usually discontinued and another product started

• Assess for extravasation; change site q48hr

• Monitor cardiac status: B/P, pulse, respiration, ECG

• Monitor renal/hepatic function tests during long-term treatment, serum potassium, periodically

Nursing diagnoses
• Cardiac output, decreased (uses)
• Knowledge, deficient (teaching)

Implementation
PO route
• Do not crush or chew ext rel products
• Cap may be opened and contents sprinkled on food; do not dissolve chew cap
• Give once a day before meals at bedtime; sus rel give with food to decrease GI symptoms

IV route
• Give by direct **IV** undiluted (Y-site, 3-way stopcock) over at least 2 min, or 3 min geriatric; discard unused sol; to prevent serious hypotension, patient should be recumbent for 1 hr or more

Syringe compatibilities: Inamrinone, heparin, milrinone

Y-site compatibilities: Aprofloxacin, dobutamine, DOPamine, famotidine, hydrALAZINE, inamrinone, meperidine, methicillin, milrinone, penicillin G potassium, piperacillin, propofol, ticarcillin

Y-site incompatibilities: Albumin, ampicillin, mezlocillin, nafcillin, oxacillin, sodium bicarbonate

Additive compatibilities: Amikacin, amiodarone, ascorbic acid, atropine, bretylium, calcium chloride, calcium gluconate, cefamandole, cefazolin, cefotaxime, cefoxitin, cephapirin, chloramphenicol, cimetidine, clindamycin, dexamethasone, diazepam, digoxin, DOPamine, epinephrine, erythromycin, gentamicin, heparin, hydrocortisone, hydromorphone, hydrocortisone sodium phosphate, insulin (regular), isoproterenol, lidocaine, magnesium sulfate, mannitol, meperidine, metaraminol, methicillin, methyldopate, methylPREDNISolone, metoclopramide, mezlocillin, morphine, moxalactam, multivitamins, naloxone, nitroglycerin, norepinephrine, oxytocin, pancuronium, penicillin G potassium, penicillin G sodium, pentobarbital, phenobarbital, phentolamine, phenytoin, piperacillin, potassium chloride, potassium phosphates, procainamide, propranolol, protamine, quinidine, sodium bicarbonate, sodium nitroprusside, theophylline, ticarcillin, tobramycin, tolazoline, vancomycin, vasopressin, vit B/C

Patient/family education
• Advise patient to increase fluids/fiber to counteract constipation
• Caution patient to avoid hazardous activities until stabilized on product and dizziness is no longer a problem
• Teach patient how to take pulse, B/P before taking product; to keep record or graph

- Instruct patient to limit caffeine consumption; to avoid alcohol, grapefruit, and OTC products unless directed by prescriber
- Advise patient to comply with medical regimen: diet, exercise, stress reduction, product therapy; to notify prescriber of irregular heartbeat, shortness of breath, swelling of feet and hands, pronounced dizziness, constipation, nausea, hypotension, **IV** calcium
- Teach patient to use as directed even if feeling better; may be taken with other CV products (nitrates, β-blockers)
- Caution patient not to discontinue abruptly; chest pain may occur
- Advise to report chest pain, palpitations, irregular heart beats, swelling of extremities, skin irritation, rash, tremors, weakness

Evaluation
Positive therapeutic outcome
- Decreased anginal pain
- Decreased dysrhythmias
- Decreased B/P

Treatment of overdose: Defibrillation, atropine for AV block, vasopressor for hypotension, **IV** calcium

---

vidarabine ophthalmic
See Appendix B

---

vigabatrin
See Appendix A, Selected New Drugs

⚠ HIGH ALERT

*vinBLAStine (VLB) (Rx)
(vin-blast'een)
Velbe ✦, vinBLAStine sulfate
Func. class.: Antineoplastic
Chem. class.: Vinca rosea alkaloid
Pregnancy category D

Do not confuse:
vinBLAStine/vinCRIStine

Action: Inhibits mitotic activity, arrests cell cycle at metaphase; inhibits RNA synthesis, blocks cellular use of glutamic acid needed for purine synthesis; a vesicant

Therapeutic outcome: Prevention of rapid growth of malignant cells; immunosuppression

Uses: Breast, testicular cancer; lymphomas; neuroblastoma; Hodgkin's, non-Hodgkin's lymphomas; mycosis fungoides; histiocytosis; Kaposi's sarcoma, Langerhan's cell histiocytosis

Dosage and routes
Adult: **IV** 0.1 mg/kg or 3-6 mg/m² qwk or q2wk, max 0.5 mg/kg or 18.5 mg/m² qwk
Child: **IV** 2.5 mg/m², then dose of 3.75, 5.0, 6.25, and 7.5 mg at 7-day intervals

Available forms: Inj powder 10 mg for 10 ml **IV** inj; sol for inj 1 mg/ml

Adverse effects
CNS: Paresthesias, peripheral neuropathy, depression, headache, **seizures**
CV: Tachycardia, orthostatic hypotension, hypertension
GI: Nausea, vomiting, ileus, *anorexia, stomatitis, constipation,* abdominal pain, GI and rectal bleeding, **hepatotoxicity,** pharyngitis
GU: Urinary retention, **renal failure,** hyperuricemia
HEMA: **Thrombocytopenia, leukopenia, myelosuppression,** agranulocytosis, granulocytosis, aplastic anemia, neutropenia, pancytopenia
INTEG: Rash, alopecia, photosensitivity, **extravasation, tissue necrosis**
META: SIADH
SYST: **Tumor lysis syndrome (TLS)**
RESP: **Fibrosis, pulmonary infiltrate, bronchospasm**

Contraindications: Pregnancy **D,** breastfeeding, infants, hypersensitivity, leukopenia, granulocytopenia, bone marrow suppression, infection

Black Box Warning: Intrathecal use

Precautions: Renal/hepatic disease, tumor lysis syndrome

Black Box Warning: Extravasation

Pharmacokinetics	
Absorption	Complete bioavailability
Distribution	Crosses blood-brain barrier slightly
Metabolism	Liver—active antineoplastic
Excretion	Biliary, kidneys
Half-life	Triphasic <5 min, 50-155 min, 23-85 hr

Pharmacodynamics	
Unknown	

Interactions
Individual drugs
Bleomycin: increased synergism
Methotrexate: increased methotrexate action
Mitomycin: increased bronchospasm

Adverse effects: *italic* = common, **bold** = life-threatening

Phenytoin: decreased phenytoin level
Radiation: increased toxicity, bone marrow suppression; do not use together

Drug classifications

Anticoagulants, NSAIDs: increased bleeding risk

Antineoplastics: increased toxicity, bone marrow suppression

CYP3A4 inducers (barbiturates, bosentan, carbamazepine, efavirenz, phenytoin, nevirapine, rifabutin, rifampin): decreased vinBLAStine effect

CYP3A4 inhibitors (aprepitant, antiretroviral protease inhibitors, clarithromycin, danazol, delavirdine, diltiazem, erythromycin, fluconazole, fluoxetine, fluvoxamine, imatinib, ketoconazole, mebefradil, nefazodone, telithromycin, voriconazole): increased toxicity

Live virus vaccines: increased adverse reactions

Drug/herb

St. John's wort: avoid use

NURSING CONSIDERATIONS
Assessment

• Monitor B/P (baseline and q15min) during administration

• Monitor CBC, differential, platelet count weekly; withhold product if WBC is <2000/mm^3 or platelet count is <75,000/mm^3; notify prescriber of results; recovery will take 3 wk; RBC, Hct, Hgb may be decreased

• Assess for dyspnea, crackles, unproductive cough, chest pain, tachypnea

• Monitor renal function tests: BUN, serum uric acid, urine CCr before, during therapy; I&O ratio; report fall in urine output of 30 ml/hr; for decreased hyperuricemia

• Monitor for cold, fever, sore throat (may indicate beginning of infection); notify prescriber if these occur

• Assess for bleeding: hematuria, guaiac, bruising or petechiae, mucosa or orifices q8hr, no rectal temp; avoid IM inj; use pressure to venipuncture sites

• Identify nutritional status: an antiemetic may need to be prescribed

• Assess for gout, joint pain, swelling, increased uric acid; allopurinol or other treatment may be used

• Assess for symptoms indicating severe allergic reactions: rash, pruritus, urticaria, itching, flushing, bronchospasm, hypotension; epinephrine and resuscitative equipment should be nearby

Nursing diagnoses

• Body image, disturbed (adverse reactions)
• Infection, risk for (adverse reactions)
• Injury, risk for (adverse reactions)
• Knowledge, deficient (teaching)

Implementation
Intermittent IV inf route

• Further dilute in 50-100 ml of NS, inf over 15-30 min

IV inj route

• Administer IV after diluting 10 mg/10 ml NaCl; give through Y-tube or 3-way stopcock or directly over 1 min

• Give by intermittent inf

• Sol should be prepared by qualified personnel only under controlled conditions

• Use Luer-Lok tubing to prevent leakage; do not let sol come in contact with skin; if contact occurs, wash well with soap and water

• Give hyaluronidase 150 units/ml in 1 ml of NaCl, warm compress for extravasation for vesicant activity treatment

Syringe compatibilities: Bleomycin, cisplatin, cyclophosphamide, droperidol, fluorouracil, leucovorin, methotrexate, metoclopramide, mitomycin, vinCRIStine

Y-site compatibilities: Allopurinol, amifostine, aztreonam, bleomycin, cisplatin, cyclophosphamide, DOXOrubicin, droperidol, filgrastim, fludarabine, fluorouracil, granisetron, heparin, leucovorin, melphalan, methotrexate, metoclopramide, mitomycin, ondansetron, paclitaxel, piperacillin/tazobactam, sargramostim, teniposide, thiotepa, vinCRIStine, vinorelbine

Y-site incompatibilities: Furosemide
Additive compatibilities: Bleomycin

Patient/family education

• Teach patient to avoid use of products containing aspirin or NSAIDs, razors, commercial mouthwash because bleeding may occur; to report symptoms of bleeding (hematuria, tarry stools)

• Instruct patient to report signs of anemia, (fatigue, headache, irritability, faintness, shortness of breath)

• Caution patient to report any changes in breathing or coughing even several mo after treatment; avoid breastfeeding; may cause male infertility

• Advise patient that contraception will be necessary during treatment; teratogenesis may occur

• Advise patient to use sunscreen, wear protective clothing and sunglasses

• Inform patient that hair may be lost during treatment; a wig or hairpiece may make patient feel better; new hair will be different in color, texture

• Advise patient to avoid vaccinations during treatment; serious reactions may occur

• Teach patient to report signs/symptoms of infection: fever, chills, sore throat; patient should avoid crowds and persons with known infections

Evaluation
Positive therapeutic outcome
• Decreased spread of malignant cells

⚡ HIGH ALERT

*vinCRIStine (VCR) 🔄 **(Rx)**
(vin-kris'teen)
Oncovin, Vincasar PFS, vinCRIStine sulfate
Func. class.: Antineoplastic—miscellaneous
Chem. class.: Vinca alkaloid

Pregnancy category D

Do not confuse:
vinCRIStine/vinBLAStine

Action: Inhibits mitotic activity, arrests cell cycle at metaphase; inhibits RNA synthesis, blocks cellular use of glutamic acid needed for purine synthesis; a vesicant

Therapeutic outcome: Prevention of rapid growth of malignant cells, immunosuppression

Uses: Lymphomas, neuroblastomas, Hodgkin's disease, acute lymphoblastic and other leukemias, rhabdomyosarcoma, Wilms' tumor, non-Hodgkin's lymphoma, malignant glioma, soft-tissue sarcoma

Dosage and routes
Adult: **IV** 0.4-1.4 mg/m^2/wk, max 2 mg
Child: **IV** 1-2 mg/m^2/wk, max 2 mg

Available forms: Inj 1 mg/ml; powder for inj 5 mg/vial

Adverse effects
CNS: Decreased reflexes, numbness, weakness, motor difficulties, CNS depression, cranial nerve paralysis, **seizures,** peripheral neuropathy
CV: Orthostatic hypotension
EENT: Diplopia
GI: Nausea, vomiting, anorexia, stomatitis, constipation, **paralytic ileus, abdominal pain, hepatotoxicity**
GU: **Renal tubular obstruction**
HEMA: **Thrombocytopenia, leukopenia, myelosuppression, anemia**

INTEG: Alopecia, extravasation
SYST: **Tumor lysis syndrome (TLS)**

Contraindications: Pregnancy **D**, breastfeeding, infants, hypersensitivity, radiation therapy

Black Box Warning: Intrathecal use

Precautions: Renal/hepatic disease, hypertension, neuromuscular disease

Black Box Warning: Extravasation

Pharmacokinetics

Absorption	Complete bioavailability
Distribution	Rapidly, widely distributed; blood-brain barrier
Metabolism	Liver
Excretion	Biliary, in feces, crosses placenta
Half-life	Triphasic <5 min, 50-155 min, 23-85 hr

Pharmacodynamics

Onset	Unknown
Peak	Unknown
Duration	1 wk

Interactions
Individual drugs
Digoxin: decreased digoxin level
Mitomycin-C: increased acute pulmonary reactions
Radiation: increased toxicity, bone marrow suppression; do not use together

Drug classifications
CYP3A4 inducers (barbiturates, bosentan, carbamazepine, efavirenz, phenytoins, nevirapine, rifabutin, rifampin): decreased vinCRIStine effect
CYP3A4 inhibitors (aprepitant, antiretroviral protease inhibitors, clarithromycin, danazol, delavirdine, diltiazem, erythromycin, fluconazole, fluoxetine, fluvoxamine, imatinib, ketoconazole, mibefradil, nefazodone, telithromycin, voriconazole): increased toxicity
Peripheral nervous system products: neurotoxicity

Drug/herb
St. John's wort: avoid use

NURSING CONSIDERATIONS
Assessment
• Monitor CBC, differential, platelet count weekly; withhold product if WBC is <4000/ mm^3 or platelet count is <75,000/mm^3; notify prescriber of results; platelets may increase or decrease

V

Adverse effects: *italic* = common, **bold** = life-threatening

- Assess neurologic status: paresthesia, weakness, cranial nerve palsies, orthostatic hypotension, lethargy, agitation, psychosis; notify prescriber
- Monitor renal function tests: BUN, serum uric acid, urine CCr before, during therapy; I&O ratio; report fall in urine output of 30 ml/hr; for decreased hyperuricemia, hyponatremia, and increased fluid retention (SIADH)
- Monitor for cold, fever, sore throat (may indicate beginning of infection)
- Identify for increased uric acid levels, joint pain in extremities; increase fluid intake to 2-3 L/day unless contraindicated

Nursing diagnoses
- Body image, disturbed (adverse reactions)
- Infection, risk for (adverse reactions)
- Injury, risk for (adverse reactions)
- Knowledge, deficient (teaching)

Implementation
◆ Do not give intrathecally: fatal
- Administer **IV** after diluting with diluent provided or 1 mg/10 ml of sterile water or 0.9% NaCl; give through Y-tube or 3-way stopcock or directly over 1 min
- Hyaluronidase 150 units/ml in 1 ml of NaCl; apply warm compress for extravasation
Syringe compatibilities: Bleomycin, cisplatin, cyclophosphamide, doxapram, DOXOrubicin, droperidol, fluorouracil, heparin, leucovorin, methotrexate, metoclopramide, mitomycin, ondansetron, vinCRIStine
Syringe incompatibilities: Furosemide
Y-site compatibilities: Allopurinol, amifostine, aztreonam, bleomycin, cisplatin, cladribine, cyclophosphamide, DOXOrubicin, droperidol, filgrastim, fludarabine, fluorouracil, granisetron, heparin, leucovorin, methotrexate, metoclopramide, mitomycin, ondansetron, paclitaxel, sargramostim, teniposide, thiotepa, vinCRIStine, vinorelbine
Y-site incompatibilities: Furosemide

Patient/family education
- Teach patient to avoid use of products containing aspirin or NSAIDs, razors, commercial mouthwash because bleeding may occur; to report symptoms of bleeding (hematuria, tarry stools)
- Instruct patient to report signs of anemia (fatigue, headache, irritability, faintness, shortness of breath)
- Caution patient to report any changes in breathing or coughing, even several mo after treatment
- Advise patient that contraception will be necessary during and 2 mo post-treatment; teratogenesis may occur
- Inform patient that hair may be lost during treatment; a wig or hairpiece may make patient feel better; new hair will be different in color, texture
- Advise patient to avoid vaccinations during treatment; serious reactions may occur
- Teach patient to report signs/symptoms of infection: fever, chills, sore throat; patient should avoid crowds or persons with known infections
- Advise patient to increase fluids, bulk in diet, exercise to prevent constipation

Evaluation
Positive therapeutic outcome
- Decreased spread of malignancies

! HIGH ALERT

vinorelbine (Rx)
(vi-nor'el-bine)
Navelbine
Func. class.: Antineoplastic—miscellaneous
Chem. class.: Semisynthetic vinca alkaloid
Pregnancy category D

Action: Inhibits mitotic spindle activity, arrests cell cycle at metaphase; inhibits RNA synthesis, blocks cellular use of glutamic acid needed for purine synthesis; a vesicant

Therapeutic outcome: Decreased spread of malignancy

Uses: Unresectable, advanced non–small-cell lung cancer (NSCLC) stage IV; may be used alone or in combination with cisplatin for stage III or IV NSCLC

Dosage and routes
Adult: **IV** 30 mg/m^2 qwk
ANC: 1000-1499, give 50% dose; <1000 hold dose; <1000 × 3 wk, discontinue

Hepatic dose
Adult: **IV** total bilirubin 2.1-3 mg/dl 15 mg/m^2 qwk; total bilirubin ≥3 mg/dl 7.5 mg/m^2/day

Available forms: Inj 10 mg/ml

Adverse effects
CNS: Paresthesias, peripheral neuropathy, depression, headache, **seizures,** weakness, jaw pain, asthenia
CV: Chest pain
GI: Nausea, vomiting, ileus, *anorexia, stomatitis,* constipation, abdominal pain, *diarrhea,* **hepatotoxicity, GI obstruction/ perforation**

HEMA: **Neutropenia, anemia, thrombocytopenia, granulocytopenia**
INTEG: *Rash, alopecia,* photosensitivity, inj site reaction, necrosis
META: Syndrome of inappropriate diuretic hormone
MS: Myalgia
RESP: Shortness of breath

Contraindications: Pregnancy **D,** breastfeeding, hypersensitivity, infants, granulocyte count <1000 cells/mm³ pretreatment

Black Box Warning: Severe neutropenia, intrathecal use

Precautions: Children, geriatric, hepatic/pulmonary/neurologic/renal disease, bone marrow suppression

Black Box Warning: Extravasation

Pharmacokinetics

Absorption	Poor bioavailability (<50%)
Distribution	Highly bound to platelets, lymphocytes
Metabolism	Liver, to metabolite
Excretion	Bile
Half-life	43 hr

Pharmacodynamics

Onset	Unknown
Peak	1-2 hr
Duration	Unknown

Interactions
Drug classifications
NSAIDs, anticoagulants: increased bleeding risk
CYP3A4 inhibitors (antiretroviral protease inhibitors, aprepitant, clarithromycin, danazol, delavirdine, diltiazem, erythromycin, fluconazole, fluoxetine, fluvoxamine, imatinib, ketoconazole, mibefradil, nefazodone, telithromycin, voriconazole): increased toxicity
CYP3A4 inducers (barbiturates, bosentan, carbamazepine, efavirenz, phenytoins, nevirapine, rifabutin, rifampin): decreased vinorelbine effect
Drug/herb
• St. John's wort: avoid use

NURSING CONSIDERATIONS
Assessment
• Monitor B/P (baseline and q15min) during administration
• Monitor CBC, differential, platelet count weekly; withhold product if WBC is <4000/mm³ or platelet count is <75,000/mm³; notify prescriber of results; recovery will take 3 wk; liver function tests: AST, ALT, bilirubin, LDH
• Assess for dyspnea, crackles, unproductive cough, chest pain, tachypnea
• Monitor renal function tests: BUN, serum uric acid, urine CCr before, during therapy, I&O ratio; report fall in urine output of 30 ml/hr; for decreased hyperuricemia
• Monitor for cold, fever, sore throat (may indicate beginning infection); notify prescriber if these occur; effects of alopecia on body image
• Assess for bleeding: hematuria, guaiac, bruising or petechiae, mucosa or orifices q8hr: no rectal temp; avoid IM inj; use pressure on venipuncture sites
• Identify nutritional status: an antiemetic may need to be prescribed
• Assess for symptoms indicating severe allergic reactions: rash, pruritus, urticaria, itching, flushing, bronchospasm, hypotension; epinephrine and resuscitative equipment should be nearby
• Assess neurologic status: numbness, pain, tingling, loss of Achilles reflex, weakness, palsies
• Assess for gout: pain, swelling, increased uric acid levels

Nursing diagnoses
• Body image, disturbed (adverse reactions)
• Infection, risk for (adverse reactions)
• Injury, risk for (adverse reactions)
• Knowledge, deficient (teaching)

Implementation
⬥ Do not give intrathecally; fatal
• Hyaluronidase 150 units/ml in 1 ml of NaCl, warm compress for extravasation for vesicant activity treatment
• Antacid before oral agent; give product after evening meal before bedtime
• Antiemetic 30-60 min before giving product and prn to prevent vomiting
Intermittent IV inf route
• Dilute to 0.5-2 mg/ml with 0.9% NaCl, 0.45% NaCl, D₅W, D₅/0.45% NaCl, LR, Ringer's; give over 6-10 min into Y-site or central line; flush line
Continuous inf
• Give 40 mg/m² q3wk after IV bol of 8 mg/m²; may be given in combination with DOXOrubicin, fluorouracil, cisplatin
Y-site compatibilities:
Amikacin, aztreonam, bleomycin, buprenorphine, butorphanol, calcium gluconate, carboplatin, cefotaxime, cisplatin, cimetidine, clindamycin, dexamethasone, enalaprilat, etoposide, famotidine, filgrastim, fluconazole,

V

fludarabine, gentamicin, hydrocortisone, lorazepam, meperidine, morphine, netilmicin, ondansetron, plicamycin, streptozocin, teniposide, ticarcillin, tobramycin, vancomycin, vinBLAStine, vinCRIStine, zidovudine

Patient/family education

• Teach patient to use liquid diet: cola, Jell-O; dry toast or crackers may be added if patient is not nauseated or vomiting

• Advise patient to rinse mouth 3-4 ×/day with water and brush teeth 2-3 ×/day with soft brush or cotton-tipped applicators for stomatitis; use unwaxed dental floss

• Inform patient that a nutritious diet with iron, vitamin supplements is necessary; avoid herbals, OTC products

• Advise patient to avoid crowds, people with infections, vaccinations

• Advise patient to use effective contraception during and for ≥2 mo after product is discontinued; avoid breastfeeding

• Teach patient hair may be lost but will grow back; new hair may be different texture, color

Evaluation
Positive therapeutic outcome

• Decreased spread of malignant cells

---

vitamin A (PO, OTC; IM, Rx)
Aquasol A, Del-Vi-A, Vitamin A
Func. class.: Vitamin, fat-soluble
Chem. class.: Retinol

Pregnancy category C (PO); X (parenteral)

Action: Needed for normal bone and tooth development, visual dark adaptation, skin disease, mucosa tissue repair; assists in production of adrenal steroids, cholesterol, RNA

Therapeutic outcome: Prevention, absence of vit A deficiency

Uses: Vit A deficiency

Dosage and routes
Adult and child >8 yr: PO 100,000-500,000 international units/day × 3 days, then 50,000/day × 2 wk; dose based on severity of deficiency; maintenance 10,000-20,000 international units for 2 mo
Child 1-8 yr: IM 5000-15,000 international units/day × 10 days
Infant <1 yr: IM 5000-15,000 international units × 10 days

Maintenance
Child 4-8 yr: IM 15,000 international units/day × 2 mo

Child <4 yr: IM 10,000 international units/day × 2 mo

Available forms: Caps 10,000, 25,000, 50,000 international units; drops 5000 international units; inj 50,000 international units/ml; tabs 10,000, 25,000, 50,000 international units

Adverse effects
CNS: Headache, **increased ICP, intracranial hypertension,** lethargy, malaise
EENT: Gingivitis, papilledema, exophthalmos, inflammation of tongue and lips
GI: Nausea, vomiting, anorexia, abdominal pain, *jaundice*
INTEG: Drying of skin, pruritus, increased pigmentation, night sweats, alopecia
META: Hypomenorrhea, hypercalcemia
MS: Arthralgia, retarded growth, hard areas on bone

Contraindications: Pregnancy **X** (parenteral), hypersensitivity to vit A, malabsorption syndrome (PO), hypervitaminosis A, parenteral, **IV** administration

Precautions: Pregnancy **C** (PO), breastfeeding, impaired renal function, children, hepatic disease, infants, alcoholism, hepatitis

Pharmacokinetics

Absorption	Rapidly absorbed
Distribution	Stored in liver, kidneys, lungs
Metabolism	Liver
Excretion	Breast milk
Half-life	Unknown

Pharmacodynamics
Unknown

Interactions
Individual drugs
Cholestyramine, colestipol, mineral oil: decreased absorption of vit A
Drug classifications
Contraceptives (oral), corticosteroids: increased levels of vit A
Drug/lab test
False increase: bilirubin, serum cholesterol

NURSING CONSIDERATIONS
Assessment

• Assess nutritional status: increase intake of yellow and dark green vegetables, yellow/orange fruits, vit A–fortified foods, liver, egg yolks

• Assess vit A deficiency: decreased growth; night blindness; dry, brittle nails; hair loss;

urinary stones; increased infection; hyperkeratosis of skin; drying of cornea
• Identify vit A deficiency by plasma vit A, carotene level
• Assess for chronic vit A toxicity: increased calcium, BUN, glucose, cholesterol, triglyceride level

Nursing diagnoses
• Knowledge, deficient (teaching)
• Nutrition, less than body requirements, imbalanced (uses)

Implementation
PO route
• Give with food (PO) for better absorption; do not give **IV** because anaphylaxis may occur, IM only
• Oral preparations are not indicated for vit A deficiency in those with malabsorption syndrome
• Store in airtight, light-resistant container
IM route
• Give deep in large muscle mass; do not use deltoid muscle for administration of >1 ml

Patient/family education
• Instruct patient that if dose is missed, it should be omitted
• Inform patient that ophth exams may be required periodically throughout therapy
• Instruct patient not to use mineral oil while taking this product because absorption will be decreased
• Advise patient to notify prescriber of nausea, vomiting, lip cracking, loss of hair, headache
• Caution patient not to take more than the prescribed amount

Evaluation
Positive therapeutic outcome
• Increase in growth rate, weight
• Absence of dry skin and mucous membranes, night blindness

Treatment of overdose: Discontinue product

---

vitamin A acid
See tretinoin

---

vitamin B₁
See thiamine

(vitamin B₁₂)
cyanocobalamin (PO, OTC; IM/SUBCUT, Rx)
(sye-an-oh-koe-bal′a-min)
Alphamin, Anacobin ✦, Bedoz ✦, Cobex, Cobolin-M Crystamine, Crysti-1000, Cyanabin ✦, Cyanoject, Cyomin, Ener-B, Hydrobexan, Hydro Cobex, Hydro-Crysti-12
Func. class.: Vitamin B₁₂, water-soluble vitamin

(vitamin B₁₂a)
hydroxocobalamin (vit B₁₂) (Rx)
(hye-drox′-o-ko-bal′-a-min)
Hydro Cobex, Hydroxycobal, LA-12, Nascobal, Neuroforter, Rubesol-1000, Rubramin PC, Shovite, Vibral LA, Vibral, Vitamin B₁₂

Pregnancy category A

Action: Needed for adequate nerve functioning, protein and carbohydrate metabolism, normal growth, RBC development and cell reproduction

Therapeutic outcome: Prevention, correction of vit B₁₂ deficiency

Uses: Vit B₁₂ deficiency; pernicious anemia; vit B₁₂ malabsorption syndrome; Schilling test; increased requirements with pregnancy, thyrotoxicosis, hemolytic anemia, hemorrhage, renal and hepatic disease

Dosage and routes
Cyanocobalamin
Adult: PO up to 1000 mcg/day; SUBCUT/IM 30-100 mcg/day × 1 wk, then 100-200 mcg/mo

Shilling test
Adult and child: IM 1000 mcg in 1 dose
Child: PO up to 1000 mcg/day; SUBCUT/IM 30-50 mcg/day × 2 wk, then 100 mcg/mo; NASAL 500 mcg qwk

Hydroxocobalamin
Adult: SUBCUT/IM 30-50 mcg/day × 5-10 days, then 100-200 mcg/mo
Child: SUBCUT/IM 30-50 mcg/day × 5-10 days, then 30-50 mcg/mo

Available forms: Cyanocobalamin: tabs 25, 50, 100, 250, 500, 1000, 5000 mcg; ext rel tabs 100, 200, 500, 1000 mcg; lozenges: 100, 250, 500 mcg; nasal gel 500 mcg/spray; inj 100, 1000 mcg/ml; hydroxocobalamin: inj 1000 mcg/ml

V

Adverse effects
CNS: Flushing, optic nerve atrophy
CV: CHF, peripheral vascular thrombosis, **pulmonary edema**
GI: *Diarrhea*
INTEG: Itching, rash, pain at inj site
META: Hypokalemia
SYST: Anaphylactic shock

Contraindications: Hypersensitivity, optic nerve atrophy

Precautions: Pregnancy **A**, breastfeeding, children

Pharmacokinetics

Absorption	Well absorbed (IM, SUBCUT)
Distribution	Crosses placenta
Metabolism	Stored in liver, kidney, stomach
Excretion	50%-90% (urine), breast milk
Half-life	Unknown

Pharmacodynamics
Unknown

Interactions
Individual drugs
Aminosalicylic acid, chloramphenicol, cimetidine, colchicine: decreased absorption
Prednisone: increased absorption
Drug classifications
Aminoglycosides, anticonvulsants, potassium products: decreased absorption
Drug/herb
Goldenseal: decreased vit B_{12} absorption
Drug/lab test
False positive: intrinsic factor

NURSING CONSIDERATIONS
Assessment
• Assess for deficiency: anorexia, dyspepsia on exertion, palpitations, paresthesias, psychosis, visual disturbances, pallor, red inflamed tongue, neuropathy, edema of legs
• Monitor potassium levels during beginning treatment in patients with megaloblastic anemia
• Monitor CBC for increase in reticulocyte count during 1st wk of therapy, then increase in RBC and hemoglobin; folic acid levels, vit B_{12} levels
• Assess nutritional status: egg yolks, fish, organ meats, dairy products, clams, oysters, which are good sources of vit B_{12}
• Monitor for pulmonary edema or worsening of CHF in cardiac patients
Nursing diagnoses
• Knowledge, deficient (teaching)
• Noncompliance (teaching) (overuse)

• Nutrition, less than body requirements, imbalanced (uses)
Implementation
PO route
• Give with fruit juice to disguise taste; administer immediately after mixing
• Give with meals if possible for better absorption; large doses should not be used because most is excreted
IM route
• Give by IM inj for pernicious anemia for life unless contraindicated
IV route
• May be mixed with TPN sol, but **IV** route is not recommended
Y-site compatibilities: Heparin, hydrocortisone sodium succinate, potassium chloride
Solution compatibilities: Dextrose/Ringer's or LR's combinations, dextrose/saline combinations, D_5W, $D_{10}W$, 0.45% NaCl, Ringer's or LR's sol, ascorbic acid
Patient/family education
• Instruct patient that treatment must continue for life if diagnosed as having pernicious anemia
• Advise patient to eat well-balanced diet from the food pyramid and comply with dietary recommendation
• Caution patient not to exceed the RDA of vit B_{12} because adverse reactions may occur
Evaluation
Positive therapeutic outcome
• Decreased anorexia, dyspnea on exertion, palpitations, paresthesias, psychosis, visual disturbances, edema of legs
• Prevention or correction of vit B_{12} deficiency

Treatment of overdose: Discontinue products

vitamin D (cholecalciferol, vitamin D_3 or ergocalciferol, vitamin D_2) (Rx, OTC)
Calciferol, Delta-D, Drisdol, Radiostol ✦, Radiostol Forte ✦, vitamin D, vitamin D_3
Func. class.: Vitamin D
Chem. class.: Fat-soluble vitamin
Pregnancy category C

Do not confuse:
Calciferol/calcitriol

Action: Needed for regulation of calcium, phosphate levels; normal bone development; parathyroid activity; neuromuscular functioning

Therapeutic outcome: Prevention of rickets, osteomalacia, normal calcium/phosphate levels

Uses: Vit D deficiency, rickets, renal osteodystrophy, hypoparathyroidism, hypophosphatemia, psoriasis, rheumatoid arthritis

Dosage and routes
Deficiency
Adult: PO/IM 12,000 international units/day, then increased to 500,000 international units/day
Child: PO/IM 1500-5000 international units/day × 2-4 wk, may repeat after 2 wk or 600,000 international units as single dose

Hypoparathyroidism
Adult and child: PO/IM 200,000 international units given with 4 g calcium tab

Available forms: Tabs 400, 1000, 50,000 international units; caps 25,000, 50,000; oral sol 8000 international units/ml; inj 500,000 international units/ml, 500,000 international units/5 ml

Adverse effects
CNS: Fatigue, weakness, drowsiness, **seizures,** headache, psychosis
CV: Hypertension, dysrhythmias
GI: Nausea, vomiting, anorexia, cramps, diarrhea, constipation, metallic taste, dry mouth
GU: Polyuria, nocturia, **hematuria, albuminuria, renal failure,** decreased libido
INTEG: Pruritus, photophobia
MS: Decreased bone growth, early joint pain, early muscle pain

Contraindications: Hypersensitivity, hypercalcemia, renal dysfunction, hyperphosphatemia

Precautions: Pregnancy **C,** CV disease, renal calculi

Pharmacokinetics

Absorption	Well absorbed
Distribution	Stored in liver
Metabolism	Liver, sun
Excretion	Bile, kidney
Half-life	12-22 hr

Pharmacodynamics

	PO	IM
Onset	Unknown	Unknown
Peak	4 hr	Unknown
Duration	15-20 days	Unknown

Interactions
Individual drugs
Cholestyramine, colestipol, phenobarbital, phenytoin: decreased effects of vit D
Verapamil: increased toxicity
Drug classifications
Antacids, diuretics (thiazide): increased toxicity

NURSING CONSIDERATIONS
Assessment
• Monitor BUN, urinary calcium, AST, ALT, cholesterol, creatinine, uric acid, chloride, magnesium, electrolytes, urine pH, phosphate—may increase; calcium should be kept at 9-10 mg/dl; vit D at 50-135 international units/dl, phosphate at 70 mg/dl; alkaline phosphatase may be decreased
• Monitor for increased blood level; toxic reactions may occur rapidly
• Assess for dry mouth, metallic taste, polyuria, bone pain, muscle weakness, headache, fatigue, tinnitus, change in LOC, irregular pulse, dysrhythmias, increased respirations, anorexia, nausea, vomiting, cramps, diarrhea, constipation; may indicate hypercalcemia
• Assess renal status: decreased urinary output (oliguria, anuria), edema in extremities, weight gain 5 lb, periorbital edema
• Assess nutritional status, diet for sources of vit D (milk, cod, halibut, salmon, sardines, egg yolk), calcium (dairy products, dark green vegetables), phosphates (dairy products)

Nursing diagnoses
• Knowledge, deficient (teaching)
• Nutrition, less than body requirements, imbalanced (uses)

Implementation
PO route
• PO may be increased q4wk depending on blood level
• Store in airtight, light-resistant container at room temperature
IM route
• Give inj deeply in large muscle mass, administer slowly, aspirate to avoid **IV** administration, rotate inj site

Patient/family education
• Advise patient to omit dose if missed; to avoid vitamin supplements unless directed by prescriber
• Inform patient of necessary foods to be included in diet
• Advise patient to keep appointments for evaluation because therapeutic and toxic levels are narrow

V

Adverse effects: *italic* = common, **bold** = life-threatening

- Instruct patient to report weakness, lethargy, headache, anorexia, loss of weight; to report nausea, vomiting, abdominal cramps, diarrhea, constipation, excessive thirst, polyuria, muscle and bone pain
- Caution patient to decrease intake of antacids and laxatives containing magnesium

Evaluation
Positive therapeutic outcome
- Calcium levels 9-10 ml/dl
- Decreasing symptoms of bone disease

vitamin E (OTC)

Amino-Opti-E, Aquasol E, Daltose ♣, E-Complex-600, E-Ferol, E-Vitamin Succinate, E-200 I.U. Softgels, Gordo-Vite E, Tocopherol, Vita-Plus E Softgels, Vitec

Func. class.: Vitamin E
Chem. class.: Fat-soluble vitamin

Pregnancy category A

Action: Needed for digestion and metabolism of polyunsaturated fats, decreases platelet aggregation, decreases blood clot formation, promotes normal growth and development of muscle tissue, prostaglandin synthesis

Therapeutic outcome: Prevention and treatment of vit E deficiency

Uses: Vit E deficiency, impaired fat absorption, hemolytic anemia in premature neonates, prevention of retrolental fibroplasia, sickle cell anemia, supplement in malabsorption syndrome

Dosage and routes
Deficiency
Adult: PO 60-75 international units/day
Child: PO 1 international unit/kg (malabsorption)

Prevention of deficiency
Adult: PO 30 international units/day
Infant: PO 5 international units/day

Topical route
Adult and child: TOP apply to affected areas as needed

Available forms: Caps 100, 200, 400, 500, 600, 1000 international units; tabs 100, 200, 400 international units; drops 50 mg/ml; chew tabs 400 units; ointment, cream, lotion, oil

Adverse effects
CNS: Headache, fatigue
CV: Increased risk of thrombophlebitis
EENT: Blurred vision
GI: Nausea, cramps, diarrhea
GU: Gonadal dysfunction
INTEG: Sterile abscess, contact dermatitis
META: Altered metabolism of hormones (thyroid, pituitary, adrenal), altered immunity
MS: Weakness

Contraindications: IV use in infants

Precautions: Pregnancy **A**, anemia, breast-feeding, hypothrombinemia

Pharmacokinetics
Absorption	20%-80% (PO)
Distribution	Widely distributed, stored in fat
Metabolism	Liver
Excretion	Bile
Half-life	Unknown

Pharmacodynamics
Unknown

Interactions
Individual drugs
Cholestyramine, colestipol, mineral oil, sucralfate: decreased absorption
Drug classification
Anticoagulants (oral): increased action of anticoagulants

NURSING CONSIDERATIONS
Assessment
- Assess nutritional status: intake of wheat germ, dark green leafy vegetables, nuts, eggs, liver, vegetable oils, dairy products, cereals
- Assess for vit E deficiency (usually in neonates): irritability, restlessness, hemolytic anemia

Nursing diagnoses
- Knowledge, deficient (teaching)
- Nutrition, less than body requirements, imbalanced (uses)

Implementation
PO route
- Chew chewable tabs well
- Sol may be dropped in mouth or mixed with food
- Store in airtight, light-resistant container
Topical route
- Apply topical to moisturize dry skin

Patient/family education
- Inform patient necessary foods to be included in diet high in vit E
- Instruct patient to omit if dose missed
- Instruct patient to avoid vit supplements unless directed by prescriber because overdose may occur

 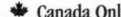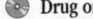

Evaluation
Positive therapeutic outcome
- Absence of hemolytic anemia
- Adequate vit E levels
- Improvement in skin lesions
- Decrease in edema

voriconazole (Rx)
(vohr-i-kahn'a-zol)
Vfend
Func. class.: Antifungal
Pregnancy category D

Action: Inhibits fungal CYP 450-mediation demethylation, needed for biosynthesis

Therapeutic outcome: Decreasing signs, symptoms of infection

Uses: Invasive aspergillosis, serious fungal infections (*Candida* sp., *Scedosporium apiospermum, Fusarium* sp.), *Monosportum, Apiospermum*

Dosage and routes
Adult/geriatric/child: PO give 1 hr before or after meals; ≥40 kg, loading dose 400 mg q12hr on day 1, then 200 mg q12hr; <40 kg, loading dose 200 mg q12hr on day 1, then 100 mg q12hr
Adult/geriatric/child: IV loading dose 6 mg/kg q12hr × 2 dose, then 4 mg/kg q12hr; may switch to oral dosing

Renal dose
Adult: PO CCr <50 ml/min, use only orally

Hepatic dose
Adult: PO 6 mg/kg q12hr × 2 doses, then 2 mg/kg q12hr or 100 mg q12hr if >40 kg; 50 mg q12hr if <40 kg

Available forms: Tabs 50, 200 mg; powder for inj, lyophilized 200 mg voriconazole, powder for oral susp 45 g (40 mg/ml after reconstitution)

Adverse effects
CNS: Headache, paresthesias, peripheral neuropathy, hallucinations, psychosis, EPS, depression, Guillain-Barré syndrome, insomnia, suicidal ideation, dizziness
CV: **Tachycardia,** hyper/hypotension, vasodilatation, **atrial dysrhythmias, atrial fibrillation, AV block, bradycardia, CHF, MI, QT prolongation, torsades de pointes**
EENT: Blurred vision, eye hemorrhage
INTEG: Burning, irritation, pain, necrosis at inj site with extravasation, dermatitis, rash, photosensitivity

GI: Nausea, vomiting, anorexia, diarrhea, cramps, **hemorrhagic gastroenteritis, acute liver failure, hepatitis, intestinal perforation, pancreatitis**
GU: Hypokalemia, azotemia, **renal tubular necrosis, permanent renal impairment, anuria, oliguria**
HEMA: Anemia, **eosinophilia,** hypomagnesemia, **thrombocytopenia, leukopenia, pancytopenia**
MISC: Respiratory disorder
SYST: **Stevens-Johnson syndrome, toxic epidermal necrolysis, sepsis**

Contraindications: Pregnancy **D**, breastfeeding, children, hypersensitivity, severe bone marrow depression, severe hepatic disease
Precautions: Renal disease **(IV)**

Pharmacokinetics
Absorption	Unknown
Distribution	Protein binding 58%
Metabolism	By CYP45 enzyme
Excretion	Via hepatic metabolism
Half-life	Unknown

Pharmacodynamics
Onset	Unknown
Peak	1-2 hr
Duration	Unknown

Interactions
Individual drugs
Cisplatin, cycloSPORINE, polymyxin B, vancomycin: increased nephrotoxicity
CycloSPORINE, phenytoin, pimozide, prednisolone, quinidine, rifabutin, sirolimus, tacrolimus, warfarin: increased effects of each specific product
Digoxin: increased hypokalemia
Drug classifications
Aminoglycosides: increased nephrotoxicity
Benzodiazepines, calcium channel blockers, ergots, HMG-CoA reductase inhibitors, non-nucleoside reverse transcriptase inhibitors, protease inhibitors, proton pump inhibitors, sulfonylureas, vinca alkaloids: increased effects of each specific product
Corticosteroids, diuretics (thiazide), skeletal muscle relaxants: increased hypokalemia
QT-prolonging drugs: increased QT prolongation
Drug/herb
Gossypol: increased nephrotoxicity
St. John's wort: do not use together
Drug/food
High-fat foods: avoid use with high-fat meals

V

Adverse effects: *italic* = common, **bold** = life-threatening

NURSING CONSIDERATIONS
Assessment
- Monitor VS q15-30min during first inf; note changes in pulse, B/P
- Monitor I&O ratio; watch for decreasing urinary output, change in specific gravity; discontinue product to prevent permanent damage to renal tubules
- Monitor blood tests: CBC, K, Na, Ca, Mg q2wk; BUN, creatinine weekly
- Monitor weight weekly; if weight increases over 2 lb/wk, edema is present; renal damage should be considered
⬥ Assess for renal toxicity: increasing BUN, serum creatinine; if BUN is >40 mg/dl or if serum creatinine >3 mg/dl, product may be discontinued or dosage reduced
⬥ Assess for hepatotoxicity: increasing AST, ALT, alkaline phosphatase, bilirubin
- Assess for allergic reaction: dermatitis, rash; product should be discontinued, antihistamines (mild reaction) or epinephrine (severe reaction) administered
- Assess for hypokalemia: anorexia, drowsiness, weakness, decreased reflexes, dizziness, increased urinary output, increased thirst, paresthesias
- Assess for ototoxicity: tinnitus (ringing, roaring in ears), vertigo, loss of hearing (rare)

Nursing diagnoses
- Infection, risk for (uses)
- Injury, risk for (uses, adverse reactions)
- Knowledge, deficient (teaching)

Implementation
- Give 1 hr before or after meals
- Store at room temperature (powder, tabs)
IV route
- Give product only after C&S confirms organism, product needed to treat condition; make sure product is used in life-threatening infections
- Reconstitute powder with 19 ml water for inj to 10 mg/ml, shake until dissolved; infuse over 1-2 hr at a conc of 5 mg/ml or less; do not admix with other products, 4.2% sodium bicarbonate inf

Patient/family education
- Teach that long-term therapy may be needed to clear infection (2 wk-3 mo depending on type of infection)
- Advise patient to notify prescriber of bleeding, bruising, or soft tissue swelling
- Teach to take 1 hr before or after meal
- Advise patient not to drive at night because of vision changes
- Advise to avoid strong, direct sunlight
- Advise that women of childbearing age should use effective contraceptive

Evaluation
Positive therapeutic outcome
- Decreased fever, malaise, rash, negative C&S for infecting organism

---

⚠ HIGH ALERT

warfarin (Rx)
(war'far-in)
Coumadin, Jantoven, warfarin sodium, Warfilone ✦
Func. class.: Anticoagulant

Pregnancy category X

Do not confuse:
Coumadin/Cardura/Compazine

Action: Interferes with blood clotting by indirect means; depresses hepatic synthesis of vit K–dependent coagulation factors (II, VII, IX, X)

Therapeutic outcome: Prevention of clotting

Uses: Antiphospholipid antibody syndrome, deep vein thrombosis, prevention or treatment of venous thrombosis, pulmonary embolism, thromboembolic complications associated with atrial fibrillation or cardiac valve replacement, after MI to reduce risk of death

Dosage and routes
Adult: PO/**IV** 2.5-10 mg/day × 3 days, then titrated to INR
Geriatric: PO/**IV** 2-10 mg/day
Child: PO/**IV** 0.2 mg/kg/day titrated to INR

Available forms: Tabs 1, 2, 2.5, 3, 4, 5, 6, 7.5, 10 mg; 5.4 mg powder for inj

Adverse effects
CNS: Fever, dizziness, fatigue, headache, lethargy
CV: Angina, chest pain, edema, hypotension, syncope
GI: Diarrhea, nausea, vomiting, anorexia, stomatitis, cramps, **hepatitis**, cholestatic jaundice
GU: **Hematuria**
HEMA: **Hemorrhage, agranulocytosis, leukopenia, eosinophilia,** ecchymosis, anemia, petechiae
INTEG: Rash, dermatitis, urticaria, alopecia, pruritus
MISC: Epistaxis, hemoptysis, mouth ulcers, taste disturbances, priapism, dyspnea
MS: Bone fractures

SYST: **Anaphylaxis,** coma, cholesterol, microembolisms, **exfoliative dermatitis, purple toe syndrome**

Contraindications: Pregnancy **X,** breastfeeding, hypersensitivity, hemophilia, leukemia with bleeding, peptic ulcer disease, thrombocytopenic purpura, hepatic disease (severe), malignant hypertension, subacute bacterial endocarditis, acute nephritis, blood dyscrasias, preeclampsia, eclampsia, hemorrhagic tendencies, surgery of CNS, eye, traumatic surgery with large open surface, bleeding tendencies of GI/GU/respiratory, stroke, aneurysms, pericardial effusion, spinal puncture, major regional/lumbar block anesthesia

Black Box Warning: Bleeding

Precautions: Alcoholism, geriatric, CHF, debilitated patients, trauma, indwelling catheters, severe hypertension, active infections, protein C deficiency, polycythemia vera, vasculitis, severe diabetes

Pharmacokinetics

Absorption	Well absorbed (PO), completely absorbed
Distribution	Crosses placenta, 99% plasma protein binding
Metabolism	Liver
Excretion	Kidney, feces (active, inactive metabolites)
Half-life	Effective ½-2½ days

Pharmacodynamics

	PO
Onset	12-24 hr
Peak	½-4 days
Duration	3-5 days

Interactions
Individual drugs
Allopurinol, amiodarone, chloral hydrate, chloramphenicol, cimetidine, clofibrate, clotrimoxazole, dextrothyroxine, diflunisal, disulfiram, erythromycin, furosemide, glucagon, heparin, indomethacin, isoniazid, mefenamic acid, metronidazole, mifepristone, phenylbutazone, quinidine, RU-486, sulfinpyrazone, sulindac, thyroid: increased warfarin action

Aprepitant, azothioprine, bosentan, carbamazepine, dicloxicillin, ethchlorvynol, factor IX/VIIa, griseofulvin, nafcillin, phenytoin, rifampin, sucralfate, sulfasalazine, thyroid, vitamin K: decreased warfarin action

Digoxin: increased hypokalemia increased toxicity

Phenytoin: increased toxicity

Drug classifications
Antidepressants (tricyclic), ethacrynic acids, HMG-CoA reductase inhibitors, NSAIDs, oxyphenbutazones, COX-2 selective inhibitors, penicillins, quinolones, salicylates, selective serotonin reuptake inhibitors, steroids, sulfonamides, thrombolytics: increased warfarin action

Barbiturates, bile acid sequestrants, contraceptives (oral), estrogens: decreased warfarin action

Sulfonylureas (oral): increased toxicity
Drug/herb
Agrimony, angelica, anise, basil, bay, bilberry, black currant, black haw, bogbean, bromelain, buchu, cat's claw, chamomile, chondroitin, cinchona bark, cranberry, danshen, devil's claw, dong quai, evening primrose, fenugreek, feverfew, garlic, ginger, ginkgo, ginseng, horse chestnut, Irish moss, kava, kelp, kelpware, khella, licorice, lovage, lungwort, meadowsweet, melatonin, motherwort, mugwort, nettle, papaya, parsley (large amounts), pau d'arco, pineapple, poplar, prickly ash, red clover, red yeast rice, safflower, saw palmetto, skullcap, tonka bean, turmeric, wintergreen, yarrow: increased risk of bleeding

Alfalfa, coenzyme Q10, flax, glucomannan, goldenseal, guar gum, St. John's wort: decreased anticoagulant effect
Drug/food
Vit K foods: decreased warfarin action
Drug/lab test
Increased: T_3 uptake, liver function tests
Decreased: uric acid

NURSING CONSIDERATIONS
Assessment
• Monitor blood studies (Hct, occult blood in stools) q3mo; partial pro-time, which should be 1½-2 × control, PTT; often done daily, APTT, ACT; platelet count q2-3day; thrombocytopenia may occur
• Monitor B/P, watch for increasing signs of hypertension
◆ Assess for bleeding: bleeding gums, petechiae, ecchymosis, black tarry stools, hematuria, epistaxis; decreased B/P may indicate bleeding and possible hemorrhage; fatal hemorrhage can occur
• Assess for fever, skin rash, urticaria
• Assess for needed dosage change q1-2wk
◆ Assess patients carefully for symptoms of Churg-Strauss syndrome (rare): eosinophilia, vasculitis, rash, worsening pulmonary symptoms, cardiac complications, neuropathy

W

Adverse effects: *italic* = common, **bold** = life-threatening

Nursing diagnoses
• Injury, risk for (uses, adverse reactions)
• Knowledge, deficient (teaching)
• Tissue perfusion, ineffective (uses)

Implementation
PO route
• Warfarin is usually given with **IV** heparin for 3 or more days, warfarin blood level may take several days
IV route
• Reconstitute with 2.7 ml of sterile water for inj; do not use solution that is discolored or has particulates
• Give over 1-2 min into peripheral vein
Y-site compatibilities: Cefazolin, ceftriaxone, DOPamine, heparin, lidocaine, morphine, nitroglycerin, potassium chloride, ranitidine

Patient/family education
• Caution patient to avoid OTC preparations unless directed by prescriber; may cause serious product interactions
• Advise patient that product may be withheld during active bleeding (menstruation), depending on condition
• Advise patient to use soft-bristle toothbrush to avoid bleeding gums, avoid contact sports, use electric razor, avoid IM inj
• Instruct patient to carry/wear emergency ID identifying product taken
• Advise patient to report any signs of bleeding: gums, under skin, urine, stools
• Teach patient to read food labels; limited intake of vit K foods (green leafy vegetables) is necessary to maintain consistent prothrombin levels

Evaluation
Positive therapeutic outcome
• Decrease of deep vein thrombosis
• Pro-time (1.3-2.0 × control)

---

xylometazoline nasal agent
See Appendix B

---

zafirlukast (Rx)
(za-feer'loo-cast)
Accolate
Func. class.: Bronchodilator
Chem. class.: Leukotriene receptor antagonist

Pregnancy category B

Action: Antagonizes the contractile action of leukotrienes (LTC_4, LTD_4, LTE_4) in airway smooth muscle; inhibits bronchoconstriction caused by antigens

Therapeutic outcome: Ability to breathe more easily

Uses: Prophylaxis and chronic treatment of asthma in adults/children >5 yr

Unlabeled uses: Chronic urticaria

Dosage and routes
Adult and child ≥12 yr: PO 20 mg bid, take 1 hr before or 2 hr after meals
Child 5-11 yr: PO 10 mg bid

Available forms: Tabs 10, 20 mg

Adverse effects
CNS: Headache, dizziness, **suicidal ideation,** fever, insomnia
GI: Nausea, diarrhea, abdominal pain, vomiting, dyspepsia, **hepatic failure, hepatitis**
HEMA: **Agranulocytosis**
MISC: Infections, pain, asthenia, myalgia, fever, increased ALT, urticaria, rash, **angioedema**

Contraindications: Hypersensitivity

Precautions: Pregnancy B, breastfeeding, children, geriatric, hepatic disease

Pharmacokinetics	
Absorption	Rapidly
Distribution	Unknown
Metabolism	Extensively by CYP450 2C9, 3A4 enzyme systems, protein binding (99%)
Excretion	Feces
Half-life	10 hr

Pharmacodynamics	
Onset	Unknown
Peak	3 hr
Duration	Unknown

Interactions
Individual drugs
Aspirin: increased plasma levels of zafirlukast
Erythromycin, theophylline: decreased plasma levels of zafirlukast
Warfarin: increased pro-time
Drug/herb
Green tea (large amounts), guarana: increased effect
Drug/food
Decreased: bioavailability of zafirlukast

NURSING CONSIDERATIONS
Assessment
• Assess respiratory rate, rhythm, depth; auscultate lung fields bilaterally; notify prescriber of abnormalities

---

 Alert   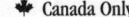 Canada Only   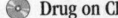 Drug on CD   * "Tall Man" lettering (See Preface)

Nursing diagnoses
- Breathing pattern, ineffective (uses)
- Knowledge, deficient (teaching)
- Noncompliance (teaching)

Implementation
- Give PO 1 hr before or 2 hr after meals; absorption may be decreased if given with food
- Give with 8 oz of water if GI upset occurs

Patient/family education
- Advise patient to check OTC medications, current prescription medications, which will increase stimulation
- Advise patient to avoid hazardous activities; dizziness may occur
- Advise patient that if GI upset occurs, to take product with 8 oz of water; avoid food if possible; absorption may be decreased
- Advise to take even if symptom free
- Advise patient to notify prescriber of nausea, vomiting, diarrhea, abdominal pain, fatigue, jaundice, anorexia, flulike symptoms (hepatic dysfunction)
- Advise patient not to use for acute asthma episodes, or to use while breastfeeding

Evaluation
Positive therapeutic outcome
- Ability to breathe more easily

zaleplon (Rx)
(zale′plon)
Sonata
Func. class.: Sedative-hypnotic, non-barbiturate
Chem. class.: Pyrazolopyrimidine

Pregnancy category C

Controlled substance schedule IV

Action: Binds selectively to ω-1 receptor of the γ-aminobutyric acid type A (GABA$_A$) receptor complex; results are sedation, hypnosis, skeletal muscle relaxation, anticonvulsant activity, anxiolytic action

Therapeutic outcome: Ability to sleep

Uses: Insomnia

Dosage and routes
Adult: PO 10 mg at bedtime; may increase dose to 20 mg at bedtime if needed; 5 mg may be used in low-weight persons
Geriatric: PO 5 mg at bedtime; may increase if needed

Available forms: Caps 5, 10 mg

Adverse effects
CNS: Drowsiness, amnesia, depersonalization, hallucinations, hyperesthesia, paresthesia, somnolence, tremor, vertigo, dizziness, anxiety, *lethargy, daytime sedation*, confusion, complex sleep-related reactions (sleep driving, sleep eating)
EENT: Vision changes, ear/eye pain, hyperacusis, parosmia
GI: Nausea, anorexia, colitis, dyspepsia, dry mouth, constipation, abdominal pain
MISC: Asthenia, fever, headache, myalgia, dysmenorrhea
SYST: Severe allergic reactions

Contraindications: Hypersensitivity, severe hepatic disease

Precautions: Pregnancy C, breastfeeding, children <15 yr, geriatric, renal/hepatic disease, psychosis, angioedema, respiratory disease, depression, sleep-related behaviors (sleep walking)

Pharmacokinetics
Absorption	Rapidly absorbed
Distribution	Extravascular tissues, crosses blood-brain barrier; crosses placenta
Metabolism	Extensively, liver to inactive metabolites
Excretion	Kidneys
Half-life	1 hr

Pharmacodynamics
Onset	Rapid
Peak	1 hr
Duration	Unknown

Interactions
Individual drugs
Cimetidine: increased action of zaleplon
Rifampin: decreased zaleplon levels
Drug classifications
CYP3A4 inhibitors/inducers: increased or decreased
Drug/herb
Black cohosh: increased hypotension
Catnip, chamomile, clary, cowslip, hops, kava, lavender, mistletoe, nettle, pokeweed, poppy, Queen Anne's lace, senega, skullcap, valerian: increased CNS depression
Drug/food
High-fat/heavy meal: prolonged absorption, sleep onset reduced

NURSING CONSIDERATIONS
Assessment
- Assess for previous product dependence or tolerance; if product dependent or tolerant, amount of medication should be restricted

- Monitor patient's mental status: mood, sensorium, affect, sleeping patterns, drowsiness, dizziness, suicidal tendencies, excessive sedation, impaired coordination

Nursing diagnoses
- Knowledge, deficient (teaching)
- Noncompliance (teaching)
- Sleep deprivation (uses)

Implementation
- Give ½-1 hr before bedtime for sleeplessness; give on empty stomach

Patient/family education
- Inform patient that product is for short-term use only
- Teach patient to take immediately before going to bed
- Advise patient that product may cause memory problems, dependence (if used for longer periods of time), changes in behavior/thinking, complex sleep-related behaviors (sleep eating/driving)
- Advise patient not to ingest a high-fat/heavy meal before taking
- Advise patient to avoid OTC preparations unless approved by a physician, to avoid alcohol ingestion or other psychotropic medications unless prescribed by a health care provider, that 1-2 wk of therapy may be required before therapeutic effects occur
- Caution patient to avoid driving, activities requiring alertness; drowsiness may occur; until medication response is known, tell patient that drowsiness may worsen at beginning of treatment
- Instruct patient not to discontinue medication abruptly after long-term use

Evaluation
Positive therapeutic outcome
- Decreased sleeplessness

---

zanamivir (Rx)
(zan-a-mee'veer)
Relenza
Func. class.: Antiviral
Chem. class.: Neuramidase inhibitor

Pregnancy category C

Action: Inhibits neuramidase enzyme needed for influenza virus replication

Therapeutic outcome: Decreased symptoms of influenza types A and B for those who have been symptomatic for no more than 2 days

Uses: Treatment of influenza types A and B

Unlabeled uses: Prophylaxis against influenza A and B infections; swine flu (H1N1)

Dosage and routes
Adult and child >7 yr: INH 2 inh (two 5-mg blisters) q12hr × 5 days, on the 1st day 2 doses should be taken with at least 2 hr between doses

H1N1 (swine flu) (unlabeled)
Adult/adolescent/child ≥7 yr: INH 2 bid × 5 days

Available forms: Blisters of powder for inhalation 5 mg

Adverse effects
CNS: Headache, dizziness, fatigue, **seizures,** self-injury, delirium (child)
EENT: Ear, nose, throat infections
GI: Nausea, vomiting, diarrhea
RESP: Nasal symptoms, cough, sinusitis, bronchitis, **bronchospasm**
SYST: Angioedema

Contraindications: Hypersensitivity

Precautions: Pregnancy **C,** breastfeeding, children <7 yr, geriatric, respiratory disease, angioedema, milk protein hypersensitivity, Reye's syndrome

Pharmacokinetics	
Absorption	4%-17% absorbed
Distribution	<10% protein binding
Metabolism	Not metabolized
Excretion	Kidneys unchanged
Half-life	2½-5 hr

Pharmacodynamics	
Unknown	

Interactions
Individual drugs
Intranasal influenza vaccine: decreased effect; separate by ≥48 hr, do not restart antiviral drugs for ≥2 wk

NURSING CONSIDERATIONS
Assessment
- Assess for symptoms of influenza A: increased temp, malaise, aches and pains
- Assess for skin eruptions, photosensitivity after administration of product
- Monitor respiratory status: rate, character, wheezing, tightness in chest
- Assess for allergies before initiation of treatment, reaction of each medication

Nursing diagnoses
- Infection, risk for (uses)
- Knowledge, deficient (teaching)

 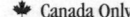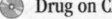

Implementation
- Give before exposure to influenza; continue for 5 days after contact
- Store in airtight, dry container

Patient/family education
- Give patient "Patient's instructions for use" and review all points before using delivery system
- Teach patient to avoid hazardous activities if dizziness occurs
- Teach patient to take product exactly as prescribed; to use for the entire 5 days
- Inform patient that this product does not reduce transmission risk of influenza to others
- Advise patients with asthma or COPD to carry a fast-acting inhaled bronchodilator since bronchospasm may occur; to use scheduled inhaled bronchodilators before using this product

Evaluation
Positive therapeutic outcome
- Absence of fever, malaise, cough, dyspnea in influenza A

---

zidovudine ⊛ (Rx)
(zye-doe′vue-deen)
Apo-Zidovudine ✦, Azidothymidine, AZT, Novo-AZT ✦, Retrovir
Func. class.: Antiretroviral
Chem. class.: Nucleoside reverse transcriptase inhibitor (NRTI)

Pregnancy category C

Action: Inhibits replication of HIV-1 by incorporating into cellular DNA by viral reverse transcriptase, thereby terminating the cellular DNA chain

Therapeutic outcome: Decreased symptoms of HIV-1 infection

Uses: Used in combination with other antiretrovirals for HIV-1 infection, human T-lymphotropic virus type I (HILV-I)

Dosage and routes
Adult: PO 600 mg/day in divided doses, either 200 mg tid or 300 mg bid in combination with other antiretrovirals; **IV** 1-2 mg/kg q4hr, initiate PO as soon as possible, up to 1000 mg
Child 6 wk-12 yr: PO 160 mg/m^2 q8hr (480 mg/m^2/day, max 200 mg q8hr) in combination with other antiretrovirals; **IV** same as adult
Neonate: PO 2-3 mg/kg/dose q6hr; **IV** 1.5 mg/kg INF over 30 min q6hr

Treatment of HIV in combination with other antiretrovirals
Adult/adolescent/child ≥30 kg: PO 300 mg bid or 200 mg tid

Perinatal transmission prophylaxis
Full-term neonate: PO 2 mg/kg or **IV** 1.5 mg/kg q6hr starting 12 hr after birth; continue up to 6 wk of age
Preterm neonate: PO 2 mg/kg or **IV** 1.5 mg/kg q12hr; if >30 wk gestation at birth, advance to q8hr at 2 wk of age; if <30 wk gestation at birth, advance to q8hr at 4 wk of age

Prevention of maternal-fetal HIV transmission
Neonatal: PO 2 mg/kg/dose q6hr × 6 wk beginning 8-12 hr after birth; **IV** 1.5 mg/kg/dose over 30 min q6hr until able to take PO
Maternal (>14 wk gestation): PO 100 mg 5 ×/day until start of labor, then during labor/delivery **IV** 2 mg/kg over 1 hr followed by **IV** INF 1 mg/kg/hr until umbilical cord clamped

Symptomatic HIV infection
Child 3 mo-12 yr: PO 160 mg/m^2 tid or 240 mg/m^2 bid; **IV** 1-2 mg/kg over 1 hr q4hr
Adult: PO 300 mg bid or 200 mg tid; **IV** 1-2 mg/kg over 1 hr q4hr

Prevention of HIV after needlestick
Adult: PO 200 mg tid plus lamivudine 150 mg bid, plus a protease inhibitor for high-risk exposure; begin within 2 hr of exposure

Available forms: Caps 100 mg; tabs 300 mg; inj 200 mg/20 ml; oral syr 50 mg/5 ml

Adverse effects
CNS: Fever, headache, malaise, diaphoresis, *dizziness, insomnia,* paresthesia, somnolence, chills, tremor, twitching, anxiety, confusion, *depression,* lability, *vertigo,* loss of mental acuity, **seizures,** malaise
EENT: Taste change, hearing loss, photophobia
GI: Nausea, vomiting, diarrhea, anorexia, cramps, *dyspepsia, constipation,* dysphagia, *flatulence,* rectal bleeding, mouth ulcer, abdominal pain, hepatomegaly
GU: Dysuria, polyuria, frequency, hesitancy
HEMA: **Granulocytopenia, anemia**
INTEG: Rash, acne, pruritus, urticaria
MS: Myalgia, arthralgia, muscle spasm
RESP: Dyspnea
SYST: **Lactic acidosis**

Contraindications: Hypersensitivity

Precautions: Pregnancy **C**, breastfeeding, children, granulocyte count <1000/mm³ or Hgb <9.5 g/dl, severe renal disease, obesity

Black Box Warning: Impaired hepatic function, anemia, lactic acidosis, myopathy, neutropenia

Pharmacokinetics

Absorption	Well absorbed (PO), completely absorbed (**IV**)
Distribution	Widely distributed—crosses placenta, CSF, protein binding 38%
Metabolism	Liver, mostly
Excretion	Kidneys
Half-life	Terminal ½-3 hr

Pharmacodynamics

	PO	IV
Onset	Unknown	Rapid
Peak	½-1½ hr	Inf end
Duration	Unknown	Unknown

Interactions
Individual drugs
Fluconazole, probenecid: increased toxicity
Ganciclovir, radiation, SMX/TMP, valganciclovir: increased bone marrow suppression
Methadone: increased zidovudine level
Drug classifications
Antineoplastics: increased bone marrow suppression

NURSING CONSIDERATIONS
Assessment
• Assess for peripheral neuropathy: tingling or pain in hands and feet, distal numbness; if these occur, product may be decreased or discontinued
• Assess for pancreatitis: abdominal pain, nausea, vomiting, elevated liver enzymes; product should be discontinued because condition can be fatal
• Assess children by dilated retinal examination q6mo to rule out retinal depigmentation
• Monitor CBC, differential, platelet count qmo; withhold product if WBC is <4000/mm³ or platelet count is <75,000/mm³; notify prescriber of results; monitor viral load, CD4 counts, LFTs, plasma HIV RNA, serum creatinine/BUN baseline, throughout treatment
• Monitor renal function tests: BUN, serum uric acid, urine CCr before, during therapy; these may be elevated throughout treatment
• Monitor temp q4hr, may indicate beginning of infection

• Monitor liver function tests before, during therapy (bilirubin, AST, ALT amylase, alkaline phosphatase) prn or qmo

Nursing diagnoses
• Infection, risk for (uses)
• Injury, risk for (adverse reactions)
• Knowledge, deficient (teaching)

Implementation
PO route
• Give on empty stomach, bid or tid
• Do not take dapsone at same time as didanosine
IV route
• Give by intermittent inf after diluting with D₅W; give over 1 hr (<4 mg/ml), do not give by direct **IV**
Y-site compatibilities: Acyclovir, allopurinol, amikacin, amphotericin B, aztreonam, ceftazidime, ceftriaxone, cimetidine, clindamycin, dexamethasone, DOBUTamine, DOPamine, erythromycin, fluconazole, fludarabine, gentamicin, heparin, imipenem/cilastatin, lorazepam, metoclopramide, morphine, nafcillin, ondansetron, oxacillin, pentamidine, phenylephrine, piperacillin, potassium chloride, ranitidine, sargramostim, tobramycin, trimethoprim/sulfamethoxazole, vancomycin
Additive incompatibilities: Blood products or protein solutions

Patient/family education
• Caution patient to take on empty stomach; to use exactly as prescribed
• Advise patient to report signs of infection: increased temp, sore throat, flulike symptoms; to avoid crowds and those with known infections
• Instruct patient to report signs of anemia: fatigue, headache, faintness, shortness of breath, irritability
• Advise patient to report bleeding; avoid use of razors or commercial mouthwash
• Inform patient that hair may be lost during therapy (rare); a wig or hairpiece may make patient feel better
• Caution patient to avoid OTC products or other medications without approval of prescriber
• Caution patient not to have any sexual contact without use of a condom; needles should not be shared; blood from infected individual should not come in contact with another's mucous membranes

Evaluation
Positive therapeutic outcome
• Decreased infection; symptoms of HIV infection

zinc
(PO, OTC; IV, Rx)
(zink sul'fate)
Orazinc, PMS Egozinc ✿, Verazinc, Zinca-Pak, Zincate, Zinc 15, Zinc-220, zinc sulfate
Func. class.: Trace element; nutritional supplement

Pregnancy category C, parenteral

Action: Needed for adequate healing, bone and joint development, taste and smell (23% zinc)

Therapeutic outcome: Replacement of zinc

Uses: Prevention of zinc deficiency, adjunct to vit A therapy

Unlabeled uses: Wound healing

Dosage and routes
Dietary supplement (elemental zinc)
Adult/adolescent pregnant females: PO 11-13 mg/day

Nutritional supplement (IV)
Adult: **IV** 2.5-4 mg/day, may increase by 2 mg/day if needed
Child to 5 yr: **IV** 50 mcg/kg/day
Adult and lactating females: PO 12-14 mg/day × 12 mo
Adult and adolescent males ≥14 yr: PO 11 mg/day
Adult females ≥19 yr: PO 8 mg/day
Adolescent females ≥14 yr: PO 9 mg/day
Child 9-13 yr: PO 8 mg/day
Child 4-8 yr: PO 5 mg/day
Child 1-3 yr: PO 3 mg/day
Infant 7-12 mo: PO 3 mg/day
Infant birth to 6 mo: PO 2 mg/day (adequate intake)

Wound healing
Adult: PO 50 mg tid until healed (elemental iron)

Available forms: Tabs 66, 110 mg; caps 220 mg; inj 1, 5 mg/ml

Adverse effects
GI: Nausea, vomiting, cramps, heartburn, ulcer formation
OVERDOSE: Diarrhea, rash, dehydration, restlessness

Precautions: Pregnancy C (parenteral), breastfeeding, hypocupremia, neonatal prematurity, neonates, renal disease

Pharmacokinetics	
Absorption	Poorly absorbed (PO), completely absorbed (**IV**)
Distribution	Widely distributed
Metabolism	Liver
Excretion	90% (feces), 10% (kidneys)
Half-life	Unknown

Pharmacodynamics
Unknown

Interactions
Drug classifications
Fluoroquinolones, tetracyclines: decreased absorption

NURSING CONSIDERATIONS
Assessment
• Monitor zinc levels during treatment

Nursing diagnoses
• Knowledge, deficient (teaching)
• Nutrition, less than body requirements, imbalanced (uses)

Implementation
PO route
• Give with meals to decrease gastric upset; restrict dairy products, caffeine, which decrease absorption
IV route
• Part of TPN

Patient/family education
• Inform patient that element must be taken for 3 mo to be effective
• Advise patient to report immediately nausea, diarrhea, rash, severe vomiting, restlessness, abdominal pain, tarry stools

Evaluation
Positive therapeutic outcome
• Absence of zinc deficiency
• Improved wound healing

ziprasidone (Rx)
(zi-praz'ih-dohn)
Geodon, Zeldox
Func. class.: Antipsychotic/neuroleptic
Chem. class.: Benzisoxazole derivative

Pregnancy category C

Action: Unknown; may be mediated through both dopamine type 2 (D_2) and serotonin type 2 (5-HT_2) antagonism

Therapeutic outcome: Decreased signs/symptoms of psychosis

Uses: Schizophrenia, acute agitation, acute psychosis, bipolar disorder, mania, psychotic depression

Dosage and routes
Adult: PO 20 mg bid with food, adjust dosage every 2 days upward to max of 80 mg bid; IM 10-20 mg; may give 10 mg q2hr, doses of 20 mg may be given q4hr, max 40 mg/day

Available forms: Tabs 20, 40, 60, 80 mg; inj 20 mg/ml

Adverse effects
CNS: EPS (pseudoparkinsonism, akathisia, dystonia, tardive dyskinesia), drowsiness, insomnia, agitation, anxiety, headache, **seizures, neuroleptic malignant syndrome,** dizziness, tremor, facial droop
CV: Orthostatic hypotension, **tachycardia, prolonged QT/QTc, sudden death, heart failure (geriatric), torsades de pointes**
EENT: Blurred vision, swollen tongue, diplopia
ENDO: Metabolic changes
GI: Nausea, vomiting, *anorexia, constipation,* jaundice, weight gain, diarrhea, dry mouth, abdominal pain
GU: Enuresis, urinary incontinence, gynecomastia, impotence, priapism
RESP: Rhinitis, dyspnea, infection, cough

Contraindications: Hypersensitivity, breastfeeding

Precautions: Pregnancy **C,** children, geriatric, renal/cardiac/hepatic disease, breast cancer, diabetes, acute MI, heart failure, QT prolongation, AV block, CNS depression, seizure disorders

Black Box Warning: Dementia

Pharmacokinetics
Absorption	Unknown
Distribution	Protein binding 90%
Metabolism	Liver, extensively to metabolite
Excretion	Unknown
Half-life	Terminal 7 hr

Pharmacodynamics
Onset	Unknown
Peak	6-8 hr
Duration	Unknown

Interactions
Individual drugs
Alcohol: increased sedation
Bepridil, chloroquine, clarithromycin, droperidol, erythromycin, grepafloxacin, halofantrine, haloperidol, methadone, moxifloxacin, pentamidine, probucol, sparfloxacin: increased QT prolongation
Carbamazepine: increased excretion of ziprasidone
Ketoconazole: increased ziprasidone level
Lithium: increased EPS
Drug classifications
Antihypertensives: increased hypotension
Antipsychotics: increased EPS
β-agonists, class IA/III antidysrhythmics, local anesthetics, phenothiazines (some), tricyclics: increased QT prolongation
CNS depressants: increased sedation
Drug/herb
Betel palm, kava: increased EPS
Chamomile, hops, kava, skullcap, valerian: increased CNS depression
Cola tree, hops, nettle, nutmeg: increased action

NURSING CONSIDERATIONS
Assessment
- Assess mental status before initial administration
- Check swallowing of PO medication; check for hoarding or giving of medication to other patients
- Monitor I&O ratio; palpate bladder if urinary output is low
- Monitor bilirubin, CBC, liver function tests, fasting blood glucose qmo
- Monitor urinalysis before, during prolonged therapy
- Assess affect, orientation, LOC, reflexes, gait, coordination, sleep pattern disturbances
- Monitor B/P standing and lying; also pulse, respirations; take these q4hr during initial treatment; establish baseline before starting treatment; report drops of 30 mm Hg; watch for ECG changes
- Assess dizziness, faintness, palpitations, tachycardia on rising
- Assess EPS, including akathisia (inability to sit still, no pattern to movements), tardive dyskinesia (bizarre movements of the jaw, mouth, tongue, extremities), pseudoparkinsonism (rigidity, tremors, pill rolling, shuffling gait)
- ⬥ Assess for neuroleptic malignant syndrome: hyperthermia, increased CPK, altered mental status, muscle rigidity
- Assess skin turgor daily
- Assess constipation, urinary retention daily; if these occur, increase bulk and water in diet

Nursing diagnoses
- Coping, ineffective (uses)
- Knowledge, deficient (teaching)
- Noncompliance (teaching)

Implementation

- Give reduced dose in geriatric
- Give antiparkinsonian agent on order from prescriber, to be used for EPS
- Provide decreased stimulus by dimming lights, avoiding loud noises
- Provide supervised ambulation until patient is stabilized on medication; do not involve in strenuous exercise program because fainting is possible; patient should not stand still for a long time

PO route

- Food increases absorption
- Store in airtight, light-resistant container

IM route

- Add 1.2 ml sterile water for inj to vial, shake vigorously until product is dissolved, do not admix

Patient/family education

- Advise patient that orthostatic hypotension may occur and to rise from sitting or lying position gradually; avoid hot tubs, hot showers, tub baths because hypotension may occur
- Advise patient to avoid abrupt withdrawal of this product; EPS may result; product should be withdrawn slowly
- Advise patient to avoid OTC preparations (cough, hay fever, cold) unless approved by prescriber, since serious product interactions may occur; avoid use with alcohol, CNS depressants; increased drowsiness may occur
- Teach patient to avoid hazardous activities if drowsy or dizzy
- Advise patient to increase fluids to prevent constipation
- Teach patient to use sips of water, candy, gum for dry mouth
- Teach patient compliance with product regimen
- Teach patient to report impaired vision, tremors, muscle twitching
- Teach patient that in hot weather, heat stroke may occur; take extra precautions to stay cool

Evaluation

Positive therapeutic outcome

- Decrease in emotional excitement, hallucinations, delusions, paranoia; reorganization of patterns of thought, speech

Treatment of overdose: Lavage if orally ingested; provide airway; *do not induce vomiting*

---

zoledronic acid (Rx)

(zoh'leh-drah'nick ass'id))

Reclast, Zometa

Func. class.: Bone-resorption inhibitor
Chem. class.: Bisphosphonate

Pregnancy category D

Action: Inhibits normal and abnormal bone resorption; potent inhibitor of osteoclastic bone resorption; inhibits osteoclastic activity, reduces bone resorption and inhibits skeletal calcium release caused by stimulating factors released by tumors; reduction of abnormal bone resorption is responsible for therapeutic effect in hypercalcemia; may directly block dissolution of hydroxyapatite bone crystals

Therapeutic outcome: Serum calcium at normal level

Uses: Moderate to severe hypercalcemia associated with malignancy; multiple myeloma; bone metastases from solid tumors (used with antineoplastics), active Paget's disease, osteoporosis, glucocorticoid-induced osteoporosis, osteoporosis prophylaxis in postmenopausal women

Dosage and routes
Hypercalemia of malignancy
Adult: IV INF 4 mg, given as a single INF over ≥15 min, may re-treat with 4 mg if serum calcium does not return to normal within 1 wk

Multiple myeloma/metastatic bone lesions
Adult: IV INF 4 mg, given over 15 min q3-4wk

Osteoporosis
Adult: IV 5 mg over 15 min or more q12mo

Active Paget's disease
Adult: IV INF 5 mg over ≥15 min

Osteoporosis prophylaxis (Reclast), postmenopausal women
Adult: IV INF 5 mg every other yr

Osteoporosis prophylaxis (Reclast) taking systemic glucocorticoids
Adult: IV 5 mg qyr

Available forms: Sol for inj 4 mg/5 ml (Reclast); inj 5 mg/100 ml (Reclast)

Adverse effects
CNS: Dizziness, headache, anxiety, confusion, insomnia, agitation
CV: Hypotension, leg edema, **atrial fibrillation,** chest pain
GI: Abdominal pain, anorexia, constipation, nausea, diarrhea, vomiting, taste change

---

GU: UTI, possible reduced renal function, **renal damage**
META: Anemia, hypokalemia, hypomagnesemia, hypophosphatemia, hypocalcemia, increased serum creatinine
MISC: *Fever, chills, flulike symptoms*
MS: Severe bone pain, *arthralgias, myalgias,* osteonecrosis of the jaw

Contraindications: Pregnancy **D**, breast-feeding, hypocalcemia, hypersensitivity to this product or bisphosphonates

Precautions: Children, geriatric, renal dysfunction, aspirin-sensitive asthma, asthmatic patients, asthma, acute bronchospasm, anemia, chemotherapy, coagulopathy, dehydration, dental disease, diabetes mellitus, renal disease, electrolyte imbalance, hypertension, hypomagnesemia, hypophosphatemia, hypovolemia, phosphate hypersensitivity, infection, multiple myeloma

Pharmacokinetics

Absorption	Rapidly cleared from circulation
Distribution	Taken up mainly by bones; plasma protein binding ~22%
Metabolism	Not metabolized
Excretion	Kidneys (~50% eliminated in urine within 24 hr)
Half-life	Terminal 167 hr

Pharmacodynamics

Onset	Unknown
Peak	15 min
Duration	Max effect 7 days

Interactions
Individual drugs
Calcium, vitamin D: decreased zoledronic acid effect
Digoxin: hypomagnesemia, hypokalemia
Infusion solutions (calcium-containing): do not mix with calcium-containing inf sol such as lactated Ringer's sol
Drug classifications
Aminoglycosides, NSAIDs, radiopaque contrast agents: increased neurotoxicity
Aminoglycosides, loop diuretics: decreased serum calcium

NURSING CONSIDERATIONS
Assessment
• Assess renal function tests and Ca, P, Mg, K, creatinine; if creatinine is elevated hold treatment
• Assess for hypercalcemia: paresthesia, twitching, laryngospasm; Chvostek's, Trousseau's signs

• Assess dental status; cover with antiinfectives for dental extraction
• Assess for atrial fibrillation

Nursing diagnoses
• Fluid volume, excess (side effects)
• Injury, risk for (uses, adverse reactions)
• Knowledge, deficient (teaching)

Implementation
• Give acetaminophen before and for 72 hr after to decrease pain
• Sol reconstituted with sterile water may be stored under refrigeration for up to 24 hr **IV**
• Administer in separate **IV** line from all other products

Zometa
• Administer after reconstituting by adding 5 ml of sterile water for inj to each vial, then add up to ≥100 ml of sterile 0.9% NaCl, D₅W, run over ≥15 min

Reclast
• No further dilution required; inf over ≥15 min at constant rate; max 5 mg

Patient/family education
• Instruct patient to report hypercalcemic relapse: nausea, vomiting, bone pain, thirst
• Advise patient to continue with dietary recommendations including calcium and vit D; take a multiple vitamin daily, 500 mg of calcium, 400 international units vit D in multiple myeloma
• Teach patient if nausea/vomiting occur, eat small meals, use lozenges or chewing gum
• Advise patient if bone pain occurs, notify prescriber to obtain analgesic
• Advise patient to avoid pregnancy
• Instruct patient to continue good oral hygiene

Evaluation
Positive therapeutic outcome
• Calcium levels decreased to normal

Treatment of overdose: Correct clinically relevant reductions in serum calcium by administering **IV** calcium gluconate; in serum phosphorus, with potassium or sodium phosphate; in serum magnesium, with magnesium sulfate

zolmitriptan (Rx)

(zole-mih-trip'tan)
Zomig, Zomig-ZMT
Func. class.: Migraine agent, abortive
Chem. class.: 5HT$_{1B}$/5HT$_{1D}$ receptor agonist
(triptan)

Pregnancy category C

Action: Binds selectively to the vascular
serotonin type 1 (5HT$_{1B}$/5HT$_{1D}$) receptor
subtype, exerts antimigraine effect; causes
vasoconstriction in cranial arteries

Therapeutic outcome: Decreased
severity, frequency of headache

Uses: Acute treatment of migraine with or
without aura

Dosage and routes:
Adult: PO start at 2.5 mg or lower (tab may
be broken), may repeat after 2 hr, max 10
mg/24 hr; NASAL 1 spray in 1 nostril at onset
of migraine, repeat in 2 hr if no relief

Available forms: Tabs 2.5, 5 mg; orally
disintegrating tabs 2.5, 5 mg; nasal spray 5 mg

Adverse effects
*CNS: Tingling, hot sensation, burning,
feeling of pressure, tightness, numbness,
dizziness, sedation*
CV: Palpitations, chest pain
GI: Abdominal discomfort, nausea, dry mouth,
dyspepsia, dysphagia
MISC: Odd taste (spray)
MS: Weakness, neck stiffness, myalgia
RESP: Chest tightness, pressure

Contraindications: Angina pectoris,
history of MI, documented silent ischemia,
ischemic heart disease, concurrent
ergotamine-containing preparations, uncontrolled hypertension, hypersensitivity, basilar
or hemiplegic migraine, risk of CV events

Precautions: Pregnancy **C**, breastfeeding,
children, postmenopausal women, men >40
yr, geriatric, risk factors for CAD, hypercholesterolemia, obesity, diabetes, impaired renal/
hepatic function

Pharmacokinetics

Absorption	Unknown
Distribution	25% plasma protein binding
Metabolism	Liver
Excretion	Urine, feces
Half-life	3-3½ hr

Pharmacodynamics

Onset	Unknown
Peak	Unknown
Duration	2-3½ hr

Interactions
Individual drugs
Cimetidine: increased half-life of zolmitriptan
Ergot: increased vasospastic effects
Fluoxetine, fluvoxamine, paroxetine, sertraline:
increased weakness, hyperreflexia, incoordi-
nation
Sibutramine: increased zolmitriptan levels
Drug classifications
Contraceptives (oral): increased half-life of
zolmitriptan
Ergot derivatives: increased vasospastic effects
MAOIs: do not use within 2 wk
Selective serotonin reuptake inhibitors: in-
creased weakness, hyperreflexia, incoordi-
nation
Drug/herb
Butterbur, feverfew: increased effect
SAM-e, St. John's wort: serotonin syndrome

NURSING CONSIDERATIONS
Assessment
• Assess tingling, hot sensation, burning,
feeling of pressure, numbness, flushing
• Assess for stress level, activity, recreation,
coping mechanisms
• Assess neurologic status: LOC, blurring
vision, nausea, vomiting, tingling in extremities
preceding headache
• Monitor ingestion of tyramine foods (pickled products, beer, wine, aged cheese), food
additives, preservatives, colorings, artifical
sweeteners, chocolate, caffeine, which may
precipitate these types of headaches
• Assess for serotonin syndrome if also taking
a selective serotonin reuptake inhibitor

Nursing diagnoses
• Knowledge, deficient (teaching)
• Noncompliance (teaching)
• Pain, acute (uses)

Implementation
• Give with fluids as soon as symptoms of
migraine occur
• Provide quiet, calm environment with
decreased stimulation for noise, bright light,
excessive talking

Patient/family education
• Teach patient to report any side effects to
prescriber
• Advise patient to use contraception while
taking product

Adverse effects: *italic* = common, **bold** = life-threatening   Z

Evaluation
Positive therapeutic outcome
- Decrease in frequency, severity of headache

---

zolpidem (Rx)
(zole-pi'dem)
Ambien, Ambien CR, Tovalt ODT, Zolpimist
Func. class.: Sedative-hypnotic
Chem. class.: Nonbenzodiazepine of imida-zopyridine class

Pregnancy category C
Controlled substance schedule IV

Action: Produces CNS depression at limbic, thalamic, hypothalamic levels of CNS; may be mediated by neurotransmitter γ-aminobutyric acid (GABA); results are sedation, hypnosis, skeletal muscle relaxation, anticonvulsant activity, anxiolytic action

Therapeutic outcome: Ability to sleep, sedation

Uses: Insomnia, short-term treatment; insomnia with difficulty of sleep onset/maintenance (ext rel)

Dosage and routes
Adult: PO 10 mg at bedtime × 7-10 days only; total dose max 10 mg; orally disintegrating 10-mg tabs use immediately before retiring; EXT REL 12.5 mg immediately before bedtime, may be useful for up to 24 wk in people 18-64 yr with primary insomnia; oral spray (Zolpimist) 10 mg (2 sprays) immediately before bedtime, max 10 mg/day
Geriatric: PO 5 mg at bedtime

Available forms: Tabs 5, 10 mg; ext rel tabs 6.25, 12.5 mg; orally disintegrating tabs 5, 10 mg; oral spray 5 mg/spray

Adverse effects
CNS: Headache, lethargy, drowsiness, daytime sedation, dizziness, confusion, light-headedness, anxiety, irritability, amnesia, poor coordination, complex sleep-related reactions (sleep driving, sleep eating), depression, somnolence, **suicidal ideation,** abnormal thinking/behavioral changes
CV: Chest pain, palpitation
GI: Nausea, vomiting, diarrhea, heartburn, abdominal pain, constipation
HEMA: **Leukopenia, granulocytopenia** (rare)
MISC: Myalgia
SYST: **Severe allergic reactions**

Contraindications: Hypersensitivity to benzodiazepines

Precautions: Pregnancy **C**, breastfeeding, children <18 yr, geriatric, anemia, renal/hepatic disease, suicidal individuals, product abuse, psychosis, seizure disorders, angio-edema, depression, respiratory disease, sleep apnea, sleep-related behavior (sleep walking)

Pharmacokinetics
Absorption	Rapidly absorbed
Distribution	Unknown
Metabolism	Liver—inactive metabolite
Excretion	Kidneys, breast milk
Half-life	2½ hr, increased in geriatric

Pharmacodynamics
Onset	PO up to 1.5 mg

Interactions
Individual drugs
Alcohol: increased action of both products
Drug classifications
CNS depressants: increased action of both products
CYP3A4 inhibitors/inducers: increased or decreased zolpidem levels
Drug/herb
Chamomile, hops, kava, skullcap, valerian: increased CNS depression
Drug/lab test
Increased: ALT, AST, serum bilirubin
Decreased: radioactive iodine uptake
False increase: urinary 17-OHCS

NURSING CONSIDERATIONS
Assessment
- Assess mental status: mood, sensorium, anxiety, affect, sleeping pattern, drowsiness, dizziness, especially geriatric; physical dependency, withdrawal symptoms: anxiety, panic attacks, agitation, seizures, headache, nausea, vomiting, muscle pain, weakness; suicidal tendencies; for indications of increasing tolerance and abuse
- Monitor B/P (lying, standing), pulse; if systolic B/P drops 20 mm Hg, hold product, notify prescriber
- Monitor I&O ratio for renal dysfunction

Nursing diagnoses
- Anxiety (uses)
- Injury, risk for (adverse reactions)
- Knowledge, deficient (teaching)

Implementation
- Do not break, crush, or chew ext rel product or orally disintegrating tab
- Give ½-1 hr before bedtime for sleeplessness; give several hr before patient is to rise (to avoid hangover)

⬥ Alert   ❋ Canada Only   💿 Drug on CD   * "Tall Man" lettering (See Preface)

- Give with food or fluids; tab may be crushed or swallowed whole
- Do not use spray with or after a meal
- Store in airtight container in cool environment

Patient/family education

- Advise patient that complex sleep-related behaviors may occur (sleep driving/eating)
- Instruct patient that product may be taken with food or fluids
- Caution patient not to use for everyday stress or longer than 3 mo unless directed by prescriber; not to take more than prescribed amount; may be habit forming; not to double or skip doses
- Caution patient to avoid OTC preparations unless approved by prescriber; alcohol and CNS depressants will increase CNS depression
- Advise patient to avoid driving, activities that require alertness, because drowsiness may occur; to avoid alcohol ingestion or other psychotropic medications; to rise slowly or fainting may occur, especially geriatric; that drowsiness may worsen at beginning of treatment
- Instruct patient not to discontinue medication abruptly after long-term use; withdrawal symptoms include vomiting, cramping, tremors, seizures
- Teach patient use of orally disintegrating tabs: place on tongue, allow to dissolve before swallowing

Evaluation
Positive therapeutic outcome

- Ability to sleep at night
- Decreased amount of early-morning awakening if taking product for insomnia

Treatment of overdose: Lavage, VS, supportive care

---

zonisamide (Rx)
(zone-is'a-mide)
Zonegran
Func. class.: Anticonvulsant
Chem. class.: Sulfonamides

Pregnancy category C

Action: May act through sodium and calcium channels, but exact action is unknown; serotonergic action

Therapeutic outcome: Decreased seizures

Uses: Epilepsy, adjunctive therapy of partial seizures

Dosage and routes
Adults and child >16 yr: PO 100 mg/day, may increase after 2 wk to 200 mg/day, may increase q2wk, max dose 600 mg/day

Available forms: Caps 25, 50, 100 mg

Adverse effects
CNS: Dizziness, insomnia, paresthesias, depression, fatigue, headache, confusion, somnolence, agitation, irritability, speech disturbance, **suicidal ideation**
EENT: Diplopia, verbal difficulty, speech abnormalities, taste perversion
GI: Nausea, constipation, anorexia, weight loss, diarrhea, dyspepsia
HEMA: **Aplastic anemia, granulocytopenia** (rare)
INTEG: Rash
SYST: **Stevens-Johnson syndrome,** metabolic acidosis

Contraindications: Hypersensitivity to this product or sulfonamides, psychiatric condition, hepatic failure

Precautions: Pregnancy **C,** breastfeeding, children <16 yr, geriatric, allergies, renal/hepatic disease

Pharmacokinetics
Absorption	Unknown
Distribution	Protein binding 40%
Metabolism	Liver
Excretion	Kidneys
Half-life	63 hr

Pharmacodynamics
Onset	Unknown
Peak	2-6 hr
Duration	Unknown

Interactions
Individual drugs
Alcohol: increased depression
Drug classifications
Products inducing CYP450 enzyme (carbamazepine, phenobarbital, phenytoin): decreased half-life of zonisamide
Drug/herb
St. John's wort: increased effect of zonisamide
Drug/food
Grapefruit: do not use together

NURSING CONSIDERATIONS
Assessment
- Assess for seizures: duration, type, intensity, precipitating factors
- Renal function: albumin conc, BUN, creatinine; serum bicarbonate baseline, periodically

◆ Assess mental status: mood, sensorium, affect, memory (long, short); suicidal thoughts/behaviors
• Assess for rash, hypersensitivity reaction

Nursing diagnoses
• Injury, risk for (uses, adverse reactions)
• Knowledge, deficient (teaching)
• Noncompliance (teaching)

Patient/family education
• Advise patient not to discontinue product abruptly; seizures may occur

• Advise patient to avoid hazardous activities until stabilized on product
• Advise patient to carry/wear emergency ID stating product use
• Teach patient to take adequate fluids; not to use grapefruit juice

Evaluation
Positive therapeutic outcome
• Decrease in severity of seizures

ALPHA-ADRENERGIC BLOCKERS

Action: α-Adrenergic blockers bind to α-adrenergic receptors, causing dilatation of peripheral blood vessels and lower peripheral resistance resulting in decreased blood pressure.

Uses: α-Adrenergic blockers are used for benign prostatic hyperplasia, pheochromocytoma, prevention of tissue necrosis, and sloughing associated with extravasation of IV vasopressors.

Adverse effects: The most common side effects are hypotension, tachycardia, nasal stuffiness, nausea, vomiting, and diarrhea.

Contraindications: Hypersensitive reactions may occur, and allergies should be identified before these products are given. Patients with myocardial infarction, coronary insufficiency, angina, or other evidence of coronary artery disease should not use these products.

Pharmacokinetics: Onset, peak, and duration vary among products.

Interactions: Vasoconstrictive and hypertensive effects of epinephrine are antagonized by α-adrenergic blockers.

NURSING CONSIDERATIONS
Assessment
- Monitor electrolytes: potassium, sodium chloride, carbon dioxide
- Monitor weight daily, I&O
- Monitor B/P with patient lying, standing before starting treatment, q4hr thereafter
- Assess for nausea, vomiting, diarrhea
- Assess for skin turgor, dryness of mucous membranes for hydration status

Nursing diagnoses
- Injury, risk for (adverse reactions)
- Sleep deprivation (adverse reactions)
- Tissue perfusion, ineffective (uses)

Implementation
PO route
- Start with low dose, gradually increasing to prevent side effects
- Give with food or milk for GI symptoms

Patient/family education
- Caution patient to avoid alcoholic beverages
- Advise patient to report dizziness, palpitations, fainting
- Instruct patient to change position slowly or fainting may occur
- Teach patient to take product exactly as prescribed; to avoid all OTC products (cough, cold, allergy) unless directed by prescriber

Evaluation
Positive therapeutic outcome
- Decreased B/P
- Increased peripheral pulses

Generic Names

phentolamine

α 1 blockers:
silodosin, tamulosin

ANESTHETICS—GENERAL/LOCAL

Action: Anesthetics (general) act on the CNS to produce tranquilization and sleep before invasive procedures. Anesthetics (local) inhibit conduction of nerve impulses from sensory nerves.

Uses: General anesthetics are used to premedicate for surgery, and for induction and maintenance in general anesthesia. For local anesthetics, refer to individual product listing for indications.

Adverse effects: The most common side effects are dystonia, akathisia, flexion of arms, fine tremors, drowsiness, restlessness, and hypotension. Also common are chills, respiratory depression, and laryngospasm.

Contraindications: Persons with CVA, increased ICP, severe hypertension, and cardiac decompensation should not use these products since severe adverse reactions can occur.

Precautions: Anesthetics (general) should be used with caution in the geriatric, children <2 yr, and those with cardiovascular disease (hypotension, bradydysrhythmias), renal/hepatic disease, and Parkinson's disease. The precaution for anesthetics (local) is pregnancy.

Pharmacokinetics: Onset, peak, and duration vary widely among products. Most products are metabolized in the liver and excreted in urine.

Interactions: MAOIs, tricyclics, and phenothiazines may cause severe hypo/hypertension when used with local anesthetics. CNS depressants will potentiate general and local anesthetics.

NURSING CONSIDERATIONS
Assessment
- Monitor VS q10min during **IV** administration, q30min after IM dose

Adverse effects: *italic* = common, **bold** = life-threatening

Nursing diagnoses
General
- Injury, risk for (adverse reactions)
- Knowledge, deficient (teaching)

Local
- Pain, acute (uses)
- Knowledge, deficient (teaching)

Implementation
- Give anticholinergic preoperatively to decrease secretions
- Administer only with resuscitative equipment nearby
- Provide quiet environment for recovery to decrease psychotic symptoms

Evaluation
Positive therapeutic outcome
- Maintenance of anesthesia
- Decreased pain

Generic Names

General anesthetics:
droperidol (high alert), etomidate, fentanyl (high alert), fentanyl/droperidol, fentanyl transdermal, fospropofol, midazolam, propofol (high alert), thiopental

Local anesthetics:
⊘ lidocaine parenteral (high alert), procaine, ropivacaine, tetracaine

---

○ ANTACIDS

Action: Antacids are basic compounds that neutralize gastric acidity and decrease the rate of gastric emptying. Products are divided into those containing aluminum, magnesium, calcium, or a combination of these.

Uses: Antacids decrease hyperacidity in conditions such as peptic ulcer disease, reflux esophagitis, gastritis, or hiatal hernia.

Adverse effects: The most common side effect caused by aluminum-containing antacids is constipation, which may lead to fecal impaction and bowel obstruction. Diarrhea occurs often when magnesium products are given. Alkalosis may occur when systemic products are used. Constipation occurs more frequently than laxation with calcium carbonate. The release of CO_2 from carbonate-containing antacids causes belching, abdominal distention, and flatulence. Sodium bicarbonate may act as a systemic antacid and produce systemic electrolyte disturbances and alkalosis. Calcium carbonate and sodium bicarbonate may cause rebound hyperacidity and milk-alkali syn-

drome. Alkaluria may occur when products are used on a long-term basis, particularly in persons with abnormal renal function.

Contraindications: Sensitivity to aluminum or magnesium products may cause hypersensitive reactions. Aluminum products should not be used by persons sensitive to aluminum. Magnesium products should not be used by persons sensitive to magnesium. Check for sensitivity before administering.

Precautions: Magnesium products should be given cautiously to patients with renal insufficiency, and during pregnancy and breastfeeding. Sodium content of antacids may be significant. Use with caution for patients with hypertension, or CHF or those on a low-sodium diet.

Pharmacokinetics: Duration is 20-40 min. If ingested 1 hr after meals, acidity is reduced for at least 3 hr.

Interactions: Products whose effects may be increased by some antacids include quinidine, amphetamines, pseudoephedrine, levodopa, valproic acid, and dicumarol. Products whose effects may be decreased by some antacids include cimetidine, corticosteroids, ranitidine, iron salts, phenothiazines, phenytoin, digoxin, tetracyclines, ketoconazole, salicylates, and isoniazid.

NURSING CONSIDERATIONS
Assessment
- Assess for aggravating and alleviating factors of epigastric pain or hyperacidity; identify the location, duration, and characteristics of epigastric pain
- Assess GI symptoms, including constipation, diarrhea, abdominal pain; if severe abdominal pain with fever occurs, these products should not be given
- Assess renal symptoms, including increasing urinary pH, electrolytes

Nursing diagnoses
- Constipation (adverse reactions)
- Diarrhea (adverse reactions)
- Pain, chronic (uses)

Implementation
- Advise patient not to take other products within 1-2 hr of antacid administration, since antacids may impair absorption of other products
- Give all products with an 8-oz glass of water to ensure absorption in the stomach
- Give another antacid if constipation occurs with aluminum products

---

Evaluation
Positive therapeutic outcome
- Absence of epigastric pain
- Decreased acidity

Generic Names
aluminum hydroxide, bismuth subsalicylate, calcium carbonate, magaldrate, magnesium oxide, sodium bicarbonate

ANTI-ALZHEIMER AGENTS

Action: Anti-Alzheimer agents improve cognitive functioning by increasing acetylcholine and inhibiting cholinesterase in the CNS. They do not cure the condition, but improve symptoms.

Uses: Anti-Alzheimer agents are used for the treatment of Alzheimer's symptoms.

Adverse effects: The most common side effects are *nausea, vomiting, diarrhea, dry mouth, insomnia, dizziness, urinary frequency, incontinence,* and *rash.* The most serious side effects are **seizures** and **dysrhythmias.**

Contraindications: Persons with hypersensitivity reactions should not use these products.

Precautions: Anti-Alzheimer agents should be used cautiously in pregnancy (C), breastfeeding, sick sinus syndrome, GI bleeding, bladder obstruction, and seizures.

Pharmacokinetics: Onset, peak, and duration vary widely among products. Most products are metabolized in the liver and excreted by the kidneys.

Interactions: Increased synergistic reactions may occur with succinylcholine, cholinesterase inhibitors, and cholinergic agonists. There may be a decrease in the action of anticholinergics, and there may be additive effects when used with cholinergic agents.

NURSING CONSIDERATIONS
Assessment
- B/P, hypo/hypertension
- Mental status: affect, mood, behavioral changes, depression, confusion
- GI status: nausea, vomiting, anorexia, diarrhea
- GU status: urinary frequency, incontinence

Nursing diagnoses
- Knowledge, deficient (teaching)
- Noncompliance (teaching)
- Thought processes, disturbed (uses)

Implementation
- Give lowest possible dose for therapeutic result; adjust dose to response
- Provide assistance with ambulation during beginning therapy if dizziness, ataxia occur

Patient/family education
- Instruct patient to report side effects, adverse reactions to healthcare provider
- Advise patient to use exactly as prescribed, at regular intervals
- Caution patient not to increase or abruptly decrease dose; serious consequences may result
- Inform patient that product is not a cure, but relieves symptoms

Evaluation
Positive therapeutic outcome
- Decrease in confusion
- Improved mood

Generic Names
donepezil, galantamine, memantine, rivastigmine

ANTIANGINALS

Action: Antianginals are divided into the nitrates, calcium channel blockers, and β-adrenergic blockers. The nitrates dilate coronary arteries, causing decreased preload, and dilate systemic arteries, causing decreased afterload. Calcium channel blockers dilate coronary arteries and decrease SA/AV node conduction. β-Adrenergic blockers decrease heart rate so that myocardial O_2 use is decreased. Dipyridamole selectively dilates coronary arteries to increase coronary blood flow.

Uses: Antianginals are used in chronic stable angina pectoris, unstable angina, and vasospastic angina. Some (i.e., calcium channel blockers and β-blockers) may be used as dysrhythmics and in hypertension.

Adverse effects: The most common side effects are *postural hypotension, headache, flushing, dizziness, nausea, edema,* and *drowsiness.* Also common are *rash, dysrhythmias,* and *fatigue.*

Contraindications: Persons with known hypersensitivity, increased ICP, or cerebral hemorrhage should not use some of these products.

Adverse effects: *italic* = common, **bold** = life-threatening

Precautions: Antianginals should be used with caution in pregnancy, breastfeeding, children, postural hypotension, renal disease, and hepatic injury.

Pharmacokinetics: Onset, peak, and duration vary widely among coronary products. Most products are metabolized in the liver and excreted in urine.

Interactions: Interactions vary widely among products. Check individual monographs for specific information.

NURSING CONSIDERATIONS
Assessment
- Monitor orthostatic B/P, pulse
- Assess for pain: duration, time started, activity being performed, character
- Assess for tolerance if taken over long period
- Assess for headache, light-headedness, decreased B/P; may indicate a need for decreased dosage

Nursing diagnoses
- Cardiac output, decreased (adverse reactions)
- Injury, risk for (uses)
- Knowledge, deficient (teaching)
- Pain, acute (uses)
- Tissue perfusion, ineffective (uses)

Implementation
- Store protected from light, moisture; place in cool environment

Patient/family education
- Instruct patient to keep tabs in original container
- Instruct patient not to use OTC products unless directed by prescriber
- Advise patient to report bradycardia, dizziness, confusion, depression, fever
- Teach patient to take pulse at home; advise when to notify prescriber
- Advise patient to avoid alcohol, smoking, sodium intake
- Advise patient to comply with weight control, dietary adjustments, modified exercise program
- Teach patient to carry/wear emergency ID to identify product being taken, allergies
- Caution patient to make position changes slowly to prevent fainting

Evaluation
Positive therapeutic outcome
- Decrease, prevention of anginal pain

Generic Names
Nitrates:
isosorbide, 💿 nitroglycerin

β-*Adrenergic blockers:*
atenolol, dipyridamole, metoprolol, nadolol, propranolol

Calcium channel blockers:
amlodipine, bepridil, diltiazem (high alert), niCARdipine, NIFEdipine, 💿 verapamil

Miscellaneous:
ranolazine

ANTIANXIETY AGENTS

Action: Benzodiazepines potentiate the action of GABA, including any other inhibitory transmitters in the CNS, resulting in decreased anxiety. Most agents cause a decrease in CNS excitability.

Uses: Anxiety is relieved in conditions such as generalized anxiety disorder and phobic disorders. Benzodiazepines are also used for acute alcohol withdrawal to prevent delirium tremens, and some products are used for relaxation before surgery.

Adverse effects: The most common side effects are dizziness, drowsiness, blurred vision, and orthostatic hypotension. Most adverse reactions are mediated through the CNS. There is potential for abuse and physical dependence with some products.

Contraindications: These products are contraindicated in hypersensitivity, acute closed-angle glaucoma, breastfeeding (diazepam), children <6 mo, and hepatic disease (clonazepam).

Precautions: Antianxiety agents should be used cautiously in geriatric or debilitated patients. Usually smaller doses are needed since metabolism is slowed. Persons with renal/hepatic disease may show delayed excretion. Clonazepam may increase the incidence of seizures.

Pharmacokinetics: Most of these agents are metabolized by the liver and excreted via the kidneys.

Interactions: Increased CNS depression may occur when given with other CNS depressants. These products should be used together cautiously. Alcohol should not be used, as fatal reactions have occurred. The serum concentration and toxicity may be increased when used with benzodiazepines.

NURSING CONSIDERATIONS
Assessment
- Assess B/P (lying and standing), pulse; if systolic B/P drops 20 mm Hg, hold product and notify prescriber; orthostatic hypotension can be severe
- Monitor renal/hepatic function tests: AST, ALT, bilirubin, creatinine, LDH, alkaline phosphatase
- Monitor physical dependency and withdrawal with some products, including headache, nausea, vomiting, muscle pain, and weakness after long-term use

Nursing diagnoses
- Anxiety (uses)
- Injury, risk for, physical (adverse reactions)
- Knowledge, deficient (teaching)

Implementation
- Give with food or milk for GI symptoms; may give crushed if patient is unable to swallow whole (tabs only, no controlled or sustained-release products)

Patient/family education
- Inform patient that product should not be used for everyday stress or long-term use; not to take more than prescribed amount since product is habit forming
- Caution patient to avoid driving and activities that require alertness since drowsiness and dizziness may occur
- Instruct patient to abstain from alcohol, other psychotropic medications unless directed by prescriber
- Caution patient not to discontinue abruptly; after extended periods, withdrawal symptoms may occur

Evaluation
Positive therapeutic outcome
- Decreased anxiety
- Increased relaxation

Generic Names

Benzodiazepines:
alprazolam, chlordiazepoxide, clonazepam, diazepam, lorazepam, midazolam, oxazepine, temazepine, triazolam

Miscellaneous:
busPIRone, doxepin, hydrOXYzine, meprobamate, paroxetine, venlafaxine

ANTIASTHMATICS

Action: Bronchodilators are divided into anticholinergics, α/β-adrenergic agonists, β-adrenergic agonists, and phosphodiesterase inhibitors. Also included in antiasthmatic agents are corticosteroids, leukotriene antagonists, mast cell stabilizers, and monoclonal antibodies. Anticholinergics act by inhibiting interaction of acetylcholine at receptor sites on bronchial smooth muscle. α/β-Adrenergic agonists act by relaxing bronchial smooth muscle and increasing diameter of nasal passages. β-Adrenergic agonists act by action on β_2-receptors, which relaxes bronchial smooth muscle. Phosphodiesterase inhibitors act by blocking phosphodiesterase and increasing cAMP, which mediates smooth muscle relaxation in the respiratory system. Corticosteroids act by decreasing inflammation in the bronchial system. Leukotriene receptor antagonists decrease leukotrienes, and mast cell stabilizers decrease histamine; both act to decrease bronchospasm.

Uses: Antiasthmatics are used for bronchial asthma; bronchospasm associated with bronchitis, emphysema, or other obstructive pulmonary diseases; Cheyne-Stokes respirations; and prevention of exercise-induced asthma. Some products are used for rhinitis and other allergic reactions.

Adverse effects: The most common side effects are tremors, anxiety, nausea, vomiting and irritation in the throat. The most serious adverse reactions are bronchospasm and dyspnea.

Contraindications: Persons with hypersensitivity, closed-angle glaucoma, tachydysrhythmias, and severe cardiac disease should not use some of these products.

Precautions: Antiasthmatics should be used with caution in pregnancy, breastfeeding, hyperthyroidism, hypertension, prostatic hypertrophy, and seizure disorders.

Pharmacokinetics: Onset, peak, and duration vary widely among products. Most products are metabolized by the liver and excreted in urine.

Interactions: Interactions vary widely among products. Check individual monographs for specific information.

NURSING CONSIDERATIONS
Assessment
- Monitor respiratory function: vital capacity, forced expiratory volume, ABGs, lung sounds, heart rate and rhythm, aggravating and alleviating factors

Nursing diagnoses
- Activity intolerance (uses)
- Airway clearance, ineffective (uses)
- Injury, risk for, physical (adverse reactions)
- Knowledge, deficient (teaching)
- Noncompliance (teaching)

Implementation
- Give inhaled product after shaking; exhale, place mouthpiece in mouth, inhale slowly, hold breath, remove, exhale slowly
- Give PO product with meals to decrease gastric irritation
- Store inhaled product in light-resistant container; do not expose to temperatures >86° F (30° C)
- Give gum, small sips of water for dry mouth

Patient/family education
- Caution patient to avoid hazardous activities; drowsiness or dizziness may occur with some products
- Instruct patient to obtain bloodwork as required; some products require blood levels to be drawn
- Advise patient to avoid all OTC medications unless approved by provider
- Instruct patient to report side effects, including insomnia, heart palpitations, light-headedness; these side effects may occur with some products

Evaluation
Positive therapeutic outcome
- Decreased severity and number of asthma attacks
- Absence of dyspnea, wheezing

Generic Names

Bronchodilators:
albuterol, arformoterol, atropine (high alert), bitolterol, dyphylline, formoterol, ipratropium, isoproterenol, levalbuterol, metaproterenol, pirbuterol, terbutaline, theophylline, tiotropium

Adrenergics:
epinephrine (high alert)

Corticosteroids:
beclomethasone, betamethasone, budesonide, cortisone, dexamethasone, flunisolide, fluticasone, hydrocortisone, methylPREDNISolone, predniSONE, trimicinolone

Leukotriene antagonists:
zafirlukast

Mast cell stabilizers:
cromolyn, nedocromil

Monoclonal antibodies:
omalizumab

ANTICHOLINERGICS

Action: Anticholinergics inhibit the muscarinic actions of acetylcholine at receptor sites in the autonomic nervous system. Anticholinergics are also known as antimuscarinic products.

Uses: Anticholinergics are used for a variety of conditions: decreasing involuntary movements in parkinsonism (benztropine, trihexyphenidyl); bradydysrhythmias (atropine); nausea and vomiting (scopolamine); and as cycloplegic mydriatics (atropine, hematropine, scopalamine, cyclopentolate, tropicamide). Gastrointestinal anticholinergics are used to decrease motility (smooth muscle tone) in the GI, biliary, and urinary tracts and for their ability to decrease gastric secretions (propantheline, glycopyrrolate).

Adverse effects: The most common side effects are dry mouth, constipation, urinary retention, urinary hesitancy, headache, and dizziness. Also common is paralytic ileus.

Contraindications: Persons with closed-angle glaucoma, myasthenia gravis, or GI/GU obstruction should not use some of these products.

Precautions: Anticholinergics should be used with caution in pregnant, breastfeeding, or geriatric patients, or in those with prostatic hypertrophy, CHF, or hypertension. Use with caution in the presence of high environmental temperature.

Pharmacokinetics: Onset, peak, and duration vary widely among products. Most products are metabolized in the liver and excreted in urine.

Interactions: Increased anticholinergic effects may occur when used with MAOIs, tricyclics, and amantadine. Anticholinergics may cause a decreased effect of phenothiazines and levodopa.

NURSING CONSIDERATIONS
Assessment
- Assess I&O ratio; retention commonly causes decreased urinary output
- Assess for urinary hesitancy, retention; palpate bladder if retention occurs
- Assess for constipation; increase fluids, bulk, exercise if this occurs
- Identify tolerance over long-term therapy; dosage may need to be increased or changed
- Assess mental status: affect, mood, CNS depression, worsening of mental symptoms during early therapy

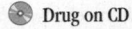

Nursing diagnoses
- Cardiac output, decreased (uses)
- Constipation (adverse reactions)
- Knowledge, deficient (teaching)

Implementation
PO route
- Give with or after meals to prevent GI upset; may give with fluids other than water
- Store at room temperature
- Give hard candy, frequent drinks, sugarless gum to relieve dry mouth

IM/IV route
- Give parenteral dose with patient recumbent to prevent postural hypotension
- Give parenteral dose slowly; keep in bed for at least 1 hr after dose; monitor VS
- Give after checking dose carefully; even slight overdose could lead to toxicity

Patient/family education
- Caution patient to avoid driving and other hazardous activities; drowsiness may occur
- Advise patient to avoid OTC medication: cough, cold preparations with alcohol, antihistamines unless directed by prescriber

Evaluation
Positive therapeutic outcome
- Decreased secretions
- Absence of nausea and vomiting

Generic Names

⬤ atropine (high alert), ⬤ benztropine, biperiden, dicyclomine, glycopyrrolate, hyoscyamine, propantheline, scopolamine (transdermal), solifenacin, trihexyphenidyl

ANTICOAGULANTS

Action: Anticoagulants interfere with blood clotting by preventing clot formation.

Uses: Anticoagulants are used for DVT, pulmonary emboli, myocardial infarction, open heart surgery, disseminated intravascular clotting syndrome, atrial fibrillation with embolization, and in transfusion and dialysis.

Adverse effects: The most serious adverse reactions are hemorrhage, agranulocytosis, leukopenia, eosinophilia, and thrombocytopenia, depending on the specific product. The most common side effects are diarrhea, rash, and fever.

Contraindications: Persons with hemophilia and related disorders, leukemia with bleeding, peptic ulcer disease, thrombocytopenic purpura, blood dyscrasias, acute nephritis, and subacute bacterial endocarditis should not use these products.

Precautions: Anticoagulants should be used with caution in pregnancy, geriatric, and alcoholism.

Pharmacokinetics: Onset, peak, and duration vary widely among products. Most products are metabolized in the liver and excreted in urine.

Interactions: Salicylates, steroids, and nonsteroidal antiinflammatories will potentiate the action of anticoagulants. Anticoagulants may cause serious effects. Check individual monographs for specific information.

NURSING CONSIDERATIONS
Assessment
- Monitor blood tests (Hct, platelets, occult blood in stools) q3mo
- Monitor PTT, which should be 1½-2 × control, PPT; daily, APTT, ACT, INR
- Monitor B/P; watch for increasing signs of hypertension
- Monitor for bleeding gums, petechiae, ecchymosis, black tarry stools, hematuria
- Monitor for fever, skin rash, urticaria
- Monitor for needed dosage change q1-2wk

Nursing diagnoses
- Injury, risk for (side effects)
- Knowledge, deficient (teaching)
- Tissue perfusion, ineffective (uses)

Implementation
- Store in tight container (PO dose)

SUBCUT route
- Give at same time each day to maintain steady blood levels
- Do not massage area or aspirate when giving SUBCUT inj; give in abdomen between pelvic bones; rotate sites; do not pull back on plunger, leave in for 10 sec; apply gentle pressure for 1 min
- Do not change needles
- Avoid all IM inj that may cause bleeding

Patient/family education
- Advise patient to avoid OTC preparations that may cause serious product interactions unless directed by prescriber
- Inform patient that product may be held during active bleeding (menstruation), depending on condition
- Caution patient to use soft-bristle toothbrush to prevent bleeding gums; avoid contact sports; use electric razor
- Instruct patient to carry/wear emergency ID identifying product taken

Adverse effects: *italic* = common, **bold** = life-threatening

• Instruct patient to report any signs of bleeding: gums, under skin, urine, stools

Evaluation
Positive therapeutic outcome
• Decrease of DVT

Generic Names

ardeparin, argatroban, **dalteparin** (high alert), danaparoid, desirudin, **enoxaparin** (high alert), fondaparinux, 🐾 **heparin** (high alert), **lepirudin** (high alert), **tinzaparin** (high alert), 🐾 **warfarin** (high alert)

ANTICONVULSANTS

Action: Anticonvulsants are divided into the barbiturates, benzodiazepines, hydantoins, succinimides, and miscellaneous products. Barbiturates and benzodiazepines are discussed in separate sections. Hydantoins act by inhibiting the spread of seizure activity in the motor cortex. Succinimides act by inhibiting spike and wave formation; they also decrease amplitude, frequency, duration, and spread of discharge in seizures.

Uses: Hydantoins are used in generalized tonic-clonic seizures, status epilepticus, and psychomotor seizures. Succinimides are used for absence (or petit mal) seizures. Barbiturates are used in generalized tonic-clonic and cortical focal seizures.

Adverse effects: Bone marrow depression is the most life-threatening adverse reaction associated with hydantoins or succinimides. The most common side effects are GI symptoms. Other common side effects for hydantoins are gingival hyperplasia and CNS effects such as nystagmus, ataxia, slurred speech, and confusion.

Contraindications: Hypersensitive reactions may occur, and allergies should be identified before these products are given.

Precautions: Persons with renal/hepatic disease should be watched closely.

Pharmacokinetics: Onset, peak, and duration vary widely among products. Most products are metabolized in the liver and excreted in urine, bile, and feces.

Interactions: Hydantoins cause decreased effects of estrogens, and oral contraceptives.

NURSING CONSIDERATIONS
Assessment
• Monitor renal function tests, including BUN, creatinine, serum uric acid, urine CCr before, during therapy
• Monitor blood tests: RBC, Hct, Hgb, reticulocyte counts weekly for 4 wk then monthly
• Monitor hepatic function tests: AST, ALT, bilirubin, creatinine
• Assess mental status, including mood, sensorium, affect, behavioral changes; if mental status changes, notify prescriber
• Assess for eye problems, including need for ophth examinations before, during, and after treatment (slit lamp, fundoscopy, tonometry)
• Assess for allergic reaction, including red, raised rash; if this occurs, product should be discontinued
• Assess for blood dyscrasias, including fever, sore throat, bruising, rash, jaundice
• Monitor toxicity, including bone marrow depression, nausea, vomiting, ataxia, diplopia, cardiovascular collapse, Stevens-Johnson syndrome

Nursing diagnoses
• Injury, risk for (uses)
• Noncompliance (teaching)
• Sleep deprivation (adverse reactions)

Implementation
PO route
• Give with food, milk to decrease GI symptoms
• Provide good oral hygiene as it is important for patients taking hydantoins

Patient/family education
• Advise patient to carry/wear emergency ID stating products taken, condition, prescriber's name, phone number
• Advise patient to avoid driving, other activities that require alertness

Evaluation
Positive therapeutic outcome
• Decreased seizure activity; document on patient's chart

Generic Names

Succinimides:
ethosuximide

Hydantoins:
fosphenytoin, 🐾 phenytoin, succinimides

Miscellaneous:
acetazolamide, carbamazepine, clonazepam, 🐾 diazepam, felbamate, gabapentin, lacosamide, lamotrigine, **magnesium sulfate** (high

alert), paraldehyde, paramethadione, phenace-mide, phenobarbitol, primidone, rufinamide, tiagabine, topiramate, valproate/valproic acid/divalproex sodium, vigabatrin, zonisamide

Barbiturates:

 phenobarbital (high alert), primidone, thiopental (high alert)

ANTIDEPRESSANTS

Action: Antidepressants are divided into the tricyclics, MAOIs, and miscellaneous antide-pressants (SSRIs). The tricyclics work by blocking reuptake of norepinephrine and serotonin into nerve endings and increasing action of norepinephrine and serotonin in nerve cells. MAOIs act by increasing concentrations of endogenous epinephrine, norepinephrine, serotonin, and dopamine in storage sites in the CNS by inhibition of MAO; increased concentra-tion reduces depression.

Uses: Antidepressants are used for depression and, in some cases, enuresis in children.

Adverse effects: The most serious adverse reactions are paralytic ileus, acute renal failure, hypertension, and hypertensive crisis, depend-ing on the specific product. Common side effects are dizziness, drowsiness, diarrhea, dry mouth, urinary retention, and orthostatic hypotension.

Contraindications: The contraindications for antidepressants are seizure disorders, prostatic hypertrophy, and severe renal/hepatic/cardiac disease depending on the type of medication.

Precautions: Antidepressants should be used cautiously in pregnant, geriatric, and suicidal patients; severe depression; schizophrenia; hyperactivity; and diabetes mellitus.

Pharmacokinetics: Onset, peak, and duration vary widely among products. Most products are metabolized in the liver and excreted in urine.

Interactions: Interactions vary widely among products. Check individual monographs for specific information.

NURSING CONSIDERATIONS
Assessment
- Monitor B/P (lying, standing), pulse q4hr; if systolic B/P drops 20 mm Hg, hold product, notify prescriber; take VS q4hr in patients with CV disease

- Monitor blood tests: CBC, leukocytes, differ-ential, cardiac enzymes if patient is receiving long-term therapy
- Monitor hepatic function tests: AST, ALT, bilirubin, creatinine
- Monitor weight weekly; appetite may increase with product
- Monitor for EPS primarily in geriatric: rigidity, dystonia, akathisia
- Assess mental status: mood, sensorium, affect, suicidal tendencies, increase in psychiat-ric symptoms (depression, panic)
- Check for urinary retention, constipation; constipation is more likely to occur in children, geriatric patients
- Assess for withdrawal symptoms: headache, nausea, vomiting, muscle pain, weakness; do not usually occur unless product was discontin-ued abruptly
- Identify alcohol consumption; if alcohol is consumed, hold dose until AM

Nursing diagnoses
- Coping, ineffective (uses)
- Injury, risk for (uses/adverse reactions)
- Knowledge, deficient (teaching)

Implementation
PO route
- Give increased fluids, bulk in diet if constipa-tion, urinary retention occur
- Give with food or milk for GI symptoms
- Give gum, hard candy, or frequent sips of water for dry mouth
- Store in airtight container at room temperature; do not refreeze
- Provide assistance with ambulation during beginning therapy since drowsiness/dizziness occurs

Patient/family education
- Teach patient that therapeutic effects may take 2-3 wk
- Advise patient to use caution in driving or other activities requiring alertness because of drowsiness, dizziness, blurred vision
- Caution patient to avoid alcohol ingestion, other CNS depressants
- Instruct patient not to discontinue medica-tion quickly after long-term use; may cause nausea, headache, malaise
- Instruct patient to wear sunscreen or large hat, since photosensitivity may occur

Evaluation
Positive therapeutic outcome
- Decreased depression

Generic Names

Tetracyclics:
mirtazapine

Tricyclics:
amitriptyline, amoxapine, clomiPRAMINE, desipramine, doxepin, imipramine, nortriptyline, trimipramine

Miscellaneous:
buPROPion, duloxetine, trazodone, venlafaxine

MAOIs:
phenelzine, tranylcypromine

SSRIs:
citalopram, escitalopram, fluoxetine, fluvoxamine, paroxetine, sertraline

---

ANTIDIABETICS

Action: Antidiabetics are divided into the insulins that decrease blood glucose, phosphate, and potassium and increase blood pyruvate and lactate and oral antidiabetics that cause functioning β-cells in the pancreas to release insulin and improve the effect of endogenous and exogenous insulin.

Uses: Insulins are used for ketoacidosis and diabetes mellitus types 1 and 2; oral antidiabetics are used for diabetes mellitus type 2.

Adverse effects: The most common side effect of insulin and oral antidiabetics is hypoglycemia. Other adverse reactions for oral antidiabetics include blood dyscrasias, hepatotoxicity, and, rarely, cholestatic jaundice. Adverse reactions for insulin products include allergic responses and, more rarely, anaphylaxis.

Contraindications: Hypersensitive reactions may occur, and allergies should be identified before these products are given. Oral antidiabetics should not be used in juvenile or brittle diabetes, diabetic ketoacidosis, or severe renal/hepatic disease.

Precautions: Oral antidiabetics should be used with caution in pregnancy, breastfeeding, geriatric, cardiac disease, and in the presence of alcohol.

Pharmacokinetics: Onset, peak, and duration vary widely among products. Oral antidiabetics are metabolized in the liver, with metabolites excreted in urine, bile, and feces.

Interactions: Interactions vary widely among products. Check individual monographs for specific information.

NURSING CONSIDERATIONS
Assessment
- Monitor blood, urine glucose levels during treatment to determine diabetes control (oral products)
- Monitor fasting blood glucose, 2 hr PP (60-100 mg/dl normal fasting level) (70-130 mg/dl—normal 2-hr level)
- Assess for hypoglycemic reaction that can occur during peak time

Nursing diagnoses
- Nutrition: more than body requirements, imbalanced (uses)

Implementation
PO route
- Give oral antidiabetic 30 min before meals
SUBCUT route
- Give insulin after warming to room temperature by rotating in palms to prevent lipodystrophy from injecting cold insulin
- Give human insulin to those allergic to beef or pork
- Rotate inj sites when giving insulin; use abdomen, upper back, thighs, upper arm, buttocks; keep a record of sites

Patient/family education
- Advise patient to avoid alcohol and salicylates except on advice of prescriber
- Teach patient symptoms of ketoacidosis: nausea, thirst, polyuria, dry mouth, decreased B/P, dry, flushed skin, acetone breath, drowsiness, Kussmaul respirations
- Teach patient symptoms of hypoglycemia: headache, tremors, fatigue, weakness; that candy or sugar should be carried to treat hypoglycemia
- Advise patient to test urine for glucose/ketones tid if this product is replacing insulin
- Advise patient to continue weight control, dietary restrictions, exercise, hygiene

Evaluation
Positive therapeutic outcome
- Decrease in polyuria, polydipsia, polyphagia
- Clear sensorium
- Absence of dizziness
- Stable gait

Generic Names

chlorproPAMIDE, glipiZIDE, glyBURIDE, **insulin aspart** (high alert), **insulin detemir** (high alert), **insulin glargine** (high alert), **insulin glulisine** (high alert), **insulin lispro** (high alert), **insulin regular** (high alert), **insulin regular concentrated** (high alert),

 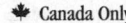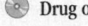

metformin, miglitol, nateglinide, pioglitazone, repaglinide, rosiglitazone, saxagliptin, sitagliptin

ANTIDIARRHEALS

Action: Antidiarrheals work by various actions including direct action on intestinal muscles to decrease GI peristalsis or by inhibiting prostaglandin synthesis responsible for GI hypermotility, acting on mucosal receptors responsible for peristalsis, or decreasing water content of stools.

Uses: Antidiarrheals are used for diarrhea of undetermined causes.

Adverse effects: The most serious adverse reactions of some products are paralytic ileus, toxic megacolon, and angioneurotic edema. The most common side effects are constipation, nausea, dry mouth, and abdominal pain.

Contraindications: The contraindications are persons with severe ulcerative colitis, and pseudomembranous colitis with some products.

Precautions: Antidiarrheals should be used with caution in pregnancy, breastfeeding, children, geriatric patients, dehydration.

Pharmacokinetics: Onset, peak, and duration vary widely among products. Most products are metabolized in the liver and excreted in urine.

Interactions: Interactions vary widely among products. Check individual monographs for specific information.

NURSING CONSIDERATIONS
Assessment
• Monitor electrolytes (potassium, sodium, chloride) if on long-term therapy
• Monitor bowel pattern before; for rebound constipation after termination of medication
• Assess response after 48 hr; if no response, product should be discontinued
• Identify dehydration in children

Nursing diagnoses
• Constipation (adverse reactions)
• Diarrhea (uses)
• Fluid volume, risk for deficient (adverse reactions)
• Knowledge, deficient (teaching)

Implementation
PO route
• Give for 48 hr only

Patient/family education
• Advise patient to avoid OTC products
• Caution patient not to exceed recommended dose

Evaluation
Positive therapeutic outcome
• Decreased diarrhea

Generic Names

bismuth subsalicylate, loperamide

ANTIDYSRHYTHMICS

Action: Antidysrhythmics are divided into four classes and miscellaneous antidysrhythmics:
• Class I increases the duration of action potential and the effective refractory period and reduces disparity in the refractory period between a normal and infarcted myocardium; further subclasses include Ia, Ib, Ic
• Class II decreases the rate of SA node discharge, increases recovery time, slows conduction through the AV node, and decreases heart rate, which decreases O_2 consumption in the myocardium
• Class III increases the duration of action potential and the effective refractory period
• Class IV inhibits calcium ion influx across the cell membrane during cardiac depolarization; decreases SA node discharge, decreases conduction velocity through the AV node
• Miscellaneous antidysrhythmics include those such as adenosine, which slows conduction through the AV node, and digoxin, which decreases conduction velocity and prolongs the effective refractory period in the AV node

Uses: Antidysrhythmics are used for PVCs, tachycardia, hypertension, atrial fibrillation, and angina pectoris.

Adverse effects: Side effects and adverse reactions vary widely among products.

Contraindications: Contraindications vary widely among products.

Precautions: Precautions vary widely among products.

Pharmacokinetics: Onset, peak, and duration vary widely among products.

Interactions: Interactions vary widely among products. Check individual monographs for specific information.

Adverse effects: *italic* = common, **bold** = life-threatening

NURSING CONSIDERATIONS
Assessment
- Monitor ECG continuously to determine product effectiveness, PVCs, or other dysrhythmias
- Assess for dehydration or hypovolemia
- Monitor B/P continuously for hypo/hypertension
- Monitor I&O ratio
- Monitor serum potassium
- Assess for edema in feet and legs daily

Nursing diagnoses
- Cardiac output, decreased (uses)
- Diarrhea (adverse reactions)
- Gas exchange, impaired (adverse reactions)
- Tissue perfusion, ineffective (uses)

Patient/family education
- Advise patient to comply with dosage schedule, even if patient is feeling better
- Instruct patient to report bradycardia, dizziness, confusion, depression, fever

Evaluation
Positive therapeutic outcome
- Decrease in B/P in hypertension
- Decreased B/P, edema, moist crackles in CHF

Generic Names

Class I:
moricizine

Class Ia:
disopyramide, procainamide, quinidine

Class Ib:
lidocaine, parenteral (high alert), mexiletine, phenytoin, tocainide

Class Ic:
flecainide, propafenone

Class II:
acebutolol, esmolol, propranolol, sotalol

Class III:
amiodarone (high alert), **dronedarone** (high alert), **ibutilide** (high alert)

Class IV:
 verapamil

Miscellaneous:
adenosine (high alert), **atropine** (high alert), **digoxin** (high alert)

Action: The antiemetics are divided into the 5-HT_3 receptor antagonists, the phenothiazines, and the miscellaneous products. The 5-HT_3 receptor antagonists work by blocking serotonin peripherally, centrally, and in the small intestine. The phenothiazines act by blocking the chemoreceptor trigger zone in the brain. The miscellaneous products work by either decreasing motion sickness or delaying gastric emptying.

Uses: Antiemetics are used to prevent nausea and vomiting due to cancer chemotherapy, radiotherapy, and surgery (5-HT_3 receptor antagonists); some of the miscellaneous products (antihistamines) work by decreasing motion sickness. Most other products are used for many types of nausea and vomiting.

Adverse effects: The most common side effects are headache, dizziness, fatigue, and diarrhea.

Contraindications: Persons developing hypersensitive reactions should not use these products.

Precautions: Antiemetics should be used cautiously in pregnancy, breastfeeding, hepatic disease, and some GI disorders.

Pharmacokinetics: Onset, peak, and duration vary widely among products. Most products are metabolized by the liver and excreted by the kidneys.

Interactions: Interactions vary widely among products. Check individual monographs for specific information. Other CNS depressants increase CNS depression.

NURSING CONSIDERATIONS
Assessment
- Assess reason for nausea, vomiting; absence of nausea and vomiting after giving product
- Monitor hypersensitivity reactions: rash, bronchospasm with some products

Nursing diagnoses
- Fluid volume, risk for deficient (uses)
- Injury, risk for, physical (uses, adverse reactions)
- Knowledge, deficient (teaching)
- Nutrition: less than body requirements, imbalanced (uses)

Implementation
- Give prophylactically, before nausea and vomiting occur, in cancer chemotherapy
- Store at room temperature vial/ampules, oral products

Patient/family education

- Caution patient to avoid hazardous activities if dizziness occurs; ask for assistance if hospitalized
- Instruct patient to rise slowly to prevent orthostatic hypotension
- Teach patient all aspects of product usage
- Teach patient conservative methods to control nausea and vomiting such as sips of water or other fluids and dry crackers

Evaluation
Positive therapeutic outcome
- Absence or decreasing nausea and vomiting after use

Generic Names

5-HT₃ antagonists:
dolasetron, granisetron, ondansetron, palonosetron

Phenothiazines:
⊕ chlorproMAZINE, prochlorperazine, promethazine, thiethylperazine

Miscellaneous:
aprepitant, dimenhyDRINATE, meclizine, metoclopramide, scopolamine, trimethobenzamide

ANTIFUNGALS (SYSTEMIC)

Action: Antifungals act by increasing cell membrane permeability in susceptible organisms by binding sterols and decreasing potassium, sodium, and nutrients in the cell.

Uses: Antifungals are used for infections of histoplasmosis, blastomycosis, coccidioidomycosis, cryptococcosis, aspergillosis, phycomycosis, candidiasis, sporotrichosis causing severe meningitis, septicemia, and skin infections.

Adverse effects: The most serious adverse reactions include renal tubular acidosis, permanent renal impairment, anuria, oliguria, hemorrhagic gastroenteritis, acute liver failure, and blood dyscrasias. Some common side effects include hypokalemia, nausea, vomiting, anorexia, headache, fever, and chills.

Contraindications: Persons with severe bone marrow depression or hypersensitivity should not use these products.

Precautions: Antifungals should be used with caution in renal/hepatic disease and pregnancy.

Pharmacokinetics: Onset, peak, and duration vary widely among products. Most products are metabolized in the liver and excreted in urine.

Interactions: Interactions vary widely among products. Check individual monographs for specific information.

NURSING CONSIDERATIONS
Assessment
- Monitor VS q15-30min during first infusion; note changes in pulse, B/P
- Monitor I&O ratio; watch for decreasing urinary output, change in specific gravity; discontinue product to prevent permanent damage to renal tubules
- Monitor blood tests; CBC, potassium, sodium, calcium, magnesium q2wk
- Monitor weight weekly; if weight increases over 2 lb/wk, edema is present; renal damage should be considered
- Assess for renal toxicity: increasing BUN, if >40 mg/dl or if serum creatinine >3 mg/dl; product may be discontinued or dosage reduced
- Assess for hepatotoxicity: increasing AST, ALT, alkaline phosphatase, bilirubin
- Assess for allergic reaction: dermatitis, rash; product should be discontinued; antihistamines (mild reaction) or epINEPHrine (severe reaction) administered
- Assess for hypokalemia: anorexia, drowsiness, weakness, decreased reflexes, dizziness, increased urinary output, increased thirst, paresthesias
- Assess for ototoxicity: tinnitus (ringing, roaring in ears), vertigo, loss of hearing (rare)

Nursing diagnoses
- Infection, risk for (uses)
- Injury, risk for (adverse reactions)
- Knowledge, deficient (teaching)

Implementation
IV route
- Give by **IV** using in-line filter (mean pore diameter >1 μm) using distal veins; check for extravasation, necrosis q8hr
- Give product only after C&S confirms organism, make sure product is used in life-threatening infections
- Provide protection from light during infusion; cover with foil
- Give symptomatic treatment as ordered for adverse reactions: aspirin, antihistamines, antiemetics, antispasmodics
- Store protected from moisture and light; diluted sol is stable for 24 hr

Patient/family education
• Teach patient that long-term therapy may be needed to clear infection (2 wk-3 mo depending on type of infection)

Evaluation
Positive therapeutic outcome
• Decreased fever, malaise, rash
• Negative C&S for infecting organism

Generic Names
amphotericin B, anidulafungin, caspofungin, fluconazole, griseofulvin, itraconazole, ketoconazole, micafungin, nystatin, posaconazole, voriconazole

---

ANTIHISTAMINES

Action: Antihistamines compete with histamines for H_1 receptor sites. They antagonize in varying degrees most of the pharmacologic effects of histamines.

Uses: Antihistamines are used to control the symptoms of allergies, rhinitis, and pruritus.

Adverse effects: Most products cause drowsiness; however, two of the newer products, loratadine and fexofenadine, produce little, if any, drowsiness. Other common side effects are headache and thickening of bronchial secretions. Serious blood dyscrasias may occur, but are rare. Urinary retention, GI effects occur with many of these products.

Contraindications: Hypersensitivity to H_1-receptor antagonists occurs rarely. Patients with acute asthma and lower respiratory tract disease should not use these products since thick secretions may result. Other contraindications include closed-angle glaucoma, bladder neck obstruction, stenosing peptic ulcer, symptomatic prostatic hypertrophy, breastfeeding, and in the newborn.

Precautions: Antihistamines must be used cautiously in conjunction with intraocular pressure since they increase intraocular pressure. Caution should also be used in pregnancy, breastfeeding, and geriatric patients and patients with renal/cardiac disease, hypertension, and seizure disorders.

Pharmacokinetics: Onset varies from 20-60 min, with duration lasting 4-12 hr. In general, pharmacokinetics vary widely among products.

Interactions: Barbiturates, opioids, hypnotics, tricyclics, and alcohol can increase CNS depression when taken with antihistamines.

NURSING CONSIDERATIONS
Assessment
• Check I&O ratio; be alert for urinary retention, frequency, dysuria; product should be discontinued if these occur
• Assess for blood dyscrasias: thrombocytopenia, agranulocytosis (rare)
• Assess for respiratory status, including rate, rhythm, increase in bronchial secretions, wheezing, chest tightness
• Assess for cardiac status, including palpitations, increased pulse, hypotension
• Assess CBC during long-term therapy, since hemolytic anemia, although rare, may occur
• Administer with food or milk to decrease GI symptoms; absorption may be decreased slightly
• Administer whole (sus rel tab)
• Provide hard candy, gum, frequent rinsing of mouth for dryness

Nursing diagnoses
• Airway clearance, ineffective (uses)

Patient/family education
• Advise patient to notify prescriber if confusion, sedation, hypotension occur
• Caution patient to avoid driving and other hazardous activity if drowsiness occurs
• Instruct patient to avoid concurrent use of alcohol and other CNS depressants
• Inform patient to discontinue a few days before skin testing

Evaluation
Positive therapeutic outcome
• Absence of allergy symptoms, itching

Generic Names
brompheniramine, budesonide, cetirizine, chlorpheniramine, cyproheptadine, desloratadine, 🔵 diphenhydrAMINE, fexofenadine, levocetirizine, loratadine, promethazine

---

ANTIHYPERTENSIVES

Action: Antihypertensives are divided into angiotensin converting enzyme (ACE) inhibitors, β-adrenergic blockers, calcium channel blockers, centrally acting adrenergics, diuretics, peripherally acting antiadrenergics, and vasodilators. β-Blockers, calcium channel blockers, and diuretics are discussed in separate sections. ACE inhibitors selectively suppress conversion of renin-angiotensin I to angiotensin II; dilatation of arterial and venous vessels occurs. Centrally acting adrenergics act by inhibiting the sympathetic vasomotor center in the CNS, which reduces impulses in the sympathetic nervous system; blood pressure, pulse rate, and cardiac output decrease. Peripherally acting antiadrenergics inhibit sympathetic vasoconstriction by inhibiting release of norepinephrine and/or depleting norepinephrine stores in adrenergic nerve endings. Vasodilators act on arteriolar smooth muscle by producing direct relaxation or vasodilatation; a reduction in blood pressure, with concomitant increases in heart rate and cardiac output, occurs.

Uses: Antihypertensives are used for hypertension and for heart failure not responsive to conventional therapy. Some products are used in hypertensive crisis, angina, and for some cardiac dysrhythmias.

Adverse effects: The most common side effects are marked hypotension, bradycardia, tachycardia, headache, nausea, and vomiting. Side effects and adverse reactions may vary widely between classes and specific products.

Contraindications: Hypersensitive reactions may occur, and allergies should be identified before these products are given. Antihypertensives should not be used in children or in patients with heart block.

Precautions: Antihypertensives should be used with caution in geriatric and dialysis patients, and in the presence of hypovolemia, leukemia, and electrolyte imbalances.

Pharmacokinetics: Onset, peak, and duration vary widely among products. Most products are metabolized in the liver, with metabolites excreted in urine, bile, and feces.

Interactions: Interactions vary widely among products. Check individual monographs for specific information.

NURSING CONSIDERATIONS
Assessment
• Monitor blood tests: neutrophil; decreased platelets occur with many of the products
• Monitor renal function tests: protein, BUN, creatinine; watch for increased levels, which may indicate nephrotic syndrome; obtain baselines in renal/hepatic function tests before beginning treatment
• Assess for edema in feet and legs daily
• Identify allergic reaction, including rash, fever, pruritus, urticaria: product should be discontinued if antihistamines fail to help

• Identify symptoms of CHF: edema, dyspnea, wet crackles, B/P
• Assess for renal symptoms: polyuria, oliguria, frequency

Nursing diagnoses
• Cardiac output, decreased (uses)
• Diarrhea (adverse reactions)
• Gas exchange, impaired (adverse reactions)
• Tissue perfusion, ineffective (uses)

Implementation
• Place patient in supine or Trendelenburg position for severe hypotension

Patient/family education
• Instruct patient to comply with dosage schedule, even if feeling better
• Advise patient to rise slowly to sitting or standing position to minimize orthostatic hypotension

Evaluation
Positive therapeutic outcome
• Decrease in B/P in hypertension
• Decreased B/P, edema, moist crackles in CHF

Generic Names

Aldosterone receptor antagonist:
eplerone

Angiotensin-converting enzyme inhibitors:
benazepril, enalapril, fosinopril, lisinopril, quinapril, ramipril, trandolapril

Angiotensin II receptor blockers:
candesartan, eprosartan, irbesartan, losartan, olmesartan, telmisartan, valsartan

Centrally acting adrenergics:
clonidine, methyldopa

Peripherally acting antiadrenergics:
doxazosin, prazosin, terazosin

Vasodilators:
ambrisentan, diazoxide, fenoldopam, hydrALAZINE, minoxidil, nitroprusside (high alert)

Antiadrenergic: Combined α/β-blocker:
labetalol

Direct renin inhibitors:
aliskiren

ANTIINFECTIVES

Action: Antiinfectives are divided into several groups, which include but are not limited to penicillins, cephalosporins, aminoglycosides, sulfonamides, tetracyclines, monobactam, erythromycins, and quinolones. These products inhibit the growth and replication of susceptible bacterial organisms.

Uses: Antiinfectives are used for infections of susceptible organisms. These products are effective against bacterial, rickettsial, and spirochete infections.

Adverse effects: The most common side effects are nausea, vomiting, and diarrhea. Adverse reactions include bone marrow depression and anaphylaxis.

Contraindications: Hypersensitive reactions may occur, and allergies should be identified before these products are given. Cross-sensitivity can occur between products of different classes (penicillins or cephalosporins). Often persons allergic to penicillins are also allergic to cephalosporins.

Precautions: Antiinfectives should be used with caution in persons with renal/hepatic disease.

Pharmacokinetics: Onset, peak, and duration vary widely among products. Most products are metabolized in the liver. Metabolites are excreted in urine, bile, and feces.

Interactions: Interactions vary widely among products. Check individual monographs for specific information.

NURSING CONSIDERATIONS
Assessment
- Assess for nephrotoxicity: increased BUN, creatinine
- Monitor blood tests: AST, ALT, CBC, Hct, bilirubin; test monthly if patient is on long-term therapy
- Monitor bowel pattern daily; if severe diarrhea occurs, product should be discontinued
- Monitor urine output; if decreasing, notify prescriber; may indicate nephrotoxicity
- Assess for allergic reaction: rash, fever, pruritus, urticaria; product should be discontinued
- Assess for bleeding: ecchymosis, bleeding gums, hematuria, stool guaiac daily
- Assess for overgrowth of infection: perineal itching, fever, malaise, redness, pain, swelling, drainage, rash, diarrhea, change in cough, sputum

Nursing diagnoses
- Diarrhea (adverse reactions)
- Infection, risk for (uses)

Implementation
- Give for 10-14 days to ensure organism death, prevention of superinfection
- Give after C&S completed; product may be taken as soon as culture is obtained

Patient/family education
- Teach patient to comply with dosage schedule, even if feeling better
- Advise patient to report sore throat, bruising, bleeding, joint pain; may indicate blood dyscrasias (rare)

Evaluation
Positive therapeutic outcome
- Absence of fever, fatigue, malaise, draining wounds

Generic Names

Aminoglycosides:
amikacin, azithromycin, clarithromycin, gentamicin, kanamycin, neomycin, streptomycin, tobramycin

Cephalosporins:
cefaclor, cefadroxil, cefazolin, cefdinir, cefditoren, cefepime, cefixime, cefonicid, cefoperazone, cefotaxime, cefprozil, ceftibuten, cefuroxime, cephalexin, cephapirin, cephradine

Fluoroquinolones:
ciprofloxacin, enoxacin, gemifloxacin, levofloxacin, lomefloxacin, norfloxacin, ofloxacin, sparfloxacin

Ketolides:
telithromycin

Miscellaneous:
adefovir dipivoxil, daptomycin, doripenem, ertapenem, meropenem, peginterferon alfa-2a, telavancin, vancomycin

Penicillins:
amoxicillin/clavulanate, ampicillin/sulbactam, cloxacillin, dicloxacillin, imipenem/cilastatin, mezlocillin, nafcillin, oxacillin, penicillin G benzathine, penicillin G, penicillin G procaine, penicillin V, piperacillin, ticarcillin, ticarcillin/clavulanate

Sulfonamides:
sulfasalazine, sulfiSOXAZOLE

Tetracyclines:
demeclocycline, doxycycline, minocycline, tetracycline

ANTILIPIDEMICS

Action: Antilipidemics are divided into three categories or subclassifications; HMG-CoA reductase inhibitors (statins), bile acid sequestrants, and miscellaneous products. The HMG-CoA reductase inhibitors work by reduction of

 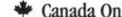

an enzyme that is responsible for the beginning step in cholesterol production. Bile acid sequestrants work by binding cholesterol in the GI system. The miscellaneous products work by various actions.

Uses: Primary hypercholesterolemia in individuals as an adjunct with other lifestyle changes.

Adverse effects: The most common side effects are headache, dizziness, fatigue, insomnia, peripheral edema, dysrhythmias, sinusitis, pharyngitis, abdominal pain, diarrhea, constipation, flatulence, and back pain.

Contraindications: Persons breastfeeding (some products) or those with hypersensitivity to any product or severe hepatic disease should not take these products. Antilipidemics are identified as pregnancy category **X** on some products.

Precautions: Some products are identified as pregnancy category **C**.

Pharmacokinetics: Pharmacokinetics and pharmacodynamics vary with each product.

Interactions: Interactions vary widely among products. Check individual monographs for specific information.

NURSING CONSIDERATIONS
Assessment
• Obtain a diet and lifestyle history, including exercise, smoking, alcohol, and stress-related activities

Nursing diagnoses
• Constipation (adverse reactions)
• Diarrhea (adverse reactions)
• Knowledge, deficient (teaching)
• Noncompliance (teaching)

Implementation
• Give as directed by health care provider; times will vary with medication used
• Provide protection from sunlight and heat

Patient/family education
• Teach patient all aspects of medication use
• Instruct patient to combine medication with lifestyle changes, including low-cholesterol diet, decreasing LDL in diet; avoid smoking, alcohol, and sedentary daily routine

Evaluation
Positive therapeutic outcome
• Decrease in triglycerides and LDL cholesterol levels

Generic Names
HMG-CoA reductase inhibitors:
atorvastatin, fluvastatin, ⊗ lovastatin, pitavastatin, pravastatin, rosovastatin, simvastatin

Bile acid sequestrants:
cholestyramine, colesevelam, colestipol

Miscellaneous:
ezetimibe, fenofibrate, fenofibric acid, gemfibrozil, niacin, niacinamide

---

ANTINEOPLASTICS

Action: Antineoplastics are divided into alkylating agents, antimetabolites, antibiotic agents, hormonal agents, and miscellaneous agents. Alkylating agents act by cross-linking strands of DNA. Antimetabolites act by inhibiting DNA synthesis. Antibiotic agents act by inhibiting RNA synthesis and by delaying or inhibiting mitosis. Hormones alter the effect of androgens, luteinizing hormone, follicle-stimulating hormone, or estrogen by changing the hormonal environment.

Uses: Antineoplastics vary widely among products and classes of products. They are used to treat leukemia, Hodgkin's disease, lymphomas, and other tumors throughout the body.

Adverse effects: Most products cause thrombocytopenia, leukopenia, and anemia. If these reactions occur, the product may need to be stopped until the problem is corrected. Other side effects include nausea, vomiting, glossitis, and hair loss. Some products also cause hepatotoxicity, nephrotoxicity, and cardiotoxicity.

Contraindications: Hypersensitive reactions may occur, and allergies should be identified before these products are given. Also, persons with severe renal/hepatic disease should not use these products unless the benefits outweigh the risks.

Precautions: Persons with bleeding, severe bone marrow depression, or renal/hepatic disease should be watched closely.

Pharmacokinetics: Onset, peak, and duration vary widely among products. Most products cross the placenta and are excreted in breast milk and in urine.

Interactions: Toxicity may occur when used with other antineoplastics or radiation.

Adverse effects: *italic* = common, **bold** = life-threatening

NURSING CONSIDERATIONS

Assessment

- Monitor CBC, differential, platelet count weekly; withhold product if WBC is <4000 or platelet count is <75,000; notify prescriber of results
- Monitor renal function tests: BUN, creatinine, serum uric acid, and urine creatinine clearance before, during therapy
- Monitor I&O ratio; report fall in urine output of 30 ml/hr
- Monitor temp q4hr (may indicate beginning infection)
- Monitor hepatic function tests before, during therapy (bilirubin, AST, ALT, LDH) monthly or as needed
- Assess for bleeding, including hematuria, guaiac, bruising or petechiae, mucosa, or orifices q8hr; obtain prescription for viscous lidocaine (Xylocaine)
- Identify jaundice of skin, sclera, dark urine, clay-colored stools, itchy skin, abdominal pain, fever, diarrhea
- Assess for edema in feet, joint pain, stomach pain, shaking
- Assess for inflammation of mucosa, breaks in skin

Nursing diagnoses

- Infection, risk for (adverse reactions)
- Nutrition: less than body requirements, imbalanced (adverse reactions)
- Oral mucous membrane, impaired (adverse reactions)

Implementation

- Check **IV** site for irritation; phlebitis
- Have epINEPHrine available for hypersensitivity reaction
- Give antibiotics for prophylaxis of infection
- Provide strict medical asepsis, protective isolation if WBC levels are low
- Provide comprehensive oral hygiene, using careful technique and soft-bristle brush

Patient/family education

- Advise patient to report signs of infection, including increased temp, sore throat, malaise
- Instruct patient to report signs of anemia, including fatigue, headache, faintness, shortness of breath, irritability
- Instruct patient to report bleeding and to avoid use of razors and commercial mouthwash

Evaluation

Positive therapeutic outcome
- Decreased tumor size

Generic Names

Alkylating agents:
bendamustine, **busulfan** (high alert), **carboplatin** (high alert), **carmustine** (high alert), chlorambucil, **cisplatin** (high alert), 🔘 **cyclophosphamide** (high alert), **dacarbazine** (high alert), lomustine, mechlorethamine, **melphalan** (high alert), oxaliplatin, thiotepa

Antimetabolites:
capecitabine, **cytarabine** (high alert), decitabine, **etoposide** (high alert), fludarabine, **fluorouracil** (high alert), mercaptopurine, 🔘 **methotrexate** (high alert), pemetrexed, pralatrexate, thioguanine (6-TG)

Antibiotic agents:
🔘 **bleomycin** (high alert), **dactinomycin** (high alert), **DAUNOrubicin** (high alert), **DOXOrubicin** (high alert), **epirubicin** (high alert), **mitomycin** (high alert), **mitoxantrone** (high alert), plicamycin

Hormonal agents:
aminoglutethimide, estramustine, flutamide, fulvestrant, goserelin, **irinotecan** (high alert), **leuprolide** (high alert), megestrol, mitotane, nilutamide, tamoxifen, testolactone, **topotecan** (high alert)

Miscellaneous agents:
alemtuzumab, anastrozole, arsenic trioxide, **asparaginase** (high alert), azacitidine, bortezomib, cetuximab, cladribine, dasatinib, erlotinib, gefitinib, gemcitabine, ibritumomab, imatinib, interferon alfa-2a, interferon alfa-2b, irinotecan, ixabepilone, lapatinib, nilotinib, panitumumab, **pentostatin** (high alert), porfimer, procarbazine, ranibizumab, rituximab, sunitinib, **vinBLAStine** (high alert), 🔘 **vinCRIStine** (high alert), **vinorelbine** (high alert)

ANTIPARKINSONIAN AGENTS

Action: Antiparkinsonian agents are divided into cholinergics, dopamine agonists, and monoamine oxidase type B. Cholinergics work by blocking or competing at central acetylcholine receptors. Dopamine agonists work by decarboxylation to dopamine or by activation of dopamine receptors. Monoamine oxidase type B inhibitors increase dopamine activity by inhibiting MAO type B activity.

Uses: Antiparkinson agents are used alone or in combination for patients with Parkinson's disease.

Adverse effects: Side effects and adverse reactions vary widely among products. The most common side effects include involuntary movements, headache, numbness, insomnia, nightmares, nausea, vomiting, dry mouth, and orthostatic hypotension.

Contraindications: Persons with hypersensitivity, closed-angle glaucoma, and undiagnosed skin lesions should not use these products.

Precautions: Antiparkinsonian agents should be used with caution in pregnancy, breastfeeding, children, renal/cardiac/hepatic disease, and affective disorder.

Pharmacokinetics: Onset, peak, and duration vary widely among products. Most products are metabolized in the liver and excreted in urine.

Interactions: Interactions vary widely among products. Check individual monographs for specific information.

NURSING CONSIDERATIONS
Assessment
- Monitor B/P, respiration
- Assess mental status: affect, behavioral changes, depression, complete suicide assessment

Nursing diagnoses
- Injury, risk for (uses)
- Knowledge, deficient (teaching)
- Mobility, impaired physical (uses)

Implementation
- Give product up until NPO before surgery
- Adjust dosage depending on patient response
- Give with meals; limit protein taken with product
- Give only after MAOIs have been discontinued for 2 wk
- Assist with ambulation during beginning therapy if needed
- Test for diabetes mellitus and acromegaly if on long-term therapy

Patient/family education
- Advise patient to change positions slowly to prevent orthostatic hypotension
- Instruct patient to report side effects: twitching, eye spasm; indicate overdose
- Advise patient to use product exactly as prescribed; if product is discontinued abruptly, parkinsonian crisis may occur

Evaluation
Positive therapeutic outcome
- Decrease in akathisia
- Improvement in mood

Generic Names

amantadine, apomorphine, benztropine, bromocriptine, cabergoline, carbidopa-levodopa, levodopa, pramipexole, rasagiline, selegiline, tolcapone, trihexyphenidyl

ANTIPLATELETS

Action: The antiplatelets are divided into the platelet aggregation inhibitors, platelet adhesion inhibitors, and the glycoprotein IIb, IIIa inhibitors. The platelet aggregation inhibitors work by action on thrombin; the platelet adhesion inhibitors work by inhibition of phosphodiesterase; and the glycoprotein IIb, IIIa inhibitors work by preventing fibrin from binding to glycoprotein IIb, IIIa receptors.

Uses: Antiplatelets are used to prevent myocardial infarction and stroke; other products are used for coronary syndromes.

Adverse effects: The most common side effects are headache, dizziness, bleeding, and diarrhea.

Contraindications: Persons developing hypersensitive reactions should not use these products.

Precautions: Antiplatelets should be used cautiously in pregnancy, breastfeeding, and bleeding disorders.

Pharmacokinetics: Onset, peak, and duration vary widely among products. Most products are metabolized by the liver and excreted by the kidneys.

Interactions: Interactions vary widely among products. Check individual monographs for specific information.

NURSING CONSIDERATIONS
Assessment
- Assess reason for use of these products
- Monitor hypersensitivity reactions with some products
- Monitor bleeding from orifices, stool urine
- Monitor blood tests: platelets, Hgb, Hct, PT/APTT, and INR

Nursing diagnoses
- Injury, risk for, physical (uses, adverse reactions)
- Knowledge, deficient (teaching)

Implementation
- Give with heparin or other aspirin (some products)

Adverse effects: *italic* = common, **bold** = life-threatening

- Store at room temperature vial/ampules, oral products

Patient/family education
- Caution patient to avoid hazardous activities if drowsiness, dizziness occurs; ask for assistance if hospitalized
- Teach patient all aspects of product usage

Evaluation
Positive therapeutic outcome
- Absence of MI, stroke, or other coronary syndromes

Generic Names

Platelet aggregation inhibitors:
cilostazol, clopidogrel, ticlopidine

Platelet adhesion inhibitors:
dipyridamole

Glycoprotein IIb, IIIa inhibitors:
eptifibatide (high alert), tirofiban (high alert)

ANTIPSYCHOTICS

Action: Antipsychotics/neuroleptics are divided into several subgroups: phenothiazines, thioxanthenes, butyrophenones, dibenzoxazepines, dibenzodiazepines, and indolones and other heterocyclic compounds. Although chemically different, these subgroups share many pharmacologic and clinical properties. All antipsychotics work to block postsynaptic dopamine receptors in the brain that are responsible for psychotic behavior, including hallucinations, delusions, and paranoia.

Uses: Antipsychotic behavior is decreased in conditions such as schizophrenia, paranoia, and mania. These agents are also effective for severe anxiety, intractable hiccups, nausea, vomiting, behavioral problems in children, and for relaxation before surgery.

Adverse effects: The most common side effects include EPS such as pseudoparkinsonism, akathisia, dystonia, and tardive dyskinesia, which may be controlled by use of antiparkinsonian agents. Serious adverse reactions such as hypotension, agranulocytosis, cardiac arrest, and laryngospasm have occurred. Other common side effects include dry mouth and photosensitivity.

Contraindications: Persons with liver damage, severe hypertension or coronary disease, cerebral arteriosclerosis, blood dyscrasias, bone marrow depression, parkinsonism, severe depression, or closed-angle glaucoma; children <12 yr; or persons withdrawing from alcohol or barbiturates should not use antipsychotics until these conditions are corrected.

Precautions: Caution must be used when antipsychotics are given to geriatric patients, since metabolism is slowed and adverse reactions can occur rapidly. Renal/hepatic disease may cause poor metabolism and excretion of the product. Seizure threshold is decreased with these products; increases in the dose of anticonvulsants may be required. Persons with diabetes mellitus, prostatic hypertrophy, chronic respiratory disease, and peptic ulcer disease should be monitored closely.

Pharmacokinetics: Onset, peak, and duration vary widely with different products and routes. Products are metabolized by the liver, are excreted in urine as metabolites, are highly bound to plasma proteins, cross the placenta, and enter breast milk. Half-life can be extended over 3 days.

Interactions: Because other CNS depressants can cause oversedation, these combinations should be used carefully. Anticholinergics may decrease the therapeutic actions of phenothiazines and also cause increased anticholinergic effects.

NURSING CONSIDERATIONS
Assessment
- Monitor bilirubin, CBC, hepatic function tests monthly, since these products are metabolized in the liver and excreted in urine
- Monitor I&O ratio: palpate bladder if low urinary output occurs, since urinary retention occurs with many of these products
- Assess affect, orientation, LOC, reflexes, gait, coordination, sleep pattern disturbances
- Assess dizziness, faintness, palpitations, tachycardia on rising
- Check B/P with patient lying and standing; wide fluctuations between lying and standing B/P may require dosage or product change, since orthostatic hypotension is occurring
- Assess for EPS, including akathisia, tardive dyskinesia, pseudoparkinsonism

Nursing diagnoses
- Sensory perception, disturbed (uses)
- Thought processes, disturbed (uses)

Implementation
- Give antiparkinsonian agent if EPS occur
- Administer liquid conc mixed in glass of juice or cola since taste is unpleasant; avoid contact with skin when preparing liquid conc or parenteral medications

 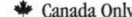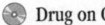

- Supervise ambulation until stabilized on medication; do not involve in strenuous exercise program, since fainting is possible; patient should not stand still for long periods
- Increase fluids to prevent constipation
- Give sips of water, candy, gum for dry mouth
- Patient should remain lying down for at least 30 min after IM inj

Patient/family education

- Advise patient to rise from sitting or lying position gradually, since fainting may occur
- Caution patient to avoid hot tubs, hot showers, or tub baths, since hypotension may occur
- Advise patient to wear sunscreen or protective clothing to prevent burns
- Advise patient to take extra precautions during hot weather to stay cool; heat stroke can occur
- Caution patient to avoid driving and other activities requiring alertness until response to medication is known
- Inform patient that drowsiness or impaired mental/motor activity is evident the first 2 wk, but tends to decrease over time

Evaluation
Positive therapeutic outcome

- Decrease in excitement, hallucinations, delusions, paranoia
- Reorganization of thought patterns, speech

Generic Names

Phenothiazines:
🔘 chlorproMAZINE, fluphenazine, perphenazine, prochlorperazine, thioridazine, thiothixene, trifluoperazine

Butyrophenone:
haloperidol

Miscellaneous:
aripiprazole, asenapine, iloperidone, loxapine, olanzapine, paliperidone, quetiapine, risperidone, ziprasidone

ANTIPYRETICS

Action: The antipyretics act on the CNS to control fever and also inhibit prostaglandin production.

Uses: Antipyretics are used to decrease fever.

Adverse effects: The most common side effects are nausea, vomiting, and rash.

Contraindications: Persons developing hypersensitive reactions should not use these products.

Precautions: Antipyretics should be used cautiously in pregnancy, breastfeeding, geriatric patients, hepatic disease, and those with certain GI disorders.

Pharmacokinetics: Onset, peak, and duration vary widely among products. Most products are metabolized by the liver and excreted by the kidneys.

Interactions: Interactions vary widely among products. Check individual monographs for specific information.

NURSING CONSIDERATIONS
Assessment

- Monitor temp frequently
- Assess reason for use and expected outcome
- Monitor hypersensitivity reactions: rash, bronchospasm with some products

Nursing diagnoses

- Injury, risk for, physical (uses, adverse reactions)
- Knowledge, deficient (teaching)

Implementation

- Give around the clock to keep fever reduced
- Store at room temperature

Patient/family education

- Teach patient all aspects of product usage

Evaluation
Positive therapeutic outcome

- Absence or decreasing fever after use

Generic Names

🔘 acetaminophen, 🔘 aspirin, choline/magnesium salicylates, choline salicylate, 🔘 ibuprofen, ketoprofen, magnesium salicylate, naproxen, salsalate

ANTIRETROVIRALS

Action: Antiretrovirals act by blocking DNA synthesis.

Uses: Antiretrovirals are used in HIV infections to slow the progression of the disease.

Adverse effects: The most common side effects are nausea, vomiting, anorexia, headache, and diarrhea. The most serious adverse reactions are nephrotoxicity and blood dyscrasias.

Contraindications: Persons with hypersensitivity should not use these products.

Precautions: Antiretrovirals should be used cautiously in pregnancy, breastfeeding, and renal/hepatic disease. Protease inhibitors should be used cautiously in diabetes.

Pharmacokinetics: Onset, peak, and duration vary widely among products. Most products are metabolized by the liver and excreted by the kidneys.

Interactions: Interactions vary widely among products. Check individual monographs for specific information.

NURSING CONSIDERATIONS
Assessment
• Monitor for signs of HIV infection: increased CD4 counts, decreased viral load
• Monitor patients with compromised renal system; since product is excreted slowly in poor renal system function, toxicity may occur rapidly

Nursing diagnoses
• Infection, risk for (uses)
• Injury, risk for (adverse reactions)
• Knowledge, deficient (teaching)
• Noncompliance (teaching)

Implementation
• Give in equal intervals around the clock
• Store at room temperature

Patient/family education
• Instruct patient to report sore throat, fever, fatigue; may indicate superinfection
• Caution patient that product does not cure condition or prevent infecting others, but controls symptoms
• Instruct patient that product must be taken around the clock, in equal intervals to maintain blood levels for duration of therapy
• Instruct patient to notify prescriber of side effects such as bruising, bleeding, fatigue, malaise; may indicate blood dyscrasias

Evaluation
Positive therapeutic outcome
• Decreased viral load
• Increased CD4 count
• Improvement in the symptoms of HIV/AIDS

Generic Names

Nonnucleoside reverse transcriptase inhibitors:
delavirdine, efavirenz, etravirine, nevirapine

Nucleoside reverse transcriptase inhibitors:
abacavir, didanosine, emtricitabine, lamivudine, stavudine, tenofovir, zalcitabine, 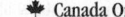 zidovudine

Protease inhibitors:
amprenavir, atazanavir, fosamprenavir, indinavir, nelfinavir, ritonavir, saquinavir, tipranavir

Fusion inhibitors:
enfuvirtide

Miscellaneous:
raltegravir

ANTITUBERCULARS

Action: Antituberculars act by inhibiting RNA or DNA, or interfering with lipid and protein synthesis, thereby decreasing tubercle bacilli replication.

Uses: Antituberculars are used for pulmonary tuberculosis.

Adverse effects: Adverse effects vary widely among products. Most products can cause nausea, vomiting, anorexia, and rash. Serious adverse reactions include renal failure, nephrotoxicity, ototoxicity, and hepatic necrosis.

Contraindications: Persons with severe renal disease or hypersensitivity should not use these products.

Precautions: Antituberculars should be used with caution in pregnancy, breastfeeding, and hepatic disease.

Pharmacokinetics: Onset, peak, and duration vary widely among products. Most products are metabolized in the liver and excreted in urine.

Interactions: Interactions vary widely among products. Check individual monographs for specific information.

NURSING CONSIDERATIONS
Assessment
• Assess for signs of anemia: Hct, Hgb, fatigue
• Monitor hepatic function tests weekly: ALT, AST, bilirubin
• Monitor renal status before treatment and monthly thereafter: BUN, creatinine, output, specific gravity, urinalysis
• Monitor hepatic status: decreased appetite, jaundice, dark urine, fatigue

Nursing diagnoses
• Infection, risk for (uses)
• Injury, risk for (adverse reactions)
• Knowledge, deficient (teaching)
• Noncompliance (teaching)

Implementation
• Give some of these agents on empty stomach, 1 hr before meals (only for isoniazid and rifampin) or 2 hr after meals
• Give antiemetic if vomiting occurs
• Give after C&S is completed; monthly to detect resistance

Patient/family education
- Teach patient that compliance with dosage schedule, duration is necessary
- Teach patient that scheduled appointments must be kept; relapse may occur
- Advise patient to avoid alcohol while taking product
- Advise patient to report flulike symptoms: excessive fatigue, anorexia, vomiting, sore throat; unusual bleeding, yellowish discoloration of skin/eyes

Evaluation
Positive therapeutic outcome
- Decreased symptoms of TB
- Negative culture

Generic Names
ethambutol, 🔹 isoniazid, pyrazinamide, rifabutin, rifampin, streptomycin

---

ANTITUSSIVES/EXPECTORANTS

Action: Antitussives suppress the cough reflex by direct action on the cough center in the medulla. Expectorants act by liquefying and reducing the viscosity of thick, tenacious secretions.

Uses: Antitussives/expectorants are used to treat cough occurring in pneumonia, bronchitis, TB, cystic fibrosis, and emphysema; as an adjunct in atelectasis (expectorants); and for nonproductive cough (antitussives).

Adverse effects: The most common side effects are drowsiness, dizziness, and nausea.

Contraindications: Some products are contraindicated in pregnancy, breastfeeding, hypothyroidism, and iodine sensitivity.

Precautions: Some products should be used cautiously with asthma and in geriatric and debilitated patients.

Pharmacokinetics: Onset, peak, and duration vary widely among products. Some products are metabolized in the liver and excreted in urine.

Interactions: Interactions vary widely among products. Check individual monographs for specific information.

NURSING CONSIDERATIONS
Assessment
- Assess cough: type, frequency, character including sputum

Nursing diagnoses
- Airway clearance, ineffective (uses)
- Breathing pattern, ineffective (uses)
- Knowledge, deficient (teaching)

Implementation
- Give decreased dosage to geriatric patients; their metabolism may be slowed
- Increase fluids to liquefy secretions
- Humidify patient's room

Patient/family education
- Advise patient to avoid driving and other hazardous activities until stabilized on this medication
- Caution patient to avoid smoking, smoke-filled rooms, perfumes, dust, environmental pollutants, cleaners that increase cough

Evaluation
Positive therapeutic outcome
- Absence of cough

Generic Names
🔹 acetylcysteine, aluminum chloride, benzonatate, 🔹 codeine, dextromethorphan, 🔹 diphenhydrAMINE, guaifenesin, hydrocodone

---

ANTIVIRALS

Action: Antivirals act by interfering with DNA synthesis that is needed for viral replication.

Uses: Antivirals are used for mucocutaneous herpes simplex virus, herpes genitalis (HSV-1, HSV-2), varicella infections, herpes zoster, and herpes simplex encephalitis.

Adverse effects: The most common side effects are nausea, vomiting, anorexia, headache, and diarrhea. The most serious adverse reactions are nephrotoxicity and blood dyscrasias.

Contraindications: Persons with hypersensitivity or immunosuppressed individuals should not use these products.

Precautions: Antivirals should be used cautiously in pregnancy, breastfeeding, and renal/hepatic disease.

Pharmacokinetics: Onset, peak, and duration vary widely among products. Most products are metabolized by the liver and excreted by the kidneys.

Interactions: Interactions vary widely among products. Check individual monographs for specific information.

Adverse effects: *italic* = common, **bold** = life-threatening

NURSING CONSIDERATIONS
Assessment
- Monitor for signs of infection, anemia
- Monitor patients with a compromised renal system; since product is excreted slowly in poor renal system function, toxicity may occur rapidly
- Monitor renal function tests: urinalysis, BUN, serum creatinine or decreased CCr may indicate nephrotoxicity; I&O ratio; report hematuria, oliguria, fatigue, weakness; check for protein in the urine during treatment
- Assess C&S before treatment; agent may be taken as soon as culture is taken; repeat C&S after treatment
- Monitor bowel pattern before, during treatment; if severe abdominal pain with bleeding occurs, agent should be discontinued
- Monitor skin reactions: rash, urticaria, itching
- Monitor hepatic function tests: AST, ALT
- Monitor blood tests: WBC, RBC, Hct, Hgb, bleeding time; blood dyscrasias

Nursing diagnoses
- Infection, risk for (uses)
- Injury, risk for (adverse reactions)
- Knowledge, deficient (teaching)

Implementation
- Give increased fluids to 3 L/day to decrease crystalluria when given **IV**
- Store at room temperature for up to 12 hr after reconstitution

Patient/family education
- Instruct patient to report sore throat, fever, fatigue; may indicate superinfection
- Caution patient that product does not prevent infecting others or cure condition but controls symptoms
- Instruct patient that product must be taken around the clock in equal intervals to maintain blood levels for duration of therapy
- Instruct patient to notify prescriber of side effects such as bruising, bleeding, fatigue, malaise; may indicate blood dyscrasias

Evaluation
Positive therapeutic outcome
- Absence or control of infection

Generic Names

acyclovir, amantadine, cidofovir, docosanol, entecavir, famciclovir, foscarnet, ganciclovir, lamivudine, maraviroc, oseltamivir, penciclovir, ribavirin, valacyclovir, valganciclovir, zanamivir

---

β-ADRENERGIC BLOCKERS

Action: β-Blockers are divided into selective and nonselective blockers. Selective β-blockers competitively block stimulation of $β_1$-receptors in cardiac smooth muscle; these products produce chronotropic and inotropic effects. Nonselective blockers produce a fall in blood pressure without reflex tachycardia or reduction in heart rate through a mixture of β-blocking effects; elevated plasma renins are reduced.

Uses: β-Blockers are used for hypertension, ventricular dysrhythmias, and prophylaxis of angina pectoris.

Adverse effects: The most common side effects are orthostatic hypotension, bradycardia, diarrhea, nausea, and vomiting. Serious adverse reactions include blood dyscrasias, bronchospasm, and CHF.

Contraindications: Hypersensitive reactions may occur, and allergies should be identified before these products are given. β-Adrenergic blockers should not be used in heart block, CHF, or cardiogenic shock.

Precautions: β-Blockers should be used with caution in pregnant and geriatric patients or in renal/thyroid disease, COPD, CAD, diabetes mellitus, and asthma.

Pharmacokinetics: Onset, peak, and duration vary widely among products. Most products are metabolized in the liver, with metabolites excreted in urine, bile, and feces.

Interactions: Interactions vary widely among products. Check individual monographs for specific information.

NURSING CONSIDERATIONS
Assessment
- Monitor renal function tests: protein, BUN, creatinine; watch for increased levels that may indicate nephrotic syndrome; obtain baselines in renal/hepatic function tests before beginning treatment
- Monitor I&O ratio, weight daily
- Monitor B/P during beginning treatment and periodically thereafter, pulse q4hr; note rate, rhythm, quality
- Monitor apical/radial pulse before administration; notify prescriber of significant changes
- Check for edema in feet and legs daily

Nursing diagnoses
- Cardiac output, decreased (uses)
- Diarrhea (adverse reactions)

- Gas exchange, impaired (adverse reactions)
- Tissue perfusion, ineffective (uses)

Implementation
- Give PO before meals and at bedtime; tab may be crushed or swallowed whole
- Give reduced dosage in renal dysfunction

Patient/family education
- Instruct patient to comply with dosage schedule, even if feeling better
- Caution patient to rise slowly to sitting or standing position to minimize orthostatic hypotension
- Advise patient to report bradycardia, dizziness, confusion, depression, fever
- Teach patient to take pulse at home; advise when to notify prescriber
- Instruct patient to comply with weight control, dietary adjustment, modified exercise program
- Advise patient to wear support hose to minimize effects of orthostatic hypotension
- Advise patient not to discontinue product abruptly; taper over 2 wk; may precipitate angina

Evaluation
Positive therapeutic outcome
- Decrease in B/P in hypertension
- Decreased B/P, edema, moist crackles in CHF

Generic Names

Selective β₁-receptor blockers:
acebutolol, atenolol, esmolol, metoprolol, nebibolol

Nonselective β₁ and β₂-blockers:
carteolol, nadolol, pindolol, ⊙propranolol, timolol

Combined α₁, β₁, and β₂-receptor blocker:
labetalol

BONE RESORPTION INHIBITORS

Action: Bone resorption inhibitors are divided into the biphosphonates and the selective estrogen receptor modulators. The biphosphonates act by absorbing calcium phosphate crystals in bone and may directly block dissolution of hydroxyapatite crystals of bone, inhibiting normal and abnormal bone resorption and mineralization. Selective estrogen receptor modulators act by reducing resorption of bone and decreasing bone turnover, mediated through estrogen receptor binding.

Uses: Bone resorption inhibitors are used for prevention and treatment of osteoporosis in postmenopausal women, treatment of Paget's disease, and treatment of osteoporosis in men.

Adverse effects: The most common side effects are nausea, vomiting, headache, bone pain, and rash.

Contraindications: Persons developing hypersensitive reactions or those with hypocalcemia should not use these products.

Precautions: Bone resorption inhibitors should be used cautiously in pregnancy, breast-feeding, the geriatric patient, renal/hepatic disease, and some GI disorders.

Pharmacokinetics: Onset, peak, and duration vary widely among products. Most products are taken up by the bones and excreted by the kidneys.

Interactions: Interactions vary widely among products. Check individual monographs for specific information.

NURSING CONSIDERATIONS
Assessment
- Assess reason for use and expected outcome
- Monitor bone density test; hormonal status (women) before starting treatment and thereafter
- Monitor hypercalcemia: paresthesia, twitching, laryngospasm; Chvostek's, Trousseau's signs

Nursing diagnoses
- Injury, risk for, physical (uses, adverse reactions)
- Knowledge, deficient (teaching)

Implementation
- Give for 6 months or more in Paget's disease
- Store at room temperature

Patient/family education
- Instruct patient to remain upright for at least 30 min after taking to prevent esophageal irritation
- Teach patient all aspects of product usage
- Inform patient to use weight-bearing exercise to increase bone density

Evaluation
Positive therapeutic outcome
- Increase in bone mass
- Absence of fractures

Generic Names

Bisphosphonates:
alendronate, etidronate, ibandronate, pamidronate, risedronate

Selective estrogen receptor modulators:
raloxifene

Adverse effects: *italic* = common, **bold** = life-threatening

CALCIUM CHANNEL BLOCKERS

Action: Calcium channel blockers inhibit calcium ion influx across the cell membrane in cardiac and vascular smooth muscle. This action produces relaxation of coronary vascular smooth muscle, dilates coronary arteries, slows SA/AV node conduction, and dilates peripheral arteries.

Uses: Calcium channel blockers are used for chronic stable angina pectoris, vasospastic angina, dysrhythmias, hypertension, and unstable angina.

Adverse effects: The most common side effects are dysrhythmias and edema. Also common are headache, fatigue, drowsiness, and flushing.

Contraindications: Persons with 2nd- or 3rd-degree heart block, sick sinus syndrome, hypotension of <90 mm Hg systolic, Wolff-Parkinson-White syndrome, or cardiogenic shock should not use these products, since worsening of those conditions may occur.

Precautions: CHF may worsen since edema may be increased. Hypotension may worsen, since B/P is decreased. Patients with renal/hepatic disease should use these products cautiously since they are metabolized in the liver and excreted by the kidneys.

Pharmacokinetics: Onset, peak, and duration vary widely with route of administration. Products are metabolized by the liver and excreted in the urine primarily as metabolites.

Interactions: Increased levels of digoxin and theophylline may occur when used with these products. Increased effects of β-blockers and antihypertensives may occur with calcium channel blockers.

NURSING CONSIDERATIONS
Assessment
• Monitor cardiac system: B/P, pulse, respirations, ECG intervals (PR, QRS, QT)

Nursing diagnoses
• Cardiac output, decreased (adverse reactions)
• Tissue perfusion, ineffective (uses)

Implementation
• Give PO before meals and at bedtime

Patient/family education
• Teach patient how to take pulse before taking product; patient should record or graph pulses to identify changes

• Advise patient to avoid hazardous activities until stabilized on this product since dizziness occurs frequently
• Inform patient of the need for compliance to all areas of medical regimen, including diet, exercise, stress reduction, and product therapy

Evaluation
Positive therapeutic outcome
• Decreased anginal pain
• Decreased B/P, dysrhythmias

Generic Names

amlodipine, clevidipine, diltiazem (high alert), felodipine, isradipine, niCARdipine, NIFEdipine, 🌀 verapamil

CARDIAC GLYCOSIDES

Action: Cardiac glycosides act by inhibiting sodium and potassium ATPase and then making more calcium available to activate contracted proteins. Cardiac contractility and cardiac output are increased.

Uses: Cardiac glycosides are used for CHF, atrial fibrillation, atrial flutter, atrial tachycardia, and rapid digitalization in these disorders.

Adverse effects: The most common side effects are cardiac disturbances, headache, hypotension, and GI symptoms. Also common are blurred vision and yellow-green halos.

Contraindications: Hypersensitive reactions may occur, and allergies should be identified before these products are given. Also, persons with ventricular tachycardia, ventricular fibrillation, and carotid sinus syndrome should not use these products.

Precautions: Persons with acute MI and those who have or may develop serum potassium, calcium, or magnesium imbalances should use these products cautiously. Also, geriatric patients and those with AV block, severe respiratory disease, hypothyroidism, or renal/hepatic disease should exercise caution when these products are prescribed.

Pharmacokinetics: Onset, peak, and duration vary widely with the route of administration. Digitoxin is inactivated by the liver, and inactive metabolites are excreted in urine. Digoxin is excreted in urine mainly as the parent product and metabolites.

Interactions: Toxicity may occur when used with diuretics, succinylcholine, quinidine, and thioamines. Increased blood levels may occur with propantheline bromide, spironolactone, quinidine, verapamil, aminoglycosides (PO), amiodarone, anticholinergics, and quinine. Diuretics may increase toxicity.

NURSING CONSIDERATIONS
Assessment
- Montior cardiac system: B/P, pulse, respirations, and increased urine output
- Monitor apical pulse for 1 min before giving product; if pulse <60, take again in 1 hr; if <60 notify prescriber
- Monitor electrolytes: potassium, sodium, chloride, calcium, magnesium; renal function tests, including BUN and creatinine; and blood tests, including AST, ALT, bilirubin
- Monitor I&O ratio, daily weights
- Monitor therapeutic product levels

Nursing diagnoses
- Cardiac output, decreased (adverse reactions)
- Tissue perfusion, ineffective (uses)

Implementation
- Give potassium supplements if ordered for potassium levels <3

Patient/family education
- Teach patient how to take pulse before taking product; patient should record or graph pulse to identify changes
- Advise patient to avoid hazardous activities until stabilized on this product since dizziness occurs frequently
- Inform patient of the need for compliance to all areas of medical regimen, including diet, exercise, stress reduction, product therapy

Evaluation
Positive therapeutic outcome
- Decreased weight, edema, pulse, respiration
- Increased urine output

Generic Names

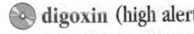 digoxin (high alert)

CHOLINERGICS

Action: Cholinergics act by preventing destruction of acetylcholine, which increases concentration at sites where acetylcholine is released. This exaggerates the effects of acetylcholine and facilitates transmission of impulses across the myoneural junction. Cholinergics may also act by stimulating receptors for acetylcholine.

Uses: Cholinergics are used for myasthenia gravis, as antagonists of nondepolarizing neuromuscular blockade, postoperative bladder distention and urinary distention, postoperative ileus.

Adverse effects: The most serious adverse reactions are respiratory depression, bronchospasm, constriction, laryngospasm, respiratory arrest, convulsions, and paralysis. The most common side effects are nausea, diarrhea, and vomiting.

Contraindications: Persons with obstruction of the intestine or renal system should not use these products.

Precautions: Caution should be used in patients with bradycardia, hypotension, seizure disorders, bronchial asthma, coronary occlusion, and hyperthyroidism, and in breastfeeding and children.

Pharmacokinetics: Onset, peak, and duration vary widely among products. Most products are metabolized in the liver and excreted in urine.

Interactions: Interactions vary widely among products. Check individual monographs for specific information.

NURSING CONSIDERATIONS
Assessment
- Monitor VS, respiration q8hr
- Monitor I&O ratio; check for urinary retention or incontinence
- Assess for bradycardia, hypotension, bronchospasm, headache, dizziness, seizures, respiratory depression; product should be discontinued if toxicity occurs

Nursing diagnoses
- Breathing pattern, ineffective (uses)
- Knowledge, deficient (teaching)
- Noncompliance (teaching)
- Urinary elimination, impaired (uses)

Implementation
- Give only with atropine sulfate available for cholinergic crisis
- Give only after all other cholinergics have been discontinued
- Give increased dosages if tolerance occurs
- Give larger doses after exercise or fatigue
- Give on empty stomach for better absorption
- Store at room temperature

Patient/family education
- Inform patient that product is not a cure; it only relieves symptoms (myasthenia gravis)
- Advise patient to carry/wear emergency ID specifying myasthenia gravis, products taken

Adverse effects: *italic* = common, **bold** = life-threatening

Evaluation
Positive therapeutic outcome
- Increased muscle strength, hand grasp
- Improved muscle gait
- Absence of labored breathing (if severe)

Generic Names

bethanechol, neostigmine, physostigmine, pyridostigmine

CHOLINERGIC BLOCKERS

Action: Cholinergic blockers inhibit or block acetylcholine at receptor sites in the autonomic nervous system.

Uses: Many cholinergic blockers are used to decrease secretions before surgery, to reverse neuromuscular blockade, and to decrease motility of the GI, biliary, and urinary tracts. Other products are used for parkinsonian symptoms, including dystonia associated with neuroleptic products.

Adverse effects: The most common side effects are dryness of the mouth and constipation, which can be prevented by frequent rinsing of the mouth and increasing water and bulk in the diet.

Contraindications: Hypersensitivity can occur, and allergies should be identified before administering these products. Persons with GI and GU obstruction should not use these products, since constipation and urinary retention may occur. They are also contraindicated in closed-angle glaucoma and myasthenia gravis.

Precautions: Caution must be used when these products are given to the geriatric patient, since metabolism is slowed. Also, persons with tachycardia or prostatic hypertrophy should use these products with caution.

Pharmacokinetics: Onset, peak, and duration vary with route.

Interactions: Increase in anticholinergic effect occurs when used with opioids, barbiturates, antihistamines, MAOIs, phenothiazines, amantadine.

NURSING CONSIDERATIONS
Assessment
- Assess I&O ratio; be alert for urinary retention, frequency, dysuria; product should be discontinued if these occur
- Assess urinary hesitancy, retention; palpate bladder if retention occurs
- Assess constipation; increase fluids, bulk, exercise
- Assess for tolerance over long-term therapy; dosage may need to be changed
- Assess mental status: affect, mood, CNS depression, worsening of mental symptoms during early therapy

Nursing diagnoses
- Mobility, impaired physical (uses)
- Pain, chronic (uses)

Implementation
- Give with food or milk to decrease GI symptoms
- Give parenteral dose with patient recumbent to prevent postural hypotension; give dose slowly, monitoring VS
- Give hard candy, gum, frequent rinsing of mouth for dryness

Patient/family education
- Caution patient to avoid driving and other hazardous activities if drowsiness occurs
- Advise patient to avoid concurrent use of cough, cold preparations with alcohol, antihistamines unless directed by prescriber
- Caution patient to use with caution in hot weather, since medication may increase susceptibility to heat stroke

Evaluation
Positive therapeutic outcome
- Absence of cramps
- Absence of EPS

Generic Names

atropine (high alert), benztropine, biperiden, glycopyrrolate, scopolamine, trihexyphenidyl

---

CORTICOSTEROIDS

Action: Corticosteroids are divided into glucocorticoids and mineralocorticoids. Glucocorticoids decrease inflammation by the suppression of migration of polymorphonuclear leukocytes, fibroblasts, increased capillary permeability, and lysosomal stabilization. They also have varied metabolic effects and modify the body's immune responses to many different stimuli. Mineralocorticoids act by increasing resorption of sodium by increasing hydrogen and potassium excretion in the distal tubule.

Uses: Glucocorticoids are used to decrease inflammation and for immunosuppression. In addition, some products may be given for allergy, adrenal insufficiency, or cerebral

---

edema. Mineralocorticoids are given for adrenal insufficiency or adrenogenital syndrome.

Adverse effects: The most common side effects include change in behavior, including insomnia and euphoria; GI irritation, including peptic ulcer; metabolic reactions, including hypokalemia, hyperglycemia, and carbohydrate intolerance; and sodium and fluid retention. Most adverse reactions are dose dependent.

Contraindications: Hypersensitivity may occur and should be identified before administering. Since these products mask infection, they should not be used in systemic fungal infections or amebiasis. Mothers taking pharmacologic doses of corticosteroids should not breastfeed.

Precautions: Caution must be used when these products are prescribed for diabetic patients since hyperglycemia may occur. Also, patients with glaucoma, seizure disorders, peptic ulcer, impaired renal function, CHF, hypertension, ulcerative colitis, or myasthenia gravis should be monitored closely if corticosteroids are given. Use with caution during pregnancy, in children, and in the geriatric patient.

Pharmacokinetics: For oral preparations the onset of action occurs between 1-2 hr, and duration can be up to 2 days, with a half-life of 2-4 days. Pharmacokinetics vary widely among products. These products cross the placenta and appear in breast milk.

Interactions: Decreased corticosteroid effect may occur with barbiturates, rifampin, and phenytoin; corticosteroid dosage may need to be increased. There is a possibility of GI bleeding when used with salicylates and indomethacin. Steroids may reduce salicylate levels. When using with digoxin glycosides, potassium-depleting diuretics, and amphotericin, serum potassium levels should be monitored.

NURSING CONSIDERATIONS
Assessment
• Monitor potassium, blood glucose, urine glucose while on long-term therapy; hypokalemia and hyperglycemia are common
• Monitor weight daily; notify prescriber if weekly gain of >5 lb since these products alter fluid and electrolyte balance
• Assess for potassium depletion: paresthesias, fatigue, nausea, vomiting, depression, polyuria, dysrhythmias, weakness
• Assess for mental status: affect, mood, behavioral changes, aggression; if severe personality changes occur, including depression, product may need to be tapered and then discontinued
• Monitor I&O ratio; be alert for decreasing urinary output and increasing edema
• Monitor plasma cortisol levels during long-term therapy (normal level is 138-635 nmol/L when drawn at 8 AM)
• Assess for infection: increased temp, WBC, even after withdrawal of medication; product masks symptoms of infection
• Assess for adrenal insufficiency: nausea, anorexia, fatigue, dizziness, dyspnea, weakness, joint pain

Nursing diagnoses
• Body image, disturbed (adverse reactions)
• Infection, risk for (adverse reactions)
• Suicide, risk for (adverse reactions)

Implementation
• Give with food or milk to decrease GI symptoms
• Give single daily or alternate-day doses in the morning before 9 AM (for replacement therapy)

Patient/family education
• Advise patient that emergency ID as steroid user should be carried/worn
• Advise patient not to discontinue this medication abruptly; adrenal crisis can result
• Teach patient all aspects of product use, including cushingoid symptoms
• Instruct patient to take with meals or a snack
• Teach patient to avoid exposure to chickenpox or measles if taking immunosuppressives

Evaluation
Positive therapeutic outcome
• Decreased inflammation

Generic Names

Glucocorticoids:
beclomethasone, betamethasone, 🔵cortisone, dexamethasone, hydrocortisone, hydrocortisone sodium phosphate, methylPREDNISolone, predniSOLONE, 🔵predniSONE, triamcinolone

Mineralocorticoid:
fludrocortisone

DIURETICS

Action: Diuretics are divided into subgroups: thiazides and thiazide-like diuretics, loop diuretics, carbonic anhydrase inhibitors, osmotic diuretics, and potassium-sparing diuretics. Each one of these subgroups differs in its mechanism of action. Thiazides and thiazide-like diuretics increase excretion of water and sodium by inhibiting resorption in the early distal tubule. Loop diuretics inhibit resorption of sodium and chloride in the thick ascending limb of the loop of Henle. Carbonic anhydrase inhibitors increase sodium excretion by decreasing sodium-hydrogen ion exchange throughout the renal tubule. Carbonic anhydrase inhibitors also decrease secretion of aqueous humor in the eye and thus decrease intraocular pressure. Osmotic diuretics increase the osmotic pressure of glomerular filtrate, thus decreasing net absorption of sodium. The potassium-sparing diuretics interfere with sodium resorption at the distal tubule, thus decreasing potassium excretion.

Uses: Blood pressure is reduced in hypertension; edema is reduced in CHF; intraocular pressure is decreased in glaucoma.

Adverse effects: Hypokalemia, hyperuricemia, and hyperglycemia occur most frequently with thiazide diuretics. Aplastic anemia, blood dyscrasias, volume depletion, and dehydration may occur when thiazide-like diuretics, loop diuretics, or carbonic anhydrase inhibitors are given. Side effects and adverse reactions vary widely for the miscellaneous products.

Contraindications: Persons with electrolyte imbalances (sodium, chloride, potassium), dehydration, or anuria should not be given these products until the problem is corrected.

Precautions: Caution must be used when diuretics are given to the geriatric patient, since electrolyte disturbances and dehydration can occur rapidly. Renal/hepatic disorders may cause poor metabolism and excretion of the product.

Pharmacokinetics: Onset, peak, and duration vary widely among the different subgroups of these products.

Interactions: Cholestyramine and colestipol decrease the absorption of thiazide diuretics. Concurrent use of thiazides with diazoxide may increase hyperuricemia, hyperglycemia, and antihypertensive effects of thiazides. Ototoxicity may occur when loop diuretics are used with aminoglycosides. Thiazide and loop diuretics may increase therapeutic and toxic effects of lithium.

NURSING CONSIDERATIONS
Assessment
- Monitor weight, I&O ratio daily to determine fluid loss; check skin turgor for dehydration
- Monitor electrolytes: potassium, sodium, chloride: include BUN, blood glucose, CBC, serum creatinine, blood pH, ABGs, uric acid, calcium; electrolyte imbalances may occur quickly
- Monitor B/P with patient lying, standing; postural hypotension may occur since fluid loss occurs from intravascular spaces first
- Assess for signs of metabolic alkalosis, including drowsiness and restlessness
- Assess for signs of hypokalemia with some products: postural hypotension, malaise, fatigue, tachycardia, leg cramps, weakness

Nursing diagnoses
- Cardiac output, decreased (adverse reactions)
- Fluid volume, excess (uses)

Implementation
- Give in AM to avoid interference with sleep if using product as a diuretic
- Give potassium replacement if potassium is less than 3 mg/dl

Patient/family education
- Teach patient to take product early in the day (diuretic) to prevent nocturia

Evaluation
Positive therapeutic outcome
- Improvement in edema of feet, legs, sacral area daily if medication is being used in CHF
- Improvement in B/P if medication is being used as a diuretic
- Improvement in intraocular pressure if medication is being used to decrease aqueous humor in the eye

---

Generic Names

Thiazides:
chlorothiazide, hydrochlorothiazide

Thiazide-like:
chlorthalidone, indapamide, metolazone

Loop:
bumetanide, furosemide, torsemide

Carbonic anhydrase inhibitors:
acetaZOLAMIDE

Potassium-sparing:
amiloride, spironolactone, triamterene

Osmotic:
mannitol

HISTAMINE H$_2$ ANTAGONISTS

Action: Histamine H$_2$ antagonists act by inhibiting histamine at H$_2$ receptor site in parietal cells, which inhibits gastric acid secretion.

Uses: Histamine H_2 antagonists are used for short-term treatment of duodenal and gastric ulcers and maintenance therapy for duodenal ulcer and for gastroesophageal reflux disease.

Adverse effects: The most serious adverse reactions are agranulocytosis, thrombocytopenia, neutropenia, aplastic anemia, and exfoliative dermatitis. The most common side effects are confusion (not with rantidine), headache, and diarrhea.

Contraindications: Persons with hypersensitivity should not use these products.

Precautions: Caution should be used in pregnancy, breastfeeding, children <16 yr, organic brain syndrome, and renal/hepatic disease.

Pharmacokinetics: Onset, peak, and duration vary widely among products. Most products are metabolized in the liver and excreted in urine.

Interactions: Antacids interfere with absorption of histamine H_2 antagonists. Check individual monographs for specific information.

NURSING CONSIDERATIONS
Assessment
- Monitor gastric pH (>5 should be maintained)
- Monitor I&O ratio, BUN, creatinine

Nursing diagnoses
- Injury, risk for (bleeding)
- Knowledge, deficient (teaching)
- Pain, chronic (uses)

Implementation
- Give with meals for prolonged product effect
- Give antacids 1 hr before or 1 hr after cimetidine
- Give **IV** slowly; bradycardia may occur; give over 30 min
- Store diluted sol at room temperature for up to 48 hr

Patient/family education
- Advise patient that gynecomastia, impotence may occur but is reversible
- Caution patient to avoid driving and other hazardous activities until patient is stabilized on this medication
- Caution patient to avoid black pepper, caffeine, alcohol, harsh spices, extremes in temperature of food
- Caution patient to avoid OTC preparations: aspirin, cough, cold preparations
- Inform patient that product must be continued for prescribed time to be effective

- Advise patient to report bruising, fatigue, malaise; blood dyscrasias may occur

Evaluation
Positive therapeutic outcome
- Decreased pain in abdomen

Generic Names
 cimetidine, famotidine, ranitidine

IMMUNOSUPPRESSANTS

Action: Immunosuppressants produce immunosuppression by inhibiting T lymphocytes.

Uses: Most immunosuppressants are used for organ transplants to prevent rejection.

Adverse effects: The most serious adverse reactions are albuminuria, hematuria, proteinuria, renal failure, and hepatotoxicity. The most common side effects are oral *Candida* infection, gum hyperplasia, tremors, and headache. The most serious adverse reactions for azathioprine are hematologic (leukopenia and thrombocytopenia) and GI (nausea and vomiting). There is a risk of secondary infection.

Contraindications: Products are contraindicated in hypersensitivity.

Precautions: Caution should be used in pregnancy and severe renal/hepatic disease.

Pharmacokinetics: Onset, peak, and duration vary widely among products. Most products are metabolized in the liver and excreted in urine.

Interactions: Interactions vary widely among products. Check individual monographs for specific information.

NURSING CONSIDERATIONS
Assessment
- Monitor renal function tests: BUN, creatinine at least monthly during treatment, 3 mo after treatment
- Monitor hepatic function tests: alkaline phosphatase, AST, ALT, bilirubin
- Monitor product blood levels during treatment
- Assess for hepatotoxicity: dark urine, jaundice, itching, light-colored stools; product should be discontinued

Nursing diagnoses
- Infection, risk for (adverse reactions)
- Injury, risk for (uses)
- Knowledge, deficient (teaching)

Adverse effects: *italic* = common, **bold** = life-threatening

Implementation
- Give for several days before transplant surgery
- Give with meals for GI upset or place product in chocolate milk
- Give with oral antifungal for *Candida* infections

Patient/family education
- Advise patient to report fever, chills, sore throat, fatigue since serious infections may occur
- Caution patient to use contraceptive measures during treatment and for 12 wk after ending therapy

Evaluation
Positive therapeutic outcome
- Absence of rejection

Generic Names
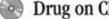 azathioprine, basiliximab (high alert), cycloSPORINE, everolimus, muromonab-CD3, sirolimus, tacrolimus

---

LAXATIVES

Action: Laxatives are divided into bulk products, lubricants, osmotics, saline laxative stimulants, and stool softeners. Bulks work by absorbing water and expanding to increase moisture content and bulk in the stool. Lubricants increase water retention in the stool, causing reabsorption of water in the bowel. Saline draws water into the intestinal lumen. Osmotics increase distention and promote peristalsis. Stimulants act by increasing peristalsis by direct effect on the intestine. Stool softeners reduce surface tension of liquid in the bowel.

Uses: Laxatives are used as a preparation for bowel, or rectal examination, for constipation, or as stool softeners.

Adverse effects: The most common side effects are nausea, abdominal cramps, and diarrhea.

Contraindications: Persons with GI obstruction, perforation, gastric retention, toxic colitis, megacolon, abdominal pain, nausea, vomiting, and fecal impaction should not use these products.

Precautions: Caution should be used in rectal bleeding, large hemorrhoids, and anal excoriation.

Pharmacokinetics: Onset, peak, and duration vary among products.

Interactions: Interactions vary widely among products. Check individual monographs for specific information.

NURSING CONSIDERATIONS
Assessment
- Monitor blood, urine electrolytes if product is used often by patient
- Monitor I&O ratio to identify fluid loss
- Determine cause of constipation; identify whether fluids, bulk, or exercise is missing from lifestyle
- Assess for cramping, rectal bleeding, nausea, vomiting; if these symptoms occur, product should be discontinued

Nursing diagnoses
- Constipation (uses)
- Diarrhea (adverse reactions)
- Knowledge, deficient (teaching)

Implementation
- Give alone only with water for better absorption; do not take within 1 hr of antacids, milk, or cimetidine
- Swallow tab whole; do not break, crush, or chew

Patient/family education
- Caution patient not to use laxatives for long-term therapy; bowel tone will be lost; that normal bowel movements do not always occur daily
- Caution patient not to use in presence of abdominal pain, nausea, vomiting
- Advise patient to notify prescriber of abdominal pain, nausea, vomiting
- Advise patient to notify prescriber if constipation is unrelieved or if symptoms of electrolyte imbalance occur: muscle cramps, pain, weakness, dizziness

Evaluation
Positive therapeutic outcome
- Decrease in constipation

Generic Names
Bulk laxatives:
calcium polycarbophil, methylcellulose, psyllium

Osmotic agents:
glycerin, lactulose

Saline laxatives:
magnesium salts, sodium biphosphate/phosphate

Stimulants:
bisacodyl, cascara sagrada, senna

Stool softeners:
docusate

 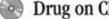

NEUROMUSCULAR BLOCKING AGENTS

Action: Neuromuscular blocking agents are divided into depolarizing and nondepolarizing blockers. They act by inhibiting transmission of nerve impulses by binding with cholinergic receptor sites.

Uses: Neuromuscular blocking agents are used to facilitate endotracheal intubation and skeletal muscle relaxation during mechanical ventilation, surgery, or general anesthesia.

Adverse effects: The most serious adverse reactions are prolonged apnea, bronchospasm, cyanosis, respiratory depression, and malignant hyperthermia. The most common side effects are bradycardia and decreased motility.

Contraindications: Persons who are hypersensitive should not be given this product.

Precautions: Caution should be used in pregnancy, breastfeeding, children <2 yr, thyroid disease, collagen disease, cardiac disease, electrolyte imbalances, dehydration, neuromuscular disease (myasthenia gravis), and respiratory disease.

Pharmacokinetics: Onset, peak, and duration vary widely among products. Most products are metabolized in the liver and excreted in urine.

Interactions: Aminoglycosides potentiate neuromuscular blockade. Check individual monographs for specific information.

NURSING CONSIDERATIONS
Assessment
- Monitor for electrolyte imbalances (potassium, magnesium); may lead to increased action of this product
- Monitor VS (B/P, pulse, respirations, airway) q15min until fully recovered; rate, depth, pattern of respirations, strength of hand grip
- Monitor I&O ratio; check for urinary retention, frequency, hesitancy
- Assess for recovery: decreased paralysis of face, diaphragm, leg, arm, rest of body
- Assess for allergic reactions: rash, fever, respiratory distress, pruritus; product should be discontinued

Nursing diagnoses
- Breathing pattern, ineffective (uses)
- Injury, risk for (adverse reactions)
- Knowledge, deficient (teaching)

Implementation
- Administer using nerve stimulator by anesthesiologist to determine neuromuscular blockade
- Administer anticholinesterase to reverse neuromuscular blockade
- Give **IV** undiluted over 1-2 min (only by qualified person, usually an anesthesiologist)
- Store in light-resistant, cool area
- Reassure if communication is difficult during recovery from neuromuscular blockade

Evaluation
Positive therapeutic outcome
- Paralysis of jaw, eyelid, head, neck, rest of body

Generic Names

atracurium, doxacurium, gallamine, mivacurium, pancuronium (high alert), pipercuronium, rocuronium, succinylcholine (high alert), tubocurarine (high alert), vecuronium (high alert)

NONSTEROIDAL ANTIINFLAMMATORIES

Action: Nonsteroidal antiinflammatories decrease prostaglandin synthesis by inhibiting an enzyme needed for biosynthesis.

Uses: Nonsteroidal antiinflammatories are used to treat mild to moderate pain, osteoarthritis, rheumatoid arthritis, and dysmenorrhea.

Adverse effects: The most serious adverse reactions are nephrotoxicity (dysuria, hematuria, oliguria, azotemia), blood dyscrasias, and cholestatic hepatitis. The most common side effects are nausea, abdominal pain, anorexia, dizziness, and drowsiness.

Contraindications: Persons with hypersensitivity, asthma, or severe renal/hepatic disease should not use these products.

Precautions: Caution should be used in pregnancy, breastfeeding, children, geriatric patients, bleeding/GI/cardiac disorders, and hypersensitivity to other antiinflammatory agents.

Pharmacokinetics: Onset, peak, and duration vary widely among products. Most products are metabolized in the liver and excreted in urine.

Interactions: Interactions vary widely among products. Check individual monographs for specific information.

Adverse effects: *italic* = common, **bold** = life-threatening

NURSING CONSIDERATIONS
Assessment
- Monitor renal, hepatic, blood tests: BUN, creatinine, AST, ALT, Hgb, before treatment, periodically thereafter
- Monitor audiometric, ophth examination before, during, and after treatment.
- Check for eye, ear problems: blurred vision, tinnitus; may indicate toxicity

Nursing diagnoses
- Knowledge, deficient (teaching)
- Mobility, impaired physical (uses)
- Noncompliance (teaching)
- Pain, chronic (uses)

Implementation
- Give with food to decrease GI symptoms; however, best to take on empty stomach to facilitate absorption
- Store at room temperature

Patient/family education
- Advise patient to report blurred vision, ringing, roaring in ears; may indicate toxicity
- Caution patient to avoid driving, other hazardous activities if dizziness, drowsiness occurs, especially in geriatric patients
- Advise patient to report change in urine pattern, increased weight, edema, increased pain in joints, fever, blood in urine; indicate nephrotoxicity
- Inform patient that therapeutic effects may take up to 1 mo

Evaluation
Positive therapeutic outcome
- Decreased pain, stiffness in joints
- Decreased swelling in joints
- Ability to move more easily

Generic Names
celecoxib, diclofenac, etodolac, fenoprofen, ibuprofen, indomethacin, ketoprofen, ketorolac, nabumetone, naproxen, piroxicam, sulindac

OPIOID ANALGESICS

Action: These agents depress pain impulse transmission at the spinal cord level by interacting with opioid receptors. Products are divided into opiates and nonopiates.

Uses: Most opioid analgesics are used to control moderate to severe pain and are used before and after surgery.

Adverse effects: GI symptoms, including nausea, vomiting, anorexia, constipation, and cramps are the most common side effects. Other common side effects include light-headedness, dizziness, and sedation. Serious adverse reactions such as respiratory depression, respiratory arrest, circulatory depression, and increased ICP may result but are less common and usually dose dependent.

Contraindications: Hypersensitive reactions occur frequently. Check for sensitivity before administering. These products should not be used if opioid addiction is suspected.

Precautions: Caution must be used when these products are given to persons with an addictive personality, since the possibility of addiction is so great. Also, persons with increased ICP may experience an even greater increase in ICP. Persons with severe heart disease, renal/hepatic disease, respiratory conditions, and seizure disorders should be monitored closely for worsening condition.

Pharmacokinetics: Onset of action is immediate by **IV** route and rapid by IM and PO routes. Peak occurs from 1-2 hr, depending on route, with a duration of 2-8 hr. These agents cross the placenta and appear in breast milk.

Interactions: Barbiturates, other opioids, hypnotics, antipsychotics, or alcohol can increase CNS depression when taken with opioids.

NURSING CONSIDERATIONS
Assessment
- Monitor I&O ratio; be alert for urinary retention, frequency, dysuria; product should be discontinued if these occur
- Assess for respiratory dysfunction: respiratory depression, rate, rhythm, character; notify prescriber if respirations are <12/min
- Assess for CNS changes: dizziness, drowsiness, hallucinations, euphoria, LOC, pupil reaction
- Assess for allergic reactions: rash, urticaria
- Assess for need for pain medication, use pain scoring

Nursing diagnoses
- Gas exchange, impaired (adverse reactions)
- Pain, acute (uses)

Implementation
- Give with antiemetic if nausea or vomiting occurs
- Give when pain is beginning to return; determine dosage interval by patient response
- Provide assistance with ambulation; patient should not be ambulating during product peak

 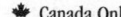

Patient/family education

• Advise patient to report any symptoms of CNS changes, allergic reactions, or shortness of breath
• Caution patient that physical dependency may result when used for extended periods
• Teach patient that withdrawal symptoms may occur, including nausea, vomiting, cramps, fever, faintness, anorexia
• Advise patient to avoid alcohol and other CNS depressants

Evaluation
Positive therapeutic outcome
• Decrease in pain

Generic Names

alfentanil, buprenorphine, butorphanol, 🌀 codeine, fentanyl (high alert), fentanyl transdermal, hydromorphone (high alert), 🌀 meperidine (high alert), methadone (high alert), 🌀 morphine (high alert), nalbuphine, oxycodone (high alert), oxymorphone (high alert), pentazocine (high alert), propoxyphene (high alert), remifentanil (high alert)

SALICYLATES

Action: Salicylates have analgesic, antipyretic, and antiinflammatory effects. The analgesic and antiinflammatory activities may be mediated through the inhibition of prostaglandin synthesis. Antipyretic action results from inhibition of the hypothalamic heat-regulating center.

Uses: The primary uses of salicylates are relief of mild to moderate pain and fever and in inflammatory conditions such as arthritis, thromboembolic disorders, and rheumatic fever.

Adverse effects: The most common side effects are GI symptoms and rash. Serious blood dyscrasias and hepatotoxicity may result when used for long periods at high doses. Tinnitus or impaired hearing may indicate that blood salicylate levels are reaching or exceeding the upper limit of the therapeutic range.

Contraindications: Hypersensitivity to salicylates is common. Check for sensitivity before administering. Persons with bleeding disorders, GI bleeding, and vit K deficiency should not use these products since salicylates increase pro-time. Children should not use these products since salicylates have been associated with Reye's syndrome.

Precautions: Caution is needed when salicylates are given to patients with anemia, renal/hepatic disease, and Hodgkin's disease. Caution should also be exercised in pregnancy and breastfeeding.

Pharmacokinetics: Onset of action occurs in 15-30 min, with a peak of 1-2 hr and a duration up to 6 hr. These products are metabolized by the liver and excreted by the kidneys.

Interactions: Increased effects of anticoagulants, insulin, methotrexate, heparin, valproic acid, and oral sulfonylureas may occur when used with salicylates. Aspirin may decrease serum concentrations of nonsteroidal antiinflammatory agents.

NURSING CONSIDERATIONS
Assessment
• Monitor renal/hepatic function tests: AST, ALT, bilirubin, creatinine, LDH, alkaline phosphatase, BUN if patient is on long-term therapy since these products are metabolized and excreted by the liver and kidney
• Monitor blood tests: CBC, Hct, Hgb, and pro-time if patient is on long-term therapy, since these products increase the possibility of bleeding and blood dyscrasias
• Assess for hepatotoxicity: dark urine, clay-colored stools, jaundiced skin and sclera, itching, abdominal pain, fever, diarrhea, which may occur with long-term use
• Assess for ototoxicity: tinnitus, ringing, roaring in ears; audiometric testing is needed before and after long-term therapy

Nursing diagnoses
• Activity intolerance (uses)
• Mobility, impaired physical (uses)
• Pain, acute (uses)
• Pain, chronic (uses)
• Sensory perception, disturbed (adverse reactions)
• Thermoregulation, ineffective (uses)

Implementation
• Give with food or milk to decrease gastric irritation; give 30 min before or 1 hr after meals with a full glass of water

Patient/family education
• Advise patient that blood sugar levels should be monitored closely, if patient is diabetic
• Caution patient not to exceed recommended dosage; acute poisoning may result
• Inform patient that therapeutic response takes 2 wk in arthritis
• Caution patient to avoid use of alcohol since GI bleeding may result

Adverse effects: *italic* = common, **bold** = life-threatening

- Advise patient to notify prescriber if ringing in the ears or persistent GI pain occurs
- Advise patient to take with full glass of water to reduce risk of lodging in esophagus

Evaluation
Positive therapeutic outcome
- Decreased pain, fever

Generic Names
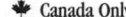 aspirin, choline salicylate, magnesium salicylate, salsalate

SEDATIVES/HYPNOTICS

Action: The sedatives/hypnotics depress the CNS; some products at the cerebral cortex, others inhibit transmitters in the CNS.

Uses: Sedatives/hypnotics are used for the treatment of sleep disorders, seizures, muscle spasms, and alcohol withdrawal.

Adverse effects: The most common side effects are nausea and drowsiness. The most serious side effects are Stevens-Johnson syndrome, blood dyscrasias, and risk of dependency.

Contraindications: Persons with hypersensitivity reactions should not use these products.

Precautions: Sedatives/hypnotics should be used cautiously in pregnancy (C) and breastfeeding.

Pharmacokinetics: Onset, peak, and duration vary widely among products. Most products are metabolized in the liver and excreted by the kidneys.

Interactions: Increased CNS depression may occur with other CNS depressants such as alcohol, opiates, antipsychotics, and antidepressants.

NURSING CONSIDERATIONS
Assessment
- Monitor mental status: affect, mood, behavioral changes, depression, confusion; seizure activity

Nursing diagnoses
- Knowledge, deficient (teaching)
- Noncompliance (teaching)
- Sleep deprivation (uses)

Implementation
- Give lowest possible dose for therapeutic result; adjust dose to response

- Provide assistance with ambulation during beginning therapy if dizziness, ataxia occur

Patient/family education
- Inform patient that these products should only be used for short-term insomnia
- Caution patient not to drive or engage in other hazardous activities while taking these products
- Instruct patient to avoid breastfeeding while taking these products
- Instruct patient to avoid alcohol or other CNS depressants as drowsiness will increase
- Teach patient that some of the products take two nights to be effective
- Advise patient to report side effects, adverse reactions to health care provider
- Instruct patient to use exactly as prescribed, at regular intervals

Evaluation
Positive therapeutic outcome
- Ability to sleep throughout the night
- Absence or decreasing seizure activity

Generic Names
Barbiturates:
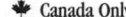 phenobarbital (high alert)

Benzodiazepines:
chlordiazepoxide, clorazepate, 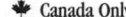 diazepam, flurazepam, lorazepam, midazolam, oxazepam, temazepam, triazolam

Miscellaneous products:
chloral hydrate, dexmedetomidine, **droperidol** (high alert), eszopiclone, hydrOXYzine, promethazine, ramelteon, zaleplon, zolpidem

SKELETAL MUSCLE RELAXANTS

Action: Most skeletal muscle relaxants inhibit synaptic responses in the CNS by stimulating receptors and decreasing neurotransmission, decreasing pain and spasticity.

Uses: Skeletal muscle relaxants are used for musculoskeletal disorders with pain or spasticity related to spinal cord injuries.

Adverse effects: The most common side effects are dizziness, weakness, fatigue, drowsiness, and headache. Some products can cause seizures, cardiovascular collapse, and severe CNS depression.

Contraindications: Persons with hypersensitivity should not use these products.

Precautions: Skeletal muscle relaxants should be used cautiously in pregnancy (C), breastfeeding, the geriatric patient, peptic ulcer, renal/hepatic disease, stroke, seizure disorder, and diabetes.

Pharmacokinetics: Pharmacokinetics vary widely among products. Check individual monographs for specific information.

Interactions: CNS depressants used with skeletal muscle relaxants may lead to increased CNS depression.

NURSING CONSIDERATIONS
Assessment
• Monitor pain: character, location, duration, alleviating/aggravating factors

Nursing diagnoses
• Injury, risk for (adverse reactions)
• Knowledge, deficient (teaching)
• Mobility, impaired physical (uses)
• Pain, acute (uses)
• Pain, chronic (uses)

Implementation
• Give when pain is beginning to return, not after pain is severe
• Store in dry area, away from heat and sunlight

Patient/family education
• Advise patient not to use with other CNS depressant unless prescriber approved
• Inform patient that many products require 1-2 mo of treatment for full effect
• Caution patient to avoid hazardous activities until response to medication is known
• Caution patient that most products should not be discontinued quickly, but tapered over 1-2 wk

Evaluation
Positive therapeutic outcome
• Decrease in pain or spasticity

Generic Names
Centrally acting:
🜨 baclofen, carisoprodol, chlorzoxazone, cyclobenzaprine, 🜨 diazepam, metaxalone, methocarbamol, orphenadrine

Direct-acting:
dantrolene

THROMBOLYTICS

Action: Thrombolytics activate conversion of plasminogen to plasmin (fibrinolysin). Plasmin is able to break down clots (fibrin).

Uses: Thrombolytics are used to treat DVT, PE, arterial thrombosis, arterial embolism, arteriovenous cannula occlusion, lysis of coronary artery thrombi after MI, and acute evolving transmural MI.

Adverse effects: Serious adverse reactions include GI, GU, intracranial, and retroperitoneal bleeding and anaphylaxis. The most common side effects are decreased Hct, urticaria, headache, and nausea.

Contraindications: Persons with hypersensitivity, active bleeding, intraspinal surgery, neoplasms of the CNS, ulcerative colitis/enteritis, severe hypertension, renal/hepatic disease, hypocoagulation, COPD, subacute bacterial endocarditis, rheumatic valvular disease, cerebral embolism/thrombosis/hemorrhage, intra-arterial diagnostic procedure or surgery (10 days), and recent major surgery should not use these products.

Precautions: Caution should be used in arterial emboli from left side of heart and pregnancy.

Pharmacokinetics: Onset, peak, and duration vary widely among products. Most products are metabolized in the liver and excreted in urine.

Interactions: Interactions vary widely among products. Check individual monographs for specific information.

NURSING CONSIDERATIONS
Assessment
• Monitor VS, B/P, pulse, respirations, neurologic signs, temp at least q4hr (increased temp is an indicator of internal bleeding), cardiac rhythm following intracoronary administration; systolic pressure increase of >25 mm Hg should be reported to prescriber
• Assess for neurologic changes that may indicate intracranial bleeding
• Assess retroperitoneal bleeding: back pain, leg weakness, diminished pulses
• Assess for allergy: fever, rash, itching, chills; mild reaction may be treated with antihistamines
• Assess for bleeding during 1st hr of treatment: hematuria, hematemesis, bleeding from mucous membranes, epistaxis, ecchymosis
• Monitor blood tests (Hct, platelets, PTT, PT, TT, APTT) before starting therapy; PT or APTT must be less than 2 times control before starting therapy; TT or PT q3-4hr during treatment

Nursing diagnoses
• Injury, risk for (uses)

Adverse effects: *italic* = common, **bold** = life-threatening

Implementation

• Administer as soon as thrombi identified; not useful for thrombi over 1 wk old
• Administer cryoprecipitate or fresh, frozen plasma if bleeding occurs
• Give loading dose at beginning of therapy; may require increased loading doses
• Give heparin after fibrinogen level is over 100 mg/dl; heparin INF to increase PTT to 1.5-2 × baseline for 3-7 days
• About 10% of patients have high streptococcal antibody titers requiring increased loading doses
• Give **IV** therapy using 0.8-μm filter
• Store reconstituted sol in refrigerator; discard after 24 hr
• Provide bed rest during entire course of treatment

Patient/family education

• Teach patient to avoid venous or arterial puncture, injection, rectal temp
• Teach patient to treat fever with acetaminophen or aspirin
• Teach patient to apply pressure for 30 sec to minor bleeding sites; inform prescriber if this does not attain hemostasis; apply pressure dressing

Evaluation
Positive therapeutic outcome
• Resolution of thrombosis, embolism

Generic Names

alteplase (high alert), anistreplase (high alert), drotrecogin alfa, streptokinase (high alert), tenecteplase (high alert), urokinase (high alert)

THYROID HORMONES

Action: Thyroid hormones increase metabolic rates, resulting in increased cardiac output, O_2 consumption, body temp, blood volume, growth, development at cellular level, respiratory rate, and enzyme system activity.

Uses: Thyroid hormones are used for thyroid replacement.

Adverse effects: The most common side effects include insomnia, tremors, tachycardia, palpitations, angina, dysrhythmias, weight loss, and changes in appetite. Serious adverse reactions include thyroid storm.

Contraindications: Persons with adrenal insufficiency, myocardial infarction, or thyrotoxicosis should not use these products.

Precautions: Caution should be used in pregnancy and breastfeeding. Geriatric patients and those with angina pectoris, hypertension, ischemia, cardiac disease, or diabetes mellitus or insipidus should be watched closely when using these products.

Pharmacokinetics: Pharmacokinetics vary widely among products. Check individual monographs for specific information.

Interactions

• Impaired absorption of thyroid products may occur when administered with cholestyramine (separate by 4-5 hr).
• Increased effects of anticoagulants, sympathomimetics, tricyclics, catecholamines may occur.
• Decreased effects of digoxin, glycosides, insulin, hypoglycemics may occur.
• Decreased effects of thyroid products may occur with estrogens.

NURSING CONSIDERATIONS
Assessment
• Monitor B/P, pulse before each dose
• Monitor I&O ratio
• Monitor weight daily in same clothing, using same scale, at same time of day
• Monitor height, growth rate if given to a child
• Monitor T_3, T_4, which are decreased; radioimmunoassay of TSH, which is increased; ratio uptake, which is decreased if patient is on too low a dosage of medication
• Assess for increased nervousness, excitability, irritability; may indicate too high a dosage of medication, usually after 1-3 wk of treatment
• Assess for cardiac status: angina, palpitation, chest pain, change in VS

Nursing diagnoses
• Body image, disturbed (adverse reactions)
• Knowledge, deficient (teaching)
• Noncompliance (teaching)

Implementation
• Give at same time each day to maintain product level
• Give only for hormone imbalances; not to be used for obesity, male infertility, menstrual conditions, lethargy
• Remove medication 4 wk before RAIU test

Patient/family education
• Advise patient that hair loss will occur in children and is temporary
• Advise patient to report excitability, irritability, anxiety; indicates overdose
• Caution patient not to switch brands unless directed by prescriber

- Caution patient that hypothyroid children will show almost immediate behavior/personality change
- Advise patient that treatment product is not to be taken to reduce weight
- Advise patient to avoid OTC preparations with iodine; read labels; to avoid iodine-containing foods: iodized salt, soybeans, tofu, turnips, some seafood, some bread

Evaluation
Positive therapeutic outcome
- Absence of depression
- Increased weight loss, diuresis, pulse, appetite
- Absence of constipation, peripheral edema, cold intolerance, pale, cool, dry skin, brittle nails, alopecia, coarse hair, menorrhagia, night blindness, paresthesias, syncope, stupor, coma, rosy cheeks

Generic Names

levothyroxine (T_4), liothyronine (T_3), liotrix, thyroid USP

VASODILATORS

Action: Vasodilators act in various ways. Check individual monographs for specific action.

Uses: Vasodilators are used to treat intermittent claudication, arteriosclerosis obliterans, vasospasm and muscular ischemia, ischemic cerebral vascular disease, hypertension, and angina.

Adverse effects: The most common side effects are headache, nausea, hypotension, hypertension, and ECG changes.

Contraindications: Some products are contraindicated in acute MI, paroxysmal tachycardia, and thyrotoxicosis.

Precautions: Caution should be used in uncompensated heart disease or peptic ulcer disease.

Pharmacokinetics: Onset, peak, and duration vary widely among products. Most products are metabolized in the liver and excreted in urine.

Interactions: Interactions vary widely among products. Check individual monographs for specific information.

NURSING CONSIDERATIONS
Assessment
- Assess bleeding time in individuals with bleeding disorders
- Assess cardiac status: B/P, pulse, rate, rhythm, character; watch for increasing pulse

Nursing diagnoses
- Cardiac output, decreased (uses)
- Knowledge, deficient (teaching)
- Tissue perfusion, ineffective (uses)

Implementation
- Give with meals to reduce GI symptoms
- Store in tight container at room temperature

Patient/family education
- Inform patient that medication is not cure, may need to be taken continuously
- Advise patient that it is necessary to quit smoking to prevent excessive vasoconstriction
- Advise patient that improvement may be sudden, but usually occurs gradually over several weeks
- Instruct patient to report headache, weakness, increased pulse, since product may need to be decreased or discontinued
- Instruct patient to avoid hazardous activities until stabilized on medication; dizziness may occur

Evaluation
Positive therapeutic outcome
- Ability to walk without pain
- Increased temp in extremities
- Increased pulse volume

Generic Names

bosentan, dipyridamole, hydrALAZINE, isoxsuprine, midodrine, minoxidil, nesiritide, papaverine

---

VITAMINS

Action: The action of vitamins varies widely among products and classes. Check individual monographs for specific action.

Uses: Vitamins are used to correct and prevent vitamin deficiencies.

Adverse effects: There is an absence of side effects or adverse reactions with the water-soluble vitamins (C, B). However, fat-soluble vitamins (A, D, E, K) may accumulate in the body and cause adverse reactions (refer to individual monographs).

Contraindications: Hypersensitive reactions may occur, and allergies should be identified before these products are given.

Pharmacokinetics: Onset, peak, and duration vary widely among products. Check individual monographs for specific information.

NURSING CONSIDERATIONS
Nursing diagnoses
- Nutrition: less than body requirements, imbalanced (uses)

Implementation
- Give PO with food for better absorption
- Store in tight, light-resistant container

Patient/family education
- Advise patient not to take more than prescribed amount

Evaluation
Positive therapeutic outcome
- Absence of vitamin deficiency

Generic Names
Fat-soluble:
phytonadione (vitamin K_1), vitamin A, vitamin D, vitamin E

Water-soluble:
ascorbic acid (C), cyanocobalamin (B_{12}), pyridoxine (B_6), riboflavin (B_2), thiamine (B_1)

Miscellaneous:
multivitamins

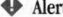 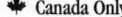

Appendix A

Selected New Drugs

abobotulinumtoxinA
Dysport
See p. 35

asenapine
Saphris
See p. 112

canakinumab
Ilaris
See p. 174

dexlansoprazole
Kapidex
See p. 304

dronedarone
Multaq
See p. 353

RARELY USED
eltrombopag
Promacta
Func. class.: Hemostatic

Uses: Idiopathic thrombocytopenic purpura that have not responded to conventional treatment; available on a limited basis

Dosage and routes
Adult: **IV** 50 mg qd on empty stomach; Asian patients should be started on 25 mg qd

Contraindications: Hypersensitivity

everolimus
Affinitor
See p. 406

febuxostat
Uloric
See p. 417

fenofibric acid
TriLipix
See p. 420

ferumoxytol
Feraheme
See p. 426

RARELY USED
fibrinogen, concentrate, human (Rx)
(fi-brin'o-gen)
Ria STAP
Func. class.: Hemostatic, orphan

Uses: Hemorrhage, afibrinogen, hypofibrinogenemia

Dosage and routes
When fibrinogen concentrate is not known
Adult/ adolescent/child: **IV** 70 mg/kg, max 5 ml/min; maintain fibrinogen level of 100 mg/dl until hemostasis is obtained

When fibrinogen concentrate is known
Adult/adolescent/child: **IV** individualized

Contraindications: Hypersensitivity

Adverse effects: *italic* = common, **bold** = life-threatening

! HIGH ALERT

fospropofol (Rx)
(fos-proe'poe-fol)
Lusedra
Func. class.: General anesthetic

Pregnancy category B

Action: Prodrug of propofol; produces dose-dependent CNS depression by activation of GABA receptor inhibition of NMDA subtype of glutamate receptors by channel gating modulation

Therapeutic outcome: Anesthesia

Uses: Induction or maintenance of anesthesia as part of balanced anesthetic technique; sedation in mechanically ventilated patients

Dosage and routes
Induction/maintenance
Adult <65 (healthy): >90 kg,* initially 577.5 mg **IV** bolus, as needed give supplemental doses up to a max of 140 mg **IV**/dose to achieve desired level of sedation, give no more frequently than q4min; *61-89 kg,* initially 6.5 mg/kg (max 577.5 mg) **IV** bolus, as needed give supplemental doses up to 1.6 mg/kg/dose (max 140 mg/dose) **IV** to achieve desired level of sedation, give no more frequently than q4min; ≤*60 kg,* initially 385 mg **IV** bolus, as needed give supplemental doses up to a max of 105 mg **IV**/dose to achieve desired level of sedation, give no more frequently than q4min

Adult <65 yr (severe systemic disease): ≥90 kg,* initially 437.5 mg **IV** bolus, as needed give supplemental doses up to a max of 105 mg **IV**/dose to achieve desired level of sedation, give no more frequently than q4min; *61-89 kg,* initially give 75% of standard dosing regimen, which is 4.875 mg/kg (max 437.5 mg) **IV** bolus, as needed give supplemental doses that are 75% of standard dosing regimen (up to 1.2 mg/kg/dose **IV,** max 105 mg/dose **IV**), give doses to achieve desired level of sedation, give no more frequently than q4min; ≤*60 kg,* initially 297.5 mg **IV** bolus, as needed give supplemental doses up to a max of 70 mg **IV**/dose to achieve desired level of sedation, give no more frequently than q4min

Geriatric: ≥90 kg,* initially 437.5 mg **IV** bolus, as needed give supplemental doses up to a max 105 mg **IV**/dose to achieve desired level of sedation, give no more frequently than q4min; *61-89 kg,* initially give 75% of standard

dosing regimen, which is 4.875 mg/kg (max 105 mg 1 dose) **IV** bolus, as needed give supplemental doses that are 75% of standard dosing regimen; give doses to achieve desired level of sedation; give no more frequently than q4min

Available forms: Inj 1050 mg/30 ml

Adverse effects
CNS: Involuntary movement, headache, jerking, fever, dizziness, shivering, tremor, confusion, somnolence, paresthesia, agitation, abnormal dreams, euphoria, fatigue, **increased intracranial pressure, impaired cerebral flow, seizures**
CV: Bradycardia, hypotension, hypertension, PVC, PAC, tachycardia, abnormal ECG, ST segment depression, **asystole, bradydysrhythmias**
EENT: Blurred vision, tinnitus, eye pain, strange taste, diplopia
GI: Nausea, vomiting, abdominal cramping, dry mouth, swallowing, hypersalivation, **pancreatitis**
GU: Urine retention, green urine, cloudy urine, oliguria
INTEG: Flushing, phlebitis, hives, burning/stinging at inj site, rash, pain of extremities
MS: Myalgia
RESP: **Apnea,** *cough, hiccups,* dyspnea, hypoventilation, sneezing, wheezing, tachypnea, hypoxia, respiratory acidosis

Contraindications: Hypersensitivity to product or soybean oil, egg, benzyl alcohol (some products)

Precautions: Pregnancy **B,** breastfeeding, children, geriatric patients, respiratory depression, severe respiratory disorders, cardiac dysrhythmias, labor and delivery, renal disease, hyperlipidemia

Pharmacokinetics

Absorption	Unknown
Distribution	Rapid, 98% protein binding
Metabolism	Liver conjugated to inactive metabolites
Excretion	Urine 7%
Half-life	1-8 min; terminal 0.81-0.88 hr

Pharmacodynamics

Onset	15-30 sec
Peak	Unknown
Duration	Unknown

 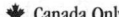

Interactions
Drug classifications
• Do not use within 10 days of MAOIs, alcohol, opioids, sedative/hypnotics, antipsychotics, skeletal muscle relaxants, inhalational anesthetics: increased CNS depression
Drug/herb
St. John's wort: increased fospropofol effect

NURSING CONSIDERATIONS
Assessment
• Assess inj site: phlebitis, burning, stinging
• Monitor ECG for changes: PVC, PAC, ST segment changes; monitor VS
• Assess CNS changes: movement, jerking, tremors, dizziness, LOC, pupil reaction
• Assess for allergic reactions: hives
• Assess for respiratory dysfunction: respiratory depression, character, rate, rhythm; notify prescriber if respirations are <10/min

Nursing diagnoses
• Injury, risk for (adverse reactions)

Implementation:
IV bolus route
• Visually inspect for particulate matter and discoloration
• Each vial is single patient/single use
• Draw from vial, discard unused portion
• Do not mix with other drugs prior to use
• Give by **IV** bolus, in free flowing peripheral **IV** line of D_5W, 5% Dextrose/0.2% NaCl, 5% Dextrose/0.45% NaCl D_5LR, LR, 0.45% NaCl, NS, 5% Dextrose/0.45% NaCl/20 mEq KCl; do not mix with other fluids; flush line with NS before and after administration
• No filtration needed
• Give only with resuscitative equipment available
• Give only by qualified persons trained in anesthesia
• Store unopened vials at room temperature

Teach patient/family:
• Teach patient that this medication will cause dizziness, drowsiness, sedation

Evaluation:
Positive therapeutic outcome
• Induction of anesthesia

Treatment of overdose: Discontinue product; administer vasopressor agents or anticholinergics, artificial ventilation

golimumab (Rx)
(goal-lim'yu-mab)
Simponi
Func. class.: Antirheumatic agent (disease modifying), immunomodulator
Chem. class.: Monoclonal antibody, DMARDS, tumor necrosis factor (TNF) modifier

Pregnancy category B

Action: Monoclonal antibody specific for human tumor necrosis factor (TNF); elevated levels of TNF are found in patients with rheumatoid arthritis

Therapeutic outcome: Decreased pain, inflammation in joints, better ROM

Uses: Rheumatoid arthritis, ankylosing spondylitis, psoriatic arthritis

Dosage and routes
Adult: SUBCUT 50 mg qmo; for RA give with methotrexate

Available forms: Inj 50 mg/0.5 ml prefilled syringe, SmartJect Auto Injector

Adverse effects
CNS: Dizziness, paresthesia
CV: Hypertension
GI: **Hepatitis**
HEMA: **Agranulocytosis, aplastic anemia, leukopenia, polycythemia, thrombocytopenia, pancytopenia**
INTEG: Psoriasis
MISC: Hypertension, **increased risk of cancer,** antibody development to this drug, **risk of infection (TB, invasive fungal infections, other opportunistic infections); may be fatal**

Contraindications: Hypersensitivity active infections

Precautions: Pregnancy **B,** breastfeeding, children, geriatric patients, CNS demyelinating disease, latent TB, CHF, hepatitis B carriers, blood dyscrasias, surgery, MS, neurological disease, diabetes, immunosuppression

Pharmacokinetics

Absorption	Unknown
Distribution	Unknown
Metabolism	Unknown
Excretion	Unknown
Half-life	Terminal 2 wk

Pharmacodynamics
Unknown

Adverse effects: *italic* = common, **bold** = life-threatening

Interactions
Drug classifications
Vaccines: do not give concurrently; immunization should be brought up to date before
treatment

Abatacept, adalimumab, anakinra, etanercept,
immunosuppressants, infliximab, rilonacept,
riuximab: increased infection

NURSING CONSIDERATIONS
Assessment
• Assess for pain, stiffness, ROM, swelling of
joints during treatment
• Check for inj site pain, swelling; usually
occur after 2 inj (4-5 days)
◆ Check for infections (fever, flulike symptoms, dyspnea, change in urination, redness/
swelling around any wounds), stop treatment if
present; some serious infections including
sepsis may occur, may be fatal; patients with
active infections should not be started on this
product

Nursing diagnoses
• Activity intolerance (uses)
• Knowledge, deficient (teaching)
• Mobility, impaired physical (uses)
• Pain, chronic (uses)

Implementation
SUBCUT route
• Do not admix with other sol or medications;
do not use filter; protect from light; give at
45-degree angle using abdomen, thighs; rotate
inj sites; discard unused portions
• Other DMARDs should be continued during
this therapy

Patient/family education
• Teach patient about self-administration if
appropriate: inj should be made in thigh,
abdomen, upper arm; rotate sites at least 1
inch from old site; do not inject in areas that
are bruised, red, hard
• Advise patient that if medication is not taken
when due, inject next dose as soon as remembered and inject next dose as scheduled

Evaluation
Positive therapeutic outcome
• Decreased inflammation, pain in joints

RARELY USED

Hylan G-F 20
(hi'lan)
Synvisc, Synvisc One

Uses: Osteoarthritis

Dosage and routes
Adult: Intraarticular (Synvisc only) 2 ml (16
mg hylan polymers) qwk × 3 injections;
Synvisc One only) 6 ml (48 hylan polymers) as
a single injection

Contraindications: Hypersensitivity to
this product or hyaluronan

---

iloperidone
Fanapt
See p. 519

---

pitavastatin (Rx)
(pit'a-va-stat'in)
Livalo
Func. class.: Antilipidemic
Chem. class.: HMG-CoA reductase inhibitor

Pregnancy category X

Action: Inhibits HMG-CoA reductase enzyme, which reduces cholesterol synthesis

Therapeutic outcome: Decreased
cholesterol levels and LDLs, increased HDLs

Uses: As an adjunct in primary hypercholesterolemia (types Ia, Ib), dysbetalipoproteinemia, elevated triglyceride levels; prevention of
cardiovascular disease by reduction of heart
risk in those with mildly elevated cholesterol

Dosage and routes
Adult: PO 2 mg/day, usual range 1-4, max 4
mg/day

Renal dose
Adult: PO CCr 30-60 ml/min 1 mg qd, max 2
mg qd; CCr <30 ml/min on hemodialysis 1 mg
qd, max 2 mg qd; CCr <30 ml/min not on
hemodialysis—not recommended

Available forms: Tabs 10, 20, 40, 80 mg

Adverse effects
CNS: Headache
GI: Constipation, diarrhea
INTEG: Rash, pruritus, alopecia
MS: Myalgia, **rhabdomyolysis**, arthralgia
RESP: Pharyngitis

Contraindications: Pregnancy **X**, breast-feeding, hypersensitivity, active liver disease, cholestasis

Precautions: Past liver disease, alcoholism, severe acute infections, trauma, severe metabolic disorders, electrolyte imbalance, seizures, surgery, organ transplant, endocrine disease, females, hypotension, renal disease

Pharmacokinetics

Absorption	Unknown
Distribution	Unknown
Metabolism	Liver
Excretion	Urine, feces
Half-life	12 hr

Pharmacodynamics
Unknown

Interactions
Individual drugs
Clofibrate, cycloSPORINE, erythromycin, gemfibrozil, niacin: increased risk of rhabdomyolysis
Colestipol: decreased action of atorvastatin
Erythromycin: increased levels of atorvastatin
Warfarin: increased action of warfarin

Drug classifications
Antifungals (azole): possible rhabdomyolysis
Contraceptives (oral): increased levels

Drug/lab test
Increased: bilirubin, alkaline phosphatase
Interference: thyroid function tests

NURSING CONSIDERATIONS
Assessment
• Assess nutrition: fat, protein, carbohydrates; nutritional analysis should be completed by dietitian before treatment
• Assess for muscle pain, tenderness; obtain CPK if these occur, product may need to be discontinued
• Monitor bowel pattern daily; diarrhea may be a problem
• Monitor triglycerides, cholesterol at baseline, throughout treatment; LDL and VLDL should be watched closely; if increased, product should be discontinued
• Monitor liver function studies q1-2mo during the first 1½ yr of treatment; AST, ALT, liver function tests may be increased
• Monitor renal studies in patients with compromised renal system: BUN, I&O ratio, creatinine
• Assess eyes via ophthalmic exam 1 mo after treatment begins, annually

Nursing diagnoses
• Diarrhea (adverse reactions)
• Knowledge, deficient (teaching)
• Noncompliance (teaching)

Implementation
• Administer total daily dose at any time of day
• Store in cool environment in airtight, light-resistant container

Patient/family education
• Inform patient that compliance is needed for positive results to occur, not to double doses
• Teach patient that risk factors should be decreased: high-fat diet, smoking, alcohol consumption, absence of exercise
• Advise patient to notify prescriber if the GI symptoms of diarrhea, abdominal or epigastric pain, nausea, vomiting; chills, fever, sore throat; muscle pain, weakness occur
• Advise patient that treatment will take several years
• Advise patient that blood work will be necessary during treatment
• Advise not to take if pregnant

Evaluation
Positive therapeutic outcome
• Decreased cholesterol levels, serum triglyceride
• Improved ratio of HDLs

plerixafor
Mozobil
See p. 816

pralatrexate
Folotyn
See p. 822

prasugrel
Effient
See p. 825

saxagliptin (Rx)
(sax-a-glip'tin)
Onglyza
Func. class.: Antidiabetic, oral
Chem. class.: Dipeptidyl-peptidase-4 inhibitor (DPP-4 inhibitor)

Pregnancy category C

Action: Slows the inactivation of incretin hormones, improves glucose homeostasis, improves glucose-dependent insulin synthesis, lowers glucagon secretions and slows gastric emptying time

Therapeutic outcome: Decrease in polyuria, polydipsia, polyphagia; clear sensorium; absence of dizziness; stable gait; blood glucose at normal level

Uses: Type 2 diabetes mellitus as monotherapy or in combination with other antidiabetic agents

Dosage and routes
Adult: PO 2.5-5 mg; may use with other antidiabetic agents (metformin, pioglitazone, rosiglitazone)

Available forms: Tabs 2.5; 5 mg

Adverse effects
CNS: Headache
ENDO: Hypoglycemia
GI: Nausea, vomiting, abdominal pain
INTEG: Urticaria, **angioedema**
MISC: Lymphopenia, peripheral edema

Contraindications: Hypersensitivity, diabetic ketoacidosis (DKA)

Precautions: Pregnancy **B**, geriatric, GI obstruction, thyroid disease, surgery, renal/hepatic disease, trauma

Pharmacokinetics

Absorption	Rapidly
Distribution	Unknown
Metabolism	Unknown
Excretion	Kidneys 24% unchanged
Half-life	Terminal 2.5 hr, 3.1 hr metabolite

Pharmacodynamics

Onset	Unknown
Peak	1-4 hr
Duration	Unknown

Interactions
Individual drugs
Aripiprazole, clozapine, fosphenytoin, olanzapine, phenytoin, quetiapine, risperidone, ziprasidone: decreased antidiabetic effect
Cimetidine, disopyramide: increased saxagliptin level
Cimetidine, fluoxetine: increased hypoglycemia
Digoxin: increased levels of digoxin

Drug classifications
ACE inhibitors, estrogens, oral contraceptives, phenothiazines, progestins, protease inhibitors, sympathomimetics, thiazide diuretics: decreased antidiabetic effect
Androgens, β-blockers, corticosteroids, fibric acid derivatives, insulins, MAOIs, salicylates: increased hypoglycemia

Drug/herb
Alfalfa, aloe, basil, bay, bilberry, bitter melon, black catechu, buchu, burdock, coriander, dandelion, eyebright (po), fenugreek, garlic, ginseng, glucomannan, glucosamine, goat's rue, gymnema, horehound, horse chestnut, jambul, myrrh, myrtle: increased antidiabetic effect
Bee pollen, blue cohosh, broom, chromium, elecampane, eucalyptus, gotu kola: decreased antidiabetic effect
Chromium, coenzyme Q-10, fenugreek: increased hypoglycemia
Glucosamine: increased hyperglycemia

NURSING CONSIDERATIONS
Assessment
• Assess for hypoglycemic reactions (sweating, weakness, dizziness, anxiety, tremors, hunger), hyperglycemic reactions soon after meals
• Monitor CBC (baseline, q3mo) during treatment; check liver function tests periodically, AST, LDH, renal studies: BUN, creatinine during treatment; glycosylated hemoglobin A1c
• Monitor blood glucose (BG) as needed

Nursing diagnoses
• Knowledge, deficient (teaching)
• Noncompliance (teaching)
• Nutrition: more than body requirements, imbalanced (uses)

Implementation
• May be taken with or without food
• Conversion from other antidiabetic agents; change may be made with gradual dosage change
• Store in tight container at room temperature

Patient/family education
- Teach patient to use regular self-monitoring of blood glucose using blood glucose meter
- Teach patient the symptoms of hypo/hyperglycemia; what to do about each
- Teach patient that product must be continued on daily basis; explain consequence of discontinuing product abruptly
- Advise patient to avoid OTC medications, alcohol, digoxin, exenatide, insulins, nateglinide, repaglinide, and other products that lower blood sugar, unless approved by prescriber
- Teach patient that diabetes is a lifelong illness; that this product is not a cure, only controls symptoms
- Teach patient that all food included in diet plan must be eaten to prevent hypo/hyperglycemia
- Teach patient to carry emergency ID

Evaluation
Positive therapeutic outcome
- Decrease in polyuria, polydipsia, polyphagia; clear sensorium; absence of dizziness; stable gait; blood glucose at normal level

---

tapentadol
Nucynta
See p. 958

---

telavancin
Vibativ
See p. 960

---

tolvaptan
Samsca
See p. 1008

---

ustekinumab
Stelara
See p. 1037

---

vigabatrin (Rx)
(vye-ga′ba-trin)
Sabril
Func. class.: Anticonvulsant
Pregnancy category C

Action: May inhibit reuptake and metabolism of GABA, may increase seizure threshold; structurally similar to GABA

Therapeutic outcome: Prevention of seizure activity

Uses: Adjunct treatment of partial seizures in adults and children ≥12 yr, infantile spasm

Dosage and routes
Partial seizures
Adult: PO 500 mg bid, titrate in 500 mg increments at weekly intervals, up to 1.5 g bid

Infantile spasm
Infant >1 mo, child ≤2 yr: PO 50 mg/kg/day in 2 divided doses titrate in 25-50 mg/kg/day increments q3days, max 150 mg/kg/day

Renal dose
Adult: PO CCr 50-80 ml/min, reduce dose by 25%
Adult: PO CCr 30-50 ml/min, reduce dose by 50%
Adult: PO CCr 10-30 ml/min, reduce dose by 75%

Available forms: powder for solution; tablet 500 mg

Adverse effects
CNS: Dizziness, irritability, lethargy, **malignant hyperthermia,** insomnia
CV: Edema
EENT: **Visual impairment**
GI: Nausea, vomiting, diarrhea, increased appetite, abdominal pain, GI bleeding, hemorrhoids, weight gain, constipation
HEMA: Anemia
INTEG: Pruritus, rash
RESP: Coughing, **respiratory depression, pulmonary embolism**

Contraindications: Hypersensitivity to this product

Precautions: Pregnancy C, breastfeeding, children <2 yr, geriatric patients, renal/hepatic disease, suicidal ideation/behavior, abrupt discontinuation

Black Box Warning: Visual disturbance

Adverse effects: *italic* = common, **bold** = life-threatening

Pharmacokinetics	
Absorption	>95%
Distribution	Widely; no protein binding
Metabolism	Not metabolized
Excretion	Urine 80% parent drug, slowed in renal disease
Half-life	7.5 hr

Pharmacodynamics	
Onset	Unknown
Peak	2 hr
Duration	Unknown

Interactions
Individual drugs
Azathioprine, chloroquine, deferoxamine, ethambutol, hydroxychloroquine, interferons, loxapine, mecasermin, rh-IGF-1, pentostatin, tamoxifen, thiothixene: Serious ophthalmic effects (glaucoma, retinopathy); avoid concurrent use

Drug classifications
CNS depressants: increased CNS depression
Corticosteroids, phenothiazines, phosphodiesterase inhibitors: Serious ophthalmic effects (glaucoma, retinopathy)

NURSING CONSIDERATIONS
Assessment
• Monitor renal studies: urinalysis, BUN, urine creatinine q3mo
• Monitor hepatic studies: ALT, AST, bilirubin
• Assess description of seizures: location, duration, presence of aura
• Assess mental status: mood, sensorium, affect, behavioral changes; if mental status changes, notify prescriber

Nursing diagnoses
• Possible injury (uses)
• Noncompliance (teaching)
• Knowledge deficit (teaching)

Implementation
PO route (tab)
• Give without regard to meals
PO route (oral solution)
• Reconstitute immediately before using
• Empty contents into a clean cup
• For each packet, dissolve 10 ml of water, conc. 50 mg/ml; do not use other liquids
• Stir until dissolved; solution should be clear
• Use calibrated oral syringe to measure correct dosage
• Discard any unused solution

Perform/provide
• Store at room temperature
• Provide assistance with ambulation during early part of treatment; dizziness occurs
• Provide seizure precautions: padded side rails; move objects that may harm patient

Patient/family education
• Teach patient to carry emergency ID stating patient's name, products taken, condition, prescriber's name and phone number
• Advise patient to avoid driving, other activities that require alertness
• Inform patient not to discontinue medication quickly after long-term use

Evaluation:
• Therapeutic response: decreased seizure activity; document on patient's chart

Appendix B

Ophthalmic, Nasal, Topical, and Otic Products

OPHTHALMIC PRODUCTS

α-ADRENERGIC BLOCKER
dapiprazole (Rx)
(da-pip'ra-zole)
Rev-Eyes

ANESTHETICS
lidocaine (Rx)
(lye'doe-kane)
Akten
proparacaine (Rx)
(proe-par'a-kane)
Alcaine, Diocaine ✤, Ophthaine,
Ophthetic
tetracaine (Rx)
(tet'ra-kane)
Minims Tetracaine ✤, Pontocaine,
Tetracaine

ANTIHISTAMINES
azelastine (Rx)
(ay-zell'ah-steen)
Optivar
emedastine (Rx)
(ee-med'-a-steen)
Emadine
epinastine (Rx)
(ep-een-as'teen)
Elestat
ketotifen (Rx, OTC)
(kee-toh-tif'en)
Zaditor
levocabastine (Rx)
(lee-voh-cab'ah-steen)
Livostin
olopatadine (Rx)
(oh-loh-pat'ah-deen)
Patanol

ANTIINFECTIVES
azithromycin (Rx)
(ay-zi-thro-my'sin)
AzaSite
besifloxacin (Rx)
(be'si-flox'a-sin)
Besivance

chloramphenicol (Rx)
(klor-am-fen'i-kole)
AK-Chlor, Chloramphenicol, Chloromycetin
Ophthalmic, Chloroptic, Chloroptic S.O.P.,
Fenicol ✤, Isopto Fenical ✤,
Pentamycin ✤
ciprofloxacin (Rx)
(sip-ro-floks'a-sin)
Ciloxan
erythromycin (Rx)
(er-ith-roe-mye'sin)
Erythromycin, Ilotycin
ganciclovir (Rx)
(gan-sye'kloe-vir)
Virgan
gatifloxacin (Rx)
(gat-ih-floks'ah-sin)
Zymar
gentamicin (Rx)
(jen-ta-mye'sin)
Garamycin Ophthalmic, Genoptic
Ophthalmic, Genoptic S.O.P., Gentacidin,
Gentamicin Ophthalmic, Gentak
levofloxacin (Rx)
(lee-voh-flock'sah-sin)
Quixin
moxifloxacin (Rx)
(mox-i-flox'a-sin)
Vigamox
natamycin (Rx)
(nat-a-mye'sin)
Natacyn
norfloxacin (Rx)
(nor-floks'a-sin)
Chibroxin
ofloxacin (Rx)
(oh-floks'a-sin)
Ocuflox

Adverse effects: *italic* = common, **bold** = life-threatening

silver nitrate 1% (Rx)
silver nitrate
sulfacetamide sodium (Rx)
(sul-fa-seet'a-mide)
AK-Sulf, Bleph-10, Bleph-10 S.O.P.,
Cetamide, Isopto Cetamide, Ocusulf-10,
Sodium Sulamyd, Sodium Sulfacetamide,
Storzsulf, Sulf-10, Sulster
tobramycin (Rx)
(toe-bra-mye'sin)
AKTob, Defy, Tobrex
trifluridine (Rx)
(trye-floor'i-deen)
Viroptic
vidarabine (Rx)
(vye-dare'a-been)
Vira-A

β-ADRENERGIC BLOCKERS
betaxolol (Rx)
(beh-tax'oh-lole)
Betoptic, Betoptic S
carteolol (Rx)
(kar-tee'oh-lole)
Carteolol HCl, Ocupress
levobetaxolol (Rx)
(lee-voh-beh-tax'oh-lohl)
Betaxon
levobunolol (Rx)
(lee-voe-byoo'no-lole)
AK Beta, Betagen
metipranolol (Rx)
(met-ee-pran'oh-lole)
OptiPranolol
timolol (Rx)
(tym'-moe-lole)
Apo-Timop ♣, Betimol, Timoptic,
Timoptic-XE

**CARBONIC ANHYDRASE
INHIBITORS**
brinzolamide (Rx)
(brin-zoh'la-mide)
Azopt
dorzolamide (Rx)
(dor-zol'a-mide)
Trusopt

CHOLINERGICS
(Direct-acting)
acetylcholine (Rx)
(ah-see-til-koe'leen)
Miochol-E

carbachol (Rx)
(kar'ba-kole)
Carbastat, Carboptic, Isopto Carbachol,
Miostat
pilocarpine (Rx)
(pye-loe-kar'peen)
Adsorbocarpine, Akarpine, Isopto Carpine,
Ocu-Carpine, Ocusert Pilo-20, Ocusert Pilo-
40, Pilagan, Pilocar, pilocarpine, Pilopine
HS, Piloptic-½, Piloptic-1, Piloptic-2,
Piloptic-3, Piloptic-4, Piloptic-6, Pilostat,
Pilopto-Carpine

CHOLINESTERASE INHIBITORS
demecarium (Rx)
(dem-e-kare'ee-um)
Humorsol
ecothiophate (Rx)
(ek-oh-thye'oh-fate)
Phospholine Iodide
isoflurophate (Rx)
(i-se'flur-e'fate)
Floropryl
physostigmine (Rx)
(fi-zoe-stig'meen)
Eserine Salicylate, Isopto Eserine

CORTICOSTEROIDS
dexamethasone (Rx)
(dex-a-meth'a-sone)
AK-Dex, Decadron Phosphate,
Dexamethasone Ophthalmic Suspension,
Maxidex, Ozurdex
fluorometholone (Rx)
(flure-oh-meth'oh-lone)
Flarex, Fluor-Op, FML, FML Forte, FML
S.O.P.
loteprednol (Rx)
(loe-tee-pred-nole)
Alrex, Lotemax
medrysone (Rx)
(me'dri-sone)
HMS
***prednisoLONE** (Rx)
(pred-niss'oh-lone)
Econopred, Econopred Plus, AK-Pred,
Inflamase Forte, Inflamase Mild, Pred-Forte
rimexolone (Rx)
(ri-mex'a-lone)
Vexol
triamcinolone (Rx)
(trye-am-sin'oh-lone)
Triesence

♦ Alert   ♣ Canada Only   🔵 Drug on CD   * "Tall Man" lettering (See Preface)

MYDRIATICS
atropine (Rx)
(a'troe-peen)
Atropine-1, Atropine Care, Atropine Sulfate
Ophthalmic, Atropisol, Isopto Atropine
cyclopentolate (Rx)
(sye-kloe-pen'toe-late)
AK-Pentolate, Cyclogyl, Cyclopentolate HCl
homatropine (Rx)
(home-a'troe-peen)
Homatropine ✤, Homatropine HBr, Isopto
Homatropine, Minims
phenylephrine (OTC)
(fen-ill-ef'rin)
AK-Dilate, AK-Nefrin, Isopto Frin, Neo-
Synephrine 2.5%, Neo-Synephrine 10%,
phenylephrine HCl, 2.5% Mydfrin,
Phenoptic Relief, Prefrin
scopolamine (Rx)
(skoe-pol'a-meen)
Isopto Hyoscine
tropicamide (Rx)
(troe-pik'a-mide)
Mydriacyl, Opticyl, Tropicacyl, Tropicamide

NONSTEROIDAL
ANTIINFLAMMATORIES
bromfenac (Rx)
(brome'fen-ak)
Xibrom
diclofenac (Rx)
(dye-kloe'fen-ak)
Voltaran
flurbiprofen (Rx)
(flure-bi'-pro-fen)
Ocufen
ketorolac (Rx)
(kee-toe'role-ak)
Acular, Acuvail
nepafenac (Rx)
(ne-pa-fen'ak)
Nevanac
suprofen (Rx)
(soo-proe'fen)
Profenal

SYMPATHOMIMETICS
apraclonidine (Rx)
(a-pra-klon'i-deen)
Iopidine

brimonidine (Rx)
(brem-on'-i-dine)
Alphagan, Alphagan P
dipivefrin (Rx)
(dye-pi'vef-rin)
Propine, AKPro
***epINEPHrine/epinephryl**
borate (Rx)
(ep-i-nef'rin)
Epifrin, Glaucon/Epinal, Eppy ✤

OPHTHALMIC DECONGESTANTS/
VASOCONSTRICTORS
lodoxamide
(loe-dox'ah-mide)
Alomide
naphazoline (Rx, OTC)
(naf-az'oh-leen)
20/20 Eye Drops, AK-Con, Albalon, Allerest
Eye Drops, Allergy Drops, Clear Eyes, Clear
Eyes ACR, Comfort Eye Drops, Degest 2,
Maximum Strength Allergy Drops,
Nafazair, naphazoline HCl, Naphcon,
Naphcon Forte, Opcon, Vasoclear, Vasocon
Regular
oxymetazoline (Rx)
(ox-i-met-ah-zoh'leen)
OcuClear, Visine L.R.
tetrahydrozoline (OTC)
(tet-ra-hye-dro'zoe-leen)
Collyrium Fresh, Eyesine, Geneye, Geneye
Extra, Mallazine Eye Drops, Murine Plus,
Optigene 3, tetrahydrozoline HCl,
Tetrasine, Tetrasine Extra, Visine
Moisturizing

MISCELLANEOUS OPHTHALMICS
bimatoprost (Rx)
(bih-mat'o-prost)
Latisse, Lumigan
latanoprost (Rx)
(la-tan'oh-prost)
Xalatan
travoprost (Rx)
(tra'voe-prost)
Travatan
unoprostone (Rx)
(yoo-noe-pros'tone)
Rescula

β-*Adrenergic blockers*
Action: Reduces production of aqueous
humor by unknown mechanism

Adverse effects: *italic* = common, **bold** = life-threatening

Uses: Ocular hypertension, chronic open angle glaucoma

Anesthetics
Action: Decreases ion permeability by stabilizing neuronal membrane

Uses: Cataract extraction, tonometry, gonioscopy, removal of foreign objects, corneal suture removal, glaucoma surgery (ophthalmic); pruritus, sunburn, toothache, sore throat, cold sores, oral pain, rectal pain and irritation, control of gagging (topical)

Antiinfectives
Action: Inhibits folic acid synthesis by preventing PABA use, which is necessary for bacterial growth

Uses: Conjunctivitis, superficial eye infections, corneal ulcers, prophylaxis against infection after removal of foreign matter from the eye

Antiinflammatories
Action: Decreases inflammation, resulting in decreased pain, photophobia, hyperemia, cellular infiltration

Uses: Inflammation of eye, eyelids, conjunctiva, cornea; uveitis, iridocyclitis, allergic conditions, burns, foreign bodies, postoperatively in cataract

Carbonic anhydrase inhibitor
Action: Converted to epINEPHrine, which decreases aqueous production and increases outflow

Uses: Open angle glaucoma, ocular hypertension

Direct-acting miotic
Action: Acts directly on cholinergic receptor sites; induces miosis, spasm of accommodation, fall in intraocular pressure, caused by stimulation of ciliary, pupillary sphincter muscles, which leads to pulling away of iris from filtration angle, resulting in increased outflow of aqueous humor

Uses: Primary glaucoma, early stages of wide angle glaucoma (less useful in advanced stages), chronic open angle glaucoma, acute closed angle glaucoma before emergency surgery; also neutralizes mydriatics used during eye exam; may be used alternately with mydriatics to break adhesions between iris and lens

Adverse effects
CNS: Headache
CV: Hypertension, tachycardia, dysrhythmias
EENT: Burning, stinging
GI: Bitter taste

Contraindications: Hypersensitivity

Precautions: Pregnancy, breastfeeding, children, aphakia, hypersensitivity to carbonic anhydrase inhibitors, sulfonamides, thiazide diuretics, ocular inhibitors, renal/hepatic insufficiency

NURSING CONSIDERATIONS
Assessment
• Monitor ophthalmic exams and intraocular pressure readings
• Monitor blood counts; renal/hepatic function tests and serum electrolytes during long-term treatment

Nursing diagnoses
• Knowledge, deficient (teaching)
• Sensory perception, disturbed: visual (uses)

Implementation
• Storage at room temperature away from light

Patient/family education
• Teach how to instill drops
• Advise patient that product may cause burning, itching, blurring, dryness of eye area

Evaluation
Positive therapeutic outcome
• Absence of increased intraocular pressure

NASAL AGENTS

NASAL ANTIHISTAMINES
olopatadine (Rx)
(oh-low-pat'uh-deen)
Patanase

NASAL DECONGESTANTS
azelastine (Rx)
(ay-zell'ah-steen)
Astelin, Astepro
desoxyephedrine (OTC)
(des-oxy-e-fed'rin)
Vicks Vapor Inhaler
ephedrine (OTC)
(e-fed'rin)
Pretz-D
epinephrine (OTC)
(ep-i-neff'rin)
Adrenalin

naphazoline (OTC)
(naff-a-zoe'leen)
Privine
oxymetazoline (OTC)
(ox-i-met-az'oh-leen)
12 Hour Nasal, Afrin 12 Hour Original,
Afrin 12-Hour Original Pump Mist, Afrin
Severe Congestion With Menthol, Afrin
Sinus With Vapornase, Afrin No-Drip 12-
Hour, Afrin No-Drip 12-Hour Extra
Moisturizing, Dristan, Duramist Plus,
Duration, Genasal, Nafrine ♣, Neo-
Synephrine 12 Hour, Nostrilla,
oxymetazoline HCl, Nasal Relief, Nasal
Decongestant Maximum Strength, Vicks
Sinex 12 Hour Long-Acting, Vicks Sinex
12-Hour Ultra Fine Mist for Sinus Relief
phenylephrine (OTC)
(fen-ill-eff'rin)
Alconefrin 12, Children's Nostril, Neo-
Synephrine, Sinex
propylhexadrine (OTC)
(proe-pil-hex'a-dreen)
Benzedrex Inhaler
pseudoephedrine (Rx, OTC)
(soo-doe-e-fed'rin)
Cenafed, Decofed, Dimetapp, Genaphed,
Sudafed, Triaminic
tetrahydrozoline (OTC)
(tet-ra-hye-dro'zoe-leen)
Tyzine, Tyzine Pediatric
xylometazoline (OTC)
(zye-loh-meh-tazz'oh-leen)
Natru-vent, Otrivin, Otrivin Pediatric Nasal

NASAL STEROIDS
beclomethasone (Rx)
(be-kloe-meth'a-sone)
Beconase AQ Nasal, Beconase Inhalation,
Vancenase AQ Nasal, Vancenase Pocket
Inhaler
budesonide (Rx)
(byoo-des'oh-nide)
Rhinocort, Rhinocort Aqua
flunisolide (Rx)
(floo-niss'oh-lide)
Nasalide, Nasarel
fluticasone (Rx)
(floo-tic'a-son)
Flonase, Veramyst
triamcinolone (Rx)
(trye-am-sin'oh-lone)
Nasacort AQ

Action: Produces vasoconstriction (rapid,
long acting) of arterioles, thereby decreasing
fluid exudation, mucosal engorgement by
stimulation of α-adrenergic receptors in
vascular smooth muscle

Therapeutic outcome: Absence of nasal
congestion

Uses: Nasal congestion

Dosage and routes
Desoxyephedrine
Adult and child >6 yr: 1-2 INH in each
nostril q2hr or less

Ephedrine
Adult: Fill dropper to the level marked, then
use in each nostril q4hr or less

Epinephrine
Adult and child >6 yr: Apply with swab,
drops, spray prn

Naphazoline
Adult and child >6 yr: 1-2 drops/spray
q6hr or less

Oxymetazoline
Adult and child >6 yr: INSTILL 2-3 gtt
or sprays to each nostril bid
Child 2-6 yr: INSTILL 2-3 gtt or sprays
0.025 SOL bid, max 3 days

Phenylephrine
Adult and child >12 yr: 2-3 drops/
spray (0.25-0.5) in each nostril q3-4hr or
less; or 2-3 drops/spray (1%) in each nostril
q4hr or less
Child 6-12 yr: 2-3 drops/spray (0.25%) in
each nostril q3-4hr
Infant >6 mo: 1-2 drops (0.16%) in each
nostril q3hr

Propylhexadrine
Adult and child >6 yr: 1-2 INH in each
nostril q2hr or less

Tetrahydrozoline
Adult and child >6 yr: 2-4 drops
(0.1%) q3-4hr prn or 3-4 sprays in each
nostril q4hr prn
Child 2-6 yr: 2-3 drops (0.05%) in each
nostril q4-6hr prn

Xylometazoline
Adult and child >12 yr: 2-3 drops/
spray (0.1%) in each nostril q8-10hr
Child 2-12 yr: 2-3 drops (0.05%) in each
nostril q8-10hr
Available forms: Nasal sol 0.025%, 0.05%
Adverse effects
CNS: Anxiety, restlessness, tremors, weakness,
insomnia, dizziness, fever, headache

Adverse effects: *italic* = common, **bold** = life-threatening

EENT: Irritation, burning, sneezing, stinging, dryness, rebound congestion
GI: Nausea, vomiting, anorexia
INTEG: Contact dermatitis

Contraindications: Hypersensitivity to sympathomimetic amines

Precautions: Pregnancy **C**, children <6 yr, geriatric, diabetes, CV disease, hypertension, hyperthyroidism, increased ICP, prostatic hypertrophy, glaucoma

NURSING CONSIDERATIONS
Assessment
• Assess for redness, swelling, pain in nasal passages before, during treatment
• Assess for systemic absorption; hypertension, tachycardia; notify prescriber; systemic absorption occurs at high doses or after prolonged use

Nursing diagnoses
• Airway clearance, ineffective (uses)
• Knowledge, deficient (teaching)
• Noncompliance (teaching)

Implementation
• Have patient tilt head back, squeeze bulb to create a vacuum, and draw correct amount of sol into dropper; insert 2 gtt of sol into nostril; repeat in other nostril
• Store in light-resistant container; do not expose to high temperature or let sol come into contact with aluminum
• Give for <4 consecutive days
• Provide environmental humidification to decrease nasal congestion, dryness

Patient/family education
• Advise patient that stinging may occur for several applications; drying of mucosa may be decreased by environmental humidification
• Caution patient to notify prescriber if irregular pulse, insomnia, dizziness, or tremors occur
• Teach patient proper administration to avoid systemic absorption
• Advise patient to rinse dropper with very hot water to prevent contamination

Evaluation
Positive therapeutic outcome
• Decreased nasal congestion

TOPICAL GLUCOCORTICOIDS

betamethasone (Rx)
(bay-ta-meth′a-sone)
Alphatrex, Beben ❧, Betacort ❧, Betatrex, Beta-Val, Betnovate ❧, Celestoderm ❧, Diprosone, Ectosonel ❧, Luxiq, Maxivate, Metaderm ❧, Psorion, Valisone

betamethasone (augmented) (Rx)
(bay-ta-meth′a-sone)
Diprolene, Diprolene AF

clobetasol (Rx)
(kloe-bay′ta-sol)
Clobex, Cormax, Dermovate ❧, Embeline E 0.05%, Temovate

desonide (Rx)
(dess′oh-nide)
Verdeso Foam

desoximetasone (Rx)
(dess-ox-i-met′a-sone)
Topicort, Topicort LP

dexamethasone (Rx)
(dex-a-meth′a-sone)
Aeroseb-Dex, Decaspray

fluocinolone (Rx)
(floo-oh-sin′oh-lone)
Fluocin, Licon, Lidemol ❧, Lidex, Lyderm ❧, Topsyn ❧, Vasoderm

flurandrenolide (Rx)
(flure-an-dren′oh-lide)
Cordran, Cordran SP, Drenison 1/4 ❧, Drenison Tape ❧

fluticasone (Rx)
(floo-tik′a-sone)
Cutivate

halcinonide (Rx)
(hal-sin′oh-nide)
Halog, Halog-E

hydrocortisone (Rx)
(hye-droe-kor'ti-sone)
Actiocort, Aeroseb-HC, Ala-Cort, Allercort, Alphaderm, Anusol HC, Bactine, Barriere-HC ❧, CaldeCORT Anti-Itch, Carmol HC, Cetacort, Cortacet ❧, Cortaid, Cortalo, Cortate ❧, Cort-Dome, Cortef ❧, Corticaine, Corticreme ❧, Cortifair, Cortizone, Cortoderm ❧, Cortril, Delcort, Dermacort, DemiCort, Dermtex HC, Emo-Cort, Epifoam, FoilleCort, Gly-Cort, Gynecort, Hi-Cor, Hycort, Hyderm ❧, Hydro-Tex, Hytone, Lacti-Care-HC, Lanacort, Lemoderm, Locoid, Locoid Lotion, My Cort, Novoehydrocort ❧, Nutracort Pharm, Pharmacort, Pentacort, Rederm, Rhulicort S-T Cort, Synacort, Sarna HC ❧, Texa-Cort, Unicort ❧, Westcort

triamcinolone (Rx)
(trye-am-sin'oh-lone)
Aristocort, Delta-Tritex, Flutex, Kenac, Kenalog, Kenonel, Triaderm, Trianide ❧, Triderm, Trymex

Action: Antipruritic, antiinflammatory

Therapeutic outcome: Decreased itching, inflammation

Uses: Psoriasis, eczema, contact dermatitis, pruritus; usually reserved for severe dermatoses that have not responded to less potent formulation

Dosage and routes
Adult and child: Apply to affected area

Adverse effects
INTEG: Acne, atrophy, epidermal thinning, purpura, striae

Contraindications: Hypersensitivity, viral infections, fungal infections

Precautions: Pregnancy **C**

NURSING CONSIDERATIONS
Assessment
• Monitor temp; if fever develops, product should be discontinued
• Monitor for systemic absorption, increased temp, inflammation, irritation

Nursing diagnoses
• Knowledge, deficient (teaching)
• Pain, chronic (uses)
• Skin integrity, impaired (uses)

Implementation
• Apply only to affected areas; do not get in eyes
• Apply and leave site uncovered or lightly covered; occlusive dressing is not recommended—systemic absorption may occur
• Use only on dermatoses; do not use on weeping, denuded, or infected area
• Cleanse area before application of product
• Continue treatment for a few days after area has cleared
• Store at room temperature

Patient/family education
• Teach patient to avoid sunlight on affected area; burns may occur
• Teach patient to limit treatment to 14 days

Evaluation
Positive therapeutic outcome
• Absence of severe itching, patches on skin, flaking

TOPICAL ANTIFUNGALS

clotrimazole (OTC)
(kloe-trye'ma-zole)
Canestew ❧, Clotrimaderm ❧, Clotrimazole, Cruex, Desenex, Lotrimin AF, Myclo ❧, Neozol ❧

econazole (OTC)
(ee-kon'a-zole)
Spectazole

ketoconazole (OTC)
(kee-toe-kon'a-zole)
Nizoral, Xolegel

miconazole (OTC)
(mye-kon'a-zole)
Absorbine Antifungal Foot Powder, Breeze Mist Antifungal, Fungoid Tincture, Lotrimin AF, Maximum Strength Desenex Antifungal, Micatin, Monistat-Derm, Ony-Clear, Tetterine, ZeaSob-AF

nystatin (OTC)
(nye-stat'in)
Mycostatin, Nodostine ❧, Nilstat, Nyoderm ❧, Nystex

selenium (OTC)
(see-leen'ee-um)
Exsel, Head and Shoulders Intensive Treatment, Selenium Sulfide, Selsun, Selsun Blue

terbinafine (OTC)
(ter-bin'a-feen)
Lamisil

tolnaftate (OTC)
(tole-naf′tate)
Absorbine Athlete's Foot Cream, Aftate for Athlete's Foot, Aftate for Jock Itch, Genaspor, Quinsana Plus, Tinactin, Ting, tolnaftate

undecylenic acid (OTC)
(un-deh-sih-len′ik)
Blis-To-Sol, Breeze Mist, Caldesene, Cruex, Decylenes, Desenex, Desenex Maximum Strength, Pedi-Pro, Phicon F, Protectol

Action: Interferes with fungal cell membrane permeability

Therapeutic outcome: Absence of itching and white patches of the skin

Uses: Tinea cruris, tinea pedis, diaper rash, minor skin irritations; amphotericin B is used for *Candida* infections

Dosage and routes
Massage into affected area, surrounding area daily or bid, continue for 7-14 days, max 4 wk

Adverse effects
INTEG: Burning, stinging, dryness, itching, local irritation

Contraindications: Hypersensitivity

Precautions: Pregnancy **B**, breastfeeding, children

NURSING CONSIDERATIONS
Assessment
• Assess skin for fungal infections: peeling, dryness, itching before, throughout treatment
• Assess for continuing infection; increased size, number of lesions

Nursing diagnoses
• Infection, risk for (uses)
• Knowledge, deficient (teaching)
• Skin integrity, impaired (uses)

Implementation
• Apply to affected area, surrounding area; do not cover with occlusive dressings
• Store below 30° C (86° F)

Patient/family education
• Instruct to apply with glove to prevent further infection; not to cover with occlusive dressings
• Teach patient that long-term therapy may be needed to clear infection (2 wk-6 mo depending on organism); compliance is needed even after feeling better
• Teach patient proper hygiene: hand-washing technique, nail care, use of concomitant top agents if prescribed

• Caution patient to avoid use of OTC creams, ointments, lotions unless directed by prescriber
• Instruct patient to use medical asepsis (hand washing) before, after each application; to change socks and shoes once a day during treatment of tinea pedis
• Advise patient to report to health care prescriber if infection persists or recurs; if blisters, burning, oozing, swelling occur
• Caution patient to avoid alcohol because nausea, vomiting, hypertension may occur
• Caution patient to use sunscreen or avoid direct sunlight to prevent photosensitivity
• Advise patient to notify prescriber of sore throat, fever, skin rash, which may indicate overgrowth of organisms

Evaluation
Positive therapeutic outcome
• Decrease in size, number of lesions

TOPICAL ANTIINFECTIVES

azelaic acid (Rx)
(a-zuh-lay′ic)
Azelex, Finacea

bacitracin (OTC)
(bass-i-tray′sin)
Bacitin ✤, Bacitracin

clindamycin (Rx)
(klin-da-my′sin)
Cleocin T, Clindets, Clindagel, ClindaMax

erythromycin (Rx, OTC)
(er-ith-roe-mye′sin)
A/T/S, Akne-Mycin, Eryderm, Erygel, Erythromycin, Staticin, T-Stat

gentamicin (Rx)
(jen-ta-mye′sin)
Gentamicin

mafenide (Rx)
(ma′fe-nide)
Sulfamylon

metronidazole (Rx)
(met-roh-nye′da-zole)
MetroGel, MetroCream, MetroLotion, Noritate

mupirocin (Rx)
(myoo-peer′oh-sin)
Bactroban

neomycin (OTC)
(nee-oh-mye′sin)
Neomycin Sulfate

 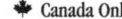

nitrofurazone (Rx)
(nye-troe-fyoor´a-zone)
Furacin, Nitrofurazone
retapamulin (Rx)
(re-tap´a-mue´lin)
Altabax
salicylic acid (Rx)
(sal´i-sil´ik)
Salitop
***silver sulfADIAZINE (Rx)**
(sul-fa-dye´a-zeen)
Flamazine ✦, Silvadene, SSD, SSD AF,
Thermazene
tretinoin (Rx)
(treh´tih-noyn)
Atralin

Action: Interferes with bacterial protein synthesis

Therapeutic outcome: Resolution of infection

Uses: Skin infections, minor burns, wounds, skin grafts, primary pyodermas, otitis externa

Adverse effects
INTEG: Rash, urticaria, scaling, redness

Contraindications: Hypersensitivity, large areas, burns, ulcerations

Precautions: Pregnancy **C**, breastfeeding, impaired renal function, external ear or perforated eardrum

NURSING CONSIDERATIONS
Assessment
• Assess for allergic reaction: burning, stinging, swelling, redness
• Assess for signs of nephrotoxicity or ototoxicity

Nursing diagnoses
• Infection, risk for (uses)
• Knowledge, deficient (teaching)
• Skin integrity, impaired (uses)

Implementation
• Apply enough medication to cover lesions completely
• Apply after cleansing with soap, water before each application; dry well
• Apply to less than 20% of body surface area when patient has impaired renal function
• Store at room temperature in dry place

Evaluation
Positive therapeutic outcome
• Decrease in size, number of lesions

TOPICAL ANTIVIRALS

acyclovir (Rx)
(ay-sye´kloe-ver)
Zovirax
penciclovir (Rx)
(pen-sye´kloe-ver)
Denavir

Action: Interferes with viral DNA replication

Therapeutic outcome: Resolution of infection

Uses: Simple mucocutaneous herpes simplex, in immunocompromised clients with initial herpes genitalis

Adverse effects
INTEG: Rash, urticaria, stinging, burning, pruritus, vulvitis

Contraindications: Hypersensitivity

Precautions: Pregnancy **C**, breastfeeding

NURSING CONSIDERATIONS
Assessment
• Assess for allergic reaction: burning, stinging, swelling, redness, rash, vulvitis, pruritus
• Assess for signs of nephrotoxicity or ototoxicity

Nursing diagnoses
• Infection, risk for (uses)
• Knowledge, deficient (teaching)
• Skin integrity, impaired (uses)

Implementation
• Apply with finger cot or rubber glove to prevent further infection
• Apply enough medication to cover lesions completely
• Apply after cleansing with soap, water before each application; dry well
• Store at room temperature in dry place

Patient/family education
• Teach patient not to use in eyes or when there is no evidence of infection
• Advise patient to apply with glove to prevent further infection
• Advise patient to avoid use of OTC creams, ointments, lotions unless directed by prescriber
• Advise patient to use medical asepsis (hand washing) before, after each application and avoid contact with eyes
• Advise patient to adhere strictly to prescribed regimen to maximize successful treatment outcome
• Advise patient to begin taking product when symptoms arise

Adverse effects: *italic* = common, **bold** = life-threatening

Evaluation
Positive therapeutic outcome
- Decrease in size, number of lesions

TOPICAL ANESTHETICS

benzocaine (OTC)
(ben'zoe-kane)
Americaine Anesthetic, Anbesol Maximum Strength, Baby Anbesol, Biozene, Boil-Ease, Children's Chloraseptic, Dermoplast, Foille, Foille Plus, Hurricaine, Lanacane, Medamint, Orabase, Oracin, Ora-Jel

dibucaine (OTC)
(dye'byoo-kane)
Dibucaine, Nupercainal

lidocaine (Rx, OTC)
(lye'doe-kane)
Anestacon, Burn-O-Jel, Dentipatch, Derma Flex, ELA-Max, Lidocaine HCl Topical, Lidocaine Viscous, Numby Staff, Solarcaine Aloe Extra Burn Relief, Xylocaine, Xylocaine 10% Oral, Xylocaine Viscous, Zilactin-L

pramoxine (OTC)
(pra-mox'een)
Itch-X, PrameGel, Prax, Tronothane

tetracaine (OTC, Rx)
(tet'ra-cane)
Pontocaine, Viractin

Action: Inhibits conduction of nerve impulses from sensory nerves

Therapeutic outcome: Decreasing inflammation, itching, pain

Uses: Oral irritation, sore throat, toothache, cold sore, canker sore, sunburn, minor cuts, insect bites, pain, itching

Dosage and routes
Adult and child: TOP apply qid as needed; RECT insert tid and after each BM

Adverse effects
INTEG: Rash, irritation, sensitization

Contraindications: Hypersensitivity, infants <1 yr, application to large areas

Precautions: Pregnancy **C,** children <6 yr, sepsis, denuded skin

NURSING CONSIDERATIONS
Assessment
- Assess pain: location, duration, characteristics before, after administration
- Assess for infection: redness, drainage, inflammation; this product should not be used until infection is treated

Nursing diagnoses
- Knowledge, deficient (teaching)
- Pain, acute (uses)

Implementation
- Store in tight, light-resistant container; do not freeze, puncture, or incinerate aerosol container

Patient/family education
- Teach patient to avoid contact with eyes
- Teach patient not to use for prolonged periods: use for <1 wk; if condition remains, prescriber should be contacted

Evaluation
Positive therapeutic outcome
- Decreased redness, swelling, pain

TOPICAL MISCELLANEOUS

docosanol (OTC)
(doh-koh'sah-nohl)
Abreva

pimecrolimus (Rx)
(pim-eh-kroh-ly'mus)
Elidel

Action: Docosanol unknown; pimecrolimus may bind with macrophilin and inhibit calcium-dependent phosphatase

Therapeutic outcome: Decreased redness, swelling, pain

Uses: Docosanol applied to fever blisters to promote more rapid healing; pimecrolimus used to treat mild to moderate atopic dermatitis in nonimmunocompromised patients ≥2 yr who are unresponsive to other treatment

Dosage and routes
Docosanol
Adult: TOP rub into blisters 5 ×/day until healing occurs

Pimecrolimus
Adult and child ≥2 yr: TOP apply thin layer 2 ×/day and rub in; use as long as needed

Adverse effects
Docosanol
None known

Pimecrolimus
INTEG: Burning

Contraindications: Hypersensitivity

Precautions: Pregnancy **C,** breastfeeding, dermal infections

 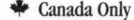

NURSING CONSIDERATIONS
Assessment
- Assess skin condition (color, pain, inflammation) before, after administration
- Assess for signs and symptoms of skin infections (redness, draining lesions); if present, avoid use of product (pimecrolimus)

Nursing diagnoses
- Skin integrity, impaired (uses)
- Infection, risk for (uses)
- Knowledge, deficient (teaching)

Implementation
- Apply to skin, rub in gently

Patient/family education
- Advise patient to avoid contact between medication and eyes
- Instruct patient to discontinue use of product when condition clears

Evaluation
Positive therapeutic outcome
- Decreased inflammation, redness

VAGINAL ANTIFUNGALS

butoconazole (OTC)
(byoo-toh-kone'ah-zole)
Femstat-3, Gynazol-1, Mycelex-3
clotrimazole (OTC)
(kloe-trye'ma-zole)
Canesten ✥, Clotriamazole, Gyne-Lotrimin 3, Gyne-Lotrimin 7, Mycelex 7, Myclo ✥
miconazole (OTC)
(mye-kon'a-zole)
Femizole-M, Monistat, Monistat 3, Monistat 7, Monistat Dual Pak, M-Zole 7 Dual Pack
nystatin (OTC)
(nye-stat'in)
Nystatin
terconazole (OTC)
(ter-kone'ah-zole)
Terazol 7, Tetrazol 3
tioconazole (OTC)
(tye-oh-kone'ah-zole)
Gyne-Trosyd ✥, Monistat 1, Vagistat-1

Action: Interferes with fungal DNA replication; binds sterols in fungal cell membranes, which increases permeability, leaking of nutrients

Therapeutic outcome: Fungistatic/fungicidal against susceptible organisms: *Candida* only

Uses: Vaginal, vulval, vulvovaginal candidiasis (moniliasis)

Dosage and routes
Butoconazole
Adult: VAG 5 g (1 applicator) at bedtime × 3-6 days

Clotrimazole
Adult: 100 mg (1 vag tab, 100 mg) at bedtime × 1 wk, or 200 mg (2 vag tab, 100 mg) at bedtime × 3 nights, or 500 mg (1 vag tab, 500 mg), or 5 g (1 applicator) at bedtime × 1-2 wk

Miconazole
Adult: 200 mg SUPP at bedtime × 3 days or 100 mg SUPP × 1 wk

Nystatin
Adult: 100,000 units/day × 2 wk

Terconazole
Adult: VAG 5 g (1 applicator) at bedtime × 7 days

Tioconazole
Adult: 1 applicator at bedtime × 1 wk

Adverse effects
GU: Vulvovaginal burning, itching, pelvic cramps
INTEG: Rash, urticaria, stinging, burning
MISC: Headache, body pain

Contraindications: Hypersensitivity

Precautions: Pregnancy, breastfeeding, children <2 yr

NURSING CONSIDERATIONS
Assessment
- Assess for allergic reaction: burning, stinging, itching, discharge, soreness

Nursing diagnoses
- Infection, risk for (uses)
- Knowledge, deficient (teaching)
- Skin integrity, impaired (uses)

Implementation
Topical route
- Administer one full applicator every night high into the vagina
- Store at room temperature in dry place

Patient/family education
- Instruct patient in asepsis (hand washing) before, after each application
- Teach patient to apply with applicator only; to avoid use of any other vaginal product unless directed by prescriber; sanitary napkin may prevent soiling of undergarments
- Instruct patient to abstain from sexual intercourse until treatment is completed; reinfection and irritation may occur

Adverse effects: *italic* = common, **bold** = life-threatening

- Advise patient to notify prescriber if symptoms persist

Evaluation
Positive therapeutic outcome
- Decrease in itching or white discharge (vaginal)

OTIC ANTIINFECTIVES

boric acid (OTC)
(bor'ik as'id)
Auro-Dri, Dri/Ear, Ear Dry
chloramphenicol (Rx)
(klor-am-fen'i-kole)
Chloromycetin Otic
ciprofloxacin (Rx)
(sip'roe-flox'a-sin)
Cetraxel

Action: Inhibits protein synthesis in susceptible microorganisms

Uses: Ear infection (external), short-term use

Adverse effects
EENT: Itching, irritation in ear
INTEG: Rash, urticaria

Contraindications: Hypersensitivity, perforated eardrum

Precautions: Pregnancy **C**

NURSING CONSIDERATIONS
Assessment
- Assess for redness, swelling, fever, pain in ear, which indicates superinfection

Nursing diagnoses
- Infection, risk for uses
- Knowledge, deficient (teaching)

Implementation
- After removing impacted cerumen by irrigation
- After cleaning stopper with alcohol
- After restraining child if necessary
- After warming sol to body temp

Patient/family education
- The correct method of instillation using aseptic technique, including not touching dropper to ear
- That dizziness may occur after instillation

Evaluation
Positive therapeutic outcome
- Decreased ear pain

Appendix C Vaccines and Toxoids

GENERIC NAME	TRADE NAME	USES	DOSAGES AND ROUTES	CONTRAINDICATIONS
avian influenza A (H5N1) virus vaccine		Prophylaxis	Adult: IM 1 ml (90 mcg) 2 doses, 28 days apart	IV
anthrax vaccine	BioThrax	Pre-/postexposure prophylaxis	**Preexposure** Adult: SUBCUT 0.5 ml at 0, 2, 4 wk, then 0.5 ml at 6, 12, 18 mo **Postexposure** Adult: SUBCUT 0.5 ml 0, 2, 4 wk, with antibiotics	Hypersensitivity
BCG vaccine	TICE BCG	TB exposure	Adult and child >1 mo: 0.2-0.3 ml Child <1 mo: Reduce dose by 50% using 2 ml of sterile water after reconstituting	Hypersensitivity, hypogamma-globulinemia, positive TB test, burns
cholera vaccine	No trade name	Immunization for cholera outside the United States	Adult and child >10 yr: IM/SUBCUT 2× of 0.5 ml, 7-30 days before traveling to cholera areas Booster is used q6mo 0.5 ml prn	Hypersensitivity, acute febrile illness
diphtheria and tetanus toxoids, adsorbed	No trade name	Induces antitoxins to provide immunity to diphtheria and tetanus	Adult and child ≥7 yr: IM (adult strength) 0.5 ml q4-8wk × 2 doses, then 3rd dose 6-12 mo after 2nd dose, booster IM 0.5 ml q10yr Child 1-6 yr: IM (pediatric strength) 0.5 ml q4wk × 2 doses, booster 6-12 mo after 2nd dose Infant 6 wk-1 yr: IM (pediatric strength) 0.5 ml q4wk × 3 doses, boost≥ 6-12 mo after 3rd dose	Hypersensitivity to mercury, thimerosal; immunocompromised patients; radiation; corticosteroids; acute illness
diphtheria and tetanus toxoids and whole-cell pertussis vaccine (DPT, DTP)	DTwP, Tr-Immunol	Prevention of diphtheria tetanus, pertussis	Adult: Booster dose q10yr Child >5 wk-6 yr: IM 0.5 ml at 2, 4, 6 mo, 1½ yr; booster needed 0.5 ml at age 6	Hypersensitivity, active infection, poliomyelitis outbreak, immunosuppression, febrile illness
diphtheria and tetanus toxoids and acellular pertussis vaccine	Acel-Imune, DTaP, Tripedia			

Continued

GENERIC NAME	TRADE NAME	USES	DOSAGES AND ROUTES	CONTRAINDICATIONS
diphtheria, tetanus, pertussis, haemophilus, polio IPV	Pentacel	Immunity to diphtheria, tetanus, pertussis, haemophilus, polio IPV	Infant >6 wk and child ≤5 yr: IM 0.5 ml at 2, 4, 6, and 15-18 mo	Hypersensitivity, polio outbreak, acute infection, immunosuppression
diphtheria, tetanus, pertussis, polio vaccine IPV	Kinrix	Immunity to diphtheria, tetanus, pertussis, polio vaccine IPV	Child: IM 0.5 ml	Hypersensitivity, polio outbreak, acute infection, immunosuppression
H1N1 influenza A (swine flu) virus vaccine	Influenza A (H1N1)	Immunity to H1N1	Adult <50 yr, adolescent, child ≥2 yr: Intranasal 1 dose (roughly 0.1 ml) into each nostril; child 2-9 repeat dose ≥4 wk later Adult, adolescent, child ≥3 yr: IM 0.5 ml as a single dose; child 3-9 yr repeat dose ≥4 wk later (Sanofi) (CSL); child 4-9 yr repeat dose ≥4 wk later (Novartis); infants ≥6 mo-child <36 mo: IM 0.25 ml, repeat in 4 wk (Sanofi) Adult: IM 0.5 ml as a single dose (GSK)	
haemophilus b conjugate vaccine, diphtheria CRM197 protein conjugate (HbOC)	HibTITER	Polysaccharide immunization of children 2-6 yr against *H. influenzae* b, conjugate	HibTITER (IM only) Child: IM 0.5 ml Child 2-6 mo: 0.5 ml q2mo × 3 inj	Hypersensitivity, febrile illness, active infection
haemophilus b conjugate vaccine, meningococcal protein conjugate (PRP-OMP)	PedvaxHIB	Immunization of child 2, 4, 6 mo	PedvaxHIB (IM only) Child 7-11 mo: Previously unvaccinated 0.5 ml q2mo inj Child 12-14 mo: Previously unvaccinated 0.5 ml × 1 inj PedvaxHIB (IM only) Child 2-14 mo: 0.5 ml × 2 inj at 2, 4 mo of age (6 mo dose not needed), then booster at 12-18 mo against invasive disease Child ≥15 mo: Previously unvaccinated 0.5 ml inj	

Vaccine	Trade Name	Use	Dosage	Contraindications
hepatitis A vaccine, inactivated	Havrix, VAQTA	Active immunization against hepatitis A virus	Adult: IM 1440 EL units (Havrix) or 50 units (VAQTA) as a single dose; booster dose is the same given at 6, 12 mo Child 2-18 yr: IM 720 EL units (Havrix) or 25 units (VAQTA) as a single dose, booster dose is the same given at 6, 12 mo	Hypersensitivity
hepatitis B vaccine, recombinant	Engerix-B, Recombivax HB	Immunization against all subtypes of hepatitis B virus	Varies widely	Hypersensitivity to this vaccine or yeast
herpes zoster virus vaccine	Zostavax	Prevention of herpes zoster	Adult ≥60 yr: SUBCUT 0.65 ml	<60 yr, child, infant, AIDS, IM/IV, leukemia, lymphoma, pregnancy
human papillomavirus recombinant vaccine, quadrivalent	Gardasil	Prevention of HPV types 6, 11, 16, 18, cervical cancer, genital warts, precancerous dysplasic lesions	Adult up to 26 yr and child >9 yr to 26 yr: IM give as 3 separate doses; 1st dose as elected; 2nd dose 2 mo after 1st dose; 3rd dose 6 mo after 1st dose	Child <9 yr, pregnancy, breastfeeding, geriatric, active disease, hypersensitivity
influenza virus vaccine	Afluria, FluMist, Fluogen, Flu-Shield, Fluviral*, Fluvirin, Fluzone, influenza virus vaccine, trivalent	Prevention of Russian, Chilean, Philippine influenza	Adult and child >12 yr: IM 0.5 ml in 1 dose Child 3-12 yr: IM 0.5 ml, repeat in 1 mo (split) unless 1978-1985 vaccine was given; also given nasal Child 6 mo to 3 yr: IM 0.25 ml, repeat in 1 mo (split) unless 1978-1985 vaccine was given; also given nasal ≥2 yr	Hypersensitivity, active infection, chicken egg allergy, Guillain-Barré syndrome, active neurologic disorders
Japanese encephalitis virus vaccine, inactivated	JE-VAX	Active immunity against Japanese encephalitis (JE)	Adult and child ≥3 yr: SUBCUT 1 ml, days 0, 7, 30; booster SUBCUT 1 ml 2 yr after last dose Child 1-3 yr: SUBCUT 0.5 ml, days 0, 7, 30; booster SUBCUT 0.5 ml 2 yr after last dose	Hypersensitivity to murine, thimerosal; allergic reactions to previous dose
Lyme disease vaccine (recombinant OspA)	LYMErix	Immunization against Lyme disease	Adult and adolescent 15-70 yr: IM 30 mcg in deltoid; repeat at 1, 12 mo after first dose	Hypersensitivity, antibiotic refractory Lyme arthritis

*Canada only.

Continued

GENERIC NAME	TRADE NAME	USES	DOSAGES AND ROUTES	CONTRAINDICATIONS
measles and rubella virus vaccine, live attenuated	M-R-Vax II	Immunity to measles and rubella by antibody production	Adult and child ≥15 mo: SUBCUT 0.5 ml (1000 units)	Hypersensitivity, immunocompromised patients, active untreated TB, cancer, blood dyscrasias, radiation, corticosteroids, pregnancy; allergic reactions to neomycin, eggs
measles, mumps, and rubella vaccine, live	M-M-R-II	Prevention of measles, mumps, rubella	Adult: SUBCUT 1 vial; 2 vials separated by 1 mo, in person born after 1957 Child >15 mo and adult: SUBCUT 0.5 ml	Hypersensitivity, blood dyscrasias, anemia, active infection, immunosuppression; egg, chicken allergy; pregnancy; febrile illness, neomycin allergy, neoplasms
measles, mumps, rubella, varicella	ProQuad	Immunity to measles, mumps, rubella, varicella	Child: SUBCUT 0.5 ml	Hypersensitivity to eggs, neomycin, cancer, radiation, corticosteroids, blood dyscrasias, active untreated TB
measles virus vaccine, live attenuated	Attenuvax	Immunity to measles by antibody production	Adult and child ≥15 mo: SUBCUT 0.5 ml (1000 units), 1 dose 15 mo, 2nd dose age 4-6 yr or 11 yr, or 12 yr	Hypersensitivity to eggs, neomycin; cancer, radiation, corticosteroids, pregnancy, immunocompromised patients, blood dyscrasias, active untreated TB
meningococcal polysaccharide vaccine	Menomune-A/C/Y/W-135, Menactra	Prophylaxis to meningococcal meningitis	Adult and child >2 yr: SUBCUT 0.5 ml	Hypersensitivity to thimerosal, pregnancy, acute illness
mumps virus vaccine, live	Mumpsvax	Active immunity to mumps	Adult and child ≥1 yr: SUBCUT 0.5 ml (20,000 units)	Hypersensitivity to eggs, neomycin; cancer, radiation, corticosteroids, pregnancy, immunocompromised patients, blood dyscrasias, active untreated TB
plague vaccine	No trade name	Active immunity to *Yersinia pestis* plague	Adult: IM 1 ml, then 0.2 ml in 4-12 wk, then 0.2 ml 5-6 mo after 2nd dose; booster 0.1-0.2 ml q6mo when in plague area	Hypersensitivity to phenol, sulfites, formaldehyde, beef, soy, casein; pregnancy, coagulation disorders
pneumococcal 7-valent conjugate vaccine	Prevnar	Immunity against *Streptococcus pneumoniae*	Child: IM 0.5 ml × 3 doses (7-11 mo); × 2 doses (12-23 mo); × 1 dose >2-9 yr	Hypersensitivity to diphtheria toxoid or this product

pneumococcal vaccine, polyvalent	Pneumovax 23, Pnu-Imune 23	Pneumococcal immunization	Adult and child >2 yr: IM/SUBCUT 0.5 ml	Hypersensitivity, Hodgkin's disease, ARDS
poliovirus vaccine, live, oral, trivalent (TOPV) poliovirus vaccine (IPV)	Orimune, IPOL	Prevention of polio	Adult and child >2 yr: PO 0.5 ml, given q8wk × 2 doses, then 0.5 ml ½-1 yr after dose 2; Infant: PO 0.5 ml at 2, 4, 18 mo; booster at 4-6 yr; may also be given: IPV at 2, 4 mo, then TOPV at 12-18 mo, booster at 4-6 yr	Hypersensitivity, active infection, allergy to neomycin/streptomycin, immunosuppression, vomiting, diarrhea
rabies vaccine, adsorbed	No trade name	Active immunity to rabies	**Preexposure** Adult and child: IM 1 ml day 0, 7, 21, or 28 days (total 3 doses); booster IM 1 ml prn q2-5yr. **Postexposure** Adult and child not vaccinated: IM 20 international units/kg of human rabies immune globulin (HRIG), give 5 total doses of 1-ml inj of rabies vaccine on days 0, 3, 7, 14, 28	Severe hypersensitivity to previous inj of vaccine, thimerosol
rabies vaccine, human diploid cell (HDCV)	Imovax Rabies, Imovax Rabies I.D.	Active immunity to rabies	**Preexposure** Adult and child: IM 1 ml day 0, 7, 21, or 28 (total 4 doses). **Postexposure** Adult and child: IM 1 ml on day 0, 3, 7, 14, 28 (total 5 doses)	No contraindications
rotavirus	RotaTeq	Prevents rotovirus	Infant: PO 3 doses given between 6 and 32 wk of age; 1st dose between 6-12 wk of age; 2nd and 3rd doses q4-10wk	Hypersensitivity, immunocompromised, blood products given within 6 wk, lymphatic disorders
rubella and mumps virus vaccine, live	Biavax II	Immunity to rubella and mumps by antibody production	Adult and child ≥1 yr: SUBCUT 0.5 ml	Hypersensitivity to eggs, neomycin; cancer, radiation, corticosteroids, pregnancy, immunocompromised patients, blood dyscrasias, active untreated TB
rubella virus vaccine, live attenuated (RA 27/3)	Meruvax II	Immunity to rubella by antibody production	Adult and child ≥1 yr: SUBCUT 0.5 ml (1000 units)	Hypersensitivity to eggs, neomycin; cancer, radiation, corticosteroids

Continued

GENERIC NAME	TRADE NAME	USES	DOSAGES AND ROUTES	CONTRAINDICATIONS
smallpox vaccine	ACAM 2000, Dry Vax	Prevention of smallpox	See package insert	No contraindications
tetanus toxoid, adsorbed/tetanus toxoid	No trade name	Tetanus toxoid: Used for prophylactic treatment of wounds	Adult and child: IM 0.5 ml q4-6wk × 2 doses, then 0.5 ml 1 yr after dose 2 (adsorbed); SUBCUT/IM 0.5 ml q4-8wk × 3 doses, then 0.5 ml ½-1 yr after dose 3, booster dose 0.5 ml q10yr	Hypersensitivity, active infection, poliomyelitis outbreak, immunosuppression
typhoid vaccine, parenteral	No trade name	Active immunity to typhoid fever	Adult: PO 1 cap 1 hr before meals × 4 doses, booster q5yr	Parenteral: Systemic or allergic reaction, acute respiratory or other acute infection, intensive physical exercise in high temperatures
typhoid vaccine, oral	Vivotif Berna Vaccine		Adult and child >10 yr: SUBCUT 0.5 ml, repeat in 4 wk, booster q3yr Child 6 mo-10 yr: SUBCUT 0.25 ml, repeat in 4 wk, booster q3yr	Oral: Hypersensitivity, acute febrile illness, suppressive or antibiotic products
typhoid Vi polysaccharide vaccine	Typhim Vi	Active immunity to typhoid fever	Adult and child ≥2 yr: IM 0.5 ml as a single dose, reimmunize q2yr 0.5 ml IM, if needed	Hypersensitivity, chronic typhoid carriers
varicella virus vaccine	Varivax	Prevention of varicella-zoster (chickenpox)	Adult and child ≥13 yr: SUBCUT 0.5 ml, 2nd dose SUBCUT 0.5 ml 4-8 wk later	Hypersensitivity to neomycin; blood dyscrasias, immunosuppression, active untreated TB, acute illness, pregnancy, diseases of lymphatic system
yellow fever vaccine	YF-Vax	Active immunity to yellow fever	Adult and child ≥9 mo: SUBCUT 0.5 ml deeply, booster q10yr Child 6-9 mo: same as above if exposed	Hypersensitivity to egg or chicken embryo protein, pregnancy, child <6 mo, immunodeficiency
zoster vaccine, live	Zostavax	Herpes zoster prevention	Reconstitute immediately after removing from freezer; give SUBCUT as a single dose; inject total amount of single-dose vial	Immunosuppression; neomycin, gelatin allergy; children, TB, pregnancy (C)

Antitoxins and Antivenins

GENERIC NAME	TRADE NAME	USES	DOSAGES AND ROUTES	CONTRAINDICATIONS
Black widow spider antivenin (*Lactrodectus mactans*)	No trade name	Black widow spider bite	Adult and child: IM 2.5 ml, 2nd dose may be given if severe; give in anterolateral thigh, obtain test for sensitivity before inj	Hypersensitivity to this product or horse serum
Crotalidae antivenom, polyvalent	No trade name	Rattlesnake bite	Adult and child: IV 20-150 ml depending on seriousness of bite, may give additional doses based on response	Hypersensitivity
Diphtheria antitoxin, equine	No trade name	Diphtheria	Adult and child: IM/slow IV 20,000-120,000 units, may give additional doses after 24 hr	Hypersensitivity
Micrurus fulvius antivenin	No trade name	East/Texas coral snake bite	Adult and child: IV 30-50 ml, give through running IV line of normal saline; give 1st 1-2 ml over 4-5 min, watch for allergic reaction	Hypersensitivity

Appendix D

Combination Products

A-200 Lice Killing Shampoo:
0.33% pyrethrins
4% piperonyl butoxide
Uses: Scabicide, pediculicide

Accuretic 10/12.5:
quinapril 10 mg
hydrochlorthiazide 12.5 mg
Uses: Antihypertensive

Accuretic 20/12.5:
quinapril 20 mg
hydrochlorthiazide 12.5 mg
Uses: Antihypertensive

Accuretic 20/25:
quinapril 20 mg
hydrochlorthiazide 25 mg
Uses: Antihypertensive

Aceta-Gesic:
acetaminophen 325 mg
phenyltoloxamine 30 mg
Uses: Pain

Activella Tablets:
estriol 1 mg
norethindrone 0.5 mg
Uses: Vasomotor symptoms (menopause)

Actonel with Calcium:
calcium carbonate 1250 mg
risedronate 35 mg
Uses: Osteoporosis

Actoplus Met:
pioglitazone 15 mg
metformin 500 mg
pioglitazone 15 mg
metformin 850 mg
Uses: Type 2 diabetes

Adderall 5 mg:
dextroamphetamine sulfate 1.25 mg
dextroamphetamine saccharate 1.25 mg
amphetamine sulfate 1.25 mg
amphetamine aspartate 1.25 mg
Uses: CNS stimulant

Adderall 7.5 mg:
dextroamphetamine sulfate 1.875 mg
dextroamphetamine saccharate 1.875 mg
dextroamphetamine aspartate 1.875 mg
amphetamine sulfate 1.875 mg
Uses: CNS stimulant

Adderall 10 mg:
dextroamphetamine sulfate 5 mg
dextroamphetamine saccharate 2.5 mg
amphetamine sulfate 2.5 mg
amphetamine aspartate 2.5 mg
Uses: CNS stimulant

Adderall 12.5 mg:
dextroamphetamine sulfate 3.125 mg
dextroamphetamine saccharate 3.125 mg
dextroamphetamine aspartate 3.125 mg
amphetamine sulfate 3.125 mg
Uses: CNS stimulant

Adderall 15 mg:
dextroamphetamine sulfate 3.75 mg
dextroamphetamine saccharate 3.75 mg
dextroamphetamine aspartate 3.75 mg
amphetamine sulfate 3.75 mg
Uses: CNS stimulant

Adderall 20 mg:
dextroamphetamine sulfate 5 mg
dextroamphetamine saccharate 5 mg
amphetamine sulfate 5 mg
amphetamine aspartate 5 mg
Uses: CNS stimulant

Adderall 30 mg:
dextroamphetamine sulfate 7.5 mg
dextroamphetamine saccharate 7.5 mg
amphetamine sulfate 7.5 mg
amphetamine aspartate 7.5 mg
Uses: CNS stimulant

Adderall XR 5 mg:
dextroamphetamine sulfate 1.25 mg
dextroamphetamine saccharate 1.25 mg
amphetamine sulfate 1.25 mg
amphetamine aspartate 1.25 mg
Uses: CNS stimulant

Adderall XR 10 mg:
dextroamphetamine sulfate 2.5 mg
dextroamphetamine saccharate 2.5 mg
amphetamine sulfate 2.5 mg
amphetamine aspartate 2.5 mg
Uses: CNS stimulant

Adderall XR 15 mg:
dextroamphetamine sulfate 3.75 mg
dextroamphetamine saccharate 3.75 mg
amphetamine sulfate 3.75 mg
amphetamine aspartate 3.75 mg
Uses: CNS stimulant

Adderall XR 20 mg:
dextroamphetamine sulfate 5 mg
dextroamphetamine saccharate 5 mg
amphetamine sulfate 5 mg
amphetamine aspartate 5 mg
Uses: CNS stimulant

Adderall XR 25 mg:
dextroamphetamine sulfate 6.25 mg
dextroamphetamine saccharate 6.25 mg
amphetamine sulfate 6.25 mg
Uses: CNS stimulant

Adderall XR 30 mg:
dextroamphetamine sulfate 7.5 mg
dextroamphetamine saccharate 7.5 mg
amphetamine sulfate 7.5 mg
amphetamine aspartate 7.5 mg
Uses: CNS stimulant

 Alert   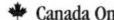 Canada Only   Drug on CD   * "Tall Man" lettering (See Preface)

Advair Diskus 100:
fluticasone 100 mcg
salmeterol 50 mcg
Uses: Corticosteroid, bronchodilator
Advair Diskus 250:
fluticasone 250 mcg
salmeterol 50 mcg
Uses: Corticosteroid, bronchodilator
Advair Diskus 500:
fluticasone 500 mcg
salmeterol 50 mcg
Uses: Corticosteroid, bronchodilator
Advicor 500:
niacin 500 mg
lovastatin 20 mg
Uses: Antilipidemic
Advicor 750:
niacin 750 mg
lovastatin 20 mg
Uses: Antilipidemic
Advicor 1000:
niacin 1000 mg
lovastatin 20 mg
niacin 1000 mg
lovastatin 40 mg
Uses: Antilipidemic
Advil Cold and Sinus Caplets:
pseudoephedrine 30 mg
ibuprofen 200 mg
Uses: Decongestant
Advil PM:
diphenhydrAMINE 38 mg
ibuprofen 25 mg
diphenhydrAMINE 200 mg
ibuprofen 200 mg
Uses: Insomnia, pain
Aggrenox:
200 mg ext rel dipyridamole
25 mg aspirin
Uses: Antiplatelet
AK-Cide Ophthalmic Suspension/Ointment:
10% sulfacetamide sodium
0.5% prednisoLONE acetate
Uses: Ophthalmic antiinfective,
antiinflammatory
Aldactazide 25/25:
spironolactone 25 mg
hydrochlorothiazide 25 mg
Uses: Diuretic
Aldactazide 50/50:
spironolactone 50 mg
hydrochlorothiazide 50 mg
Uses: Diuretic
Aldoril 15:
methyldopa 250 mg
hydrochlorothiazide 15 mg
Uses: Antihypertensive
Aldoril 25:
methyldopa 250 mg
hydrochlorothiazide 25 mg
Uses: Antihypertensive
Aldoril D30:
methyldopa 500 mg
hydrochlorothiazide 30 mg
Uses: Antihypertensive

Aldoril D50:
methyldopa 500 mg
hydrochlorothiazide 50 mg
Uses: Antihypertensive
Aleve Cold and Sinus:
naproxen 200 mg
ER pseudoephedrine 120 mg
Uses: Analgesic, adrenergic
Aleve Sinus and Headache:
naproxen 220 mg
ER pseudoephedrine 120 mg
Uses: Analgesic, adrenergic
Alka-Seltzer Original:
sodium bicarbonate 1916 mg
citric acid 1000 mg
aspirin 325 mg
Uses: Antacid, adsorbent, antiflatulent
Alka-Seltzer Plus Cold Effervescent Tablets:
acetaminophen 250 mg
chlorpheniramine 2 mg
phenylephrine 5 mg
Uses: Decongestant, analgesic, antihistamine
Alka-Seltzer Plus Night-Time Cold Liqui-Gels:
doxylamine 6.25 mg
dextromethorphan 10 mg
pseudoephedrine 30 mg
acetaminophen 325 mg
Uses: Antitussive, decongestant, antihistamine,
analgesic
Allegra-D:
fexofenadine 60 mg
pseudoephedrine 120 mg
Uses: Antihistamine, adrenergic
Allercon Tablets:
triprolidine 2.5 mg
pseudoephedrine 60 mg
Uses: Antihistamine, adrenergic
Allerest Maximum Strength Tablets:
pseudoephedrine 30 mg
chlorpheniramine 2 mg
Uses: Decongestant, antihistamine
**Allerest Allergy Sinus Relief Maximum
Strength:**
pseudoephedrine 30 mg
acetaminophen 325 mg
Uses: Antihistamine, analgesic
Allerfrim Syrup:
Per 5 ml:
triprolidine 1.25 mg
pseudoephedrine 30 mg
Uses: Antihistamine, adrenergic
Allerfrim Tablets:
triprolidine 2.5 mg
pseudoephedrine 60 mg
Uses: Antihistamine, adrenergic
All-Nite Cold Liquid:
Per 15 ml:
pseudoephedrine 30 mg
doxylamine 6.25 mg
dextromethorphan 15 mg
acetaminophen 500 mg
Uses: Decongestant, antihistamine, analgesic
Alor 5/500:
hydrocodone 5 mg

Adverse effects: *italic* = common, **bold** = life-threatening

aspirin 500 mg
Uses: Analgesic
Amaphen:
acetaminophen 325 mg
butalbital 50 mg
caffeine 40 mg
Uses: analgesic, barbiturate
Ambenyl Cough Syrup:
Per 5 ml:
bromodiphenhydramine 12.5 mg
codeine 10 mg
5% alcohol
Uses: Antihistamine, opioid analgesic
Anacin:
aspirin 400 mg
caffeine 32 mg
Uses: Analgesic
Anacin Maximum Strength:
aspirin 500 mg
caffeine 32 mg
Uses: Analgesic
Anacin PM (Aspirin Free):
diphenhydrAMINE 25 mg
acetaminophen 500 mg
Uses: Analgesic
Anaplex DM:
Per 5 ml:
brompheniramine 4 mg
dextromethorphan 30 mg
pseudoephedrine 60 mg
Uses: Decongestant, antitussive, antihistamine
Anaplex DMX:
Per 5 ml:
brompheniramine 8 mg
dextromethorphan 60 mg
pseudoephedrine 90 mg
Uses: Decongestant, antitussive, antihistamine
Anaplex HD Oral Solution:
Per 5 ml:
hydrocodone 1.7 mg
brompheniramine 2 mg
pseudoephedrine 30 mg
Uses: Antihistamine, decongestant, analgesic
Angeliq:
drospirenone 0.5 mg
estradiol 1 mg
Uses: Vasomotor symptoms (menopause)
Apresazide 25/25:
hydrALAZINE 25 mg
hydrochlorothiazide 25 mg
Uses: Antihypertensive
Apresazide 50/50:
hydrALAZINE 50 mg
hydrochlorothiazide 50 mg
Uses: Antihypertensive
Apri 28-Day:
desorgestrel 0.15 mg
ethinyl estradiol 30 mcg
Uses: Estrogen, progestin
Arthrotec:
diclofenac 50 or 75 mg
misoprostol 200 mcg
Uses: NSAID, gastric protectant

Ascriptin:
aspirin 325 mg
magnesium hydroxide 50 mg
aluminum hydroxide 50 mg
calcium carbonate 50 mg
Uses: Nonopioid analgesic, antipyretic
Ascriptin A/D:
aspirin 325 mg
aluminum hydroxide 75 mg
magnesium hydroxide 75 mg
calcium carbonate 75 mg
Uses: Analgesic
Aspirin-Free Bayer Select Allergy Sinus:
pseudoephedrine 30 mg
chlorpheniramine 2 mg
acetaminophen 500 mg
Uses: Adrenergic, antihistamine, analgesic
Aspirin Free Excedrin:
acetaminophen 500 mg
caffeine 65 mg
Uses: Analgesic
Aspirin Free Excedrin Dual:
acetaminophen 500 mg
calcium carbonate 111 mg
magnesium carbonate 64 mg
magnesium oxide 30 mg
Uses: Analgesic, antacid
Atacand HCT 16:
candesartan 16 mg
hydrochlorthiazide 12.5 mg
Uses: Antihypertensive
Atacand HCT 32:
candesartan 32 mg
hydrochlorthiazide 12.5 mg
Uses: Antihypertensive
Atripla:
efavirenz 600 mg
emtricitabine 200 mg
tenofovir 300 mg
Uses: HIV
Augmentin 250:
amoxicillin 250 mg
clavulanic acid 125 mg
Uses: Antiinfective
Augmentin 500:
amoxicillin 500 mg
clavulanic acid 125 mg
Uses: Antiinfective
Augmentin 875:
amoxicillin 875 mg
clavulanic acid 125 mg
Uses: Antiinfective
Augmentin 125 Chewable:
amoxicillin 125 mg
clavulanic acid 31.25 mg
Uses: Antiinfective
Augmentin 200 Chewable:
amoxicillin 200 mg
clavulanic acid 28.5 mg
Uses: Antiinfective
Augmentin 250 Chewable:
amoxicillin 250 mg
clavulanic acid 62.5 mg
Uses: Antiinfective

 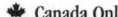

Augmentin 125 mg/5 ml Suspension:
Per 5 ml:
amoxicillin 125 mg
clavulanic acid 31.25 mg
Uses: Antiinfective
Augmentin 200 mg/5 ml Suspension:
Per 5 ml:
amoxicillin 200 mg
clavulanic acid 28.5 mg
Uses: Antiinfective
Augmentin 250 mg/5 ml Suspension:
Per 5 ml:
amoxicillin 250 mg
clavulanic acid 62.5 mg
Uses: Antiinfective
Augmentin 400 mg/5 ml Suspension:
Per 5 ml:
amoxicillin 400 mg
clavulanic acid 57 mg
Uses: Antiinfective
Auralgan Otic Solution:
5.4% antipyrine
1.4% benzocaine
Uses: Otic analgesic
Avalide:
hydrochlorthiazide 12.5 mg
irbesartan 150 mg
Uses: Antihypertensive
Avalide 300:
hydrochlorthiazide 12.5 mg
irbesartan 300 mg
Uses: Antihypertensive
Avandamet:
rosiglitazone/metformin
1 mg/500 mg
2 mg/500 mg
2 mg/1000 mg
4 mg/500 mg
4 mg/1000 mg
Uses: Diabetes mellitus
Avandaryl 4/1:
rosiglitazone 4 mg
glimepiride 1 mg
Uses: Antidiabetic
Avandaryl 4/2:
rosiglitazone 4 mg
glimepiride 2 mg
Uses: Antidiabetic
Avandaryl 4/4:
rosiglitazone 4 mg
glimepiride 4 mg
Uses: Antidiabetic
Azor:
amlodipine 5 mg
olmesartan 20 mg
amlodipine 10 mg
olmesartan 20 mg
amlodipine 5 mg
olmesartan 40 mg
amlodipine 10 mg
olmesartan 40 mg
Uses: Hypertension

Bactrim:
trimethoprim 80 mg
sulfamethoxazole 400 mg
Uses: Antiinfective
Bactrim DS:
trimethoprim 160 mg
sulfamethoxazole 800 mg
Uses: Antiinfective
Bancap HC:
acetaminophen 500 mg
hydrocodone 5 mg
Uses: Analgesic
Bellatal:
phenobarbital 16.2 mg
hyoscyamine sulfate 0.1037 mg
atropine sulfate 0.0194 mg
scopolamine hydrobromide 0.0065 mg
Uses: Barbiturate, anticholinergic
Bellergal-S:
ergotamine 0.6 mg
belladonna alkaloids 0.2 mg
phenobarbital 40 mg
Uses: α-Adrenergic blocker, anticholinergic,
barbiturate
Bel-Phen-Ergot-SR:
phenobarbital 40 mg
ergotamine tartrate 0.6 mg
belladonna alkaloids 0.2 mg
Uses: α-Adrenergic blocker, anticholinergic,
barbiturate
Benadryl Allergy Decongestant Liquid:
Per 5 ml:
diphenhydrAMINE 12.5 mg
pseudoephedrine 30 mg
Uses: Antihistamine, adrenergic
Benadryl Allergy/Sinus Headache Caplets:
diphenhydrAMINE 12.5 mg
pseudoephedrine 30 mg
acetaminophen 500 mg
Uses: Antihistamine, adrenergic, analgesic
Benadryl Decongestant
   Allergy:
pseudoephedrine 60 mg
diphenhydrAMINE 25 mg
Uses: Adrenergic, antihistamine
Benylin Expectorant Liquid:
Per 5 ml:
dextromethorphan 5 mg
guaifenesin 100 mg
5% alcohol
Uses: Expectorant, antitussive
Benylin Multi-Symptom Liquid:
Per 5 ml:
dextromethorphan 5 mg
pseudoephedrine 15 mg
guaifenesin 100 mg
Uses: Antitussive, adrenergic, expectorant
BenzaClin:
clindamycin 10%
benzoyl peroxide 5%
Uses: Antiinfective
Benzamycin:
benzoyl peroxide 5%
erythromycin 3%
Uses: Antiinfective

Adverse effects: *italic* = common, **bold** = life-threatening

Beta Tan Suspension:
Per 5 ml:
carbetapentane 30 mg
brompheniramine 4 mg
phenylephrine 7.5 mg
Uses: Antitussive
BiDil:
isosorbide 20 mg
hydrALAZINE 37.5 mg
Uses: Vasodilator
Blephamide Ophthalmic Suspension/
Ointment:
0.2% prednisoLONE
10% sodium sulfacetamide
Uses: Ophthalmic antiinfective,
    antiinflammatory
Butibel:
belladonna extract 15 mg
butabarbital 15 mg
Uses: Anticholinergic, barbiturate
Cafatine PB:
ergotamine 1 mg
caffeine 100 mg
belladonna alkaloids 0.125 mg
pentobarbital 30 mg
Uses: Migraine agent
Cafergot:
ergotamine 1 mg
caffeine 100 mg
Uses: Adrenergic blocker
Cafergot Suppositories:
ergotamine 2 mg
caffeine 100 mg
Uses: Adrenergic blocker
Caladryl:
8% calamine, camphor
2.2% alcohol
1% pramoxine
Uses: Topical antihistamine
Calcet:
calcium 152.8 mg
vitamin D 100 international units
Uses: Supplement
Caltrate 600+D:
vitamin D 200 international units
calcium 600 mg
Uses: Supplement
Cama Arthritis Pain Reliever:
aspirin 500 mg
magnesium oxide 150 mg
aluminum hydroxide 125 mg
Uses: Nonopioid analgesic,
    antacid
Capital w/Codeine:
Per 5 ml:
acetaminophen 120 mg
codeine 12 mg
Uses: Opioid analgesic
Capozide 25/15:
captopril 25 mg
hydrochlorothiazide 15 mg
Uses: Antihypertensive
Capozide 25/25:
captopril 25 mg

hydrochorothiazide 25 mg
Uses: Antihypertensive
Capozide 50/15:
captopril 50 mg
hydrochlorothiazide 15 mg
Uses: Antihypertensive
Capozide 50/25:
captopril 50 mg
hydrochlorothiazide 25 mg
Uses: Antihypertensive
Cardec DM Syrup:
Per 5 ml:
pseudoephedrine 60 mg
carbinoxamine 4 mg
dextromethorphan 15 mg
Uses: Adrenergic, antitussive
Cenafed Plus Tablets:
triprolidine 2.5 mg
pseudoephedrine 60 mg
Uses: Antihistamine, adrenergic
Cetapred Ophthalmic Ointment:
0.25% prednisoLONE
10% sodium sulfacetamide
Uses: Ophthalmic antiinfective,
    antiinflammatory
Cheracol Cough Syrup:
Per 5 ml:
codeine 10 mg
guaifenesin 100 mg
Uses: Analgesic, expectorant
Cheracol Syrup:
Per 5 ml:
codeine 10 mg
guaifenesin 100 mg
Uses: Analgesic, expectorant
Children's Cepacol Liquid:
Per 5 ml:
acetaminophen 160 mg
pseudoephedrine 15 mg
Uses: Analgesic, adrenergic
Chlor-Trimeton Allergy-D 4 Hour Relief:
pseudoephedrine 60 mg
chlorpheniramine 4 mg
Uses: Antihistamine, adrenergic
Chlor-Trimeton Allergy 12 Hour Relief
    Tablets:
pseudoephedrine 120 mg
chlorpheniramine 8 mg
Uses: Antihistamine, adrenergic
Chromagen:
ferrous fumarate 66 mg
vitamin B_{12} 10 mcg
vitamin C 250 mg
intrinsic factor 100 mg
Uses: Supplement
Cipro HC Otic:
Per 1 ml:
ciprofloxacin 2 mg
hydrocortisone 10 mg
Uses: Antiinfective/antiinflammatory
Citracal+D:
calcium 315 mg
cholecalciferol 200 international units
Uses: Osteoporosis

Claritin-D 12 Hour:
loratidine 5 mg
pseudoephedrine 120 mg
Uses: Antihistamine, adrenergic
Claritin-D 24-Hour:
loratidine 10 mg
pseudoephedrine 240 mg
Uses: Antihistamine, adrenergic
Climara Pro (transdermal)
estradiol 0.045 mg
levonorgestrel 0.015 mg
Uses: Vasomotor symptoms (menopause)
Clindex:
chlordiazepoxide 5 mg
clidinium 2.5 mg
Uses: Antianxiety, anticholinergic
Clomycin Ointment:
bacitracin 500 units
neomycin sulfate 3.5 g
polymyxin B sulfate 500 units
lidocaine 40 mg
Uses: Antiinfective, local anesthetic
Co-Apap:
pseudoephedrine 30 mg
chlorpheniramine 2 mg
dextromethorphan 15 mg
acetaminophen 325 mg
Uses: Adrenergic, antihistamine, antitussive,
   analgesic
Co-Gesic:
acetaminophen 500 mg
hydrocodone 5 mg
Uses: Analgesic
Codeprex Extended Release Suspension:
Per 5 ml:
codeine 20 mg
chlorpheniramine 4 mg
Uses: Cough, rhinitis
Codiclear DH Syrup:
Per 5 ml:
hydrocodone 5 mg
guaifenesin 100 mg
Uses: Analgesic, expectorant
Codimal:
pseudoephedrine 30 mg
chlorpheniramine 2 mg
acetaminophen 500 mg
Uses: Adrenergic, antihistamine, analgesic
Codimal DH Syrup:
Per 5 ml:
hydrocodone 1.66 mg
phenylephrine 5 mg
pyrilamine 8.33 mg
Uses: Analgesic, adrenergic
Codimal DM Syrup:
Per 5 ml:
phenylephrine 5 mg
pyrilamine 8.33 mg
dextromethorphan 10 mg
Uses: Adrenergic, antitussive
ColBenemid:
probenecid 500 mg
colchicine 0.5 mg
Uses: Antigout agent

Coldrine:
pseudoephedrine 30 mg
acetaminophen 500 mg
Uses: Decongestant, nonopioid analgesic
Col-Probenecid:
probenecid 500 mg
colchicine 0.5 mg
Uses: Antigout
Coly-Mycin S Otic Suspension:
1% hydrocortisone
neomycin base 3.3 mg/ml
colistin 3 mg/ml
0.05% thonzonium bromide
Uses: Otic antiinfective
Combigan:
brimonidine 0.2%
timolol 0.5%
Uses: Glaucoma
CombiPatch 0.05/0.14:
estradiol 0.05 mg/day
norethindrone 0.14 mg/day
Uses: Hypoestrogenism
CombiPatch 0.05/0.25:
estradiol 0.05 mg/day
norethindrone 0.25 mg/day
Uses: Hypoestrogenism
Combivent:
ipratropium bromide 18 mcg
albuterol 103 mcg/actuation
Uses: Bronchodilator
Combivir:
lamivudine 150 mg
zidovudine 300 mg
Uses: HIV
Comvax:
Per 0.5 ml:
Haemophilus B conjugate 7.5 mcg
meningococcal protein 125 mcg
hepatitis B recombinant 5 mcg
Uses: Vaccine
Congestac:
guaifenesin 400 mg
pseudoephedrine 60 mg
Uses: Expectorant, decongestant
Contac Severe Cold & Flu:
chlorpheniramine 2 mg
acetaminophen 500 mg
pseudoephedrine 30 mg
dextromethorphan 15 mg
18.5% alcohol
Uses: Decongestant, antihistamine, antitussive,
   analgesic
Cortisporin Ophthalmic/Otic Suspension:
0.35% neomycin polymyxin B 10,000 units/ml
1% hydrocortisone
Uses: Ophthalmic antiinfective,
   antiinflammatory
Cortisporin Topical Cream:
0.5% neomycin sulfate
polymyxin B 10,000 units
0.5% hydrocortisone
Uses: Topical antiinfective
Cortisporin Topical Ointment:
0.5% neomycin sulfate
bacitracin 400 units

Adverse effects: *italic* = common, **bold** = life-threatening

polymyxin B 5000 units
1% hydrocortisone
Uses: Topical antiinfective
Corzide 40/5:
nadolol 40 mg
bendroflumethiazide 5 mg
Uses: Antihypertensive
Corzide 80/5:
nadolol 80 mg
bendroflumethiazide 5 mg
Uses: Antihypertensive
Cosopt:
dorzolamide 2%
timolol 0.5%
Uses: Antihypertensive
Cough-X:
dextromethorphan 5 mg
benzocaine 2 mg
Uses: Antitussive, local anesthetic
Creon:
lipase 8000 units
amylase 30,000 units
protease 13,000 units
pancreatin 300 mg
Uses: Digestive enzyme
Cyclomydril Ophthalmic Solution:
0.2% cyclopentolate
1% phenylephrine
Uses: Mydriatic
Dallergy Tablets:
chlorpheniramine 4 mg
phenylephrine 10 mg
methscopolamine 1.25 mg
Uses: Antihistamine, adrenergic
Damason-P:
hydrocodone 5 mg
aspirin 500 mg
Uses: Analgesic
Darvocet-N 100:
propoxyphene-N 100 mg
acetaminophen 650 mg
Uses: Analgesic
Darvon Compound-65:
propoxyphene 65 mg
aspirin 389 mg
caffeine 32.4 mg
Uses: Analgesic
♣ **Darvon-N Compound:**
aspirin 375 mg
propoxyphene 100 mg
caffeine 30 mg
Uses: Analgesic
♣ **Darvon-N w/A.S.A.:**
aspirin 325 mg
propoxyphene 100 mg
Uses: Analgesic
Decadron Phosphate with Xylocaine:
Per ml:
dexamethasone 4 mg
lidocaine 10 mg
Uses: Local anesthetic
Deconamine:
pseudoephedrine 60 mg
chlorpheniramine 4 mg
Uses: Antihistamine, decongestant

Deconamine SR:
pseudoephedrine 120 mg
chlorpheniramine 8 mg
Uses: Antihistamine, decongestant
Deconamine Syrup:
Per 5 ml:
pseudoephedrine 30 mg
chlorpheniramine 2 mg
Uses: Antihistamine, decongestant
Demi-Regroton:
chlorthalidone 25 mg
reserpine 0.125 mg
Uses: Antihypertensive
Demulen 1/35:
ethinyl estradiol 35 mcg
ethynodiol diacetate 1 mg
Uses: Oral contraceptive
Demulen 1/50:
ethinyl estradiol 50 mcg
ethynodiol diacetate 1 mg
Uses: Oral contraceptive
Desogen:
ethinyl estradiol 30 mcg
desorgestrel 0.15 mg
Uses: Estrogen, progestin
Dexacidin Ophthalmic Ointment/Suspension:
Per ml:
0.1% dexamethasone
0.35% neomycin
polymyxin B 10,000 units/g
Uses: Ophthalmic, antiinfective/
    antiinflammatory
Dexasporin Ophthalmic Ointment:
Per gram:
0.1% dexamethasone
0.35% neomycin
polymyxin B 10,000 units
Uses: Ophthalmic, antiinfective/
    antiinflammatory
DHC Plus:
dihydrocodeine 16 mg
acetaminophen 356.4 mg
caffeine 30 mg
Uses: Analgesic
Di-Gel Liquid:
Per 5 ml:
aluminum hydroxide 200 mg
magnesium hydroxide 200 mg
simethicone 20 mg
Uses: Antacid, adsorbent, antiflatulent
Dihistine DH Liquid:
Per 5 ml:
pseudoephedrine 30 mg
chlorpheniramine 2 mg
codeine 10 mg
Uses: Decongestant, antihistamine, analgesic
Dilaudid Cough Syrup:
Per 5 ml:
guaifenesin 100 mg
hydromorphone 1 mg
5% alcohol
Uses: Expectorant, analgesic
Dimetapp DM Elixir:
Per 5 ml:
pseudoephedrine 5 mg

brompheniramine 2 mg
dextromethorphan 10 mg
Uses: Antihistamine, adrenergic, expectorant
Dimetapp Sinus:
pseudoephedrine 30 mg
ibuprofen 200 mg
Uses: Decongestant, analgesic
Diovan 80 HCT:
valsartan 80 mg
hydrochlorthiazide 12.5 mg
Uses: Antihypertensive
Diovan 160 HCT:
valsartan 160 mg
hydrochlorthiazide 12.5 mg
Uses: Antihypertensive
Diurigen w/Reserpine:
chlorothiazide 250 mg
reserpine 0.125 mg
Uses: Antihypertensive
Diutensen-R:
methylclothiazide 2.5 mg
reserpine 0.1 mg
Uses: Antihypertensive
Doan's PM Extra Strength:
magnesium salicylate 500 mg
diphenhydrAMINE 25 mg
Uses: Analgesic, antihistamine
Dolacet:
hydrocodone 5 mg
acetaminophen 500 mg
Uses: Analgesic
Donnatal:
phenobarbital 16.2 mg
hyoscyamine 0.1037 mg
atropine 0.0194 mg
scopolamine 0.0065 mg
Uses: Anticholinergic, barbiturate
Donnatal Elixir:
Per 5 ml:
phenobarbital 16.2 mg
hyoscyamine 0.1037 mg
atropine 0.0194 mg
scopolamine 0.0065 mg
23% alcohol
Uses: Anticholinergic, barbiturate
Donnatal Extentabs:
phenobarbital 48.6 mg
hyoscyamine 0.3111 mg
atropine 0.0582 mg
scopolamine 0.0195 mg
Uses: Anticholinergic, barbiturate
Donnazyme:
pancreatin 500 mg
lipase 1000 units
protease 12,500 units
amylase 12,500 units
Uses: Pancreatic enzymes
Dristan Cold:
pseudoephedrine 30 mg
acetaminophen 500 mg
Uses: Decongestant, analgesic
Dristan Cold Multi-Symptom Formula:
acetaminophen 325 mg
phenylephrine 5 mg

chlorpheniramine 2 mg
Uses: Analgesic, adrenergic, antihistamine
Drixoral Cold & Allergy:
pseudoephedrine 120 mg
dexbrompheniramine 6 mg
Uses: Decongestant, antihistamine
DT:
Per 5 ml:
diphtheria toxoid 2 LfU
tetanus toxoid 5 LfU
Uses: Vaccine
DTP:
Per 0.5 ml:
diphtheria toxoid 6.5 LfU
tetanus toxoid 5 LfU
pertussis 4 LfU
Uses: Vaccine
Duetact:
glimepiride 2 mg
pioglitazone 30 mg
glimepiride 4 mg
pioglitazone 30 mg
Uses: Antidiabetic
DuoDote:
atropine 21 mg
pralidoxime 0.7 ml
atropine 600 mg
pralidoxime 2 ml
Uses: Organophate toxicity
DuoNeb:
Per 3 ml:
albuterol 3 mg
ipratroprium 0.5 mg
Uses: Bronchodilator
Dura-Vent/DA:
phenylephrine 20 mg
chlorpheniramine 8 mg
methscopolamine 2.5 mg
Uses: Adrenergic, antihistamine
Durabac Forte:
acetaminophen 500 mg
caffeine 50 mg
magnesium salicylate 500 mg
phenyltoloxamine 20 mg
Uses: Analgesic, antihistamine
Duratuss AC 12:
Per 5 ml:
dextromethorphan 15 mg
diphenhydrAMINE 12.5 mg
phenylephrine 15 mg
Uses: Allergic rhinitis, common cold, flu
Dyazide:
hydrochlorothiazide 25 mg
triamterene 37.5 mg
Uses: Diuretic
Dylline-GG Tablets:
dyphylline 200 mg
guaifenesin 200 mg
Uses: Bronchodilator, expectorant
Dynafed Asthma Relief:
epHEDrine 25 mg
guaifenesin 200 mg
Uses: Adrenergic, expectorant

Dynafed Plus Maximum Strength:
pseudoephedrine 30 mg
acetaminophen 500 mg
Uses: Decongestant, analgesic
Dynex 12:
Per 5 ml:
carbetapentane 22.5 mg
phenylephrine 9 mg
Uses: Antitussive, nasal decongestant
Dyphylline GG:
dyphylline 200 mg
guaifenesin 200 mg
Uses: Bronchodilator, expectorant
Elase Ointment:
Per gram:
fibrinolysin 1 unit
desoxyribonuclease 666.6 units
Uses: Enzyme
Elixophyllin GG Liquid:
Per 5 ml:
theophylline 100 mg
guaifenesin 100 mg
Uses: Expectorant, bronchodilator
Embeda:
morphine/naltrexone
100 mg/4 mg
80 mg/3.2 mg
60 mg/2.4 mg
50 mg/2 mg
30 mg/1.2 mg
20 mg/0.8 mg
Uses: Moderate-severe pain
EMLA Cream:
lidocaine 2.5 mg
prilocaine 2.5 mg
Uses: Local anesthetic
Empirin w/Codeine #3:
aspirin 325 mg
codeine phosphate 30 mg
Uses: Analgesic
Empirin w/Codeine #4:
aspirin 325 mg
codeine phosphate 60 mg
Uses: Analgesic
♣ **Empracet-60:**
acetaminophen 300 mg
codeine 60 mg
Uses: Analgesic
Endocet:
acetaminophen 325 mg
oxycodone 5 mg
Uses: Analgesic
♣ **Endodan:**
aspirin 325 mg
oxycodone 5 mg
Uses: Analgesic
Entex PSE:
pseudoephedrine 120 mg
guaifenesin 600 mg
Uses: Adrenergic, expectorant
Epifoam Aerosol Foam:
1% hydrocortisone
1% pramoxine
Uses: Topical corticosteroid

Epzicom:
abacavir 600 mg
lamivudine 300 mg
Uses: HIV infection
Eryzole:
Per 5 ml:
erythromycin 200 mg
sulfisoxazole 600 mg
Uses: Macrolide antiinfective
Esgic-Plus:
butalbital 50 mg
acetaminophen 500 mg
caffeine 40 mg
Uses: Barbiturate, analgesic
Esimil:
guanethidine 10 mg
hydrochlorothiazide 25 mg
Uses: Antihypertensive
Estratest:
esterified estrogens 1.25 mg
methyltestosterone 2.5 mg
Uses: Vasomotor symptoms (menopause)
Estratest HS:
esterified estrogens 1.25 mg
methyltestosterone 2.5 mg
Uses: Vasomotor symptoms (menopause)
Excedrin Extra Strength:
acetaminophen 250 mg
aspirin 250 mg
caffeine 65 mg
Uses: Analgesic
Excedrin Migraine:
aspirin 250 mg
acetaminophen 250 mg
caffeine 65 mg
Uses: Migraine agent
Excedrin P.M.:
acetaminophen 500 mg
diphenhydrAMINE citrate 38 mg
Uses: Analgesic, antihistamine
Exforge:
amlodipine 5 mg
valsartan 160 mg
amlodipine 5 mg
valsartan 320 mg
amlodipine 10 mg
valsartan 160 mg
amlodipine 10 mg
valsartan 320 mg
Uses: Hypertension
Extra Strength Alka-Seltzer:
aspirin 500 mg
citric acid 1000 mg
sodium bicarbonate 1985 mg
Uses: Analgesic
Fansidar:
sulfidoxine 500 mg
pyrimethamine 25 mg
Uses: Antimalarial
Fem-1:
acetaminophen 500 mg
pamabrom 25 mg
Uses: Nonopioid analgesic

Femhrt 1/5:
norethindrone 1 mg
ethinyl estradiol 5 mcg
norethindrone 1 mg
ethinyl estradiol 5 mcg
Uses: Vasomotor symptoms (menopause)
Ferro-Sequels:
docusate sodium 100 mg
ferrous fumarate 150 mg
Uses: Laxative, hematinic
Fioricet:
acetaminophen 325 mg
caffeine 40 mg
butalbital 50 mg
Uses: Analgesic, barbiturate
Fioricet w/Codeine:
acetaminophen 325 mg
caffeine 40 mg
butalbital 50 mg
codeine 30 mg
Uses: Analgesic, barbiturate
Fiorinal:
aspirin 325 mg
caffeine 40 mg
butalbital 50 mg
Uses: Analgesic, barbiturate
Fiorinal w/Codeine:
aspirin 325 mg
caffeine 40 mg
butalbital 50 mg
codeine 30 mg
Uses: Analgesic, barbiturate
FML-S Ophthalmic Suspension:
0.1% fluorometholone
10% sulfacetamide
Uses: Ophthalmic, antiinfective/
  antiinflammatory
Gas-Ban:
calcium carbonate 500 mg
simethicone 40 mg
Uses: Antiflatulent, antacid
Gaviscon:
magnesium trisilicate 20 mg
aluminum hydroxide 80 mg
Uses: Antacid, adsorbent, antiflatulent
Gaviscon Liquid:
Per 5 ml:
aluminum hydroxide 31.7 mg
magnesium carbonate 119.3 mg
Uses: Antacid, adsorbent, antiflatulent
Gelusil:
aluminum hydroxide 200 mg
magnesium hydroxide 200 mg
simethicone 25 mg
Uses: Antacid, adsorbent, antiflatulent
Genac Tablets:
triprolidine 2.5 mg
pseudoephedrine 60 mg
Uses: Antihistamine
Genatuss DM Syrup:
Per 5 ml:
guaifenesin 100 mg
dextromethorphan 10 mg
Uses: Expectorant, antitussive

Glucovance 1.25:
glyBURIDE: 1.25 mg
metformin: 250 mg
Uses: Antidiabetic
Glucovance 2.50:
glyBURIDE: 2.5 mg
metformin: 500 mg
Uses: Antidiabetic
Glucovance 5:
glyBURIDE: 5 mg
metformin: 500 mg
Uses: Antidiabetic
Guaifenex PSE 60:
pseudoephedrine 60 mg
guaifenesin 600 mg
Uses: Decongestant, expectorant
Guaifenex PSE 120:
pseudoephedrine 120 mg
guaifenesin 600 mg
Uses: Decongestant, expectorant
Guiatuss AC:
Per 5 ml:
codeine 10 mg
guafenesin 100 mg
Uses: Analgesic, expectorant
Haley's M-O Liquid:
Per 15 ml:
magnesium hydroxide 900 mg
mineral oil 3.75 ml
Uses: Laxative
Halotussin-DM Sugar Free Liquid:
Per 5 ml:
guaifenesin 100 mg
dextromethorphan 10 mg
Uses: Expectorant, antitussive
Helidac:
In a compliance package:
bismuth subsalicylate 262.4-mg tabs
metronidazole 250-mg tabs
tetracycline 500-mg caps
Uses: Antiinfective
Humalog KwikPen Mix 50/50:
Per 1 ml:
insulin lispro protamine 50 units
insulin lispro 50 units
Uses: Antidiabetic
Humalog KwikPen Mix 75/25:
Per 1 ml:
insulin lispro protamine 75 units
insulin lispro 25 units
Uses: Antidiabetic
Humalog Mix 50/50:
insulin lispro protamine 50 units
insulin lispro (rDNA) 50 units
Uses: Antidiabetic
Humalog Mix 75/25:
insulin lispro protamine 75 units
insulin lispro (rDNA) 25 units
Uses: Antidiabetic
Humibid DM Pediatric:
dextromethorphan 15 mg
guaifenesin 300 mg
Uses: Expectorant, antitussive
Humibid DM Tablets:
dextromethorphan 30 mg

Adverse effects: *italic* = common, **bold** = life-threatening

guaifenesin 600 mg
Uses: Expectorant, antitussive
HycoClear Tuss:
Per 5 ml:
hydrocodone 5 mg
guaifenesin 100 mg
Uses: Analgesic, expectorant
Hycodan:
hydrocodone 5 mg
homatropine 1.5 mg
Uses: Analgesic, mydriatic
Hycodan Syrup:
Per 5 ml:
hydrocodone 5 mg
homatropine 1.5 mg
Uses: Analgesic, mydriatic
Hycomine Compound:
chlorpheniramine 2 mg
acetaminophen 250 mg
phenylephrine 10 mg
hydrocodone 5 mg
caffeine 30 mg
Uses: Antihistamine, analgesic, adrenergic
Hycotuss Expectorant Syrup:
Per 5 ml:
guaifenesin 100 mg
hydrocodone 5 mg
10% alcohol
Uses: Expectorant
Hydrocet:
hydrocodone 5 mg
acetaminophen 500 mg
Uses: Opioid analgesic
Hydrogesic:
hydrocodone 5 mg
acetaminophen 500 mg
Uses: Opioid analgesic
Hydropres-50:
hydrochlorothiazide 50 mg
reserpine 0.125 mg
Uses: Antihypertensive
Hyzaar:
losartan potassium 50 mg
hydrochlorothiazide 12.5 mg
potassium 4.24 mg
Uses: Antihypertensive
Imodium Advanced:
loperamide 2 mg
simethicone 125 mg
Uses: Antidiarrheal, antiflatulent
Innovar:
Per ml:
droperidol 2.5 mg
fentanyl 0.05 mg
Uses: Opioid analgesic, general anesthetic
Iofed:
brompheniramine 12 mg
pseudoephedrine 120 mg
Uses: Antihistamine, adrenergic
Iofed PD:
brompheniramine 6 mg
pseudoephedrine 60 mg
Uses: Antihistamine, adrenergic
Janumet:
metformin 500 mg

sitagliptan 50 mg
metformin 1000 mg
sitagliptan 50 mg
Uses: Antidiabetic
Kaletra Capsules:
lopinavir 133.3 mg
ritonavir 33.3 mg
Uses: HIV
Kaletra Solution:
Per 1 ml:
lopinavir 80 mg
ritonavir 20 mg
Uses: HIV
Kaletra Tablets
lopinavir 200 mg
ritonavir 50 mg
Uses: HIV
Lactinex:
Mixed culture of:
Lactobacillus acidophilus and
Lactobacillus bulgaricus
Uses: Supplement
Levell 12.5 ml Suspension:
carbetapentane 30 mg
phenylephrine 30 mg
Uses: Antitussive
Levlite:
levonorgestrel 0.100 mg
ethinyl estradiol 20 mcg
Uses: Estrogen, progestin
Levsin PB Drops:
Per ml:
hyoscyamine 0.125 mg
phenobarbital 15 mg
5% alcohol
Uses: Anticholinergic, barbiturate
Levsin w/Phenobarbital:
hyoscyamine 0.125 mg
phenobarbital 15 mg
Uses: Anticholinergic, barbiturate
Lexxel 1:
enalapril 5 mg
felodipine 5 mg
Uses: Antihypertensive
Lexxel 2:
enalapril 5 mg
felodipine 2.5 mg
Uses: Antihypertensive
Librax:
chlordiazepoxide 5 mg
clidinium 2.5 mg
Uses: Antianxiety, anticholinergic
Lida-Mantel-HC-Cream:
0.5% hydrocortisone
3% lidocaine
Uses: Antiinflammatory, analgesic
Limbitrol DS 10-25:
chlordiazepoxide 10 mg
amitriptyline 25 mg
Uses: Antidepressant, antianxiety
Lobac:
salicylamide 200 mg
phenyltoloxamine 20 mg
acetaminophen 300 mg
Uses: Skeletal muscle relaxant, analgesic

🔷 Alert   ♣ Canada Only   🔄 Drug on CD   * "Tall Man" lettering (See Preface)

Loestrin Fe 1/20:
norethindrone acetate 1 mg/tablet
ethinyl estradiol 20 mcg/tablet
  with 7 tablets of ferrous fumarate
  75 mg/container
Uses: Oral contraceptive
Loestrin Fe 1.5/30:
norethindrone acetate 1.5 mg
ethinyl estradiol 30 mcg
Uses: Oral contraceptive
Lomotil:
diphenoxylate 2.5 mg
atropine 0.025 mg
Uses: Antidiarrheal, anticholinergic
Lomotil Liquid:
Per 5 ml:
diphenoxylate 2.5 mg
atropine 0.025 mg
Uses: Antidiarrheal, anticholinergic
Lo Ovral:
ethinyl estradiol 30 mcg
norgestrel 0.3 mg
Uses: Oral contraceptive
Lopressor HCT 50/25:
metoprolol 50 mg
hydrochlorothiazide 25 mg
Uses: Antihypertensive
Lopressor HCT 100/25:
metoprolol 100 mg
hydrochlorothiazide 25 mg
Uses: Antihypertensive
Lopressor HCT 100/50:
metoprolol 100 mg
hydrochlorothiazide 50 mg
Uses: Antihypertensive
Lorcet 10/650:
acetaminophen 650 mg
hydrocodone 10 mg
Uses: Analgesic
Lorcet-HD:
hydrocodone 10 mg
acetaminophen 300 mg
Uses: Analgesic
Lorcet Plus:
acetaminophen 650 mg
hydrocodone 7.5 mg
Uses: Analgesic
Lortab 2.5/500:
hydrocodone 2.5 mg
acetaminophen 500 mg
Uses: Analgesic
Lortab 5/500:
hydrocodone 5 mg
acetaminophen 500 mg
Uses: Analgesic
Lortab 7.5/500:
hydrocodone 7.5 mg
acetaminophen 500 mg
Uses: Analgesic
Lortab 10/500:
hydrocodone 10 mg
acetaminophen 500 mg
Uses: Analgesic

Lortab Oral Sol:
Per 15 ml:
hydrocodone 7.5 mg
acetaminophen 500 mg
Uses: Analgesic
✤ **Losec 1-2-3A:**
omeprazole 20 mg
clarithromycin 500 mg
amoxicillin 1 g
Uses: Antiinfective
✤ **Losec 1-2-3M:**
omeprazole 20 mg
clarithromycin 250 mg
metronidazole 500 mg
Uses: Antiinfective
Lotrel 10/20:
amlopidine 10 mg
benazepril 20 mg
Uses: Antihypertensive
Lotrel 10/40:
amlopidine 10 mg
benazepril 40 mg
Uses: Antihypertensive
Lotrisone Topical:
0.05% betamethasone
1% clotrimazole
Uses: Local antiinfective, antiinflammatory
Lufyllin-EPG Elixir:
Per 5 ml:
dyphylline 150 mg
epHEDrine 24 mg
guaifenesin 300 mg
phenobarbital 24 mg
Uses: Bronchodilator, expectorant
Lufyllin-GG:
dyphylline 200 mg
guaifenesin 200 mg
Uses: Bronchodilator, expectorant
Lunelle Monthly Contraceptive Injection:
25 mg medroxyprogesterone
5 mg estradiol/0.5 ml
Uses: Contraceptive
Lybrel:
ethinyl estridiol 20 mcg
levonorgestrel 90 mcg
Uses: Continuous contraceptive
M-M-R-II:
measles
mumps
rubella
Uses: Vaccine, toxoid
Maalox:
aluminum hydroxide 200 mg
magnesium hydroxide 200 mg
Uses: Antacid, adsorbent, antiflatulent
Maalox Extra Strength Suspension:
Per 5 ml:
aluminum hydroxide 500 mg
magnesium hydroxide 450 mg
simethicone 40 mg
Uses: Antacid, adsorbent, antiflatulent
Maalox Plus:
aluminum hydroxide 200 mg
magnesium hydroxide 200 mg

Adverse effects: *italic* = common, **bold** = life-threatening

simethicone 25 mg
Uses: Antacid, adsorbent, antiflatulent
Maalox Suspension:
Per 5 ml:
aluminum hydroxide 225 mg
magnesium hydroxide 200 mg
Uses: Antacid, adsorbent, antiflatulent
Macrobid:
nitrofurantoin macrocrystals 25 mg
nitrofurantoin monohydrate 75 mg
Uses: Antiinfective
Malarone:
250 mg atovaquone
100 mg proguanil
Uses: Malaria
Malarone Pediatric:
62.5 mg atovaquone
25 mg proguanil
Uses: Malaria
Mapap Cold Formula:
acetaminophen 325 mg
chlorpheniramine 2 mg
pseudoephedrine 30 mg
dextromethorphan 15 mg
Uses: Bronchodilator, expectorant
Maxitrol Ophthalmic Suspension/Ointment:
Per ml:
0.35% neomycin
0.1% dexamethasone
polymyxin B 10,000 units
Uses: Ophthalmic antiinfective,
    antiinflammatory
Maxzide:
hydrochlorothiazide 50 mg
triamterene 75 mg
Uses: Antihypertensive, diuretic
Maxzide-25 MG:
hydrochlorothiazide 25 mg
triamterene 37.5 mg
Uses: Diuretic
Medigesic:
acetaminophen 325 mg
caffeine 40 mg
butalbital 50 mg
Uses: Nonopioid analgesic
Mepergan Fortis:
meperidine 50 mg
promethazine 25 mg
Uses: Analgesic, antihistamine
Mepergan Injection:
meperidine 25 mg
promethazine 25 mg
Uses: Analgesic
Metaglip 2.5:
glipiZIDE/metformin 2.5 mg/250 mg, 2.5 mg/
    500 mg, 5 mg/500 mg
Uses: Diabetes mellitus
Metimyd Ophthalmic Suspension/Ointment:
0.5% prednisoLONE
10% sodium sulfacetamide
Uses: Ophthalmic antiinfective,
    antiinflammatory
Micardis HCT 40/12.5:
telmesartan 40 mg

hydrochlorothiazide 12.5 mg
Uses: Antihypertensive
Micardis HCT 80/12.5:
telmesartan 80 mg
hydrochlorothiazide 12.5 mg
Uses: Antihypertensive
Micardis HCT 80/25:
telmesartan 80 mg
hydrochlorothiazide 25 mg
Uses: Antihypertensive
Microgestin Fe 1/20:
norethindrone 1 mg
ethinyl estradiol 20 mcg
ferrous fumarate 75 mg in container
Uses: Estrogen, progestin
Microgestin Fe 1.5/30:
norethindrone 1.5 mg
ethinyl estradiol 30 mcg
ferrous fumarate 75 mg in container
Uses: Estrogen, progestin
Midol Menstrual Complete:
acetaminophen 500 mg
pyrilamine 15 mg
caffeine 60 mg
Uses: Analgesic
Midol PMS:
acetaminophen 500 mg
pyrilamine 15 mg
pamabrom 25 mg
Uses: Analgesic
Midol, Teen:
acetaminophen 400 mg
pamabrom 25 mg
Uses: Analgesic
Midrin:
isometheptene 65 mg
acetaminophen 325 mg
dichloralphenazone 100 mg
Uses: Analgesic
Moduretic:
hydrochlorothiazide 50 mg
amiloride 5 mg
Uses: Diuretic
Monopril-HCT 10:
fosinopril 10 mg
hydrochlorothiazine 12.5 mg
Uses: Antihypertensive
Monopril-HCT 20:
fosinopril 20 mg
hydrochlorothiazine 12.5 mg
Uses: Antihypertensive
Motrin Children's Cold Suspension:
Per 5 ml:
ibuprofen 100 mg
pseudoephedrine 15 mg
Uses: Nonopioid analgesic, decongestant
Motrin Sinus Headache:
pseudoephedrine 30 mg
ibuprofen 200 mg
Uses: Adrenergic, analgesic
Mucinex D:
guaifenesin/pseudoephedrine 1200 mg/
    120 mg, 600 mg/60 mg
Uses: Expectorant, decongestant

Mucinex DM:
dextromethorphan 30 mg
guaifenesin 600 mg
Uses: Antitussive, expectorant
Murocoll-2 Ophthalmic Drops:
0.3% scopolamine
10% phenylephrine
Uses: Ophthalmic anticholinergic, mydriatic
Mycolog II Topical:
Per gram:
0.1% triamcinolone acetonide
nystatin 100,000 units
Uses: Local antiinfective, antiinflammatory
Mylanta:
aluminum hydroxide 200 mg
magnesium hydroxide 200 mg
simethicone 20 mg
Uses: Antacid, adsorbent, antiflatulent
Mylanta Double Strength Liquid:
Per 5 ml:
aluminum hydroxide 400 mg
magnesium hydroxide 400 mg
simethicone 40 mg
Uses: Antacid, adsorbent, antiflatulent
Mylanta Gelcaps:
calcium carbonate 311 mg
magnesium carbonate 232 mg
Uses: Antacid, adsorbent, antiflatulent
Naphcon-A Ophthalmic Solution:
0.25% naphazoline
0.3% pheniramine
Uses: Ophthalmic vasoconstrictor
Nasatab LA:
guaifenesin 500 mg
pseudoephedrine 120 mg
Uses: Expectorant, decongestant
NeoDecadron Ophthalmic Ointment:
0.35% neomycin
0.05% dexamethasone
Uses: Ophthalmic antiinfective, antiinflammatory
NeoDecadron Ophthalmic Solution:
0.35% neomycin
0.1% dexamethasone
Uses: Ophthalmic antiinfective, antiinflammatory
Neosporin Cream:
Per gram:
polymyxin B 10,000 units
neomycin 3.5 mg
Uses: Topical antiinfective
Neosporin G.U. Irrigant:
Per ml:
neomycin 40 mg
polymyxin B 200,000 units
Uses: Antiinfective
Neosporin Ophthalmic Ointment:
Per gram:
neomycin 3.5 mg
polymyxin B 10,000 units
bacitracin zinc 400 units
Uses: Ophthalmic antiinfective

Neosporin Ophthalmic Solution:
Per ml:
neomycin 1.75 mg
polymyxin B 10,000 units
gramicidin 0.025 mg
Uses: Ophthalmic antiinfective
Neosporin Plus Cream:
polymyxin B 10,000 units
neomycin 3.5 mg
lidocaine 40 mg
Uses: Topical antiinfective
Neosporin Topical Ointment:
Per gram:
polymyxin B 5000 units
bacitracin zinc 400 units
neomycin 3.5 mg
Uses: Topical antiinfective
Niferex-150 Forte:
ferrous sulfate 150 mg
vitamin B_{12} 25 mcg
folic acid 1 mg
Uses: Supplement
Norco:
hydrocodone 10 mg
acetaminophen 325 mg
Uses: Analgesic, opioid, nonopioid
Norco 5/325:
hydrocodone 5 mg
acetaminophen 325 mg
Uses: Analgesic, opioid, nonopioid
Norgesic:
orphenadrine 25 mg
aspirin 385 mg
caffeine 30 mg
Uses: Skeletal muscle relaxant, analgesic
Norgesic Forte:
orphenadrine 50 mg
aspirin 770 mg
caffeine 60 mg
Uses: Skeletal muscle relaxant, analgesic
Novacet Lotion:
sodium sulfacetamine 10%
sulfur 5%
Uses: Acne agent
Novafed A:
pseudoephedrine 120 mg
chlorpheniramine 8 mg
Uses: Adrenergic, antihistamine
✦**Novo-Gesic C8:**
acetaminophen 300 mg
codeine 8 mg
caffeine 15 mg
Uses: Analgesic
NuLytely:
PEG 3350/420 g
sodium bicarbonate 5.72 g
sodium chloride 11.2 g
potassium chloride 1.48 g
Uses: Laxative
NuvaRing:
ethinyl estradiol 0.015 mg/24 hr
etonogestrel 0.12 mg/24 hr
Uses: Contraceptive
Octicair Otic Suspension:
1% hydrocortisone

Adverse effects: *italic* = common, **bold** = life-threatening

neomycin 5 mg/ml
polymyxin B 10,000 units/ml
Uses: Otic antiinflammatory,
    antiinfective
Opcon-A Ophthalmic Solution:
0.027% naphazoline
0.315% pheniramine
Uses: Ophthalmic vasoconstrictor
Ornade Spansules:
phenylpropanolamine 75 mg
chlorpheniramine 12 mg
Uses: Antihistamine, decongestant
Ornex:
pseudoephedrine 30 mg
acetaminophen 500 mg
Uses: Adrenergic, analgesic
Ornex No Drowsiness Caplets:
acetaminophen 325 mg
pseudoephedrine 30 mg
Uses: Adrenergic, analgesic
Orphengesic:
orphenadrine 25 mg
aspirin 385 mg
caffeine 30 mg
Uses: Analgesic
Orphengesic Forte:
orphenadrine 50 mg
aspirin 770 mg
caffeine 60 mg
Uses: Analgesic
Ortho-cept:
ethinyl estradiol 30 mcg
desogestrel 0.15 mg
Uses: Oral contraceptive
Ortho-cyclen:
ethinyl estradiol 35 mcg
norgestimate 0.25 mg
Uses: Oral contraceptive
Ortho-Prefest:
estradiol 1 mg (15)
norgestimate 0.09 mg (15)
Uses: Vasomotor symptoms (menopause)
Ovcon-50:
ethinyl estradiol 50 mcg
norethindrone 1 mg
Uses: Oral contraceptive
♣ **Oxycocet:**
acetaminophen 325 mg
oxycodone 5 mg
Uses: Analgesic
P-A-C Analgesic:
aspirin 400 mg
caffeine 32 mg
Uses: Nonopioid analgesic
Pain-X Topical:
0.05% capsaicin
5% menthol
4% camphor
Uses: Topical analgesic
Pamprin Cramp:
acetaminophen 250 mg
pamabrom 25 mg
magnesium salicylate 250 mg
Uses: Analgesic

Pamprin Multi-Symptom:
acetaminophen 500 mg
pamabrom 25 mg
pyrilamine 15 mg
Uses: Analgesic
Panacet 5/500:
hydrocodone 5 mg
acetaminophen 500 mg
Uses: Analgesic
Panasal 5/500:
hydrocodone 5 mg
aspirin 500 mg
Uses: Analgesic
Pancrease Capsules:
amylase 20,000 units
protease 25,000 units
lipase 4500 units (microspheres)
Uses: Digestive enzyme
Pedia Care NightRest Cough-Cold Liquid:
Per 5 ml:
pseudoephedrine 15 mg
chlorpheniramine 1 mg
dextromethorphan 7.5 mg
Uses: Adrenergic, antihistamine,
    antitussive
Pediazole Suspension:
Per 5 ml:
erythromycin 200 mg
sulfiSOXAZOLE 600 mg
Uses: Antiinfective
Pepcid Complete:
calcium carbonate 800 mg
magnesium hydroxide 165 mg
famotidine 10 mg
Uses: Antiulcer agent
Percocet 2.5/325:
oxycodone 2.5 mg
acetaminophen 325 mg
Uses: Analgesic
Percocet 5/325:
oxycodone 5 mg
acetaminophen 325 mg
Uses: Analgesic
Percocet 7.5/500:
oxycodone 7.5 mg
acetaminophen 500 mg
Uses: Analgesic
Percocet 10/650:
oxycodone 10 mg
acetaminophen 650 mg
Uses: Analgesic
Percodan:
oxycodone 4.88 mg
aspirin 325 mg
Uses: Analgesic
Percogesic:
phenyltoloxamine 30 mg
acetaminophen 325 mg
Uses: Analgesic
Perdiem Granules:
Per teaspoon:
senna 0.74 g
psyllium 3.25 g
sodium 1.8 mg

 Alert   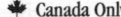 Canada Only   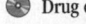 Drug on CD   * "Tall Man" lettering (See Preface)

potassium 35.5 mg
Uses: Laxative
Peri-Colace:
docusate sodium 100 mg
casanthranol 30 mg
Uses: Laxative
Peri-Colace Syrup:
Per 15 ml:
docusate sodium 60 mg
casanthranol 30 mg
Uses: Laxative
Phenerbel-S:
ergotamine tartrate 0.6 mg
belladonna alkaloids 0.2 mg
phenobarbital 40 mg
Uses: α-Adrenergic blocker,
  anticholinergic
Phenergan VC Syrup:
Per 5 ml:
phenylephrine 5 mg
promethazine 6.25 mg
Uses: Adrenergic, antihistamine
Phenergan VC w/Codeine Syrup:
Per 5 ml:
phenylephrine 5 mg
promethazine 6.25 mg
codeine 10 mg
Uses: Adrenergic, antihistamine, opioid analgesic
Phenergan w/Codeine Syrup:
Per 5 ml:
promethazine 6.25 mg
codeine 10 mg
Uses: Antihistamine, analgesic
Phenflu G:
acetaminophen 500 mg
dextromethorphan 30 mg
guaifenesin 600 mg
phenylephrine 15 mg
Uses: Analgesic, antitussive, expectorant, decongestant
Polaramine Expectorant Liquid:
Per 5 ml:
guaifenesin 100 mg
dexchlorpheniramine 2 mg
pseudoephedrine 20 mg
7.5% alcohol
Uses: Expectorant
Polycitra Syrup:
Per 5 ml:
potassium citrate 550 mg
sodium citrate 500 mg
citric acid 334 mg
Uses: Laxative
Poly-Histine Elixir:
Per 5 ml:
pheniramine 4 mg
pyrilamine 4 mg
phenyltoloxamine 4 mg
4% alcohol
Uses: Antihistamine
Polysporin Ophthalmic Ointment:
Per gram:
polymyxin B 10,000 units

bacitracin zinc 500 units
Uses: Ophthalmic antiinfective
Polysporin Topical Ointment:
Per gram:
polymyxin B 10,000 units
bacitracin zinc 500 units
Uses: Topical antiinfective
Polytrim Ophthalmic Solution:
Per ml:
trimethoprim 1 mg
polymyxin B 10,000 units
Uses: Ophthalmic antiinfective
Pravigard PAC:
aspirin 81 mg
pravastatin 20, 40, 80 mg
aspirin 325 mg
pravastatin 20, 40, 80 mg
Uses: Antihyperlipidemic, antithrombotic
Prefest:
estradiol 1 mg
norgestimate 0.09 mg
Uses: Vasomotor symptoms (menopause)
Premphase:
In a compliance package:
conjugated estrogens 0.625 mg
medroxyPROGESTERone 5 mg
Uses: Vasomotor symptoms (menopause)
Prempro:
In a compliance package:
conjugated estrogens 0.3 mg
medroxyPROGESTERone 1.5 mg
conjugated estrogens 0.45 mg
medroxyPROGESTERone 1.5 mg
conjugated estrogens 0.625 mg
medroxyPROGESTERone 2.5 mg
conjugated estrogens 0.625 mg
medroxyPROGESTERone 5 mg
Uses: Vasomotor symptoms (menopause)
Premsyn PMS:
acetaminophen 500 mg
pamabrom 25 mg
pyrilamine 15 mg
Uses: Analgesic
Prevpac:
In a compliance package:
amoxicillin 500-mg caps
clarithromycin 500-mg tabs
lansoprazole 30-mg caps
Uses: Antiinfective
Primaxin 250 mg IV for Injection:
imipenem 250 mg
cilastatin sodium 250 mg
Uses: Antiinfective
Primaxin 500 mg IV for Injection:
imipenem 500 mg
cilastatin sodium 500 mg
Uses: Antiinfective
Prinzide 10-12.5:
lisinopril 10 mg
hydrochlorothiazide 12.5 mg
Uses: Antihypertensive
Prinzide 20-12.5:
lisinopril 20 mg
hydrochlorothiazide 12.5 mg
Uses: Antihypertensive

Adverse effects: *italic* = common, **bold** = life-threatening

Prinzide 20-25:
lisinopril 20 mg
hydrochlorothiazide 25 mg
Uses: Antihypertensive

Proben-C:
colchicine 0.5 mg
probenecid 500 mg
Uses: Antigout agent

Proctofoam-HC Aerosol Foam:
1% hydrocortisone
1% pramoxine
Uses: Topical corticosteroid

Pronto Plus Lice Killing Shampoo:
piperonyl butoxide 4%
pyrethrum extract 0.33%
Uses: Lice

Propacet 100:
propoxyphene-N 100 mg
acetaminophen 650 mg
Uses: Analgesic

Pseudo-Chlor:
pseudoephedrine 120 mg
chlorpheniramine 8 mg
Uses: Antihistamine

Pseudo-Gest Plus:
pseudoephedrine 60 mg
chlorpheniramine 4 mg
Uses: Antihistamine

Pylera:
bismuth subcitrate potassium 140 mg
metronidazole 125 mg
tetracycline 125 mg
Uses: Helicobacter pylori

Quadrinal:
epHEDrine 24 mg
theophylline 65 mg
potassium iodide 320 mg
phenobarbital 24 mg
Uses: Adrenergic, bronchodilator, barbiturate

Quibron-300:
theophylline 300 mg
guaifenesin 180 mg
Uses: Bronchodilator, expectorant

Rebetron:
interferon alfa-2b 3 million units/0.5 ml
ribavirin, PO 200 mg
Uses: Biologic response modifier, antiviral

Regulace:
docusate sodium 100 mg
casanthranol 30 mg
Uses: Laxative

Renese-R:
polythiazide 2 mg
reserpine 0.25 mg
Uses: Diuretic, antihypertensive

Respahist:
pseudoephedrine 60 mg
brompheniramine 6 mg
Uses: Adrenergic, antihistamine

Respaire-60:
guaifenesin 200 mg
pseudoephedrine 60 mg
Uses: Expectorant, adrenergic

Respi-TANN:
Per 5 ml:
carbetapentane 20 mg
pseudoephedrine 30 mg
Uses: Cough suppressant, decongestant

Respi-TANN Pd:
Per 5 ml:
carbetapentane 7.5 mg
pseudoephedrine 30 mg
Uses: Cough suppressant, decongestant

Rifamate:
isoniazid 150 mg
rifampin 300 mg
Uses: Antitubercular, antileprotic

Rifater:
rifampin 120 mg
isoniazid 50 mg
pyrazinamide 300 mg
Uses: Antitubercular

Riopan Plus Suspension:
Per 5 ml:
magaldrate 540 mg
simethicone 40 mg
Uses: Antacid, adsorbent, antiflatulent

Robaxisal:
methocarbamol 400 mg
aspirin 325 mg
Uses: Skeletal muscle relaxant, analgesic

Robitussin A/C Syrup:
codeine 10 mg
guaifenesin 100 mg
35% alcohol
Uses: Antitussive, opioid analgesic

Robitussin Cold & Cough Liquigels:
pseudoephedrine 30 mg
guaifenesin 200 mg
dextromethorphan 10 mg
Uses: Antitussive, expectorant, decongestant

Robitussin-DM Liquid:
Per 5 ml:
guaifenesin 100 mg
dextromethorphan 10 mg
Uses: Expectorant, antitussive

Robitussin Maximum Strength Cough and Cold Syrup:
dextromethorphan 15 mg
pseudoephedrine 30 mg
Uses: Antitussive, adrenergic

Robitussin Night Relief Liquid:
dextromethorphan 5 mg
pyrilamine 8.3 mg
pseudoephedrine 10 mg
acetaminophen 108.3 mg
Uses: Antitussive, adrenergic

Robitussin Pediatric Cough & Cold Liquid:
Per 5 ml:
pseudoephedrine 15 mg
dextromethorphan 7.5 mg
Uses: Antitussive, adrenergic

Rolaids Calcium Rich:
magnesium hydroxide 80 mg
calcium carbonate 412 mg
Uses: Antacid, adsorbent, antiflatulent

Rondec:
pseudoephedrine 60 mg
carbinoxamine 4 mg
Uses: Adrenergic
Rondec DM Drops:
Per ml:
pseudoephedrine 25 mg
carbinoxamine 2 mg
dextromethorphan 4 mg
Uses: Adrenergic, antitussive
Rondec DM Syrup:
Per 5 ml:
pseudoephedrine 60 mg
carbinoxamine 4 mg
dextromethorphan 15 mg
Uses: Adrenergic, antitussive
Rondec Oral Drops:
Per 5 ml:
pseudoephedrine 25 mg
carbinoxamine 2 mg
Uses: Adrenergic
Roxicet 5/325:
acetaminophen 325 mg
oxycodone 5 mg
Uses: Opioid analgesic
Roxicet 5/500:
oxycodone 5 mg
acetaminophen 500 mg
Uses: Opioid analgesic
Roxicet Oral Solution:
Per 5 ml:
acetaminophen 325 mg
oxycodone 5 mg
Uses: Analgesic
Roxiprin:
aspirin 325 mg
oxycodone HCl 4.5 mg
oxycodone terephthalate 0.38 mg
Uses: Analgesic
Salutensin Demi:
hydroflumethiazide 25 mg
reserpine 0.125 mg
Uses: Antihypertensive
Sedapap-10:
acetaminophen 650 mg
butalbital 50 mg
Uses: Analgesic, barbiturate
Semprex-D:
acrivastine 8 mg
pseudoephedrine 60 mg
Uses: Adrenergic, bronchodilator
Senokot-S:
docusate 50 mg
senna concentrate 187 mg
Uses: Laxative
Septra:
sulfamethoxazole 400 mg
trimethroprim 80 mg
Uses: Antiinfective
Septra DS:
sulfamethoxazole 800 mg
trimethroprim 160 mg
Uses: Antiinfective
Ser-Ap-Es:
hydrochlorothiazide 15 mg
reserpine 0.1 mg
hydrALAZINE 25 mg
Uses: Diuretic, antihypertensive
Silafed Syrup:
Per 5 ml:
pseudoephedrine 30 mg
triprolidine 1.25 mg
Uses: Adrenergic, antihistamine
Silaminic Cold Syrup:
Per 5 ml:
phenylpropanolamine 12.5 mg
chlorpheniramine 2 mg
Uses: Antihistamine, decongestant
Sinemet 10/100:
carbidopa 10 mg
levodopa 100 mg
Uses: Antiparkinsonian
Sinemet 25/100:
carbidopa 25 mg
levodopa 100 mg
Uses: Antiparkinsonian
Sinemet 25/250:
carbidopa 25 mg
levodopa 250 mg
Uses: Antiparkinsonian
Sinemet CR 25-100:
carbidopa 25 mg
levodopa 100 mg
Uses: Antiparkinsonian
Sinemet CR 50-200:
carbidopa 50 mg
levodopa 200 mg
Uses: Antiparkinsonian
Sinus-Relief:
acetaminophen 325 mg
pseudoephedrine 30 mg
Uses: Nonopioid analgesic
Slo-Phyllin GG Syrup:
theophylline 150 mg
guaifenesin 90 mg
Uses: Bronchodilator, expectorant
Slow-Salt-K:
sodium chloride 410 mg
potassium chloride 15 mg
Uses: Potassium, sodium supplement
Solage:
mequinol 2%
tretinoin 0.01%
Uses: Antineoplastic
Soma Compound:
carisoprodol 200 mg
aspirin 325 mg
Uses: Skeletal muscle relaxant
Spec-T Lozenge:
dextromethorphan 10 mg
benzocaine 10 mg
Uses: Antitussive, topical anesthetic
Stalevo 50:
carbidopa 12.5 mg
levodopa 50 mg
entacapone 200 mg
Uses: Parkinsonism
Stalevo 100:
carbidopa 25 mg
levodopa 100 mg

Adverse effects: *italic* = common, **bold** = life-threatening

entacapone 200 mg
Uses: Parkinsonism
Stalevo 150:
carbidopa 37.5 mg
levodopa 150 mg
entacapone 200 mg
Uses: Parkinsonism
Sudafed Sinus & Cold:
pseudoephedrine 30 mg
acetaminophen 325 mg
Uses: Adrenergic, analgesic
Sudal 60/500:
pseudoephedrine 60 mg
guaifenesin 500 mg
Uses: Adrenergic, expectorant
Sudal 120/600:
pseudoephedrine 120 mg
guaifenesin 600 mg
Uses: Adrenergic, expectorant
Sultrin Triple Sulfa Vaginal Cream:
3.42% sulfathiazole
2.86% sulfacetamine
3.7% sulfabenzamide
Uses: Antiinfective
Sultrin Triple Sulfa Vaginal Tablets:
sulfathiazole 172.5 mg
sulfacetamide 143.75 mg
sulfabenzamide 184 mg
Uses: Antiinfective
Symbicort:
budesonide 80 mcg
formoterol 4.5 mcg
budesonide 160 mcg
formoterol 4.5 mcg
Uses: Asthma
Symbyax:
olanzapine 6 mg
fluoxetine 25 mg
olanzapine 6 mg
fluoxetine 50 mg
olanzapine 12 mg
fluoxetine 25 mg
olanzapine 12 mg
fluoxetine 50 mg
Uses: Bipolar disorder
Synalgos-DC:
aspirin 356.4 mg
caffeine 30 mg
dihydrocodeine 16 mg
Uses: Analgesic
Synercid:
quinupristin 150 mg
dalfopristin 350 mg
Uses: Antiinfective
Syntest H.S.:
esterified estrogens 0.625 mg
methylTESTOSTERone 1.25 mg
Uses: Vasomotor symptoms (menopause)
Taclonex:
betamethasone 0.064%
calcipotriene 0.005%
Uses: Plaque psoriasis
Talacen:
acetaminophen 650 mg

pentazocine 25 mg
Uses: Analgesic
Talwin Compound:
aspirin 325 mg
pentazocine 12.5 mg
Uses: Analgesic
Talwin NX:
pentazocine 50 mg
naloxone 0.5 mg
Uses: Analgesic, opioid antagonist
Tarka 182:
trandolapril 2 mg (immed rel)
verapamil 180 mg (sus rel)
Uses: Antihypertensive, calcium channel
blocker
Tarka 241:
trandolapril 1 mg (immed rel)
verapamil 240 mg (sus rel)
Uses: Antihypertensive, calcium channel
blocker
Tarka 242:
trandolapril 2 mg (immed rel)
verapamil 240 mg (sus rel)
Uses: Antihypertensive, calcium channel
blocker
Tarka 244:
trandolapril 4 mg (immed rel)
verapamil 240 mg (sus rel)
Uses: Antihypertensive, calcium channel
blocker
Tavist Allergy/Sinus Headache:
clemastine 0.335 mg
pseudoephedrine 30 mg
acetaminophen 500 mg
Uses: Antihistamine, adrenergic, analgesic
Tavist Sinus:
acetaminophen 500 mg
pseudoephedrine 30 mg
Uses: Analgesic, adrenergic
♣ **Tecnal:**
aspirin 330 mg
caffeine 40 mg
butalbital 50 mg
Uses: Nonopioid analgesic
Teczem:
enalapril 5 mg (ext rel)
diltiazem 180 mg (ext rel)
Uses: Antihypertensive, calcium channel
blocker
Tegrin-LT Shampoo:
0.33% pyrethrins
3.15% piperonyl butoxide
Uses: Scabicide, pediculicide
Tenoretic 50:
atenolol 50 mg
chlorthalidone 25 mg
Uses: Antihypertensive
Tenoretic 100:
atenolol 100 mg
chlorthalidone 25 mg
Uses: Antihypertensive
Terra-Cortril Ophthalmic Suspension:
1.5% hydrocortisone acetate

0.5% oxytetracycline
Uses: Ophthalmic antiinflammatory,
   antiinfective
Terramycin w/Polymycin B Sulfate Ophthalmic Ointment:
Per gram:
polymyxin B 10,000 units
oxytetracycline 5 mg
Uses: Ophthalmic antiinfective
T-Gesic:
hydrocodone 5 mg
acetaminophen 500 mg
Uses: Analgesic
Thera-Flu Cold & Cough Powder:
Per packet:
pseudoephedrine 60 mg
chlorpheniramine 4 mg
dextromethorphan 20 mg
acetaminophen 650 mg
Uses: Adrenergic, antihistamine, antitussive,
   analgesic
Timentin for Injection:
Per 3.1 g vial:
ticarcillin 3 g
clavulanic acid 0.1 g
Uses: Antiinfective
Timolide 10/25:
timolol 10 mg
hydrochlorothiazide 25 mg
Uses: Antihypertensive
Titralac Plus:
calcium carbonate 420 mg
simethicone 21 mg
Uses: Antacid, adsorbent, antiflatulent
**Tobra Dex Ophthalmic
   Suspension/Ointment:**
tobramycin 0.3%
dexamethasone 0.1%
Uses: Ophthalmic antiinfective,
   antiinflammatory
Triacin-C Cough Syrup:
Per 5 ml:
codeine 10 mg
pseudoephedrine 30 mg
triprolidine 1.25 mg
Uses: Analgesic, adrenergic, antihistamine
Tri-Hydroserpine:
hydrALAZINE 25 mg
hydrochlorothiazide 15 mg
reserpine 0.1 mg
Uses: Antihypertensive
Trinalin Repetabs:
azatadine maleate 1 mg
pseudoephedrine 120 mg
Uses: Antihistamine
TriOxin:
Per ml:
benzocaine 15 mg
chloroxylenol 1 mg
hydrocortisone 10 mg
Uses: Otic antibacterial, antifungal, anesthetic
Triple Antibiotic Ophthalmic Ointment:
Per gram:
polymyxin B 10,000 units
neomycin 3.5 mg

bacitracin 400 units
Uses: Antiinfective
**Triprolidine/Pseudoephedrine Syrup
   (generic):**
Per 5 ml
triprolidine 1.25 mg
pseudoephedrine 50 mg
Uses: Antihistamine, decongestant
**Triprolidine/Pseudoephedrine Tablets
   (generic):**
triprolidine 2.5 mg
pseudoephedrine 60 mg
Uses: Antihistamine, decongestant
Trizivir:
300 mg abacavir
150 mg lamivudine
300 mg zidovudine
Uses: HIV
Tusibron-DM Syrup:
Per 5 ml:
guaifenesin 100 mg
dextromethorphan 15 mg
Uses: Expectorant, antitussive
Tylenol Allergy Sinus, DayTime Caplet:
acetaminophen 500 mg
chlorpheniramine 2 mg
pseudoephedrine 30 mg
Uses: Antihistamine, adrenergic, analgesic
Tylenol Children's Cold:
acetaminophen 80 mg
chlorpheniramine 0.5 mg
pseudoephedrine 7.5 mg
Uses: Antihistamine, adrenergic, analgesic
**Tylenol Children's Cold Multi- Symptom
   Plus Cough Liquid:**
Per 5 ml:
acetaminophen 160 mg
dextromethorphan 5 mg
chlorpheniramine 1 mg
pseudoephedrine 15 mg
Uses: Antihistamine, adrenergic, analgesic
**Tylenol Children's Cold Plus Cough
   Chewable:**
acetaminophen 80 mg
pseudoephedrine 7.5 mg
dextromethorphan 2.5 mg
chlorpheniramine 0.5 mg
Uses: Antihistamine, adrenergic, analgesic
Tylenol Cold & Flu Severe DayTime Liquid:
dextromethorphan 5 mg
pseudoephedrine 10 mg
acetaminophen 166.7 mg
Uses: Antitussive, decongestant, analgesic
Tylenol Cold Multi-Symptom Tablets:
acetaminophen 325 mg
chlorpheniramine 2 mg
pseudoephedrine 30 mg
dextromethorphan 15 mg
Uses: Antihistamine, adrenergic, analgesic
Tylenol Cold Severe Congestion Tablets:
dextromethorphan 15 mg
guaifenesin 200 mg
pseudoephedrine 32 mg

Adverse effects: *italic* = common, **bold** = life-threatening

acetaminophen 325 mg
Uses: Antitussive, expectorant, decongestant,
   analgesic
**Tylenol Cough & Sore Throat DayTime
   Liquid:**
dextromethorphan 5 mg
acetaminophen 166.7 mg
Uses: Antitussive, analgesic
Tylenol Flu Day Non-Drowsy Gelcaps:
diphenhydrAMINE 25 mg
pseudoephedrine 30 mg
acetaminophen 500 mg
Uses: Analgesic, adrenergic, antitussive
Tylenol Flu NightTime Gelcaps:
diphenhydrAMINE 25 mg
doxylamine 2.1 mg
pseudoephedrine 30 mg
acetaminophen 500 mg
Uses: Antihistamine, decongestant, analgesic
Tylenol PM, Extra Strength:
acetaminophen 500 mg
diphenhydrAMINE 25 mg
Uses: Analgesic, antihistamine
Tylenol Severe Allergy:
diphenhydrAMINE 12.5 mg
acetaminophen 500 mg
Uses: Analgesic, antihistamine
Tylenol w/Codeine Elixir:
Per 5 ml:
acetaminophen 120 mg
codeine 12 mg
Uses: Analgesic
Tylenol w/Codeine No. 1:
acetaminophen 300 mg
codeine 7.5 mg
Uses: Analgesic
Tylenol w/Codeine No. 2:
acetaminophen 300 mg
codeine 15 mg
Tylenol w/Codeine No. 3:
acetaminophen 300 mg
codeine 30 mg
Uses: Analgesic
Tylenol w/Codeine No. 4:
acetaminophen 300 mg
codeine 60 mg
Uses: Analgesic
Tylox:
oxycodone 5 mg
acetaminophen 500 mg
Uses: Analgesic
Ultracet:
tramadol 37.5 mg
acetaminophen 325 mg
Uses: Analgesic
Unasyn for Injection 3 g:
ampicillin 2 g
sulbactam 1 g
Uses: Antiinfective
Uniretic:
moexipril 7.5 mg
hydrochlorothiazide 12.5 mg
moexipril 15 mg
hydrochlorothiazide 25 mg
Uses: Antihypertensive, diuretic

Urised:
methenamine 40.8 mg
phenylsalicylate 18.1 mg
atropine 0.03 mg
hyoscyamine 0.03 mg
benzoic acid 4.5 mg
methylene blue 5.4 mg
Uses: Antiinfective
Vanquish:
aspirin 227 mg
acetaminophen 194 mg
caffeine 33 mg
aluminum hydroxide 25 mg
magnesium hydroxide 50 mg
Uses: Nonopioid analgesic
Vaseretic 5-12.5:
enalapril 5 mg
hydrochlorthiazide 12.5 mg
Uses: Antihypertensive diuretic
Vaseretic 10-25:
enalapril 10 mg
hydrochlorothiazide 25 mg
Uses: Antihypertensive, diuretic
Vasocidin Ophthalmic Ointment:
sulfacetamide 10%
prednisoLONE 0.5%
Uses: Ophthalmic antiinfective,
   antiinflammatory
Vasocidin Ophthalmic Solution:
sulfacetamide 10%
prednisoLONE 0.25%
Uses: Ophthalmic antiinfective,
   antiinflammatory
Vasocon-A Ophthalmic Solution:
naphazoline 0.05%
antazoline 0.5%
Uses: Ophthalmic vasoconstrictor
**Vicks 44D Cough & Head Congestion
   Liquid:**
Per 5 ml:
dextromethorphan 10 mg
pseudoephedrine 20 mg
Uses: Antitussive, adrenergic
Vicks 44E Liquid:
Per 5 ml:
dextromethorphan 6.7 mg
guaifenesin 66.7 mg
Uses: Antitussive, expectorant
Vicks 44M Cold, Flu, & Cough LiquiCaps:
dextromethorphan 10 mg
pseudoephedrine 30 mg
chlorpheniramine 2 mg
acetaminophen 250 mg
Uses: Antitussive, adrenergic, antihistamine,
   analgesic
Vicks 44M Pediatric Liquid:
Per 5 ml:
pseudoephedrine 15 mg
chlorpheniramine 1 mg
Uses: Adrenergic, antihistamine, antitussive
**Vicks 44 Non-Drowsy Cold & Cough
   LiquiCaps:**
dextromethorphan 30 mg
pseudoephedrine 60 mg
Uses: Antitussive, adrenergic

 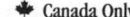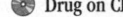

Vicks Children's NyQuil Nighttime Cough/Cold Liquid:
Per 5 ml:
pseudoephedrine 10 mg
chlorpheniramine 0.67 mg
dextromethorphan 5 mg
Uses: Adrenergic, antihistamine, antitussive
Vicks DayQuil Liquid:
dextromethorphan 3.3 mg
pseudoephedrine 10 mg
acetaminophen 108.3 mg
guaifenesin 33.3 mg
Uses: Antitussive, adrenergic, analgesic, expectorant
Vicks DayQuil Multi-Symptom Cold/Flu Relief Liquid:
dextromethorphan 33 mg
pseudoephedrine 10 mg
acetaminophen 108.3 mg
Uses: Antitussive, decongestant, analgesic
Vicks DayQull Pressure & Pain Caplet:
pseudoephedrine 30 mg
ibuprofen 200 mg
Uses: Adrenergic, analgesic
Vicks NyQuil LiquiCaps:
pseudoephedrine 30 mg
doxylamine 6.25 mg
dextromethorphan 10 mg
acetaminophen 250 mg
Uses: Adrenergic, antihistamine, antitussive, analgesic
Vicks NyQuil Multi-Symptom Cold Flu Relief Liquid:
pseudoephedrine 10 mg
doxylamine 2.1 mg
dextromethorphan 5 mg
acetaminophen 167 mg
Uses: Adrenergic, antihistamine, antitussive, analgesic
Vicodin:
acetaminophen 500 mg
hydrocodone 5 mg
Uses: Analgesic
Vicodin ES:
acetaminophen 750 mg
hydrocodone 7.5 mg
Uses: Analgesic
Vicodin HP:
acetaminophen 660 mg
hydrocodone 10 mg
Uses: Analgesic
Vicodin Tuss:
Per 5 ml:
hydrocodone 5 mg
guaifenesin 100 mg
Uses: Analgesic, expectorant
Vicoprofen:
hydrocodone 7.5 mg
ibuprofen 200 mg
Uses: Analgesic
Vytorin:
ezetimibe: 10, 10, 10, 10 mg

simvastatin: 10, 20, 40, 80 mg
Uses: Antihyperlipidemic
Yasmin 28:
ethinyl estadiol 30 mcg
dropirenone 3 mg
Uses: Oral contraceptive
YAZ:
prospirenone 3 mg
ethinyl estradiol 0.02 mg
Uses: Vasomotor symptoms (menopause)
Zegerid Capsules:
omeprazole 20 mg
sodium bicarbonate 1100 mg
omeprazole 40 mg
sodium bicarbonate 1100 mg
Uses: Gastric ulcer, GERD
Zegerid Powder (Oral Solution):
omeprazole 20 mg
sodium bicarbonate 1680 mg
omeprazole 40 mg
sodium bicarbonate 1680 mg
Uses: Gastric ulcer, GERD
Zestoretic 10/12.5:
lisinopril 10 mg
hydrochlorothiazide 12.5 mg
Uses: Antihypertensive
Zestoretic 20/12.5:
lisinopril 20 mg
hydrochlorothiazide 12.5 mg
Uses: Antihypertensive
Zestoretic 20/25:
lisinopril 20 mg
hydrochlorothiazide 25 mg
Uses: Antihypertensive
Ziac 2.5:
bisoprolol 2.5 mg
hydrochlorothiazide 6.25 mg
Uses: Antihypertensive
Ziac 5:
bisoprolol 5 mg
hydrochlorothiazide 6.25 mg
Uses: Antihypertensive
Ziac 10:
bisoprolol 10 mg
hydrochlorothiazide 6.25 mg
Uses: Antihypertensive
Ziana:
clindamycin 1.2%
tretinoin 0.025%
Uses: Acne vulgaris
Zydone:
hydrocodone 5 mg
acetaminophen 500 mg
Uses: Analgesic
Zypram:
hydrocortisone 2.35%
pramoxine 1%
Uses: Antiinflammatory
Zyrtec-D
cetirizine 5 mg
pseudoephedrine 120 mg
Uses: Antihistamine, decongestant

Adverse effects: *italic* = common, **bold** = life-threatening

Appendix E

Abbreviations and Pregnancy Categories

abd abdomen
ABG arterial blood gas
ac before meals
ACE angiotensin-converting enzyme
ACT activated clotting time
ADA American Diabetes Association
ADH antidiuretic hormone
ALT alanine aminotransferase
ANA antinuclear antibody
AP anteroposterior
APLA antiphospholipid antibody syndrome
APTT activated partial thromboplastin time
ASA acetylsalicylic acid, aspirin
ASHD arteriosclerotic heart disease
AST aspartate aminotransferase (SGOT)
AV atrioventricular
bid twice a day
BM bowel movement
BMR basal metabolic rate
B/P blood pressure
BPH benign prostatic hypertrophy
BPM beats per minute
BS blood sugar
BUN blood urea nitrogen
C Celsius (centigrade)
CAD coronary artery disease
cap capsule
Cath catheterization or catheterize
CBC complete blood cell count
CHF congestive heart failure
CHo carbohydrates
cm centimeter
CNS central nervous system
CO$_2$ carbon dioxide
cont continuous
COPD chronic obstructive pulmonary disease
CPAP continuous positive airway pressure

CPK creatinine phosphokinase
CPR cardiopulmonary resuscitation
CCr creatinine clearance
C&S culture and sensitivity
C sect cesarean section
CSF cerebrospinal fluid
CTCL cutaneous T-cell lymphoma
CV cardiovascular
CVA cerebrovascular accident
CVP central venous pressure
D&C dilatation and curettage
dir inf direct infusion
dr dram
D$_5$W 5% glucose in distilled water
DVT deep vein thrombosis
ECG electrocardiogram (EKG)
EDTA ethylenediamine tetraacetic acid
EEG electroencephalogram
EENT ear, eye, nose, and throat
EPS extrapyramidal symptoms
ESR erythrocyte sedimentation rate
ext rel extended release
FBS fasting blood sugar
FHT fetal heart tones
FSH follicle-stimulating hormone
g gram
GABA γ-aminobutyric acid
GI gastrointestinal
GPC giant papillary conjunctivitis
gr grain
GTT glucose tolerance test
gtt drops
GU genitourinary
GVHD graft-versus-host disease
H$_2$ histamine$_2$
hCG human chorionic gonadotropin
Hct hematocrit
HDCV human diploid cell rabies vaccine

Hgb	hemoglobin
H&H	hematocrit and hemoglobin
5-HIAA	5-hydroxyindoleacetic acid
HIV	human immunodeficiency virus (AIDS)
H₂O	water
HOB	head of bed
HR	heart rate
hr	hour
IBD	inflammatory bowel disease
IC	intracardiac
ICP	intracranial pressure
ID	intradermal
IgG	immunoglobulin G
IM	intramuscular
inf	infusion
INH	inhalation
inj	injection
I&O	intake and output
IPPB	intermittent positive-pressure breathing
IT	intrathecal
ITP	idiopathic thrombocytopenic purpura
IUD	intrauterine device
IV	intravenous
IVP	intravenous pyelogram
K	potassium
kg	kilogram
L	liter
lb	pound
LDH	lactic dehydrogenase
LE	lupus erythematosus
LH	luteinizing hormone
LLQ	left lower quadrant
LMP	last menstrual period
LOC	level of consciousness
LR	lactated Ringer's solution
LUQ	left upper quadrant
M	meter
m	minim
m²	square meter
MAOI	monoamine oxidase inhibitor
mcg	microgram
mEq	milliequivalent
mg	milligram
MI	myocardial infarction
min	minute
ml	milliliter
mm	millimeter
mo	month
Na	sodium
neg	negative
NGU	nongonococcal urethritis

NHL	non-Hodgkin's lymphoma
NPO	nothing by mouth (Lat. *nulla per os*)
NS	normal saline
O₂	oxygen
OBS	organic brain syndrome
OD	right eye
OR	operating room
OS	left eye
OTC	over-the-counter
OU	each eye
oz	ounce
p̄	after
P56	Plasma-Lyte 56
PaCO₂	arterial carbon dioxide tension (pressure)
PaO₂	arterial oxygen tension (pressure)
PAT	paroxysmal atrial tachycardia
PBI	protein-bound iodine
pc	after meals
PCI	percutaneous coronary intervention
PCWP	pulmonary capillary wedge pressure
PEEP	positive end-expiratory pressure
PERRLA	pupils equal, round, react to light and accommodation
pH	hydrogen ion concentration
PO	by mouth
postop	postoperative
PP	postprandial
PPHN	persistent pulmonary hypertension of the newborn
preop	preoperative
prn	as required
PT	prothrombin time
PTT	partial thromboplastin time
PVC	premature ventricular contraction
q	every
qAM	every morning
qhr	every hour
q2hr	every 2 hours
q3hr	every 3 hours
q4hr	every 4 hours
q6hr	every 6 hours
q12hr	every 12 hours
qid	four times daily
qmo	every month
qPM	every night
qs	sufficient quantity
qt	quart
qwk	every week

R right		**temp** temperature	
RAIU radioactive iodine uptake		**tid** three times daily	
RBC red blood count or cell		**tinc** tincture	
RLQ right lower quadrant		**TPN** total parenteral nutrition	
ROM range of motion		**TOP** topical	
RUQ right upper quadrant		**TSH** thyroid-stimulating hormone	
Rx prescription		**tsp** teaspoon	
SARS severe acute respiratory syndrome		**TT** thrombin time	
SCr serum creatinine		**UA** urinalysis	
SIMV synchronous intermittent mandatory ventilation		**UTI** urinary tract infection	
SL sublingual		**UV** ultraviolet	
SLE systemic lupus erythematosus		**vag** vaginal	
SOB shortness of breath		**VMA** vanillylmandelic acid	
sol solution		**vol** volume	
sp gr specific gravity		**VS** vital sign	
ss one half		**WBC** white blood cell count	
STD sexually transmitted disease		**wk** week	
SUBCUT subcutaneous		**wt** weight	
supp suppository		**yr** year	
sus rel sustained release		> greater than	
syr syrup		< less than	
T&A tonsillectomy and adenoidectomy		= equal	
tab tablet		° degree	
tbsp tablespoon		% percent	
TD transdermal		α alpha	
		γ gamma	
		β beta	

- For a list of the Institute for Safe Medicine Practices (ISMP) error-prone abbreviations, symbols, and dose designations, please see http://www.ismp.org/tools/errorproneabbreviations.pdf.
- For frequently asked questions regarding the 2010 National Patient Safety Goals, please visit The Joint Commission website at http://www.jointcommission.org/PatientSafety/NationalPatientSafetyGoals.

FDA Pregnancy Categories

A   No risk demonstrated to the fetus in any trimester

B   No adverse effects in animals, no human studies available

C   Only given after risks to the fetus are considered; animal studies have shown adverse reactions, no human studies available

D   Definite fetal risks, may be given despite risks if needed in life-threatening conditions

X   Absolute fetal abnormalities; not to be used any time during pregnancy

Note: **UK** = Unknown fetal risk (used in this text but not an official FDA pregnancy category).

Index

Entries can be identified as follows: generic name, Trade Name, DRUG CATEGORY, *Combination Product.*

Entries can be identified as follows: generic name, Trade Name, DRUG CATEGORY, *Combination Product*.

Entries can be identified as follows: generic name, Trade Name, DRUG CATEGORY, *Combination Product.*

Entries can be identified as follows: generic name, Trade Name, DRUG CATEGORY, *Combination Product.*

Entries can be identified as follows: generic name, Trade Name, DRUG CATEGORY, *Combination Product.*

Entries can be identified as follows: generic name, Trade Name, DRUG CATEGORY, *Combination Product.*

Entries can be identified as follows: generic name, Trade Name, DRUG CATEGORY, *Combination Product.*

Entries can be identified as follows: generic name, Trade Name, DRUG CATEGORY, *Combination Product.*

Entries can be identified as follows: generic name, Trade Name, DRUG CATEGORY, *Combination Product.*

Entries can be identified as follows: generic name, Trade Name, DRUG CATEGORY, *Combination Product*.

Entries can be identified as follows: generic name, Trade Name, DRUG CATEGORY, *Combination Product.*

Entries can be identified as follows: generic name, Trade Name, DRUG CATEGORY, *Combination Product.*

Entries can be identified as follows: generic name, Trade Name, DRUG CATEGORY, *Combination Product.*

Entries can be identified as follows: generic name, Trade Name, DRUG CATEGORY, *Combination Product.*

Entries can be identified as follows: generic name, Trade Name, DRUG CATEGORY, *Combination Product.*

Entries can be identified as follows: generic name, Trade Name, DRUG CATEGORY, *Combination Product.*

Entries can be identified as follows: generic name, Trade Name, DRUG CATEGORY, *Combination Product.*

Entries can be identified as follows: generic name, Trade Name, DRUG CATEGORY, *Combination Product.*

Entries can be identified as follows: generic name, Trade Name, DRUG CATEGORY, *Combination Product.*

cabazitaxel (Rx)
(ka-baz'i-tax'el)
Jevtana
Func. class.: Antineoplastic
Chem. class.: Taxane

Pregnancy category D

Action: A taxane that binds to tubulin, inhibits microtubule depolymerization, cell division, cell cycle arrest (G2/M) phase, cell proliferation; unlike other taxanes, this product may be useful for treating multidrug resistant tumors.

Therapeutic outcome: Decreased tumor size, spread of malignancy

Uses: Hormone-refractory prostate cancer in combination with prednisone in patients that have been previously treated with a docetaxel-containing regimen

Dosage and routes
Adult: **IV** INF 25 mg/m² over 1 hr on day 1, give q 3 wks with prednisone 10 mg q day, may continue for 10 cycles

Hepatic dose
Adult: **IV** INF: do not use if total bilirubin ULN ≥ or AST and/or ALT >1.5 times ULN

Available forms: Solution for injection 60 mg/1.5 ml

Adverse effects
CNS: Peripheral neuropathy, dysgeusia, dizziness, headache, fatigue, fever
CV: **Dysrhythmia,** peripheral edema, hypotension
GI: Diarrhea, nausea, vomiting, constipation, abdominal pain, dyspepsia, anorexia, mucosal inflammation
GU: **Renal failure,** dehydration, hematuria, urinary tract infection, dysuria, **obstructive uropathy,** infertility
HEMA: **Neutropenia, febrile neutropenia, anemia, leucopenia, thrombocytopenia**
MS: Back pain, arthralgia, muscle spasms
RESP: Cough, dyspnea
SYST: **Fatal infections, sepsis, anaphylaxis**

Contraindications: Hypersensitivity to this product, pregnancy **D**

Black Box Warning: Hypersensitivity to polysorbate 80, neutropenia (ANC ≤1500/mm³)

Precautions: Breastfeeding, children, diarrhea, elderly, hepatic disease, renal disease, sepsis, vomiting

Pharmacokinetics

Absorption	89-92% protein binding, primarily bound to albumin and lipoproteins
Distribution	Equally distributed between blood and plasma
Metabolism	Extensively metabolized by CYP3A4/5 in the liver and CYP2C8 to a lesser extent
Excretion	80% eliminated within 2 wks mainly in feces
Half-life	Half-life alpha, beta, gamma of 4 mins, 2 hrs, 95 hrs respectively

Pharmacodynamics
Unknown

Interactions
Individual drugs
Radiation: increased bone marrow depression

Drug classifications
Other antineoplastics: increased bone marrow depression
Strong CYP3A4 inhibitors (conivaptan, chloramphenicol, danazol, dalfopristin, delavirdine, ethinyl estradiol, fluvoxamine, imatinib, isoniazid, tipranavir, troleadomycin, zafirlukast, ketoconazole, itraconazole, clarithromycin, atazanavir, indinavir, nefazodone, nelfinavir, ritonavir, saquinavir, telithromycin, voriconazole; mild or moderate CYP3A4 inhibitors (basiliximab, fluoxetine, nicardipine, ranolazine, amiodarone, darunavir, diltiazem, miconazole, mifepristone (RU-486), posaconazole, propoxyphene, tamoxifen, erythromycin, verapamil, fluconazole: increased cabazitaxel concentrations
CYP3A4 inducers (rifampin, phenytoin, carbamazepine, rifabutin, rifapentine): decreased cabazitaxel concentrations
Vaccines: decreased immune response

NURSING CONSIDERATIONS
Assessment
- **Assess for symptoms of anaphylaxis:** hypotension, dyspnea, generalized urticaria, bronchospasm, discontinue immediately; keep emergency equipment near; usually occurs during the first or second infusion, do not use this product again, after severe hypersensitivity reactions
- Check infusion site for reactions: if given by regular **IV**, not port (redness, inflammation, warmth)

Adverse effects: *italic* = common, **bold** = life-threatening

- **Assess for bone marrow depression:** monitor CBC with differential, prior to and after one week, withhold if WBC <1500/mm³ or platelets <100,000/mm³. May not be a concern if an erythropoietin agent is given
- Assess for neurological side effects: peripheral neuropathy, dizziness, headache. During infusion of product, ice on extremities periodically, may prevent peripheral neuropathy
- Assess for musculoskeletal reactions: back pain, arthralgia, muscle spasms
- **Monitor for renal failure:** monitor BUN, creatinine and serum electrolytes; usually associated with sepsis, dehydration or obstructive uropathy; renal failure has been fatal
- **Assess for bleeding:** bruising, petechiae, hematuria, blood in emesis or stools; check mucosa orifices for stomatitis, obtain order for vicious xylocaine if needed
- Monitor temp periodically, increased temperature may indicate beginning infection
- Monitor hepatic studies: AST, ALT, bilirubin, LDH, prior to and periodically; jaundice of skin, eyes, clay-colored stools, dark urine, itching skin, abdominal pain, fever, diarrhea
- Identify effects of alopecia on body image, discuss feelings about body changes

Nursing diagnoses
- Risk for infection (adverse reactions)
- Risk for injury (adverse reactions)
- Knowledge deficit (teaching)

Implementation
- Use cytotoxic handling procedures
- Obtain neutrophil counts prior to administration, count should be >1500/ mm³
- Do not use PVC infusion containers or polyurethane infusion sets for preparation or administration
- Premedicate with diphenhydramine 25 mg **IV** or equivalent, dexamethasone 8 mg or equivalent and ranitidine 50 mg or equivalent and antiemetics
- Do not use solution that is discolored or if particulate is present, solution should be clear, yellow to brownish, discard if first or second dilution is not clear, remove immediately if solution comes in contact with skin

Intermittent IV infusion
- Two dilutions are required, both product and dilution are overfilled; *first dilution:* mix each vial of product (60 mg/1.5 ml) with the entire contents of supplied diluent (10 mg/ml); when transferring diluent, direct needle on side of vial and inject slowly to limit foaming; remove syringe and needle and gently mix by several inversions, do not shake; let stand for a few mins; *Second dilution:*

withdraw the required dose, further dilute the withdrawn product with 0.9% NaCL or D5 in a PVC free container, remove syringe and needle, mix by gently inverting the bag/bottle (final concentration 0.1-0.2 6 mg/ml), if a dose of ≥65 mg use a larger volume of infusion solution, so the concentration is max 0.26 mg/ml; do not mix with other drugs, solution may crystallize over time, discard if this occurs, us solution within 8 hrs (room temperature), 24 hrs (refrigerated); give over 1 hr, use 0.22 micrometer in-line filter

Patient/family education
- **Instruct patient to use a non hormonal form of contraception,** to notify prescriber if pregnancy is planned or suspected, pregnancy category (D); not to breastfeed
- Advise patient that hair may be lost during treatment, a wig or hairpiece may make the patient feel better, new hair will be different in color, texture
- Instruct patient to avoid receiving vaccinations while using this product
- **Teach patient to report signs of infection:** fever, sore throat, flu-like symptoms, avoid persons with known respiratory infections

Evaluation
Positive therapeutic outcome
- Decreased size, spread of malignancy

---

carglumic acid (Rx)
(kar-gloo'mik as'id)
Carbaglu
Func. class.: Metabolic agent-hyperammonemia agent

Pregnancy category: C

Action: Converts ammonia to urea, by activation of an enzyme in the liver mitochondria

Therapeutic outcome: Decreasing ammonia levels

Uses: Hyperammonemia in N-acetylglutamate synthase deficiency

Dosage and routes
Adult, adolescent, child, infant, neonate: PO 100-250 mg/kg/day divided into 2-4 doses per day, for adults round to nearest 100 mg, titrate based on plasma ammonia levels

Available forms: Tab 200 mg

Adverse effects
CNS: Fever, headache, somnolence, asthenia
EENT: Ear infection, naso-pharyngitis, tonsillitis
GI: Vomiting, abdominal pain, diarrhea, weight loss, anorexia, dysgeusia
HEMA: Anemia
INTEG: Rash
RESP: Pneumonia
SYST: Infection, influenza

Contraindications: Hypersensitivity

Precautions: Pregnancy **C**, geriatrics, breastfeeding

Pharmacokinetics
Absorption	Unknown
Distribution	Unknown
Metabolism	Unknown
Excretion	Lungs, small amount excreted in the urine and a significant portion in feces
Half-life	Terminal half-life 4.3–9.5 hrs

Pharmacodynamics
Onset	Unknown
Peak	Unknown
Duration	Plasma ammonia levels fall within 24 hours

Interactions: None

NURSING CONSIDERATIONS
Assessment
• Assess for hyperammonemia: serum ammonia

Nursing diagnoses
• Risk of injury (uses)

Implementation
PO route
• Disperse 200 mg tab/2.5 ml or more water, tabs do not dissolve completely, rinse container with additional water and administer to patient
NG Tube
• 200 mg tab/2.5 ml water or more (80 mg/ml), shake gently, draw up volume needed in oral syringe, give immediately, refill syringe with 1-2 ml of water, give immediately
• Store at room temperature, after room temperature storage, do not place in refrigerator; discard after 30 days; protect from moisture; store unopened containers in refrigerator

Patient/family education
• Teach patient reason for product and expected result
• Instruct patient to report coughing with sputum, ear pain, fever or any other symptoms following drug initiation

Evaluation
Positive therapeutic outcome
• Decreased ammonia levels

ceftaroline (Rx)
(sef-tar'oh-leen)
Teflaro
Func. class.: Cephalosporin

Pregnancy category B

Action: Inhibits cell wall synthesis through binding to essential penicillin-binding protein (PBPs)

Therapeutic outcome: Negative C&S, resolution of symptoms of infection

Uses: Acute bacterial skin/skin structure infections (ABSSI), bacterial community acquired pneumonia

Dosage and routes
Adult: IV 600 mg q 12 hrs × 5-14 days (skin/skin structure infections), × 5-7 days (bacterial community acquired pneumonia)

Renal dose
Adult: IV CCr >30-≤50 ml/min 400 mg q 12 hrs; CCr ≥15-≤30 ml/min 300 mg q 12 hrs, CCr ≤15 ml/min 200 mg q 12 hrs

Available forms: Powder for injection 400 mg, 600 mg

Adverse effects
CV: Phlebitis
ENDO: Hypokalemia
GI: Diarrhea, nausea, vomiting, constipation, abdominal pain, **pseudomembranous colitis (rare)**, elevated hepatic enzymes
INTEG: Rash, **anaphylaxis**

Contraindications: Cephalosporin hypersensitivity

Precautions: Antimicrobial resistance, breastfeeding, carbapenem/penicillin hypersensitivity, child/infant/neonate, coagulopathy, colitis, dialysis, diarrhea, geriatrics, GI disease, hypoprothrombinemia, IBS, pregnancy **B**, pseudomembraneous colitis, renal disease, ulcerative colitis, viral infection, vitamin K deficiency

Adverse effects: *italic* = common, **bold** = life-threatening

Pharmacokinetics

Absorption	Unknown
Distribution	Unknown
Metabolism	Not hepatically metabolized
Excretion	In urine 88%, feces 6%
Half-life	2.66 hrs

Pharmacodynamics

Unknown

Interactions
Drug classifications
Anticoagulants: increased prothrombin time risk

NURSING CONSIDERATIONS
Assessment
- Assess for infection: vital signs, sputum, WBC prior to and during therapy
- Assess for hypersensitivity: prior to use, obtain a history of hypersensitivity reactions to cephalosporins, carbapenems, penicillins; cross sensitivity may occur
- Obtain specimens for culture and sensitivity before beginning therapy. Begin dose and specimens are obtained
- **Assess for anaphylaxis (rare):** rash, pruritus, laryngeal edema, dyspnea, wheezing; discontinue and notify health care provider immediately, keep emergency equipment nearby
- **Monitor for pseudomembraneous colitis:** diarrhea, abdominal pain, fever, bloody stools; report immediately if these occur, may occur several weeks after terminating therapy

Nursing diagnoses
- Risk for infection (uses)

Implementation
- Visually inspect for particulate matter or discoloration if solution or container permit
- **Reconstitute:** add 20 ml of sterile water to 400 or 600 mg vial (20 ml/ml for 400 mg), (30 mg/ml for 600 mg), mix gently until dissolved: **Dilute:** in 250 ml of 0.9% NaCl, 0.45% NaCl, LR, D5, D2.5, give over 1 hr, do not admix, use within 6 hrs at room temperature or 24 hrs refrigerated
- Store reconstituted solution in the refrigerator

Patient/family education
- Explain reason for treatment and expected result
- Instruct patient to report immediately rash, itching, difficulty breathing, bloody diarrhea, fever, abdominal pain

Evaluation
Positive therapeutic outcome
- Negative C&S, resolution of symptoms of infection

dabigatran (Rx)
(da-bye-gat'ran)
Pradaxa
Func. class.: Anticoagulant-thrombin inhibitor
Pregnancy category C

Action: Direct thrombin inhibitor that inhibits both free and clot-bound thrombin, prevents thrombin-induced platelet aggregation and thrombus formation by preventing conversion of fibrinogen to fibrin

Therapeutic outcome: Decreased thrombus formation/extension, absence of emboli, post-thrombotic effects

Uses: Stroke/systemic embolism prophylaxis with non-valvular atrial fibrillation

Dosage and routes
Stroke prophylaxis
Adult: PO 150 mg BID

For conversion from an alternative anticoagulant to dabigatran
- When converting from warfarin to dabigatran, discontinue warfarin and initiate dabigatran therapy when the INR is <2.0. When converting from a parenteral anticoagulant to dabigatran, initiate dabigatran 0-2 hours before the time of the next scheduled anticoagulant dose or at the time of discontinuation of a continuously administered anticoagulant (e.g., intravenous unfractionated heparin)

For conversion from dabigatran to warfarin
Adult: CCr >50 ml/min start warfarin 3 days before discontinuing dabigatran; CCr 31-50 ml/min start warfarin 2 days before discontinuing dabigatran; CCr 15-30 ml/min start warfarin 1 day before discontinuing dabigatran

For conversion from dabigatran to parenteral anticoagulants
Adult: PO discontinue dabigatran, start parenteral anticoagulant 12 hr (CCR ≥30 ml/min), 24 hr (CCR <30 ml/min) after the last dabigatran dose

Renal dose
Adult: PO CCr 15-30 ml/min 75 mg bid

Deep vein thrombus (DVT)/
pulmonary embolism prophylaxis
(unlabeled)
Adult: PO 220 mg or 150 mg q day × 28-35 days, starting with ½ dose 1-4 hrs after surgery

Available forms: Cap 75, 150 mg

Adverse effects
CV: **Myocardial infarction**
CNS: **Intracranial bleeding**
GI: Abdominal pain, dyspepsia, peptic ulcer, esophagitis, GERD, gastritis, **GI bleeding**
HEMA: **Bleeding**
INTEG: Rash, pruritus
SYST: **Anaphylaxis (rare)**

Contraindications: Hypersensitivity, bleeding

Precautions: Abrupt discontinuation, anticoagulant therapy, breastfeeding, pregnancy **C**, children, geriatrics, labor, obstetric delivery, renal disease, surgery

Pharmacokinetics

Absorption	Protein binding 35%
Distribution	Unknown
Metabolism	Unknown
Excretion	Unknown
Half life	12-17 hrs (extended in renal disease)

Pharmacodynamics

Onset	Unknown
Peak	1 hr, high-fat meal delays peak
Duration	Unknown

Interactions
Individual drugs
Amiodarone, clopidogrel, ketoconazole, quinidine, verapamil: increased bleeding risk
Rifampin: decreased dabigatran effect
Drug classifications
Anticoagulants, thrombolytics: increased bleeding risk

NURSING CONSIDERATIONS
Assessment
• **Assess for bleeding:** blood in urine or emesis, dark tarry stools, lower back pain. Caution with arterial/venous punctures, catheters, NG tubes. Monitor vital signs frequently. The elderly are more prone to serious bleeding
• **Assess for Thrombosis/MI/Emboli:** Swelling, pain, redness, difficulty breathing, chest pain, tachypnea, cough, coughing up blood, cyanosis
• **Assess for post-thrombotic syndrome:** pain, heaviness, itching/tingling, swelling, varicose veins, brownish/reddish skin discoloration, ulcers; use of ambulation, compression stockings and adequate anticoagulation can prevent this syndrome
• Monitor serum creatinine

Nursing diagnoses
• Risk of injury (uses, adverse reactions)

Implementation
• Do not crush break, chew or empty contents of capsule
• If dose is missed take as soon as remembered if on the same day, do not administer if <6 hrs before next dose
• Take without regard to food
• Store in original package until time of use, at room temperature, discard after 30 days, protect from moisture

Patient/family education
• Explain the purpose and expected results of this product
• Instruct patient to report if bleeding is present

Evaluation
Positive therapeutic outcome
• Decreased thrombus formation/extension, absence of emboli, post-thrombotic effects

dalfampridine (Rx)
(dal-fam′pri-deen)
Ampyra
Func. class.: Neurological agent- MS
Chem. class.: Broad spectrum potassium channel blocker
Pregnancy category C

Action: Mechanism of action is not fully understood, a broad spectrum potassium channel blocker inhibits potassium channels and increased action potential conduction in demyelinated axons

Therapeutic outcome: Ability to walk at improved speed in MS

Uses: For improved walking in patients with multiple sclerosis

Dosage and routes
Adult: PO 10 mg q 12 hrs
Renal dose
Adult: PO CCr 51-80 ml/min do dosage adjustment needed, but seizure risk is unknown; CCr ≤50 ml/min, do not use

Adverse effects: *italic* = common, **bold** = life-threatening

Available forms: Extended release tab 10 mg

Adverse effects
CNS: **Seizures,** paresthesias, headache, dizziness, asthenia, insomnia
GI: Nausea, constipation, dyspepsia
GU: Urinary tract infection
MS: Back pain

Contraindications: Renal failure (CCr <50 ml/min), seizures

Precautions: Pregnancy **C,** breastfeeding, renal disease, elderly

Pharmacokinetics	
Absorption	Bioavailability 96%
Distribution	Largely unbound to plasma proteins
Metabolism	Unknown
Excretion	96% is recovered in the urine
Half-life	Unknown

Pharmacodynamics	
Onset	Unknown
Peak	3-4 hrs (fasting), longer if taken with food
Duration	Unknown

Interactions
Individual drugs
Fampridine: do not use together
Drug classifications
4-aminopyridine (4-AP) containing products: do not use together

NURSING CONSIDERATIONS
Assessment
• **Multiple sclerosis:** assess walking, including speed
• Assess for seizures: more common in those with previous seizure disorder

Nursing diagnoses
• Activity intolerance (uses)
• Injury, risk for (adverse reactions)

Implementation
• Do not break, crush, or chew; give without regard to meals
• Do not give closer together than q 12 hrs, seizures may occur
• Do not double doses, if a dose is missed, skip it

Patient/family education
• Advise patient to notify prescriber if pregnancy is planned or suspected, do not breastfeed
• Teach patient about expected results, side effects including seizures

Evaluation
Positive therapeutic outcome
• Ability to walk at improved speed in MS

---

denosumab (Rx)
(den-oh'sue-mab)
Prolia, Xgeva
Func. class.: Bone resorption inhibitor
Chem. class.: Monoclonal antibody, bone resorption

Pregnancy category C

Action: Neutralizes activity of receptor activator nuclear factor kappa-B ligand (RANKL) by binding to it and blocking its interaction with cell surface receptors, use of a RANKL inhibitor may reduce bone turnover and decrease tumor burden

Therapeutic outcome: Increased/ maintained bone density

Uses: Osteoporosis in postmenopausal women at high risk for fractures, prevention of skeletal related events in bone metastases from solid tumors

Dosage and routes
Postmenopausal osteoporosis
Adult female: Subcut 60 mg q 6 months with 1000 mg calcium and 400 international units vitamin D, max 60 mg q 6 months

Bone metastases from solid tumors
Adult: Subcut 120 mg q 4 wks, max 120 mg q 4 wks; administer with calcium and vitamin D as necessary to prevent hypocalcemia

Available forms: Solution for injection 60 mg/ml (Prolia); 120 mg/1.7 ml (Xgeva)

Adverse effects
CNS: Chills, fever, flushing, headache, vertigo, neuropathic pain
CV: Angina, **atrial fibrillation**
GI: Abdominal pain, constipation, *diarrhea,* flatulence, GERD, *vomiting, nausea*
GU: Cystitis, lactation suppression
HEMA: **Anemia, neutropenia**
INTEG: Atopic dermatitis, pruritus
META: Hypercholesterolemia, hypocalcemia, hypophosphatemia
MS: Back/bone pain, MS pain, myalgia, **osteonecrosis of the jaw**
RESP: Cough, *dyspnea*
SYST: **Infection, secondary malignancy**

Contraindications: Hypersensitivity, hypocalcemia

Precautions: Anemia, breastfeeding, child/infant/neonate, coagulopathy, diabetes mellitus, dialysis, eczema, hypoparathyroidism, immunosuppression, latex hypersensitivity, malabsorption syndrome, neonates, neoplastic disease, pancreatitis, parathyroid disease, pregnancy **C,** dental/renal/thyroid disease, TB, Vitamin D deficiency

Pharmacokinetics

Absorption	Bioavailability 62%
Distribution	Unknown
Metabolism	Unknown
Excretion	Unknown
Half-life	25.4 days

Pharmacodynamics

Onset	Unknown
Peak	Maximum serum concentration 3-21 days
Duration	Steady state 6 months

Interactions
Drug classifications
Immunosuppressives, corticosteroids: possible increased infection
Antineoplastics, corticosteroids: possible increased osteonecrosis of the jaw

NURSING CONSIDERATIONS
Assessment
• **Assess for acute acute-phase reaction:** fever, myalgia, headache, flu-like symptoms, for 72 hrs after injection, usually resolves after 72 hrs
• Monitor blood tests: serum calcium/creatinine/BUN/magnesium/phosphate
• **Assess for hypocalcemia:** paresthesia, twitching, laryngospasm, Chvostek's Trouseau's signs; preexisting hypocalcemia prior to treatment; patient with Vitamin D deficiency may require higher doses of Vitamin D
• **Assess for hypercalcemia:** nausea, vomiting, anorexia, weakness, thirst, constipation, dysrhythmias
• **Monitor dental status:** correct dental complications prior to product use, good oral hygiene should be maintained; if dental work is to be performed, antiinfectives should be given to prevent osteonecrosis of the jaw
• **Assess for infection:** Do not start treatment in those with active infections, infections should be resolved first

Nursing diagnoses
• Electrolyte imbalance, risk for (uses)

Implementation
Subcut route
• Give acetaminophen before and for 72 hrs after to decrease pain
• Do not use if particulate matter or discoloration is present; solution is clear and colorless to slightly yellow with small white/opalescent particles, remove from refrigerator and allow to warm to room temperature (15-30 mins)
• *Use of prefilled syringe with needle safety guard:* Leave green guard in original position until after administration, remove and discard needle cap immediately before injection, give by subcut injection in upper arm/thigh, or abdomen; after injection, point needle away from people and slide green guard over needle
• *Use of single-use vials:* Use 27G needle, give in upper arm/thigh, or abdomen, do not re-insert needle in vial, discard supplies as appropriate
• Avoid direct sunlight/heat, do not freeze, use within 14 days after removal from refrigerator, store unopened containers in refrigerator

Patient/family education
• Advise patient to report hypercalcemic relapse: nausea, vomiting, bone pain, thirst
• Teach patient to continue with dietary recommendations including additional calcium and vitamin D
• Advise patient to avoid use in pregnancy and breastfeeding, notify prescriber if pregnancy is planned, or suspected
• Instruct patient to use acetaminophen prior to and for 72 hrs after injection to lessen bone pain
• Explain the purpose of this product and expected results
• Advise patient to avoid OTC, Rx or herbs and supplements unless approved by prescriber
• Teach patient to use regular exercise, stop smoking and avoid alcohol to maintain bone health
• Advise patient to inform all health care providers of product use, avoid dental procedures/surgery if possible, practice good oral hygiene practices
• Teach patient that lab tests and follow-up exams will be required

Evaluation
Positive therapeutic outcome
• Increased/maintained bone density

eribulin (Rx)
(er'i-bue'lin)
Halaven
Func. class.: Antineoplastics-Non-Taxane

Pregnancy category D

Action: Potent antimitotic agent, different from taxes, vinca alkaloids, epothilones; blocks cell progression in G2-Mphase, inhibits the growth phase of microtubules and sequesters tubules leading to disruption of mitotic spindles and apoptotic cell death

Therapeutic outcome: Decreased spread and size of tumor

Uses: Metastatic breast cancer who have received at least 2 chemotherapy regimens

Dosage and routes
Adult: IV 1.4 mg/m^2 over 2-5 mins on days 1 and 8, repeat q 21 days

Recommendations for dose delay
• *For ANC < 1000/mm^3, platelets <75,000/mm^3, or grade 3 or 4 non-hematological toxicities:* Do not administer; the day 8 dose may be delayed a maximum of 1 week; *for the day 8 dose, if toxicities do not resolve to ≤ grade 2 by day 15:* Omit the dose; *for the day 8 dose, if toxicities resolve or improve to ≤ grade 2 by day 15:* Administer eribulin at a reduced dose (see below) and initiate the next cycle no sooner than 2 weeks later

Dose adjustments for hematologic toxicity
• *ANC < 500/mm^3 for >7 days or ANC <1000/mm^3 with fever or infection:* Permanently reduce dose to 1.1 mg/m^2; *platelets <25,000/mm^3 or <50,000/mm^3 requiring transfusion:* Permanently reduce dose to 1.1 mg/m^2; *if day 8 of previous cycle omitted or delayed:* Permanently reduce dose to 1.1 mg/m^2; *while receiving 1.1 mg/m^2, if recurrence of hematologic event occurs, or if day 8 of previous cycle omitted or delayed:* Permanently reduce dose to 0.7 mg/m^2; *while receiving 0.7 mg/m^2, if recurrence of hematologic event occurs, or if day 8 of previous cycle omitted or delayed:* Discontinue

Dose adjustments of eribulin for non-hematologic toxicity during treatment
• *Any Grade 3 or 4 non-hematologic toxicity:* Permanently reduce dose to 1.1 mg/m^2; *if day 8 of previous cycle omitted or delayed:* Permanently reduce dose to 1.1 mg/m^2; *while receiving 1.1 mg/m^2, if recurrence of Grade 3 or 4 non-hematologic toxicity occurs, or if day 8 of previous cycle omitted or delayed:* Permanently reduce dose to 0.7 mg/m^2; *while receiving 0.7 mg/m^2, if recurrence of Grade 3 or 4 non-hematologic toxicity occurs, or if day 8 of previous cycle omitted or delayed:* Discontinue

Available forms: Solution for injection 1 mg/2 ml

Adverse effects
CNS: Depression, dizziness, fatigue, fever, headache, insomnia, peripheral neuropathy
CV: **QT prolongation,** peripheral edema
GI: Abdominal pain, anorexia, constipation, diarrhea, dyspepsia, nausea, vomiting, weight loss
HEMA: **Anemia, neutropenia, thrombocytopenia**
INTEG: Alopecia, rash, stomatitis
META: Hypokalemia
MS: Arthralgia, myalgia, bone/back pain
RESP: Cough, dyspnea
SYST: Infection

Contraindications: Hypersensitivity, pregnancy **D**

Precautions: Bradycardia, breast-feeding, children, electrolyte imbalances, heart failure, hepatic disease, hypokalemia, hypomagnesemia, infants, infertility, neonates, neutropenia, peripheral neuropathy, QT prolongation, renal disease

Pharmacokinetics	
Absorption	Protein binding 49-65%
Distribution	Unknown
Metabolism	Inhibits CYP3A4
Excretion	Feces 82%, urine 9%
Half-life	40 hrs, increased levels in renal/hepatic disease

Pharmacodynamics
Unknown

Interactions
Individual drugs
Arsenic trioxide, astemizole, bepridil, chloroquine, cisapride, clarithromycin, dextromethorphan; quinidine, dronedarone, droperidol, erythromycin, halofantrine, haloperidol, levomethadyl, methadone, pentamidine, pimozide, posaconazole, probucol, propafenone, saquinavir, sparfloxacin, terfenadine, troleandomycin, and ziprasidone; also to a lesser degree abarelix, alfuzosin, amoxapine, apomorphine, artemether; lumefantrine, asenapine, ofloxacin, clozapine, cyclobenzaprine, dasatinib,

dolasetron, flecainide, gatifloxacin, gemifloxacin, iloperidone, lapatinib, levofloxacin, lopinavir; ritonavir, magnesium sulfate; potassium sulfate; sodium sulfate, maprotiline, mefloquine, moxifloxacin, nilotinib, norfloxacin, octreotide, ciprofloxacin, olanzapine, ondansetron, paliperidone, palonosetron, quetiapine, ranolazine, risperidone, sertindole, sunitinib, tacrolimus, telavancin, telithromycin, tetrabenazine, venlafaxine, vardenafil, vorinostat: increased QT prolongation

Drug classifications

Certain phenothiazines (chlorpromazine, mesoridazine, thioridazine), Class IA antiarrhythmics (disopyramide, procainamide, quinidine), Class III antiarrhythmics (amiodarone, bretylium, dofetilide, ibutilide, sotalol), also to a lesser degree, beta-agonists, halogenated anesthetics, local anesthetics, some phenothiazines (fluphenazine, perphenazine, prochlorperazine, trifluoperazine), tricyclic antidepressants: increased QT prolongation

NURSING CONSIDERATIONS
Assessment
• **QT prolongation:** assess for drug interactions that may occur; monitor ECG, heart rate
• Monitor blood studies: CBC and differential, serum creatinine/bun/electrolytes, liver function tests, baseline and periodically, increased AST/ALT >3 × ULN or total bilirubin >1.5 × ULN are at a greater chance of grade 4 or febrile neutropenia

Nursing diagnoses
• Injury, risk for (adverse reactions)
• Infection, risk for (adverse reactions)

Implementation
IV direct, intermittent route
• Visually inspect for particulate matter or discoloration as solution and container permit, withdraw required amount (0.5 mg/ml) from single use vial, give undiluted over 2-5 min or diluted in 100 ml 0.9% NaCl and give as intermittent infusion, do not give through line with dextrose or any other product
• Store at room temperature for 4 hours or 24 hrs refrigerated

Patient/family education
• Teach patient reason for product and expected results
• Advise patient to report side effects to health care provider
• Advise patient to avoid other medications, supplements unless approved by provider, serious drug interactions may occur

• Discuss hair loss and use of wig or hair piece
• Advise patient to notify prescriber if pregnancy is planned or suspected, avoid breastfeeding

Evaluation
Positive therapeutic outcome
• Decreasing tumor spread and size

fingolimod (Rx)
(fin-gol'i-mod)
Gilenya
Func. class.: Biologic response modifier
Chem. class.: Sphingosine 1-phosphate receptor modulator
Pregnancy category C

Action: Binds with high affinity to sphingosine 1 phosphate receptors, it blocks lymphocyte egress to lymph nodes, reducing the number of peripheral blood lymphocytes, may reduce lymphocyte migration into the CNS

Therapeutic outcome: Improved symptoms of multiple sclerosis and prevention of increasing disability

Uses: To reduce frequency of exacerbation, to delay physical disability of relapsing forms of MS

Dosage and routes
Adult: PO 0.5 mg q day

Hepatic dose
Adult: PO Child-Pugh C, total score >10: Closely monitor, fingolimod exposure is doubled

Available forms: Cap 0.5 mg
Adverse effects
CNS: Asthenia, depression, fatigue, headache, dizziness, encephalopathy, migraine, paresthesias, **stroke**
CV: AV block, bradycardia, chest pain, hypertension, palpitations
EENT: Blurred vision, vision impairment, ocular pain, macular edema
GI: Abdominal pain, anorexia, diarrhea, jaundice, vomiting, weight loss
HEMA: **Leukopenia, lymphopenia, neutropenia**
INTEG: Alopecia, pruritus
MS: Back pain
RESP: Dyspnea, cough
SYST: Infection, influenza, **secondary malignancy**
Contraindications: Hypersensitivity

Adverse effects: *italic* = common, **bold** = life-threatening

Precautions: AIDS, asthma, AV block, bradycardia, breastfeeding, dysrhythmias, cardiac disease, children, COPD, diabetes mellitus, heart failure, hepatic disease, HIV, hypertension, immunosuppression, infants, leukemia, lymphoma, neonates, pregnancy **C**, QT prolongation, respiratory insufficiency, sick sinus syndrome, syncope, uveitis

Pharmacokinetics

Absorption	Protein binding (99.7%)
Distribution	Distributed to RBCs (86%)
Metabolism	Metabolized by CYP4F2 and CYP2D6 to a lesser extent
Excretion	Excreted in urine (81% inactive metabolites)
Half-life	Terminal half-life 6-9 days

Pharmacodynamics

Onset	Unknown
Peak	12-16 hrs
Duration	Steady state 1-2 mo

Interactions
Individual drugs
Ketoconazole: increased fingolimod effect
Drug classifications
Class Ia/III antidysrhythmics: increased: risk of torsades de pointes
Antineoplastics, immunosuppressants, immune modulating therapies: increased immunosuppression
Inactive vaccines, toxoids: decreased effects
Live vaccines: increased infection risk

NURSING CONSIDERATIONS
Assessment
• **Multiple sclerosis:** Assess for improving paresthesia, muscle weakness, clonus, muscle spasms, difficulty in moving, difficulty in coordination in balance, speech, swallowing, vision problems, fatigue; prevention of increasing disability
• Monitor laboratory values: obtain before initial dose, CBC, LFTs, serum bilirubin, ophthalmologic exam, antibodies to VZ V if there is not a history of chickenpox or without vaccination, may give VZV vaccination of antibody negative patient before giving product, postpone for 1 month after vaccination; obtain ECG for evidence of bradycardia, or AV block

Nursing diagnoses
• Activity intolerance (uses)

Implementation
PO route
• Watch patient for 6 hrs after initial dose or if product is not given for >2 wks for development of bradycardia; give without regard to food
• Store at room temperature, protect from moisture

Patient/family education
• Provide med guide to patient and explain use of product and expected results
• Advise patient that continuing follow-up exams and laboratory test will be required on a regular basis
• Instruct patient to report any side effects resulting from therapy
• Teach patient to protect from moisture
• Advise patient to report chest pain, palpitations, jaundice

Evaluation
Positive therapeutic outcome
• Improved symptoms of multiple sclerosis and prevention of increasing disability

---

liraglutide (Rx)
(lir'a-gloo'tide)
Victoza
Func. class.: Antidiabetic agent
Chem. class.: Incretin mimetics
Pregnancy category C

Action: Improved glycemic control and potential weight loss via activation of the glucagon-like peptide-1 (GLP-1) receptor

Therapeutic outcome: Stable and improved serum glucose, A1C, weight loss

Uses: Type 2 diabetes mellitus in combination with diet/exercise

Dosage and routes
Adult: Subcut 0.6 mg q day × 1 wk, then increase to 1.2 mg q day, max 1.8 mg/day

Available forms: Solution for injection 18 mg/3 ml pre-filled pen

Adverse effects
CNS: Dizziness, headache
CV: Hypertension
ENDO: Hypoglycemia
EENT: Sinusitis
GI: Abdominal pain, anorexia, constipation, diarrhea, dyspepsia, nausea, vomiting, **pancreatitis**
INTEG: **Angioedema,** erythema, injection site reaction, urticaria

---

MS: Back pain
SYST: Antibody formation, infection, influenza, **secondary thyroid malignancy**

Contraindications: Hypersensitivity

Precautions: Alcoholism, breastfeeding, burns, children, cholelithiasis, type 1 diabetes mellitus, ketoacidosis, diarrhea, elderly, fever, gastroparesis, hepatic disease, hypoglycemia, infection, pancreatitis, renal disease, surgery, thyroid disease, trauma, vomiting, pregnancy **C**

Black Box Warning: Medullary thyroid carcinoma (MTC), multiple endocrine neoplasia syndrome type 2 (MEN 2), thyroid cancer

Pharmacokinetics

Absorption	Protein binding (98%)
Distribution	Binds to albumin, then released into circulation
Metabolism	Unknown
Excretion	Unknown
Half-life	12-13 hrs

Pharmacodynamics

Onset	Unknown
Peak	Peak 8-12 hrs
Duration	Unknown

Interactions
Individual drugs
Dexfenfluramine, fenfluramine, disopyramide, fluoxetine, mecasermin, octreotide, pegvisomant, salicylates: increased hypoglycemic reactions

Baclofen, cyclosporine, tacrolimus, dextrothyroxine, diazoxide, phenytoin, fosphenytoin, ethotoin, isoniazid, INH, niacin, nicotine: increased hyperglycemic reactions

Bortezomib, clonidine, alcohol, lithium, pentamidine: increased or decreased hypoglycemic reactions

Atorvastatin, acetaminophen, griseofulvin: increased or decreased effects of each specific drug

Drug classifications
Angiotensin II receptor antagonists, ACE inhibitors, other antidiabetics, beta blockers, fibric acid derivatives, MAOIs, salicylates: increased hypoglycemic reactions

Protease inhibitors, phenothiazines, atypical antipsychotics, corticosteroids, carbonic anhydrase inhibitors, estrogens, progestins, oral contraceptives, growth hormones, sympathomimetics: increased hyperglycemic reactions

Androgens, quinolones: increased or decreased hypoglycemic reactions

NURSING CONSIDERATIONS
Assessment
- Watch for hypoglycemic reactions that may occur soon after meals: hunger, sweating, weakness, dizziness, tremors, restlessness, tachycardia
- Assess for hypersensitivity to this product
- Monitor serum glucose, A1c, CBC during treatment
- **Assess for stress:** those diabetic patients exposed to stress, surgery, fever, infections may require insulin administration, temporarily
- **Assess for serious reactions:** angioedema, pancreatitis, secondary thyroid malignancy

Nursing diagnoses
- Imbalanced nutrition: more than body requirements (uses)
- Noncompliance (teaching)

Implementation
Subcut route
- Give by subcut only, inspect for particulate matter, or discoloration, do not use if unusually viscous, cloudy, discolored, or if particles are present; give q day at any time without regard to meals; pen needles must be purchased separately, use Novo Nordisk needles, prior to first use, prime, see manual for directions; give in thigh, abdomen or upper arm; lightly pinch fold of skin, insert needle at 90 degree angle or 45 degree angle if thin, release skin, aspiration is not needed, give over 6 seconds, rotate injection sites
- Storage: do not store pen with needle attached; avoid direct heat and sunlight, discard 30 days after first use, after first use may be store at room temperature or refrigerated, do not freeze

Patient/family education
- Teach patient the symptoms of hypo/hyperglycemia and what to do about each, to have glucagon emergency kit available, carry a carbohydrate source at all times
- Teach patient about side effects associated with therapy such as nausea and vomiting; upward dose titration can be delayed or ignored depending on tolerance
- Teach patient that diabetes is a life-long illness, product does not cure disease and must be continued on a daily basis
- Instruct patient to carry emergency ID with prescriber's phone number and medications taken
- Advise patient to continue with other recommendations: diet, exercise, hygiene
- Teach patient to test blood glucose using a blood glucose meter

Adverse effects: *italic* = common, **bold** = life-threatening

- Advise patient to avoid other medications, herbs, supplements unless approved by prescriber
- Advise patient to report serious skin effects, abdominal pain with nausea/vomiting
- Provide patient with written instructions if self administration is ordered

Evaluation
Positive therapeutic outcome
- Stable and improved serum glucose, A1C, weight loss

---

lurasidone (Rx)
(loo-ras′i-done)
Latuda
Func. class.: Atypical antipsychotic
Chem. class.: Benzoisothiazol derivative

Pregnancy category B

Action: May modulate central dopaminergic and serotonergic activity, high affinity for dopamine-D2 receptors, serotonin 5-HT2A receptors and partial agonist at serotonin 5-HT1A receptor

Therapeutic outcome: Decreasing hallucinations, delusions, agitation, social withdrawal

Uses: Schizophrenia

Dosage and routes
Adult: PO 40 mg q day, range 40-80 mg/day, those receiving CYP3A4 inhibitors (max 40 mg/day), do not use with strong CYP3A4 inducers/inhibitors

Hepatic/renal dose
Adult: PO Child-Pugh class B/C , CCr ≥10 ml/min-<50 ml/min max 40 mg/day

Available forms: 40 mg and 80 mg tabs

Adverse effects
CNS: Agitation, akathisia, anxiety, dizziness, drowsiness, fatigue, hyperthermia, insomnia, dystonic reactions; **neuroleptic malignant syndrome (rare)**, pseudoparkinsonism, restlessness, **seizures, suicidal ideation**, syncope, tardive dyskinesia, vertigo
CV: Angina, **AV block, bradycardia**, hypertension, orthostatic hypotension, **sinus tachycardia, stroke**
EENT: Blurred vision
ENDO: Diabetes mellitus, ketoacidosis, hyperglycemia, hyperprolactimemia
GI: Abdominal pain, diarrhea, dyspepsia, nausea, vomiting, gastritis, weight gain/loss
GU: Amenorrhea, breast enlargement, dysmenorrhea, impotence, dysuria, renal failure

HEMA: **Agranulocytosis, anemia, leucopenia, neutropenia**
INTEG: Pruritus, rash
MS: Back pain, dysarthria; **rhabdomyolysis (rare)**
SYST: **Angioedema**

Contraindications: Hypersensitivity

Precautions: Abrupt discontinuation, ambient temperature increase, breast cancer, breastfeeding, cardiac disease, children, dehydration, diabetes, ketoacidosis, driving, operating machinery dysphagia, geriatrics, heart failure, hematological/hepatic/renal disease, hypotension, hypovolemia, MI, infertility, obesity, Parkinson's disease, pregnancy **B,** seizures, strenuous exercise, stroke, substance abuse, suicidal ideation, syncope, tardive dyskinesia

Black Box Warning: Dementia: antipsychotics, such as lurasidone, are not approved for the treatment of dementia-related psychosis in geriatric patients and may increase the risk of death in this population

Pharmacokinetics

Absorption	9-19%
Distribution	99% protein binding
Metabolism	Unknown
Excretion	80% feces, 9% urine
Half-life	18 hrs

Pharmacodynamics

Onset	Unknown
Peak	1-3 hrs
Duration	Steady state 7 days

Interactions
Drug classifications
Strong CYP3A4 inhibitors: increased lurasidone effect, do not use concurrently
SSRIs, SNRIs: increased serotonin syndrome, neuroleptic malignant syndrome

NURSING CONSIDERATIONS
Assessment
- **Assess for schizophrenia:** hallucinations, delusions, agitation, social withdrawal; monitor orientation, behavior, mood prior to and periodically during therapy
- **Assess for neuroleptic malignant syndrome (rare):** fever, dyspnea, tachycardia, seizures, sweating, hyper-hypotension, muscle stiffness, pallor, report immediately
- **Monitor for blood dyscrasias:** CBC periodically, blood dyscrasias may occur

- **Monitor for serious cardiac symptoms:** AV block, stroke, bradycardia may occur
- **Assess for EPS:** restlessness, difficulty speaking, loss of balance, pill rolling, mask-like face, shuffling gait, rigidity, tremors, muscle spasms; monitor prior to and periodically during therapy; report tardive dyskinesia immediately

Nursing diagnoses
- Ineffective coping (uses)
- Noncompliance (teaching)

Implementation
- Give with a meal of at least 350 calories
- Store at room temperature, protect from moisture

Patient/family education
- Explain reason for treatment and expected results
- Teach patient to report EPS symptoms, blood dyscrasias: sore throat, fever, unusual bleeding/bruising

Evaluation
Positive therapeutic outcome
- Decreasing hallucinations, delusions, agitation, social withdrawal

pegloticase (Rx)
(peg-loe'ti-kase)
Krystexxa
Func. class.: Antigout agent
Chem. class.: Pegylated, recombinant, mammalian urate oxidase enzyme

Pregnancy category C

Action: Lowers plasma uric acid concentration by conversion of uric acid to allantoin that is readily excreted by the kidneys

Therapeutic outcome: Decrease uric acid levels; relief of pain, swelling, redness in toes, feet, knees

Uses: Chronic gout in patients experiencing treatment failure

Dosage and routes
Adult: **IV** infusion 8 mg over 2 hrs, q 2 wks

Available forms: Solution for injection 8 mg/ml

Adverse effects
CNS: Dizziness, fatigue, fever
CV: *Chest pain,* **heart failure,** hypotension
GI: *Nausea,* vomiting, diarrhea, constipation
GU: Nephrolithiasis
HEMA: **Anemia**

INTEG: Ecchymosis, *erythema, pruritus, urticaria*
MS: Back pain, arthralgia, muscle spasm
RESP: Dyspnea, upper respiratory infection
SYST: **Antibody formation, infection, anaphylaxis, infusion related reactions**

Contraindications: Hypersensitivity, G6PD deficiency

Precautions: African-American patients, breastfeeding, children/infants/neonates, pregnancy C, heart failure

Black Box Warning: Requires a specialized setting, requires an experienced clinician

Pharmacokinetics
Absorption	Unknown
Distribution	Remains primarily in intravascular space after administration
Metabolism	Unknown
Excretion	Unknown
Half-life	Elimination half-life 2 wks

Pharmacodynamics
Onset	Unknown
Peak	Unknown
Duration	Mean nadir uric acid concentration 24-72 hrs

NURSING CONSIDERATIONS
Assessment
- **Gout:** assess for pain in big toe, feet, knees, redness, swelling, tenderness lasting a few days to weeks; intake of alcohol, purines, if patient is overweight, or is taking diuretics
- Obtain uric acid levels at baseline and before administration; two consecutive uric acid levels of >6 mg/dl, may indicate therapy failure, a greater chance of anaphylaxis, and infection related reactions

Nursing diagnoses
- Pain, chronic (uses)

Implementation
- *When reconstituting,* visually inspect for particulate matter, or discoloration whenever solution/container permit, use aseptic technique, withdraw 8 mg (1 ml) of product/250 ml 0.9% NaCl or 0.45% NaCl, invert several times to mix, do not shake; discard remaining product in vial
- *Premedicate* with antihistamines and corticosteroids in all patients and acetaminophen if deemed necessary to prevent anaphylaxis and infusion site reactions

Adverse effects: *italic* = common, **bold** = life-threatening

• *Infusion:* If refrigerated, allow to come to room temperature, do not warm artificially, give over 120 mins, do not give **IV** push or bolus; use infusion by gravity feed, syringe-type pump, or infusion pump, give in a specialized setting by those that can manage anaphylaxis, or infection site reactions, monitor during and for 1 hr after infusion; if reaction occurs, slow or stop infusion, may be restarted at a slower rate, do not admix

• Store diluted product in refrigerated or room temperature for up to 4 hrs, refrigerator is preferred, protect from light, do not freeze, use within 4 hrs of preparation

Patient/family education

• Teach patient reason for infusion and expected results

• Advise patient to notify prescriber during infusion of allergic reactions, or redness, swelling pain at infusion site

• Advise patient that continuing follow-up exams and uric acid levels will be needed

Evaluation
Positive therapeutic outcome

• Decreased uric acid levels; relief of pain, swelling, redness in toes, feet, knees

---

sipuleucel-T (Rx)
(si-pu-loo'sel tee)
Provenge
Func. class.: Antineoplastic-biologic response modifiers
Chem. class.: Active cellular immunotherapy

Action: Stimulates T-cell immunity against prostatic acid phosphatase (PAP), an antigen expressed in prostatic cancer tissue

Therapeutic outcome: Decreasing size of tumor, decreasing PSA

Uses: Asymptomatic or minimally symptomatic metastatic, hormone refractory prostate cancer

Dosage and routes
Adult male: **IV** infusion: give entire contents of bag over 60 mins, q 2 wks × 3 doses; premedicate with acetaminophen and diphenhydramine 30 minutes prior to infusion to minimize acute infusion reactions

Available forms: Suspension for injection

Adverse effects
CNS: Asthenia, dizziness, fatigue, fever, flushing, headache, insomnia, paresthesia, **stroke,** tremor, chills, hot flashes
CV: Hypertension, hypoxia, sinus tachycardia

GI: Anorexia, constipation, diarrhea, weight loss, nausea, vomiting
GU: **Hematuria**
HEMA: **Anemia**
MS: Arthralgia, back/bone pain, muscle cramps, myalgia
RESP: **Bronchospasm**

Contraindications: Hypersensitivity

Precautions: Cardiac disease, chemotherapy, child/infant/neonate, immunosuppression, infusion reaction, pulmonary disease

Pharmacokinetics	
Absorption	Unknown
Distribution	T-cell stimulation at 8 wks was 8-fold higher than control
Metabolism	Unknown
Excretion	Unknown
Half-life	Unknown

Pharmacodynamics
Unknown

Interactions
Drug classifications
Antineoplastics, immunosuppressives: do not use together

NURSING CONSIDERATIONS
Assessment

• **Prostate cancer:** assess for more normal urinary patterns, hematuria, decreased tumor size

• **Bronchospasm, CV adverse reactions:** assess for ability to breathe easily, B/P, pulse, respirations, sinus tachycardia, hypertension

Nursing diagnoses

• Injury, risk for (uses, adverse reactions)

Implementation
Intermittent IV infusion route

• Premedicate with acetaminophen and antihistamine 30 mins prior to infusion
Infusion

• Visually inspect for particulate or discoloration prior to use; remove bag from container and check for leaks, do not use if leak, particulate or discoloration is present, product is slightly cloudy cream to pink color, gently mix, check for clumps of clots; must begin infusion prior to expiration date and time indicated on cell product disposition form and product label

• Infuse entire volume over 60 mins, do not use a cell filter; reactions may be treated with acetaminophen, H1/H2 blockers, low-dose meperidine, if acute reaction occurs, interrupt

---

or slow infusion, do not resume if product has been at room temperature >3 hrs
• Store in refrigerator of unopened bags, do not freeze

Patient/family education
• Instruct patient to notify health care provider of serious adverse reactions: inability to breath, blood in urine, rapid heartbeat, allergic reactions
• Discuss reasons for product and expected results

Evaluation
Positive therapeutic outcome
• Decreasing size of tumor, decreasing PSA

---

tocilizumab (Rx)
(toe'si-liz'oo-mab)
Actemra
Func. class.: DMARDs (Disease modifying anti-rheumatoid drugs)/tumor necrosis factor (TNF) modifier

Pregnancy category C

Action: Interleukin- 6 (IL-6) receptor inhibiting monoclonal antibody

Therapeutic outcome: Ability to move more easily with less pain

Uses: Rheumatoid arthritis

Dosage and routes
Adult: **IV** 4 mg/kg over 1 hr q 4 wks, may increase to 8 mg/kg q 4 wks based on clinical response, max dose 800 mg/infusion; do not initiate if ANC >2000 and platelets <100,000.

Available forms: Solution for injection 80 mg/4 ml, 200 mg/10 ml, 400 mg/20 ml

Adverse effects
CNS: Headache, dizziness
CV: Hypertension
GI: **Perforation,** abdominal pain, gastritis, mouth ulcerations
HEMA: **Neutropenia, thrombocytopenia**
INTEG: Rash, infusion reactions
RESP: Upper respiratory infections, nasopharyngitis, bronchitis
SYST: **Serious infections, anaphylaxis,** infusion-related reactions, anti-tocilizumab antibody formation

Contraindications: Serious infections, risk for GI perforation, active hepatic disease, severe neutropenia/thrombocytopenia, demyelinating disorders

Precautions: Breastfeeding, pregnancy **C**

Pharmacokinetics
Absorption	Unknown
Distribution	Unknown
Metabolism	Unknown
Excretion	Unknown
Half-life	~6 days with a single dose and ~11 days with multiple (steady state) doses

Pharmacodynamics
Unknown

Interactions
Drug classifications
Live virus vaccines: Do not use together
TNF modifiers, DMARDs, immunosuppressives: avoid use due to increased risk of infection

NURSING CONSIDERATIONS
Assessment
• **Rheumatoid arthritis:** assess ROM, pain, stiffness baseline and periodically
• Monitor blood studies: CBC, with differential, LFTs, platelet count, serum lipid profile, baseline and periodically
• Assess for infection prior to and periodically, obtain TB screening prior to beginning treatment

Nursing diagnoses
• Activity intolerance (uses)
• Injury, risk for (adverse reactions)

Implementation
Intermittent IV route
• Visually inspect for particulate matter and discoloration prior to administration whenever solution and container permit, colorless to pale yellow liquid
• From a 100 ml infusion bag or bottle, withdraw a volume of 0.9% sodium chloride injection, equal to the volume of the tocilizumab solution required for the patient's dose
• Slowly add tocilizumab from each vial into the infusion bag or bottle. Gently invert the bag to avoid foaming. Fully diluted solutions are compatible with polypropylene, polyethylene, and polyvinyl chloride infusion bags and polypropylene, polyethylene, and glass infusion bottles
• The fully diluted solutions for infusion may be stored refrigerated or room temperature for up to 24 hours and should be protected from light. Do not use unused product remaining in vials; no preservatives
• Allow the fully diluted solution to reach room temperature before infusion
• Give over 60 minutes with an infusion set. Do not administer as an **IV** push or bolus

Adverse effects: *italic* = common, **bold** = life-threatening

- Do not infuse concomitantly in the same intravenous line with other drugs

Patient/family education
- Teach patient that this treatment must continue unless safety or effectiveness is an issue; reason for use and expected result
- Advise patient to avoid use of live vaccines
- Instruct patient to report signs/symptoms of infection (including TB and Hepatitis B)

Evaluation
Positive therapeutic outcome
- Ability to move more easily with less pain

---

ulipristal (Rx)
(ue′li-pris′tal)
Ella
Func. class.: Progesterone agonist/antagonist-abortifacient

Pregnancy category X

Action: Binds to the progesterone receptor and prevents progesterone from occupying the receptor, postpones follicular rupture when taken immediately prior to ovulation

Therapeutic outcome: Absence of pregnancy

Uses: Emergency contraception

Dosage and routes
Adult/adolescent females: PO 30 mg (1 tab) as soon as possible within 120 hrs (5 days) of unprotected intercourse or a known or suspected contraception failure

Available forms: Tab 30 mg

Adverse effects
CNS: Dizziness, headache, fatigue
GI: Nausea, vomiting, abdominal pain
GU: Dysmenorrhea, breakthrough bleeding
INTEG: Acne vulgaris

Contraindications: Pregnancy **X**, children/infants/neonates, postmenopausal females

Precautions: History of ectopic pregnancy, HIV

Pharmacokinetics

Absorption	Unknown
Distribution	Protein binding >94%
Metabolism	Metabolized by CYP3A4
Excretion	Unknown
Half-life	Terminal half-life 27-38 hrs

Pharmacodynamics

Onset	Unknown
Peak	1 hr
Duration	Unknown

Interactions
Individual drugs
Bosentan, carbamazepine, felbamate, griseofulvin, oxcarbazepine, phenytoin, rifampin St. John's Wort, topiramate, bexarotene, dexamethasone, etravirine, flutamide, metyrapone, modafinil, nafcillin, nevirapine, pioglitazone, rifabutin, itraconazole, ketoconazole: decreased effect of ulipristal
Aldesleukin, IL-2, amiodarone, atazanavir, basiliximab, chloramphenicol, cimetidine, clarithromycin, dalfopristin, danazol, darunavir, delavirdine, diltiazem, dronedarone, erythromycin, fluconazole, fluoxetine, fluvoxamine, imatinib, isoniazid, lapatinib, nefazodone, nelfinavir, nicardipine, octreotide, pantoprazole, quinupristin, ranolazine, saquinavir, tamoxifen, telithromycin, tipranavir, verapamil, voriconazole, zafirlukast: increased ulipristal effect and adverse reactions
Aprepitant, fosaprepitant, efavirenz, fosamprenavir, quinine, ritonavir: increased or decreased ulipristal effect
Drug classifications
Regular hormonal contraceptive methods: decreased contraceptive action
CYP3A4 inducers, barbiturates: decreased effect of ulipristal
CYP3A4 inhibitors: increased ulipristal effect and adverse reactions
Drug/herb
St. John's Wort: decreased effect of ulipristal

NURSING CONSIDERATIONS
Assessment
- Assess need for emergency contraception, pregnancy planned or suspected, obtain pregnancy test before use (pregnancy X)
- Assess medications taken since many drug interactions may occur

Nursing diagnoses
- Noncompliance (teaching)

Implementation
- Administer without regard to food
- Store at room temperature, protect from light

Patient/family education
- Instruct patient that if vomiting occurs within 3 hours of taking the tablet, consider repeating the dose

---

- Advise patient to report to provider any side effects
- Explain reason for medication and expected results
- Advise patient to avoid use in breastfeeding

Evaluation
Positive therapeutic outcome
- Absence of pregnancy

---

vilazodone (Rx)
(vil-az'oh-done)
Viibryd
Func. class.: Antidepressant, miscellaneous

Pregnancy category C

Action: A novel antidepressant unrelated to other antidepressants, enhances serotonergic action by a dual mechanism

Therapeutic outcome: Remission of depressive symptoms

Uses: Major depression

Dosage and routes
Adult: PO 10 mg ×7 days, then 20 mg ×7 days, then 40 mg per day; if taking a potent CYP3A4 inhibitor, the max is 20 mg/day

Available forms: Tabs 10, 20, 40 mg

Adverse effects
CNS: Restlessness, dizziness, drowsiness, fatigue, mania, insomnia, migraine, **neuroleptic malignant like syndrome,** paresthesias, **seizures, suicidal ideation,** tremor, night sweats, dream disorders
EENT: Cataracts, blurred vision
GI: Nausea, vomiting, flatulence, diarrhea, xerostomia, altered taste, gastroenteritis
GU: Decreased libido, ejaculation disorder, increased frequency of urination, sexual dysfunction
HEMA: Bleeding, decreased platelets
MS: Arthralgia
SYST: Neonatal abstinence syndrome, withdrawal, **serotonin syndrome**

Contraindications: Concomitant use of MAO inhibitors or within 14 days after discontinuing a MAO inhibitor or within 14 days after discontinuing vilazodone

Precautions: Abrupt discontinuation, bipolar disorder, bleeding, operating machinery, ECT, geriatrics, hepatic disease, hyponatremia, hypovolemia, infants, labor, pregnancy **C**, substance abuse, history of seizures, serotonin syndrome, neuroleptic malignant syndrome, use with serotonin precursors (e.g., tryptophan) or serotonergic drugs, suicidal ideation and worsening depression or behavior

Black Box Warning: Child, suicidal ideation

Pharmacokinetics
Absorption	Unknown
Distribution	Protein binding 96-99%
Metabolism	Metabolized by the liver by CYP 3A4 (major) and CYP2C19 and CYP2D (minor) and non-CYP pathways
Excretion	Unknown
Half-life	25 hrs

Pharmacodynamics
Onset	Unknown
Peak	4-5 hrs
Duration	Unknown

Interactions
Individual drugs
Selegline, buspirone, dextromethorphan, fenfluramine, dexfluramine, lithium, meperidine, fentanyl, methylphenidate, dexmethylphenidate, metoclopramide, mirtazapine, nefazodone, pentazocine, phenothiazines, haloperidol, loxapine, thiothixene, molidone: increased serotonin syndrome
Drug classifications
MAO inhibitors: do not use together
SSRIs, SNRIs, serotonin receptor agonists, ergots, amphetamines: increased serotonin syndrome
Anticoagulants, thrombolytics, platelet inhibitors, salicylates: increased bleeding
CYP3A4 inhibitors: increased vilazodone levels
Drug/herb
St. John's wort: increased serotonin syndrome
Drug/food
Grapefruit juice: avoid use

NURSING CONSIDERATIONS
Assessment
- Assess mental status: orientation, mood behavior initially and periodically. Initiate suicide precautions if indicated
- Assess for history of seizures, mania
- Monitor renal, hepatic status: hyponatremia

Nursing diagnoses
- Ineffective coping (uses)
- Risk for injury (adverse reactions)
- Sexual dysfunction (adverse reactions)

Adverse effects: *italic* = common, **bold** = life-threatening

Implementation
• Administer with food, to increase absorption
• Store at room temperature, away from moisture, heat

Patient/family education
• Teach patient to take as directed, do not double doses
• Advise patient to avoid abrupt discontinuation, unless approved by prescriber
• Instruct patient not to drive or operate machinery until effects are known
• Instruct patient not to use other products unless approved by prescriber
• Advise patient to contact their prescriber if allergic reactions, personality changes (aggression, anxiety, anger, hostility), extreme sleepiness or drowsiness, feeling confused, nervous, restless or clumsiness, have numbness, tingling or burning pain in hands, arms, legs or feet, tremors, or having unusual behavior or thoughts about hurting themselves

Evaluation
Positive therapeutic outcome
• Remission of depressive symptoms